Hunter's Diseases of Occupations

Hunter's Diseases of Occupations

Tenth edition

Peter J Baxter, Tar-Ching Aw,
Anne Cockcroft, Paul Durrington and
J Malcolm Harrington

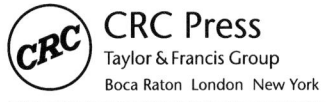

CRC Press
Taylor & Francis Group
Boca Raton London New York

CRC Press is an imprint of the
Taylor & Francis Group, an **informa** business

Chapter 15 © British Crown Copyright 2009/MOD

Cover image: Leonardo da Vinci, Studies of figures in action, Black chalk and pen and ink, c.1506-8. From The Royal Collection © 2010 Her Majesty Queen Elizabeth II.

First published in Great Britain in 1955 as Diseases of Occupations by Edward Arnold Publishers Sixth edition 1978; Seventh edition 1987; Eighth edition 1994; Ninth edition 2000

CRC Press
Taylor & Francis Group
6000 Broken Sound Parkway NW, Suite 300
Boca Raton, FL 33487-2742

© 2010 by Taylor & Francis Group, LLC
CRC Press is an imprint of Taylor & Francis Group, an Informa business

No claim to original U.S. Government works

Printed on acid-free paper
Version Date: 20161019

International Standard Book Number-13: 978-0-340-94166-9 (Pack - Book and Ebook)

This book contains information obtained from authentic and highly regarded sources. While all reasonable efforts have been made to publish reliable data and information, neither the author[s] nor the publisher can accept any legal responsibility or liability for any errors or omissions that may be made. The publishers wish to make clear that any views or opinions expressed in this book by individual editors, authors or contributors are personal to them and do not necessarily reflect the views/opinions of the publishers. The information or guidance contained in this book is intended for use by medical, scientific or health-care professionals and is provided strictly as a supplement to the medical or other professional's own judgement, their knowledge of the patient's medical history, relevant manufacturer's instructions and the appropriate best practice guidelines. Because of the rapid advances in medical science, any information or advice on dosages, procedures or diagnoses should be independently verified. The reader is strongly urged to consult the relevant national drug formulary and the drug companies' and device or material manufacturers' printed instructions, and their websites, before administering or utilizing any of the drugs, devices or materials mentioned in this book. This book does not indicate whether a particular treatment is appropriate or suitable for a particular individual. Ultimately it is the sole responsibility of the medical professional to make his or her own professional judgements, so as to advise and treat patients appropriately. The authors and publishers have also attempted to trace the copyright holders of all material reproduced in this publication and apologize to copyright holders if permission to publish in this form has not been obtained. If any copyright material has not been acknowledged please write and let us know so we may rectify in any future reprint.

Except as permitted under U.S. Copyright Law, no part of this book may be reprinted, reproduced, transmitted, or utilized in any form by any electronic, mechanical, or other means, now known or hereafter invented, including photocopying, microfilming, and recording, or in any information storage or retrieval system, without written permission from the publishers.

For permission to photocopy or use material electronically from this work, please access www.copyright.com (http://www.copyright.com/) or contact the Copyright Clearance Center, Inc. (CCC), 222 Rosewood Drive, Danvers, MA 01923, 978-750-8400. CCC is a not-for-profit organization that provides licenses and registration for a variety of users. For organizations that have been granted a photocopy license by the CCC, a separate system of payment has been arranged.

Trademark Notice: Product or corporate names may be trademarks or registered trademarks, and are used only for identification and explanation without intent to infringe.

Visit the Taylor & Francis Web site at
http://www.taylorandfrancis.com

and the CRC Press Web site at
http://www.crcpress.com

Dedication

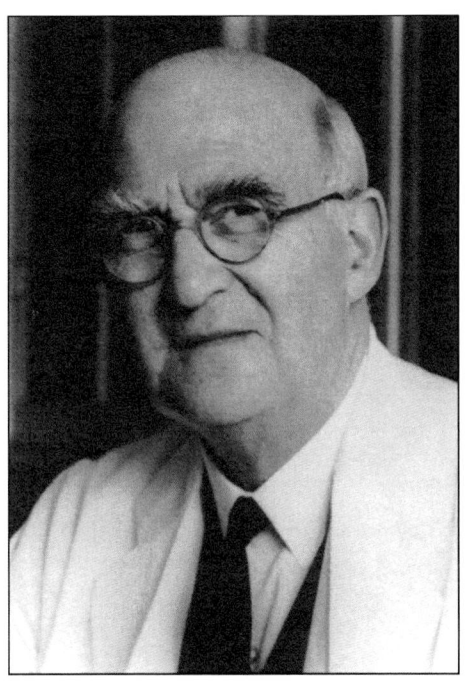

Donald Hunter CBE MD FRCP
1898–1978

Physician, The London Hospital
Senior Censor, Royal College of Physicians of London
Director, MRC Department of Research in Industrial Medicine
Founder Editor, *British Journal of Industrial Medicine*
Author, *Diseases of Occupations*

Contents

Contributors	xiii
Preface	xvii
List of abbreviations used	xix

PART ONE – GENERAL CONSIDERATIONS — 1

Section One: History and Development of Occupational Medicine — 3

1. Donald Hunter and the history of occupational health: precedents and perspectives — 5
   Joseph Melling and Tim Carter
2. The changing face of occupational diseases — 24
   Peter J Baxter, Tar-Ching Aw, Anne Cockcroft, Paul Durrington and J Malcolm Harrington

Section Two: Diagnosis of Occupational Disease — 31

3. The occupational history — 33
   Tar-Ching Aw
4. Occupational exposure to hazardous substances — 43
   John W Cherrie and Sean Semple
5. Biological monitoring — 56
   John Cocker and Howard J Mason

Section Three: Extent and Attribution of Occupational Disease — 75

6. Epidemiological methods and evidence-based occupational medicine — 77
   David Coggon
7. Attribution of disease — 89
   Anthony Newman Taylor and David Coggon
8. Compensation schemes — 96
   Anthony Newman Taylor and David Walters

Section Four: Legal Issues — 111

9. Medicolegal reports and the role of the expert witness — 113
   Diana M Kloss

PART TWO – DISEASES ASSOCIATED WITH CHEMICAL AGENTS — 123

Section One: Occupational Toxicology — 125

10. Occupational toxicology: general principles — 127
    Peter G Blain and Robert D Jefferson
11. Risks and hazards in occupational and environmental exposures — 141
    Robert L Maynard

Section Two: Metals   **149**

12   Introduction   151
    Tar-Ching Aw
13   Aluminium   153
    Perrine Hoet
14   Antimony   159
    Malcolm R Sim
15   Arsenic   160
    Malcolm R Sim
16   Beryllium   162
    Lee S Newman and Holly M Christensen
17   Cadmium   167
    Perrine Hoet
18   Chromium   173
    Tom Sorahan
19   Cobalt   175
    Perrine Hoet
20   Copper   180
    Peter Aggett
21   Gold   183
    Peter Linnett
22   Iron   185
    Peter Aggett
23   Lead   188
    Peter J Baxter and Hideki Igisu
24   Magnesium   199
    Peter Aggett
25   Manganese   201
    Grant McMillan and Finlay D Dick
26   Mercury   214
    Peter J Baxter and Hideki Igisu
27   Molybdenum   221
    Malcolm R Sim
28   Nickel   223
    Tom Sorahan
29   Phosphorus   225
    Malcolm R Sim
30   Platinum group metals   226
    Peter Linnett
31   Polonium   231
    Iain Blair
32   Silver   234
    Peter Linnett
33   Thallium   236
    Hideki Igisu and Tar-Ching Aw
34   Tin   238
    Tar-Ching Aw and Hideki Igisu
35   Tungsten   241
    Perrine Hoet
36   Uranium   243
    Iain Blair
37   Vanadium   246
    Finlay D Dick
38   Zinc   249
    Peter Aggett

Section Three: Gases — 251

- 39 Gases — 253
  Peter J Baxter
- 40 Reactive airways dysfunction syndrome and irritant-induced asthma — 310
  Jon G Ayres
- 41 Deliberate use of chemicals in warfare and by terrorists — 314
  Robert L Maynard

Section Four: Other Chemical Exposures — 319

- 42 Organic chemicals — 321
  Tiina Santonen, Antero Aitio and Harri Vainio
- 43 Pesticides and other agrochemicals — 395
  Ian Brown, Annalisa Chiodini, Chiara Somaruga and Claudio Colosio
- 44 Welding — 421
  Grant McMillan
- 45 The semiconductor industry — 444
  David Koh and Judy Sng

PART THREE – DISEASES ASSOCIATED WITH PHYSICAL AGENTS — 455

Section One: Noise — 457

- 46 Sound, noise and the ear — 459
  Richard T Ramsden and Shakeel R Saeed

Section Two: Vibration — 487

- 47 Hand–arm vibration syndrome — 489
  *Ian J Lawson, Frank Burke, Kenneth L McGeoch,
  Tohr Nilsson and George Proud*
- 48 Whole body vibration — 513
  Massimo Bovenzi and Keith Palmer

Section Three: Heat and Cold — 523

- 49 Heat and cold — 525
  E Howard N Oakley

Section Four: Barometric Pressure — 545

- 50 Diving and work at increased pressure — 547
  Stephen Watt and Andrew Colvin
- 51 Working at high altitude — 570
  Peter JG Forster
- 52 Flying and spaceflight — 591
  Mike Gibson, David Gradwell and Alyson Calder

Section Five: Radiation — 621

- 53 Ionizing radiations — 623
  Chris Sharp and Fred A Mettler Jr
- 54 Non-ionizing radiation and the eye — 644
  Michael E Boulton and David H Sliney
- 55 Extremely low frequency electric and magnetic fields — 663
  Leeka Kheifets and Gabor Mezei
- 56 Radiofrequency fields — 675
  Gabor Mezei and Leeka Kheifets

PART FOUR – DISEASES RELATED TO ERGONOMIC AND MECHANICAL FACTORS — 683

Section One: The Musculoskeletal System — 685

57 Repeated movements and repeated trauma affecting the musculoskeletal system — 687
   Cyrus Cooper and Keith Palmer

Section Two: Back and Spinal Pain — 713

58 Occupational back pain — 715
   Jos H Verbeek and Frederieke Schaafsma

PART FIVE – OCCUPATION AND TRANSMISSIBLE DISEASES — 725

Section One: Occupational Infections — 727

59 Occupational infections — 729
   Julia Heptonstall and Anne Cockcroft
60 Zoonoses — 750
   Alastair Miller and Julia Heptonstall

Section Two: Bioterrorism and Biotechnology — 771

61 Bioterrorism — 773
   Julia Heptonstall
62 Genetic modification and biotechnology — 782
   David Roomes

PART SIX – WORK AND MENTAL HEALTH — 799

Section One: Work and Stress — 801

63 Introduction to work and stress — 803
   Peter Baxter, Tar-Ching Aw and Anne Cockcroft
64 Work, stress and sickness absence: a psychosocial perspective — 804
   Maurice Lipsedge and Michael Calnan
65 Mental health at work: psychological interventions — 823
   Adrian Neal

Section Two: Work and Psychiatric Disorder — 831

66 Work and psychiatric disorder: an evidence-based approach — 833
   Nick Glozier, Max Henderson, Neil Greenberg and Simon Øverland

Section Three: Substance Abuse — 857

67 Substance abuse and the workplace — 859
   Jonathan D Chick

PART SEVEN – RESPIRATORY DISORDERS — 871

Section One: General Issues — 873

68 Imaging in occupational lung disease — 875
   Paul M Taylor
69 Work and chronic air flow limitation — 889
   David J Hendrick
70 Health effects of ultrafine/nanoparticles — 903
   Ken Donaldson, Robert J Aitken, Jon G Ayres, Brian G Miller and C Lang Tran
71 Health effects related to non-industrial workplace indoor environments — 921
   Jouni JK Jaakkola and Maritta S Jaakkola

Section Two: Organic Dust Diseases — 939

72 Occupational asthma — 941
Paul Cullinan and Anthony Newman Taylor

73 Byssinosis and other cotton-related diseases — 958
CAC Pickering and Robert Niven

74 Extrinsic allergic alveolitis — 970
Paul Cullinan and Anthony Newman Taylor

Section Three: Inorganic Dust Diseases — 983

75 Inorganic dusts: general aspects — 985
Anne Cockcroft

76 Asbestos and asbestos-related diseases — 990
David Weill and Anne Cockcroft

77 Epidemiology of asbestos-related diseases — 1000
Robin M Rudd

78 Other fibrous mineral dusts — 1011
Anne Cockcroft

79 Silica and silica-related diseases — 1014
Anne Cockcroft

80 Epidemiology of silica-related disease — 1021
Kyle Steenland

81 Other non-fibrous mineral dusts — 1029
Anne Cockcroft

82 Metal dusts and fumes — 1040
Benoit Nemery

83 Berylliosis — 1050
Holly M Christensen and Lee S Newman

PART EIGHT – OTHER EFFECTS OF WORKPLACE EXPOSURES — 1057

Section One: Occupational Diseases of the Skin — 1059

84 Occupational diseases of the skin — 1061
John English and Jason Williams

Section Two: Occupational Cancers — 1079

85 Occupational cancer: epidemiology, biological mechanisms and biomarkers — 1081
Manolis Kogevinas, J Malcolm Harrington and Roel Vermeulen

Section Three: Other Systemic Effects — 1123

86 Nephrotoxic effects of workplace exposures — 1125
Rema Saxena, Pearl Pai and Gordon M Bell

87 Neurotoxic effects of workplace exposures — 1151
Michael J Aminoff and Marcello Lotti

88 Hepatotoxic effects of workplace exposure — 1171
Thomas W Warnes and Alexander Smith

89 Workplace exposures and reproductive health — 1196
Jens Peter Bonde

90 Haemopoietic effects of workplace exposures: anaemias, leukaemias and lymphomas — 1215
Edward Gordon-Smith, Anthony Yardley-Jones and Atherton Gray

Section Four: Shift Work — **1231**

91   Shift work and extended hours of work — 1233
     Giovanni Costa, Simon Folkard and J Malcolm Harrington

Index — 1247

WEBSITE

This book has a companion website available at: www.hodderplus.com/hunters.

The website's features include:

- over 350 images from the tenth edition, including some in full colour
- Donald Hunter's original introductory chapters from the early editions of the book
- a selection of over 350 photographs from Donald Hunter's personal collection – a resource unique to this publication.

To access this content, please register on the website using the following details:

Serial number: 15gh698ert21

Contributors

Peter Aggett OBE MSc FRCP
Honorary Professor, School of Medicine and Health,
Lancaster University, Lancaster, UK

Antero Aitio MD PhD
Professor HC, Team Leader (retired), Finnish Institute of
Occupational Health, Helsinki, Finland

Rob J Aitken BA BSc(hons) PhD FiON
Director of Safenano, Institute of Occupational Medicine,
Edinburgh, UK

Michael J Aminoff MD DSc FRCP
Distinguished Professor of Neurology, School of Medicine,
University of California, San Francisco, CA, USA

Tar-Ching Aw MB PhD FRCP FRCPC FFOM FFPHM
Professor and Chair, Department of Community Medicine,
Faculty of Medicine and Health Sciences, United Arab Emirates
University, Al-Ain, UAE; Adjunct Professor, Gillings School of
Global Public Health, University of North Carolina, Chapel Hill,
USA; Visiting Professor, Canterbury Christ Church University,
Kent, UK

Jon G Ayres BSc MBBS MD FRCP FRCPE FFOM FRCPSG
Institute of Occupational and Environmental Medicine,
University of Birmingham, Edgbaston, UK

Peter J Baxter MD MSc FRCP FFOM
Consultant Physician in Occupational and Environmental
Medicine, University of Cambridge and Addenbrooke's Hospital,
Cambridge University Hospital NHS Foundation Trust,
Cambridge, UK

Gordon M Bell BSc MB ChB FRCP(E) FRCP
Renal Unit, Royal Liverpool University Hospital, Liverpool, UK

Peter G Blain CBE PhD FRCP(Lond) FRCP(Edin) FFOM FBTS FBS
Professor of Environmental Medicine, Medical Toxicology Centre,
Newcastle University, Wolfson Unit, Newcastle upon Tyne, UK

Iain Blair MA MB BChir
Department of Community Medicine, Faculty of Medicine and
Health Sciences, United Arab Emirates University, Al-Ain, UAE

Jens Peter Bonde MD PhD Dr Med Sc
Professor of Occupational Medicine and Epidemiology,
Department of Occupational and Environmental Medicine,
Copenhagen University Hospital, Copenhagen, Denmark

Michael E Boulton BSc PhD
Department of Anatomy and Cell Biology, University of Florida,
Gainesville, FL, USA

Massimo Bovenzi MD
Director and Professor of Occupational Medicine, Clinical
Unit of Occupational Medicine, Department of Reproductive,
Developmental and Public Health Sciences, University of Trieste,
Trieste, Italy

Ian Brown OBE BSc FRCP FFOM DDAM
Consultant Physician in Occupational Medicine and Toxicology,
Director of Occupational Health, University of Oxford, Honorary
Consultant Physician to the Oxfordshire Primary Care Trust
Division of Public Health, Oxford, UK

Frank Burke MBBS FRCS
Professor of Hand Surgery, Pulvertaft Hand Centre,
Derby, UK

Alyson Calder MBChB BSc MRCP FRCA
Department of Anaesthetics, Glasgow Royal Infirmary,
Glasgow, UK

Michael Calnan MSc PhD
Professor of Medical Sociology, University of Kent,
Canterbury, UK

Tim Carter MSc FRCP FFOM
Chief Medical Adviser, Maritime and Coastguard Agency,
Department of the Environment, Transport and the Regions,
London, UK

John W Cherrie BSc(Hons) PhD FFOH
Research Director, Institute of Occupational Medicine,
Edinburgh, UK

Jonathan D Chick MA MBChB MPhil DSc FRCP (Edin) FRC Psych
Consultant Psychiatrist, Royal Edinburgh Hospital; Part-time
Senior Lecturer in Psychiatry, Edinburgh University and Honorary
Professor, Health Sciences, Queen Margaret University,
Edinburgh, UK

Holly M Christensen MSPH
Axion Health Inc., Denver, CO, USA

Anne Cockcroft MD DIH FRCP FFOM
Senior Reseach Fellow, CIET group; Visiting Professor,
Autonomous University of Guerrero, Mexico

John Cocker MSc PhD
Health and Safety Laboratory, Buxton, UK

David Coggon OBE MA PhD DM FRCP FFOM FFPH FmedSci
Professor of Occupational and Environmental Medicine,
MRC Epidemiology Resource Centre, University of
Southampton, UK

Annalisa Chiodini MD PhD
Department of Occupational and Environmental Health of the University of Milan, S Paolo Hospital Unit, and International Centre for Rural Health of the University Hospital San Paolo, Milan, Italy

Claudio Colosio MD PhD
Assistant Professor of Occupational Health and Director of the International Centre for Rural Health, Department of Occupational and Environmental Health of the University of Milan, S Paolo Hospital Unit, and International Centre for Rural Health of the University Hospital San Paolo, Milan, Italy

Andrew P Colvin MRCGP MSc MFOM DRCOG DipIMC
Regional Occupational Physician Scotland and Northern Ireland, Atos Origin, Glasgow, UK

Cyrus Cooper MA DM FRCP
Director and Professor of Rheumatology, MRC Epidemiology Resource Centre (University of Southampton), Southampton General Hospital, Southampton, UK

Giovanni Costa MD
Professor of Occupational Medicine, Department of Occupational Health, University of Milan, Milan, Italy

Paul Cullinan MD FRCP FFOM
Department of Occupational and Environmental Medicine, Royal Brompton Hospital/NHLI, London, UK

Finlay Dick MD MRCGP MFOM
Senior Lecturer in Occupational Medicine, Environmental and Occupational Medicine Group, University of Aberdeen, UK

Ken Donaldson BSc(Hons) PhD DSc FIBiol FRCPath FFOM
Queens Medical Research Institute, University of Edinburgh, Edinburgh, UK

Paul Durrington MD FRCP FRCPath FAHA FACP FMedSci
Honorary Professor of Medicine, Consultant Physician, Cardiovascular Research Group, School of Biomedicine, University of Manchester, Manchester, UK

John English MBBS FRCP
Consultant Dermatologist, Nottingham University Hospital, Nottingham, UK

Simon Folkard PhD DSC HON FRCP
Visiting Professor, Paris-Descartes, France and Professor Emeritus, Swansea University, UK

Peter JG Forster MD FRCP
Honorary Consultant Physician, James Paget University Hospital, Great Yarmouth and Associate Tutor, School of Medicine, University of East Anglia, Norwich, UK

Mike Gibson PhD MPhil MB ChB FFOM DAvMED DDAM FRAES
Medical Director, Corporate Health Ltd, The Buckingham Centre, Slough, UK

Nick Glozier MA MSc MBBS MRCPsych FRANZCP PhD
Associate Professor of Psychological Medicine, Disciplines of Psychological Medicine and Sleep, Sydney Medical School, University of Sydney, Sydney, Australia and Institute of Psychiatry, Kings College London, UK

Edward Gordon-Smith MA MSc FRCPath FRCP FMedSci
Professor Emeritus of Haematology, St George's, University of London, UK

David Gradwell PhD BSc MB ChB FRCP DAvMed FRAES RAF
RAF Consultant Adviser in Aviation Medicine and Whittingham Professor in Aviation Medicine, Royal Air Force Centre of Aviation Medicine, Royal Air Force Henlow, UK

Atherton Gray MB ChB MD FRCPath FRCP
Consultant Haematologist, Great Western Hospitals NHS Foundation Trust, Swindon, UK

Neil Greenberg BSc BM MMedSc ILTM MEWI DOccMED MFFLM MD MRCPsych
Defence Professor of Mental Health, Academic Centre for Defence Mental Health, Kings College London, UK

J Malcolm Harrington CBE MSc MD FRCP FFOM FMedSci
Emeritus Professor of Occupational Medicine, University of Birmingham, Birmingham, UK

Max Henderson MBBS MSc PhD MRCP MRCPsych
Senior Lecturer in Epidemiological and Occupational Psychiatry, Institute of Psychiatry, Kings College London, UK, and Consultant Liaison Psychiatrist, Kings College Hospital, London UK

David J Hendrick MSc MD FRCP FFOM
Emeritus Professor, University of Newcastle upon Tyne, and Consultant Physician, Royal Victoria Infirmary, Newcastle upon Tyne, UK

Julia Heptonstall MSc MB BS FRCP FRCPath DTM&H
Consultant Clinical Microbiologist, Scarborough and NE Yorkshire NHS Trust, UK

Perrine Hoet MD PhD
Professor, Université Catholique de Louvain, Louvain Centre for Toxicology and Applied Pharmacology (LTAP), Brussels, Belgium

Hideki Igisu MD PhD
Director of the Fukuoka Central Health Evaluation and Promotion Center, Fukuoka, Japan

Jouni JK Jaakkola MD DSc PhD
Professor of Public Health, Institute of Health Sciences, University of Oulu, Finland and Professor of Environmental and Occupational Medicine, Institute of Occupational and Environmental Medicine, University of Birmingham, UK

Maritta S Jaakkola MD PhD
Professor of Respiratory Medicine, Respiratory Medicine Unit, Institute of Clinical Sciences, University of Oulu, Finland

Robert D Jefferson BSc MB BS FFOM CMIOSH
Consultant in Environmental Medicine and Deputy Director, Medical Toxicology Center, University of Newcastle, The Wolfson Unit, Newcastle upon Tyne, UK

Leeka Kheifets PhD
Professor, UCLA School of Public Health, Department of Epidemiology, Los Angeles, CA, USA

Diana M Kloss MBE LLB(Lond) LLM(Tulane) Hon FFOM
Barrister, Gray's Inn and Honorary Senior Lecturer, University of Manchester, Manchester, UK

Manolis Kogevinas MD PhD
Centre for Research in Environmental Epidemiology (CREAL), Municipal Institute of Medical Research (IMIM-Hospital del Mar), CIBER Epidemiologia y Salud Pública (CIBERESP), Barcelona, Spain and National School of Public Health, Athens, Greece

David Koh MBBS MSc(om) PhD FFOM FFOMI FFPH FAMS
Professor, Department of Epidemiology and Public Health, Yong Loo Lin School of Medicine, National University of Singapore, Republic of Singapore

Ian J Lawson MBBS CMIOSH FFOM FACOEM FRCP
Chief Medical Officer, Rolls-Royce plc, Derby, UK

Peter Linnett MB BS FFOM
Formerly Group Occupational Physician, Johnson Matthey plc

Maurice S Lipsedge MPhil FRCP FRCPsych FFOM(Hon)
Emeritus Consultant Psychiatrist, The South London and Maudsley NHS Trust, Visiting Senior Lecturer in the Department of Psychological Medicine within Guy's, King's and St Thomas' School of Medicine, London, UK

Marcello Lotti MD
Professor, Università degli Studi di Padova, Dipartimento di Medicina Ambientale e Sanità Pubblica, Padua, Italy

Howard J Mason MSc PhD
Health and Safety Laboratory, Buxton, UK

Robert L Maynard CBE FRCP FRCPath FFOM FBTS
Honorary Professor of Environmental Medicine, University of Birmingham, UK

Kenneth L McGeoch MB ChB MRCGP FFOM
Consultant Hand Arm Vibration Syndrome (rtd)

Grant McMillan MD MSc FRCP FRCP(Glasg) FFOM CFIOSH
Independent Occupational Physician, Honorary Senior Clinical Lecturer, University of Birmingham, UK

Joseph Melling BSc PhD
Professor, Director of the Centre for Medical History, University of Exeter, UK

Fred A Mettler Jr MD MPH
Board Certified Radiologist, US representative, United Nations Scientific Committee on the Effects of Atomic Radiations, Emeritus Professor of Radiology, University of New Mexico, Former Main Commission Member, International Commission on Radiological Protection, Albuquerque, NM, USA

Gabor Mezei MD PhD
Electric Power Research Institute, Palo Alto, CA, USA

Alastair Miller MA FRCP FRCP(Edin) DTM&H
Tropical and Infectious Disease Unit, Royal Liverpool University Hospital, Liverpool School of Tropical Medicine, Liverpool, UK

Brian G Miller BSc(Hons) PhD CStat Csci
Principal Epidemiologist, Institute of Occupational Medicine, Edinburgh, UK

Adrian Neal BA(Hons) MA ClinPsyD
Principal Clinical Psychologist (Coventry and Warwickshire NHS Partnership Trust) and Lecturer/Practitioner (Coventry and Warwick Universities Clinical Psychology Doctoral Programme)

Benoit Nemery MD PhD
Professor of Toxicology and Occupational Medicine, Department of Public Health, Katholieke Universiteit Leuven, Belgium

Lee S Newman MD MA FCCP FACOEM
Professor of Environmental and Occupational Health, University of Colorado Denver, Colorado School of Public Health, Denver, CO, USA

Anthony Newman Taylor OBE FRCP FFOM FMedSci
Deputy Principal, Faculty of Medicine, Imperial College, London, UK

Tohr Nilsson MD PhD
Associate Professor, Department of Occupational and Environmental Medicine, Sundsvalls Hospital Sweden

Robert Niven MBChB BSc MD MFOM FRCP
University of Manchester and University Hospital of South Manchester, Manchester, UK

E Howard N Oakley BA MB BCH MSc
Head of Survival and Thermal Medicine, The Institute of Naval Medicine, Alverstoke, Gosport, UK

Simon Øverland PhD PsyD
Research Centre for Health Promotion, Faculty of Psychology, University of Bergen, Norway

Pearl Pai MBChB MD FRCP
Renal Unit, Royal Liverpool University Hospital, Liverpool, UK

Keith Palmer MA BM BCh FFOM FRCP DRCOG
Professor of Occupational Medicine, MRC Epidemiology Resource Centre, University of Southampton, Southampton General Hospital, Southampton SO16 6YD, UK

CAC Pickering FRCP FFOM DIH
Professor of Occupational Medicine, North West Lung Centre, Wythenshawe Hospital, Manchester, UK

George Proud BS BDS MD FRCS
Emeritus Consultant Surgeon, Royal Victoria Infirmary, Newcastle upon Tyne, UK

Richard Ramsden MD ChB FRCS
Professor of Otolaryngology, Victoria University of Manchester, Manchester Royal Infirmary, Manchester, UK

David Roomes MRCGP MFOM LLM
Medical Director, Employee Health Management, GlaxoSmithKline, Stevenage, UK

Robin M Rudd MA MD FRCP
Consultant Physician, London Lung Cancer Group, London, UK

Shakeel R Saeed MB(BS)(Lon) FRCS(Ed) FRCS(ORL, Lon) MD (Man)
Professor of Otology/Neuro-otology, University College London Ear Institute, Consultant ENT and Skullbase Surgeon, The Royal National Throat, Nose and Ear Hospital and Royal Free Hospital, London, UK

Tiina Santonen MD PhD MSc
Team Leader, Finnish Institute of Occupational Health, Helsinki, Finland

Rema Saxena Mb ChB MRCP
Consultant Nephrologist and Physician, Renal Unit,
Royal Liverpool University Hospital, Liverpool, UK

Frederieke Schaafsma MD PhD
Independent Occupational Health Physician/Researcher,
Hunters Hill, Australia

Sean Semple BSc(Hons) MSc PhD
Senior Lecturer, Environmental and Occupational Medicine,
University of Aberdeen, Aberdeen, UK

Chris Sharp MSC FRCP FFOM DAvMED
Consultant Occupational Physician, Medical Director WorkFit-UK,
Former Member, International Commission on Radiological
Protection, WorkFit-UK Ltd, Bury St Edmunds, UK

Malcolm R Sim MBBS MSc PhD FFOM FAFOEM
Professor and Director, Monash Centre for Occupational
and Environmental Health, Department of Epidemiology and
Preventive Medicine, Monash University, Melbourne, Australia

David H Sliney PhD
Consulting Medical Physicist, Fallston, MD USA (formerly,
Program Manager, Laser/Optical Radiation Program, US Army
Center for Health Promotion and Preventive Medicine, Aberdeen
Proving Ground, MD USA)

Alexander Smith PhD
Principal Clinical Scientist, Principal Clinical Scientist, Specialist
Assay Laboratory, Department of Clinical Biochemistry, Central
Manchester Foundation Trust, Manchester, UK

Judy Sng MBBS MMed(OM) GDOM GDFM
Assistant Professor, Department of Epidemiology and Public
Health, Yong Loo Lin School of Medicine, National University of
Singapore, Republic of Singapore

Chiara Somaruga MD PhD
Department of Occupational and Environmental Health of the
University of Milan, S Paolo Hospital Unit, and International
Centre for Rural Health of the University Hospital San Paolo,
Milan, Italy

Tom Sorahan PhD DSc FFOM(Hon)
Professor of Occupational Epidemiology, Institute of Occupational
and Environmental Medicine, University of Birmingham,
Edgbaston, Birmingham, UK

Kyle Steenland PhD MS
Rollins School of Public Health, Emory University, Atlanta,
GA, USA

Paul M Taylor MB FRCP FRCR
Department of Clinical Radiology, Manchester Royal Infirmary,
Manchester, UK

C Lang Tran
Institute of Occupational Medicine, Edinburgh, UK

Harri Vainio MD PhD
Director General, Finnish Institute of Occupational Health,
Helsinki, Finland

Jos H Verbeek MD PhD
Occupational Physician, Finnish Institute of Occupational Health,
Kuopio, Finland

Roel Vermeulen PhD
Institute for Risk Assessment Sciences, Utrecht University,
Utrecht, The Netherlands

David Walters MMedSci PhD
Professor of Work Environment, Cardiff School of Social Sciences,
Cardiff University, UK

Thomas W Warnes MD FRCP
Consultant Physician, Liver Unit, Manchester Royal Infirmary,
Manchester, UK

Stephen Watt BSc MBBS FRCPEd Hon FFOM
Consultant in Respiratory and Hyperbaric Medicine,
NHS Grampian, UK

David Weill MD
Medical Director, Lung and Heart-Lung Transplant Program,
Associate Professor of Medicine, Division of Pulmonary and
Critical Care, Stanford University Medical Center, Stanford,
CA, USA

Jason Williams BSc(Hons) MB ChB(Hons) MRCP
Consultant Dermatologist, Director, Contact Dermatitis
Investigation Unit, University Department of Dermatology,
Salford Royal NHS Foundation Trust, Manchester, UK

Anthony Yardley-Jones FFOM FFOM (Irel) FRCS (Ed) FFTM RCPS (Glas) PhD DipMedAc
Consultant in Occupational Medicine, Chelsea and Westminster
Hospital, London, UK

Preface

The publication of the previous (ninth) edition of Hunter's coincided with the millennium, when in celebratory mood the preface referred to how in the previous 40 years a revolution in biomedical knowledge had led to a transformation of workplace health and safety, accelerating a decline of occupational diseases in advanced economy countries that ranked as one of the greatest triumphs of preventive health of the twentieth century. This success would not have been possible without governments legislating and providing resources to enforce controls in the workplace, with the most radical changes occurring in the 1970s.

The tenth edition goes to press at a very different time, however, with the world reeling in financial crisis and with voices calling for the regulatory 'burden' of health and safety on industry in the richest countries to be lifted. On the world scale, the concern is that the existing huge disparities in life expectancy between high and low income countries will get worse. These health inequalities stem from the circumstances in which people are born, grow, live, work and age. Despite the impressive improvements in advanced industrialized countries at the end of the twentieth century, the millennium predictions were for an *increase* in the global burden of occupational diseases, especially in those economies with large populations and undergoing rapid industrialization, such as Brazil, Russia, India and China, where the basic protections are still mostly lacking.

The need for an updated and comprehensive reference text on occupational diseases is therefore as great as ever. The early detection and diagnosis of occupational diseases depends upon knowledge of the workplace and the likely risks of exposure to workplace hazards, while the elimination of occupational diseases depends upon an effective regulatory framework, adequate risk assessments, and putting in place effective measures to control hazardous exposures. The tenth edition has new chapters on exposure and risk, and on the attribution of disease. The predominant types of work-related ill health have indeed changed over recent years in high income countries. Not all conditions encountered in the modern workforce fit the traditional pattern of defined exposures leading to specific diseases, and the sections on mental health and musculoskeletal disorders have been expanded to take into account their huge rise in prevalence and the sparse evidence base for their successful management. At the same time, it is shocking that classic 'industrial' diseases due to asbestos and silica that dominated occupational medicine in the twentieth century, including cancers, still remain as worldwide scourges, and new chapters have been included on their clinical epidemiology to highlight the continuing and serious problems they present.

Donald Hunter's original work was not only a source of reference: it stood as a bulwark against the tide of global occupational disease. We thank the many authors who have contributed to this tenth edition and whose skill, we believe, will continue to make the volume an invaluable and constant force in the goal of disease prevention. As in previous editions, the book is intended to be an accessible, up-to-date and comprehensive text on occupational and related environmental conditions written for a wide range of clinical practitioners, for consultants writing legal reports, for lawyers, and for others seeking medical guidance on the risks to health of work activities and industrial processes.

With this edition, readers will have the additional bonus of on-line access to Hunter's original chapters on the history of occupational medicine and a selection from his personal archive of photographs of patients and work processes, many of which illustrated his own editions. We anticipate that the publication of this unique material will be useful to students and many other readers interested in the history of disease.

We are grateful to Dr Paul Grime for providing us with access to the Hunter collection located at the Royal Free Hospital, London. Finally, we acknowledge the outstanding commitment and indefatigable efforts of Jo Koster, Head of Health Science Textbooks at Hodder Arnold, and Susie Bond, Project Editor, in so ably nurturing the book and bringing it to press.

Peter J Baxter
Tar-Ching Aw
Anne Cockcroft
Paul Durrington
J Malcolm Harrington

List of abbreviations used

AAOO	American Academy of Otolaryngology and Ophthalmology	BEI	biological exposure index
ABR	auditory brainstem response	BEI	biological exposure indices
ac	alternating current	BeLPT	beryllium lymphocyte proliferation test
ACD	allergic contact dermatitis	BEM	biological effect monitoring
ACGIH	American Conference of Governmental Industrial Hygienists	BHT	butylated hydroxytoluene
		BM	biological monitoring
ACh	acetylcholine	BMD	bone mineral density
AChE	acetylcholinesterase	BMI	body mass index
ACRE	Advisory Committee for Releases to the Environment	BoD	Burden of Disease
		BOHS	British Occupational Hygiene Society
ACT	acceptance and commitment therapy	BOOP	bronchiolitis obliterans organizing pneumonia
AD	Alzheimer's disease	BP	boiling point
ADME	absorption, distribution, metabolism and excretion	BSA	British Society of Audiologists
		BSO	biological safety officer
AE	alveolar echinococcosis	BSP	bromosulphophthalein
AEC	Atomic Energy Commission	BV	blood volume
ALA	amino laevulinic acid	CAA	chloroacetaldehyde
ALARP	as low as reasonably practicable	CAA	Civil Aviation Authority
ALAS	aminolaevulinic acid synthetase	CAP	concentrated ambient particles
ALL	acute lymphocytic leukaemia	CAREX	carcinogen exposure
ALP	alkaline phosphatase	CAS	Chemical Abstracts Service
ALS	amyotrophic lateral sclerosis	CAT	cognitive analytic therapy
ALT	alanine transaminase	CAWG	Compressed Air Working Group
AML	acute myeloid leukaemia	CBD	chronic beryllium disease
AMS	acute mountain sickness	CBE	chronic bronchitis and emphysema
ANA	anti-nuclear antibodies	CBE	cotton bract extract
ANCA	anti-neutrophil cytoplasmic antibodies	CBT	cognitive behavioural therapy
ANSI	American National Standards Institute	CBT	cognitive behaviour therapy
ANTU	naphthylthiourea	CCI	colour confusion index
AP	action potential	CDC	Centre for Disease Control and Prevention
AR	attributable risk		
ARS	acute radiation sickness	CDE	cotton dust extract
AST	aspartate transaminase	CDNP	combustion-derived nanoparticles
ata	atmosphere absolute	CD ROM	compact disc read-only memory devices
BAAP	British Association of Audiological Physicians	CE	cystic echinococcosis
		CEO	chloroethylene oxide
BAAS	British Association of Audiological Scientists	CFC	chlorofluorocarbons
		CFL	compact fluorescent lamp
BA	breathing apparatus	CFS	chronic fatigue syndrome
BAL	bronchoalveolar lavage	CFU	colony-forming units
BAOL	British Association of Otolaryngologists	CGH	comparative genomic hybridization
BAT	biological tolerance values	CHC	chlorinated hydrocarbon
BCC	basal cell carcinoma	CI	confidence interval

CIMAH	Control of Industrial Major Accident Hazards	EBV	Epstein–Barr virus
CLL	chronic lymphocytic leukaemia	ECG	electrocardiogram
CM	cochlear microphonic	ECM	external cardiac massage
CMV	cytomegalovirus	ECPA	European Crop Protection Association
CNS	central nervous system	EDTA	ethylenediaminatetraacetic acid
CNT	carbon nanotubes	EDXA	energy dispersive x-ray analysis
COAD	chronic obstructive airways disease	EEG	electroencephalogram
CO	carbon monoxide	EELS	electron energy loss spectrometry
COMAH	Control of Major Accident Hazards	ELF	extreme low frequency
COMARE	Committee on the Medical Aspects of Radiation in the Environment	ELV	exposure limit value
		EMAS	Employment Medical Advisory Service
COPD	chronic obstructive pulmonary disease	EMF	electromagnetic fields
COSHH	Control of Substances Hazardous to Health	EMG	electromyography
		EMLA	eutectic mixture of local anaesthetics
COSSH	Control of Substances Hazard to Health	EPA	Environmental Protection Agency
CPCs	Condensation particle counters	ERA	electric response audiometry
CR	computed radiography	ER	extraction ratio
CRFP	Council for the Registration of Forensic Practitioners	ERG	electroretinography
		ERPG	Emergency Response Planning Guidelines
CRT	choice reaction time	ESA	Employment and Support Allowance
CSE	chronic solvent encephalopathy	ESRD	end-stage renal disease
CSF	cerebrospinal fluid	ESR	erythrocyte sedimentation rate
CT	computed tomography	EtC	ethylene chlorohydrin
CTE	chronic toxic encephalopathy	EtO	ethylene oxide
CTS	carpal tunnel syndrome	ETS	environmental tobacco smoke
CWP	coal worker's pneumoconiosis	ETU	ethylenethiourea
DALY	disability adjusted life years	FAD	flavin adenine dinucleorotide
DBCP	dibromochloropropane	FCAW	flux-cored arc welding
DCS	Decompression sickness	FDA	Food and Drug Administration
DD	Dupuytren's disease	FEV1	forced expiratory volume in 1 second
DDT	dichlorodiphenyltrichlorethane	FEV1	forced expired volume in 1 second
DECOS	Dutch Expert Committee on Occupational Standards	FIOH	Finnish Institute of Occupational Health
		FISH	fluorescence in situ hybridization
DEFRA	Department for Environment, Food and Rural Affairs	FISH	fluorescent in situ hybridization
		FITS	fighter index of thermal stress
DEFRA	Department of Environment, Food and Rural Affairs	FPP	fumes from photocopiers and printers
		FR	fecundability ratio
DFG	Deutsche Forschungsgemeinschaft	FSW	friction stir welding
DFR	dislodgeable foliar residue	FTP	fitness to practise
DLCO	diffusing capacity for carbon monoxide	FVC	forced vital capacity
		GEWIS	genome-wide interactions
DMAPN	dimethylaminoproprionitrile	GGT	gamma glutamyl transferase
DMF	dimethyl formamide	GMC	General Medical Council
DMPS	differential mobility particle sizer	GMSC	Genetic Modification Safety Committee
DMSA	dimercaptosuccinic acid	GOLD	Global Initiative on Obstructive Lung Disease
DR	direct radiography		
DTPA	diethylene triamine pentoacetic acid	GWAS	genome-wide association studies
DU	depleted uranium	GWS	Gulf War syndrome
DVD	digital video devices	HACO	high altitude cerebral oedema
DVLA	Driver and Vehicle Licensing Agency	HAPO	high altitude pulmonary oedema
DWP	Department for Work and Pensions	HARN	high aspect ratio nanoparticles
EAA	extrinsic allergic alveolitis	HAVS	hand–arm vibration syndrome
EAPs	Employee assistance programmes	HBC-OCRV	health-based occupational cancer risk values
EAV	exposure action value	HCC	hepatocellular carcinoma
EBC	exhaled breath condensate	HCFC	hydrochlorofluorocarbons
EBDC	ethylenebisdithiocarbamate	HEI	Health Effects Institute

HFC	hydrofluorocarbons	IPPV	intermittent positive-pressure ventilation
HF	hexafluoride		
HFRS	haemorrhagic fever with renal syndrome	IPS	individual placement and support
HLA	human leukocyte antigen	IPSS	International Prognostic Scoring System
HLA	leukocyte associated antigens	IR	infrared radiation
HL	hearing level	ITO	indium tin oxide
HMLD	hard metal lung disease	IVF	in vitro fertilization
HPA	Health Protection Agency	JEM	job exposure matrices
HP	hypersensitivity pneumonitis	JEMs	job–exposure matrices
HPLC	high pressure liquid chromatography	KCO	gas transfer coefficient
HPS	hantavirus pulmonary syndrome	LAMMA	laser microprobe mass analysis
HRCT	high resolution computed tomography	LBP	low-back pain
HRT	hormone replacement therapy	LD50	lethal dose 50 per cent
HRV	heart rate variability	LED	light emitting diodes
HSA	human serum albumen	LEDs	light-emitting diodes
HSC	Health and Safety Commission	LET	linear energy transfer
HSE	Health and Safety Executive	LEV	local exhaust ventilation
HSL	Health and Safety Laboratory	LFT	liver function test
HTL	hearing threshold level	LMA	laryngeal mask airway
HU	Hounsfield units	LOAEL	lowest observable adverse effect level
HUS	haemolytic uraemic syndrome	LPG	liquid petroleum gas
HWE	healthy worker effect	LPS	lipopolysaccharide
Hz	Hertz	LSS	Life Span Study
IAEA	International Atomic Energy Agency	MAG	metal active gas
IARC	International Agency for Cancer Research	MAT	microscopic agglutination test
IARC	International Agency for Research in Cancer	MBI	Maslach Burnout Inventory
		MCP-1	monocyte chemotactic protein-1
IASP	International Association for the Study of Pain	MDHS	Methods for Determination of Hazardous Substances
IATA	International Air Transport Association	MDR-TB	multidrug-resistant tuberculosis
IB	incapacity benefit	MDS	myelodysplastic syndromes
ICD	irritant contact dermatitis	mEH	microsomal epoxide hydrolase
ICNIRP	International Commission on Non-ionizing Radiation Protection	MetHb	methaemoglobinaemia
		MHC	major histocompatibility complex
ICRP	International Commission on Radiological Protection	MHSWR	Management of Health and Safety at Work Regulations
IDSA	Infectious Diseases Society of America	MIG	metal inert gas
IEC	International Electrotechnical Commission	MLR	middle latency response
		MMA	manual metal arc
IEEE	Institute of Electrical and Electronic Engineers	MMMF	man-made mineral fibres
		MN	micronuclei
IESNA	Illuminating Engineering Society of North America	MNP	manufactured nanoparticles
		MPE	maximum permissible exposure
IIAC	Industrial Injuries Advisory Council	MPO	myeloperoxidase
IIA	irritant-induced asthma	MPP	methylphenyl pyridinium
IIDB	Industrial Injuries Disablement Benefit	MPTP	methyl phenyl pyridinium
IIDB	Industrial Injuries Disablement Benefits	MRI	magnetic resonance imaging
ILO	International Labor Office	MR	magnetic resonance
ILO	International Labour Office	MRR	meta-relative risk
ILO	International Labour Organisation	MRS	magnetic resonance spectrometry
INR	international normalized ratio	MSDS	material safety data sheet
IOM	Institute of Occupational Medicine	MS	mainstream smoke
IPCS	International Programme on Chemical Safety	MVOC	microbiological emissions on damped surfaces
IPD	idiopathic Parkinson's disease	MVOCs	microbial volatile compounds
IPM	Integrated pest management	MWF	metal-working fluids

NAIR	National Arrangements for Incidents involving Radioactivity	PMF	progressive massive fibrosis
NASH	non-alcoholic steatohepatitis	PMN	polymorphonuclear leukocytes
NBC	nuclear, biological and chemical	PM	particulate matter
NFCI	non-freezing cold injury	PMR	proportional mortality rates
NHL	non-Hodgkin's lymphoma	POEA	polyoxyethyleneamine
NICE	National Institute for Health and Clinical Excellence	PPB	positive pressure breathing
		PPE	personal protection equipment
		PR	prevalence ratio
NIHL	noise-induced hearing loss	PTA	pure tone audiogram
NIOSH	National Institute for Occupational Safety and Health	PTFE	polytetrafluoroethylene
		PTSD	post-traumatic stress disorder
NMR	nuclear magnetic resonance	PUO	pyrexia of unknown origin
NMSC	non-melanocytic skin cancer	PVC	polyvinyl chloride
NOAEL	no adverse effect level	QRA	quantitative risk assessment
NOAEL	no observable adverse effect level	QST	quantitative sensorineural tests
NP	nanoparticles	RADS	reactive airways dysfunction syndrome
NSADs	non-steroidal anti-inflammatory drugs	RA	rheumatoid arthritis
NSIP	non-specific interstitial pneumonitis	RAST	radioallergosorbent test
NTE	neuropathy target esterase	RBC	red blood cells
NTP	National Toxicology Program	RCS	respirable crystalline silica
OAE	Otoacoustic emissions	RCT	randomized controlled trial
OA	Osteoarthritis	REACH	Registration, Evaluation, Authorisation and Restriction of Chemicals
OC	Organochlorine		
OECD	Organisation for Economic Co-operation and Development	REA	Reduced Earnings Allowance
		REL	recommended exposure limit
OEL	occupational exposure limit	REMPAN	Radiation Emergency Medical Preparedness Assistance Network
OI	orthostatic intolerance		
OPIDP	Organophosphate-induced delayed polyneuropathy	REM	rapid eye movement
		RF	radiofrequency fields
OP	organophosphate	rms	root mean square
OP	organophosphorous compounds	RMS	root mean square
OPRA	Occupational Physicians Reporting Activity	ROS	reactive oxygen species
		RPE	respiratory protection equipment
OR	odds ratio	RR	relative risk
OSHA	Occupational Health and Safety Administration	RRs	relative risks
		RSI	repetitive strain injury
OSWAS	Ovako Working Posture Analysing System	RULA	rapid upper limb assessment
		RV	residual volume
PACS	picture archiving and communication system	SACGM	Scientific Advisory Committee for Genetic Modification
PAHs	polycyclic aromatic hydrocarbons		
PBB	polybrominated biphenyls	SAR	specific absorption rate
PB	pyridostigmine bromide	SARS	severe acute respiratory syndrome
PCBs	polychlorinated biphenyls	SBS	sick building syndrome
PCP	pentachlorophenol	SCBA	self-contained breathing apparatus
PCQ	polychlorinated quarterphenyls	SCC	squamous cell carcinoma
PCR	polymerase chain reaction	SCL	skin contamination layer
PCT	porphyria cutanea tarda	SCOEL	Scientific Committee on Occupational Exposure Limits
PD	Parkinson's disease		
PEF	peak expiratory flow	SCUBA	self-contained underwater breathing apparatus
PEFR	peak expiratory flow rate		
PEG	polyethylene glycol	SD	spatial disorientation
PEL	permissible exposure limit	SDS	safety data sheets
PEMF	pulsed electromagnetic fields	SENSOR	Sentinel Event Notification System for Occupational Risks
PEP	post-exposure prophylaxis		
PET	positron emission tomography	sg	specific gravity
PIXE	particle-induced x-ray emission	SHA	Special Hardship Allowance

SHS	secondhand smoke	TLVs	threshold limit values
SIR	standardized incidence ratio	TMA	trimethylamine
SLE	systemic lupus erythematosis	TMT	trimethyltin
SLOD DTL	Specified Level of Death Dangerous Toxic Load	TNS	tension neck syndrome
		TNT	trinitrotoluene
SMR	standardized mortality ratio	TOAE	transient otoacoustic emissions
SNC	sinonasal cancer	TOS	thoracic outlet syndrome
SNPs	single nucleotide polymorphisms	TSH	thyroid stimulation hormone
SOAE	spontaneous otoacoustic emissions	TTP	thrombotic thrombocytopenic purpura
SPECT	single-photon emission computed tomography	TTS	temporary threshold shift
SPK	superficial punctuate keratitis	TWA	time-weighted average
SPL	sound pressure levels	UNSCEAR	United Nations Scientific Committee on the Effects of Atomic Radiations
SP	summating potential		
SRR	standardized registration ratio	UROD	uroporphyrinogen decarboxylase
SRT	simple reaction time	UV	ultraviolet
SSD	surface-supplied diving	VATS	video-assisted thoracoscopic surgery
SS	sidestream smoke	VCD	vocal cord dysfunction
STEL	short-term exposure limit	VCM	vinyl chloride monomer
STSS	streptococcal toxic shock syndrome	VC	vinyl chloride
SVR	slow vertex response	VC	vital capacity
SWORD	surveillance of work-related and occupational respiratory diseases	VDU	video display units
		VLDL	very low density lipoproteins
SWS	slow wave sleep	VOCs	volatile organic compounds
TBM	tunnel boring machine	VWF	vibration white finger
TCA	trichloroacetic acid	WBGT	wet bulb globe temperature
TCDD	tetrachlorodibenzo-p-dioxin	WBV	whole body vibration
TDI	toluene diisocyanate	WCA	Work Capability Assessment
TENS	transcutaneous electrical nerve stimulation	WEL	workplace exposure limits
		WFI	work-focused interview
TET	triethyltin	WHO	World Health Organization
the CIE	International Commission on Illumination	WMSDs	work-related musculoskeletal disorders
TIC	toxic industrial chemicals		
TIG	tungsten inert gas	WTC	World Trade Center
TLCO	transfer factor for carbon monoxide	ZPP	zinc protoporphyrin
TLC	total lung capacity		

PART ONE

GENERAL CONSIDERATIONS

Section One: History and development of occupational medicine   3
Section Two: Diagnosis of occupational disease   31
Section Three: Extent and attribution of occupational disease   75
Section Four: Legal issues   111

SECTION ONE

History and development of occupational medicine

1 Donald Hunter and the history of occupational health: precedents and perspectives *Joseph Melling and Tim Carter*	5
2 The changing face of occupational diseases *Peter J Baxter, Tar-Ching Aw, Anne Cockcroft, Paul Durrington and J Malcolm Harrington*	24

Donald Hunter and the history of occupational health: precedents and perspectives

JOSEPH MELLING AND TIM CARTER

Donald Hunter: Clinician, investigator, teacher, author and historian	5
Hunter's historical perspective	6
Industrialization and risk	7
State intervention and disease prevention	10
Dangerous trades and industrial diseases	11

The medical perspective	12
The international dimension in peace and war	14
Asbestos and other toxins: Disasters waiting to happen?	16
A future history for occupational health?	18
Conclusions	20
References	21

DONALD HUNTER: CLINICIAN, INVESTIGATOR, TEACHER, AUTHOR AND HISTORIAN

Donald Hunter, the son of a Post Office engineer, was born in 1898 in East London. He trained in medicine and qualified in 1922. After a year spent researching lead poisoning at Harvard in 1926, he worked at the London Hospital from 1927 until retiring in 1963. By the 1930s, Hunter had firmly established his life-long interest in occupational health and a growing reputation as a commentator and teacher. In 1943, he became director of the Department of Industrial Medicine at the London, funded by the Medical Research Council. The following year, he became the first editor of the *British Journal of Industrial Medicine* and in 1955 he published *The Diseases of Occupations*.[1] Hunter's encyclopaedic narrative has been compared with the pioneering works of Bernardino Ramazzini and Charles Thackrah, physicians who completed monumental studies of workpeople's diseases in the eighteenth and nineteenth centuries.[2] Hunter remained deeply interested in the historical origins of occupational medicine, as well as the trends of disease and injury in the workplace.

Hunter's predecessors in Britain as authoritative writers in the field of occupational health were Thomas Arlidge (1822–99), Thomas Oliver (1852–1942) and Thomas Legge (1863–1932). They received their medical training in the Victorian period when industrial disease emerged as a serious subject for investigation. Their work is discussed below.[3] Each had some sense of historical perspective and frequently drew on a range of classical and modern sources to exemplify their studies. However, it was Hunter's own contemporaries who undertook detailed historical research on the identification and treatment of occupational diseases, particularly in the mining industries. Notable publications in the United States, often undertaken by European émigrés sympathetic to the cause of organized labour, were George Rosen's *The history of miners' diseases* (1943) and Ludwig Teleky's *History of factory and mine hygiene* (1948).[4] In the United Kingdom, renewed interest in occupational health during the 1930s was fired by a group of researchers, such as Archie Cochrane, Philip D'Arcy Hart and Ronald Lane, whose sympathies clearly lay with the social and political cause of the industrial working class.[5]

We can locate Hunter's own investigations and literary concerns, therefore, within a genre of contemporary toxicology research, historical writing and social compassion. His extensive reading was combined with the vigorous pursuit of a wide variety of cases of industrial poisoning in the east end of London and beyond. He assiduously sought out details of cases, questioning his patients on the incidence of illness among fellow employees, corresponding with other physicians on their industrial background and case history.[6] Notably, Hunter investigated the effects of methyl mercury poisoning from seed dressings on the visual cortex (later of world importance when methyl mercury effluent entered the food chain and poisoned people in Minamata, Japan). In these years, Hunter sought out intriguing cases of deformity and occupational stigmata, particularly for photographic records (presumably to show his students).[7] He was also sensitive to the geographical origins of illness. Not only were occupations, such as billiard table makers, closely examined for distinguishing signs of pneumoconiosis (lung disease) caused by silica dust from slate rather than tuberculosis, but the diverse case histories of international mining engineers with similar complaints were carefully reconstructed.[8]

In pursuing his research, Hunter had kept in touch with notable members of the Home Office's factory inspectorate, such as Edward Merewether, requesting items for the collection that Hunter was assembling.[9] In 1943, Hunter was asked if he would be willing to take charge of a research department funded by the Medical Research Council at the London Hospital.[10] London was to be one of a proposed network of university departments in industrial medicine that did not come into being, Hunter believed that Clydeside, Merseyside and Tyneside were the most obvious candidates for such centres.[11] From his department in the London Hospital, he also followed Legge's example of studies in the Great War (1914–18) by investigating industrial hazards associated with aircraft production and other essential munitions supplies during the Second World War (1939–45).

Hunter fought to raise the status of occupational health and medicine during the late 1940s. In a report on industrial medicine written in 1949, Hunter argued that England (*sic*) was the leading country in protecting workers against accidents and disease, though the scanty resources allocated by the Treasury to the Factory Department of the Ministry of Labour, deprived it of the capacity to undertake original research and limited its powers of inspection and regulation.[12] He strongly argued that the industrial physician should be closely linked to general medicine and that the university centres should forge ties within experimental pathology, pharmacology, physiology and with scientists more generally. He considered that the basic practice of industrial medicine should remain within the grasp of the general practitioner.[13]

In the 1950s, Hunter continued his research into occupational health, visiting Charles Fletcher's Pneumoconiosis Unit in Llandough Hospital (also funded by the Medical Research Council), noting privately the animosity between Fletcher's unit and the engineers at the mining school in Cardiff. He also visited the Wool (Anthrax) Disinfecting Station at Liverpool and commented on the innovative work at the Slough Industrial Health Service under Austin Eager.[14] This was one of a series of 'group occupational health services' set up in the immediate post-war years with financial support from the Nuffield Foundation. In 1955, Hunter finally published his massive work, which rapidly established a reputation as the single most authoritative English language medical reference source on occupational illness. Hunter's influence was also extended through his tireless efforts as a teacher and examiner in London, countless doctors being confronted by industrial specimens presented at oral examinations and questions posed on subjects relating to them. He continued to be an inspired teacher into the 1970s, entertaining students long after the scheduled finish of his lecture with historical exhibits produced from a large cardboard box.[15]

HUNTER'S HISTORICAL PERSPECTIVE

Hunter brought to the study of industrial illness the distinct scientific and historical perspective of British medicine in the mid-twentieth century. His survey of workplace maladies begins with a broad panorama of human history before he engages in a long narrative of progress in the industrial world. Hunter relies not only on classical texts to illuminate different periods of industrial development, but follows Rosen and others in attempting a serious economic and social history of production since the earliest years of industrialization. His historical writing bears the impress of his own time and his own text has become a significant historical document which should be read in the light of subsequent research by both economic and medical historians. Hunter acknowledges the progress made in the prevention of occupational diseases and notes the role of politics and social concern in this, but the approach he adopts has been seen by more recent historical commentators as focusing on the 'grand narrative' and the role of medical investigators in it, rather than acknowledging the views of non-specialists concerned with the harmful effects of work.[16]

Together with Rosen, Siegerist, Teleky and others, we may reasonably identify Hunter as one of the founding figures in occupational health history. In the half-century since his work was published, the discipline of historical writing has been transformed. Medical historians have been influenced by arguments in social and cultural history which have identified how different insights may be gained into familiar historical processes by examining the experiences of individuals and groups not usually included in the story. By retrieving the documents and oral testimonies left by less prominent and powerful individuals, including many of the patients treated by medical personnel, we can derive a deeper understanding of the perceptions and motives of those involved in medical treatment. Many of those who received medical attention, such as the workers suffering occupational diseases, have left few testaments and even their employers rarely spent time and resources expressing their own views of injuries or 'malingering' outside official enquiries and legal documents. It is not merely a matter of discovering new sources which might enable us to hear those who were left without a voice in older historical studies: there is also the challenge of re-reading recognized materials to trace the circumstances in which scientific knowledge itself (and its authors) became the authoritative account of the natural world and the aetiology of illness.

While there is considerable force in recent challenges to the older, more heroic, genre of medical history represented by Hunter, it can be argued that many of his judgements have withstood the test of time and scholarly criticism. Hunter's portrayal of his historical subjects may have encouraged a view of workers mainly as victims of economic change, but the empathy his writing shows with the labour force is in many ways comparable to those social historians who set out to tell a story of events 'from below'. His discussion of mining reveals interplay between society, work and health in a stark perspective as the growing scale and depth of coal mining led to the employment of women and children alongside an expanding army of adult male colliers (Figure 1.1). He discusses how public concern in the 1840s about the morality of partially clothed women and children working underground in these conditions provoked moral alarm rather than merely regard for physical welfare of those labouring in primitive conditions.

Technological change and the introduction of rock drills are similarly presented in their social context, as Hunter notes, a lethal new threat to the lungs of workers arose as unprecedented amounts of dust were generated by these 'widow makers' powered by compressed air.

More recent historical research suggests that the opening themes of the historical section of his book, in which he outlines the human condition and man's relationship to work before he provides a broad narrative of industrialization, would, if written now, be recast to include the attitudes of a wider range of people and note their distinctive contribution to the workplace, the identification of occupational hazards and the alleviation of illness. Hunter's work is, however, far more than just a record of power and attitudes of the (mainly male) medical profession of the mid-twentieth century. It is worth recalling the turbulent political struggles which marked his professional life and the intellectual battles of the years before the rise of fascism and during the cold war era in which his own major work was published. Hunter's long historical introduction to *Diseases of occupations* does present a portrait of progress in which clinical investigators played a significant and often heroic part in achieving positive change, but it is also a testimony to the social conscience of a minority of distinguished medical investigators in an age of hardship, tension and war, whose legacy remains strong.

INDUSTRIALIZATION AND RISK

Early accounts of industrial hazards include the pioneering studies by Agricola (1494–1555) and Paracelsus (1493–1541). Both investigated hazardous working conditions and the toxic hazards associated with mining labour (Figures 1.2–1.4).[17] Their concern to ameliorate the harshness of mine labour and the vulnerability of workers to human as well as environmental abuse remained a strong feature of industrial and medical commentaries into the nineteenth century. Bernadino Ramazzini (1633–1714) also paid close attention to miners' diseases, but extended his pioneering investigations across the

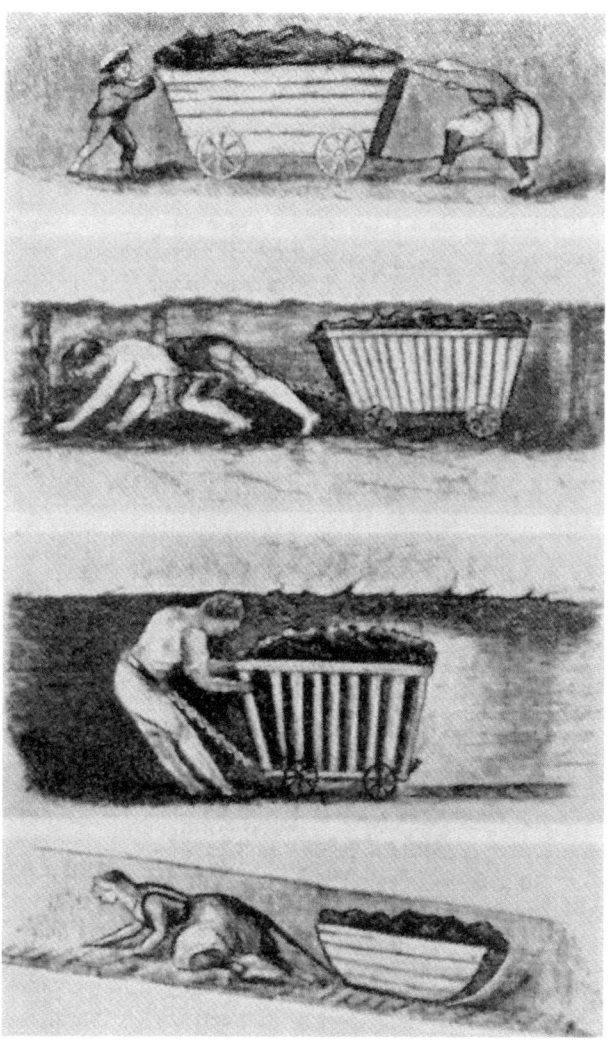

Figure 1.1 Children hauled trucks of coal and women, almost naked, were harnessed like horses to coal trucks.

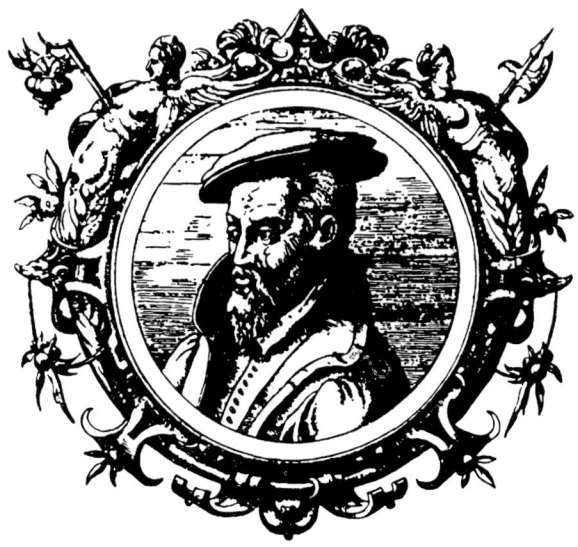

Figure 1.2 Georgius Agricola (Georg Bauer) (1494–1555).

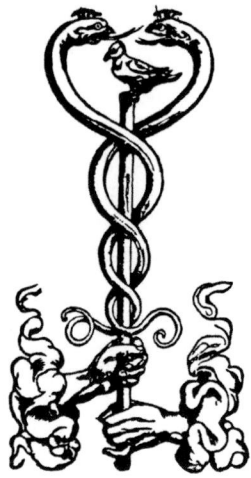

Figure 1.3 Title page of *De Re Metallica*, an illustrated treatise on mining, 1556.

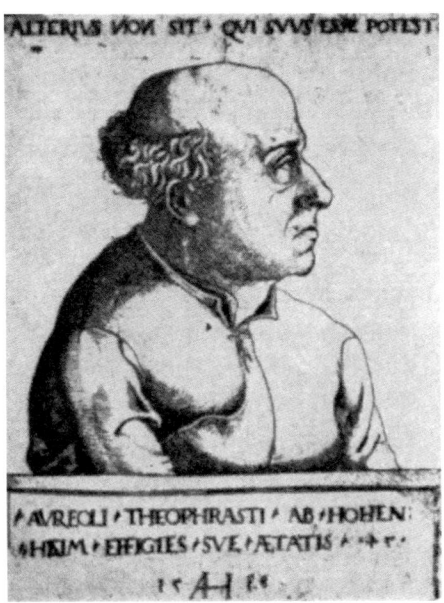

Figure 1.4 Paracelsus (1493–1541).

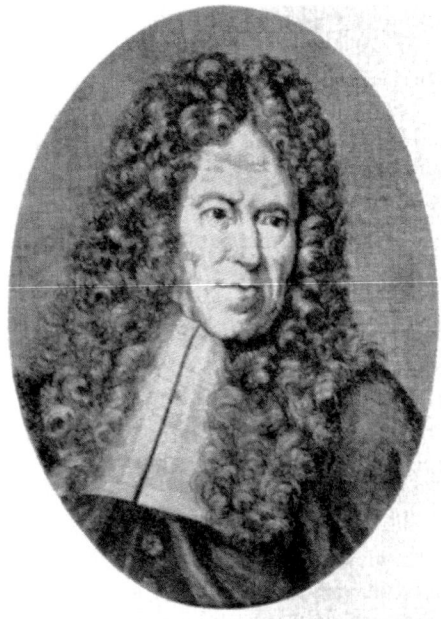

Figure 1.5 Bernardino Ramazzini (1633–1714).

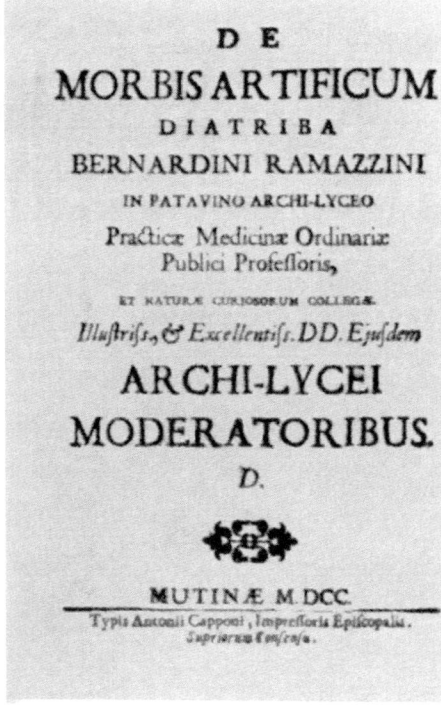

Figure 1.6 Title page of the first edition of Ramazzini's treatise: *De Morbis Artificum Diatriba*, 1713.

crafts and trades which populated the urban centres of northern Italy at the end of the seventeenth century, emphasizing the importance of personal examination of workmen and a close attention to their own accounts and experiences (Figure 1.5). Ramazzini's seminal work *Morbis artificum diatriba* offered prescient comments on the illnesses of people employed in trades such as pottery

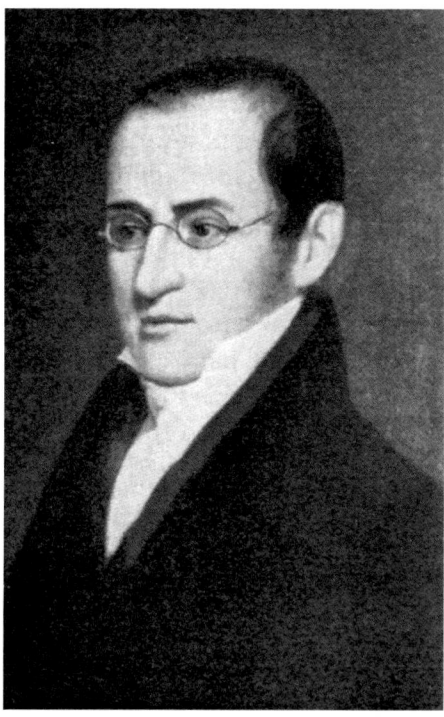

Figure 1.7 Charles Turner Thackrah (1795–1833).

in his day and also miscarriages among women living near obnoxious workshops (Figure 1.6).[18]

The search for new sources of power to fuel industrial production during the eighteenth century led to the growth of new industrial settlements and the concentration of larger groups of workers in bigger workshops and factories where economies of scale and a finer division of labour could be realized. Whereas Ramazzini composed his classical text at a time when industrial production was still dominated by relatively shallow mines and the artisan workshops of mercantile communities, Charles Turner Thackrah (1795–1833) made the first detailed study of the toxic effects of working with minerals, chemicals and organic materials in the different trades which were carried out around the mechanized industrial centre of Leeds during the 1830s (Figure 1.7).[19] Earlier investigators had addressed problems of flint dust in the pottery and ceramics workshops of Staffordshire, while lead and mercury poisoning were studied in the eighteenth century, and the exposure of boy chimney sweeps to soot led to Percival Potts' (1714–88) early recognition of cancerous warts.[20] However, it was Thackrah's celebrated study which broke new ground in seeking systematically to link the incidence of industrial disease with statistical evidence of life expectancy in different districts. Although he was one of the many commentators on the adverse effects of industrialization he most clearly quantified and detailed the health effects. Thackrah shared with other later investigators not only a deep interest in the statistical evidence gathered by census enumerators and civil registrars, but a passionate commitment to the cause of industrial and sanitation reform.

In reviewing Hunter's descriptions of these historical changes we can sketch their links with more recent studies on the industrialization of Europe and other parts of the global economy since the late eighteenth century. Concern about risks from work in pre-industrial society does seem to be limited to the writings of medical authors, with the exception of the army and navy where military campaigns were often ineffective because of illness among troops or seamen. The toll from typhus and scurvy in the eighteenth century British navy led to investigations of diet, ventilation and hygiene, notably James Lind's *Treatise on scurvy* of 1753. Social, scientific and economic factors, as well as reluctance by seamen to change their diet delayed the introduction of his recommendations for the provision of lemon juice as both prevention and cure for several decades – an early example of the interplay of many interest groups in setting the pace of prevention.[21]

The industrial revolution is now viewed differently than it was in Hunter's day. There are continuities of industrial development between the mechanical improvements of the decades after 1770 and an earlier period of 'proto' industrialization based on household and family production. The pattern of commercial, transport and trading change seen during the eighteenth and early nineteenth century did precipitate the mass movement of peoples from country to town and to longer-distance migration which we can see repeated in the industrial transformation of Asia in the past half-century. The social conditions which attended the urbanization of the British and other European populations were vividly depicted in contemporary novels as well as the parliamentary and scientific enquiries, frequently undertaken by medical men such as Thackrah, Gaskell, Kay and Greenhow.[22] Recent studies have tempered many of the bleak depictions of human misery and degradation, demographers noting the rising living standards seen particularly from the 1840s and the improvements in mortality and morbidity statistics seen after the 1870s.[23] Work processes and the relationships at work did undergo major changes with the assembly of large numbers of workers in factories and mills and the dependence on mechanical aids to increase production. Employers were driven by profits and productivity, but responded in different ways to this, with many making expedient use of low cost urban labour while a few, such as Robert Owen, established mills in rural areas and provided model working conditions with the aim of engendering both productivity and loyalty (Figure 1.8). The legal position of the employer as 'master' was strong, while that of the employee as 'servant' was weak, at least until organizations of workers, initially of craftsmen but later of all groups of workers, in trade unions developed, mainly in the teeth of concerted opposition from employers.

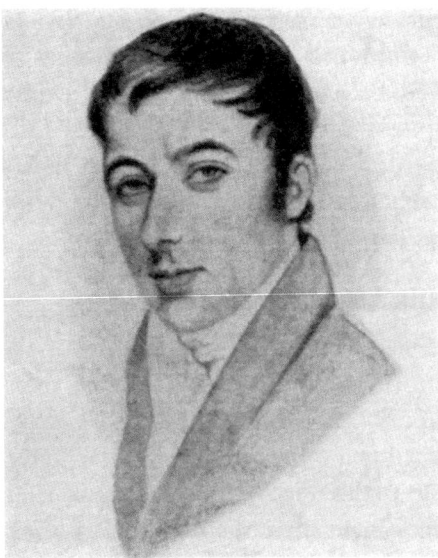

Figure 1.8 Robert Owen.

STATE INTERVENTION AND DISEASE PREVENTION

Effective factory legislation began in 1833 with the passing of an Act that could be enforced by dedicated inspectors appointed by the Home Office. This was not the first attempt to regulate but followed earlier measures that failed because of weak and corruptible local enforcement arrangements. Factory regulation at this time was a highly contested area of parliamentary business, not only between capital and labour because it was many years before workers would have the vote, but also between those who upheld the traditional agrarian structures of society and those grown newly powerful from the growth of industry. The law was initially concerned with hours and conditions of work for children and females in textile factories, although provision was also made for the appointment of surgeons to check the ages of children (Figure 1.9). The power to appoint these 'certifying surgeons' was formalized in the 1844 Factory Act when inspectors were given the power to recommend such doctors to the Home Office.[24] This was at a time when there was no unified medical profession and the inspectors had to assess suitability from first principles. In the middle part of the nineteenth century, the Factory Inspectorate with support from Robert Baker, the one medically qualified inspector, paid little attention to industrial disease, as the national priority was seen as being the prevention of disease associated with urbanization rather than that arising from work, which was sometimes seen as simply one of the consequences of employment in return for which a wage was paid. In the course of the nineteenth century, similar factory inspection regimes were set up in France, Germany, Belgium and other European countries and their empires. Inspection arrangements in the United States were created in the early twentieth century, some at state and some at federal level.

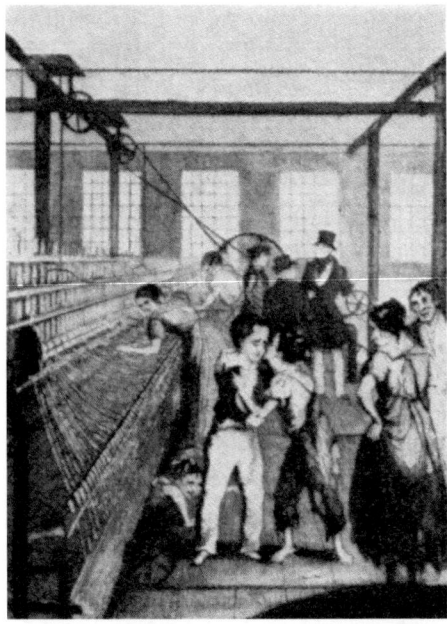

Figure 1.9 Child labour in the textile factories. The well-dressed visitors contrast with ragged apprentices. Note the small child crawling under the self-acting spinning mule. From *The life and adventures of Michael Armstrong, the factory boy* by Frances Trollope, 1840.

Statistics were themselves an important part of the story of occupational health and attempts to regulate working conditions after 1800. From 1851, decennial censuses of population included valuable information on occupations and households, while the registration of births and deaths started in 1837. These returns provided medical statisticians with materials from which to calculate mortality rates in different districts and across various occupational groups. The results based on the 1851 census were the first that could be used to measure increased mortality in towns and registration districts where dusty trades, such as ceramic manufacture and metal grinding, were based. Following Edwin Chadwick's famous *Report on the sanitary condition of the population* of 1842, the most notable and sustained investigations of the effects of work on sanitary and health statistics were carried out by Edward Greenhow (1814–88) at the instigation of John Simon at the Medical Department of the Privy Council. Greenhow examined pulmonary and other diseases among different occupational groups in meticulous studies in 1854–62 and persuasively demonstrated the link between dusty occupations and increased respiratory disease rates, though his investigations were complicated by co-morbidity from tuberculosis (although the bacillus which caused 'phthisis' had not yet been identified).[25]

Research, such as that undertaken by Greenhow, contributed to the debates on workplace health that surrounded the passage of the 1864 Factory Act, which first provided for ventilation of industrial premises outside mines. Recognition of the severe hazard presented by the metal grinding trades gradually led to the introduction of exhaust ventilation on the sandstone grindstones which caused serious lung damage or 'grinders' rot' in areas such as Sheffield and the Midlands. While factory and mine workers were subject to some state regulation, small workshops and those who were self-employed or contracted to small masters and intermediaries were notoriously unprotected throughout the nineteenth century.[26]

It was the legislation which dealt with lead poisoning in the years leading up to the Factory Act of 1891 which can reasonably be described as the foundation of both modern occupational health regulation and the use of specialist expertise in the public management of hazardous workplaces. The Act of 1891 empowered the Home Secretary (in practice his Inspectors at the Factory Department of the Home Office) to compel any trade designated as 'dangerous' to adopt special rules for the control of hazardous agents to protect workers. The last decade of the nineteenth century and the first decade of the new century deserve particular attention in the history of state attempts to regulate occupational dangers, for they saw the regulation of toxic substances and dusts, as well as establishing the reputation of several leading figures who studied these materials and advised government on their control.

DANGEROUS TRADES AND INDUSTRIAL DISEASES

The growth in government regulation of hazards at work arose in part from greater scientific understanding of the nature of the risks posed by particular substances and their widespread use as chemistry was revolutionized in the late nineteenth century. The new chemistry furnished techniques for the measurement of contaminants in the workplace and a more precise assessment of the relationship between exposure and harm to health. The effects of changes in levels of oxygen, nitrogen and carbon dioxide, as well as methane (in mines) and carbon monoxide (from fires) were investigated by innovative physiologists such as John Scott Haldane, whose field observations and experiments, often on himself in an exposure chamber, led to improvements in a range of industries, as well as in tunnels and wells.[27] Investigators in Germany, such as Lehmann, contributed to accurate measurements of toxic vapours in the atmosphere and their effects on the human body.[28] The birth of modern bacteriology and immunology with the work of Koch in Germany and Pasteur in France led to the specific identification of infectious organisms and methods of treating them from the 1880s, supplanting earlier disease theories of miasma, but also provoking wide-ranging and sustained controversies on the nature of infection.[29]

As the technologies for assessing risks and the methods for understanding diseases and their control steadily improved in the later nineteenth century, cases of poisoning affecting specific trades were more clearly identified. Three agents attracted particular attention and established the reputation of the early investigators of occupational illness in the United Kingdom and other countries: lead, phosphorus and anthrax. Lead poisoning had long been a serious problem in a range of industries including the manufacture of white lead pigment for use in paints, ceramic and pottery manufacture (lead glazes), and exposure to the element in mining and smelting operations. The employment of women in a number of these occupations led to the recognition that, as well as the abdominal, neurological and haematological effects of poisoning, they also suffered from repeated miscarriages. The Home Office established a committee to investigate white lead which recommended basic controls which were refined by later Dangerous Trades Committees and leading factory inspectors, including Thomas Legge on his appointment as first Medical Inspector of Factories in 1898. Ceramic and pottery manufacturers resisted any changes to the lead glazes, blaming their workers for poor hygiene and they maintained stubborn opposition to state interference in the early twentieth century. While significant reductions were recorded in notified cases from lead poisoning in the decade before 1914, probably as a result of more precise diagnosis, as well as the diligence of the Factory Inspectorate and increased publicity given to the problem by women's campaigners as well as health reformers, the mortality rates were little improved in the early twentieth century.[30] One indication of the persistence of problems can be found in the continuing research during the interwar years, including Hunter's period as a researcher at Harvard under Aub.

Phosphorus poisoning leading to necrosis of the jaw affected those working in the match-making industry, yellow phosphorus being used for strike-anywhere 'Lucifer' matches in the nineteenth century. 'Phossy jaw', the painful, frequently foul-smelling decay of the lower jaw led to disfigurement and death in both women and men who were involved in the making of inflammable paste and dipping of matches. Bryant and May presented themselves as model employers at their east London works until a famous industrial dispute brought the 'match girls' out on strike in 1889. Soon afterwards the press exposed the company's policy of concealing phosphorus poisoning cases by pensioning off afflicted workers. Similar problems in other countries led to proposals in 1900 for an international convention prohibiting yellow phosphorus in favour of safety matches, but the British government refused to support an international convention, seeing it as an unwarranted interference with free trade.

In contrast with the risks to the mostly unskilled females and males involved in lead and phosphorus trades, anthrax rose to prominence in Britain because of the rapid deaths from lung infection and septicaemia among the skilled men who were employed as wool sorters in the Bradford area of West Yorkshire. Suspicions had also been growing that labourers who worked with imported animal hides and hairs in places as distant as Glasgow, London and Liverpool were also suffering from a sometimes fatal skin infection associated with these materials. Dr JH Bell of

Bradford, an ophthalmic specialist, who also contributed to the identification of miners' nystagmus, achieved a national reputation in 1879–80 after linking pulmonary fatalities among wool workers with the *Bacillus anthracis* recently described in detail by Pasteur.[31] The remarkable success of Pasteur and Koch's work helped to establish the germ theory of disease among the British medical community, although heated debates continued long after about the proper role of laboratory research in tackling disease.[32] More practically, the association of anthrax with raw materials used in one of Britain's staple industries provoked fresh activism in the local labour force and a strong campaign resulted in the adoption in the early 1880s of a voluntary code of preventive measures, including the use of tables with downdraught ventilation for sorting fleeces from regions most associated with dangerous wools.

There was some improvement in recorded fatalities from anthrax and the earlier voluntary rules were extended to cover more groups of workers, tightened and made statutory (following a review by the Home Office's Committee on Dangerous Trades after 1896). The incidence of the more common skin form of 'malignant pustule' remained relatively constant, with death in about 15 per cent of cases. While Thomas Legge appears to have been convinced of the case for further legislation well before 1914, the response from the Factory Department of the Home Office can at best be described as lethargic. A contested legal decision taken on appeal to the Law Lords in 1905 that an employee infected by the bacillus should, for the purposes of compensation, be considered to have suffered an accident, helped to prompt the decision to schedule six occupational diseases as qualifying for compensation under the Workmen's Compensation Act of 1906. Anthrax remained a feature of the industrial scene in the early decades of the century. Hunter himself collected details from patients such as Elsie Mitchell, a horse hair worker aged 19 infected in 1913 and a male agricultural worker whose eye was infected after working with manure in 1921. Ever the indefatigable researcher, in 1935 Hunter interviewed the widow of a horse hair worker who had been infected in 1922 with 'filthy hair from Russia' and died. As late as 1938, Hunter examined a Harpenden man admitted to hospital with anthrax symptoms contracted at the artificial manure factory where he worked with wool processing waste or shoddy.[33]

THE MEDICAL PERSPECTIVE

In the years when the health of workers was becoming a subject of serious medical interest, three figures arose who largely defined the boundaries of occupational medicine before the Second World War. Two seminal texts were published in the decade 1892–1902. Thomas Arlidge's *Hygiene, diseases and mortality of occupations* (1892) was based on his Milroy lectures to the Royal College of Physicians delivered in 1889.[34] Originally a psychiatrist who served in an early Victorian lunatic asylum, Arlidge moved to North Staffordshire Infirmary and drew on his own encounters with cases of lead poisoning and lung disease. Arlidge also developed the methods of Thackrah and Greenhow by using census and mortality data to map the distribution of illness. Thomas Oliver was a Newcastle physician who advised the Factory Inspectorate on lead poisoning in the 1890s. His book *Dangerous trades* (1902) brought together leading authorities to describe not only industrial illnesses, but also the changing industrial technologies of the period. Oliver contributed several chapters and again made use of a mass of statistical information on mortality and morbidity.[35] Oliver resisted currently fashionable inclinations to explain the origins of industrial lung disease in bacteriological terms and emphasized the primary importance of mineral dusts (such as silica) in causing lung disease among workers. Both Arlidge and Oliver recognized the central role of the state in disease prevention, but saw workers as passive victims rather than recognizing the role of organized labour in debates on disease prevention.

Thomas Legge's *Industrial maladies* never achieved the reputation secured by his predecessors and was completed by his successor as senior medical inspector, John Bridge, after his sudden death in 1932.[36] Yet Legge (Figure 1.10) rose to early distinction and influence in a public career which his predecessors hardly contemplated. Legge was the son of a distinguished missionary in China and sinologist. He travelled widely in Europe before his appointment in 1898 to the new post of Medical Inspector of Factories, at the early age of 34 years.[37] The growth of government expertise in industrial toxicology and particularly the analysis of dust problems in the workplace which dominated the agenda for regulation until the 1960s can be dated from

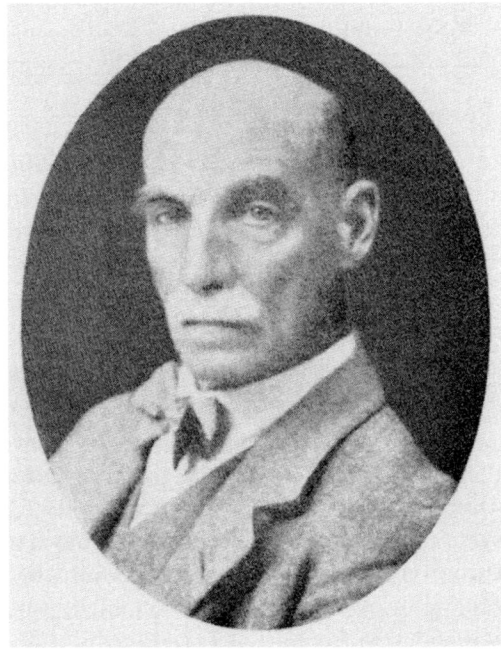

Figure 1.10 Sir Thomas Morison Legge (1863–1932), the first Medical Inspector of Factories, 1898.

his appointment. Legge's writings were influenced by the socialist and egalitarian leanings of the late nineteenth century arts and crafts movements and he frequently acknowledged the contribution of workers and their representatives to the cause of disease prevention. During the 27 years Legge served in the Home Office he investigated a wide range of diseases, undertaking systematic surveys such as that comparing the health of workers in Birmingham and at Woolwich Arsenal to isolate the effects of brassworking on health.[38] Legge continued his early interests in lead poisoning and anthrax infection, developing criteria to be used in diagnosis and supporting laboratory arrangements for anthrax investigation. His Milroy lectures of 1904 were a wide ranging review of industrial anthrax, its bacteriology, presentation, treatment and prevention. From his European visits, he became familiar with Sclavo's anthrax antiserum and subsequently served on the committee which sat during the First World War and recommended reforms which were embodied in the 1919 Anthrax Act and led to the building of the Liverpool disinfection station.[39]

In researching the effects of lead poisoning on workers, Legge struggled against the opposition of employers who sought to blame the dirty habits of their workers for poisoning to establish the primary importance of inhalation of lead particles rather than their ingestion by unclean eating habits. In collaboration with Kenneth Goadby, he refined the measurement of toxicity within the body and worked with other colleagues to restrict the hazards of lead in such booming sectors as the manufacture of lead-acid automobile batteries.[40] The contribution of government controls to the reduction in fatal lead poisoning is doubtful. The fruits of prevention and treatment were rather more apparent in anthrax where modest improvements were recorded in cases and fatality rates just before the First World War (Table 1.1). There was then a deterioration due to the use of poor quality wool to make good shortages of raw materials and to supply the enormous demand for military supplies. Long-term improvements followed legislation in 1919, but government measures probably had less impact than falling imports of more dangerous fleeces and gradual improvements in animal husbandry across the world. Legge's efforts to secure international cooperation in the control of anthrax and lead met insurmountable obstacles as outlined below.

Hunter's account of the progress of occupational medicine provides a heroic view of the pioneering efforts of enlightened individuals such as Arlidge, Oliver and Legge. Such an approach was common in many mid-twentieth century studies of medical history, where the concentration on eminent medical men tended to obscure the now current views on the impact of labour activists and interest groups and the complex political and legal context in which they were active. These physicians worked within a legislative framework which defined the terms of their involvement with industrial disease, as well as their legal responsibilities to patients and government. The passage of Workmen's Compensation legislation, in 1897 and 1906, established employers' liability for specific illnesses contracted at work, as well as accidents in industry. This placed medical knowledge in the witness box when claims were verified – at times pitting a doctor representing the employer and their insurers against another who represented the worker and their trade union, and increased the requirement for valid evidence on the causes and extent of disease affecting employees. It also narrowed the definition of occupational diseases to those conditions that were either notifiable to the Inspectorate or prescribed for compensation.

Historians have long been aware of the importance of social insurance in the building of state medical services across Europe and in other continents. In the United Kingdom, National Health Insurance was introduced in 1911, providing for the creation of 'approved societies' to administer the sickness benefits of workers and to engage panels of doctors who would attend to those insured under a state scheme funded by contributions from employers and workers as well as the Treasury. One of the concerns of nation states which created new social and health services during the late nineteenth and early twentieth centuries was the growing economic and military competition that required human, as well as industrial and territorial, resources. In this race for efficiency and supremacy, the health, and hence military potential, of 'human stock' was emphasized while eugenicists, in addition to their concerns about breeding, stressed the vital importance of maternal and infant welfare in an age when unfitness for military service could undermine the foundations of national success. Feminist historians have subsequently argued that

Table 1.1 Anthrax and lead poisoning cases, deaths and fatality rates (male and female) Britain.

Years	Anthrax			Lead poisoning		
	Cases	Deaths	Fatality rate (%)	Cases	Deaths	Fatality rate (%)
1900–1904	213	49	23	3761	131	3.4
1905–1909	290	72	25	2981	144	4.4
1910–1914	287	41	14	2741	174	6.3
1915–1919	379	54	14	1397	100	7.1
1920–1924	207	31	15	1543	104	6.7
1925–1929	199	27	13	1225	99	8.1

governments developed policies for occupational as well as public health which reflected their concerns about managing the (male) human resources of civil society. Such initiatives also reflected the gender bias and distinctive expectations of males and females in contemporary society, where adult men were expected to serve as breadwinners for the family household and to accept physical risks and working conditions from which females and children, living in a 'separate sphere', were protected. The reproductive and maternal health of fertile females was particularly emphasized by physicians, such as Arlidge and Oliver, who examined the dangers posed by lead during pregnancy and attributed poor infant mortality to working after childbirth. Women and girls were also considered to be vulnerable to mental, social and personal hazards which men were assumed to tolerate along with physical dangers or abuse at work.[41] Lady Factory Inspectors appointed from the 1890s were particularly responsible for investigating and reporting on the hazards faced by females in the workplace.[42] This topic remains controversial as other scholars have cast doubt on the claims that pre-1914 governments were particularly concerned with females in the measures passed to promote industrial health.[43]

Similar debates have surrounded the attitudes of trade unions towards compensation and safety. A common criticism of the labour unions is that they have historically shown more interest in pursuing monetary settlements for injured members than in promoting health and accident prevention in the workplace.[44] Such arguments appear to be based on an assumption that unions and their members can effectively choose whether to give priority to receiving monetary returns for injury rather than to securing safe working conditions. In practice, as writers since Ramazzini have noted, workers commonly believe they have few alternatives to tolerating hazardous working conditions and their representatives often pursue compensation payments as a necessary means of support for injured workers and their dependants. Labour leaders repeatedly expressed the largely unrealized belief that significant compensation payments would deter the employers (and their insurers) from persisting with dangerous work practices.[45] However, the lethargy of employers, the cover provided by their insurers and the apparent collusion of their medical advisers, as well as governments with poor safety standards has remained a constant feature of trade union concern since the late nineteenth century, hardly indicating widespread union tolerance of hazards in the workplace.

THE INTERNATIONAL DIMENSION IN PEACE AND WAR

In the years when nation states were introducing centralized health insurance, actuarial experts employed by insurance companies and friendly societies were assembling statistics which provided risk profiles of the working population. Statistical returns assumed a fresh importance for governments, as well as private organizations and legal experts.[46] The maintenance of the male breadwinner as the foundation for stable household income among the working population remained a theme in welfare reform and concerns about the occupational health of the workforce. International awareness of common health problems and the scope for similar approaches to resolving them certainly increased after Germany embarked on Bismarck's pioneering social insurance arrangements in the 1880s, although important differences can be seen in the way nation states addressed the question of compensation for injured workpeople and the liability of employers for different kinds of diseases. Crossnational projects, such as the building of the Alpine railway tunnels at the end of the nineteenth century, revealed the appalling hazards to which labourers were exposed, as diseases such as hookworm (ankylostomiasis) spread from the tunnels to many of the mining areas of Europe and its colonies.

Tunnelling and mining projects around the world provided a working laboratory for health researchers and contributed to the establishment in 1906 of the Permanent Commission for Occupational Health, an international grouping of occupational health experts. The huge growth in gold mining using dry drilling in siliceous rocks on the Rand of South Africa produced many cases of silicosis and these were seen in other countries, especially the United Kingdom, when miners returned home to die. Contributions to international understanding of serious respiratory illness in dusty trades were also made by the published investigations of medical experts such as Oliver and Legge. The promising moves being made towards greater international cooperation in regard to workers' injuries were interrupted by the outbreak of mass warfare in Europe in 1914, spreading to many parts of the world by 1916. Embattled states created a huge, unprecedented demand for essential war supplies, thereby introducing new risks to employees, exemplified by outbreaks of toxic jaundice among workers applying tetrachloroethane to aircraft wings and filling shells in plants handling TNT.[47] Governments responsible for munitions production were drawn into investigating and regulating conditions of work to reduce the toxic effects of chemicals used for armaments manufacture, to provide canteens and welfare services for workers away from home and to control the adverse effects of long hours on productivity and safety.[48]

At the same time, government ministers in the United Kingdom and other countries were acutely aware of the risks of labour unrest and disruption of production in the extraordinary market conditions of 'total' warfare. Concessions to organized workers included guarantees to reserve jobs for returning servicemen on the cessation of hostilities. The legacy of the war for research into and regulation of occupational hazards was a disappointing one for contemporary enthusiasts, such as the Industrial Welfare Society. The wartime research on fatigue led to the creation of the Industrial Health Research Board and was eventually incorporated into the Medical Research Council's efforts on workplace health in the interwar period, though it was not until the late 1930s and the outbreak of another international war in 1939 that fresh impetus was given to specific war-related industrial problems, where Hunter played a significant role as an investigator.[49]

Another legacy of the 1914–18 war was the creation of the League of Nations based in Geneva and its International Labour Office (ILO), which developed transnational conventions to improve labour conditions and reduce the incidence of illness at work. The ILO's conventions gave a formal status to agreements on the control of dangerous working conditions and enabled trade unions to contribute to such instruments. Dr Carozzi played a notable bridging role as both a staff member at the ILO and as secretary of the Permanent Commission for Occupational Health. Legge contributed to these innovative gatherings and sat on specialist commissions of enquiry, including one on anthrax, where other nations were unwilling to adopt the use of centralized disinfection stations, although they acknowledged the work of the United Kingdom in this area. Legge also played a key role in negotiating the convention to ban lead from interior paints. The British Government's decision to renege on its earlier undertaking to support this initiative led to Legge's widely publicized resignation from his post at the Home Office.[50] One topic on which the British Government was keen to contribute was silicosis. An international conference was convened at Johannesburg in 1930 at which national experts on silicosis exchanged views and agreed standards for classification of disease and methods of diagnosis based on South African and other international developments in radiography and pathology. As a major maritime nation, Britain also helped to draft several new ILO conventions which were important for the eradication of the worst abuses of seafarers by the global shipping industry.

President Woodrow Wilson had played a leading role in setting up the League of Nations, but the United States electorate turned their back on international commitments and Washington maintained only loose connections with the ILO through conventions and correspondence in the interwar years. Historically weaker than central governments in Europe, federal authorities played only a limited role in health and safety before the New Deal of the 1930s, although pioneering investigators such as Alice Hamilton publicized poor working conditions, especially where weakly protected immigrant and female workers were involved (Figure 1.11). The early decades of the century marked the emergence of scientific and Fordist (after Henry Ford's production line manufacture of automobiles) management practices, initially in the American automobile assembly industry, but soon transferred to other sectors and countries. These included the widespread use of timed production line operations specified and costed by 'work study' experts. The techniques of scientific or 'Taylorist' (after FW Taylor) management were vigorously criticized by early industrial psychologists such as Elton Mayo in America and by ethical employers such as Cadbury in the United Kingdom, who insisted on the importance of 'human factors' in planning production. It is also possible to detect some convergence of

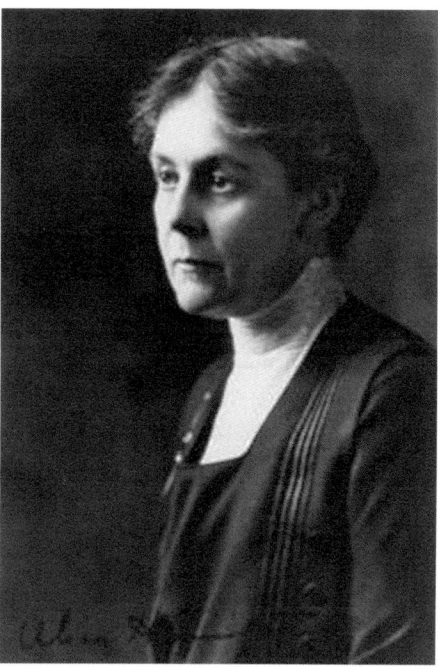

Figure 1.11 Alice Hamilton, a leading expert in the field of occupational health. Reproduced from www.nlm.nih.gov.

early 'scientific management' practices with the emerging professions of occupational psychology and industrial hygiene as firms sought to minimize labour problems by using psychometric tests for staff recruitment and to increase production by optimizing working conditions.[51] The emergence and growing employment of these specialists has remained a subject of some controversy. Criticism has come not only from trade unions who claim that these specialists tend to prioritize performance and output before employee safety, health and welfare, but also from other scientific and government experts who have questioned the methods and objectivity of such personnel. Similar criticism has been extended to those doctors in industry whose jobs were mainly structured in terms of providing support and solutions for the employer.

The international dissemination of technological and scientific information between the wars should be understood, therefore, within the strained political and industrial relations that overshadowed many societies during these years. These were also years of economic depression, industrial restructuring and rapid technological change in the global economy. The innovative use of chemicals had accelerated since the late nineteenth century, for instance using carbon disulphide in the manufacture of materials such as rayon (artificial silk), resulting in reappearance of its well-established neurological and behavioural harm in new workforces. The uses of lead featured in a variety of trades including the development of ethyl lead to slow the ignition of motor gasoline and this caused widespread poisoning where it was manufactured or blended. At the same time, traditional industries, such as coal, textiles, ceramics, steel and shipbuilding, faced harsher competition and were often slow to improve the poor conditions in their workplaces. It was a time when trade union membership had increased and spread from the craft unions to include the mass of unskilled workers, especially in the more traditional industries. By contrast, the newer sectors such as light engineering, electrical goods and parts of the consumer goods and chemical industries had supplemented their 'scientific' approaches to management with welfare provisions and were aiming to avoid a unionized workforce. In well-unionized sectors, such as coal, there was continuing pressure for compensation of industrial disease, especially of the lungs, and for preventative measures. This was at a time when some of the well-established risks, such as lead, phosphorus and anthrax, were diminishing in frequency, while others were being actively investigated. An example of this is the toxicological and chemical research in Manchester that led to improvements in the lubricating oils used for textile machinery (spinning mules) when carcinogenic polycyclic aromatic hydrocarbons were identified as the cause of skin and scrotal cancers in cotton workers.

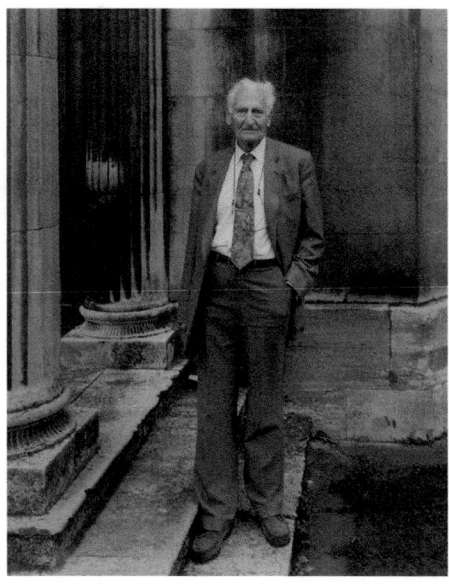

Figure 1.12 Richard Doll, a leading exponent of cancer epidemiology. Reproduced with permission from *British Medical Journal*. 1997; **314**: 695.

ASBESTOS AND OTHER TOXINS: DISASTERS WAITING TO HAPPEN?

The lung diseases linked to textiles and coal dust were gradually overshadowed by a controversy around 'the magic mineral' that became a hugely important building and transport material where serious fire risks faced manufacturers and consumers. The greatest occupational health risk of the middle and later decades of the twentieth century, and the mineral which has dominated recent debates on the national and international regulation of workplace hazards, is unquestionably asbestos. Soon after asbestos became widely used in the late nineteenth century, an early female factory inspector noted possible links to lung disease in workers.[52] These concerns resurfaced in the 1920s leading to an investigation by the Home Office's Factory Department in 1928–29. The report of this investigation by Price and Merewether set fresh standards in epidemiological analysis, demonstrating the presence of lung fibrosis or asbestosis among workers who inhaled the mineral fibres, but there was no indication of any link to cancer in workers, nor was the study designed to find one as this risk was not suspected.[53] In 1931, the report did prompt new government regulations for the control of asbestos dust and at the same time for silica.

The attitudes of the employers to these regulations and to subsequent risks have been the subject of fierce academic and courtroom controversy since the 1980s.[54] Much of the heat in these exchanges has been fuelled by the delayed rise in the incidence of cancer among people with little or no connection to the asbestos-manufacturing industry itself, but who were relatives of workers or individuals engaged in using or stripping out asbestos in buildings, transport vehicles, ships and other areas of employment where there was no perception of a risk, even at the time when cases were first appearing in heavily exposed workers. Even those living near asbestos works or consumers of their products developed disease from inhalation of the fibres.

It remains important to distinguish between known, suspected and unrecognized risks in the history of this and other industries, as well as to have a valid view on the state of knowledge at any point in time, untainted by hindsight, before making judgements about past practices. There is little doubt that the considerable risk of lung and pleural cancer was only demonstrated during the 1950s and 60s. It was during this period (rather than earlier) that we can identify efforts by the asbestos companies to suppress scientific research by Richard Doll (1912–2005) into the evidence of cancers caused by asbestos dust.[55] (Doll's pioneering studies of diseases due to asbestos and smoking were an important stimulus in the development of cancer epidemiology, in which he became a leading exponent (Figure 1.12).) Soon after this, the research of Wagner and others into the geographical pattern of mesothelioma and pleural tumours among South African crocidolite (blue asbestos) miners suggested links with the dust which blew around the streets of the mining communities, as well as with exposure in the mines.[56] The global reach of asbestos and its attendant diseases became apparent as pleural tumours were subsequently found among shipbuilding workers in the United Kingdom and the United States, where Irving Selikoff was both a leading investigator and a campaigner on behalf of those affected.

The asbestos problem became critical for governments as well as for workers, industrialists and insurers when it became apparent that the boundaries of risk within industry, and more importantly between occupational and public health hazards, were extremely difficult to draw. International scientific collaboration was needed as the different interest groups demanded new techniques and more rigorous epidemiological investigations to understand the dose–effect relationship between levels of asbestos dust and the incidence of illness. Competition as well as cooperation between leading scientists characterized the convening of medical conferences in Europe and the United States which sought to determine the hazards associated with blue and other forms of asbestos. In the 1960s and 1970s, the industry (and their medical advisers) campaigned to present chrysotile (non-blue) asbestos-containing products as essential to society and relatively safe. In particular, they emphasized the need for long-term research before enforcing any prohibition. As public regulators came under increasing pressure, bodies such as the British Occupational Hygiene Society provided standards that addressed, in a flawed analysis, the risk of asbestosis from chrysotile rather than that of cancer. The resultant controversy was sharpened by investigative journalism and media coverage (including the television documentary 'Alice: a fight for life'), forcing the British Government to introduce a battery of controls, including a licensing regime for asbestos insulation and a register of mesothelioma cases. It was the demonstration of a link between specific industrial products and public, as well as occupational, health which forced politicians to venture beyond the limited controls which had been proposed by civil servants and expert advisers.

A further and decisive blow against the continued use of asbestos and the interests of the producers came with the escalation of litigation, most particularly in the United States from the 1970s, by aggrieved plaintiffs who sought massive damages for the legacy of human and material losses which they faced from exposure to the material or from its incorporation into buildings. The scale of these claims forced the largest asbestos producer (Turner and Newall, Manchester, UK) to sell its assets and cease operations while damages also threatened the international insurance market at Lloyds with collapse at the end of the twentieth century. As a complete ban on all future use of asbestos became politically necessary in the United States and Europe, global mining and manufacture of the mineral went into steep decline, although mining continues and asbestos use persists in some lower-income regions of the world.

While the risks from asbestos overshadowed international concerns for workplace health in the later twentieth century, other occupational hazards were identified in the 'new' consumer materials of the period. Some of these toxic risks were known to earlier generations in different forms and the lesson of industrial poisoning was painfully relearned.[57] The serious risk of liver cancer presented by vinyl chloride, the raw material for PVC plastic, was identified in 1973–74 in workers who had been heavily exposed for over 20 years. Cleaners of polymerization vessels developed acro-osteolysis in their fingers and subsequent animal studies revealed disproportionate cancer rates, including the rare liver cancer angiosarcoma which was identified in exposed workers soon after the study results became available to the industry. Delays in the release of results occurred largely because of American concerns about regulatory implications, as the criticisms of historians Rosner and Markowitz make clear.[58] A familiar dilemma faced regulators in confronting the health risks from PVC production: its supporters pointed to the safety benefits of electrical insulation and other uses, as well as disruption to supplies of other essential chemical products (such as caustic soda), if PVC production was halted. Critics demanded immediate action. A compromise was adopted where producers agreed to reduce exposure levels over three years and new monitoring techniques were developed. In the longer term, the confirmation of cancer risks led to more comprehensive testing of other large volume industrial chemicals, resulting in only equivocal evidence of cancer risks in a few cases, though the principle of prior testing of substances and the need for valid risk assessments was established and later came to be incorporated into law. International bodies such as the International Agency for Cancer Research (IARC) and the International Programme on Chemical Safety also assumed a more significant role in such discussions.

Asbestos and especially its effects at low concentrations, as well as a wholly unexpected risk with vinyl chloride both focused attention on the large toll of disease that could arise from any substance with fatal effects that only become apparent after many years. This dented earlier confidence in the idea that the classic industrial poisonings were yesterday's diseases and that the major challenge of dust diseases of the lungs was now coming under control. It also led to a questioning approach to the pathology of diseases, such as the byssinosis of cotton workers delineated by Richard Schilling, where the effects of the agent in cotton and the less specific effects of pollution and smoking on the lungs had to be disentangled. Successful examples of prevention could be identified but there was now an expectation of diseases becoming apparent from new and even not so new technology, as well as uncertainty about the role of occupational sources of contamination in exacerbating or contributing to conditions that also occurred in the general population. Low level exposures also became prominent, especially as causes of cancer and mutation. The logic of a risk at any dose had been the basis on which protection against ionizing radiation had been founded for a number of years, but now there was evidence of similar patterns with asbestos and this fed into concerns about many other widely used products, such as pesticides, cosmetics and food additives. Indeed, the results of occupational epidemiology provided much of the evidence for the environmental contribution to cancers in general – a topic that remains contested.

The use of epidemiology to help frame regulations has depended on the examination of large groups of workers with comparable levels of exposure to risk whose pattern of illness could be compared either with the unexposed or with those who had a different level of exposure. A series of major studies of relatively specific risks was undertaken in the 1970s and 1980s by the Health and Safety Executive, by the Medical Research Council and by academic departments, with governmental or industry support.

The controversy surrounding asbestos and vinyl chloride coincided with a major review of state regulation of occupational safety and health in the United Kingdom by the Robens Committee. The United States had already undertaken a not dissimilar review leading to the creation of the Occupational Safety and Health Administration and the National Institute of Safety and Health in 1970. The aim of Robens was to rationalize and reduce the dense mass of regulations and inspection regimes which had developed since the nineteenth century. The 1974 Health and Safety at Work etc. Act fulfilled Robens' vision of a governance framework which separated the executive and enforcement functions of safety from the tripartite commission that decided on policy matters.[59] The new regime incorporated the recently formed Employment Medical Advisory Service (EMAS), as well as several inspectorates, into a Health and Safety Executive (HSE). EMAS's original purpose was to freely provide accurate information on occupational health to industry, trade unions and individuals, although while its connection to HSE's enforcers probably made it less palatable to employers it became better placed to function as a source of medical expertise within the new executive. Another feature of the new system was the inevitable difficulties which arose from Robens' definition of health and safety in fairly narrow occupational terms, leaving unresolved the familiar problem of drawing the boundaries of causation between workplace and the wider physical and social environment.

Since the 1974 Act, a number of new health regulations have been adopted including controls on chemicals, lead, asbestos and ionizing radiation, as well as for noise exposure, manual handling, working with pathogens and at display screens. The framework of international directives has been strengthened by European Union agreements that place penalties for non-compliance on nation states, as well as on offending employers. The agenda of occupational health and the expertise of government regulators has also changed in recent years as the historic concern with hazardous substances had to be refocused towards a range of conditions which extended from musculoskeletal pain and dermatitis to asthma, mental distress and the non-specific symptom syndromes which have been attributed to 'sick buildings', solvent exposure, pesticide use and other complicated environmental factors. As in the late nineteenth and early twentieth centuries, however, a key driver in the changing priorities and concerns of employers and governments has been the award of compensation settlements in cases of workplace stress and upper limb disorders. This has prompted defensive and preventative action by industries and their insurers.

A FUTURE HISTORY FOR OCCUPATIONAL HEALTH?

Hunter first published his major work at a point when the most lethal consequences of asbestos were still to be revealed and it was still possible to see the history of medicine as an almost unbroken trajectory of scientific improvement and heroic discovery. Within 20 years of his first edition, the bitter and escalating controversy around asbestos had blown away the notion of benign technology and consensual regulation. A few years after Hunter's work Rachel Carson's *Silent spring* was published, graphically depicting the impact of chemical production and toxic pollution on the American landscape and confirming a dawning consciousness of environmental damage which reoriented public health politics in the United States during the following three decades. The growing challenge to assumptions about the beneficial consequences of new technology and medical research was strengthened by pharmaceutical tragedies, such as the marketing of thalidomide to pregnant women and the initial reluctance of the Distillers Company to reach a compensation settlement with those families affected. We still do not know at the end of the first decade of the twenty-first century what the final toll of deaths and disability will be from the asbestos disaster.

As the promise of scientific progress and new technologies has been subjected to more critical scrutiny in the half-century since Hunter's text was published, philosophers, social scientists and historians have attempted to offer a more searching analysis of the way science itself is conducted and the terms in which knowledge about the world (and the human body) is authenticated and accepted. Social scientists have also contributed to explanations about human behaviour in the face of risks and hazards as well as to broader questions of social interaction at the workplace and individual assessment of competing responsibilities.[60] The expanding disciplines of psychology, sociology and organizational studies have also exerted greater influence over the ways in which workplace health and risks are understood and analysed. Although the diagnosis and treatment of occupational diseases had traditionally depended on a clinical examination and frequently on the sufferer's own history of their working life, industrial toxicologists had been largely concerned with the pathology of illness and establishing the nature of the link between environment and illness. In determining the provisions made for both treatment and financial maintenance of the individual worker, a range of social and political considerations has almost inevitably come into play. Governments, as well as scientists, often appeared anxious in the earlier twentieth century to preserve the distinction, however artificial in practice, between the research problem of industrial hazard and the legal and administrative procedures by which financial compensation might be decided.

Preserving these distinctions was particularly difficult when a new range of work-related ailments emerged, including asthma, dermatitis, musculoskeletal pain and mental strain where the link between illness and specific occupational conditions was less robust than in circumstances where toxins or dust might be measured with the prospect of defining clear dose–effect relationships. While an increase in prevalence might be established, the nature of individual exposure and susceptibility was much less clear. Greater reliance had to be placed on epidemiological studies of large groups of workers rather than on individual case notification.

The limitations of epidemiological studies provoked further debates about the appropriate methodologies which could be utilized in the discovery of health and illness at work. In many industries, such as oil, chemicals and pharmaceuticals, only a small number of workers were exposed to a particular hazard. Statistical testing of unusual patterns and isolated clusters of disease yielded unsatisfactory results. Researchers also found it difficult to establish valid methods to study the apparent increase in musculoskeletal and psychosocial symptoms reported in British and overseas workplaces as reports depended so heavily on subjective evaluation and self-reporting. Psychologists became contributors to HSE research projects from about 1980. Within the expanding research field of work-related psychology, divisions were also apparent between laboratory-trained personnel who followed the experimental model of study laid down during and after the 1939–45 war, and those who embraced a qualitative and more flexible social approach to the investigation of workplace attitudes and the consequences of monotony, overload and conflict in different occupations.

Most historians of work would place these trends in occupational health and the debates among experts on the nature and causes of workplace illness within the larger social and institutional context of economic and political change during the later twentieth century. Discussions about workers' welfare had moved from assessments of basic physical and mental capacity to considerations of satisfaction and fulfilment as conceptions of human well-being expanded during the long boom and rising affluence of the post-war period. European countries that developed comprehensive welfare systems funded by near-full employment and corporate bargaining between employers, unions and government embraced at least some principles of improved job fulfilment, as well as rigorous safety standards. Scandinavian research was particularly influential in a burgeoning concern with improving or 'enriching' occupational satisfaction, as well as in an escalating literature on sources of 'stress' at work and in wider society.[61] The context of these debates was radically changed in the last two decades of the twentieth century as the post-war consensus on national fiscal management and collective bargaining was disrupted in Europe and other continents by the reorganization of global production and the election of free-market conservative governments in the United Kingdom, the United States and other countries. The transformation of the global economy was confirmed by the collapse of planned economies and Soviet power, as well as the commitment of China to industrialization and world trade, in the past two decades.

These changes were reflected in renewed concern with the productivity of the workforce and with devising effective models for managing human, as well as material, resources of production. The last three decades have followed the free market ethos that has dominated in politics and business and have been marked by a cultural, as well as a political, acceptance that the idea that personal fulfilment and self-realization depends on individual responsibility for self-care and personal well-being, as well as on the conditions created by others both in the workplace and elsewhere. Public institutions, as well as private corporations came to set policy goals of transparency and accountability – reflecting increasing customer and consumer rights – as well as agreed performance targets, self-monitoring or peer assessment of performance, open-plan office spaces and technological screening of inappropriate behaviour. The collective protection offered by trade unions has been weakened by the decline of older, often male-centred sectors of production, alongside the growth of 'flexible' working, temporary and short-term contracts and self-employment. In parallel to the expansion of the practice and language of management, a significant feature of the renewed drive for productivity and controlled flexibility in global labour markets has been the erosion of the authority and autonomy of the elite professions. The titles and status of professionalism have been stretched to include less skilled and lower status groups, while the capacity of professional bodies to govern their members has been subjected to intense scrutiny by government, media and private litigants.

This changing landscape of global production and unrestricted labour markets has powerfully influenced the terms in which occupational health and safety have developed in recent decades. During the middle decades of the twentieth century, tensions between occupational medical goals and production management were apparent in large companies and organizations where much of the key research was conducted and policies were implemented. Employers promoted safety selectively and most enthusiastically where productivity gains and corporate risk reduction were most evident. This is illustrated by the unintended consequences of initiatives, such as audiometry programmes established to reduce damage to hearing from noise. While firms often ignored the representations from occupational health departments showing the need for better controls, the data recorded subsequently provided strong evidence for compensation claimants. As employment was rationalized and reorganized in the harsher competitive conditions of the late twentieth century, the problem of risk was more closely aligned to problems of output and poor performance rather than a duty of care to employees. A countervailing force appeared in the greater readiness of employees to resort to litigation on the grounds of discrimination, as well as unreasonable exposure to risk, blurring further some of the boundaries between their obligations as employees and their expectations of social responsibility from their employer. Concurrently, the 'balance' of occupational and non-work life became a familiar theme in discussions of personal and organizational stress.

Faced with the conflicting pressures and repeated demands for public engagement in questions which had previously been a domain of specific expertise, researchers into workplace health increasingly adopted broader and less technical approaches to the problem of occupational risk. This 'ecological' view of ill health rephrased many earlier concerns about the origins and causation of problems by posing questions about the nature of the health issue raised and the circumstances in which concerns began to be expressed about it. Practitioners, as well as investigators, who adopted an ecological approach now had to consider novel links between possible causes and effects in terms of the psychosocial context of the problem and the belief systems of those involved with it, as well as nature of the cause or harm that is being investigated. Rather than seek to exclude and control any stated or implicit values and subjective meanings attached to problems and policies, such studies of workplace health now often share the perspective of historians and social scientists when they study the effects of the power of different interested parties, the reasons for disputes about the significance of subjective complaints and scientific studies and the ethical and expedient basis for taking decisions about action on health concerns and risks at work.

CONCLUSIONS

An early reviewer of Donald Hunter's massive work noted his regular visits to industrial factories to fire a stream of questions at all and sundry, before departing usually with trophies to illustrate his lively lectures. These voyages of discovery into the occupational life extended to an abiding interest into the afflictions of musicians, as well as metalworkers.[62] Hunter's remarkable enterprise bears comparison with the famous surveys of Ramazzini and Oliver, for its encyclopaedic scope and detail. The work also bears the imprint of its time and the assumptions which informed occupational medicine in the first half of the twentieth century. His text offers us an authorised version of the heroic role of brilliant individual scientists and medical specialists in a progressive struggle against illness at work, confirming the fundamental importance of toxicology and studies of dust in the rise of the modern specialist and the framework of regulations introduced by government and industry. Such an approach may appear dated now that historical scholarship has challenged many of the assumptions which underlay such a grand narrative of scientific enlightenment, celebrating the role of brilliant medical men who battled selflessly against the dark forces of ignorance and vested interests. Social and political histories of occupational health have, since Hunter, uncovered the contribution of a much larger range of people and a more complex pattern of struggles, including battles along lines of labour rights, gender, ethnic immigration and rival advocates of scientific and legal expertise.

Perhaps most fundamentally, historians now seek to recover the voices of the patients and workplace witnesses who were most directly affected by disease and diagnoses. The identity of those who can be considered as the clients for expertise on occupational health risks has changed in the half-century or more since Hunter's classic text was first published. Nineteenth century commentators were acutely aware that workplace hazards and effluents were likely to affect not only the workforce but the surrounding community and to result in damage to public health. From the mid-Victorian years, responsibility for workplace and environmental health was allocated to different agencies and government departments and this overview was lost. Hunter was writing at the dawn of a new environmental politics, emanating principally from the United States, but evident also in Europe by the 1960s, that was returning to the nineteenth century model with raised awareness of the dangers presented to wider society by pollution from toxic products and discharges. Consumers, as well as producers, began to articulate their concerns in ways that compelled medical scientists, as well as policymakers, to reappraise the connections between production and public health.

The example of asbestos illustrates the fault lines in the scientific community and the employers' lethargic response to key research and government controls in the post-war years both in relation to worker and public risk. The different ways in which this story has been interpreted by historians also reveals the deep philosophical divisions which prevail among historians, as well as contemporaries in regard to the management of information and risk by some of the key players concerned with the hazards presented by such materials. Debates over the practical limits of technology for securing workers' safety provoke bitter exchanges over the legal and moral responsibility for adequate disclosure of historic risk levels. There is much less readiness than in Hunter's day to accept the veracity of pure science, although it is arguable that historical research often replicates Hunter's tendency to present history as a polarity between the forces of truth and selfish ignorance. In uncovering a multitude of new historical contributors and fresh complexities in the process of scientific enquiry, historians of workplace illness face the challenge of providing an explanation of human intervention which captures the diversity of occupational injury and political capacity described so vividly in Hunter's text. It must still be recognized, as Hunter did, that investigators using the techniques of medical science have played a leading part in the identification of health risks at work. They have worked effectively with other technical colleagues and with industry, regulators and trade unions to remove many of the more serious risks to workers. Both the agendas set for investigators and the actions that follow from the results of their investigations are, clearly, part of a social and political process involving a wide range of interest groups. Clinical vigilance and a readiness to challenge remain essential both for recognizing new risks and for ensuring that those that are known remain under control.

> **Key points**
>
> - Donald Hunter was a major contributor to occupational disease prevention as an investigator, writer and as the teacher of a generation of physicians.
> - The historical sections of Hunter's text book provide important insights into the development of occupational disease identification and prevention, as well as reflecting the historical approaches among 'practitioner historians' at the time when it was written.
> - Occupational disease recognition and prevention are now seen by historians as processes to which medical investigators make a fundamental contribution, but these processes and the guiding assumptions of investigators are decisively influenced by the social, political and economic climate of the period.
> - Successful prevention has reduced many risks to the health of workers markedly, although high levels of risk are still found, particularly in developing countries. Current concerns in developed countries now focus on conditions less specific to work and which may be seen as part of a wider environment for workers and communities.
> - Hunter's precept that constant vigilance and a readiness to try and secure remedial action remains relevant today if we are to identify and pre-empt new risks or retain control over known hazards.

REFERENCES

1. Ellis J. Donald Hunter (1898–1978). In: *Oxford dictionary of national biography*. Oxford: Oxford University Press, 2004.
2. Wright WC. Introduction to *Diseases of workers: The Latin text of 1713* by B Ramazzini, University of Chicago reprint (1940), also New York: Hafner 1964. p. xxix. Ramazzini's work was first published in 1700 and pirated from 1705 onwards. It was republished in 1746 as *Diseases of tradesmen* by Dr Robert James of London. Thackrah CT. *The effects of arts, trades, and professions on health and longevity*, 1832. Reprint: London: WH Smith/Longman, 1989.
3. Legge TM. *Industrial maladies*. Oxford: Oxford University Press, 1934. See preface by Henry SA.
4. Teleky's sympathy for state intervention is apparent in his text: 'As far as it is possible to evaluate the situation from available statistics, we find a high incidence of accidents and occupational diseases at the beginning of state intervention followed by a distinct decrease in consequence of this interaction'. Teleky L. *History of factory and mine hygiene*. New York: Columbia University Press, 1948: 282.
Rosen G. *A history of miners' diseases*. New York: Schuman's, 1943.
5. D'Arcy Hart P. Chronic pulmonary disease in South Wales coal mines: An eye witness account of the MRC surveys, 1937–42. *Social history of medicine*. 1999: 459–68.
Schilling RSF. Donald Hunter – the first editor of the British Journal of Industrial Medicine. *British Journal of Industrial Medicine*. 1977; **36**: 242.
Schilling RSF. Assessing the health of the industrial worker. *British Journal of Industrial Medicine*. 1957; **14**: 145–9. Schilling was one of the key figures in the renewed emphasis on industrial health in the 1940s.
6. Hunter Papers, Wellcome Library, PP/HUN/C 1/56, Letter Hunter to O'Loughlin of Oldchurch Hospital, 15 March 1933: 'A patient of mine employed in bath enamelling, and therefore suffering from a pulmonary silicosis, says that his work-mate, Thomas Thompson, is in No. 4 ward at your hospital suffering from the same complaint.' O'Leary to Hunter, 17 March 1933. Hunter to T Andrews (Hunter's patient and workmate of Thompson) requesting work history and Andrews to Hunter, 28 March 1933 and 30 March 1933 regarding another workplace case example.
7. Wellcome Library, London, Archives: Parkes Weber Papers, Box 137, B75/1, Hunter to Parkes Weber 9 September 1936. 'Where I most require your help is in such things as deformities of the ears in boxers and rugby football players, and ... frostbite of the tenna in Smithfield porters who carry frozen meat'.
8. Hunter Papers, Wellcome Library, PP/HUN/C 1/56. File 48: case of William Norris, 28 years levelling tables rubbing 'on sand with iron float'. Suffering from slate pneumokoniosis 15 October 1931. Hunter to CHC Touissant, Clinical Tuberculosis Officer to London Hospital, 30 October 1931, Touissant to Hunter, 3 November 1931. File 49: case of Charles Stewart. Hunter [?] to Howells, 31 August 1932 requesting case be written up for 'my folders of industrial disease ... I should be grateful for details of the mines in which he has worked and of all sources of exposure to silica. He is, of course, highly intelligent on the subject ...'.
9. Hunter Papers, PP HUN B.12, Correspondence 1943–60. Hunter to ERA Merewether, 28 January 1932, Merewether to Hunter, 29 January 1932, Hunter to Merewether, 1 February 1932.
10. PP HUN B.12, MRC Correspondence: Landsborough Thompson to Hunter 20 April 1943. Hunter was expected to devote one third of his working time to the department for his salary of £800.
11. PP HUN B.12, FJ Nattras of Newcastle to Hunter 15 March 1944, Hunter to Nattras 20 March 1944, where he argued: 'Academic work in industrial medicine must follow the scientific ideal, and must agree to exclude rigidly from its

activities all political issues. Propaganda is not excluded from such a department, but it must be undertaken with great care'.
12. PP HUN B.12, Report on Industrial Medicine by Hunter for Himsworth 29 June 1949. 'The Factory Department has 387 lay, and only 13 medical inspectors to deal with some 250 000 establishments covered by the Factories Act of 1937. ... [It] has no funds for the modern investigation of disease, cannot order x-rays, and has no laboratory facilities of its own. Neither has it any control over mines and quarries which come under a separate department ... These considerations suffice to show why the Medical Research Council entered the field of research in industrial medicine'.
13. Ibid. Hunter was not uncritical of industrial employers: 'The present-day industrialist knows that doctors in general are ignorant of conditions in industry. Too often he regards with contempt and annoyance the efforts of the medical profession to certify illness in his employees. ... It is in the same spirit that industrial firms so often aim at conditions which are just tolerable instead of setting out to design factories with the idea that they should be a joy to work in.'
14. HUN D1/1 and D1/2, Manuscript diary entries for 1947–8, mostly undated, but 15 May 1948 for the Liverpool visit.
15. Author's (TC) personal recall.
16. Pickstone JV. *Ways of knowing: A new history of science, technology and medicine*. Manchester: Manchester University Press, 2000.
17. Paracelsus. *Von de Bergsucht und anderen Bergkrankenheiten*, 1567. Agricola G. *De re metallica*, 1553. (trans. Hoover HC, Hoover LH). New York: Dover, reprinted 1950. 'The Bergmeister in order to prevent workmen from being suffocated gives no one permission to break veins or rock by fire in shaftes or tunnels where it is possible for the poisonous vapouers and smoke to permeate the veins and pass into neighbouring mines.'
'In the mines of the Carpathian Mountains women are found who have married seven husbands, all of whom this terrible consumption has carried of prematurely.'
18. Ramazzini B. *Diseases of workers*, p. 57. 'With regard to the treatment of workers of this class [potters], it is hardly ever possible to give them any remedies that would completely restore their health. For they do not ask for a helping hand from the doctor until their feet and hands are totally crippled and their internal organs have become very hard; and they suffer from yet another drawback, I mean that they are very poor and prescribe remedies that will at least mitigate the disease; but first of all they must be warned to give up their trade.' For miscarriages, Ibid, p. 137.
19. Thackrah CT 1832. Introduction by Meiklejohn A in 1989 reprint.
Cleeland J, Burt S. Charles Turner Thackrah: A pioneer in the field of occupational health. *Occupational Medicine*. 1995; **45**: 285–97.
20. Carter T. British occupational hygiene practice 1720–1920. *Annals of Occupational Hygiene*. 2004; **48**: 299–307.

Potts P. *Chirurgical observations relative to the cataract, the polypus of the nose, the cancer of the scrotum, the different kinds of ruptures and the mortification of the toes and feet*. London, 1775. 'When they get to puberty become liable to a most noisesome, painful and fatal disease ... in the inferior part of the scrotum, where it produces a superficial, painful, ragged, ill-looking sore, with hard and rising edges: the trade call it the soot wart.'
21. Lind J. *An essay on the most effectual means of preserving the health of seamen in the Royal Navy*. London, 1779. In: *Health of seamen*. London: Naval Records Society, 1965.
Vale B. The conquest of scurvy in the Royal Navy 1793–1800: A challenge to current orthodoxy. *The Mariner's Mirror*. 2008; **98**: 160–75.
22. Gaskell P. *The manufacturing population of England: Its moral, social, and physical condition and the changes which have arisen from the use of steam machinery, with an examination of infant labour*. London: Baldwin and Craddock, 1833.
Kay-Shuttleworth J. *The moral and physical conditions of the working classes of Manchester*. London: James Ridgeway, 1832.
Novels include: Dickens C., *Hard times*. Disraeli B. *Sybil*. Gaskell E. *Mary Barton, North and south*.
23. Williamson JG. English workers' living standards. A new look. *Economic History Review* 1983; XXXVI. Crafts NRF. *British economic growth during the Industrial Revolution*. Oxford: Oxford University Press, 1985, chapters 3, 4 and 6.
24. Huzzard G. The role of the certifying surgeon in the state regulation of child labour and industrial health 1833–1973. MA thesis, University of Manchester, 1976.
25. See Adisesh LA. Dr Edward Headlam Greenhow: A resume of his life and an account of his work, unpublished paper, 2004. Copy in possession of authors.
26. Knight A. On the grinders' asthma. *North of England Medical and Surgical Journal*. 1830; 170–9.
Holland GC. *Diseases of the lungs from mechanical causes*. London, 1843.
Blackburn S. *A fair day's wage for a fair day's work? Sweated labour and the origins of minimum wage legislation in Britain*. Aldershot: Ashgate, 2007.
27. Haldane JS. The air of mines. In: Oliver T (ed.). *Dangerous trades*. London: John Murray, 1902: 540–56.
28. Lehmann KB. *List of tolerable concentrations*. Munich: Munich Department of Hygiene, 1895.
29. Worboys M. *Spreading germs: Disease theories and medical practice in Britain, 1865–1900*. Cambridge: Cambridge University Press, 2000: 1–6, 232.
30. Harrison B. *Not only the dangerous trades: Women's work and health in Britain 1880–1914*. London: Taylor and Francis, 1996.
Malone C. *Women's bodies and dangerous trades in England 1880–1914*. London: Boydell, 2003, c.f. Bartrip for more sceptical note. Bartrip PWJ. *The Home Office and the dangerous trades*. Rodopi, 2002.
31. Mortimer I, Melling J. The contest between commerce and trade on one side and human life on the other. British

government policies for the regulation of anthrax infection in the wool textile trades 1880–1939. *Textile History.* 2000; **31**: 222–36.
32. Pemberton N, Worboys M. *Mad dogs and Englishmen. Rabies in Britain, 1830–2000.* London: Palgrave Macmillan, 2007.
33. Hunter Papers, PP/HUN C.1/6 Case of Elsie Mitchell, 19, from April 1913. Admitted 25 April 1913 and discharged 25 May 1913. Walter Shead, 38, infected 23 February 1921 and recovered 2 April 1921. Thomas Jevons, aged 36, died 1922, Hunter to Mrs Jevons, 9 December 1935. Robert Campbell, aged 25, admitted 13 June 1938 as 'very ill patient … laboured respiration.' He recovered seven weeks later.
34. Arlidge JT. *The hygiene, diseases and mortality of occupations.* London: Percival, 1892.
35. Oliver T. *Dangerous trades.* London: John Murray, 1902.
36. Legge (1934).
37. Waldron T. Thomas Morison Legge (1863–1932): The first medical factory inspector. *Journal of Medical Biography.* 2004; **12**: 202–209. Obituary. *Lancet.* 14 May 1932 reproduced in HSE, *The changing nature of occupational health.* London: HSE Books, 1998.
38. Legge TM. The health of brassworkers. *Appendix 1 Factories and Workshops Annual Report 1905.* London: HMSO, 1906: 388–97.
39. Legge TM. Industrial anthrax. *Milroy Lectures* 1904. *Lancet.* 1905; **i**: 689–96, 764–76, 841–6.
Report of the Departmental Committee on Anthrax. Vol. 2. Report of the committee. London: HMSO, 1918.
40. Legge TM, Goadby KW. *Lead poisoning and lead absorption.* London: Edward Arnold, 1912.
41. Harrison B. 1996. *Not only the dangerous trades. Women's work and health in Britain, 1880–1914.* London: Taylor & Francis, 1996.
42. McFeely M. *Lady inspectors: The campaign for a better workplace, 1893–1921.* Athens, GA: University of Georgia Press, 1988: 5–22 and passim.
43. Bartrip PWJ. *The Home Office and the dangerous trades. Regulating occupational disease in Victorian and Edwardian Britain.* Amsterdam and New York: Rodopi, 2002.
44. Bartrip PWJ. The rise and fall of workmen's compensation. In: Weindling P (ed). *The social history of occupational health.* London: Croom Helm, 1985: 157–79.
Bartrip PWJ, Burman S. *Wounded soldiers of industry.* Oxford: Oxford University Press, 1983. McIvor A. *Social history of work.* London: Macmillan, 2000.
45. Bufton M, Melling J. Coming up for air. Industrial silicosis and compensation provisions for workers in the United Kingdom, 1900–1939. *Social History of Medicine.* 2005; **18**: 63–86.
46. Milles D. *Dynamis.* 1993; **13**: 139–53, 141–3, 147.
Melling J. The risks of working versus the risks of not working: Trade unions, employers and responses to the risk of occupational illness in British industry, c. 1890–1940s.

London: London School of Economics Centre for Risk and Regulation Discussion Paper. 2004: 18.
47. Legge TM. Tetrachloroethane poisoning. *Chief Inspector of Factories Report 1914.* London: HMSO, 1918: 107–12.
Legge TM. Trinitrotoluene poisoning. *Chief Inspector of Factories Report 1917.* London: HMSO, 1918: pp 21–4.
48. Ineson A, Thom D. TNT poisoning and the employment of women workers in the First World War. In: Weindling P (ed.). *The social history of occupational health.* London: Croom Helm, 1985: 89–107.
49. Waldron HA. Occupational health during the Second World War: Hope deferred or hope abandoned? *Medical History.* 1997; **41**: 197–212.
50. Sir Thomas Legge resignation letter. *The Times* December 1, 1926.
51. Sellers CG. *Hazards of the job: From industrial disease to environmental health science.* Chapel Hill, NC: North Carolina University Press, 1997.
52. *Chief Inspector of Factories and Workshops Annual Report 1898.* London: HMSO, 1899: Ptii. 171.
53. Merewether ERA, Price CW. *Report on effects of asbestos dust on the lungs and dust suppression in the asbestos industry.* London: HMSO, 1930.
54. Tweedale G. *From magic mineral to killer dust.* Oxford: Oxford University Press, 2000. Bartrip PWJ. *The way from dusty death; Turner and Newall and the regulation of occupational health in the British asbestos industry 1890s–1970.* London: Athlone Press, 2001.
Melling J. An inspector calls: Perspectives on the history of occupational diseases and accident compensation in the United Kingdom. *Medical History.* 2005; **49**: 102–6.
55. Tweedale 2000: 150.
56. Mount Sinai Hospital Archives, Selikoff papers (mainly unsorted but filed by name of recipient) Gilson file: Selikoff to JC Gilson, August 3, 1965; JC Wagner to Selikoff, July 22, 1966; Selikoff to Eunic T Miner, August 3, 1966.
57. Blanc P. *How everyday products make people sick.* Berkeley: University of California Press, 2007.
58. Markowitz G, Rosner D. *Deceit and denial: The deadly politics of industrial pollution.* Berkeley: University of California Press, 2002. It should, however, be noted that the problem was only recognized because the producers funded the animal studies.
59. Safety and Health at Work: Report of the Committee 1970–72. Chair: Lord Robens. London: HMSO, 1972. Robens' background in the coal industry probably informed this model of corporate (tripartite) discussions.
60. Barnes B. *T. S. Kuhn and social science.* New York: Columbia University Press, 1982: 135.
61. Cooper CL, Levi L. Promotion of occupational and public health: The European experience and challenge. *Ergonomia.* 2006; **28**: 283–93.
62. Lane RE. Review of *Diseases of occupations. Journal of Royal Society for the Promotion of Health.* 1955; **75**: 762.

The changing face of occupational diseases

PETER J BAXTER, TAR-CHING AW, ANNE COCKCROFT, PAUL DURRINGTON
AND J MALCOLM HARRINGTON

Introduction	24
The historical legacy	24
The continuing burden of occupational diseases	25
New technologies, new hazards	26
The new wave of work-related illness	27
The future outlook	28
References	28

INTRODUCTION

Occupational diseases are all preventable, but they have exacted and continue to exact a huge human burden on a global scale. Early interventions by public health reformers around the time of the Industrial Revolution in the United Kingdom were hampered by their confusion over whether the diseases that were rife in the population were the result of the degraded and impoverished living conditions in the overcrowded industrial town slums or due to the rank factory environment, where many spent most of their waking lives.

Greater understanding of where the focus for prevention lay and the need for intervention to improve the conditions of workers grew in the late nineteenth century and the government took action to reduce acute and chronic metal poisoning arising mainly from the indiscriminate use of mercury and lead. Exposure to lead in food and drink was also widespread in the UK population and the metal was probably a common cause of undiagnosed illness. Medical science had also developed to the point of being able to diagnose, and provide a limited understanding of, the toxic manifestations of metals, including Mad Hatter's disease (mercury) and peripheral neuropathy (lead), as well as the action of lead as an abortifacient. The first medical inspector of factories, Sir Thomas Legge, was appointed in 1898 with the principal duty of stemming the lead poisoning epidemic.

The use of machinery to take over manual tasks and the introduction of drilling equipment had by the beginning of the twentieth century unwittingly precipitated increases in exposure to dust in mines and quarries, leading to increased rates of pneumoconioses, such as silicosis and coal miner's black lung. Whole mining communities fell into the grip of occupational lung diseases from mineral dusts. By the middle of the twentieth century, the chemical industry was expanding rapidly and bringing a new era of synthesized substances to revolutionize lives, but in its wake there was an unwelcome tide of novel toxic hazards, including carcinogens.

Physical hazards and extreme working environments present different risks from those of substances that can be inhaled, ingested or absorbed in the workplace. We know more about the adverse chronic effects of ionizing radiation than any other occupational hazard, in the sense that the dose–response relation for cancer is well delineated and the risk relatively precisely quantified. Deep sea fishing possibly remains the riskiest job in the UK, as was first recognized 40 years ago. In contrast, flying, deep sea diving, working at altitude or at extremes of temperature have been shorn of most of their dangers. Regulations and better work practices have also transformed the risk of back injury from mundane manual handling operations in ordinary jobs. However, the question remains for all types of occupational hazards: as human inventiveness and discovery take us into ever new worlds of work will the changes so produced inevitably present new health challenges, some of which cannot be always foreseen? If so, will the main societal role of occupational medicine in the future be, as it has been since Hunter's day, to maintain vigilant monitoring over workforces for the unexpected health consequences of ever-changing technology?

THE HISTORICAL LEGACY

Occupational health, as we know it today, is largely the product of the late twentieth century. The last edition of

Hunter's Diseases of Occupations published in 2000[1] marked the culmination of a generation of sociopolitical pressures and technological changes in occupational health and safety that began with the governments of most industrialized countries adopting radical legislation in the 1960s and 1970s which, by the end of the century, had led to a dramatic fall in the incidence of work-related ill health and injury. The whole of the twentieth century saw a revolution in public health and preventive medicine which accelerated with scientific and medical advances during a time of unprecedented material growth as the century ended. Fundamental to progress in occupational medicine over this period were developments in the medical sciences and, in particular, toxicology, but it was in the application of the new field of chronic disease epidemiology, spearheaded by epidemiologists in the United States and the United Kingdom after the Second World War, where many of the most important advances in understanding and tackling occupational diseases took place. This was the era when occupational cancer rose to prominence as epidemiologists and toxicologists identified increasing numbers of suspect human carcinogens, and public anxiety was being spurred by revelations over the toxicity of asbestos and the disastrous global legacy of the asbestos industry. The inertia of some industries to adopt costly controls to protect workers was not new, and has always been behind the need for government regulation in health and safety at work, but the uncertainties inherent in epidemiological and toxicological studies were too often cited as a justification to delay or obfuscate, rather than incorporate the lessons of research, as the asbestos saga has shown.

This edition's opening chapter is a historical panorama of occupational diseases with an interpretation that deliberately owes more to Herodotus, the father of history, than to Donald Hunter. Many Hunter readers have lamented our exclusion in recent editions of Donald Hunter's own history from the Bronze Age to the twentieth century, a tour de force occupying nearly a fifth of his book which he had already packed with fascinating historical vignettes. (This edition is accompanied by a reproduction of his chapter on the website.) Hunter marked advances in prevention with a pageant of heroic reformers and medical figures, who often ran up against stout resistance from vested interests. Colourful personalities included Sir Humphrey Davy (1778–1829), as the brilliant researcher, who achieved world fame by inventing his famous safety lamp after a brief trial of inspired experimentation, and thereby saved thousands of miners from death in gas explosions, and John Scott Haldane (1860–1936), the physician–physiologist and 'medical detective', who uncovered the toxic hazards of gases in mines by performing dangerous experiments on himself and investigating well-publicized, fatal incidents. However, Hunter's narrative neglected a whole uncharted terrain of social, political and economic history, an omission that Herodotus would have regretted.

When Donald Hunter was practising, physicians in England seeking specialist status had to pass the London Membership of the Royal College of Physicians, which at that time was a hurdle of terrifying difficulty. Hunter's book became required reading for a whole generation of candidates in case they were confronted in the pathology viva by Hunter himself as one of a number of regular and distinguished college examiners. As Seaton writes,[2] 'If you had not done this and had the misfortune to meet him, you were sunk', as he passed you a hunk of rock or a steel bit across the table. However, Donald Hunter's retirement coincided with the beginning of a long decline in occupational medicine in Britain: occupational diseases no longer feature as strongly in medical examinations, while medical undergraduates may receive hardly any teaching in the subject at all. Many occupational physicians in high income countries feel a sense of loss to their professionalism through this rapid decline in incidence of the traditional occupational diseases, which has been due only in part to effective prevention in the workplace. Globalization has brought a rise in service industries and a shift of the traditional manufacturing industries to newly industrializing countries. Yet the UK, for example, remains the sixth largest manufacturing economy in the world, with a particularly strong presence in industries such as aerospace, health and construction. This concentration of added-value manufacturing is still a one and a half times larger contributor to the economy than the financial sector. In some UK regions, however, the largest employers are the main universities or district hospitals, not foundries, steel mills or vehicle manufacturing plants. Before the Health and Safety at Work Act in 1973, the health and education sectors did not even fall under the old Factories Acts, and had never been formally inspected, let alone employed occupational health professionals. Yet no occupational health professional working in these sectors today can doubt that new challenges in work-related ill health have emerged as the old industries have moved elsewhere.

THE CONTINUING BURDEN OF OCCUPATIONAL DISEASES

Just as the worst global recession since the Second World War has shattered illusions that the global banking system had eliminated financial risk, it is premature to assume that the health risks of occupational diseases have been assigned to history in high income countries, or to forget that they are much more prevalent in the developing world, especially in the rapidly growing BRIC (Brazil, Russia, India, China) economies, where statistics are unavailable for making meaningful comparisons. Meanwhile, the Health and Safety Executive estimates that in the United Kingdom every year still more than 10 000 people die from past exposure to chemicals, fumes and dusts, a figure that far exceeds the death toll from accidents at work (200–240 annually).[3] Respiratory and skin sensitizers have become common causes of significant morbidity, and dusts may act synergistically with smoking and other causal factors in the aetiology of chronic obstructive pulmonary disease (COPD) (see Chapter 69, Work and chronic air flow limitation and Chapter 72, Occupational asthma).

Industrial carcinogens remain a special problem due to their number and the lack of adequate exposure controls in many of the smaller workplaces where they may be found. In a key study by Rushton et al.,[4] on the burden of cancer at work in the United Kingdom, occupation contributed to around 8 per cent of cancer deaths in men and almost 2 per cent in women, for six selected sites: lung, nasal sinus, bladder, non-melanoma of skin, leukaemia and mesothelioma. Asbestos contributed over half of the occupational cancer deaths, and more than half of these were due to exposures in the construction industry. Respirable crystalline silica (RCS) is judged to cause about 800 lung cancers each year in the United Kingdom, mostly in construction workers who are exposed to silica present in many common building materials.

Annually, at least 4000 people die in the United Kingdom from all diseases linked to asbestos, about twice the figure of deaths in road traffic accidents.[3] Around half of these deaths are due to mesothelioma, which is still on the increase and set to peak in incidence over the next decade. The mesothelioma epidemic is also occurring across other countries in Western Europe[5] and throughout the world.[6] Despite the use of asbestos in factories being banned in the UK since 1998, its legacy continues to give rise to exposures leading to cancer; these exposures were not envisaged early on by scientists or government agencies and have only recently featured in legislation and awareness campaigns. As asbestos production declined in the 1970s and with exposure in buildings containing asbestos supposed to be negligible, it was widely assumed that mesothelioma deaths would soon peak and then fall. However, this reckoning was based on cohorts of factory workers and ignored the exposures of tradesmen engaged in building and maintenance work – plumbers, electricians, joiners, carpenters, painters – who were mostly unaware of the hazard the asbestos in buildings presented if it became disturbed in the course of their work. An epidemiological study published in 1995[7] provided new projections of mesothelioma deaths and for the first time included the substantial contribution from these building and maintenance occupations, which to date amounts to a quarter of the total number of mesothelioma deaths. These findings raised new concerns about asbestos in buildings, such as schools, hospitals and homes, and the risk from inadvertent low but cumulative exposures, as well as brief exposures to the dust in bystanders. It was not until 2002 that the Health and Safety Executive (HSE) in the UK updated its workplace regulations to compel workplace property owners to hold registers of asbestos in their buildings, and embarked on media campaigns to raise awareness in these small groups of workers, who together numbered 1.9 million in 2009. Asbestos may be present in any building constructed or refurbished before the year 2000, amounting to at least 500 000 workplace premises in the UK.

By 2009, the death rate from mesothelioma in the United Kingdom had become the highest in the world.[8] The occupation with the highest risk was carpenters and this has been attributed to the cutting of board made from amosite (brown asbestos), which was widespread in the UK construction industry through the 1970s into the 1980s. Large amounts of amosite were imported into the UK after crocidolite (blue asbestos) had been banned in 1968, at a time when the carcinogenic potency of amosite had not been established. The mesothelioma risk of amosite is now known to be two orders of magnitude greater than that for chrysotile (white asbestos).[8]

Globally, there are an estimated 90 000 asbestos-related deaths every year and in high income countries the compensation for asbestos-related diseases is likely to reach US$300 billion over the coming years.[9] All forms of asbestos are now recognized to be carcinogenic and to date, more than 40 countries, including all member states of the European Union, have banned the use of asbestos. However, chrysotile asbestos continues to be mined and exported to developing countries by Canada and Russia, with Brazil having its own mines. The largest importer is India. Its use continues to be promoted by the industry as a safer form of asbestos for such purposes as the manufacture of asbestos cement pipes for long distance water distribution and in construction, even though substitute materials are available for all uses of asbestos. Unless international action for a worldwide ban is taken, as called for by the World Health Organization (WHO) and the International Labour Office (ILO), another asbestos disaster is looming, indeed probably already underway, this time in the developing world.[9]

NEW TECHNOLOGIES, NEW HAZARDS

Even though the health hazards of old scourges, such as asbestos and silica dusts, are now well understood, they remain important causes of occupational disease. By the 1970s, the traditional industries were already in decline in western countries, while the chemical industry had expanded rapidly since the Second World War. One chemical, vinyl chloride monomer (VCM), used in many countries in the manufacture of the highly profitable plastic PVC, had been widely assumed to be safe due to its deceptively simple chemical formula ($CH_2 = CH.Cl$), and its derivation from ethylene in the cracking of oil, but evidence from laboratory animals in 1973 showed that it could cause angiosarcoma of the liver in humans, a rare tumour and one which could therefore be easily spotted in chemical workers as a cause of death. Within months, cases of angiosarcoma had been reported in VCM workers in several countries, including the United States and the United Kingdom, and rapid action was taken to drastically reduce exposure levels in the chemical plants. This finding of an incontrovertible cancer risk in a chemical previously thought to be safe led to widespread changes in the attitude of the chemical industry and legislators to the health hazards of the large numbers of chemicals that by then had been introduced into commercial usage, the vast majority of which had not been as adequately tested for carcinogenicity as VCM.

VCM also represented the hazard of new technologies as it was one of a range of new and very useful compounds synthesized by halogenating hydrocarbons, an industrial process which started in the 1930s and grew rapidly. A whole range of chlorinated compounds were synthesized in large quantities which only later came under suspicion of being potentially toxic to humans and wildlife, with some having added dangers because of their biopersistence and their inability to be easily degraded in the environment (e.g. DDT, PCBs). Some became classified as recognized or suspect human carcinogens. The concerns of long-term health hazards arising from exposure also apply to many other chemical groups: by 2009, about 75 000 compounds were in regular commercial usage, but the vast majority of these have not been fully tested for their long-term toxicity or carcinogenicity.[10] Following the shock to the chemical industry provided by vinyl chloride, a general consensus arose that all chemicals need to be treated with caution and none should be assumed to be of low toxicity without good evidence.

During the latter part of the twentieth century, it became clear that carcinogenesis was a multistep process. Biomarkers now play a significant role in identifying key events in the process, including occupational carcinogenesis. For many carcinogenic chemicals, there has been much research interest in measuring haemoglobin adducts. In the last decade, one of the most studied genes in epidemiology has been the TP53 tumour suppressor gene (see Chapter 85, Occupational cancer: epidemiology, biological mechanisms and biomarkers). Its role in causing liver and skin tumours is a focus for much research activity. Intermediate biomarkers, such as chromosomal damage and altered DNA repair also point towards evidence of early, non-clonal and potentially non-persistent effects, which if halted or reversed, could decrease the risk of full-blown malignancy. In the past, evidence of family history susceptibility has been a crude marker for inherited susceptibility to cancer. Occupational cancer studies have not shown much evidence of family history as being an important factor, but the possible interaction between NAT2 acetylation status, benzidine exposure and the development of bladder cancer is one positive example. The role of so-called 'molecular epidemiology' in the study of cancer aetiology, so far of little practical value in occupational cancer, is likely to expand in this century.

Newer concerns over cancer have arisen with the rapid introduction of technologies such as mobile phones whose use became widespread before studies of their potential health hazard were embarked upon (Chapter 55, Extremely low frequency electric and magnetic fields). The precedent and lessons of asbestos loom large in attitudes towards synthetic fibres, in particular engineered nanomaterials, such as carbon nanotubes and nanoparticles, which have a growing number of commercial uses (see Chapter 70, Health effects of ultrafine particles).

There are now many international and national initiatives addressing occupational, environmental and consumer issues in relation to the control of toxic substances. Much better control technologies and the adoption of risk assessments under legislation, such as the Control of Substances Hazardous to Health (COSHH) in the UK have radically altered attitudes and led to far better control of exposure to chemicals, and mixtures of chemicals, in all employment sectors in recent years. In Europe, future regulations for controlling toxic substances in the workplace, including carcinogens, will flow from EU Directives and technical guidance, with the latest initiative being REACH – a new EU regulation concerning the Registration, Evaluation, Authorization and restriction of Chemicals.[11]

THE NEW WAVE OF WORK-RELATED ILLNESS

In the last two editions we included for the first time syndromes (stress, upper limb pain and lower back pain) that were beginning to change our conceptual framework of occupational disease. The dominant risk paradigm of the twentieth century which has been so successful in controlling diseases from chemical, physical and biological hazards, is based on being able to define the relationship between the degree of exposure to an agent at work and the development of a disease outcome, and then controlling the risk by eliminating or reducing exposure. Founded in toxicology, this framework became enshrined in epidemiological studies of workers in the form of exposure–response relationships and is implicit in the drawing up of risk assessments in the workplace and for a clinician to establish when a patient is suffering from an occupational disease. Diseases with high morbidity and fatality, such as chemical-induced cancers and pneumoconioses, had identifiable causes and so proved readily preventable. However, the paradigm was no longer so apt when dealing with the new wave of health problems that became the most common single cause of referral to occupational health clinics and a new burden of illness, disability and sickness absence across all employment sectors. Features of these disorders include a relationship with work that cannot be wholly explained by their assumed occupational causes and they are rarely associated with evidence of underlying pathology.[12] In one group of conditions, the symptoms can be remarkably similar, or non-specific, despite their causal exposures being very different, examples being Gulf War syndrome, exposure to organophosphates and sick building syndrome. It has become necessary to clearly distinguish between illness and disease in occupational disorders: illness is by definition a subjective state and disease is a pathological process that at least in theory is amenable to objective, external verification.[12]

We are still far from understanding the implications of these latest disorders not being a simple function of excessive exposure to noxious agents or activities, and we need more research on the role of psychological risk factors or psychologically mediated responses in these conditions, and

> **Box 2.1 Definition of terms.**[12]
>
> - **Illness.** An absence of well-being as perceived:
>   - by the affected individual (in the form of one or more symptoms); or
>   - by others (from an abnormality of function or from an abnormality of behaviour for which the affected individual cannot be held responsible).
> - **Pathology.** Abnormality of tissue structure or of biochemical or physiological function that has the potential to cause illness or death.
> - **Disease.** A combination of pathological abnormalities that are thought to be inter-related.
> - **Disorder.** A broader term encompassing both illness and disease.

how best to manage and prevent them. For example, low-back pain is becoming increasingly common and debilitating chronic low back pain is one of the six most costly health problems in developing countries – in an era when the number of jobs requiring manual handling has dramatically fallen (see Chapter 58, Occupational back pain).[13] The chapters on stress in this book also emphasize how little we currently know about the effectiveness of interventions for this problem, either at the individual or workplace level. The current explosion in information technology and computer software may yet lead to novel psychological maladaptations in workplaces and consequent increased levels of stress. We will have to look beyond the old paradigm which lends itself to reductionist biological models to one which incorporates social and behavioural factors within the workplace itself: the term 'work-related illness' has become accepted as embracing this change in thinking (see Box 2.1).

THE FUTURE OUTLOOK

The challenges facing the modern world cannot be met without the creation of new technologies with the potential to improve lives enormously. Some of these will have adverse health consequences, and in a small proportion these may be unforeseen under current regulatory approaches. The present global picture and outlook for control of occupational diseases is bleak, with many rapidly industrializing countries having inadequate legislative controls and infrastructure to protect workers from even well-known and preventable occupational health hazards. Despite the huge advances in disease prevention in industrialized countries in the last decades, or perhaps because of them, the provision of specialist advice and expertise is not keeping pace with the rapid changes in the work environment. Occupational diseases and disorders will continue to exact a significant and unnecessary burden on the societies of developed countries unless this shortfall is adequately met.

> **Key points**
>
> - Occupational diseases still present significant burdens in advanced industrialized countries, despite legislative and technological changes based on epidemiological and toxicological evidence during the late twentieth century.
> - For countries undergoing rapid industrialization, the outlook is bleak, with the prospect that occupational diseases will escalate worldwide.
> - Occupational carcinogens remain an important cause of mortality in industrialized countries. Asbestos has left a deadly legacy: tradesmen and construction workers now contribute to a significant proportion of asbestos cancer deaths. The UK now has the highest incidence of mesothelioma in the world.
> - Illnesses, such as stress, musculoskeletal disorders and non-specific fatigue syndromes, have become prominent types of work-related ill health in industrialized countries. These have substantial subjective components and their management and prevention requires strategies that incorporate social and behavioural factors.
> - Occupational medicine has an important societal role in the future to anticipate and identify the new and unforeseen health consequences arising from innovative technologies, changes in work patterns and the ageing workforce.

REFERENCES

1. Baxter PJ, Adams PH, Aw T-C et al. *Hunter's Diseases of occupations*, 9th edn. London: Arnold, 2000.
2. Seaton A. Oh no – it's Donald Hunter! *Quarterly Journal of Medicine.* 2009; 102: 827–8.
3. Health and Safety Executive. Disease reduction programme (DRP). Available from: www.hse.gov.uk/drp/index.htm.
4. Rushton L, Hutchings S, Brown T. The burden of cancer at work: Estimation as the first step to prevention. *Occupational and Environmental Medicine.* 2008; **65**: 789–800.
5. Peto J, Decarli A, La Vecchia C et al. The European mesothelioma epidemic. *British Journal of Cancer.* 1999; **79**: 666–72.
6. Lin R-T, Takahashi K, Karjalainen A et al. Ecological association between asbestos-related diseases and historical asbestos consumption: An international analysis. *Lancet.* 2007; **369**: 844–9.
7. Peto J, Matthews FE, Hodgson JT, Jones JR. Continuing increase in mesothelioma mortality in Britain. *Lancet.* 1995; **345**: 535–9.

8. Rake C, Gilham C, Hatch J *et al*. Occupational, domestic and environmental mesothelioma risks in the British population: A case-control study. *British Journal of Cancer.* 2009; **100**: 1175-83.
9. Editorial. Asbestos-related disease – a preventable burden. *Lancet.* 2008; **372**: 1927.
10. Straif K. The burden of occupational cancer. *Occupational and Environmental Medicine.* 2008; **65**: 787-88.
11. Health and Safety Executive. What is REACH? Available from: www.hse.gov.uk/reach/about.htm.
12. Coggan D. Occupational medicine at a turning point. *Occupational and Environmental Medicine.* 2005; **62**: 281-3.
13. Freburger JK, Holmes GM, Agans RP *et al*. The rising prevalence of chronic low back pain. *Archives of Internal Medicine.* 2009; **169**: 251-8.

SECTION TWO

Diagnosis of occupational disease

3 The occupational history 33
   Tar-Ching Aw
4 Occupational exposure to hazardous substances 43
   John W Cherrie and Sean Semple
5 Biological monitoring 56
   John Cocker and Howard J Mason

3

The occupational history

TAR-CHING AW

What is the occupational history?	33	Conclusion	41
Why take an occupational history?	38	Acknowledgements	41
Diagnosing an occupational disease	40	References	41

> On visiting a poor home, a doctor should be satisfied to sit on a three-legged stool, in the absence of a gilt chair, and he should take time for his examination: and to the questions recommended by Hippocrates he should add one more – What is your occupation?[1]
>
> Bernadino Ramazzini, 1713

WHAT IS THE OCCUPATIONAL HISTORY?

The occupational history

TAKING AND RECORDING INFORMATION ABOUT WORK

The occupational history refers to obtaining details from an individual about his job. It has two main components:

1. **The present job.** This includes not just the job title, but also the work tasks, chemicals used, the work environment, and availability and use of personal protective equipment. It is also important to enquire about the duration of the job, whether there is shift work, overtime work and whether the person has a second job.
2. **Previous jobs.** Similar details are required about the different jobs (paid or unpaid) that the person has done before. It is best to be systematic when obtaining the past work history; either starting from the present job and working back to the first job, or beginning from the first job and working forward to the present employment. Periods of unemployment, voluntary work locally and overseas, part-time work, casual or temporary work, and hobbies should be included, especially if these involve exposure to chemicals or contact with biological materials that might pose a risk of sensitization or infection.

A suggested template for recording the occupational history is shown in Figure 3.1.[2]

Taking the occupational history is an important part of the general medical history obtained when a patient is seen by an examining physician. Unfortunately, this is often overlooked or not taken in sufficient detail. Clinical management of a patient without information on what a person does at work can be incomplete or inadequate. This is because of a possibility of missing a condition caused by work or not recognizing the work-related nature of a common condition, such as asthma. The necessary clinical advice regarding fitness to return to work or dealing with possible occupational factors contributing to the disease will then be lacking.

In taking the occupational history, the physician should be a good listener. Much information can be obtained from a patient's description of what job activities are done at work, and how work tasks are performed. This can give an indication of workplace exposures and possible risks. In addition, the patient's occupational history may provide additional insight about a workplace, which might not be apparent even after a worksite visit. Listening to the patient may provide information on issues such as the morale of the workforce, commitment to health and safety measures by both employer and employees, and whether other workers have similar health problems.

Sometimes, evidence of significant occupational exposure or disease is discovered by chance in the course of investigations for other diseases. For example, the incidental detection of calcified pleural plaques from asbestos exposure may be detected on a chest or upper abdominal radiograph performed for other clinical reasons. In these

Fill in details of each job, listing all jobs since leaving school till the present.

Workplace (employer's name and address)	Date worked from	Date worked to	Full/part time	Type of industry	Job duties	Workplace hazards	Preventive measures and use of personal protective equipment	Time off work for illness or injury

Figure 3.1 Template for recording an occupational history.[2]

circumstances, all clinicians should make further enquiry about relevant occupational and environmental exposure.

ASKING ABOUT SYMPTOMS IN RELATION TO WORK ACTIVITIES

When a substance produces an acute effect, direct questions should show the relation between symptoms and work; a useful pointer is evidence of remissions at weekends and holiday periods. Some clinical effects may not appear until a few hours after exposure. Examples are delayed pulmonary oedema from exposure to phosgene gas, ozone or oxides of nitrogen, and occupational asthma where both an 'immediate' and 'delayed' reaction to exposure may occur and the delayed response is often more prominent (see Chapter 72, Occupational asthma). Patients may wake up breathless at night as a result of workplace exposure during the day. Caution is needed in interpreting a temporal relationship with work, because some patients with non-occupational disorders may also feel better when they are away from work or on holiday.

DELAY BETWEEN EXPOSURE AND SYMPTOMS

For chronic effects, it is not uncommon for there to be a considerable delay between first exposure to materials encountered at work and development of clinical symptoms or signs. This can be for several reasons. Sensitization of the skin or respiratory tract may not occur until an individual has worked with the sensitizing agent for some time (months or years). It may be even longer before it manifests as a clinical condition, e.g. as in occupational asthma. Once the allergic condition has developed, the effects following re-exposure to the causative agent may be immediate or occur within hours. Sometimes disease only develops after considerable cumulative exposure. For example, it usually takes at least ten years for underground coalworkers to develop evidence of coalworkers' pneumoconiosis. Once begun, the disease process may progress even after exposure ceases. In the case of occupational cancers, there is a latency period between exposure to the carcinogen and development of the cancer.

Mesotheliomas from asbestos exposure typically have a latency of 20–40 years, and the exposure at that time could have been brief. The link with previous occupational exposure may be harder to investigate when the patient has left the suspected job some years before the illness is diagnosed.

Relevant factors regarding an occupational history

THE JOB TITLE

Even when the question 'What is your job?' is asked (Ramazzini's exhortation[1]), it is recorded in medical records as a word or phrase often with very little or no information about what the job entails.

A person who states that he is a 'dentist' may convey to the physician a reasonable idea of what the job involves. However, a job title such as 'general labourer' or 'maintenance man' does not give much insight into the job activities or the possible occupational exposures. A general labourer may perform primarily manual work or may rotate between several tasks, including some with chemical exposures. A maintenance man's work may involve a variety of hazardous exposures, depending on what equipment or work process needs to be maintained.

A well-designed and properly functioning plant will operate without much danger to process workers, but when things go wrong and repairs have to be carried out, maintenance workers can be at risk. Hazardous exposures may also be encountered in 'routine maintenance'. The recognition of possible risks have led to the development of various formal procedures, such as the 'permits to work' that are required in some chemical plants or on work involving high voltage switchgear, or before doing so-called 'hot work'. The exposures of maintenance men are sometimes heavy and may be 'mixed' (i.e. to a variety of substances) and variable.

Another occupational group who often have problems with protection against occupational hazards are contract workers. These workers often have little training or experience in the job they are asked to perform. They may be migrant or even illegal workers who can be subject to exploitation by unscrupulous employers. Contract workers are often asked to perform a variety of different tasks from day to day, usually with little information, instruction and training regarding those tasks, known risks and preventive measures.

A job title may give some indication about the work tasks, but some job titles can be vague and encompass a variety of activities, while the same job title in different industries or in different countries may on occasions refer to completely different jobs. Thus, a 'general labourer' may dig holes in roads or carry bricks up ladders; they can also work in such diverse places as a chemical factory, a foundry or a cotton mill. The job title 'dresser' may indicate someone who treats seeds with pesticides, or assists a stage actor with costumes and cosmetics, or removes excess sand from metal castings, or deals with cuts and wounds in a village hospital in a developing country. A 'linesman' assists a referee in a game of soccer. A 'linesman' (or 'lineman') is also a technician who deals with electric powerlines, telephone lines or installs wiring for cable television. A process worker on an assembly line for plastic toys may not be exposed to many chemical hazards, whereas a process worker in the electronics industry can be exposed to a wide range of hazardous materials (see Chapter 45, The semiconductor industry).

History is full of interesting and often cryptic job titles. The Dictionary of Occupational Titles,[3] published by the US Department of Labor, Employment and Training Administration has a compilation and description of several hundred job titles, including puzzling jobs such as 'barrel scraper', 'dope-house operator' (may not be quite what you think it is), 'egg smeller', 'frickertron checker', 'head beater' and many more.

A good way of finding out precisely what an individual does at work, what materials he works with, and what hazards are encountered, is to ask the patient directly. The immediate supervisor at work would be another good source for such information. Even if a patient is not aware of the exact chemical that he handles daily, the availability of a trade name or a label from the container, or a copy of the material safety data sheet (MSDS) might be a starting point for finding out the hazards of the material.

'HAZARD' AND 'RISK'

'Hazard' is the potential for causing harm and 'risk' is the likelihood (or the probability) that such harm will result. The term 'risk' is now extended to include consideration of the severity of effect. If handling sheets of paper at work is just as likely to cause cuts (paper cuts) to the skin, as sharpening knives, the probability of injury from both processes is the same, but cuts from knives are more severe than 'paper cuts'. Therefore, of the two processes with equal likelihood of skin injury, sharpening knives is viewed as more risky because of the severity of the effect. The distinction between hazard and risk is important in regards to choice of suitable measures to reduce the likelihood of occupational injury or disease. Minimizing risk may be more cost-effective than eliminating hazards.

EXTENT OF EXPOSURE

A careful occupational history will indicate not only the materials a person has been exposed to, but also the extent of exposure. Recent overtime work, or weekend working can indicate acute exposure. The number of weeks or years spent on the job will give some idea of chronic exposure.

Hobbies, such as home maintenance and do-it-yourself (DIY) home improvement, may involve hazardous exposures away from the workplace. A worker in a shoe factory with contact dermatitis may suspect the adhesives at work as being responsible for his skin problems. However, this can also be the result of his hobby using glues at home for building model aeroplanes. Employers and employees can have differing views on the relative contribution of work duties versus hobbies and social activities to the development of ill health.

DETERMINING SPECIFIC EXPOSURE

When taking the occupational history, there can be uncertainty regarding the nature of the materials to which workers are exposed. This may arise in a number of ways:

Caution on chemical names

It is essential when investigating a case of possible exposure to a workplace chemical that the exact identity and nature of the chemical involved is obtained.

Benzene (C_6H_6), used in industry as a solvent and known to cause aplastic anaemia and leukaemia, is frequently confused with benzine, which is also used as a solvent, but is a mixture of liquid hydrocarbons (generally straight chain) and without the same serious haematologic effects. Another common confusion is between dioxin and dioxan (see Figure 3.2).

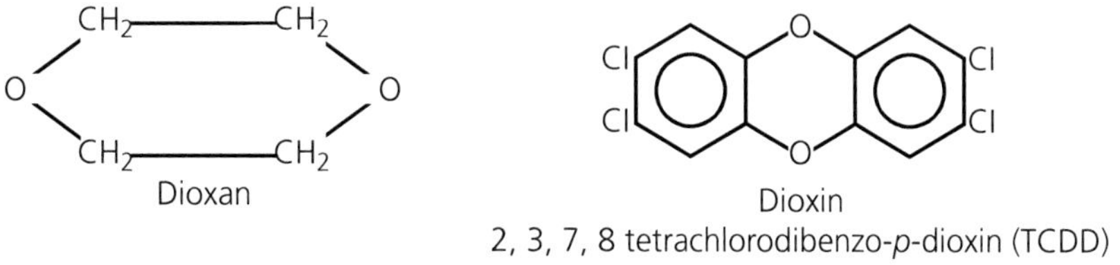

Figure 3.2

Dioxan (dioxane) has been used for many years as a solvent for fats and other materials. It has narcotic properties similar to other organic solvents and has been reported to be toxic to the liver and kidneys. Dioxin has a different chemical formula. It was the chemical released in the Seveso incident in Italy when an uncontrolled exothermic reaction resulted in workers and the surrounding population being exposed to dioxin causing chloracne, peripheral neuropathy and an increased risk of lympho-haemopoietic system malignancy.[4]

Chlordecone (Kepone™), a pesticide known to cause spermatogenic effects in occupationally exposed male workers[5,6] is sometimes confused with the similar-sounding 'dodecane'[7] – an aliphatic hydrocarbon used as a solvent. Chlordecone is no longer produced commercially, although dodecane is available and used widely.

'Methanal' is the systematic name for formaldehyde and can be confused with 'methanol', which is an alcohol.[7] The former is an irritant, allergen and carcinogen, while the latter is best known for causing optic nerve damage leading to blindness in people ingesting illicit alcohol containing more methanol than ethanol.

Patients may know only the commonly used name of a chemical that they are exposed to at work, e.g. 'trike' for trichloroethylene, or 'perk' for perchloroethylene. It can therefore be difficult for a clinician not familiar with these short names to recognize the specific chemical. Trade names are generally not helpful.

Impure chemicals

Even when the correct chemical name is obtained from the occupational history, the physician must always bear in mind that books or journals sometimes refer to the toxicity of the pure or relatively pure substance whereas, when sold commercially, chemicals will often not be pure and may well carry contaminants. For example, toluene (methyl benzene), apart from narcotic properties, does not have the same haematotoxic effects as benzene, because it is metabolized along the side chain (the methyl group), whereas benzene is metabolized on the ring, initially by the formation of an epoxide which may react with the macromolecules of the cell. Toluene is therefore recommended and used as a 'safe' substitute, but commercial toluene has been known to contain up to 15 per cent of benzene.

Formalin solution used as a tissue preservative contains formaldehyde, but methanol is also present (about 10 per cent) as a stabilizer, in addition to paraformaldehyde and formic acid. Hence, formalin solution is not pure formaldehyde.

Decomposition

When industrial processes go wrong, the chemical composition or physical properties of the materials can alter and increase the risk from exposure. Trichloroethylene, a widely used degreasing agent, if overheated, may produce phosgene gas which causes delayed pulmonary oedema. Methyl isocyanate heated above 400°C under pressure may decompose to hydrogen cyanide:[8] $CH_3NCO = H_2 + HCN + CO$. Cadmium-plated bolts do not pose a risk unless cut with an oxyacetylene, oxypropane or oxybutane torch giving rise to cadmium oxide fumes, capable of causing chemical pneumonitis (see Chapter 17, Cadmium).[9]

PHYSICAL NATURE OF MATERIALS

Metallic lead in solid form presents a physical not a toxicological hazard, but once heated to above its melting point, it is converted into fume which if inhaled will cause lead poisoning. Metallic mercury, on the other hand, is liquid at room temperature, and can vapourize easily to cause dangerous air concentrations to develop, especially in poorly ventilated rooms (see Chapter 26, Mercury).

Both toluene diisocyanate (TDI, or 2,4-tolylene diisocyanate) and methylene diphenyl diisocyanate (MDI, or diphenyl methane 4,4 diisocyanate) (see Figure 3.3) are well known as potent causes of occupational asthma (see Chapter 72, Occupational asthma). However, because TDI has a much higher vapour pressure, at room temperature, than the viscous MDI, it might be expected that MDI is safer to handle. So it is, unless the process is exothermic or involves spraying. In either of those circumstances, the advantage of the low vapour pressure of MDI in regards to safety is negated, and it has been found on a number of occasions to be a potent respiratory sensitizer.

OBTAINING FURTHER INFORMATION ON CHEMICALS

In the United Kingdom, the Control of Substances Hazardous to Health (COSHH) regulations[10] require employers to provide adequate information, instruction and training in such matters, with the result that patients may arrive at the surgery or the outpatient clinic carrying

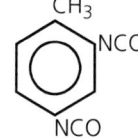

Vapour pressure 0.05 mmHg at 25°C
2.4-tolylene diisocyanate

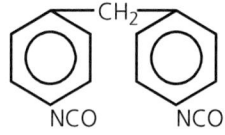

Vapour pressure 0.001 mmHg at 40°C
Diphenyl methane 4,4 diisocyanate

Figure 3.3

specially prepared leaflets (material safety data sheets) on chemicals, if they suspect that these may be responsible for their ill health. Material safety data sheets are prepared by suppliers for users and also for importers. A standard format for the preparation of such sheets is suggested by the Occupational Safety and Health Administration (OSHA) for suppliers in the United States and by European Community legislation in Europe. Most MSDS contain some data on the properties of the chemical, the possible health effects, first aid treatment and safe handling and use of the chemical. There is unfortunately often some confusing variation between MSDS produced by different organizations in different countries.

A clinician can pursue enquiries on properties and toxicity of chemicals directly with an employer, preferably through the firm's occupational physician if there is one, or from the firm's health and safety officer. In the UK, information on chemicals can also be sought from the Health and Safety Executive or from the National Poisons Information Service. Section 6 of the UK's Health and Safety at Work Act requires manufacturers, suppliers and others to provide adequate information about measures that are necessary to protect the user. An employer should therefore know about any possible harmful effects (or the absence of harmful effects) of a substance used or produced on his or her premises. Furthermore, where such information is not available, the manufacturer or supplier may be obliged to undertake research to eliminate or minimize any risks to health and safety. A patient is often able to obtain from his workplace the name and address of the supplier of a chemical or provide a copy of the MSDS.

Databases, such as Haz-Map[11] and CCINFO,[12] also provide information on hazardous chemicals and toxic effects, and websites, such as www.ilpi.com/msds, allow access to thousands of MSDSs.

USE OF PERSONAL PROTECTIVE EQUIPMENT

A patient may have been provided with, and may claim to have used for all or part of the time, some form of personal protective equipment (PPE). A careful occupational history should explore the adequacy or suitability of PPE, and the availability and use by the individual. This will give some indication as to the extent of protection provided. A 'mask' can be anything from a simple gauze pad, a filter device, to a full face respirator with an external fresh air supply, or self-contained breathing apparatus (SCBA). Similar considerations will apply to enquiries about protective measures for skin and eyes, e.g. whether gloves, an eye shield or safety spectacles, have been used and the length of time that they are used for that work cycle. Inappropriate use of, or care for, gloves can increase the risk of dermatitis instead of protecting the skin. For example, the use of powdered latex gloves in healthcare workers has been linked to allergic reactions in sensitized individuals and therefore is detrimental to health instead of preventing ill health. Use of the same pair of gloves for prolonged periods may lead to permeation of the gloves by solvents, and spillage of liquids into gloves can prolong contact between the skin of the hands and irritant or allergic substances.

SMOKING STATUS

Smoking affects the development of some occupational diseases. For example, both smoking and asbestos exposure independently increase the risk of lung cancer, and concomitant exposure to both factors multiplies the risk. This is also the case with smoking and exposure to radon gas,[13,14] as shown in studies of underground uranium miners who are exposed to radon in their work environment. While smoking increases the likelihood of byssinosis developing in cotton workers (see Chapter 73, Byssinosis and other cotton-related diseases), the evidence for smoking causing an increased risk of occupational asthma is controversial (see Chapter 72, Occupational asthma). However, smoking apparently decreases the risk of extrinsic allergic alveolitis, possibly because of impaired function of alveolar macrophages (see Chapter 74, Extrinsic allergic alveolitis).

Sometimes patients claiming compensation (or disability benefit) for occupational respiratory diseases may be reluctant to admit to smoking, or to their true level of smoking (or prepared to admit to smoking but only at home and not at work, because of restrictions in smoking at the workplace). This may be due to a concern that it may prejudice their chances of being diagnosed with an occupational condition or reduce any financial settlement or pension.

The ascertainment of current smoking status and smoking history, in addition to the occupational history, is especially important for assessing patients with respiratory disorders.

COMPENSATION

A physician may be asked by a patient about entitlement to compensation if there is an indication that his condition is work-related. The occupational history will have been instrumental in coming to a decision about any likely occupational aetiology. However, a diagnosis of an 'occupational disease' does not necessarily lead to compensation. State compensation schemes are governed by their rules regarding eligibility for benefits. For example, State benefits in the UK[15] are only payable for specific prescribed occupational diseases. Claims for benefits must also be made within a specified time frame, e.g. within five years of leaving an employment where exposure to noise resulted in occupational deafness, and within ten years of leaving a job with exposure to a sensitizer causing occupational asthma. For many prescribed conditions, no benefits are paid if the extent of disablement is assessed as <14 per cent (often referred to as the '14 per cent rule'). In Australia, Commonwealth government employees need to be assessed as having >20 per cent impairment to be eligible for hearing loss compensation.[16] How a decision is reached regarding percentage disablement is a separate issue. A patient with an occupational disease may therefore not receive state benefits despite a doctor's diagnosis of the condition and a clear occupational history of a relevant exposure, if eligibility criteria are not met.

An occupational history is also important in civil cases where a worker sues his employer or ex-employer for exposures in the workplace that have caused or contributed to ill health or injury. Again, a firm diagnosis of an occupational disease supported by an occupational history, does not necessarily guarantee that there will be financial recompense. In many countries, there is also a requirement to demonstrate negligence of the employer. In New Zealand, a 'no-fault' system[16] is in place that ensures compensation for all occupational injuries and some occupational disorders, e.g. occupational noise-induced hearing loss, without the need to prove negligence. Good doctor–patient communication is essential in making clear the distinction between obtaining an occupational history to make a clinical diagnosis versus using an occupational history as evidence to obtain compensation.

ETHICS AND CONFIDENTIALITY

Clinicians may face ethical dilemmas, including issues of confidentiality, in handling information obtained from an occupational history. For example, a worker may provide information on workplace exposure to chemicals that are deemed confidential trade secrets (such as exact ingredients and amounts of materials used for a specific process – a trade secret for the employer, but an essential piece of information for the doctor in order to assess the extent of exposure and likely contribution to ill health). A patient may describe a novel work process that is the subject of a patent application. A patient may indicate that other co-workers have ill health possibly from contact with a workplace chemical. If the outcome of identifying affected colleagues is their transfer to other jobs or ill-health retirement or redundancy, this may not be their wish nor will it necessarily be in their best interest. How should the clinician handle the information provided?

Published guidance is available on the ethical responsibilities of a doctor when there appears to be a conflict between responsibility to an individual patient and any responsibility to the employer. UK occupational physicians have access to advice from the ethics committee of the Faculty of Occupational Medicine. A helpful chapter is one on 'Relationships with others' in the Faculty of Occupational Medicine's guidance on ethics for occupational physicians.[17] Guidance on ethical issues for all physicians is also available from the British Medical Association, covering areas such as confidentiality, consent and disclosure of health information.[18]

A patient may be reluctant to reveal the identity of his/her employer. This may be because of the perceived consequences for continued employment if the employer should become aware that one of their workers has developed ill health from workplace activities or exposures. The affected worker may be torn between concerns for his health, and the need to keep his job despite the risk. From the information provided in the occupational history, the clinician can advise on individual preventive measures, but the implementation of any measures at work inevitably requires the involvement of the employer. The employer may want to know what the specific health issue is, and this may intrude into areas of confidential clinical information. The guidance resources mentioned above cover issues of patient confidentiality.

How reliable are occupational histories?

Occupational histories can be obtained during a face-to-face encounter with a patient as during a clinical consultation; or by use of an interviewer-administered or self-administered structured questionnaire. Occupational history questionnaires have been shown to provide information that is reliable and valid. They are relatively free from bias, and are acceptable to both patients and doctors.[19–21] However, the accuracy of self-reported work history appears lower in those with frequent job changes and accuracy of information is affected by number and duration of jobs.[22]

WHY TAKE AN OCCUPATIONAL HISTORY?

The two main reasons why an occupational history is important are: (1) because of the effects of work on health and (2) because of the effects of health on the safe and efficient performance of work. The value of the occupational history lies in the use of the information gathered in assessing the nature and extent of exposure to hazards in the workplace. This assessment is necessary for a physician to advise on possible occupational aetiology of a disease, and on fitness for work.

Effects of work on health

The occupational history is used when a physician has to decide if an occupational factor might have caused or contributed to a patient's illness. If there is an occupational aetiology, failure to take an adequate occupational history will lead to inappropriate management of the patient. The patient may be treated and then sent back to work in the same environment that has caused the disease, and therefore full recovery will not occur. An example is a patient with a rash that is treated with a steroid cream, and then sent back to work in an environment where exposure to the causative chemical continues. The rash may improve temporarily with treatment, but will invariably worsen with continuing contact with the causal agent.

Work can affect health in several ways:

- Occupational exposures may be a direct cause of ill health, for example exposure to hydrogen cyanide gas encountered by firefighters during their work can cause cyanide poisoning,[23] or exposure to metallic mercury in gold miners[24] or in dentists[25] causes mercury poisoning.
- Workplace exposures, while not necessarily being the sole factor causing a disease can be one of a number of contributory causes. Cigarette smoking, as mentioned earlier, multiplies the risk for lung cancer if there is exposure to asbestos fibres or radon gas. Each of these can cause lung cancer independently, but a worker who smokes, lives in a high environment radon area, and is exposed to asbestos from work activities has a much increased risk of lung cancer. Another example is that of exposure to carbon monoxide which can result from smoking, following exposure to methylene chloride[26,27] (used as a paint stripper), and working in an enclosed space such as a garage which is heated by a gas-fired heater, and has a car engine running. All these factors can act independently to increase blood carboxyhaemoglobin, but when several of these sources of carbon monoxide are present, there is an elevated risk of carbon monoxide poisoning.
- The nature of the job may worsen pre-existing non-occupational disease, e.g. hairdressing procedures or working in a kitchen can result in a worsening of endogenous eczema.
- The work environment may give easy access to potentially harmful materials, increasing the risk of their abuse. Examples of adverse health effects resulting from availability of toxic agents are effects of anaesthetic gases in anaesthetists or other health-care staff,[28,29] suicide in farm workers using pesticides,[30] and alcoholism in publicans.[31]

The effects of disease on occupation

Following a period of sickness absence, it is in a patient's and society's interest to encourage a return to work. Most patients are able to return directly to their own job after an illness or injury but some, because of residual disability, are unable to return to their former work. Many people with some impairment of function either seek work or seek to remain at work and may ask for medical advice.

The main areas where this advice is needed are:

1. The patient's condition may limit, reduce or prevent him performing the job effectively (e.g. musculoskeletal conditions that reduce mobility or diminish manipulative ability).
2. The patient's condition might be made worse by the job (e.g. excessive physical exertion in some cardiorespiratory conditions; exposure to certain allergens in individuals with asthma,[32] for example exposure to cat fur or animal dander in a vet or a technician in an animal laboratory).
3. The patient's condition is likely to make it unsafe to do the job (e.g. liability to sudden loss of consciousness while working alone and at heights).
4. The patient's condition is likely to make it unsafe for third parties, such as co-workers, visitors or members of the public. For example, a bus or train driver who is prone to episodes of unconsciousness with no warning symptoms may cause an accident affecting other crew members, passengers and the public.
5. The patient's condition might make it unsafe for the community (e.g. for consumers of the product, if a food-handler transmits infection[33]).

Some of the above areas are concerned with direct risk to the patient and some relate to risks to others, either risks to the health and safety of third parties or substantial financial risks to employers.

The occupational history will help a doctor in encouraging a timely return to appropriate work, and to retain people at work that will not harm their health. The emphasis in the UK today is on changing perceptions of fitness for work by discouraging stigmata around health and disability.[34] In the UK, proposals to reduce sickness absence include replacing the 'sick note' signed by the family physician with a 'fit note' involving discussion as necessary between the patient, the doctor, occupational health professionals and the employer.[34,35] This was implemented in April 2010.

For occupations such as drivers, divers, airline pilots and seafarers, specific guidance is published by different agencies. In the UK, the Driver and Vehicle Licensing Agency (DVLA) has produced a guide to medical standards for fitness to drive.[36] The guidance covers drivers of motor cars and motor cycles (group 1 licence holders), as well as professional drivers of large lorries (group 2, category C) and buses (group 2, category D). There are special provisions for drivers in the police force, ambulance drivers and taxi drivers. The information is updated online periodically. The latest guidance is accessible via the DVLA website (www.dvla.gov.uk). Telephone advice is also available from the DVLA for medical professionals in regards to the health status of drivers and fitness to drive. The Department of Transport has also produced a manual with advice on fitness to drive for patients with medical conditions, and this includes the basis behind the standards recommended.[37] In the United States, similar standards for commercial drivers are produced by the US Department of Transportation.[38]

For other occupations, *Fitness for Work: The Medical Aspects*[39] gives authoritative guidance using as its starting points the diseases (impairments) and disabilities from which a patient might suffer. It also has appendices on the medical standards for civil aviation, divers, offshore workers and seafarers. Advice regarding fitness for work of seafarers was updated in 1999 by Merchant Shipping Notice No. MSN 1746 issued by the Department of Environment, Transport and the Regions. The International Labour Organisation (ILO) has also produced guidelines for the medical fitness of seafarers. In the UK, NHS Plus and the Royal College of Physicians have produced national guidelines on occupational aspects of managing infected food handlers,[33] shift work in pregnancy[40] and other clinical conditions related to occupations or work activity.[41,42]

DIAGNOSING AN OCCUPATIONAL DISEASE

The occupational history is an important component for diagnosing an occupational disease. It can provide critical information on relevant occupational exposures, and on the link between the onset of symptoms and work. In general, several criteria should be met before concluding that a patient has an occupational disease.[43] The main criteria which should be satisfied are:

1. The effect, i.e. symptoms and signs, must fit with what is known about the clinical features of the suspected occupational disease. The less the features match what is expected, the less likely the diagnosis.
2. The exposure must be sufficient to cause the disease. Information on exposure may be obtained from the patient's occupational history and a description of what hazards are encountered at work. It is not sufficient just to know that there is exposure. It is essential to estimate the extent of exposure. i.e. number of substances to which the patient was exposed, intensity, frequency and duration of exposure. Sometimes, occupational hygiene data or biological monitoring records may be available and these can provide further evidence of the extent of exposure. Interpretation of exposure information for the most widely used substances can be assisted by reference to published occupational exposure standards. In the UK, the Health and Safety Executive publishes updated standards annually for about 500 substances in a document referred to as 'EH40'. This contains workplace exposure limits and biological monitoring guidance values, and is available free via the internet.[44] In the United States, there are several sets of similar standards, e.g. threshold limit values and biological exposure indices produced by the American Conference of Governmental Industrial Hygienists (ACGIH),[45] permissible exposure limits produced by the Occupational Safety and Health Administration (OSHA), and recommended exposure limits from the National Institute for Occupational Safety and Health (NIOSH). In Germany, the equivalent standards are known as MAK values.[46] In 1995, the European Commission established a Scientific Committee on Occupational Exposure Limits (SCOEL)[47] to obtain independent scientific expert opinion on chemicals in the workplace. SCOEL's efforts could contribute to harmonizing occupational hygiene standards in all European Union member countries. There are differences between the standards from the various organizations, and the basis of how they are set should be understood as a prerequisite for use. Caution must be exercised in the use of occupational hygiene monitoring results for diagnosing occupational disease. Even if exposure levels are above current workplace exposure limits (in the United Kingdom) or threshold limit values (in the United States), it does not necessarily point to the agent concerned as the cause. There are safety factors introduced in the development of exposure standards. The standards are also not purely health-based levels, but can be influenced by cost–benefit considerations. Susceptibility of exposed individuals is a factor that can cause health effects at levels of exposure even below current standards. Readings showing excursions above current standards on a single occasion may be less important than frequent measured excessive levels. The frequency and intensity of the exposures exceeding current standards demonstrate poor workplace control of exposures, and give an indication of the likelihood of the exposures causing disease. Some of the limitations in the use of exposure information as an aid for diagnosing occupational disease apply to both occupational hygiene readings, as well as biological monitoring data (see Chapter 5, Biological monitoring). Workplace exposure standards proposed by different agencies in different countries for some chemicals vary. In part, this reflects the imprecision of estimating the limit of exposure needed to protect against ill health. There is continuing debate for some substances, such as silica, about whether disease (silicosis) may develop despite exposures below the current standards (see Chapter 79, Silica and silica-related diseases).
3. The time sequence must be correct. This includes the consideration of the latent period between exposure and effect. For occupational cancers, generally a very short time interval (less than five years) between first exposure and the diagnosis of cancer suggests that the exposure may not be the relevant causative agent. For occupational asthma and allergic contact dermatitis, there may be several weeks, months or even years between first exposure and clinical manifestations. Some acute exposures produce clinical effects immediately or within minutes of exposure, e.g. hydrogen cyanide gas, or upper respiratory irritants, such as sulphur dioxide, ammonia or chlorine gas (see Chapter 39, Gases), while the time interval between exposure and effect may be several hours or one or two days for agents that cause delayed pulmonary oedema. It may appear obvious that for a diagnosis of occupational disease due to a specific agent, the exposure to that agent must precede the occurrence of clinical effects. However, there are situations where even though a disease has developed earlier in life, subsequent occupational exposures may trigger an episode or worsen the condition,

e.g. occupational asthma or contact dermatitis. In this case, a previous history of the disease does not necessarily rule out an occupational aetiology if the disease manifests again later, during working life.
4. Consideration must be given to the differential diagnosis. The examining physician should consider possible non-occupational diagnoses, as well as occupational conditions. Missing an occupational disease with its possibilities for prevention is as inappropriate as labelling a condition occupational and missing an opportunity to provide early treatment for a non-occupational disease. An example of the former is failure to recognize contact dermatitis due to a workplace agent, and an example of the latter is assuming that a peripheral neuropathy is due to n-hexane when the patient has diabetic neuropathy. The decision on whether an illness is occupational or non-occupational in an individual patient can often rest on the balance of probability in the absence of supportive or confirmatory clinical and pathological evidence. This requires good clinical diagnostic skills and an understanding of workplace activities and exposures and their effects.

CONCLUSION

The occupational history is the most effective instrument for the proper diagnosis of occupational disease.[48]

Landrigan and Baker, 1991

Key points

- The occupational history is key to determining the occupational aetiology of a disease, and is essential for advising patients on return to work.
- Taking the occupational history should be systematic and the history must be sufficiently detailed to indicate the nature and extent of workplace exposures.
- A general medical history taken during a doctor–patient consultation is incomplete without asking for information about the patient's occupation.

ACKNOWLEDGEMENTS

This chapter is updated from Chapter 1, The occupational history, by WR Lee and T-C AW, *Hunter's Diseases of Occupations*, 9th edn, 2000: 3–13.

REFERENCES

1. Ramazzini B. *Diseases of workers* (originally 1713). The classics of medicine library. Chicago, IL: University of Chicago Press, 1983.
2. Aw TC, Gardiner K, Harrington JM. *Occupational health: Pocket consultant*, 5th edn. Oxford: Blackwell Publishing, 2007.
3. National Academy of Sciences, Committee on Occupational Classification and Analysis. Dictionary of occupational titles (DOT). Last accessed March 12, 2010. Available from: www.occupationalinfo.org. Washington DC: US Department of Commerce.
4. Bertazzi PA, Bernucci I, Brambilla G *et al*. The Seveso studies on early and long-term effects of dioxin exposure: A review. *Environmental Health Perspectives*. 1998; **106**: 625–33.
5. Whorton MD. Male occupational reproductive hazards. *Western Journal of Medicine*. 1982; **137**: 521–4.
6. Jensen TK, Bonde JP, Joffe M. The influence of occupational exposure to male reproductive function. *Occupational Medicine*. 2006; **56**: 544–53.
7. Clark JOE, Hemsley W (eds). *The Rosen comprehensive dictionary of chemistry*. New York: Rosen Publishing Group, 2008.
8. Blake PG, Ijadi-Maghsoodi S. Kinetics and mechanisms of the thermal decomposition of methyl isocyanate. International *Journal of Chemical Kinetics*. 1982; **14**: 945–52.
9. Benton DC, Andrews GS, Davies HJ *et al*. Acute cadmium fume poisoning. *British Journal of Industrial Medicine*. 1966; **23**: 292–301.
10. Control of Substances Hazardous to Health Regulations, 2002. UK Statutory Instrument 2002 No. 2677. London: TSO, 2002.
11. Brown JA. HAZ-MAP: Information on hazardous chemicals and occupational diseases. Last accessed March 11, 2010. Available from: http://hazmap.nlm.nih.gov.
12. Canadian Center for Occupational Health and Safety. Last accessed March 11, 2010. Available from: http://ccinfoweb.ccohs.ca.
13. National Cancer Institute. Radon and cancer: Questions and answers. Last accessed March 11, 2010. Available from: www.cancer.gov/cancertopics/factsheet/Risk/radon.
14. Environmental Protection Agency. Radon: Health risks. Last accessed March 11, 2010. Available from: www.epa.gov/radon/healthrisks.html.
15. Department for Work and Pensions (UK). DB1: A guide to industrial injuries benefits (August 2009). Last accessed March 13, 2010. Available from: www.dwp.gov.uk/publications.
16. Carroll RL. Compensation for occupational noise induced hearing loss in Australia and New Zealand. *International Congress Series*. 2003; **1240**: 161–3.
17. Harling CC, Hunt S (eds). *FOM guidance on ethics for occupational physicians*. London: Faculty of Occupational Medicine, 2006.

18. British Medical Association. *Medical ethics today: Its practice and philosophy*, 2nd edn. London: BMJ Publishing, 2003.
19. Lewis RJ, Friedlander BR, Bhojani FA et al. Reliability and validity of an occupational health history questionnaire. *Journal of Occupational and Environmental Medicine*. 2002; **44**: 39-47.
20. Brower PS, Attfield MD. Reliability of reported occupational history information for US coal miners, 1969-1977. *American Journal of Epidemiology*. 1998; **148**: 920-6.
21. Rosenberg CR. An analysis of the reliability of self reported work histories from a cohort of workers exposed to polychlorinated biphenyls. *British Journal of Industrial Medicine*. 1993; **50**: 822-6.
22. Bourbonnais R, Meyer F, Theriault G. Validity of self reported work history. *British Journal of Industrial Medicine*. 1988; **45**: 29-32.
23. Guidotti T. Acute cyanide poisoning in pre-hospital care: new challenges. New tools for intervention. *Prehospital and Disaster Medicine*. 2005; **21**: 540-8.
24. Rodrigues AR, Souza CRB, Braga AM et al. Mercury toxicity in the Amazon: Contrast sensitivity and color discrimination of subjects exposed to mercury. *Brazilian Journal of Medical and Biological Research*. 2007; **40**: 415-24.
25. Langford NJ, Ferner RE. Toxicity of mercury. *Journal of Human Hypertension*. 1999; **13**: 651-6.
26. Amsel J, Soden KJ, Sielken RI Jr, Valdez Flora C. Observed versus predicted carboxyhaemoglobin levels in cellulose triacetate workers exposed to methylene chloride. *American Journal of Industrial Medicine*. 2001; **40**: 180-91.
27. Agency for Toxic Substances and Disease Register (ATSDR). Methylene chloride. Last accessed March 13, 2010. Available from: www.atsdr.cdc.gov.
28. Hawton K, Clements A, Simkin S, Malmberg A. Doctors who kill themselves: A study of the methods used for suicide. *Quarterly Journal of Medicine*. 2000; **93**: 351-7.
29. Blanco G, Peters HA. Myeloneuropathy and macrocytosis associated with nitrous oxide abuse. *Archives of Neurology*. 1983; **40**: 416-18.
30. Gunnell D, Eddleston M. Suicide by intentional ingestion of pesticides: A continuing tragedy in developing countries. *International Journal of Epidemiology*. 2003; **32**: 909-99.
31. Baker A. Alcohol-related deaths by occupation: What do data for England and Wales in 2001-2005 tell us about doctors' mortality. *Alcohol and Alcoholism*. 2008; **43**: 121-2.
32. Berger Z, Rom WN, Reibman J et al. Prevalence of workplace exacerbation of asthma symptoms in an urban working population of asthmatics. *Journal of Occupational and Environmental Medicine*. 2006; **48**: 833-9.
33. NHS Plus, Royal College of Physicians, Faculty of Occupational Medicine. Infected food handlers: Occupational aspects of management. A national guideline. London: Royal College of Physicians, 2008.
34. Black C. Working for a healthier tomorrow. Last accessed March 11, 2010. Available from: www.workingforhealth.gov.uk. London: TSO, 2008.
35. UK Government. Improving health and work: Changing lives. Last accessed March 11, 2010. Available from: www.workingforhealth.gov.uk. London: TSO, 2008.
36. Driver and Vehicle Licensing Authority. At a glance guide to the current medical standards for fitness to drive. Last accessed February 18, 2010. Available from: www.dft.gov.uk/dvla/medical/ataglance.aspx, 2010.
37. Carter T. *Fitness to drive: A guide for health professionals*. London: RSM Press, 2007.
38. Federal Motor Carrier Safety Administration. Medical examination report for commercial driver fitness determination. Washington DC: US Department of Transportation. Last accessed February 18, 2010. Available from: www.fmcsa.dot.gov/documents/safetyprograms/medical-report.pdf.
39. Palmer K, Cox RAF, Brown I. *Fitness for work: The medical aspects*, 4th edn. Oxford: Faculty of Occupational Medicine, Royal College of Physicians/Oxford University Press, 2007.
40. NHS Plus, Royal College of Physicians, Faculty of Occupational Medicine. Physical and shift work in pregnancy: Occupational aspects of management. A national guideline. London: Royal College of Physicians, 2009.
41. NHS Plus, Royal College of Physicians, Faculty of Occupational Medicine. Latex allergy: Occupational aspects of management. A national guideline. London: Royal College of Physicians, 2008.
42. NHS Plus, Royal College of Physicians, Faculty of Occupational Medicine. Dermatitis: Occupational aspects of management. A national guideline. London: Royal College of Physicians, 2009.
43. Aw TC. Preface to 'Information notices on occupational disease: a guide to diagnosis'. European Commission document. Last accessed March 10, 2010. Available from: http://ec.europa.eu/social/main. Luxembourg: Office for Official Publications of the European Communities, 2009.
44. Health and Safety Executive. Workplace exposure limits table. Last accessed March 13, 2010. Available from: www.hse.gov.uk.
45. American Conference of Governmental Industrial Hygienists. Threshold limit values for chemical substances and physical agents and biological exposure indices. Cincinnati, OH: ACGIH, 2009.
46. Deutsche Forschungsgemeinschaft (DFG). MAK and BAT values list, 2009. Last accessed March 13, 2010. Available from: www.dfg.de/aktuelles_presse/reden_stellungnahmen/download/mak2009.pdf.
47. European Commission (DG for Employment, Social Affairs and Equal Opportunities). The Scientific Committee on Occupational Exposure Limits (SCOEL): SCOEL Recommendations (list). Last accessed March 13, 2010. Available from: http://ec.europa.eu/social/.
48. Landrigan PJ, Baker DB. The recognition and control of occupational disease. *Journal of American Medical Association*. 1991; **266**: 676-80.

4

Occupational exposure to hazardous substances

JOHN W CHERRIE AND SEAN SEMPLE

Introduction	43	Holistic exposure assessment	48
Exposure and exposure routes	44	Control of exposure to hazardous substances	49
What is the level of exposure?	45	Attribution of a disease to an exposure	51
Exposure variability and exposure determinants	47	Conclusions	54
Inhalation exposure metrics	48	References	54
Exposure limits	48	Further reading	55

INTRODUCTION

Determining the cause of an individual's ill health or disease is one of the most important roles that a physician performs. Understanding the cause and linking exposure to disease can often be essential to the treatment and improvement of the patient's life quality. At a wider level, it can enable identification of unacceptable exposures to a workforce population and, with appropriate intervention, lead to prevention of further ill health in others. There are also sentinel cases where new hazards and new relationships between exposure and disease are discovered, leading to changes in work practices and perhaps even legislation.

Occupational hygiene offers a simple paradigm for investigating the link between exposure and disease by the processes of recognizing hazards, evaluating the degree of risk from exposure and then controlling risk to health to an acceptable level. The first element of this involves hazard identification and this can be achieved by careful review of the safety data sheets (SDS) relating to the chemicals being used in the workplace. Where there is access to the worksite then the SDSs should be available and, if not, then there are specific legal requirements on suppliers that require them to provide these. When access is not available or the patient's exposure is more historical, then a detailed occupational history is required and contact with the employer and/or investigation of a similar worksite may be fruitful in identifying the substances used in or released by the work process. A literature review of the industry or job title using websites ranging from the International Labour Organisation through to more specific searches of published scientific papers held on PubMed, or another online bibliographic database, may also provide useful insights to the substances to which the worker may have been exposed. In cases where the physician works closely with the employer and has direct access to the site then a simple 'walk-through' investigation is often the first step. Creating a list of the chemicals used and making a simple qualitative assessment of the amounts handled or processed, the degree of contact and the level of hazard as depicted by any container labels or SDS data is a useful output from such a walk-through survey.

A comprehensive understanding of how workers interact with hazardous substances in their place of work is necessary and knowledge of exposure and exposure routes is essential in making judgements about the likely causation of ill health. Exposure monitoring records may exist and, in the United Kingdom where collected, they should have been kept for a minimum of 40 years under the Control of Substances Hazardous to Health (COSHH) regulations. Where data on exposure are not available, the physician has two choices: collection of current measurements of exposure, or reconstruction and/or modelling of the past concentrations based on descriptions of the worksite, use of analogous data or mathematical models that predict how much chemical exposure would take place in a given space under the described work conditions.

Ideally, measurements of inhalation exposure in the workplace should be carried out by personal sampling, that is the attachment of the sampling device to the breathing zone of the worker – an area within a 10-cm radius of the nose and mouth. In some cases, this is not possible and static or area sampling, where the sampler is located at a fixed point, is performed. It is generally considered that, in most circumstances, static sampling will underestimate exposure of individual workers due to periodic close contact or handling of the exposure source.

Quantification of the exposure allows the process of evaluation of risk to begin. The concentration of a dust or vapour in the air can be compared to occupational exposure limits (OELs). In the United Kingdom, these are called workplace exposure limits (WELs) and are provided by the Health and Safety Executive (HSE) through the COSHH regulations for many chemicals. These limits are produced by considering toxicological and epidemiological data on health effects observed where possible after human exposure, but more often as a result of controlled exposure of animals or cellular models. The basic premise is that exposures below the WEL will limit the risk to the worker to 'acceptable levels', but it is important to be aware that not all limits are set at levels that will achieve no adverse effects and for some carcinogenic or sensitizing substances any exposure will carry some degree of risk. Other countries have their own OELs.

Treatment of the patient may be modified with knowledge of what workplace exposure has or has not caused their condition. Reduction or elimination of the exposure experienced by the worker may form one part of the medical intervention and this can have an effect on both the worker's health and also the current and future health status of other workers within the facility.

Exposure control is the final part of the role of the occupational health professional. Control of exposure to hazardous substances in the workplace is enshrined in the legislative framework of most nations. In the United Kingdom, the COSHH regulations, the Control of Lead at Work regulations and the Control of Asbestos regulations are the three principal pieces of law aimed at encouraging control of workers' exposure. All are based on a hierarchical approach to control beginning with elimination of the hazard, substitution with less hazardous materials, control by containment, ventilation and process changes and moving to the control method of last resort, namely personal protective equipment worn by the employee. There is now a wealth of guidance available to those using hazardous substances on best practice and methods of control that will lead to exposures that are less than the OELs. COSHH Essentials is a web-based tool that provides the user with targeted guidance based on easily obtainable information from the safety data sheets, the quantity and frequency of use, and how the material is being used in the workplace. The system uses simple hazard banding and exposure model estimates to recommend the type of control options that should be considered as best practice for the generic type of task being performed.

This chapter will explore in more detail how we can understand workers' exposures, both within and beyond the workplace, how to interpret measurement data and compare these to limit values and, by using illustrative examples, we will look at the process of attributing a disease to an exposure.

EXPOSURE AND EXPOSURE ROUTES

Exposure is defined as contact between an individual and a hazardous substance.[1] Workers may be exposed to hazardous substances by inhalation, inadvertent ingestion of chemical contamination, skin or eye contact and direct injection where a sharp object punctures the skin and the chemical enters directly.

Exposure occurs at the interface between the environment and the person and is measured on the outside of the body. For inhalation, exposure is conventionally defined as the concentration close to the nose or mouth multiplied by the duration of the exposure – sometimes referred to as 'cumulative' exposure. Therefore, someone exposed to a concentration of $0.1\,\text{mg/m}^3$ of benzene for four hours would have an exposure of $0.4\,\text{mg/m}^3 \times$ hour. However, to simplify the measurement and assessment of risk, it is conventional to express workplace exposure over a fixed time interval, e.g. eight hours. In the example above, the benzene exposure would be $0.05\,\text{mg/m}^3$, as an eight-hour average, i.e. 0.4 ($\text{mg/m}^3 \times$ hour) divided by 8 (hours).

Other factors may influence the amount of hazardous substance taken up into the body by inhalation, most notably the breathing rate of the worker, with a greater mass of contaminant being inhaled when a person is undertaking physical work than when they are sedentary. Although this factor will affect the risk for an individual, it is seldom taken into consideration when evaluating risk.

There is much less consensus about the definition of dermal exposure, although Schneider et al.[2] described a conceptual model of the processes involved. Chemicals that come into contact with the skin may permeate through the stratum corneum and diffuse towards the peripheral blood supply. The ideal measure of dermal exposure would be related to the potential uptake, which is mainly driven by the concentration of the chemical in the surface layers on the skin (the skin contamination layer (SCL)), the area of skin exposed and the duration of exposure. Other factors, such as the composition of the mixture of substances present in the SCL and the integrity of the stratum corneum, will also affect dermal uptake.

It is difficult to measure the concentration of chemicals in the SCL and so the mass of chemical in the SCL or the mass that impinges onto the SCL during a period of time are often used as surrogate measures of exposure. In these cases, exposure may be expressed as mass per unit area over a defined part of the body, e.g. mg/cm^2 on the torso, or as the mass on a specific body part, e.g. mg on both hands. There are no OELs for dermal exposure.

There is no consensus about how exposure by inadvertent ingestion should be assessed, although this is generally associated with hand-to-mouth contacts. Key factors involved with this type of exposure are the extent of hand contamination, the type of work, whether protective gloves are worn and personal traits of individual workers, e.g. nail biting.

For injection exposure, crude measures, such as the number of injuries per day involving contaminated objects, are often used, e.g. in the case of needle stick injuries.

The term 'aggregate' exposure refers to the risks over time from multiple sources, pathways and routes for a single chemical, and so for example, someone exposed to pesticides in their job as a farmer and then in their own garden when they spray their flowers would get aggregate exposure from these two sources. The term 'cumulative' exposure is then often used for assessments where there is exposure to a mixture of different chemicals that all have the same potential to cause an adverse health effect and some attempt is made to combine the overall exposure to produce some estimate of the overall risk. As noted earlier, the term 'cumulative' may also be used in the context of exposure in units of concentration multiplied by duration of exposure, e.g. $mg/m^3 \times$ hour, as for example might be the case in an epidemiological study investigating the relationship between the lifetime exposure to a hazardous substance, where the duration would be the working life of the individual.

In some circumstances, biomarkers may be used as an index of aggregate exposure, for example the concentration of lead in blood among workers exposed to inorganic lead compounds. These are not measures of exposure, although they are related to exposure and may offer some advantages in providing an estimate of aggregate exposure arising from more than one route. For example, blood lead will reflect exposure by inhalation and inadvertent ingestion. Considerable care has to be taken in interpreting biomonitoring data in relation to exposure because of the complex relationship between the pattern of exposure and the biological half-life of the biomarker.

WHAT IS THE LEVEL OF EXPOSURE?

Developing methods to assess the amount of contact between a worker and a chemical over a given time period has been the core of much occupational hygiene work in the past 50 years. Methods of exposure assessment can range from detailed, objective quantification using real-time direct-reading instruments through to subjective qualitative categorization into broad bands such as 'low', 'medium' and 'high'.

The first place to start is to examine what exposure monitoring information exists in the workplace. Larger worksites, in particular, may have records of regular monitoring taken as part of programmes to demonstrate compliance with legislation. Others may have sporadic records collected at the time of inspection by regulators or before/after the introduction of new processes or control equipment.

Where existing information is not available then it may be possible to measure current exposure of the worker. Depending on the chemical hazard to be assessed there are a wide range of methods available for measurement. The HSE Methods for Determination of Hazardous Substances (MDHS) series of guidance notes are freely available via the internet (www.hse.gov.uk/pubns/mdhs/index.htm). MDHS 14/3 covers sampling and analysis of total inhalable and respirable dusts,[3] while MDHS 39/4 provides guidance on sampling asbestos fibres in air and MDHS 70 details general methods for sampling airborne gases and vapours. Similar descriptions of methods for measurement of particular chemicals is provided by the US National Institute for Occupational Safety and Health (NIOSH) through their online Pocket Guide to Chemical Hazards (www.cdc.gov/niosh/npg/).

For most measurements of airborne exposures, the basic premise is in the gravimetric sampling of workplace air. This involves drawing air at a defined rate through a sampling medium which allows collection of a mass of the chemical being assessed. Simple division of the mass collected by the volume of air sampled during the collection period produces a concentration typically milligrams per cubic metre of air (mg/m^3), although units of parts per million (ppm) are more commonly given for gases and vapours by conversion using the molar constant.

For dust and particulate matter, air sampling is achieved by using a small battery-operated pump to draw air through a filter (glass fibre, PVC or PTFE are the most common types) held in a holder that selectively samples the aerosol by its size. When measuring total inhalable dust, that is the fraction of airborne dust that is inhaled through the nose and mouth, an IOM (Institute of Occupational Medicine) head (see Figure 4.1) set at a flow rate of 2.0 L/min can be used. For respirable dust (the finer fraction of dust that will reach the gaseous-exchange areas of the lung), samplers such as the cyclone (Figure 4.2) are used at flow rates of 2.2 L/min. After sampling, the filters are then reweighed and the mass increase is divided by the volume sampled, which is the product of flow-rate and duration expressed as m^3.

The approach for sampling for gases and vapours is generally similar to that for particulates with a pump pulling air at typically 50–200 mL/min through a small sampling tube with a collecting substrate, often charcoal, on which the gas or vapour is absorbed. The analysing laboratory then desorbs the chemical from the charcoal and quantifies the mass before dividing this by the volume of air sampled during the measurement period to produce a resulting concentration (e.g. mg/m^3).

Fibres, such as asbestos, are measured in a slightly different way with the concentration expressed not by mass, but as a count of the number of fibres on the filter per unit volume of air sampled (fibres/mL).

All of the above examples are suited for collection of personal sampling data and are typically employed when determining if workers are exposed at levels above or

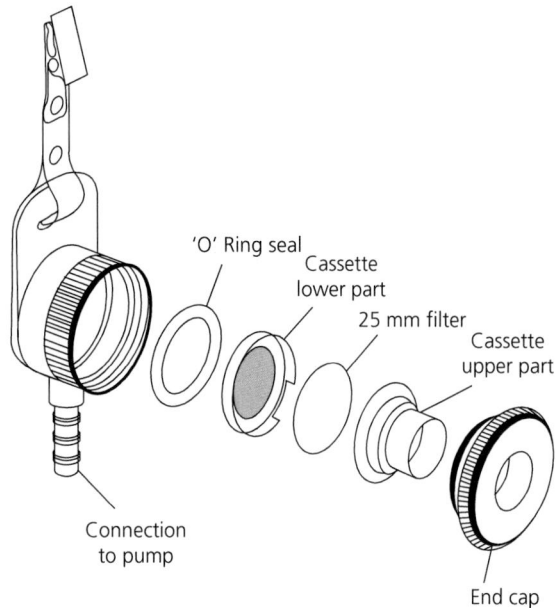

Figure 4.1 Institute of Occupational Medicine (IOM) total inhalable dust sampling head. Reproduced with permission from Ref. 3.

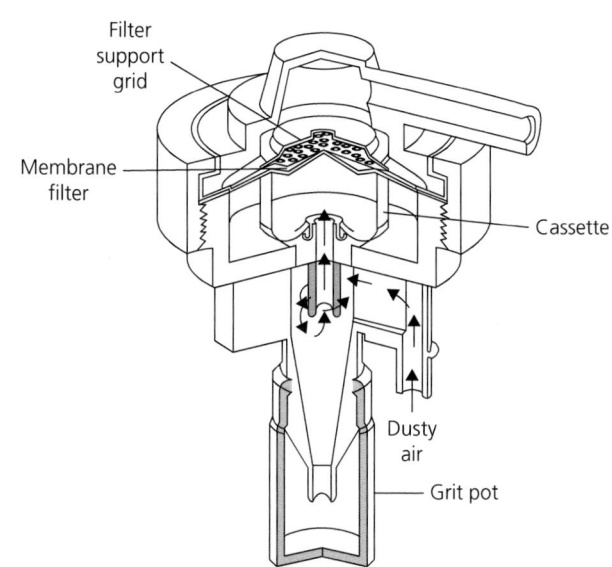

Figure 4.2 Cyclone sampler for measuring respirable dust. Reproduced with permission from Ref. 3.

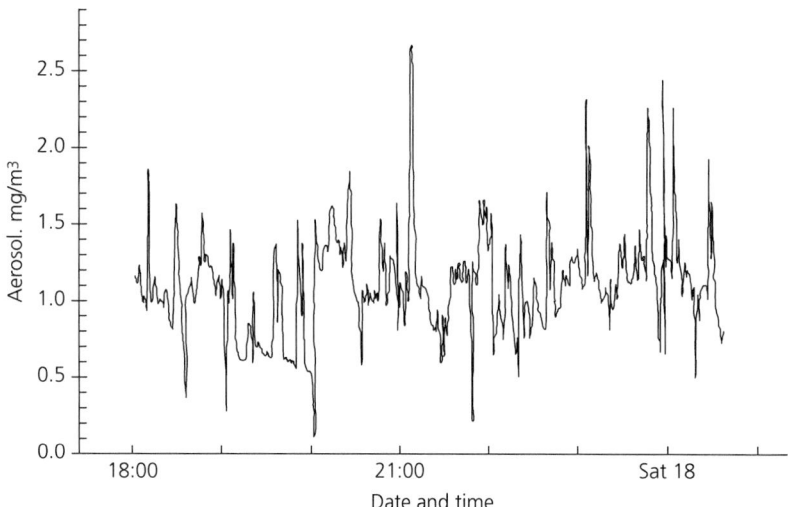

Figure 4.3 Real-time fine particulate dust exposure measured over a workshift.

below statutory limits. They all have the disadvantage that they take some time to collect and analyse, and generally involve expensive chemical analysis and involvement of a laboratory. In addition, these methods only provide information on the average concentration over the duration of the sampling and do not indicate anything to do with temporal changes and peaks of exposure while performing specific tasks. Direct reading instruments can assist when there is a need to have either immediate results or data about changes in exposure over a workshift.

Direct-reading instruments, which provide an instantaneous reading, range from simple tubes through to expensive electrochemical or photo-electric devices that can provide a log of changing concentrations in real-time. Colorimetric tubes undergo a reaction with the chemical under study to produce a colour change, with the length or intensity of this colour stain providing an instantaneous indication of the airborne concentration. There are many different types of these tubes with the media generally specific to a small number of chemicals, so proper selection is important. More accurate and sensitive portable direct reading instruments for gases and vapours using flame ionization with gas chromatography or infrared or ultraviolet photometry exist, although these instruments tend to involve large capital investment and need frequent calibration. For particulate matter measurement, small logging personal aerosol monitors can now be purchased. These operate by using light scattering methods coupled to size-selective air inlets that mechanically remove dust above a particular size.

Figure 4.3 shows the type of concentration-time output that can be generated from direct reading instruments and how these can be used to identify peaks in exposure generated from particular tasks or methods of working.

While some simple exposure assessments can be carried out using direct reading instruments by those with no special training, collection of more complex sampling data is best undertaken with the help of an experienced occupational hygienist. Input from a hygienist will help maximize the amount and quality of exposure information that can be collected with the resources available and will cover issues such as the timing and duration of sampling, how many samples should be collected to give a representative indication of exposures, the type of instruments that can be used and how to transport and analyse the resulting samples. The British Occupational Hygiene Society (BOHS) has a listing of members who carry out hygiene consultancy work in the UK. Similar occupational or industrial hygiene societies and associations exist across the world with details of national organizations available via the International Occupational Hygiene Association website (www.ioha.net).

Measurement is expensive, labour intensive and not always a practical option when the worksite has been closed or access is restricted due to geographical, political or budgetary constraints. In recent years, there has been a growing push to use existing workplace information to model exposures. Modelling can range from complex statistical examination of large datasets of previous measurements to tease out determinants of exposure through to relatively simple logic structures that utilize readily available information on the chemical properties of a material, the quantities being used, the environment within which it is being handled (confined, open, well-ventilated, outside), and the methods of application or use (contained, dispersive, low energy, high energy, etc.). The online software tool Stoffenmanager (www.stoffenmanager.nl) allows the user to enter data on each of these parameters and then produces an estimated distribution of exposure concentrations generated for the scenario provided.

Figure 4.4 shows the distribution provided for exposures to xylene during a spray painting task. The exposure distribution is broadly log-normal and so the median value, or 50th percentile is 203 mg/m^3, while the 95th percentile is over 3400 mg/m^3. Understanding 'worst case' exposures is extremely important in determining disease causation and Figure 4.4 clearly demonstrates how some workers at certain times may perform the task in a rushed manner, without the ventilation system in operation, without their usual protective equipment and perhaps with much greater quantities than they would normally use. In these cases, the exposure will be towards the upper end of the distribution and may be many times higher than the median value. There has been a great deal of recent work in understanding variability in exposure and the factors that influence both the measured level and degree of variability across a population of workers performing similarly described jobs. The British and Dutch Occupational Hygiene Society have recently published draft guidance on

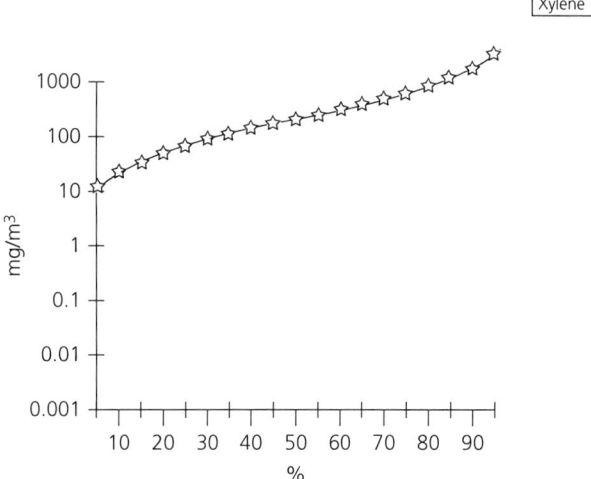

Figure 4.4 Output from the Stoffenmanager webtool showing estimated xylene concentrations for a particular task.

how to interpret exposure data in light of exposure variability and how to judge the likelihood of measurements failing to identify exposures that exceed given limits.[4]

EXPOSURE VARIABILITY AND EXPOSURE DETERMINANTS

Exposure for a single worker varies from minute to minute throughout the day as she undertakes different tasks and interacts with work equipment or processes. Two workers performing the same job in a factory will have different exposures because of differences in their work tasks, the way they do their work and their location in the plant. Workers doing a different job may have higher or lower average exposure from the first two workers, depending on how their work brings them into contact with the contaminant, their work and other exposure determinants. In all of these cases, some of the variation can be explained by exposure determinants, such as job, process, equipment, environment or other factors, and some is less clearly defined and is attributed to random influences. It is not unusual for the exposure measurements on a single day from two individuals doing the same job in the same factory to differ by more than one or two orders of magnitude. It is, therefore, very important when measuring exposure to make a careful record of the key exposure determinants, e.g. the materials handled, the way that they are handled, the presence and effectiveness of workplace control measures, the size of the workroom, the amount of general ventilation, the use of personal protection and the amount of time spent doing specific tasks or activities. In addition, the extent of the typical variation in exposure means that one or two measurements of exposure made in a specific workplace may not be particularly informative about average exposure and a more extensive dataset may be needed before clear conclusions can be made as to the extent of exposure of a group of workers in a particular workplace.

Some workers may be consistently exposed to higher or lower levels than a typical worker doing their job, either because of the way they do the work or because of the work tasks they undertake. It is important to understand these intraindividual differences in exposure when attempting to understand the role of exposure to hazardous substances in the causation of disease.

INHALATION EXPOSURE METRICS

Adverse health effects can broadly be categorized as either acute or chronic, reflecting the timescale over which the effects of exposure occur. For simplicity and practicability, exposures related to acute effects are generally measured over a 15-minute averaging period and for those related to chronic effects over an eight-hour period. For some substances, there may be both acute and chronic effects and in these cases exposure should be assessed against both time bases.

For chronic hazards, measurements would typically be made over less than eight hours and an assumption would be made about the exposure during the missing time in calculating the eight-hour average exposure. For example, a worker exposed to ethylene oxide was sampled for six hours and the measured concentration was 5 mg/m^3. If the sample had been collected over the whole of the time when the individual was exposed, i.e. the remaining two hours of his work shift did not involve any exposure, then the eight-hour average exposure would be 3.75 mg/m^3, i.e. $((5 \times 6) + (0 \times 2))/8$. If, however, the unmeasured period was judged similar to the measured period, the eight-hour average exposure would be 5 mg/m^3, i.e. $((5 \times 6) + (5 \times 2))/8$.

When a worker performs several distinct tasks, then the process of calculating a time-weighted average (TWA) is often employed. This combines the product of the exposure intensity and duration of each task and divides by the total work duration. So, for example, a baker who spends two hours decanting sacks of flour to small tubs may have an exposure to flour dust of 15 mg/m^3 for that period, followed by four hours of general baking activity, when the intensity of exposure is 2 mg/m^3 and a final two hours of bakery cleaning with an exposure of 5 mg/m^3. The time-weighted average is calculated using the equation below:

$$\text{TWA} = \frac{(15 \times 2) + (2 \times 4) + (5 \times 2)}{8} = 6 \text{ mg/m}^3$$

where measurements are made over part of a working day to investigate whether peak exposures are associated with the risk of acute ill health. For irritation, it is common to sample for 15 minutes on a number of occasions when it is likely that exposures are likely to be at their highest, e.g. during filling of drums with a volatile liquid or when cleaning a store contaminated with a toxic dust.

EXPOSURE LIMITS

Risk is most often judged by comparing the exposure to an appropriate occupational exposure limit. OELs are derived by a number of scientific and/or policy bodies and typically have legal status in the country where they were derived. Scientific limits are often set to protect the health of those exposed, i.e. exposure below these health-based OELs would not be expected to give rise to any adverse effects. Where it is either not possible to define a health-based limit or where compliance with this type of limit would be impracticable on either technological or economic grounds, a limit may be set to restrict the risks to health to some societal acceptable level.

In the European Union, health-based limits are derived by the Scientific Committee on Occupational Exposure Limits (SCOEL).[5] These limits are then implemented in each country within the EU by national legislation. Outside the EU, most countries have their own regulatory systems, although limits from different countries are often broadly comparable. A key influence on limits worldwide is the list from the American Conference of Governmental Industrial Hygienists (ACGIH). These limits, which are known as Threshold Limit Values (TLVs), were first published in the 1940s and now provide guidance on exposure levels for about 650 substances (www.acgih.org/TLV).

In the United Kingdom, the OELs are known as workplace exposure limits (WELs) and they are given legal force through the COSHH regulations. There are WELs for a few hundred of the most common chemicals used at work, which incorporates the limit values that have been agreed by the European Commission following the recommendations of the SCOEL; details are available from the HSEs website (www.HSE.gov.uk/COSHH).

OELs are straightforward to understand and make for easy management of the risks from chemicals in the workplace. However, they do not explicitly consider exposure by routes other than inhalation and they do not take account of some of the individual factors that may influence risk, e.g. genetic determinants of risk or the person's work rate and its effect on the quantity of chemical inhaled. However, despite this, they are the internationally accepted way of judging whether occupational chemical exposure is acceptable.

HOLISTIC EXPOSURE ASSESSMENT

Those involved in occupational health commonly make the mistake that the worker's exposure to chemicals stops at the factory gate or when they leave their place of work. There are several reasons why this is commonly not the case. First, there is the concept of take-home exposure where contaminated overalls or clothing is transported back to the home, where exposure continues and indeed other family members inhale or ingest the contamination within the apparent safety of their own home. Recent cases involving the spouses and children of shipbuilders and others who worked with asbestos have highlighted the potential for this take-home exposure to produce long-term health effects in those who were never directly occupationally exposed. In addition to asbestos, it is possible that other chemicals and workplace hazards, such as metals, pesticides, flour dust and animal allergens, may be transported from work to home by clothing and tools.

The worker's skills may also be in demand within the community and so they may receive additional, perhaps less well-controlled exposure to the chemical when they perform their task by doing 'homers' or self-employed work during evenings and weekends. Industrial painters are a common example of this, often working their normal workshift for their employer and then doing additional evening work for family and friends to earn extra income. It is important that the physician enquires about second jobs, home working or even hobby exposures. Farm workers exposed to pesticides during their employment may also have gardens and pick up additional exposure spraying plants with pesticides as part of their hobby, while painters exposed to solvents at work may inhale high levels of solvent maintaining an old sports car in their poorly ventilated house garage.

Dietary intake of chemicals also requires consideration and it is at this point that occupational and environmental medicine begin to overlap. For example, biological monitoring to assess off-shore workers' mercury exposure may be a poor way of identifying work exposure if the same workers have a high dietary consumption of shellfish that are known to contain mercury. Similarly, farm workers who live in rural areas may actually have greater intakes of pesticide chemicals from contaminated drinking water sources than from any direct occupational exposure. Lead piping in old domestic buildings can produce high lead intake during periods at home compared to those experienced in a well-controlled workplace.

Non-work exposure can extend beyond chemicals. Noise exposure within the home life can be important. Listening to loud music with personal head- or earphones or taking part in noisy hobbies, like shooting, can lead to noise-induced hearing loss that is additional to that produced in the workplace. Dermatitis is another 'occupational' disease that can become established or exacerbated as a result of home life exposure to chemicals and even exposure to wet tasks, including dish washing, DIY and childcare. The importance of performing a holistic assessment of the worker and their work, home and leisure environments should not be underestimated. One of the challenges for those involved in occupational medicine is to look beyond the workplace, extend the reach of their skills and to consider how the wider environment may be affecting the patient.

CONTROL OF EXPOSURE TO HAZARDOUS SUBSTANCES

Where exposures have been identified as being poorly controlled, then intervention in the workplace is called for. An occupational hygienist may be the first port of call in order to discuss the control hierarchy for the particular industry or task. Elimination of the hazard or substitution with less hazardous material may be an easy step to removing the cause of the disease. Technology moves on and newer materials or working methods may be appropriate, but the changes never implemented because of workplace inertia. Cases of illness or disease may be the prompt the company requires to review purchasing policy or consider investing in new plant that eliminates the need for a particular chemical. Engineering controls, containment and local exhaust ventilation (LEV) are the next possible steps in controlling exposure. Intervention may simply be needed to examine the maintenance and performance of existing control measures, perhaps a fan in an extraction system has stopped working or a splashguard is no longer in place causing high dermal exposure to a fluid. LEV systems are extensively used to control exposure by extracting contaminated air from close to the source before it can mix into the workroom where workers may be exposed.

Raising worker awareness through the provision of information, instruction and training is another important intervention. Making sure that workers have knowledge of the risks to their health and what steps they can take to minimize their exposure and risk can be very powerful. Other 'software' intervention methods include introducing job rotation to limit the duration of exposure to the hazard, and biofeedback-type strategies where the worker is given much more detail about the determinants of their own exposure. Visualization and real-time exposure monitoring is one such example where workers receive instant feedback about their individual dermal or inhalation exposure during particular tasks and methods of working. It can be a particularly useful educational tool in modifying workers' behaviours when handling highly toxic or hazardous materials.

Personal protective equipment (PPE) should be the intervention of last resort and should generally only be used when other control options are not possible or have failed to reduce exposures to acceptable levels.[6] Respiratory protection is widely used to reduce the risk from inhaling hazardous substances. These devices are of two basic types: breathing apparatus where the wearer is provided with clean fresh air from a cylinder worn by the individual or through a pipe connected to a source of fresh air, and respirators, where the contaminant is removed from the air by means of a filter. Both types of respiratory protection rely on a facepiece to connect the device to the wearer, either a half-facepiece covering the nose and mouth or a full-facepiece covering the whole of the front of the face. Figure 4.5 shows a selection of respirators.

PPE carries particular problems as a means of controlling exposure. For a start, PPE only protects the wearer and

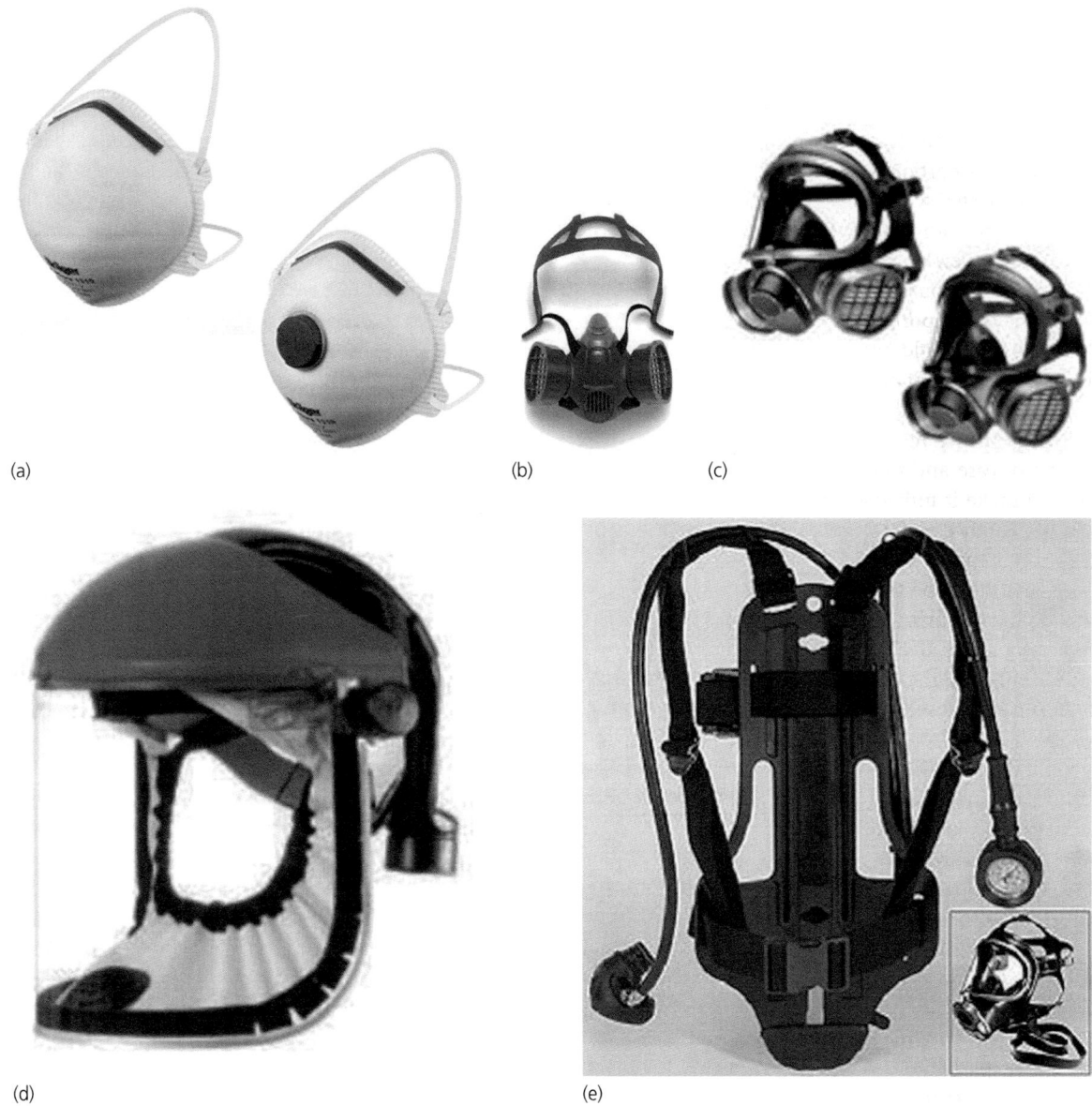

Figure 4.5 Respirators used in the workplace. (a) Disposable half-mask; (b) reusable half-mask; (c) reusable full-face masks; (d) air-fed visor; (e) breathing apparatus. Reproduced with permission from Draeger Safety UK Ltd.

not those other workers in the vicinity who do not have access to, or have decided not to wear, the same level of protection. Second, it only protects the worker while it is being worn and worn correctly. Workers will remove masks during breaks or to hold conversations and during these times no protection is afforded. Then there is the problem of proper fitting – respiratory protective equipment is typically of one size and takes little account of different face shapes and sizes to ensure a good seal between the mask and skin. Proper fit-testing of respiratory protection is extremely important if PPE is part of the workplace intervention programme. Finally, there is evidence that wearing PPE can encourage less careful working practices that actually increase exposures.

A final approach may be to remove the worker from the exposure by changing their work tasks or even recommending that they change job. The worker themselves may initiate this change once they identify the cause of their ill health. This option should be considered carefully and only when other appropriate measures in the control hierarchy have been reviewed. Simply removing the worker from the causative agent without first attempting to intervene will leave conditions unchanged and the other remaining workers exposed to the same conditions that produced the illness in the sentinel patient. In the same way that this would be deemed an unacceptable strategy for handling an outbreak of infectious disease, it should not be the primary mechanism for dealing with worker ill health.

ATTRIBUTION OF A DISEASE TO AN EXPOSURE

As discussed, there are a number of reasons why it may be necessary to attempt to attribute a causal exposure to a disease suffered by a particular individual. A high degree of confidence is needed where, for example, the person may be seeking compensation for disablement from an industrial disease or a view on causation may be needed as part of civil or criminal court proceedings. However, at a simpler level it may be important to understand whether occupational exposures could have caused a disease to assist in the clinical management of the individual.

In all cases, the attribution should be based on the person being exposed to a hazard that is accepted to cause the specific disease and that the magnitude of the risk is sufficient to make it unlikely that the disease would have arisen in the absence of the exposure. For some diseases, it is almost certain that a single agent causes the disease, e.g. mesothelioma and asbestos, although it may be less clear whether exposure during a single period of employment was solely responsible. In other cases, there may be numerous risk factors linked to the disease, none of which are necessary or sufficient causes, e.g. lung cancer where cigarette smoking and several occupational and non-occupational exposures increase risk. Despite these uncertainties, it is certain that exposure must precede onset of the disease for it to be potentially causal.

Causation in individual cases where there are multiple risk factors is generally accepted if the relative risk associated with the exposure is greater than two, which corresponds to more than half of the cases of the disease occurring in a population exposed similarly to the case being due to the exposure. This is a stringent test of causation, which relies on good information about the hazard and risks in the particular circumstances being considered.

The following list sets out a general strategy that can be followed to attempt to identify whether exposure of the case in one or more jobs is likely to have caused their disease. It is followed by three short case studies illustrating the approach.

1. Conduct a literature review to identify exposures that are known to be associated with the disease, including the likely time frame, i.e. whether exposures would be expected to be close to onset of symptoms or diagnosis (acute = days, months) or more distant (chronic = years, decades).
2. Obtain a careful occupational history from the case, taking particular care to identify relevant jobs and exposures held by the individual. As part of the work history, obtain good descriptions of the source of the hazardous substance, how the worker interacts with the source, the local controls in use, the work environment (i.e. size of the room and general ventilation), the time spent in the area by the worker, the use of personal protective equipment, such as respirators or protective gloves, and any accidental conditions that have arisen in the past. Enquire about other cases of similar disease among co-workers.
3. If possible, visit the workplace to collect more detailed information about the exposures and the circumstances where they arise.
4. Estimate exposures using any available monitoring data from the worksite, any data published in the scientific literature relating to that industry, the output from a suitable software tool such as Stoffenmanager, or from an actual simulation of the work activity in a controlled environment.
5. Identify relevant epidemiological literature that might shed light on typical relative risks for the disease and exposures in question, particularly studies where the magnitude of the exposures were similar to the case.
6. Decide whether it is possible/likely that exposure was implicated in causation, based on the exposure and the likely risk.

The following examples are intended to illustrate how this approach could be applied in practice.

Case 1: Asbestos

Mr A, a life-long non-smoker, was diagnosed with lung cancer in 2001. He had worked as a miner constructing tunnels for metro systems and roads. Between 1960 and 1978, he worked alongside a team of men who were using a caulking rope containing amosite (brown) and/or chrysotile (white) asbestos along with a cement binder. The caulking was placed between the concrete tunnel lining sections and compressed into place using a pneumatic tool. Mr A always worked at least 2–3 metres from those performing this task.

Both amosite and chrysotile are known to cause lung cancer. Mr A's diagnosis was 40 years after he was first exposed, which is again consistent with this asbestos exposure contributing to his risk. It is generally accepted that a cumulative exposure of more than 25 fibres/mL $\times$ years is associated with a more than doubling of risk for lung cancer.

The tunnels where Mr A worked were of a fairly large diameter and there tended to be some forced ventilation to provide fresh air to the workers. The caulking was not continuous, but took place about 10 per cent of the time. Up to 1970, amosite asbestos was used in the caulking rope, but for the last eight years chrysotile asbestos was used in the caulking and when it was used he wore a half-face respirator. Asbestos was no longer used in this type of work after about 1989.

The UK Health and Safety Executive have published guidance on the levels of asbestos fibres in air for a number of different work activities, although not for caulking. The nearest analogous work is machine-cutting asbestos cement boards – producing concentrations of 10 to 20 fibres/mL

Table 4.1 Mr A's estimated average exposure to asbestos from caulking.

Dates	Fibre level (fibres/mL)	Fraction time exposed	Dilution to far-field	Respiratory protection	Estimated cumulative exposure (fibre/mL × years)
1960–70	100	0.1	0.33	1	33
1970–78	15	0.1	0.33	0.1	0.05

for chrysotile. Data from work on naval shops in the late 1960s showed that men working with amosite asbestos ropes could be exposed to between 5 and 340 fibres/mL (average 100 fibres/mL). There is good evidence from other sources to substantiate that amosite products were dustier than those containing chrysotile.

Mr A's exposure was likely to have been lower than the men working with the caulking because he generally worked 2–3 metres from the task and it can thus be estimated that his personal exposure would have been about a third of their exposure. Also, the respirator would have reduced his exposure by approximately 90 per cent. Based on these assumptions, his exposure can then be estimated as shown in Table 4.1.

The majority of his exposure occurred before 1970 and there was probably sufficient cumulative exposure (33 fibres/mL × years) to more than double his risk of lung cancer, so it is reasonable to attribute his cancer to his asbestos exposure. It is generally assumed that there must be at least a ten-year gap between first exposure to asbestos and there being a risk of disease, i.e. a ten-year latency period, and this was the case for Mr A. Given that he was a non-smoker and there are no other identifiable risk factors, it seems probable that his disease was caused by his asbestos exposure.

Case 2: Organophosphates

Mr P was born in 1940 and left school at the age of 14 to work as an under-shepherd at a hill farm in the Scottish borders. In 1960, he became head shepherd and he continued in this job until 1970 when he left farming. Throughout his employment, Mr P was required to treat sheep with pesticides to prevent scab and other conditions. This was done by immersing sheep in a pool of dilute organophosphate pesticide, a process known as 'dipping' and took place four times each year during June, August, October and November. Between 2000 and 3000 sheep were dipped every year. Mr P has been diagnosed with Parkinson's disease and it has been suggested that his exposure to organophosphate compounds while dipping sheep could have caused his disease.

Mr P used a large 2000-litre dip tank. Sheep were pushed into the tank and then submerged using a T-shaped pole. He wore waterproof leggings, an oilskin jacket – which he wore back-to-front for added protection – Wellington boots and rubber gloves. He did not wear a respirator and during the summer dip the jacket was not worn because of problems with the heat. Also, Mr P was provided with one set of protective clothing each year and he reported that after a few weeks of use it was no longer completely water resistant. Occasionally, he fell into the full dip tank while dipping. Mr P also prepared the solution used in dipping by diluting concentrate organophosphate-based products. At the end of the dipping, Mr P had to clean and drain the tank.

The work involved potential dermal exposure to the concentrated and dilute dip (from direct contact and splashes), but there was little opportunity for inhalation exposure (these dips are of low volatility and there is little opportunity for a fine aerosol to form). The main focus of the exposure assessment is therefore on skin exposure. Ingestion exposure during accidental immersions of Mr P may also have contributed significantly to his overall dose, but this is difficult to quantify.

There are a number of epidemiological studies that have supported the hypothesis that pesticide exposure may increase risk of Parkinson's disease. However, the studies do not present a consistent picture and they do not provide evidence on specific compounds or even classes of compounds, such as organophosphates. In 2008, the UK Industrial Injuries Advisory Council (IIAC) examined the case for prescribing pesticide exposure and Parkinson's disease for state compensation and concluded that the evidence base was not sufficiently strong, i.e. the existing epidemiological studies do not consistently support a doubling of risk. Despite this, it is important to understand whether this man's exposure could have been implicated in causing his disease.

There are no universally accepted ways of estimating exposure to chemicals on the skin and very few measurements of dermal exposure from such situations. The most appropriate method of assessing skin exposure combines the concentration of the chemical on the skin, the area of skin exposed and the duration of exposure. This measure should be related to the amount of chemical taken up into the body through the skin.[7] Tahmaz et al.[8] developed an exposure model based on this approach for sheep dipping to assist in a study of farmers with chronic fatigue. They defined the skin exposure (E_{sk}) as the product of the concentration of the active compound (organophosphate) on the skin (C_{sk}), the duration that the skin is contaminated (t_{sk}) and the area of skin contaminated (S_{sk}). In mathematical form, this is:

$$E_{sk} = C_{sk} \times t_{sk} \times S_{sk}$$

Table 4.2 Mr P's estimated exposure to organophosphates.

Circumstances	Estimated exposure ($m^2 \times$ days)
Mr P	1400
For people with high chronic fatigue scores[8]	490–1000
People with low chronic fatigue scores[8]	30–670

The measurement units for this assessment are $m^2 \times$ days, i.e. area multiplied by the duration (concentration being dimensionless, i.e. without measurement units). For example, $100\,m^2 \times$ days skin exposure could be the result of 1000 days of exposure where $0.1\,m^2$ of skin was exposed to concentrated pesticide ($C_{sk} = 1$).

To ensure that the estimate of exposure is representative of different areas of skin that may become contaminated and the pattern of exposure, the exposure estimate was further subdivided by Tahmaz et al. into skin exposure to dilute pesticide during dipping sheep ($E_{sk,dip}$), exposure to concentrate while preparing the dilute dip ($E_{sk,conc}$), exposure while handling sheep ($E_{sk,handling}$), inhalation exposure during dipping ($E_{inhalation}$) and skin exposure on occasions where the person accidentally fell into the dipping bath ($E_{sk,falls}$). Mathematically, this is expressed as:

$$E_{sk} = E_{sk,dip} + E_{sk,conc} + E_{sk,handling} + E_{inhalation} + E_{sk,falls}$$

Each of the above terms is further elaborated in the Tahmaz et al. approach to take account of the use of protective clothing and other factors that influence the exposure. The estimated exposure can then be calculated using a computer spreadsheet.

The results from the calculation of Mr P's exposure are shown in Table 4.2, along with the range of lifetime exposures from Tahmaz et al. for 95 per cent of the farmers in that study – subdivided by whether or not they scored highly in terms of the questionnaire on chronic fatigue.

Mr P's estimated lifetime exposure was above the 95th percentile of farmers who had high chronic fatigue scores. Note that the highest estimated exposure from Tahmaz et al. was about $8500\,m^2 \times$ days.

Despite Mr P having very high exposure to organophosphate compounds during sheep dipping, it is not possible, given the current state of scientific evidence, to clearly attribute his exposure to his disease. However, it would seem prudent to advise him to avoid further exposure to organophosphate compounds at work or in other situations, such as home gardening.

Case 3: Isocyanates

Mrs I, who works in a factory making various adhesives, sealants and coatings, was diagnosed with asthma. This woman was employed on a process making a photo polymer resin product, in a fully enclosed process. One of the main raw ingredients in the process was toluene diisocyanate (TDI). During the TDI loading task, the operator wore a full-face filtering respirator, fitted with a combination gas and dust filter (note these are not recommended for use with TDI and would not provide reliable protection). She also wore cotton overalls and natural rubber (latex) gauntlets. A rubber apron was available, but was not worn. Self-contained breathing apparatus (BA) was provided for use in emergency situations and one BA set was located in the main process control room and a second set was located outside the building. The majority of Mrs I's work time was spent in the air-conditioned control room.

The company regularly undertook air monitoring for isocyanate (NCO) using the method recommended by the Health and Safety Executive (MDHS 25/3 Organic isocyanates in air). Samples were obtained using IOM sampling heads loaded with chemically impregnated glass fibre filters, treated with 1-(2-methyoxyphenyl) piperazine (1-2MP) solution. The sampling head was attached to the lapel of the operator and connected to a battery-operated personal sampling pump drawing air at 2 L/min through the filter. The samples were analysed for total isocyanate content using high performance liquid chromatography.

None of their measurements showed detectable isocyanate exposure for Mrs I, all the measurements being $<0.001\,mg/m^3$ as total NCO (the long-term occupational exposure limit is $0.02\,mg/m^3$). The only detectable isocyanate levels have been obtained for quality assurance technicians who have to extract a sample of resin for testing (maximum reading $0.004\,mg/m^3$).

An interview with Mrs I indicated that in the months before she first started to experience symptoms there had been a series of maintenance issues on the plant and that two pumps in the process had been replaced because they were leaking. No measurements of airborne isocyanate level had been made during this time, but it seems plausible that there was episodic peak exposure to TDI vapour during this time. The exposure of the quality control technician arises from a short period when the containment of the process is breached, typically 20 minutes each day. If it was assumed that the leak was continuous and that the room ventilation was sufficient to provide ten air-changes per hour then a simple calculation suggests that an eight-hour average exposure level of $0.004\,mg/m^3$ could be associated with peak exposure of about $0.1\,mg/m^3$ during the short period of sampling. Using the exposure modelling software package IH-Mod (which is freely available at: www.aiha.org/insideaiha/volunteergroups/Documents/EASCIHMOD.xls), the exposure over a full shift can be calculated. As can be seen from Figure 4.6, the concentration with a continuous leak similar to that during quality control sampling gives rise to a level of $0.2\,mg/m^3$.

There are no good exposure–response epidemiological studies for asthma associated with TDI exposure, but there is evidence that a significant proportion of exposed

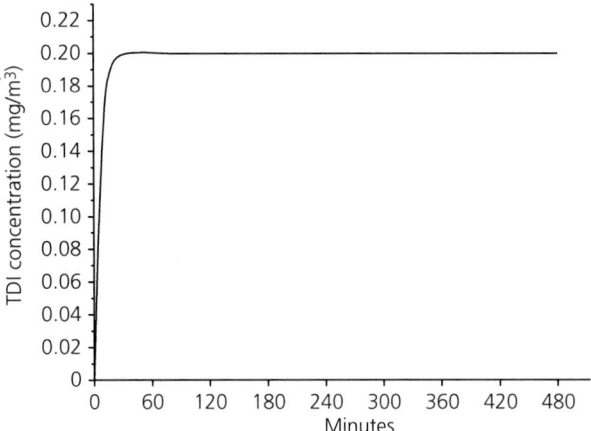

Figure 4.6 Modelled exposure to TDI from a continuous leak.

individuals may become sensitized to TDI at exposure levels above about 0.1 mg/m^3 and so it is possible that Mrs I's exposure during this time could have caused her asthma. However, confirmation of causation could be obtained from an inhalation challenge test (see Chapter 72, Occupational asthma, p. 941).

CONCLUSIONS

Understanding the relationship between disease and occupational exposure is important for the treatment and well-being of the patient. The occupational hygiene framework of identifying hazards and evaluating the risk from those hazards provides a simple method when approaching complex problems concerning attribution. There are often many sources of information available on hazards in the workplace including safety data sheets, COSHH assessments and online guidance on how specific chemicals should be handled. All of these provide the physician with the means of hazard recognition.

Discussion with the patient and the taking of a detailed occupational history are also key to identifying hazards and, often, gathering important data on likely exposure levels that can then be compared to health-based limits. Discussion can also be useful from the perspective of providing reassurance and allaying fears that specific exposures can have had an effect on health.

In some cases, the attribution of disease is not always straightforward. Some exposure–response relationships lack good quality or consistent epidemiological data on risk, indeed only a small number of substances have been classified by the Industrial Injuries Advisory Council.

While identifying the cause of a worker's disease can be useful in targeting the treatment of symptoms or improving the patient's quality of life, the real benefits of linking exposure to ill health are reaped from occupational health interventions to reduce the exposure. For most diseases, treatment of symptoms will not provide long-term help if the underlying causative exposure continues and therefore following a framework for intervention is important. For the physician who identifies illness caused by work, intervention in the workplace should also be considered as a vital public health measure. Poor working practices and high exposures will continue to cause ill health in other workers and for this reason it is necessary to remember that treating the workplace is as important as treating the worker.

Key points

- Inhalation exposure to hazardous substances is measured as the concentration in the air close to the worker's head (i.e. within 30 cm).
- Dermal exposure is often measured as the mass of chemical on the skin or the mass that impinges on to the skin during a given period of time, although the concentration on the skin would be a more appropriate measure.
- Mathematical models to estimate worker exposure are becoming more widely accepted.
- Exposure varies considerably from one person to another performing the same job and from day to day for the same worker and, as a consequence, several measurements of exposure are needed to get a reliable assessment.
- Inhalation exposure should always be controlled to an appropriate level using local ventilation or some other intervention, and should be below any relevant occupational exposure limit (OEL).
- Personal protective equipment (PPE), such as a respirator, must be carefully selected to ensure it is appropriate and comfortable for the wearer.

REFERENCES

1. International Programme on Chemical Safety. *IPCS risk assessment terminology.* Geneva: World Health Organization, 2004.
2. Schneider T, Vermeulen R, Brouwer DH *et al.* Conceptual model for assessment of dermal exposure. *Occupational and Environmental Medicine.* 1999; **56**: 765–73.
3. Health and Safety Executive. Methods for the determination of hazardous substances. 14/3 General methods for sampling and gravimetric analysis of respirable and inhalable dust. Sudbury: HSE, 2000.
4. Ogden TL. Proposed British–Dutch guidance on measuring compliance with occupational exposure limits. *Annals of Occupational Hygiene.* 2009; **53**: 775–7.
5. European Commission. Employment, Social Affairs and Equal Opportunities. Scientific Committee on Occupational Exposure Limits (SCOEL). Available from: http://ec.europa.eu/social/main.jsp?catId=153&langId=en&intPageId=684.

6. Health and Safety Executive. *Respiratory protective equipment at work. A practical guide.* Sudbury: HSE Books, 2005.
7. Cherrie JW, Robertson A. Biologically relevant assessment of dermal exposure. *Annals of Occupational Hygiene.* 1995; **39**: 387–92.
8. Tahmaz N, Soutar A, Cherrie JW. Chronic fatigue and organophosphate pesticides in sheep farming: A retrospective study amongst people reporting to a UK pharmacovigilance scheme. *Annals of Occupational Hygiene.* 2003; **47**: 261–7.

FURTHER READING

Cherrie JW, Howie RM, Semple S. *Monitoring for health hazards at work*, 4th edn. Chichester: John Wiley & Sons, 2010.

Gardiner K, Harrington JM. *Occupational hygiene*, 3rd edn. Oxford: Blackwell Publishing, 2005.

Kromhout H, Symanski E, Rappaport SM. A comprehensive evaluation of within- and between-worker components of occupational exposure to chemicals. *Annals of Occupational Hygiene.* 1993; **37**: 253–70.

Nieuwenhuijsen M. *Exposure assessment in occupational and environmental epidemiology.* Oxford: Oxford University Press, 2003.

Ramachandran G. Toward better exposure assessment strategies – the new NIOSH initiative. *Annals of Occupational Hygiene.* 2008; **52**: 297–301.

Seixas NS, Checkoway H. Exposure assessment in industry specific retrospective occupational epidemiology studies. *Occupational and Environmental Medicine.* 1995; **52**: 625–33.

5

Biological monitoring

JOHN COCKER AND HOWARD J MASON

Introduction	56	Biological effect monitoring	63
Biological monitoring	57	Conclusions	70
Setting up a biological monitoring programme	58	References	70

INTRODUCTION

Biological monitoring (BM) is based on the analysis of hazardous substances or their metabolites in biological fluids, usually urine, blood or breath. BM is a tool to assess systemic exposure and reflects absorption by all routes, inhalation, ingestion and through the skin. Often, the term 'biological monitoring' is also used to include biological effect monitoring (BEM), which reflects the early consequences of systemic exposure, although others have also used the term 'biomonitoring' to encompass BM and BEM.[1] Both BM and BEM are located on a spectrum ranging from low exposure at one end to disease, frank toxicity or death at the other (Figure 5.1). It is preferable to keep the term 'biological monitoring' for assessment of exposure separate from 'biological effect monitoring' which is an indicator of early effect and sits within 'health surveillance'. Health surveillance is the periodic clinical examination of workers designed to protect their health through the early detection of adverse effects and intervention to prevent further harm, and complements biological monitoring.

This chapter will first discuss the role and practical application of biological monitoring in the workplace, followed by an overview of the current status of biological effect monitoring.

Workers may be exposed to hazards in the workplace in the air they breathe or from contaminated surfaces and equipment. In some cases, workplace exposure can be in addition to a non-occupational hazard in the environment. Hazardous substances may enter the body via inhalation, ingestion or through the skin and the consequences largely depend on the amount absorbed and rate of absorption. Control of exposure in the workplace should prevent levels of exposure that lead to harm and monitoring techniques which provide the feedback to ensure the controls are working and being used correctly. Clearly, early detection and control of exposure is more desirable than diagnosing occupational disease after it is fully established. The objective of health professionals is to

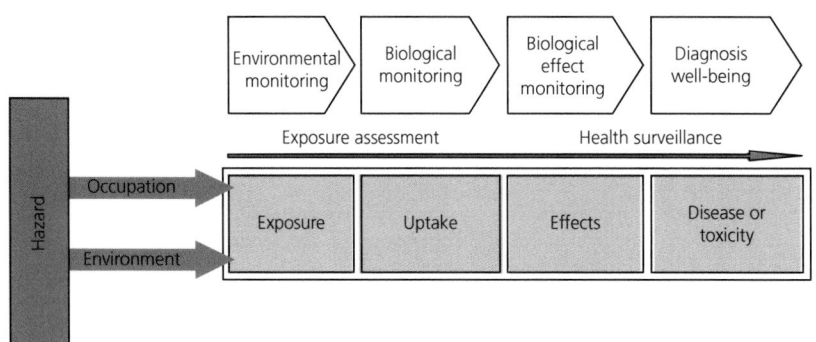

Figure 5.1 The exposure-disease paradigm.

keep systemic exposure as low as is reasonably practical and to the left of the spectrum in Figure 5.1.

Monitoring techniques can be divided into those that assess exposure and those that assess the consequences of exposure. Thus, BM relates to exposure assessment and BEM is usually part of effects assessment, and can help in the diagnosis of disease. The distinction is important because the motivation for doing the monitoring influences the way results are interpreted. A physician in the workplace may initiate BM as part of health surveillance, but the results can often only be interpreted in terms of exposure and not (directly) health. There are international differences regarding the role of BM, e.g. between Europe and the United States, with BM historically performed as a medical activity in European countries, while in the United States and now in the United Kingdom, BM also belongs within the specialism of occupational hygiene.

Biological monitoring guidance values are produced by various organizations to aid the interpretation of results, but the majority of guidance values relate to exposure assessment with the aim of controlling occupational exposure at levels below those causing noticeable health effects. In contrast, there are comparatively few biological effect guidance values.

A recent development, under the auspices of the European Centre of Ecotoxicology and Toxicology of Chemicals, has been the development of a framework for the interpretation of BM data through evaluation of their analytical integrity, their ability to describe dose (toxicokinetics), their ability to relate to effects, and an overall evaluation and weight of evidence analysis.[1] This framework may provide a rational basis to allow better use of current biomarkers and the development of novel, interpretable BM and BEM markers.

BIOLOGICAL MONITORING

Roles

Unlike air or surface monitoring which assess potential exposure, biological monitoring can help to assess actual systemic exposure, from all routes. BM is particularly useful where air monitoring alone will not give a complete picture of exposure. These roles include monitoring substances where the dermal route can contribute significantly to systemic toxicity such as those with 'Sk' or 'skin' notations in tables of exposure limits. Biological monitoring also has a role where the control of an inhalation hazard relies on personal respiratory protective equipment. In such situations, it is not very helpful to measure the ambient air levels of the substance and often difficult to measure the effectiveness of the respirators in use. A third role for biological monitoring is the overall assessment of exposure controls, including worker behaviour. The best exposure controls may not protect the worker if they are not used correctly. The individual nature of biological samples collected from workers can help provide a personal message and influence worker behaviour or give reassurance.

Legal framework

In most countries, there is a legal requirement for health surveillance of workers who may be significantly exposed to lead. In the UK, the Control of Lead at Work (CLAW 2002) regulations requires the regular monitoring of workers exposed to lead. This involves both clinical examination by an appointed physician and analysis of blood samples for lead with defined action levels based on the results. Some countries have compulsory biological monitoring for a few other substances, but the legal framework for BM usually comes under the regulations to control hazardous substances in the workplace, and biological monitoring is not compulsory.

In the UK, biological monitoring has roles under the Control of Substances Hazardous to Health (COSHH) and in particular regulation 10 (Exposure Assessment), regulation 11 (Health Surveillance) and regulations 6 and 7 (Assessing and Controlling Exposure/Risks). In the case of health surveillance, it is used when it is possible to link the results of biological monitoring to an adverse health effect. Implicit in this requirement is that a 'no-adverse effect level' has been established. However, often there is insufficient data available to do this and there are many substances in the workplace where it is not possible (e.g. carcinogens and allergens), and then the prudent approach is to try to minimize exposure to as low as possible.

In the absence of a recognized 'no-adverse effect' level for a chemical, an alternative, pragmatic approach is to establish an appropriate level based on the levels (usually the 90th percentile) seen in workplaces with good control of exposure. This approach does not require knowledge of a dose–response relationship or yield a health-based value. Instead, it allows exposure to be monitored, controlled and reduced to minimize risk of ill health, and any reduction of exposure is then reflected in reduced health risk. This approach is in line with the current approach to controlling exposure based on good occupational hygiene practice and is comparatively easy to establish. Thus, although BM is not compulsory, its simplicity and utility mean that it is increasingly being used and incorporated into codes of practice and in-house guidance for working with and controlling exposure to chemicals.

Ethics

Since BM involves the collection and analysis of biological samples from people, it is essential that the rights of the individual are protected. These rights can be protected by obtaining informed consent to collect and analyse the samples, and gaining their permission regarding who will see the results and understanding what action will be taken on the results. The programme should be discussed and agreed with all concerned, employees, employers and worker representatives. In the UK, with the exception of lead, BM is not compulsory, and workers need reassurance that their participation or non-participation will not affect their conditions of employment. To get their informed consent to participate, the purpose of the BM programme must be explained along with the type of biological samples that will be collected, and any associated risks. Workers need to be made aware of what will be analysed in the samples and reassured that no other tests (e.g. alcohol, drugs, HIV) will be performed. They need to know what action might follow depending on the BM results and what the benefits (if any) are to them as individuals. Workers should be informed that the results will be treated as personal data, treated as confidential and only revealed as grouped data without identifiers, and/or to others with specific consent, e.g. to health professionals or managers. Within the UK, the Information Commissioner has also produced guidance that relate to such issues.[2]

The programme must be supervised by a competent person, often (but not exclusively) an occupational health professional. In our experience, these arrangements do not pose any particular problems and a well-designed and executed biological monitoring programme can be an effective way of protecting workers' health.

SETTING UP A BIOLOGICAL MONITORING PROGRAMME

Guidance is available to aid setting up biological monitoring programmes for a wide range of substances and covers the basics of the ethical issues, consultation, choice of analyte, sample collection, analysis and guidance on interpreting results.[3] The main steps include:

- Define the purpose of the programme as exposure assessment or part of health surveillance.
- Appoint a competent person to oversee the programme. If the programme is for health surveillance, a health professional should be appointed.
- Select a biological monitoring strategy (who to monitor, how often, what samples to collect, when to collect them, methods to analyse them, availability of guidance for results). A competent laboratory should be employed and can help with developing the strategy. The laboratory should run appropriate internal quality control schemes and participate, if available for the analyte in question, in external quality assurance schemes.
- Consult on the programme with employees and their representatives.
- Discuss and agree the programme with the individuals concerned.
- Establish procedures for sample collection, storage, transport, analysis and quality assurance.
- Provide feedback and interpretation of the results.
- Take appropriate action on results, if required.

For many of the most common substances in the workplace, there is guidance available on the technical aspects of biological monitoring. The UK Health and Safety Executive (HSE), the American Conference of Governmental Industrial Hygienists (ACGIH) and the German Deutsche Forschungsgemeinschaft (DFG) all produce guidance documents that detail the type of sample, when to collect it, the substance to be analysed and a guidance value to aid in interpreting the results.[4-6]

Sample collection

The collection of non-invasive samples (e.g. urine, breath, saliva) is preferred, provided a validated method is available. Non-invasive samples are more acceptable to workers compared to collecting blood samples. Non-invasive sampling also reduces the risks from venepuncture and disposal of blood-contaminated material. Appropriate precautions should be taken when collecting and handling biological samples and particular attention should be taken with regulations for sending pathological samples through the post or by courier. Within the United Kingdom, appropriately packaged and labelled samples may be sent by first class post or special delivery, and the Royal Mail offers a prepaid packaging system for diagnostic biological samples. Where samples need to be sent internationally, courier rather than postal service must be used and International Air Transport Association (IATA) regulations followed, sending BM samples assigned to UN3373 or as 'exempt human specimen'.[7] In essence, sending BM samples within the UK or internationally as 'exempt human specimens', should involve primary and secondary leak-proof packaging, the latter of appropriate strength, with enough absorbent material between the packaging to absorb the entire contents and also appropriately labelled, including a return address. Any laboratory involved in BM will be able to advise on ensuring compliance with postal and transportation regulations.

Most biological monitoring is based on collection of urine samples. If the analyte is the substance to which the workers are exposed, e.g. metals, care should be taken to avoid contamination of the sample during collection. If the analytes are volatile, e.g. most solvents, care needs to be taken to avoid loss of analyte, usually by supplying a urine sample where there is little headspace remaining in the sample bottle. Most BM analytes are stable enough that refrigeration is not necessary during their transport by first class post to the laboratory.

When to sample

The optimum time for sample collection is determined by the toxicokinetics of the substance and depends mainly on the half-life of elimination. This toxicokinetic parameter also largely defines the relationship between a BM measurement and the period of exposure that it reflects.[8] Ideal sampling times are often compromised by the practicalities of sample collection in the workplace that usually dictates samples are to be collected at the 'end-of-exposure', 'end-of-shift' or prior to the start of the next shift. The route of exposure (inhalation or dermal absorption) may also have an impact on sample collection times. The apparent half-life of an inhaled substance will generally differ from the same substance if dermally absorbed, where it is subjected to a lag phase due to transit across the stratum corneum with the skin acting as a reservoir for the substance. Table 5.1 gives a generalized relationship between elimination half-life, sampling time and exposure reflected in the BM sample taken at the sampling time.

Interfering factors

Biological monitoring results can be influenced by interfering factors. These may include additional exposure through a non-occupational route, by exposure to a chemical that is also metabolized to the BM analyte being monitored, and also by altering the metabolism of the BM analyte of interest.

Sometimes, the collection of additional information by questionnaire or analysis is necessary. For example, consumption of seafood may increase total urinary mercury and total arsenic levels, but more complex analysis of the species contributing to total urinary arsenic can help attribute exposure to occupational and dietary sources.[9] Where a biomarker is derived from external exposure and also endogenously, it may be advisable to collect pre-exposure or baseline samples. Smoking can contribute to a wide range of biomarkers, including thiocyanate used to monitor exposure to cyanide and napthols.[10] Consideration should also be given to the possibility that the chosen biomarker may also be a metabolite of another substance, e.g. mandelic acid is a widely used BM metabolite of styrene, but is also formed from ethyl benzene, while carboxyhaemoglobin is formed from both carbon monoxide and dichloromethane. Alcohol and some drugs can compete for metabolism of many solvents, tending to extend their half-life of excretion. However, chronic intake of alcohol and some drugs can also induce enzymes potentially involved in metabolism of some solvents and chemicals, again altering the normal relationship between BM measurement and exposure.

Physiological factors, such as work rate, can also influence BM results for some substances where increased respiration leads to increased absorption and consequently increase systemic dose, e.g. someone exposed to xylene working moderately hard will have two to three times the respiration rate and urinary metabolite levels compared to a worker at rest with the same airborne xylene levels.

Choice of analyte

The choice of analyte will depend on the purpose of the monitoring. If the level of exposure is being assessed, then

Table 5.1 Relationship between elimination half-lives, the practical time of sampling for a biological monitoring strategy and the exposure duration that the sample reflects.

Elimination half-life in hours ($t_{\frac{1}{2}}$)	Sampling time	Exposure frame reflected by the biological monitoring sample
<2	End of exposure. With such short half-lives, the time between exposure and urine voiding becomes influential	Large uncertainty due to variable retention time of urine in bladder
2–10	End of exposure, end of shift	For $t_{\frac{1}{2}}$ of 2 hours, BM sample reflects a 35% contribution from exposure in the hour before sampling, the rest from exposure over shift. For $t_{\frac{1}{2}}$ of 10 hours, BM sample reflects a 70% contribution from exposure over the prior 24 hours, with smaller contribution (approximately 10%) from exposure in the last hour
10–100	End of exposure at the end of week or after several exposures	With increasing the $t_{\frac{1}{2}} = 10$ hours to $t_{\frac{1}{2}} = 100$ hours, the contributory influence of exposure during the 24 hours prior to sampling diminishes from 70 to 15% and the importance of exposure in the previous week increases from 20 to 60%
>100	Sampling time not critical	Contribution from exposure during the week prior to sampling decreases from 60% and with longer $t_{\frac{1}{2}}$ the influence of exposure over the previous month or months becomes more important

for inorganic substances such as metals, the element itself is usually measured. The choice for organic substances depends on the metabolism and kinetics of the substance and the possible interference from other endogenous sources. As an example, biological monitoring for toluene was once based on the analysis of its major metabolite hippuric acid, but as regulatory exposure limits for toluene were reduced the interference from dietary sources of hippuric acid made this approach no longer viable and monitoring switched to using the minor metabolite o-cresol or the measurement of toluene itself in urine.

Biomarkers that reflect flux in the toxic metabolic pathway are preferred over those that reflect detoxification and simple elimination. Examples include haemoglobin adducts after exposure to aromatic amines or alkylating reagents.

A relatively recent and comprehensive review of BM analytes and strategies for monitoring workplace chemical exposures is available.[11]

Analysis

Confidence in the results of laboratory analysis is essential. The laboratory should have analytical methods with sufficient sensitivity and specificity to accurately and reproducibly measure the analytes of interest. The laboratory should have internal quality assurance procedures and, where possible, take part in external quality assurance schemes.

Quality assurance begins with sample collection and the use of appropriate equipment to prevent contamination or loss of analyte. Samples must be unambiguously labelled and must be transported to the laboratory in a way that ensures the integrity of the sample. A few analytes may require preservatives or refrigeration prior to transport. Some analyses are within the scope of routine clinical laboratories but many may require a specialized laboratory. A good laboratory will provide sample collection equipment, packaging materials and guidance on sample collection, transport and interpretation of results.

A recent review has suggested that the potential availability of both sensitive analytical techniques and quality assurance schemes for BM means that interpretation of results has become the key, important issue.[12]

Creatinine correction

Urine concentrations of metabolites can vary widely not only due to variations in exposure, but also as a result of variations in fluid intake and insensible losses, such as sweating, which can alter urinary flow rate over a wide physiological range. Most biological monitoring is based on spot samples and it is common to make some adjustment to the analytical results to compensate for short-term concentration or dilution effects. The two most common types of adjustment are based on urine specific gravity or creatinine concentration, both of which largely adjust for the rate of urine production. However, the use of creatinine or other adjustment is not without ongoing debate.[13–15] Some authorities take the stance that no correction is the default position, others use creatinine correction as their default position, and there is ongoing work proving the value of such correction for an analyte on a case-by-case basis.[16,17]

Adjustment of analytical results for certain analytes (e.g. urine methanol) using either creatinine or specific gravity adjustment is not appropriate, where the chemical simply equilibrates between intra- and extracellular fluids, including urine. For other analytes, creatinine correction is not advised if the creatinine concentration is less than 3 mmol/L or more than 30 mmol/L suggesting the extremes of urine flow rate. Interpretation may be subject to considerable error, and a further sample is warranted.

Interpreting results: Guidance values

To aid the interpretation of BM data, various international organizations produce biological monitoring guidance values (Table 5.2). These are derived from review of data in the peer-reviewed literature and the objective, if possible, is to produce a health-based guidance value. However, for many substances, there is insufficient data to be able to derive a BM value linked to the absence of health effects from the dose–response relationship, and guidance values based on good occupational hygiene practice and 'achievability' are used instead.

Examples of health-based guidance values are the biological exposure indices (BEIs) of the ACGIH[5] and the biological tolerance values (BATs) from the DFG.[6] These are derived from dose–response relationships between a biological parameter and either the absence of health effects or, more usually, from a relationship between a biological parameter and an airborne exposure limit that is itself health based. For substances where a health-based dose–response relationship cannot be established, e.g. for many carcinogens and respiratory sensitizers, biological monitoring guidance values can be based on a relationship between a biological parameter and the airborne exposure limit. Examples of this type of guidance value are the DFG biological exposure equivalent values (EKA values).[6] An alternative approach is to base the biological monitoring guidance value on the levels of a biological parameter found in samples from workplaces employing good occupational hygiene practice, and examples are the HSE's published guidance values for carcinogens and suspect carcinogens like hexavalent chromium, methylene-bis-2-chloroaniline (MbOCA) and methylenedianiline.[4] HSE has also adopted this approach for

Table 5.2 Biological monitoring guidance values for common substances.

Substance	Analyte	Medium	Sampling time	BMGV[4]	BEI[5]	BV[6]	Health concern
Acetylcholinesterase inhibiting pesticides	Cholinesterase activity	Blood	Discretionary		70% of individual's baseline		Neurotoxicity
Aniline	Aniline	Urine	End of shift			1 mg/L (BAT)	Haematotoxic
Arsenic	Arsenic	Urine	End of shift at end of work week		35 µg/L	50 µg/L (BLW)	Cancer, haemolysis
Benzene	S-phenylmercapturic acid	Urine	End of shift		25 µg/g	25 µg/g (EKA)	Bone marrow, leukaemia
Butan-2-one (methyl ethyl ketone)	Butan-2-one	Urine	End of shift	70 µmol/L (~5 mg/L)	2 mg/L	5 mg/L (BAT)	Respiratory, eye irritation
2-Butoxyethanol	Butoxyacetic acid	Urine	End of shift	240 mmol/mol	200 mg/g	100 mg/L (BAT)	Haematotoxic
Cadmium	Cadmium	Urine	Not critical		5 µg/g	7 µg/L (BLW)	Nephrotoxic
Carbon disulphide	Thiothiazolidine-4-carboxylic acid	Urine	End of shift		0.5 mg/g	2 mg/g (BAT)	Neurotoxic
Carbon monoxide	Carboxyhaemoglobin	Blood	End of shift		3.5%	5% (BAT)	Hypoxia
	Breath carbon monoxide	Breath		30 ppm	20 ppm		
Chromium	Chromium	Urine	End of shift at end of week	10 µmol/mol (~5 µg/g)	25 µg/L	0.6 µg/L (BAR)	Respiratory and skin effects
Cobalt	Cobalt	Urine	End of shift at end of week		15 µg/L	15 µg/L	Respiratory and skin effects
N,N-dimethyl acetamide (DMA)	N-methyl acetamide	Urine	End of shift at end of week	100 mmol/mol	30 mg/g	30 mg/g (BAT)	Hepatotoxic
Dimethylformamide (DMF)	'Total' DMF	Urine	End of shift at end of week		15 mg/g	35 mg/g (BAT)	Hepatotoxic
Dichloromethane	Dichloromethane	Blood	End of shift		0.3 mg/L	0.5 mg/L (EKA)	Hypoxia
	Breath carbon monoxide	Breath		30 ppm	20 ppm		
Di-isocyanates	Di-isocyanate-derived diamines	Urine	End of exposure	1 µmol/mol			Respiratory and skin effects
Fluoride	Fluoride	Urine	Pre-shift		3 mg/g		Skeletal fluorosis
			End of shift		10 mg/g		
n-Hexane	2,5 hexanedione[a]	Urine	End of shift at end of week		0.4 mg/L		Peripheral neuropathy
Lead	Lead	Blood	Random	60 µg/dL[b] 50 µg/dL[c]	30 µg/dL	400 µg/L (BLW) 100 µg/L women <45 years	Renal, haem and neurological effects

(Continued)

Table 5.2 Continued

Substance	Analyte	Medium	Sampling time	BMGV[4]	BEI[5]	BV[6]	Health concern
Mercury	Mercury	Urine	Random	20 μmol/mol	15 μg/L	25 μg/g (BAT)	Nephrotoxic, CNS effects
4,4′-methylene-bis-2-chloroaniline (MbOCA)	'Total' MbOCA	Urine	End of shift	15 μmol/mol			Cancer
Methylenedianiline (MDA)	'Total' MDA	Urine	End of shift	50 μmol/mol			Cancer
4-methylpentan-2-one (MIBK)	4-methylpentan-2-one (MIBK)	Urine	End of shift	20 μmol/mol	2 mg/L		Irritant, CNS
Nickel metal, oxide, carbonate, sulphide	Nickel	Urine	End of shift at end of week			70 μg/L (EKA)	Cancer
Soluble nickel compounds, e.g. acetate, chloride, hydroxide, sulphate						45 μg/L (EKA)	
Polyaromatic hydrocarbons (PAHs)	1-hydroxypyrene	Urine	End of shift at end of week	4 μmol/mol			Cancer
Styrene	Mandelic acid + phenylglyoxylic acid	Urine	End of shift		400 mg/g	600 mg/g (BAT)	Irritant, CNS
Tetrachloroethylene	Tetrachloroethylene	Blood Breath	Pre-shift Pre-shift		0.5 mg/L 3 ppm		Irritant, CNS
Toluene	o-Cresol	Urine	End of shift		0.5 mg/L		Visual impairment, female reproduction
Trichloroethylene	Trichloroacetic acid	Urine	End of shift at end of week		15 mg/L		CNS
Xylene	Methyl hippuric acid	Urine	End of shift	650 mmol/mol	1.5 g/g	2 g/L	CNS

Mercury BMGV row additional values: 30 μg/dL[d], 50 μg/dL[e], 40 μg/dL[f], 25 μg/dL[g]

Results expressed as '/g' or '/mol' are expressed as /g or /mol of creatinine.
BAR, reference value for background or non-occupational exposure; BAT, biological tolerance value; BV, biological value (BAT, BAR, BKW, EKA); EKA, biological equivalent to an airborne limit.

[a] Without hydrolysis.
[b] Suspension limit.
[c] Suspension limit for young people.
[d] Suspension limit for women of reproductive capacity.
[e] Action limit.
[f] Action limit for young people.
[g] Action limit for women of reproductive capacity.

isocyanates where a dose–response for respiratory sensitization has not yet been established. The guidance value is based on the 90th percentile of data from workplaces with good control and is a practical guide to exposure control. Biological monitoring results that exceed the guidance values are unlikely to be predictive of ill health, but should stimulate an investigation of exposure controls and further monitoring. Regularly exceeding the guidance values indicates that controlling exposure could be improved.

An alternative approach was taken by the ACGIH to develop a guidance value for exposure to polycyclic aromatic hydrocarbons. It has not been possible to derive a health-based guidance value for this complex and variable mixture of carcinogens. Instead, 1-hydroxypyrene (the urinary metabolite of pyrene) is used as a marker substance and the guidance value was derived from the upper end of the distribution from non-occupational exposure. This background level approach clearly defines when biomarker levels result from occupational exposure, but controlling exposure down to these levels may be a challenge in the workplace.

Biological monitoring results reflect systemic exposure by all routes into the body, so if the values found are significantly higher or lower than anticipated for a given airborne concentration the results may indicate the route of exposure. In Figure 5.2, biological monitoring results above the dose–response line (e.g. from a BAT or BEI guidance value) derived from average inhalation exposures may indicate additional exposure due to absorption of the substance through the skin or possibly by increased absorption due to increased respiration when working hard. Conversely, if results are lower than expected, they may reflect reduced absorption due to use of respiratory protective equipment.

Where biological monitoring guidance values are not available from international authoritative or regulatory organizations it may be possible to derive in-house guidance values based on either dose–response relationships or good occupational hygiene practice with the objectives of monitoring and controlling exposure. Such types of in-house guidance values for BM are prevalent in the pharmaceutical industry and often in other sectors with strong trade associations.

BIOLOGICAL EFFECT MONITORING

Definition, examples and relationship with biological monitoring

Unlike biological monitoring (BM), biological effect monitoring (BEM) does not attempt to quantify, or act as a surrogate marker of, the absorbed dose of chemical. It reflects the combined effects of dose (current and past) and those factors in an individual which modify dose in moving to the right along a recognized toxicological pathway in the exposure-disease model (see Figure 5.1). A BEM marker should give some idea of an increased risk, or early evidence of a move towards a specific poor health outcome in an individual. Therefore, the practical use of BEM is in:

- confirming, where the potential ill-health outcome may be significant, that the risk to an exposed cohort is negligible with the current control measures in place;
- identifying that appropriate action needs to be taken to reduce the health risk for a worker, whether due to their individual work practices and subsequent exposure or physiological, genetic or other predisposing factors in that individual.

As such, it has remained in the domain of health surveillance and performed by occupational physicians, unlike BM where there has been substantial uptake in use by occupational hygienists. Also, BEM often entails the use of more invasive samples, such as blood, in comparison to BM, this increased invasiveness being permissible on the grounds that the marker is closer to a defined adverse health outcome.

The relationship between BM and BEM for an exposure is illustrated in Figure 5.3. These data are collated from routine blood lead (Pb) monitoring carried out at the UK Health and Safety Laboratory (HSL) under Control of Lead at Work Regulations (CLAW), where blood Pb is the measured BM tool and zinc protoporphyrin (ZPP) is the BEM tool reflecting the effect of absorbed Pb on

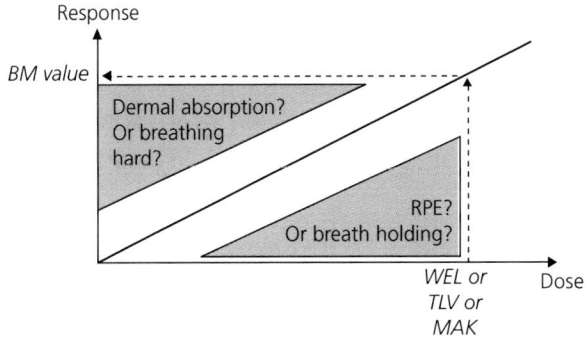

Figure 5.2 Biological monitoring idealized dose–response graph.

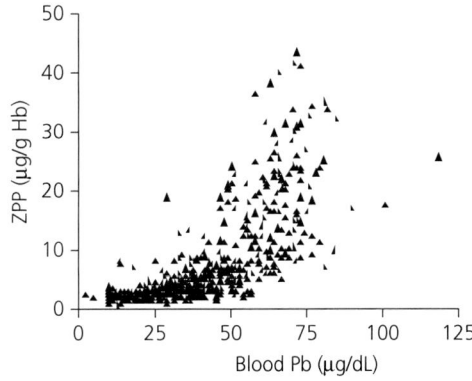

Figure 5.3 The relationship between blood lead and zinc protoporphyrin in a sample of UK workers monitored under Control of Lead at Work Regulations (CLAW) 2002.

haemopoiesis in bone marrow. Pb has a number of effects on both the production of erythrocytes, and on formed red blood cell that can ultimately lead to anaemia. Increased ZPP in blood largely reflects Pb inhibition of the insertion of the ferrous iron into protoporphyrin IX, which is a key step in the formation of the haem molecule involved in oxygen carriage by blood to tissues.

There is a significant statistical relationship between these BM and BEM markers (Figure 5.3), but it would be difficult to predict the likely blood Pb level from a ZPP measurement and vice versa in any single subject. It has sometimes been wrongly thought that BEM markers are surrogates for BM measurements reflecting absorbed dose. The variability in the relationship between blood Pb and ZPP is influenced by toxicokinetics and the pattern of exposure of the metal, and the interindividual variations in Pb transport and storage within the body, as well as at specific enzyme pathways within the bone marrow. The influence of analytical imprecision in the two measurements is relatively small compared to these biological factors. In terms of dose, blood Pb can be considered as a measure of absorbed metal, while ZPP indicates the influence in an individual of the Pb concentration at the target site(s) of interference in haemopoiesis. Figure 5.3 also shows a general feature of the relationship between BM and BEM reflecting the same exposure, in that the former is more sensitive in detecting low-level exposure than the respective BEM marker, e.g. comparison of urinary alkyl phosphates (BM) and depressions in blood cholinesterase measurements (BEM) resulting from organophosphate pesticide exposure.[18]

An ideal BEM marker should be able to measure a change in a biological parameter within an understood toxicological pathway that links exposure to clinical disease or frank toxicity. It should also be able to detect an early change, at a preferably reversible stage. However, even some well-established BEM do not necessarily fully meet such a definition. For example, urinary retinol binding protein (RBP) (or other low molecular weight proteins, such as β_2-microglobulin), has long been considered as a useful BEM marker in those exposed to cadmium.[19–21] The urinary increase in RBP is a sensitive marker of the metal's toxic effects on renal proximal tubular reabsorption. RBP can be readily measured in urine, and is sensitive to very small cadmium-induced changes in the proximal renal tubular reabsorptive process. However, the evidence is that any significant measured increase in RBP is not reversible even with complete removal of the subject from further exposure.

Biological effect monitoring, susceptibility and diagnosis

While the exposure-disease model in Figure 5.1 suggests that 'uptake', 'effect' and 'disease', and the associated analytical categories of 'biological monitoring', 'biological effect monitoring' and 'diagnosis', are clearly delineated, in practice there are grey areas and debate. There are some areas of uncertainty about where some analyses may be better considered as biological monitoring, biological effect monitoring or better defined as diagnosis of overt occupational disease.

For example, blood carboxyhaemoglobin (HbCO) could be considered a classical BEM marker for situations where there is direct exposure to carbon monoxide, from an industrial process or, often more hazardously, the use of internal combustion engines in confined spaces,[22] and through the metabolism of dichloromethane and smoking status. Circulating levels of HbCO are both a direct indicator of the reduced oxygen-carrying capacity of blood and an indirect marker of likely tissue anoxia. The relationship between HbCO and the classical toxic symptoms are well defined, so that health-based occupational limits have been readily set. Breath carbon monoxide is a non-invasive measurement that can be assessed on site using readily available instrumentation and showing a good relationship with HbCO levels.[23] Thus, in this case, the distinction between BM and BEM is arbitrary, and in higher exposures HbCO is the diagnostic test confirming possible symptoms of frank toxicity and the possible need for aggressive therapy, such as hyperbaric oxygen.

The influence of susceptibility factors on the move from exposure and frank ill health, are often linked with biological effect markers. Susceptibility factors may be protective in an individual, as well as increase the risk of possible toxicity and disease. While there are a few examples where distinct susceptibility factors can be identified as significantly altering the risk of adverse outcome (e.g. α1-antitrypsin deficiency and exposure to lung irritants[24,25]), altered risk is often related in a complex manner to a range of factors. In some cases, metabolic polymorphisms have been shown to be a risk factor for one ill-health outcome, but protective for another outcome (e.g. acetylator status for N-acetyltransferase-2 and risk of bladder and colorectal cancer when exposed to carcinogenic aromatic amines[26]). The use of biomarkers of susceptibility in occupational monitoring has raised considerable and ongoing ethical concerns, and the emphasis remains on keeping chemical exposure as low as possible to protect all workers, rather than identifying a cohort within a possible workforce who are best able to handle exposure.

An 'ideal' BEM marker would have both high sensitivity and specificity, low analytical impression and physiological variation, low cost and measureable in as non-invasive a sample as possible. These would be the same ideal characteristics for a clinical diagnostic test or test for an occupational disease. Therefore, a blurring between a BEM marker and diagnostic test is possible for the 'ideal' test, and this transfers to the real world where often tests are very much less than ideal. The difference between a test used as BEM or diagnosis may be defined by the rationale for their use and the interpretation put on the results. The value of a test used to diagnose an (occupational) disease may be expressed in terms of 'likelihood ratios' reflecting how much a positive (or negative) test is likely to change a physician's opinion of the presence (or absence) of specific disease in a patient before the test was performed. The same test used within an occupational monitoring/BEM context can be viewed as similar to 'screening' within a population where there is a significant risk of relevant ill-health outcome, where the 'positive (or negative) predictive value' of the test is more relevant in terms of the test's value. In practice, most tests are primarily developed for use in clinical diagnosis and their investigation in terms of value in occupational monitoring is secondary, often the evidence for evaluating the value of a test within occupational monitoring is scant in comparison to its clinical validation. Also, the problems of tests with less than ideal sensitivities and specificities in the context of screening in terms of false positives and negatives are well understood, which may have limited the wider spread of BEM.

In contrast, in the last 10–15 years there has been a very significant increase in the number of candidate BEM markers. This is due to the development of the experimental laboratory '-omics' disciplines (e.g. proteomics, genomics and metabolomics) in identifying changes in large numbers of proteins, enzymes and cellular control mechanisms after a toxic insult in experimental studies. Whether some or any of these potential BEM markers develop into routine occupational monitoring procedures is uncertain.

The following sections deal with BEM with regard to specific potential outcomes or sites of toxicity.

CARCINOGENS

Protein–chemical conjugates involving haemoglobin may be considered as BM markers reflecting cumulative chemical exposure over the lifetime of haemoglobin. However, DNA-chemical adducts could be considered as BEM markers, showing the potential of reactive electrophilic chemical species, or their metabolites, to become both intracellularly located and then covalently adduct to DNA with direct relevance to a potential carcinogenic pathway. Other authorities have coined the term 'biological effect dose monitors' for such DNA adducts. Over the last decade or so, a number of assays have been developed to investigate the measurements of DNA adducts in readily available nucleated cells (e.g. lymphocytes in blood) which fits within a genotoxic model of how some chemicals may cause cancer,[27–29] but their actual relationship to risk of cancer is uncertain.[30] However, both haemoglobin- and DNA-adducts reflect that an absorbed chemical can cross cell membranes to produce intracellular reactive electrophilic species capable of covalently linking to structural or functional cell elements.[27]

On an international basis, the use of haemoglobin conjugates have become an acceptable routine biomarker, highlighted by the development of guidance values for some chemicals by the DFG.[6] In contrast, DNA adducts in circulating nucleated cells remain almost exclusively within the research area. Historically, DNA-adduct analysis has relied on highly sensitive, but non-specific radiological techniques, such as ^{32}P post-labelling techniques. Recently, sophisticated chromatographic and some immunoassay-based methods have been developed.[29] However these techniques, in particular ^{32}P post-labelling, suffer from technical difficulties and complexities that would hamper their widespread adoption even if their value as risk biomarkers of cancer was better validated.

Another approach for monitoring DNA adducts takes advantage of the generally efficient DNA repair mechanisms, which leads to the urinary excretion of excised adduct-nucleic acids, e.g. urinary markers of oxidative DNA adduction.[31,32]

Further measurements in the exposure-disease model (Figure 5.1) in terms of a mutagenicity/carcinogenicity pathway have been the measurements of genotoxic BEM markers, such as DNA strand breaks, chromosomal abnormality, sister chromatid exchange, micronuclei, COMET assay, modified bases, e.g. 8-hydroxy-2'-deoxyguanosine (8-OHdG) within circulating blood lymphocytes. These markers certainly reflect alterations in genetic material, although less specific generally in relation to exposure and influenced by non-occupational lifestyle issues, especially smoking habits. Recent reviews still caution about the lack of dose–response relationships that allow some risk assessment of the relevant health end point from such measurements, and therefore their value in routine monitoring.[33–35] There is some evidence that DNA repair capacity within an individual may be an important determinant of cancer risk.[35,36] This may be related to the concept of susceptibility and polymorphism with DNA repair or metabolic enzymes systems. Some studies continue to find clear relationships between metabolic polymorphisms and evidence of DNA damage in peripheral cells[37] and actual risk of cancer in some cases, for example, polymorphism of acetylator status of NAT2 can be associated with a doubled risk of bladder cancer among individuals with high exposures to carcinogenic arylamines, with possible other metabolic polymorphisms in glutathione-S-transferases being additional risk factors.[38]

There is considerable international effort to define the relationship between biomarkers of specific chemical adduction to DNA or exposure-induced changes in DNA, genetic polymorphisms in metabolic enzyme systems and the risk of cancer. Until such progress, Hb adducts as measures of exposure have gained a higher practical use on a worldwide basis than DNA adducts. Other protein–chemical adducts, such as albumin adducts[39] have also been used in monitoring genotoxic chemical exposure. While albumin adducts reflect a shorter time frame of exposure estimation than Hb adducts, and introduce the possibility of non-invasive urine monitoring, they do not reflect that a reactive species that has become intracellularly located before covalent adduction, as albumin is an extracellular protein.

CENTRAL AND PERIPHERAL NERVOUS SYSTEM

The classical BEM markers associated with nervous system toxicity are the inhibition of the blood cholinesterase enzymes, namely plasma butyrylcholinesterase (BChE) and erythrocyte acetylcholinesterase (AChE) for anticholinergic pesticide exposure. Such pesticides inhibit AChE, mainly found at neuromuscular junctions and cholinergic synapses in the central nervous system, where its activity serves to terminate synaptic transmission. Excessive absorption of anticholinergic pesticides, namely organophosphate (OP) and carbamates, block the function of acetylcholinesterase and thus cause excessive acetylcholine to accumulate in the synaptic cleft, causing a number of symptoms in various body functions, but potentially leading to death by asphyxiation through neuromuscular paralysis.[40]

Monitoring is based on identifying an OP-induced depression in the enzyme activity of AChE and BChE. Given the extent of normal, physiological inter- and intraindividual variation, especially in BChE, OP-induced depressions are detected through comparisons with baseline, unexposed measurements or changes in serial measurements within an individual.[41] There have been attempts to produce a BChE monitoring system, based on specific activity measurements, that does not rely on serial monitoring within an individual.[42] While this more complex specific activity measurement does not show a substantial improvement in sensitivity over the simple enzyme measurement to detect OP-induced inhibition, it has value in detecting subclinical OP exposures where baseline measurements are not available.

While AChE in erythrocytes is the same enzyme as that inhibited by OPs in nervous tissue and neuromuscular junctions causing their frank toxicity, it is usually less sensitive than BChE in terms of absorption and inhibition by OPs, so BChe is often also measured, or is the sole BEM measurement. While BChE is sensitive to OP (and carbamate) inhibition, BChE inhibition has no toxicological relevance in itself and the relationship between BChE inhibition and the risk of, or actual severity of OP poisoning is weak, with very significant inhibition of BChE having been noted in the presence of minimal symptoms.[43] The relationship between erythrocyte AChE and symptoms/toxicity is much better. Thus, in this case, two BEM markers may be employed together to monitor workers using OP pesticides, with one marker a closer index of exposure and the other of toxicity. Alternative BM for anticholinergic OP exposure can be based on either a specific metabolite[44,45] or a generic group of metabolites, such as urinary alkyl phosphates, that can certainly detect OP absorption far more sensitively than using BChE depressions.[18,46,47]

RESPIRATORY AND LUNG BIOMARKERS

Respiratory sensitization and occupational asthma remains a significant occupational problem. The ability to predict, or test, whether chemicals may be respiratory sensitizers capable of producing an allergic status in exposed workers remains relatively poor.[48,49] Specific IgE measurements in sera have a long history in aiding or confirming the diagnosis of allergy or confirming sensitization to a specific chemical or protein. The sensitivity and specificity of specific IgE in reflecting symptoms or clinical diagnosis of respiratory allergy appears much better for proteinaceous allergens than low molecular weight chemicals, where the sensitivity of specific IgE tests appears poorer. The restricted availability of radiolabelled anti-human IgE and the availability of large automated analysers for immunoassays in hospital laboratories has meant that the radioallergosorbent test (RAST) has been superseded by non-isotopic commercial assays for specific IgE measurements. These commercial non-isotopic assays cover both occupational and environmental allergens that can be used to investigate an individual's sensitization status (Table 5.3), but tend to focus on commonly encountered allergens. Therefore, IgE tests add to symptom questionnaires, longitudinal peak expiratory flow monitoring in the workplace and, in the clinical setting, bronchial challenge testing that can be used to investigate an individual with asthmatic-type respiratory symptoms.[50] Specialized flow cytometry analysis also allows measurement of the T-cell populations, including the T_H1/T_H2 balance, and T-regulatory cells, which have been implicated in the mechanism underlying sensitization and symptoms of asthma.

In contrast to specific IgE, the measurement of specific IgG to proteins and low molecular weight has tended to be seen as only indicating significant, historical exposures which the immune system has recognized and responded to, without necessarily reflecting an altered increased risk of work-related respiratory disease.[51,52] However, recent evidence in a longitudinal study of paint sprayers exposed to di-isocyanates has suggested that increases in specific IgG and IgG4 appear to have a protective effect on the incidence of work-related lower and upper respiratory symptoms, respectively.[53]

Other toxic effects on the lung have been identified in the occupational context, largely through the use of symptom questionnaires and simple physiological measurements, such as FEV_1, out of a much larger armoury of diagnostic procedures used clinically. Biochemical markers were only measured in an aggressively invasive sample, such as bronchial lavage fluid, which has no role in any routine occupational monitoring strategy. However recently, interest has been stimulated in the measurement of specific lung proteins in blood plasma as biomarkers of toxicity in the lung. The change in plasma levels of these 'pneumoproteins' generally reflect the relationship between the increased synthesis or depletion of the proteins in the lung and alteration in the integrity of the blood–airspace barrier within the lung.

The proteins most investigated are the lung surfactant proteins (e.g. SP-A, SP-B and SP-D) involved in the innate immune response system of the lung, Clara cell protein

Table 5.3 Routine specific IgE tests available for a range of occupational allergens. Other, less common tests may be available through discussion with the laboratory supplying analyses.

Occupational allergens

Proteins
Laboratory animal allergens (rat, mouse, guinea pig and rabbit), urine and epithelium proteins
Alpha-amylase (*Aspergillus oryzae*) found as an additive to flour in the baking industry
Abachi wood dust. Other allergens relevant to wood dust rather than tree pollen may be available
Castor bean
Silk/silk waste
Latex, including individual allergenic components b1, b3, b5, b6.01, b6.02, b8, b9, b11
Chicken, goose feathers
Larger farm animals: cow urine/epithelia, pig urine/epithelia, sheep wool
Horse dander
Flour dust
Alcalase, savinase: bacterially derived enzymes used in cleaning products
Other enzymes, such as cellulase, papain, pepsin

Fish: e.g. trout, cod, salmon
Crustacea: e.g. crab, lobster, shrimp

Low molecular weight chemicals

Isocyanates: hexamethylene di-isocyanate (HDI), diphenylmethane di-isocyanate (MDI), toluene di-isocyanate (TDI)
Phthalic anhydride
Trimellitic anhydride
Methyltetrahydrophthalic anhydride

Maleic anhydride
Tetrachlorophthalic anhydride

Chloramine T
Ethylene oxide
Formaldehyde

(CC16) and KL-6 (Krebs von den Lungen-6). Serum levels of the immunoregulatory CC16 protein are derived from secretions of Clara cells, largely found in the bronchio-tracheal tree, with passive transudation of the CC16 through the lung–blood barrier. Decreases in serum CC16 in chronic exposure to gases and dusts reflect the sensitivity of Clara cells to toxic insult. Increases in serum SP-A or SP-D are ascribed to increased lung–blood membrane permeability by toxic insult. Such pneumoproteins continue to be investigated in the clinical context,[54] and a number of research studies relevant to occupational exposure and using serum measurements are now being published.[55–58] Whether these invasive biomarkers, using blood measurements, may move from research studies into routine occupational monitoring or health surveillance, is unclear. However, these tests do show a high degree of specificity for reflecting abnormalities in the lung.

Other recent interest has been in the analysis of exhaled breath in inflammatory lung diseases, including asthma, chronic obstructive pulmonary disease (COPD) and interstitial lung diseases.[59] Analysis of various biomarkers, including volatile chemicals and gases such as nitric oxide (NO), carbon monoxide and many non-volatile molecules, such as inflammatory markers/mediators, oxidation and nitration products in exhaled breath allows non-invasive monitoring of inflammation and oxidative stress in the respiratory tract. The measurement of NO in exhaled breath can be increasingly measured using available, relatively low cost equipment, with some devices having Food and Drug Administration (FDA) approval for monitoring asthma status.[60] While NO in exhaled breath is not specific for asthma, as it is also increased in lower respiratory tract inflammation and chronic bronchitis, an increased level may be useful in differentiating asthma from other causes of chronic cough. Its diagnostic value in distinguishing between healthy subjects with or without respiratory symptoms and patients with confirmed asthma has been identified with a specificity of 90 per cent and positive predictive value of 95 per cent using a NO cut-off of >15 ppb in exhaled breath.[60]

Furthermore, non-volatile biomarkers can be condensed from exhaled breath and analysed. The collection of this exhaled breath condensate (EBC) for analysis of non-volatiles is somewhat more difficult and involved than direct measurement of volatiles in exhaled breath. Standardized physiological conditions for collection, the development of more robust, cheaper collection equipment and high sensitivity methods for measuring the biomarkers in the EBC are necessary.[61] Thus, the technique remains at a research stage, but recent work has shown the potential for the non-invasive measurement of inflammatory markers[61–63] reflecting pathophysiology in the lung. While biomarkers in EBC are in their infancy, with their relevance and use within an occupational context still to be completely mapped out, publications with direct relevance to occupation are beginning to appear.[64–67]

RENAL MARKERS

A number of specific chemicals such as mercury, cadmium and more diffuse ill-defined chemical occupational exposures, such as solvents, have been associated with occupational exposure and renal toxicity.[68–70]

Serum creatinine, more recently cystatin C, and urinary albumin and total protein are accepted biomarkers of altered glomerular filtration rate and glomerular permeability, respectively. They are the classically used general clinical biomarkers reflecting such pathological alterations, but without any relationship to any occupational involvement of chemical exposure.

Over a number of years, there have been investigations into possible early renal biological effect markers reflecting the various renal effects of chemical exposures, and a number of markers have been suggested as of potential value.[71–73] These markers are usually urinary protein or enzymes (e.g. N-acetylglucosaminidase) reflecting direct renal cellular damage, functional changes (e.g. albumin, retinol-binding protein, transferrin), structural components (e.g. collagen/laminin fragments) or induction of protection mechanisms (e.g. metallothionein). However, currently there is no universal agreement on a validated panel of effect biomarkers that may be suitable to detect or monitor chemical-induced nephrotoxicity in the context of occupational and environmental exposure. Neutrophil gelatinase-associated lipocalin (NGAL) appears increasingly useful in clinical nephrology[74] and specifically as a sensitive marker of clinically encountered nephrotoxins, such as contrast media,[75] cisplatin.[76] Increases in urine NGAL have been found to precede changes in urinary NAG and β_2-microglobulin, or serum creatinine.[77] Even more recently, kidney injury molecule-1 (KIM-1) has been found to be a sensitive marker of tubule-interstitial damage.[78–80] Thus, NGAL and KIM-1 appear potential useful candidate damage markers in terms of monitoring occupational or environmental exposure to nephrotoxins to add to the tests historically employed.

Urinary biomarkers, such as the low molecular weight proteins, retinol-binding protein (RBP), β_2-microglobulin (with its more pH-dependent stability problems) and alpha-1-microglobulin reflect abnormality in the specific renal tubular process of protein reabsorption and are widely used to monitor the possible effects of cadmium.[17,81,82] Cadmium is a cumulative nephrotoxic where its concentration within the nephron finally overcomes defensive mechanisms and leads to measureable changes in reabsorptive processes in the proximal tubule.[20,83] Significant cadmium-induced effects appear non-reversible; however, the ability to measure very small induced changes in the proximal tubular process of low molecular weight protein reabsorption does allow exposure modification in an individual at an early stage to save the latter, grosser cadmium-induced changes due to the loss of substantial numbers of functioning nephrons.

In contrast, mercury, another acknowledged metal nephrotoxin, does not have suitable specifically associated BEM biomarkers, as with cadmium. Mercury has been associated with an immunologically mediated, rapidly presenting glomerulonephritis[84] or nephrotic syndrome,[85,86] with little clear understanding of dose–response relationships, except that it is rare in current occupational exposure conditions, and may have a large genetic component. Large increases in urine levels of high molecular weight proteins, which are not usually filtered by the glomeruli, and cellular proteins (such as NAG) are a marker of the glomerulopathic and general inflammatory nature of this mercury-associated condition, but there appears no good evidence that regular monitoring of, for example, urinary albumin can predict or identify early development of the mercury-induced glomerulonephritis. However, mercury as a general nephrotoxicant can cause some increase in the excretion of proteins and enzymes suggesting some subclinical toxicity.[87,88] There is some evidence that occupational mercury exposure leads to small reversible increases in urinary enzymes, such as urinary N-acetylglucosaminidase.[89] This probably reflects that NAG is a lysosomal enzyme involved in the normal process of exocytosis of heavy metals from renal tubular cells into forming urine, possibly together with other tubular cell membrane enzymes.

BLADDER

The bladder as a site of occupational toxicity has been sustained largely by the actual and suspected additional risk of bladder cancer in those exposed to a number of toxic chemicals, including rubber fumes, dyes and various aromatic amines, including those in cigarette smoke.[90,91] Urine cytology in normally voided urine has been historically part of health monitoring or health surveillance for current and ex-workers in high-risk industries. However, in order to get meaningful analysis, there is a need for fresh urine samples to be delivered to a centre where there is the appropriate expertise in this microscopical analysis. Centralization of hospital pathology units in the United Kingdom has increased the logistic difficulties in providing such occupational monitoring for workforces or ex-employees. Also urine cytology, while it has high sensitivity in detecting high-grade tumours, has low sensitivity in detecting low-grade tumours.[92]

There has been considerable clinical effort in investigating molecular biomarkers that might reduce the need for periodic, invasive cystoscopies or, ideally, offering a non-invasive test with better sensitivity than urine cytology. Recently, some urinary biomarkers have been suggested as fulfilling a similar role, based on the excretion of altered cellular process and components at the pre-cancerous and cancerous stages. Some commercially available biomarkers, e.g. BTA, ImmunoCyt™, NMP22 and UroVysion™, have already been approved by the US FDA for bladder cancer surveillance, while many other markers are still undergoing development for preclinical and clinical investigation. However, the clinical trial data on the majority of these markers are conflicting in terms of their diagnostic power compared against cystoscopy as the gold standard diagnosis. Individual case–control studies have produced indices of diagnostic power for one or more biomarkers, e.g. NMP22 has been shown to have

Table 5.4 A review of published sensitivities and specificities for commercially available 'new' biomarkers for bladder cancer.

Test	Sensitivity (%)	Specificity (%)
Novel commercially available biomarkers		
BTA Stat (point-of-care device)	53–78	69–87
BTA Trak (laboratory test)	51–100	73–93
NMP22 Bladder Cancer Test (laboratory test)	35–100	60–95
NMP22 BladderChek (point-of-care device)	50–65	40–90
ImmunoCyt/uCyt+	63–85	62–78
ImmunoCyt/uCyt+ and cytology	81–89	61–78
UroVysion	69–100	65–96
Traditional tests		
Cytology	12–85	78–100
Haematuria by dipstick	47–93	51–84

sensitivity and specificity of 76 and 87 per cent, respectively, in diagnosing transitional cell carcinomas, although the sensitivity does decrease significantly for the lowest staging.[93] However, a review of such studies (Table 5.4),[94] while suggesting that the novel markers tend to have better sensitivity than voided urine cytology (although traditional voided urine cytology generally has high specificity) highlighted the variation in reported sensitivity and specificity between studies for individual biomarkers. They suggested that the variation in sensitivity and specificity was due to varying case definitions between studies. The use of cross-sectional studies with cystoscopy as the 'gold standard' to validate these new bladder biomarkers has also been criticized.[95]

In general, the uptake of such tests in clinical diagnosis has been relatively low, although with wide international differences. This probably reflects that none evaluated over the last years showed remarkable improvements in sensitivity or specificity for the identification of any of the diverse types of bladder cancer in clinical practice.[92] A combination of tests may be necessary for screening in occupational cohorts at risk, in order to detect real cases of bladder cancers, without causing concern to much larger numbers of normal subjects through false-positive results.

Some of these new commercially available biomarkers (e.g. NMP22) have begun to be used in the United States, Europe and Japan in specifically monitoring occupational cohorts considered at risk. However, the evidence is scant for the value of traditional tests, such as voided urine cytology and detection of microscopic haematuria. Similarly, there is lack of evidence for the effectiveness of newer FDA-approved biomarkers, in screening current and past workers identified with occupational risk factors in order to detect bladder tumours at an early stage. This is essential for improved prognosis and long-term survival. As such, neither urine cytology nor proposed biomarkers can be considered as early markers reflecting a reversible stage.

While there is some evidence that susceptibility markers related to metabolism (NAT-2), slow metabolism and GST null/low activity may indicate some increased risk of bladder cancer in those exposed to carcinogenic arylamines.[38] Such tests of susceptibility remain in the research arena, with concerns about their ethical application and interpretation in workforces.

LIVER

The panel of liver function routinely used in clinical diagnosis has also been employed in monitoring workers exposed to hepatotoxic chemicals. These tests include alanine transaminase (ALT), aspartate transaminase (AST), gamma glutamyl transferase (GGT), alkaline phosphatase (ALP) and bilirubin.[96] Such tests reflect heptocellular damage (ALT, AST), bile duct obstruction and cholestasis (ALP, bilirubin). GGT is a microsomal enzyme widely distributed in the liver and hepatobiliary tree, as well as other organs. It is sensitive to enzyme-inducing drugs and chemicals, and can also be elevated in chronic alcohol consumption. Other tests in this standard liver function test (LFT) panel may also show some abnormalities due to chronic alcohol abuse. There is a lack of published evidence about the value of such a panel of tests in detecting early occupational hepatotoxic effects, and the frequency of idiopathic low level abnormalities in such tests unrelated to liver disease has been highlighted.[96] The prevalence of alcohol abuse in many communities means that any abnormalities in such LFT in workers, and especially the highly inducible GGT, may be unrelated to occupational exposure,[97] or that effects of occupational exposure may be masked.

If the occupational physician considers that the identification of chronic alcohol abuse is legitimately part of their role in maintaining a healthy workforce, then identification of workers with such problems can be done with better sensitivity and specificity by the measurement of serum carbohydrate-deficient transferrrin (CDT). This can also be used in the monitoring of compliance by any workers undergoing an alcohol abstinence regime.[98,99]

Serum bile acid measurements have had some use as sensitive routine liver function tests. It has also been shown that bile acids can be measured in urine, and reflect serum levels, therefore there is the potential for a non-invasive measurement of liver function,[100,101] particularly in detecting chemically induced cholestasis.

Other widely available tests for potential occupational hazards involving liver abnormality include immunoassays for antibody status in those exposed to hepatitis B or hepatitis C or determination of antibody titre in high-risk occupational groups who undergo protective immunization regimes, e.g. for leptospirosis. DNA-based detection tests offer potential advantage over tests based on antibody detection for early diagnosis of leptospirosis[102] since antibodies may only reach detectable levels several days after the onset of the infection. Polymerase chain reaction amplification techniques may well afford the capability of detecting pathogenic leptospira in urine samples, but currently such tests are not widely available.

CONCLUSIONS

Distinctions in the boundaries between the categories of BM, BEM and diagnosis are sometimes not always clear and can lead to debate about which category a biomarker may fit. However, such a debate is largely irrelevant, the focus should be on why the biomarker is being used and where it may aid in understanding and controlling any move to the right in the exposure-disease model (Figure 5.1). Any test that is used to define the extent of uptake of any chemical by any route of exposure is BM, whereas tests that are used to gauge the potential ill-health risk or substantiate the lack of increased risk in individual workers or workforces constitute BEM.

There is an ongoing increase in the routine use of BM in workplaces, allied to the availability of appropriate biomarkers to monitor chemical hazards encountered in the workplace at current levels of exposure. In reality, where the relationship between exposure and risk of ill-health is very uncertain or unknown, the application of BM to help ensure that control of exposure is as low as practical, is a reasonable strategy. Any expansion in the use and range of BEM markers has not been so noticeable. However, a significant number of potential BEM markers for various target organ toxicities are potential candidate markers. Validation data that can substantiate their use in occupational monitoring strategies are required.

The exposure-disease model and the application of biomarkers are not necessarily confined to chemical exposure, but may well have a role in exposure to physical agents and psychosocial issues, such as hand–arm vibration exposure, stress and shift work.

> ### Key points
>
> - Biological monitoring is based on the analysis of hazardous substances or their metabolites in biological fluids.
> - Biological effect monitoring reflects the early consequences of exposure.
> - BM and BEM can be helpful in programmes of health surveillance.
> - BM and BEM can aid the assessment of systemic exposure and consequences through ingestion and dermal absorption, as well as inhalation.
> - BM and BEM can provide a valuable feedback loop to aid the control (including behavioural aspects) of exposure.

REFERENCES

1. Boogaard PJ, Money CD. A proposed framework for the interpretation of biomonitoring data. *Environmental Health.* 2008; **7** (Suppl. 12): 1–6.
2. Information Commissioner Office. The Employment Practices Code, Part 4. Wilmslow: Information Commissioner Office, 2005: 73–80. Available from: www.ico.gov.uk.
3. Health and Safety Executive. Biological monitoring in the workplace. HSG 167. Sudbury: HSE Books, 1997: 1–32.
4. Health and Safety Executive. EH40/2005 Workplace exposure limits. Sudbury: HSE Books, 2005 (with amendments 2006 and 2007).
5. American Committe of Governmental Occupational Hygienists. TLVs and BEIs® based on the documentation of the threshold limit values and biological exposure indices. Cincinnati: ACGIH, 2008.
6. Deutsche Forschungsgemeinschaft. List of MAK and BAT values 2007. Report No. 42. Weinheim: Wiley VCH, 2007.
7. International Air Transport Association. Infectious substances: Shipping guidelines. The complete guide for pharmaceutical and health professions, 7th edn. Geneva: IATA, 2007. Available from: www.iata.org.
8. Droz P-O, Fiserova-Bergerova V. Biological monitoring. VI. Pharmacokinetic models in setting biological exposure indices. *Applied Ocupational and Environmental Hygiene.* 1992; **7**: 574–80.
9. Morton J, Mason H. Speciation of arsenic compounds in urine from occupationally unexposed and exposed persons in the UK using a routine LC-ICP-MS method. *Journal of Analytical Toxicology.* 2006; **30**: 293–301.
10. Yang M, Koga M, Katoh T, Kawamoto T. A study for the proper application of urinary naphthols, new biomarkers for airborne polycyclic aromatic hydrocarbons. *Archives of Environmental Contamination and Toxicology.* 1999; **36**: 99–108.
11. Lauwerys R, Hoet P. *Industrial chemical exposure: Guidelines for biological monitoring*, 3rd edn. Boca Raton: Lewis Publishers, 2001.
12. Jakubowski M, Trzcinka-Ochocka M. Biological monitoring of exposure: Trends and key developments. *Journal of Occupational Health.* 2005; **47**: 22–48.
13. Boehniger M, Lowry L, Rosenberg J. Interpretation of urine results used to assess chemical exposure with emphasis on creatinine adjustments: A review. *Journal of American Industrial Hygienists Association.* 1993; **54**: 615–27.
14. Sata F, Araki S, Yokoyama K, Murata K. Adjustment of creatinine adjusted values in urine to urinary flow rate: A study of eleven heavy metals and organic substances. *International Archives of Occupational and Environmental Health.* 1995; **68**: 64–8.
15. Berlin A, Alessio L, Sesana G *et al.* Problems concerning the usefulness of adjustment of urinary cadmium for creatinine and specific gravity. *International Archives of Occupational and Environmental Health.* 1985; **55**: 107–11.

16. Mason HJ, Williams NR, Morgan MG et al. The influence of biological and analytical variation on urine measurements for monitoring cadmium exposure. *Occupational and Environmental Medicine.* 1998; **55**: 132–7.
17. Mason H, Stevenson A, Williams N, Morgan M. Intra-individual variability in markers of proteinuria for normal subjects and those with cadmium-induced renal dysfunction: Interpretation of results from untimed, random urine samples. *Biomarkers.* 1999; **4**: 118–29.
18. Cocker J, Mason HJ, Garfitt S, Jones K. Biological monitoring of exposure to organophosphate pesticides. *Toxicology Letters.* 2002; **134**: 97–103.
19. Topping M, Forster H, Dolman C et al. Measurement of urinary retinol binding protein by enzyme linked immunosorbent assay and its application to the detection of tubular proteinuria. *Clinical Chemistry.* 1986; **32**: 1863–6.
20. Mason HJ, Davison A, Wright A et al. Relations between liver cadmium, cumulative exposure and renal function in cadmium alloy workers. *British Journal of Industrial Medicine.* 1988; **45**: 793–802.
21. Kjellstrom T, Evrin P-E, Rahnster B. Dose-response analysis of cadmium induced tubular proteinuria: A study of beta-2-microglobulin excretion among workers in a battery factory. *Environmental Research.* 1977; **13**: 303–17.
22. Gallagher G, Mason H. Carbon monoxide poisoning in two workers using an LPG forklift truck within a coldstore. *Occupational Medicine.* 2004; **54**: 483–8.
23. Wald N, Idle M, Boreham J. Carbon monoxide in breath in relation to smoking and carboxyhaemoglobin levels. *Thorax.* 1981; **36**: 366–9.
24. Berode M, Jost M, Ruegger M, Savolainen H. Host factors in occupational diisocyanate asthma: A Swiss longitudinal study. *International Archives Occupational and Environmental Health.* 2005; **78**: 158–63.
25. Sigsgaard T, Bonefeld-Jorgensen E, Hoffmann H et al. Microbial cell wall agents as an occupational hazard. *Toxicology Applied Pharmacology.* 2005; **2007** (Suppl. 2): 310–19.
26. Hengstler J, Arrand M, Herrero M, Oesch F. Polymorphisms of N-acetyltransferases, glutathione-S-transferases, microsomal epoxide hydrolases and sulphotransferases: Influence on cancer susceptibility. *Recent Results Cancer Research.* 1998; **154**: 47–85.
27. Farmer P. Monitoring of human exposure to carcinogens through DNA and protein adduct determination. *Toxicology Letters.* 1995; **82**: 757–62.
28. Peluso M, Srivatanakul P, Munnia A et al. DNA adduct formation among workers in a Thai industrial estate and nearby residents. *Science of the Total Environment.* 2008; **389**: 283–8.
29. Yong LC, Schulte PA, Kao CY et al. DNA adducts in granulocytes of hospital workers exposed to ethylene oxide. *American Journal of Industrial Medicine.* 2007; **50**: 293–302.
30. Veglia F, Loft S, Matullo G et al. DNA adducts and cancer risk in prospective studies: A pooled analysis and a meta-analysis. *Carcinogenesis.* 2008; **29**: 932–6.
31. Park E, Shigenaga M, Degan P et al. Assay of excised oxidative DNA lesions: Isolation of 8-oxoguanine and its nucleoside derivatives from biological fluids with a monoclonal antibody column. *Proceedings of the National Academy of Sciences of the United States of America.* 1992; **89**: 3375–9.
32. Marie C, Ravanat JL, Badouard C et al. Urinary levels of oxidative DNA and RNA damage among workers exposed to polycyclic aromatic hydrocarbons in silicon production: Comparison with 1-hydroxypyrene. *Environmental and Molecular Mutagenesis.* 2009; **50**: 88–95.
33. Angerer J, Ewers U, Wilhelm M. Human biomonitoring: State of the art. *International Journal of Hygiene and Environmental Health.* 2007; **210**: 201–28.
34. Knudsen LE, Hansen AM. Biomarkers of intermediate endpoints in environmental and occupational health. *International Journal of Hygiene and Environmental Health.* 2007; **210**: 461–70.
35. Au WW. Usefulness of biomarkers in population studies: From exposure to susceptibility and to prediction of cancer. *International Journal of Hygiene and Environmental Health.* 2007; **210**: 239–46.
36. Li CY, Wang LE, Wei QY. DNA repair phenotype and cancer susceptibility. A mini review. *International Journal of Cancer.* 2009; **124**: 999–1007.
37. Zhu SM, Xia ZL, Wang AH et al. Polymorphisms and haplotypes of DNA repair and xenobiotic metabolism genes and risk of DNA damage in Chinese vinyl chloride monomer (VCM)-exposed workers. *Toxicology Letters.* 2008; **178**: 88–94.
38. Yuan JM, Chan KK, Coetzee GA et al. Genetic determinants in the metabolism of bladder carcinogens in relation to risk of bladder cancer. *Carcinogenesis.* 2008; **29**: 1386–93.
39. Wang H, Chen WH, Zheng HY et al. Association between plasma BPDE-Alb adduct concentrations and DNA damage of peripheral blood lymphocytes among coke oven workers. *Occupational and Environmental Medicine.* 2007; **64**: 753–8.
40. Heath A, Vale J. Clinical presentation and diagnosis of acute organophosphate insecticide and carbamate poisoning. In: Ballantyne D (ed.). *Clinical and experimental toxicology of organophosphate and carbamate poisoning.* Oxford: Butterworth-Heinemann, 1992: 513–19.
41. Mason HJ, Lewis P. Intra-individual variation in plasma and erythrocyte cholinesterase activities and the monitoring of uptake of organo-phosphate pesticides. *Occupational Medicine.* 1989; **39**: 121–4.
42. Brock A. Inter- and intra-individual variations in plasma cholinesterase activity and substance concentration in employees of an organophosphorus insecticide factory. *British Journal of Industrial Medicine.* 1991; **48**: 562–7.
43. Mason HJ. The recovery of plasma cholinesterase and erythrocyte acetylcholinesterase after over exposure to dichlorvos. *Journal of Occupational Medicine.* 2000; **50**: 343–7.
44. Nolan R, Rick D, Freshour N, Saunders J. Chlorpyrifos: Pharmacokinetics in human volunteers. *Toxicology and Applied Pharmacology.* 1984; **73**: 8–15.

45. Byrne S, Shurdut B, Saunders D. Potential chlorpyrifos exposure to residents following standard crack and crevice treatment. *Environmental Health Perspectives.* 1998; **106**: 725-31.
46. Aprea C, Terenzoni B, De Angelis V *et al.* Evaluation of skin and respiratory doses and urinary excretion of alkylphosphates in workers exposed to dimethoate during treatment of olive trees. *Archives of Environmental Contamination and Toxicology.* 2005; **48**: 127-34.
47. Davies J, Peterson JC. Surveillance of occupational, accidental and incidental exposure to organophosphate pesticides using urine alkylphosphate and phenolic metabolite measurements. *Annals of the New York Academy of the Sciences.* 1997; **837**: 257-68.
48. Seed MJ, Cullinan P, Agius RM. Methods for the prediction of low-molecular-weight occupational respiratory sensitizers. *Current Opinion in Allergy and Clinical Immunology.* 2008; **8**: 103-9.
49. Arts JHE, Kuper CF. Animal models to test respiratory allergy of low molecular weight chemicals: A guidance. *Methods.* 2007; **41**: 61-71.
50. Tarlo SM, Balmes J, Balkissoon R *et al.* Diagnosis and management of work-related asthma: American College of Chest Physicians Consensus Statement. *Chest.* 2008; **134**: 1S-41S.
51. Park H-S, Nahm D, Kim H-Y *et al.* Role of specific IgE, IgG and IgG4 antibodies to corn dust in exposed workers. *Korean Journal of Internal Medicine.* 1998; **13**: 88-94.
52. Ott MG, Jolly AT, Burkert AL, Brown WE. Issues in diisocyanate antibody testing. *Critical Reviews in Toxicology.* 2007; **37**: 567-85.
53. Dragos M, Jones M, Malo J *et al.* Specific antibodies to diisocyanate and work-related respiratory symptoms in apprentice car-painters. *Occupational and Environmental Medicine.* 2009; **66**: 227-34.
54. Tzouvelekis A, Kouliatsis G, Anevlavis S, Bouros D. Serum biomarkers in interstitial lung diseases. *Respiratory Research.* 2005; **6**: 24.
55. Hamaguchi T, Omae K, Takebayashi T *et al.* Exposure to hardly soluble indium compounds in ITO production and recycling plants is a new risk for interstitial lung damage. *Occupational and Environmental Medicine.* 2008; **65**: 51-5.
56. Nogami H, Shimoda T, Shoji S, Nishima S. Pulmonary disorders in indium-processing workers. *Nihon Kokyuki Gakkai Zasshi.* 2008; **46**: 60-4.
57. Janssen R, Grutters J, Sato H *et al.* Analysis of KL-6 and SP-D as disease markers in bird fancier's lung. *Sarcoidosis Vasculitis and Diffuse Lung Diseases.* 2005; **22**: 51-7.
58. Tsushima K, Fujimoto K, Yoshikawa S *et al.* Hypersensitivity pneumonitis due to Bunashimeji mushrooms in the mushroom industry. *International Archives of Allergy and Immunology.* 2005; **137**: 241-8.
59. Kharitonov S, Barnes P. Biomarkers of some pulmonary diseases in exhaled breath. *Biomarkers.* 2002; **7**: 1-32.
60. Kharitonov S. Exhaled markers of inflammatory lung diseases: Ready for routine monitoring. *Swiss Medical Weekly.* 2004; **134**: 175-92.
61. Hoffmeyer F, Raulf-Heimsoth M, Bruning T. Exhaled breath condensate and airway inflammation. *Current Opinion in Allergy and Clinical Immunology.* 2009; **9**: 16-22.
62. Zietkowski Z, Tomasiak-Lozowska M, Skiepko R *et al.* High-sensitivity C-reactive protein in the exhaled breath condensate and serum in stable and unstable asthma. *Respiratory Medicine.* 2009; **103**: 379-85.
63. Chan HP, Tran V, Lewis C, Thomas PS. Elevated levels of oxidative stress markers in exhaled breath condensate. *Journal of Thoracic Oncology.* 2009; **4**: 172-8.
64. Pelclova D, Fenclova Z, Kacer P *et al.* Increased 8-isoprostane, a marker of oxidative stress in exhaled breath condensate in subjects with asbestos exposure. *Industrial Health.* 2008; **46**: 484-9.
65. Do R, Bartlett KH, Dilmich-Ward H *et al.* Biomarkers of airway acidity and oxidative stress in exhaled breath condensate from grain workers. *American Journal of Respiratory and Critical Care Medicine.* 2008; **178**: 1048-54.
66. Ono E, Mita H, Taniguchi M *et al.* Increase in inflammatory mediator concentrations in exhaled breath condensate after allergen inhalation. *Journal of Allergy and Clinical Immunology.* 2008; **122**: 768-73.
67. Gergelova P, Corradi M, Acampa O *et al.* New techniques for assessment of occupational respiratory diseases. *Bratislava Medical Journal-Bratislavske Lekarske Listy.* 2008; **109**: 445-52.
68. Nuyts G, Van Viem E, Thys J *et al.* New occupational risk factors for chronic renal failure. *Lancet.* 1995; **346**: 7-11.
69. Yaqoob M, Bell G. Occupational factors and renal disease. *Renal Failure.* 1994; **16**: 425-34.
70. Pai P, Stevenson A, Mason HJ, Bell G. Occupational hydrocarbon exposure and nephrotoxicity: A cohort study and literature review. *Postgraduate Medical Journal.* 1998; **74**: 225-8.
71. Price RG, Berndt WO, Finn WF *et al.* Urinary biomarkers to detect significant effects of environmental and occupational exposure to nephrotoxins. 3. Minimal battery of tests to assess subclinical nephrotoxicity for epidemiological studies based on current knowledge. *Renal Failure.* 1997; **19**: 535-52.
72. Taylor SA, Chivers ID, Price RG *et al.* The assessment of biomarkers to detect nephrotoxicity using an integrated database. *Environmental Research.* 1997; **75**: 23-33.
73. Finn WF, Porter GA. Urinary biomarkers: Recommendations of the Joint European United States Workshop for Future Research. *Renal Failure.* 1999; **21**: 445-51.
74. Devarajan P. Neutrophil gelatinase-associated lipocalin (NGAL): A new marker of kidney disease. *Scandinavian Journal of Clinical and Laboratory Investigation.* 2008; **68**: 89-94.
75. Hirsch R, Dent C, Pfriem H *et al.* NGAL is an early predictive biomarker of contrast-induced nephropathy in children. *Pediatric Nephrology.* 2007; **22**: 2089-95.
76. Mishra J, Mori K, Ma Q *et al.* Neutrophil gelatinase-associated lipocalin: A novel early urinary biomarker for cisplatin nephrotoxicity. *American Journal of Nephrology.* 2004; **24**: 307-15.

77. Mishra J, Ma Q, Prada A *et al*. Identification of neutrophil gelatinase-associated lipocalin as a novel early urinary biomarker for ischemic renal injury. *Journal of the American Society of Nephrology.* 2003; **14**: 2534–43.
78. Zhou Y, Vaidya VS, Brown RP *et al*. Comparison of kidney injury molecule-1 and other nephrotoxicity biomarkers in urine and kidney following acute exposure to gentamicin, mercury, and chromium. *Toxicological Sciences.* 2008; **101**: 159–70.
79. Perico N, Cattaneo D, Remuzzi G. Kidney injury molecule 1: In search of biomarkers of chronic tubulointerstitial damage and disease progression. *American Journal of Kidney Diseases.* 2009; **53**: 1–4.
80. Vaidya VS, Ramirez V, Ichimura T *et al*. Urinary kidney injury molecule-1: A sensitive quantitative biomarker for early detection of kidney tubular injury. New Orleans, LA: American Physiological Society Conference Proceedings, 2005: F517–29.
81. Elinder C-G, Edling C, Lindberg E *et al*. Beta-2-microglobulinuria among workers previously exposed to cadmium: Follow-up and dose–response analyses. *American Journal of Industrial Medicine.* 1985; **8**: 553–64.
82. Kido T, Honda R, Yamada T *et al*. Alpha-1-microglobulin determination in urine for the detection of renal tubular dysfunction caused by exposure to cadmium. *Toxicology Letters.* 1985; **24**: 195–201.
83. Savolainen H. Cadmium-associated renal disease. *Renal Failure.* 1995; **17**: 483–7.
84. Druet P, Kleinknecht D. Toxic glomerulonephritis. *La Presse Médicale.* 1989; **18**: 1840–5.
85. Becker C, Becker E, Maher J, Schreiner G. Nephrotic syndrome after contact with mercury: A report of five cases. *Archives of Internal Medicine.* 1962; **110**: 178.
86. Soo Y, Chow K, Lam C *et al*. A whitened face woman with nephrotic syndrome. *American Journal of Kidney Diseases.* 2003; **41**: 250–3.
87. Cardenas A, Roels H, Bernard A *et al*. Markers of early renal changes induced by industrial pollutants. I. Application to workers exposed to mercury vapour. *British Journal of Industrial Medicine.* 1993; **50**: 17–27.
88. Stonard M, Chater B, Duffield D *et al*. An evaluation of renal function in workers occupationally exposed to mercury vapour. *International Archives of Occupational and Environmental Health.* 1983; **52**: 177–89.
89. Mandic L, Radmila M, Jelena A, Dubravka D. Change in the iso-enzyme profiles of urinary N-acetyl-beta-D-glucosoaminidase in workers exposed to mercury. *Toxicology and Industrial Health.* 2002; **18**: 207–14.
90. Olfert SM, Felknor SA, Delclos GL. An updated review of the literature: Risk factors for bladder cancer with focus on occupational exposures. *Southern Medical Journal.* 2006; **99**: 1256–63.
91. Golka K, Wiese A, Assennato G, Bolt HM. Occupational exposure and urological cancer. *World Journal of Urology.* 2004; **21**: 382–91.
92. Volpe A, Racioppi M, D'Agostino D *et al*. Bladder tumor markers: A review of the literature. *International Journal of Biological Markers.* 2008; **23**: 249–61.
93. Jamshidian H, Kor K, Djalali M. Urine concentration of nuclear matrix protein 22 for diagnosis of transitional cell carcinoma of bladder. *Urology Journal.* 2008; **5**: 243–7.
94. Budman LI, Kassouf W, Steinberg JR. Biomarkers for defection and surveillance of bladder cancer. *Canadian Urological Association Journal.* 2008; **2**: 212–21.
95. van Tilborg AAG, Bangma CH, Zwarthoff EC. Bladder cancer biomarkers and their role in surveillance and screening. *International Journal of Urology.* 2009; **16**: 23–30.
96. McFarlane I, Bomford A, Sherwood R. *Liver disease and laboratory medicine.* Laboratory Medicine Series. McCreanor G, Marshall W (eds). London: ACB Venture Publications, 2000.
97. Fernandez-D'Pool J, Orono-Osorio A. Liver function of workers occupationally exposed to mixed organic solvents in a petrochemical industry. *Investigación Clínica.* 2001; **42**: 87–106.
98. Das SK, Dhanya L, Vasudevan DM. Biomarkers of alcoholism: An updated review. *Scandinavian Journal of Clinical and Laboratory Investigation.* 2008; **68**: 81–92.
99. Crespi V, Andreotta U, Tettamanzi E, Ferrario MM. CDT: A biological marker of alcohol abuse. *Medicina Del Lavoro.* 2007; **98**: 466–74.
100. Mason HJ, Wheeler J, Purba J *et al*. Hepatic effects of chronic exposure to mixed solvents. *Clinical Chemistry.* 1994; **40**: 1464–6.
101. Simko V, Michael S. Urinary bile acids in population screening for inapparent liver disease. *Hepato-Gastroenterology.* 1998; **45**: 1706–14.
102. Ooteman MC, Vago AR, Koury MC. Evaluation of MAT, IgM ELISA and PCR methods for the diagnosis of human leptospirosis. *Journal of Microbiological Methods.* 2006; **65**: 247–57.

SECTION THREE

Extent and attribution of occupational disease

6	Epidemiological methods and evidence-based occupational medicine *David Coggon*	77
7	Attribution of disease *Anthony Newman Taylor and David Coggon*	89
8	Compensation schemes *Anthony Newman Taylor and David Walters*	96

6

Epidemiological methods and evidence-based occupational medicine

DAVID COGGON

Introduction	77	Health outcomes other than disease or illness	86
Concepts and terminology	77	Evidence-based occupational medicine	86
Study designs	80	Further reading	87
Routine surveillance of occupational disorders	84	References	88

INTRODUCTION

Epidemiology is the branch of science that is concerned with the distribution and determinants of health outcomes in populations. The health outcomes investigated include not only diseases, but also illness (subjective absence of well-being) and disability. Determinants are predictors of the risk that an outcome will occur. They may directly cause the outcome, or while not being causal themselves, they may serve as markers for causes. For example, employment in manual work predicts a higher risk of cervical cancer, but it is not thought to cause the disease.

Along with toxicology, ergonomics and psychology, epidemiology is one of the main scientific disciplines that underpin the practice of occupational medicine. One major application is in the identification and confirmation of health hazards, in their characterization (understanding how the risk of adverse outcomes varies according to the circumstances and extent of exposure to the hazardous agent or activity), and in monitoring the effectiveness of control measures. It is also used in the prioritization of research and of interventions aimed at the prevention of occupational disorders. In addition, it can inform decisions in the management of individuals who have developed occupational diseases (e.g. whether they should change to a different job) or who have characteristics that would render them more susceptible to an occupational hazard if they undertook certain types of work. Another important use is in determining eligibility for compensation for occupational diseases, both through social security schemes and through litigation.

This chapter introduces the main concepts of occupational epidemiology and describes the methods of investigation that are used most frequently. It also outlines the methods by which epidemiological and other scientific evidence is collated so that that occupational health policy and practice can be optimized.

CONCEPTS AND TERMINOLOGY

Like most scientific disciplines, epidemiology has its own technical vocabulary. Terms are used with precise meanings that do not always correspond exactly with their usage in everyday language. To complicate matters further, not all of the meanings are universally agreed and some terms are used differently by different epidemiologists. The sections that follow describe some of the most important epidemiological concepts, where possible using standardized nomenclature.

Measures of disease and illness

CASE DEFINITION

Epidemiological investigation of a disorder requires quantification of its occurrence. Some diseases, such as cancer, are relatively all-or-none. While it may sometimes be difficult to decide whether or not a tumour is malignant, most people can be classified with some confidence as being either cases or non-cases of cancer. Many other disorders occur in a continuous spectrum of severity, in which the distinction between normality and abnormality is ill defined. For example, it is debateable at what point mild impairment of hearing on audiometry should be classed as deafness, or how much lower than the expected value forced expiratory volume in one second (FEV_1) should be before a patient is considered to have chronic obstructive pulmonary disease (COPD). However, to simplify their consideration, disorders of this type often are also classified dichotomously, so that, for example, a person is deemed either to be a case of COPD or not. Where this dichotomization is performed, the definition of a case should be unambiguous, even if somewhat arbitrary. Otherwise, findings cannot be interpreted satisfactorily.

Incidence, mortality and prevalence

Various measures are used to summarize the frequency with which disease or illness occurs in populations. The **incidence** of a disorder is the rate at which new cases occur over a defined period of time. For example, in 2004, the incidence of newly diagnosed mesothelioma among men in England was 6.2 per 100 000 per year. The **mortality** or **death rate** from a disease is the incidence of deaths for which it is thought to be the underlying cause. The **prevalence** of a disorder is the proportion of a population who are cases at a defined point in time or over a defined period. For example, the prevalence of low birthweight (<2.5 kg) in a sample of babies born over the course of two years might be 5 per cent. In contrast to incidence, which relates to an event (becoming a case), prevalence refers to a state (being a case).

Each of the above measures has its particular applications. Incidence is the index of disease occurrence that is of most immediate relevance to understanding of causation. For reasons of practicality and availability of data, mortality or prevalence may sometimes be used as a proxy for incidence in studies of causation, but care is then needed in interpretation. For example, a factor might be associated with increased mortality from a disease not because it increases people's risk of developing the disorder, but because it makes them more likely to die from it should they get it. Similarly, a factor could be associated with a higher prevalence of a disease because it delays recovery or promotes survival (i.e. people remain cases for longer) rather than because it increases incidence.

Proportional mortality

All of the measures that have been described are rates in which the occurrence of cases is related to a population 'at risk'. Sometimes, however, the size of the population that gives rise to a group of cases is unknown. For example, we may know from death certificates how many carpenters died from pleural mesothelioma in Scotland over the course of a year, but not the total population of carpenters from which these cases came. In these circumstances, the number of deaths from all causes is sometimes used as a proxy index of the population at risk. Thus, we might compare the proportion of all deaths that were ascribed to pleural mesothelioma in carpenters with that in other occupations. This use of **proportional mortality** is less satisfactory than analysis based on mortality rates insofar as the total number of deaths in a population depends on its overall (all cause) death rate, as well as its size (see Routine surveillance of occupational mortality, p. 84).

Crude and specific rates

Disease rates may be 'crude' (i.e. relating to a population in its entirety), or sex- and age-specific (i.e. relating to specific subsets of the population defined by sex and age). Because the occurrence of most disorders varies substantially by sex and age, sex- and age-specific rates usually allow more useful comparison between populations than crude rates. They can, however, be rather unwieldy, especially if there are a large number of sex and age strata in an analysis.

Standardized rates

One way of overcoming this difficulty is to summarize the sex- and age-specific rates for each population by a weighted average, the weighting factors being derived from the demographic distribution of a defined 'standard population'. This technique is known as **direct standardization**.

Another method of accounting for sex and age when summarizing disease occurrence in a population is **indirect standardization**. Here, the number of cases that occur in the study population over a defined period is compared with the number that would have been expected had the study population experienced the sex- and age-specific rates of a defined standard population. The ratio of observed to expected cases, expressed either as a decimal or as a percentage, is known as a **standardized morbidity ratio**, or if the cases are deaths, **standardized mortality ratio** (SMR).

Measures of association

Much of epidemiology involves comparing rates of disease or illness between populations. For example, to assess the risk from a chemical in the workplace, the incidence of adverse outcomes might be compared in people with different levels of exposure to the chemical. Various measures can be used to summarize associations between risk factors (characteristics or exposures that might influence or predict the risk of a health outcome) and health outcomes.

Attributable risk is the difference in risk between someone who is exposed to a risk factor and someone who is not. According to the nature of the health outcome, this might correspond to a difference in incidence, mortality or prevalence rates between exposed and unexposed populations. Attributable risk is the measure of association that is most relevant to the management of risk for the individual. For example, when deciding whether or not it is acceptable for a person with a history of asthma to work with a respiratory sensitizer, it is the attributable risk of illness and disability from undertaking the job that must be considered.

Relative risk is the ratio of risk in a person who is exposed to a risk factor to that in someone who is unexposed. This corresponds to a ratio of incidence, mortality or prevalence rates in exposed relative to unexposed populations.

An **odds ratio** compares the odds of a health outcome in people with and without an exposure (odds being defined such that a risk of $1/N$ equates to odds of $1/(N-1)$). In most circumstances, odds ratios approximate closely to relative risks. Unlike relative risks, however, they can be estimated directly from case–control studies (see Case–control studies, p. 83).

Population attributable fraction is the proportion of cases in a population that would be eliminated if risk of the health outcome in exposed people were reduced to that in the unexposed. It is useful in characterizing the impact of a causal factor in a population, and therefore in the management of risk at a population level.

The **attributable fraction in exposed persons** (AF_{exp}) is the proportion of cases among exposed members of a population that would be eliminated if their risk of the health outcome were reduced to that of the unexposed. It provides an index of the confidence with which a disease can be attributed to a causal factor in a case that has been exposed to that factor. For example, if the AF_{exp} for lung cancer from a given exposure is greater than 0.5, this implies a more than 50 per cent chance that lung cancer occurring in an exposed person would not have occurred in the absence of the exposure. AF_{exp} is thus relevant to decisions about compensation for occupational diseases. It is related to relative risk (RR) by the formula:

$$AF_{exp} = (RR - 1)/RR$$

Considerations in the design and interpretation of epidemiological studies

POPULATIONS AND SAMPLES

Epidemiological investigations normally collect and analyse data from a sample of individuals or populations with the aim of drawing conclusions that apply more widely. For example, a study might assess the association between occupational lifting and hip osteoarthritis in a sample of people selected from the general population, with the aim of characterizing the association in the population as a whole. A 'statistic' for the study sample (the relative risk of hip osteoarthritis from occupational lifting in the sample) is used to estimate a corresponding population 'parameter' (the relative risk of hip osteoarthritis from occupational lifting among people in general).

BIAS

An important consideration in the design and interpretation of epidemiological studies is the potential for 'bias'. **Bias** is a systematic tendency to underestimate or overestimate a parameter of interest because of a deficiency in the design or execution of a study. It may arise, for example, if the study sample is systematically unrepresentative of the wider population because of the way in which it has been recruited, or if the information about risk factors or health outcomes in the study sample is inaccurate. Because of the practical constraints on research in human subjects, complete elimination of bias from epidemiological studies is virtually impossible. However, studies should be designed to minimize bias and their interpretation should take into account the possible impact of any bias that remains. It should be noted that bias is specific to the parameter that is being estimated. A low response rate from people invited to take part in a study might seriously bias estimates of one parameter, while not materially influencing estimates of another.

CHANCE

Even where the method of recruitment to a study is unbiased with regard to the parameter of interest, the study sample may still be unrepresentative simply by chance. Thus, another study sample selected in a similar fashion, but perhaps a different time period, would not be expected to give exactly the same estimate for the parameter. The scope for chance variation of this type depends partly on the size of the study sample. Other things being equal, larger samples are less likely to be unrepresentative by chance than smaller samples. Therefore, studies should be designed to ensure that they have adequate size and 'statistical power'. Furthermore, the uncertainties relating to chance variation between samples must be taken into account when interpreting studies. This will be assisted by calculations of **statistical significance** or (more informatively) of **confidence intervals** around parameter estimates.

STATISTICAL SIGNIFICANCE

A test of statistical significance starts with a 'null hypothesis' about the wider population to which the findings of the study will be extrapolated (e.g. that there is no association between occupational lifting and hip osteoarthritis in this wider population). With the assumption that this null hypothesis applies, it then calculates the probability of obtaining findings as or more extreme than those observed in the study sample, simply through chance variation in sample selection. If this probability (p-value) is low, the null hypothesis becomes less tenable, and may be rejected in favour of an alternative (e.g. that occupational lifting is truly associated with hip osteoarthritis).

CONFIDENCE INTERVALS

A confidence interval around an estimate of a parameter gives a range within which, in the absence of bias, the parameter might normally be expected to lie. Most often, 95 per cent confidence intervals are derived. These are calculated in such a way that, in the absence of bias, 95 per cent of study samples would be expected to produce confidence intervals that included the true value of the population parameter. Because they are less likely to be unrepresentative by chance, larger samples tend to give tighter confidence intervals.

CONSISTENCY WITH OTHER STUDIES

Importantly, assessment of the possible contribution of chance to the findings of a study depends not only on statistical analysis of the data obtained in the study, but also on the weight of relevant evidence from other research, both epidemiological and in other disciplines. For example, an association between a chemical and cancer might be attributed to chance even though it was statistically significant (i.e. carried a low p-value), if other similar epidemiological studies had found no association and toxicological testing in animals did not suggest that the chemical was a carcinogen.

CONFOUNDING

A further consideration in epidemiological studies of causation is the potential for **confounding**. Confounding affects inferences about causation from observed statistical associations. As an example, driving a lorry might be associated with an elevated risk of bladder cancer not because the occupation is hazardous, but because lorry drivers smoke more heavily than the average. In general, confounding occurs when a **confounding factor** is associated with the risk factor under investigation, and independently determines or predicts risk of the health outcome. Depending on the nature of its association with the primary risk factor and of its relation to the health outcome, the effect of a confounding factor can be either to inflate or reduce estimates of causal impact. Various techniques are used to reduce or eliminate confounding effects in epidemiological studies, including restriction of recruitment so that exposure to a confounding factor within the study sample is uniform (e.g. recruiting only non-smokers), matching participants according to their level of exposure to the confounder, and statistical adjustment in analysis.

EFFECT MODIFICATION

Sometimes confused with confounding is **effect modification**. This occurs when the strength of the association with one risk factor (usually quantified in terms of a relative risk) varies according to the presence or level of another factor (the effect modifier). For example, the relative risk of nonmelanoma skin cancer from occupational exposure to sunlight differs according to skin colour, being lower in those with higher skin pigmentation that those with less pigmentation, e.g. in Afro-Carribeans compared to Caucasians. Effect modification is one reason why two studies of the same exposure and health outcome may produce differing estimates of risk.

STUDY DESIGNS

The most natural way to test a causal hypothesis or to quantify the impact of a cause on an outcome is to conduct a planned experiment. For ethical reasons, human experimental studies are not widely used in occupational health research – it is not usually acceptable deliberately to expose a volunteer to a hazardous agent. However, experimental studies have been used to assess the benefits of strategies to prevent illness, to investigate determinants of exposure when handling hazardous materials, such as pesticides (using an innocuous surrogate marker such as a dye), and to explore biochemical consequences of exposure to hazardous chemicals at levels well below those at which any adverse effects on health would be expected. More often, occupational studies are observational in nature. In other words, the investigator does not change participants' exposures as part of the investigation, but rather studies people as they happen to have been exposed. Some observational studies analyse data at a population level (**ecological studies**), but most collect and analyse information about individuals.

Randomized controlled experimental studies

The most widely applied experimental design in medical research overall is the randomized controlled experiment. Studies of this sort entail comparison between two or more alternative exposures, one of which may be a control involving no intervention by the investigator. Subjects who meet predefined criteria of eligibility for study are identified, and if they consent, are randomly assigned to one of the exposure groups. They are then followed up systematically, and outcomes (both beneficial and adverse) are compared according to the exposure to which they were allocated. Effects can be summarized by various measures, including attributable and relative risks/benefits. Depending on the nature of the intervention, there may be scope to reduce bias by 'blinding' participants and/or investigators to the exposure that individuals receive until the relevant health outcomes have been assessed.

Where for some reason not all participants receive the exposure to which they were assigned according to the study protocol (e.g. because of non-compliance with the requirements of the intervention), it is particularly important that outcomes be compared according to the original exposure allocation. This is because those who drop out may have withdrawn because of an adverse effect of the exposure under investigation, which otherwise would be underascertained. However, it is usually helpful to carry out a secondary analysis according to the exposure actually received. Interpretation would be circumspect if the benefits from allocation to an intervention were limited entirely to subjects who did not receive the assigned exposure as planned.

The particular strength of randomized controlled experiments is that randomization, if carried out on a sufficiently large scale, tends to ensure that exposure groups are similar with regard to potential confounding factors (including even those of which the investigator is unaware). However, if desired, even tighter control on confounding can be ensured by stratifying subjects before randomization, according to important determinants of outcome, and by 'blocking' the randomization so that within each stratum, there is always a close balance between the numbers of subjects assigned to each exposure. For example, exposures to two interventions might be randomly allocated within successive blocks of six (three to each intervention). In this way, within the matching stratum, the difference in numbers assigned to each exposure would never be greater than three.

Randomized crossover studies

A special type of randomized experiment is the randomized crossover study, a design in which each subject serves as his or her own control. The method is appropriate for investigation of short-lived effects of exposure. Again, subjects who meet specified eligibility criteria are identified and recruited (after giving informed consent). Each participant then receives each of the exposures under investigation sequentially, but in a randomly determined order (often with a 'wash-out' period between successive exposures). Outcomes are assessed during or immediately after each exposure, and are compared. Because comparisons are within rather than between participants, the method is particularly suited to investigation of subjective outcomes such as levels of pain, especially if the subject can be blinded to the exposure received.

Non-randomized controlled experiments

The benefits of randomization in control of confounding are only realized when the randomization is carried out on a sufficiently large scale. If 200 subjects are randomly allocated, half to one exposure and half to another, it is unlikely statistically that there will be a major imbalance of confounding factors between the two exposure groups. However, this does not apply where the number of units randomized is small. For example, in a study to evaluate an ergonomic intervention involving the installation of new lifting equipment in workplaces, only six workforces might be available for study. If three workforces were randomly allocated to the intervention and three to serve as a control, there could easily be important differences between the workers in the two exposure groups just by chance. In this situation, it would be better to use a non-randomized experimental design, in which allocation of the intervention to workforces was carefully planned in a way that minimized such differences between the intervention and control groups.

Sometimes non-randomized controlled experiments can be further enhanced by including a comparison of exposure groups both before and after the experimental exposure is introduced. If there are differences between the intervention and control groups before exposure, perhaps because of unrecognized confounders, these can then be controlled statistically when evaluating the impact of the intervention.

Ecological studies

Ecological studies are observational investigations which collate and analyse information about exposures and/or health outcomes at a population level. For example, a study might compare death rates from pleural mesothelioma in different countries according to their historical rates of importing asbestos and asbestos products. In occupational epidemiology, ecological studies are most often based on populations defined geographically, by occupation, by time or by combinations of these variables. They have the advantage that the data used are often readily available from routinely published statistics. However, because the information is only for populations and not individuals, it may be difficult to control for possible confounding effects. The main applications of ecological studies are in monitoring trends, and in the generation and early exploration of causal hypotheses.

Cohort studies

In a cohort study, individuals who differ in their exposure to known or suspected risk factors for a health outcome are identified. They are then followed up systematically to ascertain the subsequent occurrence of the outcome, which is compared according to the earlier presence or level of the risk factors. For example, a 'cohort' of pregnant women might be identified when they attend hospital for antenatal care, and their exposure to occupational activities during the first trimester of pregnancy assessed. They could then be followed up systematically to term, and the prevalence of outcomes, such as preterm delivery and low birthweight, compared according to their activities early in pregnancy. Where the outcome in a cohort study is the incidence of a disease (or a proxy for incidence such as mortality) estimates can be made of both attributable and relative risk.

The subjects in a cohort study may be selectively sampled according to their exposure to risk factors of interest. For example, a study might follow up a group of workers chosen because they were known to have high exposure to lead and a control group who were unexposed to the metal in their work. Alternatively, the cohort may be selected from the general population without regard to likelihood or levels of exposure. A well-known example of this approach is the Framingham study, which has followed up adult residents of the town of Framingham in Massachusetts over many years, collecting information about a wide range of risk factors (including occupational exposures) and health outcomes.[1]

Various sources of information can be used to characterize exposures in cohort studies, including employment records (giving data on job history), questionnaires, direct observation (e.g. of physical activities at work), environmental or personal monitoring of exposure to chemical or physical hazards, and measurement of relevant biomarkers in tissues and body fluids. Sometimes, the assessment of exposure is made at a single point in time and sometimes information about exposure is collected on repeated occasions over a period of time. Often in occupational cohort studies, the classification of exposures combines information on individual occupational history with generic data on patterns of exposure in different jobs (and perhaps time periods) held in the form of a 'job–exposure matrix'. Where possible, information is collected about potentially confounding exposures, as well as the risk factors of primary interest. Their effects can then be taken into account statistically when the study is analysed.

Methods for ascertaining health outcome vary according to the nature of the outcome. They include the use of health records (e.g. cancer registrations), death certificates (which give causes of death), questionnaires, physical examination and clinical investigations (e.g. spirometry, radiographs or biochemical measurements).

A major strength of the cohort study method is the assessment of exposures, which is the starting point for the investigation and often more reliable than with other study designs. The method is relatively efficient for the investigation of rare exposures, since participants can be selectively sampled according to their known or likely exposures. Furthermore, if desired, the same study can often be used to examine multiple health outcomes with little additional effort. For example, a cohort study using cancer registrations to ascertain outcome, could provide information about risk for each of a number of malignancies. On the other hand, cohort studies are less efficient for the investigation of rare health outcomes, since large numbers of people must be followed for long periods in order that the number of observed cases is sufficient for meaningful statistical analysis. Prolonged follow up may also be required where a hazardous exposure only increases the risk of a health outcome after a long latent interval. For example, most occupational cancers do not occur in excess until ten or more years after people are first exposed to the relevant carcinogen.

Two modifications to the cohort study method sometimes help to address these limitations. One involves the use of incidence or mortality rates in the general population as a comparator for disease experience in a cohort exposed to a risk factor. For example, the incidence of leukaemia in a cohort of hospital employees exposed to the sterilant, ethylene oxide, has been compared with that expected from cancer registration rates in the national population.[2] This approach is reasonable where relevant exposures in the general population are trivial in comparison with those experienced by the study cohort, and it has the advantage that the rates for the general population that are used for comparison are readily available and statistically stable (because they are based on large numbers of cases). However, it is important that the method for ascertaining cases in the study cohort be similar to that for the general population (e.g. both based on cancer registrations) or risk estimates will be liable to bias. A further limitation may be a lack of information about important confounders in the general population.

In cohort studies that compare mortality or cancer incidence with rates in the general population, risk estimates are often presented in the form of standardized mortality ratios (SMRs) or standardized incidence ratios (SIRs) based on a person-years analysis. This involves computing the time that each cohort member was at risk (i.e. under follow up and eligible to become a case if he/she developed the relevant health outcome) for different combinations of sex, age and calendar period. The person-years at risk for each combination are summed across all cohort members, and multiplied by the corresponding sex-, age- and calendar period-specific outcome rates in the comparison population to give an expected number of cases for that combination. These expected numbers are then summed across all combinations of sex, age and calendar period to derive an overall expected number of cases. The ratio of the number of cases observed to the number expected is the SMR or SIR.

The second modification is to conduct the cohort study retrospectively. With this approach, the cohort is defined according to historical criteria (e.g. all of the workers who were employed at a particular manufacturing plant for at least six months during a specified period), and eligible subjects are identified from preserved records. Health outcomes are then examined in the time since each subject fulfilled the criteria for entry to the study. To be amenable to this approach, the relevant health outcome must be ascertainable at the time the study is conducted. For example, in many countries, mortality by cause of death can be established retrospectively from death certificates and cancer incidence from records of cancer registrations. In other studies, the assessment of outcome may depend on being able to trace and contact a sufficiently large and representative proportion of the original cohort so that they can be questioned about their health during the follow-up period or examined for changes in health measures, such as pulmonary function. Importantly, the identification of the cohort should not depend on factors associated with subsequent health outcome. For example, a retrospective cohort study of lung cancer at a coke oven could be seriously biased if the records of ex-employees who were known to have died had been selectively removed from archived files.

While the main use of cohort studies in occupational medicine is to identify and characterize occupational causes of disease, they may also inform decisions in case management. For example, systematic follow up of a cohort of patients presenting with a first epileptic seizure could provide information on the risk of further seizures that was useful in deciding whether and when such individuals should be allowed to drive professionally or work at heights.

Case–control studies

In a case–control (also known as case–referent) study, people who have developed a health outcome (cases) are identified, and their past exposure to known or suspected determinants of the outcome (risk factors) is compared with that of controls who do not have the outcome. This allows estimation of odds ratios for each risk factor. For example, to assess the risk of knee osteoarthritis from prolonged kneeling, past histories of occupational kneeling might be compared in patients listed for knee surgery because of osteoarthritis and controls who do not have knee complaints.

The case–control design is best understood if it is viewed as sampling subjects from a larger, usually hypothetical, cohort study. In most cohort studies, only a small minority of subjects develop the health outcome of interest during follow up. This imbalance between cases and non-cases is statistically inefficient. In effect, a case–control study increases statistical efficiency by collecting information about all (or a substantial proportion) of the cases in a cohort, but about only a representative sample of the non-cases.

In choosing a population in which to conduct a case–control study, three criteria must be considered. First, there must be a satisfactory way of identifying and recruiting adequate numbers of cases. Second, there must be adequate heterogeneity of exposure to risk factors in the study population. Third, there must be a satisfactory way of ascertaining exposures in cases and controls. If the number of cases studied is too few or the exposures of participants are all very similar, the study will have little statistical power to detect associations with risk factors. If it is only possible to ascertain a proportion of the cases that occur in the study population over the period of investigation, then the cases studied should be representative with respect to the risk factors under investigation. If exposures cannot be ascertained satisfactorily, the study will be uninformative or misleading.

The aim in selecting controls is that their exposures to the risk factors under investigation should be representative of those in the real or theoretical cohort from which the cases derived (i.e. those people who could have been included in the study as cases had they developed the health outcome under investigation). In addition, the exposures of controls should be ascertainable in the same way and with similar accuracy as for cases. Ideally, exposures would be assessed with complete accuracy in both cases and controls, but in practice this is rarely achievable. However, if errors in exposure assessment are non-differential (i.e. similar in cases and controls), any resultant bias will be conservative (tending to obscure associations rather than to give spuriously elevated estimates of risk).

The assessment of exposures is by definition retrospective. Various sources of information may be used, including documented records, questionnaires and measurement of biomarkers. However, where biomarkers are employed, they must be indicative of exposures before the health outcome developed and unmodified by its subsequent occurrence. For example, measurement of a urinary metabolite as a marker of exposure in a case–control study of glomerulonephritis would be inappropriate if excretion of the metabolite were altered by the presence of the disease.

Suspected confounding factors can be addressed by measuring them and then adjusting statistically for their presence or level. This adjustment can sometimes be made more efficient by matching controls to cases, either individually or as a group, according to their exposure to the confounder. However, in a case–control study, matching does not of itself eliminate confounding effects and appropriate statistical analysis is still required. Where matching is employed, controls should have exposures that are representative of those in members of the source cohort from the same stratum of the matched variable.

Case–control studies have the advantage that they are statistically more efficient than cohort studies, particularly in the investigation of rare health outcomes. Moreover, they do not require prolonged follow up. However, they can be limited by difficulties in achieving unbiased retrospective assessment of exposures, especially where the ascertainment of exposure relies on subjective recall. Also, while they provide estimates of odds ratios, and therefore of approximate relative risks, they cannot be used to estimate attributable risks without additional information from other sources.

NESTED CASE–CONTROL STUDIES

As indicated above, case–control studies are sometimes 'nested' within a larger cohort investigation. This is normally done to increase efficiency or because it would be impractical to collect complete data on exposure to risk factors for all members of the cohort. For example, in a prospective cohort study of cancer incidence among workers exposed to dioxins, blood samples might be collected at baseline that could be used to measure dioxin levels in the study participants. However, because the assay for dioxins is relatively expensive, rather than performing it in every blood sample, it might be preferable to store the samples, and then carry out the measurement of dioxins only for the cancer cases that occurred during subsequent follow up and for a group of appropriately chosen controls. This could reduce costs substantially with little reduction in statistical power.

Case–cohort studies

Like nested case–control studies, case–cohort studies are a way of making cohort investigations more efficient. As in a nested case–control study, information about exposures is obtained for all of the cases that occur during the follow-up period, but for only a sample of non-cases. However, instead of sampling controls from the non-cases that were 'at risk' when each case occurred, the person-years at risk in each exposure category (and thereby the expected numbers of cases) are estimated by sampling controls at random from the total cohort.

Apart from its efficiency, especially when the assessment of individual exposures is relatively costly, the case–cohort method has the advantage that it is readily amenable to simultaneous investigation of multiple health outcomes. Furthermore, if follow up is subsequently extended, only the exposures of the new cases are required to update the analysis (this is in contrast to the nested case–control design, in which exposure would have to be characterized also for additional controls selected to match the new cases). However, bias could arise if the method for assessing the exposures of new cases differed from that carried out earlier for the baseline sample of cohort members. One reason why this might occur is that where exposure assessment is limited only to new cases, the assessor cannot easily be 'blinded' with regard to health outcome.

Case–crossover studies

Case–crossover studies are used to investigate known and suspected causes that have only a short-lived impact on the risk of a health outcome. The method is in some ways similar to that of a case–control study, but instead of comparing cases with non-cases, the exposures of cases immediately before development of the health outcome are compared with those of the same individuals at some other time. Thus, each subject serves as his or her own control (rather like in a randomized crossover experiment). A case–crossover design might be used, for example, to assess the risk of road traffic accidents from using a mobile phone while driving. Drivers who were involved in accidents would be asked about their use of a mobile phone in the minutes before the accident, and during one or more earlier control periods of similar duration.

The method is not as well developed and has not been as widely implemented as the other study designs described in this chapter. In particular, more thought is needed on the criteria by which control periods are optimally specified. By analogy with the case–control method, one might expect the control period to be representative (in terms of relevant exposures) of the times when the subject was 'at risk' of becoming a case. However, statistical efficiency may be increased if control periods are matched to case periods for one or more potential confounders. Control periods should then be representative of 'at-risk' times within the relevant stratum of matching.

A further challenge is that the subject will almost always be aware of when the relevant health outcome occurred. Thus, assessment of exposures that depends on the subject's recall cannot be blinded. This could bias estimates of risk if exposures in different time periods were not uniformly remembered. It would not be a problem, however, where the assessment of exposures was from contemporaneous records rather than from memory.

A major advantage of the case–crossover method is that, because the subject serves as his or her own control, it eliminates the potential for confounding by long-term characteristics that might complicate interpretation of a case–control study.

Cross-sectional surveys

In a cross-sectional study, information is collected from a sample of individuals at a single point in time, about health outcomes and/or exposure to possible determinants of health. The information obtained may relate to the subject's health or exposures at the time of the survey, or at some time in the past. For example, a cross-sectional study might be used to assess the current prevalence of sensorineural deafness in a sample of adults from the general population, and also their lifetime prevalence of exposure to noisy working conditions. The people studied in a cross-sectional survey may be selected without regard to their exposure, or they may be chosen because they have known exposures (e.g. to allow a comparison of health between exposed and unexposed groups).

Where information is collected about both exposures and health outcomes, the study can be used to investigate their statistical association. However, care is needed in interpretation. Because of the cross-sectional design, there may be difficulty in distinguishing the direction of cause and effect. For example, if barmen were found to drink more alcohol than other occupational groups, that could be because work in a job with ready access to alcohol encourages higher consumption. On the other hand, it could reflect a tendency for people who enjoy alcohol preferentially to seek work in bars. Also, there is a danger that selection effects may distort associations. For example, a cross-sectional comparison of the prevalence of asthma between people working with laboratory animals and unexposed controls could be misleading if people who developed allergies to animal proteins tended selectively to move to other jobs because of their symptoms. Such people would be under-represented in a cross-sectional sample of laboratory workers, leading risks to be underestimated.

Despite these limitations, cross-sectional surveys can be a valuable source of information about the occurrence of occupational illness and its causes.

ROUTINE SURVEILLANCE OF OCCUPATIONAL DISORDERS

One of the major applications of occupational epidemiology is in the routine surveillance of work-related illness and disease. Information about the occurrence of occupational disorders is used to target and prioritize control measures, and to monitor the success of preventive strategies.

The methods used to assess the frequency of occupational disorders vary according to the way in which they are related to work. Some diseases occur only as a consequence of occupational exposure (e.g. coal workers' pneumoconiosis, silicosis). For disorders of this type, the burden of disease attributable to work is indicated by its overall frequency in the population of interest. If the disease is commonly fatal, the required information could come from analysis of death certificates. If the disease normally attracts social security compensation, its incidence may be indicated in social security statistics. Otherwise, some form of reporting scheme may be required (see below).

Other disorders, although not specific to work, can nevertheless be attributed to occupation with confidence in the individual case, either because of specific clinical features (e.g. the demonstration of skin sensitization to an agent found only in the workplace), or because the relative risk and AF_{exp} for an occupational exposure are sufficiently high that attribution can reasonably be assumed in any case that has been exposed. In these circumstances, it is sufficient simply to ascertain and enumerate attributable cases. Again, social security statistics may be a useful source of information if the disorder is compensable (provided that the uptake of compensation by eligible cases is sufficiently high and does not vary importantly over time). Alternatively, attributable cases may be ascertained through a reporting scheme designed specifically for surveillance purposes. For example, in the UK, the University of Manchester has for some years operated a scheme in which cases of various occupational diseases are centrally notified by nationally representative panels of physicians.[3]

More challenging is the situation in which a disorder is caused by occupational exposures, but cannot be attributed to work with confidence in the individual case. For example, lung cancer is a hazard of work in coke ovens, but the relative risk is not so high that attribution can be assumed simply because a person with the disease has at some time worked in a coke oven. Moreover, there are no special clinical features that can establish coke ovens as the cause of lung cancer in an individual case. For hazards of this type, the burden of illness or disease that is attributable to work can be established only by controlled comparisons of risk. For example, the burden of lung cancer nationally from work in coke ovens could be estimated from a large case–control study of a nationally representative study population. Alternatively, the attributable risk of lung cancer from work in coke ovens might be estimated by comparing mortality rates in coke oven workers with those in other occupations (e.g. in a cohort study) and this risk estimate then combined with information on the national prevalence of employment in coke ovens. In practice, assessment of disease burden in this way is often far from straightforward. In particular, since individual risk varies according to the level and timing of relevant exposures, it may be difficult to extrapolate risk estimates from cohort studies of workforces, which often have been chosen for study because they have experienced unusually high exposures to a hazardous agent, to the patterns of exposure to the same agent that occur nationally. Nevertheless, if findings are interpreted with appropriate caution, useful conclusions can be drawn.

While it can be helpful to know the overall burden of a disease or illness that is attributable to an occupational exposure, it is often useful also to break down the total by, for example, occupation, industry or geographical region. This is possible with all of the approaches to monitoring that have been described.

Routine analyses of occupational mortality

One important source of information in the surveillance of occupational diseases is the routine analysis of occupational mortality at a national or regional level. Analyses of this sort have been carried out periodically in the UK for many years,[4] and have been performed also in the United States.[5,6] Their value lies not only in monitoring well-established occupational causes of mortality, but also in generating clues to previously unrecognized hazards. For example, an increased risk of infectious pneumonia following occupational exposure to metal fume first came to light in routinely generated statistics of mortality by cause among welders.[7]

Two methods of estimating risk have been applied in the routine analyses of occupational mortality carried out in the UK. In the first, the analysis focuses on deaths occurring in a period of up to five years surrounding a national census. Information about the number of deaths in a particular occupation from a specific underlying cause is obtained from death certificates (which in the UK include a record of the deceased's last full-time job). This is then compared with an expected number of deaths, calculated by applying sex- and age-specific rates for the country as a whole to the estimated numbers of people in the occupation nationally in the corresponding sex and age strata. These estimates of the populations at risk in each sex and age group are derived from information supplied by a representative subset of participants in the census. The ratio of observed to expected deaths gives a cause-specific SMR for the occupation under study.

The other method uses only information obtained from death certificates. The number of deaths by cause in each occupation is derived in the same way as for the SMR calculation described above. However, the expected number of deaths for a given occupation and cause of death is calculated by multiplying the sex- and age-specific proportions of deaths in all occupations combined that are ascribed to that cause by the number of deaths from all causes in the occupation of interest in the corresponding sex and age bands. In this case, the ratio of observed to expected deaths is a proportional mortality ratio (PMR).

Each of these methods has its strengths and limitations. A weakness of the SMR method is that data on occupation for the numerator and denominator of the risk estimate come from different sources, and this can lead to bias. For example, there is a tendency for the next of kin to promote their deceased relative when registering his or her death. Thus, a shopkeeper might be described as a company director. Where this occurs, the effect will be to inflate SMRs for more prestigious jobs. Another limitation is that SMR analyses can only be carried out for periods surrounding a census year. The PMR method is not restricted in this way, but has the disadvantage that PMRs are influenced not only by mortality from the cause of interest, but also by the overall death rate in an occupation. For example, if an occupation had unusually low death rates from common causes, such as heart disease and cancer, its PMR for a rarer cause, such as fibrosing alveolitis, could be elevated even when it was not a hazard of the occupation. These limitations must be taken into account when interpreting SMRs and PMRs from routine statistics of occupational mortality.

Similar methods of analysis can be applied to data on occupation from cancer registrations to generate standardized or proportional registration ratios (SRRs or PRRs). However, this is only possible where reliable information about occupation is available for at least the majority of cancers registered.

HEALTH OUTCOMES OTHER THAN DISEASE OR ILLNESS

In most occupational epidemiology, the health outcome investigated is a disease, illness or associated disability. However, the same study methods can often be used to look at other outcomes.

One application is in the investigation of factors influencing levels of exposure to hazardous agents. For example, a cross-sectional design might be used to explore the relation of working methods to individual uptake (dose) of a chemical pollutant, the outcome being assessed by measurement of a relevant biomarker. In this way, it was shown that a major determinant of occupational exposure to organophosphate sheep dip was whether the operator handled the concentrated product before it was diluted[8] – a finding that led to the redesign of containers with wider necks to reduce the risk of splashing.

Another area now being developed is the study of risk factors for biological effects such as cytogenetic abnormalities, that are thought to lie on, or be markers for processes on the pathway to serious disease. For example, one of the considerations that led the International Agency for Research on Cancer (IARC) to classify ethylene oxide as a human carcinogen was the demonstration that the frequency of chromosome aberrations is increased in exposed workers.[9] Such studies have the advantage that they may highlight a need to control hazardous occupational exposures at an early stage, before cases of overt disease have started to appear. Also, they may have greater statistical power than conventional studies to detect adverse effects and characterize exposure–response relationships.

EVIDENCE-BASED OCCUPATIONAL MEDICINE

Like other medical disciplines, occupational medicine is both an art and a science. While practitioners always bring their own unique personal skills and expertise to their work, their handling of occupational health problems should at the same time be consistent with the sum of relevant scientific evidence. Over recent decades, output from medical research, and specifically occupational health research, has grown rapidly, making it much more difficult for the individual practitioner to keep abreast of and assimilate new information as it becomes available. Even with the help of computerized literature searches and electronic publication of papers, there is a limit to the material that one individual can review for himself.

To address this problem, increasing emphasis is now given to formal secondary research, which attempts systematically to identify, collate and interpret published (and sometimes unpublished) scientific evidence on questions that are relevant to occupational health policy and practice. Reviews of this type initially focused mainly on the assessment of hazard and risk from occupational exposures, and were used to underpin regulatory policy, for example on exposure limits. More recently, however, the application of systematic reviews has extended to questions relevant to individual clinical decisions in the prevention and management of occupational disorders.

Methods of systematic review

As with any research study, the first step in a systematic review is to define the questions that will be addressed. An attempt is then made to identify all available evidence within prescribed limits (e.g. published in peer-reviewed papers or in specified languages) that pertains to these questions. The starting point for this is normally a search of one or more computerized databases that cover publications relevant to the focus of the review. Databases listing reports relevant to occupational medicine include Embase, Medline, PubMed, NIOSHTIC, PsycInfo and TOXLINE. The search is made by combining a series of search terms, using Boolean operators. An initial check is made to ensure that the numbers of publications identified and their titles seem appropriate, and if necessary, the search criteria are revised. The lists of publications from each database are then amalgamated, and duplicates eliminated.

Next, the titles and abstracts of the listed publications are scrutinized and those that are clearly irrelevant are eliminated. This may be done as a single exercise or in two stages (titles and then abstracts). For those publications that remain, the full text is retrieved and checked for relevance. In this way, a shortlist of relevant reports is compiled and the reference lists of these reports are checked for any additional publications that were not picked up by the original computer search. Again, abstracts and, if necessary, full texts are scanned to check for their relevance and where appropriate, the additional reports are added to the shortlist. This exercise not only guards against omission of important publications, but also serves as a check on the performance of the original search criteria. The identification of large numbers of new reports may suggest that the search criteria need revision. Each of the reports in the shortlist is then examined and summarized. The information abstracted is that which relates to the study questions and often this abstraction is facilitated by the use of a standardized format in which to record the information.

To reduce the chance of error, all stages of the process that are not automated are normally carried out independently by at least two members of the study team and any differences reconciled by discussion.

Once the required information has been abstracted, it is evaluated and synthesized. In some cases, the synthesis may extend to a formal meta-analysis in which summary estimates of outcome measures are calculated with confidence intervals. However, this is only appropriate where the design of the primary studies is sufficiently uniform, a requirement that is more often met for randomized controlled experiments than for the observational studies that are more common in occupational health research. Where studies addressing the same question produce apparently discordant results, possible explanations should be considered systematically (Table 6.1).

Some systematic reviews specify criteria in advance that will be used to grade the quality of studies, and greater weight is then given to findings from those that are classed as stronger. An attraction of this approach is that it helps to standardize assessment and interpretation, making it more reproducible. Thus, if a different group of researchers carried out the review to the same protocol, they should come to the same conclusions. However, there is a danger that evidence will be given inappropriate weight in the quest for repeatability. For example, a study showing a positive association between an exposure and disease might suffer from a bias, the effect of which was to reduce risk estimates. If the findings from this study were downgraded because of the bias, the evidence for a hazard could be assessed as weaker than it really was.

Some guidelines for systematic review have attempted to grade the strength of evidence provided by different study designs, with for example, randomized controlled experiments ranking higher than cohort studies and cohort studies higher than case–control studies. However, while in general, cohort studies are less prone to bias than case–control investigations, this is not universally true. Thus, it is better if the strength of evidence from each study is evaluated on its own merits rather than according to simple rules of thumb.

Translation into practice

Once an evidence-based review is completed, its value will only be realized if its findings are translated into policy or practice. Where the express purpose of the review is to inform regulation, this is usually straightforward, but where the aim is to guide the practice of individual healthcare workers or managers, a planned communication exercise may be required. The methods used will depend on the target audience, but may be assisted by early involvement and commitment of representatives from the groups whose practice will be affected. These representatives can then advise on the optimal methods of communication and assist in conveying findings to their constituency. A good example of this is the set of evidence-based guidelines published by NHS Plus on the management of chronic fatigue syndrome in relation to work.[10] These were drawn up following a review process that involved practising occupational physicians, and these individuals subsequently helped to disseminate the findings to their colleagues.

FURTHER READING

For readers seeking a more detailed account of epidemiological methods and the use of statistics in interpretation of epidemiological data, a number of textbooks are available.[11–14]

Table 6.1 Possible explanations for discordant results from epidemiological studies investigating the same association.

Differences in exposure	Even where exposures are defined in the same way, the mix of exposures may differ. For example, within an exposure category of >2 ppm-years, the mean exposure might be 15 ppm-years in one study, but only 2.5 ppm-years in another
Differences in health outcome	The same case definition may encompass a varying mix of cases with different causation. For example, oesophageal cancers might be mainly squamous cell tumours in one study and mainly adenocarcinomas in another
Bias	
Chance	
Confounding	
Effect modification	

> **Key points**
>
> - Epidemiology is the branch of science that is concerned with the distribution and determinants of health outcomes in populations.
> - Epidemiology is used in occupational medicine to identify, confirm and characterize health hazards in the workplace; monitor the

effectiveness of controls aimed at reducing health risks; prioritize research and interventions; inform decisions in clinical management; and determine eligibility for compensation because of occupational diseases.
- Planning of epidemiological studies and interpretation of their findings must take into consideration the possibility that results will be unrepresentative by chance or because of systematic bias or confounding.
- Various study designs are commonly employed, including randomized and non-randomized controlled experiments, ecological studies, cohort studies, case–control studies, case–cohort studies, case–crossover studies and cross-sectional surveys.
- Assessment of the overall balance of epidemiological evidence on a topic is often facilitated by formal systematic review, for which methods are now well developed.

REFERENCES

1. Felson DT, Hannan MT, Naimark A et al. Occupational physical demands, knee bending, and knee osteoarthritis: Results from the Framingham Study. *Journal of Rheumatology.* 1991; **18**: 1587–92.
2. Hagmar L, Mikoczy Z, Welinder H. Cancer incidence in Swedish sterilant workers exposed to ethylene oxide. *Occupational and Environmental Medicine.* 1995; **52**: 154–6.
3. Turner S, Lines S, Chen Y et al. Work-related infectious disease reported to the Occupational Disease Intelligence Network and The Health and Occupation Reporting network in the UK (2000–2003). *Occupational Medicine.* 2005; **55**: 275–81.
4. Drever F (ed.). Occupational health decennial supplement. (Series DS No. 10). London: HMSO, 1995.
5. Guralnick L. Mortality by occupation and cause of death among men 20 to 64 years of age, United States 1950 (vital statistics – special report 53, No. 3). Washington DC: US Dept HEW, 1963.
6. Milham S. Occupational mortality in Washington State 1950-71 (US Dept Health Educ Welfare Public Health Service publication No. 76-175). Washington DC: US Government Printing Office, 1976.
7. Coggon D, Inskip H, Winter P, Pannett B. Lobar pneumonia – an occupational disease in welders. *Lancet.* 1994; **344**: 41–3.
8. Buchanan D, Pilkington A, Sewell C et al. Estimation of cumulative exposure to organophosphate sheep dips in a study of chronic neurological health effects among United Kingdom sheep dippers. *Occupational and Environmental Medicine.* 2001; **58**: 694–701.
9. Grosse Y, Baan R, Straif K et al. Carcinogenicity of 1,3-butadiene, ethylene oxide, vinyl chloride, vinyl fluoride, and vinyl bromide. *The Lancet Oncology.* 2007; **8**: 679–80.
10. NHS Plus. Occupational aspects of the management of chronic fatigue syndrome: A national guideline. Available from: www.nhsplus.nhs.uk/.
11. Checkoway H, Pearce N, Kriebel D. *Research methods in occupational epidemiology.* Oxford: Oxford University Press, 2004.
12. Rothman KJ, Greenland S. *Modern epidemiology.* Philadelphia: Lippincott-Raven, 1998.
13. Coggon D. *Statistics in clinical practice.* London: BMJ Books, 2003.
14. Campbell MJ, Machin D. *Medical statistics – a common sense approach.* Chichester: Wiley, 1999.

7

Attribution of disease

ANTHONY NEWMAN TAYLOR AND DAVID COGGON

Introduction	89	Attribution in the individual patient	94
Causation	89	Attribution and disease registers	94
Attribution	92	References	95

Attribution: The ascribing of an effect to a cause.

Shorter Oxford English Dictionary

INTRODUCTION

Attribution of a disease to a particular cause in an individual is usually a matter of informed judgement. The judgement is based on the degree of certainty required, together with knowledge of causation in relation to the particular disease and the particular circumstances of the case. The level of certainty commonly applied, in medicine and the law, is 'on the balance of probabilities' or 'more likely than not'. As Lord Denning put it, 'If the evidence is such that the tribunal can say "we think it more probable than not", the burden of proof is discharged, but if the probabilities are equal it is not'.

Attribution of disease in the individual case implies a sufficient knowledge of causation to answer the questions:

1. Is the agent a cause of the disease, at least in certain defined circumstances?
2. If so, were the circumstances of the individual case such that the factor is more likely than not to have caused the disease to occur?

This chapter will address these two questions: disease causation and attribution in the individual case. The development of epidemiology during the past 60 years has refined our understanding of the ways in which causes relate to disease outcome, which has informed medical and legal understanding of causation and attribution.

CAUSATION

Observation can only tell us that certain events regularly follow other events. The rest is subjective inference.

David Hume, 1739

Whenever I look at my watch and see the hand pointing to ten, I hear bells beginning to ring in the church close by; but I have no right to assume ... the movement of the bells is caused by the position of the hands of my watch.

War and Peace, Tolstoy

Cause of disease: Something that at least in some circumstances, makes a disease more likely if it is introduced or less likely if it is removed.

Coggon and Martyn[1]

The characteristics which allow inference of causation have been the subject of long-standing disagreement and debate, as exemplified by the quotations above from Hume and Tolstoy. For our purpose the definition, proposed by Coggon and Martyn, provides a practical foundation: 'something which at least in some circumstances makes a disease more likely if it is introduced or less likely if it is removed'.[1] Cigarette smoking is a cause of lung cancer and high blood pressure a cause of stroke; stopping smoking reduces the risk of lung cancer and lowering blood pressure reduces the risk of stroke.

No condition has a single cause; rather all conditions have multiple causes, some of which act through one another. Aristotle distinguished necessary from sufficient causes, a distinction which can be applied to disease causation. In the absence of a necessary cause, a disease will not occur. Infection with *Mycobacterium tuberculosis* is necessary for the disease tuberculosis, as cases of tuberculosis do not occur in its absence. Similarly, inhalation of respirable crystalline silica dust is a necessary cause of silicosis. However, infection with *M. tuberculosis* is not a sufficient cause of tuberculosis: only some 10 per cent of those infected with *M. tuberculosis* will develop tuberculosis. Other factors including poverty, malnutrition, age, overcrowding, HIV infection and silicosis increase the risk for those infected with *M. tuberculosis* of developing tuberculosis. While the focus of physicians in individual cases of tuberculosis will be on the successful application of antituberculous chemotherapy, the importance of these other factors in determining the risk of tuberculosis in the population is appreciable. English mortuary registers in the 1830s showed clear evidence of the socioeconomic determinants of tuberculosis: 'the proportion of consumptive cases in gentlemen, tradesmen and labourers was 16, 28 and 30 per cent, respectively'.[2] McKeown showed that during the twentieth century, by the time streptomycin was introduced around 1950, the death rate had fallen to about 20 per cent of its level in 1900, an improvement he attributed primarily to improved nutrition in the population.[3]

Identification of a cause or combination of causes sufficient to cause a disease is uncommon other than for single gene disorders and chromosomal abnormalities. The presence of two abnormal haemoglobin genes (HbS) is sufficient to cause sickle cell disease and three copies of chromosome 21 sufficient to cause Down syndrome.

The majority of diseases are caused by a combination of factors (both genetic and environmental) which, when present, can be shown to increase the frequency of the disease, or when absent to reduce it, but which alone are neither necessary nor sufficient. Cigarette smoking is a potent cause of lung cancer, but not all cases of lung cancer have smoked cigarettes (cigarette smoking is not necessary), and only a minority of smokers develop lung cancer (cigarette smoking is not sufficient).

Investigation of a factor as a potential cause of a disease would ideally be undertaken in a representative population, half of whom were randomly allocated without their knowledge to exposure to the factor in question. This is the basis of the randomized controlled trial, whose major strength is in minimizing the problem of confounding biases (recognized and unrecognized), which can lead to false inferences of causation. Randomized controlled trials are now the bedrock underpinning decisions about the efficacy of therapeutic interventions and, in a few cases, about adverse effects of drugs. Not least for ethical reasons, such studies are usually not feasible in addressing questions of disease causation, which normally rely upon inferences from observational studies.

There are two common approaches to observational studies of disease causation:

1. Demonstration that those exposed to the putative cause develop the disease more frequently than those not exposed.
2. Demonstration that those with the disease have more frequently been exposed to the putative cause than those without the disease.

The first forms the basis of the cohort design; the second, the basis of the case–control (case–referent) design of epidemiological study.

Threats to the inference of causation

In general epidemiological studies, particularly analytical studies, are concerned with cause and effect. The essence of an epidemiological investigation is comparison within or between population samples to determine whether differences in frequency of disease are associated with the exposure or factor of interest. Cohort studies are designed to ensure that, to the extent possible, like is compared with like in all respects other than for the factor under investigation. In case–control studies, the aim is that exposure to the risk factor in the controls should be representative of exposure in the population at risk of becoming cases. Bias in a study is a systematic tendency to overestimate or underestimate a characteristic of interest, because of deficiencies in study design or execution. Bias can lead to false inferences about causation.

In thinking about potential bias in a study, it is helpful to consider three questions:

1. In what way does the study sample (healthy or unhealthy) differ from the population from which it was drawn?
2. What is the potential for inaccurate information about study participants (e.g. from errors in measurement or recall)?
3. How might such differences affect the results?

An informative example is of osteoarthritis of the hip in farmers. Farmers were over-represented among hospital patients with osteoarthritis of the hip. This did not necessarily imply that the incidence of osteoarthritis of the hip was increased among farmers, as hospital cases are not representative of the population as a whole. Cases coming to hospital are likely to include a higher proportion of more severely affected cases, and might over-represent farmers, whose livelihood depended on their physical capacity. In fact, subsequent population studies confirmed farming to be an important risk factor for osteoarthritis.

Three important sources of bias are recognized in epidemiological studies, as discussed below.

Selection bias

This arises when the sample of subjects for whom information is collected is systematically unrepresentative of the wider population about which conclusions are to be drawn with regard to the parameter (e.g. odds ratio or disease prevalence) being estimated in the study. An important example of this is the health of workforces as compared to the general population. In general, those who enter work are likely to be healthier than those not in work (healthy selection effect) and those who remain in work are healthier than those who leave work (healthy survivor effect). In a study of workers engaged in the manufacture of polyvinyl chloride (PVC), Fox and Collier[4] quantified the magnitude of these contributions to a lower than expected mortality in the workforce:

- **Selection of a healthy population for employment.** The mortality experience within five years of starting work in a factory where PVC was made was 37 per cent expected for circulatory and 21 per cent expected for respiratory disease. The standardized mortality ratio (SMR) for these conditions progressively increased with increasing duration of employment, becoming similar to the general population after 15 years.
- **Survival in employment of healthier males.** Those who had left the industry during the 15 years from first employment experienced an SMR 50 per cent higher than those who remained employed in the industry.

For cardiovascular and respiratory disease, valid comparisons of mortality experience between a workforce and the general population are likely to be difficult, particularly during the first 15–20 years of employment.

Information bias

Information bias arises from error in measuring exposure or disease. Retrospective investigation of risk factors for congenital malformations from answers to questions to their mothers is likely to be subject to recall bias: mothers whose children have congenital malformations are more likely than those whose children are without congenital malformations to recall drugs taken, infections acquired or workplace chemical exposures experienced during pregnancy.

Confounding and modifying factors

A confounder is an extraneous factor which is associated with the risk factor under investigation and which independently determines the risk of disease outcome.

A confounding factor is therefore one which:

- is associated with the disease;
- is associated with the exposure;
- is not simply an effect of the exposure.

In contrast, effect modification occurs when the strength of the association with one risk factor varies according to the presence or level of another factor (the risk modifier). For example, in a study of the association between occupational lifting and low back pain, risk estimates differed according to stature. In the shortest males, the estimated relative risk was 4.5, in those of intermediate height it was 1.6–2.4, and in the tallest males it was 1.0.[5] A similar pattern was observed in females, suggesting that stature modifies the risk of low back pain from lifting.

Observational studies are inevitably subject to potential for bias and therefore to false inference. For this reason, no single study is usually considered definitive and conclusions are therefore based on the overall weight of the evidence accumulated from several studies.

Robert Koch, the discoverer of the tubercle bacillus as the microbial cause of tuberculosis formulated four postulates which needed to be met before a causal relationship could be inferred between a particular microbe and disease:

1. The agent must be shown to be present in every case of the disease, by isolation in pure culture.
2. The agent must not be found in cases of other diseases.
3. Once cultured, the agent must be capable of reproducing the disease in experimental animals.
4. The agent must be recovered from the experimental disease produced.

The criteria are apt in the consideration of necessary, infectious causes of disease, but are not appropriate for determining non-infectious causality in chronic diseases, such as chronic obstructive pulmonary disease (COPD) where, for example, inhaled coal dust is a cause, but is not a necessary cause.

Others have explored alternative criteria, more appropriate to cancer and chronic disease. Bradford Hill is responsible for the best known criteria on which to base judgements about causal inferences from the findings of observational studies.[6] However, he emphasized that these criteria should not be applied rigidly and recognized that concepts of causation are necessarily provisional, dependent on knowledge at that time.

Of the Bradford Hill criteria, the most important are:

1. **Strength of the association**, i.e. the ratio between the incidence of disease in those exposed to the putative cause and those not exposed – relative risk (or, in case–referent studies, the ratio of the odds of being exposed in those with the disease to those without the disease). In general, the greater the relative risk or odds

ratio, the less likely it is that the observed association is due to confounding.
2. **Exposure–response gradient.** A positive relationship between disease incidence and the level of exposure to the putative cause (i.e. risk increases with higher exposures) strengthens the inference of causation from association.
3. **Consistency of findings between different studies**, undertaken in different places by different people at different times using different populations, carries considerably more weight than a single observational association.
4. **Biological plausibility.** Is there a biological mechanism through which the putative cause could cause the disease? While this is helpful, potential mechanisms have been identified for some suspected causes which have proved artefactual, and some agents can cause disease through previously unknown mechanisms.
5. **Experiment.** Can disease incidence be reduced by a reduction in exposure to the putative cause? This is the nub of a causal inference, providing the most important test of cause and effect.

The final question to be addressed having taken these others into account is: Is there any alternative hypothesis that can explain the observations equally well or better?

Demonstration of disease causation is clearest, and attribution in the individual case most confidently made, where the cause is necessary or nearly so. In these circumstances, the cause is described as specific for the condition. Such conditions include chemical poisonings, such as by lead and mercury, pneumoconiosis caused by inhaled coal and silica, mesothelioma caused by inhaled asbestos, and haemangiosarcoma of the liver caused by inhaled vinyl chloride monomer. For these diseases, the probability of causation for those exposed at work in sufficient concentration to the particular agent is comparable to that for an acute occupational injury and can approach certainty. It is not surprising that the earliest diseases to be recognized in the United Kingdom under the Workmen's Compensation Act in the early part of the twentieth century included a number of such disorders.

Other diseases (such as lung cancer, COPD, osteoarthritis (OA) of the hip), which now form the majority of diseases of occupational cause, are not specific to exposures in the workplace, but the outcome of multiple causes, none necessary or sufficient. In these circumstances, evidence for attribution to an occupational cause depends on inference from observational studies of workforces which consistently demonstrate a sufficient increase in disease incidence, not explained by chance, bias or confounding. No studies are perfect and determination that an observed association is causal is a matter of judgement, based on the strength and consistency of the evidence and its coherence. The strongest evidence for causation is a reduction in disease incidence following avoidance or removal of exposure (Figure 7.1).[7]

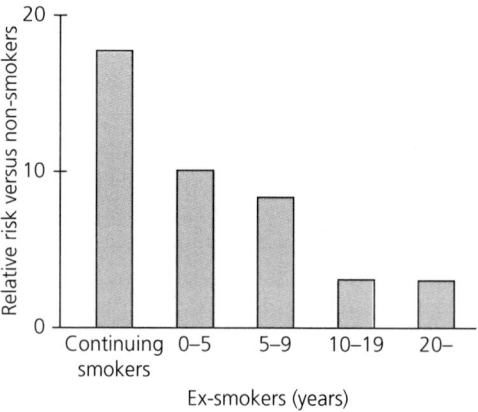

Figure 7.1 Reduction in the risk of lung cancer in British doctors in years after stopping cigarette smoking in comparison to the risk in doctors who continued to smoke. Data from Ref. 7.

ATTRIBUTION

Attribution of disease to a particular cause in the individual case depends on whether:

- the agent or exposure can cause the disease at least in some circumstances (causation);
- the circumstances of the individual case are such that the agent or exposure caused or made a sufficient contribution to the development of the disease.

The answer to the first will be based on judgement of the strength of the scientific evidence and the anwer to the second will be based on the level of probability required to accept attribution in the individual case. For this purpose, we can distinguish five levels of probability:

1. almost certainly true ('beyond reasonable doubt');
2. more likely than not ('on the balance of probabilities');
3. as likely as not;
4. less likely than not;
5. almost certainly false.

In general, the level of probability adopted for the purposes of attribution is 'more likely than not' (on the balance of probabilities).

The question of causation has been addressed in the previous section. The question of attribution will depend on potency of the causal agent in the particular circumstances of the individual case. These will include the nature and level of exposure and the presence of modifying factors.

Some diseases, such as lung cancer, can be considered as 'all or none' diseases. The effect of a cause in these conditions is to increase the probability of the occurrence of the disease. Others, such as hypertension or COPD, are 'more or less' diseases. Whereas 'all or none' diseases are or are not present, 'more or less' diseases occur in a continuum of severity, where the question is not, 'Do you or do you not have the disease?', but 'How much of the disease do you have?'.

For 'all or none' diseases, the contribution of a particular cause in the individual case can be quantified by the attributable fraction in the exposed (AF_{exp}). This is the difference in incidence rate in the exposed and unexposed as a proportion of the incidence rate in the exposed.

$$AF_{exp} = \frac{\text{Incidence in exposed} - \text{incidence in unexposed}}{\text{Incidence in exposed}}$$

It can also be considered as the proportion by which the incidence rate in the exposed would be reduced if the exposure were eliminated.

AF_{exp} can also be derived from knowledge of the relative risk (RR) by the formula:

$$AF_{exp} = \frac{RR - 1}{RR}$$

It can be seen from this that an attributable fraction in the exposed of greater than 50 per cent corresponds to an $RR > 2$. Thus, if the $RR = 2$,

$$AF_{exp} = \frac{RR - 1}{RR} = \frac{2 - 1}{2} = 50\%$$

$RR > 2$ implies that in these circumstances the occurrence of the disease in an exposed person can be attributed to the particular cause on the balance of probabilities, i.e. more likely than not: where the RR is <2, there is a less than 50 per cent chance that the particular case of disease would have been prevented if the exposure had not occurred.

This test of more likely than not has been the basis for attribution used by the Industrial Injuries Advisory Council (IIAC) in determining whether a disease should be prescribed for the purposes of statutory compensation and by the UK courts in determination of negligent damage.

An informative example is the relationship of lung cancer to asbestos exposure. In the absence of any specific identifying characteristics to distinguish a case of lung cancer caused by asbestos from one which would have occurred in the absence of asbestos exposure, attribution of lung cancer to asbestos in the individual case can only be based on the attributable fraction in the exposed and therefore the relative risk in comparison to those not exposed to asbestos. The relative risk of lung cancer for an asbestos textile worker employed in the 1950s and 1960s is more than doubled in those employed for ten years or longer, implying that 50 per cent or more of the cases of lung cancer which occurred in these workforces would not have occurred had they not worked with asbestos in these factories. Although it is not possible to be certain whether or not the individual case would not otherwise have occurred, it is more likely than not, in these circumstances, that it is attributable to asbestos exposure.

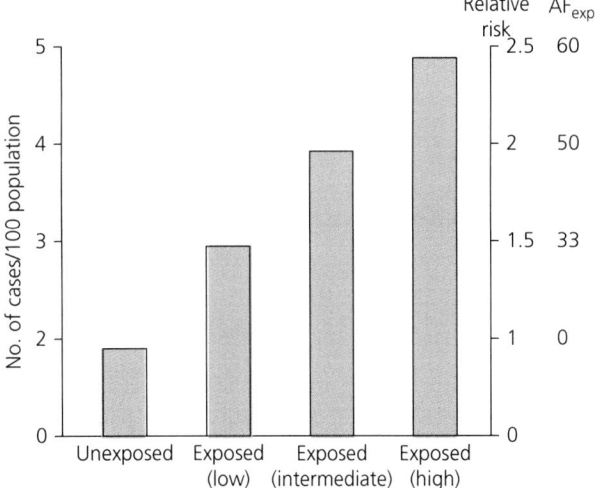

Figure 7.2 Increasing risk of disease AF_{exp} and relative risk (RR) with increasing cumulative exposure to the causal agent. At low exposure, while the risk is increased, attribution remains less likely than not (i.e. among three exposed cases it would have occurred anyway in two). At intermediate level exposure, the attribution becomes as likely as not (i.e. among four exposed cases it would have occurred in two anyway). Only at the highest level is attribution more likely than not (i.e. among five exposed cases, it would only otherwise have occurred in two).

The attributable fraction (and RR) can vary in relation to the level of exposure, usually, as with asbestos and lung cancer, increasing with increasing cumulative exposure (intensity × duration) (Figure 7.2).

'More or less' diseases

Lung cancer is an 'all or none' disease with a clear distinction between cases and non-cases. The same is not true of diseases, such as hypertension (high blood pressure) and COPD (chronic obstructive pulmonary disease characterized by low forced expiratory volume in 1 second or FEV_1) which have a continuum of severity without a clear distinction between cases and non-cases. Blood pressure and FEV_1 (a measure of limitation of airflow) are unmodally distributed in the general population and disease represents the extreme of the distribution curve. As Geoffrey Rose put it, for these conditions the question is not 'does he have it?' (an appropriate question for lung cancer), but 'how much does he have?'.

COPD can be defined (somewhat arbitrarily) in relation to the lower extreme of distribution curve. In its prescription of COPD in coal miners, IIAC took as a case definition of COPD an FEV_1 of 1 L or more below the average (mean) value for a person of the same age and height. This represented an impairment of lung function sufficient on average to be associated with a significant level of disability (inability to keep up with others of the same age when walking on the level). Studies in the United Kingdom had shown that the proportion of miners with this level of FEV_1 loss increased with increasing cumulative coal dust exposure and that at the highest levels of exposure the probability of this occurring was more than doubled (Figure 7.3).[8] From knowledge of the levels of coal dust exposure in coal miners, underground and on the surface in the UK, it was possible to identify the circumstances of exposure where the risk of this level of FEV_1 loss was more than doubled ($AF_{exp} > 50$ per cent). This was found to occur in coal miners who had worked underground for 20 years or more, which became the basis for the prescription.

More recently, it has been shown that comparable cumulative levels of exposure are also experienced by surface workers employed on the screens for 40 years (i.e. the levels of exposure are on average about one half of those underground) and prescription of COPD in coal miners has been amended to reflect this.

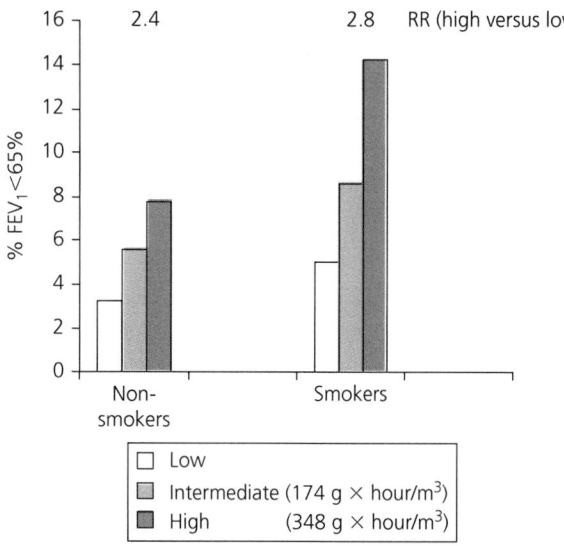

Figure 7.3 Increasing relative risk of FEV_1 <65 per cent with increasing cumulative exposure to coal mine dust. Follow up of 3380 British coal miners (mean age 47 years) with exposure of more than ten years in 20 UK coal mines with monitoring of exposure over ten years. At highest cumulative exposures, the risk is more than doubled in both non-smokers and smokers. Data from Marine et al.[8]

ATTRIBUTION IN THE INDIVIDUAL PATIENT

These principles can be applied to the question of attribution of disease to a particular cause in patients seen in clinical practice. For this purpose, it can be helpful to consider attribution of disease to an occupational cause as a hierarchy of probability of causation and associated difficulty of attribution (Figure 7.4).

Demonstration of disease causation and attribution in the individual case can be made most confidently for diseases which have followed a clearly defined accident (e.g. chemical pneumonitis following an acute inhalation accident) or for diseases with specific clinical features that link them to exposure: these include pneumoconioses and occupational asthma. Others, which now form the majority, occur at increased incidence among those with relevant occupational exposures as compared with the general population; many, such as COPD and OA hip, are common in the general population with cases of occupational cause representing a small minority. Attribution in such cases requires knowledge of the epidemiological evidence for the potency of the cause in different circumstances and whether, in the particular circumstances of the case, attribution is more likely than not. This is easier for otherwise unusual diseases, such as mesothelioma, caused by levels of exposure of asbestos above background, than for lung cancer, COPD and OA hip, where the doubling of risk occurs only in well-defined circumstances of exposure. Before attribution can be made, knowledge is needed of these circumstances together with the circumstances of exposure experienced by the individual case.

ATTRIBUTION AND DISEASE REGISTERS

The strength of good epidemiological studies is their study of populations (or a representative sample) at risk, which allows valid estimation of the level of increased risk of disease in relation to exposure. Disease registers, in contrast, depend on reporting by physicians of cases they have seen, which they consider attributable to occupation. Clearly, only cases seen by the physician and, of these, only those considered by the physician attributable to occupation,

Causation	Example
• Accident	Acute inhalation accident
• Disease with specific clinical features	Occupational asthma
• Epidemiological evidence (e.g. inference from population studies to individual case as 'more likely than not')	
▪ Easy	Mesothelioma and asbestos
▪ Difficult	Lung cancer and asbestos COPD and coal

Figure 7.4 Hierarchy of attribution.

will be reported. This can lead to two potential sources of bias, whose magnitude can be difficult to estimate: **ascertainment bias** and **attribution bias**.

The reasons for referral of cases to physicians may vary considerably between different sources of referral at different times, and physicians themselves may be unaware of this. Such differences can lead to changes (up or down) in the numbers of cases of particular conditions which come to their attention. Diseases whose relationship to occupation is more specific are more likely to be reported. Reports to the Surveillance of Work and Occupational Respiratory Disease (SWORD) voluntary reporting scheme, by chest and occupational physicians, identify many cases of occupational asbestos-related pleural disease (diffuse pleural thickening and malignant mesothelioma), but few cases of lung cancer or COPD. This is probably because diffuse pleural thickening and mesothelioma are uncommon among those not exposed to asbestos and therefore readily attributable to asbestos. In contrast, lung cancer and COPD are common in the general population and primarily attributable to a non-occupational cause, cigarette smoking. Lung cancer, particularly in cigarette smokers, is less likely to be recognized or reported as caused by asbestos than mesothelioma.

Reporting schemes, such as SWORD, have provided and continue to provide valuable information about the relative importance of diseases of occupational cause in the UK, but their limitations should be appreciated. This is of particular importance when changes in disease incidence based on reporting schemes are used for analysis of trends over time. Such changes may occur not because of changes in disease incidence, but because of alteration in the proportion of cases presenting to physicians or judged by them to be attributable to occupation.

Key points

- Attribution of disease in the individual case requires answers to the questions:
  ○ Is the agent a cause of disease at least in certain circumstances?
  ○ If so, did the circumstances of the individual case make causation likely?
- A cause of a disease can be considered as something which makes a disease more likely if introduced or less likely if removed.
- Few diseases have a single cause, but are multifactorial. For some diseases, e.g. poisonings and pneumoconiosis, the cause is specific. For the majority of disease, inference of causation comes from judgement about findings from population studies, taking due account of the potential of these studies for bias and confounding.
- In general, attribution is based on the balance of probabilities: evidence that in the particular circumstances of the case the putative cause was 'more likely than not'. This implies a relative risk of more than 2, an attributable fraction in the exposed of more than 50 per cent.

REFERENCES

1. Coggon DIW, Martyn CN. Time and chance: The stochastic nature of disease causation. *Lancet.* 2005; **365**: 1434–7.
2. Farmer P. *Infections and inequalities.* Berkeley: University of California Press, 1999.
3. McKeown T. The role of medicine: Dream mirage or nemesis? London: Nuffield Provincial Hospitals Trust, 1976.
4. Fox AJ, Collier PF. Low mortality rates in industrial cohort studies due to selection for work and survival in the industry. *British Journal of Preventive and Social Medicine.* 1976; **30**: 225–30.
5. Walsk K, Cruddas M, Coggon D. Interaction of height and mechanical loading of the spine in the development of low-back pain. *Scandinavian Journal of Work and Environmental Health.* 1991; **17**: 420–4.
6. Bradford Hill A. The environment and disease: Association or causation? *British Journal of Preventive and Social Medicine.* 1965; **58**: 295–300.
7. Doll R, Bradford Hill A. Mortality in relation to smoking. Ten years observation of British doctors. *British Medical Journal.* 1964; **1**: 1399–410.
8. Marine WM, Gurr D, Jacobsen M. Clinically important effects of dust exposure and smoking in British coal miners. *American Review of Respiratory Diseases.* 1988; **137**: 106–12.

8

Compensation schemes

ANTHONY NEWMAN TAYLOR AND DAVID WALTERS

Introduction	96	Examples of the development of disease prescription	101
Industrial injuries compensation in the United Kingdom	97	Other UK compensation schemes	104
Current pattern of claims for Industrial Injuries Benefit in the United Kingdom	97	Compensation schemes in continental Europe	105
		Compensation schemes in the United States	107
The development of UK compensation schemes	98	References	108

> Compensation: recompense for loss or damage.
>
> Shorter Oxford English Dictionary

INTRODUCTION

Statutory compensation for industrial accidents and diseases was enacted first in Germany and then in the United Kingdom in the late nineteenth and early twentieth centuries, and subsequently during the twentieth century in the great majority of countries of Western Europe, as well as in North America. The moral basis of these schemes is that workers contributing to the national good through their work should not be economically disadvantaged as a result of accident at, or disease caused by, their work. One of the earliest proponents, the nineteenth century German Chancellor Bismarck, also recognized that such a scheme could enable social peace by ameliorating potential conflict between workers and employers.

The current schemes in each country provide no fault compensation, for accidents and diseases attributed to work. However, between the United Kingdom and mainland Western European countries, there are important differences in coverage and funding.

The majority are self-governed social insurance schemes, with mandated funding by employers, based on the scheme introduced by Bismarck in Germany in the Worker's Accident Insurance in 1884, which created the first modern system of 'no fault' worker's compensation. Workmen's Compensation in the United Kingdom was also based on this principle, until the Industrial Injuries Act (1946) when government took responsibility for funding the scheme as part of the social security system. Increasing costs, particularly in relation to asbestos, have recently led several other countries to provide government funding to supplement social insurance funding.

The intention of the majority of schemes is replacement of lost earnings (at least in part) because of the inability to work, as a consequence of accident or disease caused by work. Again the UK system is different, providing benefit for physical and mental disablement, although some other countries' schemes now also include this. Coverage of many European schemes has now also broadened to include prevention and rehabilitation, as well as compensation. This is most developed in Germany where the employer's liability insurers constitute an important element of the mandatory regulatory system, as well as taking a lead in prevention and rehabilitation initiatives. A 'first principle' of the German system is 'rehabilitation before pension', with the intention of permanent reintegration into the workforce to the extent that the individual's disability allows. Sadly in the United Kingdom, despite considerable urging for more than a decade, the government has yet to introduce the means for vocational rehabilitation into the Industrial Injuries Scheme.

Which diseases are compensated can in principle be decided on the basis of 'individual proof' – attribution of disease to occupational causation in the individual case – or from a list of 'prescribed diseases', where the scientific evidence of causation in particular circumstances is sufficient to allow claimants the 'benefit of presumption'. In practice, a combination of these principles is found in different schemes. In all European countries, diseases compensated through the scheme are covered in a list. There is also a European community list. Which diseases are included in the list varies between countries, both on the basis of their determination and in their comprehensiveness. In Sweden for instance, only infectious diseases are listed; eligibility for other conditions is open and based on individual proof. Finland has an indicative list, but its system does not exclude other conditions, effectively allowing individual proof in addition to the listed conditions. On the other hand, the United Kingdom and France are more prescriptive in generally only allowing listed diseases, although in the United Kingdom individual proof exists for some conditions, such as occupational asthma (in addition to the listed prescribed causes) and dermatitis.

Eligibility of the self-employed for compensation also varies between countries. In general, social insurance schemes are more open to inclusion of the self-employed, with eligibility based on their payment of insurance premiums. The self-employed are excluded from the United Kingdom scheme.

INDUSTRIAL INJURIES COMPENSATION IN THE UNITED KINGDOM

The current scheme for the statutory compensation of accidents and diseases attributable to occupation in the United Kingdom is the Industrial Injuries Scheme, initially enacted under the National Insurance (Industrial Injuries) Act, 1946. It differs in many important respects from comparable schemes in Europe and North America.

The United Kingdom Industrial Injuries scheme is a no-fault, government-funded compensation scheme, for employed earners, which provides benefits to those disabled by accidents or suffering from listed 'prescribed diseases', i.e. attributable to occupation. In some circumstances, claimants for a prescribed disease have 'the benefit of presumption':

> Where a person has developed a disease which is prescribed in relation to him ... that disease shall, unless the contrary is proved, be presumed to be due to the nature of his employment, if that employment was in any occupation (listed in the Schedule) and he was employed on or at any time within one month immediately preceding the date on which he is treated as having developed the disease.

The 1946 Industrial Injuries Scheme provided two major benefits:

1. Industrial Injuries Disablement Benefit (IIDB), payable for 'loss of faculty' ('in proportion to loss of health, strength and the power to enjoy life attributable to industrial accident or prescribed disease') for:
   a. Accidents 'arising out of and in the course of employment' (an accident has been defined as 'an unlooked for mishap or untoward event which is not expected or designed', Lord McNaughton: Fenton v Thorley 1903).
   b. Prescribed diseases
      i. which are a recognized risk to workers in an occupation or exposed to a particular agent.
      ii. where the disease can be attributed to occupation or an agent at work on the balance of probabilities, i.e. more likely than not.

In general, attribution of a disease to a specific cause can be based on:

a. Specific clinical features
b. By inference from the results of population studies to causation in the individual patient.

In the absence of any specific characteristics to distinguish a case of disease attributable to an occupational cause from those which would have occurred in the absence of the occupational exposure, attribution in the individual case is based on an attributable fraction of more than 50 per cent in the exposed workforce, and therefore a relative risk of greater than two, when compared to those not exposed (see Chapter 7).

2. The second important benefit introduced in the 1946 Act was Special Hardship Allowance (SHA), subsequently renamed Reduced Earnings Allowance (REA). Arguably the most enlightened part of the Industrial Injuries Scheme, SHA (later REA) provided an earnings replacement benefit to enable those with occupational disease, whose health would be adversely affected by remaining in their current job, to move to other less well paid work. It provided the means to prevent disease progression to a severe and irreversible level of disability. Reduced Earnings Allowance was abolished by the government of the day in 1990, although claimants in relevant employment before 1990 remain eligible to claim.

CURRENT PATTERN OF CLAIMS FOR INDUSTRIAL INJURIES BENEFIT IN THE UNITED KINGDOM

At present some 350 000 people are in receipt of IIDB, REA or both, at a total cost of £776 million p.a. The current (2009) maximum weekly benefit is £127.10 for IIDB and £50.84 for REA. IIDB payments range from £25.42 to £127.10, the amount received based on the level of disablement that arises from the accident or prescribed disease. IIDB is not normally paid where the level of disablement is less than 14 per cent. However, for pneumoconiosis, byssinosis or mesothelioma, IIDB is paid with a minimum disablement assessment of 1 per cent. Since 2002 awards for mesothelioma and since April 2006 awards for asbestos-related lung cancers, have been paid at 100 per cent. Some 13 000 new claimants receive benefit each year, three-quarters of whom are of working age. Ninety-four per cent of accident claims,

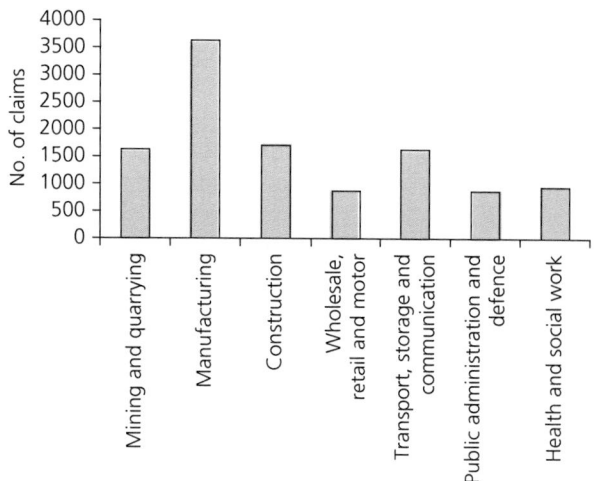

Figure 8.1 New Industrial Injuries Disablement Benefit and Reduced Earnings Allowance claims (>500) put into payment by industry.[1]

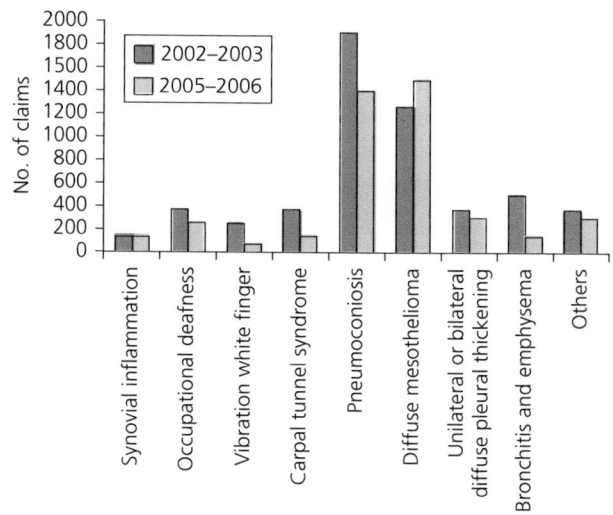

Figure 8.2 New prescribed disease claims put into payment by disease.[1]

which constitute 60 per cent of new claims, are of working age, whereas 60 per cent of new claimants for prescribed disease, which constitute 35 per cent of new claims, are over state age pension. Eighty per cent of those currently in receipt of benefit are male, with women constituting 30 per cent of new claims for prescribed disease and 7 per cent for accidents, reflecting the predominantly male workforces in industries and occupations in which the majority of accidents and prescribed diseases have occurred.

The pattern of current payments for IIDB and REA in the United Kingdom reflects the industrial history of the country during the second half of the twentieth century. Accidents are most likely to occur in manufacturing, construction and mining industries with 26 per cent of major accidents occurring in manufacturing, 16 per cent in construction and 13 per cent in mining and quarrying.[1] New benefit recipients for IIDB and REA in industries with more than 500 claims in 2005–2006 are shown in Figure 8.1.

New claims for prescribed diseases are dominated by diseases associated with mining and asbestos. Some two-thirds of new benefit recipients for a prescribed disease are for pneumoconiosis or mesothelioma. The number of new claims for the most common prescribed diseases put into benefit in 2002–2003 and 2005–2006 is shown in Figure 8.2.

Although the incidence of pneumoconiosis is falling in the United Kingdom, the incidence of mesothelioma is increasing and the long latency of both diseases makes it likely they will continue to form a large proportion of IIDB benefit recipients for many years.

THE DEVELOPMENT OF UK COMPENSATION SCHEMES

Two main types of compensation for accidents and diseases caused by work are available in English law: damages at common law in tort and benefits under the statutory industrial injuries scheme. Whereas success in the former requires proof of negligence or breach of statutory duty, the latter is a no-fault scheme, which in many instances provides the benefit of presumption in the individual case.

Statutory compensation in the United Kingdom for accidents and disease attributable to work has been available since the Workmen's Compensation Act of 1897. This scheme was replaced in 1946 by the Industrial Injuries Scheme which, in a modified form, exists today. During the long century from 1897 to the present day, workmen's compensation in the United Kingdom has adapted to the changing nature of hazardous exposures at work, the diseases associated with them and to the advances in medical technology (e.g. diagnostic x-rays), which have allowed the differentiation of occupational disease (e.g. pneumoconiosis from tuberculosis). In addition, advances in understanding the nature of occupational disease, in particular the occupational contribution to the incidence of diseases common in the population, have, more recently, allowed the inclusion of non-specific diseases (e.g. chronic obstructive pulmonary disease (COPD) in coal miners and osteoarthritis of the hip in farmers) in addition to the diseases specific to occupation, such as poisoning by lead or mercury, which have been included since 1906. The scheme of compensation has also been influenced by the development of public policy and statute: in 1897 with the first Workmen's Compensation Act, making employers liable for compensation for accidents at work, without the need to prove negligence; and the 1948 Industrial Injuries Act, which transferred responsibility for payment and administration of benefit from employers and their insurers to government, and provided benefit primarily for loss of faculty, and associated disablement, in place of loss of earnings.

Workmen's Compensation Acts (from 1897)

Statutory compensation for accidents at work and industrial diseases in the United Kingdom originated in the late nineteenth century as a statutory remedy for the failure of civil courts to provide compensation to workers injured or killed by accidents at work. At that time, fatal accidents in the United Kingdom numbered some 5000 each year, with about 1000 each year in the mining industry.

The Workmen's Compensation Act of 1897 reflected an extension of the principle of automatic compensation for those serving in the armed forces injured in war, which had its origins in Elizabethan England. Joseph Chamberlain, the architect of the 1897 Workmen's Compensation Act, referred in a speech at Birmingham Town Hall in 1894, to the victims of industrial accidents as the 'wounded soldiers of industry'. Later in the same speech, he stated that in his opinion, 'the cost of every accident in every employment is rightly a charge on the cost of production'. The subsequent 1897 Act embodied this radical new principle of automatic compensation of employees for industrial accidents, without the need to prove his employer's negligence.

Prior to the 1897 Act, employees had the right to seek compensation from their employers through the courts for accidents in the course of employment, by demonstrating negligence or breach of statutory duty. However, during the nineteenth century, the courts had accepted a number of defences which provided considerable barriers to successful action by workers. These included three in particular, known as the 'unholy trinity of defences'. (1) **Violenti non fit injuria**: accidents were an ordinary hazard of employment and by taking the job the workman was accepting the risk, expressly or by implication; (2) **contributory negligence**: negligence or want of ordinary care on the part of the workman, i.e. in order to succeed the workman had to prove his freedom from negligence; and (3) **common employment**: the employer was not liable where an injury was due to the negligence of a fellow worker in the same employment.

Of these, the defence of common employment was the most important and aroused the most antagonism and hostility. In practice, it meant an employee had a claim only if the employer had been personally negligent. In companies with a large number of employees such as railways and mines, which had the highest rates of accidental injury and death, the workman was left without the means to pursue a successful claim. Steps were first taken to abolish the defence of common employment by Act of Parliament in 1880, but it was not effectively overcome until 1897. It was during debates in and outside parliament during the 1890s that Joseph Chamberlain first advanced the principle of automatic compensation by employers for accidents at work, irrespective of cause and without the need to prove negligence. He was the architect of the first Workmen's Compensation Act of 1897, of which this was the underlying principle, taking compensation out of the courts for accidents, 'arising out of and in the course of employment', effectively abolishing legal barriers to employee's compensation.

The principle of a duty of employers to compensate employees for loss of earnings due to accidents at work, introduced in the 1897 Workmen's Compensation Act, was revolutionary in its implications: it provided the employee with the legal right to compensation at no cost to himself; it imposed on the employer a legal obligation to compensate workers for loss of earning capacity as a result of accidents at work, with the cost to be regarded as a cost of production, comparable to depreciation of capital assets; employer liability was irrespective of any negligence on the part of the employer or of the employee; and for the common law, strict liability, i.e. liability without imputation of fault was written into statute. Beveridge later described the Workmen's Compensation Act of 1897 as 'the pioneer system of social security in Britain'.

The 1897 Act did not cover industrial disease, but this omission was soon remedied. The Workmen's Compensation Act of 1906 listed six diseases for which compensation was payable: anthrax, ankylostomiasis (hookworm), poisoning by lead, mercury, phosphorus or arsenic, and their sequelae. Workers were entitled to compensation if they could establish that the disease was due to the nature of their employment and they had been engaged in that employment at any time during the 12 months preceding the date of disablement. The Home Secretary, who was responsible for the administration of the Act, was empowered to add further diseases to the schedule. In the absence of specified criteria to enable this, he set up a review committee under Herbert Samuel.

The Samuel Committee, which reported in 1907, proposed three criteria for the addition of new diseases under the Act.[2]

The disease had to be:

- outside the category of diseases already covered by the Act;
- such as to incapacitate a worker for more than one week;
- so specific to the employment that causation could be assumed in the individual case.

The important implication of the third criterion was that diseases undoubtedly associated with certain industries would not be scheduled if they were also fairly common in the general population. The committee did recognize that where a disease was common to a particular trade, but also occurred rarely outside the trade, it could be included in the schedule.

The committee used bronchitis in flax workers as an example of the difficulties of adding a disease common in the population to the schedule:

> Bronchitis, for example, is a trade disease among flax-workers; a larger proportion of that class suffer from it than of other people; but it is not specific to the

employment, for numbers of people who are not flax-workers contract it also. Unless there is some symptom which differentiates the bronchitis due to dust from the ordinary type, it is clearly impracticable to include it as a subject of compensation; for no one can tell, in any individual case, whether the flax-worker with bronchitis was one of the hundreds of persons in the town whose bronchitis had no connection with dust irritation, or whether he was one of the additional tens or scores of persons whose illness was due to that cause. To ask a court of law to decide would be to lay upon it an impossible task. If the workman were required to prove his case, he might be able to show that a larger percentage of his trade suffer from bronchitis than do the rest of the population, but he could never show that he himself was a unit in the excess, and not in the normal part, of that percentage. If it were the employer who was required to disprove a claim, he could rarely, if ever, show that the workman did not contract the illness through his employment, and he would be compelled to compensate not only those labourers whose bronchitis was in no degree an industrial disease.

The problem of statutory compensation for diseases common in the population whose risk was increased in some occupations, was the subject of continuing debate and disagreement, which was only resolved in the last quarter of the twentieth century.

On the basis of their original criteria, the Samuel Committee recommended a further 18 diseases should be included in the scheme and a further three in 1908.[3] The diseases recommended included conditions such as chrome ulceration and scrotal cancer in chimney sweeps. It did not include 'fibrous phthisis' (silicosis and silico-tuberculosis). Although recognized as a hazard of stonemasons, grinders, potters and tin miners, they considered the long latency of the disease would make it difficult to apportion liability among different employers. The committee also considered asbestos, but were unable to include it because of lack of evidence. Further diseases were subsequently added, including silicosis in 1919 through a special scheme, Workmen's Compensation (Silicosis) Act 1918, which required employers to contribute to an insurance scheme, overcoming the problem of identifying which employer was liable.

However, the operation of the Workmen's Compensation Acts was the subject of increasing dissatisfaction. Employers insured against their liability for compensation. This led to claims for compensation under the Act becoming adversarial, with high administrative costs, delay in settlement and workers being bought off by low value lump sum payments.

A Parliamentary report in 1944 expressed this dissatisfaction:

For nearly half a century the compensation of workmen for industrial injury has been a liability, imposed by law, on their employer. Under the existing scheme (the Workmen's Compensation Acts) it has been open to the employer, and in some cases obligatory on him, to insure himself against this liability; while it has been for the workman to make his claim and to take steps to enforce it, if challenged in the Courts of Law. Inevitably compensation has thus become a disputable issue between the two parties or their representatives.[4]

In his report,[5] Beveridge recognized this 'disputable' system imposed a disproportionate cost of administering the scheme compared with the payment issued in benefit to sick and injured workers.

Industrial Injuries Act, 1946

Beveridge proposed that social security should be an insurance, rather than a tax-based scheme, funded from National Insurance contributions made by employers and employees. His proposals included a new industrial injuries scheme. Enactment of the Beveridge report, including a new Industrial Injuries Act, was the responsibility of the Minister for National Insurance, Jim Griffiths, who personally initiated the inclusion of Special Hardship Allowance as an earnings replacement, in addition to disablement benefits, consequent upon 'loss of faculty'. The new Act transferred responsibility for payment and administration of benefit from employers and their insurers to government. Benefit was payable for accidents and prescribed diseases for 'loss of faculty' ('in proportion to loss of health, strength and the power to enjoy life attributable to industrial accident or prescribed disease') in place of lost earnings replacement. Loss of earnings was compensated in one provision of the Act – Special Hardship Allowance – introduced as an earnings replacement for those unable to return to prior employment. An early example of the value of Special Hardship Allowance was in making up lost earnings for those with category 2 simple coal workers' pneumoconiosis (and therefore at significant risk of progressive massive fibrosis (PMF)) who moved to 'dust approved conditions', with a reduced risk of disease progression, but less well paid work.

The 1946 Act maintained the distinction between accidents 'arising out of and in the course of employment' and prescribed (i.e. listed) diseases. The Act allowed that:

A disease or injury may be prescribed ... in relation to any insured persons, if the Minister is satisfied that:

- it ought to be treated, having regard to its causes and incidence and any other relevant considerations, as a risk of their occupation and not a risk common to all persons
- it is such that, in the absence of special circumstances, the attribution of particular cases to the nature of employment can be established or presumed with reasonable certainty.

The Dale Committee,[6] which reported in 1948 interpreted these new statutory criteria for prescription as less restrictive than the Samuel Committee criteria. They considered the meaning of a disease which is 'a risk of their occupations and not a risk common to all persons' as including both diseases specific to occupation and those diseases where the occupation 'causes a special exposure to the risk of the disease, such risk being inherent in the conditions of that employment'. They further interpreted the test of 'reasonable certainty' as being the level of proof in civil courts, i.e. 'on the balance of probability' or 'more likely than not'. This level of proof was succinctly encapsulated by Lord Denning:

> If the evidence is such that the tribunal can say 'we think it more probable than not' the burden of proof is discharged, but if the probabilities are equal, it is not.
>
> Miller v Minister of Pensions, 1947

The contentious issue of the criteria for prescription in relation to disease specificity was considered again by the Beney Committee in 1955.[7]

While the majority report of the Beney Committee agreed in principle with the conclusions of the Dale report, a minority report of three dissenting members, highlighted the failure to prescribe Raynaud's Phenomenon as evidence of the difficulty in adding new diseases to the prescribed list. They argued that,

> The fundamental difficulty is the inadequate cover for diseases common among the general public which may also be due to special occupational risk, e.g. chronic bronchitis (including emphysema) and rheumatic diseases. We consider that these diseases should be eligible for prescription and that the existing test requiring attribution of individual cases to the employment is a bar to their inclusion.

They proposed that prescription should be satisfied in relation to a disease where it was probable that more cases than not were occupational in origin, whether or not individual cases could be attributed to the nature of employment.

This proposal overcame the problem identified originally by the Samuel Committee in 1907 providing the basis for widening the scope of disease prescription to include diseases common in the population, such as chronic obstructive pulmonary disease, lung cancer and osteoarthritis of the hip, where the frequency of the disease is more than doubled in certain occupations, in certain well-defined circumstances of work, but the disease has no specific characteristics which allow the distinction of occupational from non-occupational cause.

The Dale Committee (1948) had also recommended that the Industrial Injuries Advisory Council, a recently formed tripartite committee of independent members with relevant expertise and an equal number of representatives of employers and employees, should advise the minister on which diseases should be considered for prescription.

EXAMPLES OF THE DEVELOPMENT OF DISEASE PRESCRIPTION

The development of disease prescription, particularly in relation to broadening the scope of prescription to include diseases not specific to occupation, can be shown in three examples.

Workmen's compensation and coal

The Samuel Committee had been unable to recommend prescription for silicosis, in part because it was not possible at that time to distinguish silicosis from other pulmonary diseases, particularly tuberculosis. The development of the chest radiograph in the early twentieth century allowed the differentiation of silicosis from other respiratory diseases. Silicosis was recognized as an industrial disease under the Workmen's Compensation (Silicosis) Act, 1918. The Act required employers to contribute to an insurance scheme, from which compensation would be paid, overcoming the problem, highlighted by the Samuel Committee, of identifying employer liability. It also introduced regular medical examinations authorizing medical examiners to suspend workers compulsorily at the early stages of disease, to prevent the development of incapacitating disease. Coal miners were included in the scheme in 1928, when they could demonstrate exposure to dust of silica rock and were 'totally disabled'. The scheme was further extended to include 'partially disabled' workers three years later. In 1934, the scheme was extended to include any coal miner with silicotic nodules, whether or not they were working with rock. All coal miners with radiological evidence of pneumoconiosis from coal dust exposure were included in the scheme in 1943.

Workers compensated for Coal Worker's Pneumoconiosis (CWP) were 'certified' with benefit of a weekly payment or a lump sum and compulsory suspension from mining to protect workers from further lung deterioration. The certification of large numbers of workers resulted in unforeseen social problems in South Wales as identified in 1948 by Fletcher.[8] By the end of 1945, 12 000 men had been certified in South Wales and new cases were being certified at a rate of 100 men per week. Most of these men (66 per cent) were under 50 years old and 25 per cent were under 40 years old. The majority of the men had been coal hewers and faced the prospect of being out of work with no training for alternative employment. In 1951, Hugh Jones and Fletcher[9] noted that 'at present some 5000 men with pneumoconiosis, three quarters of whom are probably capable of work, under normal industrial conditions, are unemployed'.

The nature and progression of coal worker's pneumoconiosis had become better by the 1960s. Inhaled coal dust reaching the peripheral gas exchanging parts of the lungs is removed, primarily through engulfment by scavenging macrophages, which migrate centrally to the mucociliary escalator. If the dose of respirable dust overwhelms this removal mechanism, coal dust accumulates in the lungs as centriacinar macules, which appear as rounded nodules on chest radiographs. The nodules themselves, composed of retained dust, do not cause impairment or disability. This form of the condition, characterized by retained coal dust in the lungs, was classified as simple pneumoconiosis. The severity of pneumoconiosis was graded according to the size and profusion of nodules seen on the chest radiograph. Some cases of simple pneumoconiosis developed progressive massive fibrosis, which was associated with significant disability and reduced life expectancy. During the 1940s and 1950s, PMF had been considered an atypical form of tuberculosis. However, Cochrane provided substantial evidence against this hypothesis and showed that the risk of PMF was related to the category of simple pneumoconiosis, i.e. correlated with the quantity of coal dust in the lungs.[10] His findings implied that if workers with category 2 pneumoconiosis were removed from further dust exposure, the risk of progression to PMF would be reduced. Jacobsen et al. subsequently showed that on average coal dust inhaled over a 35-year working lifetime with exposures of $4\,mg/m^2$ were associated with a 4 per cent risk of developing category 2 pneumoconiosis. Measures were put into place to reduce dust concentrations to $4\,mg/m^2$ and workers with category 2 pneumoconiosis moved to less dusty ('dust approved') working conditions. Special Hardship Allowance helped facilitate the redeployment of workers to less dusty conditions, by providing compensation for loss of earnings consequent on the move to less hazardous work. Special Hardship Allowance, which later became Reduced Earnings Allowance, was arguably the most enlightened part of the Industrial Injuries Scheme, enabling workers to remain in work while preventing further health deterioration.

Asbestos and asbestosis, lung cancer and mesothelioma

In the late nineteenth and early twentieth centuries, asbestos became increasingly widely used, primarily because of its thermal insulating properties. Subsequently, its uses broadened to include reinforcement of boarding and cement. Inhaled asbestos fibres of $>5\,\mu m$ in length, too long to be engulfed by scavenging macrophages in the lung, accumulate in the lungs to cause fibrosis (asbestosis). Asbestos fibres are also carcinogenic causing lung cancer and mesothelioma. The chronology below shows the evolution of knowledge about adverse health effects associated with asbestos:

1899: Montague Murray reports a post-mortem case of pulmonary fibrosis in an asbestos worker in the UK.
1900: Cooke reports the case of 33-year-old Nellie Kershaw who died of pulmonary asbestosis after working 20 years in the Turner and Newall asbestos textile factory in Rochdale, Lancashire, UK.[11]
1930: Merewether and Price[12] report the increased prevalence of asbestosis in the Rochdale workforce of asbestos textile workers.
1947: Merewether[13] reports excess lung cancer deaths in those with asbestosis compared to those with silicosis.
1955: Doll[14] provides definitive evidence of the increased risk of lung cancer in the Rochdale asbestos textile workforce.
1960: Wagner et al.[15] provides evidence of the association between mesothelioma and occupational and non-occupational exposure to blue asbestos (crocidolite) in NW Cape Province, South Africa.

ASBESTOSIS

Merewether and Price[12] reported an increased risk of fibrosis in asbestos textile workers, which increased in prevalence with longer duration of employment (Table 8.1).

Although remarkably high by modern standards, the number of prevalent cases of fibrosis was almost certainly an underestimate of the true size of the problem, as employees whose health was most affected by asbestos were likely no longer to be at work because of disease severity or death.

Statutory compensation of asbestosis

Asbestosis was enacted in the Workers' Compensation (Silicosis and Asbestosis) Act, 1930, which extended the provisions of the Workmen's Compensation (Silicosis) Act to asbestosis, i.e. compulsory employer liability insurance and regular medical examinations with the powers of suspension.

Asbestosis continues to be compensated as a pneumoconiosis.

MESOTHELIOMA

Mesothelioma is an uncommon respiratory cancer. Wagner et al.[15] first reported the association between mesothelioma and exposure to crocidolite (blue) asbestos

Table 8.1 Prevalence of pulmonary fibrosis in an asbestos textile factory, 1930.[12]

Years employed	Number examined	Prevalent cases of fibrosis		
		No.	%	Average age
0–4	89	0	–	–
5–9	141	36	25.5	36
10–14	84	27	32.1	40.4
15–19	28	15	53.6	43.4
20+	21	17	80.9	52.7
Totals	363	95	26.2	41.4

Table 8.2 Mesothelioma in NW Cape Province, South Africa (1960).[15]

Exposure (crocidolite)	Mesothelioma (No.)	Latency (years)
Mining or transport	10	21–43
Insulation work	4	18–29
Neighbourhood	18	35–44
Unknown	1	–

Mean age, 49 years; mean survival, 15 months.

Table 8.3 Association between pneumoconiosis (asbestos and lung cancer) and lung cancer (at post-mortem).[17]

	Deaths (No.)	Lung cancer (%)
Asbestosis	235	13.2
Silicosis	6884	1.2

Table 8.4 Causes of death in men employed in a Rochdale asbestos textile factory.[14]

Cause of death	No. of deaths	
	Observed	Expected
Lung cancer		
With asbestos	11	–
Without asbestos	0	1
Other lung diseases		
Asbestos	14	–
Other	6	8
Other cancers	4	2
Other causes	4	5
All causes	39	16 (15.4)

in the North Western Cape Province of South Africa in 1960. They observed the long latent interval between first exposure (usually >20 years) to asbestos and the onset of the disease and a short survival time post-diagnosis (<1.5 years). They also identified its occurrence both in those occupationally exposed in its extraction and use (insulation), as well as in those not occupationally exposed, who had encountered it in the neighbourhood of the mines (Table 8.2).

In the United Kingdom, there has been a high incidence of cases of mesothelioma clustered in areas historically associated with asbestos work, where railway (e.g. Swindon) and ship (e.g. Devonport and Barrow) manufacture and repair were undertaken. Before the 1960s, the Devonport dockyards used considerable quantities of crocidolite and amosite asbestos. However, from the mid-1960s, alternative insulation material was used and respiratory protection provided. Hilliard et al.[16] showed that these measures have been associated with a decrease in the number of cases of mesothelioma since the early 1990s. However, these preventative and protective measures were not implemented in the UK construction industry until the 1970s or 1980s. The incidence of mesothelioma in the United Kingdom is continuing to increase, with an increasing proportion of cases in electricians, carpenters and plumbers in the construction industry rather than in the traditional asbestos workforces in dockyards and insulation. Peto et al.[17] estimated that the peak of the UK epidemic of mesothelioma will not yet be reached until 2015–20, continuing until 2050, with some two-thirds of the cases in the UK epidemic yet to occur. A similar continuing increased incidence of mesothelioma, although at a lower level, is occurring throughout Western Europe.

Statutory compensation of mesothelioma

The prescription of mesothelioma is based on the specificity of asbestos as the cause of the disease. Mesothelioma can be caused by relatively low levels of exposure to asbestos, which is reflected in the current prescription – 'exposure to asbestos, asbestos dust or any admixture of asbestos at a level above that commonly found in the environment at large'. Claims for mesothelioma are now fast-tracked by the Department for Work and Pensions: there is no 90-day waiting period, claimants are automatically awarded 100 per cent assessments and there is no absolute requirement for corroborative evidence of occupational exposure.

LUNG CANCER

Prescription for lung cancer due to asbestos has been complex. There is a clear excess of cases of lung cancer in those with asbestosis, which was observed by Merewether in his report as HM Inspector of Factories in 1947.[13] He noted a considerably greater proportion of deaths in certified cases of asbestosis than silicosis (Table 8.3).

Subsequently Doll, in a landmark study in 1955, reported a marked excess of lung cancer deaths in men employed before the 1931 Asbestos Regulations (which had followed the Merewether and Price report) in the Turner and Newall Rochdale textile factory.[14] All cases of lung cancer were in men with asbestosis (Table 8.4).

Statutory prescription of lung cancer in asbestos workers

Lung cancer was formally prescribed in 1985 in cases of asbestosis and in cases with diffuse pleural thickening. The case for prescription of lung cancer in asbestos workers without asbestosis was more difficult due to the lack of specific clinical features to differentiate cases of lung cancer from those in the general population. It was clear, unlike mesothelioma, that the increased risk of lung cancer occurred at relatively high levels of cumulative exposure. Initially, diffuse pleural thickening was used as a surrogate for sufficient exposure to be associated with a doubling of risk of lung cancer. However, subsequent evidence indicated this was not the case but that in certain workers, such as asbestos textile workers, there was a doubling of the risk of lung cancer in those working with asbestos.

In 2006, lung cancer in the absence of asbestosis was prescribed for 'exposure to asbestos for at least five years before 1975 and ten years after 1975 in the following occupations (i) workers in asbestos textile manufacture, (ii) asbestos sprayers and (iii) asbestos insulation work, including those applying and removing asbestos-containing materials in shipbuilding'. Since 2006, cases of asbestos-related lung cancer have received 100 per cent disablement benefit.

Chronic obstructive pulmonary disease and coal workers

Cancer is an 'all or none' disease: you have cancer or you do not. In contrast, some other diseases may be 'more or less', with degrees of disease such as high blood pressure or airway narrowing in chronic bronchitis and emphysema.

Lung function can be assessed by measuring the amount of air a person can exhale during a forced expiratory manoeuvre. The total volume of air that can be exhaled is the forced vital capacity (FVC) and the volume of air that can be exhaled in 1 second is the forced expiratory volume in 1 second (FEV_1). A person with airflow limitation will have a lower FEV_1 and lower FEV_1/FVC ratio than a normal individual. In a study in 1961, Cochrane and Higgins[18] found that miners and ex-miners had lower lung function than non-miners. However, no gradient of lung function loss was observed in miners and ex-miners with increasing category of simple pneumoconiosis. In contrast, lung function was decreased in miners and ex-miners with PMF, with lung function loss increasing with increasing severity of PMF. On this basis, Cochrane considered that coal dust did not cause airway obstruction, but recognized he was using the category of simple pneumoconiosis measurements as a surrogate for airborne coal dust exposure. In 1982, Cockcroft et al.[19] found evidence that emphysema at post-mortem was considerably more frequent in coal miners than in non-miners, in individuals referred for post-mortem because of sudden death (i.e. a reason for post-mortem unrelated to occupation overcoming potential selection bias), with an odds ratio of 10.35 after adjusting for age and cigarette smoking. In a large study of UK coal miners, Marine et al.[20] in 1988 showed the proportion of coal miners with a FEV_1 <65 per cent was more than doubled in those with high, as compared to low, exposure to coal dust, in both smokers and non-smokers. This evidence together with other similar observations, particularly from the United States, provided the basis for prescription for chronic bronchitis and emphysema (now COPD) in coal workers.

In considering the terms of prescription for coal workers with COPD, the Industrial Injuries Advisory Council addressed the following questions:

- What is a disabling loss of FEV_1? A study of miners found an FEV_1 of 942 mL less than average for a man of the same age and height was associated with shortness of breath when walking with others on the level.[21]
- Is there evidence of at least a doubling of risk of this FEV_1 loss? Evidence indicated that a doubling of risk of this level of FEV_1 loss occurred at cumulative exposures to coal dust of 60–120 mg/m² per year.[20]
- What is the nature of occupational exposure in which this occurs? Hygiene data from the Institute of Occupational Medicine (IOM) in Edinburgh showed exposures for UK miners to be:

Coal face workers	2.5–6.5 mg/m²
Development operations	1.5–5.5 mg/m²
Other underground workers	1.0–3.0 mg/m²
Surface workers	0.2–0.7 mg/m²

- Can this be translated into job titles and duration of employment for purposes of prescription? IIAC translated this into 20 years employment underground in a coal mine.

Chronic bronchitis and emphysema was prescribed in 1992 as an FEV_1 of 1 L less than the average value for a man of similar age and height, in coal miners who had worked underground for 20 years, who had Category 1 Simple Coal Workers Pneumoconiosis on a chest radiograph. The requirement for Category 1 pneumoconiosis was later withdrawn. More recently, on the basis of additional evidence from IOM about coal dust exposure to surface workers, prescription has been extended to include surface screen workers, employed for 40 years, allowing a 2:1 aggregation of duration of exposure below ground and on the surface, i.e. 15 years underground plus ten years on the screens above ground qualifies for prescription.

OTHER UK COMPENSATION SCHEMES

Pneumoconiosis (Workmen's Compensation) Act, 1979

This is a state-funded scheme which provides lump sum payments to those who have developed respiratory disease through their employment, for workers unable to recover compensation through the courts or through a private no-fault compensation scheme, because their employer is no longer in business. The Act originally covered pneumoconiosis, byssinosis and mesothelioma, but has since been extended to include lung cancer with asbestosis or prescribed in relation to asbestos and bilateral diffuse pleural thickening.

To succeed, the claimant has to satisfy three criteria:

1. Disablement benefit must be payable under the industrial injuries scheme in respect of the disease in question.
2. Every relevant employer must have ceased to carry on business.
3. No action must have been brought or any claim compromised by common law.

Successful claimants under the scheme are paid lump sum compensation in addition to IIDB. The average lump sum under the scheme is £13 000 with payments made on a sliding scale based on age and level of disablement.

Diffuse Mesothelioma Scheme, 2008

The Diffuse Mesothelioma Scheme, which commenced on October 1, 2008, extends coverage for compensation for mesothelioma to those exposed to asbestos in the UK, who are otherwise unable to claim compensation. This includes the self-employed exposed to asbestos in their work and those exposed to asbestos in the home from asbestos brought home on a worker's clothes. It excludes employed earners able to claim IIDB under the 1979 Pneumoconiosis Act. Compensation is made as a lump sum payment.

In order to qualify under the scheme:

- There must be evidence to show the claimant has a malignant mesothelioma.
- The claimant must have been exposed to asbestos in the United Kingdom.
- The claim must be made within one year of diagnosis or in the case of a claim made by a dependant, within one year of the date of death.
- The third requirement, to claim within one year of death, does not apply to those diagnosed before the introduction of the scheme.

COMPENSATION SCHEMES IN CONTINENTAL EUROPE

There are broadly two main bases for the compensation systems found in continental Europe. One is modelled on the German approach with self-governed sectoral insurance associations funded by employers' contributions, providing a comprehensive prevention, rehabilitation and compensation service. In the second form, the state administers the system for compensating occupational injuries and disease as part of its wider provision for social security and levies contributions from employers to finance it.

There are further differences in the arrangements and in those responsible for governance and administration in different countries. The degree of federalization and regional autonomy differ with some countries such as Sweden and France having highly regionalized administrative structures and others, such as Germany, having a well-developed sectoral focus in addition to regionalization. The mix of public and private insurance organizations that make up the systems vary between countries. In many countries, there is now a mixture of these two approaches, with participation of both the state and private insurance systems.

In Belgium, there is a separate scheme for occupational accidents, based on private employers' insurance, and a state system for occupational diseases for industrial and commercial sector workers. This is also true in Portugal. In Denmark, private insurers carry the risk for occupational accidents, while occupational diseases are insured by specific funds financed by contributions from employers. In Norway and Finland, insurers carry the risk for both accidents and disease, but in Norway there is a state system and a private employers' insurance system which 'tops up' the state system. In some countries, the usual system of social insurance for incapacity resulting from occupational injury and disease, designed to replace lost earnings, is supplemented by additional schemes, usually resulting from agreements between trade unions, to provide additional benefits for their members. In Sweden, higher pensions are available through the labour market insurance scheme known as AFA Insurance.

Coverage of the original social insurance systems was intended for employed people in private sector industry, which remains the basis of coverage. While coverage has been extended to provide benefits for public sector employees, for part or all of those in agriculture and, in some cases, the self-employed, many of these still remain outside the general coverage of this form of social insurance and are subject to separate schemes in many countries. Workers who are unable to demonstrate a legal form of employment in relation to a claim for benefits for accident or disease while engaged in work remain ineligible for these types of benefits under most systems.

In many countries, work injury/disease insurance systems are now also involved in prevention and rehabilitation. This is most developed in Germany where the employer's liability insurers constitute an important element of the mandatory regulatory system, as well as taking a lead in prevention and rehabilitation initiatives. A 'first principle' of the German system is rehabilitation before pension, with the intention of permanent reintegration into the workforce to the extent that the individual's disability allows.

In all European countries, diseases that are compensated are covered in a list. There is also a European Union list. Which diseases are included in the list varies between countries, both on the basis of their determination and in their comprehensiveness. In Sweden, only infectious diseases are listed; eligibility for other conditions is open and based on individual proof. Finland has an indicative list, but its system does not exclude other conditions, effectively allowing individual proof in addition to the listed conditions. On the other hand, the United Kingdom and France are more prescriptive in generally only allowing listed diseases, although in the United Kingdom individual proof exists for some conditions, such as occupational asthma (in addition to the prescribed listed causes) and dermatitis.

The role of the list in determining specific cases of compensation also varies. There are two extremes of the legal and administrative principles of the different systems concerned. At one extreme is the 'open system', in which each claim for an occupational disease is treated on its own merits, as in Sweden where the occupational disease list includes only infectious diseases, with all other conditions treated individually. At the other extreme, the French list of 112 occupational diseases appended to its social security code specifies symptoms or pathological lesions required to be present, the type of work that is known to cause the condition and the time limits for compensation claims. In theory, any disease meeting the medical, occupational and administrative criteria in the list is presumed to be occupational in origin. In the other 15 EU countries, the function of the 'list' falls somewhere between these extremes in decisions concerning the eligibility of conditions. A trend evident in many countries has been the increasing recourse to 'open' systems in recent years. Despite this, well over 90 per cent of diseases recognized as occupational remain on the basis of their inclusion in the national list.

Whether the condition is on a list or identified individually as part of a mixed system, the process by which evidence is assessed and decisions taken as to its 'occupational' cause in most cases concerns two issues – the extent to which the disease can be ascribed to an occupational cause and the extent to which a claimant can show they have experienced relevant exposures. The means by which the first of these issues is resolved in most countries, as in the UK, is defined in legislation or the guidance to it. Determining the recognition of occupational associations with the cause of conditions involves review of epidemiological and other scientific/medical evidence and the achievement of broad expert agreement concerning increased risk in relation to occupational exposure. Practice in other European countries does not follow exactly the rule adopted in the UK, where decisions for prescription are based on robust epidemiological evidence of a greater than doubled risk of the disease in an exposed occupational group compared to a comparable unexposed group or the general population. However, there are broad similarities in the approach in all countries in so far as there is emphasis on the need for robust evidence of occupational risk and agreement of expert opinion.

In Belgium, Italy and Luxembourg, both the occupational risks of a disease and the occupations in which such risks occur are defined on the list of prescribed diseases appended to legislation, as in the UK. As in France, it is sufficient for individuals in these countries to demonstrate that they are suffering from a disease on the list and that they have been exposed to a relevant hazard or undertaken a job on the list. In Austria, Denmark, Finland, Germany, Switzerland, Portugal, Spain and Switzerland, the list serves as a guide to insurance organizations investigating the claim that the disease is occupationally caused; the insurance companies will seek to establish if the disease in question could have been caused by a causal agent marked on the national list, while at the same time excluding any non-occupational factors that could have caused the disease. These lead to differences in the number of claims for compensation for occupational diseases and the recognition rates for such claims between different countries.

Some clear differences emerge when comparing arrangements for work injury/disease benefits in other countries with the IIDB scheme in the UK. Partly as a consequence of its different origins, the UK approach provides for considerably lower benefits than other European systems and represents lower proportional expenditure on this form of support than is found elsewhere. Whereas the majority of schemes provide partial earnings replacement, the UK scheme compensates loss of faculty and associated disablement. Also in contrast with some other countries, it makes no provision at present for either prevention or rehabilitation. However, there are also similarities. The legacy of the industrial era is found in most systems. As long as conditions that are eligible for compensation are based on lists primarily based on the 'classic' industrial diseases, the number of claims (and therefore costs of compensation) are unlikely to increase greatly. The gender distribution of successful claimants under these systems will be predominantly male. How compensation systems deal with the predominant and very different current conditions of ill health associated with work is a major issue for all systems. While in some countries musculoskeletal disorders now feature more prominently, stress-related conditions still represent a significant challenge. The move to 'open' systems may partly address this problem, but evidence to date suggests that it does not do so entirely.

A trend evident in several countries is some reorientation of 'no-fault' compensation systems towards a closer fit with civil law models. Perceived inadequacies in levels of compensation available through social insurance combined with perceptions of injustice over employer immunity from redress under the civil law have led to these changes.

The traditional protection from actions in civil law that being part of such schemes afforded to employers in many countries, in contrast to the UK, is increasingly seen as inappropriate. At the same time, the level of individual employer contributions has become increasingly debated. Tensions in existing systems are evident and movement towards a closer alignment with the benefits available under civil law is a common international trend.

Current data on occupationally related ill health compared with the number of claims made for occupational disease and those claims recognized suggest that only a minority of those whose health is affected by their work seek compensation and in any European system, recognition of such claims rarely exceeds 50 per cent. Several explanations have been proposed, which include the limitations of the experience and ability of doctors to recognize occupational causes, ignorance of workers concerning both the hazards of their work and their entitlements to compensation and the complexity of the administration of the system for compensation. It is also important to appreciate that not only does the complexity of making a claim exclude many, but the claim process itself may also have negative consequences for recovery and return to work. While one of the great virtues of 'no-fault' systems for compensation is that they act to eliminate adversarial approaches to claims, the use of experience rating by some insurance systems destroys this advantage since it provides a strong incentive for employers to contest claims. It is also argued that the growth in precarious employment in advanced market economies has eroded the coverage of workers' compensation systems, creating administration difficulties, undermining the coverage and objectives of compulsory insurance, as well as weakening processes for making claims. There is also evidence that the costs of compensating injured workers are being shifted from workers' compensations systems to those concerned with public health or social security.

As is the case in the UK, recognition of some of these problems means that reform of the present system is planned or called for in most countries. Generally, the main thrust of such reforms is to seek to address issues of affordability and efficiency, while at the same time dealing with perceived weaknesses in cover and redress of harm. It seems unlikely that these changes to existing systems will lead to greater access to benefits for potential claimants.

COMPENSATION SCHEMES IN THE UNITED STATES

The development of workers' compensation in the United States has its origins as a response to the development by employers of defences to litigation by employees, for accidents at work, very similar in kind to 'the unholy trinity of defences' employed in the UK. These included contributory negligence, the 'fellow servant' rule (comparable to the defence of 'common employment') and the 'assumption of risk' (equivalent to *violenti non fit injuria*). Not surprisingly, therefore, much of the early development of workers' compensation in the United States was based on principles derived from the German and UK schemes.

Although workmen's compensation schemes in the United States are now insurance-based schemes, organized state by state, the federal government took the lead in the early twentieth century in providing compensation to its workforce for accidents at work. The Federal Employers' Liability Act of 1908 covered federal employees engaged in hazardous work and employees of certain carriers engaged in interstate and foreign commerce. It was adopted at the urging of President Theodore Roosevelt, who in a speech to Congress said that the 'burden of accident falls upon the hapless man, his wife and children' which was 'an outrage'.

The turning point in the development of worker's compensation legislation in the United States was the adoption by Wisconsin in 1911 of Worker's Compensation, which was the subject of considerable debate. Employers lobbied successfully for what has become known as the 'great trade off'. Employers agreed to provide medical and wage replacement benefits in exchange for the employee giving up his/her right to sue the employer. Several states subsequently adopted this model. However, it took until 1976 for all 50 states to have some form of coverage for occupational disease.

Workers' compensation schemes in the United States are no-fault schemes: in return for relinquishing the right to sue his or her employer, the employee has the right to fair and timely compensation.

The basic structures of workers' compensation in the United States and Canada are similar. A board or commission sets the rules; an insurer provides coverage on the basis of the payroll for eligible workers; cases are adjudicated in the first instance by the insurer and subsequently, if contested, by an appeals system. Despite the original intention to avoid litigation, legal advocacy remains part of the process, particularly in complicated or disputed appeals. Because of deadlines by which time an insurer must decide claims, many requests for compensation are initially rejected, forcing claimants to retain legal counsel and file lengthy appeals. The consequences for the worker can include uncompensated legal expenses and economic hardship.

Federal schemes include the Black Lung Programme for coal miners, the Longshoremen and Harbour Workers' Compensation Programme, the Federal Employers' Compensation Act, the Radiation Exposure Compensation Act and the Energy Employees' Occupational Illness Compensation Program Act. In several instances, these federal programmes replace or are intended to complement state-based compensation programmes.

In the majority of states, compensation is limited to two-thirds of previous wages and coverage of medical costs. Funding of the schemes by employers, of whom the majority are insured, is intended to internalize the cost of work-related accidents and disease, providing an incentive to employers to ensure job safety and health. However, risk pooling, the basis of insurance, blunts the financial consequences of accidents and diseases caused by work, diminishing the impact of such incentives.

All claims for compensation schemes are handled by state compensation boards. Insurers are entitled to dispute permanent disability claims. In any contested claim, the burden of proof is on the worker. This can cause considerable difficulty in substantiating the claim, particularly for conditions of long latency, where the relevant exposure occurred many years before.

Apart from federal schemes, workers' compensation varies from state to state. This is particularly the case for diseases. State schemes cover accidents without regard to fault unless self-inflicted or caused by intoxication. In most states, disease coverage was originally covered by schedules, which provided guidance for compensation boards and courts. However, the continuous need to update the schedules, and their being considered restrictive and inflexible, has led to their being generally abandoned.

Many states only compensate diseases which are 'peculiar to' or 'characteristic of' occupation, i.e. specific to occupation. This creates particular difficulty for conditions which have multiple causes and are of long latency, when it can be difficult to identify the particular workplace where the relevant exposure occurred. This is particularly true of respiratory tract diseases, such as lung cancer, which has a predominant non-occupational cause, cigarette smoking, as well as several well-recognized occupational causes, including asbestos, which is compensated uncommonly. This contrasts with mesothelioma caused by asbestos, haemangiosarcoma of the liver caused by vinyl chloride monomer and leukaemia caused by benzene, the first two of which, particularly, are more specific to occupation and more widely accepted than lung cancer. Disputes often revolve around the 'apportionment' when a worker has multiple causes of a disease, such as the estimated contribution of a worker's asbestos exposure and cigarette smoking to the development of lung cancer.

Workers' compensation in the United States is primarily a state responsibility, which has developed in a more piecemeal manner than in the UK. Its potential strengths lie in the incentives in the scheme to improve workplace health and safety through employers' insurance and rehabilitation from the responsibility for payment of medical costs. Its problems, as a fair and timely means of compensation, lie in the variation in occupational disease coverage, which in some states remains mainly restricted to diseases specific to occupation, and the frequency with which workers must appeal claims that have been rejected by insurers.

Key points

- Statutory no fault compensation schemes for accidents at work and diseases caused by work are provided in the UK, Western Europe and North America. The Industrial Injuries Benefit Scheme in the UK is funded by taxation, whereas in other countries funding is usually by social insurance schemes.
- Accident at work are in general readily recognized. Attribution of disease to work creates more problems. In the absence of specific clinical features, attribution is usually made 'on the balance of probabilities' or 'more likely than not' (i.e. an attributable fraction of more than 50 per cent).
- Diseases can in principle be compensated on the basis of 'individual proof' or from a list of 'prescribed diseases'. Different countries use different combinations of these two principles. In the UK, the great majority of compensatable diseases are set out in a prescribed list, which identifies both the disease and the circumstances in which attribution to work can be made.
- Different countries vary in the nature of the diseases they compensate. In the United States, in many states only diseases 'peculiar to' or 'characteristic of', i.e. specific to occupation, are compensated. In the UK, diseases such as lung cancer and chronic obstructive pulmonary disease are prescribed where the risk of their occurring in the workforce is at least doubled.
- Statutory compensation in the UK has developed during the past century from the prescription of disease specific to work to one of widening the inclusion of disease attributable, but not specific, to work.

REFERENCES

1. Industrial Injuries Disablement Benefit scheme. A consultation paper, January 2007. Department for Work and Pensions. London: HMSO.
2. Samuel Committee. Report of the Departmental Committee on Compensation for Industrial Diseases 1907, Cd. 3495. London: HMSO.
3. Samuel Committee. Second Report of the Departmental Committee on Compensation for Industrial Disease 1908, Cd. 4386. London: HMSO.
4. Foreword to Social Insurance Part 2 Workmen's Compensation. Proposals for an Industrial Scheme. September 1944. London: HMSO.
5. Beveridge Social Insurance and Allied Services 1942, Cmd. 6404. London: HMSO.
6. Dale Committee Report of the Departmental Committee on Industrial Disease 1948, Cmd 7557. London: HMSO.
7. Beney Committee Report of the Departmental Committee appointed to review the Diseases Provisions of the National Insurance (Industrial Injuries) Act 1955. Parliamentary papers. Cmnd 9548. London: HMSO.
8. Fletcher CM. Pneumoconiosis of coal miners. *British Medical Journal*. 1948; **1**: 1065-74.
9. Hugh Jones P, Fletcher CM. *The social consequences of pneumoconiosis among coal miners in South Wales.* London: HMSO, 1951.
10. Cochrane AL. The attack rate of progressive massive fibrosis. *British Journal of Industrial Medicine*. 1962; **19**: 52-64.
11. Cooke WE. Fibrosis of the lung due to the inhalation of asbestos dust. *British Medical Journal*. 1924; **2**: 147.
12. Merewether ERA, Price CR. Reports on effects of asbestos dust on the lungs and dust suppression in the asbestos industry. London: HMSO, 1930.
13. Merewether ERA, Chief Inspector of Factories. Annual Report of the Chief Inspector of Factories for 1947. Parliamentary papers 1948-49. Cmnd 7621. London: HMSO.
14. Doll R. Mortality from lung cancer in asbestos workers. *British Journal of Industrial Medicine*. 1955; **12**: 81-6.
15. Wagner JC, Sleggs CA, Marchand P. Diffuse pleural mesothelioma and asbestos exposure in the North Western Cape Province. *British Journal of Industrial Medicine*. 1960; **17**: 260-71.
16. Hilliard AK, Lovett JK, McGavin CR. The rise and fall in incidence of malignant mesothelioma from a British Naval Dockyard 1979-1999. *Occupational Medicine*. 2003; **53**: 209-12.
17. Peto J, Hodgson JT, Matthews FE, Jones JR. Continuing increase in mesothelioma mortality in Britain. *Lancet.* 1995; **345**: 535-9.
18. Cochrane AL, Higgins IT. Pulmonary ventilatory functions of coalminers in various areas in relation to the x-ray category of pneumoconiosis. *British Journal of Preventive and Social Medicine*. 1961; **15**: 1-11.
19. Cockcroft A, Seal RME, Wagner JC *et al.* Post mortem study of emphysema on coalworkers and non-coalworkers. *Lancet.* 1982; **2**: 600-3.

20. Marine WM, Gurr D, Jacobsen M. Clinically important respiratory effects of dust exposure and smoking in British coal miners. *American Review of Respiratory Disease.* 1988; **137**: 106–12.

21. Soutar C, Campbell S, Gurr D *et al.* Important deficits of lung function in three modern colliery populations: relations with dust exposure. *American Review of Respiratory Disease.* 1993; **147**: 797–803.

SECTION **FOUR**

Legal issues

9 Medicolegal reports and the role of the expert witness
   Diana M Kloss

9

Medicolegal reports and the role of the expert witness

DIANA M KLOSS

Introduction	113
Civil and criminal law	113
The role of the doctor in providing medicolegal reports	114
The purpose of expert medical reports	117

The form of the expert report	118
Going to court	119
References	121

INTRODUCTION

The need for a medical opinion is a daily requirement of those who work in the field of compensation for personal injury. In disputes between employers and employees, the doctor may be asked to decide whether the employee is fit for work and, if not, whether he is likely to be able to return in the foreseeable future. Doctors also regularly appear in criminal courts to give an account of the victim's injuries or to advise on the time and cause of injury. They may be asked for an opinion on the mental state of a person accused of crime. In other areas, they may be drawn into a case where relatives doubt the validity of a will signed by a testator who was allegedly incompetent, or they may become involved in child care cases. In a growing number of cases, it is the doctor who stands accused of negligence and must rely on other doctors to support what he has done, or omitted to do. This chapter will centre on medicolegal reports requested by a lawyer in a case of personal injury arising out of a work-related accident or disease and will then deal with the role of the expert medical witness appearing in a court of law.

The medical expert will be confronted with a totally different regime: a world of reasonable probabilities and reasonable doubt which is foreign to his scientific training. He may sometimes be asked to give evidence that may damage his patient, and be unable to refuse. It is important that he understand a little of the legal process and of the needs of the courts.

CIVIL AND CRIMINAL LAW

Criminal law is concerned with offences against society as a whole. Prosecution is therefore brought in almost all cases by a public official (Crown Prosecution Service in England and Wales, Procurator Fiscal in Scotland). Prosecutions for offences against the criminal law of health and safety at work are brought by the Health and Safety Executive or local authority. Crimes are divided according to the seriousness of the alleged offence. The less serious crimes are tried summarily by the magistrates courts in England and Wales, the district and sheriff courts in Scotland. The most serious crimes, such as murder and rape, are tried by a judge and jury in the Crown Court in England and Wales and the High Court in Scotland. When a defendant is found guilty by the criminal court he is punished by imprisonment, fines, probation orders etc., but although the criminal courts now also have power in some cases to order compensation to the victim, this is very much secondary to the primary function of punishment. The Criminal Injuries Compensation Board awards compensation out of public funds to the victims of crimes of violence.

Civil law is concerned with the adjudication of property rights and the award of compensation to those injured by another's unlawful act. A civil action is brought by the person who has suffered injury: the claimant (formerly known as the plaintiff) in England and Wales, the pursuer in Scotland. In England, cases of major importance are tried in the High Court; where less money is at stake, the County

Court is the proper venue. The equivalent courts in Scotland are the Court of Session and the Sheriff Court. Jury trials are rarely found in civil actions: most cases are tried by a single judge sitting without a jury. A defendant who is found liable will most commonly be ordered to pay monetary compensation or damages. Parties to civil actions have to finance themselves, unless they qualify for legal aid or are backed by a trade union or an insurance company. The loser is ordered to pay the costs of the winner, though the party who wins in a contest with a legally aided defendant cannot as a general rule recover his costs from the legal aid fund. In recent years, however, lawyers have been permitted to charge conditional fees whereby the amount of legal costs depends on the success or otherwise of the action.

In addition to the civil courts, there are a number of administrative tribunals which deal with cases in a limited area. Examples are the employment tribunals for employment disputes and the first tier tribunals for disputes over entitlement to welfare benefits. Of particular interest to doctors are medical appeal tribunals, whose work includes the determination of issues of medical assessment related to claims for industrial injuries benefits.

A vitally important distinction between the criminal and civil process is that in the criminal courts the prosecution must prove the defendant's guilt beyond a reasonable doubt, whereas in the civil action the burden is to prove liability on a balance of reasonable probabilities ('more likely than not').

In both civil and criminal courts, the British procedure is adversarial rather than inquisitorial. Each side must call evidence to support its case. The judge acts as a referee to see fair play and to make the final decision. Experts are called by both sides, not appointed by the judge, as in the civil law system adopted in most other European countries, derived from Roman law. In the United Kingdom, the coroners' courts, which deal with sudden, accidental and unnatural deaths, exceptionally follow an inquisitorial procedure.

Membership of the European Union has added an extra dimension to English and Scottish law. Since the aim of the community at its inception was primarily to create an economic community, domestic laws relating to compensation for personal injury have been unaffected. In other areas, however, where laws directly or indirectly restrict competition, sweeping changes have been directed by the Council of Ministers, the legislature of the Community. Medical and other professional qualifications obtained in one member state must be recognized in other states. The criminal law of health and safety at work and laws relating to product safety now stem mainly from Brussels, since a country which failed to achieve minimum safety standards at work or which imposed unnecessarily strict standards for consumer goods to exclude foreign imports would have an unfair advantage in an open market. Each member state must enforce Community law through its own courts and other institutions, but a reference may be made from domestic courts to the Court of Justice of the European Communities in Luxembourg.

THE ROLE OF THE DOCTOR IN PROVIDING MEDICOLEGAL REPORTS

There are two main circumstances where a medical report might be requested:

1. When a doctor has been involved in a case as an active participant and is asked to give evidence based on his knowledge of what has occurred. He may have treated the victim of a crime or accident in his surgery (office) or in hospital.
2. When the doctor is asked after the event to bring his professional skill and knowledge to bear as to how an injury was caused, its effect on the person injured or the prognosis for the future. Here, the doctor acts as an expert witness, not as a participant in the event being scrutinized by the court.

Witnesses of fact

The duty of confidentiality enshrined in the Hippocratic Oath yields to a conflicting duty to give evidence of events when called upon to do so by a court of law. Doctors, unlike lawyers, have no privilege against disclosure of their patients' secrets. A doctor who refused to obey the court's order could be punished for contempt. However, courts will sometimes rule that a doctor need not give evidence of confidential material if it is not necessary to assist the court to make a decision. The judge may be asked to peruse the relevant material in order to permit its non-disclosure.

Sometimes a claimant will be unable to decide whether he has a cause of action at all until he has seen medical evidence. He may have been told by fellow workers that he is exhibiting classic symptoms of an occupational disease, but be unsure of the medical details of his condition or of the doctor's diagnosis. Under the Civil Procedure Rules, he may apply to the court for an order that records be disclosed. The court has a discretion to restrict disclosure to the plaintiff's legal or medical advisers.

A health professional, including an occupational physician, is obliged by the Data Protection Act 1998 to disclose health records to the subject of those records, unless such disclosure would damage his physical or mental health or reveal the identity of a third party who wishes to remain anonymous. This also applies to records held by the National Health Service and foundation trusts and private hospitals, and to all medical records, both manual and held on computer.

A report of this kind should begin with factual information about the doctor, his qualifications and position, and the patient. It should state how the doctor met with the patient, giving time, place and general circumstances, together with the names of any other people present at the time. It should go on to give details of the results of the examination, and end with a summary of conclusions. At this stage, the doctor may give an opinion – for example, as to the cause of the injury or the likely prognosis for the future. This evidence may be vital later when the court has to apportion blame for the accident or fix the amount of damages.

Expert witnesses

Expert witnesses are called upon, not because they know anything about the *facts* of the case but because they can give an *opinion* as to a relevant issue. It is for the judge to decide whether someone is truly an expert. In medical cases, formal qualifications are of course important, as is experience in the relevant specialty. Any expert report, therefore, should be prefaced with the qualifications and status of the doctor. In 2000, a voluntary system of accreditation of experts of all kinds was created with the launch of the Council for the Registration of Forensic Practitioners (CRFP). The impetus for this was a number of criminal convictions which were quashed on appeal as unsafe and unsatisfactory because of the quality of expert evidence. Registration, which depends on demonstrated competence against defined standards, is voluntary. The council ceased trading in 2009. There are two other well-respected voluntary organizations created to represent and advise experts, the Expert Witness Institute and the Academy of Experts.

In 1999, a major revolution occurred in the system of civil justice in new Civil Procedure Rules (CPR), implementing reforms recommended by Lord Woolf in his report: Access to Justice. Before this, lawyers and their clients managed litigation for the most part. It was for the parties to decide which witnesses they wished to call, and experts often regarded themselves as 'hired guns', tending to be partisan in their evidence. Under the new rules, it is for the court to further the overriding objective of dealing justly with the case. This involves active management by identifying the issues at an early stage, encouraging parties to cooperate, fixing timetables and giving instructions about evidence. As regards expert evidence, though parties remain free to instruct experts as they think fit, the court has complete control over the use of evidence in court. Where the court has not sanctioned the appointment of an expert, the party may not be able to recover the costs of the expert's report, and will not permitted to rely on it in the proceedings.

Rule 35.1 states that expert evidence shall be restricted to that which is reasonably required to resolve the proceedings. Courts may refuse to give permission for any expert evidence to be called, may order that it be given in writing rather than orally in the proceedings, may limit the number of expert witnesses, or order that expert evidence may only be given by a single joint expert. This is a matter for the judge to decide and not for the parties and their lawyers. Sometimes, a party asks the judge for permission to instruct a new expert because of loss of confidence in an existing expert. In *Beck v Ministry of Defence* (2003),[1] a Flight Lieutenant in the RAF developed psychiatric illness. He was treated by an RAF general practitioner and consultant psychiatrist. He alleged that the treatment was negligent. The MOD instructed an expert psychiatrist, but lost confidence in him because he had insufficient knowledge of the MOD psychiatric referral system. They wanted a new expert, but the claimant refused to be psychiatrically examined a second time. The MOD applied to the court for permission to instruct a new expert. The Court of Appeal held that this would be granted only on condition that they disclosed to the claimant's lawyers the report of the first expert. Otherwise, the court would be encouraging the practice of 'expert shopping'. A claimant can reasonably object to having to be examined again if this is, or may be, because the conclusions of the first expert have proved more favourable to him than the defendants had anticipated.

In 2005, the Civil Justice Council approved the Protocol for the Instruction of Experts to Give Evidence in Civil Claims (the Protocol) and it was annexed to the Civil Procedure Rules as guidance for the courts. This sets out the duty of experts. They have an overriding duty to the court, which takes precedence over any obligation to the person instructing or paying them. 'Experts must not serve the exclusive interest of those who retain them'. Experts should provide opinions which are independent. A useful test of independence is that the expert would express the same opinion if given the same instructions by the opposing party.

Experts should confine their opinions to matters which are material to the disputes between the parties and provide opinions only in relation to matters which lie within their expertise. They should take into account all material facts before them at the time they give their opinion. Their reports should set out those facts and any literature or other material on which they have relied in forming their opinions. They should indicate whether an opinion is provisional, or qualified, and whether further information is required to express a final opinion.

Experts should inform those instructing them without delay (and preferably not in the middle of giving evidence) of any change in their opinions on any material matter and the reason for it. As Lord Justice Stuart-Smith said in *Vernon v Bosley (No 2)* (1997):[2]

> If a doctor whom it is proposed to call to give evidence relating to the plaintiff's expectation of life writes in any accompanying letter or subsequently that he has discovered that the plaintiff is suffering from a life-threatening disease unrelated to the accident, that letter must clearly be disclosed, if the doctor is to be called to give evidence on the question of expectation of life.

It would be the doctor's ethical duty to refuse to give evidence if he knew that a material fact was being withheld from the other side and that his evidence would therefore be misleading. The Protocol advises that experts should not be asked to, and should not, amend, expand or alter any parts of reports in a manner which distorts their true opinion, but may be invited to amend or expand their reports to ensure accuracy, internal consistency, completeness and relevance to the issues and clarity. In *Noble v Robert Thompson* (1979),[3] a psychiatrist wrote a report on a depressed mother with the hope that it would assist her in obtaining access to her children. The doctor wrote that access should not be enforced against the wishes of the children themselves. He refused to delete this when asked to do so and sued for his fee when the solicitors refused to pay. The judge gave judgement for the psychiatrist: 'It would be of no assistance to the courts if doctors were encouraged to abandon their professional approach and write reports designed to achieve particular objects, at the behest of the patient or anyone else'.

It is now mandatory for all reports to be signed and to contain the following declaration:

> I confirm that insofar as the facts stated in my report are within my own knowledge I have made clear what they are and I believe them to be true, and that the opinions I have expressed represent my true and complete professional opinion.

Part 35 Practice Direction

In addition, where there is a range of opinion on the matters dealt with in the report, the expert must summarize the range of opinions and give reasons for his own opinion. The report must also contain a statement that the expert understands his duty to the court and has complied and will continue to comply with that duty.

The House of Lords held in *Bolitho v City and Hackney Health Authority* (1998),[4] a clinical negligence claim, that as a general rule a consensus of opinion among distinguished experts in a specialty that a doctor has taken reasonable care will be accepted by the courts, but that the court has to be satisfied that such an opinion has a logical basis. As Lord Browne-Wilkinson put it:

> In particular, in cases involving, as they so often do, the weighing up of risks against benefits, the judge before accepting a body of opinion as being reasonable, responsible and respectable, will need to be satisfied that, in forming their views, the experts have directed their minds to the questions of comparative risks and benefits and have reached a defensible conclusion on the matter.

Experts should be aware that any failure by them to comply with the Civil Procedure Rules or court orders or any excessive delay for which they are responsible may result in the parties who instructed them being penalized in costs and even, in extreme cases, being debarred from placing the expert's evidence before the court. The judge can also make orders for costs directly against expert witnesses who cause significant expense to be incurred in flagrant and reckless disregard of their duties to the court (*Phillips v Symes* (2005)).[5]

Although Rule 35 obliges a party to disclose to the other an expert report on which he intends to rely at the trial, this does not extend to draft reports prepared at a preliminary stage to assist the lawyers to advise their client. The law of litigation privilege is that disclosure will not be ordered of any report prepared with a view to legal proceedings, unlike the patient's medical records which, as has already been discussed, do not attract the same privilege. In *Lee v SW Thames Regional Health Authority* (1985),[6] a child with severe burns was transported from one hospital to another in an ambulance. He was found to have suffered brain damage, probably caused by lack of oxygen. The plaintiff's lawyers asked the court to order disclosure of a memorandum prepared by the ambulance crew which had been sent to the health authority with a view to obtaining legal advice on liability. It was held that the court had no power to do this: the report was privileged. However, an accident report prepared partly to make a finding as to causation and future preventive measures and partly to prepare for legal proceedings is not privileged against disclosure (*Waugh v British Rail* (1980)).[7] The Protocol recognizes that from time to time parties instruct experts before proceedings are commenced or at any early stage in order to assess the strengths and weaknesses of a claim, without the intention of relying on those reports in litigation. Such reports are confidential and do not have to be disclosed to the other side, neither do preliminary reports made in preparation of the final report. In *Johnson v Marley Davenport Ltd* (2004),[8] the claimant suffered an accident on a construction site in which he badly damaged his head and spinal cord. A professor of forensic pathology was instructed by the claimant's solicitors to give expert advice on the possible cause of the accident, of which the claimant could remember nothing. He wrote a preliminary draft report for the purpose of a conference with the lawyers and a final report which was disclosed to the defendants. The defendants asked the court to order disclosure of the draft report, but disclosure was refused by the Court of Appeal.

Rule 35.10 removes from the ambit of privilege the lawyers' instructions to the expert, who is now required to set out in his report 'the substance of material instructions whether written or oral'. In *Lucas v Barking Havering and Redbridge Hospitals NHS Trust* (2003),[9] it was held that this did not give a right to the opposing party to see every document referred to in the expert's summary of his instructions (as, for example, a witness statement), as long as the expert's summary was complete and not misleading. However, if the expert is relying on published or unpublished literature, this must be disclosed.

A novel situation arose in *W v Egdell* (1990).[10] W was detained as a patient in a secure hospital without limit of time as a potential threat to public safety after he shot and killed five people. Ten years later, he applied to a mental health review tribunal to be discharged or transferred to a regional secure unit. His responsible medical officer, who had diagnosed him as suffering from schizophrenia which could be treated with drugs, supported the application. His solicitors instructed Dr Egdell, a consultant psychiatrist, to examine W and report on his mental condition with a view to using the report to support his application to the tribunal. In the event, Dr Egdell strongly opposed the transfer. The solicitors decided that as the report was unfavourable they would not place it before the tribunal and withdrew the application for time being. The doctor sent a copy, in breach of confidence, to the health authority, the Secretary of State and the tribunal, and the solicitors withdrew the application for the time being. It was held by the Court of Appeal as follows:

> A consultant psychiatrist who becomes aware, even in the course of a confidential relationship, of information which leads him, in the exercise of what the court considers a sound professional judgment, to fear that decisions may be made on the basis of inadequate information and with real risk of consequent danger to the public is entitled to take such steps as are reasonable in all the circumstances to communicate the grounds of his concern to the responsible authorities.

In *Kapadia v London Borough of Lambeth* (2000),[11] the claimant was pursuing a claim for disability discrimination against his employer in an employment tribunal. The employer's solicitors instructed an expert occupational physician to examine Kapadia and write a report. Kapadia gave his consent in writing, but when the case went to the tribunal he objected to the report being shown to his employer without his having the opportunity to read and approve it first. It was held that by consenting to be examined on behalf of the employers he was consenting to the disclosure in legal proceedings to the employers of a report resulting from that examination.

The Civil Proceedings Rules do not apply to employment tribunals, but the Employment Tribunals (Constitution and Rules of Procedure) Regulations 2004 follow a similar pattern. In *De Keyser v Wilson* (2001),[12] the claimant commenced proceedings against her employer in the employment tribunal for constructive dismissal. She alleged that she had a depressive illness which had been caused by stress at work. Solicitors for the employers asked that she undergo a psychiatric examination by an expert occupational physician. The letter of instruction set out a number of facts about the claimant, for example the death of her brother, a contested custody case, an adulterous affair and the criminal conviction of a man described as her lover, and invited the doctor to conclude that her illness had been caused by these events rather than her employment. The Employment Appeal Tribunal directed that the case should be allowed to proceed, but that another expert should be appointed, to be instructed in more general terms, because the instructions contained material that was irrelevant and abusive.

THE PURPOSE OF EXPERT MEDICAL REPORTS

It is suggested that the doctor should always keep clearly in mind what it is that must be proved to the court. In an action for damages for personal injury, for example, the claimant has to prove, on a balance of reasonable probabilities, first that the defendant was negligent or in breach of his statutory duties, second that the negligence of the defendant caused the claimant's injury and third that the claimant suffered some material injury to his physical or mental health. The amount of the damages (the legal term is 'quantum') will depend on the state in which the claimant is left after the accident. If a young healthy girl aged 17 years is very severely brain damaged in an accident at work caused by the negligence of her employer and dies almost immediately, her parents will receive only the statutory amount for bereavement, currently £10 000. However, if the doctors say she will live for another 20 years, though paralysed and insentient, she will be able to claim damages of £1 million or more for the necessary nursing care, special accommodation and the loss of the earnings she would have made if she had not been injured. Courts now have power to award periodic payments of damages rather than a lump sum (Courts Act 2005).

When a claimant has suffered such catastrophic injury and the damages are large, defendant insurance companies consider structured settlements. Until recently, these had to be agreed between the parties, but the Courts Act 2005 gives a discretion to the judge to order periodic rather than lump sum payments. A structured settlement involves the purchase of an annuity which then guarantees the claimant a sufficient income for the rest of his or her life, with no danger of damages running out if the doctors' predictions of life expectancy prove to be incorrect. The Inland Revenue has agreed that these payments will not be subject to income tax.

In another case, a man in his 50s is diagnosed as suffering from asbestosis due to exposure to asbestos by his employer. He is breathless and unable to work. There is a possibility that he may contract mesothelioma or lung cancer. He has been a moderate cigarette smoker all his adult life. The lawyers need from the doctor an estimate as to the percentage of disability caused by the cigarettes and a forecast of what may happen to him in the future.

Because the course of disease and injury is often unpredictable in the early stages, the doctor may write in his first report that he wishes to examine the patient again after a specified period has elapsed. Settlement of the claim may be deferred, not through lawyers' delays but to allow the full extent of the damage to become apparent. When the development of a further disability, such as epilepsy, is possible only in the longer term the lawyers may apply for an award of provisional damages. Such a settlement allows the claimant to return for more if his medical condition deteriorates after his award of damages. However, it was held in *Willson v Ministry of Defence* (1991)[13] that the mere progression of a particular disease was not appropriate for a provisional award. The plaintiff had slipped on a polished floor at work, injuring his ankle. Medical reports a year later stated that there would be degeneration of the ankle joint, that the plaintiff would remain prone to further injuries and that there was a possibility of arthritis. It was decided that this was not a suitable case for an award of provisional damages and that damages would be awarded on a lump sum basis.

Damages are of two kinds: special damages to compensate for losses up to the date of settlement or trial, and general damages to make up for future loss. By section 22 of the Social Security Act 1989 (amended in 1997), the defendant must deduct from the damages for loss of earnings paid to the claimant in respect of an accident or injury occurring after January 1, 1989 the gross amount of any relevant social security benefits paid or likely to be paid to the victim. The defendant then reimburses the Secretary of State with this sum. Relevant benefits for this purpose include attendance allowance, disablement benefit, income support, incapacity benefit, disability living and working allowance and jobseeker's allowance up to the end of the period of five years following the accident.

Causation is a particularly difficult area in which medical evidence may be vital. In cases of occupationally induced disease, evidence of research may be more important than examination of the claimant. The rate of hearing loss of workers exposed to high levels of noise in the shipyards was a central part of the evidence in *Thompson v Smiths Shiprepairers* (1984).[14] The court decided that most of the loss had occurred in the first years of exposure at a time when employers could not reasonably be expected to guard against it – a ruling that considerably lowered the awards of damages.

In *Fairchild v Glenhaven Funeral Services Ltd* (2002),[15] a worker who had been exposed to asbestos dust or fibres while working for several different employers had died of mesothelioma, a cancer caused by one or more asbestos fibres entering the pleura (or peritoneum). Did the fatal fibre or fibres which caused the cancer arise from the negligence of defendant A or defendant B or defendant C? It was impossible to identify the source of the rogue fibre and if the law demanded that degree of proof, the claimant would be bound to fail. The House of Lords held that, in such a case, it is enough for the claimant to prove that the employer's negligence *materially increased the risk* of contracting the disease. All the employers who had negligently exposed the claimant to asbestos were potentially liable. In *Barker v Corus* (2006),[16] it was held that each employer's insurance company could be liable only to pay a proportion of the damages related to the extent of the exposure for which they were responsible, but this was reversed for mesothelioma claimants by the Compensation Act 2006. The effect is that, where companies A, B and C have all been negligent in exposing a claimant to asbestos fibre, the claimant can sue any one of them for the whole of his damages. The company held liable can then sue the others for a contribution, but if they have gone out of business and no insurance policy is extant the claimant will not suffer, though he can never recover more than 100 per cent of his loss.

THE FORM OF THE EXPERT REPORT

The report should begin with the name and qualifications of the expert, the date and circumstances of his examination. The first section should deal with the history of the disease or injury. The date of birth of the patient should always be given. In an occupational injury case, the work is as important as the victim, but the lawyers will probably be asking for a separate report from an engineer on the technical aspects. In the past, lawyers were concerned about the non-admissibility of hearsay evidence, that is evidence of which the witness has no personal knowledge, but which has been reported to him. The Civil Evidence Act 1995 now permits hearsay evidence in civil proceedings, subject to safeguards.

The second section of the report should elucidate the present state of the injury. Obviously, this will be made up partly of what the patient says and partly of objective examination, such as radiographs or scans. At this stage, the doctor should consider whether there is any indication that the patient is inventing all or some of the symptoms and signs. Accusations of malingering should not be made lightly, however, although the patient cannot sue the doctor for defamation if he makes such an allegation. Later reports when injuries appear not to have responded to treatment may contain references to 'functional overlay' or 'compensationitis'. The law is that genuine psychological consequences of an injury do not preclude the award of damages: only if the patient is consciously inventing or exaggerating his symptoms is he not entitled to compensation. Defendant insurance companies may hire a photographer to catch such a claimant up a ladder repairing his roof when he is supposed to be in agony from a bad back. Courts have held that such covert surveillance is not a breach of the Human Rights Act 1998 (*Jones v University of Warwick* (2003)).[17]

At this stage in the report, the doctor should give an opinion as to the cause of the symptoms, setting out any possible alternative causes and any causes related to the conduct of the patient (e.g. obesity or cigarette smoking). As previously indicated, it is important to try to put a percentage figure on alternative causes, for example, 'the patient's smoking has contributed 50 per cent to his reduced lung function'. To write a fully comprehensive report, it is important to gain access to the patient's general practitioner and hospital records. The patient's written consent will, of course, be necessary. Some doctors follow the policy of writing a report and accompanying it with a covering letter pointing out inconsistencies or weaknesses in the patient's case. 'The patient says he has been in pain for months, but he has never visited his general practitioner during that time, nor has he been off work'. This practice is not to be encouraged. The doctor's duty to the court means that his report must be as objective as possible.

The next section should assess the effect of the disability on the patient both now and in the future. The following are important factors:

- Is there pain? Will it continue?
- Is there loss of mobility? Will it continue?
- Has the patient lost work? If still off work, how long will this continue? Will the patient be able to resume his job, or will he be permanently unfit? What job will he be able to do, if any?
- What jobs around the house is the patient unable to do? Child care? Housework? Gardening? Do-it-yourself? Will the situation improve?
- What hobbies is the patient now unable to enjoy? Will the situation improve?
- How has the disability affected the patient's general quality of life? Relationships? Enjoyment of life? What is the future likely to hold?

The report should state clearly what future complications are possible in the medical condition, if any. Arthritis? Epilepsy? Cancer? Again, the degree of risk should be estimated and the possible time scale for example, '80 per cent likelihood of arthritis within five years'. If an injury has brought forward the onset of a condition that would otherwise have remained dormant, an estimate should be made of the number of years of dormancy lost. The likely expectation of life should be given.

A typical expert report prepared for a civil court in a personal injury claim should contain the following elements:

- A coversheet with the name of the case and the case number, the name of the expert and the name of his instructing solicitors
- A table of contents
- A brief curriculum vitae of the expert
- A summary of conclusions
- The expert's instructions
- Documents examined (e.g. medical records) and other sources of evidence (e.g. any examinations or tests carried out)
- Chronology
- Scientific or technical background, with reference to relevant literature
- Opinion
- Literature citations
- Declaration that the expert acknowledges that his first duty is to the court, and the statement of truth as set out in the Practice Direction (above).

GOING TO COURT

Most actions for damages for personal injury are settled out of court. The costs of legal proceedings are such that most defendants, who are usually insurance companies, are willing to settle any claim which contains some merit. However, some claims have to be fought, because they are regarded as being without any justification or, more often, because they are in some way a test case on which other cases may depend.

The best medical expert witness from a lawyer's point of view is one who writes fair and balanced reports which he is able to defend under cross-examination. Such experts are likely to have long waiting lists. In some cases, doctors give up their medical practice in order to concentrate on medicolegal work. This may eventually be counter-productive, if the other side is able to argue that the expert is out of date or lacks recent 'hands-on' experience.

Experts are encouraged to agree reports if this is possible. It would be unusual for two eminent doctors to have totally opposing views of a particular case. The Woolf Report on civil proceedings recommends that every attempt should be made to resolve any conflict of evidence between doctors before the trial. The court may limit the parties to one expert if that is all that is necessary.

> The basic premise of my new approach is that the expert's function is to assist the court. There should be no expert evidence at all unless it will help the court, and no more than one expert in any one speciality unless this is necessary for some real purpose ... In cases where opposing experts are involved, the court already has power to direct the parties' experts to meet, before or after the experts have disclosed their reports, so as to identify and reduce areas of difference. Under the new rules the experts will be required (not simply authorized, as at present) to produce a report identifying matters agreed and outstanding areas of difference after such a meeting.[18]

As has been previously stated, the expert's role should be that of an independent adviser to the court. Lack of objectivity is to be avoided, especially if it arises from improper pressure by solicitors. As Lord Wilberforce said in *Whitehouse v Jordan* (1981):[19]

> It is necessary that expert evidence presented to the court should be, and should be seen to be, the independent product of the expert uninfluenced as to form or content by the exigencies of litigation.

It is not the function of the expert to comment in evidence about the parties' credibility as witnesses, merely to assess the likelihood of the truth of their story by objective criteria.

If the case does go to court, and the expert is called, certain practical points must be borne in mind. The first is that the expert must be available to give evidence, which may necessitate complicated arrangements if he or she is still in practice. Some solicitors follow the policy of subpoenaing their own witness, to be certain of his presence. Courts will be sympathetic to the needs of patients, but the doctor may have to wait for a considerable time before being called.

Obviously, an expert should try to make a good impression on the judge. Attire should be sober, and hands should be kept out of pockets and away from jewellery. When giving evidence, it is important to address the judge, not merely the advocate who is asking the questions. If there is to be reference to reports, these should be held in a paginated bundle, of which the judge and the other side should also have a copy. The expert should be positive and firm, yet reasonable, in approach and keep calm, especially under cross-examination. He should remember that counsel may attempt to cast doubt on his credibility by making him lose his temper or contradict himself. If the expert does not understand a question, or needs time to consider it, he should ask for it to be repeated. If he does not know the answer to a question, he should say so and not be tempted to venture speculative opinions which cannot be substantiated. It may be that in the course of the proceedings the expert's opinion has changed, because new facts have come to light. If this is the case, it is vital for him to inform his barrister before giving evidence. He should never try to tell jokes or upstage the judge when in the witness box. The judge will respect expert medical qualifications, but only if he is treated with respect.

In civil proceedings, the witness is first subjected to an examination by his own counsel. Although this should be a friendly process, it is important to answer questions, rather than volunteering information. Counsel will have planned how best to elucidate the evidence he needs. This is followed by cross-examination by counsel for the other side who is, of course, likely to be more hostile, though not discourteous, since bullying a witness can be counterproductive. Finally, a re-examination is permitted to clarify points which have been raised in cross-examination, but not to repeat the original evidence.

No one can be liable for defamation or negligence in respect of anything done in the course of judicial proceedings, which are protected by absolute privilege, that is even if the witness giving oral or written evidence to a court spoke maliciously without belief in the truth of what he was saying he cannot be sued for it, although he can be prosecuted for the crimes of perjury and contempt of court if he makes a false statement without an honest belief in its truth. It was established by the House of Lords in *Watson v M'Ewan* (1905)[20] that the same immunity attaches to statements made by the expert witness while preparing for trial.

In *Stanton v Callaghan* (2001),[21] the Court of Appeal considered how far that immunity extends. The claimant owned a house which had suffered subsidence damage. Partial underpinning was carried out, paid for by insurance, but this failed to stabilize the property. An expert surveyor, Mr Callaghan, was engaged by the claimant and reported that partial underpinning had been an inappropriate solution. He recommended total underpinning, but the insurers rejected the claim. The claimant therefore commenced proceedings against the insurance company, and Callaghan was instructed as an expert witness. Some time after the issue of proceedings, Callaghan agreed with the insurance company's expert that another and cheaper solution would be equally effective and as a result the claimant was forced to settle the claim for an amount of money which covered his legal costs, but not the costs of the remedial work. He therefore sued Callaghan for negligence. It was held that an expert is not immune from an action for negligence in respect of advice as to the merits of a party's claim in litigation, but that in this case, where the surveyor's advice was for the principal purpose of his eventually giving evidence in court, he did have immunity from civil liability.

In *Hughes v Lloyd's Bank plc* (1998),[22] in contrast, the plaintiff was injured in a road accident. She attended her general practitioner who was asked to report on the severity of her injuries for the purpose of a claim for compensation. He wrote that her condition was not serious, on the faith of which the plaintiff settled her claim for £600. It then became apparent that the injury was far more severe than the doctor had predicted and the plaintiff sued him for negligence. The Court of Appeal held that he was not immune from civil liability. When he made his report he was not an expert witness, merely a paid adviser at a preliminary stage. If he had failed to take reasonable care, he could be sued for compensation.

In *Phillips v Symes* (2004),[23] Mr Justice Peter Smith held that an expert witness can be ordered to pay costs where he has been guilty of 'flagrant reckless disregard of his duties to the court'.

The question later arose as to whether expert witnesses have immunity from the disciplinary powers of professional bodies, such as the General Medical Council (GMC). Sally Clark, a solicitor, was convicted in 1999 of the murder of two of her three infant children. At the trial, Sir Roy Meadow, an eminent paediatrician, gave evidence for the prosecution that the risk of two children in the same household dying from accidental 'cot death' was 1 in 73 million. Mrs Clark's conviction was later quashed because the prosecution had not disclosed relevant medical evidence to the defence (not because Professor Meadow's evidence was misleading), but Professor Meadow was referred to the GMC's Fitness to Practise Panel by Mrs Clark's father. They concluded that he had gone outside his field of expertise and given erroneous and misleading statistical evidence. Although he had acted in good faith, he was convicted of serious professional misconduct and his name was erased from the medical register. Professor Meadow appealed to the High Court. Mr Justice Collins held that he was not guilty of serious professional misconduct and restored his name to the register. He also held that an expert witness should, in general, be immune from fitness to practise (FTP) proceedings unless the trial judge found his shortcomings so serious that he should be referred to his professional body, if he or she had one. The GMC appealed to the Court of Appeal which held that expert witnesses did not have immunity from FTP proceedings, but agreed that Professor Meadow, though guilty of misconduct in going outside his area of expertise, was honest, though mistaken, and could not be held to be guilty of serious professional misconduct (*General Medical Council v Meadow* (2006)).[24]

Key points

- The criminal courts are primarily concerned with the punishment of offences against society as a whole, the civil courts with the adjudication of property rights and the compensation of those injured by another's unlawful act.
- Doctors are called to give evidence in courts and tribunals either as witnesses of fact, because they were involved in the case as an active participant, or as expert witnesses, called upon to give an opinion as to a relevant issue, for example, the cause of an injury and the likely prognosis.
- Although doctors, in general, owe a duty of confidence to patients and others who confide in them, courts and tribunals have power to order them to reveal confidential information without consent. The General Medical Council recognizes that disclosure in response to a court order is one of the exceptions to the duty of confidence.
- Reforms of civil procedure brought about by the Civil Procedure Rules 1999 (as amended) restrict the right of the parties to call expert evidence. In many cases, the court may order that only a single joint expert should be instructed. The 2005 Protocol sets out the duties of experts, whose overriding duty is to the court, not to the party instructing them.
- Expert witnesses have immunity from liability for defamation and negligence in respect of anything said in the course of legal proceedings, and statements made while preparing for a trial.
- However, doctors acting as an expert witness do not have immunity from Fitness to Practise Proceedings before the General Medical Council.

REFERENCES

1. [2005] 1 WLR 2206.
2. [1997] 1 All ER 614.
3. 20 July 1979, unreported.
4. [1998] AC 232.
5. [2005] 1 WLR 2043.
6. [1985] 2 All ER 385.
7. [1980] AC 521.
8. [2005] PIQR P141.
9. [2004] 1 WLR 220.
10. [1990] 1 All ER 835.
11. [2000] IRLR 699.
12. [2001] IRLR 324.
13. [1991] 1 All ER 628.
14. [1984] QB 405.
15. [2003] 1 AC 32.
16. [2006] 2 AC 572.
17. [2003] EWCA Civ 151.
18. *Access to Justice.* Final report by Lord Woolf MR to the Lord Chancellor on the civil justice system in England and Wales. London: HMSO, 1996: 139, 140.
19. [1981] 1 WLR 246.
20. [1905] AC 480.
21. [2001] QB 75.
22. [1998] PIQR 98.
23. [2005] 1 WLR 2043.
24. [2006] EWCA Civ 1390.

PART TWO

DISEASES ASSOCIATED WITH CHEMICAL AGENTS

Section One: Occupational toxicology 125
Section Two: Metals 149
Section Three: Gases 251
Section Four: Other chemical exposures 319

# SECTION ONE

Occupational toxicology

10 Occupational toxicology: general principles 127
   Peter G Blain and Robert D Jefferson
11 Risks and hazards in occupational and environmental exposures 141
   Robert L Maynard

10

Occupational toxicology: general principles

PETER G BLAIN AND ROBERT D JEFFERSON

Introduction	127	Variation in susceptibility to xenobiotics	137
Absorption and distribution of chemicals	128	Summary	138
Toxicokinetics	128	Acknowledgements	138
Kinetics of exposure	130	References	139
Detoxification and elimination	132		

INTRODUCTION

Occupational physicians are frequently involved in the assessment of health risks associated with exposure to chemicals in the workplace and this responsibility increasingly includes the public environment. Interaction with chemicals in the environment is a necessity for any living organism and human beings are no exception. As a consequence, a range of complex biochemical mechanisms has evolved in humans to protect against absorbed toxic compounds. Whenever there is a risk of exposure to hazardous chemicals, it is important that the factors affecting the absorption and distribution of chemicals in the body, the processes involved in detoxification and elimination and the influence of susceptibility are taken into consideration. An understanding of toxicology (the study of 'poisons') is essential for occupational physicians in their role as health risk managers or when investigating the exposure of workers to hazardous chemicals. Toxicology is growing rapidly as a science and demonstrates increasing relevance to the activities of all healthcare professionals. A range of standard reference texts is now available.[1]

Paracelsus is regarded as the 'father' of toxicology and credited with first recognizing the association between absorbed dose and toxicity – the dose–response relationship.[2] Although he undoubtedly understood the concept of potency, his comments on the relationship of toxic effects to the amount of chemical ingested were, in fact, intended to increase consumer confidence in the safety of novel remedies that he was marketing (he was an early snake-oil salesman!).

The dose–response relationship is a useful indicator of the toxicity of a chemical. Toxic doses in man may range from μg to g/kg body weight and chemicals may be classified according to their probable lethal human dose (Table 10.1).

In addition to intrinsic toxicity and mode of action, the dynamics of absorption, metabolism, distribution and elimination are important variables in the development of a toxic effect. Exposure in the workplace environment can be to many different chemicals, simply or as mixtures, and

Table 10.1 Toxicity rating of chemicals by probable lethal oral dose in adults.

Toxicity rating	Lethal oral dose	Typical volume
1. Practically non-toxic	>15 g/kg	More than 1 quart
2. Slightly toxic	5–15 g/kg	Between pint and quart
3. Moderately toxic	0.5–5 g/kg	Between ounce and pint
4. Very toxic	50–500 mg/kg	Between teaspoonful and ounce
5. Extremely toxic	5–50 mg/kg	Between 7 drops and teaspoonful
6. Supertoxic	<5 mg/kg	A taste (less than 7 drops)

the occupational physician must be able to recognise hazardous situations, know about the absorption and detoxification of chemicals and have a detailed knowledge of their potential toxic effects.

An additional factor is the interindividual variation in specific detoxifying enzyme activities which may differ markedly (greater or lesser) between individuals within a population. These variations constitute subgroups, or genetic polymorphisms, in the population; some subgroups are small in size (poor metabolizers of debrisoquine constitute about 10 per cent of the general population) or large (the general population are more or less equally divided into either fast or slow acetylators). Subgroups with greater activity may produce toxic metabolites more rapidly (fast acetylators are more likely to develop isoniazid hepatotoxicity), whereas poor metabolizers may be at more risk because they are unable to detoxify a chemical adequately (slow acetylators are more likely to develop an isoniazid neuropathy and poor debrisoquine metabolizers a perhexiline neuropathy). The role of interindividual variation in susceptibility to toxicity requires greater general consideration, since, in certain combinations of circumstances, it may contribute to the 'dirty worker' phenomenon. At present, most work on genetic polymorphisms relates to drug metabolism and toxicity, but the relevance to non-drug chemicals is increasingly recognized.

Within species differences in susceptibility are usually of a lesser magnitude than the variation between species. Most toxicity data are derived from animal toxicity tests and the models generated subsequently applied to man. Apart from the ethical considerations related to this use of animals, serious scientific problems may arise in extrapolating from animal models to human health risks. Ideally, data generated from animals should be supplemented or replaced with information derived from human studies.

ABSORPTION AND DISTRIBUTION OF CHEMICALS

Foreign compounds (also referred to as exogenous chemicals or xenobiotics) must be absorbed from the surrounding environment and transported to a target site in the body for a toxic effect to occur. The chemical may have to cross the many cell membranes which form a lipoprotein barrier to the extracellular environment, as well as maintaining the integrity of the cell. Specific transport mechanisms evolved to facilitate the absorption and distribution of nutrients, rather than toxic chemicals, and most xenobiotics are transported by simple methods and not complex carrier-associated processes (some compounds do enter cells on such carriers, e.g. paraquat transport into lung cells[3]). A carrier is usually specific for an endogenous substance and unless the xenobiotic compound has a very similar structure, it will not usually be able to bind to the carrier (paraquat has a similar structure to endogenous diamines, such as putrescine[4]).

Lipid solubility is a major factor determining the extent and rate of simple diffusion through a lipoprotein membrane: lipophilic molecules diffuse more readily than those that are hydrophilic. The rate of transport is dependent on the partition coefficient (i.e. the ratio of solubility in octanol/water). Non-ionized molecules are often more lipophilic and ions generally more hydrophilic, so the movement of electrolytes, such as organic acids and bases, is related to the degree of ionic dissociation and the lipid solubility of the non-ionized form of a compound.

The extent of dissociation is expressed in the Henderson–Hasselbach equation:

$$pK_a = pH - \log[A^-]/[HA]$$

or

$$pH = pK_a + \log[\text{base}]/[\text{acid}]$$

where [HA] is the concentration of the non-ionized form, [A^-] is the concentration of the ionized form and pK_a is the negative log of the dissociation constant.

The cell membrane controls the movement of chemicals in or out of the cytoplasm and several methods have been identified by which xenobiotics are transported across membranes:

- Simple diffusion down a concentration gradient is the most common and simple method, does not require expenditure of energy and is the principal mechanism for the transport of most lipid soluble, non-ionized compounds.
- Filtration allows water, ionic and hydrophilic molecules of appropriate size to pass through small pores (about 0.4 nm in diameter) in the cell membrane.
- Facilitated diffusion is carrier-mediated, transports chemicals with specific common structures across the cell membrane and at high concentrations may become saturated.
- Active transport allows the absorption of substances against a concentration gradient, but requires the expenditure of energy and so is linked to the metabolic activity of the cell.
- Phagocytosis and pinocytosis enable particulates and solutions to be taken into a cell by the extrusion or invagination of an area of the membrane and engulfing of part of the extracellular environment.

These absorption processes, although at a cellular level, influence the degree and nature of absorption through the lungs, skin and gastrointestinal tract and are, therefore, relevant at the macro level of hazard assessment.

TOXICOKINETICS

Toxicokinetics is the study of the dynamic (kinetic) relationships between the concentration of a chemical (toxicon) in body fluids and tissues and its biological effects (toxicodynamics). The investigation and management of an individual exposed to toxic chemicals require a basic knowledge of toxicokinetic concepts, alongside understanding of the mechanisms by which chemicals gain entry to the body and are biotransformed into non-toxic or possibly toxic metabolites. Toxicokinetic analysis produces a mathematical description of the dynamics of absorption, distribution and elimination of a chemical. Although this involves the descriptive use of mathematical expressions and models, it does have a practical use in evaluating the significance of blood concentrations obtained from biological monitoring and then determining the nature of exposure control (i.e. risk management). (Pharmacokinetic analysis quantifies the dynamic changes in the concentration of a drug (pharmacon) and has been incorporated into toxicokinetics as there are no fundamental differences between a drug and a toxin – the major toxic effect of a drug is often the main reason for its therapeutic use.)

The kinetic profile of a chemical can be used to estimate the body burden following workplace exposure and to predict the time required for near total elimination of a chemical from the body. Similarly, the rate at which a compound is absorbed or eliminated from the body can be quantified and applied to occupational health practice.[5,6]

Toxicokinetic concepts

The body is composed of a multitude of real 'compartments' in the form of cells, tissues and organs. However, the analysis of kinetic data necessarily models a limited number of theoretical compartments. These models are one solution to the analysis of data but it must always be remembered that models are fitted to data rather than data to models. It is sometimes difficult to be certain that a specific model accurately describes the processes involved; one method of validating a model is to perturb the system and see if the effect mirrors a similar change in the real world (e.g. decreased ventilation, hepatic metabolism, renal blood flow, etc.). Toxicokinetic concepts have led to the development of complex multicompartment models for the absorption, distribution and elimination of chemicals by the body. The simplest of these is, obviously, a single compartment model which considers the body as a homogeneous unit. More sophisticated analysis uses two, three or, occasionally, many more compartmental models (see Figure 10.1).

The rate of absorption (K_{abs}) is dependent on many parameters that are often difficult to measure individually so in the initial analysis of blood concentration data the rate of elimination (K_{el}) is determined as this often appears to be the simpler process (e.g. via the kidney). The majority of chemical substances are eliminated from blood by an apparent first-order process which is seen as an exponential decay (see Figure 10.2) and described by the mathematical equation:

$$C_t = C_0 \cdot e^{-\beta t}$$

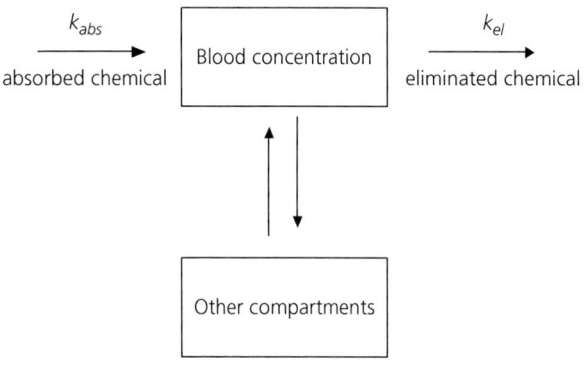

Figure 10.1 Compartmental model.

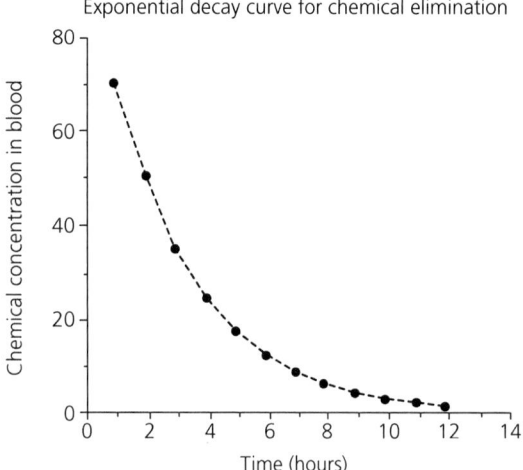

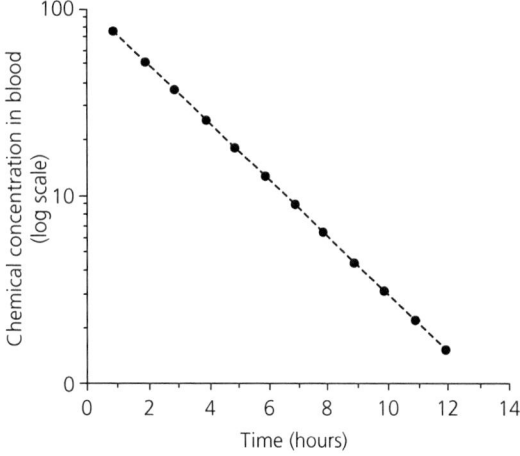

Figure 10.2 Elimination of a chemical from blood by a first-order process. The rate of elimination is linearized when log values for C_t are used.

where C_t is the plasma concentration at time t, C_0 is the plasma concentration at $t = 0$, e is the natural number (2.7182) and β is the elimination rate constant (K_{el}).

The elimination of some chemicals (e.g. phenytoin, ethanol) is non-linear and demonstrates zero order (saturation) kinetics. In first-order kinetics, a constant fraction of the chemical is eliminated in unit time. In zero-order kinetics, a constant mass of the chemical is eliminated in unit time and, consequently, the process can become saturated and toxic effects occur following a very small increase in dose.

The half life ($t_{1/2}$) of a chemical is the time period during which the blood concentration decreases by one-half and is inversely related to the elimination rate constant (β):

$$t_{1/2} = 0.693/\beta \text{ (where 0.693 is } \log_e \text{ (ln) 2)}.$$

The half-life can be determined from the slope (elimination rate) of the log plasma concentration/time graph following a single dose of a compound (Figure 10.2).

The concept of a half-life is useful for studying the uptake and elimination of compounds as it can be shown that after 3.3 half-lives the plasma concentration reaches 90 per cent of the equilibrium concentration, and 95 per cent after five half-lives. Hence, $5 \times t_{1/2}$ is the time taken for 95 per cent of a dose of chemical to be eliminated from the body after absorption, or to reach 95 per cent of its steady-state value. The half-life is also the minimum time interval between chemical exposure (or drug administration) that avoids progressive accumulation. Data about the elimination half-life of a compound can be used to assess the importance of the duration of exposure and increase the value of either blood or breath monitoring of exposed workers.

The volume of distribution (V_D) is a theoretical estimate of the extent of the distribution of a chemical in the body, provides a measure of the relative magnitude of differential tissue uptake and is expressed in units of litres or litres/kg:

$$V_D = \chi/C_0$$

where χ is the total amount of chemical (i.e. body burden, if bioavailability is 100 per cent) and C_0 is the plasma concentration at t_0.

Compounds with a large volume of distribution are widely and extensively distributed throughout the tissues of the body and the plasma concentration constitutes a small fraction of the total body burden. A small volume of distribution implies limited tissue distribution and indicates that the plasma concentration is a good indicator of the total amount in the body (chemicals with a V_D approximating to blood volume (3–5 litres) are almost totally restricted to systemic circulation); V_D is apparent and not real, so a chemical which is concentrated in a tissue (such as fat) and has a low blood concentration, will have a V_D so high that may markedly exceed the total volume of the body (e.g. >200 litres for some organic solvents).

Clearance (Cl) is the volume of the V_D that is completely cleared of a chemical per unit time (i.e. mL/min, litre/hour). Clearance is a more independent measure of elimination than half-life since it is a physiologically meaningful measure of the efficiency of elimination from the body. It provides the most reliable measurement of the elimination of a compound since clearance by a particular organ can be estimated (similar to measuring renal clearance of insulin, etc.).

In simple terms,

$$Cl = V_D \times K_{el}$$

Changes in the V_D may alter the $t_{1/2}$, but leave clearance unaltered. Chemicals with a large V_D may have a high clearance yet persist in the body and have a long $t_{1/2}$ of elimination.

The total systemic clearance is dependent on the specific clearances of each organ:

$$Cl_{systemic} = Cl_{renal} + Cl_{hepatic} + Cl_{other\ routes}$$

The clearance of a chemical by an organ (Cl_{organ}) can be measured and is principally dependent on blood flow and the degree of extraction (extraction ratio, ER) of the chemical from blood:

$$Cl_{organ} = Q \times ER$$

where Q is the organ blood flow and ER is the extraction ratio.

The ER is determined from the arterial and venous concentration difference across an organ:

$$ER = \frac{C_A - C_V}{C_A}$$

where C_A is the concentration in blood flowing into organ (arterial) and C_V is the concentration in blood flowing out of organ (venous).

For those organs with a high ER (e.g. liver, kidney), clearance will be high and directly dependent on organ blood flow. Chemicals with a high liver clearance undergo extensive first-pass metabolism (e.g. nitrites). Organs with a low ER (e.g. muscle, bone) have a clearance that is not dependent on blood flow.

KINETICS OF EXPOSURE

The principal routes of exposure in the workplace are by inhalation or skin absorption.

Inhalation kinetics

The lungs enable the efficient transfer of gases between the body and the environment. The tissue barrier separating air and blood is only 0.5–1.0 μm thick and the 300–400 million alveoli provide a large surface area for diffusion. In addition, the media on either side of this barrier are continuously renewed; the air is changed 12–15 times per minute and the pulmonary blood flows at a rate of 3.5–5 litre per minute at rest. It is not surprising, therefore, that volatile chemicals can be both efficiently absorbed from, and eliminated in, the breath.[7]

Analysis of expired air has been used to diagnose diabetes and uraemia and, more extensively, to detect ethanol consumption in motorists (although only about 1 per cent of the total body burden of ethanol is eliminated via this route). Real-time monitoring of the breath of workers exposed to volatile compounds in industry is a potentially useful non-invasive technique for determining the degree of absorption, but does require that the factors affecting the absorption, distribution, metabolism and elimination (i.e. the toxicokinetics) of compounds have been previously determined for this route in man.[8]

A number of volatile organic compounds can be identified in the breath of the normal general population[9,10] at concentrations of parts per billion (in hospital practice the inhalation kinetics of volatile compounds are of importance to the anaesthetist); in industrial workers the concentrations are generally in parts per million. Breath analysis has been used in experimental toxicology to study lipid peroxidation and in the investigation of defective intestinal absorption, but monitoring of marker metabolites in the expired breath remains a relatively unexploited technique. However, there is renewed interest in the potential of breath monitoring in the diagnosis of certain disease states.

Routine monitoring of the workplace usually assumes the level of contamination of air with a compound is a reliable indicator of worker exposure and, by implication, probable absorption of the chemical. However, this is not a direct relationship; the environmental concentration merely indicates the potential for absorption. Under continuous exposure, any change in the inhaled air concentration will have a corresponding effect on the alveolar air concentration. Increasing the duration of exposure produces a progressive increase in blood concentration towards a plateau value (equilibrium is reached). A progressive saturation of blood and tissues with the compound involves a reduction in the difference between arterial and venous blood with less of the inhaled compound moving from the alveoli to capillary blood. For volatile compounds that are highly lipophilic and selectively taken up by fatty tissues, tissue saturation is never reached in the normal exposure period in the workplace. In contrast, the elimination of such compounds from the body is extremely slow and the potential exists for progressive accumulation following frequent modest exposures.[11]

Other factors influencing the inhalation kinetics of a volatile compound include the environmental air concentration, duration of exposure, rate of alveolar ventilation, cardiac output, blood and tissue solubility and the degree of metabolism of the chemical. Volatile compounds are usually inhaled as a gas mixture with air and most are completely miscible in all proportions. The concentration of gases and volatile compounds in a mixture is expressed in terms of partial pressures, which are often incorrectly considered equivalent to concentrations; the relative concentrations of dissolved materials can be expressed in terms of partial pressures which add up to a total pressure of 100 per cent. However, a limit is set on the concentration (wt/unit vol) which this represents by the solubility of the volatile materials.

Solubility is inversely related to temperature and proportional to the pressure of the chemical in the surrounding gas. The partial pressures of constituent volatile compounds vary with the absolute pressure but, at a fixed pressure, the concentration of each gas or vapour varies directly with its partial pressure and indirectly with the total pressure of the gas/vapour mixture. A gas or vapour present at a partial pressures of 100 per cent can still have its concentration (wt/unit vol) varied over a range that is determined by the absolute pressure.

The rate of delivery of an inhaled mixture of air and a volatile compound depends upon alveolar ventilation. A doubling of alveolar ventilation from 4 litre/min to 8 litre/min produces a minimal increase in the blood concentration of a poorly water soluble substance, but an appreciable increase for highly water-soluble substances. Cardiac output has an opposing effect on alveolar concentration and this is most noticeable for highly water soluble, or extensively metabolized substances, rather than poorly soluble compounds. An increase in cardiac output results in a larger amount of the inhaled substance passing from the lungs to the blood. A decrease has the opposite result and causes a rise in alveolar concentration.[12]

An insoluble substance that does not pass into the bloodstream will increase in alveolar concentration until it is equal to the environmental air concentration, the time taken being equivalent to the lung wash-in time. A substance with an infinite solubility could in theory never increase the alveolar concentration and, although such substances do not exist, there is a broad range of solubilities. The concentration in alveolar or expired air, expressed relative to the environmental air concentration is inversely proportional to the blood solubility of a compound. Relative concentrations of >0.5 are poorly soluble and those <0.5 are highly soluble. The effect of solubility on alveolar concentration is seen in Figure 10.3.

The aerodynamic particle sizes of aerosols, mists and sprays also affect their accessibility to alveoli and large particles may be deposited in the larger airways, or in the pharynx, and swallowed.

The arterial concentration of an inhaled compound can be estimated from the alveolar concentration using the blood–air partition coefficient of the chemical (if partial pressure equilibrium is attained rapidly). This is not attained immediately, but requires a finite time that depends on the half-life of the compound:

$$t_{\frac{1}{2}} = 0.693\, V \times \frac{P_c}{F}$$

where V is the tissue volume, P_c is the tissue–blood partition coefficient and F is the rate of blood flow to the tissue.

A high relative alveolar concentration is found for compounds that undergo little metabolism. As the degree of biotransformation increases so does the level of metabolites in pulmonary blood. The combined effects of metabolism and solubility affect the blood kinetics of a

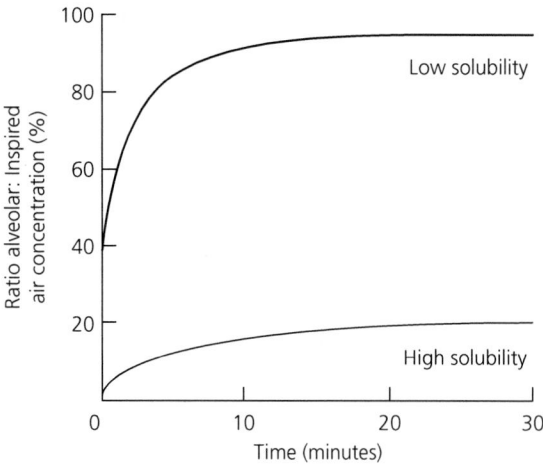

Figure 10.3 Effect of solubility on the alveolar concentration of a chemical.

chemical. Extensive metabolism can significantly undermine the usefulness of biological monitoring of exhaled breath, unless a volatile marker metabolite predominates and there is no phenotypic variation in biotransformation within the population.

Routine measurement of the breath concentrations of industrial or therapeutic chemicals is poorly utilized for monitoring exposure or assessing body burden. Rigorous kinetic analysis is essential to establish its value and reliability as a non-invasive method of assessment. The necessary technology is widely available and still simply requires more consideration.

Dermal absorption

The skin is an effective barrier to many environmental chemicals because the stratum corneum, acting to control the loss of water from the body, also functions as the principal barrier to dermal penetration by chemicals.[13] Direct absorption through the skin is a major route of exposure to pesticides and other workplace chemicals and accidental skin contamination by spillage or deposition on the skin surface can be followed by rapid systemic absorption. The lipid solubility of a chemical determines how easily it can cross the stratum corneum, the epidermis and upper dermis, and then enter the systemic circulation. Compounds with a molecular weight exceeding 500 Da cannot easily pass through the lipid layers of the stratum corneum, and hence are absorbed to a much lower extent than smaller molecules.[14] However, perturbation of the stratum corneum barrier by mechanical means, or by chemicals such as solvents, will increase percutaneous absorption. Similarly, individuals with poor barrier function originating from disease states, such as atopy, may exhibit a higher degree of percutaneous absorption. Highly lipophilic chemicals can penetrate the stratum corneum, but further penetration is limited by low solubility of the penetrant in the aqueous environment of the viable epidermis. However, lipophilic chemicals may accumulate in the stratum corneum, potentially forming a reservoir for systemic absorption after the surface dose has been removed.[15] Direct absorption through skin is utilized for pharmaceutical compounds which are rapidly metabolized by first-pass metabolism in the gut wall or liver following oral administration. The drug, in a suitable formulation, is applied to the skin and enters the systemic circulation directly bypassing initial first-pass metabolism in the liver.

Dermal absorption has been considered a passive process limited only by the physical barrier function of the stratum corneum. The skin, however, is capable of metabolizing a range of xenobiotics and studies, with whole skin homogenates and subcellular fractions, have demonstrated significant metabolic activity, albeit less than that found in liver (about 10 per cent hepatic activity). Monooxygenases (including cytochromes P450, flavin-containing monooxygenases and NAPD(H)-quinone reductases), oxidoreductases, conjugation pathways and esterase activity have all been identified in skin. Consequently, many compounds that penetrate the stratum corneum may undergo biotransformation to active metabolites before entering the systemic circulation. A limited number of *in vivo* studies in humans have indicated that metabolism takes place in the skin *in vivo* during absorption of some compounds (e.g. aldrin, glycerol trinitrate, synthetic prostaglandins and amines in oxidative hair dyes). A number of *in vitro* models of percutaneous absorption, using excised human or animal skin, have been developed in recent years, the most popular being based on static or flow through diffusion cells. A substantial number of studies have confirmed that these techniques are relatively robust[16] and give good predictions of percutaneous absorption *in vivo*.[17] The *in vitro* skin absorption test was formally adopted as a test guideline by the Organisation for Economic Co-operation and Development (OECD) in 2004.[18]

DETOXIFICATION AND ELIMINATION

Most toxic xenobiotics have no nutritional value and are metabolized primarily to reduce their potential toxicity and facilitate elimination from the body. The majority of compounds that gain entry most easily to the body are lipophilic and likely, therefore, to be retained. Before they can be excreted they must be converted into a form that is more easily eliminated. The liver is the major organ for the metabolism (biotransformation) of such compounds. There is, however, increasing evidence that other organs such as the skin, lungs, kidney and skeletal muscle may have an important capability for biotransformation, albeit at a lower level of activity than the liver (Table 10.2). Detoxification does not always occur and, for some chemicals, toxicity may be enhanced as a result of biotransformation.

The metabolism of xenobiotics is carried out by a group of relatively non-specific enzymes. The key enzyme in this system is cytochrome P450, the active site of which contains

Table 10.2 Comparative capability for biotransformation.

Organ	Approximate comparative capability for biotransformation of foreign agents (% relative to activity of liver)
Liver	100
Adrenal cortex	75
Lungs	30
Kidney	30
Testes	20
Skin	10
Gastrointestinal tract	10
Spleen	5
Heart muscle	3
Skeletal muscle	1

an iron atom that can change between divalent and trivalent oxidation states. This enzyme combines with the substrate and molecular oxygen as part of a process through which the substrate is oxidized. The group of enzymes are classified as mixed function oxidases, the specific oxidizing enzyme, cytochrome P450, having a characteristic peak in the reduced form at 450 nm in a carbon monoxide adduct difference spectrum (hence P450). The enzyme requires an electron transport chain for its reduction. This consists of a flavoprotein enzyme, cytochrome c reductase (cytochrome P450 reductase) that transfers electrons (e^-) from the flavine to cytochrome P450. Cytochrome c reductase requires NADPH as a coenzyme; microsomal oxidation requires both NADPH and O_2. Cytochrome P450 exists as a family of isoenzymes with differing and overlapping specificities and more than eight gene families have been identified.[19,20]

Cytochrome P450 is abundant in the liver, which is the primary site of protection against systemic poisons, but may occur in other parts of the body, such as the kidney, ovaries, testes and olfactory mucosa. The presence of the enzyme in the lungs, skin and gastrointestinal tract reflects a defensive role in these organs against local toxic xenobiotics. Oxidase enzyme activity is mainly associated with the smooth endoplasmic reticulum. When tissues, such as liver, are homogenized, the ER is broken down to form small vesicles known as microsomes. Microsomes are the fraction collected from centrifugation of tissue homogenate at about $100\,000\,g$ and, essentially, contain the rough and smooth endoplasmic reticulum and Golgi apparatus. There is evidence that the microsomal enzymes are associated with a lipid membrane and are lipid-dependent. Sonic vibration, or the use of hypotonic solutions, fail to solubilize them, whilst the treatment of microsomes with deoxycholic acid, which solubilizes lipid membranes, destroys the activity of oxidative enzymes.

Biotransformation of xenobiotics usually consists of two phases: phase 1, which involves oxidation (via the cytochrome P450-dependent mixed function oxygenases), reduction or hydrolysis of the parent compound, and phase 2, in which the metabolite is conjugated to glucuronic acid, glutathione, glycine, sulphate or some other endogenous compound.

In phase 1, a polar reactive group is introduced into the molecule to increase water solubility and make the compound suitable for phase 2 where the altered molecule is combined with an endogenous substrate to produce a water-soluble conjugate that is more readily excreted in the urine. Consequently, the principal function of biotransformation is to facilitate the elimination of a foreign agent by its conversion to a more polar (water soluble) metabolite and is, therefore, a detoxification mechanism. In some cases, the intermediate metabolites or final products may be more toxic than the parent compound (i.e. an entoxification). Such metabolites may be systemically toxic or, because they are produced locally by an organ, have toxic effects in the tissue of biotransformation. Most cells, particularly in the liver, have protective biochemical systems to prevent damage to vital cell processes from locally produced toxic metabolites.

In phase 1 metabolism, biotransformation may result in the formation of compounds with a variety of properties depending on whether toxicity has been increased or decreased.

INCREASED TOXICITY

Parathion, an organophosphate pesticide, is relatively non-toxic to man, but in insects is rapidly metabolized (activated) by desulphuration to paraoxon, a potent cholinesterase inhibitor. There is some evidence for variability in man of parathion activation by P450 and of activity of the enzyme, paraoxonase, which further metabolizes the paraoxon.[21]

$$(C_2H_5O)_2\overset{S}{\underset{\|}{P}}-O-\underset{Parathion}{\bigcirc}-NO_2 \rightarrow (C_2H_5O)_2\overset{O}{\underset{\|}{P}}-O-\underset{Paraoxon}{\bigcirc}-NO_2$$

Although biochemical activation may present some human hazard, it may have a useful application in the development of new pesticides or prodrugs that are converted into active products only following metabolic transformation in a target species.

DECREASED TOXICITY

Phenobarbitone is detoxified by hydroxylation of the aromatic ring to form parahydroxyphenobarbitone. Amphetamines are similarly detoxified by aromatic hydroxylation to parahydroxyamphetamines and by deamination to a benzyl methyl ketone. Both of these metabolites are less active than the parent compound.

Specific chemical reactions can occur in phase 1 metabolism.

Epoxidation

Epoxidation is the insertion of an oxygen atom between two carbon atoms. It is an important mechanism for the initial metabolism of aromatic compounds and cytochrome P450 is involved. This reaction can increase the toxicity of the parent compound, but many epoxides are unstable and undergo further reactions, such as hydroxylation. Unstable epoxides are often toxic because they bind to proteins and other macromolecules. For example, vinyl chloride is converted to an intermediate, chlorethylene oxide, which spontaneously transforms to chloracetaldehyde. The two metabolites are mutagens and considered to act as proximate carcinogens.

Vinyl chloride → Chlorethylene oxide → Chloracetaldehyde

Since both of these intermediates can bind directly with cellular macromolecules, such as DNA and proteins, it would be expected that local hepatic biotransformation of vinyl chloride is associated with liver damage. Many epidemiological studies have confirmed the association of chronic vinyl chloride exposure with the development of a hepatic angiosarcoma, an otherwise rare primary liver cancer. Carcinogenicity appeared to follow chronic exposure to relatively low levels of vinyl chloride (50–100 ppm or less). Chronic exposure to higher levels of exposure (500–1000 ppm) was more commonly associated with serious hepatotoxicity, the hepatocytes dying before malignant transformation could occur. Vinyl chloride-induced angiosarcoma of the liver can have a latency of between 15 and 40 years. As a result of stringent workplace controls limiting exposure to below 1 ppm, vinyl chloride-associated diseases are now rarely seen (see Chapter 39, Gases and Chapter 88, Hepatotoxic effects of workplace exposures).

Another example of epoxide formation is the conversion of the pesticide aldrin to dieldrin, a stable epoxide.

Aldrin → Dieldrin

Hydroxylation

Hydroxylation is the attachment of a hydroxyl group to hydrocarbon chains or rings and may follow epoxidation. An example is the metabolism of benzene epoxide, an intermediate in the biotransformation of benzene, to phenol. Benzene is initially metabolized by oxidation, primarily in the liver, with phenol as the major metabolite.

Benzene epoxide → Phenol

Other metabolites that can be formed by hydroxylation of the aromatic ring include hydroquinone, catechol and 1,2,4-trihydroxybenzene. These hydroxylated metabolites can be further oxidized to quinones and semiquinones. Urinary excretion of muconic acid, a short chain dicarboxylic acid, suggests that the benzene ring may be opened by biotransformation.

The principal target organ for benzene toxicity is bone marrow. Marrow cells contain peroxidases and mixed function oxidases capable of metabolizing benzene. The metabolites produced may bind covalently to cell macromolecules causing disruption of cell growth and replication. The specific target of benzene is probably the DNA in the pluripotential stem cells and lymphocytic cells. Cytogenetic abnormalities of bone marrow cells and circulating lymphocytes have been observed in workers exposed to benzene. Myelodysplasia may be seen in the bone marrow of individuals with chronic exposure to benzene. Benzene-induced leukaemia has a latency period of 5–15 years and in many cases is preceded by an aplastic anaemia (see Chapter 90, Haematopoeitic effects of workplace exposures).

Hydroxylation may involve the addition of one or more epoxide groups and both reactions are responsible for making several xenobiotic compounds more toxic, such as the production of the carcinogenic 7,8-diol-9,10-epoxide of benzo[a]pyrene. Benzo[a]pyrene is classified, therefore, as a procarcinogen since metabolic activation is required to convert it to a carcinogenic species.

Benzo[a]pyrene → Benzo[a]pyrene-7,8-diol-9,10-epoxide

Oxidation

Oxidation of nitrogen, sulphur or phosphorus is another important metabolic reaction in biotransformation that may increase toxicity. The oxidation of nitrogen in 2-acetylaminofluorene produces the carcinogen N-hydroxy-2-acetylaminofluorene.

2-Acetylaminofluorene (AAF) → N-Hydroxy-2-acetylaminofluorene

With parathion, the oxidative desulphuration of phosphorus produces paraoxon which is more effective than the parent compound as an inhibitor of acetylcholinesterase (see Increased toxicity, p. 133).

Dealkylation

Dealkylation is the removal of an alkyl group (such as a methyl group) and its replacement by a hydrogen atom. The reactions are carried out by mixed function oxidases. Examples include O-dealkylation of methoxychlor insecticides, N-dealkylation of the insecticide carbaryl and S-dealkylation of dimethyl mercaptan.

Reduction

Reduction of some of the major functional groups in xenobiotics is carried out by reductases. Examples include the reduction of nitro groups by nitroreductases, which are found mainly in the liver, but to a lesser extent in other organs, such as the lung and kidney. They may occur also in intestinal bacteria and reduction of xenobiotics may take place locally in the intestinal tract (e.g. dinitrotoluene).

Hydrolysis

Hydrolysis is the addition of water to a molecule prior to its division into two chemical species. Two types of compounds that undergo hydrolysis are esters (such as organophosphates) and amines, many of which are pesticides. Hydrolases occur predominantly in the liver, but also in the gastrointestinal tract, nervous tissue, blood, kidney and muscle. Aromatic esters are hydrolysed by the action of aryl esterases and alkyl esters by carboxylesterases (an example being the metabolism of synthetic pyrethroids). Esterases were originally subdivided into A, B or C esterases on the basis of their interaction with organophosphates.[22]

Depending on their degree of water solubility, the products of metabolic transformation are either excreted directly or undergo further metabolism by conjugation (phase 2 reaction).

In phase 2 reactions, the functional groups on a molecule (e.g. carboxyl, amino, hydroxyl and sulphydryl groups) are conjugated with endogenous compounds, such as glutathione, glucuronic acid, amino acids (e.g. glycine) or sugars, to form water-soluble, polar derivatives that can be more readily excreted and are less toxic. A reduction in lipid solubility decreases the ability to diffuse back across membranes.

Conjugation with glucuronic acid is the most important and most common mechanism. The enzyme UDP-glucuronyltransferase catalyses the transfer of glucuronic acid from uridine diphosphate glucuronic acid. Glucuronide conjugation products are classified by the site of bindings: a hydroxyl functional group forms an ether glucuronide, a carboxyl acid group an ester glucuronide. Glucuronides may be attached directly to nitrogen as the linking atom (e.g. aniline glucuronide) or through an intermediate oxygen atom, such as occurs in the conjugation product in N-hydroxyacetylaminoglucuronide. In contrast to the usual decrease in toxicity that results from glucuronide conjugation, this is a more potent carcinogen than the parent compound, N-hydroxyacetylaminofluorene.

Glutathione, a tripeptide of glutamic acid, cysteine and glycine, is another endogenous compound used in phase 2 reactions. The thiol groups (SH) in glutathione form covalent bonds with xenobiotic compounds and glutathione conjugates may be excreted directly, or after further metabolism to mercapturic acids (compounds with N-acetylcysteine attached). The enzyme glutathione transferase is generally required for the conjugation process and is found throughout the body.

Sulphate conjugates are completely ionized and, therefore, highly efficient in eliminating xenobiotics in the urine. The major species that form sulphate conjugates are alcohols, phenols and arylamines. Phenols are conjugated with either glucuronic acid or sulphate to form phenol glucuronide and phenol sulphate. Sulphation is a saturable pathway and so may have limited capacity for detoxification.

Other reactions can occur. Acetyltransferase involves acetylation such as in the final step in the production of mercapturic acid conjugates. Amino acids, such as glycine, form peptide conjugates. Some compounds, such as salicylic acid, can be metabolized by several different mechanisms, as well as glucuronide conjugation. Cyanide is detoxified by conjugation with sulphur to form thiocyanate (which can be monitored in blood or urine).

Most compounds undergo both metabolic transformation and conjugation, but occasionally only one of these reactions. Biotransformation may produce a metabolite that is sufficiently water soluble to be easily excreted, so that conjugation is not necessary. If the compound already possesses groups which will easily conjugate then phase 1 metabolism may not be required.

OTHER MECHANISMS

Some xenobiotics are detoxified by linkage to a large molecule, such as a protein. This produces a complex that is less toxic and which can be stored in the body. Metallothionein, a low molecular weight cysteine-rich protein, binds to heavy metals such as cadmium, zinc and copper and is found in high concentrations in the liver and kidneys.

Other sites of xenobiotic biotransformation

The liver is not always the most important site of metabolism. Reactions can occur in extrahepatic sites as a result of the activity of both microsomal and non-microsomal enzymes. For example, microsomal UDP-glucuronyltransferase is found in skin and the gastrointestinal tract. Many non-microsomal enzymes occur in plasma, the gastrointestinal tract, lungs and kidneys. Alcohol dehydrogenase in the liver, kidney and lungs oxidizes an alcohol to its aldehyde and a number of amino-oxidases and esterases are found in plasma. Bacterial flora in the gut may also have a role in xenobiotic metabolism (see above under Reduction) and first-pass metabolism by this route of exposure.

If these metabolic reactions did not occur then xenobiotics of high lipid solubility would remain and accumulate in the body with the resultant risk of toxicity. A more detailed review of the principles of biochemical toxicology can be found in standard texts.[23]

Pulmonary biotransformation

Over 40 histologically different cell types have been identified in the lungs but the susceptibility of a lung cell to toxic compounds or metabolites depends partly upon the specific biochemical activity of that cell.[24] The lungs can be the target organ for toxicity and, in some cases, there is a selective toxicity to a particular type of lung cell.[25] The level of metabolic activity of a cell depends upon its degree of specialization and the nature of the enzymes and substrates.

The lung is capable of metabolizing many xenobiotics by both phase 1 and phase 2 reactions.[26] The non-ciliated bronchiolar, or Clara cell, is the most metabolically active lung cell and has a high activity of mixed-function oxidases.[27] The mycotoxin 4-ipomeanol has been widely studied in animals as a model substrate for investigating organ-specific toxicity, since it undergoes selective metabolism and activation in the lung. It appears that the Clara cell metabolizes ipomeanol to a reactive metabolite.[28,29] Significant amounts of the cytochromes P4502B1 and P4504B1 are found in the Clara cell of the rabbit lung. In vitro these isoenzymes are effective at converting ipomeanol to its reactive metabolite. A specific Clara cell lesion is seen also following the administration of the hepatotoxin, 1-nitronaphthalene.

Carbon tetrachloride (CCl_4) is a recognized hepatotoxin-producing fatty degeneration and centrilobular necrosis of the liver (see Chapter 88, Hepatotoxic effects of workplace exposures). Biotransformation of carbon tetrachloride takes place in the liver and toxicity is believed to be linked to the production of a CCl_3^- radical that causes lipid peroxidation and irreversible damage to membrane systems. Bioactivation of CCl_4 is a classical model for free radical-induced toxicity. The first metabolic step is the formation of the trichloromethyl-free radical (CCl_3^-) by a cytochrome P450 enzyme. This free radical binds directly to microsomal lipids and other cellular macromolecules causing the breakdown of membrane structure, energy production and protein synthesis. The trichloromethyl-free radical may also undergo both anaerobic and aerobic reactions leading to the further production of toxic metabolites.

Although the liver is the target organ of toxicity for this chemical, damage to the metabolically active Clara cells, as well as types 1 and 2 alveolar epithelial and pulmonary endothelial cells, has been reported. Gould and Smuckler[30] found focal atelectasis and haemorrhages with ultrastructural changes in type 2 cells which suggested damage to the pulmonary surfactant system. Carbon tetrachloride probably also has toxic effects on lung phospholipids as the main route of elimination of unchanged carbon tetrachloride is via the breath.

The profile of the isoenzymes of cytochrome P450-dependent monooxygenases in the lung cells is important for understanding of the toxicity of substances that undergo metabolic activation. The heterogeneity of cellular distribution and the high levels of enzyme activity in certain cells can explain specific cell toxicity for some compounds (such as ipomeanol for the Clara cell), but it is not so clear why other toxins (e.g. butylated hydroxytoluene and trialkylphosphorothioates) appear to be specifically toxic to the type 1 alveolar epithelial cells. Butylated hydroxytoluene appears to be species-specific in causing murine lung damage but, despite extensive human safety evaluation, the potential for butylated hydroxytoluene in food to cause toxic lung damage in man has not been determined. Similarly, the trialkylphosphorothioates, as impurities in many organophosphorus thionates manufactured for use as pesticides (e.g. malathion), may be environmental causes of cell-specific lung damage in man. The type 1 alveolar epithelial cells do not demonstrate significant cytochrome P450 activity and their potential for xenobiotic biotransformation is unknown. It is possible that there is metabolic activation in another cell type, or even organ, and transport of the toxic metabolite to the type 1 cell. There is some evidence to suggest that certain conjugates may dissociate at a remote site after conjugation and release the toxic compound. Type 1 cells are derived from type 2, which have demonstrable metabolic capability, but in vitro the total enzyme activities of a lung preparation cannot be accounted for by the sum of just the Clara and type 2 cells. The other enzyme systems that may be involved in the activation of toxins in the lung include pulmonary flavin-monooxygenases (Clara and alveolar type 2 cells) and pulmonary prostaglandin synthetase which is capable of activating chemicals by co-oxidation with prostaglandin precursors. This pathway, in particular, could be relevant to the pulmonary toxicity of α-naphthylthiourea (ANTU) and N-methylthiobenzamide. The latter compound has a similar toxicity profile to ANTU and has been shown to be metabolized by a pulmonary flavin adenine dinucleorotide (FAD)-dependent monooxygenase. ANTU produces severe, non-haemorrhagic, pulmonary oedema with fibrin-rich pleural effusions in animals and has been used as a model for the study of the pathophysiology of pulmonary oedema. Pulmonary prostaglandin H-synthase-mediated co-oxygenation has been shown to activate procarcinogens, such as benzo[a]pyrene and aflatoxin B1.

The role of glutathione (GSH) in pulmonary detoxification has been investigated for ipomeanol and naphthalene, both of which selectively damage Clara cells in mice. GSH and GSH-S transferase concentrations are lower in the lungs than in liver and the cellular distribution is unclear, although there appears to be more activity in the Clara cells than the type 2 cells. Consequently, the protective detoxification mechanisms of the lungs are less effective than those of the liver. Low glutathione transferase activity in the lung, compared with aryl hydroxylase activity, has been associated with the increased risk of lung cancer in tobacco smokers.

The lung is a target organ for toxicity of many other compounds.[31] Some of the mechanisms involved in systemic lung toxicity have been identified in animal toxicity models. Administration of paraquat to animals causes lung fibrosis, the herbicide entering types 1 and 2 lung cells by a selective active uptake process.[32,33] Hydrazine, given intraperitoneally in mice, can produce lung tumours, and chlorphentermine, after chronic oral dosing, accumulates in the fatty tissue of the lung (and the adrenals) and causes a phospholipidosis. Polycyclic aromatic hydrocarbons may be activated in the lungs or metabolized elsewhere and transported to the lungs. There are significant species differences between animals and humans in susceptibility to the toxic effects of butylated hydroxytoluene (BHT), the trialkylphosphorothioates, ANTU, ipomeanol and paraquat.[34]

Dermal biotransformation

The importance of dermal metabolism, during absorption through the skin *in vivo*, for disposition and local toxicity is now recognized. Esterase activity in skin is exploited in the delivery of ester prodrugs; lipophilic prodrugs (containing an alkyl group ester-linked to the pharmacophore) are able to penetrate the stratum corneum. Esterase activity in the viable epidermis cleaves the ester linkage and liberates the pharmacophore. Metabolic activity plays a key role in activation of procarcinogens such as benzo[a]pyrene in the skin of experimental animals and is believed to have a similar role in humans. Metabolic activation also appears to have a key role in haptenation during skin sensitization reactions. Dermal absorption and metabolism has been assessed in tissue homogenates and in intact skin *in vitro*, using flow through diffusion systems and more recently short-term organ culture. The viability of skin in these systems and the maintenance of metabolic capacity are important but still require complete verification for all enzyme systems, especially those requiring energy. Nevertheless, expression and enzymatic activity for a wide range of enzymes in cutaneous systems has been demonstrated *in vitro* as well as *in vivo*.[35]

The degree of skin metabolism depends on the physicochemical characteristics of the compound, the rate of absorption, as well as the capacity of any metabolizing enzymes. A suitable choice of model systems is important to reflect not only absorption characteristics *in vivo*, but also metabolic capacity.[36] Metabolism may be relatively unimportant quantitatively *in vivo*, compared with metabolism by the liver, but may be highly significant when conversion to toxic metabolites causes local toxicity or where rapid detoxification follows absorption and enables the skin to act as a protective metabolic barrier against a toxic xenobiotic entering the system circulation. Furthermore, metabolic activity for the majority of cutaneous enzyme systems is highly localized in the basal layer of the epidermis and appendages. Consequently, specific activities for dermal biotransformation may be more significant than values from tissue homogenates suggest. The lower metabolic capacity of human skin compared with animals must be considered when extrapolating from animals to man in quantitative risk assessment.

VARIATION IN SUSCEPTIBILITY TO XENOBIOTICS

Disorders following occupational exposure to chemicals are well documented and some have been known for hundreds of years. In a population exposed to toxic xenobiotics in the workplace, or general environment, there is a broad range of responses between individuals. The causes of this variability, in the nature and degree of acute response or susceptibility to long-term health effects from intermittent or chronic low-dose exposure, remain largely unanswered.[37] Research into the role of genetic polymorphisms, and the contribution of epigenetic factors, in predisposing individuals to disease is beginning to identify important differences within populations. Recent advances in genetics have identified the genetic basis of many human diseases and it is probable that similar genetic mechanisms will underlie some of the effects of occupational and environmental exposures to xenobiotics.[38] Genetic polymorphisms for xenobiotic metabolism are likely to play an important role in an individual's level of susceptibility.

The clinical consequences of slow acetylator phenotype have been well studied following drug exposure and this pathway may have a role in some occupational exposures (examples include exposure to isoniazid and hydrallazine). It is also known that phenotypic variation in plasma esterases, especially cholinesterases, can contribute to the relative toxicity of some anticholinesterases by affecting both the specific toxicity of these compounds and influencing the efficiency of their metabolism and elimination. Thiomethyl transferase produces S-methylation and masks functional chemical groups, reducing water solubility and impairing further conjugation. Thiomethyl transferase is involved in the detoxification of substances, such as hydrogen sulphide and other free sulphydryl groups, including the thioesters of glutathione conjugates (a final common pathway for many toxic xenobiotics). Hydrogen sulphide has a similar toxic mechanism, as a mitochondrial poison, to cyanide and can cause an acquired defect in mitochondrial function leading to disease similar to that found in Parkinson's disease.[39] Heavy metals, such as mercury, can form toxic derivatives with the enzyme thiomethyl transferase and increased activity, such as that reported in motor neurone disease, may predispose individuals to heavy metal poisoning.

An individual's response to toxic xenobiotics is influenced by the rates of absorption, distribution, biotransformation and excretion, as well as the toxicodynamics of the chemical. The body's defences against toxic effects are complex and there are considerable interindividual (and interspecies) variations in both toxicokinetics and toxicodynamics. Many of these variations will depend on genetic polymorphisms for the specific enzymes (frequently cytochromes P450) involved in the toxic mechanisms.[1]

Epigenetics is the study of the 'all heritable and potentially reversible changes in genome function that do not alter the nucleotide sequence within the DNA' (www.answers.com/topic/epigenesis) and is a relatively new area of research in toxicology. When a cell undergoes an epigenetic change, it is the phenotype of the cell that is affected. Genetic events during embryonic development lead to the differentiation of fetal cells. The combined process of fetal development and cell differentiation is called 'epigenesis'. Epigenetics is distinct from genetics, which focuses on how traits are inherited in genes and associated DNA sequences, because in epigenetic inheritance the DNA sequence itself is not changed. Specific epigenetic processes have been identified and include paramutation, bookmarking, imprinting, gene silencing, X chromosome inactivation, transvection, many of the effects of teratogens and histone modifications. The epigenetic process often involves covalent modification of DNA by methylation.

The epigenome serves as an interface between the dynamic intra/extracellular environments and the inherited static genome. Epigenetic aberrations have similar consequences to some genetic polymorphisms and can result in variations in gene function. Recent data suggest that the epigenome is constantly changing in response to environmental signals.[36] Although our current understanding of how epigenetic mechanisms impact on the toxic action of xenobiotics is limited, it is anticipated that epigenetic factors may need to be considered in the safety assessment of chemicals. It would seem reasonable to anticipate a role in an individual's susceptibility to toxic chemicals. The notion of a dynamic epigenome implies that variations in gene function and phenotype are modulated not only by DNA sequence polymorphisms, but also by reversible, but nevertheless stable, epigenetic changes. The epigenetic pattern is cell type specific, which distinguishes it from genomic polymorphisms, and thus could create cell type specific phenotypic variations between individuals and explain some aspects of target organ specificity and idiosycratic responses.

Epigenetics provides a mechanism through which transient exposures to an environmental or occupational hazard may have persistent lifelong phenotypic effects. It may have potential implications in toxicology, for example non-genotoxic agents that have an epigenotoxic effect. Variations in epigenetic states could vary the response to toxic agents amongst individuals. Interestingly, individual variation may be tissue specific, so interindividual epigenetic variations could result from genetic differences as well as from exposures to different chemicals at critical periods throughout life. The concept is complex, but does suggest additional factors affect an individual's susceptibilty to toxicity other than genetic variations.

SUMMARY

It has been assumed to date that measurement of air concentrations of hazardous chemicals in the workplace is sufficient to adequately assess the health risks to individual workers. For most of these chemicals there are very few data on the factors affecting absorption, distribution, metabolism and elimination or the mechanism of toxicity in humans to justify this assumption. Toxicokinetic data suggest that for some compounds the degree of workplace exposure is not directly related to individual risk. Similarly, greater understanding of the mechanisms involved in the development of toxic effects in humans and the frequent discrepancies from the results of animal toxicity studies, indicate a need for more information from human studies. In addition, as with the effects on drug toxicity of genetic differences in drug metabolism, so the role of genetic polymorphisms in susceptibility to the toxic effects of hazardous chemicals must be defined. The application of more extensive human data in toxicology to the assessment of health risks in the workplace should not necessarily increase the complexity of controls, but will increase their direct relevance. Experience in the workplace can then be applied to the more contentious issues of general environmental exposure.

Key points

- The toxicokinetic profile of a chemical is an important factor in the health risk assessment process.
- Knowledge of toxic mechanisms in man enables better understanding of potential health effects.
- Interindividual variation in response to toxic exposures may have a genetic component.

ACKNOWLEDGEMENTS

The author is grateful to Dr SW Wilkison for expert advice on the dermal absorption section.

REFERENCES

1. Klaassen CD, Amdur MO, Doull J (eds). *Casarett and Doull's toxicology: The basic science of poisons.* New York: McGraw-Hill, 1996.
2. Deichmann WB, Henschler D, Holmstedt B, Keil G. What is there that is not poison? A study of the Third Defense by Paracelsus. *Archives of Toxicology.* 1986; **58**: 207–13.
3. Rose MS, Smith LL, Wyatt I. Evidence for energy-dependent accumulation of paraquat into rat lung. *Nature.* 1974; **252**: 314–15.

4. Smith LL. The identification of an accumulation system for diamines and polyamines into the lung and its relevance to paraquat toxicity. *Archives of Toxicology.* 1982; **5** (Suppl.): 1–14.
5. Woollen BH, Guest EA, Howe W *et al*. Human inhalation pharmacokinetics of 1,1,2-trichoro-1,2,2-trifluorethane (FC113). *International Archives of Occupational and Environmental Health.* 1990; **62**: 73–8.
6. Woollen BH, Marsh JR, Mahler JD *et al*. Human inhalation pharmacokinetics of chlorodifluoromethane (HCFC22). *International Archives of Occupational and Environmental Health.* 1992; **64**: 383–7.
7. Blain PG. Inhalation kinetics. In: Brewis RAL, Gibson GJ, Geddes DM (eds). *Textbook of respiratory medicine.* London: Baillière Tindall, 1990: 158–62.
8. Pietrowskie J. The application of metabolic and excretion kinetics to problems of industrial toxicology. Washington DC: US Government Printing Office, 1971.
9. Conkle JP, Camp BJ, Welch BE. Trace composition of human respiratory gas. *Archives of Environmental Health.* 1975; **30**: 290–5.
10. Krotoszynski B, Gabriel G, O'Neil H. Characterisation of human expired air; a promising investigation and diagnostic technique. *Journal of Chromatographic Science.* 1977; **15**: 239–44.
11. Fiserova Bergerova V, Vlach J, Cassady JC. Predictable 'individual differences' in uptake and excretion of gases and lipid soluble vapours. Simulation study. *British Journal of Industrial Medicine.* 1980; **37**: 42–9.
12. Kelman GR. Theoretical basis of alveolar sampling. *British Journal of Industrial Medicine.* 1982; **39**: 259–64.
13. Scott RC, Dugard PH. The properties of skin as a diffusion barrier and route of absorption. In: Greaves MW, Shuster S (eds). *Pharmacology of the skin II.* Heidelberg: Springer Verlag, 1989: 93–114.
14. Bos JD, Meinardi MMHM. The 500 Dalton rule for the skin penetration of chemical compounds and drugs. *Experimental Dermatology.* 2000; **9**: 165–9.
15. Roberts MS, Cross SE, Anissimov YG. Factors affecting the formation of a skin reservoir for topically applied solutes. *Skin Pharmacology and Physiology.* 2004; 17: 3–16.
16. van de Sandt JJM, van Burgsteden JA, Cage S *et al*. In vitro predictions of skin absorption of caffeine, testosterone, and benzoic acid: A multi-centre comparison study. *Regulatory Toxicology and Pharmacology.* 2004; **39**: 271–81.
17. Wilkinson SC, Williams FM. The relationship between *in vivo* dermal penetration studies in humans and *in vitro* predictions using human skin. In: Bronaugh RL, Maibach HI (eds). *Percutaneous absorption: Drugs, cosmetics, mechanisms, methodology,* 4th edn. New York: Taylor and Francis, 2005: 561–74.
18. Organisation for Economic Cooperation and Development. OECD guideline for the testing of chemicals TG428. *Skin absorption: In vitro method.* Paris: OECD, 2004: 1–8.
19. Nebert DW, Nelson DR, Adesnik M *et al*. The P450 superfamily: Updated listing of all genes and recommended nomenclature for the chromosomal loci. *DNA.* 1989; **8**: 1–13.
20. Nelson DR, Koymans L, Kamataki T *et al*. P450 superfamily: Update on new sequences, gene mapping accession numbers and nomenclature. *Pharmacogenetics.* 1996; **6**: 1–42.
21. Williams FM, Mutch E, Blain PG. Paraoxonase distribution in Caucasian males. *Chemico-Biological Interactions.* 1993; **87**: 155–60.
22. Aldridge WN. Two types of esterase (A and B) hydrolysing p-nitrophenylacetate, propionate and butyrate, and a method of their determination. *Biochemical Journal.* 1900; **53**: 110–17.
23. Hodgson E, Guthrie FE (eds). *Introduction to biochemical toxicology.* New York: Elsevier North Holland, 1984.
24. Sorokin SP. The cells of the lungs. In: Nettesheim P, Hanna MG, Deatherage JW (eds). Conference on morphology of experimental carcinogenesis. Washington DC: Atomic Energy Commision, 1970: 3–43.
25. Kehrer JP, Kacew S. Systematically applied chemicals that damage lung tissue. *Toxicology.* 1985; **35**: 251–93.
26. Blain PG. Toxic lung injury: Ingested agents. In: Brewis RAL, Gibson GJ, Geddes DM (eds). *Textbook of respiratory medicine.* London: Baillière Tindall, 1990: 1488–97.
27. Boyd MR. Biochemical mechanisms in chemical-induced lung injury: Roles of metabolic activation. *CRC Critical Reviews in Toxicology.* 1980; **7**: 103–76.
28. Boyd MR, Burka LT, Wilson BJ, Sasame HA. *In vitro* studies on the metabolic activation of the pulmonary toxin 4-ipomeanol by rat lung and liver microsomes. *Journal of Pharmacology and Experimental Therapeutics.* 1978; **207**: 677–86.
29. Boyd MR, Burka LT. *In vivo* studies in the relationship between target organ alkylation and the pulmonary toxicity of a chemically reactive metabolite of 4-ipomeanol. *Journal of Pharmacology and Experimental Therapeutics.* 1978; **207**: 687–97.
30. Gould VE, Smuckler EA. Alveolar injury in acute carbon tetrachloride intoxication. *Archives of Internal Medicine.* 1971; **128**: 109–17.
31. Brewis RAL, Keaney NP. Respiratory disorders. In: Davies DM (ed.). *Textbook of adverse drug reactions.* Oxford: Oxford University Press, 1986: 172–204.
32. Rose MS, Lock EA, Smith LL, Wyatt I. Paraquat accumulation: Tissue and species specificity. *Biochemical Pharmacology.* 1976; **25**: 419–23.
33. Blain PG. Aspects of pesticide toxicology. *Adverse Drug Reactions and Acute Poisoning Reviews.* 1990; **9**: 37–68.
34. Marino AA, Mitchell JT. Lung damage in mice following intraperitoneal injection of butylated hydroxytoluene. *Proceedings of the Society for Experimental Biology and Medicine.* 1972; **140**: 122–5.
35. Macpherson SE, Scott RC, Williams FM. Metabolism of pesticides during percutaneous absorption. In: Scott RC, Guy RH, Hadgraft J (eds). *Prediction of percutaneous penetration,* vol. 1. London: IBC Technical Services, 1990: 135–9.
36. Williams FM. Metabolism of xenobiotics during percutaneous absorption *in vivo* and in *in vitro* systems. In: Scott RC, Guy RH, Hadgraft J (eds). *Prediction of percutaneous penetration,* vol. 2. Southampton: IBC Technical Services, 1990: 270–8.

37. Johannessen JJ. Biomolecular appraoches to neurotoxic hazard assessment. In: Chang LW, Sukker W (eds). *Neurotoxicology: Approaches and methods*. San Diego, CA: Academic Press, 1995: 399–421.
38. Szyf M. The dynamic epigenome and its implications in toxicology. *Toxicological Sciences*. 2007; **100**: 7–23.
39. Kobayashi H, Suzuki T. Genetically determined susceptibility to environmental toxins. In: Blain PG, Harris JB (eds). *Medical neurotoxicology. Occupational and environmental causes of neurological dysfunction*. London: Arnold, 1999: 141–52.

11

Risks and hazards in occupational and environmental exposures

ROBERT L MAYNARD

Introduction	141	Explaining risk: communicating with the public	144
Hazard identification	141	Conclusions	147
Risk assessment	142	References	147
Ambient levels of carcinogens	143		

INTRODUCTION

Occupational physicians and hygienists identify hazards, estimate risks and seek to reduce both. The most direct way to assess a health risk to physical and chemical hazards arising in the workplace is through exposure assessment: this is also an essential tool by which an occupational physician can attribute a health problem to an individual's occupation. For further details, the reader is referred to Chapter 4, Occupational exposure to hazardous substances (p. 43). This companion chapter provides an introduction to the concepts of risk and hazard assessment.

A hazard may be identified as:

A phenomenon, an act, a toxic substance or a living organism that can, but does not always, pose a threat to health. For example lightning, jumping, hydrogen cyanide, a lion or a bacterium.

Risk may be defined:

Risk is the probability of an adverse effect associated with a hazard. For example, the risk of being struck by lightning or of contracting tuberculosis.

In estimating risk, it is assumed that exposure to the hazard occurs. This is important: risk may be reduced to zero if exposure to the hazard is made impossible. Removing the hazard completely achieves this, reducing exposure to the hazard can achieve this if the reduction is complete, but this is less satisfactory (and less certain) than removing the hazard itself.

HAZARD IDENTIFICATION

Many, perhaps all, occupations involve exposure to hazard. Office work involves exposure to hazard: poor ergonomic conditions, stress, danger associated with repetitive movements, such as typing, etc. Industrial work is likely to involve exposure to greater hazards: moving machinery, chemicals, high temperatures, etc. In many cases, identification of hazards involves little more than common sense: a circular saw is a rather obvious hazard, as is a hydraulic press or a conveyor belt. Chemicals pose hazards, but these are less easy to recognize. Occupational health studies and toxicological work form the bases for identifying hazardous chemicals. In the case of most chemicals, hazards can only be identified by *in vivo* – laboratory animal – toxicological studies; in the case of genotoxic carcinogens, *in vitro* mutagenicity studies may be sufficient. However, discovering that a chemical poses a hazard is very different from estimating the risk associated with exposure to that chemical. *In vivo* studies may allow exposure or dose–response relationships to be defined: extrapolating from such data to estimates of risks in man is difficult, almost always impossible. Because of this, toxicological data tend to be used for identifying levels of exposure likely to be associated with low risk. The application of safety factors (better described as uncertainty factors) to the results of *in vivo* toxicological studies has long been used for this purpose. The use of such factors should not be confused with risk estimation. If we assume that a no adverse effect level (NOAEL) can be defined or estimated in animals then dividing this by ten, to allow for unknown factors that may control for interspecies variations in sensitivity, may yield a level of exposure unlikely to have effects in man. However:

- There is no guarantee that exposure to such a level of exposure will *not* have effects in man and
- There is no guarantee that greater exposure *will* have effects in man.

The assertion that exposure to the calculated level of exposure (NOAEL/10) is unlikely to have effects, can only be based on experience with other chemicals, and experience may be misleading.

It will be obvious that hazard identification based on animal studies is less satisfactory than that based on studies in man. Human data showing adverse effects on health of occupational exposure to chemicals used to be more commonly available than at present. We should be glad to know that modern standards of occupational hygiene have reduced access to such data. For some chemicals, data can be obtained from population studies if the general public is exposed to the chemical in question. This has been the case with common air pollutants. It is a fact that such studies, often large and therefore statistically powerful, reveal effects at levels of exposure well below those shown to produce effects in animal studies, volunteer studies or smaller scale occupational studies. For example, the World Health Organization (2006) Air Quality Guidelines[1] for nitrogen dioxide and sulphur dioxide include the following recommendations:

NO_2: Annual average concentration: $40\,\mu g/m^3$
SO_2: 24-hour average concentration: $20\,\mu g/m^3$

In occupational circles, these would be regarded as very low and challenging guidelines. The reader is advised to examine the World Health Organization report for the justifications behind these figures. One important conclusion from the epidemiological studies that form the basis of the guidelines is that expected thresholds of effect may not be demonstrable at a population level. This conclusion has been generally accepted in the air pollution field and has serious implications for risk assessment. These include a move away from identification of no adverse effect levels as a substitute for quantitative risk assessment (QRA).

RISK ASSESSMENT

At its simplest, risk assessment involves deciding on whether a given level of exposure to a chemical is or is not associated with some risk of adverse effects on health. Such an assessment is of limited value unless it proves easy, or at least not too difficult, to prevent exposure entirely. As soon as questions about costs and benefits are raised, as they often are, the need for quantitative estimation of risk becomes pressing. Such estimates can be made on the basis of:

1. Real data that allow risks at relevant levels of exposure to be assessed – as in the air pollution field.
2. The use of predictive models.

The use of predictive models has been the cause of much debate among toxicologists.

Let us take an example. Studies conducted in occupational settings show that exposure to measured concentrations of some compound (for given periods) produce adverse effects. We need to be able to predict effects on exposure to lower concentrations. Thus, some form of extrapolation is needed. To the purist, extrapolation 'beyond the data' is always a risky process and one likely to be beset with errors. Some assumptions regarding the shape of the exposure (dose)–response relationship at low levels of exposure need to be made. If the mechanism of effect of the chemical is well understood, it may be possible to construct an equation that relates exposure to effects. In practice, this is very difficult and fitting a line to the available data and then producing or extending that line beyond the data is the common approach. However, we are, at once, in difficulties. Is there a threshold of effect and, if so, what is it?

Consider exposure to ozone, which may occur to workers in the chemical industry and to the general population as a ubiquitous air pollutant. Exposure to 120 ppb ($240\,\mu g/m^3$) without exercise produces a small change in indices of lung function, such as FEV_1. Exposure to 80 ppb ($160\,\mu g/m^3$), with intermittent vigorous exercise, for about six hours produces small changes in FEV_1. If we assume that the body has natural defences against the adverse effects of ozone (airway surface antioxidants such as reduced glutathione, vitamins C and E, and uric acid), we might reasonably assume that for each individual there was some level of exposure that would not produce an effect on FEV_1. This is, in fact, widely assumed. However, it is known that levels of antioxidants in the airways differ from person to person and in some hardly any exists – at least in the upper airways (nose) where measurements have been done.[2] If, in lieu of anything better, we assume that the level of antioxidant defences varies amongst people in a way that conforms to a normal distribution curve then, at a population level, the notion that a threshold of effect exists disappears. There is nothing revolutionary or surprising about this. The Probit slope, once used so widely in toxicology, is based on such assumptions and the now rather less used LD_{50} is derived from such thinking. Of course, the problem with such thinking is that the mid range of such curves inevitably tends to be better defined than the extremes of the curve and the confidence limits about the curve tend to veer away from the curve at its extremities. Even in a large toxicological study in animals one would expect to have much more confidence in the reliability of an LD_{50} value than in an $LD_{1.0}$ or LD_{99} value.

It will be appreciated that we have moved away from predicting effects on a truly mechanistic basis to predicting them on a statistical basis. Statistical models have been extensively used in quantitative risk assessment of risks associated with exposure to genotoxic carcinogens. Many such models exist. Some are entirely statistical and are based on assumptions regarding the distribution of sensitivity in the population (Probit and Logit models); others are based on assumptions regarding mechanisms of effect or, rather, characteristics of mechanisms of effect as assumed in 'one hit' or 'multi-stage' models. However, all these models are just models and their predictions of effects or risks at low levels of exposure cannot be verified. Cannot? Well – cannot as yet. It is assumed that if mechanisms of effect were perfectly understood, then a perfect model could be constructed: this is still very far away.

A very simple model has been used by the World Health Organization in predicting unit risks for carcinogens. Let us examine the derivation of the unit risk for benzene.[3] A cohort of workers studied in the United States by the National Institute for Occupational Safety and Health (NIOSH) comprised 748 workers who had been exposed to benzene in the production of rubber film material for 15 years. The cohort was followed for 25 years. Seven workers died from leukaemia. The expected number of deaths, based on national figures, was 1.25 and thus the relative risk was calculated as 5.6. The average duration of exposure was found to be 8.5 years and the average level of exposure was 30–300 mg/m^3. Peak exposures of up to 2170 mg/m^3 were recorded. So much for the data: it will be noted that the actual exposure was only rather inaccurately known and that peaks of exposure far above the average may have occurred. This raises the question of overloading of defence mechanisms by occasional very high exposures: an unresolved problem.

Now for the assumptions. It was assumed that exposure had been to 300 mg/m^3 for 8.5 years. This was taken as equivalent to a lifetime exposure of:

$$300 \times \frac{8}{24} \times \frac{240}{365} \times \frac{8.5}{70} \text{ mg/m}^3$$

i.e. 8 mg/m^3 (8000 μg/m^3).

The unit risk was calculated as the increase in risk associated with lifetime exposure to 1 μg/m^3 of benzene.

Let P_o = background risk (in this case 0.007). Then putting RR as the relative risk associated with lifetime exposure to 8000 μg/m^3 as 5.6:

$$\text{Unit risk} = \frac{P_o RR - P_o}{8000} = \frac{P_o(RR-1)}{8000} = \frac{0.007(5.6-1)}{8000}$$
$$= 4 \times 10^{-6}$$

The unit risk was more accurately defined as the 'incremental unit risk'.

It will be seen that the model used here is the simplest possible: it is entirely linear. No assumptions regarding 'one hit' or 'multi-stage' characteristics of the mechanism by which benzene causes leukaemia are included. The authors of the World Health Organization report recognized the assumptions made:

- Response (measured as relative risk) is some function of cumulative exposure.
- There is no threshold of effect for genotoxic carcinogens.
- Linear extrapolation of the dose–response curve towards zero gives the upper bound conservative estimate of the true risk function if the unknown (true) dose–response curve has a sigmoidal shape.
- There is constancy of the relative risk in the specific study situation. It was noted that in a strict sense, constancy of the relative risk means that the background age/cause specific rate at any time is increased by a constant factor. The advantage of the average relative risk method is that this needs to be true only for the average.

One important drawback of the method was noted: background rates vary from country to country and thus the incremental unit risk will also vary from one country to another. This should be borne in mind if the World Health Organization unit risk estimates are applied in calculations of benefits to health expected to be produced by reducing exposure to carcinogens.

AMBIENT LEVELS OF CARCINOGENS

It was noted by the authors of the World Health Organization report that the method outlined above was easy to use – easier than more sophisticated methods of extrapolation from the results of occupational studies to possible effects of exposure to ambient concentrations of carcinogens. The authors also pointed out that the use of more sophisticated models led to similar results to those obtained with the average relative risk model, as described above. This is an important but controversial point. The UK Department of Health Committee on the Carcinogenicity of Chemicals in Food, Consumer Products and the Environment (COC) in 1991 published a report entitled 'Guidelines for the evaluation of chemicals for carcinogenicity',[4] which included a discussion pointing out that the application of a range of models produced very different predictions of the risk (expressed as number of cases of cancer per lifetime) for a given exposure to a carcinogen. The wide range of results caused the committee to question this quantitative approach. It should be noted, again, that the accuracy of predictions produced by all such models cannot be verified. Examination of the results yielded by different models show that the mechanistic 'one hit' model produced the largest risk estimate, for a given dose, of all the models examined. This model might be used to produce a worst case estimate of risk to a specified level of exposure. In 2003, the Committee on Carcinogenicity of Chemicals in

Food, Consumer Products and the Environment agreed that if human data were available and if groups of similarly acting compounds (e.g. PAH compounds) were being considered, then the 'one hit' model might form the basis for a ranking of carcinogenic potency.[5] This is not at all the same as predicting risks, but can be useful in setting priorities for regulatory action.

EXPLAINING RISK: COMMUNICATING WITH THE PUBLIC

If estimating risk is difficult, communicating ideas about risk to the public is very difficult and failure is common. The following brief account draws heavily on a UK Department of Health Report 'Communicating about risks to public health: pointers to good practice'.[6]

People respond to information about risks, including risks to health, in a variety of ways, sometimes unpredictably. Understanding the bases of these variable responses has been seen as a useful starting point for improving risk communication. Whether this has been startlingly successful may be doubted but what more rational basis for risk communication can be proposed? We shall consider a number of points.

Lay perspectives

It is generally believed that scientists (and doctors) adopt a critical approach to evidence bearing on causality. The hypothesis-testing approach to research, as advocated by Karl Popper, identified falsification of bold hypotheses, as a reliable, perhaps the only reliable, means of making scientific progress.[7] This philosophy was embraced by distinguished scientists[8] and philosophers, but disputed by others.[9] This has led to the perception that scientists are instinctive non-believers, or falsifiers, in the causality of associations: until, that is, the hypothesis of non-causality is disproven. Put simply in this example, scientific method leads to a tendency for scientists to choose to believe that proximity of residence to high power cables is not associated with cancer until this assertion is disproven. Thus, the statistical framework used (the null, or no effect, hypothesis) can make it appear that scientists are themselves more interested in avoiding false-positive findings (type 1 errors) rather than false-negatives (type 2 errors) in situations of uncertainty. This can lead to conflict with public opinion. Many argue as follows: it is known that exposure to high concentrations of air pollutants, such as sulphur dioxide, causes bronchoconstriction, bronchoconstriction is a characteristic of asthma, therefore exposure to high concentrations of air pollutants causes asthma. Two points arise at once:

1. Is bronchoconstriction only seen in asthma?
2. Does the use of the word 'causes' imply induction of symptoms and signs associated with asthma or the induction of a permanent asthmatic state?

Many doctors would reply No to (1). Point (2) is more difficult, but many would agree that an episode of irritant-induced bronchoconstriction need not necessarily imply induction of a permanent asthmatic state. This may be disputed and reactive airways disorder syndrome (RADS) (see Chapter 40, Reactive airways dysfunction syndrome and irritant-induced asthma, p. 310) provides an example of how transient exposure to pollutants can induce long-lasting airways dysfunction. The phrase 'need not necessarily' is the key to the above assertion. Such words are commonly used and might well be used in a case such as this by many professional scientists or doctors. To the layman, their use is likely to be seen as an example of sophistry. Indeed, by including these words the assertion has been rendered vague and probably immune to falsification or, for that matter, confirmation. It seems to say: in some cases this may be true but it does not follow that it is true in all cases, or better, it does not follow that it must be true in all cases. In terms of Popperian logic, the assertion would be regarded as unscientific. An honest opinion would be that we do not know whether exposure to irritant air pollutants can, sometimes, induce asthma. The reader will have noticed a flaw in all this: asthma is not defined, except in the sense that it is not the only condition characterized by bronchoconstriction. Can asthma be defined? The layman might well say, yes of course: the diagnosis is made every day, by doctors. The respiratory physician might agree that this is certainly true, but might add that a universally acceptable definition of asthma is still awaited despite many international conferences on this subject. The layman is, by now, likely to be annoyed or alarmed: what began as an observation and an apparently simple proposition seems to have drowned in a welter of philosophical argument and dispute about terminology. He could hardly be blamed for saying: well, until the experts make up their minds, might it not be safer to assume that exposure to irritant pollutants can cause asthma? At first glance this seems a reasonable proposal; only when its implications are considered might we ask for better proof. We shall return to this point when the precautionary principle is considered.

Causality

It is widely accepted that mere association is not proof of causality. Less well known is that causality can seldom be proven. Following Popper, we may feel that causality can only be disproven. Causality is closely bound up with the concept of risk. We may say, using the example given above, that exposure to benzene is causally related to the development of leukaemia. The risk of developing leukaemia, however, as a result of a specified exposure benzene is less than 100 per cent. Why is this? Presumably individuals differ in their capacity to resist the effects of benzene: perhaps their DNA repair processes differ in efficiency. If this is the case, then increasing the exposure should increase the risk – let us assume this is so. Thus, we might argue that if the exposure was increased sufficiently all those exposed would develop leukaemia. Risk of developing leukaemia associated with a specified exposure to benzene is thus an expression of interpersonal variation. This sort of risk seems different from the risk associated with random events. Interpersonal variability has nothing to do with the likelihood of winning a lottery or being struck by lightning or throwing a double six at dice. Yet, are the risks really so different? Perhaps the binding of benzene (or some metabolic derivative) to a critical point on the DNA molecule is just an event controlled by what we describe, in lieu of a better explanation, as chance. The more often you throw the dice, the more likely it is that you will get a double six eventually (although the likelihood on each throw is unchanging); the more benzene molecules to which you are exposed, the more likely you are to develop leukaemia. Unless the association between exposure to benzene and leukaemia is causal however, the risk of developing leukaemia as a result of exposure to benzene must be zero. Deciding on causality must, therefore, precede any discussion of risk.

Discussion of causality is bedevilled by one particular misconception. This is that the nine characteristics or features of causal associations set out so clearly by Sir Austin Bradford Hill[10] are singly, or in total, tests of causality. The features defined by Bradford Hill were:

1. Strength of association
2. Consistency (of observed associations)
3. Specificity
4. The relationship in time
5. The biological gradient
6. Biological plausibility
7. Coherence of the evidence
8. The experiment
9. Reasoning by analogy.

We might contend that (8) and (9) are not features or characteristics of causal associations but, rather, lines of evidence or argument that might be advanced in support of the contention that an association is causal. It is not possible to discuss all these features here. A few points, only, will be made:

- There is no *a priori* reason why a strong association should be more likely to be causal than a weak association. But, as Bradford Hill pointed out, if a strong association is actually caused by a confounding factor closely associated with the proposed causal agent, then that factor should be easily identifiable. It follows that if the association is weak, but caused by some weak confounding factor, then that factor may be difficult to identify. This is Popperian: Bradford Hill is saying that the putative causality of a strong association is more easily falsified than that of a weak association.
- Specificity. Bradford Hill argued that a specific effect was more likely to represent the operation of causal association than a number of different effects. Put simply, if a is found to be associated with b, then the association is more likely to be causal than if a is found to be associated with b, c, d and e, etc. I accept this point, but propose a modification: if a is found to be only associated with a single mechanism of effect, then though a is found to be associated with b, c, d and e, etc., the association remains likely to be causal. In the air pollution field, the generation of free radicals has linked exposure to particulate air pollutants with a range of outcomes. The specificity of mechanism seems, to me, to support the case for causality.
- Biological plausibility. Bradford Hill argued, cogently, that this characteristic should not be demanded. An association may be demonstrated long before it can be explained. This has sometimes proved a difficulty for toxicologists who perceive that their efforts cannot refute the findings of epidemiological studies: they can only support them or fail to explain them. Of all the characteristics of causal associations discussed above, only temporal plausibility seems an inevitable requirement. The horse must be seen to precede the cart, but as Bradford Hill acknowledged, this presupposes that the cart can be confidently distinguished from the horse. This is not always easy. It was pointed out above that causality cannot, perhaps, be proven: the possibility of an undetected confounding factor playing a part can never be completely disregarded. Thus, discussion focuses on the strength of belief in the hypothesis of causality. This difficult area was not discussed by Bradford Hill. In describing levels of certainty, descriptive terms such as 'probably', 'possibly', 'unlikely' etc., are often added to the term 'causal'. These do not lend themselves to quantification, but it will be seen that uncertainty here needs to be combined with the risk estimate used to predict the likelihood of effects at an individual or population level. Attempts to refine the wording used to convey uncertainty regarding causality have sometimes led to confusion.

The following series indicates a declining level of confidence in causality:

- imprudent not to regard the association as causal;
- prudent to regard the association as causal;
- not imprudent to regard the association as causal;
- not prudent to regard the association as causal;
- imprudent to regard the association as causal.

The first of these formulations was used some time ago in a report by the Committee on the Medical Effects of Air Pollutants (COMEAP)[11] and provoked criticism that the committee was taking refuge in a double negative: so much for subtlety! Of course, it might have been easier had the committee's level of confidence in causality been scored from 1 to 5 or from 0 to 4. Why is this important? The answer is because it bears on the application of the precautionary principle as a device with which to manage risk.

The precautionary principle

Few principles are less well understood than the precautionary principle. It is well described by Foster et al.[12] The precautionary principle is designed to help the risk managers in the face of uncertainty. The government health and safety or environmental regulatory agencies are entrusted with developing policies (at a national, local or individual scale) to limit risks. They should not be confused with the scientists who attempt to define the risk in a given situation, whether they be epidemiologists or toxicologists. In essence, the precautionary principle urges the risk managers not to wait for the perfect proof before acting to reduce risk if, and this is important, inaction could lead to serious effects. What is seldom remembered is that the precautionary principle is qualified by the following points:

- **Proportionality**: measures taken should not be disproportionate to the desired level of protection and must not aim at zero risk.
- **Non-discrimination**: comparable situations should be treated similarly.
- **Consistency**: across problems and with cases where data are available.
- **Costs and benefits**: where possible these should be taken into account.
- **Examination of scientific developments**: provisional responses may be appropriate.

The cynical reader will not find it difficult to believe that these caveats were written within the European Commission. Yet they are important: without them the precautionary principle could become a charter for those pressing for action in every case of a postulated association between an alleged cause and a supposed effect.

One point of not entirely semantic confusion has been generated by equating the terms 'cautious' and 'precautionary'. The scientist assessing causality and/or risk should exercise proper scientific caution in his work. Caution is implicit in the current paradigm of research: hypothesis based, evidence driven and taking note of such guidance as is provided by Bradford Hill's work. 'Precautionary', on the other hand, applies to the work of the risk manager using the scientist's properly cautious conclusions as a basis for developing policies. The scientist undertaking risk assessment need not concern himself with 'precaution'.

Why explaining risk is difficult

Explaining anything is made easier when the recipient of the explanation trusts its provider. In the risk-communication field, trust may be lacking. It is useful to consider why this may be so:

- Experts no longer command automatic trust, irrespective of how genuine their expertise may be. The reasons for this generally accepted observation are not completely known, but scientific overconfidence, unfulfilled expectations (a cure for cancer, for example) and the entirely correct tendency for experts to modify their views as evidence changes, may all play a part. A reluctance on the part of some experts to show how they arrive at their conclusions also inspires doubt.
- Even less trusted than 'the experts' are the risk managers. Their task is a hard one in that risk management is far from an exact science and many of the factors taken into account defy precise, or at least quantitative, definition. It is certain that people want to know how a decision was taken: who contributed to it, who influenced it, who benefited from it, was it taken openly or 'behind closed doors'?
- Peoples' perceptions of risk vary with the specific risk being considered. This is sometimes described as loading of the actual risk by 'fright factors'. Much work has been undertaken to identify such factors and the following list is probably incomplete (see, for example, Slovic et al.[13]).

Perceptions leading to increased worry are listed below:

- involuntary or imposed risk;
- inequitably distributed risk;
- inescapable risk;
- unfamiliar risk;
- man-made as opposed to natural causes of risk;
- capacity to cause hidden or irreversible effects;
- risks that affect future generations;
- a form of death or illness that inspires dread, e.g. cancer;
- damage to identifiable, rather than anonymous victims;
- poorly understood by science;
- subject to contradictory statements from responsible sources or, even worse, from a single source.

These various factors combine to control the extent to which specific risks tend to be the cause of worry. We might write: worry = risk × fear (risk here being calculated or objective risk). Additionally, we might define acceptability of risk as:

$$\text{Acceptability} = \frac{1}{\text{worry}} = \frac{1}{\text{risk} \times \text{fear}}$$

The extent to which people worry about risks leads to misperceptions of the magnitude of specific risks. Overestimation of risks is common in examples such as risks from nuclear power, floods or tornados; underestimation is common with such risks as heart disease, obesity, accidents at home.

Social amplification of risks

The public's reaction or response to information about risk can be difficult to predict: sometimes the information seems to sink without trace, on other occasions something akin to panic occurs. This is discussed at some length in the Department of Health report.[6] One factor controlling this is the response of the media to an announcement about a risk to health. Media responses are themselves, seemingly, controlled by factors: media triggers. The Department of Health report identified the following:

- blame;
- secrecy and cover ups;
- human interest;
- links with high profile issues or personalities;
- signal value;
- many people potentially at risk;
- strong visual aspects;
- links to sex or crime.

These factors reflect, no doubt, upon our natures as much as upon the media *per se*: it is likely that combinations of these factors attracted interest in Rome or Athens in classical times as they do now. Signal value is an interesting factor: this implies that the event or risk is taken as indicating that 'the same thing' could happen elsewhere. Put simply: if the experts have been wrong about 'X' what else could they be wrong about?

CONCLUSIONS

'Risk' is a difficult topic. The usual paradigm of hazard identification, risk assessment, risk management is well understood, although risk communication should be added as an essential component of risk management. Each step presents problems, but those associated with the earlier steps tend to be less difficult than those occurring later. The public perceives risk differently from professional scientists and regulators: if this is not understood, risk communication can be a disaster.

Key points

- Hazard should not be confused with risk. Hazard implies the potential to cause harm. Risk specifies the likelihood of harm occurring.
- Hazard identification is usually dependent on toxicological studies; estimation of risk more often involves epidemiological approaches.
- Methods for predicting risks associated with exposure to carcinogens have been developed. Such methods, although widely used, are not without problems and the accuracy of the predictions is difficult, or impossible, to confirm.
- Causality is an important concept in assessing evidence linking exposure to chemicals with potential effects. Causality is difficult, perhaps impossible, to prove.
- The precautionary principle is often misunderstood: it is not a carte blanche for action in the presence of doubt.

REFERENCES

1. World Health Organization. Air quality guidelines. Global update 2005. Particulate matter, ozone, nitrogen dioxide and sulfur dioxide. Copenhagen: World Health Organization, 2006. Available from: www.euro.who.int/Document/E90038.pdf.
2. Housley DG, Mudway I, Kelly FJ *et al*. Depletion of urate in human nasal lavage following *in vitro* ozone exposure. *International Journal of Biochemical and Cellular Biology*. 1995; **11**: 1153–9.
3. World Health Organization. Air quality guidelines for Europe. WHO Regional Publications, European Series No 23. Copenhagen: World Health Organization, Regional Office for Europe, 1987.
4. Department of Health. Committee on the Carcinogenicity of Chemicals in Food, Consumer Products and the Environment. Guidelines for evaluation of chemicals for carcinogenicity. London: HMSO, 1991.
5. Department of Health. Committee on the Carcinogenicity of Chemicals in Food, Consumer Products and the Environment. Risks associated with exposures to low levels of carcinogenic air pollutants. COC/03/S4. London: HMSO, 2003. Available from: www.advisorybodies.doh.gov.uk/coc/airpollu.htm.
6. Department of Health. Communicating about risks to public health. Pointers to good practice. London: HMSO, 1997.
7. Popper KR. *The logic of scientific discovery*. London: Hutchinson, 1959.
8. Medawar P. *Memoir of a thinking radish*. Oxford: Oxford University Press, 1986.
9. Reichenbach H. Quoted in Popper KR. *The logic of scientific discovery*. London: Hutchinson, 1959.
10. Bradford Hill A. The environment and disease association or causation? *Proceedings of the Royal Society of Medicine*. 1965; **58**: 295–300.
11. Department of Health. Committee on the Medical Effects of Air Pollutants. Non-biological particles and health. London: HMSO, 1995.
12. Foster KR, Vecchia P, Repacholi MH. Risk management. Science and the precautionary principle. *Science*. 2000; **288**: 979–81.
13. Slovic P, Fischoff B, Lichenstein S. Facts and fears: Understanding perceived risk. In: Schwing R, Albers WA (eds). *How safe is safe enough?* New York: Plenum, 1980: 181–226.

SECTION TWO

Metals

12	Introduction *Tar-Ching Aw*	151
13	Aluminium *Perrine Hoet*	153
14	Antimony *Malcolm R Sim*	159
15	Arsenic *Malcolm R Sim*	160
16	Beryllium *Lee S Newman and Holly M Christensen*	162
17	Cadmium *Perrine Hoet*	167
18	Chromium *Tom Sorahan*	173
19	Cobalt *Perrine Hoet*	175
20	Copper *Peter Aggett*	180
21	Gold *Peter Linnett*	183
22	Iron *Peter Aggett*	185
23	Lead *Peter J Baxter and Hideki Igisu*	188
24	Magnesium *Peter Aggett*	199
25	Manganese *Grant McMillan and Finlay D Dick*	201
26	Mercury *Peter J Baxter and Hideki Igisu*	214

27	Molybdenum *Malcolm R Sim*	221
28	Nickel *Tom Sorahan*	223
29	Phosphorus *Malcolm R Sim*	225
30	Platinum group metals *Peter Linnett*	226
31	Polonium *Iain Blair*	231
32	Silver *Peter Linnett*	234
33	Thallium *Hideki Igisu and Tar-Ching Aw*	236
34	Tin *Tar-Ching Aw and Hideki Igisu*	238
35	Tungsten *Perrine Hoet*	241
36	Uranium *Iain Blair*	243
37	Vanadium *Finlay D Dick*	246
38	Zinc *Peter Aggett*	249

12

Introduction

TAR-CHING AW

Properties of metals	151
Toxicity versus essentiality	151
Diagnosis of metal poisoning	152
Acknowledgements	152
Further reading	152

PROPERTIES OF METALS

The term 'metal' refers to those elements in the periodic table (of just over a hundred elements) that have specific characteristics. They are good conductors of heat and electricity; they are bright, shiny and malleable; and they produce a ringing sound when struck. Metals lose electrons to form cations, and the resulting electropositivity gives it an affinity to bind with sulphur, chlorine and other non-metals to form compounds. Alloys are formed from a homogenous mix of metals with other elements. Examples are brass (copper and zinc), bronze (copper and tin) and steel (iron and carbon). These often have physical properties that are different from their components. The term 'superalloy' has been used for alloys with excellent mechanical strength, and the ability to resist deformation at high temperature. Many superalloys are based on nickel or cobalt. Metalloids are elements such as antimony, arsenic, polonium and tellurium. They have properties in between those of metals and non-metals. Some metalloids with doumented health effects on humans have been included in this chapter.

Gold, silver, copper, iron, tin, lead and mercury have been mined and used extensively before and during the times of the ancient Greek and Roman civilizations. Today, metals have considerable benefits for industry, for example in engineering, construction, electronics and for dental and pharmaceutical applications. However, they have also been well recognized as a cause of human health effects, and adverse effects on the environment. Measures to limit occupational exposure, while allowing safe use of metals and their compounds remains an ongoing challenge for industry.

TOXICITY VERSUS ESSENTIALITY

A number of the metals considered to be toxic in an occupational setting are essential for some metabolic processes in humans. Examples of essential metals are iron (for haem synthesis), copper (for enzymes such as ceruloplasmin and cytochrome-c oxidase), zinc (for development of skin, hair and nails), cobalt (in cyanocobalamin or vitamin B_{12}), manganese (for transferases), and magnesium (cofactor for enzymes). These metals create a dilemma in terms of the extent to which overexposure and intake should be reduced to balance toxicity against deficiency. In theory, the U-shaped relationship between dose and effect can be used to determine the ideal range for exposure and intake levels which will prevent deficiency, as well as toxicity.

The toxicity of any metal depends upon a number of factors, including:

- those related to the nature of the metal, e.g. the chemical species, including its valency and particle size;
- exposure circumstances, the route of exposure, the mode of entry to the body, other concomitant exposures, use of protective equipment; and
- the reaction of the body to the metal, and the capability for clearance.

Absorption from the lungs is generally more effective than from the gut. About 40 per cent of an inhaled dose of a metallic aerosol may be retained in the lungs, whereas usually only 10 per cent or less of an ingested dose will be absorbed. Other than particle size and solubility, relatively few factors affect uptake from the lungs. Only particles that are of respirable size of around $4\,\mu m$ or less penetrate to the alveoli and thus become available for absorption from the lungs. The uptake of metals from the gastrointestinal tract varies inversely with age. This is especially relevant in younger workers and in parts of the world where child labour continues to exist. Interactions with other constituents of the diet can affect the rate of uptake from the gut. For example, the absorption of lead varies inversely with the amount of calcium and iron in the diet and it may also be influenced by the presence of fat, protein and vitamin D in the gut. The uptake of cadmium is affected by the zinc content of the diet and that of manganese by the iron content.

Recognition of 'speciation' is fundamental to the understanding of metal toxicology. Chemical species refers to chemically identical molecular entities, such as specific compounds of a metal or specific forms or isomers of a compound. The concept of speciation includes the organic and inorganic compounds, as well as the elemental metal, and is based on the expected differences in physical, chemical and toxicological properties of different metal species. Toxicity is related to physicochemical characteristics, such as solubility and valency. As a general rule, the water-soluble forms are associated with acute toxicity, and may be cleared more easily by the body compared to water-insoluble compounds which tend to be retained for longer periods in bones and tissues. However, those forms that are slightly soluble in the biological matrix, if they allow a slow release of toxic ions, are frequently associated with chronic diseases, such as fibrosis or malignancy. Several metals can exist in different valency states, with properties differing depending on the valency. The valency of a metal refers to the maximum number of hydrogen or chlorine (or univalent) atoms that may combine with one atom of the element. It has also been defined as the number of chemical bonds formed by the atoms of a specific element. Iron, for example, can exist as ferrous (valency 2) or ferric (valency 3) forms. Chromium has a range of valencies, including trivalent, hexavalent and other rarer valency forms. Trivalent chromium is considered essential, while several hexavalent chromium compounds are toxic and carcinogenic.

DIAGNOSIS OF METAL POISONING

For a clinician faced with a case of possible metal poisoning, the diagnosis of occupational metal poisoning is not always easy, for few cases present as clear clinical entities and, usually, an occupational cause will be part of a list of different possibilities. Exposure to a metal (or, indeed, any other substance) at work does not prove that it is the cause of the patient's illness. The diagnosis often depends on the balance of probability. The higher or greater the extent and duration of occupational exposure, the more likely it is to be a cause of the illness. Epidemiological studies may provide evidence for the range of exposures that are relevant, but when an individual patient is being assessed, an additional difficulty is that there may be considerable individual variation in susceptibility. It is therefore necessary to obtain reliable information, as explained in Chapter 1, Donald Hunter and the history of occupational health: precedents and perspectives and Chapter 2, The changing face of occupational diseases, about the circumstances of exposure and their relationship to the course of the patient's illness. Also, the important difference between hazard (the inherent property of a substance to cause harm) and risk (the likelihood of harm being caused because of the way in which the substance is handled at work) should be emphasized. The clinician will also need to know what laboratory tests may be available to aid diagnosis and where such tests are best carried out. Furthermore, it may be necessary to seek specialist advice, perhaps from a university department of occupational medicine, a poisons centre or from organizations with statutory responsibility for health and safety at work, or other government agencies. In the United Kingdom, a useful contact will be the Health and Safety Executive (HSE) and the Health and Safety Laboratory (HSL), in the United States of America, the National Institute for Occupational Safety and Health (NIOSH) and the Occupational Safety and Health Administration (OSHA), and in Finland, the Finnish Institute of Occupational Health (FIOH).

> **Key points**
>
> - Some metals, such as iron, copper, zinc, cobalt, manganese and magnesium, are essential for metabolic function, although overexposure causes harm (a U-shaped dose–response relationship).
> - Metal toxicity is dependent on factors related to the agent (speciation, physical and chemical properties), the circumstances of exposure and the body's reaction.
> - A diagnosis of metal poisoning requires confirmation of the nature, extent and duration of exposure.

ACKNOWLEDGEMENTS

The editors would like to acknowledge those individuals who contributed material to the Metals chapters in the eighth and ninth editions of *Hunter's Diseases of Occupations*, some of which may persist in updated form or otherwise here.

FURTHER READING

Agricola G. *De re metallica, 1556.* Hoover HC and Hoover LH (trans). New York: Dover Publications, 1950.

Stern BS, Solioz M, Krewski D *et al.* Copper and human health: Biochemistry, genetics, and strategies for modeling dose–response relationships. *Journal of Toxicology and Environmental Health.* 2007; **10**: 157–222.

Riihimaki V, Luotamo M. *Health risk assessment report for metallic chromium and trivalent chromium.* Paris: International Chromium Development Association, 2006.

13

Aluminium

PERRINE HOET

| Introduction | 153 | Toxicity | 154 |
| Kinetics | 154 | References | 156 |

INTRODUCTION

Aluminium (Al) is the most abundant metal and the third most abundant element in the earth's crust, mainly in combination with oxygen, fluorine and silicon. It is not considered to be an essential trace element for humans.

Aluminium is a light metal, which is used more widely throughout industry than any other non-ferrous metal. Its major applications are in transportation, building and construction, packaging and electrical equipment. Aluminium and its compounds have numerous other applications, for example, in paints, fuel additives, explosives, fireworks and powder metallurgy (aluminium powder); in the manufacture of abrasives, refractories, ceramics, catalysts, paper, artificial gems, glass and heat-resistant fibres (aluminium oxides); in water purification (as alum, bentonite, zeolite); in (para)pharmaceutical products (antacids, astringents, antiperspirants, vaccines, dental products, as aluminium hydroxide and aluminium chlorohydrate) or as food additives (preservatives, fillers, colouring agents, emulsifiers, baking powders).[1–3]

Aluminium is produced from ores (primary production) and scrap (secondary production). Primary production is a two-step, energy-intensive process:

1. extraction and refining of bauxite by the Bayer process to produce alumina, $Al_2O_3.3H_2O$ (bauxite is digested at high temperature and pressure in caustic soda),
2. electrolytic reduction of alumina by the Hall–Héroult process (alumina is dissolved in molten cryolite (Na_3AlF_6) and reduced to metallic Al in electrolytic cells).[1,2]

In such settings, workers are exposed not only to aluminium, but also to caustic mist, hydrogen fluoride, particulate fluorides, perfluorocarbons, polycyclic aromatic hydrocarbons, sulphur dioxide, carbon dioxide and monoxide, and carbon dust. Exposure in secondary smelting is not well characterized; many pollutants have been identified including thermal degradation products of polyvinyl chloride, lubricants or petrol modifiers. Occupational exposures of concern appear to be inhalable dust, fluoride salts, lead, aluminium and manganese.[4,5]

Once formed, aluminium is alloyed with other materials (iron, silicon, zinc, copper, magnesium) to make an array of alloys with different properties which can be rolled, cast and extruded. Aluminium founding includes a number of different casting techniques (mainly sand and die casting), alloys, additives to melt, and binders in cores and moulds, all contributing to very heterogenous exposures. In sand foundries, exposure to high levels of total dust and silica occur, as well as exposure to furfuryl alcohol and dimethylethylamine. High levels of mineral oil mist can be measured during die casting.[5,6]

Aluminium powder is generally produced by atomization in air or inert gas, which forms particles of different shapes (irregular, spherical) and sizes (from coarse to superfine). Aluminium powders can be treated with materials such as isostearic acid or other lubricants to minimize surface oxidation or coated with polystyrene to reduce or eliminate the fire hazard.[1,2]

Welding of aluminium creates submicron-sized particles, but depending on the process and materials used, the elemental composition of total and respirable fume/dust may differ considerably.

KINETICS

Gastrointestinal absorption of aluminium is low (<0.5 per cent), but it depends on the chemical species and solubility and the simultaneous presence of ligands in the gut. Ligands such as citric acid (or other carboxylic acids) enhance uptake, while phosphate and silicon-compounds reduce it.[7–9]

Occupational exposure to aluminium fumes, dusts and powder has resulted in increased serum and urinary levels of aluminium providing indirect evidence for inhalation absorption. The bioavailability is likely to be dependent on Al species and particle size of the inhaled material. Biokinetics investigations with ^{26}Al oxide particles and occupational exposure studies suggest an inhalation absorption rate of about 1.5–2 per cent. It is suggested that inhaled nanoparticles could reach the brain through the nasal–olfactory system, bypassing the blood–brain barrier.[3,7,9]

In plasma, Al is transported in high molecular weight complexes, mainly bound to transferrin. Less than 10 per cent is associated with low molecular mass compounds (citrate). There is evidence that transferrin can mediate Al transport across the blood–brain barrier.[9,10]

About 2 per cent of Al entering the blood is retained within the body for years, but the remainder is rapidly excreted, mainly in urine (>95 per cent),[7] explaining the higher susceptibility of subjects with renal insufficiency to Al toxicity. Aluminium is distributed in the body in bone (60 per cent), lung (25 per cent), muscle (10 per cent), liver (3 per cent) and brain (1 per cent).[3]

Reported urinary half-lives in occupationally exposed subjects range from days to months or even years depending on the duration and the type of exposure. A mono-exponential decay in both urine and plasma, with half-lives of 136 and 162 days, was calculated in a welder with acute exposure.[11] In prolonged exposure, clearance is characterized by multiple half-lives. Endogenous release of Al from compartments with slow elimination kinetics (i.e. bones) and the progressive resorption of sparingly soluble particles trapped in lungs could explain why elevated urinary Al excretion can be measured for years after cessation of exposure.[12,13]

TOXICITY

Respiratory manifestations

A wide spectrum of respiratory symptoms and diseases, including interstitial fibrosis, pneumoconiosis, asthma, granulomatous disease, chronic obstructive disease, emphysema, desquamative interstitial pneumonia, and pulmonary alveolar proteinosis has been ascribed to occupational activities involving exposure to aluminium dust or fumes. Reports are often based on small numbers of cases, which limits their interpretation, and there is no consensus with regard to the causal role of aluminium in the ocurrence of these effects.

Pulmonary fibrosis has been observed, in the past, in bauxite and potroom workers, as well as in workers engaged in the manufacture of alumina abrasive.[3,14] It is very likely that simultaneous exposure to silica was the causative agent. Recent epidemiological studies provide little evidence of a serious adverse effect on the respiratory health associated with exposure to bauxite in an opencast mine or to alumina in refinery workers in present-day conditions.[15,16]

Aluminium was given prophylactically to some Canadian gold and uranium miners between 1944 and 1979, in the mistaken belief that it prevented silicosis. Men were exposed to 20 000–34 000 ppm of 'McIntyre powder', consisting of 85 per cent aluminium oxide and 15 per cent aluminium for ten minutes before each shift. Follow up over 22 years has not revealed any cases of pulmonary fibrosis and the pattern and the prevalence of respiratory disease were similar to those in gold miners who had not been exposed to aluminium.[17]

A number of cases of pulmonary fibrosis associated with occupational exposure to aluminium powder have, however, been reported.[3,18–21] As conflicting study results were published, it was speculated that factors such as particle size, density of the dust, and presence or absence of stearic acid (thought to be protective) or mineral oil (associated with fibrosis) were relevant to the development of pulmonary fibrosis.[3,14,22–24]

Krewski et al.[3] identified an airborne aluminium powder concentration of 50 mg/m^3 as a level at which adverse effects have been observed (end point: irritation). However, high-resolution computed tomography revealed lung fibrosis changes in aluminium powder workers exposed to lower levels. Biological monitoring in plasma and urine revealed higher internal exposure to Al in affected workers (33.5 μg/L plasma to 15.4 μg/L plasma) and (340.5 μg/g creatinine to 135.1 μg/g creatinine in urine).[24,25]

A number of studies have demonstrated an association between aluminium smelting and the development of an asthma-like syndrome.[3,26–31] The reported incidence varied from 0.06 to 4 per cent of exposed workers per year. It is still unclear whether 'potroom asthma' is related to exposure to respiratory irritants, such as hydrogen fluoride, particulate fluoride, chlorine, sulphur dioxide, inspirable dust exposures, carbon dust or a specific reaction to aluminium.[3,29–33] Inhalation challenges in an aluminium foundry worker[34] and an aluminium welder[35] provided evidence that aluminium can cause asthmatic reactions.

Central nervous system

The toxicity of aluminium to the central nervous system of human beings is supported by reported cases of iatrogenic aluminium intoxication. Very high plasma/serum aluminium levels caused by haemodialysis, oral consumption of large amounts of Al-containing antacids/phosphate binders by individuals with impaired renal function, as well as irrigation of the urinary bladder with massive amounts of alum to stop haemorrhaging or reconstructive otoneurosurgery with Al-containing material have resulted in encephalopathy (dialysis dementia, a degenerative neurological syndrome, characterized by the gradual loss of speech, motor and cognitive functions).

Cross-sectional studies investigating the neurological effects of Al in occupationally exposed workers have provided controversial results. Some data support the hypothesis of a relationship between chronic aluminium exposure in welders and subclinical neurological effects (impairment on neurobehavioural tests) or an increased incidence of subjective neurological symptoms. However, there is still no firm conclusion as to whether occupational aluminium exposure can result in neuropsychological disorder.[3,36–47] In an investigation on steel welders in shipyards, Riihimaki et al.[44] reported a threshold for central nervous system adverse effects in the concentration range of 108–162 μg Al/L urine and 6.75–9.5 μg/L in serum. A longitudinal study over a period of four years in welders, in the train and truck construction industry, did not support a neurotoxic effect of aluminium at a level of 88–140 μg Al/g creatinine in urine and 13–16 μg Al/L plasma (preshift samples) and a mean exposure of 15 years.[46] No neurological effects related to the exposure to aluminium were found in smelters (Al-urine, median 4.0 μg/L; range, from detection limit up to 34 μg/L), aluminium welders (median, 22.0; range, 4–255) and a small group of flake powder production workers (median, 83.0; range, 12–282).[45] Data from Letzel et al.[47] indicate that chronic exposure to Al, in an Al powder plant, at median (range) level up to 110 μg/L (5–337), 87.6 μg/g creatinine (4.6–605), and 8.7 μg/L plasma (5.1–25) did not induce measurable cognitive deficits. According to a review by Krewski et al.,[3] evidence of an association between inhalation exposure and neurological effects is limited. However, a meta-analysis on neurobehavioural data obtained by epidemiological studies in occupational settings concluded that there is concurring evidence from different studies that urinary Al concentrations below 135 μg/L have an impact on cognitive performances.[48]

Despite numerous epidemiological studies investigating the possible relationship between Al levels in drinking water and Alzheimer's disease, the association is highly controversial and although it cannot be excluded that it may play a role in the disease, the available data do not indicate that aluminium has a causal role.[49–58]

Other manifestations

Long-term dialysis and administration of aluminium containing phosphate-binders used to control hyperphosphataemia or aluminium-containing antacid drugs can cause bone toxicity (e.g. impaired mineralization, osteomalacia). Although the use of Al-containing drugs can result in aluminium overload, skeletal effects are more likely to be secondary to hypophosphataemia and phosphate depletion caused by decreased phosphorus absorption due to Al binding with dietary phosphorus.[59,60] In the general population, accumulated aluminium content in bone throughout life does not substantially influence the extent of osteoporosis or the occurrence of hip fracture.[61,62] Bone toxicity has not been documented in aluminium-exposed workers.

An excess of pulmonary and bladder cancer has been observed in aluminium production workers, and aluminium production has been recognized by the International Agency for Research on Cancer (IARC)[63] as causing human cancer. The excess risk of both lung and bladder cancers has been attributed to coal tar pitch volatiles and benzo(a)pyrene exposure in this process.[64–68] There is no evidence that aluminium metal *per se* or any of its compounds are carcinogenic.

Contact dermatitis to aluminium has been recognized and can be confirmed with patch tests,[69] but is relatively rare. Such reactions have been reported following injection of aluminium-containing vaccines.[70,71]

Medical surveillance

Workers exposed to Al dusts or fumes should be submitted to periodic health checks, including clinical examination with special attention to the lungs and central nervous system. Depending on the clinical findings from such surveillance, pulmonary function testing, periodic chest radiographs and neuropsychological testing may be considered as additional investigations.

Al concentrations <5 μg/L serum and <30 μg/L urine are generally expected in the general population. Analysis of serum concentration is performed for follow up of aluminium status in dialysis patients. Routine biological monitoring in occupationally exposed workers is recommended by some authors.[13,44,72] Samples collected immediately after a work shift are strongly related to the current exposure, whereas samples taken later after exposure (e.g. Monday morning after a weekend free from exposure) are more likely to reflect the body burden of aluminium.[12,45] The Deutsche Forschungsgemeinshaft[73] adopted 200 μg/L urine (end of shift sample) as a biological tolerance value based on a MAK value of 6 mg/m^3 for welding fumes (Al 2.34 mg/m^3). The biomonitoring action limit recommended by the Finnish Institute of Occupational Health[74] is 160 μg/L urine (Monday morning sample). However, data are scant and it is not known how well serum and urine concentrations of aluminium reflect the concentrations in the target tissues among workers exposed to different species of aluminium.[45] Moreover, because Al is ubiquitous, great care should be taken to avoid contamination at all stages of sampling and analysis.

Key points

- Aluminium (Al) is ubiquitous, but it has no known physiological function in humans.
- Accumulation of Al caused by dialysis with Al-contaminated dialysate often with concurrent intake of Al-containing drugs has resulted in encephalopathy and osteomalacia.
- A wide spectrum of respiratory effects (e.g. interstitial fibrosis, pneumoconiosis, asthma) has been ascribed to occupational activities involving exposure to Al dust or fumes; there is no consensus with regard to the causal role of Al.
- Subclinical neurological effects (impairment on neurobehavioural tests) have been reported in Al-exposed workers, however this has not been consistently observed across studies. There is no evidence for bone toxicity in Al workers.
- The possible association with Alzheimer's disease is highly controversial.

REFERENCES

1. International Aluminium Institute (IAI). International Aluminium Institute homepage. Last accessed March 2008. Available from: http://www.world-aluminium.org/Home.
2. Aluminium Federation Ltd (ALFED). Aluminium Federation homepage. Last accessed March 2008. Available from: www.alfed.org.uk/site/alfed/home.
3. Krewski D, Yokel RA, Nieboer E et al. Human health risk assessment for aluminium, aluminium oxide, and aluminium hydroxide. *Journal of Toxicology and Environmental Health. Part B, Critical Reviews.* 2007; **10** (Suppl. 1): 1–269.
4. Healy J, Bradley SD, Northage C, Scobbie E. Inhalation exposure in secondary aluminium smelting. *Annals of Occupational Hygiene.* 2001; **45**: 217–25.
5. Westberg HB, Selden AI, Bellander T. Exposure to chemical agents in Swedish aluminum foundries and aluminum remelting plants – a comprehensive survey. *Applied Occupational and Environmental Hygiene.* 2001; **16**: 66–77.
6. Westberg HB, Bellander T. Epidemiological adaptation of quartz exposure modeling in Swedish aluminum foundries: Nested case–control study on lung cancer. *Applied Occupational and Environmental Hygiene.* 2003; **18**: 1006–13.
7. Priest ND. The biological behaviour and bioavailability of aluminium in man, with special reference to studies employing aluminium^{-26} as a tracer: Review and study update. *Journal of Environmental Monitoring.* 2004; **6**: 375–403.
8. Steinhausen C, Kislinger G, Winklhofer C et al. Investigation of the aluminium biokinetics in humans: A 26Al tracer study. *Food and Chemical Toxicology.* 2004; **42**: 363–71.
9. Yokel RA, McNamara PJ. Aluminium toxicokinetics: An updated minireview. *Pharmacology and Toxicology.* 2001; **88**: 159–67.
10. Berthon G. Aluminium speciation in relation to aluminium bioavailability, metabolism and toxicity. *Coordination Chemistry Reviews.* 2002; **228**: 319–41.
11. Schaller KH, Csanady G, Filser J et al. Elimination kinetics of metals after an accidental exposure to welding fumes. *International Archives of Occupational and Environmental Health.* 2007; **80**: 635–41.
12. Lauwerys R, Hoet P. *Industrial chemical exposure. Guidelines for biological monitoring*, 3rd edn. Boca Raton, FL: Lewis, 2001.
13. Ljunggren KG, Lidums V, Bengt S. Blood and urine concentrations of aluminium among workers exposed to aluminium flake powders. *British Journal of Industrial Medicine.* 1991; **48**: 106–9.
14. World Health Organization. International programme on chemical safety. Environmental Health Criteria 194: Aluminium. Geneva: WHO, 1997.
15. Beach JR, de Klerk NH, Fritschi L et al. Respiratory symptoms and lung function in bauxite miners. *International Archives of Occupational and Environmental Health.* 2001; **74**: 489–94.
16. Musk AW, de Klerk NH, Beach JR et al. Respiratory symptoms and lung function in alumina refinery employees. *Occupational and Environmental Medicine.* 2000; **57**: 279–83.
17. Muller J, Kusiak RA, Suranyi G et al. Study of mortality of Ontario miners 1955–77, part ii. Toronto: Ontario Ministry of Labour Special Studies Branch, 1986.
18. Mitchell J. Pulmonary fibrosis in an aluminium worker. *British Journal of Industrial Medicine.* 1959; **16**: 123–5.
19. Jordan JW. Pulmonary fibrosis in a worker using an aluminium powder. *British Journal of Industrial Medicine.* 1961; **18**: 21–3.
20. McLaughlin AIG, Kazantzis G, King E et al. Pulmonary fibrosis and encephalopathy associated with the inhalation of aluminium dust. *British Journal of Industrial Medicine.* 1962; **19**: 253–63.
21. Mitchell J, Manning GE, Molyneux M et al. Pulmonary fibrosis in workers exposed to finely powdered aluminium. *British Journal of Industrial Medicine.* 1961; **18**: 10–20.
22. Corrin B. Aluminium pneumoconiosis. *In vitro* comparison of stamped aluminium powders and a granular aluminium powder. *British Journal of Industrial Medicine.* 1963; **20**: 264–7.
23. Abramson MJ, Wlodarczyk JH, Saunders NA et al. Does aluminium smelting cause lung disease? *American Review of Respiratory Disease.* 1989; **139**: 1042–57.
24. Kraus T, Schaller KH, Angerer J, Letzel S. Aluminium dust-induced lung disease in the pyro-powder-producing industry: Detection by high-resolution computed tomography. *International Archives of Occupational and Environmental Health.* 2000; **73**: 61–4.
25. Kraus T, Schaller KH, Angerer J et al. Aluminosis – detection of an almost forgotten disease with HRCT. *Journal of Occupational Medicine and Toxicology.* 2006; **1**: 4.
26. Field GB. Pulmonary function in aluminium smelters. *Thorax.* 1984; **39**: 743–51.

27. Saric M, Marelja J. Bronchial hyperreactivity in potroom workers and prognosis after stopping exposure. *British Journal of Industrial Medicine.* 1991; **48**: 653–5.
28. Barnard CG, McBride DI, Firth HM, Herbison GP. Assessing individual employee risk factors for occupational asthma in primary aluminium smelting. *Occupational and Environmental Medicine.* 2004; **61**: 604–8.
29. Taiwo OA, Sircar KD, Slade MD *et al.* Incidence of asthma among aluminum workers. *Journal of Occupational and Environmental Medicine.* 2006; **48**: 275–82.
30. Sjaheim T, Kongerud J, Soyseth V. Blood eosinophils in workers with aluminum potroom asthma are increased to higher levels in non-smokers than in smokers. *American Journal of Industrial Medicine.* 2007; **50**: 443–8.
31. Sjaheim T, Halstensen TS, Lund MB *et al.* Airway inflammation in aluminium potroom asthma. *Occupational and Environmental Medicine.* 2004; **61**: 779–85.
32. Lund MB, Oksne PI, Hamre R, Kongerud J. Increased nitric oxide in exhaled air: An early marker of asthma in non-smoking aluminium potroom workers? *Occupational and Environmental Medicine.* 2000; **57**: 274–8.
33. Fritschi L, Sim MR, Forbes A *et al.* Respiratory symptoms and lung-function changes with exposure to five substances in aluminium smelters. *International Archives of Occupational and Environmental Health.* 2003; **76**: 103–10.
34. Burge PS, Scott JA, McCoach J. Occupational asthma caused by aluminum. *Allergy.* 2000; **55**: 779–80.
35. Vandenplas O, Delwiche JP, Vanbilsen ML *et al.* Occupational asthma caused by aluminium welding. *European Respiratory Journal.* 1998; **11**: 1182–4.
36. Akila R, Stollery BT, Riihimaki V. Decrements in cognitive performance in metal inert gas welders exposed to aluminium. *Occupational and Environmental Medicine.* 1999; **56**: 632–9.
37. Bast-Pettersen R, Drablos PA, Goffeng LO *et al.* Neuropsychological deficit among elderly workers in aluminum production. *American Journal of Industrial Medicine.* 1994; **25**: 649–62.
38. Bast-Pettersen R, Skaug V, Ellingsen D, Thomassen Y. Neurobehavioral performance in aluminum welders. *American Journal of Industrial Medicine.* 2000; **37**: 184–92.
39. Rifat SL, Eastwood MR, Crapper McLachlan DR *et al.* Effect of exposure of miners to aluminium powder. *Lancet.* 1990; **336**: 1162–5.
40. Sim M, Dick R, Jusso J *et al.* Are aluminium potroom workers at increased risk of neurological disorders? *Occupational and Environmental Medicine.* 1997; **54**: 29–35.
41. Graves AB, Rosner D, Echererria D *et al.* Occupational exposure to solvents and aluminium and estimated risks of Alzheimer's disease. *Occupational and Environmental Medicine.* 1998; **55**: 627–33.
42. Buchta M, Kiesswetter E, Otto A *et al.* Longitudinal study examining the neurotoxicity of occupational exposure to aluminium-containing welding fumes. *International Archives of Occupational and Environmental Health.* 2003; **76**: 539–48.
43. Sjogren B, Iregren A, Frech W *et al.* Effects on the nervous system among welders exposed to aluminium and manganese. *Occupational and Environmental Medicine.* 1996; **53**: 32–40.
44. Riihimaki V, Hanninen H, Akila R *et al.* Body burden of aluminum in relation to central nervous system function among metal inert-gas welders. *Scandinavian Journal of Work and Environmental Health.* 2000; **26**: 118–30.
45. Iregren A, Sjogren B, Gustafsson K *et al.* Effects on the nervous system in different groups of workers exposed to aluminium. *Occupational and Environmental Medicine.* 2001; **58**: 453–60.
46. Kiesswetter E, Schaper M, Buchta M *et al.* Longitudinal study on potential neurotoxic effects of aluminium: I. Assessment of exposure and neurobehavioural performance of Al welders in the train and truck construction industry over 4 years. *International Archives of Occupational and Environmental Health.* 2007; **81**: 41–67.
47. Letzel S, Lang CJ, Schaller KH *et al.* Longitudinal study of neurotoxicity with occupational exposure to aluminum dust. *Neurology.* 2000; **54**: 997–1000.
48. Meyer-Baron M, Schaper M, Knapp G, van Thriel C. Occupational aluminum exposure: Evidence in support of its neurobehavioral impact. *Neurotoxicology.* 2007; **28**: 1068–78.
49. Martyn CN, Barker DJP, Osmond C *et al.* Geographical relation between Alzheimer disease and aluminium in drinking water. *Lancet.* 1989; **i**: 59–62.
50. Perl DP. Relationship of aluminium to Alzheimer disease. *Environmental Health Perspectives.* 1985; **63**: 149–53.
51. Crapper McLachlan DR, Lukiw WJ, Kruck TPA. New evidence for an active role of aluminium in Alzheimer disease. *Canadian Journal of Neurological Sciences.* 1989; **16**: 490–7.
52. Altmann P, Cunningham J, Dhanesha U *et al.* Disturbance of cerebral function in people exposed to drinking water contaminated with aluminium sulphate: Retrospective study of the Camelford water incident. *British Medical Journal.* 1999; **319**: 807–11.
53. Gourier-Fréry C, Fréry N, Berr C *et al.* Aluminium. Quels risques pour la santé? Synthèse des études épidémiologiques. Volet épidémiologique de l'expertise collective. In VS-Afssa-Afssaps. Saint-Maurice: Institut de Veille Sanitaire, June 2004.
54. World Health Organization. Food additives series: 58. World Health Organization, IPCS, International Programme on Chemical Safety evaluation of certain food additives and contaminants. Prepared by the Sixty-seventh meeting of the Joint FAO/WHO Expert Committee on Food Additives (JECFA). Geneva: WHO, 2007.
55. Committee on Toxicology. UK Committee on Toxicity of Chemicals in Food, Consumer Products and the Environment, Food Standards Agency. Subgroup report on the Lowermoor water pollution incident, consultation report, January 2005. Last accessed March 2008. Available from: www.advisorybodies.doh.gov.uk/cotnonfood/lsgreportjan05.pdf.

56. Becaria A, Campbell A, Bondy SC. Aluminum as a toxicant. *Toxicology and Industrial Health*. 2002; **18**: 309–20.
57. Molloy DW, Standish TI, Nieboer E *et al*. Effects of acute exposure to aluminum on cognition in humans. *Journal of Toxicology and Environmental Health. Part A*. 2007; **70**: 2011–19.
58. Rondeau V. A review of epidemiologic studies on aluminum and silica in relation to Alzheimer's disease and associated disorders. *Reviews on Environmental Health*. 2002; **17**: 107–21.
59. Cannata-Andia JB, Fernandez-Martin JL. The clinical impact of aluminium overload in renal failure. *Nephrology, Dialysis, Transplantation*. 2002; **17** (Suppl. 2): 9–12.
60. Malluche HH. Aluminium and bone disease in chronic renal failure. *Nephrology, Dialysis, Transplantation*. 2002; **17** (Suppl. 2): 21–4.
61. Hellstrom HO, Mjoberg B, Mallmin H, Michaelsson K. The aluminum content of bone increases with age, but is not higher in hip fracture cases with and without dementia compared to controls. *Osteoporosis International*. 2005; **16**: 1982–8.
62. Hellstrom HO, Mjoberg B, Mallmin H, Michaelsson K. No association between the aluminium content of trabecular bone and bone density, mass or size of the proximal femur in elderly men and women. *BMC Musculoskeletal Disorders*. 2006; **7**: 69.
63. International Agency for Research on Cancer. Monographs on the evaluation of the carcinogenic risks of chemicals to humans: 34. Polyaromatic compounds, Part 3 Industrial exposures in aluminium production, coal gasification, coke production and iron and steel founding. Lyon: IARC, 1984.
64. Romundstad P, Haldorsen T, Rennberg A. Exposure to PAH and fluoride in aluminium reduction plants in Norway. Historical estimation of exposure using process parameters and industrial hygiene measures. *American Journal of Industrial Medicine*. 1999; **35**: 164–74.
65. Gibbs GW, Armstrong B, Sevigny M. Mortality and cancer experience of Quebec aluminum reduction plant workers. Part 2: Mortality of three cohorts hired on or before January 1, 1951. *Journal of Occupational and Environmental Medicine*. 2007; **49**: 1105–23.
66. Moulin JJ, Clavel T, Buclez B, Laffitte-Rigaud G. A mortality study among workers in a French aluminium reduction plant. *International Archives of Occupational and Environmental Health*. 2000; **73**: 323–30.
67. Spinelli JJ, Demers PA, Le ND *et al*. Cancer risk in aluminum reduction plant workers (Canada). *Cancer Causes and Control*. 2006; **17**: 939–48.
68. Romundstad P, Haldorsen T, Andersen A. Lung and bladder cancer among workers in a Norwegian aluminium reduction plant. *Occupational and Environmental Medicine*. 2000; **57**: 495–9.
69. Veiren NK. Routine patch testing with aluminium trichloride. *Contact Dermatitis*. 1996; **35**: 126–33.
70. Akyol A, Boyvat A, Kundakci N. Contact sensitivity to aluminum. *International Journal of Dermatology*. 2004; **43**: 942–3.
71. Bergfors E, Bjorkelund C, Trollfors B. Nineteen cases of persistent pruritic nodules and contact allergy to aluminium after injection of commonly used aluminium-adsorbed vaccines. *European Journal of Pediatrics*. 2005; **164**: 691–7.
72. Rossbach B, Buchta M, Csanady GA *et al*. Biological monitoring of welders exposed to aluminium. *Toxicology Letters*. 2006; **162**: 239–45.
73. Deutsche Forschungsgemeinshaft. Biological exposure values for occupational toxicants and carcinogens. Critical data evaluation for BAT and EKA values, vol. 1. Weinheim: VCH, 1994.
74. Finnish Institute of Occupational Health. Biomonitoring of exposure to chemicals. Guidelines for specimen collection 2008. Last accessed March 2008. Available from: www.ttl.fi/NR/rdonlyres/71C9CA4C-D331-43A2-8BDE-96653D9F9C8C/0/BMGuideline20080101.pdf.

14

Antimony

MALCOLM R SIM

Antimony was previously one of a group of important occupational toxins, but is now largely of historical interest in the workplace setting. While this is true in most developed countries, where good workplace control has eliminated antimony as a major cause of disease, this is not necessarily the case in newly developing countries.

Antimony is a brittle, silver-white metalloid, usually obtained from the sulphide ore stibnite, which is mined in many counties worldwide. It is mixed into alloys and used in solder, sheet and pipe metal, motor bearings, castings, semiconductors and pewter, and is a byproduct of smelting lead and other metals. Antimony oxide is added to textiles, plastics, rubber, adhesives, pigments and paper to prevent them from catching fire. It is also used as a flame retardant for plastics, paints, textiles, paper, rubber and adhesives, in the form of the trioxide.

Antimony and its compounds have been found to cause several health effects in miners and other exposed workers, although these are less common now in the United Kingdom and other developed countries.[1] Such effects included irritation of mucous membranes, dermatitis (antimony spots), nose bleeds, gastrointestinal symptoms, bronchitis and a simple pneumoconiosis, characterized by fine nodular opacities close to the hilum with little effect on lung function. Antimony can also form another compound, stibine (SbH_3), which is known to cause a profound haemolytic anaemia, similar to that caused by arsine.

The International Agency for Research on Cancer (IARC) has concluded that antimony trioxide is possibly carcinogenic to humans (group 2B) on the basis of sufficient evidence in experimental animals and inadequate evidence of carcinogenicity in humans.[2] One problem with epidemiological studies of antimony-exposed workers is that the workers are often exposed to several other metals, such as arsenic, a known cause of cancer.[3] The American Conference of Governmental Industrial Hygienists (ACGIH) has set a threshold limit value (TLV) of 0.5 mg/m^3 and considers antimony to be a suspected human carcinogen.

Key points

- Antimony can cause respiratory effects such as irritation and a form of simple pneumoconiosis.
- Other effects include a type of dermatitis and gastrointestinal symptoms.
- In the form of stibine, antimony can cause a profound haemolytic anaemia.

REFERENCES

1. McCallum RI. Occupational exposure to antimony compounds. *Journal of Environmental Monitoring*. 2005; **7**: 1245–50.
2. International Agency for Research on Cancer Monographs on the Evaluation of Carcinogenic Risks to Humans. Some organic solvents, resin monomers and related compounds, pigments and occupational exposures in paint manufacture and painting, vol. 47. Lyon: IARC, 1989.
3. Jones SR, Atkin P, Holroyd C *et al*. Lung cancer mortality at a UK tin smelter. *Occupational Medicine*. 2007; **57**: 238–45.

15

Arsenic

MALCOLM R SIM

Arsenic is one of a group of previously important occupational toxins, but which is now largely of historical interest in the workplace setting. While this is true in most developed countries, where good workplace control has eliminated this group as a major cause of disease, this is not necessarily the case in newly developing countries. In addition, inorganic arsenic has become more important as a cause of disease in the environmental health setting, as its importance in the workplace has waned.

Arsenic is a metal which has been known since antiquity, but it differs from other ancient metals in that it was not extracted and used in its elemental form, but is used in compounds such as sulphides. It occurs as an impurity in the ores of other metals, such as copper, lead and zinc, and has been found in considerable quantities in some bronzes from archaeological sites. Arsenic can be found in industry in its inorganic or organic forms, but the inorganic forms have been the most important in terms of worker exposure and toxicity, especially the trivalent forms.

Most current inorganic arsenic exposure in the workplace occurs through the application of pesticides and herbicides, metal smelting, timber treatment and in the chemical and pesticide manufacturing industries. Another traditional use is in pigments such as Paris green (cupric acetoarsenite) and Scheele's green (cupric arsenite). In the middle of the nineteenth century, the use of these pigments was so common that chronic arsenical poisoning from their dusts was widespread.

Chronic, rather than acute, poisoning is the more common form of arsenic poisoning in the occupational setting and can affect many systems of the body, causing hyperpigmentation and hyperkeratosis in the skin, a sensorimotor peripheral neuropathy, megaloblastic anaemia, hepatotoxicity and liver cirrhosis. Many of these effects are caused by arsenic reacting with the thiol groups of proteins and enzymes and inhibiting their catalytic activity. While these non-malignant effects of inorganic arsenic exposure are becoming less common in developed countries, there is still concern over their impact in low to medium income countries.[1] There is no effective treatment for chronic arsenic poisoning, but removal from exposure can help to at least partially reverse some of these effects.

While the health impact of inorganic arsenic in the workplace setting is waning in many countries, arsenic has become a major cause of ill health throughout the world in many communities through contamination of drinking water. While such effects were first documented in Taiwan, in more recent times the country with the highest degree of exposure over a substantial proportion of its population is Bangladesh, where exposure occurs through drinking contaminated water from the millions of tube wells widely used in rural areas of the country. Elevated levels of arsenic in drinking water have also been documented in communities in many other countries across most continents, including India, Chile, Mongolia, Mexico and countries in Eastern Europe.[2] Arsenic in drinking water in Bangladesh has led to widespread health effects, such as arsenical keratosis and alterations in skin pigmentation in the exposed population,[3] and considerable public health concern has been raised for action to deal with this problem.[4] The contamination in Bangladesh groundwater has been thought to be naturally occurring, but recent evidence suggests that this may be contributed to by man-made ponds.[5]

Arsenic has a half-life in blood of approximately 60 hours and about 75 per cent of absorbed inorganic arsenic is excreted as methylated forms, which are less toxic than inorganic arsenic and so this *in vivo* methylation represents a true detoxification process. With normal renal function, the biological half-life of arsenic in the urine after exposure to inorganic arsenic is between one and two days. Therefore, urinary arsenic monitoring, preferably with a 24-hour sample and corrected for creatinine, is the most appropriate method for monitoring inorganic arsenic absorption in workers. Monitoring arsenic in serum, hair or nails is considered to be a less reliable method.

Arsenic has been considered by the International Agency for Research on Cancer (IARC) and has been classified as a definite (group 1) human carcinogen as there is sufficient scientific evidence to cause cancer of the lung, skin and bladder, with the mechanism thought to be via oxidative DNA damage.[6] Although cancer is currently the primary end point of interest and is usually used as the basis for setting occupational and environmental exposure limits, associations have been found between inorganic arsenic exposure and other important human diseases, such as diabetes[7] and adverse reproductive outcomes.[8]

The American Conference of Governmental Industrial Hygienists (ACGIH) has set the threshold limit value (TLV) for inorganic arsenic at 0.01 mg/m^3 and has set the biological exposure index (BEI) for inorganic arsenic and its methylated metabolites at 35 μg/L. For the latter, it is recommended that the urine sample be collected at the end of the working week.

Key points

- The main malignant effects from occupational exposure to arsenic are cancers of the lung, skin and bladder.
- Non-malignant health effects from workplace exposure are less common in developed countries, but are still a concern in low and medium income countries.
- Inorganic arsenic in drinking water is a major cause of hyperkeratosis and changes in pigmentation of the skin, and other ill effects in Bangladesh and other countries.

REFERENCES

1. Halatek T, Sinczuk-Walczak H, Rabieh S, Wasowicz W. Association between occupational exposure to arsenic and neurological, respiratory and renal effects. *Toxicology and Applied Pharmacology*. 2009; **239**: 193–9.
2. Nordstrom DK. Worldwide occurrence of arsenic in ground water. *Science*. 2002; **296**: 2143–5.
3. Tondel M, Rahman M, Magnuson A *et al*. The relationship of arsenic levels in drinking water and the prevalence rate of skin lesions in Bangladesh. *Environmental Health Perspectives*. 1999; **107**: 727–9.
4. Nickson R, McArthur J, Burgess W *et al*. Arsenic poisoning of Bangladesh groundwater. *Nature*. 1998; **395**: 338.
5. Neumann RB, Ashfaque KN, Badruzzaman ABM *et al*. Anthropogenic influences on groundwater arsenic concentrations in Bangladesh. *Nature Geoscience*. November 15, 2009. Available from: www.nature.com/ngeo/journal/vaop/ncurrent/abs/ngeo685.html.
6. Straif K, Benbrahim-Tallaa L, Baan R *et al*. A review of human carcinogens – part C: Metals, arsenic, dusts, and fibres. *Lancet Oncology*. 2009; **10**: 453–4.
7. Navas-Acien A, Silbergeld EK, Pastor-Barriuso R, Guallar E. Arsenic exposure and prevalence of type 2 diabetes in US adults. *Journal of the American Medical Association*. 2008; **300**: 814–22.
8. Rahman A, Vahter M, Smith AH *et al*. Arsenic exposure during pregnancy and size at birth: A prospective cohort study in Bangladesh. *American Journal of Epidemiology*. 2009; **169**: 304–12.

16

Beryllium

LEE S NEWMAN AND HOLLY M CHRISTENSEN

Chemical and physical properties	162	Biomarkers	163
Compounds and alloys	162	Health effects	164
Production and use	162	Prevention and treatment	164
Exposure and health effects	163	References	164

CHEMICAL AND PHYSICAL PROPERTIES

Beryllium has chemical and physical properties that make it desirable for high technology applications, but which unfortunately lead to pernicious use of this highly toxic metal. The fourth lightest element (atomic weight, 9.012), beryllium is corrosion resistant, non-sparking, non-magnetic, has a low density (1.85 g/cm^3), is heat resistant (melting point, 1278°C), and has high tensile strength and thermal conductivity. Beryllium differs chemically from other alkaline-earth metals, forming covalently bonded compounds rather than ionic.[1]

COMPOUNDS AND ALLOYS

Beryllium is found in industry in many different forms. Beryl and bertrandite ore are processed into beryllium hydroxide, which is used to produce beryllium metal, alloy and oxide. Chemical forms of beryllium include beryllium salts, sulphate, fluoride and chloride. Beryllium is most commonly alloyed with copper, aluminium and nickel.[2]

PRODUCTION AND USE

The United States is the leading producer of beryllium metals, alloys and oxide. The applications for beryllium and its alloys are widespread, including use in aerospace, the automotive industries, dental alloys, electronics, computers, nuclear weapons and telecommunications. Bertrandite is extracted via open-pit mining. The ore is leached with sulphuric acid to form beryllium sulphate, which is converted to basic beryllium carbonate by reaction with aqueous ammonium carbonate. Subsequent heating yields beryllium hydroxide, which is the basis for metal, alloy and oxide production.

Beryllium oxide is prepared by calcining beryllium hydroxide and has applications in the automotive, electronic and computer industries. As a ceramic, it is an excellent heat conductor and can be used as an electric insulator in automotive ignition systems, lasers, electronic circuits for computers, heat sinks and microwave oven components. Pure beryllium metal is used primarily in aerospace, nuclear and defence applications because of its stiffness, light weight and temperature stability. The metal is an integral part of nuclear reactor technology because it is an excellent neutron reflector and moderator. Beryllium is used in nuclear weapon triggering devices because it emits a large number of neutrons when bombarded with alpha radiation.

The most common alloy, beryllium-copper (up to 4 per cent beryllium), is obtained by fusing beryllium oxide with copper and has many desirable properties including strength, high electrical conductivity, high fatigue strength, wide temperature tolerance, high elasticity and corrosion resistance. Beryllium-copper alloys are useful in parts subject to abnormal wear or subject to extreme vibration, such as bearings, cams and gears. It is used in corrosion-resistant springs, electrical contacts, switches, relays and connectors in automobiles, computers and radar, satellite, and telecommunications equipment. Beryllium-aluminium alloy (<1–60 per cent beryllium) is used in high technology applications, such as aircraft, scientific devices on spacecraft, defence avionics packaging, high resolution medical and industrial x-ray equipment. Beryllium-nickel alloy (0.275–7 per cent beryllium) has high tensile strength and has age-hardening characteristics. It is used for diamond drill-bit matrices, watch balance wheels and airplane brakes.[3]

EXPOSURE AND HEALTH EFFECTS

Beryllium exposure assessment is focused on controlling exposure and preventing beryllium-related health effects in the workplace (see also Chapter 83, Berylliosis). Exposure to beryllium dust and fumes can cause an immune hypersensitivity reaction, dermatitis and lung diseases, including acute berylliosis, chronic beryllium disease and lung cancer. Most hazardous exposures to beryllium come from dust or fume generated by disturbing the surface of a beryllium product through machining and polishing processes. Health effects can result from exposures to beryllium metal dust, powdered and fired forms of beryllia ceramic, beryllium hydroxide, beryllium fume, and mists and dusts of soluble beryllium salts.

The dose and duration of beryllium exposure that causes adverse health effects is the subject of ongoing research. There is strong evidence, for example, that sensitization and chronic beryllium disease can occur at levels as low as $0.02\ \mu g/m^3$ lifetime weighted exposure.[4,5] Current governmental permissible exposure limits may not be sufficiently protective. Certain beryllium industrial processes and job tasks increase the risk of developing an immune response to beryllium and disease.[6–13] Even seemingly trivial and bystander exposures have caused beryllium sensitization and chronic beryllium disease.[7,8,12–22]

Because of these health effects, beryllium has been monitored in industry since the 1940s. In the United States, for example, the US Atomic Energy Commission (AEC) adopted the first beryllium permissible exposure limit (PEL). This limit was the basis for the US Occupational Safety and Health Administration (OSHA) permissible exposure limit for beryllium adopted in 1971. The limit is an eight-hour time-weighted average of $2\ \mu g/m^3$, a ceiling level of $5\ \mu g/m^3$ and a maximum peak concentration of $25\ \mu g/m^3$ for no more than 30 minutes per eight-hour workshift. The PEL is currently under review, upon recognition that cases of chronic beryllium disease (CBD) continue to occur at exposure levels 50–100 times lower than the PEL.

In the workplace, beryllium is measured using various sampling methods including area and stationary sampling, and personal breathing zone sampling. The latter is considered the preferred method. Whether particle size sampling should be performed is open to debate. It is known that the majority of beryllium particulate generated by most machining operations creates a high percentage of respirable-sized particles.

The major emission source of beryllium in the environment is from the combustion of coal and fuel oils and industrial processing of beryllium. The average concentration of beryllium in the general atmosphere in the United States is $0.03\ ng/m^3$. The median atmospheric concentration of beryllium in cities is $0.2\ ng/m^3$.[3] The ambient air standard in the United States was set at $0.01\ \mu g/m^3$ by the AEC in 1949.[23]

In the late 1940s, cases of CBD were diagnosed in residents living in the neighbourhood of a beryllium plant, in Lorain, Ohio. In an evaluation of beryllium in the community, almost all the cases resided within 0.25–0.75 miles (1.2 km) of the plant and had ambient exposures of $0.004–0.02\ \mu g/m^3$. Disease rates were comparable to rates found among beryllium plant workers. These studies helped form the basis for setting the beryllium community air standard at $0.01\ \mu g/m^3$ as a 30-day average.[24] Later, 21 community cases were reported in Reading, Pennsylvania, within 5.3 miles from a beryllium facility.[25] Eight additional cases in that same community were published recently by Maier and colleagues among individuals who never worked in the plant.[14]

BIOMARKERS

Biomarkers for beryllium include exposure, disease susceptibility, effect and disease progression. The most useful biomarkers for disease are found in the blood and lung.[26]

The most widely used beryllium biomarker is the blood beryllium lymphocyte proliferation test (BeLPT), which is commonly used to determine beryllium sensitivity. High in sensitivity, specificity and both negative and positive predictive value, beryllium-reactive blood lymphocytes proliferate when presented with beryllium antigen. The BeLPT is widely used in industry as part of workplace medical screening and surveillance. To a much lesser extent, the BeLPT can be considered a biomarker of exposure. If the test is abnormal, it is indicative of past exposure to beryllium since it is a prerequisite for this immune response. However, a negative test does not rule out past exposure.[7,8,21,27–31] Serum neopterin levels in the blood have been found to be higher in patients with CBD compared to those who are sensitized, suggesting that it may discriminate between sensitization and disease.[32,33] The most promising new test of immune response to beryllium is the beryllium ELISPOT assay which measures beryllium-stimulated T-cell production of the cytokine gamma interferon. Class II MHC HLA-DP and -DR gene variants are blood biomarkers of CBD susceptibility, but are not recommended for screening workers because of their low positive predictive value and ethical considerations. Although a high percentage of beryllium-sensitized and CBD patients carry these genes, the genes are also common in the general population.[3,23] Blood biomarkers of disease progression include markers of inflammation, such as cytokines.

Bronchoalveolar lavage (BAL) fluid obtained from the lung during bronchoscopy is used to distinguish between beryllium sensitization and CBD. The lung cells of CBD patients proliferate in response to beryllium indicating lung-specific sensitization, measured by the BeLPT using lung cells instead of blood. BAL white blood cell count and lymphocytosis in CBD patients correlate with pulmonary gas exchange and reflect disease severity.[34]

HEALTH EFFECTS

Beryllium and its alloys have a high toxic potential, predominantly targeting the lung, lymph nodes and skin, either by direct toxicity and/or its impact on the immune system. Skin lesions, including granuloma formation and ulceration, occur following direct injection of beryllium into the skin. Cutaneous contact with beryllium salts can induce contact dermatitis.

The primary route of exposure in beryllium-related respiratory diseases is through inhalation of fumes and respirable dusts of beryllium salts, metal or oxides, or beryllium alloys.[35] Exposure to high concentrations of beryllium, usually in the $25\,\mu g/m^3$ range or greater, can result in acute inflammation of the upper and lower respiratory tract and airways, tracheitis, bronchiolitis, pulmonary oedema and chemical pneumonitis.[36–38] Dermal exposure is thought to contribute to sensitization risk.

Once inhaled, beryllium particles obey general principles of particle disposition in the lung.[39,40] The chemical properties of the inhaled beryllium particle may also influence its toxicity. The solubility and the form of beryllium inhaled influence the development of an immune response and chronic disease.[41–44] Workers exposed to beryllium may develop an immune-mediated, antigen-driven immune response to beryllium without the pathologic or clinical features of CBD. These individuals are asymptomatic and have normal pulmonary function, exercise tolerance, chest radiographs, BAL and lung biopsies. The majority of those beryllium sensitized eventually develop CBD.[19,45] CBD can develop many years after exposure has ceased and typically has an indolent course and insidious onset of symptoms, including fatigue, non-productive cough, shortness of breath and chest pain. Also common is anorexia, weight loss, fevers, night sweats and arthralgia.

The International Agency for Research on Cancer classifies beryllium as a class I human carcinogen.[46,47] A preponderance of data support beryllium as a human carcinogen, especially in individuals with beryllium-related lung disease.[24,25,48–50]

PREVENTION AND TREATMENT

Primary prevention, including removal from exposure, is superior to medical treatment of CBD. Unfortunately, there is no known cure for CBD. The goals of treatment are to inhibit inflammation and slow disease progression using oral glucocorticoids as the first-line therapy. Those with more severe disease may require additional supportive measures and use of other immunosuppressive pharmaceuticals.

Key points

- Broader use of beryllium in modern industry has created an increasing public health problem globally, affecting 1–15 per cent of exposed workers.
- Chronic and acute forms of berylliosis continue to occur as a result of immunologic recognition of beryllium antigen.
- Beryllium sensitization and chronic beryllium disease can be detected in workplace surveillance programmes and can be distinguished from other granulomatous disorders using the beryllium lymphocyte proliferation test.
- Chronic beryllium disease is a latent disorder preferentially affecting the lungs and immune system, as well as other organs.
- Exposure to beryllium at levels below current permissible exposure limits results in disease, necessitating strict attention to ventilation, use of personal protective equipment, administrative controls, exposure monitoring and substitution of beryllium with safer materials whenever possible.

REFERENCES

1. Environmental Protection Agency. Toxicological review of beryllium and compounds. In: Support of summary information on the integrated risk information system (IRIS). Washington DC: EPA, 1998.
2. US Geological Survey. Mineral commodities summaries. Washington DC: USGS, 2008.
3. Agency for Toxic Substances and Disease Registry. Toxicology profile for beryllium. Atlanta, GA: ATSDR, 2002.
4. Kelleher PC, Martyny JW, Mroz MM et al. Beryllium particulate exposure and disease relations in a beryllium machining plant. *Journal of Occupational and Environmental Medicine*. 2001; **43**: 238–49.
5. Henneberger PK, Cumro D, Deubner DD et al. Beryllium sensitization and disease among long-term and short-term workers in a beryllium ceramics plant. *International Archives of Occupational and Environmental Health*. 2001; **74**: 167–76.
6. Kreiss K, Mroz MM, Zhen B et al. Epidemiology of beryllium sensitization and disease in nuclear workers. *American Review of Respiratory Disease*. 1993; **148**: 985–91.

7. Kreiss K, Wasserman S, Mroz MM, Newman LS. Beryllium disease screening in the ceramics industry. Blood lymphocyte test performance and exposure-disease relations. *Journal of Occupational Medicine*. 1993; **35**: 267-74.
8. Kreiss K, Mroz MM, Zhen B et al. Risks of beryllium disease related to work processes at a metal, alloy, and oxide production plant. *Occupational and Environmental Medicine*. 1997; **54**: 605-12.
9. Schuler CR, Kent MS, Deubner DC et al. Process-related risk of beryllium sensitization and disease in a copper-beryllium alloy facility. *American Journal of Industrial Medicine*. 2005; **47**: 195-205.
10. Stange AW, Hilmas DE, Furman FJ, Gatliffe TR. Beryllium sensitization and chronic beryllium disease at a former nuclear weapons facility. *Applied Occupational and Environmental Hygiene*. 2001; **16**: 405-17.
11. Welch L, Ringen K, Bingham E et al. Screening for beryllium disease among construction trade workers at Department of Energy nuclear sites. *American Journal of Industrial Medicine*. 2004; **46**: 207-18.
12. Newman LS, Mroz MM, Maier LA et al. Efficacy of serial medical surveillance for chronic beryllium disease in a beryllium machining plant. *Journal of Occupational and Environmental Medicine*. 2001; **43**: 231-7.
13. Rodrigues EG, McClean MD, Weinberg J, Pepper LD. Beryllium sensitization and lung function among former workers at the Nevada Test Site. *American Journal of Industrial Medicine*. 2008; **51**: 512-23.
14. Maier LA, Martyny JW, Liang J, Rossman MD. Recent chronic beryllium disease in residents surrounding a beryllium facility. *American Journal of Respiratory and Critical Care Medicine*. 2008; **177**: 1012-17.
15. Infante PF, Newman LS. Beryllium exposure and chronic beryllium disease. *Lancet*. 2004; **363**: 415-16.
16. Sackett HM, Maier LA, Silveira LJ et al. Beryllium medical surveillance at a former nuclear weapons facility during cleanup operations. *Journal of Occupational and Environmental Medicine*. 2004; **46**: 953-61E.
17. Eisenbud M, Lisson J. Epidemiologic aspects of beryllium-induced non-malignant lung disease. *Journal of Occupational Medicine*. 1983; **25**: 196-202.
18. Newman LS, Lloyd J, Daniloff E. The natural history of beryllium sensitization and chronic beryllium disease. *Environmental Health Perspectives*. 1996; **104** (Suppl. 5): 937-43.
19. Newman LS. Immunology, genetics, and epidemiology of beryllium disease. *Chest*. 1996; **109** (Suppl. 3): 40S-43S.
20. Newman LS. Significance of the blood beryllium lymphocyte proliferation test. *Environmental Health Perspectives*. 1996; **104** (Suppl. 5): 953-6.
21. Occupational Safety and Health Administration. Final rule air contaminants permissible exposure limits. Washington DC: OSHA, 1989.
22. Newman LS. Beryllium biomarkers: Application of immunologic, inflammatory, and genetic tools. In: Mendelsohn LC, Peeters JP (eds). *Biomarkers: Medical and workplace applications*. Washington DC: Joseph Henry Press, 1998: 285-300.
23. Hanifin JM, Epstein WL, Cline MJ. *In vitro* studies on granulomatous hypersensitivity to beryllium. *Journal of Investigative Dermatology*. 1970; **55**: 284-8.
24. Eisenbud M, Wanta RC, Dustan C et al. Non-occupational berylliosis. *Journal of Industrial Hygiene and Toxicology*. 1949; **31**: 282-94.
25. Lieben J, Metzner F. Epidemiological findings associated with beryllium extraction. *American Industrial Hygiene Association Journal*. 1959; **20**: 494-9.
26. Kreiss K, Newman LS, Mroz MM, Campbell PA. Screening blood test identifies subclinical beryllium disease. *Journal of Occupational Medicine*. 1989; **31**: 603-8.
27. Mroz MM, Kreiss K, Lezotte DC et al. Reexamination of the blood lymphocyte transformation test in the diagnosis of chronic beryllium disease. *Journal of Allergy and Clinical Immunology*. 1991; **88**: 54-60.
28. Stange AW, Furman FJ, Hilmas DE. The beryllium lymphocyte proliferation test: Relevant issues in beryllium health surveillance. *American Journal of Industrial Medicine*. 2004; **46**: 453-62.
29. Deubner DC, Goodman M, Iannuzzi J. Variability, predictive value, and uses of the beryllium blood lymphocyte proliferation test (BLPT): Preliminary analysis of the ongoing workforce survey. *Applied Occupational and Environmental Hygiene*. 2001; **16**: 521-6.
30. Harris J, Bartelson BB, Barker E et al. Serum neopterin in chronic beryllium disease. *American Journal of Industrial Medicine*. 1997; **32**: 21-6.
31. Maier LA, Kittle LA, Mroz MM, Newman LS. Beryllium-stimulated neopterin as a diagnostic adjunct in chronic beryllium disease. *American Journal of Industrial Medicine*. 2003; **43**: 592-601.
32. Newman LS, Bobka C, Schumacher B et al. Compartmentalized immune response reflects clinical severity of beryllium disease. *American Journal of Respiratory and Critical Care Medicine*. 1994; **150**: 135-42.
33. Balkissoon RC, Newman LS. Beryllium copper alloy (2 per cent) causes chronic beryllium disease. *Journal of Occupational and Environmental Medicine*. 1999; **41**: 304-8.
34. Kim Y. Acute beryllium disease in metal workers. *European Respiratory Journal*. 2004; **24**: 149S.
35. Hardy HL. Beryllium poisoning - lessons in control of man-made disease. *New England Journal of Medicine*. 1965; **273**: 1188-99.
36. Finkel AJ, Hamilton A, Hardy HL. *Hamilton and Hardy's Industrial toxicology*, 4th edn. Boston, MA: John Wright, 1983.
37. Martyny JW, Hoover MD, Mroz MM et al. Aerosols generated during beryllium machining. *Journal of Occupational and Environmental Medicine*. 2000; **42**: 8-18.
38. Stefaniak AB, Hoover MD, Dickerson RM et al. Surface area of respirable beryllium metal, oxide, and copper alloy aerosols and implications for assessment of exposure risk of chronic beryllium disease. *AIHA J*. 2003; **64**: 297-305.

39. Kent MS, Robins TG, Madl AK. Is total mass or mass of alveolar-deposited airborne particles of beryllium a better predictor of the prevalence of disease? A preliminary study of a beryllium processing facility. *Applied Occupational and Environmental Hygiene.* 2001; **16**: 539-58.
40. Reeves AL, Preuss OP. The immunotoxicity of beryllium. In: Dean JH, Luster MI, Munson AE (eds). *Immunotoxicology and immunopharmacology.* New York: Raven Press, 1985: 441-55.
41. McCawley MA, Kent MS, Berakis MT. Ultrafine beryllium number concentration as a possible metric for chronic beryllium disease risk. *Applied Occupational and Environmental Hygiene.* 2001; 16: 631-8.
42. Stefaniak AB, Day GA, Hoover MD *et al.* Differences in dissolution behavior in a phagolysosomal stimulant fluid for single-constituent and multi-constituent materials associated with beryllium sensitization and chronic beryllium disease. *Toxicology In Vitro.* 2006; **20**: 82-95.
43. Newman LS, Mroz MM, Balkissoon R, Maier LA. Beryllium sensitization progresses to chronic beryllium disease: A longitudinal study of disease risk. *American Journal of Respiratory and Critical Care Medicine.* 2005; **171**: 54-60.
44. International Agency for Research on Cancer. Monographs on the evaluation of the carcinogenic risk of chemicals to humans. Lyon: IARC, 1980.
45. International Agency for Research on Cancer. Meeting on the IARC working group on beryllium, cadmium, mecury, and exposures of the glass manufacturing industry. *Scandinavian Journal of Work, Environment and Health.* 1993; **19**: 360-3.
46. Mancuso TF. Occupational lung cancer among beryllium workers. In: Lemen R, Dement J (eds). *Dust and diseases.* Forest Park: Pathatox, 1979.
47. Mancuso TF. Mortality study of beryllium industry workers' occupational lung cancer. *Environmental Research.* 1980; **21**: 48-55.
48. Mancuso TF, el-Attar AA. Epidemiological study of the beryllium industry. Cohort methodology and mortality studies. *Journal of Occupational Medicine.* 1969; **11**: 422-34.
49. Infante PF, Wagoner JK, Sprince NL. Mortality patterns from lung cancer and nonneoplastic respiratory disease among white males in the beryllium case registry. *Environmental Research.* 1980; **21**: 35-43.
50. Wagoner JK, Infante PF, Bayliss DL. Beryllium: An etiologic agent in the induction of lung cancer, nonneoplastic respiratory disease, and heart disease among industrially exposed workers. *Environmental Research.* 1980; **21**: 15-34.

17

Cadmium

PERRINE HOET

Introduction	167	Health surveillance of cadmium workers	170
Metabolism	167	References	171
Toxicity	168		

INTRODUCTION

Cadmium (Cd) is one of the 'newer' metals, having been isolated by Strohmeyer in 1817. It occurs in nature mainly with zinc. It is recovered as a byproduct during the smelting of zinc and some lead ores. Primary cadmium metal production has continued to decrease from its highest levels in 1997, which roughly corresponds to the peak in worldwide NiCd battery production. Reductions in primary cadmium metal production have occurred mainly in Europe where many of the zinc/cadmium producers have shut down their cadmium refineries and now dispose of the cadmium-containing material from their zinc smelting process as hazardous waste. Asia and the Americas, on the other hand, have increased their cadmium primary production capacity from previous years, especially in Korea.[1]

Cadmium and cadmium compounds are utilized in five major product areas which include NiCd batteries (about 80 per cent of its use), pigments, stabilizers, coatings, and minor uses which include specialized alloys and electronic compounds. The major classes of products where cadmium is present as an impurity are non-ferrous metals (zinc, lead and copper), iron and steel, fossil fuels (coal, oil, gas, peat and wood), cement and phosphate fertilizers.[1]

In occupational settings, workers may be exposed to Cd through the inhalation of oxide fumes generated during heating or welding of Cd-containing materials, or inhalation of particles of metal, oxide and pigment dust.

The major non-occupational route of cadmium intake for non-smokers is ingestion through food or water. This is largely due to the presence of trace amounts of cadmium in foodstuffs of natural origin or to the use of phosphate fertilizers or sludge on agricultural soils. Smoking typically doubles the daily absorption of Cd by inhalation of cadmium oxide fumes.

METABOLISM

Cadmium is poorly absorbed from the gut ($<$5 per cent); its bioavailability is, however, dependent on the composition of the diet (low Ca, Fe, Zn and protein contents tend to increase Cd absorption) and the source of Cd (soil and seafood Cd are less absorbed than ionic Cd; rice-associated Cd appears to be more absorbed than that of other sources). In individuals with depleted iron stores, bioavailability could increase up to 5–10 per cent (mainly in women). Absorption rate after inhalation ranges from 10 to 50 per cent, depending on the particle size and solubility.[2]

In blood, about 70–90 per cent of Cd is bound in the red cells; in plasma, Cd is predominantly bound to proteins of high molecular weight (albumin or larger). In tissues, cadmium is largely bound to metallothionein which is a zinc storage protein containing between 30 and 35 per cent of cysteine. The high proportion of sulphur-containing amino acids enables it to bind heavy metals, each molecule being able to bind seven divalent cations, usually zinc or copper, but also cadmium, mercury and a number of other metals. Its synthesis is induced by the presence of zinc, cadmium, copper and mercury.

Cadmium has a long biological half-life (about 10–20 years) and with continued exposure, it accumulates with age. The body burden in smokers is higher than in non-smokers.

After long-term low-level exposure, about half the body burden of cadmium is localized in the kidneys and liver, a third of the total being in the kidneys mainly in the renal cortex. At higher levels of exposure, a greater proportion of the body burden is found in the liver. The ratio between the cadmium concentration in the kidney and that in the liver decreases with the intensity of exposure. Cadmium is excreted in the urine, largely as a cadmium–metallothionein complex, but the rate of excretion is low (hence the long biological half-life) unless there is concomitant kidney damage. Small amounts of cadmium may also appear in the bile, saliva, hair and nails.[2–4]

TOXICITY

Respiratory manifestations

Acute effects may be noted after the inhalation of cadmium oxide fumes which are generated from welding or brazing on cadmium or its alloys. Because of its low boiling point (765°C) by comparison to other metals such as zinc, Cd fumes are generated in potentially toxic concentrations in Cd alloy production and welding, during oxyacetylene cutting of Cd-coated steel and rivets and in the smelting, melting and refining of metals that contain Cd. There is generally a lag period of up to ten hours after the inhalation of the fumes before any untoward effects become apparent. The patient then notices retrosternal pain, dyspnoea and cough. With heavy exposure, pulmonary oedema may develop after one or two days. The first stage is very similar to 'metal fume fever' (see Chapter 44, Welding), but it is essential not to confuse both conditions, since the lung effects from Cd exposure can include delayed pulmonary oedema and possibly death. Subjects who survive acute cadmium poisoning may recover without damage, although some authors have reported delayed development of lung impairment.[2]

Long-term occupational exposure has been reported in earlier studies to cause emphysema and dyspnoea. Other studies, however, have not shown a cadmium-related impaired respiratory function.[2,5] Lung function tests, which have sometimes been reported to be abnormal in cadmium workers, do not seem to show any dose–response relationship and are certainly not as sensitive indicators of cadmium damage as the excretion of tubular proteins (see under Kidney manifestations).[6]

Anosmia was also noted to be a common finding in early reports. More recent investigations observed olfactory disorders in workers exposed to cadmium levels much lower than those reported in the past. A statistically significant correlation was found between olfactory dysfunction and cadmium concentrations in the blood and urine, but not between olfactory dysfunction and the duration of exposure. It was postulated that the action of the metal was due to an elective tropism for the olfactory epithelium and not to a non-specific irritant effect on the nasal cavity. These effects occurred in the absence of renal toxicity. Primary olfactory neurons may therefore represent early targets for cadmium toxic action. It seems most likely that cigarette smoking, which is a considerable source of cadmium, can intensify this dysfunction.[7–9]

Kidney manifestations

The kidney is generally considered to be the principal target organ affected by chronic exposure to Cd. An early sign of cadmium poisoning is tubular proteinuria. The increased excretion of low molecular weight (LMW) proteins (such as retinol binding protein (RBP), β2-microglobulin (β2-MG), α1-microglobulin (α1-MG) (or protein HC) or a urinary enzyme leakage such as N-acetyl-β-D-glucosaminidase (NAG)) is particularly characteristic of this tubular toxicity. The proteinuria may be accompanied by other evidence of tubular damage, such as calciuria, aminoaciduria, glycosuria and phosphaturia. Hypercalciuria might be responsible for the increased incidence of renal stones reported in some cadmium-exposed workers.[2,4,10–12]

Less commonly, an increased urinary excretion of high molecular weight (HMW) proteins (albumin, immunoglobulin G or transferrin) can occur indicating an effect of Cd on the glomerulus which can develop with or without tubular LMW proteinuria.[2]

Many other parameters have been investigated and suggested as early biomarkers of Cd nephrotoxicity (e.g. enzymes (intestinal alkaline phosphatase, alanine aminopeptidase, lactate dehydrogenase, glutathione-S-transferase), other proteins (Tamm–Horsfall glycoprotein, cystatin C, Clara cell protein, kidney injury molecule-1), extracellular matrix components (laminin, fibronectin, proteoglycans), tubular antigens or serum antibodies, eicosanoids, thromboxane B_2, kallikrein activity, sialic acid, glycosaminoglycans, cytokines). Changes in renal biomarkers of unknown health significance and predictive value can occur at very low levels; the health significance of most of these biomarkers and their predictive value for the development of end-stage renal failure are largely unknown.

Cadmium-induced LMW proteinuria is presently the only renal effect of Cd with documented health risk significance. The critical concentration of cadmium in the renal cortex associated with increased incidence of LMW proteinuria is estimated to be about 200 ppm, equivalent to a urinary Cd excretion of about 10 μg Cd/g creatinine. When the concentration of Cd in urine exceeds 10 μg/g creatinine, the risk of developing tubular proteinuria is well established. This risk increases almost linearly with the urinary Cd concentration from an expected prevalence of tubular proteinuria around 10 per cent for CdU (cadmium in urine) values slightly above 10 μg/g creatinine to more than 20 per cent when CdU values exceed 20 μg/g creatinine.[13] This threshold has been considered as clinically relevant because several studies have indicated that ongoing overexposure with CdU >10 μg/g creatinine may lead to irreversible renal damage, an exacerbation of the age-related decline in the glomerular filtration rate and a decrease in the filtration reserve capacity.[2] Cd-induced microproteinuria is often considered as irreversible, except at the incipient stage of the intoxication where a partial or complete reversibility has been found in some studies. In some studies on exposed workers, microproteinuria was reversible when reduction or cessation of exposure occurred, while tubular damage was still mild (β2-MG <1500 μg/g creatinine) and CdU had never exceeded 20 μg Cd/g creatinine.[14]

Although the concept of a critical concentration refers to the total amount of cadmium in the renal cortex, it is only the small amount of the metal not bound to metallothionein that is capable of causing nephrotoxicity. It has been suggested that the concentration of free cadmium which will produce β2-microglobulinuria is 2 ppm or 1 per cent of the critical concentration of the total cadmium concentration in the kidney. There is some evidence that factors, such as the capacity to synthesize metallothionein and ageing, may decrease the critical concentration of cadmium which is associated with the development of tubular damage. Workers that have higher plasma metallothionein antibody levels might more readily develop cadmium-induced renal dysfunction.[15,16]

Bone manifestations

High cadmium exposure is known to cause bone damage. 'Itai-itai disease' was the name given to an outbreak of osteomalacia found in postmenopausal multiparous women in Japan. The women in whom the condition was first noted lived in an area where crops had become contaminated with cadmium from water that had drained through an old zinc mine and had been used for irrigation. The women had pains in the back and legs (itai-itai literally means 'ouch-ouch') and some developed pathological fractures. Vitamin D and other nutritional deficiencies are thought to be cofactors in the aetiology of itai-itai disease. The metabolic changes in cadmium-induced osteomalacia have been described by Stanbury and Mawer.[17]

Environmental exposure to cadmium has been associated with an increased loss of bone mineral density in both sexes, leading to osteoporosis and increased risk of fractures, especially in the elderly and in females.[2,18–24] Data on workers are scant, although there is some evidence supporting the existence of an association between cadmium at low exposure level and alterations in the vitamin D metabolic pathway[25] or bone mineral density.[26] However, more supporting evidence on this relationhip is required.

Whether disturbances in the calcium balance and the effects on the skeleton are mediated directly on bone or are secondary to kidney damage is still unclear. Several mechanisms have been postulated. A direct effect of cadmium on bone metabolism (with impairment of bone formation and/or increased bone resorption) and loss of bone calcium is a first possibility. The second putative mechanism includes several factors resulting from kidney damage. Increased calciuria, caused by cadmium-induced tubular damage is a possibility. Moreover, kidney damage may cause other changes capable of disturbing bone metabolism: loss of phosphate, reduced hydroxylation of 25-OH-vitamin D, and acidosis. The increase in parathyroid hormone secretion secondary to kidney damage may further aggravate bone disease.[2,27–29]

Other manifestations

Cadmium exposure has been linked to lung and prostate cancer in humans. In 1993, a Working Group of the International Agency for Research on Cancer[30] concluded that there was sufficient evidence in humans for the carcinogenicity of cadmium and cadmium compounds on the lung. More recent studies have indicated the importance of confounding exposures, such as arsenic, and do not support the hypothesis that cadmium compounds are human lung carcinogens.[2,31–33] The association between cadmium exposure and prostate cancer was not confirmed in more recent reviews.[33,34] A recent meta-analysis indicated that exposure to cadmium appears to be associated with renal cancer, but this conclusion is tempered by the inability of studies to assess cumulative cadmium exposure from all sources including smoking and diet.[35]

Cadmium does not appear to be directly genotoxic. Indirect effects of cadmium are mediated by the generation of reactive oxygen species (ROS). Cadmium also modulates gene expression and signal transduction and reduces activities of proteins involved in antioxidant defences. Several studies have shown that it interferes with DNA repair.[36–40]

It has been suggested that cadmium in the environment may be involved in the aetiology of hypertension.[41] In experimental animals, exposure to cadmium modifies a number of mechanisms that regulate cardiovascular function, but there are some important differences between species.[42] In epidemiological studies, cadmium workers do not have an increased prevalence of hypertension. The role of cadmium in the aetiology of hypertension in those who are exposed to it only in the general environment is uncertain.

Neurobehavioural disturbances have been dose-dependently associated with CdU in cadmium-exposed workers. The possibility of a promoting role by increased cadmium body burden in the development of peripheral neuropathy in the elderly has been raised.[43,44] At present, this remains speculative.

Yellowing of the teeth has been associated with long-term ingestion and/or inhalation of cadmium.[45,46] However, studies reporting these effects are subject to a number of uncertainties, including the measurements of cadmium exposure, the magnitude of confounding by other toxicants and the evaluation of the effect.

Although cadmium can accumulate in the liver, inhalation of Cd fumes does not appear to have significant effects on the liver. Liver damage is not a prominent feature of chronic cadmium poisoning.

HEALTH SURVEILLANCE OF CADMIUM WORKERS

Biological monitoring of cadmium workers is necessary to prevent excessive uptake leading to renal damage.[3,47] The interrelationships between cadmium exposure and cadmium concentration in blood and urine are complex and reflect the accumulation of cadmium in liver and kidney over considerable periods of time. The maximum value of CdB (blood cadmium), which is about twice as high in smokers than non-smokers, is generally below 3 μg/L in European subjects not occupationally exposed to cadmium. In workers, after the start of exposure Cd concentration in blood increases linearly then levels off when an equilibrium is reached. Blood Cd is a useful indicator of recent exposure. After long-term high Cd exposure, an increasing proportion of blood Cd will be related to body burden. After cessation of exposure, CdB may reflect the body burden and the decrease of CdB displays an initial fast component with a half-life of three to four months and a slow component with a half-life of about ten years.[2,3,14,40,48,49]

In subjects with no occupational or environmental exposure, concentrations of Cd in urine are normally below 1–2 μg/g creatinine. The urinary excretion of Cd is influenced by smoking habits, but not to the same extent as blood Cd levels. At low exposure levels (general environmental exposure), the amount of Cd absorbed may be insufficient to saturate all the body binding sites (e.g. induced metallothionein). Urinary excretion increases in proportion to the amount of Cd stored in the body and not proportionally to the exposure levels. In such circumstances, there is a significant correlation between urinary Cd and Cd in kidney. In high exposure conditions, the Cd binding sites become progressively saturated and any further absorption of cadmium cannot be retained in the kidney: it is rapidly excreted in the urine. In these situations, the urinary Cd concentration would be a better reflection of current exposure levels. The relative influence of the body burden and recent exposure on CdU depends on the exposure intensity. If exposure continues and kidney damage occurs, urinary Cd excretion is increased even more. Eventually, the amount of Cd that can be released from the kidney decreases progressively and the urinary Cd concentration follows the same trend. In newly exposed subjects, a latent period may thus be observed before Cd in urine correlates with exposure.[2,3]

In workers, the critical CdU level (based on LMW microproteinuria) is around 10 μg/g creatinine. However, for several reasons, including the long biological half-life of Cd, the possible interaction with other causes of renal dysfunction (e.g. diabetes) and the fact that no treatment to remove Cd from its storage sites is presently available, it seems prudent to recommend that occupational exposure to Cd does not result in CdU levels exceeding 5 μg Cd/g creatinine[3,4,50] or possibly even as stringent as 2 μg Cd/g creatinine.[3]

The assessment of renal function relies on the measurement of the excretion of both LMW and HMW proteins. Increased excretion of LMW proteins indicates tubular damage and failure of reabsorption, whereas excretion of HMW proteins, such as albumin, reflects glomerular damage. Measurement of urinary β2-MG has been widely used as an indicator of tubular function. This protein is, however, degraded rapidly in the bladder when urinary pH is less than 5.5. RBP is stable at all urinary pH values and is therefore a more suitable indicator for tubular function (see Chapter 5, Biological monitoring). Protein HC and NAG are other biomarkers of Cd-induced subclinical tubular dysfunction.[2] The levels of plasma metallothionein antibody have been suggested as a biomarker of susceptibility to renal dysfunction in occupational cadmium exposure.[15]

The following guidelines for interpreting CdU, β2-MG and RBP measurements in workers exposed to Cd have been recommended:[13]

- CdU between 2 and 5 μg/g creatinine: sign of an increased body burden. Exceptionally, such levels can also be found in heavy smokers. At this stage, periodic screening for tubular dysfunction is usually not recommended.
- CdU between 5 and 10 μg/g creatinine: risk of developing tubular proteinuria remains unlikely, except perhaps in particularly vulnerable subjects or in subjects who have been exposed in the past and progressively lose their body burden of Cd. Screening for tubular proteinuria is recommended in subjects who persistently show an urinary Cd above 5 μg/g creatinine.
- CdU exceeding 10 μg/g creatinine: risk of developing tubular proteinuria well established.

A persistent increase of urinary LMW proteins over intervals of months or years may be a sign of irreversible degenerative changes likely to compromise renal function. Several stages can be identified from incipient tubular damage to overt nephropathy with decreased renal function (adapted from Ref. 13):

- <300 μg/g creatinine: normal;
- 300–1000 μg/g creatinine: incipient cadmium tubular damage with a possibility of reversibility after removal from exposure. No change in GFR (glomerular filtration rate);
- 1000–10 000 μg/g creatinine: irreversible tubular proteinuria which may lead to accelerated decline in GFR with age.
- >10 000 μg/g creatinine: overt cadmium nephropathy usually associated with decreased GFR.

There is presently insufficient evidence to support periodic surveillance for bone effects.

It is possible to measure cadmium concentrations in liver and kidney *in vivo* using neutron activation analysis. This technique is non-invasive, produces negligible amounts of radiation and uses transportable equipment. However, it is presently a research tool, and not recommended for periodic assessment of exposed individuals.[51,52]

Key points

- Cadmium (Cd) has no beneficial function in humans and is toxic at low dose.
- Cd accumulates in the body, in particular in the liver and kidneys, and has a very long biological half-life. Smokers have a higher body burden than non-smokers.
- Acute cadmium oxide inhalation exposure occurs rarely, but may result in metal fume fever and pulmonary oedema, a much more severe condition.
- Long-term exposure to Cd affects primarily the kidney, especially the proximal tubules resulting in a Fanconi-like syndrome, and the skeletal system leading to bone demineralization.
- Regulatory bodies have concluded that there is sufficient evidence to classify Cd as a human carcinogen. However, the possible confounding by concomitant exposure to arsenic has been evoked.

REFERENCES

1. International Cadmium Association website. Last accessed March 2008. Available from: www.cadmium.org.
2. European Chemicals Bureau. European risk assessment: Cadmium and cadmium oxide, 2003. Available from: http://ecb.jrc.it/.
3. Lauwerys R, Hoet P. *Industrial chemical exposure. Guidelines for biological monitoring*, 3rd edn. Boca Raton: Lewis, 2001: 54-69.
4. Friberg L, Elinder C, Kyellstrom T. *Cadmium and health: Toxological and epidemiological appraisal*, vol. I. Boca Raton: CRC Press, 1986.
5. Parkes WR. *Occupational lung disorders*, 3rd edn. London: Heinemann, 1994.
6. Edling C, Elinder CG, Randma E. Lung function in workers using cadmium containing solders. *British Journal of Industrial Medicine*. 1986; **43**: 657-68.
7. Mascagni P, Consonni D, Bregante G *et al*. Olfactory function in workers exposed to moderate airborne cadmium levels. *Neurotoxicology*. 2003; **24**: 717-24.
8. Rydzewski B, Sulkowski W, Miarzynska M. Olfactory disorders induced by cadmium exposure: A clinical study. *International Journal of Occupational Medicine and Environmental Health*. 1998; **11**: 235-45.
9. Sulkowski WJ, Rydzewski B, Miarzynska M. Smell impairment in workers occupationally exposed to cadmium. *Acta Otolaryngologica*. 2000; **120**: 316-18.
10. Kawada T, Koyama H, Suzuki S. Cadmium, NAG activity, and β_2-microglobulin in the urine of cadmium pigment workers. *British Journal of Industrial Medicine*. 1989; **46**: 52-5.
11. Lauwerys R, Bernard AM. Cadmium and the kidney. *British Journal of Industrial Medicine*. 1986; **43**: 433-5.
12. Jarup L. Cadmium overload and toxicity. *Nephrology, Dialysis, Transplantation*. 2002; **17** (Suppl. 2): 35-9.
13. Bernard A. Renal dysfunction induced by cadmium: Biomarkers of critical effects. *Biometals*. 2004; **17**: 519-23.
14. Roels HA, Hoet P, Lison D. Usefulness of biomarkers of exposure to inorganic mercury, lead, or cadmium in controlling occupational and environmental risks of nephrotoxicity. *Renal Failure*. 1999; **21**: 251-62.
15. Chen L, Jin T, Huang B *et al*. Critical exposure level of cadmium for elevated urinary metallothionein – an occupational population study in China. *Toxicology and Applied Pharmacology*. 2006; **215**: 93-9.
16. Chen L, Jin T, Huang B *et al*. Plasma metallothionein antibody and cadmium-induced renal dysfunction in an occupational population in China. *Toxicological Sciences*. 2006; **91**: 104-12.
17. Stanbury SW, Mawer EB. Metabolic disturbances in acquired osteomalacia. In: Cohen RD, Lewis B, Albert KCMM, Denman AM (eds). *The metabolism and molecular basis of acquired disease*, vol. 2. London: Baillière Tindall, 1990: 1717-82.
18. Alfven T, Jarup L, Elinder CG. Cadmium and lead in blood in relation to low bone mineral density and tubular proteinuria. *Environmental Health Perspectives*. 2002; **110**: 699-702.
19. Alfven T, Elinder CG, Hellstrom L *et al*. Cadmium exposure and distal forearm fractures. *Journal of Bone and Mineral Research*. 2004; **19**: 900-5.
20. Akesson A, Bjellerup P, Lundh T *et al*. Cadmium-induced effects on bone in a population-based study of women. *Environmental Health Perspectives*. 2006; **114**: 830-4.
21. Jarup L, Alfven T. Low level cadmium exposure, renal and bone effects – the OSCAR study. *Biometals*. 2004; **17**: 505-9.
22. Staessen JA, Roels HA, Emelianov D *et al*. Environmental exposure to cadmium, forearm bone density, and risk of fractures: Prospective population study. Public Health and Environmental Exposure to Cadmium (PheeCad) Study Group. *Lancet*. 1999; **353**: 1140-4.
23. Zhu G, Wang H, Shi Y *et al*. Environmental cadmium exposure and forearm bone density. *Biometals*. 2004; **17**: 499-503.
24. Jin T, Nordberg G, Ye T *et al*. Osteoporosis and renal dysfunction in a general population exposed to cadmium in China. *Environmental Research*. 2004; **96**: 353-9.
25. Chalkley SR, Richmond J, Barltrop D. Measurement of vitamin D3 metabolites in smelter workers exposed to lead

and cadmium. *Occupational and Environmental Medicine.* 1998; **55**: 446–52.
26. Jarup L, Alfven T, Persson B et al. Cadmium may be a risk factor for osteoporosis. *Occupational and Environmental Medicine.* 1998; **55**: 435–9.
27. Kazantzis G. Cadmium, osteoporosis and calcium metabolism. *Biometals.* 2004; **17**: 493–8.
28. Berglund M, Akesson A, Bjellerup P, Vahter M. Metal–bone interactions. *Toxicology Letters.* 2000; **112–113**: 219–25.
29. Coonse KG, Coonts AJ, Morrison EV, Heggland SJ. Cadmium induces apoptosis in the human osteoblast-like cell line Saos-2. *Journal of Toxicology and Environmental Health. Part A.* 2007; **70**: 575–81.
30. International Agency for Research on Cancer. Monographs on the evaluation of carcinogenic risks to humans, vol. 58. Beryllium, cadmium, mercury, and exposures in the glass manufacturing industry. Lyon: IARC, 1993.
31. Sorahan T, Lancashire RJ. Lung cancer mortality in a cohort of workers employed at a cadmium recovery plant in the United States: An analysis with detailed job histories. *Occupational and Environmental Medicine.* 1997; **54**: 194–201.
32. Sorahan T, Esmen NA. Lung cancer mortality in UK nickel-cadmium battery workers, 1947–2000. *Occupational and Environmental Medicine.* 2004; **61**: 108–16.
33. Verougstraete V, Lison D, Hotz P. Cadmium, lung and prostate cancer: A systematic review of recent epidemiological data. *Journal of Toxicology and Environmental Health. Part B, Critical Reviews.* 2003; **6**: 227–55.
34. Sahmoun AE, Case LD, Jackson SA, Schwartz GG. Cadmium and prostate cancer: a critical epidemiologic analysis. *Cancer Investigation.* 2005; **23**: 256–63.
35. Il'yasova D, Schwartz GG. Cadmium and renal cancer. *Toxicology and Applied Pharmacology.* 2005; **207**: 179–86.
36. Bertin G, Averbeck D. Cadmium: Cellular effects, modifications of biomolecules, modulation of DNA repair and genotoxic consequences (a review). *Biochimie.* 2006; **88**: 1549–59.
37. Filipic M, Fatur T, Vudrag M. Molecular mechanisms of cadmium induced mutagenicity. *Human and Experimental Toxicology.* 2006; **25**: 67–77.
38. Giaginis C, Gatzidou E, Theocharis S. DNA repair systems as targets of cadmium toxicity. *Toxicology and Applied Pharmacology.* 2006; **213**: 282–90.
39. Verougstraete V, Lison D, Hotz P. A systematic review of cytogenetic studies conducted in human populations exposed to cadmium compounds. *Mutation Research.* 2002; **511**: 15–43.
40. Waisberg M, Joseph P, Hale B, Beyersmann D. Molecular and cellular mechanisms of cadmium carcinogenesis. *Toxicology.* 2003; **192**: 95–117.
41. Staessen J, Bulpitt CJ, Roels H et al. Urinary cadmium and lead concentrations and their relation to blood pressure in a population with low exposure. *British Journal of Industrial Medicine.* 1984; **41**: 241–8.
42. Boscolo P, Carmignani M. Mechanisms of cardiovascular regulation in male rabbits chronically exposed to cadmium. *British Journal of Industrial Medicine.* 1986; **43**: 605–10.
43. Viaene MK, Roels HA, Leenders J et al. Cadmium: A possible etiological factor in peripheral polyneuropathy. *Neurotoxicology.* 1999; **20**: 7–16.
44. Viaene MK, Masschelein R, Leenders J et al. Neurobehavioural effects of occupational exposure to cadmium: A cross sectional epidemiological study. *Occupational and Environmental Medicine.* 2000; **57**: 19–27.
45. Friberg L. Health hazards in the manufacture of alkaline accumulators with special reference to chronic cadmium poisoning. *Acta Medica Scandinavica.* 1950; **138** (Suppl. 240): 1–124.
46. Liu YZ, Huang JX, Luo CM et al. Effects of cadmium on cadmium smelter workers. *Scandinavian Journal of Work and Environmental Health.* 1985; **11** (Suppl. 4): 29–32.
47. Lauwerys R, Roels H, Regniers M et al. Significance of cadmium concentrations in blood and in urine in workers exposed to cadmium. *Environmental Research.* 1979; **20**: 375–91.
48. Olsson IM, Bensryd I, Lundh T et al. Cadmium in blood and urine – impact of sex, age, dietary intake, iron status, and former smoking – association of renal effects. *Environmental Health Perspectives.* 2002; **110**: 1185–90.
49. Jarup L, Persson B, Elinder CG. Blood cadmium as an indicator of dose in a long-term follow-up of workers previously exposed to cadmium. *Scandinavian Journal of Work and Environmental Health.* 1997; **23**: 31–6.
50. Kido T, Nordberg G, Roels H. Cadmium-induced renal effects. In: De Broe M, Porter G, Bennett W, Verpooten G (eds). *Clinical nephrotoxins. Renal injury from drugs and chemicals,* 2nd edn. Amsterdam: Kluwer Academic, 2003: 507–30.
51. Al-Haddad IK, Chettle DR, Fletcher JR, Fremlin JH. A transportable system for measurement of kidney cadmium *in vivo. International Journal of Applied Radiation and Isotopes.* 1981; **32**: 109–12.
52. Grinyer J, Byun SH, Chettle DR. *In vivo* prompt gamma neutron activation analysis of cadmium in the kidney and liver. *Applied Radiation and Isotopes.* 2005; **63**: 475–9.

18

Chromium

TOM SORAHAN

Introduction	173	Monitoring of workers exposed to chromium	174
Metabolism and action	173	References	174
The carcinogenicity of chrome compounds	174		

INTRODUCTION

Chromium is a hard, silver white metal which is used for chrome plating and in the manufacture of special steels, such as stainless steel and ferrochrome. A number of its compounds are important as mordants in dyeing silk, wool and other textiles, as tanning agents and as pigments. Those chromium compounds which are commercially important occur in two valency states: trivalent (including chromic oxide and chromic sulphate) and hexavalent (including chromium trioxide, chromic acid and the dichromates of a number of metals). The trivalent compounds are generally considered to be virtually non-toxic, whereas the hexavalent salts are irritant, corrosive and, in some instances, carcinogenic.

METABOLISM AND ACTION

Chromium is an essential element; it is required for normal carbohydrate metabolism and it potentiates the action of insulin. Its hexavalent salts can be absorbed from the lungs, the gut and, to a certain extent, through the intact skin. Trivalent chromium, however, is very poorly absorbed. Chromium is rapidly excreted in the urine with a half-life of between 15 and 41 hours.

All chrome compounds are sensitizers and may cause contact dermatitis; some may be a cause of occupational asthma. Chrome ulcers (chrome holes) are circular, well-demarcated lesions which look as if they have been punched out of the skin (Figure 18.1). They are only slightly painful and tend to heal spontaneously, but may be troublesome if secondarily infected. They can, however, be treated adequately with a 10 per cent solution of calcium EDTA. Long-term exposure to chromium compounds may cause perforation of the cartilaginous nasal septum (Figure 18.2) and occasionally lead to chronic rhinitis and chronic bronchitis. It may also induce conjunctivitis, keratitis and ulcerations on the eyelids.

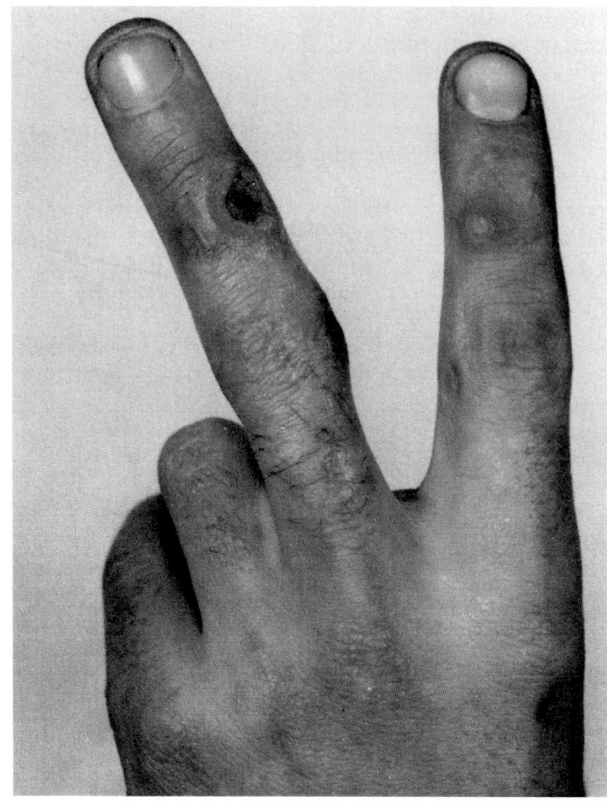

Figure 18.1 Chrome ulcers in various stages of activity on the hand of a fitter who worked in a chromium plating shop maintaining the plating tanks. Courtesy of Professor RI McCallum.

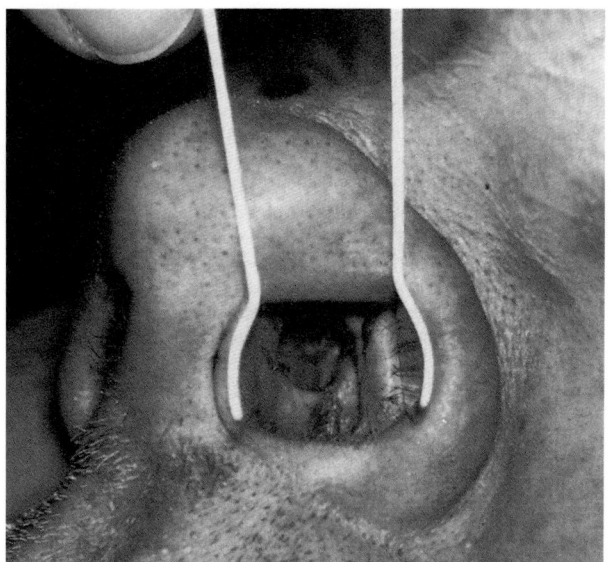

Figure 18.2 Healed nasal perforation from inhalation of the vapour from a chrome-plating tank. Courtesy of the late Professor RI McCallum.

The inhalation of large concentrations of hexavalent chromium compounds may cause coughing, wheezing, inspiratory pain, fever and loss of weight. Prolonged skin contact may lead to local irritation and, if skin damage is extensive, enough of the compound may be absorbed to cause renal damage and death.

THE CARCINOGENICITY OF CHROME COMPOUNDS

The most serious consequence of exposure to chromium compounds is the risk of developing lung cancer (see Chapter 85, Occupational cancer: epidemiology, biological mechanisms and biomarkers). The carcinogenicity of hexavalent chromium compounds is well established and markedly elevated lung cancer rates have been found in workers engaged in primary chromate production, in the chrome pigment production industry, and in chrome plating.[1] The direct evidence relating to stainless steel welders and workers in the ferrochromium industries is inconclusive. The human evidence relating to trivalent chromium is also inconclusive.

In short-term tests, hexavalent chromium produces mutations in bacterial systems without prior activation and, *in vitro*, the mutagenic potential of soluble and slightly soluble compounds does not differ. Trivalent chromium has a limited mutagenic effect, although it has been shown to be 20 times more potent in decreasing the fidelity of DNA synthesis *in vitro* than the hexavalent form.

It may be that, in fact, the trivalent form of the metal is the proximate carcinogen having been produced by intracellular reduction of the hexavalent form. The apparent inactivity *in vivo* is thought to result from poor absorption. Bound to certain ligands, trivalent chromium is able to cross cell membranes. The carcinogenic effect may not be due to the trivalent form at all, however, but to some reactive intermediate formed during the reduction of hexavalent chromium, perhaps a pentavalent compound.[2]

Lung cancer was prescribed in 1986 under the Social Security Act for occupations involving the use or handling of or exposure to the dust of zinc chromate, calcium chromate or strontium chromate (see Chapter 8, Compensation schemes).

MONITORING OF WORKERS EXPOSED TO CHROMIUM

Special attention should be given to the skin and nose of chrome workers. It may also be prudent to conduct periodic tests of lung function if cases of asthma are suspected.

The chromium concentration in the urine at the end of a work shift is an index of recent exposure to soluble hexavalent chromium compound. Levels in unexposed people are below 12 nmol/L in blood and 0.2–3 mmol/mol creatinine in urine.[3]

> **Key points**
>
> - Chromium is an essential element.
> - Heavy chrome exposure can cause chrome ulcers.
> - Hexavalent chromium compounds are potent human lung carcinogens.

REFERENCES

1. Cross HJ, Faux SP, Sadhra S *et al. Criteria document for hexavalent chromium.* Paris: International Chromium Development Association, 1997.
2. Norseth R. The carcinogenicity of chromium and its salts. *British Journal of Industrial Medicine.* 1986; **43**: 649–51.
3. McAughey JJ, Samuel AM, Baxter PJ, Smith NJ. Biological monitoring of occupational exposure in the chromate production industry. *Science of the Total Environment.* 1988; **71**: 317–22.

19

Cobalt

PERRINE HOET

| Introduction | 175 | Medical surveillance | 177 |
| Toxicity | 176 | References | 178 |

INTRODUCTION

Cobalt (Co) is a silvery grey, magnetic metal mainly recovered as a byproduct from copper and silver mining. The main mining centres are in Central Africa, Canada, Russia, Australia and Central America. Cobalt is a transition element occurring in four valences (0, +2, +3 and +4), the divalent oxidation state being the most common. It is an essential element and central to the action of vitamin B_{12}.

Cobalt has a wide application in many sectors: metallurgy (super alloys, high speed and high strength steels, prosthetics, spring alloys), magnetic alloys, chemicals (batteries, tyres, paint dryers, soaps, pigments, catalysts in the petroleum and the textile industry, adhesives, electroplating, agriculture and medicine), cemented carbides, electronics, ceramics and enamels (colours in pottery, enamels, glass and china).[1]

The metal form of cobalt is used in the manufacture of superalloys which are alloys developed for applications where elevated temperatures and high mechanical stress are encountered, principally used in jet engines. It is also used in magnetic alloys and alloys that are required for purposes requiring hardness, wear resistance and corrosion resistance. Recently, cobalt oxide has been used in the active ingredient of lithium ion rechargeable batteries. In nickel-cadmium and nickel metal hydride batteries, several cobalt compounds are used as additives, for either the positive or negative electrode. Radioactive cobalt (^{60}Co) is used as a source of high energy gamma radiation in radiotherapy and industrial radiography.[1]

The main use of cobalt is in hard metals. Exposure to cemented carbides and cobalt-diamond tools should be distinguished from the other types of exposure to cobalt. Hard metals are materials in which metallic carbides are bound together or cemented by a soft and ductile metal binder, usually cobalt or nickel.[2] Hard metals usually consist of more than 80 per cent tungsten carbide (WC) particles and less than 10 per cent cobalt metal, although the cobalt content can be more (up to 25 per cent) depending on the application. These powders are compacted and heated at high temperature in a process called sintering, hence the term 'sintered carbides' or 'cemented carbides'. Other constituents – chromium, titanium, tantalum, vanadium, niobium, etc. – may be added. Hard metals have a hardness almost that of diamond and are used to make machine parts that require high heat resistance, or to make tools used for drilling, cutting, machining or grinding. Exposure to hard metal dust takes place at all stages of the production of hard metals, but the highest levels of exposure have been reported to occur during the weighing, grinding and finishing phases.[2] The continuous recycling of coolants, used with hard metals, has been shown to result in increased concentrations of dissolved cobalt in the metal-working liquid and hence a greater potential for exposure to (ionic) cobalt in aerosols from these fluids.[2] Although they do not contain WC, cobalt-containing diamond tools are often considered in the same category. They are also produced by powder metallurgy, whereby microdiamonds are impregnated in a matrix of compacted, extrafine cobalt powder and the proportion of cobalt in such tools is higher (up to 90 per cent) than in hard metals. Diamond polishers have been reported to inhale metallic Co, iron and silica.

The absorption from the gut varies considerably from 5 to 45 per cent, and about 30 per cent of an inhaled dose of cobalt oxide is absorbed. The solubilization and bioavailability of cobalt in the extracellular milieu was shown to increase in the presence of WC.[3] Cobalt does not accumulate in any specific organ, except in the lungs when inhaled in the form of insoluble particles. In blood, cobalt ions bind strongly to proteins, mainly albumin. It is mainly (80 per cent) excreted in the urine, the remainder in the faeces.[2]

TOXICITY

Respiratory disorders that have been related to occupational exposure to cobalt involve the upper respiratory tract (inflammation of the nasopharynx), the bronchial tree (bronchial asthma) and the parenchyma with the development of an interstitial lung disease, the so-called 'hard metal lung disease' (HMLD) which may cover several clinical pictures from hypersensitivity pneumonitis or desquamative alveolitis to interstitial lung fibrosis (see Chapter 82, Metal dusts and fumes).

In its most typical clinical presentation, interstitial lung disease consists of a giant-cell interstitial pneumonia (GIP), characterized by the presence of 'cannibalistic' multinucleated giant cells in air spaces and bronchoalveolar lavage. The process by which these giant cells are produced and the role of Co, if any, in this process are still unknown.[2,4–7] Typical symptoms are wheezing, shortness of breath and chest tightness, and lung function tests show restrictive effects (reduced FVC) with a reduction in the diffusion capacity. The chest radiograph may be normal or show a nodular, reticulonodular or reticular pattern. High resolution computed tomography (HRCT) findings have been described in a small number of patients. Reported abnormalities include patchy lobular ground-glass opacities, reticulation, centrilobular nodularity, honeycombing, bronchiectasis, and large peripheral cystic spaces in the mid and upper lung zones.[8,9]

The alveolitis usually improves spontaneously when the subject is no longer exposed to cobalt, but if exposure continues, irreversible pulmonary fibrosis may develop gradually and may lead to cor pulmonale and death.[5,10]

The disease has only been diagnosed in workers in the hard metal and diamond polishing industries and also in dental technicians, where exposure is mixed, being not only to cobalt metal, but also to different carbides, diamond or other particles.[2,11–13] Experimental findings, both *in vitro* and *in vivo*, indicate that the biological reactivity of the mixture of cobalt powder with different carbides is much higher than that of pure cobalt powder.[3] There is no evidence for the occurrence of typical HLMD in workers exposed to cobalt alone. An epidemiological study in a large cobalt refining plant did not find evidence of parenchymal disease among workers highly exposed to pure cobalt.[14] Based on a 13-year surveillance programme (from 1988 to 2001) of these workers, FEV_1 was found to decrease over time, but only in association with smoking. It was calculated that an exposure resulting in urinary cobalt levels of 10, 20 or 40 µg/g creatinine (which is roughly equivalent to a time-weighted average exposure at 10, 20 or 40 µg/m^3) would cause, for a 30-year-old smoking worker, an additional decrement of 64, 84 or 103 mL of FEV_1 after ten years of work at this plant.[15] Another investigation on current and former workers who had worked more than ten years in a cobalt plant found no chronic respiratory diseases, except asthma.[16] Simultaneous exposure to cobalt and other substances is probably necessary to cause HMLD. It is conceivable that the individual susceptibility to develop HMLD is related to an innate or acquired inability to deal with oxidant injury. The existence of genetic susceptibility to HMLD has been suggested because of the very low prevalence of the disease (less than 1 per cent) and the lack of correlation with the intensity or duration of exposure.

There is ample evidence that cobalt causes bronchial asthma. Cobalt asthma is associated in some, but not all cases, with circulating cobalt-specific IgE and generalized bronchial hyperresponsiveness; a type 1 allergic reaction is therefore suspected.[17] Occupational asthma has been recorded in all industry sectors with exposure to cobalt, either alone or in association with other constituents.[16,18,19] There is strong evidence that all cobalt species that are significantly soluble in biological media can cause asthma. Cross-respiratory sensitization between nickel and cobalt compounds has been reported.

In 1990, the International Agency for Research on Cancer (IARC)[20] concluded that cobalt and cobalt compounds were possibly carcinogenic to humans (group 2B), with inadequate evidence of carcinogenicity in humans, and sufficient evidence for the carcinogenicity of cobalt metal powder in experimental animals (see Chapter 85, Occupational cancer: epidemiology biological mechanisms and biomarkers). Further evidence in respect of carcinogenicity of cobalt compounds came in 1996 when the National Toxicology Program in the United States reported that a two-year inhalation bioassay with cobalt sulphate in rats had shown an increased lung cancer incidence.[21] In 1998, the European Union classified cobalt metal and all metal compounds as category 2 carcinogens, i.e. 'may cause cancer in experimental animals'. Since the 1990 IARC evaluation, several epidemiological studies addressed cancer risks among workers exposed to dusts containing cobalt with or without tungsten carbide in hard metal production facilities. Those conducted in France provided evidence of an increased lung cancer risk related to exposure to hard-metal dust containing cobalt and tungsten carbide, taking into account potential confounding by smoking and other occupational carcinogens.[22–25] Hence, in 2003, cobalt metal with tungsten carbide was re-evaluated as probably carcinogenic to humans (group 2A) on the basis of limited evidence in humans for increased risk of lung cancer and sufficient evidence in experimental animals for the carcinogenicity of cobalt sulphate and of cobalt metal powder. The evidence of carcinogenicity for exposure to cobalt in the absence of tungsten carbide was considered inadequate, so that with sufficient evidence in experimental animals for the carcinogenicity of cobalt sulphate and of cobalt metal powder, the overall evaluation of cobalt metal without tungsten carbide was possibly carcinogenic to humans (group 2B). Cobalt sulphate and other soluble cobalt (II) salts were evaluated as possibly carcinogenic to humans (group 2B).[2] There is insufficient information for cobalt oxides and other compounds.[26]

Co(II) ions are genotoxic *in vitro* and *in vivo*, Co metal is genotoxic *in vitro*. Hard metal dust is proven to be genotoxic *in vitro* and *in vivo*. The production of reactive oxygen species and/or DNA repair inhibition are mechanisms possibly involved.[26,27] Contrary to what is generally assumed for most metals, the biological activity of cobalt metal is not exclusively mediated by the ionic form dissolved in biological media.[27]

Cobalt and cobalt compounds have skin-sensitizing properties which may lead to occupational contact dermatitis, particularly of the hands.[28–32] Concurrent reaction to cobalt, nickel and chromate may occur.[33,34]

At one time, cobalt salts were added to beer as a foam stabilizer and a number of outbreaks of congestive cardiomyopathy were linked to that use. Those affected suffered from an abrupt onset of left ventricular failure with pericardial effusion and polycythaemia. It was generally considered that the aetiology was multifactorial since the amount of cobalt consumed, even by the most heavy drinkers, was far less than that given therapeutically for anaemia. The fact that the condition was seen almost exclusively in heavy drinkers suggested that there was a synergistic action between the cobalt in the beer, the direct effects of alcohol on the myocardium and an inadequate intake of proteins and vitamins.[35] Isolated cardiomyopathy cases have been reported among workers exposed to cobalt or hard metals.[36] Cumulative exposure to cobalt in cobalt production workers was found to be associated with echocardiographic changes indicating altered left ventricular relaxation and early ventricular filling, but not associated with clinically significant cardiac dysfunction.[37] A possible mechanism for the findings could be the accumulation of cobalt in the myocardium, the result being an increase in myocardial stiffness and the inhibition of cellular respiration due to inhibition of mitochondrial dehydrogenase.[36,37]

Cobalt has an effect on thyroid function. It inhibits tyrosine iodinase which prevents the synthesis of thyroxine. This, in turn, leads to an oversecretion of thyroid-stimulating hormone and to thyroid hyperplasia.

Cobalt also mimicks hypoxia and induces the production of erythropoietin, leading to polycythaemia.

MEDICAL SURVEILLANCE

Workers exposed to pure cobalt powder or to cobalt-containing dusts should be submitted to periodic health checks, including clinical examination with special attention to the lungs and skin. Pulmonary function testing and periodic chest radiographs may be considered in the surveillance programme. The retention time of cobalt in the human body is short. Excretion is biphasic, a rapid phase of elimination lasts approximately two days after which a second phase of prolonged and low-level elimination follows. Where exposure is to soluble cobalt compounds (e.g. salts), to the metal or to hard metal dust, measurement of cobalt in the urine at the end of the working week will give an indication of the extent of recent exposure. However, when exposure is to cobalt oxides, the urinary concentration of cobalt does not correlate well with recent exposure.[38,39]

For unexposed people, the level of urinary cobalt is generally $<2\,\mu g/g$ creatinine, and the level in blood $<1\,\mu g/L$.[2,39] Elevated levels have been reported in cobalt metal, oxide and salt production workers, hard metal workers, battery plant workers, pottery painters, as well as in dental technicians.[4,15,40–42] Metal-on-metal hip and knee arthroplasties can cause increased blood and urine levels.[43–46]

In Germany,[47] exposure equivalents for carcinogenic materials (Expositionsäquivalente für krebserzeugende Arbeitsstoffe (EKA)) are derived for substances in carcinogen categories 1 to 3. These substances are not given biological tolerance values (BAT) because it is considered that, at present, it is not possible to specify safe levels of such substances in biological materials. However, the relationship between the concentration of the substance in the workplace air and that of the substance (or metabolite) in biological materials is investigated for the occupational medical detection and quantification of the individual exposure to the substance. For cobalt, the EKA values are 15, 30, 60 and 300 μg/L urinary cobalt (sampling time not fixed) for 0.025, 0.05, 0.10 and 0.50 mg/m^3 cobalt in air. The biological exposure indices (BEI) recommended by the American Conference of Governmental Industrial Hygienists (ACGIH)[48] for cobalt are 15 μg/L urine and 1 μg/L blood (end of shift at end of work-week samples), corresponding to an atmospheric exposure level of 0.02 mg/m^3 (TLV-TWA, inhalable fraction).

Exhaled breath condensate (EBC), a fluid formed by cooling exhaled air, is postulated to be a suitable matrix to assess target tissue dose and the effects of inhaled cobalt and tungsten. It was speculated that Co-EBC reflects not only exposure, but also the amount of the element retained in the lung and eliminated with exhaled air after its interaction with – and possibly damage to – resident cells.[49] However, this technique is still at an exploratory stage and generally not available for routine surveillance of cobalt-exposed workers.

Key points

- Cobalt is an essential element necessary for the formation of vitamin B$_{12}$.
- Following inhalation exposure to Co, the main target organ is the respiratory tract. Fibrosing alveolitis (hard metal disease) has been reported in hard metal workers and in diamond polishers, but not in workers exposed to other cobalt species. Exposure to cobalt alone can cause asthma and allergic contact dermatitis.
- Cobalt metal with tungsten carbide (hard metal) is considered as probably carcinogenic to humans, cobalt without tungsten carbide, cobalt sulphate and other soluble salts as possibly carcinogenic to humans.
- Other target organs include the thyroid, the haematopoietic system and the myocardium.

REFERENCES

1. Cobalt Development Institute website. Last accessed March 2008. Available from: www.thecdi.com.
2. International Agency for Research on Cancer. Monographs on the evaluation of carcinogenic risks to humans, vol. 86. Cobalt in hard metals and cobalt sulfate, gallium arsenide, indium phosphide and vanadium pentoxide. Lyon: IARC, 2006.
3. Lison D, Lauwerys R, Demedts M et al. Experimental research into the pathogenesis of cobalt/hard metal lung disease. *European Respiratory Journal.* 1996; **9**: 1024-8.
4. Cullen A. Respiratory diseases from hard metal or cobalt exposure. A continuing enigma. *Chest.* 1984; **86**: 513-14.
5. Fishbein EA. Clinical findings amongst hard metal workers. *British Journal of Industrial Medicine.* 1992; **49**: 17-24.
6. Lison D. Human toxicity of cobalt-containing dust and experimental studies on the mechanism of interstitial lung disease (hard metal disease). *Critical Reviews in Toxicology.* 1996; **26**: 585-616.
7. Nemery B, Abraham JL. Hard metal lung disease: Still hard to understand. *American Journal of Respiratory and Critical Care Medicine.* 2007; **176**: 2-3.
8. Dunlop P, Muller NL, Wilson J et al. Hard metal lung disease: High resolution CT and histologic correlation of the initial findings and demonstration of interval improvement. *Journal of Thorac Imaging.* 2005; **20**: 301-4.
9. Gotway MB, Golden JA, Warnock M et al. Hard metal interstitial lung disease: High-resolution computed tomography appearance. *Journal of Thorac Imaging.* 2002; **17**: 314-18.
10. Ruokonen EL, Linnainmaa M, Seuri M et al. A fatal case of hard-metal disease. *Scandinavian Journal of Work and Environmental Health.* 1996; **22**: 62-5.
11. Meyer-Bisch C, Pham QT, Mur JM. Respiratory hazards in hard metal workers: A cross sectional study. *British Journal of Industrial Medicine.* 1989; **46**: 302-9.
12. Nemery B, Casier P, Rousels D et al. Survey of cobalt exposure and respiratory health in diamond polishers. *American Review of Respiratory Disease.* 1992; **145**: 610-16.
13. Lison D. Lung fibrosis reported in a dental technician. *AIHAJ.* 2000; **61**: 158-9.
14. Swennen B, Buchet JP, Stanescue D et al. Epidemiological survey on workers exposed to cobalt oxides, cobalt salts and cobalt metal. *British Journal of Industrial Medicine.* 1993; **50**: 835-42.
15. Verougstraete V, Mallants A, Buchet JP et al. Lung function changes in workers exposed to cobalt compounds: A 13-year follow-up. *American Journal of Respiratory and Critical Care Medicine.* 2004; **170**: 162-6.
16. Linna A, Oksa P, Palmroos P et al. Respiratory health of cobalt production workers. *American Journal of Industrial Medicine.* 2003; **44**: 124-32.
17. Shirakawa T, Kusaka T, Fujimura N et al. The existence of specific antibodies to cobalt in hard metal asthma. *Clinical Allergy.* 1988; **18**: 451-60.
18. Leysens B, Aurerx J, Van Den Eeckhout A et al. Cobalt-induced bronchial asthma in diamond polishers. *Chest.* 1989; **88**: 740-4.
19. Kusaka Y, Iki M, Kumagai S. Epidemiological study of hard metal asthma. *Occupational and Environmental Medicine.* 1996; **53**: 188-99.
20. International Agency for Research on Cancer. Monographs on the evaluation of carcinogenic risks to humans, vol. 52. Chlorinated drinking-water, chlorination by-products; some other halogenated compounds; cobalt and cobalt compounds. Lyon: IARC, 1991.
21. National Toxicology Program. Technical report on the toxicology and carcinogenesis studies of cobalt sulfate heptahydrate in rats and mice (inhalation studies). National Institutes of Health publication No 96-3951, 1996.
22. Moulin JJ, Wild P, Mur JM et al. A mortality study of cobalt production workers: An extension of the follow-up. *American Journal of Industrial Medicine.* 1993; **23**: 281-8.
23. Lasfargues G, Wild P, Moullin JJ et al. Lung cancer mortality in a French cohort of hard metal workers. *American Journal of Industrial Medicine.* 1994; **26**: 585-95.
24. Moulin JJ, Wild P, Romazini S et al. Lung cancer risk in hard-metal workers. *American Journal of Epidemiology.* 1998; **148**: 241-8.
25. Wild P, Perdrix A, Romazini S et al. Lung cancer mortality in a site producing hard metals. *Occupational and Environmental Medicine.* 2000; **57**: 568-73.
26. De Boeck M, Kirsch-Volders M, Lison D. Cobalt and antimony: Genotoxicity and carcinogenicity. *Mutation Research.* 2003; **533**: 135-52.
27. Lison D, De Boeck M, Verougstraete V, Kirsch-Volders M. Update on the genotoxicity and carcinogenicity of cobalt compounds. *Occupational and Environmental Medicine.* 2001; **58**: 619-25.
28. Athavale P, Shum KW, Chen Y et al. Occupational dermatitis related to chromium and cobalt: Experience of dermatologists (EPIDERM) and occupational physicians (OPRA) in the UK over an 11-year period (1993-2004). *British Journal of Dermatology.* 2007; **157**: 518-22.
29. Dotterud LK, Smith-Sivertsen T. Allergic contact sensitization in the general adult population: A population-based study from Northern Norway. *Contact Dermatitis.* 2007; **56**: 10-15.
30. Hindsen M, Persson L, Gruvberger B. Allergic contact dermatitis from cobalt in jewellery. *Contact Dermatitis* 2005; **53**: 350-1.
31. Macedo MS, Avelar Alchorne AO, Costa EB, Montesano FT. Contact allergy in male construction workers in Sao Paulo, Brazil, 2000-2005. *Contact Dermatitis.* 2007; **56**: 232-4.
32. Warshaw EM, Ahmed RL, Belsito DV et al. Contact dermatitis of the hands: Cross-sectional analyses of North American Contact Dermatitis Group Data, 1994-2004. *Journal of the American Academy of Dermatologists.* 2007; **57**: 301-14.
33. Hegewald J, Uter W, Pfahlberg A et al. A multifactorial analysis of concurrent patch-test reactions to nickel, cobalt, and chromate. *Allergy.* 2005; **60**: 372-8.

34. Ruff CA, Belsito DV. The impact of various patient factors on contact allergy to nickel, cobalt, and chromate. *Journal of the American Academy of Dermatologists.* 2006; **55**: 32-9.
35. Alexander CS. Cobalt-beer myopathy. *American Journal of Medicine.* 1972; **53**: 395-417.
36. Seghizzi P, D'Adda F, Borleri D et al. Cobalt myocardiopathy. A critical review of literature. *Science of the Total Environment.* 1994; **150**: 105-9.
37. Linna A, Oksa P, Groundstroem K et al. Exposure to cobalt in the production of cobalt and cobalt compounds and its effect on the heart. *Occupational and Environmental Medicine.* 2004; **61**: 877-85.
38. Lauwerys R, Hoet P. *Industrial chemical exposure guidelines for biological monitoring*, 3nd edn. London: Lewis Publishers, 2001.
39. Lison D, Buchet J-P, Swennen B et al. Biological monitoring of workers exposed to cobalt metal, salts, oxides and hard metal dust. *Occupational and Environmental Medicine.* 1994; **5**: 447-50.
40. Burgaz S, Demircigil GC, Yilmazer M et al. Assessment of cytogenetic damage in lymphocytes and in exfoliated nasal cells of dental laboratory technicians exposed to chromium, cobalt, and nickel. *Mutation Research.* 2002; **521**: 47-56.
41. Kraus T, Schramel P, Schaller KH et al. Exposure assessment in the hard metal manufacturing industry with special regard to tungsten and its compounds. *Occupational and Environmental Medicine.* 2001; **58**: 631-4.
42. Yokota K, Johyama Y, Kunitani Y et al. Urinary elimination of nickel and cobalt in relation to airborne nickel and cobalt exposures in a battery plant. *International Archives of Occupational and Environmental Health.* 2007; **80**: 527-31.
43. Daniel J, Ziaee H, Pradhan C et al. Blood and urine metal ion levels in young and active patients after Birmingham hip resurfacing arthroplasty: Four-year results of a prospective longitudinal study. *Journal of Bone and Joint Surgery. British volume* 2007; **89**: 169-73.
44. Luetzner J, Krummenauer F, Lengel AM et al. Serum metal ion exposure after total knee arthroplasty. *Clinical Orthopaedics and Related Research.* 2007; **461**: 136-42.
45. Williams S, Schepers A, Isaac G et al. The 2007 Otto Aufranc Award. Ceramic-on-metal hip arthroplasties: A comparative *in vitro* and *in vivo* study. *Clinical Orthopaedics and Related Research.* 2007; **465**: 23-32.
46. Witzleb WC, Ziegler J, Krummenauer F et al. Exposure to chromium, cobalt and molybdenum from metal-on-metal total hip replacement and hip resurfacing arthroplasty. *Acta Orthopaedica.* 2006; **77**: 697-705.
47. Deutsche Forschungsgemeinshaft. List of maximum concentration at the workplace and biological tolerance values. Report No.43. Commission for the Investigation of Health Hazards of Chemical Compounds in the Work Area. Berlin: VCH, 2007.
48. American Conference of Governmental Industrial Hygienists. Threshold limit values for chemical and physical agents and biological exposure indices. Cincinnati: ACGIH, 2007.
49. Goldoni M, Catalani S, De Palma G et al. Exhaled breath condensate as a suitable matrix to assess lung dose and effects in workers exposed to cobalt and tungsten. *Environmental Health Perspectives.* 2004; **112**: 1293-8.

20

Copper

PETER AGGETT

| Properties and uses | 180 | Exposure and health effects | 181 |
| Essentiality and metabolism | 180 | References | 182 |

PROPERTIES AND USES

Copper was one of the first metals to have been used by man and its use in bronze, a mixture of nine parts copper with one part tin, has defined a stage of human civilization. This started, possibly 10 millennia ago, but certainly the alloy was being used in the Aegean littoral about 7000 years ago. Copper is the third most widely used metal after iron and aluminium.[1–3]

Copper's malleability, ductility, thermal conductivity and resistance to corrosion underpinned its early usage as the native metal, as bronze and as other alloys such as those with zinc (brass) and nickel. Subsequently, its electrical conductivity and biostatic effects extended its domestic, commercial and industrial exploitation.

Thus, copper is used in the following applications: in coinage, either as copper coins or as a coating or alloy with nickel cupronickel or zinc; piping and plumbing systems; as a roofing material (exposed copper becomes green as the metal forms the pale green carbonate, verdigris); guttering, doors and similar architectural features; bronze statuary; cooking utensils; electroplating; kitchen and domestic fittings; work surfaces; stills; furniture and domestic fittings; door fittings, electrical wiring and electronic applications; photography; wood preservatives, often as the arsenate; as an anti-fouling agent on boat hulls; pigments, for example, in paints and glass; fireworks; munitions; and as in the manufacture of rayon, textiles, paper and tyres.

The metal is used as a self-disinfecting and bacteriostatic surface. Copper sulphate is used in topical sterilizing agents and as a water treatment, and it has been used as a fungicide and algaecide, for example in Bordeaux mixture which is a mixture of copper sulphate 0.05–2 per cent with soda lime (i.e. a mixture of calcium hydroxide with sodium or potassium hydroxide). A similar compound of copper sulphate is an accepted pesticide in organic farming. Additionally, copper is used as a food supplement in animal husbandry, not simply as a nutrient, but also as an intestinal microbiocidal to alter the intestinal microflora. This may improve the energy efficiency of growth in the livestock, usually pigs, and may also lead to atypical concentrations of copper in pig carcass livers. In some areas where local soil characteristics limit the uptake of copper by plants, copper salts may be included in fertilizers.[1–3]

Metallic copper occurs naturally, but most copper is obtained from sulphide minerals of copper: chalcopyrite, bornite, covellite and chalcocite. Other mineral sources are the carbonates azurite and malachite, and the chloride and oxide, cuprite. The principal sources are pit mines in Chile and the Sonora Desert, but there are many other mines throughout the world, particularly in Africa. Global copper supplies are thought to be at risk of running out in the next 50 years, so increased recovery of copper from existing artefacts may become a source of occupational exposure.

ESSENTIALITY AND METABOLISM

Copper is an essential nutrient.[1] It has two biologically relevant oxidation (valency) states: Cu (I) and Cu (II) which are exploited in redox enzyme activities. Cuproenzymes include oxidases and electron transport systems, such as cytochrome-c-oxidase. Thus, copper underpins the synthesis of adrenalin and noradrenalin, neurotransmitters, encephalins and neuropeptides; substrate metabolism and mitochondrial respiration; antioxidant activity via superoxide dismutase; cross-linking of collagen for the formation of connective tissue and the organic matrix of bone; the absorption and distribution of iron, and haemoglobin synthesis; efficient muscle contractibility; and the formation of melanin.

Copper is absorbed by a carrier-mediated process and by passive diffusion in the proximal small intestine. Absorbed copper is carried in the portal circulation bound to albumin, amino acids and a specific carrier, transcuprein, to the liver where it is taken up by the hepatocytes and is incorporated into apocaeruloplasmin to form caeruloplasmin. The liver contains at least four pools of copper, one is the cuproenzymes, another is caeruloplasmin which is the major means for systemic distribution of copper, the third pool is a depot of copper bound to a cysteine-rich protein, metallothionein, and which is probably a reserve of the element, and the fourth pool is that of copper principally accrued from recirculated caeruloplasmin from which copper is transferred to a pool destined for biliary excretion. The regulation and exchange of copper between these pools within the liver is unknown.

Copper is distributed peripherally mostly bound to caeruloplasmin (70–80 per cent) from which copper is taken up by endocytosis. The role of caeruloplasmin is not absolutely clear. It is a copper donor, but in individuals with acaeruloplasminaemia copper metabolism is unaffected, so the residual 20–30 per cent of circulating copper which is bound to albumin, transcuprein and amino acids is also available to peripheral tissues, and can compensate the absence of caeruloplasmin.

The major route of copper excretion is in the bile, in which it is associated with low molecular-weight copper-binding components, as well as macromolecular binding species. Reabsorption of biliary copper is negligible, but the reason for this is unclear. At high intakes of copper, intestinal uptake and transfer is downregulated by reduced expression of enterocytic copper carriers, and by the induction of metallothionein which binds copper and blocks its transfer to the body. Urinary losses of copper are small.[1]

EXPOSURE AND HEALTH EFFECTS

Mining and extraction of copper causes exposure to copper particulates, as does processing and working on the metal. Copper powder is pink-red, but it turns green on exposure to moist air; prolonged exposure to this may cause an asymptomatic superficial discolouration of the exposed skin, hair and the tongue, and of the teeth. Occasionally, copper dust induces a contact dermatitis. Copper in copper carbonate and oxide minerals can be released by gastric acid from ingested dust and particles, and might increase systemic exposure. Copper in copper sulphide and other complexes is not released by gastric acid and is thought not to pose such a risk. Some workers exposed to high atmospheric levels of copper, estimated to provide 200 mg/day (the recommended dietary intake is around 2.0 mg/day) have developed elevated serum copper levels and hepatomegaly.[2,3]

However, such exposure is seldom limited to copper alone, and simultaneous exposure to arsenic, nickel, silica, lead, cadmium, zinc and iron needs to be considered in the assessment of occupational exposure. Workers using Bordeaux mixture have developed diffuse pulmonary linear and nodular interstitial fibrosis and granulomatous disease of the lungs and liver.

Exposure to fumes causes metal fume fever and may occur during smelting, brassing, welding, and working on preserved woods; and from the burning of coal and waste incineration. Exposure standards to atmospheric copper dust have been set at 0.5–1 mg Cu/m^3 and to copper fumes at 0.1–0.2 mg Cu/m^3.

Water can leach copper from copper conduits, particularly if it is acid. The metallic, bitter and salty taste of copper in water can be detected by healthy adults at concentrations of 2.5–3.5 mg copper/L which is just below the threshold for the onset of gastrointestinal effects of nausea, abdominal pain and vomiting which are associated with drinking water containing 4–5 mg copper/L. This threshold does not, of course, represent actual exposure levels, and in some areas higher concentrations are tolerated. The regulatory upper limit for copper in drinking water has been set at 3 mg copper/L.[1,4]

Suicidal drinking of copper solutions involving doses of 20–70 g of copper is associated with the above gastrointestinal features which progress to haematemesis, diarrhoea, headache, dizziness, and, some hours later, more severe systemic features, such as tachycardia, respiratory difficulty, intravascular haemolysis, haematuria, gastrointestinal haemorrhagic necrosis, hepatocellular necrosis and liver failure, hypovolaemic shock, and acute tubular necrosis and kidney failure, coma and death. The stools and vomit may be green.

In young children, similar copper overload syndromes have been described: Indian childhood cirrhosis (ICC) and idiopathic copper toxicosis (ICT). The former arises from drinking milk that has been heated or stored in brass vessels first described in India, classically buffalo milk, and the latter from high copper content in water supplies, for example local well water, in North America and Europe. Both are associated with progressive hepatic inflammation, steatosis, fatty infiltration, necrosis, fibrosis, cirrhosis and liver failure. These appear to be ecogenetic conditions in that affected individuals have a genetic susceptibility to a high exposure to copper.[1] It is not known if such populations, or other individuals who are heterozygous for the copper overload syndrome, Wilson disease, are at increased risk when exposed to copper occupationally.

The diagnosis of these conditions depends on history. There are no reliable markers of copper excess. Serum copper or caeruloplasmin concentrations are tightly controlled and are more responsive to elevations during infection and stress than they are to increased body burdens which are predominantly in the liver. Thus, liver biopsy is needed for a definitive diagnosis of systemic overload.

Acute ingestion of copper can be managed by early gastric lavage if possible. In this situation, serum copper values may be of prognostic value. Concentrations below 3 mg/L (50 μmol/L) suggest moderate toxicity, and levels above 8 mg/L (125 μmol/L) indicate severe poisoning. Treatment with standard systemic metabolic support and with the chelator D-penicillamine (25 mg/kg body weight daily) will reduce the copper load, in both acute and chronic copper overload. Other treatments include unithiol and N-acetyl cysteine.[3,5]

> **Key points**
>
> - Systemic copper toxicity can arise via inhalation and ingestion of particulates and salts in solution.
> - Industrial exposure often involves potentially toxic co-exposure to other metals.
> - Inhalation of copper fumes and salts causes metal fume fever and pulmonary fibrosis.
> - Acute oral toxicosis includes necrosis of the gastrointestinal tract, liver and kidneys with resultant organ failure.
> - Chronic systemic copper toxicosis is associated with progressive hepatic fibrosis and failure.
> - Treatment includes D-penicillamine, Unithiol, and N-acetyl cysteine.

REFERENCES

1. Stern BR, Solioz M, Krewski D et al. Copper and human health: Biochemistry, genetics, and strategies for modelling dose–response relationships. *Journal of Toxicology and Environmental Health. Part B, Critical Reviews.* 2007; **10**: 157–222.
2. International Programme on Chemical Safety. Copper Environmental Health Criteria 200. Geneva: World Health Organization, 1998.
3. Barceloux DG. Copper. *Journal of Toxicology. Clinical Toxicology.* 1999; **37**: 217–30.
4. Araya M, Olivares M, Pizarro F et al. Gastrointestinal symptoms and blood indicators of copper load in apparently healthy adults undergoing controlled copper exposure. *American Journal of Clinical Nutrition.* 2003; **77**: 646–50.
5. Walshe JM. Treatment of Wilson's disease: The historical background. *Quarterly Journal of Medicine.* 1996; **89**: 553–5.

21

Gold

PETER LINNETT

Introduction	183	Medical surveillance	183
Properties and uses	183	Environmental risks	184
Occupational toxicology	183	References	184
Exposure limits	183		

INTRODUCTION

Gold has been found in countries throughout the world and, though present as a trace element in many ore bodies, the important sources are South Africa, Australia, North America and South America. Due to its high value, there is considerable recycling and refining of this precious metal.

Many hazards are associated with the mining of gold, including silicosis, barotraumas, noise-induced hearing loss, hand and arm vibration and heat exhaustion, as well as those due to public health issues in underdeveloped countries which may include losses of mercury in the recovery process.[1] Refining of gold may be accompanied by exposure to toxic contaminants, e.g. mercury, cadmium, selenium and lead, depending on the source of the metal ore and processes used.[2,3] Chlorine may be used, for example in the Miller process by which base metals and silver are removed from molten gold as metal chlorides, some of which are corrosive. If platinum is present, highly allergenic chloroplatinates may accumulate in the condensates from this process. Electrorefining uses a solution of gold chloride or gold cyanide. Lead oxides are used in fire assay and in cupellation for concentration of gold. Gold is very dense and, even with small volumes, there are considerable manual handling challenges particularly in handling molten metal and heavy moulds.

PROPERTIES AND USES

Gold, a precious metal and therefore resistant to corrosion, has a high lustre and the depth of the gold colour depends on other metals in the alloys which provide strength and hardness. It is malleable, ductile and electroconductive.

For thousands of years, gold has been valued and used for jewellery and as a monetary unit and for investment. It is applied as decorative finishes on fine ceramic and glassware and on conductive surfaces in electronics. As it is biologically inert, the metal is used for medical and dental prostheses, although gold compounds, such as aurothiomalate, may be used therapeutically for rheumatoid arthritis.

OCCUPATIONAL TOXICOLOGY

Metallic gold is biologically inactive, but gold compounds may be toxic, e.g. gold cyanide used for plating solutions, and cases of dermatitis have been attributed to this, as well as gold sodium thiosulphate. Cyanide salts are used in the extraction of gold and other metals, and fatalities from cyanide poisoning have been reported in these extraction processes (see also Chapter 39, Gases). Aurothiomalate is nephrotoxic and therefore when used for therapy requires close monitoring of the patients.

Splashes of gold chloride during the electrorefining process result in a temporary purple discolouration of the underlying skin which is shed by normal desquamation.

EXPOSURE LIMITS

There is no exposure limit for gold.

MEDICAL SURVEILLANCE

There is no indication for medical surveillance of workers exposed only to gold metal or fume. However, the recovery and refining processes and the manufacture of gold products may be associated with other exposures, e.g. chlorine, lead, mercury, cadmium, and medical surveillance may be appropriate for these.

ENVIRONMENTAL RISKS

Gold being a noble metal and resistant to corrosion does not have an adverse environmental effect.

> **Key point**
>
> - Risks associated with gold are those of the extractive process and contamination of the refining and fabrication processes by other contaminants, such as mercury and lead.

REFERENCES

1. Weeks JL. Health hazards of mining and quarrying. In: Stellman JM (ed.). *Encyclopaedia of occupational health and safety*, vol. III. Geneva: International Labour Office, 2001: 74.51–74.54.
2. Malm O. Gold mining as a source of mercury exposure in the Brazilian Amazon. *Environmental Research*. 1998; **77**: 73–8.
3. Donaghue M. Mercury toxicity due to the smelting of placer gold recovered by mercury amalgam. *Occupational Medicine*. 1998; **48**: 413–15.

22

Iron

PETER AGGETT

| Properties and uses | 185 | Exposure and health effects | 186 |
| Essentiality and metabolism | 185 | References | 186 |

PROPERTIES AND USES

Iron is the fourth most abundant element, comprising about 5 per cent of the Earth's crust and it is the most widely used metal; 90–95 per cent of metal production is devoted to iron for use, usually alloyed with carbon and silicon as steel, in construction, engineering, vehicle and shipping manufacture. Correspondingly, about 90 per cent of mining activity is applied to the extraction of iron, most commonly from hematite and magnetite which are iron oxides. The metal is then released by the reduction of the ores in blast furnaces at 2000°C, impurities are removed by the addition of limestone (calcium carbonate).[1]

ESSENTIALITY AND METABOLISM

Iron is a biologically essential element. Organisms have evolved means of exploiting its two oxidation (valency) states, ferrous (FeII) and ferric (FeIII) iron, and controlling the potential damage that ionic iron species could do to tissues. Adult humans contain 2.5–4.0 mg of iron, males having larger depots than females. Most iron is used in haemoglobin in red cells and in myoglobin in muscles which distribute and store oxygen, respectively. In these compounds, iron is incorporated in haem which in turn is encased in globin, the juxtaposition of which enables it to bind oxygen and carbon dioxide reversibly, according to prevailing gas tensions and pH conditions.[1]

Haem is in other enzymes such as cytochromes a, b, c, cytochrome c oxidase, the cytochrome P450 system, peroxidizes including iodoperoxidases, catalase and sulphite oxidase. Iron-sulphur compounds are in aconitase, aldehyde and xanthine dehydrogenases, NADH and succinate dehydrogenases, and tyrosine, tryptophan and phenylalanine hydroxylases, as well as prolyl hydroxylase. Collectively, these demonstrate the element's involvement with the citric acid cycle, oxidative phosphorylation, mixed function oxidase systems, neurotransmitter synthesis, pyridine metabolism, collagen synthesis and thyroid function, and antioxidant activity. Even so, only about 1 per cent of systemic iron is present in enzymes, the largest pools are haemoglobin (60–70 per cent) and myoglobin (10 per cent). Variable amounts (0.5–1.5 mg) are in depots in the liver and in the reticuloendothelial system, in which iron is bound to ferritin, or to haemosiderin which is degraded ferritin.

Iron has a low margin of safety and, given its environmental ubiquity and its potential systemic toxicity, systems have evolved mechanisms to limit the amount of iron they take up, and to minimize the possibility of free iron causing systemic tissue damage. Thus, in humans, the intestinal uptake and transfer of the element is regulated according to the systemic need for iron, which is to compensate adventitious losses in shed skin and epithelia, hair and menstruation, with the additional need in young people of meeting their requirements for growth. Consequently, the intestine is set to absorb a relatively small amount of dietary iron.[2,3] This regulation is effected by down-regulation of iron uptake into the enterocytes, and by reducing the transfer of iron out of the intestinal mucosa into the portal circulation. Iron that is taken up into the gut mucosa, but which is not transferred systemically is retained bound as ferritin and is lost when the enterocytes are desquamated. These processes are controlled principally by feedback from the liver mediated by a low molecular weight protein, hepcidin.[3] The inherited iron overload syndromes, the haemochromatoses, of which there are probably six, two of dominant inheritance and four with autosomal recessive inheritance, all involve defects in this regulatory control and feedback.[2,4]

In the circulation, iron is distributed by transferrin; this takes up iron from specific carriers at the enterocytic basolateral membrane and distributes it to the hepatocytes. Iron in the Kupfner cells of the liver arises from the breakdown of erythrocytic haemoglobin by the reticuloendothelial system. The systemic pool of iron and its turnover is also tightly regulated, and there is no means of specifically excreting iron. The only way that the body loses iron is through the adventitious losses mentioned above.

Intracellular iron is mainly bound in ferritin. In situations of iron overload, ferritin is degraded to haemosiderin which can be further degraded within the lysosomes. Iron in ferritin can be released when it is needed, but once ferritin has been degraded to haemosiderin, it is only released during lysosomal breakdown of the protein. This can result in 'free' iron in the liver and tissues, which in turn can cause oxidative damage to membrane lipids, proteins, nucleic acids and other components. The resultant inflammation and fatty degeneration may progress to necrosis and fibrosis, leading to liver cirrhosis, and similar functional and architectural damage in the heart, adrenals and endocrine organs. Classically, this degree of overload occurs only in people with one of the haemochromatoses, or in patients who have secondary iron overload from repeated transfusions for the management of defective haemoglobin synthesis or haemolytic anaemias.[2,4]

EXPOSURE AND HEALTH EFFECTS

There is no good evidence that occupational iron toxicosis occurs. However, the estimated carrier frequency for the major form of haemochromatoses is 0.1 and there is interest in the possibility that heterozygous individuals, particularly males, may be at an increased risk of excessive systemic accumulation of iron. However, although such individuals may have serum ferritin concentrations at the upper end of the reference ranges, there is no evidence that they have iron overload, nor an increased risk from occupational exposure to iron.[1]

African iron overload, previously called Bantu siderosis,[2] is an ecogenetic disorder caused by a combination of a genetic defect affecting iron metabolism and increased exposure to iron. The former is a suspected propensity to accumulate iron caused by a defect distinct from those causing the haemochromatoses, and the source of iron is classically the consumption of beer that has been stored in ungalvanised steel containers. However, exposure may also come from iron cooking pots. In contrast to haemochromatoses, in African iron overload, the excess iron is in both the hepatocytes and Kupfner cells, as is seen in transfusion overload, and both heterozygotes and homozygotes appear to be affected.[2] It is not known if occupational exposure to iron is a risk factor for African iron overload.

Chronic exposure to large doses of iron interferes with the intestinal uptake and absorption of zinc and copper. It is speculated that this interaction may cause systemic defects in the utilization of these elements causing deficiency features, such as growth retardation and anaemia. However, these considerations apply principally to children rather than the workforce.[5]

Most cases of acute iron toxicity occur accidentally and also predominantly in children.[6] There are no systematic dose–response data for acute toxicity. Doses in the order of 20 mg elemental iron/kg body weight are said to precipitate intestinal features, whereas systemic manifestations occur at a threshold around 40–60 mg/kg, and exposures in the order of 100 mg/kg body weight are usually lethal. Features include initial nausea, vomiting and loose stools resulting from corrosive damage and haemorrhagic necrosis of the gastrointestinal mucosa. Four to six hours later, the loss of the gastrointestinal barrier may result in fluid loss leading to early hypovolaemic shock and increased systemic uptake of iron. The increased iron load causes multiorgan damage, particularly affecting the liver. This may take 12–48 hours to develop. The shock worsens, and metabolic acidosis, coagulopathies and cardiovascular collapse may progress to death. After recovery, intestinal scarring may lead to strictures and mechanical obstruction.

Treatment[6,7] is with induced vomiting or gastric lavage. These are useful if they can be done within two hours of ingestion. Further management involves supportive measures for shock, acidosis and chelators such as desferroxamine (15–30 mg/kg) with which there is most experience for acute poisoning. Secondary iron overload may also be managed with desferroxamine or with deferiprone.[8]

> ### Key points
>
> - Iron salts can cause metal fume fever, otherwise occupational toxicity is uncommon.
> - A common cause of toxicity is the ingestion of iron salts used as nutritional supplements.
> - Acute high exposures cause severe gastrointestinal necrosis with haemorrhage, hypovolaemic shock and systemic organ failure.
> - Chronic exposure to excess iron might induce zinc and copper deficiencies.
> - Treatment is with desferroxamine or deferiprone.

REFERENCES

1. Expert Group Vitamins and Minerals. Safe upper levels for vitamins and minerals: Iron. London: Food Standards Agency, 2003: 275–86.
2. Andrews NC. Disorders of iron metabolism. *New England Journal of Medicine.* 1999; **341**: 1986–95.

3. Ganz T. Hepcidin: A regulator of iron absorption and iron recycling by macrophages. *Clinical Haematology.* 2005; **18**: 171–82.
4. Pietrangelo A. Hereditary hemochromatosis – a new look at an old disease. *New England Journal of Medicine.* 2004; **350**: 2383–97.
5. Fischer WC, Kordas I, Stoltzfus RJ, Black RE. Interactive effects of iron and zinc on biochemical and functional outcomes in supplementation trials. *American Journal of Clinical Nutrition.* 2005; **82**: 5–12.
6. Mills KC, Curry SC. Acute iron poisoning. *Emergency Medicine Clinics of North America.* 1994; **12**: 397–413.
7. Porter JB. Practical management of iron overload. *British Journal of Haematology.* 2001; **115**: 239–52.
8. Cohen AR, Galanello R, Piga A *et al.* Safety profile of the oral iron chelator deferiprone: A multi-centre study. *British Journal of Haematology.* 2000; **108**: 305–12.

23

Lead

PETER J BAXTER AND HIDEKI IGISU

Introduction	188	Inorganic lead poisoning	192
Historical aspects	188	Investigation of lead poisoning	194
Present-day exposures	189	Treatment	194
The uptake of lead	190	Organic lead poisoning	195
Distribution of lead in the body	190	Evaluating lead exposure	195
Biochemical effects of lead	191	References	197

INTRODUCTION

Lead is a bluish-grey metal with the symbol Pb, atomic number 82 and atomic weight 207.2. Due to the high specific gravity (sg 11.34), ease of casting and fabrication, low melting point (327.4°C), resistance to corrosion and opacity to x-rays, it has had a wide range of uses, such as soldering, printing type, ammunition, brass, piping and shielding against x-rays.[1,2] Inorganic lead has been used in paint pigments, glass and ceramics. Among organic lead compounds, tetraethyl lead was used extensively as an antiknocking agent in gasoline. Because of the health problems caused by lead, its use in, for example, solder, printing type and water pipes, has been replaced by other materials. Use of tetraethyl lead in petrol for cars has ceased in high economy countries.

In advanced economy countries, lead poisoning no longer occupies the predominant position it once held, and few physicians will see a case during their working lifetime. By contrast, in developing countries, lead poisoning is still commonplace, and on a worldwide scale it remains the most common of the occupational poisonings. However, it is essential that physicians who encounter lead workers have an understanding of the clinical effects of lead and can detect symptoms of poisoning at an early stage, as faulty work practices with lead can in some instances be extremely hazardous to health. Concerns over exposure to low levels of lead fume or dust in small workshops are justified and regular blood lead monitoring is usually required, as elevated blood lead levels are easily attained in the absence of sufficient awareness of the hazard lead working can present.

HISTORICAL ASPECTS

Lead has been used for at least 6000 years and is a most attractive metal for cultures that employ simple technology. It is easy to extract from its principal ores, has a low melting point so that it can be cast and moulded with ease, is malleable and so can be worked without undue effort. It can easily be joined together with moderate heat and it resists corrosion by the elements. Moreover, galena (lead sulphide), which was the ore from which lead was derived in antiquity, contains variable amounts of silver. Indeed, it was for its silver and not its lead that galena was first mined and the so-called 'silver mines' of the ancient world were, in fact, lead mines.

During the mediaeval period in Europe, the practice developed of adulterating wines of modest vintage with lead and this must have caused much harm. The pernicious habit persisted well into the eighteenth century and there were also a number of epidemics of lead poisoning attributable to the drinking of wines that were (accidentally or deliberately) contaminated with lead. The 'Devonshire colic' was extensively investigated in 1767 by Sir George Baker who showed, by a mixture of observation and experimentation, that it was caused by lead being incorporated into the Devonshire cider during the course of its production, from the cider pounds and presses which had lead in their structure.

In Europe, the eighteenth and nineteenth centuries were the heyday for lead poisoning and there are dozens of remarkable accounts of the conditions to which lead workers were subjected. Most workers in the lead trades could expect to develop symptoms of some sort and, in the potteries, women who dipped the wares into lead glazes had a stillbirth rate which might approach 60 per cent. Lead poisoning also afflicted great numbers of the general population who were exposed to contaminated water supplies and to adulterated food.

Because of its widespread occurrence, physicians in the nineteenth century became expert on lead poisoning, perhaps none more so than Tanquerel des Planches whose *'Traite des maladies de plomb ou saturnines'* in 1839 was a synthesis of his experience with more than 120 patients with lead poisoning whom he had treated in Paris. One of the features of lead poisoning that Tanquerel described was the blue line on the gums which was described in the *Lancet* the following year by Burton and which has since been known (in English-speaking countries at least) as the burtonian line; clearly, Burton had not read the *Traite*!

Concern about occupational lead poisoning in the second half of the nineteenth century contributed to the establishment of the Medical Inspectorate of Factories. Thomas Legge devoted much energy to reducing the toll from this disease, which he accomplished with considerable success.

In more recent years, much has been written about lead poisoning, but perhaps the most influential work has been that of Robert Kehoe who first put forward the notion that, if the blood lead concentration was kept below 80 mg/dL, the probability of a worker contracting lead poisoning was remote. Although this concept has been challenged in recent years, with the possibility that 'subclinical' forms of lead poisoning might occur, experience has tended to support Kehoe's point of view and it is only in recent years that the maximum blood lead concentration considered safe for male lead workers has been lowered from 80 mg/dL.

PRESENT-DAY EXPOSURES

Worldwide, about 2.5 million tonnes of lead are produced each year, almost half of which is consumed in the United States. Workers engaged in primary or secondary lead smelting may have heavy exposures and they may also be exposed at the same time to other metals, such as arsenic or cadmium. Primary lead smelting is the process by which lead is extracted from its ore, usually lead sulphide (galena). High temperatures are used and, although large amounts of respirable lead oxide fume are evolved, the processes are usually well enclosed and ventilated. Secondary smelting involves the melting of scrap lead to reclaim the metal. This is usually carried out at temperatures below 500°C, with little evolution of lead oxide fume provided that temperature control is effective. The 'dross' (oxidized lead) that is skimmed off the surface of the molten metal may, however, give rise to considerable quantities of lead-bearing dust which may be inhaled or ingested by workers. Lead in any of its forms may be processed by secondary smelting and breaking down lead storage batteries is a main source.

There is still a demand for lead in the building industry. Significant quantities of lead were used in the manufacture of motor vehicles, although the practice has now been mostly phased out. Repairing car radiators involved rebuilding them using lead, but the trade has almost ceased with the introduction of radiators made from plastic, although it lives on in the restoration of radiators in antique vehicles and aeroplanes.

Airborne lead dust, sufficient to cause poisoning, may be produced during the manufacture of lead batteries, paints and colours, lead compounds, rubber products and glass, and during the dry disking, grinding and cutting by power tools of lead. Exposure may also arise from 'sanding down' (rubbing down) and from the application of lead paints and glazes, unless they are low solubility lead compounds. Stained glass workers and roofers who renovate ancient buildings and churches may be exposed to large amounts of fine, oxidized lead dust when removing weathered lead. Archaeologists and paleopathologists can also have inadvertent exposure to the dust when handling old lead coffins. Poisoning from the inhalation of lead oxide fume may occur in the demolition industry where lead-painted metalwork is cut up with gas-powered burning torches. Figure 23.1 shows the use of local extraction and personal protective wear to protect against lead dust and fume.

Firearms instructors and members of rifle clubs have also been found to have increased lead absorption resulting from exposure to lead dust from bullets and lead azide fume from the explosive charge. Some enthusiasts have been known to make their own bullets on the kitchen stove.

Lead compounds, such as dibasic lead phthalate, lead chlorosilicate and basic lead carbonates, are frequently incorporated into polyvinyl chloride (PVC) plastics when thermal stability and high tensile strength are needed. Some exposure to lead may occur during the manufacture of these plastics, although there is no risk from the finished materials.

Organic lead compounds have been added to petrol as anti-knock agents for over half a century. The most important additives are tetraethyl and tetramethyl lead; the former is extremely toxic, but the latter is less so. Exposure may result from the handling of these compounds in refineries or during the cleaning out of tanks that have contained leaded petrol. Because of the strict control measures in industrialized countries, lead poisoning among workers who put the additives into petrol is exceptionally rare. Poisoning has also been reported when leaded petrol has been inadvertently used as a solvent in the manufacture of cheap shoes or as a degreasing agent. A few cases of organic lead poisoning have also occurred in those who habitually sniff petrol.

The International Agency for Research on Cancer (IARC) has determined that inorganic lead compounds are probably carcinogenic to humans (group 2A), and that organic lead compounds are not classifiable as to their carcinogenicity to humans (group 3).[3]

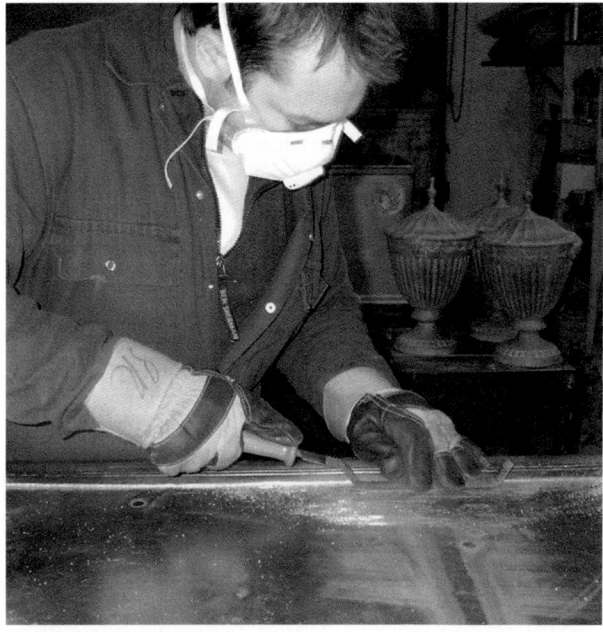

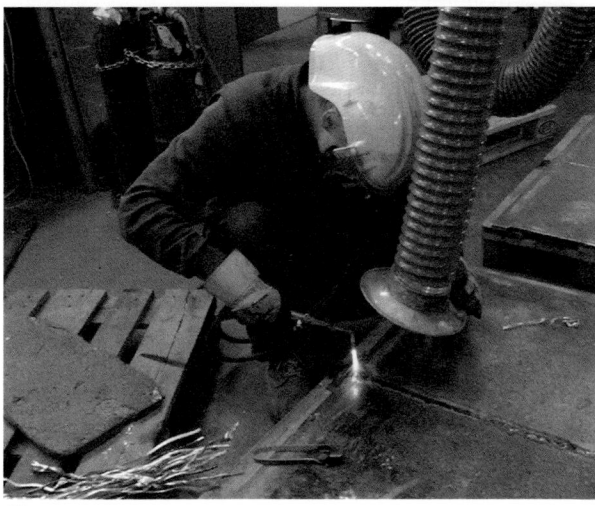

Figure 23.1 Working with lead metal and controlling exposure from (a) lead dust (gloves and mask) and (b) lead fume (local extraction and air stream helmet). For colour plate, see website (www.hodderplus.com/hunters).

THE UPTAKE OF LEAD

Lead can be absorbed through any route (respiratory, gastrointestinal and dermal), but the major route for elemental and inorganic lead is the respiratory and gastrointestinal tracts, whereas organic lead, such as tetraethyl lead, may be absorbed through the skin as well. Lead particles deposited in the upper airways are cleared by mucociliary movements and passed into the gastrointestinal tract where absorption takes place, whereas those in the lower respiratory tract are absorbed directly. Lead deposited deep in the lungs may be completely absorbed.[1] About 6–19 per cent of lead in the gut is absorbed, but it may be higher in children or in fasting adults.[2]

The rate of absorption from both gut and lungs depends upon the solubility of the lead compound in body fluids; lead chromate is highly insoluble, whereas lead oxide is highly soluble and for this reason the toxicity of the chromate is considerably less than the oxide.

At one time, it was customary to give lead workers a pint of milk a day in order to protect them against the toxic effects of the metal. This well-meant gesture would have had little protective effect, however, for the presence of calcium in the gut cannot influence the uptake of lead from the lung and, moreover, the large amounts of lactose in the milk might have had the effect of actually increasing the uptake from the gut. Nevertheless, it was commonly observed that the general health of lead workers improved when they were given milk to drink – almost certainly a comment on their poor diet.

Inhalation is still the major route of entry for those with occupational lead exposure, but the risk from ingestion tends sometimes to be overlooked. Ingestion is often the principal route of entry, particularly where good standards of personal hygiene are not followed. Lead workers who are allowed to eat or drink in their workplace without first carefully washing their hands are unnecessarily increasing the risk they run, as are those who smoke at work. Inorganic lead compounds are not significantly absorbed through the skin, but organic ones may be.

DISTRIBUTION OF LEAD IN THE BODY

Once absorbed, lead is distributed in the body independently of the route of absorption. Most of the lead in blood is in erythrocytes. Approximately 94 per cent of the total body burden of lead is in the bones in adults.[2] Pregnancy, lactation, menopause and osteoporosis may increase bone resorption and may increase blood lead levels. Organic lead compounds are dealkylated by P450 enzymes in the liver and converted to inorganic lead. The main routes of excretion of lead are urine and faeces. Renal clearance is positively related to blood lead levels at least in the range of 25 to 80 μg/dL. The elimination half-lives of inorganic lead are approximately 30 days in blood and 27 years in bone.[2]

Lead circulates in the blood bound to haemoglobin molecules, and substantially less than 5 per cent of the total blood lead is in the plasma; clinicians should therefore request blood lead and not serum lead analyses in a suspected case of lead poisoning. Lead has a long biological half-life and the total body burden increases with time. For the sake of simplicity, the total body burden can be considered to consist of three pools: a rapidly exchangeable pool in the blood and soft tissues, an intermediate pool in the soft tissues, and the skeletal pool. The skeletal pool may be further subdivided into an intermediate exchangeable pool in the marrow and the trabecular bone, and a very slowly exchangeable pool in the compact bone and dentine. By far the greatest part of the total body burden is in the skeletal tissues.

The rapidly exchangeable pool in the blood is toxicologically the most important, although it represents only about 2 per cent of the total body burden and has a biological half-life of about 30 days. The blood lead concentration is the most commonly used index of lead exposure, but it should be remembered that it reflects only recent exposure and is not necessarily related in any way to the total body burden.

Lead is excreted through the kidney and the urinary lead concentration was used for many years to estimate exposure until reliable methods of blood lead analysis became available. Furthermore, there is a considerable circadian variation in excretion but, although urinary lead analyses no longer have a role in the monitoring of inorganic lead exposure, they are the most useful form of monitoring exposure to organic lead. A small amount of lead is excreted into the bile to appear in the faeces, but most of the lead in faeces is that which was ingested but not absorbed.

Small amounts of lead are also eliminated in other body fluids, e.g. sweat, saliva and breast milk, but they are not important routes of excretion compared with urine.

Tetraethyl lead is dealkylated in the liver to the triethyl form which then spontaneously dealkylates to the diethyl form. Diethyl lead is excreted into the bile and is further dealkylated in the gut to ionic lead. Diethyl lead is the only metabolite of the tetraethyl form that appears in the urine.

BIOCHEMICAL EFFECTS OF LEAD

Lead has two important biochemical properties that largely determine its toxic manifestations. First, it has a very high affinity for sulphydryl (-SH) groups and thus is able to inhibit the activity of enzymes which depend upon -SH groups for their proper functioning. Two enzymes that are inhibited by lead are of particular interest. They are delta-aminolaevulinic acid dehydratase (ALAD) and ferrochelatase, and both are concerned with haem synthesis (Figure 23.2).

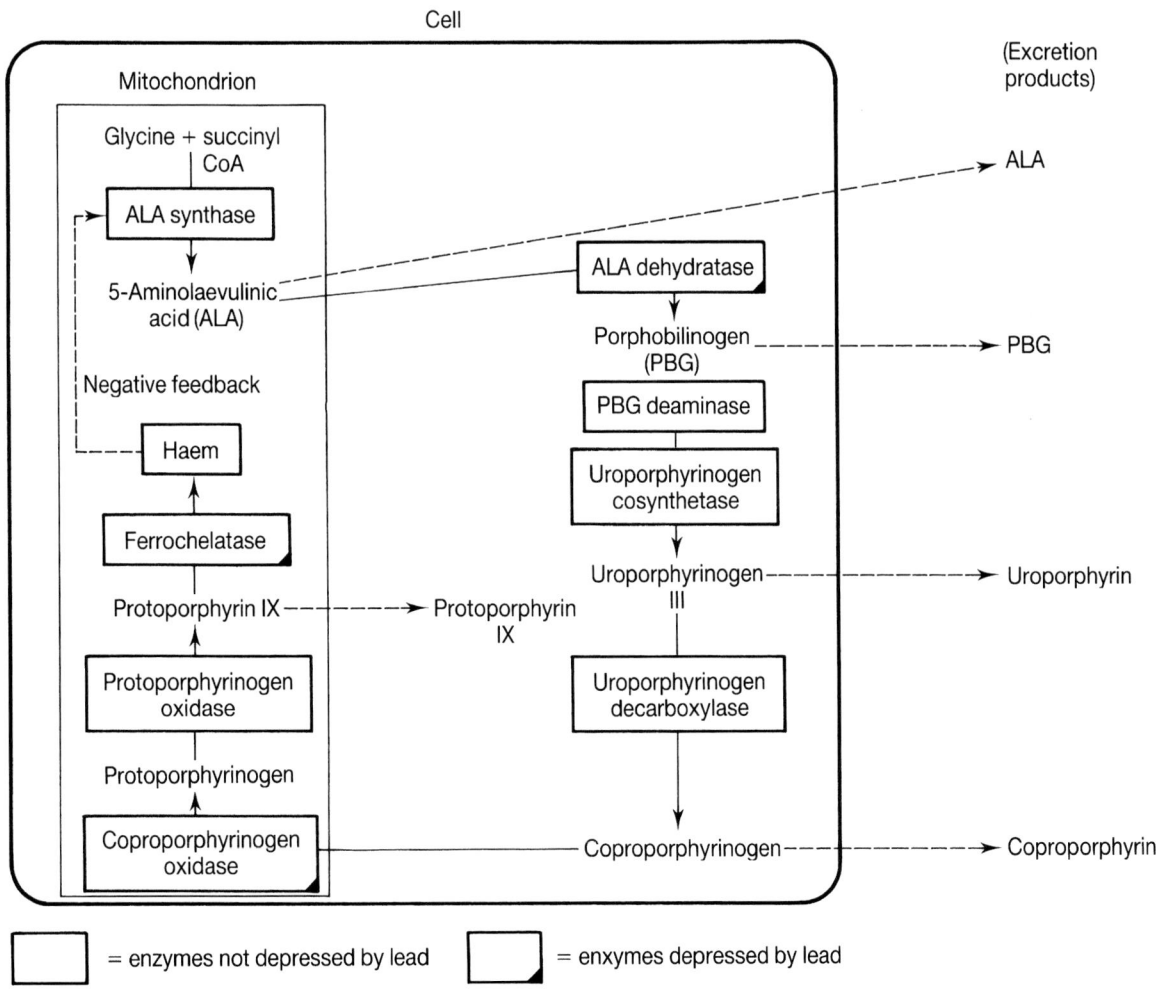

Figure 23.2 Haem synthesis.

Second, the metabolism of lead mimics that of calcium in many respects and it is able competitively to inhibit the action of calcium at some important sites, such as the synapse, and during mitochondrial respiration. It is this feature of its metabolism that determines its bone-seeking properties.

INORGANIC LEAD POISONING

Lead gradually accumulates until critical body burdens are reached, when symptoms may appear suddenly and progress rapidly, although subclinical manifestations (e.g. depression of ALAD activity, reduced motor nerve conduction velocity) will have been demonstrable earlier. The outline of haem synthesis is shown in Figure 23.2, beginning with the reaction of glycine and succinyl coenzyme A to form delta-aminolaevulinic acid (ALA). Two molecules of ALA move from the mitochondrium into the cell where they condense to form porphobilinogen (PBG) through the action of ALAD; from PBG are formed a series of porphyrinogens and porphyrins. The molecule then moves back into the mitochondrium where final rearrangement of the side chains produces protoporphyrin IX. The incorporation of ferrous iron into protoporphyrin IX, through the action of ferrochelatase, leads to the formation of haem. Normal functioning of this synthetic pathway is essential for the production of both haemoglobin and the oxidative enzymes in all body tissues.

Depression of ALAD and of ferrochelatase, results in increased amounts of ALA in the urine and increased amounts of protoporphyrin in the circulating red cells. Because of the ferrochelatase suppression, protoporphyrin forms a metal chelate with zinc instead of with iron, giving increased amounts of zinc protoporphyrin (ZPP). Other stages of the synthetic pathway are also affected and large amounts of coproporphyrin III are excreted in the urine.

The rate-limiting enzyme in this series is ALA synthase, so decreased formation of haem has the effect of increasing the amount of ALA formed. This process produces what is essentially a lead-induced porphyria. Depression of haem synthesis in many tissues (not only the erythropoietic) leads to progressive impairment of their ability to synthesize oxidative enzymes. There may also be competitive inhibition by ALA of transmission by gamma-aminobutyric acid (GABA), a putative brain neurotransmitter. The similarity in their chemical structures is shown below:

$$NH_2CH_2COCH_2CH_2COOH$$
5-aminolaevulinic acid (ALA)

$$NH_2CH_2CH_2CH_2COOH$$
gamma-aminobutyric acid (GABA)

This pattern of effects is unique to lead poisoning and may be a useful adjunct in arriving at the diagnosis. The effects on ALAD occur at very low blood lead levels (less than 20 μg/dL; 1 mmol/L) and somewhere around 85 per cent of the activity of this enzyme may be suppressed before an increase in ALA in the blood is observed. Frank anaemia is usually a late phenomenon in lead poisoning. The mild anaemia of lead poisoning is mainly due to the impairment of haem synthesis, but there is also some evidence that red cell life span is somewhat shortened.[4] This may be due to an increase in the mechanical or osmotic fragility of the red cells which, in turn, may be related to a loss of potassium caused by the inhibition of Na-K-ATPase.[5]

Symptoms and signs of overexposure to inorganic lead

Classically, the patient with lead poisoning presents with a history of abdominal pain, colic and constipation. However, in high economy countries, not many patients now reach that stage. More likely, they will complain of the premonitory symptoms of undue fatigue, lassitude, generalized aches and pains in the muscles and joints with, perhaps, some abdominal discomfort. A few patients have diarrhoea; some may have a bad taste in the mouth. Because these symptoms are non-specific, the diagnosis of lead poisoning is not immediately considered, but a careful occupational history will be an important pointer. The diagnosis is a clinical one and the term 'lead poisoning' should not be used for asymptomatic workers who simply have abnormal biological tests. In the absence of clinical symptoms and signs, the term 'excessive lead absorption' may be more appropriate.

Cardiovascular system

In the British Regional Heart Study, a very weak but statistically significant positive association was found between blood lead and both systolic and diastolic blood pressure.[6] The data also indicated that an estimated mean increase of 1.45 mmHg in systolic blood pressure occurs for every doubling of blood lead concentration. In a recent systematic review, Navas-Acien *et al.* concluded that the evidence is sufficient to infer a causal relationship of lead exposure with hypertension and that the evidence is suggestive, but not sufficient, to infer a causal relationship of lead exposure with clinical cardiovascular outcomes (e.g. coronary heart disease).[7]

Kidneys

Lead is nephrotoxic, and when occupational exposures were considerably greater, renal damage was common (see Chapter 86, Nephrotoxic effects of workplace exposures). The early effects of lead poisoning on the kidneys are directed against the cells of the proximal tubule, but with continued exposure, severe and progressive renal insufficiency may develop with interstitial fibrosis and secondary hypertension. Lead workers formerly had an increased mortality from cerebrovascular disease, but recent studies suggest that this is no longer the case.[8] In adults with lead poisoning, renal effects are not likely to loom large in the clinical picture, but in children, renal tubular dysfunction, leading to a Fanconi-like syndrome, with aminoaciduria, glycosuria and hyperphosphaturia is much more common.

Toxic effects are uncertain over the range of blood lead level 20–50 μg/dL, but when the blood lead level exceeds 50 μg/dL, clear functional or pathological changes, including proteinuria, excretion of enzymes (e.g. *N*-acetyl-beta-D-glucosaminidase) in urine, and a lowered glomerular filtration rate may be observed.[2] It was suggested that a low burden of lead (blood levels <5 μg/dL) may act as a cofactor with more established renal risk factors to increase the risk for chronic kidney disease and the rate of progression.[9]

Nervous system

Lead can affect the central, peripheral and autonomic nervous system. Mild changes in the central nervous system are characterized by progressive fatigue and lethargy. This is often first noted by family members and may become so severe as to disturb the patient's work and social life. It is not unusual to hear the spouse complain that the patient has 'changed'; he or she may lose interest in domestic and social activities and may come home from work, sit down and immediately fall asleep.

Severe encephalopathy with impaired consciousness, confusion and bizarre neurological signs is rare in adults in the developed countries, but is a common mode of presentation of lead poisoning in children. Occasionally, patients with inorganic lead poisoning may have psychiatric symptoms and the condition resembles a mixed affective organic state. It would be very unusual if these were presenting symptoms following occupational exposure, but the possibility that exposure to lead may exacerbate pre-existing psychiatric symptoms should be borne in mind.

In typical poisoning in adults with lead (metallic or inorganic), the major symptoms and signs are abdominal pain, anaemia and muscle weakness (peripheral neuropathy). Abdominal pains are often associated with abnormalities of intestinal movements (constipation and/or diarrhoea, and its repetition), which may reflect autonomic dysfunction. The pain is not necessarily so severe as to be referred to as 'colic'. Neuropathy is predominantly motor, tending to be in the muscles most often used, often asymmetric, while sensory involvement is rare. In adults, the weakness is more common in the upper extremities than in the lower extremities. Extensors of fingers may be first impaired and then wrist extensors causing 'wrist drop' (Figure 23.3), but it is rarely encountered in developed countries today. Muscle weakness and atrophy may not be limited to the fingers and wrist: thenar and interosseous muscles may also be involved. Even upper arm and proximal muscles

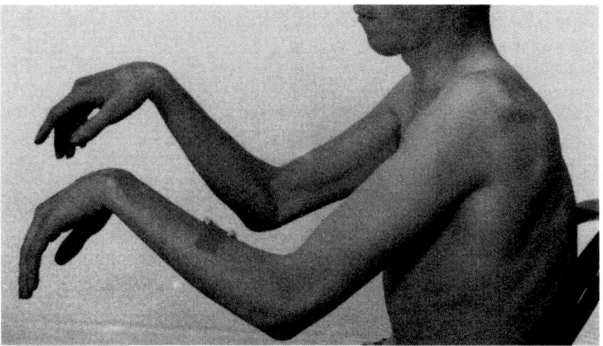

Figure 23.3 Lead palsy in a ship-breaker. He had bilateral wrist drop which took several months to recover. Courtesy of the late Professor RI McCallum.

may show weakness. Weakness in lower extremities, which is more commonly seen in children, may be present as 'foot drop'.[10]

Overt impairment of the brain (encephalopathy) occurs in one- to three-year-old children who have compulsive ingestion (pica) of lead-containing materials, such as wall chips in old, run-down houses. Adults who consume a large amount of 'moonshine' (whisky made in lead-lined stills)[11] and some Ayurvedic medicines may develop lead encephalopathy.[12] Rarely, occupational exposure to inorganic lead causes apparent encephalopathy.[13] Most of the patients have anaemia. The severity of symptoms range from confusion, disorientation to repeated seizures, coma and death.[11] Lateralizing neurologic signs (focal seizures, hemiparesis, positive Babinski sign on one side) were seen in 35 per cent of patients reported by Whitfield *et al*.[11] Most seizures were refractory to standard anti-convulsants, but many of them responded dramatically to intravenous administration of $CaNa_2EDTA$. Changes observed on magnetic resonance imaging (MRI) in one patient, also resolved after treatment with British anti-lewisite (BAL).[11]

Exposures to organic lead (tetraethyl lead) may occur occupationally and intentionally (sniffing leaded petrol).[14] Encephalopathy may appear several hours to weeks after the exposure, with headaches, excessive salivation, vomiting, irritability, insomnia, delusions and hallucinations. Tremor and ataxia are often seen. Death may follow coma. However, in occupational intoxication with tetraethyl lead, once recovery starts, it often takes place rapidly and may be complete within two months.[15]

With much less severe exposures to lead, subclinical encephalopathy may be detected by a neuropsychological test in children. For instance, Canfield *et al*. reported that blood lead concentrations less than 10 μg/dL are inversely associated with intelligence quotient determined at the ages of three and five years.[16] It has not been clarified whether such an association exists in adults. Nevertheless, low to moderate exposure in adults had been associated with symptoms of malaise, fatigue, irritability, lethargy, headache and decreased libido, as well as decreased neurobehavioural test scores.[17] Analysing data from 21 environmental and occupational studies from 1996 to 2006, Shih et al. concluded that there is moderate evidence for an association between psychiatric symptoms and lead dose, but only at high levels of current occupational lead exposure or with cumulative dose in environmentally exposed adults. Further work is needed to confirm if chronic lead exposure is related to a syndrome of mild cognitive impairment.[18]

Reproductive system

Lead may lower the fertility of men having blood lead levels higher than 30–40 μg/dL.[2] Sperm abnormalities may appear when the blood lead level is higher than 40 μg/dL.[2]

Endocrine system

At blood lead levels higher than 40–60 μg/dL, serum thyroxine may be lowered and thyroid-stimulating hormone (TSH) may not be appropriately released.[2] Delayed puberty (manifesting as delayed appearance of pubic hair and breast development) has been found in girls with higher blood lead levels.[19]

Musculoskeletal system

Arthralgia has been recognized as a manifestation of acute lead poisoning for well over 100 years, but is usually a non-specific symptom. Lead also interferes with normal urate metabolism and may precipitate attacks of gout sometimes associated with nephropathy.[20] The condition affects those who consume large quantities of home-distilled spirits, which may contain significant quantities of lead derived from solder within the still – hence 'saturnine gout'.

INVESTIGATION OF LEAD POISONING

There are few clinical signs to aid the diagnosis of lead poisoning. The patient may be pale and there may be some muscle weakness if there is a peripheral neuropathy; wrist drop is one of the classic signs of lead poisoning, but is now rare (Figure 23.3). A burtonian or blue line may be present on the dental margin of the gums. It is caused by bacterial deposition of lead sulphide, is associated with poor dental hygiene and is absent from the edentulous. It indicates lead exposure, not lead poisoning. There may be general tenderness of muscles and joints, and on palpation of the abdomen. The pallor of lead poisoning is not caused by anaemia, but by cutaneous vasoconstriction.

Laboratory investigations are important in the diagnosis of lead poisoning. About a century ago, the appearance of basophilic granules in the red blood cells was recognized as a concomitant, almost as a sign, of lead poisoning. By the 1920s, before the advent of microchemistry, the stippled cell count was used to monitor the exposure of lead workers. That has now been replaced by the biochemical measures described below. Stippled cells are not unique, as was at one time thought, but may be found, for example, in severe secondary anaemia, malignant disease and malaria. The importance of stippled cells today is that the haematologist may spot them in the blood film of a patient 'under investigation' and alert the clinician to consider the possibility of lead poisoning. In lead poisoning, iron entering the erythrocyte precursors is not fully utilized and accumulates. This non-haem iron, together with ferruginous micelles, fragments of damaged mitochondria, and some RNA is believed to comprise the basophilic granules (see Chapter 90, Haemopoietic effects of workplace exposures: anaemias, leukaemias and lymphomas).

A band of increased density may be seen on radiographs at the growing ends of the long bones and the phalanges in children with lead poisoning, but not in adults. This increased density is caused by an alteration in the architecture of the bone and not by deposition of lead. This may be comparable to 'growth arrest lines'. In severe cases, there may be changes in the shape of the bone, which revert gradually to normal once the child is removed from exposure and recovers.

TREATMENT

The basis of the treatment of lead intoxication is immediate removal from any source of exposure to lead. If symptoms are mild, further treatment is unnecessary and the blood lead level will gradually fall towards normal and should be monitored periodically. The process may take up to several months, so blood testing every few days is unnecessary and the clinician should not be anxious provided the patient's condition is improving. If the condition is more severe, treatment with chelating agents should be considered, but should be based on occurrence of severe symptoms and not on biochemical or haematological measurements. In some countries, chelation is carried out simply because the blood lead level is high: there is no evidence that this confers any long-term benefit and there is always the risk of an adverse reaction to the drug.

The agents most commonly used for chelation are penicillamine and sodium calcium edetate. Penicillamine is given orally, 1 g/day for adults in divided doses for five days. If after a few days the blood lead level rises again and the symptoms recur, the course of treatment might have to be repeated. Sodium calcium edetate is used at 50–75 mg/kg per day in two divided doses as a slow intravenous infusion for five days.[11] This will relieve colic within a few hours. With both drugs, the full blood count should be tested at the beginning and end of each treatment period. Because of their nephrotoxicity, the urine should be tested for proteinuria and haematuria, although renal disturbance is unlikely with the doses and the relatively short duration of therapy in acute lead poisoning. During the course of treatment, 24-hour specimens of urine should be taken to monitor the rate of lead excretion; this should be continued for five to seven days after the end of treatment. Blood lead concentrations should be estimated at 48 hours and at five days, by which time symptoms will usually have subsided.

After treatment, it is important that no further exposure occurs until symptoms have completely remitted and the patient's blood lead concentration has returned to an acceptable level, preferably below 40 μg/dL (2.0 mmol/L). It follows that once workers have developed symptoms they must be carefully supervised thereafter. If they require further treatment, it is prudent that they should not have any further exposure to lead.

If symptoms persist or recur, it may be necessary to repeat the chelation, or perhaps use one of the newer chelating agents, such as 3-dimercaptopropane sulphonate (DMPS) or dimercaptosuccinic acid (DMSA), both of which are derivatives of dimercaprol (BAL).

ORGANIC LEAD POISONING

Poisoning with tetraethyl lead causes a toxic organic psychosis and so the picture is dominated by psychiatric symptoms which may appear suddenly. There is nothing in the clinical picture that is pathognomonic of organic lead poisoning and the diagnosis is made by establishing exposure. Occupational cases are uncommon and, as noted previously, usually occur in those who have been cleaning out tanks in which leaded petrol has been stored or who have been using leaded petrol inappropriately as a solvent or degreasing agent – tetraethyl lead is well absorbed through the skin. Occasionally, cases are seen arising from the abuse of solvents containing organic lead compounds.

Tetraethyl lead decomposes slowly in air, rapidly in bright sunlight, to yield needle-like crystals of tri-, di- and monoethyl lead compounds with a garlic-like odour. In their dry state, they may be dispersed mechanically in air to be inhaled or deposited on the skin. Their inhalation induces vigorous, often paroxysmal sneezing, irritation of the upper respiratory tract and, in sufficient dosage, mild organo-lead poisoning. In contact with warm, moist skin or unprotected ocular membranes, they induce itching, burning and transient redness.

The symptoms found in inorganic lead poisoning do not occur in organic lead poisoning, although patients may have some abdominal discomfort and anorexia. It is, however, important to remember that both forms of lead poisoning may occur together, particularly in workers involved in the demolition or refurbishment of leaded-fuel storage tanks, which may be lead painted. The blood lead is usually not raised above 50 μg/dL (2.5 mmol/L) and sometimes not elevated at all, and ZPP and porphyrin levels are usually within normal limits. A raised urinary lead is the most important confirmatory laboratory test.

Poisoning is not seen at concentrations below 150 μg/dL (0.7 mmol/L), but may occur at concentrations above 350 μg/dL (1.8 mmol/L). The use of chelating agents in the treatment of organic lead poisoning is of little value and symptomatic therapy, such as with diazepam, is required. Adequate sedation (which may need to be prolonged) and nutritional support are important and, because sedation is symptomatic, it should be used only as long as is necessary to control symptoms. Complete recovery is usual, but the illness may be prolonged and characterized by periodic and sudden psychotic relapses. The main features of a clinical case are shown in Figure 23.4.

EVALUATING LEAD EXPOSURE

In the United Kingdom and the United States, most lead workers and establishments working with lead come under specific regulations and there are criteria laid down for deciding whether lead exposure is going to be significant enough to warrant this legal requirement. In the UK, the Control of Lead at Work Regulations and accompanying Approved Code of Practice provides detailed stipulations on working with lead, including medical surveillance. Physicians monitoring the workers under these regulations have to be appointed by the Health and Safety Executive.[21] In the UK and other countries, the general physician seeing a patient who has been working with lead should obtain further advice from the statutory health and safety body of their country, or from an occupational physician, when they suspect that the exposure may be causing ill health.

Among the methods to evaluate lead exposure in workers, lead levels in whole blood are the most widely used because of their relative ease and accuracy. The blood lead concentration in the normal UK population is less than 10 μg/dL (0.5 mmol/L). Occupationally exposed workers can have levels much higher than this, but acute poisoning seldom occurs if the blood lead level is below 80 μg/dL (4 mmol/L), as described above. Data on the correlation between the clinical effects of lead and blood lead concentrations have been summarized in publications such as the International Programme on Chemical Safety (IPCS) Environmental Health Criteria on inorganic lead.[22] Abdominal colic and renal effects are unlikely to arise if blood leads are below 100 μg/dL, and the risk of developing significant anaemia is small below 50 μg/dL. As far as severe neurological effects are concerned, life-threatening encephalopathy is unlikely to occur at blood levels below 100–120 μg/dL in adults (80–100 μg/dL in children). There are no firm quantitative data for the development of the classical sign of peripheral neuropathy.

Mr A.T.

Petrol refinery work at .... since 1969. Aged 47 years.

Occupational history

– 1975	Worked on plant extracting sulphur compounds.
1975 – present	On TEL plant, adding TEL into large covered tanks.

Work is carried out in covered workplace.

TEL arrives in drums and is pumped under pressure into opening of tank.

Spills occur 'many times' on to head, face and arms.

Wears gloves, boots and long-sleeved cotton overalls, which are often splashed.

Provided with a 'filter mask'.

Medical history

Symptoms began with numbness in head and hands
Developed: dizziness, headaches and vertigo
Later: blurred vision, especially in dim twilight
Heard strange sounds
Insomnia: could not sleep well because felt disturbed and agitated

Investigations

Date	Blood lead (μg/dl)	Urine lead (μg/dl)
1986	40	173
13.02.89	41	131
18.02.89	11	259
22.02.89	7	655
05.07.89	3	475
12.02.90	33	141
03.10.90	27	130
08.01.91	–	414

Figure 23.4 A case report of a man with tetraethyl lead (TEL) poisoning. Courtesy of Professor WR Lee.

Suspension levels

Lead workers may need to be removed from continuing exposure to lead if the blood levels rise too high. In the UK, there is a statutory requirement for doing this in asymptomatic men with blood lead levels greater than 60 μg/dL (3 mmol/L) and women of reproductive capacity with blood lead levels above 30 μg/dL (1.5 mmol/L), and for young people (under 18 years) with blood lead levels above 50 μg/dL (2.5 mmol/L). All such cases are reportable by the employer to the Health and Safety Executive and poisoning by lead or compound of lead is also a prescribed disease (see Chapter 5, Biological monitoring).

A woman of reproductive age who has a medical or physical condition that would make it impossible for her to conceive (e.g. she is sterilized, or had a hysterectomy, or is post-menopausal), would be suspended at 60 μg/dL (3.0 mmol/L). The reason for this higher level is that 30 μg/dL is set to protect the developing fetus, which does not apply in this situation.

The blood lead should be urgently repeated to confirm the level and the suspended worker can continue working (away from lead exposure) until the level falls, usually over a period of two weeks or more. There is a concession to workers who may have been in the lead industry for many years and who have built up a large body burden of lead (not a likely eventuality in the UK nowadays) which could take a long time to fall below the suspension level of 60 μg/dL. They may be asymptomatic, with normal levels of ZPP. Further official guidance should be sought on their management.

Action levels

Action levels are also laid down which warn the employer that the blood lead concentration is reaching the suspension level and action needs to be taken to control exposure with the aim of reducing the worker's blood lead below the action level. The action levels are for women of reproductive capacity 25 μg/dL (1.25 mmol/L), young people (aged 16 and 17) 40 μg/dL (2.0 mmol/L), and for any other employee 50 μg/dL (2.5 mmol/L).

The frequency of blood testing for lead depends upon the levels found and is stipulated in the information provided with the regulations on medical surveillance.

A high blood lead is not synonymous with lead poisoning, so additional tests may be useful. The ZPP level in the normal population is usually less than 2.0 mg/g Hb. It begins to rise when blood lead concentrations reach the range 35–45 μg/dL (1.75–2.25 mmol/L) in males or 25–35 μg/dL (1.25–1.75 mmol/L) in females. Levels rise rapidly at blood lead concentrations higher than 50 μg/dL (2.5 mmol/L). In lead poisoning, the ZPP level will be above 20 mg/g Hb, often at least one order of magnitude greater. The only other common condition that causes a rise in ZPP is iron deficiency anaemia. It is important, however, to remember that the ZPP does not immediately increase following lead exposure as it depends upon the formation of new red cells, and lag periods of up to two months have been reported. For recent exposures, it is better to measure urinary ALA concentrations. Normal values for subjects not exposed to lead are less than 5 mg ALA/g creatinine (4 mg/mmol creatinine) and the increase consequent upon lead exposure reflects that of ZPP. The lag period is only two weeks and levels in people suffering from lead poisoning will be above 20 mg ALA/g creatinine (16 mg/mmol creatinine). If the exposure period is less than two weeks, it may be possible to have the blood ALAD activity measured: the normal level is greater than 6 European units.

At blood lead concentrations lower than those which cause frank neuropathy, motor nerve conduction velocity, especially of the slower fibres, is reduced.[23] There is no evidence of a dose–effect relationship. Changes in performance in psychometric tests have been reported in lead workers with blood lead levels below 70 μg/dL (3.5 mmol/L). There is almost no consistency in the pattern of changes observed and, although some improvement in test scores is reported following a reduction in exposure,[24] the changes are of little long-term significance and the subjects are not themselves aware of any deterioration in their performance. These changes in the peripheral and central nervous systems are, however, of little value in the diagnosis of acute lead poisoning.

A recent advance is in making a distinction between recent and longer-term cumulative doses. Blood lead represents the former,[25] and a biological marker of cumulative dose is the bone lead level which can be measured by K-shell x-ray fluorescence. The bone (e.g. tibia) is irradiated by x-ray to provoke emission of photons of lower energy (fluorescence) and the fluorescence characteristic of lead is determined.[26] Since most lead is finally accumulated in bones, bone lead is a good index of exposures over a long period and it can be determined non-invasively. Utilizing this and magnetic resonance spectrometry (MRS), another non-invasive method applicable to the brain, Weisskopf et al. assessed metabolites in the hippocampus and suggested that glial changes may be a sensitive indicator of cumulative exposure to lead in adults.[25]

At present, however, x-ray fluorescence is available only in a limited number of institutions. Repeated measures of blood lead over time of exposure can be used to derive time-integrated indices, i.e. integrated blood lead (IBL) or cumulative blood lead index (CBLI). These are mathematically the area under the curve of a graph of blood lead versus time. Such indices have been demonstrated to be well correlated with tibia lead levels.[26]

Kosnett et al. consider that there is a growing body of evidence that establishes the potential for hypertension, effects on renal function, cognitive dysfunction and adverse female reproductive outcomes in adult workers with blood lead concentrations regularly below 40 μg/dL.[27] These and other authors[28,29] are concerned that while the effects of lead at low levels are reversible, repeated occupational exposure (as measured by tibia lead levels) is cumulative in the body and can lead to chronic health effects. Accepting that regulations and their action or suspension levels are an integral part of modern-day controls on exposure, it would nevertheless be prudent for the physician to recommend all employers and lead workers to adopt work practices and control measures that aim to keep the blood lead concentration below 30 μg/dL.

Key points

- Clinical lead poisoning has become increasingly rare in inorganic lead workers in advanced economy countries, but it remains common in other parts of the world. Regular environmental and blood lead monitoring is needed to prevent excess lead absorption by inhalation and ingestion.
- Blood lead action levels and suspension levels are laid down in Lead Regulations in the UK and doctors have to be specially appointed to undertake the monitoring of lead workers. Appointed doctors have powers to suspend workers in accordance with the Lead Regulations.
- Organic lead exposure, e.g. tetraethyl lead, is much less common in industry and clinical poisoning is marked by a toxic organic psychosis and encephalopathy. The symptoms found in inorganic lead poisoning do not occur in organic lead poisoning and sometimes the blood lead is not raised at all.
- In classical inorganic or metallic lead poisoning, the major symptoms and signs are abdominal pain, colic, constipation, anaemia and wrist drop (peripheral neuropathy). More commonly, workers will present with fatigue, lassitude and generalized aches and pains.
- Because of the lack of knowledge on the health effects of lead at lower levels of exposure, it would be prudent to ensure that the blood lead level in individual workers is kept below 30 μg/dL.

REFERENCES

1. American Conference of Governmental Industrial Hygienists. Lead and inorganic compounds: Tetraethyl lead. In: Documentation of the TLVs and BEIs with Other Worldwide Occupational Exposure Values CD-ROM. Cincinnati, OH: ACGIH, 2005.
2. Agency for Toxic Substances and Disease Registry. US Public Health Service. Toxicological profile for lead. Atlanta, GA, ATSDR, 2007. Available from: www.atsdr.cdc.gov/toxprofiles/tp13.pdf.
3. International Agency for Research on Cancer. Inorganic and organic lead compounds. Summary of data reported and evaluation. IARC Monographs on the Evaluation of Carcinogenic Risks to Humans, vol. 87. Lyon: IARC, 2006. Available from: http://monographs.iarc.fr/ENG/Monographs/vol87/index.php.
4. Leiken S, Eng G. Erythrokinetic studies of the anemia of lead poisoning. *Pediatrics*. 1963; **31**: 996–1002.
5. Secci GC, Alessio L, Cambiogghi G. Na/K-ATPase activity of erythrocyte membrane. *Archives of Environmental Health*. 1973; **27**: 399–400.

6. Pocock SJ, Shaper AG, Ashby D et al. The relationship between blood lead, blood pressure, stroke, and heart attacks in middle-aged British men. *Environmental Health Perspectives.* 1988; **78**: 23-30.
7. Navas-Acien A, Guallar E, Silbergeld EK, Rothenberg SJ. Lead exposure and cardiovascular disease – a systematic review. *Environmental Health Perspectives.* 2007; **115**: 472-82.
8. Gerhardsson I, Lundstrom NG, Nordberg G, Wall S. Mortality and lead exposure: A retrospective study of Swedish smelter workers. *British Journal of Industrial Medicine.* 1986; **43**: 707-12.
9. Ekong EB, Jaar BG, Weaver VM. Lead-related nephrotoxicity: A review of the epidemiologic evidence. *Kidney International.* 2006; **70**: 2074-84.
10. Cory-Schlecta DA, Schaumburg HH. Lead, inorganic. In: Spencer PS, Schaumburg HH (eds). *Experimental and clinical neurotoxicology*, 2nd edn. New York: Oxford University Press, 2000: 708-20.
11. Whitfield CL, Ch'ien LT, Whitehead JD. Lead encephalopathy in adults. *American Journal of Medicine.* 1972; **52**: 289-98.
12. Atre AL, Shinde PR, Shinde SN et al. Pre- and posttreatment MR imaging findings in lead encephalopathy. *American Journal of Neuroradiology.* 2006; **27**: 902-3.
13. Kumar S, Jain S, Aggarwal CS, Ahuja GK. Encephalopathy due to inorganic lead exposure in an adult. *Japanese Journal of Medicine.* 1987; **26**: 253-4.
14. Valpey R, Sumi SM, Copass MK, Goble GJ. Acute and chronic progressive encephalopathy due to gasoline sniffing. *Neurology.* 1978; **28**: 507-10.
15. Schaumburg HH. Lead, organic. In: Spencer PS, Schaumburg HH (eds). *Experimental and clinical neurotoxicology*, 2nd edn. New York: Oxford University Press, 2000: 720-1.
16. Canfield RL, Henderson CR Jr, Cory-Slechta DA et al. Intellectual impairment in children with blood lead concentrations below 10 µg per deciliter. *New England Journal of Medicine.* 2003; **348**: 1517-26.
17. Balbus-Kornfeld JM, Stewart W, Bolla KI, Schwartz BS. Cumulative exposure to inorganic lead and neurobehavioural test performance in adults: An epidemiological review. *Occupational and Environmental Medicine.* 1995; **52**: 2-12.
18. Shih RA, Hu H, Weisskopf MG, Schwartz BS. Cumulative lead dose and cognitive function in adults: A review of studies that measured both blood lead and bone lead. *Environmental Health Perspectives.* 2007; **115**: 483-92.
19. Selevan SG, Rice DC, Hogan KA et al. Blood lead concentration and delayed puberty in girls. *New England Journal of Medicine.* 2003; **348**: 1527-36.
20. Batumen V, Maesaka JK, Haddad B et al. The role of lead in gout nephropathy. *New England Journal of Medicine.* 1981; **304**: 520-3.
21. Health and Safety Executive. The control of lead at work regulations. Approved code of practice and guidance, 3rd edn. Sudbury: HSE Books, 2002.
22. International Programme on Chemical Safety (IPCS). Inorganic lead. Environmental Health Criteria 165. Geneva: World Health Organization, 1995.
23. Seppalainen AM, Hernberg S, Kock B. Relationship between blood levels and nerve-conduction velocity. *Neurotoxicology.* 1979; **1**: 313-32.
24. Baker EL, White RF, Pothier LJ et al. Occupational lead neurotoxicity: Improvement in behavioural effects after reduction of exposure. *British Journal of Industrial Medicine.* 1985; **42**: 507-16.
25. Weisskopf MG, Hu H, Sparrow D et al. Proton magnetic resonance spectroscopic evidence of glial effects of cumulative lead exposure in the adult human hippocampus. *Environmental Health Perspectives.* 2007; **115**: 519-23.
26. Hu H. Bone lead as a new biologic marker of lead dose: Recent findings and implications for public health. *Environmental Health Perspectives.* 1998; **106** (Suppl. 4): 961-7.
27. Kosnett MJ, Wedeen RP, Rothenberg SJ et al. Recommendations for medical management of adult lead exposure. *Environmental Health Perspectives.* 2007; **115**: 463-71.
28. Schwartz BS, Hu H. Adult lead exposure: Time for a change. *Environmental Health Perspectives.* 2007; **115**: 451-4.
29. Silbergeld EK, Weaver EM. Exposure to metals: Are we protecting the workers? *Occupational and Environmental Medicine.* 2007; **64**: 141-2.

24

Magnesium

PETER AGGETT

| Properties and uses | 199 | Exposure and health effects | 199 |
| Essentiality and metabolism | 199 | References | 200 |

PROPERTIES AND USES

Magnesium comprises 2 per cent of the earth's crust and as such is the eighth most abundant element. It is an alkaline earth metal and its salts are highly soluble in water. Its major industrial uses are in alloys with aluminium, to produce light and strong materials employed in manufacturing automobiles, missiles, aircraft and ships, and in containers of all sizes down to cans. It is used in refining steel and titanium, and in the extraction of uranium. Its reactivity with oxygen in air is exploited in flares and fireworks and magnesite (magnesium carbonate) is used as furnace linings for the production of metal, glass and cement. Magnesium salts, such magnesium hydroxide, are used as an antacid (milk of magnesia), and the sulphate has historical popular usage in topical applications to wounds and pustules, and as a laxative (Epsom salts).[1]

There are many potential magnesium ores, such as magnesite, dolomite, calcite, talc, serpentine and olivine. Dolomite and magnesite are mined extensively throughout the world. Magnesium is also commercially produced as magnesium chloride by electrolysis of seawater.

ESSENTIALITY AND METABOLISM

Magnesium is a biologically essential nutrient and is the second most abundant intracellular cation, after calcium. Its affinity for phosphate ligands lends it to the stabilization of biological molecules, such as nucleic acids and nucleotides, particularly adenosine triphosphate. The magnesium–ATP complexes and similar nucleotide complexes are cofactors for a wide variety of enzyme activities involving energy transfer, phosphorylation, and the active transport of compounds and cations (e.g. sodium, potassium, calcium, copper, iron and zinc) across membranes.[1]

Magnesium is ubiquitous in the body: 40 per cent of systemic magnesium is in soft tissue and 60 per cent is in the skeleton. At customary intakes (200–600 mg daily), magnesium is absorbed by specific carrier-mediated pathway across the enterocytes, and by a paracellular route driven by solvent drag. About 50 per cent of the daily intake is absorbed, and this is in essence unregulated, though it might increase in response to vitamin D. The element is distributed in the circulation principally (70–80 per cent) unbound, of which about half is ionized; the remainder is bound to proteins, particularly albumin. There is a rapid exchange of the cation between pools. The mechanisms and regulation of the systemic distribution and uptake of magnesium are becoming better understood.[2] Overall, homeostasis is achieved by renal adaptation; with increasing body burdens of magnesium renal clearance of the element is increased and when systemic needs increase, renal excretion is reduced. Magnesium is reabsorbed in the thick part of the ascending loop of Henle, and this is influenced by calcitonin, thyroxin, glucocorticoids, glucagon and angiotensin. On typical dietary intakes, 95 per cent of the filtered load of magnesium is reabsorbed.[1,2]

EXPOSURE AND HEALTH EFFECTS

There is very little evidence of occupational systemic magnesium toxicity occurring in otherwise healthy individuals.[1,3] Excessive intakes, usually of medicines and unlicensed products, may cause adverse effects in individuals with renal dysfunction, and even in healthy individuals excessive ingestion of magnesium laxatives and antacids may cause diarrhoea, which is probably an osmotic effect of the metal cation and of the accompanying sulphate or chloride anions. With larger exposure, other features appear, including nausea, vomiting, abdominal pain, parasthesia, muscle weakness, reduced blood pressure, bradycardia and paralytic ileus. Biochemical features include hypermagnesaemia, metabolic alkalosis and hypokalaemia. The neuromuscular phenomena, and intestinal ileus arise from disturbances of calcium metabolism and they respond to a controlled intravenous infusion of calcium.[3]

Inhalation of magnesium oxide fumes from burning magnesium may cause metal fume fever; classically with fever, chills, nausea or vomiting and muscle pain 12 hours after exposure, lasting up to 48 hours.[1]

Key points

- Magnesium salts can cause metal fume fever.
- Magnesium toxicity is unusual in healthy individuals, but the risk is increased in those with impaired renal function.
- Magnesium salts cause gastrointestinal symptoms predominated by diarrhoea.
- Systemic features of magnesium excess include neuromuscular symptoms, alkalosis and hypokalaemia which arise from altered calcium-dependent functions.
- Treatment is by calcium infusion.

REFERENCES

1. Expert Group Vitamins and Minerals. Safe upper levels for vitamins and minerals, magnesium. London: Food Standards Agency, 2003: 287–92.
2. Alexander RT, Hoenderop JG, Bindels RJ. Molecular determinants of magnesium homeostasis: Insights from human disease. *Journal of the American Society of Nephrology.* 2008; **19**: 1451–8.
3. Kontani M, Hara A, Ohta S, Ikeda T. Hypermagnesemia induced by massive cathartic ingestion in an elderly woman without pre-existing renal dysfunction. *Internal Medicine.* 2005; **44**: 448–52.

25

Manganese

GRANT McMILLAN AND FINLAY D DICK

Introduction	201	Manganism	204
Sources	201	Pathology and resulting central nervous system dysfunction in manganism	204
Characteristics	201	Diagnostic features of manganism	204
Principal uses and sources of occupational exposures	201	Imaging	206
Metabolic activity	202	Occupational manganism	207
Exposure	202	Workplace exposure limits	208
Absorption, transport, distribution and homeostasis	203	Health surveillance	208
Mutagenicity, teratogenicity and carcinogenicity	203	Treatment	208
Acute effects on health	203	References	209
Chronic effects on health	203		

INTRODUCTION

Manganese is relatively non-toxic to the adult human, but exposures can cause serious disease of the respiratory and central nervous systems.

SOURCES

Manganese (Mn), a ubiquitous naturally occurring element found in rocks, soil, water and food, is the twelfth most abundant element in the Earth's crust, about 0.1 per cent of it. It is the fourth most widely used metal in the world in terms of tonnage, yet does not occur naturally as the free metal. Some 46 million tons of manganese ore are extracted annually (2008) from shallow underground mines or open pits – some of colossal size. Ninety per cent is used in steel production. Commercially important ores include those containing pyrolusite (MnO_2), the main manganese ore, and the much less commonly found rose-red to pink rhodochrosite ($MnCO_3$).[1] The principal producers of manganese ore are South Africa (23 per cent), China (23 per cent), Australia (18 per cent), Gabon (13 per cent), Brazil (11 per cent), India (8 per cent) and Ukraine (4 per cent).[2]

CHARACTERISTICS

After mining, the ore must be milled and further processed before it can be used commercially. The metal is whitish-grey in colour, very hard but ordinarily too brittle to be of structural value itself yet, paradoxically, has proved over centuries to be an irreplaceable alloying material imparting strength and hardness to iron and steel.

PRINCIPAL USES AND SOURCES OF OCCUPATIONAL EXPOSURES

Mining and preliminary treatment of ore

Manganese ore must be mined, milled, separated from other minerals, dried, sometimes crushed or ground again, often packed and mixed with other minerals before it can be refined for commercial use. Considerable amounts of airborne dust are liable to be produced during all these processes, with the attendant risk of exposure unless effective dust suppression and other protective measures are taken.

Refining manganese and making iron and steel

The ore must be refined. Pure manganese used for the production of non-ferrous alloys is produced by hydrometallurgical and electrolytic processes. Blast or electric furnaces are used to process the much greater quantities of ore required in the manufacture of basic iron and in steelmaking. In the former, it is added directly to the furnace charge. For steelmaking, alloys such as ferro-manganese (50–80 per cent Mn), silicomanganese (60–70 per cent Mn) and spiegeleisen (10–35 per cent Mn) are made containing industry-specified amounts of manganese, iron ore, carbon and silica oxide. The furnaces are tapped into pots and moulds. After cooling, the alloy ingots may be cut for easier handling and/or are often crushed or milled for transport. This allows better control of formulation during steel manufacture when specified quantities of such alloys are added to the furnace charge to impart the properties (including hardness and wear resistance, stiffness and strength) which equip them for particular fabrication or manufacturing tasks. No substitute for manganese has been found to provide these essential qualities of steel.

Occupational exposures to manganese oxide compounds may occur at each and any of these stages in manufacture.[3] The composition and structure of the aerosol particles in the emissions are complex and vary from process to process. The compositional complexity of these particles is such that toxicological investigations of the kinetics of pure compounds may not easily be associated with the work situation exposures.[4]

Fabrication and manufacture

As welding to join steel components is such a widely used process and manganese compounds are always present in fume arising from it, it is probably now the greatest source of industrial exposure to manganese in terms of the number of people who work with or close to the process. Most steel welding consumables which are melted to form the joint contain less than 6 per cent manganese, but those used on joining high manganese steels – such as those used on railway crossing points or in the process of hardfacing (used for toughening surfaces such as the 'biting edge' of bulldozer blades) – contain much higher concentrations. Selective distillation of the fume in the arc can increase the proportion of manganese in it to seven-fold that found in the consumable. There is further potential for occupational exposure to inorganic manganese and its compounds in manufacture and/or use of a wide range of other products, for example:

- **Manganese chloride**: dry cell batteries, supplemental trace element in animal feed, catalyst for chlorination of organic compounds, precursor of other manganese compounds.
- **Manganese dioxide**: dry cell batteries, porcelain and glass-bonding materials, amethyst glass production, incendiaries, fireworks, matches, the starting material for other manganese compounds.
- **Manganese sulphate**: fertilizer, ceramics, glazes, varnishes, fungicide, livestock nutritional supplement.
- **Potassium permanganate**: produced by the electrolytic oxidation of MnO_2 in potassium hydroxide (KOH) is used as a disinfectant, anti-algal agent, water purifier; in metal cleaning, bleaching and tanning; and as a preservative for fruit and flowers.
- **Manganese ethylene-bis-dithiocarbamate** (MANEB): which is widely applied to edible crops as a fungicide against many foliage diseases and is therefore a potential source of manganese in soil and in food crops.
- **Methylcyclopentadienyl manganese tricarbonyl**: (MMT) is used to improve combustion in boilers and motors and may be used as a substitute for lead as an anti-knock agent in petrol/gasoline.
- **Manganese dipyridoxyl diphosphate** and other manganese compounds have been recommended to replace gadolinium complexes as tissue-specific contrast agents.

METABOLIC ACTIVITY

Manganese is an essential trace element for humans.[5] It acts across a broad spectrum of activities within or as a cofactor for enzymes, such as superoxide dismutase and xanthine oxidase.[6]

EXPOSURE

Exposure to manganese may be dietary, background environmental and occupational.

Diet is the prime source of manganese for those not occupationally exposed. Examples of common sources are grains, nuts, milk products, meat, poultry, fish, eggs, fruits, leafy green vegetables and tea. Water is usually not a principal source. Dietary deficiency disease has not been reported.

Some manganese compounds, for example $MnCl_2$ and $MnSO_4$, are soluble in water and therefore exposure to manganese may result from the ingestion of drinking water which has been contaminated by natural sources[7] or buried waste, e.g. batteries. This may be of particular importance to children's intellectual function.[8]

All humans have background exposure to manganese as it occurs in almost all types of soil. Erosion is the most important natural source of manganese in the air. Anthropogenic sources include the combustion of fossil fuels and emission of manganese from industrial processes. Above average background exposures are most likely to occur in those who work or live near a mine, ore mill, smelter, factory or other site where significant amounts of manganese are released into the air. Almost all manganese-related disease is related to occupational exposures.

ABSORPTION, TRANSPORT, DISTRIBUTION AND HOMEOSTASIS

Manganese compounds may be absorbed into the body through the gastrointestinal tract and the lung, can cross the intact blood–brain barrier[9] and penetrate the placenta.[10] The route of exposure can influence the distribution, metabolism and potential for toxicity of manganese-containing compounds.[11] The respiratory inhalation route is usually much more important than the oral route for risk assessment of occupational exposures.[11,12] A direct neuronal route from the nose to the brain, circumventing the blood–brain barrier, has been demonstrated in animal studies, but not in humans.[13–15]

There is a paucity of information on the rate and degree of absorption of inhaled and respirable particles containing inorganic manganese. Both relate significantly to the respiratory load; the solubility of the particles,[11,16] which is affected by structure and formulation – notably the degree of oxidation; the capacity of manganese transport systems across the alveolar membrane and beyond, including through the blood–brain barrier; and the availability of these systems in the face of competition, notably from iron.[17–19] In animal studies relative iron deficiency has been shown to increase susceptibility to manganese loading in the brain and elsewhere,[15,19,20] whereas iron overloading is associated with decreased uptake.[21] This may have an as yet unexplored practical effect on the risks of toxicity associated with some occupational exposure to manganese-containing compounds, e.g. some steel welders have been shown to be iron overloaded.[22]

Absorbed manganese is rapidly eliminated from blood, initially mainly to the liver which seeks to maintain homeostatic control between absorption and requirement and where excesses are stored in the first instance. It is then widely distributed in the body. Some 98 per cent of excess amounts of manganese are excreted in the bile for disposal in faeces with the remainder being excreted in urine. Homeostatic mechanisms can be overwhelmed by excess exposure and absorption through the lungs and/or gastrointestinal tract and/or by liver dysfunction. This may result in accumulation of manganese in the brain (see below Acute effects on health).

MUTAGENICITY, TERATOGENICITY AND CARCINOGENICITY

Expert review indicates that relatively high doses of manganese affect DNA replication and repair in bacteria, and cause mutations in microorganisms and mammalian cells, although the Ames test does not appear to be particularly responsive to manganese.[10] In mammalian cells, manganese causes DNA damage and chromosome aberrations.

Manganese deficiency can affect fertility adversely and be teratogenic – but this is unlikely to be a practical problem in humans as deficiency is rare. Large amounts of manganese salts also affect fertility in mammals, can penetrate the placenta and are toxic to the embryo and fetus. It has been stated that pregnant women should not be exposed to manganese at the workplace.[10]

Information on cancer due to organic and inorganic compounds of manganese exposure is scanty, but the results available do not demonstrate that manganese is carcinogenic.[10,23,24]

ACUTE EFFECTS ON HEALTH

Acute injury or illness due to manganese exposure appears to be rare. Exposure to freshly formed oxides of manganese may cause metal fume fever (which is described in Chapter 44, Welding, fumes and inhalational fevers). Inhalation of particulate manganese compounds has been linked causally to the development of pneumonitis, an association first reported in a group of British workers manufacturing potassium permanganate.[25] A statistical association was observed between deaths from pneumonia and manganese exposure in Norwegian ferroalloy plants.[26] Iron deficiency, resulting in skin lesions, has been observed in manganese mine workers and attributed to the cumulative effects of high levels of manganese in the drinking water in addition to dust, in the workplace.[7]

Solutions of potassium permanganate >1:5000 are corrosive and mistaken ingestion carries the risk of local and possibly life-threatening burns of the upper gastrointestinal tract.[27] Manganese may be absorbed through damaged skin, for example following burning with a hot acid solution containing 6 per cent manganese.[28] Manganese has also been implicated in the development of allergic contact dermatitis in a worker handling aluminium alloy which contained manganese.[29] The acute onset of clinical neurological or psychotic symptoms was described over 40 years ago in a small number of mine labourers exposed to high concentrations of dust from drilling rock containing manganese compounds.[30]

CHRONIC EFFECTS ON HEALTH

Long-lasting observed effects of overexposure to manganese include asthma and impaired lung function[7,31] and the development of the serious mood and movement disorder termed 'manganism'. It has been hypothesized that manganese exposure, especially during employment as a welder, might also cause or accelerate the development of Parkinson's disease (PD). This and wider aspects of occupational manganism are considered in detail later in this section.

A rare manifestation of manganese poisoning known as Morvan's fibrillary chorea has been postulated in a case report from Germany, but there is no definite proof.[32] One group has reported that there may be toxic effects on the cardiovascular system.[33]

MANGANISM

The clinical manifestations of manganism are well documented, largely due to the work of Huang and colleagues who have followed up a number of workers affected by manganese intoxication over many years.[34–37] It is a slowly progressive, disabling, neurological complex of signs and symptoms characterized by neuropsychiatric and extrapyramidal dysfunction attributed to deposition of manganese in the brain, selectively within the basal ganglia. There is evidence of individual hypersusceptibility (see under Workplace exposure limits, p. 208).

Clinical manganism was first described in 1837 by John Couper, Regius Professor of Materia Medica in the University of Glasgow in Scotland.[38] The victims were workers employed to grind 'black oxide of manganese' in that city's St Rollox Chemical Works, the largest industrial chemicals complex in the world at that time. It was used as a catalyst in the production of chlorine in a new process to manufacture bleaching powder much less expensively than elsewhere. This material was required in vast quantities in the manufacture of linen and paper, two of Scotland's main industries at that time. The savings which resulted gave Scotland a great commercial advantage and greatly enhanced its trade and wealth. Couper remarks, 'the surface of their bodies is, of course, constantly covered with the manganese; the air which they breathe is loaded with it in the form of fine powder, and they are exposed, from neglect of cleanliness, to swallow portions of it along with their food'.

Little more was written about manganism until 1901 when Von Jaksch described similar symptoms, including very marked uncontrollable laughter, in three men who worked together in a factory making potassium permanganate – where they were employed as grinders of manganese dioxide by stamping on it wearing wooden shoes amidst much dust – and attributed their illness to their work.[39] Elsewhere, the illness of four men who had been exposed for several months to air filled with fine dust as they ground 'brownstone' (manganese dioxide) was reported.[40] They had mask-like faces, fell if they tried to walk backwards, 'on stepping downstairs were compelled, after losing control of several steps, to take two or three plunging steps forward', and many other clinical features of classical manganism as described today.

Subsequent reports described similar effects in workers in a range of workplaces and processes including manganese mines, ore crushers and separating mills, ferromanganese and silicomanganese plants, and in welders. Some research groups have attributed subclinical effects to exposure. It has been hypothesized that exposure to manganese may accelerate the onset of Parkinson's disease. These remain controversial areas[41–44] and are discussed under Occupational manganism (p. 207).

PATHOLOGY AND RESULTING CENTRAL NERVOUS SYSTEM DYSFUNCTION IN MANGANISM

The causal relationship between exposure to manganese and specific effects on the nervous system was established in 1919[45] when, for the first time, detailed clinical, laboratory and epidemiological information were brought together.

The brain normally contains very little manganese. Manganism is due to overexposure to manganese, usually over a protracted period, and, put simply, to it accumulating in and damaging principally dopamine receptor cells in the basal ganglia deep in the brain. This provides specific appearances on magnetic resonance imaging (MRI) of the basal ganglia (see below under Diagnostic features of manganism). In contrast to idiopathic Parkinson's disease (IPD), dopamine generation is left intact (as demonstrated by the absence of a good response to L-dopa medication). In consequence, there is dysfunction of dopamine and other neurotransmitter-dependent facilitating and inhibiting chains which exert controls over movement. It is not yet understood how mood and cognitive function are affected.

Following cessation of exposure, manganese is cleared slowly from the brain with a variable time course. Within neurons, it is sequestered within mitochondria and these can clear a manganese load only very slowly. With inhalation exposure, the lungs may act as a reservoir of manganese to be absorbed once external exposure has ceased. All these factors may contribute to the progression of clinically apparent manganism even after cessation of manganese exposure.

DIAGNOSTIC FEATURES OF MANGANISM

It can be useful to consider manganism as having up to four stages. This should not be taken to imply that the disease will present at stage 1 as stages may be bypassed, nor that the stages will form a continuum as there is insufficient consistent evidence to reach a firm conclusion on that point.

Progress is usually slow, extending over years before the full blown syndrome is apparent, with the rate and extent of progression related loosely to the level of dose of manganese received, but subject to the vagaries of individual susceptibilities in those who appear to be doing the same or similar work. These may be constitutional or due perhaps to differences in working and hygiene habits, alcohol intake and/or coexistent liver disease.

Advanced manganism is a chronic crippling disease with permanent disability, particularly with regard to the use of the legs, but does not appear to be life-shortening.

Manganism bears a superficial similarity to idiopathic Parkinson's disease but, as summarized in Table 25.1, can be distinguished from it by careful clinical examination and appropriate imaging investigations.[46–51] Differentiating these two conditions is an important practical consideration for several reasons, but possibly none more vital than preventing further exposure if manganism is shown to be the correct diagnosis as the longer the delay the more likely it is that symptoms will persist or worsen. In practice, in the current state of knowledge it may be thought prudent to at least consider preventing occupational exposure to manganese in all those found to have idiopathic Parkinson's disease as the possibility of an additive effect cannot be excluded and no safe threshold has been established.[52]

Stage 1

Subclinical performance deficits may be the first manifestations. These may be undetectable without special neuropsychological testing and occur at exposures much lower than those at which clinical manganism has been observed. It is important to be able to detect the disease at this stage as this will allow intervention by stopping exposure. Reviewers have concluded that insufficient soundly based evidence of a consistent pattern of significant test outcomes or of a dose–response relationship has been published to permit subclinical identification of occupational manganism in isolation, as part of a continuum of disease or as a basis for health surveillance of potentially exposed workers.[42,53] That said, the published conclusions drawn in some of the studies cast sufficient doubt on the level of protection afforded by the then extant occupational exposure standards to have prompted changes in regulatory action (see under Workplace exposure limits, p. 208).

Stage 2

There is often a prodromal clinical period with insidious onset of non-specific symptoms. It is not seen in idiopathic Parkinson's disease. Diagnosis relies on awareness to include manganism in the differential diagnosis then recognizing a source of exposure through taking and using a good occupational history.

Table 25.1 Key features differentiating idiopathic Parkinson's disease and manganism.[46–51]

Topic	Idiopathic Parkinson's disease	Manganism
Exposure history	Postulated environmental influences, e.g. pesticide exposure	Must have history of excess occupational or environmental exposure to manganese
	May have incidental exposure to manganese	May have regression of symptoms after removal from exposure
Early	Non-specific complaints, including discomfort in the limbs, paraesthesia and fatigue	May be prodromal psychiatric 'manganese madness' (but this stage may be bypassed)
Established	Asymmetric	Not asymmetric
	Resting tremor	No resting tremor
		Speech impairment
		Gait dysfunction – cock gait or slapping broad-based gait
		Balance dysfunction with propensity to fall backwards when displaced
Treatment trial	Responds to L-dopa and other dopamine-mimetic drugs that stimulate the D_2 dopamine receptors (levadopa and the synthetic dopamine agonists)	Failure to have sustained response to L-dopa and other dopaminomimetrics. Response in early stages may be placebo effect. Mixed views on chelation
Imaging	MRI usually normal. Substantia nigra may appear smudged and there may be some non-specific atrophy, but neither are sufficiently specific or severe to be of diagnostic value	May be abnormal with diagnostic bilateral signal changes in T_1-weighted images if concentrations are high
	Fluorodopa PET abnormal with reduced uptake in the striatum, particularly in the posterior putamen	18 Fluorodopa PET scan normal

MRI, magnetic resonance imaging; PET, positron emission tomography.

Symptoms include the onset of general weakness, irritability, anxiety, nervousness, anorexia, headache, sleep problems and confusion. These may be accompanied by or progress to loss of libido and/or autonomic symptoms, such as impotence, bladder and sphincter dysfunction. Specific to the disease, there may be 'manganic madness' and 'locura manganica' – disorientation, indifference and apathy, lethargy, emotional lability such as uncontrollable laughter or tears, impulsive/compulsive behaviour, aggressive/hostile behaviour, bouts of excitability, excessive and incoherent garrulity, hallucinations, illusions and delusions,[54,55] accompanied by heaviness or stiffness in the lower limbs. The emotional symptoms may be the first indication of toxicity.

Stage 3

The intermediate clinical stage is marked by the appearance of more specific signs and symptoms related to dysfunction of the basal ganglia. This may be the first indication if the subtle changes of the first stage have been missed and, as appears to happen in some cases, the second stage has been 'bypassed'. The voice becomes quiet and monotonous; speech is slow and halting without tone or inflection; the face vacant, mask-like, dull and expressionless with a fixed stare. The victim may be euphoric with, perhaps, uncontrolled laughter or crying. Tremor may develop at this or the next stage. It is less common than in idiopathic Parkinson's disease and, when present, it tends to be fine (as against coarse) and is described as postural, intentional or kinetic because it accompanies voluntary movements, rather than occurring at rest.

In this and the final stage, the movement disorder is dominated by dystonia and increasing bradykinesia (movement and gestures are slow and awkward) perhaps with a waving movement of the arms. Forward walking gait is normal at this third stage, but the patient is unable to run and can walk backwards only with difficulty, sometimes with retropulsion. Adiadochokinesia (an inability to perform rapidly alternating movements, such as pronation and supination or flexion and extension) may develop, but neurological examination often reveals no changes except, in some cases, exaggeration of the tendon reflexes.

If exposure to manganese is terminated soon after the neurological effects appear, the individual often recovers but some speech and balance problems may remain. In some cases, clinical progression continues even ten years after cessation of exposure, and after tissue concentrations and T_1-weighted images on MRI have returned to normal.

Stage 4

The final clinical stage may be seen only a few months later. The patient's condition deteriorates noticeably and various disorders, especially those affecting the gait, grow steadily more pronounced. The patient's mind works only slowly. There may be a postural tremor, frequently in the lower limbs but even generalized. As the disease progresses, walking and turning round become increasingly difficult and the handwriting becomes irregular with some words illegible. Soon the patient cannot walk backwards, falling if this is attempted; has difficulty in maintaining his balance with his feet together and in walking downhill, going uncontrollably faster and faster until he has to run and then will fall over if he cannot catch hold of something to stop and steady him. Attempts to counter this unsteadiness may result in a broad-based slapping gait. Alternatively, as a result of increasing muscular rigidity, there may be development of the characteristic 'cock gait' – slow, spasmodic, unsteady, walking or strutting on extended feet and toes, putting weight on the metatarsus, with elbow flexion and a straight spine. Tendon reflexes become exaggerated. Sensorial functions remain normal. At this stage, the disease becomes evolutive and irreversible or may worsen even after withdrawal from exposure,[39,55] although some affected workers may show limited recovery.[55,56]

IMAGING

Imaging of the brain using MRI and, to detail the function of dopamine cells, positron emission tomography (PET) with fluorodopa (a radioactive form of levodopa) can contribute to the diagnosis of manganism and assist in differentiating it from idiopathic Parkinson's disease, although this may be difficult in the early stages.

The arrangement of electrons in the manganese ion (Mn^{2+}) results in it having a large magnetic moment allowing it to be imaged by MRI scan to provide evidence of its accumulation and deposition in the brain. Characteristically, in manganese intoxication, the scan will show a high signal in the globus pallidus on T_1-weighted images, but with no alteration on the T_2-weighted image. It is likely that this reflects recent manganese exposure rather than toxicity.[57] Patients with idiopathic Parkinson's disease have normal T_1-weighted MRI images. Functional imaging of patients with manganism, using 18-fluorodopa-labelled PET, does not show the reduced striatal uptake typically seen in idiopathic Parkinson's disease,[58] so normal uptake favours the diagnosis of manganism rather than IPD.

These typical manganese accumulation images may be seen in patients with occupational overexposure to manganese (even without symptoms), liver disease (and thus accumulated manganese), and those receiving total parenteral nutrition with excess manganese intake. The signals must be differentiated from increased intensities due to other causes such as fat, iron deposits, haemoglobin breakdown products, melanoma, lesions of neurofibromatosis and calcification.

The T1 changes in the MRI in manganism tend to start to disappear within some eight months of withdrawal from the source of manganese accumulation, despite there being permanent neurological damage and even progressing clinical manifestations of the intoxication.

OCCUPATIONAL MANGANISM

The occupational groups in which manganism has been described include miners, ore mill workers, smelter workers, workers exposed to high doses of manganese dioxide in the manufacture of dry batteries, enamellers and potters, those coating welding electrodes, and welders using these and other manganese-containing consumable electrodes or filler metals.

Mining was the original major cause of manganism but, usually, this is now a much more controlled environment where dust exposure is minimized. Cases, usually from mines using dry methods of extraction, especially dry drilling, were described in Silesia,[59] Morocco,[54] Chile,[55,60,61] Cuba,[62] Egypt[30] and India.[63,64]

By 1924, there had been so many cases associated with ore crushing, sorting and grinding in Germany that factory regulations had been modified to prevent the workers coming into contact with 'brownstone' ore dust containing manganese dioxide. Reports of adverse effects of exposure to these and associated processes were seen elsewhere, for example in baggers in Singapore[65,66] and in a range of tasks in mills in the United States,[67–72] notably after concern in the 1930s and 1940s that more than 90 per cent of the manganese ore used there was imported prompted a successful national campaign to stimulate domestic production of manganese.

Whereas studies may not have provided definitive evidence of manganism in workers involved in the production of manganese salts and oxides[73–75] or manganese-containing enamels,[76] it does seem to have occurred, mainly but not always at the subclinical stage, in workers exposed to high concentrations of powders rich in manganese compounds during the manufacture of dry cell batteries.[77–79] Rarely, cases may have occurred in those exposed to manganese compounds while making, glazing or firing pottery and other ceramics.[80,81]

Exposure to manganese compounds through work in smelting and ferromanganese foundries and other steel works has been linked to development of clinical and/or subclinical manganism.[34–37,82–97] Manufacture of cast iron, which may contain small concentrations of manganese, or its recycling, can expose foundry workers to excessive amounts and has been said to be associated with reversible non-specific neurological symptoms of manganism.[98]

Metal cutting and arc welding have been centres of attention as putative causes of clinical and subclinical manganism and/or causing or accelerating the onset of idiopathic manganism. Several thousand lawsuits that allege neurological effects in current or former welders had been filed in courts throughout the United States by 2005.[99]

'Welding' is an occupation that involves highly diverse environments and mixed exposures to numerous chemicals. Moreover, those who describe themselves as 'welders' may actually be more involved with metal cutting or other processes allied to welding rather than joining metal – the traditional and correct usage of 'welding'. This is an important distinction as it is thought likely that, unlike particles from other processes, a substantial proportion of the manganese compound-containing particles in fume from welding have a complex shell-core structure which may seal manganese within the core to a degree which reduces its bioavailability (see Chapter 44, Welding).

Of the 45 workers said to have had clinical manganism in case and group study reports in the literature between 1965 and 2005, a maximum of 29 (and possibly only 15) had been engaged in welding as a joining process.[42] The other processes through which the workers may have been exposed to fumes and dust containing manganese compounds included hard facing and arc burning, cutting or gouging. It has been asserted that only five of the 29 met sufficient criteria for manganism to even just cross the diagnostic threshold and even then they carry a degree of doubt with them.[42]

Individual[100] and group studies[101] have been reported seeking to determine that some workers exposed to welding fume are at risk of developing subclinical manganism, i.e. neuropsychological effects of occupational exposure to manganese. It has been said that some of the studies are flawed.[102] The results of more focused analysis of data[103] do not weigh sufficiently to tip the balance of the conclusions of an earlier meta-analysis that a convincing argument has yet to be made for there to be a causal relationship between occupational exposure to manganese as the source of an individual's cognitive, sensory or motor impairments based on neuropsychological testing or symptom reports.[104] It would, however, be imprudent to dismiss the warnings which have been sounded and not to act to minimize exposure and introduce effective exposure monitoring and health surveillance for those employed in welding and cutting.

As mentioned earlier, a hypothesis was advanced that employment as a welder was causally associated with early onset of Parkinson's disease.[105–107] The suggestion was that manganese in the fume was the causative agent. A number of large case–control studies of occupational risk factors for Parkinson's disease,[108–112] cohort studies of welders[113,114] and literature reviews[41–43] have been conducted. These have failed to find evidence of an increased risk of Parkinson's disease among welders or any other evidence to support the hypothesis that manganese causes Parkinson's disease. In fact, the evidence leads to the conclusion that manganese-induced parkinsonism and Parkinson's disease are distinct and separate disease entities.

WORKPLACE EXPOSURE LIMITS

Neither a dose–response curve for manganism nor a threshold for exposure effects on the central nervous or respiratory systems has been defined. This is due in part to species differences rendering data from most existing animal studies of limited relevance for the risk assessment of chronic low level manganese exposure in humans; the marked variation in exposures to manganese compounds which can occur between different people doing the same job, and differences observed in individual susceptibility to the effects of exposure. Such hypersusceptibility has been reported in infants and people of advanced age,[115] patients with iron deficiency anaemia,[116] liver dysfunction including rarer conditions such as portal-systemic shunt,[117] hereditary haemorrhagic telangiectasia[118] and genetic polymorphism CYP2DL.[119]

In the face of growing concern about the significance of reported subclinical effects, several prudent authorities have reduced their recommended or mandated standards for tolerable exposure to airborne manganese. The American Conference of Governmental Industrial Hygienists (ACGIH) has assigned respirable manganese the threshold limit value of 0.2 mg/m^3 as a time-weighted average.[120] The UK work exposure limit (WEL) for manganese has been set at 0.5 mg/m^3 (eight-hour time-weighted average),[121] while the German maximale Arbeitsplatz-Konzentration (MAK value) or maximum concentration at the workplace[122] for manganese (inhalable fraction) is 0.5 mg/m^3.

HEALTH SURVEILLANCE

There is so far no reliable and practicable health surveillance regime for exposed workers to detect at a very early, hopefully reversible, stage any signs of excessive absorption of manganese or its accumulation in the central nervous system.

Clinical methods are certain to be insufficiently sensitive, although technology, such as laser-based systems to quantify tremor in workers exposed to low levels of manganese, may have been inadequately explored and have undeveloped potential to assist in detection.[123]

Biomarkers and biological monitoring are not yet helpful. Concentrations of manganese in biological samples, such as blood and urine, do not correlate sufficiently with exposure, absorption or effect to permit reliable individual biological monitoring,[124] but may distinguish between exposed and unexposed groups.[125]

Brain imaging using MRI has been suggested as a monitoring tool. This would involve significant time and expense – perhaps too much for it to be used as a screening tool. While research has indicated a possible continuum of appearances from normality to clinical stages in workers occupationally exposed to manganese, the degree of variability is too high for this to be applied usefully.[126]

Neurobehavioural tests do not yet meet requirements. The literature on a manganese neuropsychological/behavioural effect is quite consistent and offers potential for development of a reliable surveillance tool. This would require better structured, more comparable evaluation methods with the proven ability to detect and track changes at an early, reversible stage than are available at the time of writing. A core battery of tests has been suggested for evaluation.[127]

Overall, there is insufficient good quality evidence for recommending health surveillance of workers exposed to manganese. There may, however, be benefit in checking for anaemia in those occupationally exposed as those who are iron deficient are more likely to absorb manganese.[116]

TREATMENT

The management of suspected manganism in an exposed worker should include withdrawal from further exposure and action to protect others. The treatment of manganese intoxication is challenging and therapeutic options are limited. There is no recognized standard regime.

Beneficial effects have been reported with levodopa,[128] but others have found that in true manganism it was not effective at all or any apparent benefit was not lasting.[129,130] It seems likely that the apparent improvement which some authors observed was due to a placebo effect.[129] Indeed, that lack of response may be used to assist in the diagnosis of manganism. Mena reported great improvement in one manganese miner treated with 5-OH tryptophan, but no follow-up data were provided on this patient.[128]

Some have advocated treating severe cases by removing manganese from the body by chelation. Promising results have been reported with CaNa$_2$EDTA[131,132] but, where removing manganese from the body has been achieved, this has not been associated with improvement in signs and symptoms.[133–136] Others have used p-amino salicylic acid (PAS) with some success in animal studies and treatment of humans with severe chronic exposure,[137,138] with a significant persisting alleviation of effects of intoxication over a 17-year follow up of one woman treated.[139]

> **Key points**
>
> - Manganese is an essential trace element.
> - It is the fourth most widely used metal in the world; 90 per cent is used in steelmaking.
> - Many potential sources of exposures with welding steel make it now probably the most ubiquitous.
> - It is relatively non-toxic to adults.
> - It can cause respiratory disease and the specific central nervous system disorder of manganism – as distinct from Parkinson's disease.

REFERENCES

1. International Manganese Institute. About manganese. Last accessed August 14, 2009. Available from: www.manganese.org/about_mn/introduction.
2. Global Infomine. Last accessed January 27, 2010. Available from: www.infomine.com/commodities/manganese.asp.
3. Johnsen HL, Hetland SM, Saltyte Benth J et al. Quantitative and qualitative assessment of exposure among employees in Norwegian smelters. *Annals of Occupational Hygiene.* 2008; **52**: 623–33.
4. Gunst S, Weinbruch S, Wentzel M et al. Chemical composition of individual aerosol particles in workplace air during production of manganese alloys. *Journal of Environmental Monitoring.* 2000; **2**: 65–71.
5. Aggett PJ. Physiology and metabolism of essential trace elements: An outline. *Clinics in Endocrinology and Metabolism.* 1985; **14**: 513–43.
6. Barceloux DG. Manganese. *Journal of Toxicology. Clinical Toxicology.* 1999; **37**: 293–307.
7. Boojar MM, Goodarzi F, Basedaghat MA. Long-term follow-up of workplace and well water manganese effects on iron status indexes in manganese miners. *Archives of Environmental Health.* 2002; **57**: 519–28.
8. Wassermann GA, Liu X, Parvez F et al. Water manganese exposure and children's intellectual function in Araihazar, Bangladesh. *Environmental Health Perspectives.* 2006; **114**: 124–9.
9. Yokel RA, Crossgrove JS. Manganese toxicokinetics at the blood–brain barrier. *Research Report (Health Effects Institute).* 2004; **119**: 7–58 (discussion 59–73).
10. Gerber GB, Léonard A, Hantson PH. Carcinogenicity, mutagenicity and teratogenicity of manganese compounds. *Critical Reviews in Oncology/Haematology.* 2002; **42**: 25–34.
11. Roels H, Meiers G, Delos M et al. Influence of the route of administration and the chemical form on the absorption and cerebral distribution of manganese in rats. *Archives of Toxicology.* 1997; **71**: 223–30.
12. Dobson AW, Erikson KM, Aschner M. Manganese neurotoxicity. *Annals of the New York Academy of the Sciences.* 2004; **1012**: 115–28.
13. Brenneman KA, Wong BA, Buccellato MA et al. Direct olfactory transport of inhaled manganese ($^{54}MnCl_2$) to the rat brain: Toxicokinetic investigations in a unilateral nasal occlusion model. *Toxicology and Applied Pharmacology.* 2000; **169**: 238–48.
14. Oberdörster G, Sharp Z, Atudorei V et al. Translocation of inhaled ultrafine particles to the brain. *Inhalation Toxicology.* 2004; **16**: 437–45.
15. Thompson K, Molina RM, Donaghey T et al. Olfactory uptake of manganese requires DMT1 and is enhanced by anemia. *FASEB Journal.* 2007; **21**: 223–30.
16. Dorman DC, Struve MF, James RA et al. Influence of particle solubility on the delivery of inhaled manganese to the rat brain: Manganese sulphate and manganese tetroxide pharmacokinetics following repeated (14-day) exposure. *Toxicology and Applied Pharmacology.* 2001; **170**: 79–87.
17. Antonini JM, Santamaria AB, Jenkins NT et al. Fate of manganese associated with the inhalation of welding fumes: Potential neurological effects. *Neurotoxicology.* 2006; **27**: 304–10.
18. Aschner M, Aschner JL. Manganese transport across the blood–brain barrier: Relationship to iron homeostasis. *Brain Research Bulletin.* 1990; **24**: 857–60.
19. Chua AC, Morgan EH. Effects of iron deficiency and iron overload on manganese uptake and deposition in the brain and other organs of the rat. *Biological Trace Element Research.* 1996; **55**: 39–54.
20. Heilig E, Molina R, Donaghy T et al. Pharmacokinetics of pulmonary manganese absorption: Evidence for an increased susceptibility to manganese loading in iron deficient rats. *American Journal of Physiology. Lung Cellular and Molecular Physiology.* 2005; **288**: L887–93.
21. Brain JD, Heilig E, Donaghey TC et al. Effects of iron status on transpulmonary transport and tissue distribution of Mn and Fe. *American Journal of Respiratory Cell and Molecular Biology.* 2006; **34**: 330–7.
22. Doherty MJ, Healy M, Richardson SG, Fisher NC. Total body iron overload in welder's siderosis. *Occupational and Environmental Medicine.* 2004; **61**: 82–5.
23. Hobbesland A, Kjuus H, Thelle DS. Study of cancer incidence among 6363 male workers in four Norwegian ferromanganese and silicomanganese producing plants. *Occupational and Environmental Medicine.* 1999; **56**: 618–24.
24. Hobbesland A, Kjuus H, Thelle DS. Study of cancer incidence among 8530 male workers in eight Norwegian plants producing ferrosilicon and silicon metal. *Occupational and Environmental Medicine.* 1999; **56**: 625–31.
25. Lloyd Davies TA. Manganese pneumonitis. *British Journal of Industrial Medicine.* 1946; **3**: 111–35.
26. Hobbesland A, Kjuus H, Thelle DS. Mortality from nonmalignant respiratory diseases among male workers in Norwegian ferroalloy plants. *Scandinavian Journal of Work and Environmental Health.* 1997; **23**: 342–50.
27. Southwood T, Lamb CM, Freeman J. Ingestion of potassium permanganate crystals by a three-year-old boy. *Medical Journal of Australia.* 1987; **146**: 639–40.
28. Laitung JK, Mercer DM. Manganese absorption through a burn. *Burns, Including Thermal Injury.* 1983; **10**: 145–6.
29. Leis Dosil VM, Cabeza Martinez R, Suarez Fernandez RM, Lazaro Ochaita P. Allergic contact dermatitis due to manganese in an aluminium alloy. *Contact Dermatitis.* 2006; **54**: 67–8.
30. Abd El Naby S. Neuropsychiatric manifestations of chronic manganese poisoning. *Journal of Neurology, Neurosurgery, and Psychiatry.* 1965; **28**: 282–8.
31. Wittczak T, Dudek W, Krakowiak A et al. Occupational asthma due to manganese exposure: A case report. *International Journal of Occupational Medicine and Environmental Health.* 2008; **21**: 81–3.
32. Huag BA, Schoenle PW, Karch BJ et al. Morvan's fibrillary chorea. *Clinical Neurology and Neurosurgery.* 1989; **91**: 53–9.

33. Jiang Y, Zheng W. Cardiovascular toxicities upon manganese exposure. *Cardiovascular Toxicology.* 2005; **5**: 345–54.
34. Huang CC, Chu NS, Lu CS et al. Chronic manganese intoxication. *Archives of Neurology.* 1989; **46**: 1104–6.
35. Huang CC, Lu CS, Chu NS et al. Progression after chronic manganese exposure. *Neurology.* 1993; **43**: 1479–83.
36. Huang C-C, Chu N-S, Lu C-S, Calne DB. Cock gait in manganese intoxication. *Movement Disorders.* 1997; **12**: 807–8.
37. Huang CC, Chu NS, Lu CS et al. Long-term progression in chronic manganism: Ten years of follow-up. *Neurology.* 1998; **50**: 698–700.
38. Couper J. On the effects of black oxide of manganese when inhaled into the lungs. *British Annals of Medical Pharmacology.* 1837; **1**: 41–2.
39. Von Jaksch R. *Wiener Klinische Runschau.* 1901; 729.
40. Embden H. *Deutsche Medizinische Wochenschrift.* 1901; **27**: 795.
41. Jankovic J. Searching for a relationship between manganese and welding and Parkinson's disease. *Neurology.* 2005; **64**: 2021–8.
42. McMillan G. Is electric arc welding linked to manganism or Parkinson's disease? *Toxicological Reviews.* 2005; **24**: 237–57.
43. Santamaria AB, Cushing CA, Antonini JM et al. State-of-the-science review: Does manganese exposure during welding pose a neurological risk? *Journal of Toxicology and Environmental Health. Part B, Critical Reviews.* 2007; **10**: 417–65.
44. Perl DP, Olanow CW. The neuropathology of manganese-induced Parkinsonism. *Journal of Neuropathology and Experimental Neurology.* 2007; **66**: 675–82.
45. Edsall DL, Wilbur FP, Drinker CK. The occurrence, course and prevention of chronic manganese poisoning. *Journal of Industrial Hygiene.* 1919; **1**: 183–93.
46. Olanow CW, Alberts M, Djang W, Stajich J (eds). MR imaging of putamenal iron predicts response to dopaminergic therapy in parkinsonian patients. In: *Early markers in Parkinson's and Alzheimer's diseases.* Berlin: Springer-Verlag, 1990: 99–109.
47. Hughes AJ, Ben-Shlomoa Y, Daniel SE, Lees AJ. What features improve the accuracy of clinical diagnosis in Parkinson's disease: A clinicopathologic study. *Neurology.* 1992; **42**: 1142–6.
48. Olanow CW. Magnetic resonance imaging in parkinsonism. *Neurologic Clinics.* 1992; **10**: 405–20.
49. Wenning GK, Ben-Shlomo Y, Daniel SE, Lees AJ. What clinical features are most useful to distinguish multiple system atrophy from Parkinson's disease. *Journal of Neurology, Neurosurgery, and Psychiatry.* 2000; **68**: 434–40.
50. Olanow CW. Manganese-induced parkinsonism and Parkinson's disease. *Annals of New York Academy of the Sciences.* 2004; **1012**: 209–23.
51. Cersosimo MG, Koller WC. The diagnosis of manganese-induced parkinsonism. *Neurotoxicology.* 2006; **27**: 340–6.
52. Haber LT, Maier A. Scientific criteria used for the development of occupational exposure limits for metals and other mining related chemicals. *Regulatory Toxicology and Pharmacology.* 2002; **36**: 262–79.
53. Kristiansen J, Frost P, Lund SP et al. Occupational manganese exposure in Denmark. Proceedings of FORCE Technology International Conference on Health and Safety in Welding and Allied Processes, May 9–11, 2005, Copenhagen, Denmark.
54. Rodier J. Manganese poisoning in Moroccan miners. *British Journal of Industrial Medicine.* 1955; **12**: 21–35.
55. Mena I, Marin O, Fuenzalida S, Cotzias GC. Chronic manganese poisoning. Clinical picture and manganese turnover. *Neurology.* 1967; **17**: 128–36.
56. Casamajor L. An unusual form of mineral poisoning affecting the nervous system: Manganese. *Journal of the American Medical Association.* 1913; **60**: 646–9.
57. Nelson K, Golnick J, Korn T, Angle C. Manganese encephalopathy: Utility of early magnetic resonance imaging. *British Journal of Industrial Medicine.* 1993; **50**: 510–13.
58. Kim Y. Neuroimaging in manganism. *Neurotoxicology.* 2006; **27**: 369–72.
59. Schlockow. *Deutsche Med Wchnsch* 1879, cited by McNally WD. Industrial manganese poisoning. *Industrial Medicine.* 1935; **4**: 581–99.
60. Schuler P, Oyanguren H, Maturana V et al. Manganese poisoning. Environmental and medical study at a Chilean mine. *Industrial Medicine and Surgery.* 1957; **26**: 167–73.
61. Hochberg F, Miller G, Valenzuela R et al. Late motor deficits of Chilean manganese miners: A blinded control study. *Neurology.* 1996; **47**: 788–95.
62. Penalver R. Diagnosis and treatment of manganese intoxication. Report of a case. *Archives of Industrial Health.* 1957; **16**: 64–6.
63. Balani SG, Umarji GM, Bellare RA, Merchant HC. Chronic manganese poisoning – a case report. *Journal of Postgraduate Medicine.* 1967; **13**: 116–21.
64. Chandra SV, Seth PK, Mankeshwar JK. Manganese poisoning: Clinical and biochemical observation. *Environmental Research.* 1974; **7**: 374–80.
65. Chia SE, Foo SC, Gan SL et al. Neurobehavioural functions among workers exposed to manganese ore. *Scandinavian Journal of Work, Environment and Health.* 1993; **19**: 264–70.
66. Chia SE, Gan SL, Chua LH et al. Postural stability among manganese exposed workers. *Neurotoxicology.* 1995; **16**: 519–26.
67. Canavan MM, Cobb S, Drinker CK. Chronic manganese poisoning: Report of a case with autopsy. *Archives of Neurology and Psychiatry.* 1934; **32**: 501–12.
68. Flinn RH, Neal PA, Reinhart WH, Dalla Valle JM. Chronic manganese poisoning in an ore-crushing mill. *Public Health Bulletin.* 1940; **247**: 77.
69. Flinn RH, Neal PA, Fulton WB. Industrial manganese poisoning. *Journal of Industrial Hygiene and Toxicology.* 1941; **23**: 374–87.

70. Tanaka S, Lieben J. Manganese poisoning and exposure in Pennsylvania. *Archives of Environmental Health.* 1969; **19**: 674–84.
71. Greenhouse AH. Manganese intoxication in the United States. *Transactions of the American Neurological Association.* 1971; **96**: 248–9.
72. Cook DG, Fahn S, Brait KA. Chronic manganese intoxication. *Archives of Neurology.* 1974; **30**: 59–64.
73. Roels H, Lauwerys R, Buchet JP et al. Epidemiological survey among workers exposed to manganese: Effects on lung, central nervous system, and some biological indices. *American Journal of Industrial Medicine.* 1987; **11**: 307–27.
74. Roels H, Lauwerys R, Genet P et al. Relationship between external and internal parameters of exposure to manganese in workers from a manganese oxide and salt producing plant. *American Journal of Industrial Medicine.* 1987; **11**: 297–305.
75. Crump KS, Rousseau P. Results from eleven years of neurological health surveillance at a manganese oxide and salt producing plant. *Neurotoxicology.* 1999; **20**: 273–86.
76. Deschamps FJ, Guillaumot A, Raux S. Neurological effects in workers exposed to manganese. *Journal of Occupational and Environmental Medicine.* 2001; **43**: 127–32.
77. Emara AM, El-Shawabi SH, Madkour OI, El-Samra GH. Chronic manganese poisoning in the dry battery industry. *British Journal of Industrial Medicine.* 1971; **28**: 78–82.
78. Roels HA, Ghyselen P, Buchet JP et al. Assessment of the permissible exposure level to manganese in workers exposed to manganese dioxide dust. *British Journal of Industrial Medicine.* 1992; **49**: 25–34.
79. Roels HA, Ortega Eslava MI, Ceulemans E et al. Prospective study on the reversibility of neurobehavioral effects in workers exposed to manganese dioxide. *Neurotoxicology.* 1999; **20**: 255–71.
80. Hine CH, Pasi A. Manganese intoxication. *Western Journal of Medicine.* 1975; **123**: 101–7.
81. Blodgett E. Potters and manganese toxicity. Last accessed October 25, 2007. Available from: www.ceramic-materials.com/cermat/education/139.html.
82. Smyth LT, Ruhf RC, Whitman NE, Dugan T. Clinical manganism and exposure to manganese in the production and processing of ferromanganese alloy. *Journal of Occupational Medicine.* 1973; **15**: 101–9.
83. Saric M, Markicevic A, Hrustic O. Occupational exposure to manganese. *British Journal of Industrial Medicine.* 1977; **34**: 114–18.
84. Jonderko G, Ciesielski M, Gabryel A et al. Psychological and neurological disturbances and an increased accident rate among workers exposed to high manganese concentration. *Applied Psychology.* 1979; **28**: 33–6.
85. Wang J-D, Huang C-C, Hwang Y-H et al. Manganese induced parkinsonism: An outbreak due to an unrepaired ventilation control system in a ferromanganese smelter. *British Journal of Industrial Medicine.* 1989; **46**: 856–9.
86. Iregren A. Psychological test performance in foundry workers exposed to low levels of manganese. *Neurotoxicology and Teratology.* 1990; **12**: 673–5.
87. Cizinsky G, Hagman M, Iregren A et al. Manganese exposure in Swedish steel smelter plants – a health hazard to the nervous system. *Scandinavian Journal of Work, Environment and Health.* 1991; **17**: 275–81.
88. Hua MS, Huang CC. Chronic occupational exposure to manganese and neurobehavioral function. *Journal of Clinical and Experimental Neuropsychology.* 1991; **13**: 495–507.
89. Wennberg A, Iregren A, Struwe G et al. Manganese exposure in steel smelters a health hazard to the nervous system. *Scandinavian Journal of Work, Environment and Health.* 1991; **17**: 255–62.
90. Wennberg A, Hagman M, Johansson L. Preclinical neurophysiological signs of parkinsonism in occupational manganese exposure. *Neurotoxicology.* 1992; **13**: 271–4.
91. Beuter A, Mergler D, de Geoffroy A et al. Diadochokinesimetry: A study of patients with Parkinson's disease and manganese exposed workers. *Neurotoxicology.* 1994; **15**: 655–64.
92. Mergler D, Huel G, Bowler R et al. Nervous system dysfunction among workers with long-term exposure to manganese. *Environmental Research.* 1994; **64**: 151–80.
93. Lucchini R, Bergamaschi E, Smargiassi A et al. Motor function, olfactory threshold, and haematological indices in manganese-exposed ferroalloy workers. *Environmental Research.* 1997; **73**: 175–80.
94. Gibbs JP, Crump KS, Houck DP et al. Focused medical surveillance: A search for subclinical movement disorders in a cohort of US workers exposed to low levels of manganese dust. *Neurotoxicology.* 1999; **20**: 299–313.
95. Lucchini R, Apostoli P, Perrone C et al. Long-term exposure to 'low levels' of manganese oxides and neurofunctional changes in ferroalloy workers. *Neurotoxicology.* 1999; **20**: 287–97.
96. Sinczuk-Walczak H, Jakubowski M, Matczak W. Neurological and neurophysiological examinations of workers occupationally exposed to manganese. *International Archives of Occupational and Environmental Health.* 2001; **14**: 329–37.
97. Bast-Pettersen R, Ellingsen DG, Hetland SM, Thomassen Y. Neuropsychological function in manganese alloy plant workers. *International Archives of Occupational and Environmental Health.* 2004; **77**: 277–87.
98. Lander F, Kristiansen J, Lauritsen JM. Manganese exposure in foundry furnacemen and scrap recycling workers. *International Archives of Occupational and Environmental Health.* 1999; **72**: 546–50.
99. Finley B, Santamaria AB. Current evidence and research needs regarding the risk of manganese-induced neurological effects in welders. *Neurotoxicology.* 2005; **26**: 285–9.

100. Bowler RM, Koller W, Schilz PE. Parkinsonism due to manganism in a welder. Neurological and neuropsychological sequelae. *Neurotoxicology*. 2006; **26**: 327–32.
101. Bowler RM, Gysens S, Diamond E et al. Neuropsychological sequelae of exposure to welding fumes in a group of occupationally exposed men. *International Journal of Hygiene and Environmental Health*. 2003; **206**: 517–29.
102. Lees-Haley PR, Grieffenstein MF, Larrabee GJ, Manning EL. Methodological problems in the neuropsychological assessment of effects of exposure to welding fumes and manganese. *Clinical Neuropsychologist*. 2004; **18**: 449–64.
103. Park RM, Bowler RM, Eggerth DE et al. Issues in neurological risk assessment for occupational exposures: The Bay Bridge welders. *Neurotoxicology*. 2006; **27**: 373–84.
104. Lees-Haley PR, Rohling ML, Langhinrichsen-Rohling J. A meta-analysis of the neuropsychological effects of occupational exposure to manganese. *Clinical Neuropsychologist*. 2006; **20**: 90–107.
105. Racette BA, McGee-Minnich L, Moerlin SM et al. Welding-related Parkinsonism: Clinical features, treatment and pathophysiology. *Neurology*. 2001; **56**: 8–13.
106. Racette BA. Reply to comments on Reference 21. *Neurology*. 2001; **57**: 936.
107. Racette BA, Tabbal SD, Jennings D et al. Prevalence of parkinsonism in a large sample of Alabama welders. *Neurology*. 2005; **64**: 230–5.
108. Tsui JK, Calne DB, Wang Y et al. Occupational risk factors in Parkinson's disease. *Canadian Journal of Public Health*. 1999; **90**: 334–7.
109. Park J, Yoo C-I, Sim CS et al. Occupations and Parkinson's disease: A multi-center case–control study in South Korea. *Neurotoxicology*. 2005; **26**: 99–105.
110. Marsh GM, Gula MJ. Employment as a welder and Parkinson disease among heavy equipment manufacturing workers. *Journal of Occupational and Environmental Medicine*. 2006; **48**: 1031–46.
111. Dick FD, De Palma G, Ahmadi A et al. Environmental risk factors for Parkinson's disease and parkinsonism: The Geoparkinson study. *Occupational and Environmental Medicine*. 2007; **64**: 666–72.
112. Tanner CM, Ross GW, Jewell SA et al. Occupation and risk of parkinsonism: A multicenter case–control study. *Archives of Neurology*. 2009; **66**: 1106–13.
113. Fryzek JP, Hansen J, Cohen S et al. A cohort study of Parkinson's disease and other neurodegenerative disorders in Danish welders. *Journal of Occupational and Environmental Medicine*. 2005; **47**: 466–72.
114. Fored CM, Fryzek JP, Brandt L et al. Parkinson's disease and other basal ganglia or movement disorders in a large nationwide cohort of Swedish welders. *Occupational and Environmental Medicine*. 2006; **63**: 135–40.
115. Cooper WC. The health implications of increased manganese in the environment resulting from the combustion of fuel additives: A review of the literature. *Journal of Toxicology and Environmental Health*. 1984; **14**: 23–46.
116. Mena I, Horiuchi K, Burke K, Cotzias GC. Chronic manganese poisoning. Individual susceptibility and absorption of iron. *Neurology*. 1969; **19**: 1000–6.
117. de la Fuente-Fernandez R. Portal systemic shunts, manganese, and Parkinsonism. *Journal of Neurology, Neurosurgery, and Psychiatry*. 2004; **75**: 1081–2.
118. Yoshikawa K, Matsumoto M, Hamanaka M, Nakagawa M. A case of manganese-induced parkinsonism in hereditary haemorrhagic telangiectasia. *Journal of Neurology, Neurosurgery, and Psychiatry*. 2003; **74**: 1312–14.
119. Zheng YX, Chan P, Pan ZF et al. Polymorphism of metabolic genes and susceptibility to occupational chronic manganism. *Biomarkers*. 2002; **7**: 337–46.
120. ACGIH. 2009 TLVs® and BEIs® based on the documentation of the threshold limit values for chemical substances and physical agents and biological exposure indices. Cincinnati, OH: Signature Publications, 2009.
121. Health and Safety Executive. EH 40/2005. Workplace exposure limits. Last accessed August 24, 2009. Available from: www.hse.gov.uk/coshh/table1.pdf.
122. Deutsche Forschungsgemeinschaft (DFG). List of MAK and BAT values 2009: Maximum concentrations and biological tolerance values at the workplace. Report 45. Weinheim: Wiley-VCH, 2009.
123. Beuter A, Lambert G, MacGibbon B. Quantifying postural tremor in workers exposed to low levels of manganese. *Journal of Neuroscience Methods*. 2004; **139**: 247–55.
124. Smith D, Gwiazda R, Bowler R et al. Biomarkers of Mn exposure in humans. *American Journal of Industrial Medicine*. 2007; **50**: 801–11.
125. Cowan DM, Fan Q, Yan Zon Y et al. Manganese exposure among smelting workers: Blood manganese–iron ratio as a novel tool for manganese exposure assessment. *Biomarkers*. 2009; **14**: 3–16.
126. Lucchini R, Albini E, Placidi D et al. Brain magnetic resonance imaging and manganese exposure. *Neurotoxicology*. 2000; **21**: 769–76.
127. Zoni S, Albini E, Lucchini R. Neuropsychological testing for the assessment of manganese neurotoxicity: A review and a proposal. *American Journal of Industrial Medicine*. 2007; **50**: 812–30.
128. Mena I, Court J, Fuenzalida S et al. Modification of chronic manganese poisoning: Treatment with L-dopa or 5-OH tryptophane. *New England Journal of Medicine*. 1970; **282**: 5–10.
129. Lu C-S, Huang C-C, Chu N-S, Calne DB. Levodopa failure in chronic manganism. *Neurology*. 1994; **44**: 1600–2.
130. Koller WC, Lyons KE, Truly W. Effect of levodopa treatment for parkinsonism in welders: A double-blind study. *Neurology*. 2004; **62**: 730–3.
131. Peñalver R. Diagnosis and treatment of manganese intoxication; report of a case. *AMA Archives of Industrial Health*. 1957; **16**: 64–6.

132. Hernandez EH, Discalzi G, Valentini C *et al.* Follow-up of patients affected by manganese-induced Parkinsonism after treatment with CaNa2EDTA. *Neurotoxicology.* 2006; **27**: 333-9.
133. Calne DB, Chu NS, Huang CC *et al.* Manganism and idiopathic parkinsonism. Similarities and differences. *Neurology.* 2004; **44**: 1583-6.
134. Discalzi G, Pira E, Hernandez EH *et al.* Occupational Mn parkinsonism: Magnetic resonance imaging and clinical patterns following CaNa2-EDTA chelation. *Neurotoxicology.* 2000; **21**: 863-6.
135. Ono K, Komai K, Yamada M. Myoclonic involuntary movement associated with chronic manganese poisoning. *Journal of Neurological Science.* 2002; **199**: 93-6.
136. Crossgrove JS, Zheng W. Review of manganese toxicity upon overexposure. *NMR in Biomedicine.* 2004; **17**: 544-53.
137. Zheng W, Jiang YM, Zhang Y *et al.* Chelation therapy of manganese intoxication with para-aminosalicylic acid (PAS) in Sprague-Dawley rats. *Neurotoxicology.* 2009; **30**: 240-8.
138. Ky SQ, Deng HS, Xie PY, Hu W. A report of two cases of chronic serious manganese poisoning treated with sodium para-aminosalicylic acid. *British Journal of Industrial Medicine.* 1992; **49**: 66-9.
139. Jiang YM, Mo XA, Du FQ *et al.* Effective treatment of manganese-induced occupational Parkinsonism with p-aminosalicylic acid: A case of 17-year follow-up study. *Journal of Occupational and Environmental Medicine.* 2006; **48**: 644-9.

26

Mercury

PETER J BAXTER AND HIDEKI IGISU

Introduction	214	Mercury poisoning	217
Historical aspects	214	Laboratory diagnosis	218
Present-day exposures to mercury	215	Treatment of mercury poisoning	218
Uptake of mercury	216	Evaluating mercury exposure	219
Distribution in the body	216	References	219
Excretion	217		

INTRODUCTION

Mercury (Hg) is a metal that is liquid at room temperature under normal pressure, with a high specific gravity (sg 13.59 at 20°C), high expansion coefficient and large surface tension.[1] Many metals can be mixed with mercury to form amalgams. The various uses of mercury include thermometers, electrical appliances (lamps, switches, batteries), extracting gold, and the restoration of teeth (dental amalgam).[1] It has found its way into the manufacture of energy-saving, compact fluorescent lamps (CFLs), as it makes the bulb's inner phosphor coating fluoresce, and the recycling of these presents an opportunity for occupational exposure, as broken bulbs emit mercury vapour. Mercury is present as inorganic or organic compounds, with the latter containing at least one covalent carbon–mercury bond. Because of its toxicity, the use of mercury and mercury compounds is decreasing sharply. Among the inorganic compounds, mercuric sulphide (HgS) is used as a pigment (vermilion). In the past, inorganic mercury was used widely as a medicine (disinfectant, laxative and diuretic). Methyl mercury, a typical organic mercury compound, was used in the past as a fungicide. Dimethyl mercury may be used as a standard in nuclear magnetic resonance in mass spectrometry.[1] Environmental pollution by mercury has occurred from industrial sources and toxic waste in the past, but active volcanoes are ever present emitters of mercury on land and under the sea.

HISTORICAL ASPECTS

Mercury, like lead, was one of the metals of antiquity and it also has a long history of inflicting harm upon those who use it or work with it. The quicksilver mines in Spain, which the Romans exploited, had an even more terrible reputation than the lead mines, and all the uses to which mercury was put until recent times involved great risk to health. Mercury gilding and the silvering of mirrors were two especially dangerous occupations. Gold or silver was amalgamated with mercury and applied to a manuscript or to glass and the mercury was allowed to vaporize with or without the application of heat. Exposures of artist or artisan were consequently considerable. Ramazzini, in his *De Morbis Artificum Diatriba*, had something to say about both gilders and mirror makers. Of the former he states:

> We all know what terrible maladies are contracted from mercury by goldsmiths, especially those employed in gilding silver and copper objects ... craftsmen of this sort very soon become subject to vertigo, asthma and paralysis. Very few of them reach old age, and even when they do not die young their health is so terribly undermined that they pray for death.

Of the mirror makers, he wrote:

> They learn by experience just like gilders how malignant is mercury when, as is the custom, they coat with quicksilver huge sheets of glass so that the other side may give a clearer reflection. Those who make mirrors become palsied and asthmatic from handling mercury.

Kussmaul's classic work of 1861 on mercury poisoning was based on his experience among the silverers of mirrors in Fürth and Nuremberg. Mirrors were backed with an amalgam of tin and mercury. The working conditions were so bad that he was hardly able to find an adult male in the trade with a single tooth in his head. In addition to salivation and stomatitis, he described reddening of the pharynx (Kussmaul's sign) and ulceration of the buccal mucosa and palate. He described how the condition advanced in three clinical stages: erethism (abnormal irritability), tremor and cachexia. Publication of his findings led to stringent regulations which resulted in the mercurial silvering of mirrors being abandoned altogether. During the nineteenth century, mercurial poisoning was so common among hat makers, who used mercuric nitrate in the carotting of felt – a process in which the hairs obtained from rabbit pelts were flattened and meshed together to form felt, that phrases such as 'hatter's shakes' and 'mad as a hatter' passed into common use. As an aside, the Mad Hatter in Alice in Wonderland almost certainly did not have mercurial poisoning despite the many assertions that he did. The toxicity of mercury became clearer during the eighteenth century, when the use of mercurial ointments to treat syphilis became popular. When the patient complained of excessive salivation or his teeth began to blacken and fall out, his physician could be sure that he was complying with the therapeutic regimen and that large amounts of mercury were being absorbed. Ramazzini noted that the surgeons who themselves rubbed ointment into their patients were by no means immune from its harmful effects.

Mercury is unique among all the toxic metals in that it has accounted for several epidemics of environmental poisoning. The best known of these, but by no means the most serious, was Minamata disease which was first noted at the end of 1953 when an unusual neurological disorder began to affect the villagers living on Minamata Bay on the southwest coast of the most southerly of the main islands of Japan. It was commonly referred to as 'kibyo', that is, the mystery illness. Both sexes and all ages were affected, and the signs and symptoms were those of a polyneuropathy with cerebellar ataxia, dysarthria, deafness and disturbance of vision. The prognosis for the condition was poor; many patients became disabled and bed-ridden and the case fatality rate was about 40 per cent. The elucidation of the cause of the disease owed much to the work of Donald Hunter and his colleagues, who first reported cases of occupational methyl mercury poisoning[2] in a British factory manufacturing mercury seed dressings. Four workers were affected among 16 who were exposed to dusts containing methyl mercury (nitrate and iodide salt). Three to four months after first exposure, they began to have sensory difficulties in the extremities and loss of peripheral vision, with problems walking and speaking. On examination, visual field constriction, ataxia, dysarthria, hearing impairment and sensory disturbance (vibration and two-point discrimination) were observed. In one autopsied case, localized atrophy in the cerebrum (area striata) and cerebellar atrophy associated with profound loss of granular cells were found.[3] It was subsequently suggested by Douglas McAlpine that Minamata disease resembled this syndrome and a source of organic mercury should be sought. It was eventually confirmed that the fishermen and their families who were the main victims of the disease, had been intoxicated with methyl mercury due to the consumption of contaminated fish.[4] The first case was officially reported in 1956 from the Minamata Bay area (Kumamoto Prefecture), and in 1964–65 in the Agano River basin (Niigata Prefecture) where the pollution was less severe than in the Minamata area. In each area, it was caused by discharges of methyl mercury into the sea from a factory. Tsubaki,[5] who examined many patients in the Niigata area, emphasized the following as important symptoms and signs: sensory impairment (bilateral, marked in extremities), ataxia and dysequilibrium, weakness, perioral sensory impairment, abnormalities in eye movement, narrowing of the visual fields and hearing difficulty.

Importantly, there was a cluster of births of children with cerebral palsy in mothers suffering from Minamata disease – clear evidence of a teratogenic effect of methyl mercury.

The largest outbreak of organic mercury poisoning occurred in 1971–72, when at least 6000 people were poisoned and 459 persons died in Iraq, where in the midst of a famine they had knowingly consumed toxic wheat and barley seeds that had been treated with methyl mercury.[6] In the United States, a family was poisoned by eating contaminated meat from a hog which had been inadvertently fed on seed grains dressed with methyl mercury.[7] Four children showed very severe neurological disturbances 22 years later. The two eldest had cortical blindness or constricted visual fields, diminished hand proprioception, choreoathetosis and attention deficits. The two youngest suffered from quadriplegia, blindness and severe mental retardation. One of them, who was exposed at age 8 and died aged 30, had brain mercury levels over 50 times those of the control patients, whereas mercury levels in systemic organs were comparable with controls. These and other similar incidents have led to the use of organic mercury as a seed dressing being prohibited in most countries.

PRESENT-DAY EXPOSURES TO MERCURY

The toxicity of mercury is so well known nowadays in high economy countries that exposure to mercury metal and its compounds in industrial processes has become sufficiently well controlled to pose few problems to the limited number of workers involved in its use. Mercury is still a serious hazard in developing countries, for example in gold extraction in remote prospecting areas using liquid mercury (vapour hazard). Inadvertent high exposure to workers can still occur through a failure in control measures or awareness, or in the general population as a result of accidental contamination of offices or homes, as well as to a failure to adequately decontaminate industrial buildings or laboratories before being put to other uses.[8–10]

Next to dietary sources, such as fish, the main source of exposure to mercury in the general population is from dental amalgam.[11] Mercury vapour is released from dental amalgam fillings into the oral cavity from where it is inhaled and absorbed by the lungs. Blood and urine mercury concentrations in amalgam bearers are usually below one-tenth of the critical values described above and inside the range found in the general population, although small increases are detectable after dental procedures involving fillings.[12] However, some people have been found to have high mercury uptake from their fillings equivalent to the work exposure limit (see below), when removal of the fillings has been recommended.[13] Thus, dental fillings may have a bearing on the monitoring of workers and others exposed to mercury vapour or mercury compounds at work.

Mixing of dental amalgams is no longer done by hand and should no longer present a mercury hazard in modern, well-equipped dental surgeries. Pregnant dentists or dental nurses do not need to be restricted from dental practice as long as best occupational hygiene practice is followed.[14]

UPTAKE OF MERCURY

Mercury is encountered in many different forms, as the metal, and as mercurous, mercuric or organic compounds, the last of which are grouped into alkyl, aryl and alkoxyl categories. The different forms have very different properties which help to determine their uptake, distribution and toxicity; the elemental, inorganic and alkyl forms are much the most toxic.

Mercury and its compounds generally cross biological membranes with ease and they may be absorbed by any of the three common routes: inhalation, ingestion and the skin.

Inhalation

Mercury vapour and compounds are well absorbed from the lung (80 per cent of inhaled mercury is absorbed), and so the inhalation of vapour, aerosol or dust poses a high risk. This applies particularly to the metal itself which has a relatively high vapour pressure at room temperature: saturated air contains 20 mg/m^3 of mercury (2.37 ppm) at 25°C, i.e. 1000 times the UK workplace exposure limit. Few of those who regularly come into contact with elemental mercury, such as laboratory workers and dental nurses, realize that the metal vaporizes at room temperature and is readily absorbed through the lungs. Compounds of mercury are also rapidly absorbed through the lungs.

Ingestion

The organic compounds of mercury are more readily absorbed from the gut than are the inorganic. Metallic mercury may be swallowed safely because only 0.01 per cent of an ingested dose is absorbed. Ingested methyl and phenyl mercury are taken up quickly and virtually completely. About

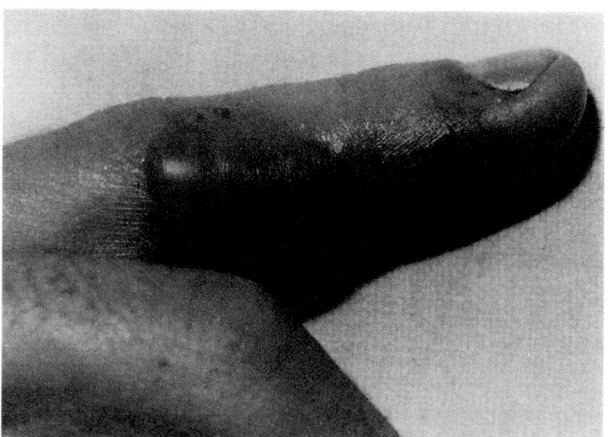

Figure 26.1 Blister on the finger of a chemist who worked with butyl mercury nitrate. Courtesy of the late Professor RI McCallum.

10 per cent of an ingested dose of mercuric salts is absorbed, but uptake of mercurous salts is about 80 per cent less. Many inorganic and aryl compounds including bichloride, nitrate, phenyl and butyl salts are corrosive when swallowed.

The skin

Mercury vapour is not absorbed through the skin, but soluble and insoluble mercury compounds, both inorganic and organic, appear to be absorbed at similar rates. Absorption is, however, too slow to cause acute poisoning but may lead to chronic intoxication.

Some organic mercury compounds, such as phenyl or butyl salts, can cause chemical burns and blistering (Figure 26.1).

DISTRIBUTION IN THE BODY

After uptake, any form of mercury may undergo chemical changes, such as oxidation and reduction. For instance, metallic mercury is oxidized in erythrocytes and lungs and converted into a divalent cation (Hg^{++}). Absorbed inorganic mercury compound may be reduced and excreted in the expired air as metallic mercury. Organic mercury compounds, such as phenyl mercury and alkoxy mercury, may be rapidly converted to Hg^{++}.[15] Methyl mercury entered into the brain may be demethylated into the inorganic form and may persist within the brain over a long period.[16,17]

Mercury has a great affinity for thiol groups and is distributed bound to sulphur-containing ligands. Its affinity for thiol groups explains a number of its toxic effects for, like lead, it is able to combine with, and inhibit the action of, enzymes containing -SH groups. Following the absorption of elemental mercury, it is transformed intracellularly into the divalent ionic form; the aryl, alkoxy and alkyl compounds also tend to release divalent mercuric ions in the tissues. In the blood, inorganic mercury is distributed almost equally between the red cells and the plasma, whereas the alkyl compounds (such as methyl mercury) are concentrated 10- or 20-fold in the red cells. The principal target organs for mercury are the central nervous system and the kidney. Within the kidney, mercury binds to metallothionein and the resultant metal protein complex may protect against the toxic effects of the free metal, and only when the metallothionein receptors are saturated does renal damage occur. The blood–brain barrier is crossed rapidly and readily by elemental mercury and by alkyl mercury compounds, but not so well by inorganic compounds. The post-mortem findings in a man who developed classical signs of mercurialism after working for 18 months filling mercury thermometers, and who died 16 years later after a slow but incomplete recovery, are interesting. While there was no histological evidence of mercury toxicity, mercury was detected in lysosomal dense bodies in many nerve cells. It is not clear, however, how the presence of neuronal mercury was related to the mental and psychological state of the patient.[18]

By contrast, inorganic mercury accumulates rapidly in the cortex of the kidney, but more slowly in the brain. These differences in distribution obviously contribute to the different toxic effects exerted by the various mercury compounds, but it is not merely a matter of tissue concentration. Methyl mercury concentrations in the kidney, for example, are considerably higher than those in the central nervous system but, whereas the brain may be severely affected in methyl mercury poisoning, renal damage occurs only rarely.[19]

EXCRETION

Mercury is excreted in the urine and faeces and may also be found in the sweat, saliva and breast milk. The concentration of mercury in breast milk may be as much as 5 per cent of the concentration in the blood and so be a risk to breast-fed infants of mothers who are exposed to mercury. Organomercury compounds are excreted in bile and reabsorbed from the gut. The half-life of mercury compounds in the body is about 70 days; thus, the excretion of absorbed material is slow and there is a tendency for the metal to accumulate with time. The urinary excretion of mercury shows considerable circadian variation and urinary concentrations are not always a good indicator of acute exposure, but are used for the monitoring of exposed workers over a period of time. Blood mercury concentration, on the other hand, reflects absorption well, once equilibrium has been achieved,[20] and is a suitable marker for acute exposure.

MERCURY POISONING

Acute poisoning

Acute poisoning usually results from the accidental or deliberate ingestion of mercury compounds and seldom from occupational exposure. The toxicity of inorganic compounds is proportional to their solubility in the gastric juices and, for example, the ingestion of less than 100 mg of mercuric chloride (corrosive sublimate) may cause severe symptoms. Soon after taking it, vomiting and abdominal pain may develop and watery diarrhoea, haematemesis, and then shock cause death. Even without these, oliguria (renal tubular dysfunction) associated with unconsciousness may occur in 48 hours. In severe cases, acute papillary necrosis will occur. A chemical colitis may develop after 24–72 hours with the passage of bloody diarrhoea containing mucosal slough. There may be shock, oedema, tremor and ataxia. Specific diagnostic tests are of limited value, but will demonstrate raised blood mercury levels and increased urinary and faecal excretion. Poisoning from the inhalation of large amounts of mercury, including the vapour from exploding mercury lamps, may cause an acute, life-threatening chemical pneumonitis with cough, dyspnoea, retrosternal pain, basal, late-inspiratory crackles, abnormal blood gases and patchy shadowing on chest radiograph. In severe cases, there may be fever, expectoration of blood-stained sputum and pulmonary oedema.

Chronic poisoning

The classic symptoms of chronic mercury poisoning (noted by Kussmaul) are tremor, gingivitis and erethism (Greek *erethismos*, irritate). In addition, there may be evidence of renal damage and organic damage to the central nervous system. The earliest findings are usually gingivitis, hypersalivation (mercurial ptyalism) and an unpleasant, bitter, metallic taste in the mouth. A bluish line on the dental margin of the gums, similar to that seen in lead workers, and a slate-grey or reddish, punctate pigmentation of the buccal mucosa are sometimes described, but rarely seen. Gingivitis is most marked in those with poor oral hygiene and may be severe enough to cause loosening or loss of teeth. Tremor, generally considered to be the first neurological indication of poisoning by elemental mercury or its inorganic compounds, is usually present at rest especially in the hands. It may be slight and accompanied by mild motor retardation (mercurial micro-parkinsonism). There is often an intentional component to the tremor, resembling that seen in cerebellar disease, which may seriously impair the ability to carry out fine and complex movements, such as handwriting. The tremor in mercury poisoning may fluctuate in severity and be accompanied by ataxia resulting in difficulties in walking and in speaking. In poisoning with methyl mercury, cerebellar ataxia and dysarthria predominate, sometimes with constriction of the visual fields as the result of damage to the visual cortex. The clinical picture may resemble parkinsonism, multiple sclerosis or cerebellar disease, but nystagmus is not a feature. Inability to release an object gripped in the hand has also been reported but, unlike the situation found in myotonia, it persists after repeated movements. When the term 'erethism' was first coined, towards the end of the eighteenth century, it was used to describe the whole range of symptoms of mercury poisoning, but it is now reserved for the psychogenic manifestations. It is a form of toxic organic psychosis characterized by excessive timidity, morbid irritability, mental hyperactivity and outbursts of temper. There may be other features such as impairment of memory, difficulty in concentration, depression and somnolence. Short-term memory may also be slightly impaired in workers exposed to mercury who are otherwise normal.[21] Mercury poisoning may present as a peripheral neuropathy which is predominantly sensory and is most common in those with organic mercury poisoning. Prolonged distal latencies in nerve conduction have been reported in some asymptomatic mercury workers and the neurophysiological changes correlate with time-integrated urinary mercury concentrations.[22] In advanced cases, there are paraesthesiae of the extremities and around the mouth. In fatal cases, the dorsal and ventral roots of the spinal cord have been found to have undergone axonal degeneration and to have suffered a loss of myelin (see Chapter 87, Neurotoxic effects of workplace exposures).[23]

The usual effect on the kidneys is tubular damage. Necrosis is more common in inorganic than organic poisoning. The glomerulus may also be damaged, leading to albuminuria in workers who have been exposed to mercury for many years. Rarely, a nephrotic syndrome may present as a manifestation of inorganic mercury poisoning.[24] Poisoning by mercury or a compound of mercury is a prescribed disease in the United Kingdom (see Chapter 8, Compensation scheme).

LABORATORY DIAGNOSIS

The finding of mercury in the urine or blood of those exposed to elemental mercury or to its inorganic or organic compounds confirms that absorption has occurred. Blood mercury concentrations in those exposed to methyl mercury are a good index of exposure. If poisoning has occurred, the blood mercury concentration may be well above 95 μmol/L and the urinary level above 120 nmol/mmol creatinine for inorganic compounds and 15 nmol/mmol creatinine for organic compounds.

Diagnosis of organic mercury poisoning depends on its characteristic clinical picture and diagnostic radiology, especially magnetic resonance imaging (MRI).[25] In cases of methyl mercury or dimethylmercury intoxication, MRI may reveal atrophic changes in the occipital lobe, cerebellum and post-Rolandic region in the cerebrum.

TREATMENT OF MERCURY POISONING

Acute poisoning by elemental, inorganic and organic mercury compounds is a medical emergency and is dealt with in texts on poisoning. The purpose of treatment is to encourage the excretion of mercury and to limit gastrointestinal and renal damage. First-aid treatment involves the administration of four glasses of milk as an emulsient. If there is corrosive damage to the oropharynx as in the case of mercurous and mercuric chlorides, attention must be paid to the patency of the airway. Emergency cricothyroidotomy may be required if the airway cannot be secured by endotracheal intubation. A stomach tube should be passed and gentle (bearing in mind the corrosive action of some mercury compounds) gastric lavage carried out using, preferably, warm, 10 per cent sodium bicarbonate solution. If organo-mercury is involved, between three and six sachets of the basic anion-exchange resin cholestyramine should be administered before the tube is withdrawn, as sequestration of bile salts increases faecal excretion of these compounds. Chelation therapy should be started, using oral penicillamine (1–4 g daily, in four divided doses). It has been suggested[26] that in chronic mercury poisoning, although penicillamine may hasten the excretion of an easily mobilized extracellular fraction, it does not increase the excretion of mercury over a long period of time. Care must be exercised as the chelation of mercury may enhance its passage across the blood–brain barrier and for this reason the use of dimercaprol (BAL) is contraindicated in poisoning with organic mercury compounds.[27] It is, however, extremely effective in the treatment of acute poisoning with inorganic mercurials when given by intramuscular injection. The recommended dose is 2.5 mg/kg body weight, repeated at four-hour intervals for two days; after this, the injections are given twice daily for ten days or until recovery is complete. In the absence of these drugs, intravenous administration of 100 mL of 5 per cent sodium sulphate or 500–1000 mL of Ringer–Locke solution may be helpful. There is some evidence that alkaline diuresis, as described for salicylate poisoning in standard medical textbooks, with physiological saline, 5 per cent dextrose and 1.26 per cent bicarbonate solution affords the kidney some protection against mercury damage and might prevent the onset of anuria. This technique, however, is not without serious risk and ought to be carried out under continuous observation of fluid replacement and of electrolyte and acid-base status, as in an intensive care or high dependency unit.

Inhalation of large quantities of mercury vapour may lead to the onset of chemical pneumonitis 24–48 hours after exposure which may require treatment with bronchodilators. Intercurrent infection will necessitate the use of appropriate antibiotics. If the condition is severe and respiratory failure threatens, mechanical ventilation with positive end-expiratory pressure will be required. If the risk of permanent damage is high, it would be prudent to give steroids prophylactically, but these have no proven value once the condition has developed.

There is no effective treatment for chronic mercury poisoning. Penicillamine and BAL may be tried, but are unlikely to alter the course of the illness, and the neurological effects of intoxication may never completely reverse. Mercaptopropionyl glycine has been used for the treatment of organic mercury poisoning in Japan. This drug produces a sustained increase in urinary excretion, but has little effect on the clinical picture.[28]

EVALUATING MERCURY EXPOSURE

For workers exposed to inorganic mercury, the Health and Safety Executive workplace exposure limit (eight-hour time-weighted average (TWA))[29] is 25 µg/m^3 with a corresponding urine value of 20 µmol/mol creatinine and a blood threshold of 45 nmol/L mercury. The monitoring of workers exposed to mercury is generally based upon the periodic measurement of mercury in the urine. Urine levels provide a measure of low level or cumulative exposure and are usually preferred over blood levels, which are more appropriate measures after acute exposures to inorganic mercury vapour. This also applies to people in the general population who may have become accidentally exposed to vapour from liquid mercury. Mild and reversible proteinuria is the most sensitive clinical indicator of mercury vapour toxicity, followed by non-specific symptoms and changes in plasma lysomal enzyme, and in more advanced cases, objective tremor and psychomotor disturbances.[11] An apparent threshold for these effects is 20 µmol/mol creatinine in the urine and 45 nmol/L in the blood, i.e. the equivalent of the current UK workplace exposure limit (exposures should therefore be kept well below this).[29] The first clinical symptoms in workers (rarely seen anymore in high economy countries) are proteinuria and slight hand tremor. Testing the urine for reversible proteinuria by a simple dipstick method was widely used in routine exposure monitoring and was surprisingly sensitive to increases in exposure.

In evaluating mercury levels found in an unexposed working population in the UK, the upper 95 per cent limits for urinary mercury are <2 µmol/mol creatinine for unexposed people; the equivalent unexposed blood range is 0.6–19 nmol/L (Health and Safety Executive, unpublished data). These limits are also useful when checking individuals who may have had a brief, inadvertent exposure to mercury vapour and who need reassurance.

Pregnancy and work with mercury is contraindicated on general precautionary grounds unless a risk assessment shows that exposure can be kept to negligible levels. There are no consistent findings of adverse reproductive effects in laboratory animals or in epidemiological occupational studies for elemental mercury exposure (see Chapter 89, Workplace exposures and reproductive health), but methyl mercury is teratogenic in humans.[30]

Although mercury is being phased out of thermometers and sphygmomanometers in hospitals, breakages leading to spillages may still occur. Airborne concentrations of mercury vapour are usually low and insignificant in these small spills, which can be dealt with by a spills kit for removing liquid mercury. Large spillages in a home or workplace will require exposure assessment and specialist treatment.[31]

Key points

- Acute inorganic mercury poisoning is rare in modern industry due to awareness of the hazards of metallic mercury vapour and mercury compounds. Organic mercury, such as methyl mercury, is no longer used in seed dressings, following incidents of mass organic mercury poisoning around the world.
- Clinicians need to be aware of the effects of chronic overexposure to low levels of mercury, the first clinical symptoms of which are classically proteinuria and tremor. Measuring urinary mercury is a simple and effective means of monitoring inorganic mercury exposure and checking the control of exposure to metallic mercury vapour. With accidental exposure to mercury vapour in, for example, incidents in laboratories or after breakages of mercury-containing equipment, testing for blood mercury levels soon after the event are the best guide to exposure.
- The apparent threshold for early clinical findings in chronic mercury exposure is 20 µmol/mol creatinine in the urine and 45 nmol/L in the blood, which correspond to the current UK workplace exposure limit (25 µg/m^3 eight-hour TWA), so actual exposures should be kept consistently below this level.
- Mercury spillages should always be cleaned up using special spillage kits or otherwise expertly removed for toxic waste disposal. Accumulation of mercury in the fabric of old laboratory buildings or dental surgeries has presented exposure issues to workers who subsequently use the same work areas.

REFERENCES

1. Agency for Toxic Substances and Disease Registry. Toxicological profile for mercury. US Department of Health and Human Services. Atlanta, GA: ATSDR, 1999: 1–611.
2. Hunter D, Bomford RR, Russell DS. Poisoning by methylmercury compounds. *Quarterly Journal of Medicine.* 1940; **9**: 193–213.
3. Hunter D, Russell DS. Focal cerebral and cerebellar atrophy in a human subject due to organic mercury compounds. *Journal of Neurology, Neurosurgery, and Psychiatry.* 1954; **17**: 235–41.
4. Takeuchi T, Eto K. *The pathology of Minamata disease. A tragic story of water pollution.* Fukuoka: Kyushu University Press, 1999.
5. Tsubaki T. Recent problems for the diagnosis of Minamata disease. *Advances in Neurological Sciences.* 1974; **18**: 882–9.

6. Bakir F, Damluji SF, Amin-Zaki L et al. Methylmercury poisoning in Iraq. *Science*. 1973; **181**: 230–41.
7. Davis LE, Kornfeld M, Mooney HS et al. Methylmercury poisoning: Long-term clinical, radiological, toxicological, and pathological studies of an affected family. *Annals of Neurology*. 1994; **35**: 680–8.
8. Agocs MM, Etzel RA, Parrish RG et al. Mercury exposure from interior latex paint. *New England Journal of Medicine*. 1990; **323**: 1096–101.
9. Centers for Disease Control. Mercury exposure in a residential community – Florida, 1994. *Morbidity and Mortality Weekly Reports*. 1995; **44**: 436–43.
10. Orloff KG, Ulirsch G, Wilder L et al. Human exposure to elemental mercury in a contaminated residential building. *Archives of Environmental Health*. 1997; **52**: 169–72.
11. International Programme on Chemical Safety (IPCS). Inorganic mercury. Environmental Health Criteria, 181. Geneva: World Health Organization, 1991.
12. Halbach S. Amalgam tooth fillings and man's mercury burden. *Human and Experimental Toxicology*. 1994; **13**: 496–501.
13. Barregård L, Sällstein G, Järvolm B. People with high mercury uptake from their own dental amalgam fillings. *Occupational and Environmental Medicine*. 1995; **52**: 124–8.
14. Lindbolm M-L, Ylöstalo P, Sallmén M et al. Occupational exposure in dentistry and miscarriage. *Occupational and Environmental Medicine*. 2007; **64**: 127–33.
15. Kark RAP. Clinical and neurochemical aspects of inorganic mercury intoxication. In: Vinken PJ, Bruyn GW (eds). *Handbook of clinical neurology. Intoxications of the nervous system. Part I.* Amsterdam: Elsevier, 1994: 367–411.
16. Kulig K. A tragic reminder about organic mercury. *New England Journal of Medicine*. 1998; **338**: 1692–4.
17. Marsh DO. Organic mercury: Clinical and neurotoxicological aspects. In: Vinken PJ, Bruyn GW (eds). *Handbook of clinical neurology. Intoxications of the nervous system. Part I.* Amsterdam: Elsevier, 1994: 413–29.
18. Hargreaves RJ, Evans JG, Janota I et al. Persistent mercury in nerve cells 16 years after metallic mercury poisoning. *Neuropathology and Applied Neurobiology*. 1988; **14**: 443–52.
19. Clarkson TW. The pharmacology of mercury compounds. *Annual Review of Pharmacology*. 1972; **12**: 375–406.
20. Buchet JP, Roels A, Bernard A, Lauwerys R. Assessment of renal function of workers exposed to inorganic lead, cadmium or mercury vapor. *Journal of Occupational Medicine*. 1980; **22**: 741–50.
21. Smith PJ, Langold GD, Goldberg J. Effects of occupational exposure to elemental mercury on short term memory. *British Journal of Industrial Medicine*. 1983; **40**: 413–19.
22. Levine SP, Cavender GD, Langold GD, Albers JW. Elementary mercury exposure: Peripheral neurotoxicity. *British Journal of Industrial Medicine*. 1982; **39**: 136–9.
23. Takeuchi T, Morikawa N, Matsumoto H et al. A pathologic study of Minamata disease in Japan. *Acta Neuropathologica*. 1962; **2**: 40–57.
24. Kazantzis G, Schiller KFR, Asscher AW et al. Albuminuria and the nephrotic syndrome following exposure to mercury and its compounds. *Quarterly Journal of Medicine*. 1962; **31**: 403–18.
25. Korogi Y, Takahashi M, Okajima T et al. MRI findings of Minamata disease – Organic mercury poisoning. *Journal of Magnetic Resonance Imaging*. 1998; **8**: 308–16.
26. Gledhill RF, Hopkins AP. Chronic inorganic mercury poisoning treated with *N*-acetyl-D-penicillamine. *British Medical Journal*. 1972; **29**: 225–8.
27. Magos L. Effect of 2,3-dimercaptopropanol (BAL) on urinary excretion and brain content of mercury. *British Journal of Industrial Medicine*. 1968; **25**: 152–4.
28. Tsubaki T, Trukayama K. *Minamata disease*. Amsterdam: Elsevier, 1977.
29. Health and Safety Executive. Mercury Criteria Document Summaries. EH64, 1995 supplement. Sudbury: HSE Books, 1995.
30. International Programme on Chemical Safety (IPCS). Methylmercury. Environmental Health Criteria, 101. Geneva: World Health Organization, 1990.
31. Baughman TA. Elemental mercury spills. *Environmental Health Perspectives*. 2006; **114**: 1147–52.

27

Molybdenum

MALCOLM R SIM

Along with arsenic, phosphorus and antimony, molybdenum is one of a group of previously important occupational toxins, but which is now largely of historical interest in the workplace setting. While this is true in most developed countries, where good workplace control has eliminated them as major causes of disease, this is not necessarily the case in newly developing countries. In addition, some of these substances, such as inorganic arsenic, have become more important as causes of disease in the environmental health setting, as their importance in the workplace has waned.

Molybdenum is a silver-white metal which is mined mainly in the form of molybdenum ore ($MoSO_2$). It is an essential element for humans and is required for the enzyme xanthine oxidase. It is used as a hardener in steels, in the production of some special alloys, ceramics and pigments, and in electrical wire. Other sources of occupational exposure include fertilizers, coal-powered electricity generation, and as a byproduct of copper smelting, pigments and paints. It forms many soluble and insoluble compounds, including molybdenum trioxide (MO_3), sulphides and halides.

Most evidence for toxicity comes from animal studies, with effects in several body systems, including anaemia, stunted growth, deformities of the bones and joints and degeneration of the central nervous system. In humans, the type of toxic effect is dependent upon the molybdenum compound involved and the duration of exposure. Acute exposure to molybdenum trioxide is known to be irritant to mucous membranes of the eyes, nose and throat, while chronic exposure is thought to cause a type of hard metal lung disease and allergic alveolitis.[1] There may also be other, as yet, unrecognized health effects from molybdenum exposure. For example, a recent study has found evidence for adverse effects on sperm concentration and morphology and molybdenum exposure in a dose–response relationship, after adjusting for the effect of potential confounders and other metals.[2]

The International Agency for Research on Cancer (IARC) has concluded that there is limited evidence for the carcinogenicity of metal alloys containing cobalt, chromium and molybdenum in experimental animals;[3] however, a case–control study has found an association between occupational exposure to molybdenum and lung cancer.[4] The American Conference of Governmental Industrial Hygienists (ACGIH) has set a threshold limit value (TLV) for molybdenum of 5 mg/m^3 for soluble compounds and 10 mg/m^3 for insoluble compounds, the latter being the nuisance dust level.

> **Key points**
>
> - Occupational exposure to molybdenum is known to cause mucous membrane irritation.
> - There is also evidence for longer term effects in the respiratory system, such as hard metal disease.
> - There is limited evidence that molybdenum causes cancer.

REFERENCES

1. Ott HC, Prior C, Herold M et al. Respiratory symptoms and bronchoalveolar lavage abnormalities in molybdenum exposed workers. *Wiener Klinische Wochenschrift.* 2004; **116** (Suppl. 1): 25–30.
2. Meeker JD, Rossano MG, Protas B et al. Cadmium, lead, and other metals in relation to semen quality: Human evidence for molybdenum as a male reproductive toxicant. *Environmental Health Perspectives.* 2008; **116**: 1473–9.

3. International Agency for Research on Cancer Monographs on the Evaluation of Carcinogenic Risks to Humans. Cobalt in hard metals and cobalt sulfate, gallium arsenide, indium phosphide and vanadium pentoxide, vol. 86. Lyon: IARC, 2006.

4. Droste JH, Weyler JJ, Van Meerbeeck JP *et al.* Occupational risk factors of lung cancer: A hospital based case-control study. *Occupational and Environmental Medicine.* 1999; **56**: 322–7.

28

Nickel

TOM SORAHAN

| Nickel carbonyl | 224 | References | 224 |

Nickel is a hard silvery metal. It was first isolated by Cronstedt in 1751 and takes its name from 'Old Nick' because of the 'devilish' difficulties it caused during the refining of Saxony copper ores.

It is a transition metal and is thus capable of having a number of oxidation states with markedly different properties. Some of the water insoluble or slightly soluble salts are soluble in biological matrices. Nickel forms important alloys, a number of oxides and also organometallic compounds. Nickel tetracarbonyl is remarkable in being a gaseous metallic compound at ambient temperatures. Although nickel tetracarbonyl was known to be acutely toxic, little was known of any other hazards associated with the refining or use of nickel until in 1923 when a case of nasal cancer at a refinery in Wales saw the beginning of modern nickel toxicology. The cancer problem was subsequently noted in other refineries processing sulphuride ores at high temperatures.

Nickel is widely distributed in the Earth's crust. Mining, crushing and grinding and flotation followed by pyrometallurgy and then electrodeposition, or the carbonyl process are used to recover the metal.[1]

Ninety per cent of nickel is used in alloys, mostly stainless steel, but the high nickel alloys (containing around 30–50 per cent nickel) are important in the aero engine industry, desalination plants and where corrosion resistance is needed. Other uses include plating, foundry work and catalysts. Electroplated nickel silver (EPNS) is used on cutlery. Nickel powders find application in rechargeable batteries and other uses include the coating of fibres and foam for use in electronics. In combination with other metal oxides, nickel oxide forms commercially important alloys, called spinels.

Markedly increased risks of pulmonary and nasal sinus cancer have been found to be associated with high temperature oxidation of nickel matte and nickel–copper matte and with electrolytic refining of nickel. The problem in some of these refinery studies was first thought to be associated with arsenic exposure or nickel carbonyl gas, but more recently the cancer effects have been attributed to the very high levels of dust and fume pertaining in these early workplaces.[2] A major epidemiological study[3] concluded that nickel sulphides (especially the subsulphide) and oxides involved in the processes were the principal culprits. A later cohort study of workers at the Kristiansand refinery in Norway has found that soluble nickel salts, such as nickel sulphate, are also human lung carcinogens, but it is possible that the role of arsenic has not been fully accounted for in this study.[4]

The National Toxicology Program in the United States undertook an animal inhalation study, and exposed both rats and mice to three different nickel compounds.[5] The investigators found that nickel subsulphide was the most potent metal species, nickel oxide less so and nickel sulphate, which is a soluble salt, did not cause cancer under the conditions of the study. Modern processes technology has essentially eliminated the exposure of workers to the hazards. There is no firm direct evidence of any excess cancer risk in user industries, including welding of stainless steel, nickel plating and the production of nickel alloys.

Primary sensitization may result from close and prolonged contact which may be occupational or domestic, especially skin piercing with the subsequent use of nickel in 'sleepers' to maintain the patency of the skin. The skin reaction may be local or remote.[6] Sensitized people may subsequently react to contact with nickel at work or in clothing or jewellery. Since the introduction of automation and improved hygiene in the workplace, as well as new legislation limiting nickel in jewellery, 'nickel itch' is now less common, but occupational nickel contact dermatitis has been observed in people handling nickel-plated instruments or tools. Clinical diagnosis is by patch tests and the lymphocyte proliferation test.

Asthma may be associated with the inhalation of droplets of soluble nickel and also possibly the fine nickel oxide fume resulting from welding of nickel-containing alloys. As with dermatitis, if a causal relationship is clearly established, then affected workers should be removed from further exposure.[7]

Ingestion of soluble nickel is toxic and has occurred in the workplace, due to accidental contamination of the drinking water supply.[8]

Biological monitoring cannot differentiate between inhalation or ingestion. It is not therefore recommended as a routine procedure in the absence of skilled interpretation, except in nickel carbonyl poisoning where it has a health guidance value and in exposure to soluble nickel, such as in nickel platers.[9]

NICKEL CARBONYL

Nickel tetracarbonyl gas was discovered by Ludwig Mond and co-workers in 1888. It is formed when carbon monoxide is passed over finely divided nickel at ambient temperatures and it decomposes at 180°C to deposit nickel metal of extremely high purity. This is the basis of the Mond process. The gas is acutely dangerous and similar in toxicology to phosgene. Its use is limited to a few refineries and to coating applications.

It has an immediate acute effect including giddiness, nausea and headache followed after an interval of 12–18 hours by a severe chemical pneumonitis. Treatment is discussed in Chapter 39, Gases.

Poisoning by nickel carbonyl is a prescribed disease in the United Kingdom (see Chapter 8, Compensation schemes).

Key points

- Nickel is widely distributed in the earth's crust.
- Nickel is extracted for use in alloys.
- Some nickel processes have shown clear excess risks of lung cancer and nasal cancer.

REFERENCES

1. Habashi F (ed). Nickel. In: *Handbook of extractive metallurgy*. Weinheim: Wiley-VCH, 1997: 716–90.
2. International Agency for Research on Cancer. Monographs on the evaluation of carcinogenic risks to humans: 49. Chromium, nickel and welding. Lyon: IARC, 1990.
3. Doll R. Report of the International Committee on nickel carcinogenesis in man. *Scandinavian Journal of Work and Environmental Health*. 1990; **16**: 1–82.
4. Anderson A, Berge SR, Engeland A, Norseth T. Exposure to nickel compounds and smoking in relation to incidence of lung and nasal cancer among nickel refinery workers. *Occupational and Environmental Medicine*. 1996; **53**: 708–13.
5. Dunnick JK, Elwell MR, Radovsky AE *et al*. Comparative effects of nickel subsulfide, nickel oxide or nickel sulphate hexahydrate chronic exposures in the lung. *Cancer Research*. 1995; **55**: 5251–6.
6. Maibach HI, Menné T (eds). Nickel and the skin. In: *Immunology and toxicology*. Boca Raton, FL: CRC Press, 1989: 117–32.
7. Bright P, Burge PS, O'Hickey SP *et al*. Occupational asthma due to chrome and nickel electroplating. *Thorax*. 1997; **52**: 28–32.
8. Sunderman FW Jr, Dingle B, Hopfer SM *et al*. Acute nickel toxicity in electroplating workers who accidentally ingested a solution of nickel sulphate and chloride. *American Journal of Industrial Medicine*. 1988; **14**: 257–66.
9. Kiilunen M, Utela J, Rantanen T *et al*. Exposure to soluble nickel in electrolytic nickel refining. *Annals of Occupational Hygiene*. 1997; **41**: 167–88.

29

Phosphorus

MALCOLM R SIM

Phosphorus is among a group of previously important occupational toxins, but which are now largely of historical interest in the workplace setting. While this is true in most developed countries, where good workplace control has eliminated them as major causes of disease, this is not necessarily the case in newly developing countries.

Phosphorus is highly reactive, as it oxidizes extremely rapidly on contact with air. There are three allotropes of phosphorus: white (or yellow), red and black, of which the white variety is the most toxic. In modern industry, phosphorus and its compounds have many uses including the manufacture of munitions and other incendiary devices, the production of fertilizers, detergents, animal foods, pharmaceuticals and pesticides. They are also used in engraving, electropolishing, photography, metal cleaning, as scale inhibitors in water treatment and in the manufacture of semiconductors, so exposure may occur in many industries.

The use of white phosphorus in match-making began in 1832 and ushered in what Donald Hunter referred to as 'the greatest tragedy in the whole story of occupational disease'. This was phosphorus-induced necrosis of the jaw, known as 'phossy jaw'. The onset of the disease was slow, taking an average of about five years for the symptoms to develop after first exposure. Phossy jaw was an extremely painful and disfiguring condition with the mandible becoming necrotic and the formation of abscesses which discharged foul-smelling pus. The mortality rate was about 20 per cent, usually due to septicaemia. Surgical removal of the mandible was often required. A complete ban on white phosphorus was slow to be introduced, one of the last countries being the United States in 1931, although the Berne Convention of 1906 prohibited the manufacture and import of all white phosphorus matches into Europe.

Phossy jaw is now very uncommon and when it does occur, such as in the manufacture of munitions, it is a much milder disease. Interestingly, osteonecrosis in the oral cavity, with features similar to those of phossy jaw, has recently been found to occur in patients treated with bisphosphonate for multiple myeloma or secondary cancer in bone,[1] which demonstrates the importance of retaining knowledge of what might be considered historical occupational diseases, which may recur in modern times in new guises.

Another important effect of white phosphorus is burning on contact with the skin and such burns must be washed as rapidly as possible with a solution of a suspension of 5 per cent sodium bicarbonate and 3 per cent copper sulphate in 1 per cent hydroxyethyl cellulose.[2] The resultant blackened appearance facilitates the removal of the phosphorus particles from the skin. Phosphoric acid and phosphoric compounds are irritant to the eyes, the mucous membranes and the respiratory tract. On this basis the American Conference of Governmental Industrial Hygienists (ACGIH) has set a threshold limit value (TLV) of $1\,\text{mg/m}^3$ and a short-term exposure limit (STEL) of $3\,\text{mg/m}^3$.

Key points

- Phosphorus causes 'phossy jaw', an important disease in the history of occupational medicine, which has now virtually disappeared as an occupational disease.
- Phosphorus is also a potent cause of skin burns, which require specialist treatment.
- Some patients treated with bisphosphonate for cancer have been found to develop a type of bone necrosis with features similar to phossy jaw.

REFERENCES

1. Ashcroft J. Bisphosphonates and phossy-jaw: Breathing new life into an old problem. *Lancet Oncology*. 2006; **7**: 447–9.
2. Chou TD, Lee TW, Chen SL *et al*. The management of white phosphorus burns. *Burns*. 2001; **27**: 492–7.

30

Platinum group metals

PETER LINNETT

Introduction	226	Iridium	228
Platinum	226	Ruthenium	228
Palladium	227	Osmium	229
Rhodium	228	References	229

INTRODUCTION

Six elements constitute the group collectively referred to as the platinum group elements (PGE) or metals (PGM). They are platinum (Pt), palladium (Pd), rhodium (Rh), iridium (Ir), ruthenium (Ru) and osmium (Os). They occur together in mineral bodies in variable ratios.

Platinum was first identified as a precious metal in 1751 and was present as a contaminant of silver (plata) from South America from which it derives its name.[1]

Early reports indicate that the PGM existed as native metals in rich ore bodies in South America and the Urals. They are now found in complex mineral bodies, especially the copper and nickel sulphide ore bodies of South Africa, Siberia and Canada in which there may also be present several other metals and metalloids, e.g. arsenic which has well-known toxic properties. Recovery of the PGM involves mining, crushing and milling of the ore, then concentration by a hydrometallurgical or pyrometallurgical route followed by refining. The process risks are common to extraction of several metals,[2] but the hazards during refining are specific to platinum.

PGM are rare metals and, as they have high value, there is considerable recovery and recycling of the metals from industrial use[3] and consequently minimal loss to the environment.

PLATINUM

Platinum is a bright, silver-coloured, very dense metal which is malleable, ductile and electroconductive and has exceptional catalytic properties. It is corrosion resistant and resistant also to molten glass. It is a rare metal and more valuable than gold.

Its properties determine the major uses for platinum as catalysts for the chemical (e.g. nitric acid, silicone production), petrochemical (reforming and isomerization) and pharmaceutical industries, as well as for catalysis of exhaust emissions from the internal combustion engine – autocatalyst which uses about 46 per cent of Pt produced.[3] Other uses include fuel cells, thermocouples and chemical sensors, lining of moulds for the production of glass, coating of turbine blades and tips for spark plugs. Being a noble metal and biologically inert, platinum is used in medical implants, e.g. vascular stents, pacemaker electrodes and dental prostheses, but certain complex Pt compounds are effective as cytotoxic agents, e.g. cisplatin, carboplatin, oxaliplatin for the treatment of solid tumours. Platinum has long been used for investment and jewellery and there is increasing consumption in electronics.

Occupational toxicology

Separation of the PGM from each other and other metals, e.g. gold, is achieved by a chemical approach. The metals, though resistant to corrosion, are soluble in aqua regia (concentrated nitric acid and hydrochloric acid) and also in concentrated hydrochloric acid supplemented by chlorine. Chloroplatinic acid (H_2PtCl_6) is thus produced. This is an extremely potent allergen causing symptoms of type I allergic reactions, including asthma, rhinitis and urticaria.

Chloroplatinate salts produced by subsequent treatment of the liquors are equally allergenic and platinum refinery workers have a very high risk of becoming sensitized to these salts.[4,5] The risk of naive workers being sensitized has been as high as 50 per cent in the first five years of employment,[6] although the risk has been reduced by new technologies, such as solvent extraction and improved containment of liquors and suppression of airborne aerosols and powders. The allergenicity is restricted to the halogeno-complex salts of platinum, such as ammonium hexachloroplatinate (yellow salt) which is reduced thermally to the non-toxic metal, while other neutral platinum compounds such as tetraammine platinum dichloride are non-allergenic.[6,7]

Occupational exposures to platinum compounds

Exposure to the halogeno-complex salts of platinum occurs mainly in the refining of platinum and precious metals and production of platinum catalysts. All workers associated with these activities may be at risk of sensitization. Chloroplatinic acid may be used for coating of electrodes and in specific manufacturing processes, e.g. silicone production. Small quantities are used in research laboratories.

Medical surveillance

Personal risk factors have been studied at pre-placement medical examination. Originally, atopy was considered to be relevant but this has not been confirmed, although smoking is a significant risk factor.[6,8–10] Some human leukocyte-associated antigens (HLA) have also been studied and shown to correlate with sensitization.[11] Eczema and dermatitis is aggravated by the work conditions and rapidly leads to sensitization and asthma is aggravated by the irritant environment during refining.

Medical surveillance of workers exposed to chloroplatinates is directed to the early identification of sensitization. This includes direct questioning for symptoms of respiratory and dermal sensitization, as well as skin prick testing with a standardized dilute solution of sodium hexachloroplatinate 10^{-3} g Pt salt/mL.[12–14] The suggested frequency of testing is at least annually, but should be more frequent if the exposure levels are high and if there is a high rate of sensitization in the exposed workforce.

Immediate cessation of exposure following diagnosis of sensitization by skin prick test prevents the development of asthma.[13,15] Investigation of occupational asthma in the absence of a positive skin prick test requires monitoring of peak flow[16] and confirmation by specific bronchial challenge. In cohort studies, specific IgE has been shown to correlate with skin prick test, but only for grouped results and the complicated test is not useful for investigation of an individual.

Refining of platinum is associated with exposure to other respiratory irritants, e.g. chlorine and ammonia which will aggravate pre-existing respiratory disorders especially asthma. Appropriate respiratory surveillance is required for this.[13]

Biological monitoring in workers exposed to chloroplatinates has not been found to correlate with evidence of absorption with sensitization.[17] A significant confounder may be the presence of PGM in dental prostheses. Platinum in blood has been determined in nurses in an oncology unit who administer platinum-containing chemotherapy, but this reflects exposure and not sensitization.

Exposure limits

The UK workplace exposure limit for platinum salts is 0.002 mg/m^3 with a notation that the halogeno-platinum compounds are sensitizers. Even at the exposure limit, the risk of sensitization is significant and stringent control measures need to be maintained to minimize exposure, as well as to conduct medical surveillance. Only the complex chlorides of the halogeno-platinum compounds are used in any significant amount. There is limited use of the other halogenated Pt compounds in research and development laboratories.

Environmental risks

The environmental risk posed by release of platinum into the environment, particularly from autocatalysts, was reviewed by the International Programme on Chemical Safety of the World Health Organization in the 1991 Environmental Health Criteria 125 – Platinum.[18] The levels of platinum in the environment are too low to be a risk to human health.

PALLADIUM

Palladium like platinum is a lustrous, malleable, ductile and electroconductive metal with good catalytic properties. It is used as a catalyst in the chemical industries, as well as in autocatalysts. Significant amounts are used in electronic components.[3] Palladium is used in dental prostheses with geographic variations in the amount used.

Occupational toxicology

Reports on patch testing from dermatology clinics indicate a high potential for people who are allergic to nickel to react also to palladium chloride, though not to palladium metal.[19,20] As there have been positive patch test cases with no previous exposure to palladium compounds, a cross-reactivity between nickel and palladium has been suggested. Cross-reactivity between palladium and cobalt may also occur. Palladium chloride may induce sensitization in guinea pigs by repeated open application, but this does not occur with the metal. Cases of stomatitis have been attributed to the presence of palladium in the alloys of dental prostheses.[19] A case of asthma has been reported in a worker exposed to palladium tetraammine dichloride.[21]

Occupational exposures to palladium compounds

Exposure to palladium compounds occurs in the refining process and production of chemical process catalysts and autocatalysts. Palladium plating solutions are used in the electronics industry. Dental technicians may be exposed to metal dusts in the preparation of dental prostheses, but no adverse consequences have been reported.

Medical surveillance

Routine medical surveillance for people exposed to palladium compounds has not been prescribed. In many occupational situations, exposure to palladium compounds occurs together with exposure to platinum compounds. These workers will normally be under regular medical surveillance for platinum exposure. In some cases, e.g. the electronics industry, platinum may not be present, although salts of other metals may be used. Increased attention should be paid to dermal health with special concern for cross-reactivity to palladium chloride in people who are allergic to nickel.

Exposure limits and environmental risks

There are no workplace exposure limits for palladium compounds. The environmental concerns about the potential effects of palladium released from autocatalysts was reviewed in the IPCS Environmental Heath Criteria 226 – Palladium and palladium compounds. The environmental levels are very low and do not pose a risk to the community.[19]

RHODIUM

Rhodium is a bright, lustrous metal resistant to corrosion with good catalytic properties. It is harder than platinum and more difficult to work with. It is used for thermocouple wires, in jewellery often as a surface plating to provide a hard bright finish and in the glass industry for production of thin glass sheets for flat screens.

Rhodium compounds have a deep rose hue. Its major use is in the production of autocatalysts.[3]

There are a few reports of dermatitis attributed to rhodium compounds.

The occupational exposure limit assigned to rhodium compounds of 0.001 mg/m^3 has not been supported by epidemiology. The value was extrapolated from the limit value for platinum and, as rhodium has half the atomic weight of platinum, it was assigned half the exposure limit value of platinum compounds.

No specific medical surveillance has been advised for workers exposed only to rhodium compounds; however, many of them will have mixed exposures to other PGM and will be subject to medical surveillance for platinum compounds.

There have been no reviews of the environmental risks. Rhodium is rarer than platinum and is considerably more valuable so losses to the environment are minimized and environmental levels are insignificant.

IRIDIUM

Iridium is a hard shiny metal. It is resistant to corrosion and has a high melting point.

It is used in chlor-alkali production for anode coating. Iridium crucibles are used for the production of high purity crystals for electronics. Its resistance to heat has encouraged the use of iridium tips in spark plugs for internal combustion engines and iridium compounds may be used as process catalysts in the chemical industry.

Positive skin prick test reactions to iridium salts have been reported.

There are no workplace exposure limits set for iridium.

No specific medical surveillance has been advised for workers exposed only to iridium compounds; however, many of them will have mixed exposures to other PGM and will be subject to medical surveillance for platinum compounds.

There have been no reviews of the environmental risks from iridium. Environmental levels are insignificant.

RUTHENIUM

Ruthenium may be used as a catalyst and is also used in the electronics industry in the production of resistor chips and hard disks.[3] Ruthenium tetroxide is used as a fixative in electron microscopy.

There are no reports of adverse reactions in workers exposed to ruthenium metal or its compounds, but fumes of ruthenium tetroxide are corrosive, affecting the cornea and conjunctiva, as well as the respiratory mucosa.

No medical surveillance has been recommended, but many ruthenium workers will also be under surveillance for concomitant exposure to platinum salts.

No studies have been made of environmental levels of this rare metal.

OSMIUM

Osmium metal is silvery blue in colour and very hard. It is recovered in the refining process as a fine grey powder which oxidizes in air to produce osmium tetroxide. It is therefore stored in a sealed container with an inert atmosphere. It may be used with iridium to produce a very hard alloy, osmiridium. Osmium tetroxide in air forms osmic acid. It is used in electron microscopy and in histology for staining fat especially in neural tissue.

Toxicology

Osmium tetroxide is very irritant to the respiratory tract. Acute exposure causes conjunctivitis and corneal oedema with the effect of causing the appearance of haloes around bright lights. Impaired vision lasts for one or two days. Inhalation causes severe pain in the nose with rhinorrhoea and difficulty in breathing. Transient haematuria, proteinuria and pyuria have been reported. Chronic exposure has been associated with corneal ulceration and opacification, as well as contact dermatitis.

Occupational exposures

Major exposures may occur in refining of PGM and release of osmium tetroxide. Minor exposure episodes may occur in electron microscopy and in histology laboratories.

Exposure limits

No workplace exposure limits have been set for osmium.

Medical surveillance

Routine medical surveillance has not been advised. Symptomatic treatment is suggested for acute exposures.

Environmental risks

Environmental risks due to this very rare metal have not been investigated.

Key points

Platinum

- Halogeno-complex salts of platinum are potent type I allergens.
- Platinum metal and neutral platinum compounds are non-allergenic.
- Skin prick testing is an integral component of medical surveillance with positive reactions predictive of asthma if exposure to allergenic salts is continued.

Palladium

- Nickel-sensitive subjects often react to patch test with palladium chloride, but not to palladium metal.

Osmium

- Osmium tetroxide causes corneal oedema and is a respiratory irritant.

REFERENCES

1. McDonald D, Hunt L. *A history of platinum and its allied metals*. London: Johnson Matthey, 1982.
2. Allison S. Processing ore. In: Stellman JM (ed.). *Encyclopaedia of occupational health and safety*, vol. III. Geneva: International Labour Office, 2001: 82.10–11.
3. Platinum Today. The world's leading authority on platinum group metals. Last accessed September 2009. Available from: www.platinum.matthey.com.
4. Hunter D, Milton R, Perry KMA. Asthma caused by the complex salts of platinum. *British Journal of Industrial Medicine*. 1945; **2**: 92–8.
5. Pepys J, Pickering CAC, Hughes EG. Asthma due to inhaled chemical agents – complex salts of platinum. *Clinical Allergy*. 1972; **2**: 391–6.
6. Linnett PJ, Hughes EG. 20 years of medical surveillance on exposure to allergenic and non-allergenic platinum compounds: The importance of chemical speciation. *Occupational and Environmental Medicine*. 1999; **56**: 191–6.
7. Cleare MJ, Hughes EG, Jacoby B, Pepys J. Immediate (type I) allergic responses to platinum compounds. *Clinical Allergy*. 1976; **6**: 183–95.
8. Venables KM, Dally MB, Nunn AJ *et al*. Smoking and occupational allergy in workers in a platinum refinery. *British Medical Journal*. 1989; **299**: 939–42.
9. Calverley AE, Rees D, Dowdeswell RJ *et al*. Platinum salt sensitivity in refinery workers: Incidence and effects of smoking and exposure. *Occupational and Environmental Medicine*. 1995; **52**: 661–6.

10. Niezborala M, Garnier G. Allergy to complex platinum salts: A historical prospective cohort study. *Occupational and Environmental Medicine.* 1996; **53**: 252–7.
11. Newman Taylor AJ, Cullinan P, Lympany PA *et al.* Interactions of HLA phenotype and exposure intensity in sensitization to platinum salts. *American Journal of Respiratory and Critical Care Medicine.* 1999; **160**: 435–8.
12. Hughes EG. Medical surveillance of platinum refinery workers. *Journal of the Society of Occupational Medicine.* 1980; **30**: 27–30.
13. Linnett PJ. Concerns for asthma at pre-placement assessment and health surveillance in platinum refining – a personal approach. *Occupational Medicine.* 2005; **55**: 595–9.
14. Merget R, Schultze-Werninghaus G, Bode F *et al.* Quantitative skin prick and bronchial provocation tests with platinum salt. *British Journal of Industrial Medicine.* 1991; **48**: 830–7.
15. Merget R, Caspari C, Dierkes-Globisch A *et al.* Effectiveness of a medical surveillance program for the prevention of occupational asthma caused by platinum salts. A nested case-control study. *Journal of Allergy and Clinical Immunology.* 2001; **107**: 707–12.
16. British Occupational Health Research Foundation. Occupational asthma: Identification, management and prevention: evidence based review and guidelines. Last accessed September 2009. Available from: www.bohrf.org.uk/content/asthma.htm.
17. Merget R, Kulzer R, Kniffka A *et al.* Platinum concentrations in sera of catalyst production workers are not predictive of platinum salt allergy. *International Journal of Hygiene and Environmental Health.* 2002; **205**: 1–5.
18. World Health Organization. Environmental health criteria 125 – Platinum. Geneva: World Health Organization, 1991.
19. World Health Organization. Environmental health criteria 226 – Palladium. Geneva: World Health Organization, 2002.
20. Todd DJ, Burrows D. Patch testing with pure palladium metal in patients with sensitivity to palladium chloride. *Contact Dermatitis.* 1992; **26**: 327–31.
21. Daenen M, Rogiers P, Van de Walle C *et al.* Occupational asthma caused by exposure to palladium. *European Respiratory Journal.* 1999; **13**: 213–16.

31

Polonium

IAIN BLAIR

Introduction	231	Health effects	232
Uses	231	Studies	232
Exposure, absorption and toxicity	231	References	232
Exposure levels	232		

INTRODUCTION

Polonium (Po) is a rare, unstable radioactive element that was discovered in 1898 by Marie Curie and named after her native land of Poland. Polonium has 25 known isotopes, all of which are radioactive. Polonium-210, an alpha emitter, is the most widely distributed isotope and it decays directly to its daughter isotope lead-206, with a half-life of 138 days. Polonium dissolves in dilute acids and will readily form compounds including oxides and halides. It vapourizes in a few hours at 55°C. Polonium can be detected and measured by alpha-particle spectroscopy.

Polonium is found in uranium ores at about one part in $10.^{10}$ These amounts are not harmful. Polonium is present in tobacco smoke from tobacco leaves grown with phosphate fertilizers. Synthetic polonium can be created in nuclear reactors by bombarding bismuth with neutrons. About 100 g are produced each year in this way, nearly all in Russia.

USES

A single gram of polonium-210 generates 140 watts of power and because of this property it has been used as a heat source for space travel. As a source of charged particles polonium-210 is used in anti-static devices. When mixed with beryllium, it is a source of neutrons that can be used as a trigger for nuclear weapons. Because of its very high toxicity, polonium has been used as a poison (see under Health effects, p. 232).

EXPOSURE, ABSORPTION AND TOXICITY

Following ingestion about 10 per cent of polonium is absorbed into the bloodstream and is subsequently cleared by the kidneys with a biological half-life of 30–50 days. Clearance may be accelerated using chelating agents,[1] although significant amounts of polonium-210 are deposited in tissues within a few hours of ingestion.

The main hazard is its intense radioactivity (166 TBq/g). Alpha particles emitted by polonium will readily damage tissue if it is ingested or inhaled, but do not penetrate the skin and so are not hazardous if the polonium remains outside the body. The median lethal dose (LD_{50}) for acute radiation exposure is about 4.5 Sv and this dose can be delivered by ingesting about 50 ng of polonium or inhaling about 10 ng.

The general population is naturally exposed to small amounts of polonium in food, water, tobacco smoke and as decay products of indoor radon. Increased exposure to polonium-210 from environmental sources is unlikely, although polonium-210 is present in devices that are easily available. Potentially lethal amounts of polonium are present in anti-static devices that are readily available in photographic stores or by mail order. Polonium-210 from a static eliminator source contaminated equipment and flooring at a soft-drink manufacturing plant.[2] Disposal of solid radioactive waste at a waste disposal facility did not appear to result in increased environmental levels of polonium.[3] Follow up of a large cohort of workers employed at a nuclear plant between 1944 and 1972 when polonium-210 operations were being conducted did not show any excess mortality. Among workers specifically monitored for polonium-210, mortality was less than expected, although more lung cancers were observed. No dose–response trends were observed.[4]

EXPOSURE LEVELS

Maximum exposure levels for polonium in food and for the workplace have been published by national and international authorities including the US Nuclear Regulatory Commission,[5] the International Commission on Radiological Protection[6] and the Food and Agriculture Organization of the United Nations.[7] For example, the maximum allowable body burden for ingested polonium-210 is only 1.1 kBq, which is equivalent to a particle weighing only 6.8 pg. The maximum permissible workplace concentration of airborne polonium-210 is about 10 Bq/m^3.

HEALTH EFFECTS

Alexander Litvinenko, a Russian living in London, died in November 2006 after being poisoned with polonium-210 a few weeks earlier. Litvinenko was probably the first person ever to die of the acute alpha-radiation effects of polonium-210.

Following ingestion, polonium distributes widely through the tissues of the body leading to whole body radiation exposure. Most exposure occurs in the first 30 days. After a minimum lethal dose, no initial illness would result due to the time it takes for exposure to accumulate, but death would be expected from the poisoning within two or three months. However, Litvinenko was ill on the day he was poisoned, was seriously ill on day 11 and died on day 23. This indicates that he was poisoned with many times the lethal dose of polonium-210 with the initial burden of exposure falling on the gastrointestinal tract. Two other people who were with Litvinenko on the day of the presumed poisoning became ill about 36 days after Litvinenko, which is consistent with absorption of a sublethal dose.

There are unsubstantiated reports that Irène Joliot-Curie, the Nobel prize winning chemist and daughter of Marie Curie, died from leukaemia in Paris in 1956 as a result of exposure to polonium in a laboratory accident ten years earlier. Similarly, it has been suggested that four deaths among staff at a research institute in Israel between 1957 and 1969 were due to a polonium leak.

STUDIES

Following the death of Litvinenko, there has been intense interest in the radiotoxicity of polonium-210 on the human body. A large number of people were identified who may have had low-level exposure as a result of working at or visiting places that were contaminated with polonium-210. Many of these provided samples for measuring 24-hour urinary excretion of polonium-210. By applying biokinetic models, it was possible to calculate intakes by ingestion or inhalation and the resulting radiation doses. Of the 695 people examined, 560 had urinary levels of 30 mBq per day or less which is the natural background level. Eighty-five had levels greater than this, but had received an estimated dose of less than 1 mSv, 34 had received an estimated dose of more than 1 mSv but less than 6 mSv, and 16 had received an estimated dose of 6 mSv or more. For those who had received doses of more than 1 mSv, it was estimated that their lifetime risk of death from cancer was increased by between 0.03 and 0.5 per cent.[8]

Extrapolating from animal studies indicates that ingestion (or inhalation) of a few tenths of a milligram of polonium-210 is likely to be fatal to all exposed persons. Such intakes will cause fatal damage to the bone marrow and other organs, including the kidneys and liver. Deaths will occur within about a month with levels of >1 MBq/kg body mass, but will occur over a longer period for lower exposures. Below 0.02 MBq/kg body mass, deaths from deterministic effects are not expected to occur, but the risk of cancer could be significant.[9]

One study has estimated that Litvinenko might have ingested between 27 and 1408 MBq (0.2–8.5 μg).[10] A second study concluded that 0.1–0.3 GBq absorbed into the bloodstream of an adult male would probably be fatal within one month. Assuming 10 per cent absorption into the bloodstream, this would correspond to ingestion of 1–3 GBq. There would be reductions in white cell count due to bone marrow failure complicated by damage to other organs, such as the kidneys and liver. Damage to these other organs would most probably be fatal even if the bone marrow could be rescued.[11]

Key points

- The general population is naturally exposed to small amounts of polonium in food, water, tobacco smoke and indoor radon.
- Synthetic polonium has commercial uses.
- Polonium is highly toxic when ingested or inhaled due to the emission of alpha particles.
- Alexander Litvinenko was fatally poisoned with polonium-210 in November 2006.

REFERENCES

1. National Council on Radiation Protection and Measurements. Report No. 65: Management of persons accidentally contaminated with radionuclides. National Council on Radiation Protection and Measurements, Bethesda, MD, USA. Accessed November 2008. Available from: www.ncrponline.org/AboutNCRP/About_NCRP.html.

2. Wallace JD, Williamson MR. Contamination of a soft-drink manufacturing plant by 210Po. *Health Physics*. 1990; **58**: 469–75.
3. Arthur WJ III, Markham OD. Polonium-210 in the environment around a radioactive waste disposal area and phosphate ore processing plant. *Health Physics*. 1984; **46**: 793–9.
4. Wiggs LD, Cox-DeVore CA, Voelz GL. Mortality among a cohort of workers monitored for 210Po exposure: 1944–1972. *Health Physics*. 1991; **61**: 71–6.
5. United States Nuclear Regulatory Commission. Last accessed November 2008. Available from: www.nrc.gov/reading-rm/doc-collections/cfr/part020/appb/.
6. International Commission on Radiological Protection (ICRP). Last accessed November 2008. Available from: www.icrp.org/index.asp.
7. Food and Agriculture Organization of the United Nations. Radionuclide contamination of foods: FAO recommended limits. Last accessed November 2008. Available from: www.fao.org/DOCREP/U5900T/u5900t08.htm#radionuclide%20contamination%20of%20foods:%20fao%20recommended%20limits.
8. Health Protection Agency. Followup of public health surveillance following polonium 210 incident. Last accessed January 2010. Available from: www.hpa.org.uk/web/HPAweb&HPAwebstandard/HPAweb_C/1195733719534.
9. Scott BR. Health risk evaluations for ingestion exposure of humans to polonium-210. *Dose Response*. 2007; **5**: 94–122.
10. Li WB, Gerstmann U, Giussani A *et al*. Internal dose assessment of 210Po using biokinetic modeling and urinary excretion measurement. *Radiation and Environmental Biophysics*. 2008; **47**: 101–10.
11. Harrison J, Leggett R, Lloyd D *et al*. Polonium-210 as a poison. *Journal of Radiological Protection*. 2007; **27**: 17–40.

Silver

PETER LINNETT

Introduction	234	Exposure limits	235
Properties and uses	234	Medical surveillance	235
Occupational toxicology	234	References	235
Other occupational exposures	235		

INTRODUCTION

Silver is a precious metal which occurs throughout the world sometimes in its native form, but also in mixed ore bodies especially with lead and zinc ores. Thus, the initial recovery of silver from a mixed ore is also associated with the risks attributable to the other minerals, e.g. lead, cadmium, selenium and tellurium.

Impure silver is melted and cast into anodes for electro-refining using a nitrate liquor. Pure silver is collected on titanium anodes, while impurities collect in anode slimes which require further treatment.

PROPERTIES AND USES

Silver is a soft white metal which takes a high polish. It is ductile and malleable. Pure silver has the highest electrical and thermal conductivity of all metals with the lowest contact resistance. Silver metal is used in jewellery, silverware, electronic components, solders and dental amalgams. Silver halides react to light and have extensive use in photography, including x-ray plates. Silver and silver compounds have bactericidal properties and other uses include catalysts, window coatings, mirrors, electroplating and sanitation.[1]

OCCUPATIONAL TOXICOLOGY

Ingestion is the most common route for acute absorption. Soluble compounds cause acute gastric irritation. Other effects are decreased blood pressure, diarrhoea and decreased respiration. Respiratory effects following inhalation of soluble compounds include irritation of the upper and lower respiratory tracts, although this may not be due to the silver component of the compounds so much as the chloride or nitrate ion.

Chronic absorption of soluble silver compounds, which may be due to self-medication with colloidal silver or silver-coated pills, results in widespread deposition of silver throughout all organs of the body. The clinical condition is termed 'argyria'. The dermal manifestation is a gradual darkening of the skin to a bluish grey colour. Microscopy of the skin has shown that there is silver deposition in the basement membrane with a profusion of melanocytes. This pigmentation is irreversible. The normal tanning reaction on exposure to sunlight is enhanced by the profusion of melanocytes. The sclera become dark blue-grey and silver is deposited in Descemet's membrane deep to the cornea and may be detected by slit-lamp examination. The impairment of night vision with haloes around lights may be reported. Although there is widespread pigmentation in all tissues and organs, there is an absence of adverse systemic effects and argyria is mainly a cosmetic impairment. There is no effective treatment for argyria which is irreversible.

In occupational settings, fine particles of soluble compounds may enter the eye and stain the conjunctiva and caruncle. Ocular burns with silver nitrate may result in permanent blemishes on the sclera. In the absence of generalized effects, the localized ocular effect is termed 'argyrosis'.

Splashes of silver nitrate are common in workplaces where it is used. The compound is corrosive and causes a chemical burn. Copious irrigation of the affected area with water is required. If the burn is superficial, there is initial erythema. On exposure to light, the colour then deepens to black. The skin dries and following the process of desquamation is replaced by normal healthy skin. If the silver compound is in contact with subcuticular tissues, there will be staining deep to the epidermis. Such cases have been reported from the excessive use of silver sulphadiazine for the treatment of wounds and burns.

Intradermal or implantation of splinters of silver metal during the fabrication of metal products may result in localized pigmentation causing a cosmetic change with no systemic effect.[2]

OTHER OCCUPATIONAL EXPOSURES

Refining of silver may be accompanied by exposure to fumes of other metals. Melting of scrap silver may release fumes of, for example, cadmium which have been incorporated in alloys to impart strength to the silver which is otherwise soft. Adequate extraction ventilation and filtration of the exhaust is required.

Silver solders may also contain cadmium and should only be used with adequate ventilation.

EXPOSURE LIMITS

The American Conference of Governmental Industrial Hygienists (ACGIH) exposure limit[3] for silver metal is 0.1 mg/m^3 and for soluble silver compounds it is 0.01 mg/m^3. This reflects the differences in absorption of silver from soluble compounds compared with the limited absorption from insoluble compounds and metallic silver.

MEDICAL SURVEILLANCE

No specific measures have been advised for medical surveillance for silver exposure. Compliance with the exposure limits will prevent systemic absorption and argyria. Examination of the sclera and mucous membranes of workers handling soluble silver compounds may indicate if there is some staining, although early changes are very subtle and difficult to identify.

Biological monitoring has been performed and determination of silver in blood has demonstrated that workers exposed to soluble silver compounds as in plating processes have higher levels than those whose exposure is to silver metal or fume alone.[4] The levels reported were not associated with argyria and routine biological monitoring has not been recommended as integral to a medical surveillance programme.

Most cases of argyria now reported are the result of self-medication.

Key points

- Chronic absorption of soluble silver compounds leads to argyria with widespread deposition of silver in all organs.
- In the skin, there is deposition of silver in the basement membrane with a profusion of melanocytes resulting in an exaggerated tanning response.

REFERENCES

1. Drake PL, Hazelwood KJ. Exposure-related health effects of silver and silver compounds: A review. *Annals of Occupational Hygiene*. 2005; **49**: 575–85.
2. Sarsfield P, White JE, Theaker JM. Silverworkers finger: An unusual occupational hazard mimicking a melanocytic lesion. *Histopathology*. 1992; **20**: 73–5.
3. American Conference of Governmental Industrial Hygienists (2007) Threshold limit values for chemical substances and physical agents and biological exposure indices. Cincinnati: ACGIH.
4. Armitage SA, White MA, Wilson HK. The determination of silver in whole blood and its application to biological monitoring of occupationally exposed groups. *Annals of Occupational Hygiene*. 1996; **40**: 331–8.

33

Thallium

HIDEKI IGISU AND TAR-CHING AW

Thallium is a soft, malleable, bluish-white metal with the symbol 'Tl', atomic number 81, atomic weight 204.38 and specific gravity 11.85.[1,2] Although the annual global production of thallium reduced from 15 to 10 tons between 1995 and 2004,[3] its use is wide-ranging, including semiconductors, optical fibres, optical lens, imitation jewellery, fireworks and as a rodenticide. Radioisotope ^{201}Tl is used for cardiac imaging. In addition, due to recent research and development activities, the use of thallium may greatly expand in the future as a material for high-temperature superconductors.[3] Since thallium and many thallium salts are highly toxic and yet tasteless and odourless, accidental or intentional thallium poisoning has occurred.[4,5] Cases with clinical effects that may have resulted from occupational thallium exposure have been described.[6] These include a worker engaged alone in the production of a 'new type of special glass' containing thallium.[7] The worker deployed to replace him also succumbed to similar effects.

Thallium can be absorbed through the gastrointestinal tract, respiratory tract and skin, and is then rapidly distributed to all organs.[1,2] It passes through the placenta and blood–brain barrier. In the early phase of poisoning, its concentration is high in the kidneys, but low in adipose tissue and the brain, but the cerebral concentration increases subsequently.[2] In an autopsied case (from a patient who died nine days after taking 5–10 g of thallium nitrate), the thallium concentration exceeded 100 mg/g in the colon, testis, cardiac ventricles, pituitary and several regions of the brain (thalamus, corpus striatum, cerebellar cortex and cerebral cortex).[8]

Thallium may be excreted into the gastrointestinal tract, kidneys, hair, skin, sweat, saliva and breast milk.[2,9] Reabsorption takes place in the gastrointestinal tract (mainly the colon). The biological half-life in humans is estimated to be approximately ten days, but can be as long as 30 days.[2]

Characteristic features of thallium poisoning are gastrointestinal disturbance, neurological impairment and alopecia. In acute poisoning, initial symptoms are nausea, vomiting and abdominal pain, which may be associated with the passage of bright red blood *per rectum*. Tachycardia and hypertension may result from autonomic (vagus nerve) dysfunction. Characteristic symptoms of paraesthesia and pains in the lower limbs, reflecting polyneuropathy, appear after several days. Decrease of sensation in the distal extremities and weakness, especially in the lower limbs, may be present. There can be difficulties with swallowing and speech, as well as other cranial nerve effects (e.g. optic nerve, ocular movement and facial muscle dysfunction). Central nervous system involvement leads to seizures, unconsciousness, ataxia and involuntary movements. Alopecia appears approximately two weeks later. It is usually most evident in the scalp, but hair in other parts of the body can also be lost. This latent period for alopecia to appear corresponds to the maturation period of the new epithelial cells of the hair matrix.[9] Mees lines (transverse white stripes) in the nails appear three to four weeks later. In subacute or chronic poisoning, the onset is associated with loss of appetite, headache, irritability, insomnia and loss of body weight.

The lethal dose varies from 6 to 40 mg/kg, but on average is between 10 and 15 mg/kg. Death occurs within 10–12 days if not treated. In extreme cases, death occurs within hours.[2]

Thallium poisoning should be considered if there is a history of exposure, and the clinical effects are gastrointestinal disturbances followed by neurological impairment and then alopecia. Alopecia is seen only two to three weeks after the neurological signs have appeared. Microscopic examination of the hair root by polarized light may show black discolouration at the base, but this is non-specific. Determination of thallium in urine and saliva can provide an important clue for the diagnosis. Blood thallium levels may be elevated, but it does not reflect the tissue concentration because thallium is rapidly taken up by the cells.

To treat thallium poisoning, Prussian blue is administered orally, dissolved in 10–15 per cent mannitol,

250 mg/kg body weight, per day in three to four divided doses. Prussian blue forms an insoluble complex with thallium, suppresses its reabsorption and enhances excretion of thallium via faeces. Without treatment, the excretion half-life of thallium is approximately eight days, but the administration of Prussian blue shortens it to three days.[2]

In the early stages (within 48 hours after exposure), charcoal haemoperfusion and haemodialysis is used, although it has been suggested that haemodialysis can be effective even in the third week of poisoning.[10] Forced diuresis may also be effective. Chelators, such as dimercaprol, EDTA and penicillamine, are not effective and dithiocarbamate is contraindicated because it enhances the distribution of thallium into the brain. Following recovery from thallium overexposure, hair growth usually reappears, whereas neurological disturbances, such as ataxia, tremor, dementia and mental signs, often persist.

Key points

- Thallium has wide-ranging applications, with a potential for use in high-temperature semiconductors.
- Thallium poisoning is characterized by gastrointestinal effects, neurological impairment and alopecia.
- The lethal dose for thallium is from 6 to 40 mg/kg body weight.
- Oral administration of Prussian blue and mannitol is used for treating thallium poisoning.

REFERENCES

1. American Conference of Governmental Industrial Hygienists. Thallium and soluble compounds. In: Documentation of the TLVs and BEIs with other worldwide occupational exposure values, CD-ROM, 2005.
2. World Health Organization. International programme on chemical safety. Environmental health criteria 182: Thallium. Geneva: WHO, 1996.
3. US Geological Survey. Thallium statistics. Available from: http://minerals.usgs.gov/ds/2005/140/thallium.pdf.
4. Moore D, House I, Dixon A. Thallium poisoning. Diagnosis may be elusive but alopecia is the clue. *BMJ* 1993; **306**: 1527–9.
5. Meggs WJ, Hoffman RS, Shih RD et al. Thallium poisoning from maliciously contaminated food. *Clinical Toxicology.* 1994; **32**: 723–30.
6. Richeson EM. Industrial thallium intoxication. *Industrial Medicine and Surgery.* 1958; **27**: 607–19.
7. Hirata M, Taoda K, Ono-Ogasawara M et al. A probable case of chronic occupational thallium poisoning in a glass factory. *Industrial Health.* 1998; **36**: 300–303.
8. Davis LE, Standefer JC, Kornfeld M et al. Acute thallium poisoning: Toxicological and morphological studies of the nervous system. *Annals of Neurology.* 1981; **10**: 38–44.
9. Tromme I, Van Neste D, Dobbelaere F et al. Skin signs in the diagnosis of thallium poisoning. *British Journal of Dermatology.* 1998; **138**: 321–5.
10. Misra UK, Kalita J, Yadav RK et al. Thallium poisoning: Emphasis on early diagnosis and response to haemodialysis. *Postgraduate Medical Journal.* 2003; **79**: 103–5.

34

Tin

TAR-CHING AW AND HIDEKI IGISU

Introduction	238	Organic tin compounds	238
Inorganic tin compounds	238	References	239

INTRODUCTION

Tin is a malleable, silvery-white metal with the symbol 'Sn', atomic number 50, atomic weight 118.69, melting point 232°C and a boiling point of >2000°C.[1] Metallic tin is used for protective coatings including tin-plated steel containers to preserve food, in the manufacture of solder, and in alloys such as bronze, brass, pewter and gunmetal. Tin compounds exist in two valency states – valency II (stannous compounds) and valency IV (stannic compounds). Stannous chloride is used as a stabilizer in soaps and perfumes, as a mordant for textiles, and in toothpaste with stannous fluoride to prevent dental caries. Organotins, which have at least one covalent carbon–tin bond, are deployed mainly as stabilizers for polyvinyl chloride polymers, catalysts in the production of polyurethane foams, and as biocides.[2] Triphenyltin is used in disinfectants, molluscides and anti-fouling agents in marine paints.

INORGANIC TIN COMPOUNDS

Acute effects following consumption of foods contaminated with inorganic tin include nausea, vomiting and diarrhoea. There is no evidence that inorganic tin damages the immune or the nervous system or that it is mutagenic or carcinogenic in humans.[1] Chronic exposure to dusts or fumes of inorganic tin such as stannic oxide causes a benign form of pneumoconiosis (stannosis) in which widespread mottling appears on a chest x-ray due to the high radiodensity of tin, but lung function is not compromised despite the x-ray changes. Patients with stannosis are also asymptomatic.

ORGANIC TIN COMPOUNDS

Organotins, in comparison to the inorganic tin compounds, are relatively toxic to humans. Tri-organotin compounds are more toxic than mono- and di-organotin compounds, with the toxicity of trialkyltins decreasing with an increase in the number of carbon atoms in the alkyl chain. Organotin compounds are skin and eye irritants. Tributyltin, dibutyltin and dioctyltin are immunotoxic in rodents, and organotins have been shown to be embryotoxic and teratogenic in laboratory animals, with cleft palate and other facial malformations as the most common abnormalities. Alterations of enzyme activities in sex hormone synthesis and haematological effects by organotins have been reported *in vitro* and *in vivo*, but there is no evidence of similar effects in humans.[1]

By contrast, the neurotoxicity of organotins, especially triethyltin (TET)[3,4] and trimethyltin (TMT),[5,6] has been clearly shown in humans, as well as in animals. Lethal poisoning due to TET or TMT has also been observed in humans. TET and TMT are colourless liquids under normal pressure, and the boiling point is relatively low for TMT (18°C). Both compounds are soluble in organic solvents but not in water, and they can be absorbed via the respiratory and gastrointestinal tracts, as well as through the skin. Poisoning by TET or TMT has occurred following occupational exposure.

Triethyl tin

In 1954 in France, approximately 1000 people took stalinon (an oral preparation containing 15 mg of diethyltin diiodide) to treat a variety of clinical conditions, such as staphylococcal skin infections, osteomyelitis and acne. As a result, more than 200 individuals were poisoned and there were approximately 100 deaths.[3,7] Impurities identified in stalinon were monoethyltin triiodide and triethyltin iodide. Triethyltin iodide, approximately 1.5 mg per capsule, was believed to be the primary cause of the poisoning. Judging from these cases, oral intake of 70 mg of triethyltin iodide over eight days will lead to tin intoxication. The clinical features of poisoning are severe headache approximately four days from initial exposure and absorption, with associated vomiting, dizziness, dysuria and visual disturbances, such as photophobia. Loss of appetite, hypothermia, somnolence and mental signs may also be seen. Disturbance in consciousness leading to coma may occur in severe cases. On spinal tap, the cerebrospinal fluid pressure is often elevated, but cell count, sugar and protein concentrations in the cerebrospinal fluid are normal. Death may follow coma, epileptic attacks or cardiopulmonary insufficiency.

Triethyl tin has been well recognized as a cause of cytotoxic brain oedema.[8] In laboratory animals, vacuoles occur diffusely in white matter. These are associated with splitting of myelin lamellae, but no changes in major chemical compositions of the myelin are observed. In human cases of TET poisoning, the main signs reflect diffuse leukoencephalopathy without any localized abnormalities. Fundoscopy and cerebrospinal fluid pressure may be normal.[3] The severe headaches and vomiting reported are most likely due to increased intracranial pressure.

From the effects observed in animals, magnetic resonance imaging (MRI) (especially T_2-weighted images) may be a useful tool for following up patients with TET intoxication,[9] although experience of the use of MRI in affected humans is limited. In a Japanese worker intoxicated with TET while engaged in manufacturing a large amount of tetraethyltin over a period of about ten days, the organotin level was elevated in whole blood, but not in serum or urine.[7]

There is no specific antidote for TET poisoning. In cases of stalinon poisoning, surgical decompression to relieve the increased cerebrospinal fluid pressure was considered the only clinically effective treatment.[3]

As for prognosis, complete recovery may take place, but in many cases it takes a long time and the recovery may be incomplete, leaving disabilities including paraparesis and visual disturbances. In the case of the affected Japanese worker, it took approximately six months before the cerebrospinal fluid pressure returned to normal.[7]

Trimethyl tin

Pathological lesions are limited to the nervous system with the major affected site being the limbic system.[6,10] The clinical picture appears to reflect this, presenting as aggressiveness, hyperphagia, disturbed sexual behaviour, disorientation, memory impairment and complex partial seizures. Animals given TMT also show aggressiveness, seizures, learning and memory impairment, and self-mutilation (biting their own tail). Central nervous system changes in affected animals revealed changes in the hippocampus, cerebral cortex[6] and the cerebellum.[11] The clinical presentation includes nystagmus and ataxia. Tinnitus and hearing difficulty may develop due to impairment of the brainstem and/or inner ear.

In the case of two individuals who consumed contaminated wine (containing an unknown quantity of TMT), tinnitus began within 10 minutes and abnormal behaviour, such as agitation, occurred three hours after drinking the wine.[10] It is uncertain how much of the alcohol consumed contributed to the behavioural effects.

Determination of organotins in urine may provide an important clue for the diagnosis. In six workers exposed to TMT vapour, while cleaning a tank in Germany, urinary organotin levels reached a peak within four to ten days.[11] (A mean normal urine level for tin has been reported at $16.6\,\mu g/L$.[12]) Electroencephalography (EEG) may show abnormalities in the temporal regions (spikes and/or slowing of EEG waves). Complete recovery occurs in mild cases, but clinical abnormalities often persist. In the above six workers, one died and two remained seriously disabled following the incident.[11] In a 23-year-old postgraduate student accidentally exposed to TMT while performing laboratory experiments, memory impairment and EEG abnormalities (slow waves in the temporal region) were observed 43 months later, but with no MRI changes.[13] Hence, the prognosis is poor for severely affected individuals.

Key points

- Tin exists as the pure metal (inorganic stannous (valency II) and stannic (valency IV) compounds) and as organotins.
- Exposure to inorganic tin dust leads to 'stannosis' – a benign effect despite widespread mottling on chest x-ray.
- Organotins are generally more toxic than inorganic tin compounds. They are irritant to the skin and eyes, and are neurotoxic.

REFERENCES

1. Agency for Toxic Substances and Disease Registry, US Public Health Service. Toxicological profile for tin and tin compounds. 2005: 23–248. Accessed on October 18, 2009. Available from: www.atsdr.cdc.gov/toxprofiles/tp55.html.
2. American Conference of Governmental Industrial Hygienists. Tin, organic compounds. In: *Documentation of the TLVs and BEIs with other worldwide occupational exposure values*. CD-ROM. Cincinnati, OH: ACGIH, 2005.

3. van Heijst ANP. Triethyltin (PIM 588). International Programme on Chemical Safety 1997. Accessed on October 26, 2009. Available from: www.inchem.org/documents/pims/chemical/pim588.htm.
4. Krinke GJ. Triethyltin. In: Spencer PS, Schaumburg HH (eds). *Experimental and clinical neurotoxicology*, 2nd edn. New York: Oxford University Press, 2000: 1206-8.
5. van Heijst ANP. Trimethyltin compounds (PIM G019). International Programme on Chemical Safety 1999. Available from: www.inchem.org/documents/pims/chemical/pimg019.htm.
6. Krinke GJ. Trimethyltin. In: Spencer PS, Schaumburg HH (eds). *Experimental and clinical neurotoxicology*, 2nd edn. New York: Oxford University Press, 2000: 1211-14.
7. Nishikawa M, Tsukiyama K, Matsumoto I *et al.* A case of alkyltin compounds intoxication. *Clinical Neurology.* 1965; **5**: 88-94.
8. Kimelberg HK. Current concepts of brain edema. Review of laboratory investigations. *Journal of Neurosurgery.* 1995; **83**: 1051-9.
9. Barnes D, McDonald WI, Tofts PS *et al.* Magnetic resonance imaging of experimental cerebral oedema. *Journal of Neurology, Neurosurgery, and Psychiatry.* 1986; **49**: 1341-7.
10. Kreyberg S, Torvik A, Bjorneboe A *et al.* Trimethyltin poisoning: Report of a case with postmortem examination. *Clinical Neuropathology.* 1992; **11**: 256-9.
11. Besser R, Krämer G, Thümler R *et al.* Acute trimethyltin limbic-cerebellar syndrome. *Neurology.* 1987; **37**: 945-50.
12. Goyer AG, Clarkson TW. Toxic effects of metals. In: Klaassen CD (ed.). *Casarett and Doull's Toxicology: The basic science of poisons*, 6th edn. New York: McGraw-Hill, 2001: 811-67.
13. Feldman RG, White RF, Eriator II. Trimethyltin encephalopathy. *Archives of Neurology.* 1993; **50**: 1320-4.

35

Tungsten

PERRINE HOET

Tungsten (wolfram) is a naturally occurring element. Two kinds of tungsten-bearing mineral rocks, called wolframite and scheelite, are mined commercially. Tungsten is an extremely hard metal and highly resistant to heat. It is used in the filaments of incandescent light bulbs and in the steels for producing metal tools. Most of the tungsten used in industry is in the manufacture of sintered tungsten carbide (cemented carbides). In this process, a mixture of powders, including tungsten carbide, cobalt, nickel or chromium metal, are shaped into the form of cutting tools and then heated at high temperatures to produce machine tools that are almost as hard as diamond. Some of the soluble compounds of tungsten, such as tungsten molybdenate, are used in the textile industry as mordants or fireproofing agents, and some of the highly coloured tungsten salts are used as pigments in paints, inks, ceramics and textiles.

In the hard metal manufacturing industry, there is exposure to:

- tungsten carbide in the forming, pressing and sintering workshops;
- a combination of tungsten carbide, tungsten oxide and tungsten metal in the tungsten carbide production workshop;
- tungsten metal alone in the powder processing department.

Grinders are exposed to tungstenate during wet grinding, and to tungsten oxide and carbide when dry grinding is carried out. Despite its low solubility, tungsten carbide is bioavailable. The bioavailability increases in the order: tungsten metal, tungsten carbide, tungstenate. Tungsten concentrations in urine of hard metal-producing workers were shown to vary greatly between the different workshops. The highest tungsten concentrations excreted in urine were found in grinders who had a mean value of 94.4 μg/g creatinine and a maximum value of 177.5 μg/g creatinine. High urinary tungsten concentrations were also detected in workers from the departments producing tungsten carbide (mean, 42.1 μg/g creatinine; maximum, 79.9 μg/g creatinine) and heavy alloys (mean, 24.9 μg/g creatinine; maximum, 84.8 μg/g creatinine). The 95th percentile for the general population is 1 μg/g creatinine.[1]

Exhaled breath condensate (EBC), obtained by cooling exhaled air under condition of spontaneous breathing, has also been proposed as a matrix to assess target tissue dose and effects of inhaled cobalt and tungsten.[2]

The main hazard associated with the use of tungsten carbide is hard metal disease (see Chapter 19, Cobalt and Chapter 82, Metal dusts and fumes). Although cobalt probably plays a critical role in the pathogenesis of hard metal lung disease (HMLD), it is suggested that tungsten carbide has a contributory synergistic effect. Animal experiments have shown that pure tungsten carbide is inert.[3] In lung biopsy samples from patients with HMLD, tungsten particles were found to be mainly distributed in centrilobular fibrosing lesions, suggesting that inhaled hard metal was trapped at the bronchioles and triggered the inflammation seen in HMLD.[4]

A case of tungsten-induced occupational asthma, with immediate hypersensitivity reaction at the scratch test has been reported.[5] However, tungsten as a cause of allergy is rare.

> **Key points**
>
> - Tungsten (wolfram) has no beneficial function in humans yet reported.
> - Tungsten and its compounds show low toxicity, but data are scant.

REFERENCES

1. Kraus T, Schramel P, Schaller KH et al. Exposure assessment in the hard metal manufacturing industry with special regard to tungsten and its compounds. *Occupational and Environmental Medicine.* 2001; **58**: 631-4.
2. Goldoni M, Catalani S, De Palma G et al. Exhaled breath condensate as a suitable matrix to assess lung dose and effects in workers exposed to cobalt and tungsten. *Environmental Health Perspectives* 2004; **112**: 1293-8.
3. Lasfargues G, Lison D, Maldague P, Lauwerys R. Comparative study of the acute lung toxicity of pure cobalt powder and cobalt–tungsten carbide mixture in rat. *Toxicology and Applied Pharmacology.* 1992; **112**: 41–50.
4. Moriyama H, Kobayashi M, Takada T et al. Two-dimensional analysis of elements and mononuclear cells in hard metal lung disease. *American Journal of Respiratory and Critical Care Medicine.* 2007; **176**: 70-7.
5. Miyamoto T, Inoue S, Watanabe T. A case of immediate hypersensitivity reaction with tungsten. *Allergy.* 2005; **60**: 415–16.

36

Uranium

IAIN BLAIR

Introduction	243	Health effects	244
Uses	243	References	245
Exposure, absorption and toxicity	243		

INTRODUCTION

Refined uranium is a silver-grey weakly radioactive metal that is 70 per cent more dense than lead, but not as dense as gold or tungsten. Uranium is found naturally in low concentrations in soil, rock and water and is more plentiful than tin or silver. The worldwide production of uranium in 2006 amounted to 39 603 tonnes of which 28 per cent was mined in Canada and 23 per cent in Australia. Other important uranium mining countries are Russia, Niger, Namibia and Kazakhstan. In nature, uranium is mostly the isotope uranium-238 (>99 per cent), with small amounts of uranium-235 and very small amounts of uranium-234. Uranium isotopes have very long half-lives. They decay slowly through a series of decay products by emitting alpha particles.

USES

Historically, uranium was a byproduct of radium production, which was used to make luminous paints for clock and aircraft dials. It was used as a colourant in the glass and pottery-glazing industries.

Contemporary uses for uranium rely on its unique nuclear properties. Uranium-235 is naturally fissile and can produce a sustained nuclear chain reaction which is exploited in nuclear reactors and nuclear weapons. One kilogram of uranium-235 can produce as much energy as 1500 tonnes of coal and as little as 7 kg can be used to make an atomic bomb.

To be used as a nuclear fuel, uranium must be enriched, so that the uranium-235 concentration is increased to between 3 and 5 per cent. The enrichment process produces large amounts of uranium that is depleted of uranium-235, but with correspondingly more uranium-238, so-called depleted uranium (DU).

When alloyed with 1–2 per cent of other elements, DU produces a very dense, low cost, material that is easily machined or cast. It has many uses in the defence industry, including ammunition, armour plate and counterweights in various devices.

The use of DU has become controversial following the widespread use of DU munitions by the United States, United Kingdom and other countries during recent wars in Iraq, the Balkans and Afghanistan. Although less radioactive, DU behaves chemically and toxicologically like natural uranium. The toxicity of DU has been studied mostly as a health issue for military personnel, but many tons of DU have been left in war-affected areas where the local civilian populations continue to be exposed to DU mainly in the form of dust. Although no conclusive epidemiological data have linked DU exposure with specific human health effects, such as cancer, DU remains controversial because of unanswered questions about potential long-term health effects (see under Health effects, p. 244).

EXPOSURE, ABSORPTION AND TOXICITY

Exposure to uranium and its radioactive decay products including radon gas may occur during the mining and processing of uranium ore, the enrichment of uranium for reactor fuel or as a result of transport or storage accidents. Excessive worker exposure to uranium is unlikely in workplaces where good occupational hygiene measures are in place.

Military personnel and local civilians may be exposed in areas where DU munitions have been used. Exposure may also occur in areas where soil and groundwater have high levels of naturally occurring uranium. The main routes of exposure are by inhaling dust, ingesting contaminated water and food, or in the case of DU munitions, through injury causing open wounds and embedded fragments.

Absorption of uranium from the gastrointestinal tract is low and depends on the solubility of the particular uranium compounds. Over 95 per cent is eliminated in the faeces and two-thirds of the absorbed fraction is filtered by the kidney and excreted in the urine in 24 hours. Uranium within the body deposits at bone surfaces and is slowly cleared via blood and kidneys with a half-life of up to one year. Inhaled uranium particles may be retained in the lung and may lead to irradiation damage and lung cancer as they are slowly absorbed into the bloodstream. Exposure to uranium can be monitored by measuring urinary uranium excretion. Chelation is ineffective.

Uranium is weakly radioactive, but of greater significance is its chemical toxicity which it shares with other heavy metals. The health effects of uranium which are known from animal studies and human epidemiology include lung cancer, kidney damage and DNA damage. Uranium is less toxic than lead.

The World Health Organization (WHO)[1] and most national regulatory agencies[2] have set minimum, recommended or permissible exposure limits for soluble and insoluble uranium compounds by ingestion and inhalation. These limits consider both renal toxicity and radiation exposure and apply to both the general population and the workplace. Levels are also available for air and drinking water. The levels vary depending on the methodology that is used and the levels of risk and uncertainty that are deemed acceptable. For example, the WHO recommends that the general public's intake of soluble uranium compounds should not exceed $0.5\,\mu g/kg$ of body weight per day by ingestion and $1\,\mu g/m^3$ by inhalation. Occupational exposure to soluble and insoluble uranium compounds, as an 8-hour time-weighted average should not exceed $0.05\,mg/m^3$.

HEALTH EFFECTS

Epidemiological studies have shown an association between uranium mining and lung cancer. It is exposure to radon gas and other radioactive decay products rather than uranium *per se* that explains this association.[3,4] Radon exposure also explains the increase in lung cancer seen in other groups of miners. Uranium miners may also have an increased risk of developing leukaemia as a consequence of radon exposure,[5] although this outcome may require lengthy occupational exposure to longer-lived radionuclides and gamma-radiation.[6]

Only a few humans have had sufficiently large acute intakes of uranium compounds to lead to kidney failure. Studies of these few cases indicate that kidney failure is likely to occur within a few days at concentrations above about $50\,\mu g$ uranium per gram of kidney. The levels of kidney uranium that may cause minor kidney dysfunction in humans are not well established, but are considered to be at least ten-fold less than the value of $3\,\mu g$ uranium per gram of kidney that has often been used as the basis for occupational exposure limits. Acute exposures that lead to concentrations of about $1\,\mu g$ uranium per gram kidney have been associated with minor kidney dysfunction, but the levels that can occur for short periods without causing long-term kidney damage have not been defined.

Epidemiological studies have examined the health of workers potentially exposed in uranium-processing plants and community studies have examined health outcomes in populations living near uranium plants. Lack of exposure data, confounding factors and the expected 'healthy worker' effect make interpretation of the results difficult. Generally, there is no consistent evidence for any increase in cancer or serious kidney disease due to uranium exposure in these settings.

Incidents involving acute or subacute exposure to uranium have occurred in a variety of settings. Workers at a uranium-processing plant where there was poor dust control had evidence of increased urinary uranium levels and impaired renal function.[7] Following the uranium enrichment process, large quantities of depleted uranium hexafluoride (HF) are produced and have to be stored indefinitely in steel containers. Inevitably accidental releases occur. In one such release in 1986, one worker died from HF inhalation and 31 other workers were exposed and showed evidence of short-term kidney damage. None, however, had lasting kidney toxicity from the uranium exposure. Magdo and others reported nephrotoxicity with raised beta-2-microglobulin excretion rate in a three-year-old child as a result of drinking water from a well at their home in Connecticut with naturally elevated concentrations of uranium (866 and $1160\,\mu g/L$).[8]

Depleted uranium has been widely studied as a possible contributory factor in 'gulf war syndrome': the immune system disorders and other wide-ranging symptoms reported in about 25 per cent of combat veterans of the 1991 Gulf War. There have been several authoritative reports and a precautionary approach is advised.[9]

Thirty-five American Gulf War I veterans who had significant DU-retained shrapnel burden as a result of combat were assessed 16 years after initial exposure. They continued to have elevated concentrations of urinary uranium with minor abnormalities of renal tubular function and bone formation, but without clinically significant related health effects.[10]

A follow-up study after eight years of 2499 firefighters, police officers and hangar workers who were potentially exposed to uranium from the balance weights of a crashed aircraft in the 1992 Amsterdam air disaster found no evidence of higher urinary uranium concentration or disturbed renal function.[11]

Animal studies suggest that DU is a teratogen and there is some evidence that human parental DU exposure may be associated with an increased risk of abnormality in their progeny.[12] Persistent chromosome abnormalities have been reported in a cohort of uranium miners.[13]

Key points

- Uranium is a very dense, weakly radioactive metal which, when enriched, is used in nuclear reactors and nuclear weapons. Depleted uranium-238 is used in the defence industry and is controversial because of its potential health effects.
- Exposure to uranium can occur in various settings by inhalation, ingestion or embedded fragments.
- Although poorly absorbed, like other heavy metals, uranium is toxic to kidney and other tissues.
- Inhaled uranium particles may lead to irradiation damage and lung cancer.
- In epidemiological studies, the health effects of uaranium exposure are often confounded by radon exposure.

REFERENCES

1. World Health Organization. Depleted uranium. Accessed November 2008. Available from: www.who.int/ionizing_radiation/env/du/en/.
2. Agency for Toxic Substances and Disease Registry. Minimal risk levels (MRLs) for hazardous substances. Accessed November 2008. Available from: www.atsdr.cdc.gov/mrls/index.html.
3. Tomasek L, Rogel A, Tirmarche M et al. Lung cancer in French and Czech uranium miners: Radon-associated risk at low exposure rates and modifying effects of time since exposure and age at exposure. *Radiation Research.* 2008; **169**: 125–37.
4. Grosche B, Kreuzer M, Kreisheimer M et al. Lung cancer risk among German male uranium miners: A cohort study, 1946–1998. *British Journal of Cancer.* 2006; **95**: 1280–7.
5. Rericha V, Kulich M, Rericha R et al. Incidence of leukemia, lymphoma, and multiple myeloma in Czech uranium miners: A case–cohort study. *Environmental Health Perspectives.* 2006; **114**: 818–22.
6. Möhner M, Lindtner M, Otten H, Gille HG. Leukemia and exposure to ionizing radiation among German uranium miners. *American Journal of Industrial Medicine.* 2006; **49**: 238–48.
7. Shawky S, Amer HA, Hussein MI et al. Uranium bioassay and radioactive dust measurements at some uranium processing sites in Egypt – health effects. *Journal of Environmental Monitoring.* 2002; **4**: 588–91.
8. Magdo HS, Forman J, Graber N et al. Grand rounds: Nephrotoxicity in a young child exposed to uranium from contaminated well water. *Environmental Health Perspectives.* 2007; **115**: 1237–41.
9. The Royal Society Working Group on the Health Hazards of Depleted Uranium Munitions. The health effects of depleted uranium munitions: A summary. *Journal of Radiological Protection.* 2002; **22**: 131–9.
10. McDiarmid MA, Engelhardt SM, Dorsey CD et al. Surveillance results of depleted uranium-exposed Gulf War I veterans: Sixteen years of follow-up. *Journal of Toxicology and Environmental Health.* 2009; **72**: 14–29.
11. Bijlsma JA, Slottje P, Huizink AC et al. Urinary uranium and kidney function parameters in professional assistance workers in the Epidemiological Study Air Disaster in Amsterdam (ESADA). *Nephrology, Dialysis, Transplantation.* 2008; **23**: 249–55.
12. Hindin R, Brugge D, Panikkar B. Teratogenicity of depleted uranium aerosols: A review from an epidemiological perspective. *Environmental Health.* 2005; **4**: 17. Available from: www.ehjournal.net/content/pdf/1476-069X-4-17.pdf.
13. Mészáros G, Bognár G, Köteles GJ. Long-term persistence of chromosome aberrations in uranium miners. *Journal of Occupational Health.* 2004; **46**: 310–15.

37

Vanadium

FINLAY D DICK

Introduction	246	Treatment	247
Sources	246	Health surveillance	247
Uses	246	References	247
Health effects	246		

INTRODUCTION

This transition metal was discovered in Mexico in 1801 by del Rió[1] and called vanadium by Sefström, who purified vanadium oxide in 1830.[2] Vanadium is found in the blood of sea cucumbers and sea squirts.[3] Whether vanadium is an essential element for humans remains unclear.[4]

SOURCES

Commercially important vanadium ores include carnotite, patronite and vanadinite and the main reserves are in South Africa, Russia, China and the United States.[1] The primary source of vanadium is vanadium-bearing steel slag, with vanadium ores as a secondary source. Crude oil contains trace amounts of vanadium[5] with Venezuelan oil being (relatively) vanadium rich. Oil combustion concentrates vanadium in the residual oil fuel ash which can contain up to 40 per cent vanadium by mass. As a consequence, this ash has commercial value and 8 per cent of world vanadium production comes from refining such ash.[1]

USES

Owing to its hardness, fatigue resistance and corrosion resistance vanadium has been widely employed, as ferrovanadium, in the production of steel alloys used in the manufacture of high speed hard steel tools and in aviation. It is used as a catalyst in sulphuric acid production, in the manufacture of yellow pigments, in microelectronics, ceramics and batteries. It is a highly reactive metal and so it is not found as the pure metal in nature.

Exposure to vanadium as vanadium oxide dust can occur during vanadium refining and manufacture of steel alloys. Industrial boiler cleaning is an important occupational exposure owing to the high level of vanadium in the residual oil fuel ash.

HEALTH EFFECTS

Vanadium pentoxide (V_2O_5) is a skin and respiratory irritant which may cause respiratory and skin sensitization. Acute exposure leads to eye and skin irritation, rhinitis, epistaxis, a metallic taste, pharyngitis, a productive cough, breathlessness, chest pain, haemoptysis and pneumonitis.[4] Some have reported fine tremor,[6,7] but the evidence for this is inconclusive.[3] Many authors describe exposed workers as having a greenish-black or greenish-yellow tongue,[3,6–9] although this is thought to be an index of exposure rather than toxicity.[8,9]

Lees observed that workers exposed to residual oil fuel ash showed reductions in both FEV_1 and FVC and suggested that such changes would resolve over ten days.[9] In contrast, Kiviluoto[10] found no evidence of impaired lung function in workers exposed to relatively low vanadium in air levels (0.01–0.04 mg/m^3), but exposures had previously been much higher at 0.1–3.9 mg/m^3. A study of US boiler makers exposed to relatively low levels of vanadium (median full shift dose estimate 53.2 µg) found an excess of upper and lower respiratory symptoms among boiler makers when compared with utility workers.[11] Vanadium exposure has been associated with the development of occupational asthma in workers in a vanadium pentoxide plant exposed to Na_3VO_3 vapour, NH_4VO_3 powder and V_2O_5 fumes and dust,[12] and one case report has described a metal fume fever-like syndrome in a man exposed to a catalyst containing vanadyl pyrophosphate dust.[13] Skin sensitization to vanadium, confirmed on patch testing, has also been described in a worker in a vanadium pentoxide manufacturing plant exposed to dust containing vanadium.[3] Vanadium interferes with iron metabolism and haem synthesis causing elevated zinc protoporphyrin (ZPP).[14] Barth et al.[15] suggested that vanadium pentoxide has short-term effects on cognitive function, but these findings have yet to be replicated.

In 2006, vanadium pentoxide was classified as a 'possible human carcinogen' (2B) by the International Agency for Research on Cancer (IARC) based on animal studies showing an excess of lung adenomas and cancer.[16] This assessment has, however, been disputed.[17] Recent work has shown increased DNA damage in a group of workers exposed to vanadium pentoxide dust with median serum vanadium of 2.2 μg/L.[18]

TREATMENT

Treatment for overexposure to vanadium or its compounds is mainly supportive.

There are no specific antidotes that have been shown to be effective in humans.

Measuring exposure

The current United States Occupational Safety and Health Administration (OSHA) exposure limit for vanadium respirable dust (as V_2O_5) is $0.5\,mg/m^3$ and the exposure limit for vanadium fume (as V_2O_5) is $0.1\,mg/m^3$.[19] The American Conference of Governmental Industrial Hygienists (ACGIH) has assigned respirable vanadium pentoxide a threshold limit value of $0.05\,mg/m^3$ as an eight-hour time-weighted average based on the upper and lower respiratory tract irritancy of vanadium pentoxide.[20] The UK work exposure limit (WEL) for vanadium pentoxide is $0.05\,mg/m^3$ (eight-hour time-weighted average).[21] There is currently no German maximale Arbeitsplatz-Konzentration or maximum concentration at the workplace (MAK value) assigned for vanadium.[22]

HEALTH SURVEILLANCE

Biological monitoring may be undertaken using post-shift urinary vanadium at the end of the working week. Creatinine-adjusted urinary vanadium is highly correlated with serum vanadium values.[23] Vanadium is rapidly excreted in the urine[24] and in workers with long-term exposure most vanadium is excreted within 24 hours.[23] Ingested vanadium is largely excreted unabsorbed in the faeces.[4] Blood and serum values of around 1 nmol/L and urinary vanadium values of 10 nmol/L have been proposed as likely normal values in unexposed populations, although these will be influenced by environmental factors such as residency near steel works or oil-burning power stations.[25]

> **Key points**
>
> - Vanadium pentoxide (V_2O_5) is a skin and respiratory irritant.
> - Industrial boiler cleaning is an important occupational exposure owing to the high level of vanadium in the residual oil fuel ash.
> - Vanadium exposure has been associated with occupational asthma.
> - Skin sensitization to vanadium has very rarely been described.
> - Treatment for overexposure to vanadium is mainly supportive.
> - Vanadium pentoxide is classified as a 'possible human carcinogen' (group 2B) by the International Agency for Research on Cancer (IARC).

REFERENCES

1. Monakhov IN, Khromov SV, Chernousov PI, Yusfin YS. The flow of vanadium-bearing materials in industry. *Metallurgist*. 2004; **48**: 381–5.
2. Dutton WF. Vanadiumism. *Journal of the American Medical Association*. 1911; **56**: 1648.
3. Sjöberg S-G. Health hazards in the production and handling of vanadium pentoxide. *Archives of Industrial Hygiene and Occupational Medicine*. 1951; **3**: 631–46.
4. Barceloux DG. Vanadium. *Clinical Toxicology*. 1999; **37**: 265–78.
5. McTurk LC, Hirs CHW, Eckardt RE. Health hazards of vanadium-containing residual oil ash. *Industrial Medicine and Surgery*. 1956; **25**: 29–36.
6. Wyers H. Some toxic effects of vanadium pentoxide. *British Journal of Industrial Medicine*. 1946; **3**: 177–82.
7. Williams N. Vanadium poisoning from cleaning oil-fired boilers. *British Journal of Industrial Medicine*. 1952; **9**: 50–5.
8. Lewis CE. The biological effects of vanadium: II. The signs and symptoms of occupational vanadium exposure. *AMA Archives of Industrial Health*. 1959; **19**: 497–503.
9. Lees REM. Changes in lung function after exposure to vanadium compounds in fuel oil ash. *British Journal of Industrial Medicine*. 1980; **37**: 253–6.
10. Kiviluoto M. Observations on the lungs of vanadium workers. *British Journal of Industrial Medicine*. 1980; **37**: 363–6.
11. Woodin MA, Liu Y, Neuberg D et al. Acute respiratory symptoms in workers exposed to vanadium-rich fuel-oil ash. *American Journal of Industrial Medicine*. 2000; **37**: 353–63.

12. Irsigler GB, Visser PJ, Spangenberg PAL. Asthma and chemical bronchitis in vanadium plant workers. *American Journal of Industrial Medicine.* 1999; **35**: 366–74.
13. Vandenplas O, Binard-van Cangh F, Gregoire J et al. Fever and neutrophilic alveolitis caused by a vanadium based catalyst. *Occupational and Environmental Medicine.* 2002; **59**: 785–7.
14. Missenard C, Hansen G, Kutter D, Kramer A. Vanadium induced impairment of haem synthesis. *British Journal of Industrial Medicine.* 1989; **46**: 744–7.
15. Barth A, Schaffer AW, Komaris C et al. Neurobehavioural effects of vanadium. *Journal of Toxicology and Environmental Health. Part A.* 2002; **65**: 677–83.
16. International Agency for Research on Cancer. Vanadium pentoxide. IARC Monographs on the Evaluation of Carcinogenic Risks to Humans, vol. 86. Lyon: World Health Organization, International Agency for Research on Cancer, 2006: 227–92. Last accessed September 20, 2009. Available from: www.monographs.iarc.fr/ENG/Monographs/vol86/mono86-10.pdf.
17. Duffus JH. Carcinogenicity classification of vanadium pentoxide and inorganic vanadium compounds. The NTP study of carcinogenicity of inhaled vanadium pentoxide, and vanadium chemistry. *Regulatory Toxicology and Pharmacology.* 2007; **47**: 110–4.
18. Ehrlich VA, Nersesyan AK, Hoelzl C et al. Inhalative exposure to vanadium pentoxide causes DNA damage in workers: Results of a multiple end point study. *Environmental Health Perspectives.* 2008; **116**: 1689–93.
19. United States Department of Labor Occupational Safety and Health Administration. Chemical sampling information: Vanadium, respirable dust (as V_2O_5). Last accessed October 19, 2009. Available from: www.osha.gov/dts/chemicalsampling/data/CH_275100.html.
20. American Conference of Governmental Industrial Hygienists. 2009 TLVs and BEIs based on the documentation of the threshold limit values for chemical substances and physical agents and biological exposure indices. Cincinnati, OH: ACGIH, 2009: ISBN: 978-1-882417-95-7.
21. Health and Safety Executive. Workplace exposure limits. EH 40/2005. Last accessed August 24, 2009. Available from: www.hse.gov.uk/coshh/table1.pdf.
22. Deutsche Forschungsgemeinschaft (DFG). List of MAK and BAT values 2009: Maximum concentrations and biological tolerance values at the workplace, Report 45. Weinheim: Wiley-VCH, 2009: ISBN 978-3-527-32596-2.
23. Kiviluoto M, Pyy L, Pakarinen A. Serum and urinary vanadium of workers processing vanadium pentoxide. *International Archives of Occupational and Environmental Health.* 1981; **48**: 251–6.
24. White MA, Reeves GD, Moore S et al. Sensitive determination of urinary vanadium as a measure of occupational exposure during cleaning of oil fired boilers. *Annals of Occupational Hygiene.* 1987; **31**: 339–43.
25. Sabbioni E, Kuèera J, Pietra R, Vesterberg O. A critical review on normal concentrations of vanadium in human blood, serum and urine. *Science of the Total Environment.* 1996; **188**: 49–58.

38

Zinc

PETER AGGETT

Properties and uses	249	Exposure and health effects	250
Essentiality and metabolism	249	References	250

PROPERTIES AND USES

Zinc is the twenty-fifth most abundant element in the Earth's crust and is the fourth most widely used metal. Zinc is more reactive with oxygen than either iron or steel, and it is therefore used to coat (galvanize) these to protect them from oxidation and corrosion. Half of zinc's production is used for galvanizing. It is also used in alloys, such as: brass; wrought zinc (zinc, copper and titanium) for example in roofing; 'nickel silver' typewriter metal and other die casting alloys with copper, aluminium and magnesium; catalysts, batteries and, with a copper coating, in coins. Other uses include pigments, medicines, ointments and topical lotions such as calamine, eye drops (zinc sulphate), cosmetics, deodorants containing zinc chloride and anti-dandruff shampoos with zinc pyrithione. Organic zinc is used as a fungicide and zinc phosphide, which releases phosphine, as a rodenticide. It is also found as feed additives and in over-the-counter mineral supplements.[1,2]

Zinc occurs naturally in soils and in most rocks as the sulphide (ZnS) in blende and sphalerite, which accounts for 95 per cent of that used commercially. Other sources include calamine, zinc spar, wilemite and zincite (zinc oxide). Many of these ores also contain copper, lead, iron and silicate.

ESSENTIALITY AND METABOLISM

Zinc is an essential trace element. It has a single oxidation state and therefore does not transfer electrons, but it readily acts as a Lewis acid, and forms complexes with oxygen, nitrogen and sulphur donors. These characteristics enable it to have catalytic, structural and regulatory roles in enzymes, and structural and regulatory roles in other proteins, histones, nucleic acids (zinc finger proteins) and receptor binding. The metal is involved in over 200 enzymes representing all classes of activity and involving every metabolic pathway and function in the body, including for example protein digestion and synthesis, vision, carbohydrate metabolism, bone health, free radical protection, cell turnover and new tissue synthesis.

Zinc is absorbed predominantly in the proximal, but also throughout the small intestine. There are specific carrier-mediated pathways and also diffusional routes for its uptake and transfer. It is distributed in the circulation to the liver, and systemically from the liver bound to albumin, transferrin and alpha-2-macroglobulin. Zinc is in pancreatic and biliary, and other intestinal secretions. This contributes to an enteropancreatic circulation of zinc, within which the intestinal reabsorption of the secreted zinc is an important regulator of systemic zinc accumulation and an important component of zinc homeostasis. Thus the principal route of zinc loss is in the faeces, which also contain unabsorbed dietary zinc.[1,3]

No specific systemic zinc store has been identified. It accumulates in the liver where it induces and binds to a low molecular weight cysteine-rich protein, metallothionein. At high exposures or when the system has no need for zinc, its systemic accumulation is further regulated by down-regulation of the mucosal zinc transporters to reduce uptake and the induction of enterocytic metallothionein which blocks transfer of the element and traps it in the mucosa.[3]

EXPOSURE AND HEALTH EFFECTS

There are few reports of zinc toxicity, particularly as a result of occupational exposure.[2,4] Contact dermatitis to zinc salts occurs and prolonged or repeated exposure might cause a papular folliculitis. Acute exposure to zinc from drinking contaminated food or water, such as drinks that have been stored in galvanized containers causes acute nausea, vomiting, abdominal pain and faintness.[2,4,5] Zinc sulphate solutions may cause simply upper gastrointestinal discomfort and symptoms; zinc chloride is more corrosive and can cause pharyngitis and oesophagitis, as well as haemorrhagic gastritis. These effects are ameliorated by the simultaneous ingestion of food. The metallic taste of zinc solutions is evident at 15 mg Zn/L. The regulatory limits for the zinc content of water supplies are around 5 mg Zn/L. High acute exposures can lead to renal damage and pancreatitis.[2,4]

Prolonged oral exposure to zinc interferes with the metabolism of copper, and to a lesser extent, iron. The mechanisms for this are thought to involve competition at carrier sites and, in the case of copper, the induction of intestinal metallothionein which blocks its onward transfer to the body. In some instances, this has led to symptomatic copper deficiency manifest by hypocupraemia, impaired iron metabolism, anaemia, leukopenia, neutropenia, reduced erythrocytic superoxide dismutase activity, and reduced caeruloplasmin.[1,6] This intake of zinc at which this phenomenon occurs depends on the effects of the dietary matrix on the availability of zinc to interact with the gut mucosa; it is probably in the region of 30–50 mg of elemental zinc daily which is about three to five times the daily requirement. Some workers galvanizing metals have been reported to have reduced circulating copper levels, but no other clear evidence of an increased systemic load of zinc or other features of clinically significant copper deficiency.[7]

Zinc salts, such as the oxide, are volatile at low temperatures.[1,2] White fumes of zinc oxide are produced when the metal is being worked in welding and galvanizing. This can precipitate metal fume fever. Inhalation of zinc chloride has been associated with pneumonitis and adult respiratory distress syndrome.[8] Inhalation exposure to particles can produce nasopharyngeal damage and inflammation, as well as upper gastrointestinal effects. These are variably described as Brass founder's ague, zinc chills, Spelters' shakes, metal shakes and zinc fever: common with those using non-ferrous metals or ferrous alloys.

There is limited experience with treating systemic overload of zinc. The recommended chelator is calcium disodium ethylenediaminetetraacetate (CaNa$_2$EDTA).[2]

Key points

- Occupational zinc toxicity is principally metal fume fever.
- Exposure from drinks stored in galvanized containers is a common cause of zinc toxicity.
- Acute exposure is associated with gastrointestinal symptoms and acute high exposure is associated with renal and pancreatic damage.
- Chronic exposure impairs normal copper and iron metabolism and simulates deficiencies of these.
- Treatment is seldom needed. The recommended chelator is calcium disodium ethylenediaminetetraacetate (CaNa$_2$EDTA).

REFERENCES

1. International Programme on Chemical Safety. Zinc: Environmental Health Criteria 221. Geneva: World Health Organization 2001. Last accessed September 2009. Available from: www.who.int/ipcs/publications/ehc/ehc_221/en/index.html.
2. Barceloux DG. Zinc. *Journal of Toxicology. Clinical Toxicology.* 1999; **37**: 279–92.
3. Cousins RJ, Liuzzi JP, Lichten LA. Mammalian zinc transport, trafficking, and signals. *Journal of Biological Chemistry.* 2006; **281**: 24085–9.
4. Fox MRS. Zinc excess. In: Mills CF (ed.). *Zinc in human biology.* New York: Springer-Verlag, 1989: 365–70.
5. Brown MA, Thom IV, Orth GL *et al.* Food poisoning involving zinc contamination. *Archives of Environmental Health.* 1964; **8**: 657–60.
6. Yadrick MK, Kenney MA, Winterfeldt EA. Iron, copper, and zinc status: response to supplementation with zinc or zinc and iron in adult females. *American Journal of Clinical Nutrition.* 1989; **49**: 145–50.
7. El Safty A, El Mahgoub K, Helal S, Abdel Maksoud N. Zinc toxicity among galvanisation workers in the iron and steel industry. *Annals of the New York Academy of Sciences.* 2008; **1140**: 256–62.
8. Hjortsø E, Qvist J, Bud MI *et al.* ARDS after accidental inhalation of zinc chloride smoke. *Intensive Care Medicine.* 1988; **14**: 17–24.

SECTION THREE

Gases

39	Gases *Peter J Baxter*	253
40	Reactive airways dysfunction syndrome and irritant-induced asthma *Jon G Ayres*	310
41	Deliberate use of chemicals in warfare and by terrorists *Robert L Maynard*	314

# 39

Gases

PETER J BAXTER

Introduction	253	Investigation of gassing incidents	265
Definitions	254	Gases in the ambient air	265
Classification of gases according to their health effects	255	Properties and effects of industrial gases	268
Characteristics of hazardous gases	255	Primary irritant gases	278
Occupational exposure to gases in industry	256	Irritant or other gases with systemic toxic effects	284
Exposure to gases in the outdoor and indoor air	256	Gases with mainly anaesthetic action: general anaesthetics	298
Exposure to gases in major industrial incidents	256	Geothermal power	302
Exposure to gases in fires	258	References	304
Principles of first aid and treatment in gassing incidents	262		

INTRODUCTION

Inhalation accidents have been a threat to workers since early times from encounters with gases in fires, mines and fermentation processes. Volcanic and geothermal gases formed the earliest atmosphere of the Earth. Scientists laid the foundations of the chemical industry with the isolation and identification of individual gases. One of the foremost of these, Joseph Priestley (1733–1804), while working as a schoolmaster in England, is credited with the discovery of 'alkaline air' (ammonia), vitriolic acid air (sulphur dioxide), nitrous oxide, nitrogen dioxide and methane, as well as isolating what he called 'dephlogisticated air' in 1774. Lavoisier, after meeting Priestley, gave the latter the name oxygen and demonstrated its role in respiration and combustion, though the disputed claim for priority for its discovery is one of the most famous episodes in the history of chemistry.

Early experience with gases in manufacturing industries inevitably included avoidable deaths among workers from leaks or as a result of faulty working practices; today, however, deaths from occupational exposure to gases are rare in high economy countries, even though inhalation incidents are not uncommon. In the United Kingdom during the period 1990–3, a total of 1180 inhalation incidents was reported to SWORD, a national scheme for the surveillance of work-related and occupational respiratory diseases involving occupational and chest physicians. Gases and combustion products comprised by far the largest group of agents (45 per cent), with chlorine and oxides of nitrogen the most commonly reported gases.[1] Irritant gases (unspecified, 42 per cent) again dominated reporting in 1992–2001.[2]

Flammable and toxic gases stored in large quantities under pressure are an important cause of disaster. In 1974, an explosion at a chemical plant in Flixborough, England, caused by a leak of cyclohexane vapour, had an explosive force equivalent to 32 tonnes of TNT, destroying the plant and killing 28 workers on site, with extensive damage to houses and shops as far as 10 km away. This event profoundly influenced the approach to regulating major hazards (see under Exposure to gases in major industrial incidents, p. 256). In 1984, over 500 people died in Mexico City when a liquid petroleum gas plant exploded. Even greater hazards are posed by the release of a cloud of toxic irritant gas, which may cause death or pulmonary injury in populations for many kilometres downwind, as highly toxic irritant gases can be extremely dangerous in even very dilute concentrations. The disaster at Bhopal, India, in 1984, involving the release of methyl isocyanate was the world's worst industrial incident of this kind, resulting in over 10 000 deaths either immediately or subsequently from their lung injuries, while hundreds of thousands have been reported to be suffering from disabling chronic respiratory symptoms. These incidents have led to a concerted and successful worldwide effort by national and international agencies to reduce the hazard of accidental toxic releases during chemical manufacture, storage and transport.[3]

Chemical and other industrial installations may also become military or terrorist targets. The first recorded mass civilian casualty incident due to a toxic release in warfare was during the London Blitz, when 47 people were overcome by ammonia gas. They were sheltering in a brewery cellar which received a direct hit in a heavy air raid and a fragment of flying metal pierced a pipe of an ammonia condenser.[4] The use of gases as military weapons has a long history, but in modern combat dates from the First World War (see Chapter 41, Deliberate use of chemicals in warfare and by terrorists).

In recent years, renewed attention has been given to air pollution and respiratory health with the recognition of the effects that exhaust emissions from the growing number of motor vehicles are having on air quality. Carbon dioxide, carbon monoxide, sulphur dioxide and nitrogen oxides are produced in the combustion of fossil fuels, whether as coal or petroleum products, and so are common pollutants of the outdoor and indoor air. The worst episodes of air pollution occurred during the era when coal burning was the prime source of energy. The most dramatic of these was the London smog of December 1952 when there were an estimated 4000 excess deaths over a five-day period provoked by a dense blanket of pollutants which included smoke and sulphur dioxide. This episode was a defining moment in Clean Air legislation in the UK, eventually followed by many other countries in the world.

DEFINITIONS

A gas is any gaseous substance that is above its critical temperature and therefore is not capable of being liquefied by pressure alone. A vapour is the gaseous form of a substance which may condense at high concentrations, or is capable of being liquefied by pressure alone; aerosol (particulate) forms may coexist with the vapour. A vapour diluted with air behaves like a gas, as long as none of the substance is available in the liquid form. The same sampling devices can be used for the collection of gases and vapours.

Not all industrial 'gases', however, are true gases according to this definition. Examples are chlorine, ammonia, propane and butane which when handled in bulk are liquefied under pressure. Examples of 'true' or 'permanent' gases that require cooling as well as pressure to turn them into liquids are oxygen, nitrogen and methane.

Aerosols are solid or liquid particles dispersed in the atmosphere as dust, fumes, smoke, mists and fogs. Stability is an essential characteristic.

A fume, as strictly defined, is the solid particles generated by condensation from the gaseous state, generally after volatilization from melted substances and often accompanied by a chemical reaction such as oxidation. A cloud, or mist, of acid droplets (e.g. formed by the contact of hydrogen chloride gas with moist air) is often, but technically incorrectly, referred to as a fume.

The concentrations of gases and vapours in the air can be expressed in three main ways:

1. As the ratio of the volume of the gas to the volume of air in which the gas is contained usually expressed in parts per million (ppm) or parts per billion (ppb);
2. As the mass of gas in a specified volume of air usually expressed as mg or μg per cubic meter (mg/m^3 or μg/m^3);
3. In physiological terms as the partial pressure of a gas, such as in the oxyhaemoglobin dissociation curve.

The mass concentration as expressed above will be dependent on the ambient temperature and pressure. The volume mixing ratio is independent of the ambient temperature and pressure, if ideal gas behaviour is assumed. The two systems of units are interchangeable using a conversion formula:

$$\text{Concentration in ppm} = \frac{\text{molecular volume}}{\text{molecular weight}} \times \text{concentration (as mg/m}^3 \text{ or } \mu\text{g/L)}$$

where molecular volume $= 22.41 \times T/273 \times 10^{13}/P$ L (T is the ambient temperature (K) and P is the atmospheric pressure (in millibars).)

From a toxicological standpoint, the pathophysiological response on exposure to a gas is not dependent on the mass of the molecules, but on the number present. It is therefore more appropriate in this chapter to express the concentration in the air as ppm or ppb, but in many official publications mg or μg/m^3 are used instead. This can give rise to considerable confusion.

The available human evidence may or may not be adequate for determining a no observable adverse effect level (NOAEL) or a lowest observable adverse effect level (LOAEL) on exposure to a gas. Workplace exposure limits (WELs) are concentrations of hazardous substances in the air, approved by the UK Health and Safety Commission (HSC). UK employers have a responsibility to ensure that these limits are not exceeded in order to protect the health of workers. WELs are not necessarily purely health based, and are set by committees generally faced with a situation of uncertainty and who take scientific data from a wide range of sources, where available, and also consider the economic and engineering feasibility of achieving a limit when setting a new WEL. This is why published WELs for exposure to a gas in the workplace can be higher than the LOAEL derived from published data. Nevertheless, WELs do reflect a level at which most people at work will be reasonably well protected. WELs and the measured concentration of a gas in the workplace are therefore very useful as an aid to interpreting symptoms in a worker who may or may not be especially susceptible to a particular irritant gas, for example, because they suffer from asthma. All the exposure limits cited for individual gases in this chapter are taken from published Health and Safety Commission Workplace Exposure Limits, unless indicated otherwise.

CLASSIFICATION OF GASES ACCORDING TO THEIR HEALTH EFFECTS

Most of the common gases described in this chapter may be categorized according to the original classification of Henderson and Haggard.[5]

Irritant gases

As a rule, the irritant gases are substances which chemically are regarded as corrosive. They injure surface tissues and induce inflammation of the air passages and the parenchymal region. Primary irritants are those which have little or no systemic toxic effect in the concentrations that cause death. Secondary irritants produce systemic toxic effects in addition to the surface tissue irritation.

Workers may sometimes be exposed to a mixture of irritant gases, for example in welding. In these circumstances, there is little information on how different gases interact, but additive or synergistic effects should be allowed for when comparing the concentrations of gases in the air to their work exposure limits. Thus, if the effects of the different gases are believed to be additive, the mixed exposure should be assessed using the formula:

$$C_1/L_1 + C_2/L_2 + C_3/L_3$$

where C_1, C_2, etc., are the concentration of contaminants in the air and L_1, L_2, etc., are the corresponding exposure limits. The sum of the C/L fractions should not exceed unity.

Asphyxiant gases

This group of gases interferes with the supply and utilization of oxygen in the body. Simple asphyxiants, for example methane and hydrogen, exclude oxygen from the lungs. Chemical asphyxiants cause death by preventing the transportation of oxygen by the blood (e.g. carbon monoxide) or inhibit cellular respiration (e.g. hydrogen cyanide). Many simple asphyxiants are odourless and are not readily detectable. They are not given occupational exposure standards and the best means of ensuring safety is by monitoring the oxygen content of the air. Under normal atmospheric pressures, the oxygen content of the air should not be allowed to fall below a minimum of 18 per cent by volume.

Gases with a drug-like action

This group includes anaesthetic gases, hydrocarbons and solvents. They can have systemic effects after they have been absorbed through the lungs into the blood.

Thus, in this chapter, gases have been classified as follows:

1. asphyxiant gases: simple asphyxiants, chemical asphyxiants;
2. irritant gases: primary irritants with little or no systemic toxic effects, secondary irritants which produce systemic effects;
3. low-irritancy gases with a systemic drug-like action.

CHARACTERISTICS OF HAZARDOUS GASES

The general characteristics of gases which most relate to their health hazard are their density, water solubility and flammability. The air has a relative molecular mass of about 29 and the relative density of a gas compared with air is important in determining its tendency to disperse or accumulate at normal temperature and atmospheric pressure. When released from an industrial point source, denser than air gases, such as carbon dioxide or chlorine, can displace the air and flow under gravity or be blown by the wind along the ground, adding to their danger to workers and the population in the vicinity.

Flammable gases also have lower and upper flammable (explosive) limits within which the resultant mixture with air may ignite. When ignited in a confined space an explosion may result, but in an unconfined space, such as the open air, the consequence may be a flash fire. Most flammable gas clouds cease to be dangerous when diluted to about 2 per cent by volume. Alarm levels for flammable gases are set at 20 per cent of the lower explosive/flammable level so as to avoid the risk. Liquefied petroleum gases are stored or transported by road, rail and sea in large amounts and are major fire and explosion hazards. The flammability limits of flammable gases are usually much higher than the toxic levels, except for gases which spontaneously ignite on contact with air (pyrophoric gases), such as silane. Other exceptions are the flammable, simple asphyxiant gases such as hydrogen and methane whose lower flammable limits are exceeded before they can cause asphyxia by displacing air.

The localization of the effects of irritant gases in the respiratory tract depends upon the water solubility and concentration of the gas. At low-to-moderate concentrations of highly soluble gases, such as ammonia, hydrogen chloride, hydrogen fluoride and hydrogen bromide, injury is greatest from the nasopharynx to the bronchi. Nose breathing of these gases may confine injury to the nasal passages. For less water-soluble gases, for example, nitrogen dioxide, the main localization is from the proximal to the distal acinus. At high concentrations of soluble gases, or if the gases are dissolved in fine aerosols, damage may extend throughout the respiratory tract. Solubility will also determine whether the gas will be rapidly taken up by suspended droplets in the workplace atmosphere, for example hydrogen chloride and hydrogen fluoride will readily combine with water to form hydrochloric and hydrofluoric acids, respectively. Acid gases rarely exist in a purely gaseous state, but in a form that is partitioned between the gas and aqueous phases. Inhalation kinetics are dealt with further in Chapter 10, Occupational toxicology: general principles.

Hydrogen chloride and sulphur dioxide, being soluble in water, readily form acid aerosols. Occupations, such as battery-making and galvanizing, used to be associated with dental erosion in people working above acid baths,[6] but the condition is now seen more commonly in low economy countries where exposures to aerosols are less controlled.

OCCUPATIONAL EXPOSURE TO GASES IN INDUSTRY

In practice, zero exposure to chemical agents at work is an unattainable goal in industry and instead exposure limits are set to protect the worker. Under UK legislation the Health and Safety Executive defines a work exposure limit as the concentration that is not likely to be injurious, averaged over a reference period. These limits for many gases are long-term time-weighted average (TWA) (eight hours) and short-term exposure limit (STEL) (15 minutes) for peak exposures.[7] STELs are typically used to protect against effects which may occur rapidly, such as irritation of the eyes or nose/throat. A worker's sense of smell is not a reliable guide to the presence of a gas, let alone a safe level. Apart from individual variability some gases, for example hydrogen sulphide and hydrogen cyanide, actually induce olfactory fatigue at higher and more dangerous concentrations. Nevertheless, information on olfactory levels may be useful for a clinician when taking a patient's history. Objective measures of exposure require the use of chemical sensors or infrared detectors, colorimetric detection tubes and other specialized measuring devices.

EXPOSURE TO GASES IN THE OUTDOOR AND INDOOR AIR

The main sources of outdoor air pollution in high economy countries are motor vehicle emissions. Primary pollutants are those released directly into the air, and include carbon monoxide and nitric oxide, as well as benzene and particulate material. Diesel engines burn an excess of air and so produce little carbon monoxide, but they do give out more nitrogen dioxide and fine particles. The main single sources of sulphur dioxide in the UK are coal-fuelled electric power stations. Secondary pollutants are those formed by chemical changes to the primary pollutants. Thus, nitrogen dioxide is produced by rapid atmospheric oxidation of nitric oxide emitted by motor vehicles, and subsequently may undergo photochemical oxidation to form ozone. Important combustion sources of gases in the home are gas cookers, which produce much higher concentrations of nitrogen dioxide inside houses compared with the ambient air, and faulty gas or paraffin heaters emitting carbon monoxide. Ambient air quality standards for pollutants set on health criteria alone are almost invariably lower than occupational exposure standards, including for gases. No standards have yet been established for indoor air.

A different concept again is the exposure to gases as pollutants of indoor air in offices and homes. No limits or guideline values have as yet been set for indoor air and in such cases where workers are being inadvertently exposed to gases in indoor or outdoor ambient air, then separate air quality criteria should be applied, not occupational exposure limits, which are inappropriate for this type of exposure.[8] Carbon dioxide levels are sometimes used in office buildings as a surrogate measure of the rate of air exchange.

EXPOSURE TO GASES IN MAJOR INDUSTRIAL INCIDENTS

Major chemical disasters can be caused by large vapour or flammable gas explosions, fires and toxic releases. The accidental release of gases and chemicals during their distribution by pipeline, water, rail or road can also have severe consequences.[9] The gases that most often feature in toxic releases from plants are chlorine, ammonia, sulphuric acid, hydrogen chloride, phosgene, hydrogen sulphide and nitrous fumes.

In modern industry, with control measures in place, the plant operative, engineer or technician is only likely to receive heavy exposure to an industrial gas through a failure in the plant or other inadvertent event. Occupational exposure limits are set for workers who receive repeated daily exposures to hazardous substances on the basis of eight-hour work days over a working lifetime and are set to protect as far as is reasonably practicable against acute and chronic effects. They are obviously not set to protect against risks of unconsciousness, incapacitation or intolerable irritation which would greatly reduce the chances of escape in an emergency arising from a chemical release or a fire.

Information on the effects in humans of a single exposure to substantially higher levels of toxic gases and vapours under these life-threatening circumstances is sparse and consists mainly of case reports almost invariably without the recording of the level or duration of the acute exposure. Yet it is following just such inadvertent incidents that the physician will be consulted for advice, as the consequences may be life-threatening or lead to concerns about long-term respiratory or systemic health effects. Toxicity data relating to routes of exposure other than inhalation, such as contact with the skin in some gases, should be treated with caution unless it is known that the toxicokinetics and sites of action for the different routes are comparable. Knowledge of the long-term effects of single exposures, such as carcinogenicity, teratogenicity and other target organ damage, is very inadequate. Extrapolation from single exposure studies in animals to humans is also fraught with problems, such as species difference.

The ultimate harm caused by an acute high exposure to a toxic gas will depend primarily upon the concentration of gas and the period of exposure.[10] Experimental studies suggest the following general relationship may hold for acute lethality for many gases and vapours:

$$\text{toxic load} = \text{concentration}^n \times \text{time}$$

where n is any number other than zero. Thus the toxicity of an inhaled irritant gas is not necessarily the product of the concentration in the inhaled air and duration of exposure, which is known as Haber's rule, a simple relationship that applies to some gases and vapours. For hydrogen chloride $n = 1$, sulphur dioxide $n = 2$, and hydrogen sulphide $n = 4$. For chlorine, $n = 2$, and so for incidents involving exposure to chlorine lasting between 5 and 20 minutes, it is the concentration which is more important than the duration in determining the effects on health.[10] In practice, most releases will last a short time until emergency measures at the plant bring the release under control, but the risk of death and risk of dangerous dose for chlorine, ammonia ($n = 2$), hydrogen fluoride ($n = 1$) and sulphur dioxide, can be calculated for different time periods and exposure conditions (Table 39.1). These irritant gases have a similar toxic mechanism acting on the respiratory tract and lungs.

Unplanned releases of gases may lead to exposure off-site in a sudden large release from a tank failure or a pressurized leak of long enough duration. For emergency planning for such an eventuality and for land use planning around a major hazard site (all part of a 'safety case' which has to be prepared before a plant under the Control of Industrial Major Accident Hazards (CIMAH) Regulations is allowed to operate) can be derived by using animal data (e.g. LC_{50} data over a known duration) to estimate the specified level of toxicity for land use planning purposes, which the Health and Safety Executive calls the LUP SLOT and defines as the concentration at which there is:

- severe distress to almost everyone on the area;
- substantial fraction of the exposed population requires medical attention;
- some people are seriously injured requiring prolonged treatment;
- highly susceptible people are possibly killed.

A similar procedure can be used to derive a toxic load equation to predict exposure conditions for any other specified level of toxicity, such as the mortality of 50 per cent of an exposed population: this is known as the Specified Level of Death Dangerous Toxic Load (SLOD DTL).[11] For land use planning, allowance needs to be made for the proportion of the population indoors, as this will provide a level of protection compared to being outdoors.

Any assessment of the toxic impact of a release into the general population must take into account the presence

Table 39.1 Health effects levels for the most common irritant gases

	Occupational exposure limit (ppm)		'n' value	SLOT DTL (ppm^n.min)	SLOD DTL (ppm^n.min)	ERPG-1 (ppm)	ERPG-2 (ppm)	ERPG-3 (ppm)
	15 min	8 h						
Ammonia	35	25	2	3.78×10^8	1.03×10^9	25	150	750
Chlorine	0.5	–	2	1.08×10^5	4.84×10^5	1	3	20
Hydrogen chloride	5	1	1	2.37×10^4	7.65×10^4	3	20	150
Hydrogen cyanide	10	–	2	1.92×10^5	4.32×10^6	NA	10	25
Hydrogen fluoride	3	1.8	1	1.2×10^4	4.1×10^4	3	20	50
Hydrogen sulphide	10	5	4	2×10^{12}	1.5×10^{13}	0.1	30	100
Nitrogen dioxide	5	3	2	9.6×10^4	6.24×10^5	1	15	30
Sulphur dioxide	5	2	2	4.655×10^6	7.448×10^7	0.3	3	15

SLOD DTL, Dangerous toxic load for significant likelihood of death (mortality of 50% population); SLOT DTL, Dangerous toxic load for specified level of toxicity (land use planning value).
ERPG levels: Exposure up to 1 hour without causing in most people:
  ERPG-1, More than mild transient and irreversible effects.
  ERPG-2, Irreversible effects or effects that may affect the ability to take preventive action.
  ERPG-3, Life-threatening effects.

of the young, old, pregnant and individuals with pre-existing illness, particularly those who may be already suffering from acute or chronic respiratory conditions at the time of the release. Little information is available about the susceptibility of these vulnerable groups, and the toxicity data used for these planning criteria contain significant uncertainty.

The American Industrial Hygiene Association's Emergency Response Planning Guidelines (ERPGs) are another attempt at setting community exposure limits for use in community emergency response planning for anticipating the adverse health impacts from chemical release emergencies; they are planning tools, as there is usually no time for making exposure measurements and acting upon these in an actual release.[12] One use of such data, for example, would be to model the health consequences in a population living near a plant who would be told in an emergency to shelter inside their houses in the event of an unplanned gas release. The ERPGs are maximum airborne concentrations below which nearly all individuals could be exposed up to one hour without experiencing or developing:

ERPG 1. More than mild, transient adverse health effects or without perceiving a clearly defined objectionable odour;
ERPG 2. Irreversible or other serious health effects or symptoms that could impair an individual's ability to take preventive action;
ERPG 3. Life-threatening health effects.

Experience in making evacuation decisions in actual chemical emergencies is still very limited.[13]

In accordance with the EC Seveso Directive 1982 (revised as Seveso II in 1996), the UK introduced the Control of Industrial Major Accident Hazards (CIMAH) Regulations 1984 which included a requirement for emergency planning to be undertaken for on-site and off-site air releases at plants storing or using dangerous substances in larger than the threshold quantities laid down in the regulations; these chemicals include commonly used toxic or flammable gases.[14] The CIMAH regulations were superseded by the Control of Major Accident Hazards (COMAH) regulations in 1999, which treat risks to the environment as seriously as those to people. Chlorine is the most widely used gas for which emergency planning and land use planning to mitigate the effects of a major incident on the local population is undertaken; it is an example of a denser than air, highly corrosive gas that can cause injury to the respiratory tract ranging from irritation to incapacity or death from bronchospasm, laryngeal oedema or toxic pulmonary oedema.[15] Fortunately, no large-scale releases of chlorine gas have occurred in recent times, the last being in Romania in 1936 when 40 people were killed. While engineering measures directed towards successful containment of stored gases, such as chlorine, are clearly proving to be successful, small-scale releases of gases and other chemicals do inevitably occur from fixed sites or during their transportation. Thus, in the United States, one of the few countries with comprehensive reporting, chlorine remains the most common substance involved in hazardous chemical releases resulting in personal injury.

Computer models of the dispersion of chlorine and other dense gases can be applied to determine risk contours, so that the impact of a gas release on a nearby populated area can be predicted for different likely wind and weather conditions (Figure 39.1). The outer contour defines the consultation distance around major hazard sites, outside of which the risk to the population is not deemed as significant. The probability and size of preventable releases can be estimated to determine the serious but reasonably foreseeable event, such as a fracture of a liquid gas pipe or failure of a road tanker delivery coupling to a storage tank (Figure 39.2). Plotting the concentration contours for a predicted plume on to maps of the area around a plant is a useful planning guide for police, fire brigade and ambulance services, as COMAH requires on-site and off-site response plans to be prepared by emergency services as part of the consent process. Engineers can provide well-established failure rates for tanks, pipes and process functions, including human factors, which are used to quantify risks using gas dispersion modelling. In the UK, the Buncefield explosion and fire in 2005, not long after the fatal Texas City refinery explosion in the same year, led to an important re-evaluation of the operation of COMAH and the interested reader is referred to the Major Incident Investigation Board Report for further information.[16]

EXPOSURE TO GASES IN FIRES

The main threats to life in fires are toxic gases, heat and oxygen deficiency.[17] The temperature in a room in a house fire can easily reach 500–1000°C, and as many as 400 toxic compounds can be demonstrated in the smoke. The principal toxic constituents of smoke are soot, carbon monoxide, carbon dioxide, nitrogen oxides, hydrogen cyanide, hydrogen chloride, sulphur dioxide, hydrogen fluoride, hydrogen sulphide, isocyanates, acrolein, benzene, phenol, formaldehyde and a range of chlorinated hydrocarbons. Carbon monoxide is an important factor in 50–80 per cent of all fire fatalities. The role of hydrogen cyanide is less clear, although it is formed in many fires especially those involving wool, silk, nylon and polyurethane products.[17,18]

The chemistry involved in combustion reactions is extremely complex, even in the simplest example, such as the burning of a jet of natural gas or methane in oxygen or air, when numerous reactive species, including free radicals (such as OH, O and CH_3) are produced which eventually form mainly carbon dioxide, water and large particles of carbon (soot).

$$CH_4 + 2O_2 = CO_2 + 2H_2O$$

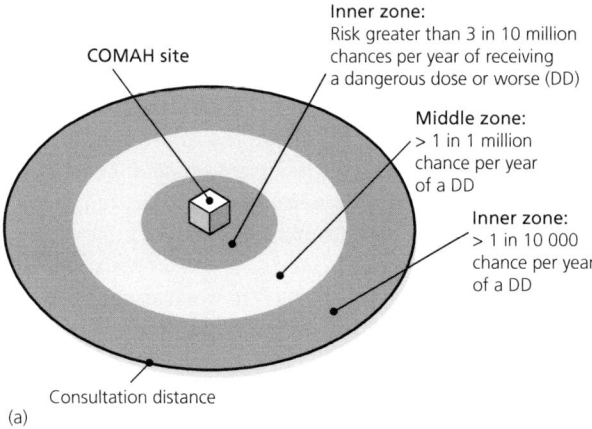

Level of sensitivity	Development in inner zone	Development in middle zone	Development in outer zone
1	DAA	DAA	DAA
2	AA	DAA	DAA
3	AA	AA	DAA
4	AA	AA	AA
Sensitivity level 1	Example	Factories	
Sensitivity level 2	Example	Houses	
Sensitivity level 3	Example	Vulnerable members of society, e.g. primary schools, old people's homes	
Sensitivity level 4	Example	Football ground/large hospital	

(b)

Figure 39.1 Consultation distance and zones, with land use planning 'sensitivity levels' (a) and decision matrix (b). AA, advise against the development; DDA, do not advise against the development. *Source:* Health and Safety Executive, quoted in Ref. 16.

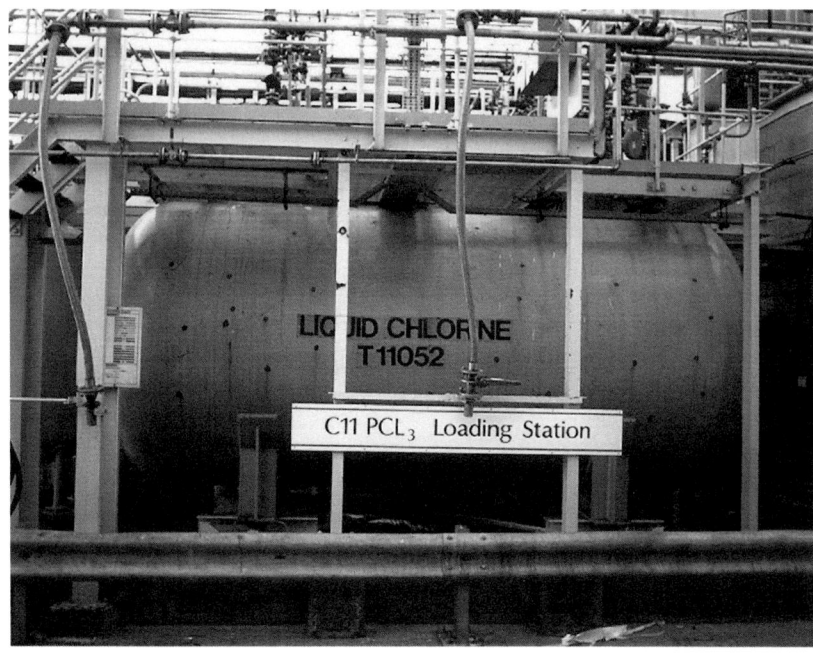

Figure 39.2 Chlorine storage tank in a chemical factory.

Smoke comprises a mixture of gases, liquid and solid particles which arise as combustion and pyrolysis products. Predicting the products of combustion (oxidative degeneration) and pyrolysis (thermal decomposition) of burning materials and hence determining in retrospect the effects of exposure of firemen or other victims to the constituents of a smoke plume is not straightforward. Some general principles can be considered.[18] Materials consumed by fires contain carbon, hydrogen and oxygen as their main elements, and hence the bulk of all combustion products will consist of compounds formed from these, for example carbon monoxide and carbon dioxide. The next important elements are halogens (mostly chlorine) and nitrogen, with smaller amounts of elements such as sulphur and phosphorus. Almost all the inorganic anions are released as the irritant acid gases, hydrogen chloride and hydrogen fluoride, if fluorine is present. For the nitrogen present the products depend upon the availability of oxygen: in well-ventilated fires oxides of nitrogen are released, but in large fires in buildings, where the ventilation is poorer, a larger proportion of the nitrogen is released as hydrogen cyanide. Organic compounds may form a number of partially decomposed products, for example formaldehyde, acrolein, crotonaldehyde and possibly free radicals that add to the irritancy of the smoke. Other compounds, such as decomposition products from isocyanates, styrene and phenol, may also be important.[18] Fires in warehouses storing chemicals will potentially release a cocktail of irritants and toxic substances which may greatly add to the hazard of the fire plume.

Polyvinyl chloride (PVC) is the most widely used plastic and fires involving large amounts of this material at storage sites and recycling installations are not uncommon and attract notoriety because they are difficult for the fire services to put out while they generate toxic plumes.[19] At over 300°C, PVC decomposes to form hydrogen chloride and carbon monoxide together with small amounts of about 50 various hydrocarbons. About 50 per cent of the polymer's weight comes off as hydrogen chloride, and the irritancy of the plume is added to by the presence of acrolein, ammonia, sulphur dioxide, nitrogen dioxide, aldehydes and particles. Phosgene is produced only in rare circumstances. There is now no doubt that dioxins are formed whenever chlorinated plastics are burned: in a large-scale plastics fire typically involving 500–1000 tonnes of PVC as much as 1–2 kg of dioxins could be produced.[19]

In February 1991, during the Gulf War, about 600 naturally pressurized oil wells were set alight in Kuwait.[20] Close to the fires the smoke rained oil drops which coated large areas of desert. The plume contained carbon dioxide, carbon monoxide, sulphur dioxide and particles, including soot. The major health concern revolved around the particle fallout that contained elemental carbon, rock/soil particles, metal oxides, silicates, vanadium, nickel and polycyclic aromatic hydrocarbons. Exposure studies and air monitoring started too late to ascertain the health risk to ground troops or the general population. Aplastic anaemia has been reported in a Gulf War veteran and a Kuwaiti child exposed to the fumes.[21] Fortunately, the fires were extinguished by November 1991, and since then the debate on whether there were any chronic ill effects from this incident has not been resolved. In contrast, the massive unplanned explosion and fire at a large fuel storage site in Buncefield, England, which supplied London Heathrow airport, in 2005 set off a blaze and a huge plume of smoke on 11 December that traversed southern England and was blown across the English Channel to France until it was extinguished on 14 December. Analysis of the plume using a special aircraft showed that it mainly comprised harmless soot particles as the burning was very complete; fortunately the weather allowed the buoyant plume to remain aloft and no significant particulate air pollution occurred at ground level.[16] There were 660 firefighters deployed during the burn phase, about three-quarters of whom reported inhaling smoke, but no major acute health symptoms were identified in a comprehensive occupational health surveillance programme.

Even if not directly fatal themselves, carbon monoxide and hydrogen cyanide singly or in combination may lead to the rapid incapacitation of the individual who is then unable to escape.[18] The other toxic gases can cause acute airways and lung injury or may obscure vision through causing eye irritation. An elevated carbon dioxide level will induce hyperventilation and hyperpnoea, and increase exposure to the combustion gases. In most fires, these toxic factors are usually more important to survival than heat. However, intense fires can lead to severe burning from hot convected air or thermal radiation and in some fires direct burning from the heat of the flame can be the cause of death. Thermal injury to the airways and lungs is not as common as toxic damage, since the upper respiratory tract rapidly conducts heat away from the inspired air. Nevertheless air containing hot, respirable particles or steam can cause injury as deep as the bronchioles. Less important is oxygen depletion except in major conflagrations or in intense building fires.

Firefighters

In the past, many firefighters did not always use respiratory protection equipment, but nowadays as the equipment and training have improved, breathing apparatus and chemical suits are routinely donned at fires emitting toxic smoke (Figure 39.3). As a result, firefighters are now much less likely to be exposed to the injurious effects of smoke than in the past. However, accidental inhalation exposure may occur if the firefighters make a faulty judgement on their assessment of the fire conditions, or if the smoke plume unexpectedly blows towards unprotected firefighters, or if an immediate rescue of a victim has to be made. Skin contamination by noxious combustion products may also occur when the protective clothing is removed unless decontamination procedures are adequate.

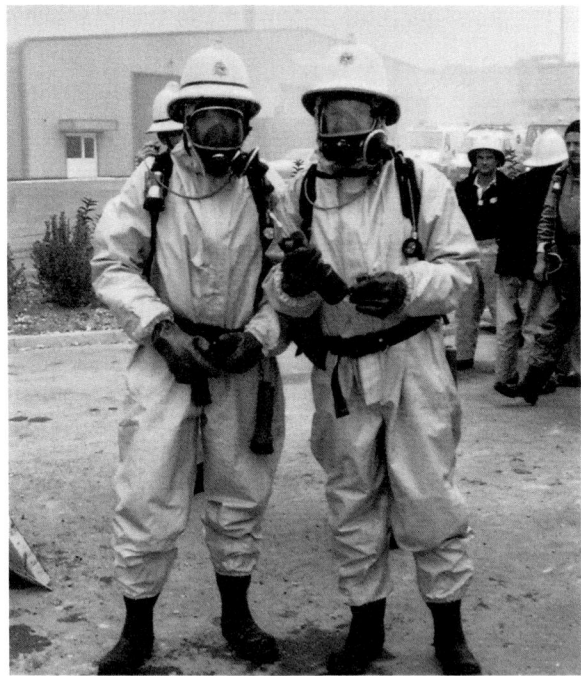

Figure 39.3 Firefighters at a plastics (PVC) fire. The breathing apparatus and chemical suits protect the firemen from smoke which contains hydrogen chloride and carbon monoxide together with other combustion and pyrolysis products.

The effects of single and repeated inhalation exposures to smoke therefore need to be considered. A fire victim will have a history of smoke exposure and the skin and clothing may be stained by smoke. The possibility of inhalation injury must be considered if there is production of carbonaceous sputum, reactive conjunctivitis and a hoarse voice. If the skin on the face and in the inside of the mouth or pharynx has been badly burned, then thermal injury to the airways and lungs should be suspected; oedema of the glottis and larynx may develop rapidly and upper airways intubation with continuous positive airways ventilation should be urgently considered. Smoke can cause a chemical tracheobronchitis, the inflammation of the airways being associated with denudation of airway epithelium, ulceration and oedema with cellular infiltration. The inflammatory changes may give rise to an increase in airways reactivity even in patients without a previous history of asthma, and despite an apparently full clinical recovery the patient may go on to develop mild airways obstruction which can persist for months.[22] Firefighters who have received acute exposure to smoke should therefore be considered for early referral for an assessment of lung function as it may be advisable to begin early treatment with inhaled anti-inflammatory drugs.

Reports of neurological symptoms following smoke exposure are uncommon. A group of firemen heavily exposed to the fumes of toluene diisocyanate for several hours developed persistent poor memory, personality change, emotional instability or depression;[23] however, no further incidents of a similar nature appear to have been reported. However, medical attendants should be alert to the possibility of injury to other organs as well as the lungs in fire victims, particularly as it may be impossible to confirm the identity of materials and other combustion and pyrolysis products in fires, for example at warehouses or chemical plants.

In the 1970s and 1980s, the concerns of firefighters that they were at high risk of premature death became a subject of epidemiological investigation and a greater awareness of the hazards led to an improvement in measures to protect the firefighter from smoke and toxic substances inhalation.[24] The extensive and routine use of respiratory equipment to protect against smoke exposure is now widely adopted and so the exposure to hazardous chemicals and particulate pollution should be, in theory at least, much reduced compared with in the past. No consistent trend of ill health in firefighters has been demonstrated despite suggestions in earlier studies of a more rapid loss of lung function than expected and an increase in non-specific respiratory symptoms. The risk of cancer of the respiratory tract may be theoretically increased by respiratory irritants impairing ciliary clearance mechanisms, thereby enhancing uptake of carcinogens adsorbed on particles, or from direct exposure to inhaled carcinogenic chemicals or polycyclic aromatic hydrocarbons in smoke.[25] Overall, the findings on cancer mortality studies in firefighters show no consistent trends.[26]

An analysis of the deaths occurring in on-duty US firefighters in the 11 years up to 1994 (excluding the terrorist attack on September 11, 2001) found that the risk of death from coronary heart disease was substantially higher during certain emergency firefighting duties compared with non-emergency duties; one-third of the deaths from heart disease occurred while firefighting, which takes up no more than 5 per cent of the average firefighter's time. The evidence from other studies shows that firefighters have a low risk of heart disease, so the findings starkly reflect the well-known link between psychological and physical stress with fatal heart disease.[27]

In 2001, 344 firefighters died in the events of September 11 at the World Trade Center (WTC) in New York City. A study of the 10 116 firefighters involved found increases in acute and chronic respiratory symptoms (cough, wheeze, phlegm production) related to exposure to the WTC dust in the debris. The high alkalinity of the resuspended WTC concrete dust (pH 9.0–11.0) and the smoke which were abundant in the two days after the attack were thought to be responsible for provoking bronchial hyper-reactivity, persistent cough and increased risk of asthma. The extent of wearing respiratory protection was unclear.[28]

Nuclear reactor incidents

The processing of uranium involves a variety of hazardous substances. Hydrazine, chlorine and ammonia are used in nuclear power facilities and may be released into the atmosphere in an incident and threaten local populations. In 1985, a uranium processing plant in Gore, Oklahoma, released a cloud of hydrogen fluoride. A plume from a nuclear reactor incident may contain radioactive inert gases which are fission products of uranium. At Three Mile Island in 1979, very slight amounts of krypton-85 and xenon-133, together with iodine-131, were emitted following core damage to this commercial reactor. In the fire in the graphite reactor at Chernobyl in 1986, which lasted for several days, several million curies of these gases, together with radioactive iodine-131 and -133, caesium, strontium and plutonium, were released in radioactive clouds that blew across Europe, making this event the worst nuclear accident in the world.[29] During the following eight days, the iodine-131 was absorbed by the thyroid glands of people living nearby. More than 350 000 people were relocated. Since 1990, a marked rise in cases of thyroid cancer in children has occurred in the Belarus region around Chernobyl, a condition which fortunately has a good survival rate with early treatment.[30]

PRINCIPLES OF FIRST AID AND TREATMENT IN GASSING INCIDENTS

Regardless of the kind of gas involved, the victim should be moved immediately to fresh air and given life support. If breathing has stopped or cardiac arrest has supervened then cardiopulmonary resuscitation should be begun. If hydrogen cyanide poisoning is suspected, then a manual resuscitator should be used to maintain respiration so that mouth-to-mouth resuscitation is avoided.

Simple asphyxiant gases or lack of oxygen will cause loss of consciousness without irritation of the eyes or mucous membranes of the respiratory tract, but complications may include patchy consolidation of the lungs. Unless the hypoxia is severe, the victim will recover consciousness in fresh air. If the patient is breathing and if oxygen is available, 100 per cent oxygen should be given by oronasal mask until more specific treatment can be instituted. The treatment of overexposure to anaesthetically active gases is similar. Oxygen reverses hypoxaemia and accelerates the elimination of carbon monoxide and helps to support persons poisoned by cyanide or hydrogen sulphide.

Inhalation of irritant gases and smoke gives rise to similar effects on the respiratory tract ranging from mild irritation to mucous membranes lining the airways, leading to cough and bronchospasm, to severe non-cardiogenic pulmonary oedema and respiratory failure. Sensory irritant potency depends upon the interactions between the substance and irritancy nerve receptors. Acid gases, such as the halogens and hydrogen halides, dissociate forming high concentrations of hydrogen ions that, along with the chemical nature of the reactive base, give rise to the tissue response. The irritant potency is mostly accounted for by acidity, associated with a range of properties, such as aqueous and lipid solubility, and other tissue components that may compete with receptor stimulation. Other pathophysiological mechanisms will relate to the special properties of individual gases, such as free radical formation with chlorine. The stimulation of nerve receptors in the airways triggers subjective sensations such as cough, chest tightness and breathlessness and also reflex responses that can provoke bronchoconstriction, increased mucous secretion and vascular engorgement, all of which may contribute to symptoms. These effects can be very rapid following even a single, brief exposure.

Irritant gases in high concentrations may kill the victim outright after a few deep breaths and before pulmonary oedema has had time to develop, an effect probably due to oxygen having been displaced from the air: there may be no sign of a death struggle. Exposure of the eyes or skin to corrosive gases should be treated by thorough irrigation or washing with water or sterile physiological (0.9 per cent) saline, and all contaminated clothing must be removed.

Victims of gassing accidents should be initially considered to be hypoxic. Central cyanosis (a blue colouration of the tongue and mucous membranes) is a variable clinical finding and when present is a sign of central hypoxia, although hypoxia may occur in the absence of cyanosis. Methaemoglobinaemia is another cause of cyanosis and hypoxia. In poisoning by carbon monoxide and hydrogen cyanide, the skin retains its pink colour even in the presence of tissue hypoxia.

Even in the absence of clinically obvious signs of hypoxia or respiratory distress, the patient can nevertheless be severely hypoxic and may collapse on slight exertion. This was first emphasized in First World War casualties in the management of phosgene gassing on the battlefield, and which was attributed to the increased efflux of pulmonary oedema fluid during exertion.[31] In hospital, arterial blood gases should be tested at the earliest opportunity to assess the degree of hypoxaemia (PaO_2), partial pressure of carbon dioxide ($PaCO_2$), and acid-base state. Hypoxaemia is treated with oxygen therapy, but in advanced respiratory failure the patient may require endotracheal intubation and mechanical ventilation. Positive end-expiratory pressure is recommended in the presence of pulmonary oedema (acute chemical pneumonitis).[32] The possibility of laryngeal oedema causing respiratory obstruction should not be forgotten, for example after ammonia exposure, but it may also be present in fire victims if burns are present on the face and around the mouth and lips, or if soot is found in the anterior nares and larynx.

High concentration oxygen treatment (100 per cent given by a tight fitting oronasal mask or intermittent positive-pressure ventilation (IPPV) and hyperbaric oxygen in severe cases) is essential in carbon monoxide poisoning despite a normal PaO_2, as the oxygen will compete with carbon monoxide for haemoglobin binding sites and reduces the half-life of carboxyhaemoglobin from about 320 to 80 minutes. Pulse oximetry can be misleading in carbon monoxide poisoning as it detects carboxyhaemoglobin as oxyhaemoglobin, and thus may overestimate the actual concentration of oxyhaemoglobin; erroneous readings may also arise in methaemoglobin states.[33] The use of hyperbaric oxygen should be urgently considered in cases of poisoning by the chemical asphyxiant gases (carbon monoxide, hydrogen sulphide and hydrogen cyanide). Most experience of this treatment has been gained with carbon monoxide.

Skin burns from corrosive or acid gases and vapours should be treated as for chemical burns. Hydrofluoric acid burns may also need the administration of local and parental calcium antidotes. Contaminated clothes, jewellery, boots, etc., should be removed, and all affected areas should be washed or showered with water for at least ten minutes. Eye irrigation may also be needed. It is widely assumed that burns caused by corrosive gases and vapours will cause damage similar to thermal burns, for example irritation, erythema and bullae formation, but there is a dearth of hard facts on this in the literature. Certain agents, such as methyl bromide and vesicant warfare agents (e.g. mustard gas, see Chapter 41, Deliberate use of chemicals in warfare and by terrorists), are recognized as causing bullae formation, but erythematous lesions which may progress to intraepidermal or subepidermal vesicles (bullae) with sweat gland necrosis can also occur in some cases of coma caused by carbon monoxide poisoning. The mechanism of bullae formation in human skin is not understood. Bullae can occur in prolonged coma from various causes, for example in barbiturate poisoning, and could be caused by pressure, hypoxia or direct toxic effects to the tissues.

Cold injury from the accidental contact of the unprotected skin with the liquid, vapour or gas of very cold liquefied gases resembles the local effects of severe cold which are described in Chapter 49, Heat and cold, together with their treatment. The damage to the skin can be similar to heat burns, or to frostbite if exposure of unprotected parts is prolonged or severe.

The hospital management of victims of poisoning by irritant gases such as chlorine is outlined in Table 39.2. It should be noted that the treatment of the high permeability pulmonary oedema caused by irritant gases has not been well studied. In response to damage to the capillary endothelium, water accumulates in the interstitial space and then in the alveoli. The value of diuretics has not been confirmed and these should be used cautiously, if at all. Glucocorticosteroids may not be of value. Chest infection is common after severe gassing because of the denuded bronchial epithelium; vigorous antibiotic therapy is often required. The oedema fluid can have a higher protein content than in cardiogenic oedema, which may more readily coagulate and the residual coagulum then becomes the skeleton on which lung fibrosis develops.[34]

Convulsions caused by certain gases, e.g. methyl bromide, should be treated with anticonvulsant drugs as appropriate, although more intensive therapy may be needed if they prove resistant.

Even mild gassing incidents can induce severe anxiety if individuals suddenly experience respiratory symptoms such as acute tightening of the chest and difficulty breathing, especially if they are asthma sufferers. Further alarm can be generated if their or other lives are perceived to be at imminent risk. Health professionals called to such incidents need to be aware that affected individuals may subsequently suffer post-traumatic distress syndrome or other emotional disturbances requiring psychological support. Several of the physical conditions arising from inhalation of toxicants are described below.

Acute lung injury and acute respiratory distress syndrome

The inhalation of irritant agents may produce a common reaction in the lungs of rapid onset referred to as high permeability pulmonary oedema, or pulmonary oedema of non-cardiogenic origin, otherwise known as chemical pneumonitis. Pathologically, there is diffuse alveolar damage.[35] Mild cases recover rapidly and most without residual effects, but many authorities would nowadays regard chemical pneumonitis as belonging to the less severe end of a clinical spectrum of acute lung injury that extends to acute respiratory distress syndrome at the other. Acute respiratory distress syndrome is diagnosed in acute lung injury after inhaling a toxic fume or gas if there is acute lung injury and severe refractory hypoxaemia – using the PaO_2 to FiO_2 ratio.[36]

Bronchiolitis obliterans

This rare and life-threatening form of fixed obstructive lung disease is due to damage to the epithelium of the small airways and usually manifests itself pathologically as a proliferation of tufts or plugs of granulation tissue in the lumen of bronchioles. Diffuse alveolar damage and epithelial injury of the bronchioles may occur together after inhalation exposure to a single noxious agent leading to inflammation or fibrosis narrowing or blocking the airway. Bronchiolitis obliterans is a recognized complication in gassing accidents involving nitrogen dioxide, and sporadic cases have been reported after incidents with fire smoke, sulphur dioxide, ammonia, chlorine, hydrogen chloride, phosgene, hydrogen sulphide, hydrogen selenide and hydrogen bromide.[35]

Diagnosis is made on the basis of the history, fixed airway obstruction with normal diffusing capacity, and typical findings on high resolution computed tomography (HRCT). The diagnosis is likely to be missed in the initial stages, and mistakenly identified as asthma, bronchitis, emphysema or bronchiectasis.

Table 39.2 Chlorine poisoning: Hospital management.

Immediate decontamination on arrival at hospital (ideally decontamination should occur at the scene of the incident):	Remove all contaminated clothing and thoroughly wash skin and eyes as necessary
Assessment of patient:	Examine mucous membrane, eyes, and skin for signs of corrosive injury Check lung sounds, peak flow and vital signs: if patient is known to have been heavily exposed or has a cough or difficulty in breathing at rest perform baseline chest x-ray examination Take brief medical history, with particular attention to any history of respiratory or cardiovascular disease

Initial treatment:	*Oxygen*: all patients identified as being at risk (see Assessment of patient, above) should initially receive 100% oxygen. Oxygen concentration may subsequently be adjusted to the need of the patient
	Bronchodilators: salbutamol or terbutaline, used by nebulizer, may help relieve respiratory difficulties
	Dose: Salbutamol Adults 2.5–5 mg as required
	                              Children 2.5–5 mg as required
	            Terbutaline Adults 2.5–10 mg as required
	                              Children up to 200 mg/kg
	Corticosteroids have not been proved to produce improvement in chlorine poisoning but have caused pronounced improvement after smoke inhalation. If patient exposed less than 4 hours previously and at risk of pulmonary injury (as defined above) steroids should be given
	Dose: Methyl prednisolone Adults 2 g i.v. stat (or equivalent)
	                                          Children 400 mg i.v. stat (or equivalent)
	Laryngeal oedema: give corticosteroids (dosage as above) if patient develops laryngeal oedema. Obtain early and expert help from anaesthetist as tracheal intubation may be needed. If tracheal intubation is not needed, then a trial of continuous positive airway pressure by mask or hood may be attempted. In less severely poisoned patients non-invasive ventilation may be tried for a short period and continued if there is improvement.
	Skin burns should be treated as thermal burns
	Eye damage requires ophthalmic referral

Monitoring:	Monitor respiratory function, particularly respiratory rate and arterial blood gases regularly Pulmonary oedema may occur up to 24 hours after exposure Patients who are well 24 hours after exposure may be discharged
Pulmonary oedema:	If pulmonary oedema occurs, give oxygen by face mask If pO_2 still cannot be maintained above 60 mmHg, or the respiratory rate >40 bpm, intubate the trachea and start mechanical ventilation with positive end expiratory pressure. Intravenous fluids should be given with great caution as fluid overload is extremely dangerous in such patients: if this occurs diuretics such as frusemide are indicated

Reactive airways dysfunction syndrome and irritant-induced asthma

Irritant-induced asthma and vocal cord dysfunction (or irritable larynx syndrome) are conditions classified as reactive airways dysfunction syndrome (RADS) when they arise after exposure to a toxic gas. Gases reported to induce RADS following unplanned high exposure at work form a long list which includes hydrogen sulphide, nitrogen dioxide, sulphur dioxide (and sulphuric acid), ammonia, chlorine, ethylene oxide, phosgene, welding fumes and smoke.[35] The term was coined by Brooks in 1968 to describe a syndrome of respiratory symptoms after gas or chemical exposure at work.[37] Occupational health practitioners are quite likely to have patients referred to them at some time with suspected reactive airways dysfunction syndrome following an inadvertent exposure to an irritant substance at work, and so a detailed account of this important condition is given in Chapter 40, Reactive airways dysfunction syndrome and irritant-induced asthma.

Hypoxic brain injury

Simple asphyxiant gases will reduce the inspired oxygen concentration and cause hypoxic hypoxia, or low blood levels of oxygen. Acute, severe hypoxic hypoxia does not usually lead to brain damage or long-term neurological signs and symptoms unless accompanied by cardiac arrest, when the neurological picture resembles global ischaemia as seen after cardiac arrest from any cause.

Hydrogen cyanide and hydrogen sulphide inhibit cellular respiration and induce histotoxic hypoxia. As before, poisoning by these agents does not usually cause brain damage unless hypotension supervenes, when injury to the cerebral cortex and hippocampus may arise in a distribution resembling that seen in global ischaemia after cardiac arrest. Both gases are potent and immediate depressors of blood pressure, however, and the 'knock down' which occurs in sudden apnoea with hydrogen sulphide poisoning may possibly be the result of cardiac hypotension or cardiac standstill.

The action of carbon monoxide is undoubtedly more complex than either of these agents, but the mechanism is poorly understood. Focal damage to the globus pallidus and substantia nigra is more often seen in severe carbon monoxide poisoning, as is delayed neurological deterioration associated with the late destruction of white matter and demyelination. However, much the same pattern of injury may arise occasionally in patients who have suffered global ischaemia from other causes, including cyanide poisoning.[38]

The electroencephalogram, magnetic resonance imaging and computed tomography scans may all be normal in some patients with permanent hypoxic injury.

INVESTIGATION OF GASSING INCIDENTS

In all gassing accidents, investigations should be undertaken to determine or confirm the agent involved together with the degree of exposure whenever possible. Where biological tests for specific gases are available for verifying exposure, these are mentioned in the subsequent text. It is important that this task is done as part of the overall management of the patient and not as an afterthought. Thus, blood (5 mL EDTA (ethylenediaminatetraacetic acid)) and urine (50 mL universal container) samples should always be stored and collected at the earliest opportunity in case investigative tests are required later.

The post-mortem appearances are often non-specific. Corrosive gases will cause macroscopic injury to the airways. Pulmonary oedema, however, may be found in rapid hypoxic and anoxic deaths from any cause as well as from gassing by irritant, corrosive gases, and is due to increased capillary permeability. In asphyxiated victims, the viscera may show little change apart from congestion, oedema and petechial haemorrhages; conjunctival petechiae may also be present. Aerosol propellants, anaesthetic gases, carbon monoxide and hydrogen cyanide are volatile or unstable and may be lost from post-mortem blood.

Survivors of gassing accidents should always be followed up for the development of short- and long-term psychological and physical sequelae. Accidental exposures to gases in industry may be life-threatening and there are few follow-up studies of incidents in the literature. Pulmonary function testing should be undertaken after exposure incidents involving irritant gases, and referral for neurological and neuropsychological investigations should be considered in all patients who have experienced a severe exposure to a simple or chemical asphyxiant gas, with or without a period of unconsciousness.

GASES IN THE AMBIENT AIR

Air is a mixture of gases, the average composition of which stays remarkably constant (Table 39.3) and sustains life on Earth. This constancy is the outcome of a climate system that is fully coupled to the cycles of plate tectonics, weathering, erosion and biological activity. Fears over global warming led to the Kyoto Protocol agreement in 1997 that came into force in 2005; 187 countries have ratified the protocol, which requires industrialized nations to cut total anthropogenic emissions of the greenhouse gases carbon dioxide, methane, nitrous oxide and sulphur hexafluoride, and two groups of greenhouse gases: hydrofluorocarbons and perfluorocarbons. The Montreal Protocol (1987) required countries to phase out the manufacture of chlorofluorocarbons (CFCs) for all uses by 2010 to protect the stratospheric ozone layer that shelters Earth's surface from harmful ultraviolet radiation. The stable CFCs synthesized by the chemical industry for use as refrigerants, propellants and solvents, eat away at the ozone; they were initially replaced by hydrochlorofluorocarbons (HCFCs) and then by the hydrofluorocarbons (HFCs), which do not. Unfortunately, HFCs are powerful greenhouse gases and are covered

Table 39.3 Composition of the Earth's atmosphere

Gas	Vol (%)
Nitrogen (N_2)	78.094
Oxygen (O_2)	20.946
Argon (Ar)	0.934
Carbon dioxide (CO_2)	0.035
Neon (Ne)	1.82×10^{-3}
Helium (He)	5.24×10^{-4}
Methane (CH_4)	1.72×10^{-4}
Krypton (Kr)	1.14×10^{-4}
Hydrogen (H_2)	5×10^{-5}
Nitrous oxide (N_2O)	3.1×10^{-5}
Xenon (Xe)	0.86×10^{-5}
Ozone (O_3)	up to 10^{-5}
Carbon monoxide (CO)	up to 10^{-5}
Radon (Rn)	6×10^{-18}
Water (average)	0.1–4

by the Kyoto Protocol, as mentioned above. HFC emissions have been rising rapidly as demand for refrigerators and air conditioning grows in countries such as China. Occupational exposure to CFCs will potentially continue long after 2010 because of the continuing use of old air conditioning and fire-fighting systems that contain them.

Methyl bromide, a fumigant pesticide, is also being phased out under the Montreal Protocol.

Oxygen lack

Oxygen-deficient atmospheres can be encountered in mines and other underground or confined spaces. The main danger of suddenly entering an atmosphere devoid of oxygen is that it will lead to an almost immediate loss of consciousness without warning; even very quiet breathing will produce sudden loss of consciousness within 50 seconds when all the remaining oxygen in the lungs has gone.[39]

It is the partial pressure of oxygen, not its percentage, which is of physiological importance, but gas measuring instruments and alarms record volume concentrations. A drop of 3–4 per cent of oxygen by volume is of little physiological significance in humans, but it will extinguish a candle flame. (A candle flame will continue to burn at levels of atmospheric pressure well below those at which humans will be asphyxiated: it will not go out until 10 per cent of normal pressure.) The level of oxygen has to fall to 13 per cent volume (equivalent to a 33 per cent asphyxiant gas in air mixture) before symptoms become very noticeable.

The effects of low oxygen concentration (oxygen (per cent vol. in air)) are as follows:

- 16–13 per cent: Dizziness and shortness of breath on exertion; pulse rate accelerated and volume of breathing increased. Ability to maintain attention is diminished but it can be restored with conscious mental effort.
- 13–10 per cent: Judgement faulty. Rapid fatigue and fainting on exertion. Severe injuries cause no pain. Emotional lability.
- 10–6 per cent: Nausea and vomiting. Loss of ability to perform any vigorous muscular movements or even to move at all.
- <6 per cent: Loss of consciousness with fainting or coma. Rapidly fatal.

Oxygen excess

Industrial and medical oxygen supplies can enrich atmospheres in a room to dangerous levels. At 25 per cent oxygen in air, even damp vegetation will continue to burn once a fire has started, and substances which do not normally burn easily in air may burn vigorously. Lubricants must never be used on oxygen equipment as they may react explosively with pressurized oxygen. Even in the open air, oxygen may remain trapped in clothing which can then be readily ignited and cause severe burns. Oxygen and other compressed gases should only be used in well-ventilated areas.

Anaerobic fermentation

Natural biological processes produce toxic gases in the absence of oxygen. In anaerobic fermentation, bacteria that are methanogens or sulphate reducers remove hydrogen ions in the form of methane or hydrogen sulphide, respectively. Excessive or abnormal colonic gas production has been hypothesized to play a role in the pathogenesis of irritable bowel syndrome[40] and inflammatory bowel disease.[41] About a litre of human flatus is produced a day and typically contains nitrogen (68 per cent), oxygen (less than 1 per cent), carbon dioxide (9 per cent), hydrogen (16 per cent) and methane (6 per cent), while the malodorous gases (ammonia, skatole, hydrogen sulphide) comprise less than 1 per cent of the total. In contrast, the rumen of animal species such as the cow, sheep, goat and deer contain mostly methanogenic bacteria.

Fermentation of human or animal excrement releases toxic gases which can be a threat to sewer workers or workers in confined spaces on farms and in swine confinement buildings, among others (Figure 39.4). Farm animal-house air can be contaminated by ammonia, hydrogen sulphide and carbon dioxide. The mixing or pumping of slurry, for example in cowsheds, can release lethal amounts of hydrogen sulphide into enclosed spaces.

Anaerobic fermentation of sheep intestines and their contents can cause hydrogen sulphide keratoconjunctivitis in sausage makers, the same condition that Ramazzini recorded in workers who emptied 'jakes' (privy vaults). 'Sewer gas' is methane with small amounts of hydrogen sulphide and it also occurs in septic tanks and cesspits. JS Haldane investigated a fatal incident in a sewer in East Ham, London in 1895 and proved the deaths had been caused by hydrogen sulphide gas; he had shown earlier using bacteriological experiments that sewer gas or 'miasma' was not a cause of typhoid.[42] The smell of putrefaction had a long history of being associated with disease and being known as 'miasma' or bad air, and it was a central tenet of Edwin Chadwick and other nineteenth century sanitarians. At the time of his epidemiological investigations into cholera, the celebrated pioneer of anaesthesia in England, John Snow (1813–58), used his knowledge of gases and the properties of air to support the overthrow of this ancient belief. In doing so, he used statistics from the registrar general to show that male workers in the 'offensive trades', i.e. malodorous ones involving animal remains, such as rendering and bone boiling, had lower mortality rates than the male general population.[43]

Gases from decaying fish can be a hazard to workers unloading catch from poorly refrigerated and unventilated holds. Decay of organic matter generally provides hydrogen sulphide, ammonia, methane and carbon dioxide; levels of

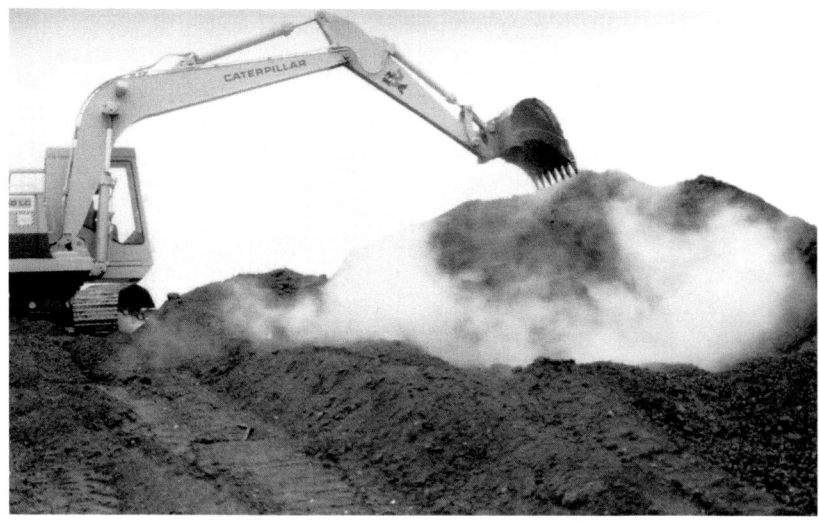

Figure 39.4 Gas clouds released from untreated sewage sludge being added to topsoil on a toxic waste reclamation site. A machine driver collapsed from the gas which turned out to be ammonia.

carbon monoxide in air can sometimes also be dangerously elevated in manure storage areas. Bacterial action on nitrogenous compounds may form nitrogen dioxide, and fermentation of silage can produce high concentrations of this gas within two days of silo filling. Carbon dioxide and methane concentrations, if elevated, depress oxygen levels, or oxygen may be depleted anyway. Following gassing accidents in confined spaces, it is important to measure as soon as possible for oxygen depletion and elevated levels of carbon dioxide, as well as the full range of gases mentioned above, to determine what was responsible for the incident.

A condition occasionally, but not exclusively, reported in hog farmers is organic dust toxic syndrome, which may present as an acute systemic illness characterized by fever, malaise, aches and pains in the limbs, vomiting and a dry cough. The onset is within a few hours of heavy exposure to endotoxin-producing Gram-negative bacteria, as may occur in swine confinement buildings. The condition, which resolves completely within 72 hours, should not be confused with the toxic effects of gases produced by fermentation. Pig farming exposes workers to a mixture of ammonia, organic dusts and high levels of endotoxins, and the types of disinfectants in regular use can contain respiratory sensitizers.[44]

Confined spaces

Confined spaces include trenches, pits, tanks, sewers, tunnels and also submarines and spacecraft. Working in enclosed spaces with inadequate natural ventilation is a well-known cause of death from asphyxia due to oxygen deficiency or from a build up of toxic gases and vapours, such as carbon dioxide, carbon monoxide, methane, ammonia, hydrogen sulphide, petroleum vapour and liquid petroleum gas. Toxic substances can accumulate where workers are welding or flame-cutting. In addition, the presence of flammable gases such as butane, propane and petrol, all of which are normally heavier than air, can be responsible for explosions in tanks. The risk of fire and explosion may be increased by enrichment of the air by oxygen in the event of a leak from an oxygen cylinder forming part of welding equipment. A fatal explosion occurred in 2007 in a compartment of a British nuclear submarine beneath the Arctic ice when an oxygen generator canister exploded after becoming contaminated with grease.

Oxygen deficiency in pits can arise from an ingress of methane or absorption of oxygen by certain constituents of soils. The rotting of vegetation and the rusting of metalwork inside tanks also consume oxygen. Manholes, tunnels and trenches in limestone soils can partly fill with carbon dioxide formed by the action of acid groundwater. Apparently safe atmospheres can become suddenly dangerous if the residues and sludges in tanks or in sewers are disturbed by the worker walking in them, or by water surges following sudden heavy rainfall. Underground spaces may be in ground which is contaminated or near old refuse tips, or they may be connected to sewers. In the construction industry, pipe-freezing work is carried out using liquid nitrogen to solidify soil to enable drilling to be performed in wet conditions and fatalities have occurred from the cold gas pushing out the available air.

In order to avoid gassing accidents, safe systems of work must be adhered to and these often require the use of electronic monitors or detector tubes to test for toxic, flammable and asphyxiating gases before initial entry to a confined space and while the work continues. The space should be well ventilated before entry, otherwise appropriate breathing apparatus has to be worn. In the UK, safe working practices are followed under the Confined Spaces Regulations (1997).[45]

There is no formal medical examination laid down for workers in confined spaces in the UK, but the competent person who carries out the risk assessment under the Regulations[45] will need to consider the physical suitability of the individuals involved and to check that they are of suitable build. Medical advice on an individual's suitability may be needed. A history of claustrophobia, fits, blackouts and fainting attacks would be reasons for exclusion, as are chronic respiratory problems such as asthma, bronchitis or exertional dyspnoea, and other evidence of lack of fitness to wear breathing apparatus. The presence of heart disease or severe hypertension might also be a contraindication. Physical limitations, such as deafness, lack of a sense of smell, visual defects, and problems with balance (e.g. Menière's disease) should also be considered. Prospective workers with limited mobility from back or joint trouble, certain physical handicaps or psychiatric problems may also be unsuitable.

Routine sewer work is normally safe as long as standard measures to detect toxic and flammable gases and oxygen-deficient atmospheres are performed. However, the possibility of unusually toxic substances entering sewage systems must always be borne in mind.

> In an unusual incident in Aberdeen, Scotland, a group of 26 workers went down a sewer to investigate an unusual smell, and 14 became unwell. The symptoms, which included cough, chest discomfort, breathlessness and fatigue, developed over several days. The more severely affected also complained of thirst, sweating, irritability and loss of libido. Five workers with persistent symptoms were investigated and in one a desmopressin test was abnormal and he was diagnosed as suffering from cranial diabetes insipidus; other endocrine organ tests included thyroid function, follicular stimulating hormone, luteinizing hormone, prolactin and testosterone which were all normal. The causal agent and its possible source were not identified, but the coincidence of autonomic symptoms and diabetes insipidus suggested that the gas exposure was responsible. Organic sulphur compounds with intense odours, such as dimethyldisulphide, were also considered.
>
> Watt et al.[46]

This episode shows the importance of all workers donning full positive-pressure breathing apparatus when investigating unusual problems in sewers.

Mines

'Black damp' was the name given to the residual gas encountered in mines where the oxygen has been removed by natural chemical oxidative processes such as in the oxidation of coal, timber and iron sulphide.[47] It typically contains 12–15 per cent carbon dioxide but can be higher, with the rest of the gas as nitrogen. 'Fire damp' is methane which is present under pressure in coal seams and may be given off with carbon dioxide and nitrogen accompanied by audible hissing noises during mining. The main hazard is explosion. The introduction of a form of safety lamp by Sir Humphrey Davy in 1812 was a sensation, making the inventor internationally celebrated, as it markedly reduced the risk of catastrophic explosions in mines. The flame of the lamp is surrounded by a fine metal gauze that offers little resistance to gases, but which leads heat away from them so effectively that the flame cannot cross it. The oil flame gave warning of the presence of fire damp (1–4 per cent methane makes the flame burn taller, so the concentration of methane can be estimated from its height) and is also extinguished before the oxygen levels fall to dangerous levels. After an explosion of methane and coal dust, the mixture of gases produced in the mine is called 'afterdamp': it can contain toxic levels of carbon monoxide, responsible for the deaths of miners and rescuers in numerous mining disasters. JS Haldane showed that odourless carbon monoxide was the main cause of death in explosions of methane and coal dust and it was due to his advocacy that it became a legal requirement for canaries to be kept at all coal mines to give warning of the presence of carbon monoxide, which would otherwise not be detectable using the safety lamp alone.[42,47]

PROPERTIES AND EFFECTS OF INDUSTRIAL GASES

Simple asphyxiant gases

METHANE (CH_4)

[CAS No. 74-82-8]
Relative density: 0.56
Flammability in air: 5.0–15.4 per cent (vol.)

Methane is a colourless flammable gas with a non-detectable or a sickly sweet oily odour which is normally too faint to provide warning of its presence. The main global sources of methane are rice paddies and wetlands from the anaerobic fermentation of organic material, but it is released from coal mining, biomass burning, the leakage of natural gas from the earth, as well as pipelines and well-heads, landfills and enteric fermentation in mammals (mainly ruminants). Total global emissions of methane are about 500 million tonnes a year, two-thirds of which come from anthropogenic sources. It is second only to carbon dioxide as a cause of global warming. Natural gas contains methane as a major constituent combined with significant amounts of ethane, propane and butane, together with diethyl sulphide as a deodorant. Some natural gas sources contain substantial amounts of mercury, which can be an occupational hazard.[48] Coal gas, which it replaced as a fuel, contains methane together with hydrogen and a little carbon monoxide and ethylene plus small amounts of carbon dioxide, nitrogen, oxygen, ammonia and hydrogen sulphide. Marsh gas is mostly methane with a little hydrogen, carbon dioxide and nitrogen. It has been widely believed that marsh gas can undergo a spontaneous combustion, producing a pale, ghostly light (Will o' the Wisp or Jack o' Lantern), but another fermentation product is likely to be responsible.

One minute it darted like a kingfisher, and the next it entirely disappeared. At times it grew as big as an ox's head, and then straightaway shrank to a cat's eye ... finally ... it returned to frisk in the reeds.

George Sand 1848[49]

Mixtures of methane and air do not ignite spontaneously, otherwise flames would be seen around the tails of cows. Methane burns with a hot, yellowish flame and not cold, bluish-white. Fermentation may also produce traces of phosphine, PH_3, but this does not ignite spontaneously in air either, although it commonly contains an impurity, phosphoretted hydrogen, P_2H_4, which does.

As methane is much lighter than air it does not form an explosion hazard in the open as it readily disperses, but the gas can accumulate as an upper layer in the air of poorly ventilated spaces where it may cause asphyxia by displacing oxygen or, at much lower concentrations, become an explosive risk if ignited by a flame or spark. Methane blasts in coal mines are not uncommon tragedies in Russia and China due to safety breaches: in 2007 at the Ulanovskaya mine in Russia 110 miners died in the worst mining accident in 60 years, followed by 38 deaths in a blast later that year in the same region. A major incident involving methane took place at Abbeystead, England, in 1984 when 34 local residents and eight employees were visiting the valve house at the local water pumping station. The pipe system had been drained down and, unknown to the engineers, methane gas from the surrounding methane-rich soils had permeated the pipes. When the pumping began, the methane entered the atmosphere of the valve house and exploded, killing 16 people. Carboniferous geological strata are methane rich and soil emissions may increase with rapid falls in atmospheric pressure. The air near the ground in oil-rich regions may contain as much as 1 per cent methane.

Another important methane mixture is landfill gas produced by putrefaction of municipal and other wastes buried in an excavation and covered with clay and topsoil. Huge amounts of landfill gas may be generated containing typically a methane/carbon dioxide mixture in the ratio 60:40. Volatile organic compounds may also enter and add to the toxicity of the gas. The gas can migrate long distances through the ground and cause a hazard to workers by flooding into trenches. Nearby residential areas may be at risk from soil gas. To help avoid these hazards, special vents are incorporated into landfill sites to provide adequate escape for the copious amounts of gas produced (Figure 39.5).

CARBON DIOXIDE (CO_2)

[CAS No. 124-38-9]
Exposure limits:
   LTEL (8 h TWA) 5000 ppm or 0.5 per cent
      (9000 mg/m^3)
   STEL (10 min) 15 000 ppm or 1.5 per cent
      (27 000 mg/m^3)
Relative density: 1.53

Joseph Priestley was the first to establish the biological properties of this gas and in 1772 came upon the art of manufacturing carbonated water, which was made popular by Joseph Schweppes who started a business in Bristol in 1794. The dangers of carbon dioxide were, however, known to wine producers in Roman times, if not earlier. Today, carbon dioxide is encountered in numerous ways, for example as a refrigerant, in fire extinguishers, arc welding, breweries and wineries, flue gases, fermentation processes which deplete oxygen (including in unventilated mines, wells, tunnels) and in the manufacture and use of dry ice. It is often regarded as a simple asphyxiant, yet it has been known since the turn of the last century that it has a toxic action which is independent of oxygen deficiency. The toxic

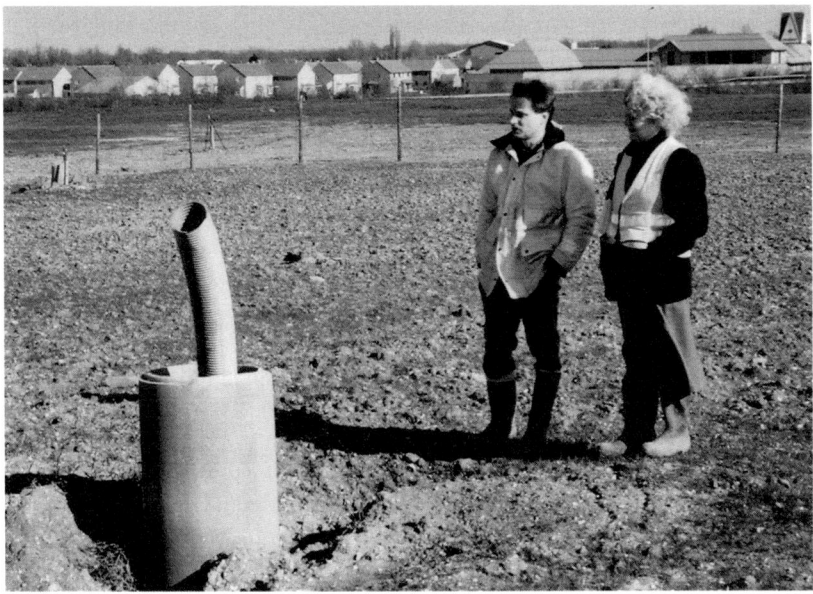

Figure 39.5 Methane outlet on a municipal waste landfill site. Note the proximity of local housing (hazard of soil seepage of gas).

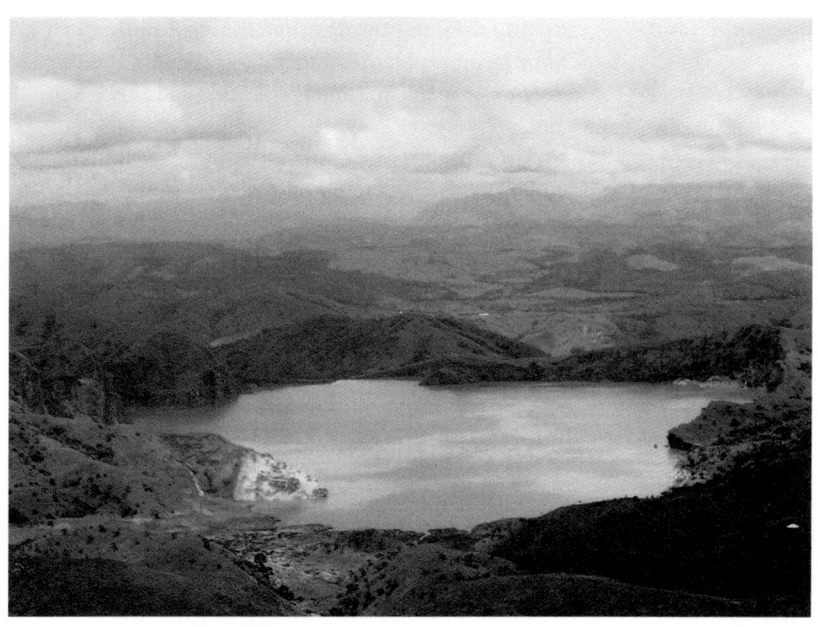

Figure 39.6 Lake Nyos, Cameroon. On August 21, 1986, carbon dioxide was suddenly degassed from the lake and flowed down into the adjacent valleys in this remote region. The lake, 200 m deep, is replenished from a bottom spring rich in carbon dioxide. This event was the first recorded exposure of a population to a wide-scale release of carbon dioxide.

properties of carbon dioxide were demonstrated on a large scale in the disaster at Lake Nyos, Cameroon, in 1986, where over 1700 people were killed when as much as a quarter of a million tonnes of carbon dioxide held in the depths of the lake under hydrostatic pressure were suddenly released and flowed down into the nearby valleys (Figure 39.6). The water was saturated with dissolved gas ready for some modest disturbance to trigger its rapid rise to the surface and exsolution. The sparse medical findings and the accounts of survivors strongly suggested that the carbon dioxide had mixed with air to give rise to prolonged states of coma due to carbon dioxide narcosis in many of the victims.[50] Skin bullae were another unusual finding. This unprecedented massive release contrasts with incidents in industry when isolated deaths from carbon dioxide are normally attributed to oxygen lack or simple asphyxia, and there are no characteristic findings on autopsy.

Carbon dioxide is dangerous because it is colourless and odourless, but when breathed from an anaesthetic machine it has a faintly acid smell. The effects of breathing the gas are very characteristic.[51] A 2–3 per cent carbon dioxide level in air will pass unnoticed at rest, but tidal volume is increased by 30 per cent and the minute volume by 5 per cent; on exertion there may be marked shortness of breath. At 3 per cent carbon dioxide in air, breathing becomes noticeably deeper and more frequent at rest, with the effect becoming more marked until at 5 per cent carbon dioxide in air there is severe dyspnoea, which limits exposure for most people. Subjects complain of headache and are sweaty and have a bounding pulse. At 10 per cent carbon dioxide in air, respiratory distress develops rapidly with loss of consciousness in 10–15 minutes, even though the oxygen concentration is reduced to 19 per cent only. Exposures to carbon dioxide levels above 15 per cent are intolerable, and rapid loss of consciousness ensues after a few breaths of a mixture of 30 per cent carbon dioxide in air. Even at this level, the oxygen concentration is 15 per cent, not enough to cause loss of consciousness from hypoxia, but death will occur if the carbon dioxide level is maintained. Thus, it is important to note that monitoring oxygen in air is an inadequate guide to the carbon dioxide hazard; carbon dioxide should be directly measured. A working or living area should be immediately evacuated when concentrations exceed 1.5 per cent by volume (the occupational short-term exposure limit value). Experimental studies show that carbon dioxide exerts a narcotic action at the higher concentrations through a disturbance of acid-base balance resulting in a fall in pH of arterial blood and the cerebrospinal fluid.[51]

Industrial carbon dioxide poisoning is a rare occurrence. Survival after severe intoxication by carbon dioxide has been described (in a patient in Bristol in 1972):

A 34-year-old male worker was overcome by an accidental release of the gas from a fire extinguishing system, filling the room 'like a cold, thick fog.' There were two others present, one died and the other managed to rescue the patient and save himself. The patient was given artificial respiration, but breathed by himself within a very short time whilst remaining deeply unconscious. On admission to hospital within 15–20 minutes of the accident he was still deeply unconscious, but was maintaining a free airway. He had a respiratory rate of 24 per minute, but was grossly hypernoeic, flushed and markedly vasodilated. He was normotensive, with a heart rate of 120 per minute, and his chest was clear. He became rousable after 35 minutes in the hospital whilst being treated with oxygen through an MC mask. Soon he was rational, and complained of headache and feeling stiff all over. He developed pre-renal uraemia, which spontaneously resolved over several days, and he was eventually discharged well.

Brighten[52]

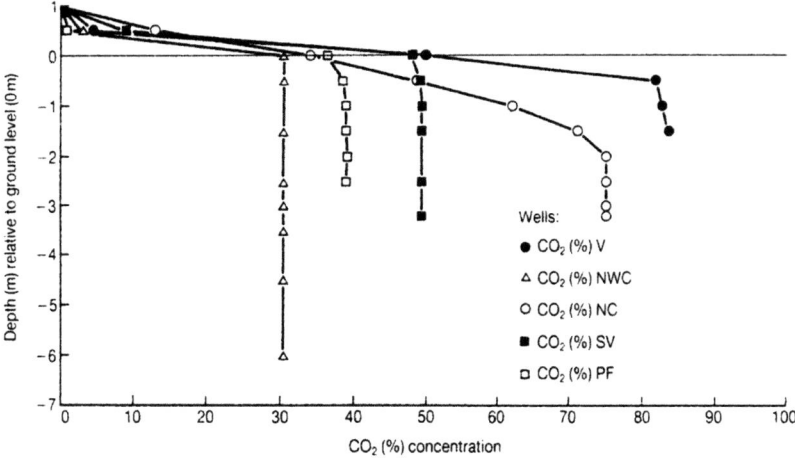

Figure 39.7 Carbon dioxide concentrations measured with an infrared analyser in five domestic water wells in Vulcano, Sicily. Carbon dioxide measured from the top of the well above ground level to the water surface. The carbon dioxide concentration is lethal (>30 per cent) in all the wells within 1 m of the top and a worker would lose consciousness almost immediately on entry using a ladder. On this volcanic island, carbon dioxide diffuses into wells from the soil. Courtesy of Jean Claude Baubron.

Soil gas emissions in volcanic and geothermal areas can be a silent hazard to workers. In Mammoth Mountain, California, a popular ski resort, park rangers have been overcome due to an unsuspected increase in gas flow associated with volcanic unrest.[53] In the largest island of the Azores, San Miguel, the town of Furnas is built in an active caldera where soil gas emissions have overwhelmed workers digging roads. The phenomenon is not new, with Loudon reporting in 1832 on the famous 'Valley of Death' in Java which contained the skeletal remains of many wild animals and birds that had strayed into the layer of carbon dioxide floating above the ground.[51] Drilling boreholes in certain urban areas in Italy associated with old volcanism has triggered hazardous gas blowouts that need to be capped, placing emergency workers and other people at risk.[54]

The danger of entering an enclosed space containing carbon dioxide is illustrated by the concentration gradient of the gas in wells on Vulcano, Sicily, a volcanic island with areas which have strong ground emissions of carbon dioxide (Figure 39.7). The breathing zone of a worker entering such a well by ladder will be at a narcotic level of carbon dioxide without warning and within a very short descent (less than 2 m) below the top. The worker would lose consciousness after a few breaths and fall to the bottom of the well. The carbon dioxide gradient is so steep that there would be no opportunity for the worker to become aware himself that he was hyperventilating before consciousness was lost. Spaces where carbon dioxide may build up can therefore be much more dangerous than is commonly supposed because of diffusion of the gas. It has been known from ancient times (in wine production) that the flame of a candle can be used to give adequate warning of the presence of lethal levels of carbon dioxide. A vertically held lit candle or oil lamp is normally extinguished when the oxygen level falls to 17.6 per cent in the presence of nitrogen, but carbon dioxide has a stronger effect, causing the flame to be extinguished at 18.8–18.9 per cent (or 8–10 per cent carbon dioxide).

Carbon dioxide levels can be used to measure the quality of indoor air. At a ventilation rate of 4.6 m^3/min per person the carbon dioxide level in an office would be expected to be approximately 800–1000 ppm in the absence of unvented combustion sources. Higher levels of carbon dioxide would indicate the need to increase ventilation to improve the outdoor air supply.[55]

ARGON A (A OR Ar)

[CAS No. 7440-37-1]
Relative density: 1.4

Argon is the most abundant 'rare' gas in the atmosphere and, together with helium and neon, makes up nearly 1 per cent of air: all three gases are of inorganic origin. Argon is inactive, colourless and odourless. It is used in the control of high technology refining and semiconductor processes. It is also used in lamps, as a shielding gas in welding, and in many gas-filled devices.

HELIUM (He)

[CAS No. 7440-59-7]
Relative density: 0.14

Helium is colourless, inert, non-flammable and very light. It is found with natural gas deposits in the United States and Poland. Extraction from air is not commercially viable. It is used as a shielding gas in welding, in electric lighting tubes, as a substitute for nitrogen in diving gas mixtures and as a balloon gas.

HYDROGEN (H₂)

[CAS No. 1333-74-0]
Deuterium D_2 or $^2H_2$
Relative density: (H_2) 0.07

Hydrogen is very light, colourless and flammable. It is used for hydrogenation of fats and in chemical synthesis. Deuterium is a heavier stable isotope of hydrogen and is used as a tracer. Hydrogen burns with a bluish, non-luminous flame.

KRYPTON (Kr)

[CAS No. 7439-90-9]
Relative density: 2.9

Krypton is a rare gas present in the atmosphere at about 1 ppm. It is colourless, non-flammable and has applications in electrical equipment. Its radioactive isotope ^{85}Kr is used in respiratory and cardiac studies.

NEON (Ne)

[CAS No. 7440-01-9]
Relative density: 0.7

Neon is a rare gas present in the atmosphere at about 18 ppm. It is colourless and non-flammable, used in fluorescent tubes, and as a cryogenic refrigerant.

XENON (Xe)

[CAS No. 7440-63-3]
Relative density: 4.5

Xenon is a rare gas present in the atmosphere at about 0.086 ppm. It is colourless, non-flammable and is used for specialized lighting.

NITROGEN (N₂)

[CAS No. 7727-37-9]
Relative density: 0.97

Nitrogen is the major constituent of air, comprising about 78 per cent by volume. It is very widely used as an inerting agent and in freezing processes of many varieties including food, earth freezing in civil engineering projects and metal shrinkage in machinery manufacture. Because the uses are ubiquitous, nitrogen is not infrequently implicated in anoxic deaths or incidents. Under increased pressure, it induces narcosis.

Liquid nitrogen and argon are commonly stored in cylinders in laboratory areas, and may have to be transported in the confined space of a lift. One litre of liquid nitrogen will form ~700 litres of gas at room temperature.

A sudden loss of nitrogen into an unventilated area could rapidly lead to an oxygen-depleted atmosphere and the worst scenario would be if the full contents of a vessel are released to atmosphere over a short period of time: the hazard can be determined using an oxygen depletion calculator or by a simple calculation, described below.

Calculate the worst scenario on the basis that the full contents of the vessel are released to atmosphere over a short period of time:

$$\% O_2 = \frac{100 \times V_o}{V_f}$$

where for argon and nitrogen

$$V_o = 0.2095 (V_f - V_g)$$

and for oxygen

$$V_o = 0.2095 (V_f - V_g) + V_g$$

V_g = maximum gas release which is the liquid volume capacity of the vessel $V \times$ gas expansion

V_f = room volume

Gas expansion being for

nitrogen 682.7
oxygen 842.1
argon 823.8

An example of such a calculation is:

LC 200 containing 200 liquid litres of nitrogen in a room 20 m $\times$ 20 m $\times$ 3 m
$V_r = 20 \times 20 \times 3 = 1200$ cubic metres
$V_g = 200$ litres $\times 682.7 = 136\,540$ litres
    $= 136.5$ cubic metres
$V_o = 0.2095 (1200 - 136.5) = 222.80$
$\% O_2 = 100 \times 222.8/1200 = 18.6\%$

If the calculation suggests an oxygen content in the atmosphere lower than 18 per cent, then either

- site the vessel outside the building and pipe gas to the point of use; or
- pipe the pressure release valve and bursting disc to vent gas outside the building; and/or
- fit a permanent oxygen monitor;
- ensure personnel use/wear personal monitors;
- fit a forced ventilation system triggered by the permanent oxygen monitor.

Source: British Compressed Gas Association, guidance note GN11

Chemical asphyxiant gases

CARBON MONOXIDE (CO)

[CAS No. 630-08-0]
Exposure limits:
   LTEL (8 h TWA) 30 ppm (35 mg/m^3)
   STEL (15 min) 200 ppm (232 mg/m^3)
Relative density: 0.97
Flammability range: 12.5–74.2 per cent (vol.)

Carbon monoxide is a colourless, odourless, non-irritating gas which is slightly soluble in water and burns in air with a bright blue flame. It is the most widely encountered toxic gas in industry and the general environment, commonly as the result of incomplete combustion of fossil fuels. Although Ramazzini (1633–1714) remarked on the danger of gases from burning coal and Harmant in France gave the first clinical description of coal gas poisoning in 1775, it was Leblanc in 1842 who identified carbon monoxide as the toxic agent. The potential for dangerous exposures to carbon monoxide arises in metal production in iron foundries, steel works and electrical arc furnaces; in the chemical industry, in the manufacture of methanol, the catalytic cracking of hydrocarbons, around gas generating and purification plant, and in the synthesis of carbon black. Vehicle exhausts may pose hazards from carbon monoxide to workers in roll-on/roll-off vehicle ferries, as well as in multi-storey car parks and enclosed garages.

Typical carbon monoxide concentrations in gas mixtures are: blast furnace gas 20–25 per cent; coal and coke oven gas 7–16 per cent; petrol or LPG (liquid petroleum gas) engine exhaust gas 1–10 per cent; and diesel engine exhaust gas 0.1–0.5 per cent. Water gas is formed by passing steam through a bed of white-hot coke and consists of carbon monoxide and hydrogen. A mixture of carbon monoxide and nitrogen, known as producer gas, is used to fire metal-making furnaces and is produced by passing air over hot coke.

Potentially dangerous sources of carbon monoxide in homes and workplaces are faulty heaters that produce excessive fumes or burn in a restricted air supply, whether using natural gas, propane, butane, coal, coke or wood. Reducing ventilation in buildings in the winter to conserve heat may unwittingly elevate carbon monoxide levels in the indoor air to hazardous levels. Carbon monoxide from faulty gas appliances kills nearly 30 people in the UK every year, and at least 100 are known to suffer ill health from this cause. The elderly and the very young are most at risk. In the United States, approximately 600 accidental deaths due to carbon monoxide poisoning are reported each year, while the number of intentional carbon monoxide-related deaths is between five and ten times higher. The use of catalytic converters in car exhausts has reduced carbon monoxide emissions, making suicide more difficult by inhaling exhaust gases in an enclosed space; death may in certain circumstances be more likely due to carbon dioxide instead.

Propane-fuelled equipment is commonly believed to be safe, but hazardous emissions of carbon monoxide have been reported in indoor environments with the use of ice resurfacing machines[56] and in forklift trucks with poorly adjusted carburettors.[57]

Carbon monoxide is a chemical asphyxiant because it combines with haemoglobin with an affinity some 250 times that of oxygen to form carboxyhaemoglobin (COHb). Carbon monoxide also increases the oxygen affinity of haemoglobin and causes the oxygen dissociation curve to shift to the left by impeding the release of oxygen to the tissues. With 50 per cent saturation of the blood with COHb the oxygen pressure must fall to less than half the usual value in order to dissociate half the oxygen present.[58] The clinical manifestations of poisoning and tissue hypoxia are known to be greater than can be accounted for by loss of the oxygen-carrying capacity of the blood alone. Experimental studies suggest that carbon monoxide exerts a direct action by combining with other haem-containing proteins in cells such as cytochrome oxidase, myoglobin and cytochrome P450. The interaction with cytochrome oxidase may result in mitochondrial dysfunction and a prolonged impairment of oxidative metabolism. An alternative hypothesis is that carbon monoxide damages mitochondria by provoking the release of free nitric oxide. Central nervous system injury may also be due to reoxygenation injury as a result of the production of partially reduced oxygen species, which in turn can oxidize essential proteins and nucleic acids, and induce brain lipid peroxygenation.

Normal metabolism produces some endogenous carbon monoxide and the normal COHb concentration is less than 1 per cent. Tobacco smoke contains carbon monoxide and it is the most common cause of an elevated blood COHb. Cigarette smokers on average have a COHb level of 5–6 per cent and heavy smokers can have levels in excess of 10 per cent. Typically urban non-smokers will have levels of 1–2 per cent COHb. A level greater than 5 per cent in non-smokers and 10 per cent in most smokers suggests a source of carbon monoxide in the inhaled air. Levels in excess of 10 per cent can sometimes be found in groups such as drivers, firefighters, garage employees and dock workers, especially if they are smokers.[58]

The proportions of COHb and oxyhaemoglobin in blood depend upon the partial pressure of carbon monoxide and oxygen. Several empirical equations have been proposed for estimating per cent COHb at different levels of exposure to carbon monoxide in combination with sedentary, light or heavy work and which take into account the duration of exposure, pulmonary ventilation and the COHb present before inhalation of contaminated air. The relation is not necessarily a simple one and therefore exposure should be assessed measuring both COHb and the levels of carbon monoxide in the air, but the following formula first proposed by Forbes and others[59] may be used:

% COHb = k × % CO in air × minutes of exposure

The constant k is 3 for an individual at rest, 5 for light activity, 8 for light work, and 11 for heavy work. More refined formulae, such as Coburn–Forster–Kane equations,[60] are also available. Figure 39.8 can be used to predict COHb in an individual with a continuing exposure to a specified concentration of carbon monoxide at different levels of exertion.

Performance of light-to-moderate work (up to 70 per cent of maximum aerobic capacity) is not affected at low levels of carbon monoxide, that is COHb levels of 4–6 per cent, but short-term maximal exercise duration is reduced in young healthy men. The effect is small and is only likely to be of concern for competing athletes. Subtle impairment of mental functioning has been reported in volunteers when COHb levels exceed about 5 per cent. These changes include impairment of memory, learning ability, attention span, coordination and abstract thinking.[58]

A less well-known hazard arises from the use of methylene chloride (dichloromethane), a widely used solvent and a main ingredient of commonly used removers of paint and varnish from wood. Dichloromethane is readily absorbed through skin contact and in the lungs as a vapour and is metabolized in the liver. Carbon monoxide is an important metabolite of dichloromethane and forms COHb: peak levels can occur within three hours of exposure associated with elevated alveolar carbon monoxide levels, and there is a return to pre-exposure levels in 24–48 hours after the exposure has ceased.[61] Approximately 5 per cent COHb saturation is obtained following exposure of non-smokers to 200 ppm dichloromethane for four to eight hours. High exposure to this solvent by inhalation as a result of stripping paint in an inadequately ventilated working area for two to three hours may result in levels of COHb high enough to precipitate angina or myocardial infarction in workers with pre-existing cardiovascular disease.[62]

Clinical features of carbon monoxide poisoning

Acute poisoning

Exposure to carbon monoxide resulting in levels of 10–30 per cent COHb may produce throbbing headaches and mild exertional dypnoea. At 30–50 per cent, additional symptoms include dizziness, nausea, weakness and collapse. Acute heavy exposures may result in loss of consciousness without warning, followed by coma, convulsions and death. Fatal levels of COHb in healthy people are usually in excess of 50 per cent; anaemia predisposes to carbon monoxide poisoning. The classic cherry pink colour of the skin is a rare sign, and if present suggests a carboxyhaemoglobin level over 20 per cent, but venous blood frequently looks arterial. Carboxyhaemoglobin levels in heparinized blood samples are measured by dedicated co-oximeters or by spectrophotometry by second derivative.[63] In post-mortem blood, gas chromatographic analysis is the preferred method because of the breakdown of haemoglobin.

There is no diagnostic symptom complex for carbon monoxide poisoning and the diagnosis can be easily missed. The clinical presentation can vary widely, with vomiting, headaches, malaise, weakness, fatigue, chest pain, palpitations and dyspnoea. It is as well to know that the signs and symptoms of non-lethal exposure may mimic those of a non-specific viral illness.[64] While blood carboxyhaemoglobin concentrations are diagnostic, the levels are not a good guide to prognosis and the clinical condition is more important, especially if the patient is or has been

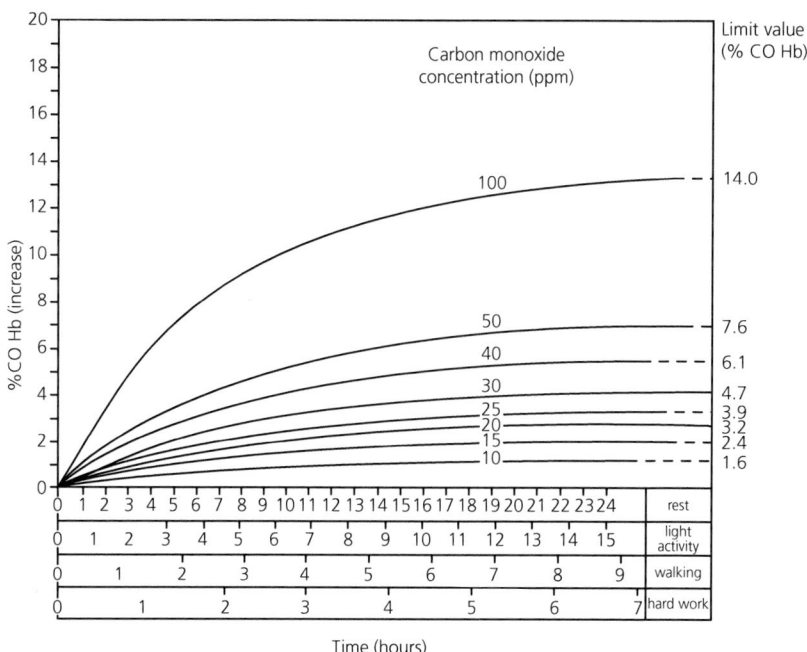

Figure 39.8 Uptake of carbon monoxide by blood. Adapted from Ref. 72, with permission.

unconscious. This is because tissue hypoxia through unmeasured tissue uptake of carbon monoxide is the primary insult and it correlates poorly with carboxyhaemoglobin levels. Without adequate treatment, 10–30 per cent of severely poisoned patients may develop late neuropsychiatric manifestations 3–240 days after exposure.[64] The prevention of this adverse outcome is the main reason for advocating aggressive early treatment.

The half-life of COHb is normally about four hours (longer if induced by methylene chloride exposure), but without treatment coma can last for 24 hours or longer. The relatively short half-life of COHb means that by the time the patient is seen, measurement of COHb may not be a good guide to the initial exposure. Therapy is directed towards reducing the half-life of COHb which falls to 80 minutes when the patient is given 100 per cent oxygen at sea level. Most authorities now advocate giving hyperbaric oxygen where there is access to a hyperbaric chamber.[65] Hyperbaric oxygen at 2.5 atmospheres (252 kPa) reduces the half-life to 20 minutes and increases the amount of oxygen dissolved in the blood to a concentration sufficient to meet the needs of the body even without functioning haemoglobin.

Hyperbaric oxygen should be considered for pregnant women and for patients who have evidence of:

- a period of unconsciousness;
- neurological or psychiatric symptoms;
- cardiac complications;
- carboxyhaemoglobin levels above 40 per cent.

Neuropsychiatric damage can be immediate or a clear period of several days may be followed by the development of neuropsychiatric symptoms within the next two to three weeks or longer. Carbon monoxide has a predilection for the 'watershed' areas of the brain where there is a meagre blood supply: the basal ganglia, with their high oxygen consumption, are most often affected. Other commonly affected areas are the cerebral white matter, hippocampus and cerebellum.

Neurological manifestations such as vegetative state, akinetic mutism, parkinsonism, agnosia, visual impairment, and amnestic-confabulatory states have all been described.[64,66,67] The patient can develop changes in personality typified by increased irritability, verbal aggressiveness, violence, impulsiveness and moodiness. Up to 40 per cent of patients develop memory impairment, and 33 per cent can suffer late deterioration of personality. Depression and suicidal tendencies are also reported. Although many patients improve after some months, a proportion will be found not to have improved three years later.[68] The syndrome of delayed neurological sequelae is more characteristic of carbon monoxide poisoning than other types of anoxia, and the cause remains speculative, but it seems likely that carbon monoxide has a specific cytotoxic action. Bilateral necrosis of the globus pallidus is common, and lesions may also be found in the basal ganglia, hippocampus and white matter on computerized axial tomography or magnetic resonance imaging (MRI),[69,70] but delayed neurological sequelae may also occur in the absence of such findings. Positron emission tomography scanning can detect regions of the brain affected by ischaemia in the acute poisoning stage, and which may be at risk of late complications, but the technique is no better at predicting the eventual outcome.[71] Neuropsychometric assessment will show impairment in acute poisoning and may reveal cognitive deficiency consistent with organic brain damage in the delayed syndrome. The diagnosis of delayed neurological sequelae may be missed, and the patient assumed to have even made a good recovery, until a return to work reveals a failure to perform to the expected level.

The neurological examination should include tests of fine movement and balance (finger–nose movement; Romberg's test, normal gait and heel–toe walking), testing of short-term memory, and the ability to subtract 7 serially from 100.

Ambient air exposure to carbon monoxide

By far the principal source of carbon monoxide in the general outdoor atmosphere is general pollution by vehicle exhausts. Uptake of carbon monoxide from multiple sources, such as smoking and traffic, is not additive. Smokers who already have a carboxyhaemoglobin level above the equilibrium value that would be reached by breathing air in their surroundings are liable to act as 'source', breathing out carbon monoxide rather than absorbing more. Air quality standards therefore in effect protect non-smokers from peak concentrations close to heavy traffic. The most important adverse health impact from environmental exposure to carbon monoxide is the effect on people with angina and disease from the coronary arteries. In the EU, the air quality standard has been set at a level at which the carboxyhaemoglobin should not exceed 2.5 per cent in people breathing the air over a prolonged period, that is, 10 ppm measured as a running eight-hour average.[72] This level equates to 25 ppm for one hour, 50 ppm for 30 minutes and 87 ppm for 15 minutes when breathing at maximum levels of activity. The reader should note that this standard is substantially below the work exposure limit for an eight-hour period, and its rationale is about the need to ensure the adequate protection of people who suffer from ischaemic heart disease if they are likely to come into contact with the gas.

Recent studies indicate that even a circulating blood concentration of COHb of 2–3.9 per cent is associated with impairment of cardiovascular function in patients with angina pectoris, who may show detectable changes in the cardiac ischaemic threshold on light-to-moderate exercise (as assessed on the electrocardiogram (ECG) by a reduction in time to the ST end point) and an earlier development of angina pectoris.[73] In healthy workers, there is no clear evidence that these levels of COHb (or indeed levels as high as 10 per cent COHb) impair the functioning of the central nervous system. Nevertheless, deterioration in physical work (maximum work capacity or maximum aerobic capacity) can be demonstrated with increasing levels of COHb. It is possible that healthy individuals are able to adapt to the mild hypoxia of chronic exposure to carbon monoxide. Experimental studies have shown that carbon monoxide has an atherogenic effect in rabbits and rats, but it is not generally accepted that low-level occupational exposures contribute to atherosclerosis in man; more information is needed on the effects of carbon monoxide on vascular endothelium and lipid metabolism. An epidemiological study of a cohort of bridge and tunnel workers regularly exposed to traffic fumes concluded that carbon monoxide may be a contributory factor in increasing cardiovascular mortality, but the mechanism was not clear.[74]

There is no available evidence to suppose that carbon monoxide is mutagenic or carcinogenic, but exposure is suspected to be a contributory factor for low birthweight in the babies of pregnant women who smoke. The teratogenic effects of carbon monoxide have been attributed to the transfer of carbon monoxide across the placenta and a consequently reduced oxygen supply to the fetus. Studies have predicted significant changes in fetal oxygenation as a result of maternal carboxyhaemoglobin levels of about 5 per cent. Severe acute exposures have caused fetal death; and developmental and other neurological abnormalities have been recorded in live births.[75]

The pregnant worker should avoid occupational exposure to carbon monoxide or methylene chloride (dichloromethane) and exposure to carbon monoxide should be especially prevented in workers with symptomatic ischaemic heart disease. It is also important to appreciate that the effects of carbon monoxide in people living or working at high altitude (or at a reduced partial pressure of oxygen) are greater than at sea level.

HYDROGEN CYANIDE (HCN)

[CAS No. 74-90-8]
Exposure limit: (STEL 15 min) 10 ppm (11 mg/m^3)
Relative density: 0.95
Flammability limits: 6–41 per cent (vol.)

As well as hydrogen cyanide, the gaseous cyanides include cyanogen $(CN)_2$, once used as a fumigant, and cyanogen chloride (CICN), a fumigant and industrial intermediate. Exposure to cyanide in industry may also be the result of the accidental or intentional ingestion of cyanide salts (e.g. sodium, potassium, calcium and copper cyanide) and from exposure to the vapour of nitrites, such as acrylonitrile (vinyl cyanide) and acetonitrile (methyl cyanide). Cyanide salts are used widely for metal cleaning or hardening, in metal refining, gold extraction and film recovery and electroplating. Historically, hydrogen cyanide used to be widely used as a fumigant, but today its main industrial usage is in the production of acrylonitrile and methyl methacrylate. The gas is also evolved when acids come into contact with cyanide salts. Firemen may be exposed to the gas in fires involving the combustion of nitrogen-containing synthetic materials. The main route of poisoning by hydrogen cyanide is inhalation, although in solution it can also readily penetrate the skin.

At room temperature, hydrogen cyanide is a clear, highly volatile liquid (boiling point 26°C). The gas has a characteristic odour of bitter almonds which is recognizable at 2–5 ppm, but its detection by odour is unreliable; at higher concentrations, it causes olfactory fatigue. At 18–36 ppm, warning symptoms of poisoning may occur, such as irritation of the eyes, nose and throat, dizziness, nausea, general weakness and headaches, flushed or occasionally pale skin, and palpitations. Rapid and sudden loss of consciousness and cessation of breathing may occur on exposure to levels over 100 ppm. Levels of hydrogen cyanide above cyanide plating baths normally vary around 1–5 ppm and workers do not complain of symptoms; headache and vertigo may be reported at slightly higher concentrations.

Cyanide paralyses mitochondrial respiration by binding reversibly with enzymes containing ferric ions, in particular cytochrome aa3, thereby blocking intracellular respiration. Its direct action on the respiratory centre may also induce respiratory failure.

Victims of acute poisoning present with headache, dizziness and vertigo. There may be marked agitation and confusion, with nausea and vomiting. Dyspnoea is accompanied by hyperpnoea due to lactic acidosis. Acute cyanide poisoning induces sustained seizures, endogenous catecholamine release and cardiovascular shock. On examination, the external findings may be normal with a pink appearance even when the blood pressure is immeasurable. The diagnosis can be confirmed by measuring cyanide in a sample of heparinized whole blood. Cyanide is concentrated in the red blood cells and plasma cyanide measurements are not recommended. Concentrations greater than 50 mmol/L are associated with altered consciousness, and the lethal level is above 100 mmol/L. Blood thiocyanate is a metabolite which can be measured after the acute event. Other useful tests include plasma lactate and arterial blood gases. In fatal cases, there are no specific pathological changes and in particular the blood remains well oxygenated.

The treatment of cyanide poisoning remains controversial because the effectiveness of the recommended antidotes, and so the treatment of choice, is not proven. Immediate first-aid measures include removing the patient to fresh air, keeping the patient warm and at rest, and removing contaminated clothing. Contaminated skin should be washed thoroughly. Oxygen should be administered if available. First-aiders should wear suitable protective clothing, including impervious gloves, to avoid skin absorption of cyanide. Where there is the potential for a large release of hydrogen cyanide, first-aiders should be trained in the use of self-contained or airline breathing apparatus for the rescue of victims. However, in most

Table 39.4 Overall outline of first-aid treatment for cyanide poisoning.

Speed is essential. Obtain immediate medical attention	
Protect yourself and the casualty from further exposure during decontamination and treatment	
Inhalation	Remove patient from exposure. Keep warm and at rest. Oxygen should be administered. If breathing has ceased apply artificial respiration using oxygen and a suitable mechanical device such as a bag and mask. Do not use mouth-to-mouth resuscitation
Skin contact	Remove all contaminated clothing immediately. Wash the skin with plenty of water. Treat patient as for inhalation
Eye contact	Immediately irrigate with water for at least 10 minutes. Treat patient as for inhalation
Ingestion	Do not give anything by mouth. Treat patient as for inhalation

Source: Health and Safety Executive.

biological laboratories the amount of cyanide in routine use does not normally warrant this precaution.

The UK Health and Safety Executive (HSE) issued new advice on the first-aid treatment of cyanide poisoning at work in 1997, since when little has changed. The HSE no longer recommends the use of any antidote in the first-aid treatment of cyanide poisoning and does not require employers to keep supplies. Instead, the administration of oxygen is regarded as the most useful initial treatment using a bag and mask device connected to an oxygen supply. The latest advice is summarized in Table 39.4. There is growing animal and human evidence that oxygen is itself an antidote to cyanide or improves the response to treatment with specific antidotes.

The main antidotes recommended in the UK are amyl nitrite and dicobalt edetate. A conservative approach to their use is recommended. Any patient exposed to hydrogen cyanide who reaches hospital fully conscious will probably not need treatment with antidotes, their use being reserved for the patient who is unconscious or who has a clear history of exposure to cyanide and has deteriorating physical signs.[76] To be effective, the antidotes should be administered immediately the diagnosis of cyanide poisoning is made, but the problem is that the uninitiated could readily mistake an ordinary collapse for poisoning. Accidental cyanide poisoning is rare in British industry today, but the risk of suicide bids from swallowing cyanide in solid form or in liquids, such as acetonitrile, is also a possibility of which occupational physicians need to be aware.

The rationale of treatment is the rapid fixation of cyanide ion which can be achieved by direct fixation with the antidote dicobalt edetate or by inducing methaemoglobin formation with amyl nitrite. The resultant methaemoglobin binds strongly with cyanide as cyanmethaemoglobin. Experience with gassing incidents suggests that after the unconscious casualty has been removed from further exposure, he should be observed for any deterioration of vital signs before administering cyanide antidotes as patients often recover spontaneously and quickly from apparently severe poisoning. A rapid method of diagnosing cyanide poisoning is to test the patient's breath for hydrogen cyanide with a gas detector tube. Amyl nitrite by inhalation and oxygen delivered by face mask are relatively safe and may be administered if the patient is conscious. A capsule of amyl nitrite is broken into a handkerchief and the patient inhales the vapour for 15–30 seconds. This process must be repeated every two to three minutes until the capsule is exhausted. There is, however, little scientific evidence that it is of significant benefit. If the patient is comatose, or starts to become drowsy and has the features of cyanide poisoning, then dicobalt edetate (300 mg in 20 mL glucose solution) may be administered by slow intravenous injection over 3–4 minutes. The second-line treatment, if there is no return to consciousness, is to give sodium thiosulphate (12.5 g – i.e. 25 mL of 50 per cent solution) intravenously over 5–6 minutes. Dicobalt edetate is a chelating agent that combines with cyanide to form an inert complex, cobalticyanide. This antidote is not innocuous and if administered in the absence of cyanide will cause cobalt poisoning, hence the need to be cautious about its use. Thiosulphate is a sulphur donor and accelerates the detoxification of cyanide by assisting in its conversion to the non-toxic thiocyanate.

If the patient is not breathing, then artificial respiration should be commenced using a manual resuscitator. Mouth-to-mouth artificial respiration may put the first aider at risk of absorbing cyanide from the patient's mouth or breath. The manual methods of artificial ventilation, such as Holger–Nielsen, are no longer recommended because they have poor efficiency and cause problems in maintaining an adequate airway.

Hydrogen cyanide may be formed when cyanides come into contact with acids. The cyanogen halides cyanogen chloride (CNCl) and cyanogen bromide (CNBr) also have local irritant effects on the eyes and respiratory tract and can cause inflammation of the bronchioles and pulmonary oedema, as well as having a similar toxic action as hydrogen cyanide. The cyanonitriles have a slower rate of intoxication than cyanide gas or cyanide salts as the cyanide is released when they are metabolized by the body over several hours; they also have their own toxic properties. Cyanide is not produced in the metabolism of isocyanates or diisocyanates.

Despite evidence that hydrogen cyanide can be inhaled in fires, the use of dicobalt edetate is not routinely recommended in the treatment of fire casualties. The relatively safer antidotes amyl nitrite and sodium thiosulphate, as well as hyperbaric oxygen, have been used to treat fire casualties in hospital, but amyl or sodium nitrite reduce blood oxygenation by displacing oxygen from carboxyhaemoglobin, and so may add to the oxygen-depriving effects of carbon monoxide. Hydroxocobalamin (the precursor of vitamin B_{12}), which reacts with cyanide to form cyanocobalamin, is being increasingly advocated by some experts as an alternative in smoke inhalation victims.[77] As it is relatively safer to use than the other drugs, it is being actively considered by some countries as the drug of choice in cyanide poisoning in general.[78]

The evidence for chronic health effects arising from long-term exposure to cyanides at work is limited. Workers may experience recurrent mild acute, or subacute, symptoms if exposures are not being adequately controlled.[79] In the clinical setting, a neurotoxicological role for cyanide has been suggested in tobacco amblyopia, and tropical ataxic neuropathy associated with the ingestion of certain types of cassava which have not been adequately prepared before cooking. Cyanides are mostly metabolized to thiocyanates in the body, and a toxic side effect of thiocyanate administration was found to be goitre when it was advocated in the past for the treatment of hypertension. Evidence for goitre, but not for neurological complications, has been reported in association with chronic cyanide exposure in a group of electroplating workers.[80]

PRIMARY IRRITANT GASES

CHLORINE (Cl_2)

[CAS No. 7782-50-5]
Exposure limits:
 LTEL not available
 STEL (15 min) 0.5 ppm (1.5 mg/m^3)
Relative density: 2.47

Chlorine is a greenish, highly irritant gas with a pungent odour; it is moderately soluble in water. It is widely used in the manufacture of chemicals, the bleaching of pulp and paper, for disinfecting water and in waste treatment. Workers may also be exposed in the production of chlorine by diaphragm cell or mercury electrolytic cell processes. Chlorine is used in the manufacture of polyvinyl chloride and thousands of organochlorine compounds, most of which do not occur in nature and persist in the environment, the most toxicologically potent being the 'dioxins'.

Chlorine was discovered by the Swedish pharmacist, CW Scheele, in 1774, who was the first to observe its bleaching properties. Chlorine-based bleaching agents have been used in the pulp industry for more than a century. Chlorine dioxide was first synthesized in 1811 by Humphrey Davy, but was not introduced in the pulp and paper industry until 1946. This gas is at least as toxic as chlorine.[81] Exposure to workers and occasionally the public is by the accidental release of chlorine from closed systems under pressure. In the UK, it is the most common hazardous chemical stored in large quantities at industrial installations. In the United States, railroad tanker incidents during transit are infrequent but may lead to large-scale releases of chlorine with substantial injury and deaths; wherever possible hazardous materials should be re-routed away from densely populated areas.

There are two mechanisms of action of chlorine, both involving the generation of free radicals. The chlorine atom itself is a free radical; when released, it reacts with other molecules to oxidize them. The second pathway is via the indirect generation of reactive oxygen species, by first reacting with water in the respiratory tract to form hypochlorous acid and hydrochloric acid:

$$Cl_2 + H_2O \leftrightarrow HCl + HOCl$$

The hypochlorous acid is a strong oxidizing agent and on dissolution releases hydrochloric acid and reactive oxygen species, both of which initiate inflammatory responses:

$$HOCl \leftrightarrow HCl + \dot{O}$$

Despite its widespread commercial exploitation since before the First World War, human data on dose–effect relations are sparse and instead the results of animal experiments extrapolated to man are used to estimate lethal or dangerous concentrations of chlorine gas. Its odour can be detected by most people at 0.2 ppm and by some at 0.02 ppm. For irritant or potentially inflammatory effects on the upper and lower airways in fit individuals and subjects with some degree of pre-existing airway hyperresponsiveness, a NOAEL is 0.5 ppm over six to eight hours. In susceptible individuals, significant changes in lung function occur at 1 ppm after four to eight hours. Exposures in the range 15–150 ppm may be dangerous after 5–10 minutes, particularly at the higher end of this range or in susceptible individuals, for example with chronic respiratory disease. At 400–500 ppm, the gas is estimated to be fatal in 50 per cent of active healthy people exposed for 30 minutes, and exposure to 1000 ppm will be fatal after a few breaths.

The effects of chlorine are mainly confined to the respiratory system.[82] Because of its moderate solubility, it will act in the upper and lower respiratory tract. Acute exposure to raised concentrations in air can cause immediate irritation of the mucous membranes of the eyes, nose and throat, producing cough, choking, substernal pain and tightness. Abdominal pain, nausea and vomiting have also been reported in inhalation incidents. Upper respiratory tract obstruction from laryngeal oedema should always be considered, but the most frequently encountered severe effect is toxic pneumonitis with interstitial oedema which leads to impairment of gas diffusion and hypoxaemia; a restrictive and obstructive defect in lung function may be due to bronchospasm or interstitial oedema. Death may occur from respiratory failure or cardiac arrest due to non-cardiogenic pulmonary oedema. Irritation and necrosis of the skin can be caused by contact with a jet of gas, but mild erythema resembling first-degree burns may follow lesser exposure. Most mildly affected patients will settle quickly with rest, but symptomatic treatment for cough and soreness of eyes and throat may need to be given. Symptomless casualties should rest for at least eight hours and be told to report any change in their health to a doctor. The treatment of severe chlorine poisoning is as for irritant gases in general (see under Principles of first aid and treatment in gassing incidents, p. 262).

After acute gassing incidents with chlorine, persistent reactive airways dysfunction syndrome may occur: bronchial hyper-responsiveness may persist for at least 18–24 months.[83] Pre-existing bronchial hyper-responsiveness may also be aggravated in some individuals for weeks or months afterwards. In most people, however, the evidence of a deterioration in airway function is transient. More studies are needed to determine whether chronic low-level exposures to chlorine can lead to long-term respiratory effects.[84,85] The recent follow-up studies of acute chlorine gassing among pulp mill and other groups of workers do indicate that the health effects of major incidents involving the accidental release of the gas may be much more extensive and persistent than was previously supposed for irritant exposures.[86]

Several studies have reported a relationship between indoor chlorination swimming pools and the prevalence of wheeze, asthma, hay fever, rhinitis and atopic eczema in swimmers and swimming pool attendants.[87] Chlorination of public swimming pools results in free chlorine reacting with nitrogenous compounds (sweat and urine) introduced by bathers to form chloramines, especially nitrogen trichloride with dichloramine (NH_2Cl_2) and monochloramine (NH_2Cl). These can be in the atmosphere in the form of droplets or gas and are irritant in their own right, but they may also decompose to form hydrochloric acid and ammonia. The main putative agent is considered to be nitrogen trichloride (NCl_3), which is an upper airway irritant as powerful as chlorine and may build up in the air of indoor pools.[88] Few direct measurements of NCl_3 have been made. Free chlorine and hypochlorite are unlikely to be present in the swimming pool atmosphere. A similar type of problem can arise in the processing of green salads in water containing hypochlorite.[89]

Cleaners have suffered near fatal pulmonary oedema from chlorine liberated by the mishandling of standard household bleaches (5.25 per cent sodium hypochlorite solution – NaOCl), for example by mixing bleach with a cleaning agent containing acids, such as phosphoric acid, when chlorine gas and water are released.[90] Another hazard may arise in the chlorination of swimming pools using hydrochloric acid and sodium hypochlorite if the two chemicals are accidentally mixed in a way to cause a release of a cloud of chlorine gas.[91] Mixing bleach with a solution of ammonia produces monochloramine and dichloramine, and an accident, involving cleaning agents has led to a mass casualty event involving inhalation of chlorine gas.[92]

There is no evidence that chlorine is carcinogenic or that typical industrial exposures affect reproductive outcome. The use of chlorine to disinfect drinking water has been one of the greatest public health advances of the twentieth century, saving countless lives, but chlorine reacts with organic matter in untreated water to form trihalomethanes – of which chloroform is the most common – and these are potentially carcinogenic.[93] Spatial epidemiological studies have not identified a significant risk.

PHOSGENE (COCl2)

[CAS No. 75-44-5]
Exposure limit:
    LTEL (8 h TWA) 0.02 ppm (0.08 mg/m^3)
    STEL (15 min) 0.06 ppm (0.25 mg/m^3)
Relative density: 3.48

Phosgene is a colourless, relatively insoluble gas.[94] At low concentrations (1 ppm), it smells like new-mown hay, but is pungent and irritating at higher levels. The gas dissolves in water and moist air to form carbon dioxide and hydrogen chloride, but only a small amount will hydrolyse in the upper and lower airways when inhaled, most of the reaction taking place in the alveoli. It is not reported to affect the skin. The danger of phosgene is that it may cause only mild transient irritation of the mucous membranes of the eyes and respiratory tract at concentrations which can nevertheless cause delayed and fatal damage to lung tissue, the symptoms of which may not begin until 30 minutes to 48 hours later. In having a latent asymptomatic period following exposure, the gas resembles nitrogen dioxide, but the mechanism of its toxicity is unknown.

Exposure is usually confined to the chemical industry where it is used in many organic syntheses requiring chlorination, such as in the manufacture of isocyanates, polyurethane and polycarbonate resins. Gassing may occur from accidental releases from plant. It may also arise whenever a volatile chlorine compound or its vapour comes into contact with a flame or very hot metal and this could give rise to dangerous exposures in confined spaces; for example, welders in the hold of a ship in Sweden welding steel plates which had been degreased by trichloroethylene all suffered pulmonary oedema. In fires, polystyrene may burn to form phosgene, as well as chlorine.

The odour of phosgene is recognizeable at concentrations exceeding 0.5 ppm, above which level it is probably dangerous to inhale the gas for prolonged periods. At exposures above 10–20 ppm for 1–2 minutes severe lung injury can follow, and inhalation of 90 ppm is said to be rapidly fatal. The main feature of phosgene poisoning is massive pulmonary oedema.[94] In most fatal cases, pulmonary oedema reaches a maximum in 12 hours followed by death in 24–48 hours. The trachea and bronchi are usually normal in appearance, which contrasts with chlorine poisoning in which there is typically damage to the epithelial lining with desquamation. Exposure to high concentrations may also cause severe conjunctivitis and subsequent turbidity of the cornea. Chronic bronchitis and emphysema have been reported as a consequence of acute exposure.

No animal studies are available on the carcinogenicity of phosgene. No information is available on its reproductive toxicity or carcinogenicity in humans.[94] Because it is a highly reactive electrophilic compound it would be expected to bind in biological systems at the point of contact and so systemic absorption of unchanged phosgene by the inhalation or dermal route of exposure is not likely to be significant.

A notable escape of phosgene gas from storage tanks occurred in Hamburg in 1928, leaving at least 11 people dead and 250 casualties.

Hydrogen halides

The irritant effect of hydrogen halides arises from the fact that they behave as strong acids in aqueous media, i.e. they dissociate forming high concentrations of hydrogen ions. Hydrochloric acid, hydrofluoric acid, hydrobromic acid and hydroiodic acid all behave as very strong acids and for equal molar concentrations they are expected to behave very similarly in their capacity to release hydrogen ions and cause irritation to the respiratory system. Incidents involving inhalation of high concentrations of hydrogen chloride in the workplace can lead to reactive airways dysfunction syndrome; it seems plausible that high levels of exposure to hydrogen bromide and hydrogen iodide would have similar consequences.

HYDROGEN CHLORIDE (HCl)

[CAS No. 7647-01-0]
Exposure limit:
  LTEL (8 h TWA) 1 ppm (2 mg/m^3)
  STEL (15 min) 5 ppm (7.6 mg/m^3)
Relative density: 1.27

Hydrogen chloride is a colourless to light yellow gas which has a sharp, suffocating odour perceptible at 0.8 ppm. It is highly soluble in water and will produce a mist containing hydrochloric acid in moist air. Occupational exposure will therefore usually be to a mixture of gas and aerosol. It has a wide range of uses in the chemical industry. In parallel with chlorine consumption anhydrous HCl is used in the synthesis of vinyl chloride and other chlorinated hydrocarbons, and in steel pickling. Hydrogen chloride is also formed in the exhaust gases of many types of missile.

A NOAEL for irritant or potentially inflammatory effects on the lower respiratory tract and outer eye is a concentration in the air of 1 ppm.[95] The maximum levels of exposure that can be sustained over several hours are 10–50 ppm, although partial tolerance does occur. A lethal level in air is often quoted as 500–1000 ppm for short exposures, but this is probably an overestimate of toxicity. The gas is highly irritant to the eye, causing conjunctival irritation and superficial corneal damage; on contact with the skin, it will dissolve in the perspiration and produce epidermal inflammation. Repeated elevated exposures to the mist may cause ulceration of the nasal septum. Inhalation can cause choking, coughing, laryngeal oedema and non-cardiogenic pulmonary oedema depending upon the severity of exposure. Chronic, elevated exposures to the mist can give rise to the discolouration and erosion of teeth, particularly the incisors. It is some 30 times less irritant to the respiratory tract than chlorine and major incidents involving the public have not been recorded.[92]

Hydrogen chloride was one of the first gases to have its factory emissions controlled by legislation with the passing of the Alkali Acts in 1863. The alkali industry of the nineteenth century manufactured sodium sulphate which was used in glass making and to produce alkalis, such as sodium carbonate and sodium hydroxide. The Leblanc process was based upon the reaction of common salt with sulphuric acid, and the unwanted byproduct hydrogen chloride was discharged into the air around the factories where it blighted vegetation over wide areas.[96] Hydrogen chloride is one of the most common gases emitted by volcanoes and it readily dissolves in rainwater to form acid rain. The gas is also formed in voluminous white clouds when liquid lava flows into sea water.

Hydrogen chloride is emitted from a variety of industrial sources including incinerators and coal-burning power plants. It is not one of the major ambient air pollutants. It undergoes rapid dry deposition from the air and low ambient air levels do not seem to pose a direct health risk. Subjects with asthma do not appear to respond with adverse respiratory effects on exercising while breathing air containing less than 2 ppm hydrogen chloride.[95] Limited experimental and epidemiological studies do not provide any evidence that the gas is a human carcinogen.[97] There are concerns that co-exposure to hydrogen chloride and formaldehyde may enhance the known carcinogenicity of formaldehyde possibly by the formation of bis(chloromethyl) ether (BCME), a human and animal lung carcinogen, but the amounts of this carcinogen formed by this mechanism are probably too low to be significant.

There are no studies on the potential effects of the gas on human reproduction.

Compounds which hydrolyse to hydrochloric acid

The following gases are highly soluble in water and hydrolyse to hydrochloric acid; the treatment of overexposure is the same as hydrogen chloride and for irritant gases in general (see under Principles of first aid and treatment in gassing incidents, p. 262).

BORON TRICHLORIDE (BCl$_3$)

[CAS No. 10294-34-5]
Exposure limit: not established
Relative density: 4.1

Boron dichloride is a colourless gas which will form a mist in moist air to give hydrochloric acid and boric acid. It has a sharp odour and is non-flammable. It is used in metal refining and as a catalyst.

DICHLOROSILANE (SiH$_2$Cl$_2$)

[CAS No. 4109-96-0]
Exposure limit: not established
Relative density: 3.5

Dichlorosilane is colourless and produces a mist in moist air. It is used in the semiconductor industry for the deposition of silicon.

NITROSYL CHLORIDE (NOCl)

[CAS No. 2696-92-6]
Exposure limit: not established
Relative density: 2.3

Nitrosyl chloride is a reddish brown, non-flammable, highly irritant gas. It is used in diazo reactions and other organic preparations. It reacts rapidly with water to form hydrogen chloride and nitrogen oxides which makes it a highly dangerous irritant gas with both immediate and delayed effects on mucous membranes and lungs.

Other hydrogen halides

Both of these gases are more corrosive than hydrogen chloride.

HYDROGEN BROMIDE (HBr)

[CAS No. 10035-10-6]
Exposure limit:
   STEL (15 min) 3 ppm (10 mg/m^3)
Relative density: 3.5

Hydrogen bromide is a colourless, fuming, corrosive and non-flammable gas with a strong acidic odour. It is used as a chemical reagent in the manufacture of inorganic bromides, in organic synthesis, in the processing of ores and as an alkylation catalyst.

It is usually met in solution as aqueous hydrobromic acid to a strength of 48 per cent HBr.

Because of its high solubility, the major irritant effects of acute exposure are confined to the eyes (conjunctivae) and the upper respiratory tract. Knowledge on the effects of the gas in humans is sparse. Evidence from animal studies suggests that its effects are similar in character to, but less severe than, those seen in exposure to a similar concentration of hydrogen chloride.[98] A NOAEL based on this comparison is 2 ppm. Exposure to 2–6 ppm for several minutes causes nasal and throat irritation, but no eye irritation.

Other severe exposures to hydrogen bromide have been rarely reported. These have been as a result of inadvertent pyrolysis of fire extinguisher compounds and home fumigant agents containing methyl bromide.

No studies on the carcinogenicity of hydrogen bromide are available.

HYDROGEN IODIDE (HI)

[CAS No. 10034-85-2]
Exposure limit: not established
Relative density: 4.5

Hydrogen iodide is a colourless, corrosive, very dense, fuming gas and the most unstable of the hydrogen halides. It is used as a reducing agent and in the preparation of iodides. The anhydrous hydrogen iodide produces aqueous hydroiodic acid when dissolved in water, which is a strong acid that is corrosive and reacts strongly with bases.

Human data on the effects of hydrogen iodide are too sparse and so a notional NOAEL for irritation of the respiratory tract is based on the other hydrogen halide gases, which is 1 ppm.

Fluorine and hydrogen fluoride

FLUORINE (F$_2$)

[CAS No. 7782-41-4]
Exposure limit:
   LTEL not available
   STEL (15 min) 11 ppm (1.6 mg/m^2)
Relative density: 1.31

Fluorine is a pale yellow acrid gas which is highly reactive and rarely exists in the elemental state in nature. It is more toxic than hydrogen fluoride. Its effects on the eyes and respiratory tract resemble hydrogen fluoride, but gaseous fluoride is capable of reacting with the skin to induce severe thermal or chemical burns depending upon the duration of exposure.

The element fluorine is widely distributed in the environment, being present in virtually all rocks, normal soils, surface waters, seawater and air. Low concentrations of fluoride in drinking water (about 1 ppm) are beneficial in preventing dental caries, but excessive ingestion or inhalation of fluoride over prolonged periods causes fluorosis in humans and livestock. Since 1974, chlorofluorocarbons (CFCs or 'freons') have been implicated in stratospheric ozone depletion. Hydrofluorocarbons (HFCs) are less destructive of ozone, but they and CFCs are 'greenhouse' gases.

HYDROGEN FLUORIDE (HF)

[CAS No. 7664-39-3]
Exposure limit:
 LTEL 1.8 ppm (1.5 mg/m^3)
 STEL (15 min) 3 ppm (2.5 mg/m^3)
Relative density: 1.86

Hydrogen fluoride, or anhydrous hydrofluoric acid, is a colourless, corrosive liquid which boils at 19.4°C and reacts in moist air to form a mist. Its main uses are in the manufacture of fluorocarbons, the etching and polishing of glass and as a fluoridating agent in organic and inorganic reactions; it is handled in the form of gaseous hydrogen fluoride or as an aqueous solution of hydrofluoric acid which on contact with the skin can cause severe burns.

Industrial exposure to fluoride may also arise in mining and use of fluoride-containing materials. Fluorspar (CaF_2) is mined in many countries (in Derbyshire, England, local deposits are known as 'Blue John') and is used throughout the world as a flux in high temperature smelting and refining processes for the production of metals and alloys. It is reacted with concentrated sulphuric acid to produce hydrogen fluoride. Cryolite ($_3NaF\ AlF_3$) used to be mined in Greenland until deposits became exhausted and is now produced by chemical synthesis instead: it is used in the manufacture of aluminium. Fluorapatite ($CaF_{2-3}Ca_3(PO_4)_3$) is present in rock phosphate which is mined in vast quantities in the production of phosphate fertilizers, phosphoric acid and phosphorus.

Exposure to hydrogen fluoride and silicon tetrafluoride, as well as fluoride particles, may occur in a wide range of processes. Silicon tetrafluoride is also produced when hydrofluoric acid is used to etch glass, and in water this toxic gas hydrolyses to form fluosilicic acid (H_2SiF_6) which is the agent most commonly used to fluoridate water. Processes with the potential to create large fluoride emissions include: phosphate fertilizer production, which involves the crushing and drying of phosphate rock; the manufacture of bricks, tiles, pottery and cement products when fluoride is released during the firing of clays containing fluoride; glass enamel and glass fibre production; metal casting; steel and petroleum refining; coal combustion; and aluminium production. Calcium fluoride and other inorganic fluorides are used as fluxing agents in arc welding. In uranium processing plants, isotopes of uranium are separated using the extremely corrosive solid uranium hexafluoride; emissions of fluoride compounds are usually negligible, but a cloud of hydrogen fluoride was released from a uranium plant in Gore, Oklahoma, in 1985, killing one worker and affecting numerous others.

In 1989, an accidental release of about 24 tonnes of hydrogen fluoride occurred over a 48-hour period at a petroleum plant in Texas; 94 local residents were hospitalized and many others suffered from the irritant effects of the gas 'fog'.[99]

Acute health effects of hydrogen fluoride and fluorides

In industrial exposures to gaseous and particulate fluoride, absorption of fluoride is mainly through the respiratory tract. Of fluoride in the body, 99 per cent is found in the skeleton since fluoride is not retained in soft tissue and is not metabolized. There is rapid renal excretion of an acutely absorbed dose so that about half is lost in the urine in a few hours. Only a very small amount is excreted in sweat or in the faeces. Occupational fluoride exposure has not been shown to cause liver or kidney injury and evidence is inadequate to implicate hydrogen fluoride and fluoride-derived gases as carcinogens or teratogens.

The maximum concentration of hydrogen fluoride in air tolerated by humans for one minute is about 120 ppm when it causes smarting of the skin, conjunctivitis and irritation of the respiratory tract.[100] The gas has a sour taste. At 60 ppm, there are no skin symptoms but irritation of the eyes and nose with discomfort in the pharynx and trachea is present. A level of 30 ppm can be tolerated for several minutes.[101] In magnitude of acute toxicity, studies of human volunteers and experimental animals suggest that the halide gases hydrogen fluoride, hydrogen chloride and hydrogen bromide are of the same order;[98] their high water solubility ensures a rapid absorption in the nose and upper respiratory tract.

Inadvertent inhalation of high levels of hydrogen fluoride can cause rapid death from intense inflammation of the respiratory tract and gross haemorrhagic pulmonary oedema. Inhalation of hydrogen fluoride and fluorine and most fluorine-derived gases may cause coughing, choking and chills lasting 12 hours after exposure.[102,103] After an asymptomatic period of one or two days, pulmonary oedema may develop followed by regression over a period of 10–30 days. Advice to patients who have been in gassing accidents involving fluorine gases should therefore be cautious and should include the need for admission to hospital for 24–48 hours' observation.

The NOAEL for irritant effects on the face, eye and respiratory airways is 1 ppm.[104,105]

Chronic fluoride toxicity – osteofluorosis

Osteofluorosis was first recognized as an occupational disease in Danish cryolite workers in 1932, since when cases have been reported in aluminium production, magnesium foundries, fluorspar processing and superphosphate manufacture. The accumulation of fluoride in the skeletal tissues is associated with pathological bone formation. The condition appears to be identical to endemic skeletal fluorosis found in parts of the world where drinking water contains fluoride in excess of 5–10 ppm and which was first described several years after the report of the first case of occupational fluorosis was published.[106]

The disease is detected by osteosclerotic changes in spongey and other bones on the radiograph. There may be no symptoms even in the presence of radiological changes, or back stiffness and vague joint pains are reported in the absence of such changes. Initially, there may be increased density of vertebral and pelvic bones but as the disease advances the bone contours and trabeculae become uneven and blurred. The bones of the extremities show irregular periosteal thickening with calcification of ligaments and muscular attachments. The cortex of the long bones is thick and dense and the medullary cavity is diminished. Radiological thickening of the bone may cause confusion with Paget's disease or osteoblastic metastases. In severe cases, exostoses and osteophytes develop and calcification of ligaments, tendons and muscle insertions may lead to fusion of the spine and the development of a 'poker back' which clinically resembles ankylosing spondylitis.

Diagnosis is based upon the radiological findings and a history of prolonged fluoride exposure, together with raised urinary fluoride levels. Urinary excretion may remain high for several years after long-term heavy industrial exposure. There is evidence that the condition at least partially regresses if occupational exposure ceases, unless exposure has been prolonged in a patient suffering from poor nutrition.

The daily limit that may be ingested without risk of developing the skeletal fluorosis is 4–5 mg of fluoride,[100] and in areas of endemic fluorosis, the level of ingestion often exceeds 8 mg daily. In industrial situations, absorption higher than 20–25 mg daily used to occur due to the inhalation of fluoride dust and gases. The current eight-hour time-weighted average work exposure limit for gaseous and particulate fluorides (as fluorine) is 1.5 mg/m^3, which is intended to protect workers against developing fluorosis.[107] Inorganic fluoride exposure at 3.4 mg/m^3 has resulted in an increase in bone density in workers. Persistent urinary concentrations of fluorides above 5–7 ppm are quoted in the literature as reflecting unsafe exposure, while the urinary biological exposure limits published by the American Conference of Governmental Industrial Hygienists (ACGIH) are 18 mol/mmol creatinine pre-shift and 60 mol/mmol creatinine post-shift.

Plasma fluoride levels correlate with concentrations of inhaled hydrogen fluoride, but they are not used for routine monitoring.[104]

Workers exposed to fluorides are not at risk of developing dental fluorosis as the mottling occurs when enamel is being laid; beyond 12–14 years of age, a person's permanent teeth can no longer be mottled, whatever the fluoride intake. Roholm, however, described three different family cases of dental fluorosis arising in the children of female cryolite workers in which the exposure to fluoride was believed to have been through the mother's breast milk.[106] The manifestations of dental fluorosis range from chalky white flecks on the teeth in mild forms to brown discolouration and pitting in the severe cases (Figure 39.9). There are many parts of the world dependent on groundwater supplies for drinking which are contaminated by fluorides in geological strata. Developing, particularly

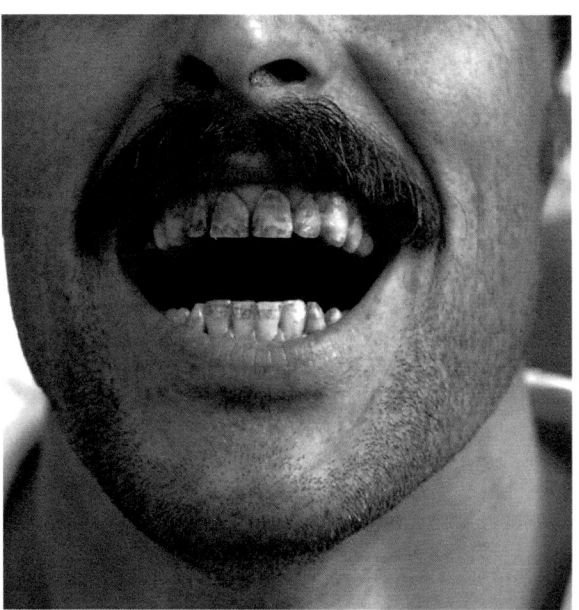

Figure 39.9 Dental fluorosis in a fisherman brought up on the volcanic islands of the Azores. Until recently, his village water supply came from a spring fed by groundwater contaminated with fluoride (>5 ppm).

permanent, teeth are extremely sensitive to fluorides during their formation.

Pot room asthma in aluminium production

Aluminium is produced by the reduction of alumina (Al_2O_3) which is obtained from bauxite, an ore produced mainly in South America and Australia. Since 1936, reports of asthmatic symptoms in pot room workers engaged in the manufacture of aluminium have suggested that respiratory irritants in the working atmosphere (hydrogen fluoride, sulphur dioxide and fluoride particles) may cause asthma or chronic obstructive pulmonary disease. Despite numerous studies, the relation between exposure agents and disease is not resolved, but exposure to irritant gases, such as hydrogen fluoride, can cause a bronchial inflammatory reaction and a reactive airway dysfunction syndrome.[108]

The traditional Hall–Heroult process for producing aluminium was invented over a century ago and involved the extraction of alumina ore from bauxite and then placing the ore in a reduction cell, or 'pot'. Bauxite, the chief ore of aluminium, contains aluminium oxides and hydroxides with fluorides present as impurities. The prebake method uses carbon anodes prepared from calcine, petroleum pitch and coal pitch. In the prebake process, the carbon anodes burn out releasing carbon dust, sulphur dioxide, carbon dioxide and carbon monoxide. In the Soderberg process, on the other hand, carbon paste is dropped into a steel casing hanging over the pot and the ore is baked *in situ* using separate, vertically placed, anodes.

The manufacture of carbon anodes in the carbon plant is associated with the release of polycyclic aromatic hydrocarbons from coal tar pitch volatiles and substantial exposure to these in the past has been found to be associated with an excess risk of lung cancer in several epidemiological studies.[109] Gaseous and particulate fluoride are given off in the two reduction processes.[110]

Exposure of susceptible individuals to the pot room atmosphere may provoke bronchial hyper-reactivity or precipitate symptoms in those with subclinical asthma, but the mechanism is probably irritant rather than allergic. The syndrome tends to persist in some individuals even after stopping exposure. A study of Norwegian pot room workers over six years of follow up found an increased decline in FEV_1.[111]

Occupational systemic poisoning by fluorides

Acute systemic toxicity may arise from the ingestion of fluoride salts, e.g. sodium fluoride, or from absorption of fluoride in hydrofluoric acid burns.[112] There is no single cause of death in fluoride poisoning. Fluoride causes enzyme inhibition involving vital functions, such as the origin and transmission of nerve impulses. Calcium complex formation, with a rapid fall in plasma calcium, may interfere with blood clotting and cell membrane permeability. Deaths associated with profound hypocalcaemia, hypermagnesaemia and hyperkalaemia have all been reported. In addition, there may be specific organ injury involving cell damage and necrosis. Terminally, there is a shock-like syndrome in which tetany is a prominent characteristic. There is no specific antidote, but the slow infusion of intravenous calcium gluconate may be life-saving.[112]

Accidental exposure of the skin to hydrofluoric acid solutions can cause severe, deep tissue injury. The treatment is beyond the scope of this chapter, but it relies on immediate removal of contaminated clothing, thorough washing of the skin with water and rigorous topical application of 2.5 per cent calcium gluconate gel which should always be available for use at locations where workers may be exposed. In hospital, subcutaneous injections of 5 per cent calcium gluconate solutions may be necessary. Systemic effects from skin burns may be fatal; in one patient, as little as 2.5 per cent of the body surface area was affected.[113]

The first-aid procedures in the event of exposure to hydrofluoric acid are shown in Table 39.5.

Other gases which hydrolyse to hydrofluoric acid

The following gases hydrolyse to hydrofluoric acid. Their effects and treatment of overexposure are as for hydrogen fluoride.

BORON TRIFLUORIDE (BF_3)

[CAS No. 7637-07-2]
Exposure limits: not available
Relative density: 2.4

Boron trifluoride is colourless and forms a mist in moist air to give hydrogen fluoride and boric acid. It is highly corrosive and has severe irritant effects on body tissues. It has a sharp odour and is non-flammable. It is used mainly as a catalyst in many chemical processes.

CHLORINE TRIFLUORIDE (ClF_3)

[CAS No. 7790-91-2]
Exposure limits: not available
Relative density: 3.2

Chlorine trifluoride is extremely reactive. The utmost care must be taken in ensuring that no contact with living tissue

Table 39.5 Recommendations on first-aid procedures for hydrofluoric acid poisoning.

Skin contact	Remove contaminated clothing while protecting your hands with suitable gloves
	Flood the skin with plenty of water for at least 5–10 minutes
	Apply calcium gluconate gel on and around the affected area and continually massage it into the skin until at least 15 minutes after pain is relieved. Cover the area with a dressing soaked in the gel and lightly bandage. These procedures an be continued during transit to hospital
	Send the patient urgently to the Emergency Department of the local hospital
Eye contact	Flush the eye with water for at least 20 minutes. This can be continued during transit to hospital.
Gassing	Remove the casualty from the contaminated area and place in fresh air
	If necessary resuscitate the casualty
	If suitably trained give oxygen
	Send to the hospital Emergency Department
Swallowing	Never attempt to induce vomiting
	If the casualty is conscious rinse out their mouth with water
	Send to the hospital Emergency Department

Source: Health and Safety Executive.

is possible. It is used for specialized purposes, such as rocket propellants and fluorinating agents.

CARBONYL FLUORIDE (COF)

[CAS No. 353-50-4]
Exposure limit: not established
Relative density: 2.29

Carbonyl fluoride is a colourless, pungent gas used mainly for the preparation of organic fluorine compounds. It is also produced during the thermal decomposition of polytetrafluoroethylene (PTFE).

PERCHLORYL FLUORIDE (ClO_3F)

[CAS No. 7616-94-6]
Exposure limits:
    STEL (15 min) 6 ppm (26 mg/m^3)
Relative density: 3.6

Perchloryl fluoride is a colourless, stable, non-flammable, sweet-smelling gas. It is a strong oxidizing agent used in fluorination processes and for rocket fuels.

PHOSPHORUS PENTAFLUORIDE (PF_5)

[CAS No. 7647-19-0]
Exposure limit: not established
Relative density: 4.5

Phosphorus pentafluoride is a colourless gas with a sharp odour. It produces a mist in contact with moist air. With large quantities of water it will ultimately yield phosphoric acid. It is used in laboratory and experimental work.

PHOSPHORUS TRIFLUORIDE (PF_3)

[CAS No. 7783-55-3]
Exposure limit: not established
Relative density: 3.0

Phosphorus trifluoride is a colourless gas. It is odourless at concentrations which can cause toxic effects. It is used in specialized small chemical processes for the fluorination of some metals. The gas is highly toxic, but only slowly hydrolyses to hydrogen fluoride.

SILICON TETRAFLUORIDE (SiF_4)

[CAS No. 7783-61-1]
Exposure limit: not established
Relative density: 3.6

Silicon tetrafluoride is a colourless non-flammable gas with an overwhelming odour, and produces a dense white mist in air. It is used to manufacture fluosilicic acid (H_2SiF_6) and thence cryolite and aluminium fluoride. Fluosilicic acid has the same general effect as hydrogen fluoride and the treatment is the same.

SULPHUR TETRAFLUORIDE (SF_4)

[CAS No. 7783-60-0]
Exposure limits: not available
Relative density: 3.8

Sulphur tetrafluoride is a very reactive, colourless and corrosive gas with a sharp odour. It is rapidly hydrolysed to hydrogen fluoride and thionyl fluoride, which in turn is slowly hydrolysed further into hydrogen fluoride and sulphur dioxide. It is used to batch produce fluorinated compounds by replacing oxygen with fluorine.

TETRAFLUOROHYDRAZINE (N_2F_3)

[CAS No. 10036-47-2]
Exposure limit: not established
Relative density: 3.7

Tetrafluorohydrazine is a colourless gas with a musty odour and which slowly hydrolyses to hydrazine and hydrogen fluoride. Hydrazine is suspected of being a potential carcinogen in man. Tetrafluorohydrazine is used for the preparation of specialized fluorides.

OXYGEN DIFLUORIDE (OF_2)

[CAS No. 7783-41-7]
Exposure limit: not established
Relative density: 1.9

Oxygen difluoride is a highly toxic, colourless gas with a foul smell. It is a very strong oxidizing agent used in the preparation of complex fluorides.

SULPHUR HEXAFLUORIDE (SF_6)

[CAS No. 2551-62-4]
Exposure limit:
    LTEL (8-h TWA) 1000 ppm (6070 mg/m^3)
    STEL (15 min) 1250 ppm (7590 mg/m^3)
Relative density: 5.1

This is an inert, heavy, colourless and odourless gas used by the electrical supply industry to insulate high voltage circuit breakers and cables. It is also frequently added to emissions to track the spread of pollution. The gas may also be used in loudspeakers and gas-filled cushions in the soles of trainer shoes. It is harmless except in a confined space where it displaces air, but electric sparking in the presence of oxygen will produce the irritant breakdown products sulphur oxyfluoride, sulphur dioxide and sulphuryl fluoride. A group of repair workers were inadvertently exposed to these gases by inhalation and suffered severe irritant effects.[114] It is one of the most potent greenhouse gases known.

NITROGEN TRIFLUORIDE (NF₃)

[CAS No. 7783-54-2]
Exposure limits: not available
Relative density: 2.46

This gas is used as an oxidizing agent in rocket fuel and in fluorination reactions. Its principal hazard on inhalation is that it readily oxidizes haemoglobin to form methaemoglobin.

SULPHURYL DIFLUORIDE (SO₂F₂)

[CAS No. 2699-79-8]
Exposure limits:
   LTEL (8-h TWA) 5 ppm (21 mg/m³)
   STEL (15 min) 10 ppm (42 mg/m³)
Relative density: 3.7

Sulphuryl difluoride is a colourless, odourless nonflammable gas with minimal smell. Its main use is as a fumigant. Overexposure has been reported to cause respiratory tract irritation, nausea and vomiting with crampy abdominal pain.

The following gases contain fluorine and are usually relatively inert, but they can undergo pyrolysis to produce respiratory irritants.

Fluorinated hydrocarbons

These gases are more widely known by their trade names. They are heavy, colourless, usually non-flammable and are used as refrigerants, specialized solvents and aerosol propellants. The usage of CFCs grew rapidly in the 1950s and 1960s as aerosol spray can propellants and blowing agents for foam insulation and foam packaging containers. CFCs are not biologically reactive and, being insoluble in water, are not removed from the air by rain. In the stratosphere, they undergo photodissociation, the chlorine atom reacting with ozone to form chlorine monoxide (CIO) and oxygen. The destruction of the ozone layer by CFCs has been recognized since 1974, but the dramatic discovery by investigators from the British Antarctic Survey of an ozone hole above Antarctica in 1985 led scientists to confirm that the depletion was due to the increase of CFCs and related halocarbons (especially methyl chloroform-1,1,1,-trichloroethane and halons). There are now plans to phase out the worldwide usage of the fully hydrogenated CFCs (see under Gases in the ambient air, p. 265).

Although CFCs chiefly pose an occupational hazard by displacing oxygen in confined spaces, they are not all as innocuous as has been supposed. Most cause narcosis at high concentrations and skin contact with the compounds with low boiling points can cause skin irritation or frostbite. In animal studies mixtures of over 1 per cent (vol.) cause respiratory depression, bronchoconstriction and reduced pulmonary compliance. The pyrolysis products of CFCs include chlorine, hydrogen chloride, hydrogen fluoride and phosgene, and these may be a hazard to firefighters. CFC-22 (chlorodifluoromethane) has been reported to cause cardiac arrhythmias (palpitations) in hospital workers who sprayed tissue with an aerosol preparation in order to 'speed up' the work of a cryostat machine,[115] but these adverse effects have not been found in studies of refrigerator repairmen. CFC-113 (Freon-113 or Genetron-113) has been implicated in fatalities from cardiac arrhythmia, asphyxiation or both in those working in confined spaces or in poorly ventilated areas.

The following gases are representative of the group and include some related compounds.

DICHLORODIFLUOROMETHANE (FREON-12, GENETRON-12) (CCl₂F₂)

CHLOROTRIFLUOROMETHANE (FREON-13, GENETRON-13) (CClF₃)

TETRAFLUOROMETHANE (FREON-14) (CF₄)

This substance occurs naturally in significant traces in natural gas and is a potent greenhouse gas, being inert like silicon hexafluoride.

DICHLOROFLUOROMETHANE (FREON-21) (CHCl₂F)

CHLORODIFLUOROMETHANE (CFC-22; FREON-22) (CHClF₂)

Exposure limit:
   LTEL (8-h TWA) 1000 ppm (3590 mg/m³)
   STEL – none

FLUOROFORM (FREON-23) (CHF₃)

1,1,2-TRICHLORO-1,2,2-TRIFLUOROETHANE (FREON-113) (CCl₂FCClF₂)

1,2-DICHLOROTETRAFLUOROETHANE (FREON-114, GENETRON-114) (C₂Cl₂F₄)

HEXAFLUOROETHANE (FREON-116) (C₂F₆)

CHLOROPENTAFLUOROETHANE (GENETRON-115) (C₂ClF₅)

1,1-DIFLUOROETHYLENE (GENETRON-1132A) (H₂C: CF₂)

1,1-DIFLUORO-1-CHLOROETHANE (GENETRON-142B) (H₃CCClF₂)

1,2-DIBROMOTETRAFLUOROETHANE (FLUOROCARBON-114B2) (C₂Br₂F₄)

1,1,1,2-TETRAFLUOROETHANE (HCFC-134A)

Exposure limit:
   LTEL 1000 ppm (4240 mg/m³)

This is used as a new ozone-sparing propellant, and has been used in asthma inhalers, for example. No human data on its health effects are available. At high concentrations in animal studies, delayed fetal development has been found. For a review of the health effects of the fully halogenated chlorofluorocarbons, see Ref. 116.

Substitutes for the phased out chlorofluorocarbons are the partially halogenated hydrochlorofluorocarbons (HCFCs), the most important being 1,1-dichloro-2,2,2-trifluoroethane (HCFC 123) and 1-chloro-1,2,2,2-tetrafluoroethane (HCFC 124). These have only recently become available for commercial and industrial use.[117,118] An outbreak of liver disease has recently been reported in workers who received repeated accidental exposure to a mixture of these two compounds.[119] They were drivers of an overhead gantry in a secondary smelting depot and were exposed to a leaking air-cooling system in their cabin. Three out of nine workers presented with acute hepatitis, the remainder progressively developed varying degrees of liver abnormalities. Liver biopsy showed hepatocellular necrosis which was prominent in perivenular zone three and focally extending from portal tracts to portal tracts and centrilobular areas. Autoantibodies against human liver cytochrome P4502E1 and P58 protein disulphide isomerase isoform (P58) were found in the serum of five of the workers.[119]

BROMOTRIFLUOROMETHANE (HALON 1301) (CF$_3$Br)

[CAS No. 75-63-8]
Exposure limits: not available
    STEL (15 min) 1200 ppm (7430 mg/m^3)

This gas is commonly used as a fire extinguishant in computer and high technology facilities. A group of workers exposed in an accidental discharge of a halon fire-extinguishing system reported irritation symptoms of the eyes, nose and throat, and light-headedness, but there may also have been exposure to irritant breakdown products of halon 1301 and Freon-22.[120]

SULPHUR DIOXIDE (SO$_2$)

[CAS No. 7446-09-5]
Exposure limits:
    LTEL (8-h TWA) 2 ppm (5.3 mg/m^3)
    STEL (15 min) 5 ppm (13 mg/m^3)
Relative density: 2.26
Ambient air quality standard: 100 ppb (15 min)

Sulphur dioxide is a colourless, highly irritating, non-flammable toxic gas. It is a common pollutant of urban air, wherever fossil fuels are burnt. Being moderately soluble in water, it will dissolve easily in the layer of fluid on the surface of the epithelium of the nasal passages and upper airways. The upper respiratory tract and the large bronchi are the major site of absorption and toxicity of sulphur dioxide, but at high concentrations it behaves like other soluble irritant gases in causing acute lung injury and damage to the front of the eye.[121] Survivors of gassing incidents with sulphur dioxide may develop reactive airways dysfunction syndrome.

Sulphur dioxide from anthropogenic sources, such as coal- or oil-fired power stations, is oxidized in the atmosphere to sulphate at a rate of about 1–5 per cent per hour,[122] but it can be faster in the presence of catalysts, such as metals or their particulate compounds in a plume. Sulphate is much more soluble than the gas and readily forms fine sulphuric acid aerosols or combines with rainwater and cloud droplets to produce acid rain, often at long distances from the source of the pollution. Acid rain has no direct health impact, but it blights vegetation, acidifies surface waters and corrodes buildings. The major natural sources of sulphur dioxide are volcanic activity, and the oxidation of dimethyl sulphide released from marine organisms.

Occupational exposures to the gas may arise in petroleum processing, wood pulping, food preservation, sulphuric acid production, and in paper mills. The uses of sulphur dioxide include bleaching and refrigeration. Quite high exposures to sulphur dioxide are common in many smelting operations since most ores contain sulphide; it is also a contaminant of the air of non-ferrous metal foundries. Explosions of sulphide dust may occur when blasting in massive sulphide ores, and workers may become exposed to dangerously elevated concentrations of sulphur dioxide in such accidents.[123,124] Particulate matter will arise during many industrial processes, as well as in the combustion of fossil fuels, and the respiratory effects of the accompanying particle concentrations may also need to be considered.

Sulphur dioxide concentrations of 3–5 ppm in the air are easily noticeable and at these levels a few sensitive individuals will show a fall in pulmonary function at rest.[125] Healthy individuals do not respond to sulphur dioxide below 1 ppm, but may respond on exercise or deep breathing at levels of 1–5 ppm; healthy individuals may show an effect with an increase in airflow resistance when exposed to concentrations of 4–5 ppm or higher for five minutes. Asthma sufferers, on the other hand, are especially sensitive to sulphur dioxide and can respond at rest to short-term concentrations of about 0.4 ppm and very sensitive subjects as low as 0.2 ppm, although no discernible threshold exists. The odour threshold is in excess of 1 ppm and so this criterion does not provide warning of potentially harmful lower levels. In the past, regular exposures in industry to over 30 ppm have been recorded, but marked irritation of the eyes, throat and upper respiratory tract usually occur at concentrations around 10 ppm. The maximum concentration that healthy individuals can endure for a few minutes is 150 ppm,[125] a level which can be fatal in the elderly asthma sufferer.[126]

'Dark-room disease' is a term coined for radiographers reporting eye and upper respiratory irritation during the course of working in x-ray film processing under poorly ventilated conditions. Although the precise cause has not been ascertained, a study showed that the main airborne contaminants were sulphur dioxide and acetic acid at concentrations of about 0.1 ppm, as well as detectable glutaraldehyde.[127] With the introduction of automated film development and processing, this condition is now rarely encountered.

Much attention has been paid to sulphur dioxide as one of the main pollutants in smogs that occurred in cities in the nineteenth century and the first half of the twentieth century as a result of the widespread burning of coal in homes and factories. In the London smog of 1952, many deaths occurred in London when daily black smoke (particulate matter) concentration exceeded 5000 µg/m³ and was associated with very high levels of sulphur dioxide: 4000 µg/m³ (1.5 ppm). With changing patterns of energy production, the emissions of the gas have been much reduced. In the United Kingdom, the highest levels' peak levels may be mainly found 30–40 km downwind of fossil-fuel power stations where the plume may fumigate at ground level.[128] At low concentrations, sulphur dioxide is thought to act on contact with the nose, throat and bronchi by stimulating neural reflexes which cause the smooth muscle of the airways to contract. This causes a reflex cough, irritation and a feeling of chest tightness. Other mechanisms contributing to airway narrowing include the development of mucosal oedema, vascular congestion of the mucosa and increased airways excretions. Although exposure studies have focused on asthma sufferers, it is likely that similar effects may be observed in patients with other chronic lung diseases. The evidence for longer-term effects and whether exposure to sulphur dioxide actually causes lung disease rather than only provoking attacks of asthma, remains conflicting.

Pre-employment health screening in workplaces where exposure to sulphur dioxide may be high enough to affect susceptible individuals should aim to advise patients with asthma or other chronic lung disease to seek alternative employment, although the occupational physician should carefully evaluate individual cases.

A proportion of the population are, when exposed to inhaled irritants over time, prone to develop mucous gland hyperplasia and chronic obstructive pulmonary disease. Epidemiological studies of smelter and pulp mill workers exposed to sulphur dioxide at regular concentrations of 1–5 ppm or over have shown inconclusive results on measures of respiratory symptoms or chronic reduction in pulmonary function. Because of its irritant properties, sulphur dioxide has been thought possibly to act as a co-carcinogen in the causation of lung cancer. Studies of workers in copper smelters have shown an increased risk in relation to exposure to arsenic, but no independent effect of sulphur dioxide was seen.[129] There is little information available on teratogenic effects, but the gas is not considered to be a human carcinogen.[97]

'Smelter disease' has been recognized in workers replacing pipes in sulphuric acid manufacturing plants. Characterized by dyspnoea, diarrhoea, colicky pain, muscle pain and dermatitis, it was attributed to sulphur dioxide in the past, but it is due to mercury fume exposure when burning through the pipes containing sludge.[130]

Sodium metabisulphite is widely used in the food and beverage industry and in the fishing industry as a preservative. It may have an irritant effect on the airways through a mechanism leading to the release of sulphur dioxide when it is dissolved in water.

SULPHUR TRIOXIDE (ANHYDRIDE OF SULPHURIC ACID) (SO₃)

[CAS No. 7446-11-9]

Oleum ('fuming sulphuric acid') is a complex mixture of sulphuric acid and sulphur trioxide. Sulphur trioxide can exist as a gas, liquid or solid, and is used primarily as a sulphating or sulphonating agent, for example in the manufacture of detergents, dyestuffs, drugs and insecticides. Dense clouds of sulphuric acid mist are formed when sulphur trioxide comes into contact with moisture in the air.

Sulphuric and other inorganic acid mists

Erosion of the enamel of the teeth has been reported with occupational exposure to sulphuric and other strong inorganic acid mists (nitric, hydrochloric and phosphoric acids).[6] They are irritating to mucous epithelia and provoke respiratory symptoms and changes in pulmonary function and, at high concentrations, death.[131] Acid mists may also cause pulmonary irritation by adhering to fine particles. There is sufficient evidence that occupational exposure to strong inorganic mists containing sulphuric acid is carcinogenic; laryngeal and lung cancer have been implicated in certain strong acid processes.[97,132]

An interesting incident demonstrating the impact of factory emissions containing concentrated sulphuric acid aerosols occurred in Japan between 1960 and 1969 when asthmatic symptoms were reported in about 600 individuals living within 5 km of a titanium dioxide plant during this period.[133]

AMMONIA (NH₃)

[CAS No. 7664-41-7]
Exposure limits:
    LTEL (8-h TWA) 25 ppm (18 mg/m³)
    STEL (15 min) 35 ppm (25 mg/m³)
Relative density: 0.59
Flammability limits in air: 15–28 per cent (vol.)

Anhydrous ammonia is a colourless gas with a distinctive pungent odour. It is extremely soluble in water, forming a caustic alkaline solution of ammonium hydroxide. Ammonia is one of the most widely used industrial gases, as a catalyst and reagent, and has been used for many years as a refrigerant and in the manufacture of fertilizers. Although the gas is lighter than air, it can behave paradoxically, as in an accidental release from storage in liquid form under pressure by undergoing rapid cooling to form a dense cloud that hugs the ground.

Most people will recognize the odour of ammonia at 30–50 ppm. At or above 50 ppm, the gas is irritant to the eyes and mucous membranes of the respiratory tract, although partial tolerance does develop. Being readily hydroscopic, it is absorbed by the mucous coating of the upper respiratory tract. Human data are sparse, but the only clearly established effect arising from exposure to low concentrations

(<200 ppm) in humans is irritation of the skin, eyes and upper respiratory tract. There is no evidence that ammonia is genotoxic, carcinogenic or reprotoxic. Exposure to concentrations up to 500 ppm for a few minutes can be tolerated by healthy adults, but at this level there is cough, hoarseness and tightness of the throat, as well as marked eye irritation and conjunctivitis. At estimated levels of between 5000 and 10 000 ppm, ammonia is likely to damage the lower respiratory tract and be life-threatening, and concentrations in excess of 10 000 ppm may be rapidly fatal.[134,135] At life-threatening levels, the gas causes chemical burns of the nose, mouth and throat which become red and raw, and corneal burns. The tracheal epithelium and bronchi may become denuded of epithelium. Pulmonary oedema by itself or with subsequent bronchopneumonia is the main cause of death, but fatalities can also be caused by the very rapid onset of acute laryngeal oedema which initially can manifest itself by hoarseness and dyspnoea.[136,137]

The strongly irritant nature of ammonia has led to the oft-repeated view that laryngeal spasm is a frequent cause of death in gassing accidents, but it is more likely to be due to rapid onset of laryngeal oedema. Although spasm of the glottis could persist long enough to induce asphyxia, the spasm would normally relax during unconsciousness and then breathing would recommence.

Apart from respiratory tract irritation, injury to the eyes at high concentrations can be severe. Irrigation of the eyes should be instituted immediately after exposure to prevent rapid absorption of ammonia by the eye. Ophthalmic sequelae include corneal opacities, cataract and glaucoma. A jet of anhydrous ammonia on to the moist skin can cause second-degree burns, as will splashes of liquid ammonia. The literature reports a case of severe gastritis continuing for months after a gassing accident.[137]

There is good evidence that some individuals who have survived an acute gassing incident may go on to develop permanent respiratory disability with complications such as progressive airway obstruction, diminishing diffusion capacity (low transfer factor), bronchiolitis obliterans, bronchiectasis, and continuing cough and sputum.

In contrast, exposure to ammonia in pig farmers is around a few ppm. Respiratory symptoms are common in these workers. However, exposure to dust, disinfectants and endotoxins may contribute to the respiratory irritants in the air of livestock confinement buildings.[44,138]

Alkyl amine gases

The following aliphatic amine gases are used widely in industrial processes and pharmaceutical manufacturing:

MONOMETHYLAMINE (CH_3NH_2)

DIMETHYLAMINE ($CH_3)_2NH$

[CAS No. 124-40-3]
Exposure limits:
  STEL (15 min) 6 ppm (11 mg/m^3)
  LTEL (8-h TWA) 2 ppm (3.8 mg/m^3)

TRIMETHYLAMINE ($CH_3)_2N$

[CAS No. 75-50-3]
Exposure limits: not available

They are flammable, highly soluble, alkaline, colourless gases which have a fishy odour at low concentrations and an ammoniacal odour at higher concentrations. They are all denser than air and act as irritants to the eyes, nose, throat, respiratory tract and skin. Trimethylamine (TMA) is a major component of the odour produced by decaying fish. In fish odour syndrome, an uncommon inherited autosomal recessive condition, the oxidation of trimethylamine in the body is impaired. Unoxidized trimethylamine is increased in urine, breath, sweat and other secretions, causing the fish smell.[139]

OZONE (O_3)

[CAS No. 10028-15-6]
Exposure limits:
  STEL (15 min) 0.2 ppm (0.40 mg/m^3)
Relative density: 1.66

Ozone is a faintly bluish gas with a characteristic pungent odour. Because it is irritant to mucous membranes and as it is only moderately soluble in water, it readily penetrates to the small airways and alveoli, even with brief exposure, and at elevated concentrations causes pulmonary oedema. Exposure to moderately elevated levels of ozone causes a measurable fall in FEV_1 and FVC (forced vital capacity) associated with symptoms in susceptible adults, and children. These changes are compatible with an inflammatory bronchiolitis causing reflex inhibition of respiration. They are related to the duration of exposure and to exercise and have been recorded at concentrations as low as 0.08 ppm over periods of 6.6 hours.[140] There is no evidence that asthma sufferers or subjects with chronic obstructive pulmonary disease are more sensitive to ozone than others. Distinct irritation to the eyes and respiratory tract occurs at 0.5 ppm and prolonged exposure to this concentration is reported to cause pulmonary oedema or could increase susceptibility to respiratory infections (bacterial and viral). Even brief exposure to 1 ppm is inadvisable as it may cause severe cough and malaise. The lethal level is not known precisely but inhalation of 50 ppm for 30 minutes is regarded as a potentially fatal exposure.

Ozone is used in industry as an oxidizing agent in chemical reactions, for water fumigation and for the bleaching of synthetic and natural fibres, oils, paper and flour. It is also generated by electrical storms and by discharges in electrical equipment, for example during processes involving arc welding or emission of ultraviolet radiation. In offices with poor ventilation electrostatic photocopiers which utilize the action of high intensity discharge lamps, and laser printers, particularly older models, may produce sufficient ozone to cause symptoms such as headache and eye and throat irritation in some workers. Laser printers have ozone filters and it is important that the machines are regularly serviced according to the manufacturer's instructions.

The mechanism of ozone in the lung has been one of the most extensively studied.[140] The cells most susceptible to damage are type 1 cells which line the alveoli and form part of the barrier for gaseous exchange between the air and the blood. With their loss and exposure of the basement membrane, stimulation of inflammatory cascades and increased fluid leak from the capillaries occur, together with an increase in macrophages, neutrophils and alveolar surface protein in the interstitial and alveolar spaces. This is accompanied by the release of surfactant and other secretions by the epithelial type 2 cells, which like the Clara cells, normally produce surfactant which prevents alveolar collapse and helps to keep the alveoli 'dry'. Biochemical changes induced in the lung by inhaled oxidants of free radical nature, such as ozone and nitrogen oxides are complex and not understood, but include lipid peroxidation. Both the upper and lower respiratory tract have a considerable range of protective antioxidants, with intracellular reduced glutathione (GSH) being one of the major ones of the lower respiratory tract. Clara cells have a major role in chemical detoxification by being a major site for the metabolism of inhaled and systemically administered chemicals by means of GSH, NADPH and P-450 monooxygenases; they also provide the bulk of the antioxidant molecules of the liquid lining of the airways.[140]

Much attention has been focused on ozone as the major oxidant in photochemical smog. In terms of producing inflammation of the respiratory tract, ozone is the most toxic of the common air pollutants. Ozone may also increase bronchial responsiveness to allergens in atopic asthmatic subjects[140] and the response to other bronchoconstrictor pollutants, such as sulphuric acid or sulphur dioxide. The UK Department of Health has advised that those healthy or asthmatic individuals who are particularly sensitive to ozone should limit heavy exercise in the open air in the afternoon, the time of day when ozone levels reach a peak during periods of poor air quality, if peak hourly levels are likely to exceed 0.1 ppm.[140]

There is no information in humans on whether long-term exposure to levels of ozone at the current occupational exposure standard (0.2 ppm) can cause chronic pulmonary health effects or adverse reproductive effects. In practice, most industrial exposures tend to be brief and related to attending specific processes; hence only a STEL has been established. Monitoring methods should be in place to detect leaks so that ozonators can be shut down if abnormal operating conditions prevail. Leak detection by nose is not satisfactory because even slight leaks cause the sensation of smell to be numbed.

Nitrogen oxides

NITRIC OXIDE (NO)

[CAS No. 10102-43-9]
Exposure limits: under review
    LTEL (8-h TWA) 25 ppm (31 mg/m^3)
    STEL (15 min) 35 ppm (44 mg/m^3)
Relative density: 1.04

Certain conditions, e.g. septic shock, result in enhanced endogenous synthesis of nitric oxide via induction of a nitric oxide synthase in endothelial and vascular smooth muscle cells, leading to vasodilatation and hypotension. A 40 ppm NO/air inspired mixture acts as a highly selective pulmonary vasodilator and reduces pulmonary hypertension. Its therapeutic properties are under study in patients requiring assisted ventilation, as in adult respiratory distress syndrome. Endogenous nitric oxide production probably accounts for most of the methaemoglobin in the blood of normal subjects. At 40 ppm nitric oxide, the increase in methaemoglobin is small and clinically insignificant, but at over 100 ppm methaemoglobinaemia and pulmonary oedema are the principal hazards of the gas. Much of the toxicity is accounted for by the formation of nitrogen dioxide, which is not a vasodilator.

NITROGEN DIOXIDE (NO$_2$)

[CAS No. 1010244-0]
Exposure limits: under review
    LTEL (8-h TWA) 3 ppm (5.7 mg/m^3)
    STEL (15 min) 5 ppm (9.6 mg/m^3)
Relative density: 2.62

Nitric oxide is a colourless and odourless gas which rapidly oxidizes in air to nitrogen dioxide, a reddish-brown gas with a pungent odour apparent to most people at about 0.5 ppm. Both are found in nitrous fumes produced by fuming nitric acid, but nitric oxide is non-irritant, while nitrogen dioxide is the more hazardous. Nitrogen dioxide is non-flammable and hydrolyses in water to form nitrous and nitric acid. Nitric oxide and nitrogen dioxide are formed in the combustion of fossil fuels or from biomass burning, the amount depending upon the nitrogen content of the fuel and the combustion temperature. Some fuels, such as natural gas, contain negligible amounts of nitrogen, but nitrogen oxides are also formed during the combustion of all fuels in the regions of peak flame temperature. In the United Kingdom, some 50 per cent of the atmospheric nitrogen dioxide is produced by motor vehicles and some 25 per cent by power stations. The most significant indoor source of nitrogen dioxide is cooking with gas. Like ozone, nitrogen dioxide is an oxidant gas with free radical properties and these may be responsible for its injurious effects on the pulmonary parenchyma by damaging cell membranes and proteins, although the gas is considerably less irritant than ozone. The formation of nitrous and nitric acid in dissolved nitrogen dioxide may also injure the airways. Individuals with mild asthma are more sensitive than unaffected people to exposure to nitrogen dioxide. At relatively high concentrations, the gas causes acute inflammation of the airways. Nitrogen dioxide reduces mucociliary clearance and in animal studies has been shown to affect the immune cells of the airways and increase susceptibility to bacterial and viral respiratory infections.[141,142]

In the indoor environment, the burning of natural gas as a cooking fuel in homes is an important source of nitrogen dioxide as are paraffin space heaters: indoor air concentrations may readily exceed those outside the home. An unvented gas cooker may typically provide peak levels of 200–400 ppb in a kitchen.

In industry, nitrogen dioxide is released as a byproduct whenever nitric acid acts on metals or on organic materials, such as in the nitration of cotton or other cellulose, and in the manufacture of many chemicals. Certain welding operations also produce nitrogen dioxide. Fermentation of silage will produce high concentrations of gas within two days of silo filling and exposure to farmers entering the confined silo space may give rise to acute fatalities or the respiratory effects of exposure to nitrogen dioxide known as 'silo fillers' disease'. The hazard from oxides of nitrogen in silos was first reported from the United States where farmers commonly silage maize stalks.[143,144] Under certain growth conditions, for example drought or in soils with elevated nitrates, the content of nitrate in the grass or maize stalks used for silage may be increased enough to release an abundance of nitrous acid during fermentation which then breaks down into oxides of nitrogen. Warning signs to farmers are dead birds or rodents and a yellow-brown haze around the silage surface. Elevated carbon dioxide and reduced oxygen concentrations may also occur at the same time. Similar reactions can arise if silage grass is treated with ammonium salts. To prevent the build up of gases, silos should have adequate mechanical ventilation. Nitro-explosive fumes contain oxides of nitrogen, and when dynamite or gun cotton burn quietly instead of detonating, nearly the whole of the nitrogen is given off as nitric oxide instead of free nitrogen. Thus, numerous inhalation accidents have occurred in mining and tunnelling from the imperfect detonation of nitro-explosives, or from dynamite catching fire in poorly ventilated spaces. Armed services personnel may also be exposed to the fumes in gun-pits, armoured vehicles, ships' magazines and turrets.

Increased airways resistance has been measured in healthy human volunteers exposed to two-hour concentrations as low as 2.5 ppm of nitrogen dioxide. Asthma sufferers may respond at concentrations as low as 0.3 ppm when exercising and exposure may enhance their response to common allergens.[145] The main danger of nitrogen dioxide is that it is only a mild upper respiratory tract irritant so that exposure to up to 50 ppm may produce no immediate symptoms to warn of its potential hazard. However, exposure to 4–25 ppm may result in severe cough, haemoptysis and chest pain. Exposure for less than an hour to 100–150 ppm can result in fatal pulmonary oedema arising between 3 and 72 hours later, with the initial irritant effects comprising throat irritation, cough, headaches, tightness in the chest and sweating, all of which may pass off within 30 minutes. Thus, people who are believed to have received significant exposure should be admitted to hospital and placed under observation for 48 hours. At more elevated concentrations, a few breaths can produce severe and immediate hypoxaemia which may be fatal. In less severe cases, the delayed symptoms will be dyspnoea, chest pain with haemoptysis, and headache followed by an uneventful recovery in most patients, although the cough may last several weeks.

Apollo astronauts were accidentally exposed in an incident to an average of 250 ppm of nitrogen dioxide for 4 minutes before splashdown. They developed chest symptoms and evidence of pneumonia over the next day.

Poisoning by oxides of nitrogen is a prescribed disease.

The initial treatment of nitrogen dioxide poisoning is as for non-cardiac pulmonary oedema induced by irritant gases. However, with this gas a second episode of pulmonary oedema may occur, and following apparent recovery bronchiolitis obliterans (see above under Bronchiolitis obliterans, p. 263) may develop after an asymptomatic period that can last up to six weeks.[146]

Nitrogen dioxide exposure should always be considered in workers who have suffered an acute onset of pulmonary symptoms with haemoptysis associated with minimal evidence of preceding respiratory irritation. Such incidents have also involved ice hockey players and spectators due to nitrogen dioxide emitted by malfunctioning combustion engines in ice surfacing machines that use propane.[147] Symptoms attributed to high levels of nitrogen dioxide have been reported in blast furnace workers when the slag is under cooling conditions (cold blast furnace syndrome).

Methaemoglobin determinations should be routinely performed: in an accident involving the deaths of three men entering a silo that had been filled with corn the previous day post-mortem blood samples showed a methaemoglobinaemia in the range of 38–44 per cent in the three men.[148]

Information on the effects of chronic low-level occupational exposures is currently inadequate. A meta-analysis of epidemiological studies of the effects of exposure to nitrogen dioxide in the indoor air from domestic gas cookers on respiratory disease in children was inconclusive.[140] Nitrogen dioxide is not considered to be carcinogenic or teratogenic.[141]

HYDROGEN SULPHIDE (H_2S)

[CAS No. 778306-4]
Exposure limits:
    STEL (15 min) 10 ppm (14 mg/m^3)
    LTEL (8-h TWA) 5 ppm (7 mg/m^3)
Relative density: 1.19
Flammability limits: 4.3–46 per cent (vol.)

Hydrogen sulphide is a colourless gas which burns in air with a pale blue flame and is moderately soluble in water. It is rapidly converted to sulphur dioxide in the atmosphere by a reaction with hydroxyl groups and carbonyl sulphide. In the body, the sulphide ion is oxidized to thiosulphate and sulphate in the liver and kidneys and is mostly eliminated in the urine. The toxic effects of the gas are caused through the inhibition of cytochrome oxidase and through a direct depressant effect on the respiratory centre of the brain.[149] At high concentrations, hydrogen sulphide is very poisonous, but recent research has found that at low levels it normally behaves in the body as a cell messenger emitted in red blood cells.

Hydrogen sulphide poisoning is a frequently met hazard in the oil, gas and petrochemical industries where the risks of exposure are well known. Less well recognized are the dangers from the release of hydrogen sulphide as a result of the fermentation of proteinous material, e.g. the decay of 'trash' fish in boat holds and on farms which store slurry and liquid manure. It may also be found in dangerous concentrations in the vicinity of fumaroles and the craters of volcanoes, as well as in geothermal and hot spring areas (Figure 39.10). Occupations associated with hydrogen sulphide exposure include carbon disulphide production, viscous rayon production, sewer and tunnel work and mining, petroleum production or processing, rubber vulcanizing, pulp industry, sulphuric acid production, tanning and glue manufacture. Its characteristic smell of rotten eggs is normally readily detectable below 1 ppm: the threshold of detection of the gas is 0.02 ppm and the rotten egg smell is detectable at levels several times higher. However, the sense of smell to hydrogen sulphide is soon lost at over 20 ppm and so the worker may have little, if any, warning of the presence of the gas at dangerous concentrations. Inhalation of concentrations of 10 ppm hydrogen sulphide has no effect on pulmonary function in exercising healthy subjects[150] and levels of 20 ppm can be tolerated for some hours without harm (Figure 39.10), and there is no cumulative action.

Hydrogen sulphide is an irritant to the upper airways, but asthma sufferers do not appear to so readily respond to low levels of hydrogen sulphide as they may do to sulphur dioxide.[150] An exposure study of asthma patients who required regular medication, but excluding patients with severe asthma, found that an effect on airways resistance (but not FEV_1 or FVC) was discernible in two of ten subjects exposed to a concentration at 2 ppm, a level which is regarded as a lowest observed adverse effect level.[151,152]

On volcanoes, scientists can be totally unaware of hydrogen sulphide because its smell may be undetectable, even at low levels, in mixtures of fumarolic gases for reasons which are not clear. As with other toxic gases, a safe system of work that includes air monitoring is essential. While the toxic hazard of hydrogen sulphide depends on the duration of exposure as well as its concentration, levels above 500 ppm should be regarded as very dangerous and immediate evacuation from a contaminated atmosphere should begin well below this level.

The symptoms of acute intoxication ($>$1000 ppm) are rapid breathing and distress, with nausea and vomiting, and these may be rapidly followed by loss of consciousness usually in association with cessation of breathing. Loss of consciousness without warning can occur on sudden exposure to a high concentration of hydrogen sulphide ($>$2000 ppm) after only one or two breaths ('knock down') and there is a high probability of death unless emergency resuscitation is commenced. Hydrogen sulphide is also a pulmonary irritant and brief exposures above 500 ppm may cause acute non-cardiogenic pulmonary oedema; this potentially fatal complication can occasionally occur with prolonged exposures at concentrations exceeding 250 ppm.[153]

Eye irritation has been reported in workers exposed to 10–20 ppm hydrogen sulphide for six to seven hours.[152] Exposure at concentrations greater than 50 ppm for one hour or more may severely damage eye tissues.[152] Hydrogen sulphide keratoconjunctivitis is usually a feature of subacute intoxication by the gas that may arise after prolonged

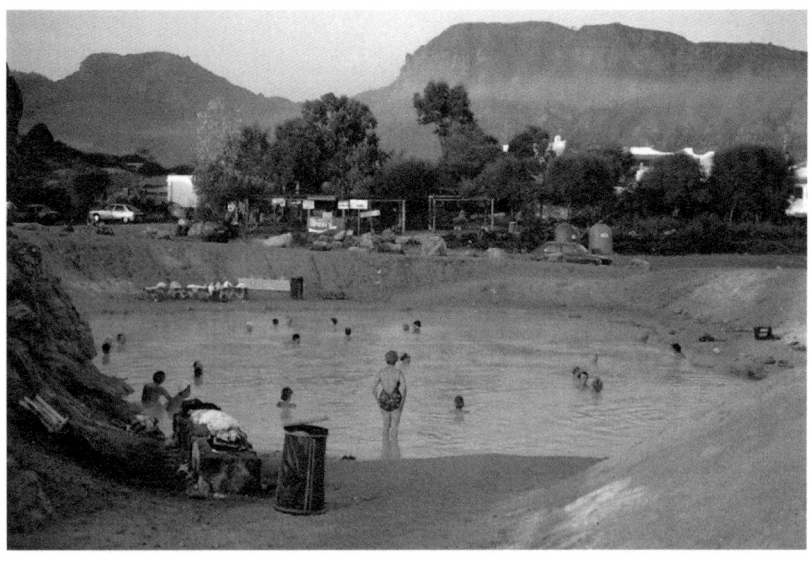

Figure 39.10 Bathers in a volcanic mudpool on Vulcano Island, Italy. Hydrogen sulphide concentrations up to 20 ppm can be measured above the surface of the water.

exposure above 50–60 ppm, the symptoms being related to blepharitis and irritant conjunctivitis with lacrimation and photophobia. Sensations of grittiness or pain in the eye are associated with superficial punctate corneal erosions. Usually, the eyes recover within 24 hours following removal from exposure, or after treatment with chloramphenicol eye ointment, but corneal ulceration has been recorded.

With prompt first aid and hospital treatment, the overall fatality rate from hydrogen sulphide poisoning with loss of consciousness is low and recovery is normally complete.[153] However, in a small minority of patients, neurological sequelae may be found after an episode of unconsciousness. There is no specific treatment for hydrogen sulphide poisoning and the use of nitrite therapy is controversial. There is no specific finding at autopsy. Blood sulphide concentrations can be measured in fatal and non-fatal poisonings using an ion-selective electrode method,[154] but blood and urine thiosulphate are believed to be more reliable by most laboratories,[155,156] although experience remains limited. As sulphaemoglobin is not formed *in vivo* by hydrogen sulphide, sulphaemoglobinaemia is not evidence of exposure to the gas.[157]

Evaluating the long-term effects of hydrogen sulphide poisoning is complicated when case reports often lack good information on exposure levels, in particular, the presence or absence of other gases, such as ammonia and carbon monoxide, which may be present due to fermentation processes. There is also a dearth of good follow-up studies. Reports of interstitial fibrosis and chronic disability following pulmonary oedema (pneumonitis) are uncommon.[158] Clinical experience and animal experiments suggest that neurological damage due to hydrogen sulphide poisoning is similar to hypoxic brain damage from any other cause, and case reports of delayed sequelae as in carbon monoxide poisoning are rare.[159] However, there is a group of patients occupationally exposed to hydrogen sulphide who present with non-specific symptoms, such as hypersusceptibility to gas smells and other strong odours, fatigue, lack of energy, poor memory, irritability, decreased libido and disturbances of equilibrium. There may even be signs of vestibular dysfunctioning on clinical investigation. Ahlborg[160] concluded that the majority of these patients have suffered repeated episodes of intoxication without loss of consciousness. They may also fall into the category of those patients who develop non-specific symptoms following chemical exposure incidents. There is insufficient evidence in the literature to justify the entity of cumulative or chronic hydrogen sulphide intoxication at prolonged exposures at 50–100 ppm, and such levels above the occupational exposure standard should not be regularly encountered anyway in modern industry.

Chronic exposures to low levels in the environment, such as in geothermal areas, as well as at workplaces, have not been shown to be harmful, although its unpleasant smell can be a considerable nuisance. The New Zealand city of Rotorua sits on a geothermal field, and the air is polluted by low levels of hydrogen sulphide, but there is an absence of scientific data on which to base opinions on the carcinogenicity, teratogenicity or reproductive effects of the gas in this or other locations.[161,162] The World Health Organization has issued a guideline concentration limit in ambient air of 7 μg/m^3 (30-minute averaging period), based on odour annoyance.[8,152] Natural gas may contain as much as 50 per cent hydrogen sulphide that must be removed through refining. In 1950, an escape of hydrogen sulphide from a refining plant into the local neighbourhood occurred in Poza Rica, Mexico, resulting in 320 hospitalized persons and 22 deaths.[163]

Malodorous sulphur compounds

Hydrogen sulphide and methyl mercaptan are present in the breath of individuals with halitosis as a result of proteolytic activity by microorganisms residing on the tongue and teeth. Both substances, together with dimethyl sulphide and dimethyl disulphide are the principal air pollutants emitted by pulp mills. For safety reasons, odorants are added to natural domestic gas, namely diethyl sulphide, tertiary butyl mercaptan, ethyl mercaptan and methyl ethyl sulphide. Evidence for health effects of low level exposure to reduced sulphur compounds in the ambient air rests in studies of communities in the vicinity of sulphate paper mills in Finland, where concentrations of total reduced sulphur compounds in excess of 40 mg/m^3 (one-hour or daily means) have been associated with daily reported symptoms of headache, depression, tiredness and nausea.[164] Dimethyl sulphide is allegedly the principal component of foetor hepaticus.[165]

CARBONYL SULPHIDE (COS)

[CAS No. 463-58-1]
Exposure limit: not established
Relative density: 2.1
Flammability range: 12–29 per cent (vol.)

The most abundant sulphur species in the atmosphere is carbonyl sulphide, being naturally produced from soil decomposition, wetlands and marshes, etc. The gas is often encountered with hydrogen sulphide in processes involving the destructive distillation of coal and the purification of petroleum. It is a colourless gas with an odour of rotten eggs that decomposes in moist air to carbon dioxide and hydrogen sulphide. The gas is less irritant to the lungs than hydrogen sulphide and probably acts in the same way on the central nervous system to cause respiratory paralysis.

SILANE (SiH$_4$)

[CAS No. 7803-62-5]
Exposure limits:
    LTEL (8-h TWA) 0.5 ppm (0.67 mg/m^3)
    STEL (15 min) 1 ppm (1.3 mg/m^3)
Relative density: 1.1

Silane is a colourless gas with a repulsive odour and even at low concentrations is spontaneously flammable in air at room temperature. When silane burns in pipelines carrying the gas, silicon oxide dust is formed. The main use of silane is in the semiconductor industry as a source of high purity silicon where, because of its fire hazard, it has to be used under special control technology with the result that human exposure has tended to be minimal. There is little information on the effects of human exposure, but as it will form silicic acid in the presence of moisture, it is assumed that silane will have an irritant effect on the eyes, mucous membranes and respiratory tract.

METHYL MERCAPTAN (METHANETHIOL) (CH_3SH)

[CAS No. 74-93-1]
Exposure limits: not available
Relative density: 1.7
Flammability limits: 3.9–21.8 per cent

Methyl mercaptan (methanethiol) is colourless and flammable with a very foul odour detectable at very low concentrations. It is reported to have similar toxic properties to hydrogen sulphide, being capable of causing central respiratory paralysis and pulmonary oedema. In a rare case of death by overexposure, acute severe haemolytic anaemia and methaemoglobinaemia were found in the comatose victim, although this effect was probably unique to the patient who, in addition, suffered from glucose-6-phosphate dehydrogenase deficiency.[166]

HYDROGEN SELENIDE (H_2Se)

[CAS No. 7783-07-5]
Exposure limits: not available
Relative density: 2.8

Hydrogen selenide is an irritant gas capable of causing pulmonary oedema. In one reported case of acute poisoning, the effects were acute severe cough and wheeze which were followed by a lasting obstructive lung disorder.[167] Effects of chronic selenium exposure include extreme lassitude and fatiguability, garlic odour on the breath, tremor, excess perspiration, abdominal pain and vomiting, and a metallic taste in the mouth. The gas is used in the preparation of selenides and is important as a doping gas in the semiconductor industry, but routine biological monitoring for selenium is not undertaken.

IRRITANT OR OTHER GASES WITH SYSTEMIC TOXIC EFFECTS

ARSINE (AsH_3)

[CAS No. 778442-1]
Exposure limit:
    LTEL (8-h TWA) 0.05 ppm (0.16 mg/m^3)
Relative density: 2.69

Arsine is a colourless, non-irritating gas with a garlicky odour and is moderately soluble in water. Apart from its use in the manufacture of semiconductors in the microelectronics industry, its evolution is almost always accidental.[168] It can be produced by the action of water on a metallic arsenide, and an ore contaminated with arsenic will liberate arsine when treated with acid. Poisoning may arise in metal smelting and extraction, but exposure may also occur in galvanizing, soldering, etching and lead plating, as well as in the disposal of toxic waste containing arsenic or arsenides.

The gas may lead to incidents in the most unexpected ways. In a classical incident off the British coast involving the *Asiafreighter*, a cylinder of arsine stored in the ship's hold leaked through a cylinder valve: four crew members who inspected the hold were inadvertently exposed to the gas and suffered severe poisoning, but exchange transfusion was life-saving, the diagnosis having been made by a physician-toxicologist over the telephone.[169] The occupational and general physician should be alert to arsine poisoning and its characteristic features. The gas is a powerful haemolytic agent and its effects are usually fatal if exposure is severe enough to cause anuria, unless the diagnosis is made quickly and exchange transfusion is employed as a mainstay of treatment.

The presenting symptoms are nausea, vomiting and headache which can arise 2–24 hours after a casual exposure to arsine which may have lasted only 1–2 minutes. There may be no olfactory or other warning of the presence of the gas. Exposure to only 3–10 ppm of arsine in air can produce symptoms after several hours of exposure and 25–50 ppm for 30 minutes is potentially lethal in humans. Early on, the victim may pass dark red urine, and the combination of haemoglobinuria (without intact red blood cells in the urine), jaundice and abdominal pain should alert one to the diagnosis. The abdominal pain and jaundice typically arise in 24–48 hours; and anuric or oliguric renal failure sets in by 72 hours.

Other causes of haemoglobinuria to be considered in the differential diagnosis are leptospirosis, malaria and paroxysmal nocturnal haemoglobinuria. Other chemical agents capable of causing haemoglobinuria include potassium chlorate, pyrogallic acid and stibine gas.

Diagnosis is made on the history of exposure and the finding of elevated urinary arsenic.

Because acute poisoning produces rapid and fulminant haemolysis, many body organs, particularly the kidney, are at risk from the sludging of red cell debris within the microcirculation, hypoxia and the direct effect of arsine, but the mechanisms involved are not fully understood. There is reticulocytosis and leukocytosis with an elevated plasma haemoglobin, and methaemoglobin may form in the plasma and urine. Renal failure from severe tubular necrosis is the main clinical complication and requires treatment with exchange transfusion to remove the arsine adequately.[170] In mild cases of haemoglobinuria, forced diuresis is recommended. Recovery from the acute tubular necrosis may be followed by the development of chronic renal failure with glomerular sclerosis, atrophic tubules and interstitial fibrosis. A wide spectrum of clinical manifestations may arise including damage to the liver, myocardium, nervous system and bone marrow.

A chronic form of poisoning from low-level exposure to arsine has been described in workers engaged in the cyanide extraction of gold and in zinc smelting. This gave rise to severe anaemia, mildly elevated serum bilirubin and raised urinary arsenic.[168]

STIBINE (SbH₃)

[CAS No. 7803-52-3]
Exposure limits: not available

Stibine is a highly toxic, colourless gas which is formed when an acid reacts with a metal containing antimony as an impurity, or when nascent hydrogen comes into contact with metallic antimony or a soluble antimony compound. The gas is not used in industry and its evolution is unintentional. Exposure may occur in metallurgy or chemical laboratories but, unlike arsine, it has an extremely unpleasant odour. Stibine poisoning is rare in industry. The manifestations of poisoning and the physiological action of the gas resemble arsine, but are less fulminant. Haemolysis, myoglobinuria, haematuria, renal failure, nausea, vomiting and headache have been reported after inhalation. Antimony trioxide is used as a fire retardant in plastics manufacture, and the release of stibine from PVC cot mattresses was considered, and later discounted, as a cause of sudden infant death syndrome. Urine antimony measurements may be used as a guide to overexposure to the gas in workers.

GERMANE (GeH₄)

[CAS No. 7782-65-2]
Exposure limits:
  LTEL (8-h TWA) 0.2 ppm (0.64 mg/m^3)
  STEL (15 min) 0.6 ppm (1.9 mg/m^3)
Relative density: 2.6

Germane is flammable and colourless and has a pungent odour. Unlike its cousin arsine, it is not encountered as an incidental product in ore or scrap processing. It is used to deposit pure germanium in semiconductor manufacturing.

The toxicity of the family appears to be in the order Ge, As, Sb. Although germane produces haemolysis, no industrial poisonings have been reported. By analogy with arsine, any victim of significant exposure should be removed to an intensive care facility and assessment of blood, kidney and cerebral function continued for some days.

PHOSPHINE (PH₃)

[CAS No. 7803-51-2]
Exposure limit:
  LTEL (8-h TWA) 0.1 ppm (0.14 mg/m^3)
  STEL (15 min) 0.2 ppm (0.28 mg/m^3)
Relative density: 1.18

Phosphine or hydrogen phosphide is a colourless, flammable gas which can auto-ignite at ambient temperatures if it contains other phosphorus anhydrides as impurities. Pure phosphine will auto-ignite above 38°C and forms an explosive mixture in air at concentrations greater than 1.8 per cent by volume. The pure gas is considered odourless, but impurities will give it a characteristic smell of dead fish or garlic which may be imperceptible at low, but hazardous, concentrations.[171]

Phosphine is used as an intermediate in the synthesis of organophosphines and organic phosphonium derivatives. It is widely used in its pure form as a dopant in the manufacture of semiconductors, but it has chiefly gained notoriety through its use as a fumigant against insects and rodents in grain stores, in grain elevators and on board ships. It is an unwanted byproduct in various metallurgical reactions and in the manufacture of acetylene using impure calcium carbide. It may also be generated when water or acids come into contact with metals containing phosphide as a contaminant, such as ferrosilicon and spheroidal graphite iron.

Aluminium phosphide is a common poison used in suicide in India where it is widely used to fumigate stored grains. When consumed, it reacts with hydrochloric acid in the stomach to liberate phosphine, where it can become an unsuspecting hazard to pathologists performing autopsies as the gas will escape when the stomach is opened. Phosphine may arise transiently in the anaerobic degradation of phosphorus-containing matter, as in marsh gas, but is otherwise rare in nature.

Aluminium or magnesium phosphide pellets are inserted into the cargo of wheat on board ships for fumigation purposes. The moisture causes a chemical reaction which releases phosphine and leaves a harmless residue of aluminium hydroxide. Peak concentrations will arise in a sealed hold during a voyage and it is necessary that the gas is dissipated by opening the hatches to the air for at least 24 hours before the cargo is discharged. Acute poisoning incidents used to be reported with grain cargoes if the gas escaped into living or working areas of the ship.[172] If the cargo is too dry, the gas is liberated after the hold is opened when the phosphide pellets come into contact with moist air: workers in the mill processing of the discharged cargo can then be affected.

Initial symptoms of exposure to low concentrations of the phosphine include headache, weakness, fainting, pain in the chest, cough, chest tightness and difficulty in breathing. With prolonged exposure, nausea, vomiting and diarrhoea may occur. The main hazard is pulmonary oedema which usually occurs within 24 hours, but may be delayed for up to two days. Central nervous system signs and symptoms, progressing to convulsions, coma and death, have been reported; so too, have gastrointestinal symptoms such as nausea, vomiting, diarrhoea and severe epigastric pain.[171] Unlike arsine, phosphine does not cause haemolysis, but a case of purpura ascribed to phosphine poisoning is known.[169] However, some sources of exposure to phosphine may also lead to exposure to arsine whose haemolytic effects should therefore be sought. Chronic poisoning does not appear to have been recorded.

The reported maximum concentration that can be tolerated for several hours is 7 ppm. A level of 2000 ppm is regarded as rapidly fatal and the maximum exposure that can be tolerated for 30–60 minutes without serious effects is 100–200 ppm. Recovery from phosphine poisoning is usually complete.[171]

The evidence for genotoxic effects of phosphine in humans is inconclusive.[173]

METHYL BROMIDE (BROMOMETHANE) (CH₃Br)

[CAS No. 74-83-9]
Exposure limits:
   LTEL (8-h TWA) 5 ppm (20 mg/m^3)
   STEL (15 min) 15 ppm (59 mg/m^3)
Relative density: 3.36
Flammability limits: 10–16 per cent (but practically non-flammable)

Methyl bromide (bromomethane) is a colourless, odourless and relatively insoluble gas, but it is said to have a faintly detectable sweet odour at high concentrations. The gas has been widely used as a fumigant, but it is being phased out. It is highly toxic against mammals, insects, mites and pathogenic organisms in soil and compost.[174] Thus, it has been used to fumigate soil in compost under gas-proof sheets; fruit in ships' holds or freight containers; and in aircraft and special fumigation chambers. Fire extinguishers containing methyl bromide are no longer manufactured.

Methyl bromide is the most abundant gaseous bromine species in the atmosphere, being emitted from a wide range of natural as well as industrial sources. Atom for atom, bromine is about 50 times more effective than chlorine in destroying stratospheric ozone, and hence countries are moving to cease production and importation of methyl bromide, although it is proving difficult to find substitutes for some specialized applications.

Sporadic cases of acute poisoning may still occur but, because of its severe toxicity and low warning properties, only qualified operators are normally permitted to undertake fumigant work with this gas and they are well versed in the dangers and protective measures.

Occupational exposure is by inhalation or skin absorption. Although the hazards are well known, serious exposure incidents continue to occur due to lapses in the standard protective measures laid down for working with this gas. At low but dangerous concentrations, it has no irritating effects, thus dangerous exposure may occur without adequate warning, with onset of symptoms usually delayed from 30 minutes up to 48 hours later. Symptoms of mild exposure can come on within a few hours and include headache, eye and nose irritation, cough, nausea and malaise. At high exposures, the gas typically causes injury to the central nervous system as well as the lungs, producing headache, nausea, vomiting, pulmonary oedema (up to 30 hours after exposure), tremors and convulsions followed by coma; the convulsions may not respond to standard anticonvulsant therapy. Health effects may also arise from chronic exposure to lesser concentrations, resulting in nervous system involvement with manifestations such as numbness (especially of the feet), visual disturbance (including optic atrophy), mental confusion, psychiatric disturbances and tremor.[174]

Exposure above 25 ppm is dangerous and acute central nervous system symptoms with possible permanent effects on the vision, hearing and balance are reported to occur above 120 ppm. Concentrations greater than 250 ppm are associated with pulmonary oedema, coma and convulsions. Exposure of the skin to high concentrations of vapour or liquid produces erythema with blister formation and severe burns, particularly if the gas or liquid is trapped under clothing. Blisters are usually large and surrounded by areas of redness and swelling; they may take a long time to heal. Severe inflammation of the eyes induced by the vapour may lead to conjunctivitis and temporary blindness.

First-aiders must not use mouth-to-mouth resuscitation. Treatment of acute poisoning should concentrate on controlling the convulsions and, if there is no response to drug therapy, muscular paralysis and positive pressure ventilation should be considered early on. The toxic mechanism is unknown and no specific antidotes are recognized, but the administration of dimercaprol and glutathione have been suggested.[174–176]

Regular users of methyl bromide should notify the local hospital of the hazard and appropriate treatment measures. Biological monitoring should be undertaken by measuring serum bromide levels. According to the UK Health and Safety Executive, a level of serum bromide of 0.18 mmol/L (1.45 mg/dL) or more suggests occupational exposure, and above 0.35 mmol/L (2.8 mg/dL, equivalent to a concentration of 28 ppm methyl bromide in air) symptoms may arise, but dietary intake of bromide should also be excluded as a cause of increased levels.[177] The toxic symptoms of methyl bromide are not directly related to the levels of circulating bromide and so the results must be interpreted with caution.

Methyl bromide is a methylating agent and is mutagenic in short-term tests, but it is not carcinogenic in rodents.[178]

Poisoning by methyl bromide is a prescribed disease.

METHYL CHLORIDE (CHLOROMETHANE) (CH₃Cl)

[CAS No. 74-87-3]
Exposure limits:
   LTEL (8-h TWA) 50 ppm (105 mg/m^3)
   STEL (15 min) 100 ppm (210 mg/m^3)
Relative density: 1.78
Flammability limits: 10.7–17.4 per cent

Methyl chloride is a colourless, flammable and sweet-smelling gas which is widely used in the chemical industry, for example to produce methyl silicone polymers and resins, as a methylating agent in the production of butyl rubber and tetramethyl lead and as a blowing agent for polystyrene foams. The gas is a natural source of chlorine in the atmosphere, being released from the oceans and biomass burning.

The effects of methyl chloride and methyl iodide are similar to methyl bromide in that their primary target organs are the brain, liver, kidneys and lungs. All three are mutagens and potential carcinogens, and methyl chloride is a suspect occupational teratogen. However, the evidence for carcinogenicity or teratogenicity in humans is inadequate.

Because methyl chloride is almost odourless, hazardous levels of exposure may occur with little warning. In mild poisoning, there is a staggering gait, dizziness, headaches, nausea and vomiting resembling acute alcoholism, followed by recovery. In more severe poisoning, symptoms and signs include vertigo, confusion, drowsiness, seizures, ataxia and diplopia; these effects may last for weeks and even months or lead on to coma and death.

METHYL ISOCYANATE (NCOCH$_3$)

[CAS No. 624-83-9]
Exposure limits: as NCO
    LTEL (8-h TWA) 0.02 mg/m^3
    STEL (15 min) 0.07 mg/m^3
Relative density: 2

Methyl isocyanate is not a widely used chemical, but it gained worldwide notoriety after its disastrous release from the Union Carbide pesticide plant in Bhopal in India in 1984.[179] It was being used in the chemical synthesis of carbaryl pesticides, and had been stored in liquid form in two steel tanks. The cause of the incident is still not known, but at 00:30 on December 3, 1984 an exothermic reaction took place in one of the storage tanks, resulting in the escape over a few hours of 40 tonnes of methyl isocyanate. A dense cloud of methyl isocyanate flowed over an area of the city about 40 km^2 at a time when there was a temperature inversion and a light wind. It is considered that more than 10 000 people were killed and hundreds of thousands injured in the disaster.

Respiratory involvement was the most common serious health problem, with many victims suffering breathlessness, cough, throat irritation or choking, chest pain and haemoptysis. Death was mostly from bronchial necrosis or pulmonary oedema. Eye reactions were also prominent, and included severe watering, photophobia, lid oedema and corneal ulceration.

A follow-up study of survivors after three years reported an increased risk of eye infections and hyper-responsive phenomena, possibly related to immune disturbance.[180] A cross-sectional survey conducted ten years after the gas leak suggested that many survivors had symptoms commensurate with persistent small airways obstruction and with obliterative bronchiolitis.[181]

There was scarcely any toxicological information available on the effects of methyl isocyanate in humans at the time of the incident. Unfortunately, follow-up studies of the survivors have been too few to adequately document the potential long-term pulmonary changes, as well as the adverse effects to other organs, including teratogenicity.

ETHYLENE OXIDE (CH$_2$CH$_2$O)

[CAS No. 75-21-8]
Exposure limit:
    LTEL (8-h TWA) 5 ppm (9.2 mg/m^3)
Relative density: 1.49
Flammability limits in air: 3.0–80 per cent (vol.)

The main use of ethylene oxide is as a chemical intermediate in the production of ethylene glycol, polyester fibres and detergents, but it has been used on a much smaller scale since the 1950s as a sterilizing agent for medical supplies and foodstuffs. Most hospital gas sterilizers are automatic general purpose sterilizers and many of these use ethylene oxide, the gas being mixed with dichlorodifluoromethane to reduce the flammability and explosion risk. Exposures in hospitals and production facilities in Europe and North America are today generally well controlled using exhaust systems, and air levels should be routinely monitored using sensor and alarm systems. The odour detection level is at least 500 ppm and is therefore of no value in warning the worker of significant exposure.[182]

Ethylene oxide is a narcotic and depresses the central nervous system, as well as being a primary irritant of the respiratory tract. Acute exposure to high concentrations leads to nausea, vomiting and headache; also reported are excitement, muscular weakness, sleeplessness and diarrhoea. Four men were exposed to an intermittently leaking sterilizer (around 500 ppm) for between two and eight weeks, and three developed a reversible peripheral neuropathy, and one reversible acute encephalopathy. Irreversible neuropathy and encephalopathy have been described in other operators of leaking sterilizers at similar levels of intermittent exposure.[182]

The gas condenses to a liquid at 10°C and is infinitely soluble in water. Excessive exposure to the vapour causes irritation of the eyes, while contact of the skin with even dilute solutions may cause erythema, oedema, blistering and necrosis. Allergic contact dermatitis has also been reported.

Ethylene oxide is considered to have potential for causing cancer and adverse reproductive effects in humans. It is a highly reactive epoxide and a direct alkylating agent, as well as being a recognized animal carcinogen associated with leukaemia and brain cancer in rodents. Chromosome aberrations and sister chromatid exchange have been found in studies of exposed workers. Epidemiological studies have not equivocally demonstrated an association with human cancer, in particular of the haemopoietic system, but it is viewed as a human carcinogen by the International Agency for Research on Cancer (IARC).[183,184]

Medical surveillance of exposed workers using complete blood count and differential was recommended in the United States (lymphocytosis had been reported in symptomatically exposed workers), but no longer. Ethylene oxide is a potent sensitizing agent: occupational asthma associated with measurable IgE antibodies to ethylene oxide used to sterilize latex gloves and adsorbed on to the glove powder has been reported in a healthcare worker.[185]

HEXAFLUOROACETONE (F_3CCOCF_3)

[CAS No. 684-16-2]
Exposure limit:
   LTEL (8-h TWA) 0.1 ppm (ACGIH)
Relative density: 5.7

Hexafluoroacetone is colourless, non-flammable, fumes in moist air, and has a stale smell. It is very reactive and is used to prepare a variety of chemicals.

It is irritating to mucous membranes and especially to the lung. Chronic exposure has been shown to lead to cumulative effects in the testes, kidney and bone marrow of experimental animals. It is teratogenic in rats.

DIBORANE (B_2H_6)

[CAS No. 19287-45-7]
Exposure limit:
   LTEL (8-h TWA) 0.1 ppm (0.12 mg/m^3)
Relative density: 0.96
Flammability limits in air: 0.9–98.0 per cent

As well as a doping agent for semiconductor manufacture, diborane has uses in organic syntheses and in rocket fuel. It is a colourless gas with a sickly sweet odour. The ability to detect the odour is rapidly lost with exposure. It is spontaneously flammable in air, but because its ignition temperature (40–50°C) is above room temperature it may remain for several days in air at room temperature without igniting. Diborane is used as a dopant gas, a catalyst in polymer manufacture, and as a rubber vulcanizer. It is hydrolysed to boric acid in the moisture of the respiratory tract and exposure can cause dizziness, headache, drowsiness, chest tightness, cough and nausea. Severe poisoning with boranes is marked by convulsions and pulmonary oedema. The gas is also irritant to the eyes and skin and should be treated with the same respect as phosgene or chlorine.

The other boron hydrides are pentaborane and decaborane. These are more toxic than diborane and they can be readily absorbed through the skin and conjunctivae, as well as by inhalation. Boranes are neurotoxic.

NICKEL CARBONYL (TETRACARBONYLNICKEL) ($Ni(CO)_4$)

[CAS No. 13463-39-3]
Exposure limit: as nickel
   LTEL (10 min) 0.1 mg/m^3
Relative density: at 50°C, 5.95
Lower flammability limit in air: 2 per cent (vol.)

Nickel carbonyl is actually a liquid with a boiling point at 43°C, but its vapour is highly toxic. It has a 'brick dust' odour detectable at 1–3 ppm. Nickel carbonyl is prepared by passing carbon monoxide over finely divided nickel. In the Mond process, the gas is used to isolate nickel from its ore. The effects of occupational exposure to nickel carbonyl have only been documented in workers engaged in the Mond process which has also been associated with an elevated incidence of carcinoma of the nasal cavities, lung and pharynx.

Acute inhalation effects of nickel carbonyl fall into two categories, immediate and delayed. The immediate response includes headache, dizziness, nausea, vomiting and dyspnoea, which may resolve within a day in mild cases on removal from exposure. The worker should be kept under observation or admitted to hospital because symptoms of pulmonary oedema may arise 12–120 hours after exposure. The patient becomes febrile and cyanosed with a rapid pulse and develops a leukocytosis. Delirium may precede other central nervous system changes, such as cerebral oedema. Death may follow in 4–11 days after exposure. Exposure to 30 ppm for 30 minutes is said to be potentially lethal in humans.

Nickel carbonyl is rapidly absorbed by the lungs and nickel levels rise in the blood and urine soon after exposure. Measurement of nickel in the blood and urine is an important guide for diagnosis and management. In severe cases, therapy with chelating agents to remove nickel from the body is recommended (e.g. disulfuram), as well as treatment with oxygen and corticosteroids. Concomitant poisoning by carbon monoxide from the Mond process should be excluded by measuring carboxyhaemoglobin.[186]

Poisoning by nickel carbonyl is a prescribed disease.

GASES WITH MAINLY ANAESTHETIC ACTION: GENERAL ANAESTHETICS

The inhalational anaesthetics consist of gases and volatile liquids. The first deliberate use of an inhaled gas to produce anaesthesia for the performance of surgical operations was in animals, being carried out by Henry Hill Hickman in 1823 using carbon dioxide, but his work went unrecognized by medical opinion at the time. (Later in the century, carbon dioxide was tried out on humans, but was found to be unsuitable as it induced convulsions at anaesthetic concentrations.) The first general anaesthetic to be used in surgery was diethyl ether in 1846 by William Morton in the Massachusetts General Hospital and later that year in a leg amputation performed by Robert Liston at University College Hospital, London. This agent was subsequently replaced by chloroform as the most widely used inhalational agent following its introduction by Sir James Simpson and John Snow in 1847. Snow was later to achieve fame in public health when he ordered the removal of the Broad Street pump handle in the cholera epidemic of 1854. Joseph Priestley discovered nitrous oxide in 1772 and in 1800 Humphrey Davy had proposed the use of the gas as an anaesthetic: surprisingly, it was not adopted until much later. Cyclopropane was popular for induction anaesthesia in children until the 1980s.

As for volatile agents, trichloroethylene later became popular in obstetrics, but it has now been discontinued in the United States and in the United Kingdom. Since 1956, the CFC halothane ($CF_3CHClBr$) has been one of the most popular agents. Isoflurane has been used since 1971 and, because about 2 per cent of the gas inhaled is biotransformed compared with 18 per cent of halothane, it is considered safer for patients. Other agents in use are enflurane and the newer agents, desflurane and sevoflurane. Fluorinated anaesthetics undergo metabolic breakdown in the liver to inorganic fluoride with potential for nephrotoxicity, but this is not a consideration for the occupational exposure of anaesthetists. Airway irritation may occur in patients with halogenated anaesthetics particularly when used for inhalation induction of anaesthesia.

Most concern over the health effects of anaesthetic gases has centred on the hazard to the reproductive system in anaesthetists and operating theatre staff. This was first highlighted in 1968 in a report describing a marked increase in spontaneous abortions among a group of female anaesthetists in the former USSR. The combined results of subsequent epidemiological studies in Denmark, the United States and the United Kingdom seemed at first to confirm this finding and in addition raised the possible risk of congenital abnormalities in pregnant women and in the offspring of male anaesthetists. In 1976, the UK Department of Health released a circular advising the use of scavenging systems in operating theatres. By 1980, the considered opinion was that spontaneous abortions in operating room staff were likely to be linked with exposure to inhalational agents. However, in the mid-1980s detailed evaluation of the evidence available then did not show support for any of the risks raised.[187,188] The current prudent view is that exposure to anaesthetic gases should be kept to a minimum and active or passive scavenging should be incorporated into operating theatre design (Figure 39.11). A meta-analysis of the epidemiological studies based on data in the pre-scavenging era indicated an increased risk of spontaneous abortion.[189] Some of the earlier reports of adverse reproductive outcome may have been related to much higher exposures than occur today. Even now, high levels of nitrous oxide can be achieved in poorly ventilated delivery rooms where a mixture of half nitrous oxide and half oxygen (Entonox, BOC Gases) is used for analgesia. These high levels could impair mood and cognitive functions in staff, but in a study of more typical average time-weighted exposure levels (nitrous oxide 58 ppm and halothane 1.4 ppm average) no changes were found.[190] However, high levels of nitrous oxide may impair fertility in female staff.[191]

Suspicion that the health of anaesthetists is poorer than other medical specialists keeps recurring and studies have suggested a higher risk of suicide, lymphomas and reticuloendothelial tumours, as well as an increased rate of early retirement on grounds of ill health.[192] A mortality study of British anaesthetists found a doubling of deaths from suicide compared with other men in social class 1, but the rate was not significantly different from that among doctors as a whole.[192] It may be speculated that adverse health effects could be related to job factors, such as sustained mental stress, long hours or inadequate time to rest and eat.

Occupational hygiene studies in the UK showed that the geometric mean time-weighted average exposure to nitrous oxide among anaesthetists is 94 ppm in unscavenged theatres compared with 32 ppm in scavenged theatres, the corresponding means for halothane being 1.7 ppm and 0.7 ppm. Active scavenging systems are much more effective than passive ones.[193] A further study by the Health and Safety Executive in 14 veterinary practices showed similar results, although the duration of exposure of veterinarians and nurses was shorter than in hospital operating room

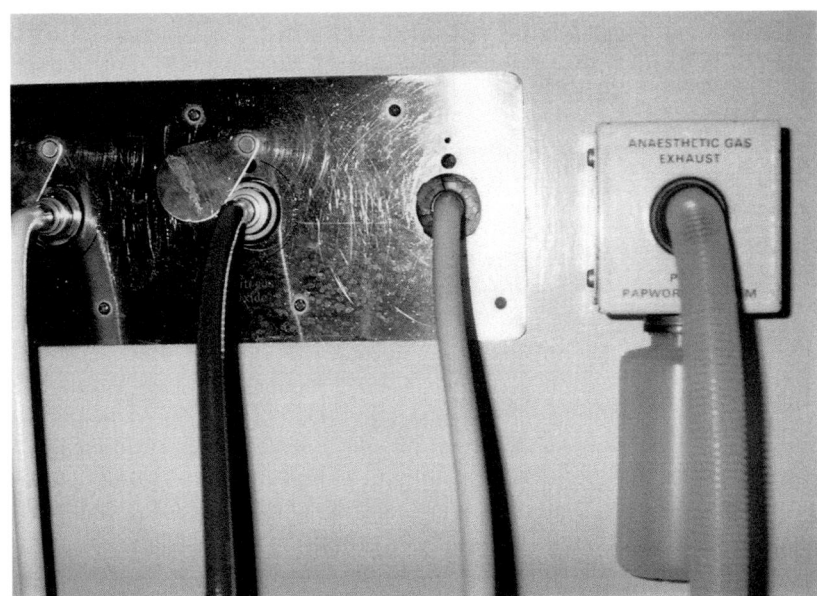

Figure 39.11 Wall gas connections for operating theatre anaesthetic gas machine showing scavenging outlet.

staff; halothane is the most common inhalational agent used in veterinary practice.[194] Dental practices may also operate with inhalational agents for only a few hours a week. A high level of efficient forced general ventilation is important for reducing exposure levels by removing contaminants not handled by scavenging. Leakages readily occur from mask use, and intubation is to be preferred whenever it is clinically feasible.

Occupational exposure standards for anaesthetic gases were introduced in the UK in 1996, and these are equally applicable to manufacturing facilities, as well as hospitals.[195] These are (8-h TWA): halothane 10 ppm (82 mg/m^3), enflurane 50 ppm (383 mg/m^3) and isoflurane 50 ppm (383 mg/m^3). As anaesthetic gases are toxic agents, they all call for consideration under the Control of Substances Hazardous to Health Regulations. In hospitals, compliance with the occupational exposure standards is achievable through balanced supply and extract ventilation with high rates of air change in, for example, delivery rooms and recovery areas, as well as by the use of gas scavenging equipment in operating theatres.

NITROUS OXIDE (N_2O)

[CAS No. 10024-97-2]
Exposure limit:
  LTEL (8-h TWA) 100 ppm (183 mg/m^3)
Relative density: 1.5

Nitrous oxide is a stable, toxic gas which has been shown experimentally to interfere with DNA synthesis by inactivating vitamin B_{12}, a coenzyme for methionine synthase activity. It is normally used for short periods, as in intensive care, because it may cause megaloblastic changes in the bone marrow if exposure goes on for longer than 24 hours. Excessive occupational exposure to the gas in dentists has been reported to cause measurable bone marrow changes from depression of vitamin B_{12} activity.[196] Agranulocytosis and subacute combined degeneration of the spinal cord have also occurred after repeated exposure in patients. Experimental studies of nitrous oxide in animals indicate that at subanaesthetic levels it may reduce fetal weight and growth, but there is no evidence of teratogenicity or mutagenicity. However, a study of female dental assistants suggested that exposure to high levels of unscavenged nitrous oxide may impair fertility as measured by an increased time before conception.[191] Nitrous oxide neuropathy has been reported in abusers of the gas. Abusers may develop addictive behaviour, tolerance and psychological dependence, and anaesthetists are an at-risk group because of their access to the gas. Deaths have occurred in healthcare workers who have tried to obtain a 'high' without using supplementary oxygen. (Nitrous oxide abuse has also been reported in the restaurant trade where it is used in power-whipped cream dispensers and as a non-tainting foaming agent for dairy products.) Overall, there is no convincing evidence that exposure to nitrous oxide in the workplace has caused developmental defects in the fetus or any other reproductive health effects, but this lack of evidence should not foster complacency in its usage.

Other common anaesthetically active gases

ACETYLENE (ETHYNE) (C_2H_2)

[CAS No. 74-86-2]
Exposure limit: not established
Relative density: 0.9

Acetylene is a colourless, highly flammable gas. It is regarded as a simple asphyxiant, but marked intoxication will occur at 20 per cent mixture in air. Very pure acetylene has a pleasant sweet smell, but commercial acetylene smells of garlic. It burns at a very high temperature with oxygen, up to approximately 3500°C.

Acetylene is used in the manufacture of many organic chemicals and polymers. Its fierce flame is used for oxyacetylene cutting and welding and wherever there is an application for great heat.

CYCLOPROPANE (C_3H_6)

[CAS No. 79-19-4]
Exposure limit: 400 ppm (ACGIH)
Relative density: 1.4

Cyclopropane is colourless, flammable and smells like ether. It is used for chemical synthesis and was popular as a general anaesthetic, mainly in children.

DIMETHYL ETHER (CH_3OCH_3)

[CAS No. 115-10-6]
Exposure limits:
  LTEL (8-h TWA) 400 ppm (766 mg/m^3)
  STEL (15 min) 500 ppm (958 mg/m^3)
Relative density: 1.6

Dimethyl ether is colourless, flammable and is used as a refrigerant and as a fuel gas in welding. It has a lesser anaesthetic action than diethyl ether.

METHYL VINYL ETHER ($CH_3OCH:CH_2$)

[CAS No. 109-92-2]
Exposure limit: not established
Relative density: 2.0

The principal physiological effect of this gas is its anaesthetic action, but it is much less than that produced by dimethyl ether.

2,2-DIMETHYL PROPANE $C(CH_3)_4$

[CAS No. 463-82-1]
Exposure limit: not established
Relative density: 2.5

2,2-Dimethyl propane is a colourless, flammable gas. It is used in the manufacture of synthetic rubber.

ETHANE (CH_3CH_3)

[CAS No. 74-84-0]
Exposure limit: not established
Relative density: 1.0

Ethane is colourless, odourless and flammable. It is regarded as a simple asphyxiant, and is used as a low temperature refrigerant and an anti-knock agent.

ETHYL CHLORIDE (CHLOROETHANE) (C_2H_5Cl)

[CAS No. 75-00-3]
Exposure limits:
    LTEL (8-h TWA) 50 ppm (124 mg/m^3)
Relative density: (gas) 2.2

Ethyl chloride is colourless and flammable, with an ethereal odour. It is used as a refrigerant, a local spray anaesthetic and as a specialized solvent. At 40 000 ppm (4 per cent) it produces stupor and eye irritation almost at once.

ETHYLENE (CH_2CH_2)

[CAS No. 74-85-1]
Exposure limit: not established
Relative density: 0.98

Ethylene is a colourless, flammable and sweet-smelling gas which is regarded as a simple asphyxiant. It is used in horticulture for ripening fruit and increasing plant growth rates, and in specialized welding. It is an important feedstock in the production of ethylene oxide and many polymers.

ISOBUTANE ($CH(CH_3)_3$)

[CAS No. 75-28-7]
Exposure limit: not established
Relative density: 2.1

Isobutane is the simplest isoalkane. It is a colourless, flammable gas which is mainly used as an intermediate in the production of aviation fuel and various organic chemicals.

ISOBUTYLENE (($CH_3)_2CCH_2$)

[CAS No. 75-28-5]
Exposure limit: not established
Relative density: 1.9

Isobutylene is a colourless, flammable gas used in the manufacture of butyl rubber.

Liquefied petroleum gases

N-BUTANE ($CH_3CH_2CH_2CH_3$)

[CAS No. 106-97-8]
Exposure limits:
    LTEL (8-h TWA) 600 ppm (1450 mg/m^3)
    STEL (15 min) 750 ppm (1810 mg/m^3)
Relative density: 2.1
Flammability limits: 1.8–8.4 per cent (vol.)

Butane is a colourless, flammable gas with a mild aromatic odour, widely used in the petrochemical industry and as a fuel.

PROPANE ($CH_3CH_2CH_3$)

[CAS No. 744-98-6]
Exposure limit: not established
Relative density: 1.5
Flammability limits: 2.2–9.5 per cent (vol.)

Propane is colourless and flammable. It is widely used as a fuel gas, in welding, as a solvent and as a refrigerant.

PROPYLENE (CH_3CHCH_2)

[CAS No. 115-07-1]
Exposure limit: not established
Relative density: 1.5
Flammability limits: 2.0–11.1 per cent (vol.)

Propylene is a colourless, flammable gas. It is a widely used chemical feedstock. On July 11, 1978 a road tanker carrying liquefied petroleum gas ran into the Los Alfaques camping ground on the east coast of Spain and overturned, with the fuel that remained in liquid form flowing over the campsite. Ignition of the fuel soon occurred forming an open flammable cloud fire. One hundred and two people died on the site, and there were 148 casualties with burns, at least 122 of whom were severe, requiring urgent hospital treatment.

VINYL BROMIDE (CH_2CHBr)

[CAS No. 693-60-2]
Exposure limit: not available.
Relative density: 3.79
Flammability limits: 9–14 per cent (vol.)

Vinyl bromide is a colourless, flammable gas with a pleasant smell. It is a chemical intermediate, a flame retardant and is used to manufacture acrylic fibres. Easily polymerized, it is used as a fire retardant in plastics. It behaves like an anaesthetic gas, inhalation of very high concentrations leading to coma and death. Liquid splashes are irritant to the eyes and skin. The gas is mutagenic and induces liver angiosarcoma and hepatocellular carcinoma in laboratory animals exposed through inhalation; it is regarded as 'probably carcinogenic to humans' by the IARC.

VINYL CHLORIDE (CH$_2$CHCl)

[CAS No. 75-01-4]
Maximum exposure limits:
  LTEL (8-h TWA) 3 ppm (7.8 mg/m^3)
Relative density: 2.21
Flammability limits: 4–22 per cent (vol.)

The main use of vinyl chloride monomer (VCM) is to manufacture PVC, the most widely used plastic polymer. Production took off after the Second World War. Polymerization is a batch process undertaken in autoclaves. In the past, workers entered the autoclaves after each batch to clean them from inside; unfortunately, VCM was regarded as very safe and many workers failed to use adequate respiratory protection. As a result, very high levels of exposure to VCM occurred until 1974, when the first human cases of angiosarcoma of the liver were reported in these heavily exposed workers.

Health problems associated with these high exposures had begun to be recognized in the mid-1960s. Acro-osteolysis typically affected the terminal phalanges of the hands, giving rise to 'pseudo-clubbing', with clinical and radiological appearances which resemble those seen in some patients with hyperparathyroidism. Other bones could also be affected by osteolysis. Scleroderma and Raynaud's phenomenon were also reported. These three conditions are now considered to be able to arise independently of one another with VCM exposure.

Animal studies were undertaken to reproduce osteolysis experimentally and these unexpectedly led to the discovery that VCM caused angiosarcoma of the liver, with the first report of the tumour in VCM workers emerging from the United States in 1974. Since then, many cases associated with the industry have been reported worldwide. Angiosarcoma of the liver is an extremely rare tumour in the general population,[197] but sporadic cases without obvious causal factors arise in all age groups. Almost all of the occupational tumours have been reported in highly exposed VCM autoclave workers, although many other chemical workers had some contact with VCM before its dangers were known and its usage came under strict control (in 1974 in the United Kingdom and the United States). Hepatic injury from this chemical also produces non-cirrhotic periportal fibrosis and portal hypertension. Workers exposed in the PVC manufacturing industry before 1974 are at potential risk of manifesting these problems.

The adverse effects of VCM are unlikely to be seen arising from present-day working conditions in the United Kingdom and the United States, but an increasing number of workers worldwide are exposed to VCM, many of whom live in countries where exposure is less strictly regulated. Chemical firms should ensure that general practitioners retain a history of exposure to VCM in the individual's medical record, in case they develop symptoms that could be referable to VCM exposure. There are, however, no valid routine screening tests of use in the early detection of angiosarcoma of the liver or periportal fibrosis, including special imaging. There is presently insufficient evidence to implicate VCM exposure in humans as a causal factor in primary cancers at other sites such as lung and brain.

In the United Kingdom, angiosarcoma of the liver (but not hepatocellular carcinoma), osteolysis, VCM-related Raynaud's phenomenon and VCM-related scleroderma are all independently prescribed diseases.

Heating plastic packaging film will form thermal degradation products which may be associated with symptoms known as 'meat wrappers' asthma'. All heated plastics will generate carbon monoxide, but PVC also gives off hydrogen chloride and plasticizers such as di-octyl phthalate and di-octyl adipate. The polyolefin plastics (polyethylene and polypropylene) can produce formaldehyde and acrolein. The degradation products are normally quickly dispersed and diluted, but attention needs to be paid to the correct operation of manual heating sealing machines to ensure temperature regulation, and the cleanliness and maintenance of the sealing head. Inhalation incidents have been reported in PVC film manufacture if the film is accidentally overheated.

VINYL FLUORIDE (CH$_2$CHF)

[CAS No. 75-02-5]

Vinyl fluoride, a chemical intermediate, is regarded as 'probably carcinogenic in humans' by the IARC.

GEOTHERMAL POWER

The possibility of using hydrothermal energy to produce heat and electricity arises in parts of the world where there is active volcanism or where magma (liquid rock) lying close to the Earth's surface forms shallow bodies of hot rocks and fluids (Figure 39.12). The world's first geothermal steam field was built at Larderello, Italy, in 1904 and today the world's largest, the Geysers, California, produces nearly 2000 megawatts of electricity. In Reykjavik, Iceland, all the hot water needs of the city are provided by geothermal sources.

The occupational and environmental problems of utilizing geothermal power must be assessed separately in different parts of the world as the technology needed to generate electricity from steam turbines using geothermal energy and the toxic compounds arising in geothermal fluids may vary widely.[198] In the steam fields in Utah and California, hydrogen sulphide, ammonia, carbon dioxide, methane and radon-222 are the chief gases emitted. Of these, hydrogen sulphide is the most important, but in fields elsewhere in the world it may be only a minor component. Leaks from geothermal steam wells may expose workers to gases and toxic compounds, such as mercury, arsenic, boron, selenium, lead, cadmium and fluoride. Steam leaving turbines is passed through a condenser and it is the 'non-condensable' gases and toxic compounds that

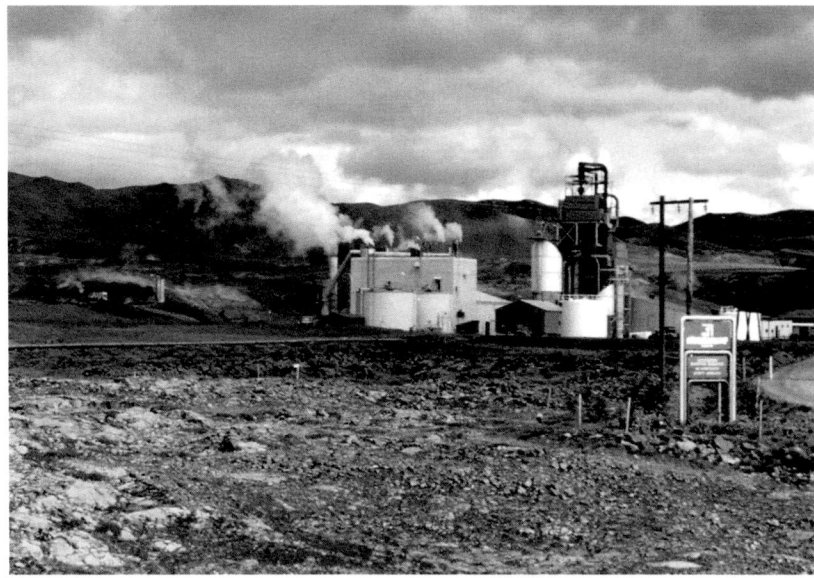

Figure 39.12 The Icelandic Diatomite Plant at Lake Myvatn uses geothermal steam to dry algal deposits dredged from the lake bottom, and power is fed directly from the nearby Krafla geothermal power plant. Elsewhere in the world, diatomaceous earth (kieselguhr) is obtained by open-cast mining.

will enter cooling towers and a proportion of these will escape into the air (Figure 39.13). The drift from the cooling tower may waft around and be deposited in the vicinity. Workers may also be exposed to hazardous gases and entrained substances from leaks inside the plant or by working on or near drilling rigs. Carbon dioxide may pose a risk of asphyxiation in confined spaces, and accidental blow-outs of wells can occur.

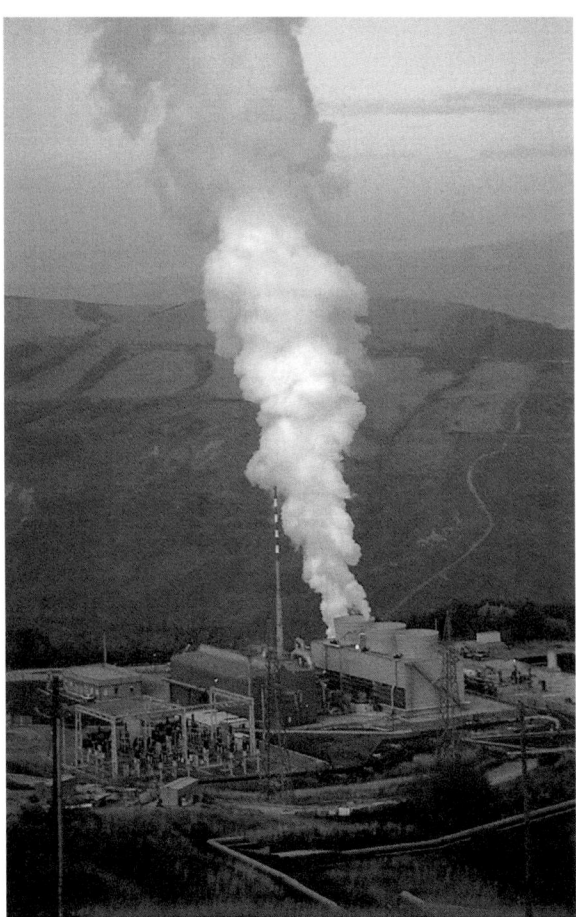

Figure 39.13 Steam venting from a geothermal power plant in Tuscany, Italy. Mount Amiata is an extinct volcano where mercury ore was mined until 1980.

Key points

- Inhalation incidents involving gases are still common in industry in all countries.
- Chlorine remains the most common gas stored under pressure and is the most frequent gas cited in major toxic hazard planning.
- Gases, such as carbon monoxide, hydrogen sulphide and nitrogen dioxide can present as occupational hazards in a wide range of settings and a high degree of vigilance is needed.
- Anaesthetic gases are potential health hazards if exposure to healthcare workers is not adequately controlled.
- Workers in emerging economies may still be exposed to the carcinogenic hazards of gases, such as vinyl chloride, and the risk of explosion disasters from the build up of flammable gases in deep mines.

REFERENCES

1. Sallie B, McDonald C. Inhalation accidents reported to the SWORD Surveillance Project 1990-1993. *Annals of Occupational Hygiene.* 1996; **40**: 211-21.
2. McDonald JC, Chen Y, Zekveld C, Cherry NM. Incidence by occupation and industry of acute work related respiratory diseases in the UK, 1992-2001. *Occupational and Environmental Medicine.* 2005; **62**: 836-42.
3. Organization for Economic Co-operation and Development. OECD Monograph No. 81. Health aspects of chemical accidents. Paris: OECD, 1994.
4. Caplin M. Ammonia-gas poisoning. Forty-seven cases in a London shelter. *Lancet.* 1941; **ii**: 95-6.
5. Henderson Y, Haggard HW. *Noxious gases*, 2nd edn. New York: Reinhold, 1943.
6. Wiegand A, Attin T. Occupational dental erosion from exposure to acids - a review. *Occupational Medicine.* 2007; **57**: 169-76.
7. Health and Safety Executive. EH40/2005 (as consolidated with amendments October 2007). List of approved workplace exposure limits. Last accessed May 2010. Available from: www.hse.gov.uk/coshh/table1.pdf.
8. World Health Organization. Air quality guidelines for Europe, 2nd edn. Copenhagen: WHO, 2000.
9. Health and Safety Commission. Advisory Committee on Dangerous Substances. Major hazard aspects of the transport of dangerous substances. London: HMSO, 1991.
10. Illing HPA. Assessment of toxicity for major hazards: Some concepts and problems. *Human Toxicology.* 1989; **8**: 369-74.
11. Health and Safety Executive. Assessment of the dangerous toxic load (DTL) for specified level of toxicity (SLOT) and significant likelihood of death (SLOD). Last accessed May 2010. Available from: www.hse.gov.uk/hid/haztox.htm.
12. American Industrial Hygiene Association. The AIHA 2007 emergency response planning guidelines and workplace environmental exposure level handbook. Fairfax: AIHA, 2007.
13. Kinra S, Lewendon G, Nelder R et al. Evacuation decisions in a chemical air pollution incident: Cross-sectional survey. *British Medical Journal.* 2005; **330**: 1471-5.
14. Health and Safety Executive. The control of industrial major accident hazards regulations (CIMAH): Further guidance on emergency plans. London: HMSO, 1985.
15. Baxter PJ, Davies PC, Murray V. Medical planning for toxic releases into the community: The example of chlorine gas. *British Journal of Industrial Medicine.* 1989; **46**: 277-85.
16. Buncefield Major Incident Investigation Board. The Buncefield incident, 11 December 2005, the final report, vols 1 and 2. 2008. Available from: www.buncefieldinvestigation.gov.uk/reports/index.htm.
17. National Research Council. Fire and smoke: Understanding the hazards. Washington DC: National Academy Press, 1986.
18. Purser DA. Toxicity assessment of combustion products. In: *SFPE handbook of fire protection engineering*, 3rd edn. Boston: National Fire Protection Association, 2002: 2.83-2.171.
19. Baxter PJ, Heap BJ, Rowland MGM, Murray VSG. Thetford plastics fire, October 1991: The role of a preventive medical team in chemical incidents. *Occupational and Environmental Medicine.* 1995; **52**: 694-8.
20. Hobbs PV, Radke LF. Airborne studies of the smoke from the Kuwait oil fires. *Science.* 1992; **256**: 987-90.
21. Stern SCM, Kumar R, Roberts IAG. Aplastic anaemia after exposure to burning oil. *Lancet.* 1995; **346**: 183.
22. Kinsella J, Carter R, Reid WH et al. Increased airways reactivity after smoke inhalation. *Lancet.* 1991; **337**: 595-7.
23. Axford AT, McKerrow CB, Jones AP, Le Quesne PM. Accidental exposure to isocyanate fumes of a group of firemen. *British Journal of Industrial Medicine.* 1976; **33**: 65-71.
24. Guidotti TL, Clough VM. Occupational health concerns of firefighting. *Annual Review of Public Health.* 1992; **13**: 151-71.
25. Guidotti TL. Evaluating causality for occupational cancers: The example of firefighters. *Occupational Medicine.* 2007; **57**: 466-71.
26. Howe GR, Burch JD. Fire fighters and risk of cancer: An assessment and overview of the epidemiologic evidence. *American Journal of Epidemiology.* 1990; **132**: 1039-50.
27. Kales SN, Soteriades ES, Christophi CA, Christiani DC. Emergency duties and deaths from heart disease among firefighters in the United States. *New England Journal of Medicine.* 2007; **356**: 1207-15.
28. Landrigan P, Lioy PJ, Thurston G et al. Health and environmental consequences of the World Trade Center disaster. *Environmental Health Perspectives.* 2004; **112**: 731-9.
29. Medvedev ZA. *The legacy of Chernobyl.* London: Blackwell, 1990.
30. Beverstock K, Williams D. The Chernobyl accident 20 years on: An assessment of the health consequences and the international response. *Environmental Health Perspectives.* 2006; **114**: 1312-17.
31. Marrs TC, Maynard RL, Sidell FR. *Chemical warfare agents. Toxicology and treatment.* Chichester: Wiley, 1996.
32. Kales SN, Christiani DC. Acute chemical emergencies. *New England Journal of Medicine.* 2004; **350**: 800-8.
33. Williams AJ. Assessing and interpreting arterial blood gases and acid-base balance. *British Medical Journal.* 1998; **317**: 1213-16.
34. Pritchard JS. Pulmonary oedema. In: Weatherall DJ, Ledingham JGG, Warrell DA (eds). *Oxford textbook of medicine*, 3rd edn. Oxford: Oxford University Press, 1996: 2495-505.
35. Wright JL, Churg A. Diseases caused by gases and fumes. In: Churg A, Green FHY (eds). *Pathology of occupational lung disease*, 2nd edn. Baltimore: Williams and Wilkins, 1998: 57-75.
36. Wheeler AP, Bernard GR. Acute lung injury and the acute respiratory distress syndrome: A clinical review. *Lancet.* 2007; **369**: 1553-65.
37. Brooks SM. Occupational asthma. *Chest.* 1985; **87** (Suppl.): 218-22.

38. Aver RA, Benveniste H. Hypoxia and related conditions. In: Graham DI, Lantos PL (eds). *Greenfield's Neuropathology*, 6th edn. London: Arnold, 1997: 263–314.
39. Haldane JS, Priestley JG. *Respiration*. Oxford: Clarendon Press, 1935.
40. King TS, Elia M, Hunter JO. Abnormal colonic fermentation in irritable bowel syndrome. *Lancet*. 1998; **352**: 1187–9.
41. Cummings J, Pitcher M. Hydrogen sulphide: A bacterial toxin in ulcerative colitis? *Gut*. 1996; **39**: 1–4.
42. Goodman M. *Suffer and survive. The extreme life of Dr JS Haldane*. London: Simon and Schuster, 2007.
43. Smith GD. Commentary: Behind the Broad Street pump: Aetiology, epidemiology and prevention of cholera in mid-19th century Britain. *International Journal of Epidemiology*. 2002; **31**: 920–32.
44. Preller L, Heederik D, Boleij JSM et al. Lung function and chronic respiratory symptoms of pig farmers: Focus on exposure to endotoxins and ammonia and use of disinfectants. *Occupational and Environmental Medicine*. 1995; **52**: 654–60.
45. Health and Safety Executive. Safe work in confined spaces. Confined Spaces Regulations 1997. Approved Code of Practice Regulations and Guidance. Norwich: HMSO, 1997.
46. Watt MK, Watt SJ, Seaton A. Episode of toxic gas exposure in sewer workers. *Occupational and Environmental Medicine*. 1997; **54**: 277–80.
47. Haldane J. The air of mines. In: Oliver T (ed.). *Dangerous trades*. London: John Murray, 1902: 540–56.
48. Boogaard PJ, Houtsma A-T AJ, Journée HL, Van Sittert NJ. Effects of exposure to elemental mercury on the nervous system and the kidneys of workers producing natural gas. *Archives of Environmental Health*. 1996; **51**: 108–14.
49. Sand G. *La petite fadette*. Paris: Garnier Flammarion, 1967.
50. Baxter PJ, Kapila M, Mfonfu D. Lake Nyos disaster, Cameroon, 1986: The medical effects of large scale emission of carbon dioxide? *British Medical Journal*. 1989; **298**: 1437–41.
51. Stupfel M, Le Guern F. Are there biomedical criteria to assess an acute carbon dioxide intoxication by a volcanic emission? *Journal of Volcanology and Geothermal Research*. 1989; **39**: 247–64.
52. Brighten P. A case of industrial carbon dioxide poisoning. *Anaesthesia*. 1976; **31**: 406–9.
53. Farrar CD, Sorey ML, Evans WC. Forest-killing diffuse CO_2 emissions at Mammoth Mountain as a sign of magmatic unrest. *Nature*. 1995; **376**: 675–7.
54. Barberi F, Carapezza M, Ranaldi M, Tarchini L. Gas blowout from shallow boreholes at Fiumicino (Rome): Induced hazard and evidence of deep CO_2 degassing on the Tyrrhenian margin of Central Italy. *Journal of Volcanology and Geothermal Research*. 2007; **165**: 17–31.
55. Norbäck D, Björnsson E, Janson C et al. Asthmatic symptoms and volatile organic compounds, formaldehyde, and carbon dioxide in dwellings. *Occupational and Environmental Medicine*. 1995; **52**: 388–95.
56. Centers for Disease Control. Carbon monoxide poisoning at an indoor ice arena and bingo hall. *Morbidity and Mortality Weekly Report*. 1996; **45**: 265–7.
57. Fawcett TA, Moon RE, Fracica PJ et al. Warehouse workers' headache. Carbon monoxide poisoning from propane-fueled forklifts. *Journal of Occupational Medicine*. 1992; **34**: 12–15.
58. World Health Organization. Carbon monoxide: Environmental Health Criteria, 13. Geneva: WHO, 1979.
59. Forbes WH, Sargent F, Roughton FJW. The rate of carbon monoxide uptake by normal men. *American Journal of Physiology*. 1945; **143**: 594–608.
60. Coburn RF, Forster RE, Kane PB. Considerations of the physiological variables that determine the blood carboxyhaemoglobin concentration in man. *Journal of Clinical Investigation*. 1965; **44**: 1899–910.
61. Illing HPA, Shillaker RO. *Dichloromethane (methylene chloride)*. Toxicity Review 12. Health and Safety Executive. London: HMSO, 1985.
62. Stewart RD, Hake CL. Paint-remover hazard. *Journal of the American Medical Association*. 1976; **235**: 398–401.
63. Barnett K, Wilson JF. Quantification of carboxyhaemoglobin in blood: External quality assessment of techniques. *British Journal of Biomedical Science*. 1998; **55**: 123–6.
64. Ernst A, Zibrak JD. Carbon monoxide poisoning. *New England Journal of Medicine*. 1998; **339**: 1603–8.
65. Thom SR, Taber RL, Mendiguren II et al. Delayed neuropsychologic sequelae after carbon monoxide poisoning: Prevention by treatment with hyperbaric oxygen. *Toxicology*. 1995; **25**: 474–80.
66. Hardy KR, Thom SR. Pathophysiology and treatment of carbon monoxide poisoning. *Clinical Toxicology*. 1994; **32**: 613–29.
67. Choi IS. Delayed neurologic sequelae in carbon monoxide poisoning. *Archives of Neurology*. 1983; **40**: 433–5.
68. Sidney Smith J, Brandon S. Morbidity from acute carbon monoxide poisoning at three-year follow-up. *British Medical Journal*. 1973; **1**: 318–32.
69. Sawada Y, Takahasi M, Ohashi N. Computerised tomography as an indication of long-term outcome after acute carbon monoxide poisoning. *Lancet*. 1980; **i**: 783–4.
70. Vieregge P, Klostermann W, Blüm RG, Borgis KJ. Carbon monoxide poisoning: Clinical, neurophysiological, and brain imaging observations in acute disease and follow-up. *Journal of Neurology*. 1989; **236**: 478–81.
71. De Reuck J, Decoo D, Lemahieu I et al. A positron emission tomography study of patients with acute carbon monoxide poisoning treated by hyperbaric oxygen. *Journal of Neurology*. 1993; **240**: 430–4.
72. Department of the Environment. Expert Panel on Air Quality Standards: Carbon monoxide. London: HMSO, 1994.
73. Allred EN, Bleecker ER, Chaitman BR et al. Short-term effects of carbon monoxide exposure on the exercise performance of subjects with coronary heart disease. *New England Journal of Medicine*. 1989; **321**: 1426–32.

74. Stern FB, Halperin WE, Hornung RW et al. Heart disease mortality among bridge and tunnel officers exposed to carbon monoxide. *American Journal of Epidemiology.* 1988; **128**: 1276-88.
75. Norman CA, Halton DM. Is carbon monoxide a workplace teratogen? A review and evaluation of the literature. *Annals of Occupational Hygiene.* 1990; **34**: 335-47.
76. Peden NR, Taha A, McSorley PD et al. Industrial exposure to hydrogen cyanide. *British Medical Journal.* 1986; **293**: 538.
77. Houeto P, Hoffman JR, Imbert M et al. Relation of blood cyanide to plasma cyanocobalamin concentration after a fixed dose of hydroxocobalamin in cyanide poisoning. *Lancet.* 1995; **346**: 605-8.
78. Cummings TF. The treatment of cyanide poisoning. *Occupational Medicine.* 2004; **54**: 82-5.
79. Blanc P, Hogan M, Mallin K et al. Cyanide intoxication among silver reclaiming workers. *Journal of the American Medical Association.* 1985; **253**: 367-71.
80. El Ghawabi SH, Gaafar MA, El-Saharti AA et al. Chronic cyanide exposure: A clinical, radio isotope and laboratory study. *British Journal of Industrial Medicine.* 1975; **32**: 215-19.
81. Toren K, Blanc PD. The history of pulp and paper bleaching: Respiratory health effects. *Lancet.* 1997; **349**: 1316-18.
82. World Health Organization. Chlorine and hydrogen chloride. Environmental Health Criteria, 21. Geneva: WHO, 1982.
83. Bherer L, Cushman R, Courteau J-P et al. Survey of construction workers repeatedly exposed to chlorine over a 3-6 month period in a pulpmill: II. Follow-up of affected workers by questionnaire, spirometry, and assessment of bronchial responsiveness 18-24 months after exposure ended. *Occupational and Environmental Medicine.* 1994; **51**: 225-8.
84. Wegman D, Eisen EA. Acute irritants, more than a nuisance. *Chest.* 1990; **97**: 773-5.
85. Schwartz DA, Smity DD, Lakshminarayan S. The pulmonary sequelae associated with accidental inhalation of chlorine gas. *Chest.* 1990; **97**: 820-5.
86. Kennedy SM, Enardson DA, Janssen RG, Chan-Yeung M. Lung health consequences of reported accidental chlorine gas exposures among pulpmill workers. *American Review of Respiratory Disease.* 1991; **143**: 74-9.
87. Nieuwenhuijsen M. The chlorine hypothesis: Fact or fiction? *Occupational and Environmental Medicine.* 2007; **64**: 5-6.
88. Massin N, Bohadana AB, Wild P et al. Respiratory symptoms and bronchial responsiveness in lifeguards exposed to nitrogen trichloride in indoor swimming pools. *Occupational and Environmental Medicine.* 1998; **55**: 258-63.
89. Hery M, Gerber JM, Hecht G et al. Exposure to chloramines in a green salad processing plant. *Annals of Occupational Hygiene.* 1998; **42**: 437-51.
90. Centers for Disease Control. Chlorine gas toxicity from mixture of bleach with other cleaning products – California. *Morbidity and Mortality Weekly Report.* 1991; **40**: 619-29.
91. Deschamps D, Soler P, Rosenberg N et al. Persistent asthma after inhalation of a mixture of sodium hypochlorite and hydrochloric acid. *Chest.* 1994; **105**: 1895-6.
92. Pascuzzi TA. Mass casualties from acute inhalation of chloramine gas. *Military Medicine.* 1998; **163**: 102-4.
93. Sim M, Fairley C, McIver J. Drinking water quality: New challenges for an old problem. *Occupational and Environmental Medicine.* 1994; **53**: 649-51.
94. International Programme on Chemical Safety (IPCS). Phosgene. Environmental Health Criteria, 193. Geneva: WHO, 1997.
95. Stevens B, Koenig JQ, Rebolledo V et al. Respiratory effects from the inhalation of hydrogen chloride in young adult asthmatics. *Journal of Occupational Medicine.* 1992; **34**: 923-9.
96. Brimblecombe P. *The big smoke.* London: Routledge, 1987.
97. International Agency for Research on Cancer. Monographs on the Evaluation of Carcinogenic Risks to Humans, 54. Occupational exposures to mists and vapours from strong inorganic acids, and other industrial chemicals. Lyon: IARC, 1992.
98. Stavert DM, Archuleta DC, Behr MJ, Lehnert BE. Relative toxicities of hydrogen fluoride, hydrogen chloride and hydrogen bromide in nose- and pseudo-mouth-breathing rats. *Fundamental and Applied Toxicology.* 1991; **16**: 636-55.
99. Wing JS, Sanderson LM, Brender JD et al. Acute health effects in a community after a release of hydrofluoric acid. *Archives of Environmental Health.* 1991; **46**: 155-60.
100. World Health Organization. Fluorine and fluorides. Environmental Health Criteria, 36. Geneva: WHO, 1984.
101. Turner RM, Fairhurst S. *Toxicology of substances in relation to major hazards: Hydrogen fluoride.* London: HMSO/Health and Safety Executive, 1990.
102. Machle W, Thamann F, Kitzmiller K, Cholak J. The effects of the inhalation of hydrogen fluoride. I. The response following exposure to high concentrations. *Journal of Industrial Hygiene.* 1933; **16**: 129-45.
103. Chela A, Reig R, Sanz P et al. Death due to hydrofluoric acid. *American Journal of Forensic Medicine and Pathology.* 1989; **10**: 47-8.
104. Lund K, Ekstrand J, Boe J et al. Exposure to hydrogen fluoride: An experimental study in humans of concentrations of fluoride in plasma, symptoms, and lung function. *Occupational and Environmental Medicine.* 1997; **54**: 32-7.
105. Largent EJ, Columbus A. The metabolism of fluorides in man. *Archives of Industrial Health.* 1960; **21**: 318-23.
106. Grandjean P. Occupational fluorosis through 50 years: Clinical and epidemiological experiences. *American Journal of Industrial Medicine.* 1982; **3**: 227-36.
107. Dinman B, Elbow D, Bonny MJ et al. A 15 year retrospective study of fluoride excretion and bone radiopacity among aluminium smelter workers – Pt 4. *Journal of Occupational Medicine.* 1976; **18**: 21-5.
108. Abramson MJ, Wlodarczyk JH, Saunders NA, Hensley MJ. Does aluminium smelting cause lung disease? *American Review of Respiratory Disease.* 1989; **139**: 1042-57.

109. Armstrong B, Tremblay C, Baris D, Therault G. Lung cancer mortality and polynuclear aromatic hydrocarbons: A case-cohort study of aluminium production workers in Arvida, Quebec, Canada. *American Journal of Epidemiology*. 1994; **139**: 250–62.
110. Burgess WA. *Recognition of health hazards in industry: A review of materials and processes*, 2nd edn. New York: Wiley, 1995.
111. Søyseth, Boe J, Kongerud J. Relation between decline in FEV_1 and exposure to dust and tobacco smoke in aluminium pot room workers. *Occupational and Environmental Medicine*. 1997; **54**: 27–31.
112. Upfal M, Doyle C. Medical management of hydrofluoric acid exposure. *Journal of Occupational Medicine*. 1990; **32**: 726–31.
113. Tepperman PB. Fatality due to acute systemic fluoride poisoning following a hydrofluoric acid skin burn. *Journal of Occupational Medicine*. 1980; **22**: 691–2.
114. Kraut A, Lilis R. Pulmonary effects of acute exposure to degradation product of sulphur hexafluoride during electrical cable repair work. *British Journal of Industrial Medicine*. 1990; **47**: 829–32.
115. Speizer FE, Wegman DH, Ramirez A. Palpitation rates associated with fluorocarbon exposure in a hospital setting. *New England Journal of Medicine*. 1975; **292**: 624–6.
116. International Programme on Chemical Safety (IPCS). Fully halogenated chlorofluorocarbons. Environmental Health Criteria, 113. Geneva: WHO, 1990.
117. International Programme on Chemical Safety (IPCS). Partially halogenated chlorofluorocarbons (methane derivatives). Environmental Health Criteria, 126. Geneva: WHO, 1991.
118. International Programme on Chemical Safety (IPCS). Partially halogenated chlorofluorocarbons (ethane derivatives). Environmental Health Criteria, 139. Geneva: WHO, 1992.
119. Hoet P, Graf M-LM, Bourd M *et al*. Epidemic of liver disease caused by hydrochlorofluorocarbons used as ozone-sparing substitutes of chlorofluorocarbons. *Lancet*. 1997; **350**: 556–9.
120. Holness DL, House RA. Health effects of halon 1301 exposure. *Journal of Occupational Medicine*. 1992; **34**: 722–5.
121. Charan NB, Myers CG, Lakshminarayan S, Spencer TM. Pulmonary injuries associated with acute sulfur dioxide inhalation. *American Review of Respiratory Disease*. 1979; **119**: 555–60.
122. Eatough DJ, Caka FM, Farber RJ. The conversion of SO_2 to sulfate in the atmosphere. *Israeli Journal of Chemistry*. 1994; **34**: 301–14.
123. Harkonen H, Nordmann H, Korhonen O, Winblad I. Long-term effects of exposure to sulfur dioxide. Lung function four years after a pyrite dust explosion. *American Review of Respiratory Disease*. 1983; **128**: 890–3.
124. Piirila PL, Nordmann H, Korrhonen OS, Winblad I. A thirteen-year follow-up of respiratory effects of acute exposure to sulfur dioxide. *Scandinavian Journal of Work, Environment and Health*. 1996; **22**: 191–6.
125. World Health Organization. Sulfur oxides and suspended particulate matter. Environmental Health Criteria, 8. Geneva: WHO, 1979.
126. Huber AL, Loving TJ. Fatal asthma attack after inhaling sulfur fumes. *Journal of the American Medical Association*. 1991; **266**: 2225.
127. Scobie E, Dabill DW, Groves JA. Chemical pollutants in x-ray film processing departments. *Annals of Occupational Hygiene*. 1996; **40**: 423–35.
128. Department of the Environment. Expert Panel on Air Quality Standards: Sulphur dioxide. London: HMSO, 1995.
129. Enterline PE, Marsh GM, Esmen NA *et al*. Some effects of cigarette smoking, arsenic, and SO_2 on mortality among US copper smelter workers. *Journal of Occupational Medicine*. 1987; **29**: 831–8.
130. Koizumi A, Aoki T, Tsukada M *et al*. Mercury, not sulphur dioxide, poisoning as cause of smelter disease in industrial plants producing sulphuric acid. *Lancet*. 1994; **343**: 1411–12.
131. Turner RM, Fairhurst S. *Toxicology of substances in relation to major hazards. Sulphuric acid mist*. London: HMSO, 1992.
132. Coggan D, Pannett B, Wield G. Upper aerodigestive cancer in battery manufacturers and steel workers exposed to mineral acid mists. *Occupational and Environmental Medicine*. 1996; 53: 445–9.
133. Kitagawa T. Cause analysis of the Yokkaichi asthma episode in Japan. *Journal of the Air Pollution Control Association*. 1984; **34**: 743–6.
134. Payne MP, Delic J, Turner RM. *Toxicology of substances in relation to major hazards: Ammonia*. London: HMSO, 1990.
135. World Health Organization. Ammonia. Environmental Health Criteria, 54. Geneva: WHO, 1986.
136. Leung CM, Foo CL. Mass ammonia inhalational burns – experience in the management of 12 patients. *Annals of the Academy of Medicine, Singapore*. 1992; **21**: 624–9.
137. De la Hoz R, Schlueter DP, Rom WN. Chronic lung disease secondary to ammonia inhalation injury: A report on three cases. *American Journal of Industrial Medicine*. 1996; **29**: 209–14.
138. Dongham KJ, Reynolds SJ, Whitten P *et al*. Respiratory dysfunction in swine production facility workers: Dose-response relationships of environmental exposures and pulmonary function. *American Journal of Industrial Medicine*. 1995; **27**: 405–18.
139. Ayesh R, Mitchell SC, Zhang A, Smith RL. The fish odour syndrome: Biochemical, familial and clinical aspects. *British Medical Journal*. 1993; **307**: 655–7.
140. Department of the Environment: Expert Panel on Air Quality Standards. Ozone. London: HMSO, 1994.
141. International Programme on Chemical Safety. Nitrogen oxides. Environmental Health Criteria, 188, 2nd edn. Geneva: WHO, 1997.
142. World Health Organization. Oxides of nitrogen. Environmental Health Criteria, 4. Geneva: WHO, 1977.
143. Grayson RR. Silage gas poisoning: Nitrogen dioxide pneumonia, a new disease in agricultural workers. *Annals of Internal Medicine*. 1956; **45**: 393–408.

144. Ramirez RJ, Dowell AR. Silo-filler's disease: Nitrogen dioxide induced lung injury. *Annals of Internal Medicine.* 1971; **74**: 569-76.
145. Department of the Environment: Expert Panel on Air Quality Standards. Nitrogen dioxide. London: HMSO, 1996.
146. Hatton DV, Leach CS, Nicogossian AE, Di Ferrante N. Collagen breakdown and nitrogen dioxide inhalation. *Archives of Environmental Health.* 1977; **32**: 33-6.
147. Brauer M, Spengler JD. Nitrogen dioxide exposures inside ice skating rinks. *American Journal of Public Health.* 1994; **84**: 429-33.
148. Fleetham JA, Tunnicliffe BW, Munt PW. Methemoglobinemia and the oxides of nitrogen. *New England Journal of Medicine.* 1978; **298**: 1150.
149. World Health Organization. Hydrogen sulfide. Geneva: WHO, 1981.
150. Bhambani Y, Burnham R, Snydmiller G et al. Effects of 10 ppm hydrogen sulfide inhalation on pulmonary function in healthy men and women. *Journal of Occupational and Environmental Medicine.* 1996; **38**: 1012-17.
151. Jappinen P, Vilkka V, Marttila O, Haahtela T. Exposure to hydrogen sulphide and respiratory function. *British Journal of Industrial Medicine.* 1990; **47**: 824-8.
152. World Health Organization. Hydrogen sulphide: Human health aspects. Geneva: WHO, 2003.
153. Arnold IMF, Dufresne RM, Alleyne BC, Stuart PJW. Health implication of occupational exposure to hydrogen sulfide. *Journal of Occupational Medicine.* 1985; **27**: 373-6.
154. Jappinen P, Tenhunen R. Hydrogen sulphide poisoning: Blood sulphide concentration and changes in haem metabolism. *British Journal of Industrial Medicine.* 1990; **47**: 283-5.
155. Kage S, Takekawa K, Kurosaki K et al. The usefulness of thiosulfate as an indicator of hydrogen sulfide poisoning: Three cases. *International Journal of Legal Medicine.* 1997; **110**: 220-2.
156. Kangas J, Savolainen H. Urinary thiosulphate as an indicator of exposure to hydrogen sulphide vapour. *Clinica Chimica Acta.* 1987; **164**: 7-10.
157. Finch CA. Methemoglobinemia and sulfhemoglobinemia. *New England Journal of Medicine.* 1948; **239**: 470-8.
158. Parra O, Monso E, Gallego M, Morera J. Inhalation of hydrogen sulphide: A case of subacute manifestations and long term sequelae. *British Journal of Industrial Medicine.* 1991; **48**: 286-7.
159. Tvedt B, Skyberg K, Aaserud O et al. Brain damage caused by hydrogen sulfide: A follow-up study of six patients. *American Journal of Industrial Medicine.* 1991; **20**: 91-101.
160. Ahlborg G. Hydrogen sulfide poisoning in shale oil industry. *Archives of Industrial Hygiene and Occupational Medicine.* 1951; **3**: 247-66.
161. Bates MN, Garrett N, Graham B, Read D. Air pollution and mortality in the Rotorua geothermal area. *Australia and New Zealand Journal of Public Health.* 1997; **21**: 581-6.
162. Bates MN, Garret N, Graham B, Read D. Cancer incidence, morbidity and geothermal air pollution in Rotorua, New Zealand. *International Journal of Epidemiology.* 1998; **27**: 10-14.
163. McCabe LC, Clayton GD. Air pollution by hydrogen sulfide in Poza Rica, Mexico. *Archives of Industrial Hygiene and Occupational Medicine.* 1952; **6**: 199-213.
164. Partti-Pellinen K, Marttila O, Vilkka V et al. The South Karelia air pollution study: Effects of low-level exposure to malodorous sulphur compounds on symptoms. *Archives of Environmental Health.* 1996; **51**: 315-20.
165. Tangerman A, Meuwese-Arends MT, Jansen JBMJ. Foetor hepaticus. *Lancet.* 1994; **343**: 1569.
166. Schults WT, Fountain EN, Lynch EC. Methanethiol poisoning. *Journal of the American Medical Association.* 1970; **211**: 2153-4.
167. Schecter A, Shanske W, Stenzler A et al. Acute hydrogen selenide inhalation. *Chest.* 1980; **77**: 554-5.
168. Fowler BA, Weissberg JB. Arsine poisoning. *New England Journal of Medicine.* 1974; **291**: 1171-4.
169. Wilkinson SP, McHugh P, Horsley S et al. Arsine toxicity aboard the Asiafreighter. *British Medical Journal.* 1975; **3**: 559-63.
170. Hesdorffer CS, Milne FJ, Terblanche J, Meyers AM. Arsine gas poisoning. The importance of exchange transfusions in severe cases. *British Journal of Industrial Medicine.* 1986; **43**: 353-5.
171. World Health Organization. Phosphine and selected metal phosphides. Environmental Health Criteria, 73. Geneva: WHO, 1988.
172. Wilson R, Lovejoy FH, Jaeger RJ, Landrigan P. Acute phosphine poisoning aboard a grain freighter. *Journal of the American Medical Association.* 1980; **244**: 148-50.
173. Barbosa A, Bonin AM. Evaluation of phosphine genotoxicity at occupational levels of exposure in New South Wales, Australia. *Occupational and Environmental Medicine.* 1994; **51**: 700-5.
174. International Programme for Chemical Safety (IPCS). Methyl bromide. Environmental Health Criteria, 166. Geneva: WHO, 1995.
175. Yang RS, Witt KL, Alden CJ, Corkerham LG. Toxicology of methyl bromide. *Reviews of Environmental Contamination and Toxicology.* 1995; **142**: 65-85.
176. Behrens RH, Dukes DCD. Fatal methyl bromide poisoning. *British Journal of Industrial Medicine.* 1986; **43**: 561-2.
177. Health and Safety Executive. Fumigation using methyl bromide. Guidance note CS12. London: HMSO, 1991.
178. Garnier R, Rambourg-Schepens M-O, Müller A, Hallier E. Glutathione transferase activity and formation of macromolecular adducts in two cases of acute methyl bromide poisoning. *Occupational and Environmental Medicine.* 1996; **53**: 211-15.
179. Mehta PS, Mehta AS, Mehta SJ, Makhijani AB. Bhopal tragedy's health effects: A review of methyl isocyanate toxicity. *Journal of the American Medical Association.* 1990; **264**: 2781-7.
180. Andersson N, Ajurani MK, Mahashabde S et al. Delayed eye and other consequences from exposure to methyl isocyanate: 93% follow-up of exposed and unexposed

cohorts in Bhopal. *British Journal of Industrial Medicine.* 1990; **47**: 553–8.

181. Cullinan P, Acquilla S, Ramana Dhara V. Respiratory morbidity 10 years after the Union Carbide gas leak at Bhopal: A cross-sectional survey. *British Medical Journal.* 1997; **314**: 338–42.

182. World Health Organization. Ethylene oxide. Environmental Health Criteria, 55. Geneva: WHO, 1985.

183. Steenland K, Stayner L, Grief A *et al.* Mortality among workers exposed to ethylene oxide. *New England Journal of Medicine.* 1991; **324**: 1402–7.

184. Shore RE, Gardner MJ, Pannett B. Ethylene oxide: An assessment of the epidemiological evidence on carcinogenicity. *British Journal of Industrial Medicine.* 1993; **50**: 971–97.

185. Verraes S, McChel O. Occupational asthma induced by ethylene oxide. *Lancet.* 1995; **346**: 1434.

186. Kurta DL, Dean BS, Krenzelok EP. Acute nickel carbonyl poisoning. *American Journal of Emergency Medicine.* 1993; **11**: 64–6.

187. Tannenbaum TN, Goldberg RJ. Exposure to anesthetic gases and reproductive outcome. *Journal of Occupational Medicine.* 1985; **27**: 659–68.

188. Spence AA. Environmental pollution by inhalation anaesthetics. *British Journal of Anaesthesia.* 1987; **59**: 96–103.

189. Boivin J-F. Risk of spontaneous abortion in women occupationally exposed to anaesthetic gases: A meta-analysis. *Occupational and Environmental Medicine.* 1997; **54**: 541–8.

190. Stollery BT, Broadbent DE, Lee WR *et al.* Mood and cognitive functions in anaesthetists working in actively scavenged operating theatres. *British Journal of Anaesthesia.* 1988; **61**: 446–55.

191. Rowland AS, Baird DD, Weinberg CR *et al.* Reduced fertility among women employed as dental assistants exposed to high levels of nitrous oxide. *New England Journal of Medicine.* 1992; **327**: 993–7.

192. Neil HAW, Fairer JG, Coleman MP *et al.* Mortality among male anaesthetists in the United Kingdom, 1957–83. *British Medical Journal.* 1987; **295**: 360–1.

193. Gardner RJ. Inhalation anesthetics – exposure and control: A statistical comparison of personal exposures in operating theatres with and without anaesthetic gas scavenging. *Annals of Occupational Hygiene.* 1989; **33**: 159–73.

194. Gardner RJ, Hampton J, Causton JS. Inhalation anaesthetics – exposure and control during veterinary surgery. *Annals of Occupational Hygiene.* 1991; **35**: 377–88.

195. Health and Safety Commission: Health Service Advisory Committee. Anaesthetic agents: Controlling exposure under COSHH. London: HMSO, 1995.

196. Sweeney B, Bingham RM, Amos RJ *et al.* Toxicity of bone marrow in dentists exposed to nitrous oxide. *British Medical Journal.* 1985; **291**: 567–9.

197. Elliott P, Kleinschmidt I. Angiosarcoma of the liver in Great Britain in proximity to vinyl chloride sites. *Occupational and Environmental Medicine.* 1997; **54**: 14–18.

198. Nicholson K. *Geothermal fluids: Chemistry and exploration techniques.* Berlin: Springer, 1993.

# Reactive airways dysfunction syndrome and irritant-induced asthma

JON G AYRES

Introduction	310	Prognosis	312
Terminology and definitions	310	Pathology	312
Epidemiology	311	References	313
Clinical picture	311		

INTRODUCTION

Exposure to chemicals or gases in the workplace during a spill or leak can lead to acute severe pulmonary injury and at high concentrations to death through alveolar leak and pulmonary oedema, the classic example being silo-filler's disease due to nitrogen dioxide, or acute pneumonitis/chemical pneumonia. In these cases, the exposure is clear, the effects immediate and often devastating and the long-term prognosis is usually easy to determine. However, such exposures can lead to effects which are less life-threatening and the term 'reactive airways dysfunction syndrome' (RADS) was coined by Brooks in 1985[1] to describe a syndrome of respiratory symptoms occurring after chemical or gas exposure in the workplace.

TERMINOLOGY AND DEFINITIONS

Brooks used the term 'RADS' to define an asthma-like state occurring shortly after a high exposure to a chemical or gas, usually in the workplace. He described fairly strict criteria for the definition of RADS describing it as an asthmatic-like state occurring within 24 hours of an acute, very high-dose exposure and which was characterized by the presence of bronchial hyper-responsiveness to methacholine in an individual with no pre-existing lung disease. However, in the early 1990s the issue of persistent (repeated) lower-dose exposure to chemicals or gases resulting in airways disease was raised. As a consequence, in 1995 a consensus statement on asthma in the workplace[2] recommended that the term 'irritant-induced asthma' (IIA) could be used in this context embracing both classical RADS and the consequences of lower-dose exposures. This was achieved by relaxation of the Brooks' RADS criteria to produce the following more comprehensive criteria:

- absence of previous respiratory complaints;
- onset of asthma symptoms within 24 hours of a single exposure to a high concentration of respiratory irritant gas (or by implication a fuming chemical);
- persistence of asthma symptoms for at least three months after exposure;
- symptoms associated with increased bronchial responsiveness and/or the presence of airflow obstruction with reversibility to bronchodilator in the absence of previous lung disease.

This definition covers all forms of IIA, including classical RADS and low-dose exposure to irritants over time. This issue of a changing definition was highlighted in a review of this area[3] where it was recognized that in a number of reported cases authors included multiple acute exposures as causing IIA, some allowing up to a week after exposure for the onset of symptoms to occur, and some allowing lesser degrees of exposure – so-called low-dose RADS or 'not so sudden IIA' in their definition of IIA.[4] The possibility of exposures such as those which are recognized to lead to RADS/IIA could cause a stepwise worsening of patients with pre-existing respiratory disease is equally plausible, perhaps even more so, but does not fall under these definitions. However, in the context of considering the health effect of the specific ambient exposures considered here this should be regarded as possible although difficult to prove particularly where litigation is an issue.

The likelihood that repeated exposure to chemicals or gases might cause more than simple short-term irritancy symptoms and to more established airways disease fits with reports of asthma developing in cleaners and workers exposed to solvents[5,6] and with the finding that 18 per cent of cases of occupational asthma reported to the SHIELD scheme in the West Midlands were due to irritants such as cleaning agents.[7] A wider European survey[8] also showed similar associations between persistent respiratory symptoms (cough, wheeze and breathlessness) in workers exposed to irritants. In the occupational setting, small but above normal exposures have been reported to result both in accelerated fall in FEV_1 over time and enhanced bronchial responsiveness.[9]

EPIDEMIOLOGY

Prevalence

Because of the variation of definitions over the time since RADS was first described, clear information on the epidemiology is difficult to secure, in particular in terms of prevalence and prognosis.[10] Much of the published literature in this area has been as case reports or short case series which do not allow prevalence data to be defined, although do identify causal agents. Depending upon the diagnostic criteria used, estimates of the prevalence of RADS or IIA range from 2 to 3 per cent[1,11] to 18 per cent from the UK's SWORD reporting scheme[12] to 23 per cent for a range of occupational populations, although most estimates lie in the 3–6 per cent range.[10] Even then, there are issues with what population to use as a denominator – the total workforce exposed or the total workforce within that industry, although using those exposed as the true denominator is both logistically better when reporting a series and more logical as those unexposed will not have had the chance to develop symptoms. For example, one report of approximately 3000 people exposed to a pesticide spill (metam sodium: monoalkyl dithiocarbamate which part decomposes to methyl isocyanate) showed that 30 individuals (1 per cent of those exposed) fulfilled the criteria for IIA. In this study, the authors included those with exacerbation of pre-existing asthma,[13] which again raises the issue of variation in diagnostic criteria.

Causal agents

The most important causal agents are gases, with chlorine the most reported, but including also sulphur dioxide and nitrogen dioxide,[10] a pattern which applies to both RADS and IIA. Between 1989 and 2003 in the United Kingdom, over 330 cases of chlorine exposure causing respiratory symptoms were reported to the SWORD database, mostly as inhalation accidents, but 69 (20 per cent) of those exposed to chlorine were reported to have developed asthma as did 26 (20 per cent) of those exposed to hydrochloric acid. The occupational group in which exposures were most likely to occur was chemical, gas and petroleum operators (10 per cent for chlorine, 8.5 per cent for hydrogen chloride). In some cases, the exposure is not simple, the best example being those individuals developing RADS who were rescue workers at the World Trade Center disaster,[14] where no clear individual causal agent could be implicated, although alkalinity of the aerosol (pH 10) might have played a part.[15] While the majority of cases of RADS and IIA (around 80 per cent) occur in the workplace, a significant number occur in the home or in the wider environment.[10] As most of these events are reported *post hoc*, it is very rare for measured levels of exposure to have been reported so attempts at dose–response relationships are not possible.

Risk factors

The most important causal factor is the dose of the agent, as the nearer individuals are to a spill the greater is the risk of developing RADS[16,17] which was also the key factor in determining the risk of developing RADS after exposure to World Trade Centre dust.[14] Characteristically, males are more represented in the RADS literature with approximate gender equality for IIA, the average age for both being in the late 30s.[10] Atopy does not appear to be a risk factor, although in much of the literature, atopy was not reported which makes generalizations insecure.[10] Whether current cigarette smoking is a risk factor for either RADS or IIA is unclear.

CLINICAL PICTURE

In someone with RADS, by definition, symptoms should begin within 24 hours of exposure, although in some for whom there is good evidence for causality there is delay in onset of symptoms of a few days. This is likely to be due to acceptance of minor symptoms as 'normal' or to the fact that the development of inflammation in some individuals is only at a later stage sufficient to induce symptoms. Symptoms are dominated by breathlessness and cough which are reported in over two-thirds of cases, but wheeze and chest tightness are reported in just under a half.[10] Upper airway irritation, eye irritation and mucus production are seen in fewer cases, usually between 10 and 20 per cent. Clinical signs if present are non-specific with only occasional wheeze being heard in some cases. Lung function in RADS is either normal or shows a mild obstructive pattern, whereas in IIA (when recorded, which is more often the case not reported) lung function is more likely to be normal.[10] In some affected individuals, particularly those in whom cough is the main symptom, good quality lung function can be impossible to obtain, as forced expiration results in coughing before expiration is complete. Bronchodilator reversibility has not often been recorded in these individuals, although frequently symptomatic relief over short time periods is reported by patients with use of beta-agonist bronchodilators.

Vocal cord dysfunction (VCD) may also be present following single exposures, a diagnosis which is difficult to make.[18] Clinically, individuals complain of wheezy breathlessness or cough, classically inspiratory and often with inspiratory or throat tightness. Dysphonia is a common associated complaint. Diagnosis is made by direct laryngoscopy while inhaling an irritant which the individual knows will cause symptoms, the classical appearance being paradoxical adduction of either the false or true cords (or both). Deformation of the flow volume loop with truncation of the expiratory peak and flattening of the inspiratory limb if found is a helpful finding, although in most cases this test is normal.

Treatment of RADS is based on that used in conventional asthma therapy largely depending on inhaled steroids and relief beta-agonists, but the response is often poor.[10] One study found that patients with RADS showed considerably less improvement when treated with inhaled β_2-agonists alone than did patients with classical sensitization-associated occupational asthma with a latency period.[19] In the reported literature, around one-third of patients are reported to be taking inhaled steroids which would support the view that they may have limited benefit.[10] The role of oral steroids is debatable, although anecdotally they may be of some help; supportive evidence for benefit has been demonstrated in a mouse model.[20]

Treatment of IIA has not been subject to critical assessment, but the condition is often more refractory to conventional asthma treatment much as in classical RADS. Treatment of VCD is also difficult, as inhaled therapy is rarely effective.

PROGNOSIS

In classical RADS, the tendency is for improvement to occur over time, although in many individuals symptoms continue for years. There is much less evidence about what happens with IIA more broadly, although the impression is that this is a much more permanent state of affairs. However, there are as yet no longitudinal studies of outcome in either of these particular groups. Prognosis can be assessed by persistence of symptoms or by changes in measures of bronchial hyper-responsiveness. Overall, duration of symptoms is poorly recorded in the literature[10] often because the case was reported before symptoms had ceased, the reason for publication being the need to report the causal agent before the long-term outlook had become clear. Consequently, attempts to define likely average duration of symptoms or rates of change in symptoms over time for prognostic purposes should be regarded with caution. However, in one follow-up study, normalization of both FEV_1 and PC_{20} to methacholine was seen in approximately a quarter of subjects two and a half years post-exposure.[21] This makes advice on return to work difficult although it appears that, in contrast to individuals with occupational asthma, patients with RADS do not necessarily develop a recurrence of their symptoms when re-exposed to a low level of the substance that initiated their problem. Consequently, a worker with RADS may be able to return to work if they can tolerate the prevailing exposure levels in their workplace.[22]

PATHOLOGY

Thus, both single high-dose and repeated lower-dose exposures to relevant agents (alone or as complex mixtures) may result in persistent airway symptoms, but whether this is through the same mechanism(s) is not known. Cumulative exposure over years may result in a chronic inflammatory response,[23] but while there is some suggestion that in RADS histologically there is less eosinophilic infiltration and more fibrosis,[1] in general such differences are difficult to interpret as the reported literature on the histology of RADS is very limited. Nevertheless, the pattern of relative steroid resistance might suggest a condition which in some individuals may be more akin to the picture of chronic obstructive pulmonary disease or bronchitis than to asthma.[24]

It is possible that specific exposures, such as exposures to chlorine, may induce specific pathological responses.[16,25] One worker underwent bronchial biopsies on four occasions following exposure to chlorine.[26] The histology revealed initial epithelial desquamation with a fibrinous exudate followed later by proliferation of basal cells, subsequent regeneration of the epithelium leading to collagen deposition in the submucosa and basement membrane thickening,[27] which might explain the attenuated airflow reversibility seen in RADS. Animal models have confirmed these stages[28] but, interestingly, inflammatory cells do not seem to play an essential role. However, this proposed model is not consistently supported in larger studies.[29] There is no information on the histopathology of RADS occurring in rescue workers involved in the World Trade Center disaster.[14]

> **Key points**
>
> - Reactive airways dysfunction syndrome and irritant-induced asthma are linked conditions associated with single high exposures or repeated lower-dose exposures to a range of substances, most commonly gases such as chlorine and chemicals.
> - More than 60 agents have now been implicated in the development of these conditions. In some cases, the acute exposure was to a mixture of substances where the mixture itself rather than any specific single component may have been the driver of effect such as has been suggested for workers exposed during the World Trade Center disaster.

- These conditions are likely to be more common than is usually believed, but information on outcome is limited.
- The prognosis is poorly understood with relatively little information available to advise employees affected by the condition and their employers.
- The response to anti-asthma therapy is disappointing with limited benefit from inhaled steroids, but good short-lived relief from short-acting bronchodilators.

REFERENCES

1. Brooks SM, Weiss MA, Bernstein IL. Reactive airways dysfunction syndrome (RADS): Persistent asthma syndrome after high level irritant exposures. *Chest.* 1985; **88**: 376-84.
2. Chan-Yeung M. ACCP Consensus Statement on Assessment of Asthma in the Workplace. *Chest.* 1995; **108**: 1084-113.
3. Brooks SM, Hammad Y, Richards I et al. The spectrum of irritant-induced asthma: Sudden and not-so sudden and the role of allergy. *Chest.* 1998; **113**: 42-9.
4. Tarlo SM. Workplace irritant exposures: Do they produce true occupational asthma? *Annals of Allergy, Asthma and Immunology.* 2003; **90** (Suppl.): 19-23.
5. Medina-Ramon M, Zock JP, Kogevinas M et al. Asthma symptoms in women employed in domestic cleaning: A community-based study. *Thorax.* 2003; **58**: 950-4.
6. Rosenman KD, Reilly MJ, Schill DP et al. Cleaning products and work-related asthma. *Journal of Occupational and Environmental Medicine.* 2003; **45**: 556-63.
7. Gannon PF, Burge PS. The SHIELD scheme in the West Midlands Region, United Kingdom. *British Journal of Industrial Medicine.* 1993; **50**: 791-6.
8. Kogevinas M, Anto JM, Sunyer J et al. Occupational asthma in Europe and other industrialised areas: A population-based study. European Community Respiratory Health Survey Study Group. *Lancet.* 1999; **353**: 1750-4.
9. Gautrin D, Leroyer C, Infante-Rivard C et al. Longitudinal assessment of airway caliber and responsiveness in workers exposed to chlorine. *American Journal of Respiratory and Critical Care Medicine.* 1999; **160**: 1232-7.
10. Shakeri MS, Dick FD, Ayres JG. Which agents cause reactive airways dysfunction syndrome (RADS)? A systematic review. *Occupational Medicine.* 2008; **58**: 205-11.
11. Tarlo SM, Broder I. Irritant-induced occupational asthma. *Chest.* 1989; **96**: 297-300.
12. Ross DJ, McDonald JC. Asthma following inhalation accidents reported to the SWORD project. *Annals of Occupational Hygiene.* 1996; **40**: 645-50.
13. Cone JE, Wugofski L, Balmes JR et al. Persistent respiratory health effects after a metam sodium pesticide spill. *Chest.* 1994; **106**: 500-8.
14. Prezant DJ, Weiden M, Banauch GI et al. Cough and bronchial responsiveness in firefighters at the World Trade Center site. *New England Journal of Medicine.* 2002; **347**: 806-15.
15. Lioy PJ, Weisel CP, Millette JR et al. Characterisation of the dust/smoke aerosol that settled east of the World Trade Center (WTC) in lower Manhattan after the collapse of the WTC, 11 September 2001. *Environmental Health Perspectives.* 2002; **110**: 703-14.
16. Jajosky RA, Harrison R, Flattery J et al. Surveillance of work-related asthma in selected US states - California, Massachusetts, Michigan, and New Jersey, 1993-1995. *Morbidity and Mortality Weekly Report. Surveillance Summaries.* 1999; **48**: 1-20.
17. Renisch F, Harrison RJ, Cussler S et al. Physician reports of work-related asthma, 1993-1996. *American Journal of Industrial Medicine.* 2001; **39**: 72-83.
18. Newman KB, Mason UG, Schmaling KB. Clinical features of vocal cord dysfunction. *American Journal of Respiratory and Critical Care Medicine.* 1995; **152**: 1382-6.
19. Gautrin D, Boulet LP, Boutet M et al. Is reactive airways dysfunction syndrome a variant of occupational asthma? *Journal of Allergy and Clinical Immunology.* 1994; **93**: 12-22.
20. Das R, Blanc PD. Chlorine gas exposure and the lung: A review. *Toxicology and Industrial Health.* 1993; **9**: 439-55.
21. Malo JL, Cartier A, Boulet LP et al. Bronchial hyperresponsiveness can improve while spirometry plateaus two to three years after repeated exposure to chlorine causing respiratory symptoms. *American Journal of Respiratory and Critical Care Medicine.* 1994; **150**: 1142-5.
22. Alberts WM, Do Pico GA. Reactive airways dysfunction syndrome. *Chest.* 1996; **109**: 1618-26.
23. Kipen HM, Blume R, Hutt D. Asthma experience in an occupational and environmental medicine clinic. Low-dose reactive airways dysfunction syndrome. *Journal of Occupational Medicine.* 1994; **36**: 1133-7.
24. Balmes J. Occupational airways disease from chronic low-level exposures to irritants. *Clinics in Chest Medicine.* 2002; **23**: 727-35.
25. Chan-Yeung M, Lam S, Kennedy S, Frew AJ. Persistent asthma after repeated exposure to high concentrations of gases in pulp mills. *American Journal of Respiratory and Critical Care Medicine.* 1994; **149**: 1676-80.
26. Lemière C, Malo JL, Boutet M. Reactive airways dysfunction syndrome due to chlorine: Sequential bronchial biopsies and functional assessment. *European Respiratory Journal.* 1997; **10**: 241-4.
27. Boulet LP, Laviolette M, Turcotte H et al. Bronchial subepithelial fibrosis correlates with airway responsiveness to methacholine. *Chest.* 1997; **112**: 45-52.
28. Demnati R, Fraser R, Ghezzo H et al. Time-course of functional and pathological changes after a single high acute inhalation of chlorine in rats. *European Respiratory Journal.* 1998; **11**: 922-8.
29. Glindmeyer H, Lefante J, Freyder L et al. Relative rate of new onset asthma among workers exposed to irritant chemicals. *American Journal of Respiratory and Critical Care Medicine.* 1997; **155**: A258.

41

Deliberate use of chemicals in warfare and by terrorists

ROBERT L MAYNARD

Introduction	314	Occupational health issues	318
Terrorism	315	References	318

INTRODUCTION

The use of chemicals as a means of causing deliberate injury or death has a long history. Until the First World War, chemicals, though often used or considered for use, had had little impact on the outcome of battles. This was because the compounds used lacked toxicity and the means available for distributing them were primitive. Irritant substances, e.g. ethylbromoacetate and chloracetone, were deployed by French forces in 1914 with little effect, but on April 22, 1915 German forces launched the first and perhaps most successful large-scale attack with chemicals yet recorded. The chemical used was chlorine: released from cylinders brought up to the front line and making use of a favourable wind. One hundred and sixty-eight tons of chlorine were discharged from 5730 cylinders along a 6-km front at Ypres. The effect was very significant: the gas was effective for up to 5 km downwind and 15 000 casualties, including 5000 dead, were produced.[1] French troops retired in disorder. This attack was allegedly completely unexpected, although Alan Clark throws doubt on this in his work, *The donkeys*.[2] He records that the *Bulletin of the French Army* (March 30, 1915) and later reports (April 15 and 16) suggested that a gas attack by German forces was being prepared. Such warnings were clearly ignored and unprotected troops were exposed. Never again was a single gas attack so effective: protective equipment and drills were rapidly developed and by the end of the First World War, although phosgene and sulphur mustard were used on an extraordinary scale, there was never any likelihood of gas producing a breakthrough at well-defended locations. The scale of use of chemicals in the First World War is often forgotten: in all, about 113 000 tons of chemicals were used, including 12 000 tons of mustard gas (sulphur mustard). Despite their lack of effectiveness as far as winning battles was concerned, chemicals produced many casualties: up to 400 000 mustard gas casualties in all, with 14 000 British mustard gas casualties produced during the first three months of use of this weapon beginning on June 12, 1917, again at Ypres.

Italian forces used sulphur mustard against unprotected Ethiopian troops in 1936: again this resulted in many casualties. Iraq used sulphur mustard against Kurdish civilians in the 1980s: casualties were treated in a number of European cities, including London; the author was involved in their care.

Organophosphorus compounds (nerve agents) were produced on a large scale in Germany during the Second World War. These compounds were much more toxic than First World War chemical weapons: the LD_{50} of sarin (GB) being about 0.01 mg/kg i.v. and that of VX about 0.007 mg/kg i.v. However, these weapons were not used despite great urging by senior members of the German Government. No satisfactory explanation for their not being used has been produced. A lack of material is not the explanation: 12 000 tons of Tabun (GA) were produced by Germany. Nerve agents were used by Iraq during the Iran–Iraq war and against Kurdish unprotected civilians at Halabja. As would be expected, this resulted in many deaths. Thereafter, little was heard of these agents until 1995 when sarin (GB) and VX were used by terrorists in Japan. These incidents are considered in detail below.

What lessons can be learned from the above history? It is clear that chemicals have great potential as weapons, that this is known and that a number of groups (nations and terrorists) have sought to use them in this way. It is also clear that chemicals are likely to be most effective against unprotected troops or civilians. That chemicals would be used on a large scale in war seems unlikely, indeed attempts to destroy chemical weapons and to prohibit their use are proceeding rapidly.[3] Those at greatest risk today are probably civilians targeted by terrorist groups and, importantly, those asked to rescue victims and care for them. It is with this aspect of the deliberate use of chemicals to cause injury and death that this chapter deals.

TERRORISM

Terrorism is by no means a recently developed activity. Terrorist organizations see themselves as fighting for a cause and, in general, may not feel bound by international agreements regarding the 'normal usages of warfare'. In particular, terrorist groups may show little reluctance regarding attacks on civilians and, indeed, may focus on these rather than on better protected military targets. The range of weapons available to terrorist groups is wide: explosives being the most frequently used. That chemicals have been so little used is difficult to explain: access to chemicals by purchase or theft is not difficult and dispersion of chemicals can be readily managed. Though it may be unprofitable to speculate as to why chemicals have not been much used, it would be decidedly unwise to ignore the possibility that they could be used and to fail to prepare to deal with the consequences of their use. The incidents in Japan are likely to have been noted and perhaps studied by other terrorist organizations. Recent events (early–mid 2007) in Iraq suggest that bulk carriers of chlorine have been targeted by terrorist groups. A completely successful defence against the use of chemicals by terrorists is difficult or perhaps impossible to achieve: this, again, makes preparations for dealing with the consequences of such use importance.

Chemicals that might prove attractive to terrorists

It will be understood that all countries which perceive that they may be at significant risk of attack by terrorists will have prepared lists of chemicals that they anticipate might be used. Such lists are, for obvious reasons, classified and no attempt will be made here to predict their contents. However, it is obvious to all, including, presumably, terrorist organizations, that the so-called classical chemical warfare agents might prove attractive and certain toxic industrial chemicals (TIC) might be chosen for use as have been recently reviewed by Marrs et al.[4] Only a brief account of classical chemical warfare agents not dealt with in other chapters of this book will be provided here.

Organophosphorus nerve agents

Nerve agents comprise a group of highly toxic compounds with the general formula:

$$\begin{array}{c} R_1 \\ \diagdown O \\ P \diagup\!\!\!\diagup \\ \diagup \diagdown \\ R_2 X \end{array}$$

Sarin (GB) has the formula:

$$\begin{array}{c} CH_3 \\ | \\ CH_3CHO O \\ \diagdown \diagup\!\!\!\diagup \\ P \\ \diagup \diagdown \\ CH_3 F \end{array}$$

and is volatile (vapour pressure at 20°C = 2.10 mmHg).

VX has the formula:

$$\begin{array}{c} CH_3CH_2O O CH(CH_3)_2 \\ \diagdown \diagup\!\!\!\diagup \diagup \\ P \\ \diagup \diagdown \diagdown \\ CH_3 SCH_2CH_2N CH(CH_3)_2 \end{array}$$

and is not volatile (vapour pressure at 20°C = 0.00044 mmHg).

Nerve agents bind to and inhibit, effectively irreversibly, the enzyme acetylcholinesterase and thus cause an accumulation of acetylcholine at central and peripheral sites of transmission of nerve impulses. This leads to increased secretion from glands (salivary, nasal mucosal glands, bronchial glands), bradycardia, contraction of the pupil (miosis) and skeletal muscle twitching. Death is caused by inhibition of the medullary respiratory centres and depolarizing blockade of the diaphragm. Nerve agents may be absorbed by the lung and across the skin: a volunteer at Porton Down died in 1952 after sarin was placed on his forearm under clothing that prevented evaporation. At high concentrations, collapse occurs rapidly and death follows quickly. Low level exposure causes miosis, eye pain, conjunctival injection and headache. Fortunately, antidotes exist: atropine to block the effects of acetylcholine at muscarinic receptors and oximes (e.g. pralidoxime mesylate P2S) to reactivate the inhibited acetylcholinesterase. Diazepam is useful in preventing convulsions. These drugs should be given as soon as possible by intravenous or intramuscular injection. Autoinjection devices containing 2 mg of atropine, 500 mg of P2S and 5 mg of a diazepam–lysine conjugate (Avizafone) are commercially available. Assisted ventilation is essential in all severely poisoned casualties. Exposure to nerve agents is unlikely to cause delayed peripheral neuropathy (OPIDN), but the intermediate syndrome may occur and long-lasting effects on the electroencephalogram (EEG) and on memory function have been reported.[5]

Sulphur mustard

'Mustard gas' is a liquid of low volatility (vapour pressure at 20°C = 0.0650 mmHg). The structural formula is:

$$S\begin{cases} CH_2 - CH_2 - Cl \\ CH_2 - CH_2 - Cl \end{cases}$$

It is rather immiscible with water.

Exposure to the liquid and to the vapour causes intense, but delayed, eye irritation and skin blistering. Blisters may contain up to a litre of fluid, but this fluid does not pose a hazard to the patient or to attendants: mustard binds rapidly to proteins. Sulphur mustard has a radiomimetic effect: damaging bone marrow and the airway and gut epithelium. Its lethality is low, but patients require weeks of care to make a full recovery. Eye damage may cause delayed keratitis leading to blindness. No antidote is known and management is supportive. Eye damage can be severe and sticking of the eyelid margins can be a problem. Vaseline to prevent this and saline irrigation are useful. Hoscine (0.25 per cent) drops to relieve spasm of the iris are also helpful. Photophobia may be severe. Ascorbate and citrate eye drops have been recommended. In cases of bone marrow depression advice regarding bone marrow stimulation with colony-stimulating factors should be sought. Skin lesions are slow in healing and flamazine cream can be useful in preventing secondary infections. Caring for a patient exposed to a high concentration of sulphur mustard: temporarily blinded, coughing sloughed respiratory epithelium, with widespread skin blisters and a collapsing bone marrow is a major challenge. Despite this, the death rate in the First World War was <2 per cent. Other classical chemical warfare agents (hydrogen cyanide, chlorine and phosgene, and arsenical compounds) are dealt with in Chapter 8, Gases.

One group of compounds that might prove attractive to terrorists are the so-called riot control agents. Of these CS (sometimes called CS gas though it is usually encountered as a finely divided powder dispersed as an aerosol) is perhaps the best known. Riot control agents are remarkable in that they cause intense and incapacitating eye irritation, but are characterized by remarkably large LD_{50} values. The intravenous LD_{50} of CS in the male mouse is 48 mg/kg and yet the TC_{50} (concentration intolerable to 50 per cent of the population) is 3.6 µg/L. Exposure to the aerosol produces no lasting effects and the acute effects on the eye disappear rapidly on the patient being removed from the source of exposure. Eye damage as a result of spraying directly into the eye can occur.

Japanese experience with nerve agents deployed by terrorists

Okumura and colleagues[6] have provided a disturbing account of the consequences of the release of sarin (GB) by the Aum Shinnikoy cult on the Tokyo subway on March 20, 1995. This account should be read by all interested in this area.[6] Only a brief summary, in note form, is provided here.

- On March 20, five terrorists punctured plastic bags containing an impure preparation of sarin on Tokyo subway trains.
- Twelve people died, 5654 were affected, 999 people were admitted to hospital, 4643 needed treatment (the large numbers are estimates and vary according to source).
- Atropine was used as the major antidote and atropine eye drops proved useful – this had been questioned in earlier accounts.
- Oxime (2-PAM, pralidoxime chloride) was not thought to have been life saving, although it was used.
- Secondary contamination led to medical and paramedical staff being affected.
- A 'field test' for sarin failed to identify or detect the agent.
- Long-term effects, including visual disturbances, eye discomfort, headache, fatigue and vestibulocerebellar disturbance, were reported. Measures of visual evoked potentials (P300 and VEP) and heart rate variability (R–R interval) also showed long-lasting effects. Post-traumatic stress disorder (PTSD) questionnaire scores were high. That medical and paramedical staff were affected by off-gassing of sarin from patients was notable and in some ways surprising. Casualties had been exposed only to vapour (not to liquid) and yet enough was retained on clothing to produce secondary effects. It should also be noted that though the number dying was low, some thousands of people attended hospitals. This overloading of medical facilities is likely to occur as a result of the use of chemicals and to be a serious logistical problem in a terrorist incident. That the medical and paramedical staff coped as well as they did with a frightening and unique challenge can only be a matter for congratulation regarding their training and dedication.

Dealing with a terrorist incident involving the use of chemicals

The key to success is teamwork. Emergency services, medical services and local authorities need to combine to (1) assess risks, (2) plan how to deal with incidents and (3) exercise their plans. Detailed accounts of this have been provided by Baker[7] and by Roberts and Maynard.[8] Here, we focus on patient care, but other issues including provision of appropriate protective equipment and chemical detectors for first responders are also very important. Modelling the dispersion of chemicals is also vital for planning. Real-time modelling of dispersion during an incident is difficult, but may be possible, especially if the area affected has been studied in advance. Much, of course, depends on the nature of the incident. In Tokyo, a chemical was released in a closed (not outdoor) environment and it is likely that the release, though not instantaneous as would be produced by an explosion, was short-lived. A slow release, for example, from cylinders or a tanker is also possible and this would present a different set of problems.

In approaching chemical casualties a number of golden rules should be noted:

1. Attendants and rescue workers must be protected – if not, they may soon become casualties.
2. Casualties must be decontaminated before admission to hospitals or other facilities where unprotected staff are working.
3. Life supporting care is the first priority.
4. Specific antidotes are few but, if available, should be given as soon as possible.
5. The identity of the chemical producing the casualties may not be known at first and treatment of effects will be needed. For example, lung injuring agents may cause bronchospasm. Management of effects does not, in general, depend on knowing the exact identity of the causative agent.

Decontamination of casualties

Removing a casualty's clothing may remove 80 per cent of liquids or powder contamination. This, then, is the first step towards decontamination. Water is the key decontaminant. If a little dilute bleach can be added to the water, this will improve decontamination by aiding hydrolysis. The logistical problems of decontaminating a few hundred casualties are formidable and need to be addressed by planning and exercises. Crowd control is critically important and close liaison between the police and resource services is needed. It should be noted that in Tokyo the majority of subjects made their own way to hospital undecontaminated. In many countries, mobile decontamination units have been developed and facilities for showering and reclothing in clean garments are provided. Preventing hypothermia is obviously important and some facilities provide warmed water. Decontamination of collapsed patients presents special problems: at its simplest a 'bucket and sponge' approach is satisfactory. Decontamination using solid decontaminants, such as fullers' earth, is now not generally recommended.

Separating the contaminated (or potentially contaminated) from the decontaminated is important. In many countries, the incident area is divided into 'hot', 'warm' and 'cold' zones. In the hot zone, there is a risk of primary contamination by the released chemical or chemicals: only well-protected staff can enter this area. In the warm zone, the risk to staff is from contaminated patients: the level of protection needed by staff will be less than in the hot zone. In the cold zone, only decontaminated patients are allowed and here the risk to staff is small and only normal clinical measures, e.g. gloves, are needed. Maintaining the integrity of these zones is clearly important.

Medical care at the scene

The organization of medical care at the scene of a chemical incident is a hotly debated topic. Some authorities recommend dispatching a medical team to the scene with a consultant in intensive care to take charge of casualty management.[7] Others argue that holding medical staff at hospitals and allowing paramedics to take the lead at the scene is more appropriate. The former approach is adopted in Paris, the latter in London. Whichever staff are present at the scene, they must be trained in the rapid identification of the effects of chemicals. It is important to note that the incident may not be known to involve chemicals and recognizable effects may provide the first clue to this. Having an experienced clinical toxicologist at the scene would clearly help. However, such trained medical staff are few and form a resource that should be carefully deployed. Sending medical staff into the hot zone is also debated: the level of protective equipment sometimes recommended may significantly reduce the diagnostic skills of even senior doctors and closed circuit breathing apparatus plus an impermeable protective suit may make such tasks as intubation and establishing an intravenous line difficult. This leads to the question of what level of protection needs to be worn. If the nature of an incident is unknown, there is likely to be a tendency to overprotect staff.

What drugs can be given in the hot zone?

It has already been noted that there are very few effective antidotes of proven value in chemical poisoning. This is sometimes forgotten and it is imagined that medical staff at the scene of an incident will have a battery of effective drugs with which to treat casualties.

In fact, the effects of only two chemicals that might be used by terrorists can be treated by means of antidotes. Casualties exposed to nerve agents causing collapse and impairment of respiration should be treated at once with atropine and oxime. Delay can be fatal and provision of autoinjection devices that can be used to give an intramuscular injection through clothing is important. This should be done as soon as the diagnosis is made. A patient with breathing difficulties, who has small pupils and who is salivating or twitching needs atropine and oxime at once. The second cause of poisoning that calls for rapid antidote therapy is cyanide. Exposure to hydrogen cyanide is rapidly fatal and the likelihood that rescuers will reach patients at risk of dying sufficiently quickly to give an antidote is low. Whether Kelocyanor® or the combination of sodium nitrite and sodium thiosulphate is used, the antidote must be given intravenously. This presents difficulties in the hot zone. Cyanide casualties who survive exposure and who are breathing spontaneously on being brought out into the fresh air do not need antidote therapy: this is unlike the case of nerve agent poisoning where antidote therapy is needed for some time. It is important to stress again that support for ventilation and the provision of oxygen is critically important for patients with breathing difficulties. Oxygen can be provided and masks attached to low-weight cylinders, with special heads and valves, allow a number of patients to be treated simultaneously. Light ventilators are also available: the ComPac ventilator (Smiths Medical International, St Paul, MN, USA) is a good example of a battery-driven portable device that can supply air filtered through a respirator canister. Oxygen-enriched air can also be provided by portable ventilators connected to light-weight oxygen cylinders.

Much of the thinking outlined above comes from the military field and important differences between the military (battlefield) and civilian (terrorist incident) scenario should be noted. Military doctors do not deal with babies and children or with old or perhaps already ill subjects. Planning should include these groups: dose schedules for babies and children need to be developed and such obvious things as the length of the needle of autoinjection devices are easily overlooked. Treating seriously ill casualties in a contaminated environment is a great challenge and there is a strong case for moving casualties to a more satisfactory environment as soon as possible.

OCCUPATIONAL HEALTH ISSUES

Staff from the emergency services, as well as doctors and paramedical staff may be placed at significant risk at the scene of a terrorist incident. The following hazards need to be considered:

- Physical stress imposed by rescue work. Wearing protective equipment imposes a significant physiological penalty in terms of heat stress, dehydration and exhaustion. Staff should be rotated through difficult conditions and adequate periods for rest and recovery should be provided. Staff undertaking such work should be physically fit.
- Exposure to chemicals may occur and casualties among healthcare workers and rescue workers should be expected. Training in the use of protective equipment is vitally important: the duration of safe use of such equipment should be noted and each person's time in protective equipment should be monitored. The operational period possible in closed circuit breathing apparatus may be short. Protective equipment must be checked for damage before use. Removing contaminated protective clothing is potentially dangerous and drills to allow this to be done safely should be developed.
- Healthcare workers and rescue staff are likely to be exposed to intense mental stress. This should be monitored. Staff may suffer from post-traumatic stress disorder and advice should be taken regarding professional counselling.

Key points

- The use of chemicals by terrorists is a very real threat in many countries today.
- A terrorist incident involving the use of chemicals will present formidable difficulties for medical and paramedical staff, including occupational physicians. The key to success under such conditions is planning and training. This needs to be rigorous and repeated.
- Cadres of specially trained staff working to established protocols are important and research needs to be done to develop both better therapies and procedures. In many countries, this research is underway.
- Measures to prevent the chemical contamination of healthcare workers and rescuers are essential.
- Terrorist incidents are very stressful for all responders, and staff may suffer from post-traumatic stress disorder and require specific support.

REFERENCES

1. Prentiss AM. *Chemicals in war*. New York: McGraw-Hill, 1937.
2. Clark A. *The donkeys: A history of the British expeditionary force in 1915*. London: Pimlico, 1991.
3. Pearson GS. The total prohibition of chemical weapons. In: Marrs TC, Maynard RL, Sidell F (eds). *Chemical warfare agents: Toxicology and treatment*, 2nd edn. Chichester: John Wiley, 2007: 633–62.
4. Marrs TC, Maynard RL, Sidell F (eds). *Chemical warfare agents: Toxicology and treatment*, 2nd edn. Chichester: John Wiley, 2007.
5. Marrs TC. Toxicology of organophosphate agents. In: Marrs TC, Maynard RL, Sidell F (eds). *Chemical warfare agents: Toxicology and treatment*, 2nd edn. Chichester: John Wiley, 2007: 191–222.
6. Okumura T, Nomura, T, Suzuki T et al. The dark morning: The experiences and lessons learned from the Tokyo subway sarin attack. In: Marrs TC, Maynard RL, Sidell F (eds). *Chemical warfare agents: Toxicology and treatment*, 2nd edn. Chichester: John Wiley, 2007: 277–86.
7. Baker DJ. The management of casualties following toxic agent release: The approach adopted in France. In: Marrs TC, Maynard RL, Sidell F (eds). *Chemical warfare agents: Toxicology and treatment*, 2nd edn. Chichester: John Wiley, 2007: 261–76.
8. Roberts G, Maynard RL. Responding to chemical terrorism: Operational planning and decontamination. In: Marrs TC, Maynard RL, Sidell F (eds). *Chemical warfare agents: Toxicology and treatment*, 2nd edn. Chichester: John Wiley, 2007: 175–90.

SECTION FOUR

Other chemical exposures

42	Organic chemicals	321
	Tiina Santonen, Antero Aitio and Harri Vainio	
43	Pesticides and other agrochemicals	395
	Ian Brown, Annalisa Chiodini, Chiara Somaruga and Claudio Colosio	
44	Welding	421
	Grant McMillan	
45	The semiconductor industry	444
	David Koh and Judy Sng	

42

Organic chemicals

TIINA SANTONEN, ANTERO AITIO AND HARRI VAINIO

Introduction	321	Phenol and phenol derivatives	357
Hydrocarbons	322	Epoxides	360
Alcohols	336	Cyclic acid anhydrides	362
Aldehydes	338	Isocyanates	364
Ketones	339	Chlorinated hydrocarbons	365
Ethers	340	Sulphur-containing substances	374
Carboxylic acids and their derivatives	346	Acknowledgements	376
Esters	347	References	376
Nitrogen-containing hydrocarbons	348		

INTRODUCTION

Organic chemicals are a vast group of widely different entities. They differ in their inherent acute, long-term and organ toxicity, as well as reproductive toxicity, carcinogenicity and sensitizing and irritant properties. They are traditionally divided, by their chemical nature, into groups such as alcohols, carboxylic acids, ethers, etc. While this classification may be useful, many organic chemicals contain more than one active group and could thus be listed under many headings in such listings, and more importantly, may show characteristics of different groups. Most chemicals also have several different synonyms, the identification of which is not always straightforward. A unique identification system is provided by the Chemical Abstracts Service (CAS) registry numbers. Often, it is easiest to find information on a specific chemical by searching databases using the CAS number. Therefore, the CAS numbers have been given in this chapter.

It is a formidable task to characterize, even crudely, the hazardous characteristics of all these different individual chemicals. Several approaches have tried to solve the problem by structure–activity analyses, but at present, such approaches cannot be considered reliable. Even if at some time in the future, we have all the statutory animal and *in vitro* tests done on every chemical that is produced on a large scale – as the European Union legislation on Registration, Evaluation, Authorisation and Restriction of Chemicals (REACH) intends to do – we still have the nagging uncertainty of the reliability of our models, notably of the species to species extrapolation, and also the even larger number of chemicals that are produced at small amounts, but to which people are still exposed.

This chapter can provide only a superficial perspective on the world of organic chemicals. The individual chemicals presented here in detail have been selected on the basis of their widespread use or known existence as workplace contaminants, and since they are known to exert toxicological hazards capable of causing occupational diseases. Some chemicals, which have been important occupational toxicants in the past but have, thanks to different national or international bans and restrictions, lost their position as commonly used industrial chemicals are presented in the text only briefly. These include carcinogenic 2-naphthylamine and benzidine. Even if some chemicals are not covered in this text, it does not mean that they may not be toxicologically important. Since our knowledge is advancing and new chemicals are constantly being introduced, new hazardous chemicals or new health hazards of 'old' chemicals may become evident. It is therefore of utmost importance for an occupational physician not to consider texts as representing the final word on chemically induced health hazards, but instead, to keep his mind and eyes open, and to be aware of new findings on the effects of all chemicals.

HYDROCARBONS

Aliphatic hydrocarbons

Hydrocarbons are substances consisting of carbon and hydrogen. They are divided into aliphatic and aromatic hydrocarbons, aromatic hydrocarbons being based on specific ring structure. Aliphatic hydrocarbons can exist as open-chain compounds, such as *n*-hexane, or as cyclic compounds, such as cyclohexane. Aliphatic hydrocarbons may form branched isomers, like 2-methylhexane, which is also called isoheptane. Examples of aliphatic hydrocarbons are given in Table 42.1.

The simplest aliphatic hydrocarbons are methane, ethane, propane and butane. These are saturated hydrocarbons belonging to the group of alkanes, which are also known as paraffins. They have a molecular formula of C_nH_{2n+2}. In the case of methane, n = 1, ethane, n = 2, etc. Methane is a principal component of natural gas, and it is also formed in the decay of organic matter. It can act as a simple asphyxiant. Propane and butane are widely used as domestic and industrial fuels and in aerosol propellants, and are extremely flammable gases. As the number of carbons in the carbon chain of alkanes increases, so does the boiling point. While the lightest alkanes are gases, alkanes heavier than butane exist as liquids at room temperature. Alkanes with their boiling points are presented in Table 42.2.

Alkenes are a group of compounds with a carbon–carbon double bond in their hydrocarbon chain. The simplest alkene is ethene, which is commonly known as

Table 42.1 Examples of aliphatic hydrocarbons with their molecular structures and main hazards.

Group	Compound	Molecular formula	Molecular structure	Main hazards
Alkanes (straight chain)	Methane (CAS 74-82-8)	CH_4	CH_4	Simple asphyxiant, extremely flammable
	Propane (CAS 74-98-6)	C_3H_8	$H_3C\diagdown\diagup CH_3$	Extremely flammable, acute CNS effects at high concentrations
	n-Hexane (CAS 110-54-3)	C_6H_{14}	$H_3C\diagdown\diagup\diagdown\diagup CH_3$	CNS effects, polyneuropathy
Alkanes (branched)	Isobutane (2-methylpropane) (CAS 75-28-5)	C_4H_{10}	$H_3C-CH(CH_3)-CH_3$	Highly flammable
	2-Methylpentane (isohexane) (CAS 73513-42-5)	C_6H_{14}	$H_3C-CH(CH_3)-CH_2-CH_3$	Highly flammable
Alkanes (cyclic)	Cyclohexane (CAS 110-82-7)	C_6H_{12}	(hexagon)	Highly flammable, irritant, CNS effects
Alkenes	Ethylene (CAS 74-85-1)	C_2H_4	$H_2C=CH_2$	Highly flammable
	Propylene (CAS 115-07-1)	C_3H_6	$H_2C=CH-CH_3$	Highly flammable
Dienes	1,3-Butadiene (CAS 106-99-0)	C_4H_6	$H_2C=CH-CH=CH_2$	Cancer
Alkynes	Acetylene (CAS 74-86-2)	C_2H_2	$HC\equiv CH$	Highly flammable, simple asphyxiant

CNS, central nervous system.

Table 42.2 Alkanes and their boiling points.

Alkane	Boiling point (°C)
Methane	−162
Ethane	−89
n-Propane	−42
n-Butane	−0.5
n-Pentane	36
n-Hexane	69
n-Heptane	98
n-Octane	126
n-Nonane	151
n-Decane	174

ethylene. Alkenes have a molecular formula of C_nH_{2n}. Ethylene is followed by propene (propylene) and butenes (1-butene, 2-butene and isobutylene). Like corresponding alkanes, ethylene, propylene and butenes are highly flammable gases. With increasing chain length, the boiling points of alkenes increase.

In contrast to alkenes, dienes contain two carbon–carbon double bonds in their hydrocarbon chain. Rubber is a natural polymer of isoprene (2-methyl-1,3-butadiene). 1,3-butadiene is a compound used in the manufacture of synthetic rubbers like styrene-butadiene rubber and polybutadiene rubber.

Alkynes contain a carbon–carbon triple bond in their hydrocarbon chain. They have a general molecular formula of C_nH_{2n-2}. The simplest alkyne is acetylene, which is commonly used as a welding gas. Like alkanes and alkenes, the first compounds in this series are highly flammable gases at room temperature, whereas higher homologues are liquids. Acetylene has a low toxicity, but it may act as a simple asphyxiant by lowering the oxygen content of the air in confined spaces.

Generally, many aliphatic hydrocarbons may cause acute central nervous system depression at high exposure levels. Some of them, like methane and acetylene, work as simple asphyxiants. In occupational medicine, the most important compounds in this group are n-hexane and 1,3-butadiene, which are discussed in detail below.

n-HEXANE

[CAS No. 110-54-3]

n-Hexane is a volatile, colourless liquid with a characteristic disagreeable odour and a high vapour pressure. It is produced from the refining of crude oil, and has been used in special glues, for example in shoe-making, as a solvent in certain processes and as a laboratory chemical. Gasoline contains small amounts of n-hexane. Exposure to n-hexane in workplaces occurs primarily via inhalation.

Clinical effects and epidemiology

n-Hexane is not irritating and its acute toxicity is low. Acutely it may result in central nervous system (CNS) depression at exposure levels of approximately 1000–5000 ppm (3500–17 000 mg/m^3). (In this chapter, the ppm to mg/m^3 conversion is performed assuming a temperature of 20°C and an atmospheric pressure of 101.3 kPa, used in most European countries.) Its main hazards are, however, related to long-term exposure resulting in neurotoxicity. n-Hexane has been shown to induce peripheral neuropathy in humans, which was first observed in the shoe-manufacturing industry in Japan and Italy. In an early epidemiological study carried out in sandal manufacturing in the 1960s, 93 cases of polyneuropathy (both sensory and sensorimotor neuropathy) were diagnosed out of 296 examined workers.[1] Exposure levels were said to range from 500 to 2500 ppm (1700–9000 mg/m^3). Common signs and symptoms of n-hexane polyneuropathy include numbness in the distal portions of the extremities, muscle weakness, hypoactive reflexes, coldness, reddishness and roughness of the skin. Numbness in the feet and hands are the first symptoms to appear, followed by weakness in the lower legs and feet. The severity of the symptoms depends on the exposure: occupational exposure to 500 ppm (1700 mg/m^3) may result in overt neuropathy, whereas subclinical reductions in nerve conduction velocities may be observed after a few years of exposure at air levels of <100 ppm (<350 mg/m^3).[2–4]

Muscle wasting and atrophy have been reported in individuals with severe n-hexane neurotoxicity, although CNS symptoms may not be present. In EMG examination, abnormalities in conduction velocity, distal latency and action potential amplitudes have been reported.[4] The findings may be subclinical. Biopsies of peripheral nerves may show demyelination and infiltration of leukocytes. After cessation of exposure, gradual improvement may be seen. A follow-up study[5] of shoe manufacture workers diagnosed in the past with n-hexane polyneuropathy showed some improvement in motor nerve conduction velocities and distal latencies one year after the cessation of exposure. However, sensory nerve conduction velocities and distal latencies, while improved from those at diagnosis, were still statistically significantly worse than in controls. The neurotoxicity of n-hexane is caused by one of its metabolites, 2,5-hexanedione, which is formed by P450-mediated oxidative metabolism.[4] The mechanism of action of n-hexane polyneuropathy may involve formation of lysine adducts and cross-linking, resulting in neurofilament accumulation, axonal swelling and ultimate axonal degeneration.[4]

Methyl ethyl ketone (MEK) and methyl iso-butylketone (MiBK) have been shown to enhance the neurotoxicity of n-hexane via metabolic interaction.[4] It has also been suggested that acetone potentiates n-hexane neurotoxicity by decreasing the body clearance of 2,5-hexanedione.[6]

Metabolism and monitoring

n-Hexane is metabolized by mixed function oxidases in the liver to a number of metabolites including the neurotoxicant 2,5-hexanedione. Most of the absorbed n-hexane is excreted as metabolites in urine, with 2,5-hexanedione as the major metabolite. n-Hexane exposure can therefore be monitored by measuring 2,5-hexanedione in the urine.

Management and diagnosis

Diagnosis of n-hexane neuropathy is based on typical symptoms, neurophysiological examination (ENMG) and the assessment of exposure. Other possible causes of polyneuropathy, e.g. long-term alcohol abuse, diabetes, neurotoxic drugs, vitamin B_1, B_6 and B_{12} deficiencies, and inflammatory, infectious or malignant diseases causing polyneuropathy, must be excluded. Biological monitoring can be used in the assessment of current exposure and the management of n-hexane-related health risks.

1,3-BUTADIENE

[CAS No. 106-99-0]

1,3-Butadiene is a colourless gas, with a mild aromatic odour and an odour threshold between 0.4 and 1.7 ppm (1 and 4 mg/m^3). The main industrial uses of 1,3-butadiene include the manufacture of synthetic rubbers, such as styrene-butadiene rubber (SBR) and polybutadiene rubber, manufacture of thermoplastic resins like acrylonitrile-butadiene-styrene (ABS), and manufacture of styrene-butadiene latex. It is also used as a chemical intermediate, e.g. in the production of the nylon precursor hexamethylenediamine. The industrial use of butadiene occurs in closed systems. However, 1,3-butadiene is also found in cigarette smoke and in the combustion products of fossil fuels, and hence it is one of the impurities found in urban air.

Clinical effects and epidemiology

1,3-Butadiene has low acute toxicity. The main hazard related to butadiene is its carcinogenicity. Inhaled butadiene is metabolized in the body to active epoxide metabolites (1,2-epoxy-3-butene, 1,2,3,4-diepoxybutane and the monoepoxide diol, which are responsible for its carcinogenic effects.[7] The International Agency for Research on Cancer (IARC) has classified 1,3-butadiene as a known human carcinogen (group 1) on the basis of sufficient epidemiological and toxicological evidence.[8]

The most convincing evidence on butadiene carcinogenicity in humans comes from the large cohort studies of styrene-butadiene rubber manufacturing workers in the United States and Canada, which show a relationship between estimated cumulative butadiene exposure and leukaemia.[9–11] This relationship remained after correction for other confounding exposures, i.e styrene and dimethyldithiocarbamate. Although there are uncertainties related to dose–response relationships of butadiene-induced cancer, there is some indication of the role of peak exposures in the development of leukaemia. Peak exposure intensities of ≥ 100 ppm (230 mg/m^3) may be of importance in causing an increased cancer risk.[9,10]

Based on animal tests, butadiene may cause harm to the developing fetus.[7] Therefore, exposure during pregnancy should be avoided.

Metabolism and monitoring

The first step in 1,3-butadiene metabolism is the formation of epoxybutene (Figure 42.1). Further metabolism of epoxybutene can, however, proceed by a number of different pathways, with possible conjugation with glutathione, hydrolysis to monoepoxide diol, or further epoxidation to diepoxybutane. There are considerable species differences in the metabolism of butadiene, shown by diepoxybutane levels in the mouse exceeding those in the rat by up to 160-fold in some tissues at equivalent butadiene exposure levels.[7] This may explain the species differences in the carcinogenicity of butadiene. In humans, butadiene is metabolized to epoxybutene with subsequent hydrolysis to monoepoxy diol. There are no data on the formation of diepoxybutane in humans in vivo. However, considerable interindividual variation in the metabolism of butadiene has been observed, which raises the possibility that some humans may be quantitatively comparable to the mouse in terms of the production of diepoxybutene. Human low-level 1,3-butadiene exposure has been monitored by measuring haemoglobin adducts in the blood of exposed workers.[12,13] This method is, however, mainly used for research purposes.

Management and diagnosis

The management of butadiene-related cancer risks is mainly related to monitoring and controlling exposure to 1,3-butadiene to as low as technically feasible.

There are no unique diagnostic features for butadiene-caused leukaemias (nor indeed for almost all occupational malignancies). If there is a suspicion regarding butadiene as a cause of leukaemia in an individual, consideration should be given to the extent of exposure, and other possible exposures and risk factors for the disease.

Aromatic hydrocarbons

Aromatic hydrocarbons consist of unsaturated cyclic hydrocarbon compounds based on a benzene ring. Thus, benzene is the simplest member of this group. Other important compounds in this group include toluene, xylene and styrene, which have widespread use and well-documented central nervous system toxicity. These substances are discussed in detail below.

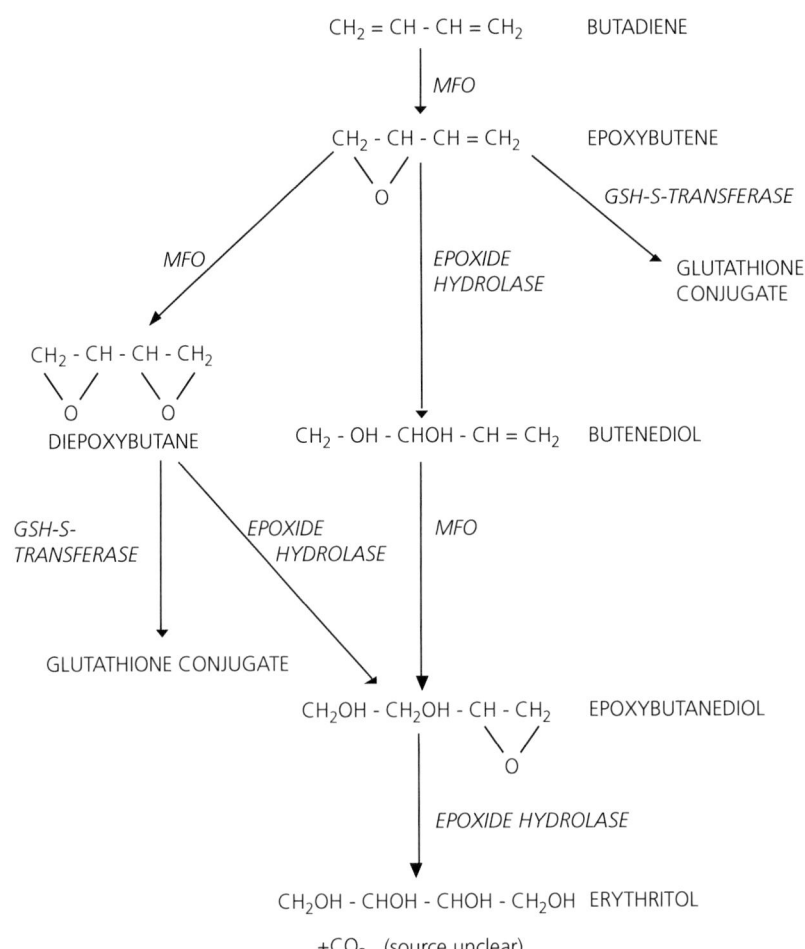

Figure 42.1 Metabolic routes for butadiene (from Ref. 7).

Other significant compounds in this group are ethylbenzene, cumene and vinyl toluene. Irritation and central nervous system effects are the main hazards related to these substances. Similar to styrene, ethylbenzene is metabolized to mandelic acid and phenylglyoxylic acid. Urinary mandelic acid can be used for the biomonitoring of ethylbenzene exposure.

BENZENE

[CAS No. 71-43-2]

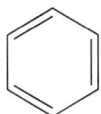

Benzene is a clear colourless liquid with a vapour pressure of 10 kPa at room temperature. Crude oil is the main natural source of benzene. Motor fuel and coal tar also contain benzene. In motor fuel, benzene exists usually at concentrations of 1–5 per cent. Exposure to benzene has occurred especially in the petroleum industry. Benzene is used also as an intermediate for chemical synthesis; it forms the basis for the production of a great variety of aromatic and cycloaliphatic compounds such as ethylbenzene, cumene, cyclohexane, nitrobenzenes, alkylbenzenes, chlorobenzene and maleic anhydride.[14] Only very small quantities are used nowadays as a laboratory reagent or as a solvent. Cigarette smoke also contains benzene.

Clinical effects and epidemiology

Occupational exposure to benzene occurs mainly by inhalation, but it is also well absorbed through the skin. Acute (few hours) exposure to benzene at exposure levels of >50–150 ppm (160–500 mg/m^3) can cause headache, weakness and drowsiness.[14] However, the most relevant health hazard of benzene in occupational settings is related to its long-term toxicity to the haemopoietic system.

Haematotoxicity

Benzene has been shown to induce haematotoxic effects varying from depression of white and red blood cell counts to potentially life-threatening aplastic anaemia and leukaemia. Decreases in white and red cell counts have been seen after long-term exposure to levels of >10–20 ppm (30–60 mg/m^3) of benzene. These effects on blood cell counts have usually been reversible, whereas aplastic anaemia resulting from bone marrow failure may be irreversible. According to recent studies,[15,16] the most sensitive reaction in humans to long-term benzene exposure is lymphocytopenia. When compared to controls, statistically lower lymphocyte counts have been reported in workers exposed to benzene levels of 1–31 ppm (3–100 mg/m^3).[15,16]

Leukaemia

Benzene is classified by IARC as a group 1 carcinogen[17] because of its ability to cause leukaemia in humans. Acute myeloid leukaemia (AML) has been shown to be related to benzene exposure. Also an association between benzene exposure and other types of haematological malignancies, such as multiple myeloma and non-Hodgkin's lymphoma, has been suggested.[18,19] Leukaemias caused by benzene have often been associated with predisposing myelodysplasia or aplastic anaemia.

Estimates on the exposure–response relationships of benzene-induced cancer vary between different studies, with some studies suggesting significant increases at cumulative exposures of <40 ppm years (e.g. exposure to 1 ppm concentration for 40 years) and some only at dose levels of 200 ppm years.[20,21] Other studies have suggested the role of high peak exposures.[22] The latency period for benzene-induced leukaemia may be up to ten years.[23]

Mechanisms behind benzene haematotoxicity and leukaemia are still unclear, but may include oxidative stress induced by benzene metabolites (especially phenolic metabolites, but also benzene oxide, trans, trans muconaldehyde), which may result in DNA damage in bone marrow cells.[24] Benzene is regarded as a genotoxic carcinogen since it has been shown to induce chromosomal aberrations and micronuclei in animal tests. However, most of the bacterial tests for gene mutations for benzene have been negative.[14,25,26] Genetic differences in benzene-metabolizing enzymes (especially CYP2E1) may affect the sensitivity of different individuals to benzene toxicity.

Metabolism and monitoring

Once absorbed, benzene is rapidly distributed throughout the body (Figure 42.2). Because of its lipophilicity, lipid-rich tissues have been found to contain the highest levels of benzene.[26] Benzene is metabolized to a number of metabolites by the cytochrome P450 mixed-function oxidase system. CYP2E1 is one of the most important isoenzymes metabolizing benzene. It has been shown that oxidative metabolism of CYP2E1 is needed for the induction of haematotoxic and genotoxic effects of benzene. Since ethanol is able to induce CYP2E1, alcohol consumption can enhance benzene toxicity.

Excretion of benzene metabolites occurs mainly in the urine, whereas after inhalation unchanged benzene is rapidly

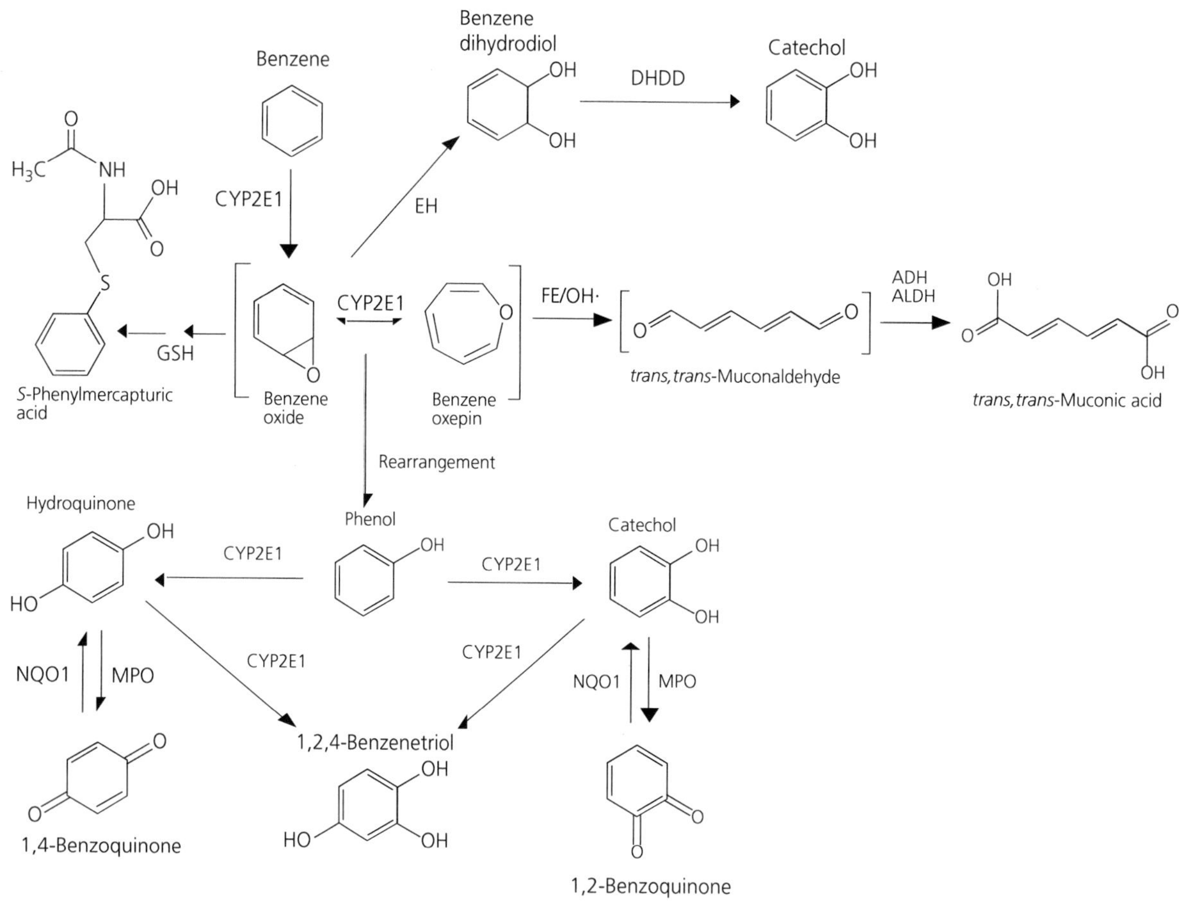

Figure 42.2 Metabolism of benzene.[25]

eliminated in exhaled air. The main metabolites measured in urine include *S*-phenyl mercapturic acid, *trans, trans*-muconic acid, phenol and phenolic metabolites. *Trans, trans*-muconic acid is commonly used for biological monitoring of benzene exposure, but at low exposure levels diet may interfere with the assessment since sorbic acid present in diet is also metabolized to *trans, trans*-muconic acid. *S*-phenyl mercapturic acid is not as sensitive to dietary effects and it has been shown to correlate well with blood benzene levels.[27] Since cigarette smoke contains benzene, smoking is one of the confounding factors in the interpretation of biomonitoring results.

Management and diagnosis

Monitoring and controlling of exposure to levels as low as technically feasible is important in the prevention of benzene-caused cancers. At the dose levels following modern standards for controlling exposure (e.g. to below the American Conference of Governmental Industrial Hygienists (ACGIH) threshold limit value (TLV) of 0.5 ppm (1.6 mg/m^3)), risks of developing health effects are likely to be very low.

If AML has been diagnosed, the classical circumstances that might support benzene as a potential cause are:[23]

- occurrence of certain forms of myelodysplastic syndrome;
- defects in chromosome 5 or 7;
- a substantial exposure history with a cumulative dose of at least 40 ppm-years during the preceding ten years;
- a poor response to anti-leukaemic chemotherapy.[23]

Confounding aetiologic factors include heavy cigarette smoking, previous exposure to chemotherapy or radiation, or certain underlying constitutional disorders, such as Down's syndrome or pernicious anaemia.[23] However, the occurrence of *de novo* AML and myelodysplasias in the general population increases dramatically with advancing age and these diseases may exhibit similar chromosomal changes as those found in benzene-caused AMLs in younger individuals, even without any specific history of hazardous exposures.[23]

TOLUENE, XYLENE AND STYRENE

Toluene (CAS No. 108-88-3), xylene (CAS No. 1330-20-7, mixed isomers) and styrene (CAS No. 100-42-5) are well-known and widely used aromatic hydrocarbons with a benzene ring-based structure. Toluene has one methyl group bound to benzene ring, whereas xylene has two methyl groups allowing three different isomers: *ortho-*, *meta-* and *para-*isomers. Styrene has a vinyl group with a double bond bound to benzene ring making it possible to form polymers.

Toluene (methyl benzene) is a volatile, highly flammable liquid with a vapour pressure of 3 kPa at 20°C. It has a sweet benzene-like odour. Toluene is produced by different petroleum conversion processes. The main use of commercial toluene is as an intermediate in the production of other chemicals, but it is also widely used as a solvent in paints, thinners, adhesives, inks and as an extraction solvent in the production of pharmaceutical and other chemical products.[28] Significant exposure to toluene may occur in painting, gluing (for example, in car or boat upholstery) or in rotogravure printing.

Xylene (dimethylbenzene) is a colourless liquid with a sweet benzene-like odour. Technical xylene is a mixture of xylene isomers with 4–20 per cent *o*-xylene, 44–60 per cent *m*-xylene and 12–20 per cent *p*-xylene. Some technical grades may also contain ethylbenzene and small amounts of benzene or toluene as an impurity. Xylene has a vapour pressure 0.8 kPa at 20°C. Like toluene, it is produced by petroleum conversion processes. Xylene is used as a solvent in a variety of different applications, but also to a great extent for further separation into the three isomers through distillations and fractionated crystallization. Separated isomers are used for the production of other chemicals, e.g. *ortho-*xylene is used for the synthesis of phthalic acid anhydride, and *para*-xylene for the production of dimethylterephthalate and terephthalic acid, which are then used for the production of polyethyleneterephthalate (PET). All three isomers are also raw materials for the synthesis of vitamins, pharmaceuticals and flavouring agents. Significant exposure to xylene may occur in painting, especially in spray painting with xylene.

Styrene (vinyl benzene) is a colourless to slightly yellow volatile liquid with a sweet and pungent odour. It has a vapour pressure of 0.6 kPa at 20°C. On exposure to light and air styrene polymerizes, but it can also oxidize to form certain aldehydes and ketones. Styrene is mainly produced commercially from crude oil. The main use of styrene is as a precursor to polystyrene, an important synthetic material. It is also used in the production of co-polymers, e.g. acrylonitrile–butadiene–styrene, styrene–acrylonitrile, methyl methacrylate–butadiene–styrene and in the production of styrene–butadiene rubber (SBR) and related latices (e.g. SB latex). In the production of glass-reinforced plastics, styrene is added to unsaturated polyester resins to act as a cross-linking agent and reactive diluent. It also acts as a solvent for the resins. Significant styrene exposure may occur in glass-reinforced plastic plants and in boat manufacturing.

All three compounds are well absorbed by inhalation. Dermal absorption also occurs and it contributes to total systemic exposure.

Clinical effects and epidemiology

Acute effects

The main target organ for these compounds is the central nervous system. In uncontrolled situations, all three compounds can easily form air concentrations resulting in acute central nervous system effects like headache, dizziness, drowsiness and drunkenness. Dose–response relationships on these acute effects are presented in Table 42.3. Accidental high-level exposures have also caused liver and kidney changes.[28–30]

Solvent-induced, long-term neurotoxicity

Long-term, low-level exposure to solvents may cause chronic neurotoxicity, which may become evident as so-called 'chronic solvent encephalopathy' (CSE) or 'chronic toxic encephalopathy' (CTE).[31] Symptoms related to chronic toxic encephalopathy are unspecific, including fatigue, poor memory, difficulties in concentration, emotional lability and depression.[32] Memory is suggested to be the first mental property to be impaired in chronic toxic encephalopathy.[32] The most persistent dysfunction in chronic toxic encephalopathy seems to be difficulties in tasks demanding working memory processing, which is a good predictor of the CSE status.[33] The memory deficits in CTE may resemble those seen in moderate or severe Parkinson's disease.[33]

Other neurobehavioural disorders related to CTE include possible defects in colour vision and visual perception. CSE patients may have impaired colour discrimination ability, despite their eyes and their other visual functions being normal.[34] Visual search performance may also be impaired when compared to healthy controls.[35]

Since occupational exposure to solvents usually involves mixtures of different solvents, it is difficult in epidemiological studies to show associations between a specific solvent exposure and long-term CNS effects. However, rotogravure printers are exposed almost purely to toluene and past exposure levels may have been considerable. There are some studies suggesting an increased risk of organic brain syndrome in these toluene-exposed workers. A higher frequency of organic brain syndrome in subjects exposed to toluene for more than 12 years has been observed.[36] In another study,[37] toluene-exposed workers had substantially more neurasthenic symptoms and scored lower in psychometric tests. However, in more recent studies no significant effects have been seen in rotogravure printers.[38,39] It appears that at low exposure levels in modern industry, the risk of long-term CNS effects from toluene is low.

Workers occupationally exposed to solvent mixtures including xylene have been reported to have neurophysiological and psychological disorders,[30] but since xylene is one of several different components of the solvent mixtures, it is difficult to attribute these effects to xylene alone.

Since high styrene exposures have occurred in the glass-reinforced plastics industry, there are many studies evaluating the neuropsychological effects of long-term styrene exposure. In some of these studies, effects on neurological and neuropsychological function have been seen but the results have been variable.[29,40] Benignus and co-workers[41] conducted a meta-analysis of several studies on styrene exposure and effects on reaction times (simple and choice reaction times: in simple reaction time (SRT), the subject must simply react to a predefined stimulus as quickly as possible, whereas in choice reaction time (CRT), the subject must first select between options before deciding whether to respond or not and how to respond) and colour

Table 42.3 Acute effects of toluene, xylene and styrene and their dose-response relationships.[28-30]

	Toluene	Xylene	Styrene
Eye or mucosal irritation	>75–100 ppm (300–400 mg/m³)	>460 ppm (2000 mg/m³)	Slight: >200 ppm (900 mg/m³) Severe: >375 ppm (1600 mg/m³)
Mild CNS effects	>75–100 ppm (300–400 mg/m³): headache, dizziness, feeling of intoxication and sleepiness. Impaired performance in neuropsychological tests	200–300 ppm (900–1300 mg/m³): slight effects on neuropsychological performance, including increased reaction times 700 ppm (3000 mg/m³): headache, dizziness, feeling of intoxication and sleepiness	>200 ppm (900 mg/m³): impairment in neuropsychological test performance 400–600 ppm (1700–2600 mg/m³): headache, dizziness, feeling of intoxication and sleepiness
Serious CNS effects and death	≥5000 ppm (20 000 mg/m³): unconsciousness and death	>5000 ppm (22 000 mg/m³): unconsciousness and death	800 ppm (3500 mg/m³): signs and symptoms of pronounced CNS depression ≥2500–5000 ppm (11 000–22 000 mg/m³): unconsciousness and death

vision (using a colour confusion index that measures the ability to discriminate between colours). According to this analysis, eight years of exposure to 20 ppm (90 mg/m^3) of styrene was estimated to produce a 6.5 per cent increase in CRT, whereas no significant effect was observed on SRT. An increase in colour confusion index (CCI) was seen; with similar exposures estimated to cause a 2.23 per cent increase in CCI, which is the same as the expected effect of 1.7 additional years of age in men.

Aromatic hydrocarbon solvents and ototoxicity

Organic solvents have also been suggested to induce ototoxicity. A review found the incidence of sensorineural hearing loss to be higher than expected in noise-exposed workers who were also exposed to solvents.[42] Aromatic hydrocarbon solvents are among the best studied occupational toxicants suggested to cause ototoxic effects in humans.

The most convincing data on the ototoxicity of industrial chemicals are those relating to styrene. Exposure to low levels of styrene and noise was studied in a cross-sectional study in Sweden.[43,44] According to the results, noise exposure (past and current) and urine mandelic acid levels (the biological marker for styrene exposure) were significantly related to the incidence of hearing loss; the odds ratios for hearing loss were 2.44 times greater for each mmol of mandelic acid per gram of creatinine, 1.18 times greater for each dB of current noise exposure, and 1.19 times greater for each year of age. Workers exposed to noise and styrene had significantly poorer pure-tone thresholds in the high-frequency range (3–8 kHz) than the controls or, for example, noise-exposed workers. Supporting results have been obtained in a Polish study in which hearing loss was observed in 76 per cent of the workers exposed to styrene and noise or styrene and toluene, in 57 per cent of the styrene-only group, 56 per cent in the noise-only group, and 33 per cent in the unexposed group. Hearing loss was observed in styrene-exposed workers (seen as higher mean audiometric thresholds, especially at 2–6 kHz, but also at 8 kHz frequencies).[45] Noise levels ranged from 78 to 86 dB and styrene levels in the styrene-exposed groups were from 11 to 38 ppm (48–160 mg/m^3) on average.

According to recent studies, styrene may also affect balance. Toppila and co-workers[46] evaluated the effects of low concentrations of styrene on balance among Finnish fibreglass-reinforced plastic boat manufacturers. They found impairment in postural stability in those working as laminators.

There are also some data suggesting an association between toluene exposure and an increase in the occurrence and severity of noise-induced hearing loss. Prevalence of hearing loss caused by toluene was evaluated in a study involving 124 rotogravure printing workers exposed to various levels of noise and an organic solvent mixture of toluene, ethyl acetate and ethanol.[47] Forty-nine per cent of the workers had hearing loss. Age and urinary hippuric acid (the biologic marker for toluene in urine) were significantly related to hearing loss. The odds ratio estimates for hearing loss were 1.76 times greater for each gram of hippuric acid per gram of creatinine.

Other long-term hazards

Styrene has caused lung tumours (mainly adenomas) in cancer bioassays in mice. In humans, no clear and consistent epidemiological evidence for the causal link between cancer and exposure to styrene exists. Mutagenicity of styrene is equivocal, although some studies show that styrene may be weakly clastogenic in humans. The possible genotoxicity and carcinogenicity of styrene is considered to be mediated through reactive metabolites, especially styrene 7,8 oxide (SO) and 4-vinylphenol (4-VP). Clara cells in mice bronchioles can metabolize styrene to these active metabolites. Since Clara cells are not as abundant in humans as in mice, there has been discussion regarding whether or not these carcinogenic effects seen in mice are relevant in humans. The IARC has classified styrene as a group 2B carcinogen.[48]

Based on animal studies, all these aromatic solvents may cause developmental toxicity.[28–30] The effects seen include decreases in birthweight, delayed development and developmental neurotoxicity. In the case of toluene, data on pregnant women sniffing toluene showed low birthweight and neurological dysfunction in their offspring.

These aromatic solvents have a degreasing effect on the skin of humans, resulting in dermatitis on repeated skin exposure. They are not known to be skin sensitizers.

Metabolism and monitoring

Toluene

Most of absorbed toluene is metabolized in the liver by the P450 system and excreted in urine (Figure 42.3). Around 20 per cent of absorbed toluene is eliminated in expired air. Toluene is metabolized via benzyl alcohol and benzaldehyde to benzoic acid, which is then conjugated with glycine and excreted in the urine as hippuric acid. If insufficient glycine is available, the benzoic acid may be conjugated with glucuronic acid to form benzoylglucuronide. Small amounts of toluene undergo ring hydroxylation to form o-, m- and p-cresol, which are excreted in the urine as sulphate or glucuronide conjugates.[28]

Toluene exposure can be monitored by measuring blood toluene levels or hippuric acid levels in urine. Although good correlation between toluene air levels and concentration of hippuric acid in post-shift urine samples have been demonstrated, background levels of hippuric acid formed as a product of endogenous metabolism, and metabolism of substances present in food may decrease the sensitivity of the method. At exposure levels below 100 ppm as eight-hour time-weighted average (TWA) (380 mg/m^3), urine hippuric acid cannot be used to separate an exposed person from an unexposed one.[49] In some developing countries, low urinary hippuric acid background levels are found, and so it can be used as a biological marker for toluene exposure even at exposure levels lower than 100 ppm (380 mg/m^3).[28]

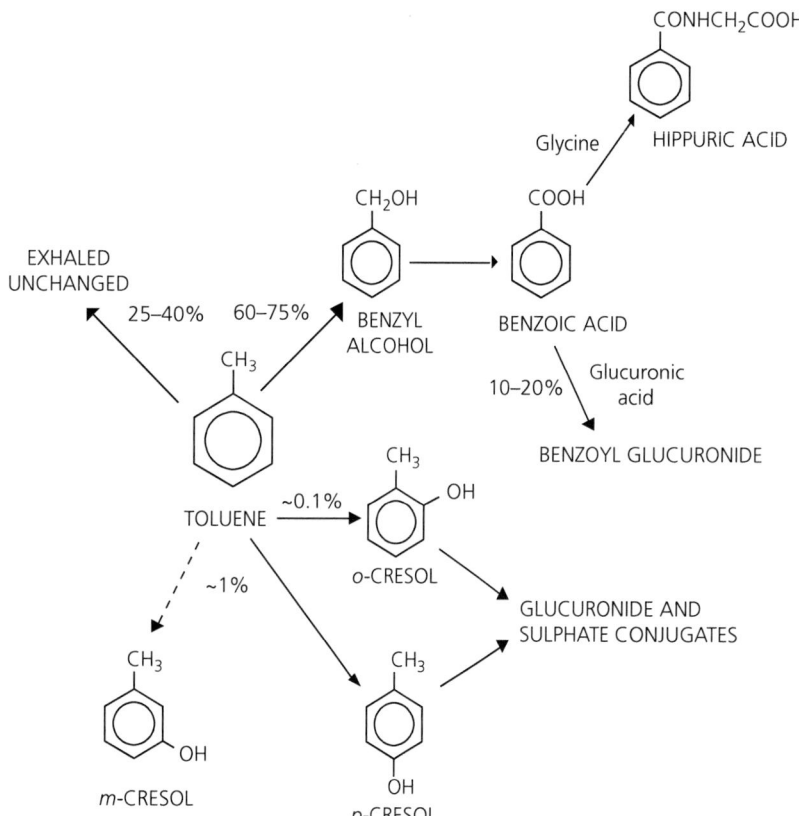

Figure 42.3 Metabolism of toluene.[50]

Styrene

Styrene can be metabolized via several different metabolic pathways, which have all been identified both in rodents and in humans, although there are species differences in their relative importance. The most important pathway involves cytochrome P450-mediated oxidation to styrene-7,8-oxide (SO). Specific P450 isoforms involved in the production of SO include CYP2E1, CYP2B6 and CYP2C8 in the liver and CYP2F2/1 and CYP2E1 in the lung.[29] SO is either further conjugated with glutathione to give mercapturic acid or hydrolysed by epoxide hydrolase to phenylglycol, which is further metabolized to mandelic, phenylglyoxylic and hippuric acids. Mandelic acid or combined urine levels of mandelic and phenylglyoxylic acids can be used to monitor styrene exposure (Figure 42.4).

Xylene

Absorbed xylenes are excreted mainly as metabolites in urine (Figure 42.5). Metabolism of xylenes in humans includes primarily side-chain oxidation to form methylbenzoic acid, which is subsequently conjugated mainly with glycine and excreted in urine as methylhippuric acid. More than 90 per cent of xylene is transformed to methylhippuric acid and excreted in urine.

Urinary methylhippuric acid has proved to be a robust measure of the amount of xylene taken up in the body and is therefore routinely used in many countries for the biomonitoring of xylene exposure.

Management and diagnosis

Chronic nervous system damage including CSE caused by long-term, low-level exposure has aroused significant controversy worldwide.[51–53] Therefore, the diagnosis and status of chronic solvent encephalopathy as an occupational disease varies in different countries. For example, in Scandinavian countries, chronic solvent encephalopathy is accepted as an occupational disease, with the diagnosis being based on a history of long-term, high-level exposure to solvents, specific signs and symptoms and exclusion of the other possible aetiological factors.

Neurotoxic symptoms of CSE can be screened by questionnaires,[54] including the Q16 questionnaire[55] and Euroquest (EQ).[56,57] Neuropsychological testing forms the basis of the diagnosis of solvent-caused organic brain disease. In some cases, neuroimaging (magnetic resonance imaging (MRI), single photon emission computed tomography (SPECT)) findings[58,59] and changes in colour vision tests may support the diagnosis. Other diseases, which may cause similar signs and symptoms, have to be considered in the differential diagnosis. These include clinical depression and other diseases resulting in organic brain disease, such as degenerative brain diseases, cerebrovascular

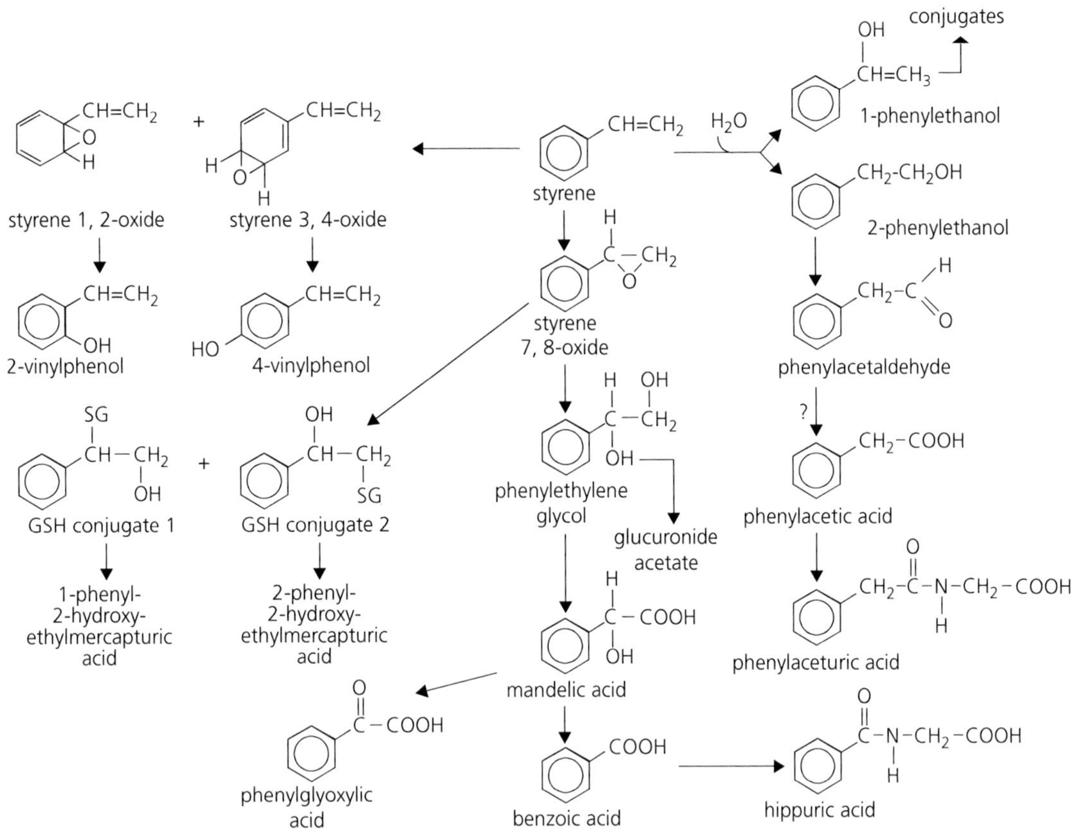

Figure 42.4 Metabolism of styrene.[60]

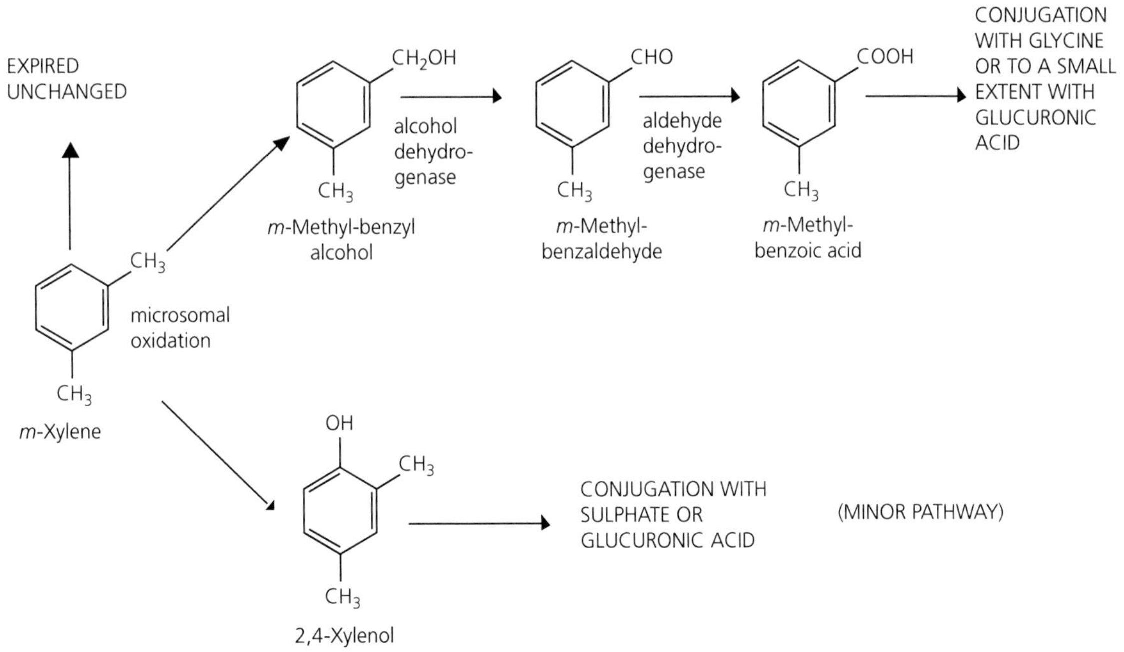

Figure 42.5 Metabolism of m-xylene.[30]

disease, brain injuries, tumours and infections, vitamin B_{12} deficiency, disturbances in cerebrospinal fluid circulation and effects caused by other toxic agents, for example alcohol and medicines. The progression of CSE usually stops after the cessation of exposure. If clear progression of organic brain disease occurs after the cessation of exposure, other aetiological causes for the disease should be considered.

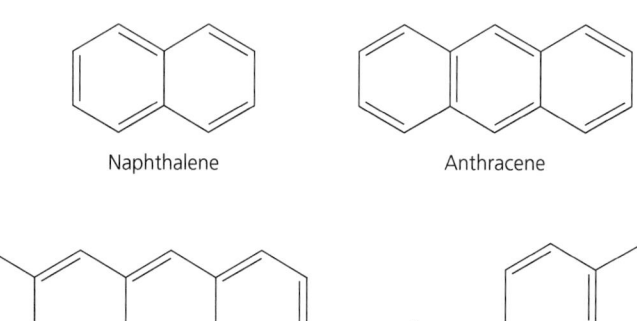
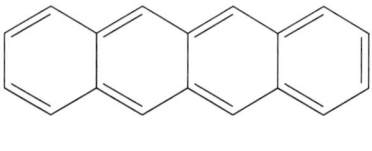
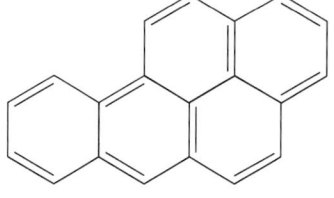

Figure 42.6 Polycyclic aromatic hydrocarbons: molecular structures of naphthalene, anthracene, naphthacene and benzo[a]pyrene.

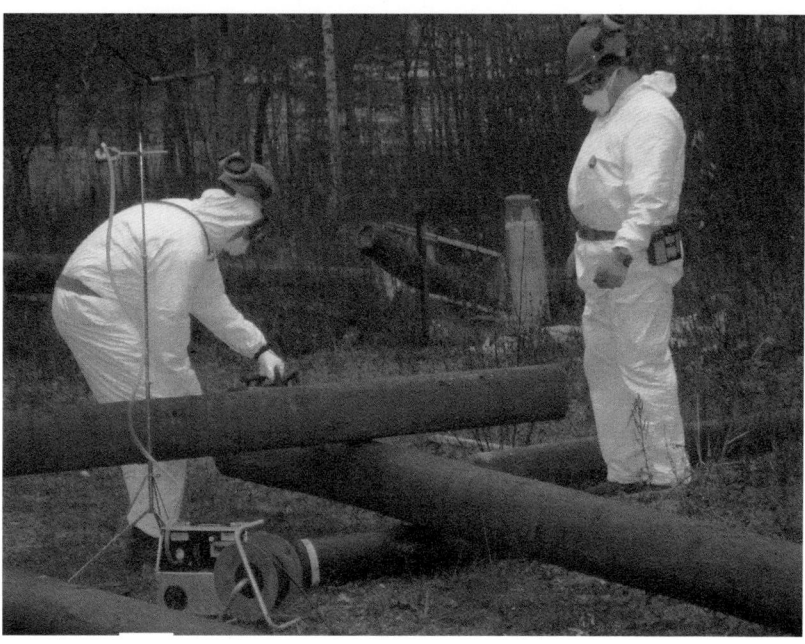

Figure 42.7 Handling of wood impregnated with creosote may result in significant polycyclic aromatic hydrocarbon exposure, unless appropriate personal protective measures are used. In this example, exposure is prevented by full-body protective clothing and respiratory protection. Reproduced with permission from the Finnish Institute of Occupational Health. For colour plate, see website (www.hodderplus.com/hunters).

Polycyclic aromatic hydrocarbons

Polycyclic aromatic hydrocarbons (PAHs) are formed in incomplete combustion processes. They exist almost always as mixtures of several different compounds, except single compounds such as naphthalene, which has been widely used in moth repellents for clothing.

PAHs consist of two or more fused benzene rings, the simplest being naphthalene, anthracene and naphthacene (Figure 42.6). The most well-known PAH compound is benzo[a]pyrene. Industry, traffic and heating produce PAH compounds in the environment. Thus, all individuals are exposed to PAHs via the environment, from cooking food, and from tobacco smoke.

Industrially important mixtures containing polycyclic aromatic hydrocarbons include coal tar creosote, which is used for wood impregnation (Figure 42.7), coal tar pitch and its distillation products, bitumen used for road paving, heating oils and diesel oils. Bitumen and diesel oil produced from crude oil contain 10–100 times less PAHs than creosote produced from coal tar.

Occupational exposure to PAHs occurs via the inhalation of fumes or aerosols containing PAHs, or via skin contact. Most PAH compounds have low vapour pressure and exist in particulate phase in workplace air, but some lighter PAHs, like naphthalene and phenanthrene, are found almost exclusively in gaseous phase. Occupations in which exposure to PAH mixtures may occur are listed in Table 42.4.

NAPHTHALENE

Naphthalene (CAS 91-20-3) is used as an intermediate for phthalic anhydride production and in the production of azo dyes and naphthalene sulphonic acids. The use of naphthalene as a moth repellent and insecticide has decreased in Europe since the introduction of chlorinated compounds, such as p-dichlorobenzene,[61] but it is still used for the production of moth balls in other countries. Naphthalene is a

Table 42.4 Occupations in which there is significant exposure to polycyclic aromatic hydrocarbons.[62]

Occupation
Coke oven work
Coal gasification
Foundry work
Aluminium production
Impregnation of wood with creosote
Handling of creosote-impregnated wood
Asphalt and pavement work
Use of coal tar in roofing
Chimney sweeping
Graphite electrode production
Petroleum refineries
Smokehouses (for smoked meat and fish)

white solid, which has a vapour pressure (sublimation pressure) of 10 Pa at room temperature. It has a characteristic odour with a very low odour threshold of 0.08 ppm (0.4 mg/m^3).

Clinical effects and epidemiology

Non-cancer effects

The acute toxicity of PAHs varies from moderate to low. Systemic toxicity, other than carcinogenicity, is very rare. The only PAH compound known to cause significant acute or systemic toxicity in humans is naphthalene.

Naphthalene causes haemolytic anaemia. It has caused several poisoning accidents when naphthalene-containing moth balls have been eaten. Serious poisonings after dermal or inhalation exposures have been described mainly in small children who have been exposed to naphthalene via moth ball-treated nappies, clothing or blankets.[61,62] The lethal oral dose of naphthalene in humans is 5–15 g in adults. The first signs and symptoms of naphthalene poisoning include nausea, vomiting, diarrhoea, dark urine, pallor, fever and abdominal pain. On clinical examination, the liver and spleen may be enlarged and jaundice may be present. On haematology, fragmentation of red blood cells with anisocytosis and poikilocytosis, and reduction in haemoglobin and haematocrit levels are seen. More severe reactions include Heinz body formation, haemoglobinuria and mild methaemoglobinaemia. Individuals who are deficient in G-6-PD (glucose 6-phosphate dehydrogenase) are particularly sensitive to haemolytic anaemia produced by naphthalene.[63] Occupational exposure has not, however, been reported to cause naphthalene poisoning or haemolytic anaemia.

PAH mixtures, like coal tar pitch and coal tar creosote, have been shown to induce phototoxicity in humans. The symptoms appear when PAH-exposed skin parts are exposed to sunlight. Skin irritation, dermatitis, hyperpigmentation and even blisters may be observed.

In animal tests, different PAHs have been reported to have immunosuppressive effects. The relevance of these effects to human exposures is, however, unclear.

Carcinogenicity of PAHs

The main hazard related to polycyclic aromatic hydrocarbons is their potential mutagenicity and carcinogenicity. The first occupational cancers caused by PAHs were described in 1775 when Sir Percival Pott described scrotal cancers in chimney sweeps exposed to soot. The ability of individual PAHs to induce cancer varies. Since human exposure to PAHs is almost exclusively a mixed exposure, data on the carcinogenicity of the individual PAHs come from animal tests. Although some individual PAHs are extensively tested, there are many PAH compounds for which the toxicological data are very limited. The IARC has recently classified several PAH compounds according to their carcinogenicity; the results of the IARC classification are shown in Table 42.5.

Many PAH compounds have shown mutagenic activity in mutagenicity tests. The mechanism of the carcinogenicity of PAH compounds is considered to be related to the formation of DNA binding species, mainly diol epoxides in the body resulting in mutagenicity.[64]

Naphthalene has caused nasal cancers in carcinogenicity tests in animals after inhalation exposure. Naphthalene is, however, not genotoxic and it has been suggested that the mechanism of naphthalene-caused nasal cancers is mainly related to local tissue damage. This may, therefore, be relevant for humans only at high exposure levels that cause considerable local nasal irritation.[62]

The carcinogenicity of several work tasks involving significant PAH exposures has been studied in epidemiological studies. In the case of coal gasification, epidemiological studies have consistently shown an excess of lung cancer associated with gas production.[64] Also, most of the epidemiological studies have provided evidence of an excess risk for lung cancer among coke production workers.[64,65] Additionally, in the case of aluminium production, an association between cancer and PAH exposure has been demonstrated.[64,65] A recent meta-analysis of PAH exposure and lung cancer estimated the risk equivalent to a relative risk of 1.06 for a working lifetime at 1 μg/m^3 exposure to benzo[a]pyrene for exposures in the coke ovens, gas works and aluminum industries.[65] All these work tasks have been recently evaluated by the IARC and designated as carcinogenicity group 1 (carcinogenic to humans).[64,100] Other work tasks evaluated by the IARC and assigned to carcinogenicity group 1 because of the PAH exposure include coal tar distillation, paving and roofing with coal tar pitch, and chimney sweeping.[64,100]

Creosote has been shown to induce local skin cancers in mice at the site of application.[66] In cohort studies of Swedish and Norwegian wood impregnators and in Finnish round-timber workers, increased risks for lip and skin cancers have been observed.[66–68] However, epidemiological data on the carcinogenicity of creosote are still

Table 42.5 Carcinogenicity classification of different polycyclic aromatic hydrocarbons according to a recent IARC evaluation.[64]

Group	Polycyclic aromatic hydrocarbons
1	Benzo[a]pyrene
2A	Cyclopenta[cd]pyrene, dibenz[a,h]anthracene, dibenzo[a,l]pyrene
2B	Naphthalene, benz[j]aceanthrylene, benz[a]anthracene, benzo[b]fluoranthene, benzo[j]fluoranthene, benzo[k]fluoranthene, benzo[c]phenanthrene, chrysene, dibenzo[a,h]pyrene, dibenzo[a,i]pyrene, indeno[1,2,3-cd]pyrene, 5-methylchrysene
3	Acenaphthene, acepyrene (3,4-dihydrocyclopenta[cd]pyrene), anthanthrene, anthracene, 11H-benz[bc]aceanthrylene, benz[l]aceanthrylene, benzo[b]chrysene, benzo[g]chrysene, benzo[a]fluoranthene, benzo[ghi]fluoranthene, benzo[a]fluorene, benzo[b]fluorene, benzo[c]fluorene, benzo[ghi]perylene, benzo[e]pyrene, coronene, 4H-cyclopenta[def]chrysene, 5,6-cyclopenteno-1,2-benzanthracene, dibenz[a,c]anthracene, dibenz[a,j]anthracene, dibenzo[a,e]fluoranthene, 13H-dibenzo[a,g]fluorene, dibenzo[h,rst]pentaphene, dibenzo[a,e]pyrene, dibenzo[e,l]pyrene, 1,2-dihydroaceanthrylene, 1,4-dimethylphenanthrene, fluoranthene, fluorene, 1-methylchrysene, 2-methylchrysene, 3-methylchrysene, 4-methylchrysene, 6-methylchrysene, 2-methylfluoranthene, 3-methylfluoranthene, 1-methylphenanthrene, naphtho[1,2-b]fluoranthene, naphtho[2,1-a]fluoranthene, naphtho[2,3-e]pyrene, perylene, phenanthrene, picene, pyrene, triphenylene

International Agency for Research on Cancer (IARC) classification: Group 1, carcinogenic to humans; group 2A, probably carcinogenic to humans; group 2B, possibly carcinogenic to humans; group 3, not classifiable for its carcinogenicity.

quite limited. The IARC has classified creosote as probably carcinogenic to humans (IARC group 2B[64]). Other PAH-containing mixtures classified by IARC for their carcinogenicity include coal tar pitch, coal tars and soots (group 1[69]), diesel engine exhausts (group 2A[70]) and bitumen (group 2B[69]).

Metabolism and monitoring

PAH compounds are absorbed through the lungs and skin. The metabolism of PAH is complex: parent compounds are converted via intermediate epoxides to phenols, diols and tetrols, which can then be conjugated with sulphuric or glucuronic acids or with glutathione. PAH metabolites and their conjugates are excreted in urine and faeces. Urinary 1-hydroxypyrene, which is the metabolism product of pyrenol, has been commonly used as a biological marker of exposure to PAH compounds. 1-Naphthol has been used as a marker of naphthalene exposure.

Management and diagnosis

Management of PAH-related cancer risks is mainly related to good industrial hygienic practice and monitoring and controlling of the exposure to PAHs to as low as technically feasible. Special attention should be paid to avoidance of skin exposure. Urinary 1-hydroxypyrene measurement is especially important when exposure occurs mainly via the skin.

There are no identified special features in PAH-induced cancers. If suspicion on the aetiological role of PAH exposure for the cancer (especially lung or skin cancer) arises, consideration should take account of the extent of the long-term exposure to PAHs, and other possible confounding exposures and aetiological factors that may be responsible for the disease (smoking, sun exposure, etc.).

Hydrocarbon mixtures

There are a number of hydrocarbon mixtures consisting of different aliphatic and aromatic hydrocarbons, the final properties of the mixture depending on its special hydrocarbon composition. Many different hydrocarbon mixtures are produced by distillation of crude oil. These include:[71]

- Petroleum solvents, which can be divided on the basis of their distillation ranges to:
  - special boiling-point solvents, which are mixtures of C-5 to C-9 normal- and branched-chain paraffins and cycloparaffins with a boiling range of 30–160°C;
  - white spirits, used extensively as industrial solvents, which have longer chain-length (C-7 to C-12) and higher boiling range (150–220°C) and contain various amounts of aromatic compounds; and
  - high boiling point (BP) aromatic solvents (BP 160–300°C) containing more than nine carbon atoms per molecule.
- gasolines, kerosene and other fuel oils (such as diesel fuel, jet fuel)
- lubricant base oils, greases and waxes
- bitumen.

Of the petroleum solvents, white spirits are the most important due to their toxicological properties and widespread use.

The main health hazards related to gasoline include its potential carcinogenicity due to its benzene content and central nervous system depressant properties at high exposure levels.

Table 42.6 Three different types of white spirits, which can be separated by their different production processes (modified from Ref. 74).

Type of white spirit	CAS	Production process	Aromatic content	Benzene content	Description
1	64742-82-1	Hydro-desulphurized	<25	<0.1	Hydrocarbons with carbon numbers predominantly in the 7–12 range and boiling points in the range of 90 to 230°C
2	64741-92-0	Solvent extracted	<5	<0.02	Predominantly aliphatic hydrocarbons with carbon numbers predominantly in the 7–12 range and boiling points in the range of 90 to 230°C
3	64742-48-9	Hydrogenated (hydrotreated)	<1	<0.002	Hydrocarbons (mainly aliphatics and cycloalkanes) with carbon numbers predominantly in the 6–13 range and boiling points in the range of 65 to 230°C

Kerosene and other fuel oils have also been studied for carcinogenicity, but the results are inconclusive. Certain types of fuel oils may contain significant amounts of polycyclic aromatic hydrocarbons in addition to aliphatic and aromatic hydrocarbons, but the PAH content of, for example, kerosene and diesel fuel is less than 5 per cent.[72] The IARC has determined that residual (heavy) fuel oils and marine diesel fuel are possibly carcinogenic to humans (group 2B). However, evidence on the carcinogenicity of distillate (light) fuel oils or distillate (light) diesel fuels is inconclusive (IARC group 3).[73]

Bitumen (asphalt) is a complex mixture of naphthenic, aliphatic and/or aromatic hydrocarbons and heterocyclic compounds containing sulphur, nitrogen and oxygen. It is mainly used for paving roads. It has been studied extensively for the possible carcinogenicity of its vapours and aerosols formed during paving. These vapours and aerosols also contain polycyclic aromatic hydrocarbons.[69]

WHITE SPIRITS

White spirits are colourless liquids with boiling points between 130 and 230°C and vapour pressures between 0.1 and 1.4 kPa at 20°C (Table 42.6). They are mixtures of saturated aliphatic and alicyclic hydrocarbons (mainly C7–C12) and aromatic hydrocarbons (C7–C12). In the past, they have contained benzene, but modern white spirits usually contain very little or no benzene. The most widely used quality of white spirit (white spirit type 1, stoddard solvent, CAS 8052-41-3) contains 80–85 per cent (by weight) aliphatic and alicyclic alkanes and 15–20 per cent (by weight) aromatic hydrocarbons.[74]

The various types and grades of white spirit are produced from straight-run naphtha and straight-run kerosene, which are refinery streams obtained from the distillation of crude oil. Fractional distillation into appropriate boiling ranges and different kind of treatments are used to obtain the desired type of white spirit. The current trend in western countries is towards increased use of low aromatic white spirits.

Straight-run white spirit (type 0, CAS 64742-88-7) is a white spirit that has not been treated beyond the process of distillation. Types 1, 2 and 3 are further divided into three technical grades defined by flash point: 'low flash' white spirit, 'regular flash' white spirit and 'high flash' white spirit.

White spirits are widely used in paints and varnishes, in cleaning products and as a degreasing and extraction solvent. The main use is in paints and as a paint diluent. The odour threshold of white spirit is quite low; vapours can be detected at air levels of 0.5–5 mg/m^3. Exposure to white spirits occurs mainly through inhalation, but absorption through the skin may also occur.[74]

Clinical effects and epidemiology

Vapours of white spirit can cause eye and mucous membrane irritation at air levels of 600 mg/m^3 (100 ppm). At higher levels, dizziness, drowsiness, headache and nausea may be induced. In controlled volunteer studies, exposure to white spirit for seven hours at 600 mg/m^3 or more has resulted in impaired balance and increased reaction times.[74] Skin exposure may result in defatting of the skin from repeated exposure.

According to several studies in painters, white spirits may cause chronic solvent encephalopathy. The clinical picture of the disease is the same as described in the case of aromatic hydrocarbon solvents, with symptoms including fatigue, poor memory, difficulties in concentration, emotional lability and depression.[31,74,75] The incidence of symptoms increases with increasing number of years of exposure.[75] Impaired performance in neuropsychological tests may be seen. Chronic solvent encephalopathy induced by white spirits may also be associated with defects in colour vision and visual perception, which has been suggested in studies of patients with a diagnosis of chronic solvent encephalopathy.[34,35]

In the past, white spirits contained small amounts of benzene. However, nowadays benzene levels are very minimal or negligible. The carcinogenicity of white spirit has not been fully evaluated.

Metabolism and monitoring

Since white spirits are complex mixtures of several different hydrocarbons with varying composition, general metabolic pathways or specific monitoring methods cannot be provided for white spirits.

Management and diagnosis

The diagnosis of chronic solvent-induced encephalopathy follows the principles described above under Toluene, xylene and styrene, p. 327.

ALCOHOLS

Alcohols share the common property of an -OH group in a carbon chain; primary alcohols in the form of R-CH$_2$OH, secondary alcohols R$_1$R$_2$CHOH and tertiary alcohols R$_1$R$_2$R$_3$C-OH. With increasing chain length, the volatility, water solubility and skin penetration capacity of the alcohol decrease. Toxicity per mole absorbed increases with increasing chain length, but methanol is an important exception.

Alcohols are very extensively used as solvents and also as building blocks in organic synthesis.

The acute toxic effects of alcohols, notably of the low-boiling alcohols, such as methanol, ethanol and propanols, is mostly due to the ingestion of large quantities, but adverse effects have also been described after occupational inhalation and dermal exposure. The common and most apparent effect of alcohols on humans, is the effect on the central nervous system.

METHANOL

[CAS No. 67-56-1]

Methanol is a clear, colourless, volatile flammable liquid with a mild alcoholic odour. It is, as measured by production volume, one of the most used organic chemicals. It is used in the production of acetic acid and formaldehyde and as a starting material for the synthesis of methyl-*tert*-butyl ether (MTBE), which is an octane-enhancing and oxygen-donating additive in automotive gasoline. Methanol has also been used as a gasoline additive.

Clinical effects and epidemiology

After exposure, methanol has an acute depressive effect on central nervous system function. This is followed by a symptom-free latent period lasting usually 12–24 hours, occasionally up to two days. Thereafter, dizziness, headache, nausea, vomiting, gastrointestinal pain, blurred vision and pain and light-sensitivity of the eyes follow. The late symptoms are caused by the accumulation of the toxic metabolite, formic acid, which causes a metabolic acidosis (low blood pH, anion gap, compensatory low arterial pCO_2). Untreated metabolic acidosis may lead to death. The ocular effects are likely to be induced by inhibition of the cytochrome oxidase by formate.

The damage to the retina may be permanent and varies from slight visual disturbance to complete blindness. In mild cases, visual disturbances may disappear with time.

Epidemics with high mortality have been described from the ingestion of illicitly distilled spirits containing methanol.[76–78] There are case reports and case series of serious, even fatal methanol poisoning following inhalation, and even dermal exposure.[79–81]

Limited testing in animals has revealed no carcinogenic effects of methanol in animals. Methanol is not genotoxic. Oral and inhalation exposure (usually at exposure levels >10 000 ppm; 13 000 mg/m^3) to methanol induced teratogenesis (usually neural and ocular defects, cleft palate, hydronephrosis, deformed tails and limb (paw and digit) anomalies) in mice. This effect apparently is not mediated by the action of formate.[82–86]

Metabolism and monitoring

Methanol is oxidized by alcohol dehydrogenase to formaldehyde, and this is further oxidized by aldehyde dehydrogenase to formic acid (Figure 42.8). Formic acid is the actual toxic species: it induces metabolic acidosis, and in humans is cleared slowly, with the half-times generally being between three and ten hours, but cases with a half-time of 77 hours have been reported.[87,88]

Management and diagnosis

Methanol intoxication should be suspected when a patient with a history of exposure to methanol presents with metabolic acidosis, with or without effects on vision. Diagnosis may be aided by the analysis of methanol and formate in serum. Elevated concentration of formate in serum is not

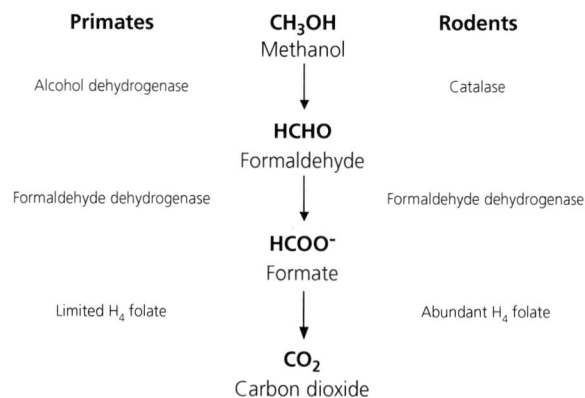

Figure 42.8 Metabolism of methanol in primates (including humans) and rodents.[89]

specific for methanol intoxication (there may have been exposure to formate itself), but it is useful in the monitoring of the efficacy of treatment and also in the assessment of the need for haemodialysis.

The traditional management of methanol poisoning makes use of the fact that the toxicity of methanol is due to the oxidation of methanol to formate: this reaction is blocked by administration of ethanol, which competitively and effectively blocks methanol oxidation. The same effect may be achieved by administration of methylpyrazole (fomepizole). Fomepizole has recently gained popularity over ethanol as the main therapeutic choice, as it is easier to maintain the therapeutic concentration with fomepizole than with ethanol – for which there is a wide variation in the clearance kinetics.[90]

Formate may be removed from the body by haemodialysis. It has been recommended that haemodialysis should be started if the blood methanol concentration exceeds 50 mg/dL (15.8 mmol/L).[87]

In addition to the methods chosen to decrease the generation of formate from methanol, the metabolic acidosis has to be corrected by use of sodium bicarbonate. Furthermore, it may be advantageous to facilitate the conversion of formic acid to carbon dioxide by the administration of folinic acid.

Occupational exposure to methanol may be assessed through biological monitoring by the analysis of methanol in urine.[91] As an alternative, analysis of urinary formate has also been suggested.[92] However, meaningful interpretation is only possible if the sample is collected in the morning after the exposure (16 hours after the cessation of the exposure) because of accumulation in the body over time.

ETHYLENE GLYCOL

[CAS No. 107-21-1]

HO~~~OH

Ethylene glycol is a clear, colourless, odourless, relatively non-volatile, viscous liquid. It is used primarily in the production of polyesters for fibres and films, and polyethylene terephthalate. It is also used in a broad range of products, including paints, lacquers and resins, adhesives, coolants and hydraulic brake fluids, automotive antifreeze/coolants, and as a component of de-icing fluids for aircraft, runways and taxiways.[93,94]

Clinical effects and epidemiology

Numerous case reports on ethylene glycol poisoning, several with fatal outcome, have been described after ingestion of ethylene glycol; published minimal lethal doses in humans have ranged from approximately 0.3 to 1.4 g/kg body weight. Signs of toxicity following ingestion are due mainly to effects on the central nervous system: inebriation, lethargy, seizures and coma. These are followed by metabolic acidosis, hyperkalaemia, hypocalcaemia, concomitant with tachycardia and hypertension. Finally, haematuria, renal tubular necrosis and renal failure may develop.[93,94]

Following inhalation exposure, ethylene glycol toxicity observed in humans has been low, nose and throat irritation being the major findings. Notably, metabolic acidosis and renal effects have not been reported after inhalation exposure. Ethylene glycol is a mild irritant to the eyes and skin. Contact dermatitis has not been reported.

In experimental animals, ethylene glycol is not mutagenic and limited carcinogenicity testing has not shown evidence of carcinogenicity. Ethylene glycol is teratogenic in rats and mice at doses lower than those overtly toxic to the dams.

Metabolism and monitoring

Ethylene glycol is effectively absorbed from the gastrointestinal tract and by inhalation. Dermal absorption is slower and less complete, but has reached 20–30 per cent in six hours in experimental animals.[93] Ethylene glycol is oxidized by alcohol dehydrogenase to glycol aldehyde, and subsequently to glycolic acid, formic acid and oxalic acid (Figure 42.9).

Acidosis and subsequent renal toxicity after high oral doses of ethylene glycol is caused by metabolites of ethylene glycol, notably by oxalic acid, which crystallizes in the kidneys. Cytotoxicity of other metabolites, such as glycoaldehyde, glycolic acid, and glyoxylic and formic acids, may contribute to the renal damage (with the acids contributing to the acidosis).

Management and diagnosis

Ethylene glycol poisoning should be suspected in cases with metabolic acidosis with anion and osmolal gap. A diagnosis may be reached from the analysis of oxalic acid and ethylene glycol in urine or blood.

As the renal toxicity ensues from the action of metabolites, toxicity may be prevented by the inhibition of ethylene

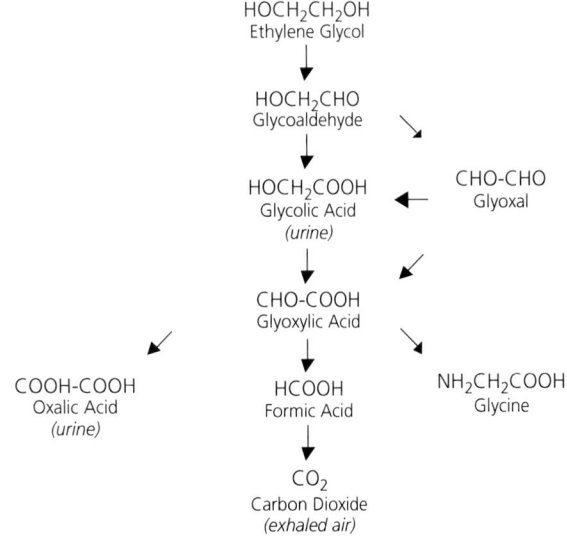

Figure 42.9 Metabolism of ethylene glycol.[94]

glycol metabolism. The treatment includes correction of the acidosis, hyperkalaemia and hypocalcaemia, treatment of seizures, and inhibition of the metabolism of ethylene glycol with ethanol infusion, or fomepizole. Ethylene glycol and the toxic metabolites may be removed by haemodialysis.[95]

ALDEHYDES

Aldehydes have the common structure R-CHO. They react avidly especially with thiols and amines. Because of the reactivity, many of them are irritants or even corrosive, and in experimental systems, genotoxic and cytotoxic. Also because of the reactivity, they tend to have a short half-life, and their effects are mostly limited to the site of entry. Exposure to liquid aldehydes tends to cause contact eczema by irritation or sensitization.

FORMALDEHYDE

[CAS No. 50-00-0]

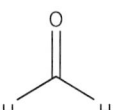

Formaldehyde is a flammable, colourless and readily polymerized gas at ambient temperature with a pungent, suffocating odour. Formaldehyde solution (formalin) is a clear, colourless liquid with a pungent odour. The most common commercially available form of formalin is a 30–50 per cent aqueous solution containing methanol. Formaldehyde is used mainly as an intermediate in the chemical industry for the production of resins for the wood, paper and textile processing industries and in the synthesis of methylene dianiline, diphenylmethane diisocyanate, hexamethylenetetraamine, trimethylol propane, neopentylglycol, pentaerythritol and acetylenic agents. Aqueous solutions of formaldehyde are employed as germicides, bactericides and fungicides. Tobacco smoke, release from urea-formaldehyde foam insulation, formaldehyde-containing disinfectants and preservatives in consumer products, as well as from engine exhausts are important sources of formaldehyde exposure. Formaldehyde is also a product of intermediary metabolism.[96,97]

It is quickly metabolized and even at high inhalation exposure levels, elevated concentrations of formaldehyde have not been observed in the blood. Thus, the most likely targets for formaldehyde action are the sites of immediate contact, i.e. the respiratory tract epithelium and the skin.

Clinical effects and epidemiology

Irritation of the eyes and respiratory tract by formaldehyde has been observed consistently in clinical studies and epidemiological surveys, usually when the concentration of formaldehyde in the air exceeds approximately 0.1 ppm (0.1 mg/m^3). At higher concentrations, formaldehyde may also contribute to the induction of obstructive effects on lung function, which are usually quantitatively minor and reversible.[96] The respiratory effects of formaldehyde may be mediated by an immunological mechanism, but respiratory sensitization to formaldehyde is apparently rare.

Dermal exposure to formaldehyde in solution causes skin irritation and can provoke contact eczema through irritation, but also through an immunological mechanism affecting susceptible individuals. Contact dermatitis may be elicited in sensitized individuals following exposure to formaldehyde at concentrations as low as 30 mg/L.[98]

A large number of epidemiological studies have investigated the possible role of formaldehyde as a causative agent for cancer in different parts of the respiratory tract and of leukaemia. In October 2009, IARC concluded that 'there is sufficient evidence in humans of an increased incidence of nasopharyngeal carcinomas among formaldehyde-exposed people', and the epidemiological evidence on leukaemia has become stronger with new studies. For both cancer types, the group 1 classification is supported by strong mechanistic evidence.[99,100]

Inhalation exposure to formaldehyde induced squamous cell carcinoma in the nasal cavity in rats. Formaldehyde is genotoxic *in vitro*; it also induced protein–DNA crosslinks and cellular proliferation in respiratory epithelium in experimental animals after inhalation exposure. It is likely that both genotoxicity and cell proliferation contribute to the carcinogenic action of formaldehyde.[96,99,100]

Metabolism and monitoring

Formaldehyde is rapidly absorbed from the respiratory tract and metabolized mainly to formic acid and carbon dioxide. Part of the inhaled formaldehyde undergoes intermediary metabolism. Elevated formaldehyde levels in the plasma or urine have not been demonstrated after inhalation exposure to formaldehyde in humans or experimental animals.

GLUTARALDEHYDE

[CAS No. 111-30-8]

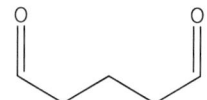

Glutaraldehyde is a colourless, oily liquid which crosslinks with proteins and, in aqueous solutions, partially polymerizes to form oligomers. Glutaraldehyde is used as an immersion disinfectant in a 1 or 2 per cent aqueous solution for sterilizing endoscopes and other surgical instruments; as a hardener in x-ray film processing; for the prevention of microbial growth and metal corrosion in circulating water systems, including off-shore operations; as a biocide in the petroleum, pulp and paper industries; and as a preservative in industrial cleaning agents for example, in the food, beverage and tobacco manufacturing industries, and in retail detergents. It is used to disinfect animal housing and bird cages in the form of sprays and by fogging, and to control microorganisms in fish farming. Aqueous solutions of glutaraldehyde are used to soften leathers and to improve their resistance to water, alkalis and mould. It is also used as a tissue fixative in histology and electron and light microscopy. Glutaraldehyde is allowed as a preservative for cosmetics in Europe, but not in the form of aerosols or sprays.[101]

Clinical effects and epidemiology

Glutaraldehyde is an irritant at high concentrations and is corrosive to the skin, eyes and respiratory membranes. The irritative effect is accentuated by the presence of bicarbonate which is added to the glutaraldehyde solutions in use to improve their efficacy as a disinfectant.

In some patients with glutaraldehyde-induced contact dermatitis, there is a positive reaction in patch testing, indicating an immunological mechanism. Immunological processes may also be involved in the respiratory effects (asthma, rhinitis) of glutaraldehyde.[102,103]

In experimental animals, glutaraldehyde is positive in genotoxicity studies *in vitro*, but usually negative in *in vivo* studies. Exposures causing maternal toxicity induce embryo- and fetotoxicity, but teratogenicity has not been reported.[101]

KETONES

The basic structure of ketones is $R_1R_2C=O$. The most commonly used ketones are acetone, methylethylketone, methyl isobutylketone, cyclohexanone, 4-hydroxy-4-methyl-2-pentanone, isophorone, mesityl oxide and acetophenone. Ketones are very extensively used notably as solvents, as they dissolve organic compounds. Ketones are irritating to the mucous membranes and skin. They induce central nervous system depression. Ketones have no sensitizing potential; they are generally not mutagenic, or toxic to reproduction, and have not been shown to be carcinogenic.

ACETONE

[CAS No. 67-64-1]

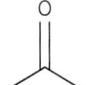

Acetone is the simplest of ketones. It is a clear and colourless liquid with a strong 'fruity' odour. Acetone is extensively used as an industrial solvent, and in inks, paints, varnishes and other consumer products. It is a starting material for the synthesis of other ketones, such as isophorone and methyl isobutylketone, and other organic chemicals, for example methyl methacrylate and bisphenol A. Acetone is quite volatile, and thus use of acetone may lead to substantial inhalation exposure.

Acetone is produced endogenously in intermediary metabolism mainly from fatty acid oxidation, and its concentration may be high among patients with uncontrolled diabetes mellitus. Fasting and strenuous exercise also elevate body acetone concentrations.

Clinical effects and epidemiology

Acetone has low toxicity. At high concentrations, acetone vapour can cause CNS depression, cardiorespiratory failure and death. Eye and nose irritation have been reported at concentrations $\geqslant 250$ ppm (600 mg/m^3), with headache, dizziness, mood changes and 'confusion' at 1000 ppm (2400 mg/m^3). Vomiting and fainting have been reported in workers exposed to acetone vapour at concentrations $>12\,000$ ppm (29 000 mg/m^3) for approximately four hours. Experimental exposure to 250 ppm (600 mg/m^3) of acetone was reported to induce changes in neurobehavioural tests.[104]

Acetone is negative in mutagenicity tests, only slight developmental effects were observed in rats and mice at exposure levels in excess of 6600 ppm (16 000 mg/m^3). No carcinogenicity studies are available on acetone, but it has been used extensively as a negative control in skin painting carcinogenicity studies.

Metabolism and monitoring

Acetone is metabolized to acetate and formate; these are intermediate steps in metabolic pathways (e.g. to fatty acids, amino acids and in gluconeogenesis). Acetone is mainly excreted unchanged by exhalation, and as the ultimate step in its catabolism, to carbon dioxide. Small amounts of acetone are also excreted in urine.

Acetone induces the cytochrome P450 2E1 enzymes, and may thus effect the metabolism of chemicals that rely on this pathway (e.g. ethanol, benzene, *N*-nitrosodimethylamine, *N*-nitrosodiethanolamine, haloalkanes).

METHYLETHYL KETONE

[CAS No. 78-93-3]

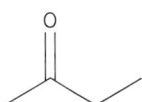

Methylethyl ketone (MEK) is a highly flammable, volatile, clear, colourless liquid that is stable under ordinary conditions. The primary use of methylethyl ketone, accounting for approximately 63 per cent of all use in the United States, is as a solvent in protective coatings. It is also used as a solvent in adhesives, printing inks, paint removers, in the production of magnetic tapes, and in dewaxing lubricating oil. Methylethyl ketone is used as a chemical intermediate in several reactions, including condensation, halogenation, ammonolysis and oxidation. Small amounts of methylethyl ketone are used as a sterilizer for surgical instruments, hypodermic needles, syringes, and dental instruments; as an extraction solvent for hardwood pulping and vegetable oil; and as a solvent in pharmaceutical and cosmetic production.[105] MEK is also found in tobacco smoke and exhaust gases from gasoline engines.

MEK is more irritating than acetone to mucous membranes. It has low acute toxicity, but it potentiates the neurotoxicity of n-hexane and methyl-n-butylketone (see under n-Hexane, p. 323) and the liver and kidney toxicity of carbon tetrachloride and trichloromethane. The mechanism for the latter may be induction of cytochrome P450, although an inducing effect of MEK on this enzyme activity is not observed at low exposure levels.[106] The mechanism could be the same for the potentiation of hexacarbon neurotoxicity, but this has not been clearly demonstrated.[107]

MEK is readily absorbed via the respiratory tract, and metabolized to 2-butanol, 2-hydroxy-2-butanone, and 2,3-butanediol and further to products that are incorporated in intermediary metabolism. Smaller amounts are exhaled unchanged; MEK is also found in urine at low levels.

METHYL ISOBUTYL KETONE

[CAS No. 108-10-1]

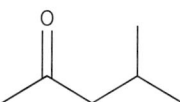

Methyl isobutyl ketone (MiBK) is a clear liquid with a sweet odour. The primary use of methyl isobutyl ketone is as a solvent in protective coatings. It is also used as a solvent in specialty adhesives, in ink formulations, in dewaxing mineral oil, and in textile coatings and leather finishing. As a process solvent, methyl isobutyl ketone is used in the separation and purification of certain metal ions, such as zirconium from hafnium; in the extraction and purification of antibiotics and other pharmaceuticals; and in the manufacture of insecticides and other pesticides. It is also used in purifying stearic acid, refining tall oil and extracting rosin from softwood, especially pine.[108] It is used as a carrier in riot control sprays, for example CS gas.

Exposures to MEK in the range of 25–50 ppm (260–530 mg/m^3) have been reported to cause respiratory tract irritation. Inhalation exposure to concentrations in excess of 1000 ppm (11 000 mg/m^3) causes central nervous system depression.

METHYL n-BUTYL KETONE (2-HEXANONE)

[CAS No. 591-78-6]

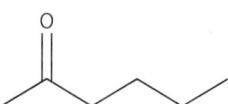

Methyl-n-butyl ketone (MnBK) is a clear, colourless, volatile liquid with a sharp odour. It is metabolized to 2-hexanol, 5-hydroxy-2-hexanone, and then to 2,5-hexanedione. This is the metabolite responsible for hexane neuropathy (see under n-Hexane, p. 323). Consistent with this finding, many cases of peripheral neuropathy have been reported among workers exposed to 2-hexanone;[109–111] the disease has also been reproduced in experimental animals.

Hexanone, and also 2,5-hexanedione, have induced adverse testicular effects in rodents.[109]

ETHERS

Ethers have the general formula R_1–O–R_2, the simplest of them being dimethyl and diethyl ethers (CH_3OCH_3, $C_2H_5OC_2H_5$). Ethers are used as solvents, and intermediates in synthetic processes.

CHLOROMETHYLMETHYLETHER AND BIS(CHLOROMETHYL)ETHER

Chloromethylmethylether   Bis(chloromethyl)ether

Chloromethylmethylether (CMME) (CAS No. 107-30-2) is a colourless liquid with a characteristic odour. It is a direct-acting alkylating agent and it has been extensively used as a cross-linking agent in ion exchange resins and as an intermediate in chemical syntheses. It is a potent irritant to mucous membranes. In 1968, it was demonstrated to be a potent carcinogen in experimental animals. The impurity bis(chloromethyl)ether (BCME) (CAS No. 542-88-1), which occurred in technical chloromethylmethylether, was an even more potent carcinogen. Bis(chloromethyl)ether can form spontaneously from the reaction of hydrochloric acid with formaldehyde. Several studies, starting in the 1970s, have convincingly demonstrated that exposure to technical chloromethylmethylether – apparently always containing BCME as an impurity at a level of a few per cent – is a very potent carcinogen in humans, causing lung cancer, usually of the microcellular type.[100,112–114] IARC concluded in 1987 that bis(chloromethyl)ether and technical chloromethylmethylether are carcinogenic to humans;[17] they induce cancer of the lung.[100] The homologues bis(2-chloroethyl)ether and bis(2-chloro-1-methylethyl)ether were not classifiable as to their carcinogenicity to humans.[115,116]

METHYL-tert-BUTYLETHER

[CAS No. 1634-04-4]

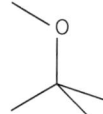

Methyl-tert-butylether (MTBE) is a volatile, colourless liquid at room temperature with a terpene-like odour. It is used as an octane enhancer and oxygen provider in gasoline, and to a small extent, as a solvent.[117] Following the introduction of two separate fuel programmes in the

United States requiring the use of gasoline oxygenates, consumers in some areas complained about headache, eye and nose irritation, cough, nausea, dizziness and disorientation. Epidemiological studies of occupationally and non-occupationally exposed people, and studies of exposed volunteers, have not been able to identify a basis for these complaints.[118]

Inhalation exposure to methyl-*tert*-butyl ether increased the incidence of hepatocellular adenomas in female mice and that of renal tubular tumours in male rats in a non-dose-related manner. In a gavage study in rats, MTBE increased the incidence of Leydig-cell tumours of the testis in males, and of lymphomas and leukaemias in females. The IARC concluded from these carcinogenicity data that there is limited evidence for the carcinogenicity of MTBE in experimental animals. MTBE does not appear to be genotoxic, and does not induce adverse developmental effects in experimental animals at exposure levels that are not overtly toxic to the dams.[117,119]

MTBE is oxidatively demethylated to formaldehyde and t-butanol (TBA). Formaldehyde is rapidly biotransformed (and has not been measured *in vivo* following MTBE exposures) further to formic acid, CO_2, or becomes incorporated into the one-carbon pool. The biotransformation of TBA yields 2-methyl-1,2-propanediol and α-hydroxyisobutyric acid (Figure 42.10).

Concentration of *tert*-butyl alcohol in morning urine specimens (16 hours after the cessation of the exposure) may be used for biomonitoring of MTBE.[120,121]

tert-AMYLMETHYLETHER

[CAS No. 994-05-8]

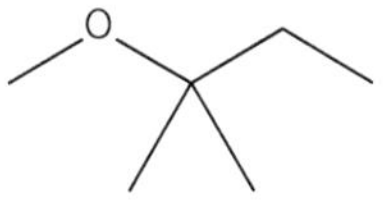

tert-Amylmethylether (TAME) is clear, colourless and volatile liquid. Like MTBE, it is used as an octane-enhancer and oxygen donor in gasoline, and as a component of an ether mixture added to gasoline. The proportion of TAME in gasoline may exceed 10 per cent.[122] The advantage of TAME over MTBE is that it is less volatile, and since it is less water soluble, it is not an equal threat to groundwater. TAME is slightly irritating to the eyes and respiratory tract, and at high concentrations, narcotic. In a 78-week gavage study in rats, with limited data reported, statistically non-significant increases were observed for tumours at several sites, and a significant increase was observed for lymphomas and leukaemias combined.[123] Noting the non-mutagenicity of TAME, and the uncertainties in the assessment of the only available carcinogenicity study, the European Union decided not to use carcinogenicity as the end point for the risk assessment of TAME.[122] In developmental toxicity studies in mice, cleft palate was observed in mice at inhalation exposure levels that only induced hepatic enlargement in the dams. In rats, weight reduction of the litters was observed at inhalation exposure levels that also induced maternal weight reduction. Based on these findings, the European Union did not consider there to be sufficient evidence to classify TAME as hazardous to human reproduction.[122] TAME is metabolized to several metabolites (2-methyl-2,3-butanediol, 2-hydroxy-2-methylbutyric acid and 3-hydroxy-3-methylbutyric acid), after an initial hydrolysis of the ether bond to *tert*-amyl alcohol. Concentration of *tert*-amyl alcohol in morning urine specimens may be used for biomonitoring.[120,121]

Glycol ethers

Glycol ethers, also called 'cellosolves', and chemically more appropriately called 'alkoxyalcohols' are condensation products of a glycol, such as ethylene glycol or propylene glycol, and an alcohol, such as methanol, ethanol or propanol. Because of their physicochemical characteristics, notably solubility both in water and in organic solvents, and low vapour pressure, they have found very extensive use as solvents in paints, lacquers, resins and pesticides. Glycol ethers are also present in consumer products, such as perfumes and household chemicals.

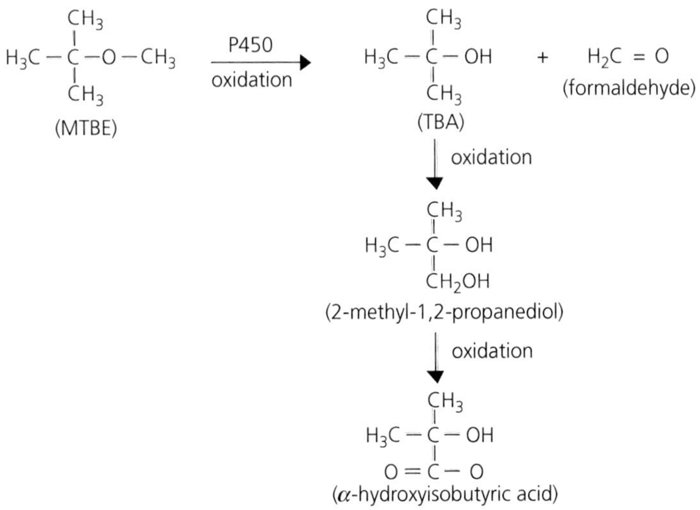

Figure 42.10 Metabolism of methyl-*tert*-butyl ether.[119]

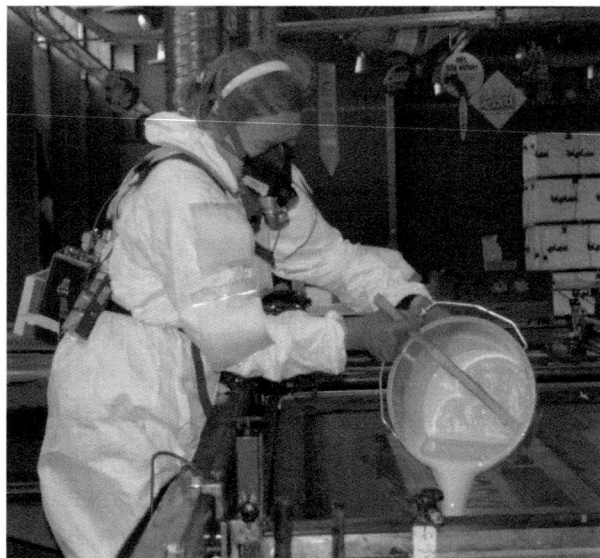

Figure 42.11 Glycol ethers like ethoxyethanol and its acetate can be used as a diluent in paints for serigraphy. Their dermal absorption may become significant if proper skin protection is not used. In this picture, the proportion of glycol ether absorbed through the lungs is estimated by personal air sampling in a situation in which skin absorption is prevented. At the end of the work day, urine samples are collected to indicate the absorbed dose. Reproduced with permission from the Finnish Institute of Occupational Health. For colour plate, see website (www.hodderplus.com/hunters).

Many glycol ethers are readily absorbed through the skin, and as the volatility of glycol ethers is low, in many instances, dermal absorption may be more significant than the respiratory uptake at work. While alkoxyalcohols in general have low acute toxicity, some of them are toxic to reproduction, and some cause haemolysis (Figure 42.11).

The first glycol ethers to enter the market were the simplest ones, ethyleneglycol ethers of methanol and ethanol. These, however, proved to be toxic to reproduction, and should by now no longer be used anywhere. They have been replaced by ethers with longer-chain alcohols, such as butanol, and derivatives of propylene glycol rather than ethylene glycol.

In addition to glycol ethers, their acetates (such as methoxyethanol acetate versus methoxyethanol) also have been extensively used. In most cases, the acetates are very readily hydrolysed to the parent glycol ethers by the action of carboxylesterases, and present practically identical toxicity as the parent glycol ethers themselves.

METHOXYETHANOL (ETHYLENEGLYCOL MONOMETHYL ETHER)

Methoxyethanol (CAS No. 109-86-4) and methoxyethylacetate (CAS No. 110-49-6) are stable flammable liquids with a slight odour at normal room temperature and pressure.

2-Methoxyethanol has been used in paints, coatings, inks, varnishes, cleaners, polishes, brake fluids and jet fuels, as a solvent, as a chemical intermediate and as a solvent coupler of mixtures and water-based formulations.

Clinical effects and epidemiology

2-Methoxyethanol is of low to moderate acute toxicity following oral, inhalation or dermal exposure. It has low potential for causing skin or eye irritation and has not been shown to be a skin sensitizer. Effects on haematological parameters, notably on red blood cell counts, have been observed in humans occupationally exposed to methoxyethanol/acetate. In addition, available data are suggestive of effects on spermatogenesis in men employed in occupations involving exposure to 2-methoxyethanol. Increased risk of spontaneous abortions has been observed in studies among women exposed to alkoxyethanols. It is not possible to discern the effect of methoxyethanol exposure in these studies.

Haematological effects were observed among men exposed to methoxyethanol at exposures where no effects on sperm counts were observed.[124] These men were apparently not exposed to other alkoxyalcohols or chemicals known to affect the bone marrow. A clear-cut haematotoxic effect was observed in workers exposed to 2-methoxyethanol at a time-weighted average concentration of 36 ppm (113 mg/m^3). A recovery towards normal was noted at an exposure level of 2.7 ppm (8.4 mg/m^3) and full recovery occurred at 0.55 ppm (1.7 mg/m^3).[125]

In laboratory animals, the key adverse health effects following repeated exposure to 2-methoxyethanol are haematological effects, and reproductive and developmental toxicity, including both effects on fertility and teratogenicity. Testicular degeneration and effects on the blood were observed following oral and inhalation exposure of rats to the lowest dose tested.[126] Methoxyethanol is considered toxic to reproduction.[127,128]

Metabolism and monitoring

Methoxyethanol is readily absorbed via the respiratory tract, but also through the skin (Figure 42.12). In occupational settings, the dermal absorption may be the major route of absorption.[129] Methoxyethyl acetate is hydrolysed by esterase activity to methoxyethanol. Methoxyethanol is metabolized by alcohol dehydrogenase and aldehyde dehydrogenase to methoxyacetaldehyde and methoxyacetic acid. A minor metabolic pathway leads to ethylene glycol and formic acid (and helps explain oxaluria reported in cases of acute intoxication after large oral doses of methoxyethanol). Methoxyacetic acid is apparently the ultimate toxic species both for the haematological and reproductive toxicity. Because of the possibility of extensive dermal absorption, the best estimate of exposure at the workplace is by biological monitoring, i.e. analysis of

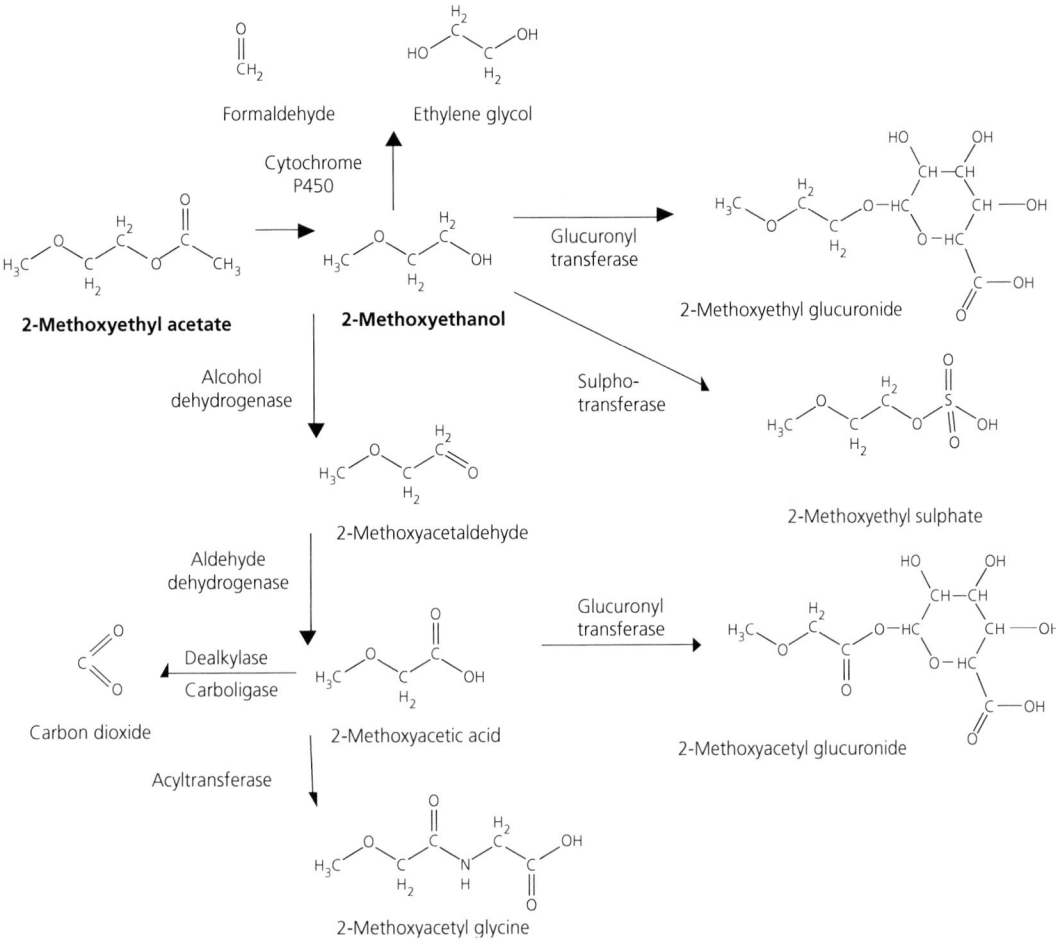

Figure 42.12 Metabolism of methoxyethanol.[126]

methoxyacetic acid in the urine in a post-shift specimen collected towards the end of the working week.[130–133]

ETHOXYETHANOL (ETHYLENEGLYCOL MONOETHYL ETHER) AND ETHOXYETHYL ACETATE

Ethoxyethanol (CAS No. 110-80-5) and ethoxyethyl acetate (CAS No. 11-15-9) are stable flammable liquids with a slight odour at normal room temperature and pressure. They have been used in paints, coatings, inks, cleaners, polishes, brake fluids and jet fuels, as well as a solvent, chemical intermediate and solvent coupler of mixtures and water-based formulations. Ethoxyethyl acetate is readily hydrolysed to ethoxyethanol, and has practically identical effects at equimolar exposure levels.

Because of the risk to reproduction, ethoxyethanol has been widely abandoned; however, it is not self-evident that its use has completely stopped in different parts of the world.

Clinical effects and epidemiology

While some cases of acute intoxication by ethoxyethanol after ingestion of large doses have been described, ethoxyethanol and its acetate have low acute toxicity in occupational settings. They have low irritant potential, and there are no data to indicate that they cause dermal or respiratory sensitization.

Three studies point to a possibility that ethoxyethanol induces semen abnormalities following occupational exposure.[134–136] Two other studies, one of which was performed in workers involved in silk screening with a reasonably pure exposure to ethoxyethanol, indicated that the exposure induced a deficit in erythropoiesis.[137,138]

While studies in exposed humans are quite limited and often involve mixed exposure with regard to both these end points, they are amply supported by studies in experimental animals, which clearly demonstrate that ethoxyethanol causes sperm abnormalities in males and is embryotoxic, fetotoxic and teratogenic in different animal species at exposure levels that are not overtly toxic to the dams – and after both inhalation and dermal exposure.[139] Similarly, the effect on haematopoiesis is demonstrated convincingly in experimental animals.[139]

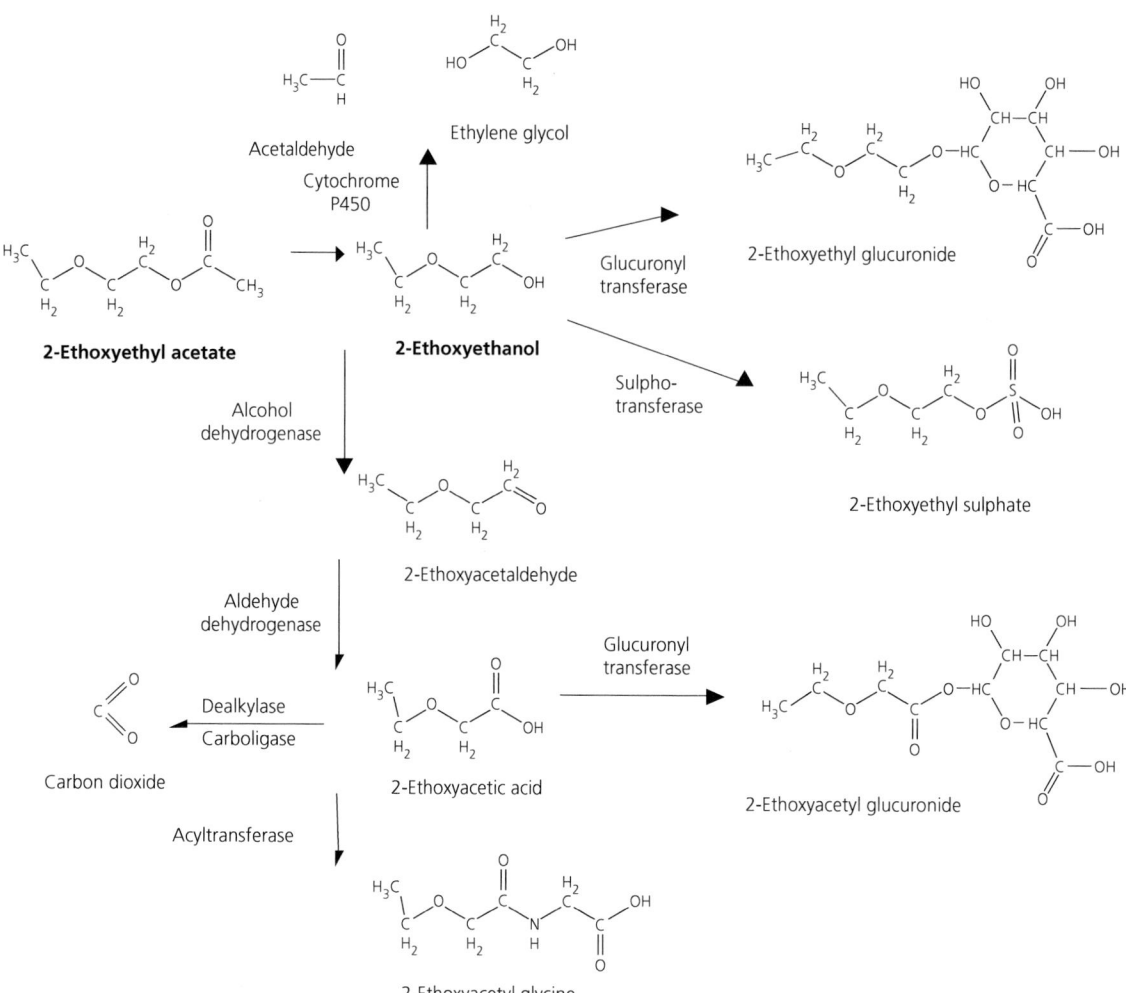

Figure 42.13   Metabolism of ethoxyethanol.[139]

Metabolism and monitoring

Ethoxyethanol is readily absorbed via the respiratory tract, but also through the skin. In occupational settings, dermal absorption may be the major route of absorption.[140] Ethoxyethyl acetate is hydrolysed by esterase activity to ethoxyethanol. Ethoxyethanol is metabolized by alcohol dehydrogenase and aldehyde dehydrogenase to ethoxyacetaldehyde and ethoxyacetic acid (Figure 42.13). Ethoxyacetic acid is apparently the ultimate toxic species both for haematological and reproductive toxicity. Therefore, and because of the possibility of extensive dermal absorption, the best estimate of exposure at the workplace is by biological monitoring, i.e. analysis of ethoxyacetic acid in a post-shift specimen of urine collected towards the end of the working week.

BUTOXYETHANOL (ETHYLENEGLYCOL MONOBUTYL ETHER)

2-Butoxyethanol (CAS No. 111-76-2) is a colourless liquid with a mild ether-like odour. It is widely used as a solvent in surface coatings (paints and varnishes), paint thinners, printing inks and glass- and surface-cleaning products (including those used in the printing and silk-screening industries), and as a chemical intermediate.[141]

Clinical effects and epidemiology

Statistically significant minor changes in haematocrit and mean corpuscular haemoglobin concentration were observed in a group of people occupationally exposed to average concentrations of 2-butoxyethanol of 0.6 ppm (3 mg/m^3).[142,143]

Nasal and eye irritation were observed at exposures between 100 and 180 ppm (500–900 mg/m^3) 2-butoxyethanol for two to four hours. When two males and two females were exposed to 2-butoxyethanol at 100 ppm (500 mg/m^3) for eight hours, the effects included vomiting and headache, with no clinical signs of haemolysis.[144]

Haemoglobinuria, erythropenia, metabolic acidosis, hypotension, pulmonary oedema, albuminuria and hepatic abnormalities have been reported in individuals who had attempted suicide by ingesting cleaning solutions containing

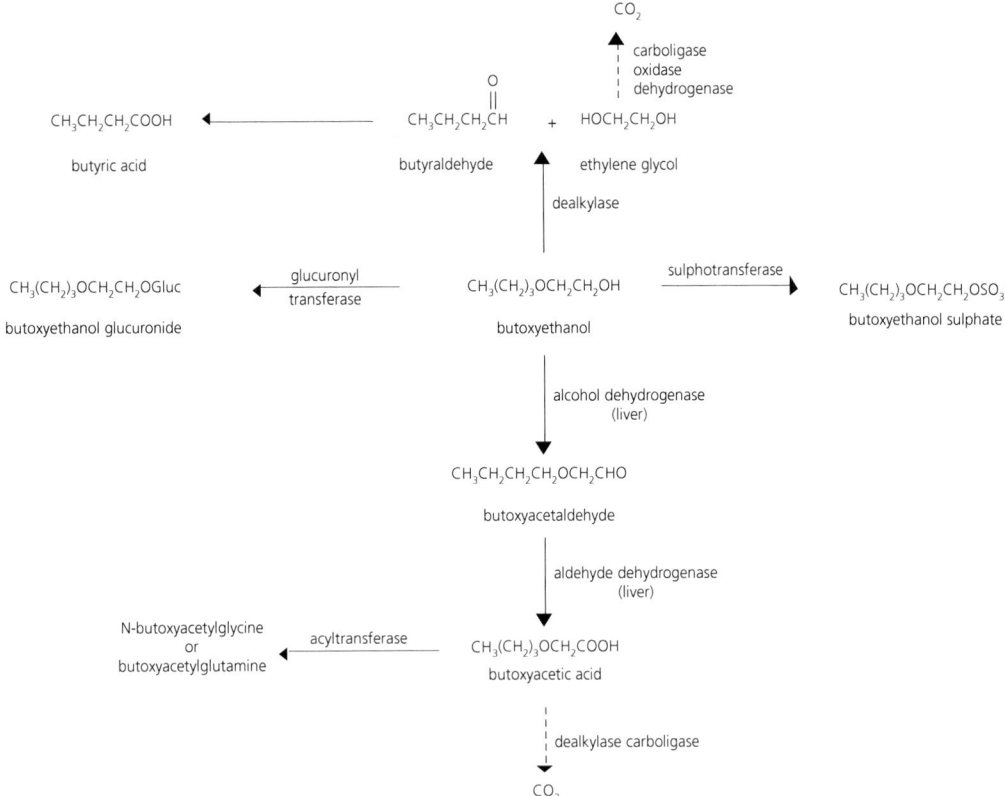

Figure 42.14 Metabolism of 2-butoxyethanol.[155]

2-butoxyethanol.[145–150] Effects characteristic of poisoning with ethylene glycol (a metabolite of 2-butoxyethanol in humans) such as coma, metabolic acidosis, and renal function changes have been reported in several cases and in cross-sectional studies.[143,145,151] 2-Butoxyethanol is apparently not a skin sensitizer.[152]

Good studies on the carcinogenicity of butoxyethanol in humans are not available. In long-term studies on carcinogenicity, exposure to 2-butoxyethanol induced a dose-related increase in the incidence of haemangiosarcomas of the liver in male mice and a dose-related increase in the incidences of combined forestomach squamous-cell papillomas or carcinomas (mainly papillomas) in female mice. No clear-cut carcinogenic effect was observed in rats. The IARC has included butoxyethanol in group 3, i.e. 'not classifiable'.[141]

In contrast to methoxy- and ethoxyethanol, there is no indication that butoxyethanol is toxic to reproduction. Tests on genotoxicity are similarly negative; however, the intermediate in butoxyethanol metabolism, butoxyaldehyde, is weakly genotoxic.

Metabolism and monitoring

Butoxyethyl acetate (CAS No. 112-07-2) is readily hydrolysed by esterases to butoxyethanol. The main metabolites of butoxyethanol are butoxyaldehyde and butoxyacetic acid, the formation of which is catalysed by alcohol and aldehyde dehydrogenases (Figure 42.14). De-ethylation of butoxyethanol produces ethyleneglycol as a minor metabolite. The haemolytically active species is butoxyacetic acid.

In humans, the generation of butoxyacetic acid from butoxyethanol is slower than in rodents, and in addition, rodent erythrocytes are more sensitive than humans to the haemolytic effect of butoxyacetic acid.

For butoxyethanol, the contribution of dermal absorption to total body exposure has been estimated by different authors to be between 25 and 75 per cent of total absorption.[153,154] Since butoxyethanol is readily absorbed through the skin, biological monitoring methods have been developed for the assessment of exposure to butoxyethanol. This is performed by the analysis of butoxyacetic acid (the metabolite responsible for the main toxicological effects) in urine.[91,143]

METHOXYPROPANOL (PROPYLENEGLYCOL METHYLETHER)

[CAS No. 107-98-2 and CAS No. 1589-47-5]

1-methoxy-2-propanol
α-isomer

2-methoxy-1-propanol
β-isomer

Commercially produced propyleneglycol methylether (PGME) is a colourless liquid with a characteristic odour.

It is a mixture of two isomers, 1-methoxy-2-propanol, also called α-isomer, i.e. secondary alcohol, and 2-methoxy-1-propanol, also called β-isomer, i.e. primary alcohol. This is important, as the two isomers have distinct metabolic differences, and are also toxicologically different. In many countries, limits have been set for the maximal proportion of the β-isomer allowed in the commercial product.

Propyleneglycol methylethers are soluble in water and solvents, are not very volatile, have low irritation capacity, and have no offensive smell. They have found extensive use as solvents for surface coatings, inks, lacquers, paints, resins, dyes, agricultural chemicals, oils and greases.[156–158]

Clinical effects and epidemiology

In experimental inhalation exposure, no irritation or discomfort was observed at concentrations of 100 ppm (370 mg/m^3), with slight discomfort reported at 150 ppm (560 mg/m^3).[159] No data on reproductive or long-term effects in humans are available.

Inhalation exposure to 1000 ppm PGME for two years induced renal tubular adenomas in male Fischer rats; this was accompanied by renal accumulation of α-2 microglobulin and hyaline-drop degeneration.[160] This phenomenon has been considered to be specific to male rats and thus not fully relevant to humans.[161] No increased incidence of tumours in other tissues of rats or mice were observed.

PGME had no effect on the fertility, did not affect sperm quality in rats, was not embryo- or fetotoxic in mice, rats or rabbits and did not induce teratogenesis.[162–165] The β-isomer in contrast was fetotoxic and teratogenic,[166] and decreased testicular and epididymal sperm counts in rats.[167] It has been thought that the difference in the toxicity of the α-isomer and β-isomer is due to the formation of the methoxypropionic acid from the latter, but not from the former (see below). It is the alkoxyacid which apparently is the cause of the reproductive, developmental and even haematotoxic effects of methoxy-, ethoxy- and butoxyethanols, but methoxypropionic acid only caused developmental effects at exposure levels that also were toxic to the dams.[168] It has been proposed that if the content of the β-isomer in PGME is below 0.5 per cent, it is unlikely to cause reproductive toxicity.[168] 2-Methoxy-1-propanol (but not 1-methoxy-2-propanol) is classified as reproductive toxicity category 2 by the European Union.[127,128]

Metabolism and monitoring

Like ethyleneglycol ether acetates, propyleneglycolethylether acetate is rapidly hydrolysed *in vivo* and *in vitro* to PGME; the two seem to be toxicologically equivalent.[169,170]

At low exposures, most of inhaled PGME is metabolized to carbon dioxide and exhaled. At increasing doses, PGME is increasingly conjugated with glucuronic acid and sulphate. A smaller fraction is *O*-demethylated to propylene glycol. PGME is also excreted in urine unchanged. Oxidation to methoxypropionic acid apparently does not take place.[171] The β-isomer is mainly oxidized by alcohol dehydrogenase to methoxypropionic acid. Direct conjugation with glucuronic acid and metabolism to carbon dioxide are minor pathways.

As dermal exposure may significantly contribute to the total exposure, biomonitoring is useful for the assessment of exposure. Analysis of total 1-methoxy-2-propanol in urine is the best validated urinary marker of exposure.[172,173]

CARBOXYLIC ACIDS AND THEIR DERIVATIVES

Carboxylic acids form a large and heterogeneous group of chemicals, with the generic formula R–COOH. This family includes aliphatic acids, saturated and unsaturated, all of which may be mono- or polycarboxylic, as well as aromatic acids. Carboxylic acids may contain substituents other than carbon, oxygen and hydrogen. Acids containing halogens have important industrial applications, and many are of occupational health interest.

Carboxylic acids are generally soluble in water; the solubility decreasing with increasing molecular mass. The most conspicuous characteristic of carboxylic acids from the human health point of view is that they are strongly irritating or even corrosive to the mucous membranes and the skin. Systemic adverse effects from carboxylic acids are rare in occupational settings, although serious and fatal intoxications have been described after oral and dermal exposure. The main toxicological feature in such cases is usually metabolic acidosis with its sequelae, such as hyperkalemia and hypocalcaemia. Several case reports have been published describing fatal intoxications due to dermal exposure to monochloroacetic acid [CAS No. 79–11–8]. The poisoning cases have involved epidermal and superficial dermal burns, with disorientation, agitation, cardiac failure, metabolic acidosis, rhabdomyolysis, renal insufficiency and cerebral oedema occurring within a few hours.[174–180]

FORMIC ACID

[CAS No. 64-18-6]

$$\text{H}-\overset{\overset{\displaystyle O}{\|}}{\text{C}}-\text{OH}$$

Formic acid is a colourless, fuming liquid, with a pungent odour. It is used in dyeing and finishing of textiles and paper, treatment of leather, electroplating and brewing, silvering glass, and as an intermediate in the manufacture of many chemicals, as a silage additive and prophylactic in animal feeds.[179]

Clinical effects and epidemiology

Human data on the toxicity of formic acid are limited. Severe burns have been reported after dermal exposure to undiluted formic acid.[180,181]

Acute poisoning after oral or dermal exposure has resulted in metabolic acidosis, intravascular haemolysis and haemoglobinuria.[180–185] Many cases of fatal formic acid poisoning after ingestion exposure have been described; a dose of 60 g has invariably led to death.[182,186] Ocular toxicity, similar to methanol intoxication, has been observed in animals treated with formic acid. In inhalation studies in rats and mice, microscopic examination showed lesions (squamous metaplasia, necrosis, degeneration, inflammation) of the nose, larynx and pharynx at concentrations of 60 ppm (120 mg/m^3) and higher. Formic acid is immediately transformed to formate in the body. Formate tested negative in bacterial mutagenicity tests using different Salmonella strains.[187] Formic acid has apparently not been studied for carcinogenicity in experimental animals. In a limited developmental toxicity study, formic acid was not teratogenic, while methanol, causing similar blood formic acid concentrations, induced brain abnormalities.[84]

Metabolism and monitoring

Formate is partly metabolized in the one carbon pool and is partially excreted unchanged in the urine. The concentration of formate in urine has been used for the biological monitoring of formate exposure.[92]

Management and diagnosis

Formate intoxication is rare, and as a distinction from methanol poisoning, it is likely that there are symptoms at the point of entry: skin burns and severe gastric discomfort. Poisoned patients also have metabolic acidosis and usually haemolysis. Vision may be affected. A diagnosis may be made by the analysis of methanol and formate in blood. Elevated blood levels of formate, but not of methanol, suggest formic acid poisoning.

Formate poisoning has been successfully treated with haemodialysis, intravenous bicarbonate, administration of folinic acid to facilitate the incorporation of formate to the one carbon pool, and general supportive measures.[181,184]

ESTERS

Esters are condensation products of an acid and an alcohol, and have a general formula R_1COOR_2; the simplest ester being methylformate CH_2OOCH_3. Esters comprise a very large group of chemicals, the acid moiety may be an alkane, alkene or an aromatic compound, and similarly, the alcohol part may vary. Small molecular weight esters are soluble in water and readily volatile. With an increasing molecular size, both these characteristics decrease. Esters are extensively used as solvents. They are generally inert, with their most important adverse effects usually being narcotic effects at high concentrations, and eye and airway irritation, also skin irritation, from liquid esters. Other than irritation, toxicity is mostly due to the acid part of the molecule.

ACRYLIC ACID ESTERS

Ethyl acrylate   Methyl methacrylate

Acrylic acid (CAS No. 140-88-5) and methacrylic acid (CAS No. 80-62-6) esters readily polymerize and are used extensively for polymer production.

Methyl methacrylate is commonly used in a mixture with pre-polymerized oligomers to prepare medical and dental prostheses and orthodontic devices that are often finished with the technician's bare hands to obtain the desired dimensions before final hardening of the product. In this respect, dental uses of the monomer differ from industrial application, which do not generally require manual handling of monomer-containing products. Thus, it is understandable that reports on adverse effects from methyl methacrylate come mainly from its use in dentistry.

Clinical effects and epidemiology

Acrylic and methacrylic esters are irritating to the eyes, respiratory tract and the skin.

Methyl methacrylate is well known to cause allergic contact dermatitis, typically at the fingertips, spreading along the nail walls, with painful desquamation.[188–190] Among dental laboratory technicians, the most common allergens include methyl methacrylate, 2-hydroxyethyl methacrylate and ethyleneglycol dimethacrylate.[191] Sensitization to a large number of other acrylates has also been described in a variety of occupations with skin contact to monomer-containing products. Acrylate derivatives to which sensitization has been demonstrated include methylmethacrylate, ethylmethacrylate, 2-hydroxyethyl methacrylate, 2-hydroxypropyl methacrylate, N,N-dimethylaminoethyl methacrylate, glycidyl methacrylate, tetrahydrofurfuryl methacrylate, ethyleneglycol dimethacrylate, diethyleneglycol dimethacrylate, triethyleneglycol dimethacrylate, polyethyleneglycol dimethacrylate, urethane dimethacrylate, ethyl acrylate, hydroxyethyl acrylate, hydroxypropyl acrylate, phenoxyethoxy ethylacrylates, hexandediol diacrylate and trimethylolpropane triacrylate.[192–197]

In addition to dentistry, occupations with reported cases include manufacture of printed circuit boards,[198] opticians working with polymethyl(meth)acrylate[199] and optical fibre manufacture (UV-curable acrylate resin coating).[200]

Skin exposure to methyl methacrylate (usually in the presence of dermatitis) may lead to neurological damage. In an early study, 17 per cent of a group of dental technicians, their assistants, and students of the Dental Technician Institute in Finland reported current or previous hand dermatitis, and 25 per cent reported other finger symptoms, such as whitening, numbness, coldness or pain.[201] Slowed distal sensory conduction velocity from digits I, II and III of the right hand, and also of the radial aspects of the digits II and III of the left hand was observed among the dental technicians. These findings represent mild axonal degeneration on the areas with the closest and most frequent contact with methyl methacrylate.[202] Finger paraesthesia may also develop without overt dermatitis.[203]

Asthma, rhinitis and conjunctivitis have been reported among workers exposed to acrylates, methacrylates and cyanoacrylates. Hypersensitivity pneumonitis has also been observed in methacrylate-exposed dental techncians.[204–209] Available epidemiological evidence does not point to a carcinogenic effect of methyl methacrylate.[210,211] The IARC has categorized it into group 3 (i.e. not classifiable).

Methyl methacrylate has been tested in rats and mice for carcinogenicity by inhalation; IARC concluded that there is evidence suggesting lack of carcinogenicity.[210] For ethyl acrylate, the IARC concluded that there is sufficient evidence of carcinogenicity in animals (group 2B).[212] Many acrylates, including methyl methacrylate, are mutagenic to bacteria and/or mammalian cells *in vitro*, but are mostly negative in genotoxicity tests *in vivo*. Methyl methacrylate was not toxic to reproduction in experimental animals.[210]

Metabolism and monitoring

Acrylates are absorbed effectively through the respiratory tract and also the skin. They are metabolized rapidly. For several (meth)acrylate esters, metabolism yields small amounts of thioethers, indicating electrophilic metabolites. No validated biomonitoring methods exist for acrylates.

Management and diagnosis

The main means of diagnosing allergic contact dermatitis is by patch testing. However, the group of acrylates is large and varied, and not all possible allergens are available commercially as test reagents. Therefore, the products to which the patient has been exposed, should also be included in the test series – as is also true for diagnosing most cases of occupational contact dermatitis.[192] Challenge tests have been used for the diagnosis of acrylate-induced rhinitis and asthma, when the clinical picture and history do not provide a conclusive diagnosis.[204–209] However, caution must be exercised in ensuring that, especially for bronchial provocation tests, these are performed in hospital settings with access to immediate emergency support in the event that a severe allergic reaction results from the challenge. Methyl methacrylate-induced axonal damage may be present in the absence of contact dermatitis. The diagnosis is based on the clinical picture and history; nerve conduction velocity determinations may be considered. Axonal damage in dental personnel is a difficult clinical management problem, because acrylates penetrate standard gloves, and truly effective protective gloves tend to affect manual dexterity. This poses a dilemma in regards to providing occupational medical advice on continuing or changing vocation for affected individuals.

NITROGEN-CONTAINING HYDROCARBONS

Amides

Amides are of the general form $R_1CONR_2R_3$, the simplest of them being formamide -$HCONH_2$. Dimethylacylamides, such as dimethylformamide, and dimethylacetamide are used extensively. They are miscible in water in all ratios, and are soluble in organic solvents. They are chemically stable, with low vapour pressure, and they are used as solvents, in acrylic and cellulose triacetate fibre production, polyurethane coating, electronics industry, varnishing, surface coating, polyamide coating, absorbents, cleaners, extractants, and in pharmaceuticals and plant protection products.[213–216]

DIMETHYLFORMAMIDE

[CAS No. 68-12-2]

N,N-dimethylformamide (DMF) is a colourless liquid at room temperature with a faint amine odour. It is extensively used in the chemical industry as a solvent, an intermediate catalyst, and as a paint stripper and additive.[214,215,217]

Clinical effects and epidemiology

The liver is the target organ for the toxicity of DMF in humans. Symptoms include alcohol intolerance, abdominal pain, nausea, vomiting, diarrhoea, anorexia and jaundice. Objective findings include elevated levels of serum alanine-aminotransferase, aspartate aminotransferase, alkaline phosphatase, gammaglutamyl transferase and bilirubin. Although histopathological changes have not been extensively studied, enlarged Kupffer cells, hepatocellular necrosis and fatty degeneration have been described.[213,214]

Alcohol intolerance, characterized by flushing of the face, dizziness, nausea and tightness of the chest, has been widely reported among DMF-exposed workers after alcohol consumption, and is apparently an effect that occurs at low exposure levels.[213] While it is difficult to establish with any certainty the lowest concentration of DMF at which increases in these subjective symptoms first appear, they have been associated with mean or median levels of 10 ppm (30 mg/m^3). In a recent study, some workers reported symptoms upon exposure to concentrations for which the median value was as low as 1.2 ppm (3.6 mg/m^3).[218]

Low sperm motility, but with no variation in sperm morphology or semen volume, was related to urinary concentrations of N-methylformamide (NMF) among workers exposed to DMF in a synthetic leather factory

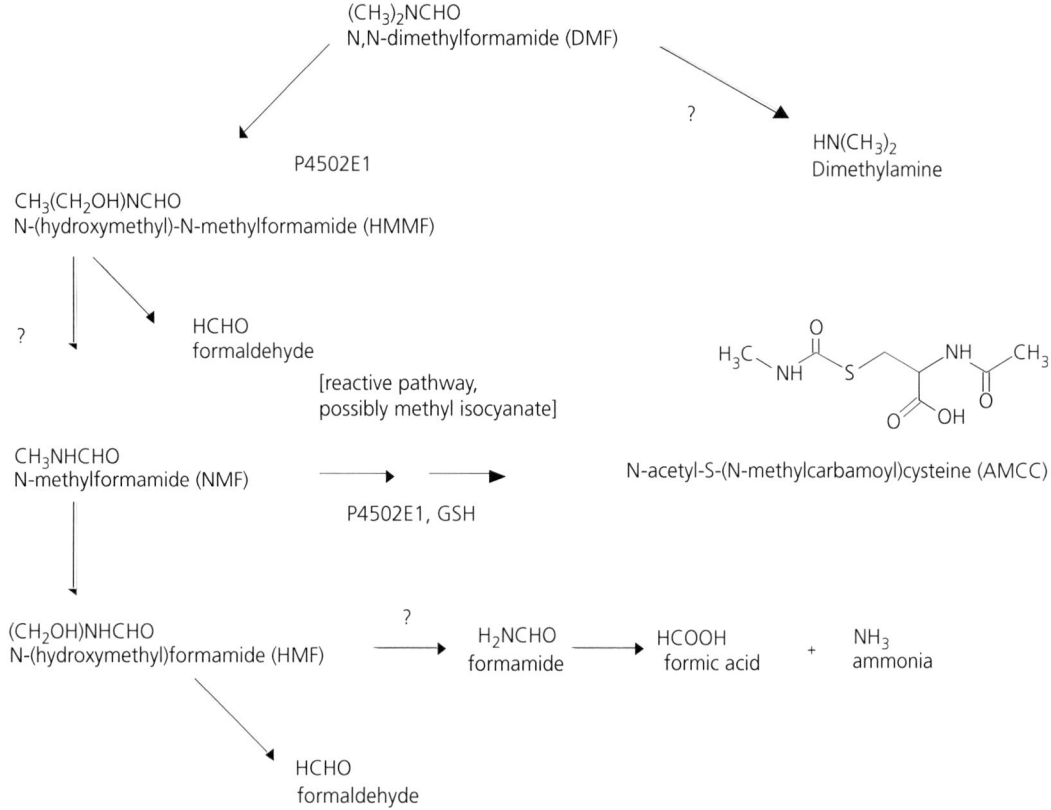

Figure 42.15   Metabolic pathways of N,N-dimethylformamide.[213]

in Taiwan. There was no relationship with the airborne concentrations of DMF, and the reasons for this may be dermal absorption from splashes, or to the mediation of the effect by an active metabolite, instead of to the parent compound.[219] Although several experimental studies have indicated that DMF may adversely affect sperm quality, these effects have only been seen at exposure levels considerably higher than those inducing hepatic damage. The irritation potency of DMF is low; no consistent information is available on any sensitizing capacity. An early study reported an increased incidence of testicular tumours in men exposed to DMF; later studies have not been able to confirm this finding.[213,217]

The IARC evaluated data on the carcinogenicity of dimethylformamide in experimental animals, and concluded that based on adequate findings in one study on rats and one using mice, there was evidence suggesting lack of carcinogenicity.[217] However, a subsequent study reported that inhalation exposure to dimethylformamide led to an increased incidence of liver adenomas and carcinomas in both rats and mice.[220] Dimethylformamide has been extensively studied for genotoxicity *in vivo* and *in vitro*, with consistently negative results.[215] Fetotoxic and teratogenic effects have been reported in several animal studies at doses that are toxic to the dams, but also in some studies at doses that are not overtly toxic to the dams.[221] In the European Union, dimethylformamide has been classified as being toxic to reproduction in category 2.[128]

Metabolism and monitoring

Dimethylformamide is effectively absorbed by the respiratory and also dermal route. Dermal absorption is significant not only for liquid dimethylformamide, but also for the gaseous form. Dermal exposure may be more important than respiratory exposure in occupational settings.[222,223]

Dimethylformamide is hydroxylated to N-hydroxymethyl-N-methylformamide, which is the main metabolite in humans (Figure 42.15). A minor further oxidation pathway, also catalysed by cytochrome P450 2E1, leads through N-methylformamide (or maybe directly) to a reactive intermediate, probably methyl isocyanate, and further via glutathione conjugation, to N-acetyl-N-methylcarbamoyl)cysteine (AMCC).[224,225] This minor pathway, and probably the intermediate methyl isocyanate, is responsible for the liver toxicity of dimethylformamide. This notion is supported by the finding that individuals with heritable lack of glutathione S-transferase T1 are at a considerable higher risk to hepatic damage, when exposed to dimethylformamide at work.[226]

Because of the likelihood of dermal absorption, biological monitoring of exposure to dimethylformamide is a useful tool for exposure and risk assessment. Most often, N-methylformamide is measured in after-shift urine specimens. In the analytical methods used, because the main metabolite HMMF is converted to N-methylformamide, the sum of the two metabolites is measured. These metabolites have the advantage in that the precursor of the putative toxic metabolite is being measured.[91] Analysis of N-methylcarbamoylated haemoglobin (lysine or N-terminal valine) in blood has also been proposed as a long-term indicator of exposure to N-methylformamide,[227–229] but the experience is very limited, and the analytical technique more demanding.

Prevention

In keeping with the importance of dermal exposure in the uptake of dimethylformamide at work, it was noted that in synthetic leather production, protection of the skin was more effective than respiratory protection against absorption of dimethylformamide.[223]

N,N-DIMETHYLACETAMIDE

[CAS No. 127-19-5]

Dimethylacetamide (DMAA) is used in the production of acrylic fibres and polyurethane elastane yarns (Spandex™ or Lycra™) as the spinning solvent. DMAA may also be used as a solvent for production of x-ray and photographic products, reactor solvent for cosmetic and pharmaceutical intermediates, aramid fibres, polyamide films and polymers, resins and polymers, miscellaneous organic chemicals, and liquid treatment fibres and as a solvent in production of photoresistant stripping compounds.[216]

Clinical effects and epidemiology

The irritation potency of DMAA is low; no consistent information is available on any sensitizing capacity. Like dimethylformamide, the main effect of DMAA in occupationally exposed people, is liver damage.[216,230–232] Liver damage has generally been observed from elevated levels of enzymes in blood reflecting damage to hepatic function and liver cellular integrity; alcohol intolerance has not been reported.

In experimental animals, fetotoxic and teratogenic effects have been reported in several studies at doses that are toxic to the dams. Fetotoxicity and teratogenicity were also observed in inhalation studies in rats at exposure levels that did not induce hepatic damage, although there was slight decrease in weight gain of the dams,[233] and also in oral studies in the absence of overt dam toxicity.[216] In the European Union, dimethylacetamide has been classified as being toxic to reproduction in category 2.[128] DMAA is consistently negative in genotoxicity studies, and in limited testing for carcinogenicity, no consistent elevation of tumour incidence has been observed.[216]

Metabolism and monitoring

DMAA is extensively absorbed via the cutaneous route even from the vapour phase.[234,235] It is metabolized mainly to N-methylacetamide, and to a minor extent also to hydroxymethylacetamide, acetamide and S-acetamidomethylmercapturic acid.[216,235]

Management and diagnosis

Because of the likelihood of dermal exposure, biological monitoring of exposure to dimethylacetamide is a useful tool for exposure and risk assessment. N-methylacetamide is usually measured in after-shift urine specimens.[235–238]

ACRYLAMIDE AND *N*-METHYLACRYLAMIDE

[CAS No. 79-06-1 and CAS No. 1187-59-3]

Acrylamide is a white crystalline solid which sublimes slowly at room temperature. Its vapour pressure is 0.9 Pa. The main use is in the production of polyacrylamides which are used in waste water treatment, paper and pulp processing and mineral processing. The monomer content of polyacrylamides is usually less than 0.1 per cent. In research laboratories, acrylamide is used to produce polyacrylamide electrophoresis gels used for the separation of nucleic acids.

Acrylamide has been used also as a grouting agent. In the European Union, its production for this purpose ended at the end of the 1990s.[239] N-methylacrylamide is also a grouting agent, with a potential to regenerate acrylamide.[239] The extent to which this occurs is not known and may depend on environmental conditions. Also, the use of N-methylacrylamide for grouting has ceased in Western Europe, but in some parts of the world it may still be used.

Since the vapour pressure of acrylamide is low, occupational exposure to acrylamide occurs via the respiratory route mainly when aerosols are generated, or also through the skin.

Clinical effects and epidemiology

The main concerns related to acrylamide are its neurotoxicity, carcinogenicity and mutagenicity. Based on animal studies, it is also a reproductive toxicant affecting the fertility of male rats and mice.[128,239]

Skin irritation, rashes and peeling of the skin have been reported in workers exposed to acrylamide solutions.[240] In the same study, 38 out of 71 (54 per cent) workers occupationally exposed to aqueous acrylamide monomer in the manufacture of monomeric and polymeric acrylamide reported skin peeling of the hands, and on clinical examination this finding was observed in 16 of the 71 workers (23 per cent).[240] In the control group, the incidence was 2/51 (4 per cent). Erythema was reported in 23 per cent of exposed workers compared with none in the control group. In animal studies, acrylamide has been clearly positive in skin sensitization tests, but in humans skin sensitization appears to be rare.[239]

Neurotoxic effects of acrylamide

There are several studies in animals showing the development of peripheral neuropathy after repeated exposure to acrylamide.[239] Also, in occupationally exposed workers, neurotoxic effects have been described.[240] In a Chinese factory producing monomeric and polymeric acrylamide, neurotoxic effects were experienced by the workers. Symptoms including numbness of hands and feet, lassitude, sleepiness, muscle weakness, clumsiness of hand, anorexia, unsteady gait and coldness of hands and feet; difficulty in grasping and stumbling and falling were reported significantly more in workers than in a control group. Peeling of the skin and excessive sweating of the hands were the first effects described. Other symptoms, like muscle weakness of the legs, numbness and tingling of hands and feet appeared only after a few months of exposure. On clinical examination, signs observed in exposed workers included impairment of vibration sense, pain, diminished touch and altered propioception. Some workers had muscular atrophy, and diminished or loss of reflexes in the extremities. In electroneuromyographic studies, findings suggestive of partial denervation and axonal degeneration were also seen in some workers who did not have any apparent clinical signs of neurotoxicity.[240]

In the late 1990s, two incidents of significant occupational and environmental acrylamide exposure occurred in Scandinavia in tunnel construction when N-methyloacrylamide-based grouting agents were used.[241,242] The first incident occurred in Hallandsås in 1997 during the construction of a railway tunnel. Due to leakage of the chemical, a nearby creek was also contaminated by acrylamide and N-methyloacrylamide resulting in fish deaths and neurological symptoms in cows that drank water from the creek. Some of the tunnel construction workers were suspected of being heavily exposed and regular medical examinations, including neurophysiological and dermatological assessment and analysis of acrylamide haemoglobin adducts were performed. The results of this study showed exposure-related signs and symptoms of peripheral nervous system dysfunction. An association of symptoms with acrylamide-haemoglobin adduct levels was demonstrated. More than half of the symptomatic workers showed improvement in the symptoms and signs of peripheral nervous system dysfunction after six months of follow up, and after 12 and 18 months almost all were asymptomatic showing reversibility of the acrylamide neuropathy after cessation of exposure.[241] Similar results were also obtained in Norwegian tunnel construction workers showing slight demyelinating and axonal changes in peripheral nerves which were reversible after a year of follow up.[242]

Carcinogenicity and mutagenicity

Data on the carcinogenicity of acrylamide is based on animal experiments showing an increase in the incidence of several types of tumours in different organs.[239,243,244] No clear evidence of acrylamide carcinogenicity is available from epidemiological studies in exposed workers, although two most recent updates of epidemiological cohort studies found increased rates of pancreatic cancer, which were, however, not clearly related to increasing exposure levels.[245,246] The IARC evaluation is 2A (probably carcinogenic to humans).[243] There are substantial data available showing that acrylamide is a genotoxic substance.[239,244] It has also been shown to induce heritable genetic damage.

Attempts have been made to estimate the potential carcinogenicity risk of low level acrylamide exposure. One of the most recent estimates is from the Dutch Expert Committee on Occupational Standards (DECOS), which has calculated so-called health-based occupational cancer risk values (HBC-OCRVs) for acrylamide.[244] Based on the results of animal studies, the committee estimated that an acrylamide exposure of $0.4\,\mu g/m^3$ (time-weighted average) for 40 years leads to a cumulative excess cancer incidence of 10^{-5}, and at $40\,\mu g/m^3$ to an excess cancer incidence of 10^{-3}.

Metabolism and monitoring

Once absorbed, acrylamide undergoes a complex metabolism involving direct conjugation with glutathione and the formation of an epoxide intermediate glycidamide.[239] The main urinary metabolites include acrylamide-based mercapturic acid N-acetyl-S-(propionamide)-cysteine (APC), glycidamide-based mercapturic acids N-acetyl-S-(carbamoylethyl)-1-cysteine and N-(R,S)-acetyl-S-2-carbamoyl hydroxyethyl-1-cysteine (GAMA).[247,248] All of these have been suggested as markers for biological monitoring of acrylamide exposure.[247,248] Acrylonitrile exposure and smoking are potential confounding factors in biological monitoring especially when N-acetyl-S-(propionamide)-cysteine (APC) is used as a biomarker.[248] Since the excretion of acrylamide into urine is rapid, urine biomarkers represent very recent exposure (Figure 42.16).

Haemoglobin adducts have been used as a biological marker for acrylamide exposure, but the invasive nature of blood sampling and complex analytical methodology limit the routine application of this approach.

Management and diagnosis

Diagnosis of acrylamide-induced polyneuropathy is based on typical symptoms, neurophysiological examination and the assessment of exposure. Other possible causes of polyneuropathy, e.g. long-term alcohol abuse, diabetes, neurotoxic drugs, vitamin B_1, B_6 and B_{12} deficiencies, and some inflammatory, infectious or malignant diseases, must be excluded. According to current knowledge, the signs and symptoms of acrylamide-induced neuropathy are at least partially reversible after the cessation of exposure.

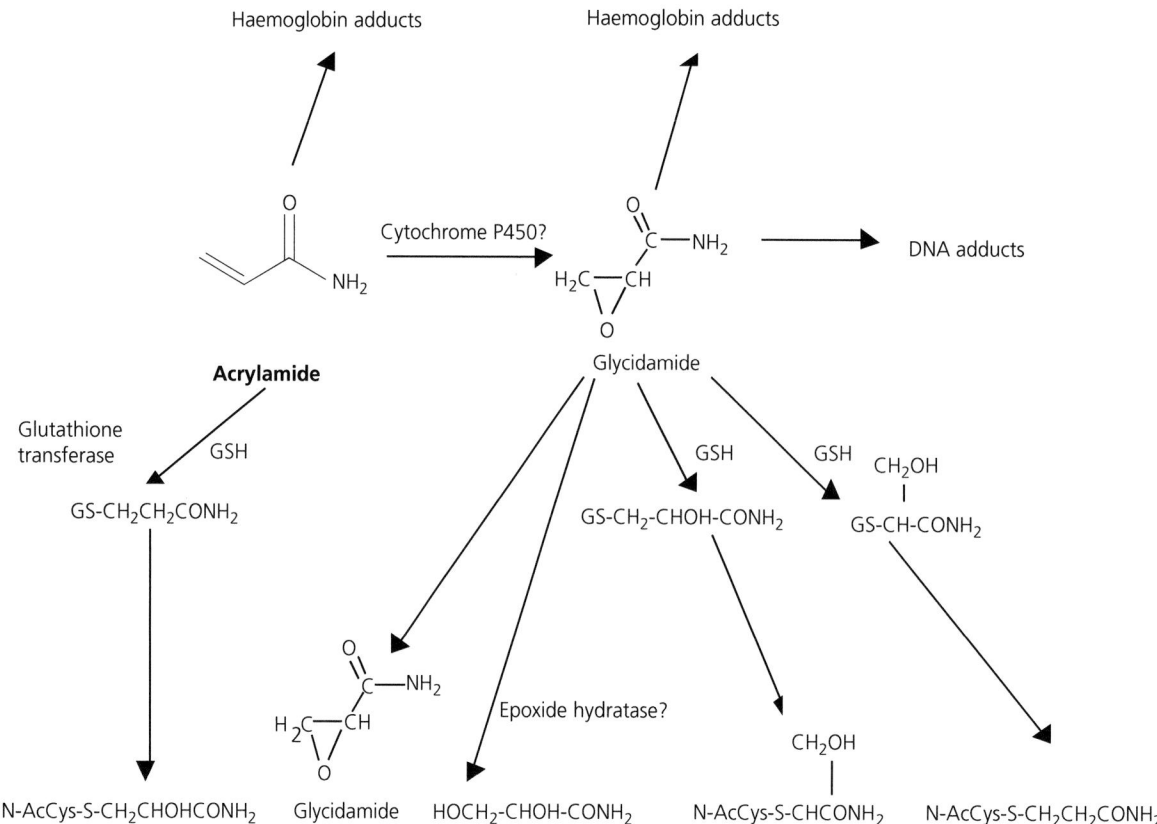

Figure 42.16 Acrylamide. Metabolism of acrylamide.[243] Urinary metabolites are shown on the bottom row.

Nitriles

ACRYLONITRILE AND ACETONITRILE

[CAS No. 107-13-1 and CAS No. 75-05-8]

Nitriles are organic chemicals with one or more cyanide (-CN) groups bound in a hydrocarbon chain. Common, widely used nitriles include acrylonitrile and acetonitrile. Acrylonitrile is used in the production of nitrile–butadiene rubber, acrylonitrile–butadiene–styrene and styrene–acrylonitrile polymers. Acetonitrile is used as a solvent, laboratory chemical and in the chemical or pharmaceutical industry in the production of other chemicals or pharmaceuticals. Acrylo- and acetonitrile have high vapour pressures and therefore they can lead to significant air concentrations and a risk of inhalation exposure in uncontrolled situations.

Clinical effects and epidemiology

Although some nitriles, for example acrylonitrile and acetonitrile, may release cyanide in the body, the toxicity of nitriles varies. Acrylonitrile is over ten times more toxic than acetonitrile. Symptoms of acrylonitrile or acetonitrile poisoning resemble that of cyanide poisoning, but manifest slower than the symptoms of cyanide poisoning. Initial symptoms of acrylonitrile poisoning occur at air levels of 20–100 ppm (44–220 mg/m^3) and include headache, irritation, dizziness, nausea and vomiting.[249] At higher dose levels, symptoms of cyanide poisoning including weakness, convulsions and respiratory failure, may become evident, but these may be delayed by 15 minutes up to several hours after exposure. Liver failure due to acrylonitrile poisoning has also been described.

Based on animal experiments, acrylonitrile is suspected of being carcinogenic to humans.[250] In a rat cancer bioassay, it has caused a range of tumours including those of the central nervous system, ear canal, gastrointestinal tract and mammary glands both by ingestion and by inhalation. Tumours have been reported at non-toxic doses and at periods as early as 7–12 months following onset of exposure.[250] Acrylonitrile is considered as a genotoxic carcinogen. There is no clear epidemiological evidence of the carcinogenicity of acrylonitrile in humans.

Metabolism and monitoring

Acrylonitrile or acetonitrile do not accumulate in the body.[250] Acrylonitrile is metabolized primarily either by conjugation with glutathione to form N-acetyl-S-(2-cyanoethyl)cysteine or oxidation by cytochrome P450 2E1. Oxidative metabolism of acrylonitrile leads to the formation of genotoxic 2-cyanoethylene oxide, which is either

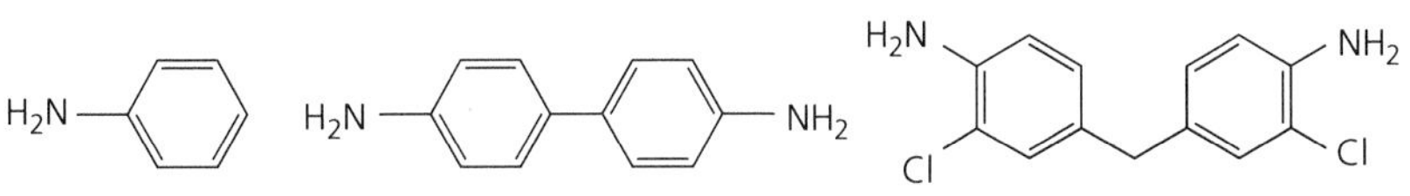

Figure 42.17 Molecular structures of aniline, benzidine and MOCA (4,4′-methylenebis(2-chloroaniline).

Aniline
CAS No. 62-53-3

Benzidine
CAS No. 92-87-5

MOCA
CAS No. 101-14-4

conjugated with glutathione to form cyanide and thiocyanate or directly hydrolysed by epoxide hydrolase. Also, acetonitrile metabolism follows an oxidative pathway by cytochrome P450 resulting in the formation of cyanohydrin, which then spontaneously decomposes to hydrogen cyanide and formaldehyde.[251] Elimination occurs via the urine.

Management and diagnosis

Diagnosis of nitrile poisoning is based on history and characteristic symptoms. Treatment of severe nitrile poisoning follows the procedures for the treatment of cyanide poisoning. Administration of oxygen is essential and may suffice for less severe cases of poisoning. Amyl nitrite (0.2 mL ampoule) can be given by inhalation repeatedly (maximum of six times). Because of the slow release of cyanide ions, patients have to be followed up for a sufficiently long time and antidotes may be needed even several hours after the poisoning. Intravenous antidotes which may be used in severe poisoning include hydroxycobalamine, 4-dimethylaminophenol, sodium thiosulphate and dicobalt edetate. However, treatment protocols differ between countries.

Aromatic amines

Aromatic amines are aromatic hydrocarbons in which one or more hydrogen atoms are replaced with an amino (-NH$_2$) group. It is a large group of compounds with different uses. A common toxicological property of these substances is their ability to cause methaemoglobinaemia. Several aromatic amines are known or suspected carcinogens, typically causing urinary tract carcinomas.

ANILINE

Aniline (Figure 42.17) is the simplest member of this group of compounds. It is a colourless oily liquid with a characteristic amine odour. Its vapour pressure at ambient temperature is 40 Pa. Aniline is used mainly as a chemical intermediate in the production of methylene dianiline (MDA) and in the production of rubber chemicals and dyes. Exposure to aniline in occupational settings may occur by inhalation and by skin exposure. Aniline is well absorbed after oral, dermal and inhalation exposure.

Clinical effects and epidemiology

Critical health hazards related to aniline are its acute toxicity due to the formation of methaemoglobin and its suspected carcinogenicity.

Methaemoglobinaemia

Methaemoglobinaemia is caused by the oxidation of the iron in the haem group of the haemoglobin molecule from the ferrous state to the ferric state resulting in inability of haem to transport oxygen effectively.[252] Normally, methaemoglobin levels are <1 per cent. Spontaneous formation of methaemoglobin is normally counteracted by protective enzyme systems – NADH methaemoglobin reductase, in which cytochrome b reductase plays a major role and NADPH methaemoglobin reductase (minor pathway). Initial symptoms of methaemoglobinaemia can be seen at methaemoglobin levels of approximately 15 per cent.[252] Hereditary deficiencies of cytochrome b5 reductase or inherited abnormal haemoglobin variants (HbM) can result in abnormally high methaemoglobin levels with a higher susceptibility to chemical agents capable of inducing methaemoglobinaemia. Also, some medicines can increase the levels of methaemoglobin. For example, the mechanism for nitrites used as an antidote for cyanide poisoning is through methaemoglobin formation. Methaemoglobin has an affinity for circulating cyanide, and is able to bind to cyanide before it affects cellular respiration.

Signs and symptoms of occupational aniline poisoning were frequently reported in the past when aniline was produced and used in poorly controlled circumstances. Since the first manifestation of aniline poisoning is an intense cyanosis, the victims of poisoning were referred to as 'blue boys'.[253] Other signs and symptoms characteristic for aniline poisoning include headache, dizziness, nausea, vomiting, chest and abdominal pain, weakness, seizures and cardiac dysrhythmias. Also, photophobia and visual disturbances can be seen. There is an aniline odour on the breath and on the sweat. The urine is dark in colour owing to the presence of haemoglobin. A Heinz-body haemolytic crisis may follow the development of methaemoglobinaemia after two to seven days.[253] Anaemia can follow long-term exposure to aniline (as well as other methaemoglobinaemia-causing agents). The average lethal inhalation dose in humans is reported to be 25 mg/L air or 0.35–1.43 g/kg body weight, whereas 0.4–0.6 mg/L air may be borne without much harm for 0.5–1 hour, but 0.1–0.25 mg/L for several hours produces slight symptoms. In long-term exposure, effects may be seen at even lower exposure levels.[254] The oral no-effect dose of aniline for methaemoglobin formation in an adult man after a single exposure has been estimated to approximate 15 mg/man (about 0.21 mg/kg body weight),[254] the mean oral lethal dose being between 15 and 30 g.[255]

Other effects

Aniline has been positive in genotoxicity tests measuring the induction of chromosomal aberrations and micronuclei.[253,254] In animal tests, it has caused spleen carcinomas in rats.[256,257] In humans, bladder cancer has been suggested after exposure, for example in aniline dye manufacturing, but these are most probably attributable to exposure to chemicals other than aniline.[17,253] The IARC has categorized aniline as group 3 (not classifiable as to its carcinogenicity to humans).

Metabolism and monitoring

Aniline is metabolized by acetylation and hydroxylation. Acetylation is mediated by N-acetyltransferase and results in the formation of acetanilide, which may be either deacetylated back to aniline or 4-hydroxylated to 4-hydroxyacetanilide. The glucuronide and sulphate conjugates of 4-hydroxyacetanilide represent the major urinary metabolites of aniline.[253] About 50 per cent of Europeans have genetically lower activity of N-acetyltransferase; these are called 'slow acetylators' in contrast to 'fast acetylators'. In these individuals, the reaction of aniline to acetanilide is retarded in favour of formation of phenylhydroxylamine, nitrosobenzene and aminophenol. Since this is the principal route by which aniline produces methaemoglobinaemia, these individuals may be more susceptible to aniline toxicity.[258]

Occupational exposure to aniline can be biomonitored by measuring urinary aniline in post-shift samples.[259]

Management and diagnosis

Treatment of methaemoglobinaemia is based on the administration of oxygen and intravenous administration of methylene blue, which acts as a reducing agent converting oxidized iron in haem from ferric back to its normal ferrous state. The usual recommended initial dose for methylene blue as an antidote is 1–2 mg/kg of 1 per cent solution given intravenously, but additional doses may be needed depending on the speed of clinical response.[260] The total dose administered should not exceed 7 mg/kg. In patients with G6PD deficiency, treatment may cause haemolytic anaemia and will therefore not be effective.[261] The use of hyperbaric oxygen has also been considered together with other life-supporting measures.[260]

Toluidines

o-, p-, m-Toluidines are aromatic amines, in which one hydrogen atom of aniline is substituted with a methyl group. They are mainly used as intermediates in the production of other chemicals.[262–264] Toluidines are also able to induce methaemoglobinaemia, m-toluidine being the most potent isomer in this respect.[262–264] The IARC has classified o-toluidine in group 1, as it has caused urinary bladder tumours in workers.[100,262–265] p- and m-Toluidine have not been sufficiently tested for their carcinogenic potential to be known.[263,264]

Benzidine and naphthylamines

Aromatic amines also include substances with two combined aromatic rings. Naphthylamines are based on naphthalene with one hydrogen atom replaced by an amine-group. In benzidine, two aromatic structures are linked together (Figure 42.17). 2-Naphthylamine and benzidine have been used in the past, for example in the manufacturing of azo dyes, but because of their carcinogenicity, they have been replaced by less toxic substances and prohibited by law in many countries. Workers exposed to 2-naphthylamine and benzidine have been reported to suffer from an excess of bladder tumours,[17] which were first described at the turn of the twentieth century. Their carcinogenicity was subsequently also confirmed in animal experiments.[17] They are classified as group 1 by the IARC.[100] In contrast, 1-naphthylamine has not demonstrated carcinogenic activity.[17] A rubber chemical, N-phenyl-2-naphthylamine (CAS No. 90-30-2) is partly dephenylated in the body to 2-naphthylamine and it has therefore been examined for its potential carcinogenicity. It has been found negative in animal mutagenicity and carcinogenicity assays.[17,266,267] This is supported by animal data indicating only very small (at maximum 1 per cent) conversion rates to 2-naphthylamine.[267] The IARC has classified it as group 3.

4,4-Methylenedianiline (CAS No. 101-77-9)

4,4′-Methylenedianiline (MDA) is used as an intermediate in the production of 4,4′-methylenediphenylisocyanate (see under Isocyanates, p. 364). The target organ for MDA toxicity is the liver. It has been described to cause jaundice after oral, dermal and inhalation exposure. Jaundice caused by MDA was termed 'Epping jaundice' after an incident in 1965 in the Epping area in the United Kingdom when 84 people suffered ill effects caused by eating bread baked with flour contaminated by MDA.[268] Regardless of several reports of acute liver disease caused by MDA, no human fatalities have been described. MDA is a skin sensitizer. It has also demonstrated mutagenic activity in animal tests and caused liver and thyroid cancers in animals.[269] The IARC has classified MDA as group 2B.[270] There is no clear evidence of MDA carcinogenicity in exposed workers.

Chloroanilines and MOCA (4,4′-methylenebis (2-chloroaniline))

If one or more hydrogen atoms in an aromatic amine are substituted by chlorine, different kinds of chloroanilines are formed. 2-Chloroaniline, 3-chloroaniline and 4-chloroaniline are used as intermediates for the production of other chemicals. All these isomers are haematotoxic and can cause methaemoglobinaemia, with 4-chloroaniline causing the most severe effects.[271] 4-Chloroaniline has shown genotoxicity in various systems, and has also shown carcinogenic activity in animal tests, with the induction of unusual and rare tumours of the spleen in male rats.[271] The results of assays for 2- and 3-chloroaniline are inconsistent and indicate weak or no genotoxic effects.

3,4-Dichloroaniline is a chemical in which two hydrogen atoms of aniline are substituted by chlorine. It is used as an intermediate in chemical production. This compound is acutely toxic and causes methaemoglobinaemia. It has demonstrated skin-sensitizing properties in guinea pigs, but no case reports on sensitization in humans have been published.[272]

MOCA (4,4′-methylenebis(2-chloroaniline)) (Figure 42.17) was introduced in the mid-1950s for the production of high-performance polyurethane mouldings. Although its use has decreased, it is still used in some applications in the rubber and plastics industries and in polyurethane production. It is well absorbed by all routes of exposure, and skin exposure may be significant in occupational settings. MOCA has been demonstrated in animal tests as a genotoxic and carcinogenic substance producing tumours in different organs in animals, including transitional-cell carcinomas of the urinary bladder and urethra in dogs.[273] Human epidemiological data on the carcinogenicity of MOCA are limited. IARC has classified MOCA as group 1 based on epidemiological and mechanistic (genotoxicity) data.[100] MOCA is metabolized to glucuronide and acetyl conjugates and excreted in the urine as a free compound or as glucuronide or acetyl metabolites, the main metabolite in the urine being n-glucuronide MOCA. N-hydroxy-MOCA is the main toxic, DNA reactive, intermediate of MOCA metabolism. MOCA can be biomonitored by measuring total MOCA (free and conjugated MOCA) in the urine.[274] DNA adduct analyses, to measure the levels of biologically active MOCA in the body, have been developed but are not in routine use.[275]

Phenylhydrazine

Phenylhydrazine (CAS No. 100-63-0) is a substance used worldwide mainly as a chemical intermediate in the pharmaceutical, agrochemical and chemical industries. It is composed of a hydrazine (diamine) group attached to a benzene ring. Phenylhydrazine is an acutely toxic chemical. Toxic effects seen mainly in animal tests include methaemoglobin formation, destruction of red blood cells, reduction in erythrocyte count, increased reticulocyte count and the formation of Heinz bodies. There are a number of case reports of skin sensitization to phenylhydrazine and its hydrochloride salt in humans.[276] Phenylhydrazine has shown mutagenic activity in genotoxicity tests and it is clearly carcinogenic in mice following oral dosing, inducing tumours of the vascular system.[276]

Aliphatic amines

Aliphatic amines are organic chemicals with an amino (NH_2) group in an aliphatic hydrocarbon chain.

Ethanolamine, diethanolamine and triethanolamine are aliphatic amines (Figure 42.18), which are used in many different applications including production of cosmetics, detergents, soaps, corrosion control inhibitors, and in pharmaceutical applications. They are also widely used in the metal industry in metal-working fluids. They are colourless viscous liquids or crystalline solids with a faint ammonia-like odour and with low vapour pressure at ambient temperatures. Exposure to ethanolamines may occur by all routes of exposure.

Clinical effects and epidemiology

The main hazard related to ethanolamines is their ability to cause sensitization. Occupational skin sensitization due to ethanolamines has been described in the metal industry after contact to ethanolamines in metal-working fluids.[277,278] Monoethanolamine seems to be the most common allergen in metal-working fluids. Geier *et al.*[277] tested over 200 metal workers who were suspected of having allergic dermatitis due to metal-working fluids with the current metal-working fluid (MWF) series and 155 with the historical MWF series. The results show that among the current MWF allergens, monoethanolamine ranked highest as a contact allergen with 11.6 per cent positive reactions. Diethanolamine (3.0 per cent) and triethanolamine (1.1 per cent), and diglycolamine (CAS No. 929-06-6) (1.9 per cent) elicited positive reactions far less frequently.

Ethanolamines are also highly irritating and corrosive. Case reports have referred to asthma caused by monoethanolamine,[279–281] diethanolamine[282] and triethanolamine.[281]

Metabolism and monitoring

Ethanolamine is metabolized in the liver and excreted in urine as urea, glycine, serine, choline and uric acid.[283] Part of the ethanolamine is excreted in urine unmetabolized. Nine to twenty per cent of ethanolamine is excreted via exhaled air. Diethanolamine is excreted predominantly unchanged with a half-life of approximately one week in urine. Ethanolamine and diethanolamine are incorporated

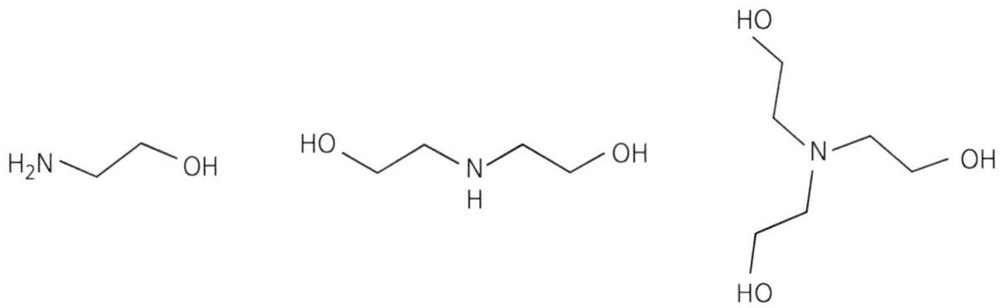

Ethanolamine
CAS 141-43-5

Diethanolamine
CAS 111-42-2

Triethanolamine
CAS 102-71-6

Figure 42.18 Molecular structures of ethanolamine, diethanolamine and triethanolamine.

in the body in phospholipids.[283] Triethanolamine is not incorporated in phospholipids and is readily eliminated in urine.[283,284] Urinary triethanolamine can be used for biological monitoring. However, urinary limit values indicative of safe exposure have not been established.

Management and diagnosis

The management of sensitization caused by ethanolamines is based on prevention of exposure by appropriate protective clothing and gloves, and follow up and prevention of air contamination with ethanolamines. Diagnosis of ethanolamine-caused skin sensitization is based on a history of exposure and patch-testing. Diagnosis of ethanolamine-caused asthma is based on work-related symptoms, serial peak-flow readings, and on an exposure chamber challenge with the suspected agent, if necessary.

Heterocyclic nitrogen compounds

This group of compounds includes substances whose common chemical feature is a ring structure with nitrogen as a part of the ring.

Examples of heterocyclic nitrogen compounds are piperazine, pyrrolidone and its derivatives N-methyl pyrrolidone and N-vinylpyrrolidone. Many piperazine derivatives are successful medicines. Piperazine is used in the pharmaceutical industry and in the manufacture of plastics and resins. Pyrrolidone derivatives are widely used industrial chemicals.

N-METHYLPYRROLIDONE AND N-VINYLPYRROLIDONE

[CAS No. 872-50-4 and CAS No. 88-12-0]

N-Methylpyrrolidone   N-Vinylpyrrolidone

N-methylpyrrolidone (NMP) is a colourless liquid with a vapour pressure of 39 Pa at 20°C. It is widely used nowadays as a solvent, for example, for extraction purposes in the petrochemical industry, as a remover of graffiti, as a paint stripper, and for stripping and cleaning applications in the microelectronics fabrication industry, as well as a reactive medium in polymeric and non-polymeric chemical reactions. It is also used as a formulating agent in pigments, dyes and inks; in insecticides, herbicides and fungicides; and in the pharmaceutical and cosmetics industry.[285] There are no known natural sources of N-methylpyrrolidone.

N-vinylpyrrolidone (NVP) is a colourless to light yellow liquid with a relatively low vapour pressure at ambient temperatures (12 Pa at 20°C). It is used in the production of polyvinylpyrrolidone (used for pharmaceuticals, cosmetics and food additives) and co-polymers (used as viscosity improvers in oils and in water-borne paints and adhesives), and as a reactive thinner in UV-cured inks and lacquers and in the manufacture of contact lenses.[286]

In occupational settings, exposure to N-methyl- and N-vinylpyrrolidone can occur through inhalation, especially when aerosols are formed or when heated. Both compounds are also well absorbed through the skin.[286,287]

Clinical effects and epidemiology

NMP can cause skin irritation and dermatitis. Its use as a cleaner or as a paint stripper has been described to result in redness, swelling, thickening and painful vesicles of the skin.[285,288] At high air levels, eye irritation and headache have also been reported.[289] Headaches and irritation of the skin, eyes and the upper airways have been reported among graffiti removers exposed to mixtures of NMP and glycol ethers.[290] In animal tests, NMP has caused developmental toxicity resulting in delayed development, malformations and early fetal resorptions after oral exposure.[291] Fetal toxicity has also been observed after inhalation or dermal exposure, but mainly at maternally toxic levels.[292,293] No epidemiological data on the effects of NMP in humans are available.

N-vinylpyrrolidone can cause respiratory tract irritation when inhaled. It has also caused liver damage in animals at relatively low exposure levels. In long-term inhalation exposure studies in animals, it has resulted in tumour formation in the liver, larynx and nasal cavity at exposure levels close to those experienced at occupational settings.[286] The mechanism of tumour formation is unclear, but in the absence of evidence to the contrary, these tumours must be considered of relevance to humans. The IARC has allocated NVP to group 3.[294]

Metabolism and monitoring

Since NMP is well absorbed through the skin, biological monitoring may be valuable in the assessment of exposure.[287] NMP is hydroxylated to 5-hydroxy-N-methyl-2-pyrrolidone (5-HNMP), which is oxidized to N-methylsuccinimide (MSI) and further hydroxylated to 2-hydroxy-N-methylsuccinimide (2-HMSI). All these metabolites can be found in the urine of exposed workers.[285] 2-Pyrrolidone (2-P) is a urinary metabolite which is probably formed by demethylation of NMP.[295]

5-HNMP in plasma or urine is recommended for biomonitoring of NMP exposure.[296]

No information on the metabolites of N-vinylpyrrolidone in humans is available. According to animal experiments, it is metabolized to polar metabolites and excreted mainly in the urine.[286]

Management

Management of the health risks from NMP and NVP is based on the monitoring and control of exposure. Attention should be paid to dermal exposure.

N-NITROSAMINES

N-Nitrosodimethylamine

N-Nitrosopiperidine

N-Nitrosomorpholine

N-Nitrosodiethanolamine

N-nitrosamines are an extensive group of chemicals, many of which have been demonstrated to be carcinogenic in several animal species, probably by a genotoxic mechanism. There is no reason to think that humans would be resistant to N-nitrosamine-induced cancer, but clear-cut epidemiological proof of the carcinogenicity of N-nitrosamines as a group, or of individual N-nitrosamines in humans, is lacking. The carcinogenic potency in experimental animals of N-nitrosamines varies widely, some being very potent, inducing cancer even after a single dose. Exposure to N-nitrosamines may be occupational, dietary and also endogenous: amines may be nitrosated in the body to yield nitrosamines.

Early studies indicated the presence of volatile N-nitrosocompounds in azo dye production, fish processing, fish meal production, cutting fluid manufacture and use, rubber industry, and leather tanning.[297–299] N-nitrosodimethylamine (CAS No. 62-75-9), N-nitrosodiethylamine, N-nitrosopiperidine (CAS No. 100-75-4) and N-nitrosomorpholine (CAS No. 59-89-2) were detected in practically all breathing zone air samples in a rubber vehicle sealing plant.[300] Similarly, these plus N-nitrosobutylamine, were detected in more than half of some 700 air samples collected in rubber industries in France.[301] As in the American study, the highest concentrations were observed for N-nitrosodimethylamine. N-nitrosodimethylamine and N-nitrosomorpholine were also detected in rubber industries in Germany, Poland, Holland, the United Kingdom and Sweden.[302] Low concentrations of N-nitrosodimethylamine, N-nitrosomethylethylamine, N-nitrosodiethylamine, N-nitrosodi-n-propylamine, N-nitrosodiisopropylamine, N-nitrosodi-n-butylamine, N-nitrosopiperidine, N-nitrosopyrrolidine and N-nitrosomorpholine were detected in rubber industries in Italy.[303] Volatile N-nitrosoamines (notably N-dimethylnitrosamine, N-nitrosomethylethylamine) were detected in the air in eight foundries using the Ashland procedure for core production.[304] Varying, even high concentrations of N-nitrosodiethanolamine (CAS No. 1116-54-7) have been detected in metal cutting/machining fluids.[305–309]

Clinical effects and epidemiology

N-nitrosodimethylamine ingested at a large dose has caused extensive, even fatal, liver damage but aside from this, there are few data on the toxicity or carcinogenicity of N-nitrosamines in humans. However, exposure to volatile N-nitrosamines in the rubber industry is well documented, and there are several epidemiological studies demonstrating excess cancer. Tobacco smoke contains at least seven N-nitrosoamines, which are considered specific for tobacco smoke[310] and it is likely that these proven animal carcinogens contribute to the elevated cancer risk among smokers.

N-dimethyl- and N-diethylnitrosamine, and N-nitrosomorpholine cause liver damage in experimental animals. N-nitrosodiethanolamine is relatively non-toxic in experimental animals, and causes only very limited liver damage.[17,311]

N-nitrosodimethylamine has induced tumours in some 20 animal species after oral, inhalation and parenteral administration. N-diethylnitrosamine has been tested for carcinogenicity in more than 40 animal species, and caused tumours in all of them. N-nitrosodiethanolamine is a potent carcinogen; it consistently induced liver tumours in rats, and nasal cancer in rats and hamsters. N-nitrosomorpholine induced liver tumours in rats and mice, and tumours of the trachea and nasal cavity in hamsters. N-nitrosopiperidine induced tumours in mice, rats, hamsters and monkeys.[17,311,312]

Thus, there is a marked variation in the target organ for carcinogenic effects between different animal species. Although several alkylnitrosamines are hepatotoxic, there is no direct relationship between hepatotoxicity and carcinogenicity.

Metabolism and monitoring

N-nitrosoamines are activated to genotoxic species by dealkylation, catalysed by CYP2E1 (the same isoenzyme oxidizes ethanol), producing a direct-acting carbonium species, which is considered to be the ultimate carcinogen, and which alkylates DNA.

PHENOL AND PHENOL DERIVATIVES

PHENOL

[CAS No. 108-95-2]

Phenol is a colourless to yellow or light pink solid, which absorbs water easily and liquefies. It has an unpleasant odour with an odour threshold of 0–05 ppm (0.2 mg/m^3). It is a weak acid. Phenol is a widely used industrial chemical. Its main uses are in the production of bisphenol A, phenol resins, alkylphenols, caprolactam, salicylic acid, nitrophenols, diphenyl ethers, halogen phenols and other chemicals. A small amount serves as a component in cosmetics and medical preparations. It can also be used for the production of paints and lacquers, adhesives, impregnating agents and biocides.

Clinical effects and epidemiology

Phenol is a corrosive and acutely toxic chemical. It can cause serious poisoning by skin absorption, inhalation of vapours or by ingestion.[313] Skin contact following spillage of phenolic solutions can lead to rapid absorption, collapse and death within 30 minutes.[313] Death has resulted from the absorption of phenol through a skin area as small as 400 cm^2.[313] Because of the analgesic properties of phenol, the sensation of pain due to local exposure to phenol may be diminished leading to less awareness of contact with the chemical and thus resulting in higher degrees of local damage. Affected skin areas turn brown and gangrenous. Prolonged exposure may result in deposition of a dark pigment in the skin (ochronosis). Clinical features of phenol poisoning include shock, collapse, coma, convulsions, cyanosis, damage to internal organs and death. Cardiac manifestations including different kinds of arrhythmias are also typical. A recent case report describes a 47-year-old male who had 90 per cent phenol spilled over his left foot and shoe (3 per cent of body surface area). After a $4\frac{1}{2}$-hour exposure, clinical manifestations included confusion, vertigo, faintness, hypotension, ventricular premature beats, atrial fibrillation, dark-green urine, swelling, blue-black discoloration and numbness of the affected area. His peak serum phenol level was 21.6 mg/L, which was considered to be in the fatal range.[314]

Metabolism and monitoring

After absorption, phenol is rapidly distributed in body tissues. In the body, it is extensively metabolized to its sulphate and glucuronide conjugates which are excreted in the urine. Exposure to phenol can be assessed by measuring urinary total (free and conjugated) phenol.

Management and diagnosis

In the management of phenol-related health risks, special emphasis should be given to accident prevention and avoidance of dermal exposure. If a spillage resulting in skin contact has occurred, aggressive decontamination of the skin is essential. Polyethylene glycol (PEG) and isopropyl alcohol have been shown to be effective in minimizing phenol-induced skin damage. PEG and isopropyl alcohol with water treatment can also significantly reduce systemic phenol absorption.[315,316]

Phenol derivatives

There is a wide variety of phenol derivatives with different toxicological profiles. These include for example chlorophenols, which have been used as biocides and pesticides, cresol (o-, p-, m-cresol) and resorcinol, as well as nonylphenol and bisphenol A. Some phenol derivatives have been shown to produce skin toxicity resulting in vitiligo. These include p-tert-butylphenol and certain catechol derivatives (4-tert-butylcatechol) and hydroquinone.

CHLOROPHENOLS

Chlorophenols are a group of chemicals in which one to five chlorine atoms have been added to the phenol molecule (Figure 42.19). Thus, five basic types of chlorophenols are monochlorophenols, dichlorophenols, trichlorophenols, tetrachlorophenols and pentachlorophenol. There are 19 different chlorophenols altogether. Chlorophenols have been used as biocides and pesticides and as chemical intermediates in the production of other chemicals. In North America and in Scandinavia, mixtures of chlorophenols, containing mainly 2,3,4,6-tetra-, penta- and 2,4,6-trichlorophenols, have been widely used as wood preservatives, but after national restrictions this use has declined. Chlorophenols have, however, contaminated many old sawmill sites. In a Finnish study, exposure of workers to chlorophenols in the clean up of these contaminated sawmill sites has been generally low.[317]

Chlorophenols can be absorbed into the body by all routes of exposure. In occupational settings, skin absorption may be significant. Chloracne, acquired porphyria cutanea tardia, hyperpigmentation, folliculitis, keratosis

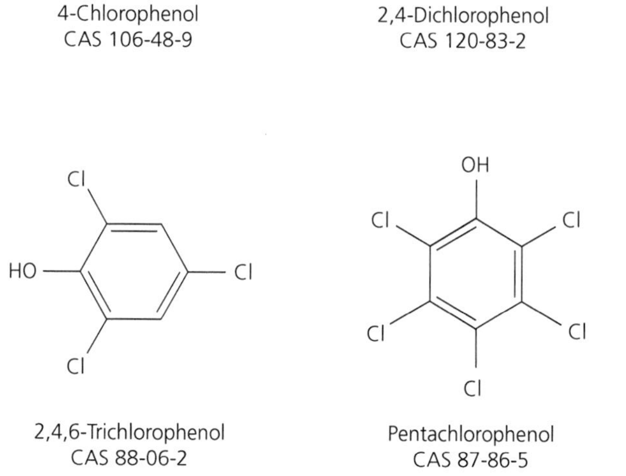

4-Chlorophenol
CAS 106-48-9

2,4-Dichlorophenol
CAS 120-83-2

2,4,6-Trichlorophenol
CAS 88-06-2

Pentachlorophenol
CAS 87-86-5

Figure 42.19 Molecular structures of 4-chlorophenol, 2,4-dichlorophenol, 2,4,6-trichlorophenol and pentachlorophenol.

and hirsutism have been observed in workers employed in the manufacture of 2,4-DCP- and 2,4,5-TCP-based herbicides.[318,319] However, since chlorophenols may contain other chlorinated compounds, especially 2,3,7,8-tetrachlorodibenzo-p-dioxin (TCDD; see under Chlorinated dioxins and furans and related compounds, p. 370) as impurities, it is difficult to ascribe these effects specifically to chlorophenols. Acute toxicity of chlorophenols varies between the individual compounds, pentachlorophenol being the most toxic with an estimated lethal oral dose for humans about 30 mg/kg body weight.[320] It decouples of oxidative phosphorylation resulting in a general increase of metabolic activity.

Pentachlorophenol has shown carcinogenic activity in animal tests, causing for example liver tumours in mice. According to the IARC's evaluation, there is sufficient evidence in experimental animals for the carcinogenicity of pentachlorophenol.[321] Also 2,4,6-trichlorophenol has shown increased incidences of cancer in carcinogenicity tests in mice. The epidemiological evidence on the carcinogenicity of chlorophenol exposure is limited, although in some studies significant associations with several types of cancer, e.g. with soft-tissue sarcoma and non-Hodgkin's lymphoma have been suggested.[322,323] Potential co-exposure to TCDD complicates the interpretation of these studies. IARC has classified combined exposures to polychlorophenols or to their sodium salts as possibly carcinogenic to humans (group 2B).[321]

Exposure to chlorophenols can be assessed by measuring the levels of chlorophenols in urine.[324]

CRESOL AND RESORCINOL

Of cresol isomers, o-cresol (CAS No. 95-48-7) is widely used as an intermediate in the production of other different chemical products including plastics, resins and pesticides.[325] Cresols are corrosive substances. p-Cresol has been associated with occupational vitiligo.[326] Resorcinol (CAS No. 108-46-3) is used in the rubber industry as a chemical intermediate. It has also been used in antiseptics and in keratolytic topical medications in low concentrations. This chemical has caused skin sensitization after medicinal use and also in exposed workers, but in general resorcinol-caused sensitization seems to be rare.[327] Resorcinol has been associated with thyroid effects, including hypothyroidism and goitre mainly after medicinal use (mainly for treating skin ulcers), but some older studies report these effects also in workers exposed to unknown levels of resorcinol.[327]

4-tert-BUTYLPHENOL

4-tert-Butylphenol (CAS No. 98-54-4) is used as an intermediate for phenol resins and polycarbonate resins. It can also be used as a raw material for construction components and floors in buildings. 4-tert-butylphenol is a well-known cause of vitiligo.[326] There are several reports on occupational vitiligo in workers from 4-tert-Butylphenol producing factories.[327]

Vitiligo may become evident a few months to several years after the beginning of exposure. Depigmented patches occur especially at the skin of exposed body sites, such as the hands and forearms, although in some cases it can also be seen at body sites covered by clothing.[328] Some reports have suggested liver and thyroid effects in exposed workers.

The mechanism by which 4-tert-butylphenol and other phenol derivatives cause occupational vitiligo is still uncertain, but probably relates to their structural similarity with the melanin precursor tyrosine. This structural similarity to tyrosine possibly leads to a tyrosinase-related protein-1-mediated mechanism in which the generation of reactive oxygen species causes melanocyte death (apoptosis).[328]

NONYLPHENOL AND BISPHENOL A

[CAS No. 25154-52-3 and CAS No. 80-05-7]

Bisphenol A is used especially in the production of polycarbonates and epoxy resins. Bisphenol A diglycidyl ether (see below under Epoxides), derived from bisphenol A and epichlorohydrin, is the building block of epoxy resins. Other uses of bisphenol A include the manufacture of phenoplast resins, unsaturated polyester resins, can coatings and PVC.[329]

Nonylphenol (and branched 4-nonylphenol (CAS No. 84852-15-3)) are used in the production of nonylphenol ethoxylates and in the plastics industry for the production of phenol and formaldehyde resins. Nonylphenol ethoxylates are used nowadays in many different applications, for example in cleaning and washing agents, cosmetics and construction materials, and as additives in paints.[330]

There are a number of case reports of individuals showing skin sensitization following exposure to epoxy resins derived from bisphenol A. However, it is unclear whether bisphenol A itself or related epoxy resins (see under Bisphenol A diglycidyl ether, p. 361) was the underlying cause of the sensitization.[329] Bisphenol A in the presence of UV light may elicit skin reactions in humans, and positive results for photosensitization have also been obtained in animal tests.[329]

Other hazards related to both of these compounds include irritation (bisphenol A) and corrosivity (nonylphenol) and possible reproductive toxicity. In animal tests, both compounds have shown endocrine modulating (oestrogenic/anti-androgenic) activity, with a potency of 3–6 orders of magnitude less than that of oestradiol.[329–330] Bisphenol A has caused adverse effects in fertility especially in mice.[331] Also, nonylphenol has caused minor effects, compatible with possible oestrogenic activity, in the reproductive system of offspring in multi-generation studies.[330,332] The relevance of these findings to humans is unclear.

EPOXIDES

An epoxide is a compound containing an oxirane ring, i.e. a ring with an oxygen bridge between two adjacent carbon atoms. Oxirane rings are highly strained and reactive especially towards any nucleophilic chemical structure, such as water, amines, aldehydes, alcohols and carboxylic acids. This reactivity is the basis for the uses of epoxides, and also for their biological effects.[333]

ETHYLENE OXIDE

[CAS No. 75-21-8]

At room temperature and normal atmospheric pressure, ethylene oxide is a colourless, highly reactive, and flammable gas with a characteristic ethereal odour. It is mainly used for the synthesis of ethylene glycol (used as anti-freeze), and for the synthesis of polyester resin and solvents. High exposures are encountered in its minor use as a sterilant for hospital supplies, and a fumigant for furs and some food items.

Clinical effects and epidemiology

Ethylene oxide is an ocular, respiratory and dermal irritant and a sensitizing agent. Cataracts have been reported after exposure to ethylene oxide. Sensorimotor polyneuropathy has been reported in a few cases of workers exposed to relatively high concentrations.[334]

An important occupational health concern from ethylene oxide exposure is cancer of lymphohaematopoietic origin. In an extensive study on 18 000 employees at 14 industrial facilities where ethylene oxide was used as a sterilant, there was no overall increase in the risk of mortality from non-Hodgkin's lymphoma or multiple myeloma. However, associations were observed between cumulative exposure and mortality from lymphoid tumours (i.e. non-Hodgkin's lymphoma, multiple myeloma and chronic lymphocytic leukaemia) in men.[335] Results from other cohort studies of ethylene oxide exposure did not point clearly or consistently to an increased risk for these cancers. An increase in breast cancer has not been consistently reported in other studies; however, an internal analysis in a study of 7500 women showed a significant exposure–response relationship between ethylene oxide exposure and breast cancer incidence. The IARC working group considered the epidemiological evidence on causal association between ethylene oxide exposure and cancer to be 'limited'.[100,336]

Mice exposed to ethylene oxide by inhalation showed an increased incidence of alveolar and bronchiolar lung tumours, tumours of the Harderian gland, malignant lymphomas, uterine adenocarcinomas and mammary carcinomas. Rats similarly exposed by inhalation, showed an increased incidence of mononuclear-cell leukaemia, brain tumours, peritoneal mesotheliomas located in the region of the testis and subcutaneous fibromas.

Ethylene oxide induces a dose-related increase in the amount of haemoglobin adducts in humans and rodents and DNA adducts in rodents. It is mutagenic and clastogenic at different phylogenetic levels and it induces heritable translocations in the germ cells of rodents. It also induces a dose-related increase in the frequency of sister chromatid exchange, chromosomal aberrations, and micronucleus formation in lymphocytes of exposed workers.[334]

As an overall evaluation of all the data available, noting especially the consistent results on adduct formation and genotoxicity in exposed humans, the IARC working group classified ethylene oxide as 'carcinogenic to humans' (group 1).[100,336]

Epidemiological studies, while not conclusive, point to an association between exposure to ethylene oxide and spontaneous abortions.[334,337]

In experimental animals, ethylene oxide is fetotoxic in the presence and absence of maternal toxicity at concentrations higher than those associated with cancer and other non-cancer end points (e.g. neurological effects). It is teratogenic only at very high concentrations (above about 1600 mg/m^3).[334]

Metabolism and monitoring

Ethylene oxide is rapidly taken up via the lungs, distributed and metabolized to ethylene glycol and to glutathione conjugates. It can also be absorbed through the skin from the gas phase and from aqueous solutions. Ethylene oxide is an alkylating agent that directly reacts with DNA.[330,334,336] DNA and haemoglobin adducts have been demonstrated in exposed humans. However, quantitative information on the association of these findings with exposure (or health risks) is very limited. Because of the short half-time of ethylene oxide in blood/exhaled air, the application of these analyses for biomonitoring is problematic.

PROPYLENE OXIDE AND 1,2-BUTYLENE OXIDE (1,2-EPOXYBUTANE)

[CAS No. 75-56-9 and CAS No. 106-88-7]

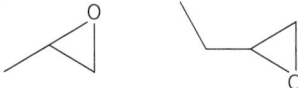

Propylene oxide   1,2-Epoxybutane

Alkane oxiranes with longer chain length (than ethylene oxide) share the irritating propensity of epoxides, but is less marked with longer alkyl chains; at the same time, the volatilit also decreases. In addition to irritation and a slight narcotic effect, little information is available on the adverse effects of these epoxides in humans. Polyneuropathy, similar to that observed in humans, has been reported in experimental animals after exposure to propylene oxide and butylene oxide.[338]

Propylene oxide is a colourless, highly volatile liquid at room temperature and normal atmospheric pressure. It is highly flammable. Inhalation exposure to propylene oxide induced nasal tumours in rats and mice, and less consistently tumours in other organs. Propylene oxide administered by oral gavage to rats produced tumours of the forestomach. Propylene oxide was consistently mutagenic in several *in vitro* test systems, and also induced cytogenetic changes in experimental animals *in vivo*. Haemoglobin adducts, but not cytogenetic effects or DNA damage, has been reported in exposed humans.[339–342] Propylene oxide caused reproductive toxicity (decreased fetal weight and delayed ossification) with no teratogenic effects in rats, only at doses overtly toxic to the dams.[343]

Epoxybutane is a colourless liquid with a characteristic odour. It induced degenerative changes in the nasal mucosa in rats and mice in two-year inhalation studies. It also induced a low frequency of nasal adenomas in male and female rats, as well as alveolobronchiolar carcinomas in male rats.[344] The IARC working group considered these data to provide limited evidence of carcinogenicity in animals, but based on extensive data demonstrating genotoxic activity concluded that epoxybutane is possibly carcinogenic to humans (rather than the 'not classifiable' normally deduced from limited evidence in animals in the absence of epidemiological data).[345]

EPICHLOROHYDRIN

[CAS No. 106-89-8]

Epichlorohydrin is a colourless liquid, the vapour of which forms explosive mixtures with air. It is strongly irritating to the eyes and the skin; it may penetrate rubber gloves to the extent that it can cause marked dermal irritation of the underlying skin. Obstructive lung damage and increased small airways resistance, in addition to irritant effects, have been reported among workers exposed to epichlorohydrin.[346]

Epidemiological studies on four small populations exposed to epichlorohydrin gave inconsistent results with regards to lung cancer risk and epichlorohydrin exposure. Epichlorohydrin induced tumours in rats after inhalation and oral exposure, and noting the chemical reactivity of epichlorohydrin and its direct activity in a wide range of genetic tests, IARC classified it under group 2A.[347]

BISPHENOL A DIGLYCIDYL ETHER

[CAS No. 1675-54-3]

Bisphenol A diglycidyl ether (BADGE) is the building block of epoxy resins; it is synthesized from epichlorohydrin and bisphenol A. Epoxy resins are used extensively for sealing, encapsulating, making castings and pottings, and formulating lightweight foams. Resins are used as binders in the preparation of laminates of paper, polyester cloth, fibreglass cloth and wood sheets. Epoxy resins have outstanding adhesive properties.[348] Fully hardened resin has low toxicity; it is the monomers and oligomers with free epoxide groups that are responsible for the different aspects of epoxy resin toxicity.

The key toxic characteristic of BADGE is contact dermatitis (Figure 42.20), which has been amply demonstrated in numerous case reports; it is apparently the most common causative agent for epoxy resin-induced contact

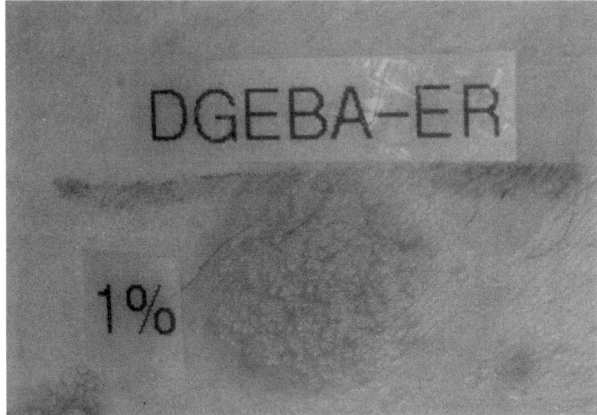

(a)

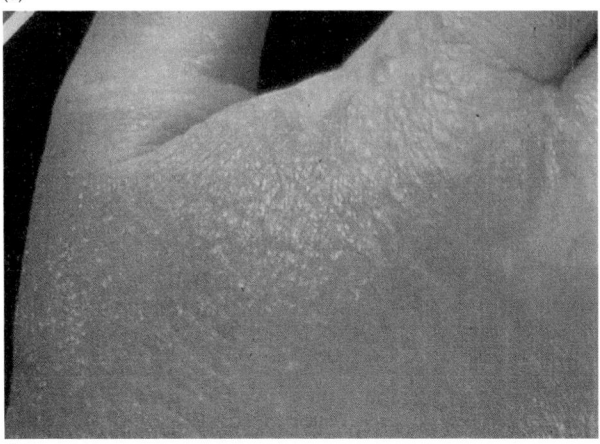

(b)

Figure 42.20 (a) Allergic patch test reaction to epoxy resin; (b) allergic contact dermatitis from epoxy resin. Reproduced with permission from the Finnish Institute of Occupational Health. For colour plate, see website (www.hodderplus.com/hunters).

dermatitis (other possibilities being reactive diluents, amine hardeners and epoxy acrylates).[349–351] It also elicits sensitization in experimental animals. Cases of contact urticaria have also been described after exposure to BADGE.[352] Carcinogenicity studies with BADGE have given conflicting results, the IARC evaluation being 'limited evidence in experimental animals'.[353]

Workers exposed to BADGE exhibited elevated urinary concentrations of bisphenol A.[354] Bisphenol A has oestrogenic and anti-androgenic characteristics in studies on endocrine disruption.[355,356] It is not clear whether this has significance from the human health point of view. However, in one study, blood concentrations of FSH, but not of LH or testosterone, were lower in workers exposed to BADGE than in referents.[354] BADGE did not give rise to developmental toxicity in standard experimental tests.[353,357]

CYCLIC ACID ANHYDRIDES

Cyclic acid anhydrides are a group of reactive chemicals, which are used in the manufacture of polyester and alkyd resins and plasticizers and as epoxy resin hardeners. At room temperature, cyclic anhydrides are powders or crystals, and exposure is mostly to dusts. Hot processes, such as hardening of epoxy resins, welding or burning of painted metals, or curing of the paints, may also involve exposure to fumes.

Cyclic acid anhydrides in use, and with similar clinical effects, include phthalic, hexahydrophthalic, methyl hexahydrophthalic, tetrahydrophthalic, methyl tetrahydrophthalic, tetrachlorophthalic and tetrabromophthalic hydrides, as well as trimellitic, maleic, himic, succinic, dodecenylsuccinic, chlorendic anhydrides and pyromellitic dianhydride (Figure 42.21).

Clinical effects and epidemiology

Exposure to cyclic acid anhydrides causes irritation of the skin, eyes and the respiratory tract as an immediate effect after direct contact. Trimellitic anhydride especially is a very potent eye irritant. Irritation is caused by exposure to both dusts and to vapours.[358]

Contact dermatitis and a positive result on prick testing has been reported in a worker exposed to dodecenylsuccinic anhydride, and in another worker exposed to methyl hexahydrophthalic anhydride. Contact urticaria has been reported in a few cases after exposure to chlorendic, phthalic, maleic, methyl tetrahydrophthalic and methylhexahydrophthalic anhydrides. Urticaria usually occurs after direct dermal contact, but also cases induced by inhalation exposure have been reported.

Occupational asthma and rhinitis have been described after exposure to many different cyclic anhydrides. Typically, after an exposure of 1–35 months, the worker develops rhinitis and asthma. The diagnosis has been based on the exposure, symptoms and a cause–effect relationship supported by immunological tests or challenge tests. The disease is apparently an IgE-mediated immediate-type asthma.[359] In patients with asthma related to the anhydrides, induction of specific IgE antibodies to phthalic anhydride, trimellitic, maleic, methyltetrahydrophthalic, tetrachlorophthalic, hexahydrophthalic, methylhexahydrophthalic, himic and chlorendic anhydride has been detected.[360–374] Cross-reactivity between some acid anhydrides has been reported.[360,369,375,376]

Specific IgG antibodies against trimellitic anhydride-human serum albumin have been correlated with late-onset occupational asthma due to trimellitic anhydride.[368,377–380]

The potency to induce respiratory sensitization varies between different cyclic anhydrides, phthalic and tetrachlorophthalic apparently being less potent than trimellitic, methyltetrahydrophthalic, methylhexahydrophthalic or hexahydrophthalic anhydrides (Table 42.7).

Metabolism and monitoring

Cyclic anhydrides are metabolized to the corresponding carboxylic acids. The concentrations of phthalic and methyltetrahydro-, hexahydro- and methylhexahydrophthalic acids in the urine have been reported to be related to the time-weighted average concentrations in the breathing zone air. Their analysis thus offers the possibility for biological monitoring.[381–384] The information, however, at present is limited and reliable prediction of sensitization risk in an individual from urinary carboxylic acid concentrations is not possible.

Anhydrides react with proteins with lysine residues, and the conjugates are a likely mediator of the immunological response. A relationship between the concentration of the protein conjugates, and air-borne exposure to hexahydro- and methylhexahydrophthalic anhydride has also been demonstrated.

Management and diagnosis

For some cyclic anhydrides, information is available of concentrations likely to induce sensitization (Table 42.7). Individuals already sensitized are likely to develop symptoms at considerably lower exposures, and it is not likely that people once sensitized will be able to carry out tasks with exposure to anhydrides. Cross-reactivity between different anhydrides has been reported.

Diagnosis is based on exposure, and exposure-related symptoms. Specific IgE and also IgG concentrations in the serum are often elevated among exposed groups; and positive skin prick test results have also been reported. However, no reliable information is available on the sensitivity or specificity of these analyses. Positive challenge tests have been reported, but these tests have been seldom used for investigating effects of cyclic anhydrides.[358,359]

Phthalic anhydride (CAS 85-44-9)

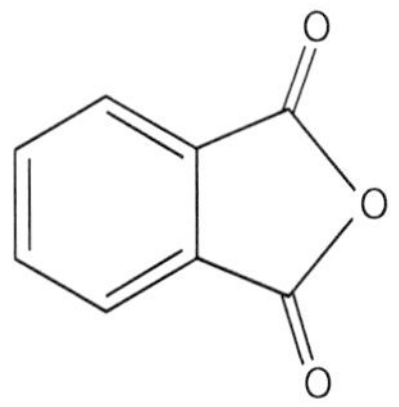

Trimellitic anhydride (CAS 552-30-7)

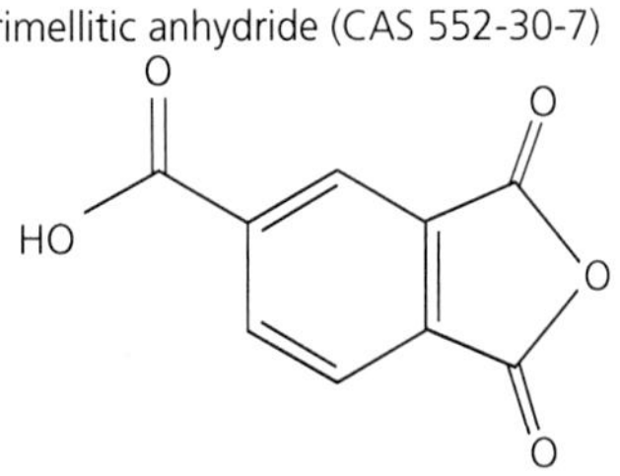

Maleic anhydride (CAS 108-31-6)

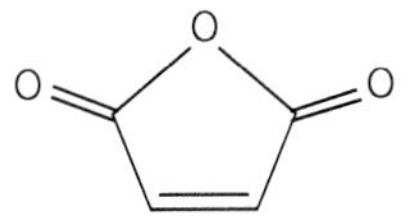

Hexahydrophthalic anhydride (CAS 85-42-7)

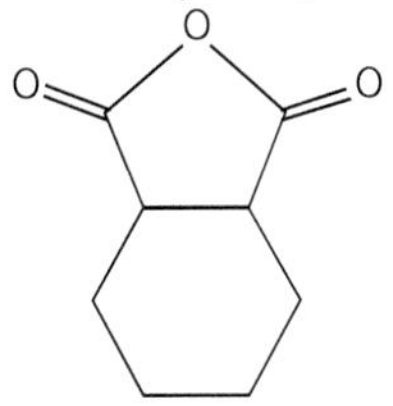

Methylhexahydrophthalic anhydride (CAS 25550-51-0)

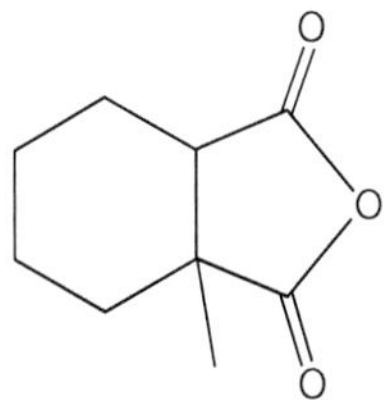

Methyltetrahydrophthalic anhydride (CAS 19438-64-3)

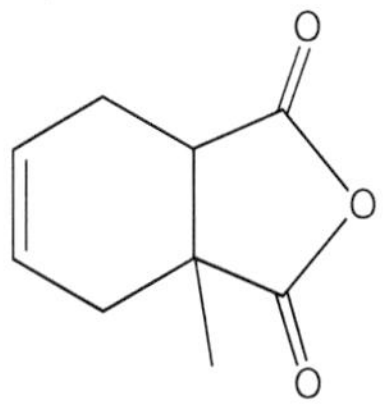

Tetrahydrophthalic anhydride (CAS 85-43-8)

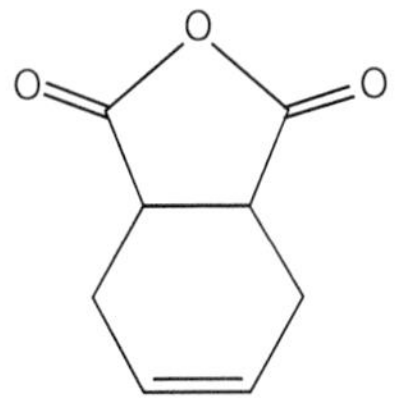

Tetrachlorophthalic anhydride (CAS 117-08-8)

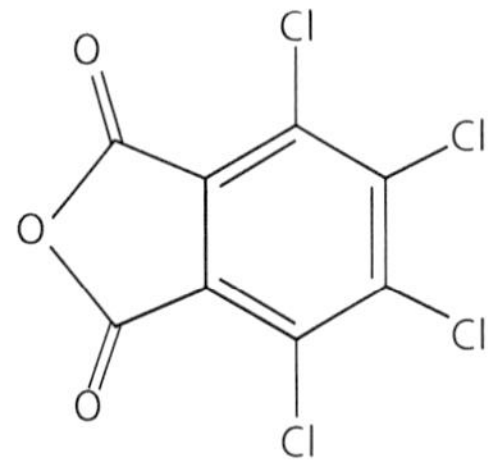

Pyromellitic dianhydride (CAS 89-32-7)

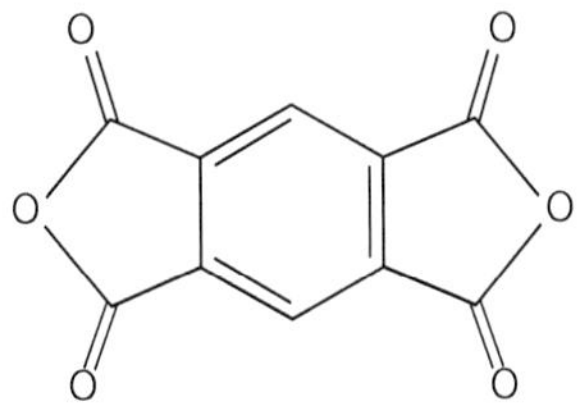

Himic anhydride (CAS 826-62-0)

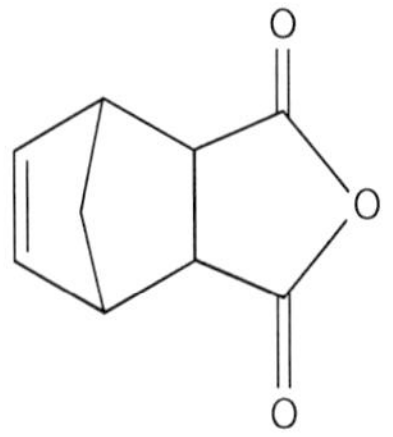

Succinic anhydride (CAS 108-30-5)

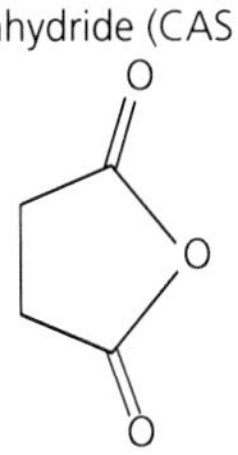

Dodecenyl succinic anhydride (CAS 25377-73-5)

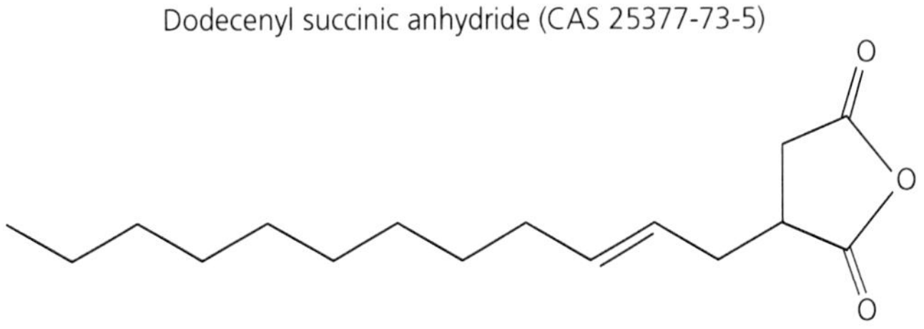

Chlorendic anhydride (CAS 115-27-5)

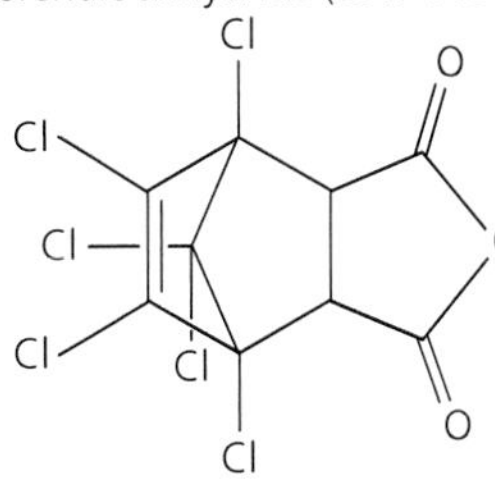

Tetrabromophthalic anhydride (CAS 632-79-1)

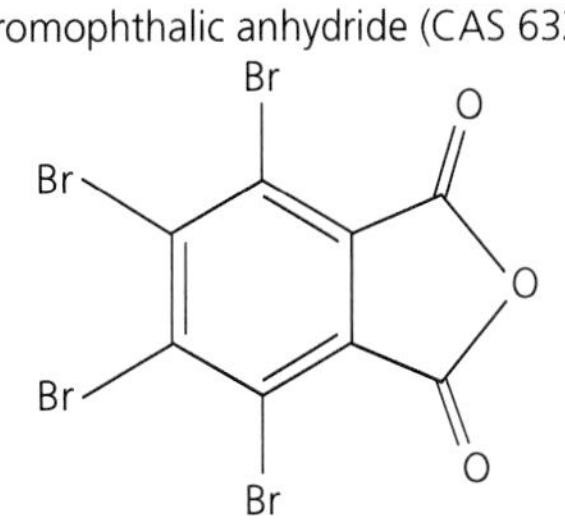

Figure 42.21 Examples of cyclic acid anhydrides.

ISOCYANATES

Isocyanates are a varied group of chemicals, with the isocyanate group (N=C=O) as the common structural element (Table 42.8). They are reactive and can be irritating to the skin and mucous membranes. There are several thousand different diisocyanates, but relatively few are used extensively. Commerically, the most important isocyanates are shown in Table 42.8. Pre-polymerized oligomers of the diisocyanates, which still contain free isocyanate groups, are increasingly being used. Aliphatic isocyanates, such as HDI, are mostly used in paints and coatings (e.g. car paints) due to the excellent resistance to abrasion and superior weathering characteristics, such as gloss and colour retention. Aromatic isocyanates are used as foams, adhesives, sealants, elastomers and binders. Polyurethane foams are a major end use of aromatic isocyanates.[385] Exposure to isocyanates is also possible in tasks which involve heating of polyurethanes or polyurethane-coated products, such as welding, flame cutting, and sawing. Methyl isocyanate (CH_3NCO; CAS No. 624-83-9) is an intermediate in the synthesis of carbamate pesticides; it has also been used in the production of rubbers and adhesives.

Table 42.7 Exposure levels for cyclic anhydrides which have been reported to induce sensitization.[358,359]

Acid anhydride	Exposure level ($\mu g/m^3$)	Critical effect
Phthalic anhydride	1500–17 400	Sensitization, asthma
Tetrachlorophthalic anhydride	140–590	Sensitization, work-related asthma symptoms
Trimellitic anhydride	10–40	Sensitization, work-related symptoms
Hexahydrophthalic anhydride and methyl hexahydrophthalic anhydride	10–50	Sensitization
Methyltetrahydrophthalic anhydride	5–20	Sensitization, rhinitis, conjunctivitis, asthma

Clinical effects and epidemiology

Exposure to isocyanates causes respiratory tract irritation, sensitization and asthma; cases of hypersensitivity pneumonitis have also been described. They also cause skin irritation and contact dermatitis. Diisocyanates are the most common chemical cause of occupational asthma in many countries.

Methyl isocyanate was the cause of the Bhopal incident, where approximately 42 tonnes was accidentally released from an underground storage facility in a densely populated area in India. An estimated 8000 people were killed initially, and another 9000 later. The principal health effects were irritation and corrosion of the respiratory tract. Among the survivors, several studies have reported residual adverse effects on respiratory function.[386–389]

Table 42.8 The most important isocyanates currently in commercial use.

2,4-Toluene diisocyanate (TDI)
CAS 584-84-9

2,6-Toluene diisocyanate (TDI)
CAS 91-08-7

4,4-Methylenediphenyl isocyanate (MDI)
CAS 101-68-8

1,6-Hexamethylenediisocyanate (HDI)
CAS 822-06-0

Isophorone diisocyanate (IPDI)
CAS 4098-71-9

Polymeric MDI
CAS 97568-33-7

The concentrations of isocyanates in the air that are likely to induce respiratory sensitization are not known. It is also not clear if it is the time-weighted average concentration or transient high peak levels that are more important. However, a very high frequency of asthma developed in a new wood-treating facility using MDI and MDI pre-polymer, where the plant was designed to minimize worker exposure. Preventive measures included engineering controls and a comprehensive personal protection programme, as the management was aware that diisocyanate-induced asthma had been reported from other wood-processing facilities.[390] The cases occurred despite the preventive measures implemented.

Dermal exposure may contribute significantly to the development of asthma.[385,390]

While different isocyanates may differ as to their potency to induce asthma, it seems clear that any reactive isocyanate has such potential; the pre-polymerized oligomers included. It is likely that a determinant of the irritation/sensitization potential is the N=C=O group, and a relevant indicator of exposure is the number of N=C=O structures instead of the concentration of the whole chemical in air samples.[385]

In many patients with isocyanate asthma, the symptoms persist even when the exposure is considerably diminished, or stopped completely.[391–393] Patients with elevated levels of IgE antibodies seem to have a more favourable prognosis with fewer and less severe symptoms on follow up.[394]

Metabolism and monitoring

Isocyanates are mainly absorbed via the respiratory tract, but absorption through the skin is also possible, notably in contact with liquid isocyanates. Isocyanates are readily metabolized to the corresponding amines, which are rapidly excreted in the urine as such, and as acetylated products. Biological monitoring methods, based on the analysis of the amines in post-shift urine have been published for MDI and TDI, but not for the aliphatic isocyanates HDI and IPDI.[395,396]

Management and diagnosis

Measurement of isocyanates in the air is complicated, especially for the isocyanates that have low volatility. They partition between the gas and the aerosol phase; both phases being capable of causing sensitization and provoking an asthmatic attack in the already sensitized individuals. Thus, the measurement should comprise both the gaseous and aerosol-carried components of the isocyanate(s), and all chemical species containing these groups should be measured.

The diagnosis of isocyanate-induced asthma depends on a history of symptoms and their relationship to exposure. Demonstration of lung function changes at work may be conclusive. Serial peak flow readings taken at and away from work can indicate a pattern of declines in FEV_1/FVC (forced expiratory volume in 1 second over forced vital capacity) typical of asthma (Figure 42.22). Analysis of specific IgE has a high specificity, but low sensitivity to

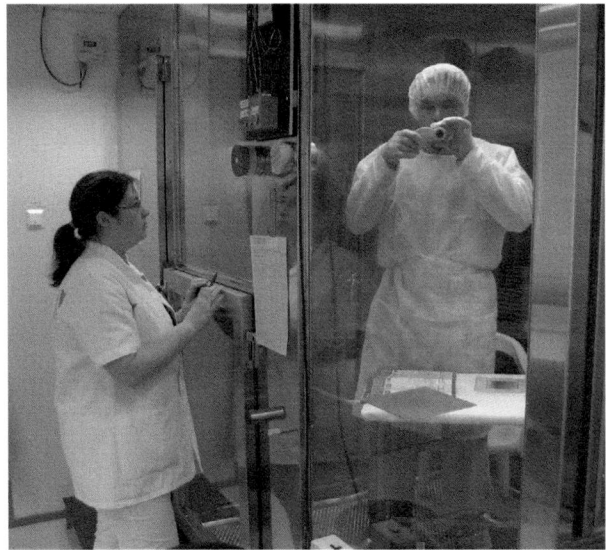

Figure 42.22 Bronchial provocation test carried out in special test chambers can be used for the diagnosis of, for example, isocyanate asthma. Reproduced with permission from the Finnish Institute of Occupational Health.

detect isocyanate-induced asthma. IgG analysis is neither specific nor sensitive. Inhalation provocation tests may be performed, but should be limited to specialized units usually in hospital settings.[397] Urinary analysis of the amines generated in the metabolism of aromatic isocyanates (TDI, MDI) have been used for biological monitoring.[396,398]

CHLORINATED HYDROCARBONS

Halogenated hydrocarbons include both aliphatic and aromatic compounds in which one or more hydrogen atoms are replaced by a halogen. Chlorine is the relevant halogen for the compounds in this section.

The most common and toxicologically relevant aliphatic halogenated hydrocarbons are tri- and tetrachloroethenes, methylene chloride, chloroform, carbon tetrachloride and vinyl chloride. In addition to the toxicological hazards described below, they may also generate highly toxic phosgene gas when heated.

TRICHLOROETHENE AND TETRACHLOROETHENE

[CAS No. 79-01-6 and CAS No. 127-18-4]

Trichloroethene (trichloroethylene) is a colourless liquid with a characteristic chloroform-like odour. The odour threshold lies between 20 and 30 ppm. It has a vapour pressure of 8.6 kPa at 20°C. The main use of trichloroethene is in cleaning of metal parts. According to industry data, 82 per cent of trichloroethene is used for metal degreasing, 9 per cent in adhesives, 6 per cent for consumer uses and 3 per cent for other uses (e.g. extraction, leather preparation, pharmaceuticals).[399] In Europe, use of trichloroethene in metal cleaning has decreased over the past few years.[392]

Tetrachloroethene (tetrachloroethylene, perchloroethylene) is a colourless liquid with an ethereal odour. It has a vapour pressure of 1.9 kPa at 20°C. The major uses of tetrachloroethene are as a chemical intermediate and as a dry cleaning agent. Other uses include metal cleaning and extraction processes.[400]

Exposure to trichloroethene or tetrachloroethene in occupational settings may occur by inhalation or through the skin.[399,401]

Clinical effects and epidemiology

Acute exposure to high trichloroethene concentrations causes central nervous system (CNS) depression. Concentrations of >5000 ppm causes narcosis and potentially serious arrhythmias including ventricular tachycardia. In controlled volunteer studies, marked changes in visual-motor performance and subjective symptoms like dizziness, light-headedness and lethargy have been observed following acute exposure to trichloroethene for two hours at 1000 ppm, whereas exposure to 300 ppm caused only slight, non-significant changes in tests measuring visual-motor performance.[399] Alcohol potentiates the acute neurotoxicity of trichloroethene.[402] The consumption of alcohol following exposure to trichloroethene may cause 'degreaser's flush'. This is a transient redness of the face and neck, often accompanied by chest discomfort and dyspnoea. It only affects a minority of exposed individuals, and the mechanism is uncertain.

Acute inhalation of high concentrations of tetrachloroethene induces CNS depression, dizziness, fatigue, headache, loss of coordination and narcosis, and liver damage with some deaths having been reported. CNS depression and mild respiratory tract irritation may occur at air levels of 690 mg/m^3.[401] In addition, subclinical deficits in vision, cognitive and motor function have occurred in a randomized exposure chamber study at 340 mg/m^3.[403] Both trichloroethene and tetrachloroethene can irritate the skin and mucous membranes, and cause occupational dermatitis due to their defatting properties. Based on animal data and human experience, they are unlikely to cause skin or respiratory sensitization.[399,401]

Long-term exposure to trichloroethene or tetrachloroethene has been suggested to cause chronic solvent encephalopathy (see under Toluene, xylene and styrene, p. 327). A cohort of nearly a hundred metal degreasers showed a significantly increased risk of psycho-organic syndrome from solvent exposure characterized by cognitive impairment, personality changes and reduced motivation, vigilance and initiative.[404] In this study, there was an odds ratio of 5.6 (CI, 0.93–34.3) for psycho-organic syndrome in the medium-exposed group and 42.2 (CI, 1.9–66.6) in the most highly exposed group of workers. None of four other potential confounders (arteriosclerotic disease, neurologic/psychiatric disease, alcohol abuse and current solvent exposure) had any significant association with psycho-organic syndrome.[404]

Exposure-related effects on neuropsychological performance have also been observed in dry cleaners exposed to tetrachloroethene. Impairments in visual reproduction, pattern memory and pattern recognition have been seen in dry cleaners with high chronic exposure.[405] These impairments of visually mediated function were consistent with the impairment of visuospatial functions observed in the patients diagnosed earlier with tetrachloroethene encephalopathy. Effects on visuospatial function were consistently found in subjects employed as dry cleaners for an average of 14.6 years and exposed to an estimated tetrachloroethene eight-hour TWA air concentration of 280 mg/m^3. Effects of tetrachloroethene on colour vision have also been reported.[406]

In animal experiments, trichloroethene has caused midfrequency hearing loss in animal tests.[407] Synergistic effects with noise on hearing thresholds have been reported in animals.[408] In humans, specific evidence on the effects of trichloroethylene on hearing is lacking. One report suggests ototoxic effects in jet engine repair workers resulting in balance disturbances. However, they may have also been exposed to other neurotoxicants.[409]

The carcinogenicity of trichloroethene has been investigated in a number of long-term animal studies. These studies provide clear evidence on trichloroethene's carcinogenicity in rodents. It has induced hepatocellular and lung tumours in mice and kidney tumours in rats.[399] Recent epidemiological studies provide support for the carcinogenicity of trichloroethene. Associations between trichloroethene exposure and kidney cancers, liver and biliary tract cancers, and lymphomas have been suggested.[410] Two recent cohort studies show statistically significant associations between kidney cancer and increasing trichloroethene exposure.[411,412]

Trichloroethene has been shown to have genotoxic potential. However, there are still uncertainties related to mode of action and metabolites responsible for trichloroethene-induced cancers. The available data support the likelihood that toxicity is due to multiple metabolites through several modes of actions.[413] The IARC has classified trichloroethene as class 2A. Some studies have tried to characterize specific mutations related to trichloroethene-induced renal cancers. Currently, however, no specific pattern of mutations in trichloroethene cancers has been identified.

Tetrachloroethene has caused liver and kidney tumours in animal carcinogenicity tests. Epidemiological evidence on the association between occupational exposure to tetrachloroethene and cancer is limited. However, because of the strong animal evidence and the evidence of the genotoxicity of its main metabolites, the IARC has classified tetrachloroethene as group 2A.[414,415]

Metabolism and monitoring

Trichloroethene is predominantly cleared from the body after metabolism, accounting for 50–99 per cent of the absorbed dose. The major metabolic pathway for trichloroethene involves the initial conversion of trichloroethylene by cytochrome P450 to a transient epoxide, which subsequently undergoes intramolecular rearrangement to form trichloroacetaldehyde. Trichloroacetaldehyde is hydrolysed to form chloral hydrate, which is converted by alcohol dehydrogenase and chloral hydrate dehydrogenase to trichloroethanol and trichloroacetic acid, respectively. Other minor metabolites, which have been suggested to be of relevance for trichloroethene-induced cancers include dichloroacetic acid (DCA) and S-(1,2-dichlorovinyl)-L-cysteine (DCVC), which may be involved in liver and kidney carcinogenicity of trichloroethene, respectively.[413]

Unmetabolized trichloroethene is mostly exhaled, whereas metabolites of trichloroethene are predominantly eliminated in urine. Urine trichloroacetic acid (U-TCA) is commonly used to assess exposure to trichloroethene.

Most (98–99 per cent) of absorbed tetrachloroethene is excreted unchanged in exhaled air, regardless of exposure route. The rest is metabolized by two main pathways, cytochrome P450-mediated oxidative route and glutathione-S-transferase (GST)-mediated conjugation. The major metabolite detected in human blood and human urine is trichloroacetic acid (TCA), formed by cytochrome P450-dependent oxidation of tetrachloroethene to epoxide intermediate, but even TCA is formed only in small quantities. The second pathway involves conjugation of tetrachloroethene with glutathione and is associated with generation of reactive metabolites via initial cleavage to S-(1,2,2-trichlorovinyl)-L-cysteine and further degradation of the cysteine conjugate by beta-lyase to a reactive dithioketene and ultimately dichloroacetic acid. Metabolites derived from P450 metabolism, specifically TCA and DCA, have been linked to hepatotoxicity and liver tumorigenesis, whereas reactive metabolites formed through the GSH conjugation pathway have been associated with tetrachloroethene-induced renal toxicity and carcinogenicity.[416]

The available data indicate that tetrachloroethene concentrations in blood and exhaled air give a reliable impression of the exposure over the previous several days. Trichloroacetic acid is a less suitable exposure indicator, as it is also the major metabolite of trichloroethene and trichloroethane, which are often present as impurities in tetrachloroethene, or can be used in the same location as tetrachloroethene.[401] Tetrachloroethene in urine has also been suggested for biomonitoring of tetrachloroethene.[417]

Management and diagnosis

The diagnosis of chronic solvent-induced encephalopathy follows the principles described under Toluene, xylene and styrene, p. 327.

Management of tri- and tetrachloroethene-related risks is mainly related to monitoring and controlling of exposure to as low as technically feasible.

METHYLENE CHLORIDE

[CAS No. 75-09-2]

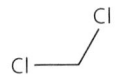

Dichloromethane

Methylene chloride is a clear, highly volatile liquid with a characteristic ether-like odour. It is used because of its good solvent properties in many different applications. One of the most widespread applications is its use as a paint remover. This use is likely to decrease in Europe due to the planned restrictions on methylene chloride use in paint removers. Methylene chloride is well absorbed by inhalation or through the gastrointestinal tract. Absorption through the skin also occurs.

Clinical effects and epidemiology

Since methylene chloride is a highly volatile liquid, it can result in high air concentrations especially when it is used in closed spaces. There are several poisoning cases described in the literature, which have been caused by methylene chloride use in confined spaces.[418] Acute exposure to air levels of 700 mg/m^3 causes slight central nervous system effects (behavioural disturbances), with more significant effects being seen at concentrations in excess of 2000 mg/m^3.[418] Methylene chloride is metabolized in the body to carbon monoxide resulting in elevated carboxyhaemoglobin (CO-Hb) levels. Exposure to 100 or 530 mg/m^3 for 7.5 hours leads to CO-Hb levels of 3.4 and 5.3 per cent, respectively, in human volunteers.[418] Fatal poisonings are considered to be due to the narcotic effects of methylene chloride rather than directly due to carbon monoxide poisoning.[418–421] Poisoning cases in which methylene chloride has been heated resulting in the formation of phosgene have been also described in the literature.[422,423]

Methylene chloride has caused cancer in mice bioassays. According to current knowledge, this effect is related to the specific metabolism of methylene chloride in mice, and the cancer risk in humans is low.[418] No epidemiological data on the carcinogenicity of methylene chloride in humans are available. IARC classification is that methylene chloride is possibly carcinogenic to humans (2B).[424]

Metabolism and monitoring

When inhaled, most of the absorbed methylene chloride is exhaled unchanged and the remainder is metabolized to carbon monoxide, carbon dioxide and inorganic chloride.[418] At lower doses, the main route of metabolism is mediated by cytochrome P450, whereas at high-dose levels ($\geq$1800 mg/m^3) this route is saturated and the metabolism is transferred to involve glutathione transferase (GST) resulting in the formation of formaldehyde, formate and finally carbon dioxide. In mice, the GST pathway is the major pathway.

Methylene chloride can be monitored by measuring the solvent itself in exhaled air or blood, or by analysis of carbon monoxide in exhaled air, or by measuring carboxyhaemoglobin (CO-Hb) in blood, which is currently the preferred method. Smoking is a significant confounding factor in increasing CO-Hb levels.

Management and diagnosis

Because of the high volatility and acute toxicity, methylene chloride should always be handled only in well-ventilated areas. Diagnosis of methylene chloride poisoning is based on a history, symptoms and carboxyhaemoglobin measurement. Treatment is symptomatic including administration of oxygen and follow up of liver, nervous system and renal functions.

VINYL CHLORIDE

[CAS No. 75-01-4]

Vinyl chloride is a colourless, flammable gas with a slightly sweet odour and was previously used as an anaesthetic agent. It is now mainly used for the production of polyvinyl chloride (PVC) plastics in closed systems. It is not known to occur naturally, but is present in cigarette smoke. The level of residual vinyl chloride (VC) in polyvinyl chloride has been regulated since the late 1970s in many countries and nowadays the release of VC from the thermal degradation of PVC is either not detectable or is at very low levels.[425] Exposure to vinyl chloride occurs mainly by inhalation.

Clinical effects and epidemiology

Vinyl chloride has low acute toxicity, but long-term exposure causes severe adverse effects including a specific type of cancer, liver angiosarcoma, in humans.

Prior to the mid-1950s, exposure levels in PVC production could easily exceed 1000 ppm and a specific syndrome called 'vinyl chloride illness' was described in workers. Symptoms included headache, dizziness, earache, blurred vision, fatigue, nausea, sleeplessness, breathlessness, stomach ache, pain in the liver/spleen area, pain and tingling sensation in the arms and legs, cold sensation in the extremities, loss of appetite, loss of libido and weight loss.[425] Specific findings in the skin and bones caused by vinyl chloride included acro-osteolysis accompanied by scleroderma-like changes in the fingers and peripheral circulatory changes resembling Raynaud's disease. Acro-osteolysis is caused by the decalcification of the terminal phalanges of the hands and feet, which may be reversible after cessation of exposure. Also Raynaud's disease caused by vinyl chloride may show some improvement after cessation of the exposure.[425] In a study[426] on 725 workers exposed to significant VC levels, 3 per cent developed acro-osteolysis, 10 per cent Raynaud-type phenomenon and 6 per cent sclerodermoid skin lesions. Genetic susceptibility has been suggested as a possible reason for variability in the clinical picture.

Exposure to VC is also associated with hepatomegaly and/or splenomegaly.[425] Early histological lesions in VC workers showed focal hepatocellular hyperplasia and hyperplasia of sinusoidal cells along with hyperplasia of hepatocytes.[427] Later effects preceding angiosarcoma include subcapsular fibrosis, progressive portal fibrosis and a borderline increase of intralobular connective tissue, all associated with focal stimulation and proliferation of sinusoidal lining cells and hepatocytes.

The ability of vinyl chloride to cause liver angiosarcoma is well known. A recent meta-analysis of two recently updated multicentre cohorts and six smaller studies evaluated the relationship of cancer mortality and vinyl chloride exposure.[428] Six studies suggested an increased risk of liver cancer. For four of these studies, excesses persisted when known cases of angiosarcoma of the liver were excluded. It was noted however, that these results may have been influenced by the underdiagnosis of angiosarcoma. Also increased standardized mortality ratios (SMRs) were suggested for brain cancer, soft tissue sarcomas and lymphatic and haematopoietic neoplasms. Mortality from other neoplasms, including lung cancer, did not appear to be increased according to this meta-analysis. Gennaro and co-workers[429] recently published a reanalysis of updated mortality experience among Italian vinyl chloride and PVC workers exposed in a large petrochemical plant in Porto Marghera between July 1950 and July 1985. In this study, elevated risks for liver cancer, including angiosarcoma, haemolymphopoietic system cancers and lung cancer, were observed in exposed workers. The IARC concluded in 2009 that vinyl chloride causes angiosarcoma of the liver and hepatocellular carcinoma.[100]

The mechanism for liver cancer caused by vinyl chloride has been well studied. Mechanistic events resulting to cancer include:[430,431]

- metabolic activation to form chloroethylene oxide;
- DNA binding of the chloroethylene oxide to form exocyclic etheno adducts;
- ability of these adducts to cause base mutations; and
- effects of such mutations on proto-oncogenes/tumour suppressor genes at the gene and gene product levels.

Specific mutations associated with vinyl chloride-induced liver tumours include G>A transitions at codon 13 of Ki-ras proto-oncogene and A>T transversions in tumour suppressor protein p53.[431] Also serum anti-*p53* antibodies have been found in angiosarcoma patients and in some workers with occupational exposure to VC.[431]

There are some published risk estimates of cancer risk from VC at low exposure levels based on different sets of data.[430] According to these estimates, an angiosarcoma risk of approximately 3×10^{-4} for exposure to 1 ppm vinyl chloride over an entire human working lifetime has been suggested.

Metabolism and monitoring

Vinyl chloride undergoes rapid oxidative metabolism to yield reactive metabolites, the most reactive being chloroethylene oxide (CEO) and its derivative chloroacetaldehyde (CAA).

CEO is formed by cytochrome P450 isoenzyme CYP2E1 and detoxified by epoxide hydrolase and glutathione-S-transferase.[431] Polymorphism of the genes of these xenobiotic metabolizing enzymes may affect the cancer susceptibility of individual exposed workers. According to current knowledge, CEO is the most biologically relevant metabolite and it is likely that VC biotransformation into CEO occurs in the hepatocytes, thus allowing the epoxide to reach and hit the adjacent sinusoidal lining cells that are the target for angiosarcomas. This results in the formation of exocyclic etheno adducts identified in exposed animals and in humans.[430,431]

Management and diagnosis

At current exposure levels in PVC manufacturing (≤1 ppm), the risk for cancer is low, but because of the assumed linear dose–response relationship it is not excludable. Liver angiosarcoma is an uncommon tumour type and therefore if the occupational history shows possible vinyl chloride exposure, the possibility of occupational cancer must be considered. Since there is increasingly more information on specific features of VC-induced liver cancers including specific mutations, these may provide some new tools for the differential diagnosis of VC-induced cancers in future. The prognosis of angiosarcoma of the liver is poor.

The risk of non-cancer effects from VC exposure is related to high-dose exposures and these are unlikely to occur from current work processes.

CHLOROFORM AND CARBON TETRACHLORIDE

[CAS No. 67-66-3 and CAS No. 56-23-5]

Chloroform is a clear, colourless, volatile liquid with a characteristic, ether-like odour. Its main use is in HCFC-22 production. HCFC-22 is used in refrigerant applications (decreasing use) and increasingly as the feedstock for fluoro-polymers, such as polytetrafluoroethylene (PTFE). Earlier use of chloroform as an anaesthetic has been largely discontinued in the western world. Worldwide, chloroform is also used in pesticide formulations, as a solvent for fats, oils, rubber, alkaloids, waxes, gutta-percha (a rubber-like latex from tropical trees used for wire insulation, and for root canal fillings in dentistry) and resins, as a cleansing agent, in fire extinguishers, and in the rubber industry.[432]

Carbon tetrachloride is a colourless, volatile liquid with a characteristic sweet odour. It has been used especially in the production of chlorofluorocarbons (CFCs) used widely as refrigerants and propellants, but this use has decreased in recent years due to restrictions on the use of CFC compounds. It has also had many other uses as a grain fumigant, pesticide, solvent, metal degreaser, fire extinguisher and flame retardant, and in the production of paint, ink, plastics, semiconductors and petrol additives, but many of these uses have decreased or stopped.[433]

Both substances are well absorbed through the lungs, skin and gastrointestinal tract.

Clinical effects and epidemiology

Chloroform has been used in the past to induce and maintain medical anaesthesia. Induction levels were approximately 24–73 g/m³ and maintenance levels 12–48 g/m³ air. This practice was discontinued because chloroform anaesthesia caused deaths due to respiratory effects and arrhythmias and cardiac failure. In addition, jaundice and hepatic dysfunction resulting in lethal liver necrosis have been described after chloroform anaesthesia.[432] Some reports suggest toxic liver jaundice and hepatitis in workers exposed to varying levels of chloroform for less than six months to four years.[434,435] In animal tests, chloroform has caused liver damage and increased kidney weight after repeated inhalation exposure at high doses.[432]

The liver and kidney are also target organs for carbon tetrachloride toxicity. Symptoms of acute intoxication after accidental or suicidal high level exposure are independent of the route of intake and include nausea, vomiting, headache, dizziness and dyspnoea. Liver damage appears after 24 hours or more, but kidney damage is evident often only after two to three weeks following the poisoning.[433] No association between occupational, long-term low-level exposure to carbon tetrachloride and liver disease has been described.

Both substances have induced cancer in animals. Chloroform has been negative in genotoxicity tests and its carcinogenicity (hepatic and renal cancers) is most likely secondary to hepatotoxicity and nephrotoxicity observed in animal tests at high dose levels.[432] In addition, carbon tetrachloride has been mainly negative in genotoxicity tests and hepatomas and hepatocellular carcinomas seen in long-term cancer bioassays in animals have been observed mainly at the dose levels producing liver toxicity.[433] No clear epidemiological evidence on their carcinogenicity in humans is available.

Metabolism and monitoring

Chloroform is metabolized mainly by CYP2E1. The end-product of oxidative metabolism by CYP2E1 is carbon dioxide and reactive intermediates include phosgene.

Carbon tetrachloride is metabolized by cytochrome P450 enzymes (CYP2E1 and CYP2B1/2B2), leading to the formation of reactive trichloromethyl and trichloromethylperoxyl radicals, which can further react to form phosgene.[432,433]

Management and diagnosis

Liver and kidney diseases caused by chloroform and carbon tetrachloride are mainly related to high level accidental exposures or anaesthesia (chloroform). The treatment of acute carbon tetrachloride or chloroform poisoning is symptomatic, including follow up of liver and kidney function. N-acetylcysteine and pyridoxine (administered orally) may provide some protection against carbon tetrachloride-caused hepatic injury, if administered early following acute exposure.[260]

CHLOROBENZENES

Chlorobenzenes, like 1,4-dichlorobenzene and hexachlorobenzene, are examples of aromatic halogenated hydrocarbons. 1,4-Dichlorobenzene (CAS No. 106-46-7) is a substance used in the chemical industry for the production of other chemicals, but also in moth repellants, air fresheners and toilet blocks. The main health concern related to 1,4-dichlorobenzene is its ability to cause liver tumours in mice.[436] The mechanism of this effect is unknown, but appears to be related to high experimental doses.

Hexachlorobenzene (CAS No. 118-74-1) is an environmental contaminant released from a number of sources, including the use of some chlorinated pesticides, incomplete combustion, old waste removal sites and inappropriate manufacture and disposal of waste from the manufacture of chlorinated solvents, chlorinated aromatics and chlorinated pesticides.[437] Hexachlorobenzene caused poisoning of more than 600 people in Turkey when they consumed bread made from wheat that was contaminated with hexachlorobenzene used as a fungicidal seed dressing in the 1950s. The clinical manifestations were porphyria cutanea tarda with disturbances in porphyrin metabolism, dermatological lesions, hyperpigmentation, hypertrichosis, enlarged liver, thyroid gland and lymph nodes, osteoporosis and arthritis.[437] Acquired hepatic porphyrias have also been described following exposure to vinyl chloride, some halogenated biphenyls, chlorinated naphthalenes, and organophosphate and organochlorine pesticides. Hexachlorobenzene has been carcinogenic in animal tests producing liver tumours. IARC classified it under group 2B.[438]

Chlorinated dioxins and furans, and related compounds

2,3,7,8-Tetrachlorodibenzo-p-dioxin

Table 42.9 Relative toxicity of dioxin-like compounds.[439]

Compound	CAS No.	TEF
Chlorinated dibenzo-p-dioxins		
2,3,7,8-TCDD	1746-01-6	1
1,2,3,7,8-PeCDD	40321-76-4	1
1,2,3,4,7,8-HxCDD	57653-85-7	0.1
1,2,3,6,7,8-HxCDD	57653-85-7	0.1
1,2,3,7,8,9-HxCDD	19408-74-3	0.1
1,2,3,4,6,7,8-HpCDD	35822-46-9	0.01
Octachlorodibenzodioxin	3268-87-9	0.0003
Chlorinated dibenzofurans		
2,3,7,8-TCDF	51207-31-9	0.1
1,2,3,7,8-PeCDF	57117-41-6	0.03
2,3,4,7,8-PeCDF	57117-31-4	0.3
1,2,3,4,7,8-HxCDF	70648-26-9	0.1
1,2,3,6,7,8-HxCDF	57117-44-9	0.1
1,2,3,7,8,9-HxCDF	72918-21-9	0.1
2,3,4,6,7,8-HxCDF	60851-34-5	0.1
1,2,3,4,6,7,8-HpCDF	67562-39-4	0.01
1,2,3,4,7,8,9-HpCDF	55673-89-7	0.01
Octachlorodibenzofuran	39001-02-0	0.0003
Non-ortho substituted PCBs		
PCB 77 (3,4,3',4'-tetraCB)	32598-13-3	0.0001
PCB 81 (3,4,5,3'-tetraCB)	70362-50-4	0.0003
PCB 126 (3,4,5,3',4'-pentaCB)	57465-28-8	0.1
PCB 169 (3,4,5,3',4',5'-hexaCB)	32774-16-6	0.03
Mono-ortho substituted PCBs		
105 (2,3,4,3',4'-pentaCB)	32598-14-4	0.00003
114 (2,3,4,5,4'-pentaCB)	74472-37-0	0.00003
118 (2,4,5,3',4'-pentaCB)	31508-00-6	0.00003
123 (3,4,5,2',4'-pentaCB)	65510-44-3	0.00003
156 (2,3,4,5,3',4'-hexaCB)	38380-08-4	0.00003
157 (2,3,4,3',4',5'-hexaCB)	69782-90-7	0.00003
167 (2,4,5,3',4',5'-hexaCB)	52663-72-6	0.00003
189 (2,3,4,5,3',4',5'-heptaCB)	39635-31-9	0.00003

TEF, toxicity equivalence factor.

2,3,7,8-Tetrachlorodibenzofuran

TCDD (more accurately, 2,3,7,8-tetrachlorodibenzo-p-dioxin (CAS No. 1746-01-6), is the most potent of a large group of halogenated chemicals, which share qualitatively similar toxicological properties, while differing widely in their potency. The key to the toxicity of these chemicals is the planar molecular configuration, with 3–4 halogen atoms at the corners. This molecular form fits a receptor molecule in the body, and this is apparently the reason for the unique toxicity of these compounds.

While the most studied group is compounds with chlorine substituents, other halogenated compounds have similar effects. One of the best studied is polybrominated biphenyls (PBBs), previously used as flame retardants. The most toxic of these compounds are listed in Table 42.9, with an estimated relative toxicity for each as assessed by WHO in 1998 and 2005.[439]

Dioxins cause chloracne, peripheral neuropathy, liver damage, hepatic porphyria and hypercholesterolaemia. Changes in the immune system and glucose metabolism have been described in adults, as well as alterations in thyroid hormone levels, and possible changes in neurobehavioural tests, and infection resistance.[440,441]

The best information on cancer and dioxins comes from cohorts exposed to dioxin-contaminated herbicides in herbicide production.[440] In these cohorts, the risk of cancer at all sites was elevated and showed a relationship with the estimated intensity of the exposure. The cancer types that show the most consistent relationship to dioxin exposure, are cancer of the lung, non-Hodgkin's lymphoma and soft tissue sarcoma. The best studied dioxin, 2,3,7,8-tetrachlorodibenzodioxin, is clearly a carcinogen in experimental animals. The mechanism of carcinogenicity apparently is tumour promotion through modification of cellular replication and apoptosis. The IARC evaluation is group 1 for 2,3,7,8-TCDD and 2,3,4,7,8-pentachlorodibenzodioxin.[100] Recently, the IARC group 1 classification was extended also to 2,3,4,7,8-pentachlorodibenzofuran (CAS No. 51207-31-9) and 3,4,5,3',4'-pentachlorobiphenyl, which are indicator chemicals for a larger class of dioxin-like chlorinated dibenzofurans and dioxin-like polychlorinated biphenyls.[100]

From a meta-analysis of studies performed (but not all published), it was concluded that there was an elevated frequency of all malformations among babies born to mothers exposed to Agent Orange (containing dioxins) during the Vietnam war.[442] The data are strongest for spina bifida and anencephaly.[443] Exposure to TCDD was related to semen quality and serum testosterone levels in exposed men.[444,445] In experimental animals, TCDD is toxic to reproduction and to development; the developing fetus seems to be orders of magnitude more sensitive to TCDD than adult animals. The spectrum of malformations induced varies between species.

POLYCHLORINATED BIPHENYLS

Polychlorinated biphenyls (PCBs) have been produced commercially since 1929 (Figure 42.23). They have been used in plasticizers, surface coatings, inks, adhesives, flame retardants, pesticide extenders, paints and microencapsulation of dyes for carbonless duplicating paper, as well as dielectric fluids in transformers and capacitors. Many countries have severely restricted or banned the production of PCBs and at present, occupational exposure should be limited to waste disposal. The pyrolysis of PCB mixtures produces hydrogen chloride and polychlorinated dibenzofurans (PCDFs), and pyrolysis of mixtures containing chlorobenzenes also produces polychlorinated dibenzodioxins (PCDDs). Commercial PCBs are mixtures of (theoretically) 209 different isomers and the trade names used include Aroclor, Pyranol, Pyroclor (United States), Phenochlor, Pyralene (France), Clopehn, Elaol (Germany),

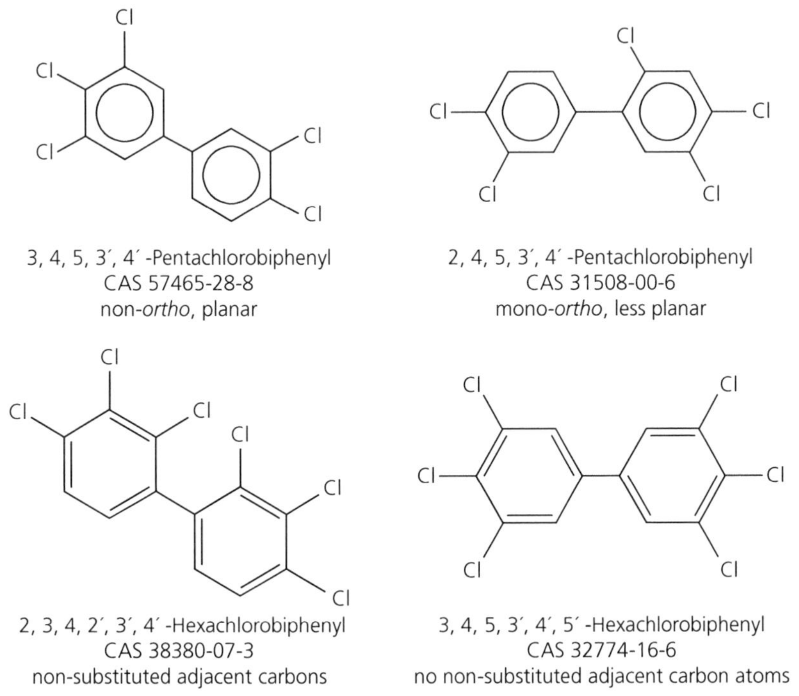

3, 4, 5, 3', 4' -Pentachlorobiphenyl
CAS 57465-28-8
non-*ortho*, planar

2, 4, 5, 3', 4' -Pentachlorobiphenyl
CAS 31508-00-6
mono-*ortho*, less planar

2, 3, 4, 2', 3', 4' -Hexachlorobiphenyl
CAS 38380-07-3
non-substituted adjacent carbons

3, 4, 5, 3', 4', 5' -Hexachlorobiphenyl
CAS 32774-16-6
no non-substituted adjacent carbon atoms

Figure 42.23 Molecular structures of various polychlorinated biphenyls.

Kanechlor, Santotherm (Japan), Fenchlor, Apirolio (Italy) and Sovol (Russia).[441]

Clinical effects and epidemiology

Some PCB compounds are structurally close to dioxins and also exhibit dioxin-like toxicity, albeit at a much lower potency than TCDD (see Table 42.9). Heat transfer fluids and dielectric fluids, which have been exposed to heat, are likely to also contain furans/dioxins.

'Yusho disease' was the term given to clinical effects of PCBs that occurred following ingestion of rice oil contaminated with Kanechlor 400 (a heat-transfer medium containing PCB). Two well-recognized public health incidents of Yusho disease occurred in southern Japan in 1968, and central Taiwan in 1979. PCDFs and PCQs (polychlorinated quarterphenyls) also detected in the contaminated oil may be largely responsible for the health effects.

In occupational exposure to high concentrations of PCB, skin rashes occurred a few hours after the exposure. Furthermore, itching, burning sensations, irritation of the conjunctivae, pigmentation of the fingers and nails, and chloracne were found after exposure to high PCB concentrations. Chloracne is one of the most prevalent findings among PCB-exposed workers. Liver disturbances are also a constant finding after occupational exposure to high levels of PCB. In addition, immunosuppressive changes, neurological and unspecific psychological or psychosomatic effects, such as headache, dizziness, depression, sleep and memory disturbances, nervousness, fatigue and impotence have been described, although the causal relationship to exposure to PCB is not well established.[446] Reproductive/developmental effects, such as effects on sperm motility, fetal growth rate (lower birthweight, smaller head circumference) and development (shorter gestational age, neuromuscular immaturity), and neurological functions of the offspring (impaired autonomic function, increased number of abnormally weak reflexes, reduced memory capacity, lower IQ scores, and attention deficit) have also been associated with exposure to PCB.[441] However, it is uncertain if these effects are directly caused by PCB.

PCBs have low acute toxicity in experimental animals. In long-term studies, adverse effects have been described, notably on the liver, skin, kidneys, as well as on the immunological and endocrine system. Fetotoxicity has been described at high doses; neurodevelopmental effects have been observed in monkeys at doses that are not toxic to the mother.[441]

PCB isomers, notably those with more than 50 per cent chlorination, as well as commercial mixtures of highly chlorinated PCB, consistently induced tumours in experimental animals,[17,441] apparently through a mechanism that does not involve direct genotoxic action. The IARC evaluation is group 2B for polychlorinated biphenyls; the non-*ortho*-substituted planar, dioxin-like PCB 126, however, was classified as a group 1 carcinogen.[100]

Metabolism and monitoring

PCBs are absorbed by ingestion, inhalation and readily by the dermal route. They are metabolized by hydroxylation, but there are marked differences in the rate of metabolism between different congeners. PCBs that are highly chlorinated and lack adjacent non-substituted carbon atoms (e.g. 2,4,6 and 3,5 substituted PCBs) are metabolized only very slowly and accumulate in adipose tissue.[447] The body burden of PCBs may be assessed from the determination of PCB in serum.

Hydrochlorofluorocarbons

In hydrochlorofluorocarbons (HCFC), there is at least one hydrogen atom left unsubstituted in a structure composed of an alkane chain (usually 1–3 carbons); the rest of hydrogen atoms being substituted by chlorine and fluorine. The most commonly encountered HCFCs are chlorodifluoromethane (HCFC 22, CHF_2Cl), dichlorotrifluoroethane (HCFC 123, $CHCl_2CF_3$), chlorotetrafluoroethane (HCFC 124, $CHClFCF_3$), dichlorofluoroethane (HCFC 141b, CH_3CFCl_2) and chlorodifluoroethane (HCFC 142b, CH_3CF_2Cl).[448]

Partially substituted hydrochlorofluorocarbons were introduced as a substitute for completely substituted chlorofluorocarbons, when the ozone-depleting and global warming potential of the latter led to their ban under the Montreal protocol. (The Montreal protocol on substances that deplete the ozone layer was an international agreement signed under the Vienna convention in 1985 to restrict the use of chlorofluorocarbons and other halogenated chemicals, for environmental protection.) However, even HCFC have some ozone-depleting and global warming properties, and the amendments of the Montreal protocol dictate restriction and ultimate phasing out also of HCFCs.[449]

In contrast to fully substituted chlorofluorocarbons, HCFCs are to a varying extent metabolized in the body. The toxicity of HCFCs in animals, even from long-term studies, is low. The main health concerns have been their potential to induce cardiac arrhythmias, and for some PCBs the issue of carcinogenicity has also been raised as a cause of concern.

CHLORODIFLUOROMETHANE

[CAS No. 75-45-6]

Chlorodifluoromethane (HCFC22) is a non-flammable gas (at room temperature and normal atmospheric pressure), colourless and practically odourless. It is used as a refrigerant, aerosol propellant and blowing agent for polystyrene. It is an intermediate in the production of tetrafluoroethylene.[450]

Clinical effects and epidemiology

Increased palpitations were reported in a limited study among people exposed to HCFC22, but the study is very difficult to interpret. In a 24-hour electrocardiogram (ECG) recording of a small number of people exposed to HCFC12 and 22, no clear-cut connection between the exposure and different arrhythmias was observed.[451]

In mice and dogs, exposure to HCFC22 in most studies at concentrations in excess of $1000\,g/m^3$ has been reported to increase the sensitivity of the animals to adrenaline-induced arrhythmias.[450] Based on findings of an increased incidence of subcutaneous fibromas and Zymbal gland tumours in male rats, and no evidence of carcinogenicity in mice or female rats, the IARC concluded that the evidence of carcinogenicity of HCFC22 in experimental animals is limited.[452] HCFC22 induced base-pair substitution mutations in *Salmonella typhimurium*, but was otherwise negative in genotoxicity testing. High concentrations of HCFC22 induced eye malformations in rats.

Metabolism and monitoring

HCFC22 is absorbed from the respiratory tract. It is not significantly metabolized; it is excreted unchanged in exhaled air, the bulk of the absorbed amount being excreted within a few minutes.

DICHLOROTRIFLUOROETHANE

[CAS No. 306-83-2]

Dichlorotrifluoroethane (HCFC123) is a non-flammable volatile liquid with a faint ethereal odour. The principal use for HCFC123 is as a refrigerant in commercial and industrial air-conditioning installations, in fire extinguishers, as a foam-blowing agent, and in metal and electronics cleaning.[453]

Clinical effects and epidemiology

Four case series convincingly demonstrate that repeated occupational exposure to HCFC123 leads to liver damage.[454–457] This effect has also been seen in experimental animals. No reports are available on cardiac arrhythmias in humans exposed to HCFC123. In dogs, exposure to HCFC combined with an adrenaline challenge induced fatal arrhythmias. In a carcinogenicity study in rats, there was an increased incidence of hepatocellular adenomas in females and males, of cholangiofibromas in females administered the highest dose, and of pancreatic acinar cell adenomas and Leydig cell adenomas in males. With the exception of clastogenicity reported *in vitro*, studies on mutagenicity were negative. All tumour types observed were benign; HCFC123 is apparently non-mutagenic *in vivo*, and the carcinogenic mechanism is therefore probably not through a genotoxic mechanism. However, in the view of the International Programme on Chemical Safety (IPCS) of the World Health Organization (WHO), the elevated incidence of several types of tumours raises a concern for possible carcinogenicity in humans.[453]

HCFC123 did not show teratogenicity or other reproductive toxicity in experimental animals.

Metabolism and monitoring

HCFC123 is metabolized by cytochromes P450 reductively and oxidatively. Both reaction pathways lead to the metabolites trifluoroaldehyde and trifluoroacetic acid that are common to halothane ($CHClBrCF_3$), a known hepatotoxic anaesthetic.

CHLOROTETRAFLUOROETHANE

[CAS No. 63938-10-3]

Chlorotetrafluoroethane (HCFC124) is a non-flammable, colourless and odourless gas. It is used as a blowing agent for polystyrene and polyolefin foams and as a blend in refrigerants.

Clinical effects and epidemiology

Human health effects from exposure to HCFC124 have not been reported. The main effects seen in experimental studies are lethargy and other signs of depression of the central nervous system. No liver toxicity was observed in rats in 90-day or two-year studies at exposure levels up to 50 000 ppm. Benign mammary fibroadenomas were observed in female rats exposed to 50 000 ppm for two years. HCFC124 was not genotoxic and did not result in adverse developmental or fertility effects in animals. Inhalation exposure to 2.5 per cent or more of HCFC124 to dogs increased the sensitivity of the animals to adrenaline-induced arrhythmias.[458–461]

Metabolism and monitoring

HCFC124 is metabolized by cytochrome P450 IIE1 to trifluoroaldehyde and trifluoroacetic acid (which are the hepatotoxic metabolites from halothane produced by the oxidative pathway); however, to a much smaller extent than HCFC123.[461]

1,1-DICHLORO-1-FLUOROETHANE

[CAS No. 1717-00-6]

1,1-Dichloro-1-fluoroethane (HCFC141b) is a non-flammable volatile liquid with a faint ethereal odour. It was developed as a substitute for CFC-11, a fully halogenated chlorofluorocarbon mainly for use as a blowing agent for polyurethane and polyisocyanurate insulating foams and as a solvent in electronic and other precision cleaning applications. It is being phased out following the Montreal protocol.[462]

Clinical effects and epidemiology

No information on adverse effects after occupational exposure of humans to HCFC141b is available; a six-hour experimental inhalation exposure to 1000 ppm did not lead to adverse effects.

In experimental animals, HCFC141b induced narcosis at concentrations of approximately 40 000 ppm. HCFC141b was not hepatotoxic; it did not induce teratogenesis or other adverse effects on reproduction. HCFC141b caused Leydig cell hyperplasia and adenomas in male rats, but induced no malignant tumours in either female or male rats. It was negative in tests for bacterial mutagenicity, but gave both negative and positive results in cytogenetic studies in vitro. It did not induce micronuclei in mouse bone marrow in vivo.

HCFC141b increases the sensitivity of dogs to adrenaline-induced arrhythmias at inhalation exposure levels of 10 000 ppm.[463–467]

Metabolism and monitoring

HCFC141b is metabolized slowly by cytochrome P450 IIE1 to 2,2-dichloro-2-difluoroalcohol, and to an even smaller extent, further to 2,2-dichloro-2-difluoroacetic acid. In contrast to the metabolites (trifluoroacetaldehyde and trifluoroacetate) of HCFC123, no binding to proteins of these metabolites was observed.[468]

1-CHLORO-1,1-DIFLUOROETHANE

[CAS No. 1717-00-6]

1-Chloro-1,1-difluoroethane (HCFC142b) is a flammable, colourless and odourless gas mainly used as a blowing agent and in the production of fluoropolymers. Small amounts are used as a component of refrigerant fluids. Its use is being phased out in compliance with the Montreal protocol.[469]

Clinical effects and epidemiology

No information on the toxicity of HCFC142b in humans is available. It caused anaesthesia at high concentrations in experimental animals, but with no morphological adverse effects in the central nervous system. It was not hepatotoxic, did not induce teratogenesis or other reproductive toxicity, and was not carcinogenic to rats.[469] It was mutagenic to Salmonella, but did not induce cytogenetic abnormalities in mouse bone marrow in vivo.

HCFC141b sensitized dogs to the arrhythmogenic effect of adrenaline at inhalation exposure levels of 25 000 ppm.[470]

Metabolism and monitoring

HCFC142b is mostly excreted unchanged. Dechlorination has however been observed in vitro and chlorodifluoroacetic acid has been reported as a metabolite. The metabolic pathways are analogous to those responsible for halothane liver toxicity.[471,472]

SULPHUR-CONTAINING SUBSTANCES

CARBON DISULPHIDE

[CAS No. 75-15-0]

S=C=S

Carbon disulphide is a clear, colourless or faintly yellow, liquid. It is mainly used in the production of viscose fibre and cellophane film. Other uses include the manufacture of carbon tetrachloride (apparently only very small amounts produced and used at present), sodium sulphite, mineral flotation agents, xanthates, mercaptans and thioureas. Carbon disulphide is also used as a solvent for fats, lipids, resins, rubbers, sulphur monochloride and white phosphorus.[473]

Clinical effects and epidemiology

Single or long-term exposure to high levels of carbon disulphide led to the recognition of chronic carbon disulphide intoxication, characterized by psychoses, polyneuropathy of the lower extremities, gastrointestinal disturbances, myopathy of the calf muscles, neurasthenic syndrome, optic neuritis and atherosclerotic vasculoencephalopathy.[473,474]

In exposure conditions not leading to overt intoxication, the peripheral and central nervous systems appear to be the critical target for carbon disulphide-induced toxicity. The effects include reduced conduction velocity in the peripheral nerves and impaired performance in psychomotor testing.[473,475] Brain nuclear magnetic resonance (NMR) images usually show multiple high signal intensities in the basal ganglia and subcortical white matter suggesting a vascular event particularly in the small

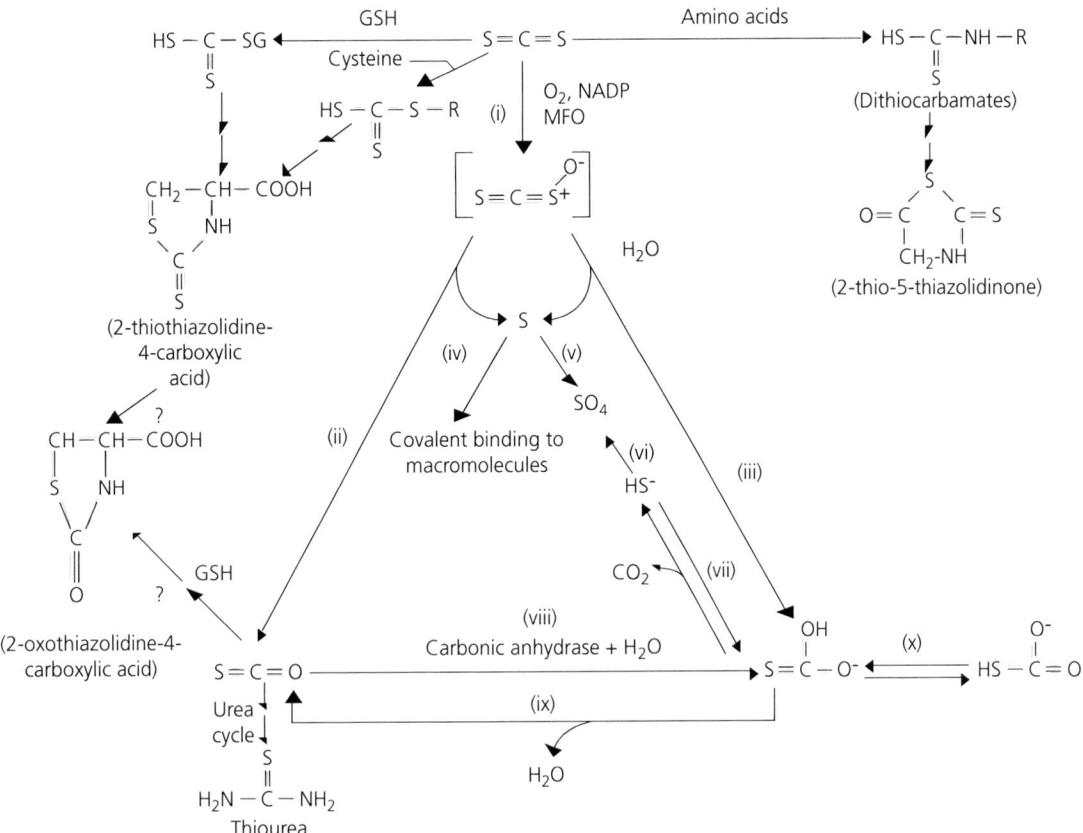

Figure 42.24 Metabolism of carbon disulphide.[494]

vessels.[476–478] NMR of the brain also revealed cerebral effects even among workers whose neuropsychological testing results have not been adversely affected.[479]

Increased mortality from cardiovascular disease after exposure to carbon disulphide was described in the 1970s in a rayon producing facility. When the exposure was lowered to below 10 ppm (30 mg/m^3), this effect was not observed.[480,481] Several larger studies have since verified the potential of carbon disulphide to cause cardiovascular mortality, notably at levels in excess of 30 mg/m^3.[473,482,483] However, at these low exposure levels, i.e. less than 30 mg/m^3, some studies have demonstrated a decrease in carotid artery elasticity.[484,485]

Carbon disulphide exposure also leads to elevated serum cholesterol levels and blood pressure, both recognized as risk factors for cardiovascular disease.[473,486] While some studies have reported elevated cholesterol levels at estimated exposure levels of <30 mg/m^3,[487] cholesterol levels were not elevated among workers, where exposures have mainly remained below 3 ppm (10 mg/m^3),[488] and also in workers with an average of 20 years of exposure at mean exposure levels of 5 ppm (15 mg/m^3).[489]

Carbon disulphide exposure potentiates the effect of noise on hearing loss[490] and induces ophthalmologic effects, including those on colour vision and damage to the blood vessels of the retina.[473,491]

Cancer has not been well studied in the epidemiological studies on carbon disulphide-exposed worker groups. In the limited studies available, there is no consistent picture of an increase in any specific cancer type.[473] No adequate carcinogenicity studies have been published on carbon disulphide in experimental animals. The database to assess the genotoxicity of carbon disulphide is limited. In bacterial mutagenicity assays, it has been negative, while mammalian cell studies are equivocal. The available limited data on genotoxicity *in vivo* are generally negative.

While there are several reports of reduced libido and/or impotence in male workers exposed to carbon disulphide in the viscose rayon industry, there is no clear evidence of effects on male fertility or on fetal development.[492] An exploratory study reported an increased frequency of spontaneous abortions among female workers of a company producing rayon fibre;[493] conflicting reports on the study have been published thereafter. In experimental animals, no effect on semen quality has been reported. Fetotoxicity has been clearly demonstrated at dose levels toxic to the mother only, and teratogenicity is seen mostly at dose levels higher than those needed to produce fetotoxicity.[128,473]

Metabolism and monitoring

Carbon disulphide is absorbed by inhalation and via the skin. It is extensively metabolized (Figure 42.24) and the main metabolites are thiocarbamide, thiothiazolidine-carboxylic acid (TTCA), and 2-thio-5-thiazolidine. Analysis of TTCA in urine is an established means for biomonitoring.[91,495,496]

Management and diagnosis

Carbon disulphide causes serious adverse health effects at occupational exposure limits that are close to, or even below the exposure guideline, 5 ppm (15 mg/m^3), adopted in many countries and also recommended in Europe.[496] This exposure guideline may well be inappropriate, and may need review and revision. Thus, regular monitoring of occupational exposure is essential to ensure that levels remain well below 5 ppm. Carbon disulphide is absorbed through the skin, and in the viscose industry this may be the main route of exposure. A well-established method for biomonitoring of the exposure to carbon disulphide is the analysis of 2-thiothiazolidine-4-carboxylic acid in urine.

Key points

- Organic substances comprise a multitude of compounds, which contain at least one carbon–carbon bond.
- Limited or no data are available on the human health effects to many organic compounds. The only way to predict possible adverse health effects for such compounds is to extrapolate from data on animals, *in vitro* systems and other sources. Irrespective of the basic similarity in the response to chemicals between animals and humans, this extrapolation remains uncertain. For end points such as central nervous system toxicity, there are no valid animal models.
- For most chemicals, exposure at work is likely to be much higher than exposure from the environment. Health effects from new chemicals are thus most likely to become apparent among occupationally exposed people.
- At low-level exposures, a major health concern is carcinogenicity. This chapter mainly relies on the authoritative assessments of carcinogenic hazards by the International Agency for Research on Cancer.
- This text, as all texts on chemically induced adverse health effects, only reflects what is known today, and should be reviewed periodically.
- For heavy metals with a long half-life in the body, biological monitoring has long been used successfully in the estimation of body burden and health risk. For organic chemicals, meaningful biological monitoring requires reliable information on the metabolic pathways and kinetics in humans.

ACKNOWLEDGEMENTS

The authors are grateful to Dr Ari Kaukiainen for his valuable comments related to chronic solvent encephalopathy. Ms Piia Anttila is thanked for her help with tables and figures. They thank Mr Mauri Mäkelä for his comments on polycyclic aromatic hydrocarbons. The authors are grateful to Mr Mauri Mäkelä, Dr Kristiina Alanko, Dr Juha Laitinen, Mrs Katri Suuronen and Dr Esko Toppila for providing illustrations for the text.

The editors thank Dr RD Jefferson for his careful review and helpful comments on earlier drafts of this chapter.

REFERENCES

1. Yamamura Y. *n*-Hexane polyneuropathy. *Folia Psychiatrica et Neurologica Japonica*. 1969; **23**: 45–57.
2. IPCS. *n*-Hexane. Environmental Health Criteria, vol. 122. Geneva: International Programme on Chemical Safety. 1991: 164. Available from: www.inchem.org/documents/ehc/ehc/ehc122.htm.
3. Sanagi S, Seki Y, Sugimoto K, Hirata M. Peripheral nervous system functions of workers exposed to n-hexane at a low level. *International Archives of Occupational and Environmental Health*. 1980; **47**: 69–79.
4. Agency for Toxic Substances and Disease Registry. Toxicological profile for *n*-hexane. US Department of Health and Human Services, Public Health Service. 1999. Available from: www.atsdr.cdc.gov/toxprofiles/tp113.html.
5. Valentino M. Residual electroneurographic modifications in subjects with *n*-hexane induced polyneuropathy: A follow-up study. *La Medicina del Lavoro*. 1996; **87**: 289–96.
6. Ladefoged O, Perbellini L. Acetone-induced changes in the toxicokinetics of 2,5-hexanedione in rabbits. *Scandinavian Journal of Work, Environment and Health*. 1986; **12**: 627–9.
7. European Union. 1,3-Butadiene. European Union Risk Assessment Report. 2002: 194. Luxembourg: European Union. Available from: http://ecb.jrc.ec.europa.eu/documents/existing-chemicals/risk_assessment/report/butadienereport019.pdf.
8. International Agency for Research on Cancer. 1,3-Butadiene, ethylene oxide and vinyl halides (vinyl fluoride, vinyl chloride and vinyl bromide). IARC Monographs on the Evaluation of Carcinogenic Risks to Humans, vol. 97. Lyon: IARC, 2008. Available from: www.thelancet.com/journals/lanonc/article/PIIS1470-2045%2807%2970235-8/fulltext#article_upsell.
9. Cheng H, Sathiakumar N, Graff J et al. 1,3-Butadiene and leukemia among synthetic rubber industry workers: exposure-response relationships. *Chemico-biological Interactions*. 2007; **166**: 15–24.
10. Delzell E, Macaluso M, Sathiakumar N, Matthews R. Leukemia and exposure to 1,3-butadiene, styrene and dimethyldithiocarbamate among workers in the synthetic rubber industry. *Chemico-biological Interactions*. 2001; **135–136**: 515–34.

11. Graff JJ, Sathiakumar N, Macaluso M et al. Chemical exposures in the synthetic rubber industry and lymphohematopoietic cancer mortality. *Journal of Occupational and Environmental Medicine*. 2005; **47**: 916–32.
12. Albertini RJ, Sram RJ, Vacek PM et al. Biomarkers for assessing occupational exposures to 1,3-butadiene. *Chemico-biological Interactions*. 2001; **135–136**: 429–53.
13. Swenberg JA, Christova-Gueorguieva NI, Upton PB et al. 1,3-Butadiene: Cancer, mutations, and adducts. Part V: Hemoglobin adducts as biomarkers of 1,3-butadiene exposure and metabolism. *Research Report (Health Effects Institute)*. 2000; 191–210 (discussion 211–19).
14. European Union. Benzene. European Union Risk Assessment Report. pp. 587. Luxembourg: European Union. Available from: http://ecb.jrc.ec.europa.eu/documents/existing-chemicals/risk_assessment/report/benzenereport063.pdf.
15. Dosemeci M, Rothman N, Yin SN et al. Validation of benzene exposure assessment. *Annals of the New York Academy of Sciences*. 1997; **837**: 114–21.
16. Rothman N, Li GL, Dosemeci M et al. Hematotoxicity among Chinese workers heavily exposed to benzene. *American Journal of Industrial Medicine*. 1996; **29**: 236–46.
17. International Agency for Research on Cancer. Overall evaluations of carcinogenicity: An updating of IARC Monographs vols 1–42. IARC Monographs on the Evaluation of Carcinogenic Risks to Humans. Supplement 7. Lyon: IARC, 1987: 440. Available from: http://monographs.iarc.fr/ENG/Monographs/suppl7/index.php.
18. Kirkeleit J, Riise T, Bratveit M, Moen BE. Increased risk of acute myelogenous leukemia and multiple myeloma in a historical cohort of upstream petroleum workers exposed to crude oil. *Cancer Causes and Control*. 2008; **19**: 13–23.
19. Smith MT, Jones RM, Smith AH. Benzene exposure and risk of non-Hodgkin lymphoma. *Cancer Epidemiology, Biomarkers and Prevention*. 2007; **16**: 385–91.
20. Hayes RB, Yin SN, Dosemeci M et al. Benzene and the dose-related incidence of hematologic neoplasms in China. Chinese Academy of Preventive Medicine–National Cancer Institute Benzene Study Group. *Journal of the National Cancer Institute*. 1997; **89**: 1065–71.
21. Rinsky RA, Smith AB, Hornung R et al. Benzene and leukemia. An epidemiologic risk assessment. *New England Journal of Medicine*. 1987; **316**: 1044–50.
22. Collins JJ, Ireland B, Buckley CF, Shepperly D. Lymphohaematopoeitic cancer mortality among workers with benzene exposure. *Occupational and Environmental Medicine*. 2003; **60**: 676–9.
23. Natelson EA. Benzene-induced acute myeloid leukemia: A clinician's perspective. *American Journal of Hematology*. 2007; **82**: 826–30.
24. Snyder R. Benzene's toxicity: A consolidated short review of human and animal studies by HA Khan. *Human and Experimental Toxicology*. 2007; **26**: 687–96.
25. Agency for Toxic Substances and Disease Registry. Toxicological profile for benzene. US Department of Health and Human Services, Public Health Service. Atlanta, GA: ATSDR, 2007. Available from: www.atsdr.cdc.gov/toxprofiles/tp3.html.
26. International Programme on Chemical Safety. Benzene. Environmental Health Criteria, vol. 150. Geneva: IPCS, 1993: 156. Available from: www.inchem.org/documents/ehc/ehc/ehc150.htm.
27. Einig T, Dehnen W. Sensitive determination of the benzene metabolite S-phenylmercapturic acid in urine by high-performance liquid chromatography with fluorescence detection. *Journal of Chromatography. A*. 1995; **697**: 371–5.
28. European Union. Toluene. European Risk Assessment Report, vol. 30. Luxembourg: EU, 2003: 283. Available from: http://ecb.jrc.ec.europa.eu/documents/existing-chemicals/risk_assessment/report/toluenereport032.pdf.
29. European Union. Styrene. European Union Risk Assessment Report, draft. Luxembourg: EU, 2007. Available from: http://ecb.jrc.ec.europa.eu/documents/existing-chemicals/risk_assessment/report/styrenereport034.pdf.
30. International Programme on Chemical Safety. Xylenes. Environmental Health Criteria, vol. 190. Geneva: IPCS, 1997: 147. Available from: www.inchem.org/documents/ehc/ehc/ehc190.htm.
31. Edling C, Ekberg K, Ahlborg G Jr et al. Long-term follow up of workers exposed to solvents. *British Journal of Industrial Medicine*. 1990; **47**: 75–82.
32. Chouaniere D, Wild P, Fontana JM et al. Neurobehavioral disturbances arising from occupational toluene exposure. *American Journal of Industrial Medicine*. 2002; **41**: 77–88.
33. Akila R, Muller K, Kaukiainen A, Sainio M. Memory performance profile in occupational chronic solvent encephalopathy suggests working memory dysfunction. *Journal of Clinical and Experimental Neuropsychology*. 2006; **28**: 1307–26.
34. Paallysaho J, Nasanen R, Mantyjarvi M et al. Colour vision defects in occupational chronic solvent encephalopathy. *Human and Experimental Toxicology*. 2007; **26**: 375–83.
35. Ojanpaa H, Nasanen R, Paallysaho J et al. Visual search and eye movements in patients with chronic solvent-induced toxic encephalopathy. *Neurotoxicology*. 2006; **27**: 1013–23.
36. Larsen F, Leira HL. Organic brain syndrome and long-term exposure to toluene: A clinical, psychiatric study of vocationally active printing workers. *Journal of Occupational Medicine*. 1988; **30**: 875–8.
37. Orbaek P, Nise G. Neurasthenic complaints and psychometric function of toluene-exposed rotogravure printers. *American Journal of Industrial Medicine*. 1989; **16**: 67–77.
38. Seeber A, Schaper M, Zupanic M et al. Toluene exposure below 50 ppm and cognitive function: A follow-up study with four repeated measurements in rotogravure printing plants. *International Archives of Occupational and Environmental Health*. 2004; **77**: 1–9.

39. Zupanic M, Demes P, Seeber A. Psychomotor performance and subjective symptoms at low level toluene exposure. *Occupational and Environmental Medicine*. 2002; **59**: 263–8.
40. Rebert CS, Hall TA. The neuroepidemiology of styrene: A critical review of representative literature. *Critical Reviews in Toxicology*. 1994; **24** (Suppl.): S57–106.
41. Benignus VA, Geller AM, Boyes WK, Bushnell PJ. Human neurobehavioral effects of long-term exposure to styrene: A meta-analysis. *Environmental Health Perspectives*. 2005; **113**: 532–8.
42. Barregard L, Axelsson A. Is there an ototraumatic interaction between noise and solvents? *Scandinavian Audiology*. 1984; **13**: 151–5.
43. Morata TC, Johnson AC, Nylen P et al. Audiometric findings in workers exposed to low levels of styrene and noise. *Journal of Occupational and Environmental Medicine*. 2002; **44**: 806–14.
44. Johnson AC, Morata TC, Lindblad AC et al. Audiological findings in workers exposed to styrene alone or in concert with noise. *Noise and Health*. 2006; **8**: 45–57.
45. Sliwinska-Kowalska M, Zamyslowska-Szmytke E, Szymczak W et al. Ototoxic effects of occupational exposure to styrene and co-exposure to styrene and noise. *Journal of Occupational and Environmental Medicine*. 2003; **45**: 15–24.
46. Toppila E, Forsman P, Pyykko I et al. Effect of styrene on postural stability among reinforced plastic boat plant workers in Finland. *Journal of Occupational and Environmental Medicine*. 2006; **48**: 175–80.
47. Morata TC, Fiorini AC, Fischer FM et al. Toluene-induced hearing loss among rotogravure printing workers. *Scandinavian Journal of Work, Environment and Health*. 1997; **23**: 289–98.
48. International Agency for Research on Cancer. Styrene. In: Some traditional herbal medicines, some mycotoxins, naphthalene and styrene. IARC Monographs on the Evaluation of Carcinogenic Risks to Humans, vol. 82. Lyon: IARC, 2002: 437–550. Available from: http://monographs.iarc.fr/ENG/Monographs/vol82/mono82-9.pdf.
49. Lauwerys R. Toluene. In Human Biological Monitoring of Industrial Chemicals Series. Ispra: Industrial Health and Safety, 1983.
50. International Programme on Chemical Safety. Toluene. Environmental Health Criteria, vol. 52. Geneva: 1986. Available from: www.inchem.org/documents/ehc/ehc/ehc52.htm.
51. Dick FD. Solvent neurotoxicity. *Occupational and Environmental Medicine*. 2006; **63**: 221–6.
52. Ridgway P, Nixon TE, Leach JP. Occupational exposure to organic solvents and long-term nervous system damage detectable by brain imaging, neurophysiology or histopathology. *Food and Chemical Toxicology*. 2003; **41**: 153–87.
53. Spurgeon A. Watching paint dry: Organic solvent syndrome in late-twentieth-century Britain. *Medical History*. 2006; **50**: 167–88.
54. Williamson A. Using self-report measures in neurobehavioural toxicology: Can they be trusted? *Neurotoxicology*. 2007; **28**: 227–34.
55. Lundberg I, Hogberg M, Michelsen H et al. Evaluation of the Q16 questionnaire on neurotoxic symptoms and a review of its use. *Occupational and Environmental Medicine*. 1997; **54**: 343–50.
56. Carter N, Iregren A, Soderman E et al. EUROQUEST – A questionnaire for solvent-related symptoms: Factor structure, item analysis and predictive validity. *Neurotoxicology*. 2002; **23**: 711–17.
57. Chouaniere D, Cassitto MG, Spurgeon A et al. An international questionnaire to explore neurotoxic symptoms. *Environmental Research*. 1997; **73**: 70–2.
58. Heuser G, Mena I, Alamos F. NeuroSPECT findings in patients exposed to neurotoxic chemicals. *Toxicology and Industrial Health*. 1994; **10**: 561–71.
59. Thuomas KA, Moller C, Odkvist LM et al. MR imaging in solvent-induced chronic toxic encephalopathy. *Acta Radiologica*. 1996; **37**: 177–9.
60. Agency for Toxic Substances and Disease Registry. Toxicological profile for styrene. Draft for public comment September 2007. US Department of Health and Human Services, Public Health Service. 2010. Available from: http://www.atsdr.cdc.gov/ToxProfiles/tp.asp?id=421&tid=74.
61. European Union. Naphthalene. European Risk Assessment Report, vol. 33. Luxembourg: EU, 2003. Available from: http://ecb.jrc.ec.europa.eu/DOCUMENTS/Existing-Chemicals/risk_assessment/report/naphthalenereport020.pdf.
62. International Programme for Chemical Safety. Selected non-heterocyclic polycyclic aromatic hydrocarbons. Environmental Health Criteria, vol. 202. Geneva: IPCS, 1998. Available from: www.inchem.org/documents/ehc/ehc/ehc202.htm.
63. Gosselin RE, Smith RP, Hodge HC. *Clinical toxicology of commercial products*, 5th edn. London: Williams & Wilkins, 1984.
64. International Agency for Research on Cancer. Some non-heterocyclic polycyclic aromatic hydrocarbons and some related industrial exposures (in preparation). IARC Monographs on the Evaluation of Carcinogenic Risks to Humans, vol. 92. Lyon: IARC, 2008. Available from: http://monographs.iarc.fr/ENG/Meetings/92-pahs.pdf.
65. Armstrong B, Hutchinson E, Unwin J, Fletcher T. Lung cancer risk after exposure to polycyclic aromatic hydrocarbons: A review and meta-analysis. *Environmental Health Perspectives*. 2004; **112**: 970–8.
66. International Programme on Chemical Safety. Coal tar creosote. Concise International Chemical Assessment Document, vol 62. Geneva: IPCS, 2004. Available from: www.inchem.org/documents/cicads/cicads/cicad62.htm.
67. Karlehagen S, Andersen A, Ohlson CG. Cancer incidence among creosote-exposed workers. *Scandinavian Journal of Work, Environment and Health*. 1992; **18**: 26–9.
68. Pukkala E. *Cancer risk by social class and occupation: A survey of 109,000 cancer cases among Finns of working age*. Basel: Karger, 1995: 277.

69. International Agency for Research on Cancer. Bitumens, coal-tars and derived products, shale-oils and soots. IARC Monographs on the Evaluation of Carcinogenic Risks to Humans. Polynuclear Aromatic Compounds, part 4, vol. 35. Geneva: IARC, 1987: 271.
70. International Agency for Research on Cancer. Diesel and gasoline engine exhausts and some nitroarenes. IARC Monographs on the Evaluation of Carcinogenic Risks to Humans, vol. 46. Geneva: IARC, 1989.
71. International Programme for Chemical Safety. Petroleum products, selected. Environmental Health Criteria, vol. 20. Geneva: IPCS, 1982. Available from: www.inchem.org/documents/ehc/ehc/ehc020.htm.
72. Agency for Toxic Substances and Disease Registry. Toxicological profile for fuel oils. US Department of Health and Human Services, Public Health Service. Atlanta, GA: ATSDR, 1995. Available from: www.atsdr.cdc.gov/toxprofiles/.
73. International Agency for Research on Cancer. Occupational exposures in petroleum refining; Crude oil and major petroleum fuels. IARC Monographs on the Evaluation of Carcinogenic Risks to Humans, vol. 45. Lyon: IARC, 1989: 322. Available from: http://monographs.iarc.fr/ENG/Monographs/vol45/volume45.pdf.
74. International Programme for Chemical Safety. White spirit. Environmental Health Criteria, vol. 187. Geneva: IPCS, 1996. Available from: www.inchem.org/documents/ehc/ehc/ehc187.htm.
75. Kaukiainen A, Riala R, Martikainen R et al. Solvent-related health effects among construction painters with decreasing exposure. *American Journal of Industrial Medicine*. 2004; **46**: 627–36.
76. Brahmi N, Blel Y, Abidi N et al. Methanol poisoning in Tunisia: Report of 16 cases. *Clinical Toxicology*. 2007; **45**: 717–20.
77. Hovda KE, Hunderi OH, Tafjord AB et al. Methanol outbreak in Norway 2002–2004: Epidemiology, clinical features and prognostic signs. *Journal of Internal Medicine*. 2005; **258**: 181–90.
78. Paasma R, Hovda KE, Tikkerberi A, Jacobsen D. Methanol mass poisoning in Estonia: Outbreak in 154 patients. *Clinical Toxicology*. 2007; **45**: 152–7.
79. LoVecchio F, Sawyers B, Thole D et al. Outcomes following abuse of methanol-containing carburetor cleaners. *Human and Experimental Toxicology*. 2004; **23**: 473–5.
80. Van Kampen RJ, Krekels MM, Derijks HJ, Peters FP. [Serious intoxication after inhaling methanol]. *Nederlands Tijdschrift voor Geneeskunde*. 2006; **150**: 1298–302.
81. Soysal D, Yersal Kabayegit O, Yilmaz S et al. Transdermal methanol intoxication: A case report. *Acta Anaesthesiologica Scandinavica*. 2007; **51**: 779–80.
82. Bolon B, Dorman DC, Janszen D et al. Phase-specific developmental toxicity in mice following maternal methanol inhalation. *Fundamental and Applied Toxicology*. 1993; **21**: 508–16.
83. Bolon B, Welsch F, Morgan KT. Methanol-induced neural tube defects in mice: Pathogenesis during neurulation. *Teratology*. 1994; **49**: 497–517.
84. Dorman DC, Bolon B, Struve MF et al. Role of formate in methanol-induced exencephaly in CD-1 mice. *Teratology*. 1995; **52**: 30–40.
85. Rogers JM, Brannen KC, Barbee BD et al. Methanol exposure during gastrulation causes holoprosencephaly, facial dysgenesis, and cervical vertebral malformations in C57BL/6J mice. *Birth Defects Research. Part B, Developmental and Reproductive Toxicology*. 2004; **71**: 80–8.
86. Rogers JM, Mole ML. Critical periods of sensitivity to the developmental toxicity of inhaled methanol in the CD-1 mouse. *Teratology*. 1997; **55**: 364–72.
87. Hantson P, Haufroid V, Wallemacq P. Formate kinetics in methanol poisoning. *Human and Experimental Toxicology*. 2005; **24**: 55–9.
88. Hovda KE, Mundal H, Urdal P et al. Extremely slow formate elimination in severe methanol poisoning: A fatal case report. *Clinical Toxicology*. 2007; **45**: 516–21.
89. International Programme for Chemical Safety. Methanol. Environmental Health Criteria, vol. 196. Geneva: IPCS, 1997: 180. Available from: www.inchem.org/documents/ehc/ehc/ehc196.htm.
90. Barceloux DG, Bond GR, Krenzelok EP et al. American Academy of Clinical Toxicology practice guidelines on the treatment of methanol poisoning. *Journal of Toxicology. Clinical Toxicology*. 2002; **40**: 415–46.
91. Lauwerys RR, Hoet P. *Industrial chemical exposure: Guidelines for biological monitoring*, 3rd edn. Boca Raton, FL: Lewis Publishers, 2001.
92. Liesivuori J, Savolainen H. Urinary formic acid as an indicator of occupational exposure to formic acid and methanol. *American Industrial Hygiene Association Journal*. 1987; **48**: 32–4.
93. International Programme for Chemical Safety. Ethylene glycol: Human health aspects. Concise International Chemical Assessment Document, vol. 45. Geneva: IPCS, 2002. Available from: www.inchem.org/documents/cicads/cicads/cicad45.htm.
94. Agency for Toxic Substances and Disease Registry. Draft toxicological profile for ethylene glycol (September 2007). US Department of Health and Human Services, Public Health Service. Atlanta, GA: ATSDR, 2007: 264. Available from: www.atsdr.cdc.gov/toxprofiles/tp96.pdf.
95. International Programme for Chemical Safety. Ethylene glycol. Poisons Information Monograph, vol. 227. Geneva: IPCS, 2001. Available from: www.inchem.org/documents/pims/chemical/pim227.htm.
96. International Programme for Chemical Safety. Formaldehyde. Concise International Chemical Assessment Document, vol. 40. Geneva: IPCS, 2002: 72. Available from: www.inchem.org/documents/cicads/cicads/cicad40.htm
97. Organisation for Economic Co-operation and Development. Formaldehyde. OECD SIDS. Geneva: UNEP Publications, 2002: 395. Available from: www.chem.unep.ch/irptc/sids/oecdsids/formaldehyde.pdf.
98. Health Canada. Formaldehyde. Canadian Environment Protection Act, 1999. Priority Substances List Assessment

99. International Agency for Research on Cancer. Formaldehyde. In: Formaldehyde, 2-butoxyethanol, and 1-tert-butoxypropan-ol. IARC Monographs on the Evaluation of Carcinogenic Risks to Humans, vol. 88. Lyon: IARC, 2006: 37–325. Available from: http://monographs.iarc.fr/ENG/Monographs/vol88/index.php.
    Report. Minister of Public Works and Government Services Canada, 2001: 102. Available from: www.hc-sc.gc.ca/ewh-semt/alt_formats/hecs-sesc/pdf/pubs/contaminants/psl2-lsp2/formaldehyde/formaldehyde-eng.pdf.
100. International Agency for Research on Cancer. A review of human carcinogens, part F: chemical agents and related occupations. Highlights and summary of evaluations. IARC Monographs on the Evaluation of Carcinogenic Risks to Humans, vol. 100F. Lyon: IARC, 2009. Available from: http://monographs.iarc.fr/pdfnews/WG-100F.pdf.
101. Organisation for Economic Co-operation and Development. Glutaraldehyde, CAS No: 111-30-8. OECD SIDS. Geneva: UNEP Publications, 1998: 83. Available from: www.chem.unep.ch/irptc/sids/OECDSIDS/111308.pdf.
102. Curran AD, Burge PS, Wiley K. Clinical and immunologic evaluation of workers exposed to glutaraldehyde. *Allergy*. 1996; **51**: 826–32.
103. Di Stefano F, Siriruttanapruk S, McCoach J, Burge PS. Glutaraldehyde: An occupational hazard in the hospital setting. *Allergy*. 1999; **54**: 1105–9.
104. International Programme on Chemical Safety. Acetone. Environmental Health Criteria, vol. 207. Geneva: IPCS, 1998: 159. Available from: www.inchem.org/documents/ehc/ehc/ehc207.htm.
105. US Environment Protection Agency. Methyl ethylketone. Chemical summary. Washington DC: US EPA, 1994. Available from: www.epa.gov/chemfact/.
106. Liira J, Elovaara E, Raunio H *et al*. Metabolic interaction and disposition of methyl ethyl ketone and *m*-xylene in rats at single and repeated inhalation exposures. *Xenobiotica*. 1991; **21**: 53–63.
107. International Programme on Chemical Safety. Methyl ethyl ketone. Environmental Health Criteria, vol. 143. Geneva: IPCS, 1992: 161. Available from: www.inchem.org/documents/ehc/ehc/ehc143.htm.
108. US Environment Protection Agency. Methyl isobutylketone. Chemical summary. Washington DC: US EPA, 1994. Available from: www.epa.gov/chemfact/.
109. Agency for Toxic Substances and Disease Registry. Toxicological profile for 2-hexanone. US Department of Health and Human Services, Public Health Service. Washington DC: ATSDR, 1992: 92. Available from: www.atsdr.cdc.gov/toxprofiles/tp44.html.
110. Allen N, Mendell JR, Billmaier DJ *et al*. Toxic polyneuropathy due to methyl *n*-butyl ketone. An industrial outbreak. *Archives of Neurology*. 1975; **32**: 209–18.
111. Billmaier D, Allen N, Craft B *et al*. Peripheral neuropathy in a coated fabrics plant. *Journal of Occupational Medicine*. 1974; **16**: 665–71.
112. Nishimura K, Miyashita K, Yoshida Y *et al*. [An epidemiological study of lung cancer among workers exposed to bis(chloromethyl)ether]. *Sangyo Igaku*. 1990; **32**: 448–53.
113. Gowers DS, DeFonso LR, Schaffer P *et al*. Incidence of respiratory cancer among workers exposed to chloromethyl-ethers. *American Journal of Epidemiology*. 1993; **137**: 31–42.
114. Weiss W, Nash D. An epidemic of lung cancer due to chloromethyl ethers. 30 years of observation. *Journal of Occupational and Environmental Medicine*. 1997; **39**: 1003–9.
115. International Agency for Research on Cancer. Bis(2-chloroethyl)ether. In: Re-Evaluation of Some Organic Chemicals, Hydrazine and Hydrogen Peroxide. IARC Monographs on the Evaluation of Carcinogenic Risks to Humans, vol. 71. Lyon: IARC, 1999: 1265–9. Available from: http://monographs.iarc.fr/ENG/Monographs/vol71/mono71-66.pdf.
116. International Agency for Research on Cancer. Bis(2-chloro-1-methylethyl)ether. In: Re-Evaluation of Some Organic Chemicals, Hydrazine and Hydrogen Peroxide. IARC Monographs on the Evaluation of Carcinogenic Risks to Humans, vol. 71. Lyon: IARC, 1999: 1275–9. Available from: http://monographs.iarc.fr/ENG/Monographs/vol71/mono71-69.pdf.
117. European Union. Tert-butyl methyl ether. European Union Risk Assessment Report, vol 19. Luxembourg: European Communities, 2002: 282. Available from: http://ecb.jrc.ec.europa.eu/documents/existing-chemicals/risk_assessment/report/mtbereport313.pdf.
118. International Programme on Chemical Safety. Methyl tertiary-butyl ether. Environmental Health Criteria, vol. 206. Geneva: IPCS, 1998: 199. Available from: www.inchem.org/documents/ehc/ehc/ehc206.htm.
119. International Agency for Research on Cancer. Methyl tert-butyl ether. In: Some Chemicals that Cause Tumours of the Kidney or Urinary Bladder in Rodents and Some Other Substances. IARC Monographs on the Evaluation of Carcinogenic Risks to Humans, vol. 73. Lyon: IARC, 1999: 339–83. Available from: http://monographs.iarc.fr/ENG/Monographs/vol73/mono73-18.pdf.
120. Vainiotalo S, Kuusimaki L, Pekari K. Exposure to MTBE, TAME and aromatic hydrocarbons during gasoline pump maintenance, repair and inspection. *Journal of Occupational Health*. 2006; **48**: 347–57.
121. Vainiotalo S, Riihimaki V, Pekari K *et al*. Toxicokinetics of methyl tert-butyl ether (MTBE) and tert-amyl methyl ether (TAME) in humans, and implications to their biological monitoring. *Journal of Occupational and Environmental Hygiene*. 2007; **4**: 739–50.
122. European Union. 2-Methoxy-2-methylbutane (TAME). European Union Risk Assessment Report. Luxembourg: EU, 2002: 168. Available from: http://ecb.jrc.ec.europa.eu/documents/existing-chemicals/risk_assessment/report/tamereport413.pdf.
123. Belpoggi F, Soffritti M, Minardi F *et al*. Results of long-term carcinogenicity bioassays on tert-amyl-methyl-ether

124. Shih TS, Hsieh AT, Liao GD et al. Haematological and spermatotoxic effects of ethylene glycol monomethyl ether in copper clad laminate factories. *Occupational and Environmental Medicine*. 2000; **57**: 348–52.
125. Shih TS, Hsieh AT, Chen YH et al. Follow up study of haematological effects in workers exposed to 2-methoxyethanol. *Occupational and Environmental Medicine*. 2003; **60**: 130–5.
126. International Programme on Chemical Safety. Selected alkoxyethanols: 2-methoxyethanol. Concise International Chemical Assessment Document, vol. 67. Geneva: IPCS, 2008. Available from: www.who.int/ipcs/publications/cicad/methoxyethanol.pdf.
127. European Union. Commission Directive 2004/73/EC of 29 April 2004. Adapting to technical progress for the twenty-ninth time. Council Directive 67/548/EEC on the approximation of laws, regulations and administrative provisions relating to the classification, packaging and labelling of dangerous substances. *Official Journal of the European Union*. 2004; **L152**: 1–311.
128. European Commission. Joint Research Centre. Institute for Health and Consumer Protection. European Chemical Substances Information System (ESIS), 2008. Available from: http://ecb.jrc.it/esis/.
129. Chang HY, Lin CC, Shih TS et al. Evaluation of the protective effectiveness of gloves from occupational exposure to 2-methoxyethanol using the biomarkers of 2-methoxyacetic acid levels in the urine and plasma. *Occupational and Environmental Medicine*. 2004; **61**: 697–702.
130. Groeseneken D, Veulemans H, Masschelein R, Van Vlem E. An improved method for the determination in urine of alkoxyacetic acids. *International Archives of Occupational and Environmental Health*. 1989; **61**: 249–54.
131. Groeseneken D, Veulemans H, Masschelein R, Van Vlem E. Experimental human exposure to ethylene glycol monomethyl ether. *International Archives of Occupational and Environmental Health*. 1989; **61**: 243–7.
132. Veulemans H, Groeseneken D, Masschelein R, van Vlem E. Survey of ethylene glycol ether exposures in Belgian industries and workshops. *American Industrial Hygiene Association Journal*. 1987; **48**: 671–6.
133. Shih TS, Liou SH, Chen CY, Chou JS. Correlation between urinary 2-methoxy acetic acid and exposure of 2-methoxy ethanol. *Occupational and Environmental Medicine*. 1999; **56**: 674–8.
134. Welch LS, Schrader SM, Turner TW, Cullen MR. Effects of exposure to ethylene glycol ethers on shipyard painters: II. Male reproduction. *American Journal of Industrial Medicine*. 1988; **14**: 509–26.
135. Ratcliffe JM, Schrader SM, Clapp DE et al. Semen quality in workers exposed to 2-ethoxyethanol. *British Journal of Industrial Medicine*. 1989; **46**: 399–406.
136. Veulemans H, Steeno O, Masschelein R, Groeseneken D. Exposure to ethylene glycol ethers and spermatogenic disorders in man: A case–control study. *British Journal of Industrial Medicine*. 1993; **50**: 71–8.
137. Kim Y, Lee N, Sakai T et al. Evaluation of exposure to ethylene glycol monoethyl ether acetates and their possible haematological effects on shipyard painters. *Occupational and Environmental Medicine*. 1999; **56**: 378–82.
138. Loh CH, Shih TS, Liou SH et al. Haematological effects among silk screening workers exposed to 2-ethoxy ethyl acetate. *Occupational and Environmental Medicine*. 2003; **60**: E7.
139. International Programme on Chemical Safety. Selected alkoxyethanols: 2-ethoxyethanol and 2-propoxyethanol. Concise International Chemical Assessment Document. Geneva: IPCS, 2008. Available from: www.who.int/ipcs/publications/cicad/ethoxy_propoxyethanol.pdf.
140. Chen HI, Liou SH, Hsieh MH et al. Hematological follow-up of an intervention program adding rubber glove-wearing to local ventilation for 2-ethoxyethanol acetate-exposed workers. *Journal of Occupational Health*. 2007; **49**: 285–93.
141. International Agency for Research on Cancer. 2-Butoxyethanol. In: Formaldehyde, 2-Butoxyethanol, and 1-Tert-butoxypropan-ol. IARC Monographs on the Evaluation of Carcinogenic Risks to Humans, vol. 88. Lyon: IARC, 2006: 329–414. Available from: http://monographs.iarc.fr/ENG/Monographs/vol88/index.php.
142. International Programme on Chemical Safety. Selected alkoxyethanols: 2-Butoxyethanol. Concise International Chemical Assessment Document, vol 67. Geneva: IPCS, 2005: 51. Available from: www.inchem.org/documents/cicads/cicads/cicad67.htm.
143. Haufroid V, Thirion F, Mertens P et al. Biological monitoring of workers exposed to low levels of 2-butoxyethanol. *International Archives of Occupational and Environmental Health*. 1997; **70**: 232–6.
144. Carpenter CP, Keck GA, Nair JH 3rd et al. The toxicity of butyl cellosolve solvent. *Archives of Industrial Health*. 1956; **14**: 114–31.
145. Rambourg-Schepens MO, Buffet M, Bertault R et al. Severe ethylene glycol butyl ether poisoning. Kinetics and metabolic pattern. *Human Toxicology*. 1988; **7**: 187–9.
146. Gijsenbergh FP, Jenco M, Veulemans H et al. Acute butylglycol intoxication: A case report. *Human Toxicology*. 1989; **8**: 243–5.
147. Bauer P, Weber M, Mur JM et al. Transient non-cardiogenic pulmonary edema following massive ingestion of ethylene glycol butyl ether. *Intensive Care Medicine*. 1992; **18**: 250–1.
148. Gualtieri J, DeBoer M, Harris C, Corley R. Repeated ingestion of 2-butoxyethanol: Case report and literature review. *Journal of Toxicology and Clinical Toxicology*. 2003; **41**: 57–62.
149. Gualtieri J, Harris C, Roy R et al. Multiple 2-butoxyethanol intoxications in the same patient: Clinical findings, pharmacokinetics, and therapy. *Journal of Toxicology and Clinical Toxicology*. 1995; **33**: 550–1.
150. McKinney PE, Palmer RB, Blackwell W, Benson BE. Butoxyethanol ingestion with prolonged hyperchloremic

metabolic acidosis treated with ethanol therapy. *Journal of Toxicology. Clinical Toxicology.* 2000; **38**: 787–93.
151. Collinot JP, Collinot JC, Deschamps F *et al.* Evaluation of urinary D-glucaric acid excretion in workers exposed to butyl glycol. *Journal of Toxicology and Environmental Health.* 1996; **48**: 349–58.
152. Greenspan AH, Reardon RC, Gingell R, Rosica KA. Human repeated insult patch test of 2-butoxyethanol. *Contact Dermatitis.* 1995; **33**: 59–60.
153. Johanson G, Boman A. Percutaneous absorption of 2-butoxyethanol vapour in human subjects. *British Journal of Industrial Medicine.* 1991; **48**: 788–92.
154. Corley RA, Bormett GA, Ghanayem BI. Physiologically based pharmacokinetics of 2-butoxyethanol and its major metabolite, 2-butoxyacetic acid, in rats and humans. *Toxicology and Applied Pharmacology.* 1994; **129**: 61–79.
155. Agency for Toxic Substances and Disease Registry. Toxicological profile for 2-butoxyethanol and 2-butoxyethanol acetate. US Department of Health and Human Services, Public Health Service. Atlanta, GA: ATSDR, 1998: 357. Available from: www.atsdr.cdc.gov/toxprofiles/tp118.html.
156. Cragg S, Boatman R. Glycol ethers: Ethers of propylene, butylene glycols, and other glycol derivatives. In: Bingham E, Chorssen B, Powell C (eds). *Patty's Toxicology*, 5th edn. New York: John Wiley, 2001: 271–395.
157. Organisation for Economic Co-operation and Development. 1-Methoxypropanol-2-ol (PGME). OECD SIDS. Geneva: UNEP Publications, 2003: 102. Available from: www.chem.unep.ch/irptc/sids/OECDSIDS/107982.pdf.
158. European Union. 1-Methoxy-propan-2-ol (PGME) Part 1, Environment. European Union Risk Assessment Report, vol. 66. Luxembourg: European Union, 2006: 44. Available from: http://ecb.jrc.ec.europa.eu/documents/existing-chemicals/risk_assessment/report/pgmeenvreport406.pdf.
159. Emmen HH, Muijser H, Arts JH, Prinsen MK. Human volunteer study with PGME: Eye irritation during vapour exposure. *Toxicology Letters.* 2003; **140–141**: 249–59.
160. Spencer PJ, Crissman JW, Stott WT *et al.* Propylene glycol monomethyl ether (PGME): Inhalation toxicity and carcinogenicity in Fischer 344 rats and B6C3F1 mice. *Toxicologic Pathology.* 2002; **30**: 570–9.
161. Capen C, Dybing E, Rice J, Wilbourn J (eds). *Species differences in thyroid, kidney and urinary bladder carcinogenesis*, vol. 147. Lyon: IARC, 1999.
162. Carney EW, Crissman JW, Liberacki AB *et al.* Assessment of adult and neonatal reproductive parameters in Sprague–Dawley rats exposed to propylene glycol monomethyl ether vapors for two generations. *Toxicological Sciences.* 1999; **50**: 249–58.
163. Doe JE, Samuels DM, Tinston DJ, de Silva Wickramaratne GA. Comparative aspects of the reproductive toxicology by inhalation in rats of ethylene glycol monomethyl ether and propylene glycol monomethyl ether. *Toxicology and Applied Pharmacology.* 1983; **69**: 43–7.

164. Hanley TR Jr, Calhoun LL, Yano BL, Rao KS. Teratologic evaluation of inhaled propylene glycol monomethyl ether in rats and rabbits. *Fundamental and Applied Toxicology.* 1984; **4**: 784–94.
165. Hanley TR Jr, Young JT, John JA, Rao KS. Ethylene glycol monomethyl ether (EGME) and propylene glycol monomethyl ether (PGME): Inhalation fertility and teratogenicity studies in rats, mice and rabbits. *Environmental Health Perspectives.* 1984; **57**: 7–12.
166. Merkle J, Klimisch HJ, Jackh R. Prenatal toxicity of 2-methoxypropylacetate-1 in rats and rabbits. *Fundamental and Applied Toxicology.* 1987; **8**: 71–9.
167. Lemazurier E, Lecomte A, Robidel F, Bois FY. Propylene glycol monomethyl ether. A three-generation study of isomer beta effects on reproductive and developmental parameters in rats. *Toxicology and Industrial Health.* 2005; **21**: 33–40.
168. Carney EW, Pottenger LH, Johnson KA *et al.* Significance of 2-methoxypropionic acid formed from beta-propylene glycol monomethyl ether: Integration of pharmacokinetic and developmental toxicity assessments in rabbits. *Toxicological Sciences.* 2003; **71**: 217–28.
169. Miller RR, Hermann EA, Young JT *et al.* Propylene glycol monomethyl ether acetate (PGMEA) metabolism, disposition, and short-term vapor inhalation toxicity studies. *Toxicology and Applied Pharmacology.* 1984; **75**: 521–30.
170. Domoradzki JY, Brzak KA, Thornton CM. Hydrolysis kinetics of propylene glycol monomethyl ether acetate in rats *in vivo* and in rat and human tissues *in vitro*. *Toxicological Sciences.* 2003; **75**: 31–9.
171. Miller RR, Hermann EA, Young JT *et al.* Ethylene glycol monomethyl ether and propylene glycol monomethyl ether: Metabolism, disposition, and subchronic inhalation toxicity studies. *Environmental Health Perspectives.* 1984; **57**: 233–9.
172. Jones K, Dyne D, Cocker J, Wilson HK. A biological monitoring study of 1-methoxy-2-propanol: analytical method development and a human volunteer study. *Science of the Total Environment.* 1997; **199**: 23–30.
173. Devanthery A, Dentan A, Berode M, Droz PO. Propylene glycol monomethyl ether (PGME) occupational exposure. 1. Biomonitoring by analysis of PGME in urine. *International Archives of Occupational and Environmental Health.* 2000; **73**: 311–15.
174. Kulling P, Andersson H, Bostrom K *et al.* Fatal systemic poisoning after skin exposure to monochloroacetic acid. *Journal of Toxicology. Clinical Toxicology.* 1992; **30**: 643–52.
175. Pirson J, Toussaint P, Segers N. An unusual cause of burn injury: Skin exposure to monochloroacetic acid. *Journal of Burn Care and Rehabilitation.* 2003; **24**: 407–9; discussion 402.
176. Kusch GD, McCarty LP, Lanham JM. Monochloroacetic acid exposure: A case report. *Polish Journal of Occupational Medicine.* 1990; **3**: 409–14.

177. Nayak SG, Satish R, Gokulnath. An unusual toxic cause of hemolytic-uremic syndrome. *Journal of Toxicological Sciences.* 2007; **32**: 197-9.
178. Rogers DR. Accidental fatal monochloroacetic acid poisoning. *American Journal of Forensic Medicine and Pathology.* 1995; **16**: 115-16.
179. Health Council of the Netherlands. Formic acid. Health-based Reassessment of Administrative Occupational Exposure Limits. Report 2000/15OSH/149. The Hague: Health Council of the Netherlands, Committee on Updating of Occupational Exposure Limits, 2005: 25. Available from: www.gezondheidsraad.nl/sites/default/files/00@15OSH149.pdf.
180. Sigurdsson J, Bjornsson A, Gudmundsson ST. Formic acid burn – local and systemic effects. Report of a case. *Burns, including Thermal Injury.* 1983; **9**: 358-61.
181. Chan TC, Williams SR, Clark RF. Formic acid skin burns resulting in systemic toxicity. *Annals of Emergency Medicine.* 1995; **26**: 383-6.
182. Rajan N, Rahim R, Krishna Kumar S. Formic acid poisoning with suicidal intent: A report of 53 cases. *Postgraduate Medical Journal.* 1985; **61**: 35-6.
183. Verstraete AG, Vogelaers DP, van den Bogaerde JF et al. Formic acid poisoning: Case report and *in vitro* study of the hemolytic activity. *American Journal of Emergency Medicine.* 1989; **7**: 286-90.
184. Moore DF, Bentley AM, Dawling S et al. Folinic acid and enhanced renal elimination in formic acid intoxication. *Journal of Toxicology. Clinical Toxicology.* 1994; **32**: 199-204.
185. Westphal F, Rochholz G, Ritz-Timme S et al. Fatal intoxication with a decalcifying agent containing formic acid. *International Journal of Legal Medicine.* 2001; **114**: 181-5.
186. Jefferys DB, Wiseman HM. Formic acid poisoning. *Postgraduate Medical Journal.* 1980; **56**: 761-2.
187. National Toxicology Program. Technical report on studies of formic acid (CAS No: 64-18-6) administered by inhalation to F344/N rats and B6C3F1 mice. National Toxicology Program, Technical Report Series No. 19. Washington DC: Public Health Service, National Institutes of Health, 1992: 62. Available from: http://ntp.niehs.nih.gov/ntp/htdocs/ST_rpts/tox019.pdf.
188. Rajaniemi R. Clinical evaluation of occupational toxicity of methylmethacrylate monomer to dental technicians. *Journal of the Society of Occupational Medicine.* 1986; **36**: 56-9.
189. Kanerva L, Estlander T, Jolanki R, Tarvainen K. Occupational allergic contact dermatitis caused by exposure to acrylates during work with dental prostheses. *Contact Dermatitis.* 1993; **28**: 268-75.
190. Kanerva L, Mikola H, Henriks-Eckerman ML et al. Fingertip paresthesia and occupational allergic contact dermatitis caused by acrylics in a dental nurse. *Contact Dermatitis.* 1998; **38**: 114-16.
191. Rustemeyer T, Frosch PJ. Occupational skin diseases in dental laboratory technicians. I. Clinical picture and causative factors. *Contact Dermatitis.* 1996; **34**: 125-33.
192. Aalto-Korte K, Alanko K, Kuuliala O, Jolanki R. Methacrylate and acrylate allergy in dental personnel. *Contact Dermatitis.* 2007; **57**: 324-30.
193. Organisation for Economic Co-operation and Development. Glycidyl methachrylate. OECD SIDS. Geneva: UNEP Publications, 2002: 79. Available from: www.chem.unep.ch/irptc/sids/OECDSIDS/106912.pdf.
194. Organisation for Economic Co-operation and Development. 2-Hydroxyethyl methachrylate. OECD SIDS. Geneva: UNEP Publications, 2005: 132. Available from: www.chem.unep.ch/irptc/sids/OECDSIDS/868779.pdf.
195. Organisation for Economic Co-operation and Development. Hydroxyethyl acrylate. OECD SIDS. Geneva: UNEP Publications, 2006: 142. Available from: www.chem.unep.ch/irptc/sids/OECDSIDS/818611.pdf.
196. Organisation for Economic Co-operation and Development. Hydroxypropyl acrylate. OECD SIDS. Geneva: UNEP Publications, 2006: 112. Available from: www.chem.unep.ch/irptc/sids/OECDSIDS/25584832.pdf.
197. European Union. Methyl methacrylate. European Union Risk Assessment Report, vol. 22. Luxembourg: EU, 2003: 181. Available from: http://ecb.jrc.ec.europa.eu/documents/existing-chemicals/risk_assessment/report/methylmethacrylatereport024.pdf.
198. Kanerva L, Tarvainen K, Jolanki R et al. Airborne occupational allergic contact dermatitis due to trimethylolpropane triacrylate (TMPTA) used in the manufacture of printed circuit boards. *Contact Dermatitis.* 1998; **38**: 292-4.
199. Kanerva L, Estlander T, Jolanki R. Optician's occupational allergic contact dermatitis, paresthesia and paronychia caused by anaerobic acrylic sealants. *Contact Dermatitis.* 2001; **44**: 117-19.
200. Jolanki R, Kanerva L, Estlander T et al. Allergic contact dermatitis from phenoxyethoxy ethylacrylates in optical fiber coating, and glue in an insulin pump set. *Contact Dermatitis.* 2001; **45**: 36-7.
201. Rajaniemi R, Tola S. Subjective symptoms among dental technicians exposed to the monomer methyl methacrylate. *Scandinavian Journal of Work and Environmental Health.* 1985; **11**: 281-6.
202. Seppalainen AM, Rajaniemi R. Local neurotoxicity of methyl methacrylate among dental technicians. *American Journal of Industrial Medicine.* 1984; **5**: 471-7.
203. Baran RL, Schibli H. Permanent paresthesia to sculptured nails. A distressing problem. *Dermatology Clinics.* 1990; **8**: 139-41.
204. Savonius B, Keskinen H, Tuppurainen M, Kanerva L. Occupational respiratory disease caused by acrylates. *Clinical and Experimental Allergy.* 1993; **23**: 416-24.
205. Lindstrom M, Alanko K, Keskinen H, Kanerva L. Dentist's occupational asthma, rhinoconjunctivitis, and allergic contact dermatitis from methacrylates. *Allergy.* 2002; **57**: 543-5.

206. Braun D, Wagner W, Zenner HP, Schmahl FW. Disabling disturbance of olfaction in a dental technician following exposure to methyl methacrylate. *International Archives of Occupational and Environmental Health.* 2002; **75** (Suppl.): S73-4.
207. Scherpereel A, Tillie-Leblond I, Pommier de Santi P, Tonnel AB. Exposure to methyl methacrylate and hypersensitivity pneumonitis in dental technicians. *Allergy.* 2004; **59**: 890-2.
208. Quirce S, Baeza ML, Tornero P et al. Occupational asthma caused by exposure to cyanoacrylate. *Allergy.* 2001; **56**: 446-9.
209. Piirila P, Kanerva L, Keskinen H et al. Occupational respiratory hypersensitivity caused by preparations containing acrylates in dental personnel. *Clinical and Experimental Allergy.* 1998; **28**: 1404-11.
210. International Agency for Research on Cancer. Methyl methacrylate. In: Some Industrial Chemicals. IARC Monographs on the Evaluation of Carcinogenic Risks to Humans, vol. 60. Lyon: International Agency for Research on Cancer, 1994: 445-74. Available from: http://monographs.iarc.fr/ENG/Monographs/vol60/mono60-18.pdf.
211. Tomenson JA, Bonner SM, Edwards JC et al. Study of two cohorts of workers exposed to methyl methacrylate in acrylic sheet production. *Occupational and Environmental Medicine.* 2000; **57**: 810-17.
212. International Agency for Research on Cancer. Ethyl acrylate. In: Re-Evaluation of Some Organic Chemicals, Hydrazine and Hydrogen Peroxide. IARC Monographs on the Evaluation of Carcinogenic Risks to Humans, vol. 71. Lyon: International Agency for Research on Cancer, 1999: 1447-57. Available from: http://monographs.iarc.fr/ENG/Monographs/vol71/mono71-99.pdf.
213. International Programme on Chemical Safety. N,N-dimethylformamide. Concise International Chemical Assessment Document, vol 31. Geneva: IPCS, 2001: 56. Available from: www.inchem.org/documents/cicads/cicads/cicad31.htm.
214. International Programme on Chemical Safety. Dimethylformamide. Environmental Health Criteria, vol. 114. Geneva: IPCS, 1991: 124. Available from: www.inchem.org/documents/ehc/ehc/ehc114.htm.
215. Organisation for Economic Co-Operation and Development. Dimethylformamide. OECD SIDS. Geneva: UNEP Publications, 2004: 287. Available from: www.chem.unep.ch/irptc/sids/oecdsids/dimethylform.pdf.
216. Organisation for Economic Co-Operation and Development. N,N-dimethylacetamide (DMAC). OECD SIDS. Geneva: UNEP Publications, 2004: 95. Available from: www.chem.unep.ch/irptc/sids/OECDSIDS/127-19-5.pdf.
217. International Agency for Research on Cancer. Dimethylformamide. In: Re-Evaluation of Some Organic Chemicals, Hydrazine and Hydrogen Peroxide. IARC Monographs on the Evaluation of Carcinogenic Risks to Humans, vol. 71. Lyon: IARC, 1999: 545-74. Available from: http://monographs.iarc.fr/ENG/Monographs/vol71/mono71-23.pdf.
218. Wrbitzky R. Liver function in workers exposed to N,N-dimethylformamide during the production of synthetic textiles. *International Archives of Occupational and Environmental Health.* 1999; **72**: 19-25.
219. Chang HY, Shih TS, Guo YL et al. Sperm function in workers exposed to N,N-dimethylformamide in the synthetic leather industry. *Fertility and Sterility.* 2004; **81**: 1589-94.
220. Senoh H, Aiso S, Arito H et al. Carcinogenicity and chronic toxicity after inhalation exposure of rats and mice to N,N-dimethylformamide. *Journal of Occupational Health.* 2004; **46**: 429-39.
221. Hellwig J, Merkle J, Klimisch HJ, Jackh R. Studies on the prenatal toxicity of N,N-dimethylformamide in mice, rats and rabbits. *Food and Chemical Toxicology.* 1991; **29**: 193-201.
222. Mraz J, Nohova H. Absorption, metabolism and elimination of N,N-dimethylformamide in humans. *International Archives of Occupational and Environmental Health.* 1992; **64**: 85-92.
223. Wang SM, Shih TS, Huang YS et al. Evaluation of the effectiveness of personal protective equipment against occupational exposure to N,N-dimethylformamide. *Journal of Hazardous Material.* 2006; **138**: 518-25.
224. Mraz J, Jheeta P, Gescher A et al. Investigation of the mechanistic basis of N,N-dimethylformamide toxicity. Metabolism of N,N-dimethylformamide and its deuterated isotopomers by cytochrome P450 2E1. *Chemical Research in Toxicology.* 1993; **6**: 197-207.
225. Mraz J, Simek P, Chvalova D et al. Studies on the methyl isocyanate adducts with globin. *Chemico-biological Interactions.* 2004; **148**: 1-10.
226. Luo JC, Cheng TJ, Kuo HW, Chang MJ. Abnormal liver function associated with occupational exposure to dimethylformamide and glutathione S-transferase polymorphisms. *Biomarkers.* 2005; **10**: 464-74.
227. Mraz J, Duskova S, Galova E et al. Biological monitoring of N, N-dimethylformamide. Reference value for N-methylcarbamoyl adduct at the N-terminal valine of globin as a biomarker of chronic occupational exposure. *International Archives of Occupational and Environmental Health.* 2002; **75** (Suppl.): S93-6.
228. Mraz J, Cimlova J, Stransky V et al. N-Methylcarbamoyl-lysine adduct in globin: A new metabolic product and potential biomarker of N,N-dimethylformamide in humans. *Toxicology Letters.* 2006; **162**: 211-18.
229. Kafferlein HU, Ferstl C, Burkhart-Reichl A et al. The use of biomarkers of exposure of N,N-dimethylformamide in health risk assessment and occupational hygiene in the polyacrylic fibre industry. *Occupational and Environmental Medicine.* 2005; **62**: 330-6.
230. Spies GJ, Rhyne RH Jr, Evans RA et al. Monitoring acrylic fiber workers for liver toxicity and exposure to dimethylacetamide. 2. Serum clinical chemistry results of dimethylacetamide-exposed workers. *Journal of Occupational and Environmental Medicine.* 1995; **37**: 1102-7.

231. Jung SJ, Lee CY, Kim SA et al. Dimethylacetamide-induced hepatic injuries among spandex fibre workers. *Clinical Toxicology*. 2007; **45**: 435–9.
232. Lee CY, Jung SJ, Kim SA et al. Incidence of dimethylacetamide induced hepatic injury among new employees in a cohort of elastane fibre workers. *Occupational and Environmental Medicine*. 2006; **63**: 688–93.
233. Okuda H, Takeuchi T, Senoh H et al. Developmental toxicity induced by inhalation exposure of pregnant rats to N,N-dimethylacetamide. *Journal of Occupational Health*. 2006; **48**: 154–60.
234. Nomiyama T, Omae K, Ishizuka C et al. Dermal absorption of N,N-dimethylacetamide in human volunteers. *International Archives of Occupational and Environmental Health*. 2000; **73**: 121–6.
235. Perbellini L, Princivalle A, Caivano M, Montagnani R. Biological monitoring of occupational exposure to N,N-dimethylacetamide with identification of a new metabolite. *Occupational and Environmental Medicine*. 2003; **60**: 746–51.
236. Borm PJ, de Jong L, Vliegen A. Environmental and biological monitoring of workers occupationally exposed to dimethylacetamide. *Journal of Occupational Medicine*. 1987; **29**: 898–903.
237. Kennedy GL Jr, Pruett JW. Biologic monitoring for dimethylacetamide: Measurement for 4 consecutive weeks in a workplace. *Journal of Occupational Medicine*. 1989; **31**: 47–50.
238. Spies GJ, Rhyne RH Jr, Evans RA et al. Monitoring acrylic fiber workers for liver toxicity and exposure to dimethylacetamide. 1. Assessing exposure to dimethylacetamide by air and biological monitoring. *Journal of Occupational and Environmental Medicine*. 1995; **37**: 1093–101.
239. European Union. Acrylamide. European Union Risk Assessment Report, vol. 24. Luxembourg: European Commission, 2002: 207. Available from: http://ecb.jrc.ec.europa.eu/documents/existing-chemicals/risk_assessment/report/acrylamidereport011.pdf.
240. He FS, Zhang SL, Wang HL et al. Neurological and electroneuromyographic assessment of the adverse effects of acrylamide on occupationally exposed workers. *Scandinavian Journal of Work, Environment and Health*. 1989; **15**: 125–9.
241. Hagmar L, Tornqvist M, Nordander C et al. Health effects of occupational exposure to acrylamide using hemoglobin adducts as biomarkers of internal dose. *Scandinavian Journal of Work, Environment and Health*. 2001; **27**: 219–26.
242. Kjuus H, Goffeng LO, Heier MS et al. Effects on the peripheral nervous system of tunnel workers exposed to acrylamide and N-methylolacrylamide. *Scandinavian Journal of Work, Environment and Health*. 2004; **30**: 21–9.
243. International Agency for Research on Cancer. Acrylamide. In: Some Industrial Chemicals, IARC Monographs on the Evaluation of Carcinogenic Risks to Humans, vol. 60. Lyon: IARC, 1994: 389–433. Available from: http://monographs.iarc.fr/ENG/Monographs/vol60/mono60-16.pdf.
244. Health Council of the Netherlands (DECOS). Health Council of the Netherlands. Acrylamide. Health-based calculated occupational cancer risk values, vol. 2006/05OSH. The Hague: Health Council of the Netherlands, 2006: 70. Available from: www.gezondheidsraad.nl/sites/default/files/06@05OSH.pdf.
245. Marsh GM, Lucas LJ, Youk AO, Schall LC. Mortality patterns among workers exposed to acrylamide: 1994 follow up. *Occupational and Environmental Medicine*. 1999; **56**: 181–90.
246. Swaen GM, Haidar S, Burns CJ et al. Mortality study update of acrylamide workers. *Occupational and Environmental Medicine*. 2007; **64**: 396–401.
247. Boettcher MI, Angerer J. Determination of the major mercapturic acids of acrylamide and glycidamide in human urine by LC-ESI-MS/MS. *Journal of Chromatography. B, Analytical Technologies in the Biomedical and Life Sciences*. 2005; **824**: 283–94.
248. Bull PJ, Brooke RK, Cocker J et al. An occupational hygiene investigation of exposure to acrylamide and the role for urinary S-carboxyethyl-cysteine (CEC) as a biological marker. *Annals of Occupational Hygiene*. 2005; **49**: 683–90.
249. International Programme on Chemical Safety. Acrylonitrile. Health and Safety Guide, vol 1. Geneva: IPCS, 1986. Available from: www.inchem.org/documents/hsg/hsg/hsg001.htm.
250. International Programme on Chemical Safety. Acrylonitrile. Concise International Chemical Assessment Document, vol. 39. Geneva: IPCS, 2002. Available from: www.inchem.org/documents/cicads/cicads/cicad39.htm.
251. International Programme on Chemical Safety. Acetonitrile. Environmental Health Criteria, vol. 154. Geneva: IPCS, 1993. Available from: www.inchem.org/documents/ehc/ehc/ehc154.htm.
252. Umbreit J. Methemoglobin – it's not just blue: A concise review. *American Journal of Hematology*. 2007; **82**: 134–44.
253. European Union. Aniline. European Risk Assessment Report, vol 50. Luxembourg: European Commission, 2004: 222. Available from: http://ecb.jrc.ec.europa.eu/documents/existing-chemicals/risk_assessment/report/anilinereport049.pdf.
254. Jenkins FP, Robinson JA, Gellatly JB, Salmond GW. The no-effect dose of aniline in human subjects and a comparison of aniline toxicity in man and the rat. *Food and Cosmetics Toxicology*. 1972; **10**: 671–9.
255. Hathaway GJ, Proctor NH, Hughes JP. *Chemical hazards of the workplace*, 4th edn. New York: Van Nostrand Reinhold, 1996.
256. National Cancer Institute. Bioassay of aniline hydrochloride for possible carcinogenicity. CAS No. 142-04-1. NCI Technical Report Series, vol 130. Bethesda, MD: US Department of Health, Education and Welfare, 1978: 55. Available from: http://ntp.niehs.nih.gov/ntp/htdocs/LT_rpts/tr130.pdf.
257. CIIT. 104-Week chronic toxicity study in rats. Aniline hydrochloride. Final report. Virginia: Hazleton Laboratories, 1982.

258. Lewalter J, Korallus U. Blood protein conjugates and acetylation of aromatic amines. New findings on biological monitoring. *International Archives of Occupational and Environmental Health.* 1985; **56**: 179-96.
259. Teass AW, DeBord DG, Brown KK et al. Biological monitoring for occupational exposures to o-toluidine and aniline. *International Archives of Occupational and Environmental Health.* 1993; **65**: S115-18.
260. Rumack B. POISINDEX. Information system, CCIS, vol. 136. Englewood, CO: Micromedex, 2008.
261. Liao YP, Hung DZ, Yang DY. Hemolytic anemia after methylene blue therapy for aniline-induced methemoglobinemia. *Veterinary and Human Toxicology.* 2002; **44**: 19-21.
262. Organisation for Economic Co-Operation and Development. o-Toluidine. OECD SIDS. Initial Assessment Report. Geneva: UNEP Publications, 2006. Available from: www.chem.unep.ch/irptc/sids/OECDSIDS/95534.pdf.
263. Organisation for Economic Co-Operation and Development. p-Toluidine. OECD SIDS. Initial Assessment Report. Geneva: UNEP Publications, 2007: 207. Available from: www.chem.unep.ch/irptc/sids/OECDSIDS/106490.pdf.
264. Organisation for Economic Co-Operation and Development. m-Toluidine. OECD SIDS. Initial Assessment Report. Geneva: UNEP Publications, 2003: 178. Available from: www.chem.unep.ch/irptc/sids/OECDSIDS/108441.pdf.
265. International Agency for Research on Cancer. ortho-Toluidine. In: Some Industrial Chemicals. IARC Monographs on the Evaluation of Carcinogenic Risks to Humans, vol. 77. Lyon: IARC, 2000: 267-322. Available from: http://monographs.iarc.fr/ENG/Monographs/vol71/mono71-26.pdf.
266. International Programme on Chemical Safety. N-phenyl-1-naphtylamine. Concise International Chemical Assessment Document, vol 9. Geneva: IPCS, 1998. Available from: www.inchem.org/documents/cicads/cicads/cicad9.htm.
267. Weiss T, Bruning T, Bolt HM. Dephenylation of the rubber chemical N-phenyl-2-naphthylamine to carcinogenic 2-naphthylamine: A classical problem revisited. *Critical Reviews in Toxicology.* 2007; **37**: 553-66.
268. Kopelman H, Robertson MH, Sanders PG, Ash I. The Epping jaundice. *British Medical Journal.* 1966; **1**: 514-16.
269. European Union. 4,4'-Methylenedianiline. European Risk Assessment Report, vol. 9. Luxembourg: European Commission, 2001. Available from: http://ecb.jrc.ec.europa.eu/documents/existing-chemicals/risk_assessment/report/mdareport008.pdf.
270. International Agency for Research on Cancer. 4,4'-Methylenedianiline and its dihydrochloride. In: Some Chemicals Used in Plastics and Elastomers. IARC Monographs on the Evaluation of Carcinogenic Risks to Humans, vol. 39. Lyon: IARC, 1986: 347-68. Available from: http://monographs.iarc.fr/ENG/Monographs/vol39/volume39.pdf.
271. International Programme on Chemical Safety. 4-Chloroaniline. Concise International Chemical Assessment Document, vol. 48. Geneva: IPCS, 2003. Available from: www.inchem.org/documents/cicads/cicads/cicad46.htm.
272. European Union. 3,4-Dichloroaniline. European Union Risk Assessment Report, vol. 65. Luxembourg: European Commission, 2006: 132. Available from: http://ecb.jrc.ec.europa.eu/documents/existing-chemicals/risk_assessment/report/34dichloroaniline_dcareport048.pdf.
273. International Agency for Research on Cancer. Occupational exposures of hairdressers and barbers and personal use of hair colourants; some hair dyes, cosmetic colourants, industrial dyestuffs and aromatic amines. IARC Monographs on the Evaluation of Carcinogenic Risks to Humans, vol. 57. Lyon: IARC, 1993: 427. Available from: http://monographs.iarc.fr/ENG/Monographs/vol57/index.php.
274. Robert A, Ducos P, Francin JM. Biological monitoring of workers exposed to 4,4'-methylene-bis-(2-orthochloroaniline) (MOCA). I. A new and easy determination of 'free' and 'total' MOCA in urine. *International Archives of Occupational and Environmental Health.* 1999; **72**: 223-8.
275. Kaderlik KR, Talaska G, DeBord DG et al. 4,4'-Methylene-bis(2-chloroaniline)-DNA adduct analysis in human exfoliated urothelial cells by 32P-postlabeling. *Cancer Epidemiology, Biomarkers and Prevention.* 1993; **2**: 63-9.
276. International Programme on Chemical Safety. Phenylhydrazine. Concise International Chemical Assessment Document, vol. 19. Geneva: IPCS, 2000. Available from: www.inchem.org/documents/cicads/cicads/cicad_19.htm.
277. Geier J, Lessmann H, Dickel H et al. Patch test results with the metalworking fluid series of the German Contact Dermatitis Research Group (DKG). *Contact Dermatitis.* 2004; **51**: 118-30.
278. Geier J, Lessmann H, Schnuch A, Uter W. Contact sensitizations in metalworkers with occupational dermatitis exposed to water-based metalworking fluids: Results of the research project 'FaSt'. *International Archives of Occupational and Environmental Health.* 2004; **77**: 543-51.
279. Gelfand HH. Respiratory allergy due to chemical compounds encountered in the rubber, lacquer, shellac, and beauty culture industries. *Journal of Allergy and Clinical Immunology.* 1963; **34**: 374-81.
280. Kabe J. [Bronchial asthma and asthma-like dyspnea caused by inhalation of simple chemicals]. *Arerugi.* 1971; **20**: 444-50.
281. Savonius B, Keskinen H, Tuppurainen M, Kanerva L. Occupational asthma caused by ethanolamines. *Allergy.* 1994; **49**: 877-81.
282. Piipari R, Tuppurainen M, Tuomi T et al. Diethanolamine-induced occupational asthma, a case report. *Clinical and Experimental Allergy.* 1998; **28**: 358-62.
283. Knaak JB, Leung HW, Stott WT et al. Toxicology of mono-, di-, and triethanolamine. *Reviews of Environmental Contamination and Toxicology.* 1997; **149**: 1-86.
284. Stott WT, Waechter JM, Rick DL, Mendrala AL. Absorption, distribution, metabolism and excretion of intravenously and dermally administered triethanolamine in mice. *Food and Chemical Toxicology.* 2000; **38**: 1043-51.

285. International Programme on Chemical Safety. *N*-Methyl-2-pyrrolidone. Concise International Chemical Assessment Document, vol. 35. Geneva. IPCS, 2001. Available from: www.inchem.org/documents/cicads/cicads/cicad35.htm.
286. European Union. 1-Vinyl-2-pyrrolidone. European Union Risk Assessment Report, vol. 39. Luxembourg: European Commission, 2003: 116. Available from: http://ecb.jrc.ec.europa.eu/documents/existing-chemicals/risk_assessment/report/vinylpyrrolidonereport040.pdf.
287. Bader M, Keener SA, Wrbitzky R. Dermal absorption and urinary elimination of *N*-methyl-2-pyrrolidone. *International Archives of Occupational and Environmental Health*. 2005; **78**: 673–6.
288. Leira HL, Tiltnes A, Svendsen K, Vetlesen L. Irritant cutaneous reactions to *N*-methyl-2-pyrrolidone (NMP). *Contact Dermatitis*. 1992; **27**: 148–50.
289. Beaulieu H, Schmerber K. M-pyrol (NMP) use in the microelectronics industry. *Applied Occupational and Environmental Hygiene*. 1991; **6**: 874–80.
290. Langworth S, Anundi H, Friis L *et al.* Acute health effects common during graffiti removal. *International Archives of Occupational and Environmental Health*. 2001; **74**: 213–18.
291. Saillenfait AM, Gallissot F, Langonné I, Sabaté JP. Developmental toxicity of *N*-methyl-2-pyrrolidone administered orally to rats. *Food and Chemical Toxicology*. 2002; **40**: 1705–12.
292. Becci PJ, Knickerbocker MJ, Reagan EL *et al.* Teratogenicity study of *N*-methylpyrrolidone after dermal application to Sprague-Dawley rats. *Fundamental and Applied Toxicology*. 1982; **2**: 73–6.
293. Saillenfait AM, Gallissot F, Morel G. Developmental toxicity of *N*-methyl-2-pyrrolidone in rats following inhalation exposure. *Food and Chemical Toxicology*. 2003; **41**: 583–8.
294. International Agency for Research on Cancer. *n*-Vinyl-2-pyrrolidone and polyvinylpyrrolidone. In: Re-Evaluation of Some Organic Chemicals. Hydrazine and Hydrogen Peroxide, 71. Lyon: IARC, 1999: 1181–7. Available from: http://monographs.iarc.fr/ENG/Monographs/vol71/mono71-57.pdf.
295. Carnerup MA, Spanne M, Jonsson BA. Levels of *N*-methyl-2-pyrrolidone (NMP) and its metabolites in plasma and urine from volunteers after experimental exposure to NMP in dry and humid air. *Toxicology Letters*. 2006; **162**: 139–45.
296. Akesson B, Jonsson BA. Biological monitoring of *N*-methyl-2-pyrrolidone using 5-hydroxy-*N*-methyl-2-pyrrolidone in plasma and urine as the biomarker. *Scandinavian Journal of Work, Environment and Health*. 2000; **26**: 213–18.
297. Fine DH. Exposure assessment to preformed environmental *N*-nitroso compounds from the point of view of our own studies. *Oncology*. 1980; **37**: 199–202.
298. Fajen JM, Fine DH, Rounbehler DP. *N*-Nitrosamines in the factory environment. *IARC Scientific Publications* 1980; 517–30.
299. Fajen JM, Rounbehler DP, Fine DH. Summary report on *N*-nitrosamines in the factory environment. *IARC Scientific Publications*. 1982; 223–9.
300. Reh BD, Fajen JM. Worker exposures to nitrosamines in a rubber vehicle sealing plant. *American Industrial Hygiene Association Journal*. 1996; **57**: 918–23.
301. Oury B, Limasset JC, Protois JC. Assessment of exposure to carcinogenic *N*-nitrosamines in the rubber industry. *International Archives of Occupational and Environmental Health*. 1997; **70**: 261–71.
302. de Vocht F, Burstyn I, Straif K *et al.* Occupational exposure to NDMA and NMor in the European rubber industry. *Journal of Environmental Monitoring*. 2007; **9**: 253–9.
303. Iavicoli I, Carelli G. Evaluation of occupational exposure to *N*-nitrosamines in a rubber-manufacturing industry. *Journal of Occupational and Environmental Medicine*. 2006; **48**: 195–8.
304. Ducos P, Gaudin R, Maire C *et al.* Occupational exposure to volatile nitrosamines in foundries using the 'Ashland' core-making process. *Environmental Research*. 1988; **47**: 72–8.
305. Jarvholm B, Zingmark PA, Osterdahl BG. *N*-nitrosodiethanolamine in commercial cutting fluids without nitrites. *Annals of Occupational Hygiene*. 1991; **35**: 659–63.
306. Jarvholm B, Zingmark PA, Osterdahl BG. High concentration of *N*-nitrosodiethanolamine in a diluted commercial cutting fluid. *American Journal of Industrial Medicine*. 1991; **19**: 237–9.
307. Monarca S, Scassellati Sforzolini G, Spiegelhalder B *et al.* Monitoring nitrite, *N*-nitrosodiethanolamine, and mutagenicity in cutting fluids used in the metal industry. *Environmental Health Perspectives*. 1993; **101**: 126–8.
308. Eisenbrand G, Fuchs A, Koehl W. *N*-nitroso compounds in cosmetics, household commodities and cutting fluids. *European Journal of Cancer Prevention*. 1996; **5** (Suppl. 1): 41–6.
309. Ducos P, Gaudin R, Francin JM. Determination of *N*-nitrosodiethanolamine in urine by gas chromatography thermal energy analysis: Application in workers exposed to aqueous metalworking fluids. *International Archives of Occupational and Environmental Health*. 1999; **72**: 215–22.
310. Hecht SS. DNA adduct formation from tobacco-specific *N*-nitrosamines. *Mutation Research*. 1999; **424**: 127–42.
311. Lijinsky W. *N*-nitrosocompounds. In: Bingham E, Chorssen B, Powell C (eds). *Patty's Toxicology*, 5th edn. New York: John Wiley, 2001: 633–81.
312. International Agency for Research on Cancer. *N*-Nitrosodiethanolamine. In: Some Industrial Chemicals. IARC Monographs on the Evaluation of Carcinogenic Risks to Humans, vol. 77. Lyon: IARC, 2000: 403–38. Available from: http://monographs.iarc.fr/ENG/Monographs/vol77/mono77-16.pdf.
313. European Union. Phenol. European Union Risk Assessment Report, vol. 64. Luxembourg: European Commission, 2006: 226. Available from: http://ecb.jrc.ec.europa.eu/documents/existing-chemicals/risk_assessment/report/phenolreport060.pdf.

314. Bentur Y, Shoshani O, Tabak A et al. Prolonged elimination half-life of phenol after dermal exposure. *Journal of Toxicology. Clinical Toxicology.* 1998; **36**: 707–11.
315. Monteiro-Riviere NA, Inman AO, Jackson H et al. Efficacy of topical phenol decontamination strategies on severity of acute phenol chemical burns and dermal absorption: *In vitro* and *in vivo* studies in pig skin. *Toxicology and Industrial Health.* 2001; **17**: 95–104.
316. Hunter DM, Timerding BL, Leonard RB et al. Effects of isopropyl alcohol, ethanol, and polyethylene glycol/industrial methylated spirits in the treatment of acute phenol burns. *Annals of Emergency Medicine.* 1992; **21**: 1303–7.
317. Priha E, Ahonen I, Oksa P. Control of chemical risks during the treatment of soil contaminated with chlorophenol, creosote and copper-chrome-arsenic-wood preservatives. *American Journal of Industrial Medicine.* 2001; **39**: 402–9.
318. Bleiberg J, Wallen M, Brodkin R, Applebaum IL. Industrially acquired porphyria. *Archives of Dermatology.* 1964; **89**: 793–7.
319. Bond GG, McLaren EA, Brenner FE, Cook RR. Incidence of chloracne among chemical workers potentially exposed to chlorinated dioxins. *Journal of Occupational Medicine.* 1989; **31**: 771–4.
320. Agency for Toxic Substances and Disease Registry. Toxicological profile for chlorophenols. US Department of Health and Human Services, Public Health Service. Atlanta, GA: ATSDR, 1999. Available from: www.atsdr.cdc.gov/toxprofiles/tp107.html.
321. International Agency for Research on Cancer. Polychlorophenols and their sodium salts. In Re-Evaluation of Some Organic Chemicals, Hydrazine and Hydrogen Peroxide, 71. Lyon: IARC, 1999: 769–816. Available from: http://monographs.iarc.fr/ENG/Monographs/vol71/mono71-34.pdf.
322. Demers PA, Davies HW, Friesen MC et al. Cancer and occupational exposure to pentachlorophenol and tetrachlorophenol (Canada). *Cancer Causes Control.* 2006; **17**: 749–58.
323. Hoppin JA, Tolbert PE, Herrick RF et al. Occupational chlorophenol exposure and soft tissue sarcoma risk among men aged 30–60 years. *American Journal of Epidemiology.* 1998; **148**: 693–703.
324. Lindroos L, Koskinen H, Mutanen P, Jarvisalo J. Urinary chlorophenols in sawmill workers. *International Archives of Occupational and Environmental Health.* 1987; **59**: 463–7.
325. Organisation for Economic Co-operation and Development. *o*-Cresol. OECD SIDS. Initial Assessment Report. Geneva: UNEP Publications, 2005: 47. Available from: www.chem.unep.ch/irptc/sids/OECDSIDS/95487.pdf.
326. Boissy RE, Manga P. On the etiology of contact/occupational vitiligo. *Pigment Cell Research.* 2004; **17**: 208–14.
327. International Programme on Chemical Safety. Resorcinol. Concise International Chemical Assessment Document. Geneva: IPCS, 2006. Available from: www.inchem.org/documents/cicads/cicads/cicad71.htm.
328. Organisation for Economic Co-operation and Development. *p*-tert-Butylphenol. OECD SIDS. Initial Assessment Report. Geneva: UNEP Publications, 2002: 135. Available from: www.chem.unep.ch/irptc/sids/OECDSIDS/98544.pdf.
329. European Union. 4,4′-isopropylidenediphenol (bisphenol-A). European Risk Assessment Report, vol. 37. Luxembourg: European Commission, 2003: 290. Available from: http://ecb.jrc.ec.europa.eu/documents/existing-chemicals/risk_assessment/report/bisphenolareport325.pdf.
330. European Union. 4-nonylphenol (branched) and nonylphenol. European Union Risk Assessment Report, vol. 10. Luxembourg: European Commission, 2002: 227. http://www.bfr.bund.de/cm/252/4_nonylphenol_und_nonyl phenol.pdf.
331. National Toxicology Program. Bisphenol-A: (CAS No. 80-05-7). Reproductive and fertility assessment in CD-1 mice when administered in the feed. United States Department of Health and Human Services. NTP Report, Public Health Service. Bethesda, MD: National Institutes of Health, 1985. Available from: http://ntp.niehs.nih.gov/index.cfm?objectid=071c89f0-f76a-d393-446c76e3f5ac28ea.
332. National Toxicology Program. Reproductive toxicity of nonylphenol (CAS 84852-15-3) administered by gavage to Sprague–Dawley rats. Public Health Service. Bethesda, MD: National Institutes of Health, 1997. http://ntp.niehs.nih.gov/index.cfm?objectid=071D9342-AE22-E76C-6C82D206806B591F.
333. Waechter J, Veenstra G. Epoxy compounds – Olefin oxides, aliphatic glycidyl ethers and aromatic monoglycidyl ethers. In: Bingham E, Chorssen B, Powell C (eds). *Patty's Toxicology*, 5th edn. New York: John Wiley, 2001: 993–1085.
334. International Programme on Chemical Safety. Ethylene oxide. Concise International Chemical Assessment Document, vol. 54. Geneva: IPCS, 2003: 57. Available from: www.inchem.org/documents/cicads/cicads/cicad54.htm.
335. Steenland K, Stayner L, Deddens J. Mortality analyses in a cohort of 18 235 ethylene oxide exposed workers: Follow up extended from 1987 to 1998. *Occupational and Environmental Medicine.* 2004; **61**: 2–7.
336. Grosse Y, Baan R, Straif K et al. Carcinogenicity of 1,3-butadiene, ethylene oxide, vinyl chloride, vinyl fluoride, and vinyl bromide. *Lancet Oncology.* 2007; **8**: 679–80.
337. Gresie-Brusin DF, Kielkowski D, Baker A et al. Occupational exposure to ethylene oxide during pregnancy and association with adverse reproductive outcomes. *International Archives of Occupational and Environmental Health.* 2007; **80**: 559–65.
338. Ohnishi A, Murai Y. Polyneuropathy due to ethylene oxide, propylene oxide, and butylene oxide. *Environmental Research.* 1993; **60**: 242–7.
339. International Agency for Research on Cancer. Propylene oxide. In: Some industrial chemicals. IARC Monographs on

the Evaluation of Carcinogenic Risks to Humans, vol. 60. Lyon: IARC, 1994: 181-213. http://monographs.iarc.fr/ENG/Monographs/vol60/mono60-9.pdf.
340. Boogaard PJ, Rocchi PS, van Sittert NJ. Biomonitoring of exposure to ethylene oxide and propylene oxide by determination of hemoglobin adducts: Correlations between airborne exposure and adduct levels. *International Archives of Occupational and Environmental Health.* 1999; **72**: 142-50.
341. Czene K, Osterman-Golkar S, Yun X et al. Analysis of DNA and hemoglobin adducts and sister chromatid exchanges in a human population occupationally exposed to propylene oxide: A pilot study. *Cancer Epidemiology, Biomarkers and Prevention.* 2002; **11**: 315-18.
342. Albertini RJ, Sweeney LM. Propylene oxide: Genotoxicity profile of a rodent nasal carcinogen. *Critical Reviews in Toxicology.* 2007; **37**: 489-520.
343. Okuda H, Takeuchi T, Senoh H et al. Effects of inhalation exposure to propylene oxide on respiratory tract, reproduction and development in rats. *Journal of Occupational Health.* 2006; **48**: 462-73.
344. National Toxicology Program. Toxicology and carcinogenesis studies of 1,2-epoxybutane (CAS No. 106-88-7) in F344/N rats and B6C3F1 mice (inhalation studies). NTP Technical Report Series No. 329. Department of Health and Human Services. Technical Report Series: Public Health Service. Bethesda, MD: National Institutes of Health, 1988: 176. Available from: http://ntp.niehs.nih.gov/ntp/htdocs/LT_rpts/tr329.pdf.
345. International Agency for Research on Cancer. 1,2-Epoxybutane. In: Re-Evaluation of Some Organic Chemicals, Hydrazine and Hydrogen Peroxide. IARC Monographs on the Evaluation of Carcinogenic Risks to Humans, vol. 71. Lyon: IARC, 1999: 629-40. Available from: http://monographs.iarc.fr/ENG/Monographs/vol71/mono71-27.pdf.
346. Luo JC, Kuo HW, Cheng TJ, Chang MJ. Pulmonary function abnormality and respiratory tract irritation symptoms in epichlorohydrin-exposed workers in Taiwan. *American Journal of Industrial Medicine.* 2003; **43**: 440-6.
347. International Agency for Research on Cancer. Epichlorohydrin. In: Re-Evaluation of Some Organic Chemicals, Hydrazine and Hydrogen Peroxide. IARC Monographs on the Evaluation of Carcinogenic Risks to Humans, vol. 71. Lyon: IARC, 1999: 603-28. Available from: http://monographs.iarc.fr/ENG/Monographs/vol71/mono71-26.pdf.
348. Waechter J, Veenstra G. Epoxy compounds – aromatic diglycidyl ethers, polyglycidyl ethers, glycidyl ethers, and miscellaneous epoxy compounds. In: Bingham E, Chorssen B, Powell C (eds). *Patty's Toxicology*, 5th edn. New York: John Wiley, 2001: 1087-145.
349. Jolanki R, Kanerva L, Estlander T et al. Occupational dermatoses from epoxy resin compounds. *Contact Dermatitis.* 1990; **23**: 172-83.
350. Jolanki R, Estlander T, Kanerva L. 182 patients with occupational allergic epoxy contact dermatitis over 22 years. *Contact Dermatitis.* 2001; **44**: 121-3.
351. Kanerva L, Jolanki R, Tupasela O et al. Immediate and delayed allergy from epoxy resins based on diglycidyl ether of bisphenol A. *Scandinavian Journal of Work, Environment and Health.* 1991; **17**: 208-15.
352. Kanerva L, Pelttari M, Jolanki R et al. Occupational contact urticaria from diglycidyl ether of bisphenol A epoxy resin. *Allergy.* 2002; **57**: 1205-7.
353. International Agency for Research on Cancer. Bisphenol A diglycidyl ether. In: Re-Evaluation of Some Organic Chemicals, Hydrazine and Hydrogen Peroxide. IARC Monographs on the Evaluation of Carcinogenic Risks to Humans, vol. 71. Lyon: IARC, 1999: 1285-9. Available from: http://monographs.iarc.fr/ENG/Monographs/vol71/mono71-71.pdf.
354. Hanaoka T, Kawamura N, Hara K, Tsugane S. Urinary bisphenol A and plasma hormone concentrations in male workers exposed to bisphenol A diglycidyl ether and mixed organic solvents. *Occupational and Environmental Medicine.* 2002; **59**: 625-8.
355. Nakazawa H, Yamaguchi A, Inoue K et al. In vitro assay of hydrolysis and chlorohydroxy derivatives of bisphenol A diglycidyl ether for estrogenic activity. *Food and Chemical Toxicology.* 2002; **40**: 1827-32.
356. Stroheker T, Picard K, Lhuguenot JC et al. Steroid activities comparison of natural and food wrap compounds in human breast cancer cell lines. *Food and Chemical Toxicology.* 2004; **42**: 887-97.
357. Hyoung UJ, Yang YJ, Kwon SK et al. Developmental toxicity by exposure to bisphenol A diglycidyl ether during gestation and lactation period in Sprague-Dawley male rats. *Journal of Preventive Medicine and Public Health.* 2007; **40**: 155-61.
358. Keskinen H. Cyclic acid anhydrides. The Nordic Expert Group for Criteria Documentation of Health Risks from Chemicals and The Dutch Expert Committee on Occupational Standards, vol. 136. Stockholm: Nordic Council of Ministers, 2004: 74. Available from: https://gupea.ub.gu.se/dspace/bitstream/2077/4327/1/ah2004_15.pdf.
359. International Programme on Chemical Safety. Cyclic acid anhydrides. Human health aspects. Concise International Chemical Assessment Document, vol. 75. Geneva: IPCS, 2008. Available from: www.who.int/ipcs/publications/cicad/cicad75.pdf.
360. Drexler H, Weber A, Letzel S et al. Detection and clinical relevance of a type I allergy with occupational exposure to hexahydrophthalic anhydride and methyltetrahydrophthalic anhydride. *International Archives of Occupational and Environmental Health.* 1994; **65**: 279-83.
361. Howe W, Venables KM, Topping MD et al. Tetrachlorophthalic anhydride asthma: Evidence for specific IgE antibody. *Journal of Allergy and Clinical Immunology.* 1983; **71**: 5-11.
362. Liss GM, Bernstein D, Genesove L et al. Assessment of risk factors for IgE-mediated sensitization to tetrachlorophthalic anhydride. *Journal of Allergy and Clinical Immunology.* 1993; **92**: 237-47.

363. Maccia CA, Bernstein IL, Emmett EA, Brooks SM. *In vitro* demonstration of specific IgE in phthalic anhydride hypersensitivity. *American Review of Respiratory Disease.* 1976; **113**: 701–4.
364. Moller DR, Gallagher JS, Bernstein DI *et al.* Detection of IgE-mediated respiratory sensitization in workers exposed to hexahydrophthalic anhydride. *Journal of Allergy and Clinical Immunology.* 1985; **75**: 663–72.
365. Nielsen J, Welinder H, Schutz A, Skerfving S. Specific serum antibodies against phthalic anhydride in occupationally exposed subjects. *Journal of Allergy and Clinical Immunology.* 1988; **82**: 126–33.
366. Nielsen J, Welinder H, Horstmann V, Skerfving S. Allergy to methyltetrahydrophthalic anhydride in epoxy resin workers. *British Journal of Industrial Medicine.* 1992; **49**: 769–75.
367. Rosenman KD, Bernstein DI, O'Leary K *et al.* Occupational asthma caused by himic anhydride. *Scandinavian Journal of Work, Environment and Health.* 1987; **13**: 150–4.
368. Sale SR, Roach DE, Zeiss CR, Patterson R. Clinical and immunologic correlations in trimellitic anhydride airway syndromes. *Journal of Allergy and Clinical Immunology.* 1981; **68**: 188–93.
369. Topping MD, Venables KM, Luczynska CM *et al.* Specificity of the human IgE response to inhaled acid anhydrides. *Journal of Allergy and Clinical Immunology.* 1986; **77**: 834–42.
370. Welinder H, Nielsen J, Gustavsson C *et al.* Specific antibodies to methyltetrahydrophthalic anhydride in exposed workers. *Clinical and Experimental Allergy.* 1990; **20**: 639–45.
371. Welinder HE, Jonsson BA, Nielsen JE *et al.* Exposure–response relationships in the formation of specific antibodies to hexahydrophthalic anhydride in exposed workers. *Scandinavian Journal of Work, Environment and Health.* 1994; **20**: 459–65.
372. Welinder H, Nielsen J, Rylander L, Stahlbom B. A prospective study of the relationship between exposure and specific antibodies in workers exposed to organic acid anhydrides. *Allergy.* 2001; **56**: 506–11.
373. Yokota K, Johyama Y, Yamaguchi K *et al.* Specific antibodies against methyltetrahydrophthalic anhydride and risk factors for sensitization in occupationally exposed subjects. *Scandinavian Journal of Work, Environment and Health.* 1997; **23**: 214–20.
374. Zeiss CR, Wolkonsky P, Pruzansky JJ, Patterson R. Clinical and immunologic evaluation of trimellitic anhydride workers in multiple industrial settings. *Journal of Allergy and Clinical Immunology.* 1982; **70**: 15–18.
375. Lowenthal M, Shaughnessy MA, Harris KE, Grammer LC. Immunologic cross-reactivity of acid anhydrides with immunoglobulin E against trimellityl-human serum albumin. *Journal of Laboratory and Clinical Medicine.* 1994; **123**: 869–73.
376. Welinder H, Nielsen J. Immunologic tests of specific antibodies to organic acid anhydrides. *Allergy.* 1991; **46**: 601–9.
377. Patterson R, Addington W, Banner AS *et al.* Antihapten antibodies in workers exposed to trimellitic anhydride fumes: A potential immunopathogenetic mechanism for the trimellitic anhydride pulmonary disease–anemia syndrome. *American Review of Respiratory Disease.* 1979; **120**: 1259–67.
378. Patterson R, Zeiss CR, Pruzansky JJ. Immunology and immunopathology of trimellitic anhydride pulmonary reactions. *Journal of Allergy and Clinical Immunology.* 1982; **70**: 19–23.
379. Patterson R, Zeiss CR, Roberts M *et al.* Human antihapten antibodies in trimellitic anhydride inhalation reactions. Immunoglobulin classes of anti-trimellitic anhydride antibodies and hapten inhibition studies. *Journal of Clinical Investigation.* 1978; **62**: 971–8.
380. Turner ES, Pruzansky JJ, Patterson R *et al.* Detection of antibodies in human serum using trimellityl-erythrocytes: Direct and indirect haemagglutination and haemolysis. *Clinical and Experimental Immunology.* 1980; **39**: 470–6.
381. Jonsson B, Welinder H, Skarping G. Hexahydrophthalic acid in urine as an index of exposure to hexahydrophthalic anhydride. *International Archives of Occupational and Environmental Health.* 1991; **63**: 77–9.
382. Lindh CH, Jonsson BA, Welinder H. Biological monitoring of methylhexahydrophthalic anhydride by determination of methylhexahydrophthalic acid in urine and plasma from exposed workers. *International Archives of Occupational and Environmental Health.* 1997; **70**: 128–32.
383. Pfaffli P. Phthalic anhydride as an impurity in industrial atmospheres: Assay in air samples by gas chromatography with electron-capture detection. *Analyst.* 1986; **111**: 813–17.
384. Yokota K, Johyama Y, Kunitani Y *et al.* Methyltetrahydrophthalic acid in urine as an indicator of occupational exposure to methyltetrahydrophthalic anhydride. *International Archives of Occupational and Environmental Health.* 2005; **78**: 413–17.
385. Bello D, Woskie SR, Streicher RP *et al.* Polyisocyanates in occupational environments: A critical review of exposure limits and metrics. *American Journal of Industrial Medicine.* 2004; **46**: 480–91.
386. Andersson N, Ajwani MK, Mahashabde S *et al.* Delayed eye and other consequences from exposure to methyl isocyanate: 93% follow up of exposed and unexposed cohorts in Bhopal. *British Journal of Industrial Medicine.* 1990; **47**: 553–8.
387. Broughton E. The Bhopal disaster and its aftermath: A review. *Environmental Health.* 2005; **4**: 6.
388. Cullinan P, Acquilla SD, Dhara VR. Long term morbidity in survivors of the 1984 Bhopal gas leak. *National Medical Journal of India.* 1996; **9**: 5–10.
389. Dhara VR, Dhara R, Acquilla SD, Cullinan P. Personal exposure and long-term health effects in survivors of the Union Carbide disaster at Bhopal. *Environmental Health Perspectives.* 2002; **110**: 487–500.

390. Petsonk EL, Wang ML, Lewis DM et al. Asthma-like symptoms in wood product plant workers exposed to methylene diphenyl diisocyanate. *Chest.* 2000; **118**: 1183-93.
391. Moller DR, Brooks SM, McKay RT et al. Chronic asthma due to toluene diisocyanate. *Chest.* 1986; **90**: 494-9.
392. Banks DE, Rando RJ, Barkman HW Jr. Persistence of toluene diisocyanate-induced asthma despite negligible workplace exposures. *Chest.* 1990; **97**: 121-5.
393. Pisati G, Baruffini A, Bernabeo F et al. Rechallenging subjects with occupational asthma due to toluene diisocyanate (TDI), after long-term removal from exposure. *International Archives of Occupational and Environmental Health.* 2007; **80**: 298-305.
394. Piirila PL, Nordman H, Keskinen HM et al. Long-term follow-up of hexamethylene diisocyanate-, diphenylmethane diisocyanate-, and toluene diisocyanate-induced asthma. *American Journal of Respiratory and Critical Care Medicine.* 2000; **162**: 516-22.
395. Dalene M, Skarping G, Lind P. Workers exposed to thermal degradation products of TDI- and MDI-based polyurethane: biomonitoring of 2,4-TDA, 2,6-TDA, and 4,4'-MDA in hydrolyzed urine and plasma. *American Industrial Hygiene Association Journal.* 1997; **58**: 587-91.
396. Rosenberg C, Nikkila K, Henriks-Eckerman ML et al. Biological monitoring of aromatic diisocyanates in workers exposed to thermal degradation products of polyurethanes. *Journal of Environmental Monitoring.* 2002; **4**: 711-16.
397. Bernstein DI, Jolly A. Current diagnostic methods for diisocyanate induced occupational asthma. *American Journal of Industrial Medicine.* 1999; **36**: 459-68.
398. Persson P, Dalene M, Skarping G et al. Biological monitoring of occupational exposure to toluene diisocyanate: Measurement of toluenediamine in hyrolysed urine and plasma by gas chromatography-mass spectrometry. *British Journal of Industrial Medicine.* 1993; **40**: 1111-18.
399. European Union. Trichloroethylene. European Risk Assessment Report, vol. 31. Luxembourg: European Commission, 2004: 336. Available from: http://ecb.jrc.ec.europa.eu/documents/existing-chemicals/risk_assessment/report/trichloroethylenereport018.pdf.
400. European Union. Tetrachloroethylene. Part 1. Environment. European Risk Assessment Report, vol. 57. Luxembourg: European Commission, 2005: 154. Available from: http://ecb.jrc.ec.europa.eu/documents/existing-chemicals/risk_assessment/report/tetraenvreport021.pdf.
401. International Programme on Chemical Safety. Tetrachloroethene. Concise International Chemical Assessment Document, vol. 68. Geneva: IPCS, 2006. Available from: www.inchem.org/documents/cicads/cicads/cicad68.htm.
402. Ferguson RK, Vernon RJ. Trichloroethylene in combination with CNS drugs. Effects on visual-motor tests. *Archives of Environmental Health.* 1970; **20**: 462-7.
403. Altmann L, Bottger A, Wiegand H. Neurophysiological and psychophysical measurements reveal effects of acute low-level organic solvent exposure in humans. *International Archives of Occupational and Environmental Health.* 1990; **62**: 493-9.
404. Rasmussen K, Arlien-Soborg P, Sabroe S. Clinical neurological findings among metal degreasers exposed to chlorinated solvents. *Acta Neurologica Scandinavica.* 1993; **87**: 200-4.
405. Echeverria D, White RF, Sampaio C. A behavioral evaluation of PCE exposure in patients and dry cleaners: A possible relationship between clinical and preclinical effects. *Journal of Occupational and Environmental Medicine.* 1995; **37**: 667-80.
406. Cavalleri A, Gobba F, Paltrinieri M et al. Perchloroethylene exposure can induce colour vision loss. *Neuroscience Letters.* 1994; **179**: 162-6.
407. Crofton KM, Lassiter TL, Rebert CS. Solvent-induced ototoxicity in rats: An atypical selective mid-frequency hearing deficit. *Hearing Research.* 1994; **80**: 25-30.
408. Muijser H, Lammers JH, Kullig BM. Effects of exposure to trichloroethylene and noise on hearing in rats. *Noise and Health.* 2000; **2**: 57-66.
409. Kilburn KH. Neurobehavioral and respiratory findings in jet engine repair workers: A comparison of exposed and unexposed volunteers. *Environmental Research.* 1999; **80**: 244-52.
410. Scott CS, Chiu WA. Trichloroethylene cancer epidemiology: A consideration of select issues. *Environmental Health Perspectives.* 2006; **114**: 1471-8.
411. Raaschou-Nielsen O, Hansen J, McLaughlin JK et al. Cancer risk among workers at Danish companies using trichloroethylene: A cohort study. *American Journal of Epidemiology.* 2003; **158**: 1182-92.
412. Zhao Y, Krishnadasan A, Kennedy N et al. Estimated effects of solvents and mineral oils on cancer incidence and mortality in a cohort of aerospace workers. *American Journal of Industrial Medicine.* 2005; **48**: 249-58.
413. Caldwell JC, Keshava N. Key issues in the modes of action and effects of trichloroethylene metabolites for liver and kidney tumorigenesis. *Environmental Health Perspectives.* 2006; **114**: 1457-63.
414. International Agency for Research on Cancer. Dry cleaning, some chlorinated solvents and other industrial chemicals. IARC Monographs on the Evaluation of Carcinogenic Risks to Humans, vol. 63. Lyon: IARC, 1995.
415. Mundt KA, Birk T, Burch MT. Critical review of the epidemiological literature on occupational exposure to perchloroethylene and cancer. *International Archives of Occupational and Environmental Health.* 2003; **76**: 473-91.
416. Lash LH, Parker JC. Hepatic and renal toxicities associated with perchloroethylene. *Pharmacological Reviews.* 2001; **53**: 177-208.
417. Gobba F, Righi E, Fantuzzi G et al. Perchloroethylene in alveolar air, blood, and urine as biologic indices of low-level exposure. *Journal of Occupational and Environmental Medicine.* 2003; **45**: 1152-7.

418. International Programme on Chemical Safety. Methylene chloride. Environmental Health Criteria, vol. 164. Geneva: International Programme on Chemical Safety, 1996. Available from: www.inchem.org/documents/ehc/ehc/ehc164.htm.
419. Leikin JB, Kaufman D, Lipscomb JW et al. Methylene chloride: report of five exposures and two deaths. American Journal of Emergency Medicine. 1990; **8**: 534-7.
420. Manno M, Rugge M, Cocheo V. Double fatal inhalation of dichloromethane. Human and Experimental Toxicology. 1992; **11**: 540-5.
421. Zarrabeitia MT, Ortega C, Altuzarra E et al. Accidental dichloromethane fatality: A case report. Journal of Forensic Science. 2001; **46**: 726-7.
422. Gerritsen WB, Buschmann CH. Phosgene poisoning caused by the use of chemical paint removers containing methylene chloride in ill-ventilated rooms heated by kerosene stoves. British Journal of Industrial Medicine. 1960; **17**: 187-9.
423. Snyder RW, Mishel HS, Christensen GC 3rd. Pulmonary toxicity following exposure to methylene chloride and its combustion product, phosgene. Chest. 1992; **101**: 860-1.
424. International Agency for Research on Cancer. Dichloromethane. In: Re-Evaluation of Some Organic Chemicals, Hydrazine and Hydrogen Peroxide. IARC Evaluations of Carcinogenic Risks to Humans. Lyon: IARC, 1999. Available from: http://monographs.iarc.fr/eng/monographs/vol71/volume71.pdf.
425. International Programme on Chemical Safety. Vinyl chloride. Environmental Health Criteria, vol. 215. Geneva: IPCS, 1999. Available from: www.inchem.org/documents/ehc/ehc/ehc215.htm.
426. Lelbach WK, Marsteller HJ. Vinyl chloride-associated disease. Ergebnisse der inneren Medizin und Kinderheilkunde. 1981; **47**: 1-110.
427. Tamburro CH, Makk L, Popper H. Early hepatic histologic alterations among chemical (vinyl monomer) workers. Hepatology. 1984; **4**: 413-18.
428. Boffetta P, Matisane L, Mundt KA, Dell LD. Meta-analysis of studies of occupational exposure to vinyl chloride in relation to cancer mortality. Scandinavian Journal of Work, Environment and Health. 2003; **29**: 220-9.
429. Gennaro V, Ceppi M, Crosignani P, Montanaro F. Reanalysis of updated mortality among vinyl and polyvinyl chloride workers: Confirmation of historical evidence and new findings. BMC Public Health. 2008; **8**: 21.
430. Bolt HM. Vinyl chloride - a classical industrial toxicant of new interest. Critical Reviews in Toxicology. 2005; **35**: 307-23.
431. Dogliotti E. Molecular mechanisms of carcinogenesis by vinyl chloride. Annali dell'Istituto Superiore di Sanità. 2006; **42**: 163-9.
432. International Programme on Chemical Safety. Chloroform. Concise International Chemical Assessment Document, vol. 58. Geneva: IPCS, 2004. Available from: www.inchem.org/documents/cicads/cicads/cicad58.htm.
433. International Programme on Chemical Safety. Carbon tetrachloride. Environmental Health Criteria, vol. 208. Geneva: IPCS, 1999. Available from: www.inchem.org/documents/ehc/ehc/ehc208.htm.
434. Bomski H, Sobolewska A, Strakowski A. [Toxic damage of the liver by chloroform in chemical industry workers]. Internationales Archiv für Arbeitsmedizin. 1967; **24**: 127-34.
435. Phoon WH, Goh KT, Lee LT et al. Toxic jaundice from occupational exposure to chloroform. Medical Journal of Malaysia. 1983; **38**: 31-4.
436. European Union. 1,4-dichlorobenzene. European Union Risk Assessment Report, vol. 48. Luxembourg: European Commission, 2004: 160. Available from: http://ecb.jrc.ec.europa.eu/documents/existing-chemicals/risk_assessment/report/14dichlorobenzenereport001.pdf.
437. International Programme on Chemical Safety. Hexachlorobenzene. Environmental Health Criteria, vol. 195. Geneva: IPCS, 1997. Available from: www.inchem.org/documents/ehc/ehc/ehc195.htm.
438. International Agency for Research on Cancer. Hexachlorobenzene. In: Some Thyrotropic Agents. IARC Monographs on Evaluation of Carcinogenic Risks to Humans, vol. 79. Lyon: IARC, 2001: 493-568. Available from: http://monographs.iarc.fr/ENG/Monographs/vol79/mono79-18.pdf.
439. Van den Berg M, Birnbaum LS, Denison M et al. The 2005 World Health Organization reevaluation of human and mammalian toxic equivalency factors for dioxins and dioxin-like compounds. Toxicological Sciences. 2006; **93**: 223-41.
440. International Agency for Research on Cancer. Polychlorinated dibenzo-para-dioxins and polychlorinated dibenzofurans. IARC Monographs on the Evaluation of Carcinogenic Risks to Humans, vol. 69. Lyon: IARC, 1997: 666. Available from: http://monographs.iarc.fr/ENG/Monographs/vol69/index.php.
441. International Programme on Chemical Safety. Polychlorinated biphenyls. Human health aspects. Concise International Chemical Assessment Document. Geneva: IPCS, 2003: 58. Available from: www.who.int/ipcs/publications/cicad/en/cicad45.pdf.
442. Ngo AD, Taylor R, Roberts CL, Nguyen TV. Association between Agent Orange and birth defects: Systematic review and meta-analysis. International Journal of Epidemiology. 2006; **35**: 1220-30.
443. Schecter A, Constable JD. Commentary: Agent Orange and birth defects in Vietnam. International Journal of Epidemiology. 2006; **35**: 1230-2.
444. Dhooge W, van Larebeke N, Koppen G et al. Serum dioxin-like activity is associated with reproductive parameters in young men from the general Flemish population. Environmental Health Perspectives. 2006; **114**: 1670-6.
445. Mocarelli P, Gerthoux PM, Patterson DG Jr et al. Dioxin exposure, from infancy through puberty, produces endocrine disruption and affects human semen quality. Environmental Health Perspectives. 2008; **116**: 70-7.

446. International Programme on Chemical Safety. Polychlorinated biphenyls and terphenyls. Environmental Health Criteria, vol. 140. Geneva: IPCS, 1993: 682. Available from: www.inchem.org/documents/ehc/ehc/ehc140.htm.
447. Mukerjee D. Halogenated biphenyls. In: Bingham E, Chorssen B, Powell C (eds). *Patty's Toxicology*, 5th edn. New York: John Wiley, 2001: 323–447.
448. United Nations Environment Programme. HCFCs controlled under the Montreal Protocol. Geneva: UNEP, 2008. Available from: www.uneptie.org/ozonaction/topics/hcfclist.htm#footnote1.
449. United Nations. Montreal protocol on substances that deplete the ozone layer. Montreal, September 16, 1987. Decision XIX/6 – Adoption of adjustments. New York: United Nations, 2007. http://untreaty.un.org/English/CNs/2007/1001_1100/1096E.pdf.
450. International Programme on Chemical Safety. Partially halogenated chlorofluorocarbons (methane derivatives). Environmental Health Criteria, vol. 126. Geneva: IPCS, 1991: 97. Available from: www.inchem.org/documents/ehc/ehc/ehc126.htm.
451. Antti-Poika M, Heikkila J, Saarinen L. Cardiac arrhythmias during occupational exposure to fluorinated hydrocarbons. *British Journal of Industrial Medicine*. 1990; **47**: 138–40.
452. International Agency for Research on Cancer. Chlorodifluoromethane. In: Some Halogenated Hydrocarbons and Pesticide Exposures. IARC Monographs on the Evaluation of Carcinogenic Risks to Humans, vol. 41. Lyon: IARC, 1986: 237–52. Available from: http://monographs.iarc.fr/ENG/Monographs/vol41/volume41.pdf.
453. International Programme on Chemical Safety. 2,2-Dichloro-1,1,1-trifluoroethane (HCFC-123). Concise International Chemical Assessment Document. Geneva: IPCS, 2000: 31. Available from: www.inchem.org/documents/cicads/cicads/cicad23.htm.
454. Hoet P, Graf ML, Bourdi M et al. Epidemic of liver disease caused by hydrochlorofluorocarbons used as ozone-sparing substitutes of chlorofluorocarbons. *Lancet*. 1997; **350**: 556–9.
455. Takebayashi T, Kabe I, Endo Y et al. Exposure to 2,2-dichloro-1,1,1-trifluoroethane (HCFC-123): A causal inference. *Journal of Occupational Health*. 1998; **40**: 334–8.
456. NICNAS. 2,2-Dichloro-1,1,1-trifluoroethane (HCFC-123). Priority Existing Chemical No. 4. Secondary Notification Assessment. Full Public Report. Canberra: Commonwealth of Australia, 1999: 127. Available from: www.nicnas.gov.au/Publications/CAR/PEC/PEC4s/PEC_4s_Full_Report_PDF.pdf.
457. Boucher R, Hanna C, Rusch GM et al. Hepatotoxicity associated with overexposure to 1,1-dichloro-2,2,2-trifluoroethane (HCFC-123). *AIHA J*. 2003; **64**: 68–79.
458. International Programme on Chemical Safety. Partially halogenated chlorofluorocarbons (ethane derivatives). Environmental Health Criteria, vol. 139. Geneva: IPCS, 1992: 130. Available from: www.who.http://www.inchem.org/pages/ehc.html.
459. Malley LA, Carakostas M, Elliott GS et al. Subchronic toxicity and teratogenicity of 2-chloro-1,1,1,2-tetrafluoroethane (HCFC-124). *Fundamental and Applied Toxicology*. 1996; **32**: 11–22.
460. Malley LA, Frame SR, Elliott GS et al. Chronic toxicity, oncogenicity, and mutagenicity studies with chlorotetrafluoroethane (HCFC-124). *Drug and Chemical Toxicology*. 1998; **21**: 417–47.
461. Harris JW, Jones JP, Martin JL et al. Pentahaloethane-based chlorofluorocarbon substitutes and halothane: Correlation of *in vivo* hepatic protein trifluoroacetylation and urinary trifluoroacetic acid excretion with calculated enthalpies of activation. *Chemical Research in Toxicology*. 1992; **5**: 720–5.
462. Organisation for Economic Co-operation and Development. 1-Chloro-1,2,2,2-tetrafluoroethane. OECD SIDS. Geneva: UNEP Publications, 2005: 95. Available from: www.chem.unep.ch/irptc/sids/OECDSIDS/INDEXCHEMIC.htm.
463. Organisation for Economic Co-operation and Development. 1,1-Dichloro-1-fluoroethane (HCFC). OECD SIDS. Geneva: UNEP Publications, 2003: 62. Available from: www.chem.unep.ch/irptc/sids/OECDSIDS/INDEXCHEMIC.htm.
464. Brock WJ, Trochimowicz HJ, Millischer RJ et al. Acute and subchronic toxicity of 1,1-dichloro-1-fluoroethane (HCFC-141b). *Food and Chemical Toxicology*. 1995; **33**: 483–90.
465. Rusch GM, Millischer RJ, de Rooij C et al. Inhalation teratology and two-generation reproduction studies with 1,1-dichloro-1-fluoroethane (HCFC-141b). *Food and Chemical Toxicology*. 1995; **33**: 285–300.
466. Millischer RJ, de Rooij CG, Rush GM et al. Evaluation of the genotoxicity potential and chronic inhalation toxicity of 1,1-dichloro-1-fluoroethane (HCFC-141b). *Food and Chemical Toxicology*. 1995; **33**: 491–500.
467. Maeng SH, Kim HY, Chung HW et al. Micronuclei induction by 13 week-inhalation of 1,1-dichloro-1-fluoroethane in Sprague–Dawley rats. *Toxicology Letters*. 2004; **146**: 129–37.
468. Loizou GD, Anders MW. Gas-uptake pharmacokinetics and biotransformation of 1,1-dichloro-1-fluoroethane (HCFC-141b). *Drug Metabolism and Disposition*. 1993; **21**: 634–9.
469. Organisation for Economic Co-operation and Development. 1-Chloro-1,1-difluoroethane. OECD SIDS. Geneva: UNEP Publications, 2004: 79. Available from: www.chem.unep.ch/irptc/sids/oecdsids/indexchemic.htm.
470. Reinhardt CF, Azar A, Maxfield ME et al. Cardiac arrhythmias and aerosol 'sniffing'. *Archives of Environmental Health*. 1971; **22**: 265–79.
471. Van Dyke RA. Dechloriation mechanisms of chlorinated olefins. *Environmental Health Perspectives*. 1977; **21**: 121–4.
472. Dodd DE, Brashear WT, Vinegar A. Metabolism and pharmacokinetics of selected halon replacement candidates. *Toxicology Letters*. 1993; **68**: 37–47.
473. International Programme on Chemical Safety. Carbon disulfide. Concise International Chemical Assessment

474. International Programme on Chemical Safety. Carbon disulfide. Environmental Health Criteria, vol. 10. Geneva: International Programme on Chemical Safety, 1979: 100. Available from: www.inchem.org/documents/ehc/ehc/ehc010.htm.
    Document, vol. 46. Geneva: IPCS, 2002: 42. Available from: www.inchem.org/documents/cicads/cicads/cicad46.htm.
475. Godderis L, Braeckman L, Vanhoorne M, Viaene M. Neurobehavioral and clinical effects in workers exposed to CS(2). *International Journal of Hygiene and Environmental Health*. 2006; **209**: 139–50.
476. Cha JH, Kim SS, Han H et al. Brain MRI findings of carbon disulfide poisoning. *Korean Journal of Radiology*. 2002; **3**: 158–62.
477. Huang CC. Carbon disulfide neurotoxicity: Taiwan experience. *Acta Neurologica Taiwanica*. 2004; **13**: 3–9.
478. Nishiwaki Y, Takebayashi T, O'Uchi T et al. Six year observational cohort study of the effect of carbon disulphide on brain MRI in rayon manufacturing workers. *Occupational and Environmental Medicine*. 2004; **61**: 225–32.
479. Cho SK, Kim RH, Yim SH et al. Long-term neuropsychological effects and MRI findings in patients with CS2 poisoning. *Acta Neurologica Scandinavica*. 2002; **106**: 269–75.
480. Partanen T, Hernberg S, Nordman CH, Sumari P. Coronary heart disease among workers exposed to carbon disulphide. *British Journal of Industrial Medicine*. 1970; **27**: 313–25.
481. Nurminen M, Hernberg S. Effects of intervention on the cardiovascular mortality of workers exposed to carbon disulphide: A 15 year follow up. *British Journal of Industrial Medicine*. 1985; **42**: 32–5.
482. Pepllonska B, Sobala W, Szeszenia-Dabrowska N. Mortality pattern in the cohort of workers exposed to carbon disulfide. *International Journal of Occupational Medicine and Environmental Health*. 2001; **14**: 267–74.
483. Kotseva K, Braeckman L, De Bacquer D et al. Cardiovascular effects in viscose rayon workers exposed to carbon disulfide. *International Journal of Occupational and Environmental Health*. 2001; **7**: 7–13.
484. Braeckman L, Kotseva K, Duprez D et al. Vascular changes in workers exposed to carbon disulfide. *Annals of the Academy of Medicine, Singapore*. 2001; **30**: 475–80.
485. Kotseva K, Braeckman L, Duprez D et al. Decreased carotid artery distensibility as a sign of early atherosclerosis in viscose rayon workers. *Occupational Medicine*. 2001; **51**: 223–9.
486. Chang SJ, Chen CJ, Shih TS et al. Risk for hypertension in workers exposed to carbon disulfide in the viscose rayon industry. *American Journal of Industrial Medicine*. 2007; **50**: 22–7.
487. Kotseva K. Occupational exposure to low concentrations of carbon disulfide as a risk factor for hypercholesterolaemia. *International Archives of Occupational and Environmental Health*. 2001; **74**: 38–42.
488. Tan X, Chen G, Peng X et al. Cross-sectional study of cardiovascular effects of carbon disulfide among Chinese workers of a viscose factory. *International Journal of Hygiene and Environmental Health*. 2004; **207**: 217–25.
489. Takebayashi T, Nishiwaki Y, Uemura T et al. A six year follow up study of the subclinical effects of carbon disulphide exposure on the cardiovascular system. *Occupational and Environmental Medicine*. 2004; **61**: 127–34.
490. Chang SJ, Shih TS, Chou TC et al. Hearing loss in workers exposed to carbon disulfide and noise. *Environmental Health Perspectives*. 2003; **111**: 1620–4.
491. Wang C, Tan X, Bi Y et al. Cross-sectional study of the ophthalmological effects of carbon disulfide in Chinese viscose workers. *International Journal of Hygiene and Environmental Health*. 2002; **205**: 367–72.
492. Vanhoorne M, Comhaire F, De Bacquer D. Epidemiological study of the effects of carbon disulfide on male sexuality and reproduction. *Archives of Environmental Health*. 1994; **49**: 273–8.
493. Hemminki K, Niemi ML. Community study of spontaneous abortions: Relation to occupation and air pollution by sulfur dioxide, hydrogen sulfide, and carbon disulfide. *International Archives of Occupational and Environmental Health*. 1982; **51**: 55–63.
494. Agency for Toxic Substances and Disease Registry. Toxicological profile for carbon disulfide. pp. 219. US Department of Health and Human Services, Public Health Service. Atlanta, GA: ATSDR, 1996. Available from: www.atsdr.cdc.gov/toxprofiles/tp82.html.
495. Riihimaki V, Kivisto H, Peltonen K et al. Assessment of exposure to carbon disulfide in viscose production workers from urinary 2-thiothiazolidine-4-carboxylic acid determinations. *American Journal of Industrial Medicine*. 1992; **22**: 85–97.
496. SCOEL. Recommendation from the Scientific Committee on Occupational Exposure Limits for Carbon Disulphide. SCOEL/SUM/82, March 2008: 15. Available from: http://ec.europa.eu/social/keyDocuments.jsp?pager.offset=0&langId=en&mode=advancedSubmit&policyArea=0&subCategory=0&year=0&country=0&type=0&advSearchKey=scoel.

Pesticides and other agrochemicals

IAN BROWN, ANNALISA CHIODINI, CHIARA SOMARUGA AND CLAUDIO COLOSIO

Introduction	395
Classification of pesticides	396
The mechanisms for pesticide toxicity	397
Epidemiology and incidence of pesticide poisoning	403
Clinical effects of pesticide toxicity	403
The management of acute pesticide poisoning	409
The monitoring of exposure	412
The importance of training for pesticide operators	416
Conclusions	416
Appendix. Recommended biological effect monitoring strategy for occupational exposure to organophosphates (OPs)	417
References	417

INTRODUCTION

Pesticides are chemicals used to control noxious or unwanted living species ('pests'). In order to be active against living organisms, pesticides must necessarily have some biological activity and, in order to reach their target, they are deliberately released into the environment. Therefore, since their toxicity may not be specific to the target organism, their use can endanger non-target species, including man. Pest control is essential in modern agriculture and it is estimated that, without such control, up to 50 per cent of the total agricultural production might be lost, particularly in tropical climates. Pesticides are widely used, with the highest use rates in tropical countries, where the growing season lasts the whole year, and where agriculture is a major source of income. On a worldwide scale, pesticide usage has doubled every ten years from 1945 to the 1980s, after which a slow-down occurred, due to changes in plant protection strategies and growing concerns for environmental and human health. The highest plant protection product users per capita in the world are the Central American countries, where large landholders favour monocultures or single crops, for example, bananas. In a similar way, pesticides are used in the United States, France and Brazil by cereal, fruit and other produce growers and in countries with a large population but a small land area for the exploitation of intensive cultivation, for example, Japan.

Pesticides are used:

- In public health, e.g. in mosquito control in public areas, or in the disinfection of hospitals. In tropical countries, an important use is in the prevention of vector-borne diseases, with practices such as 'indoor residual application'; with the periodic treatment of the internal walls and surfaces of tropical and subtropical houses, application on mosquito nets, or the treatment of aircraft. Use in aircraft, especially those flying from tropical countries to areas where vector-borne diseases are not endemic, is to prevent long-range migration of vectors and disease.
- By the public, for example in controlling insects in the domestic environment.
- In several formulations and products to protect materials from biological degradation (e.g. paints, wood and furniture treatment, paper production, leather tanning, photographic industry, and boat production and maintenance). Based on the large-scale use of these compounds, the term 'plant protection product' or 'agrochemical' refers only to one of the possible uses (agriculture), but it does not adequately describe many other functions that these compounds may have globally.

Bio-pesticides are those derived from natural materials, such as animals, plants, bacteria and some minerals. They fall into three major classes:

1. **Microbial pesticides** which consist of a microorganism (e.g. a bacterium, fungus, virus or protozoan) as the active ingredient. The most widely used microbial pesticides are subspecies and strains of *Bacillus thuringiensis*.

2. **Plant pesticides** that plants may produce from genetic material that has been added to the genome of the plant (genetic modification or manipulation).
3. **Biochemical pesticides** which are naturally occurring substances that control pests by non-toxic mechanisms. They include substances such as insect sex pheromones that interfere with mating, as well as various scented plant extracts that attract insect pests into traps.

Integrated pest management (IPM) programmes are a series of pest management evaluations, decisions and controls which rely on comprehensive information on the life cycles of pests. IPM is a tiered approach which starts from defining 'action thresholds', points at which pest populations or environmental conditions indicate that pest control action must be taken. Once pest control is required and preventive methods are no longer enough, IPM programmes provide for effective, less harmful pest control, from highly targeted chemicals or mechanical control to (if less risky controls are not effective) additional pest control methods including specific pesticides.[1]

With regard to health risks in organic farming, products of biological origin may have different properties from 'conventional' agrochemicals, but they cannot be considered 'risk free'. Pesticides such as natural pyrethrum derivatives or some essential oils are not completely safe, and some pesticides with complex molecules may possess sensitizing properties.

The use of different compounds to control pests is reported in ancient Greek and Roman texts, highlighting that since the beginning of agricultural production, the need for plant protection was important. Seed treatment, fumigation and tree banding were the first practices performed, based on easily available products, such as plant or animal derivatives, and minerals.[2] Examples of these uses are seed treatment with ashes, or macerated pounded roots and leaves of wild cucumber for mildew control, use of soaking lupin flowers as herbicides, the practice of smearing pruning knives with bear's blood or fat or using fumes from various vegetables, locusts, animal faeces, bones or horns as insect repellents. Among the substances used from antiquity, alum, antimony, arsenical compounds, chalk, cobalt, copper sulphate, sodium sulphate, iron and iron salts, lime, mercury and sulphur derivatives are listed.[3]

In 1874, the first chemical pesticide was synthesized, known properly as 1,1,1-trichloro-2,2-bis[4-chlorophenyl] ethane or the dichlorodiphenyltrichloroethane (DDT), but this compound did not find any commercial use until 1939, when Muller and co-workers discovered its insecticidal properties.[4] After 1939, its production and use grew and DDT found use either in public health, mainly against the Anopheles mosquito in an effort to eradicate malaria, and since 1946, in agriculture for the protection of cotton, deciduous fruits, cereals and potatoes. The effective insecticidal activity, together with low acute toxicity to humans, brought about a continuous increase in the use of DDT, including private indoor use and treatment of human external parasites, such as pediculosis. During the second half of the 1960s, the first concern for the bioaccumulation potential of DDT arose, and the suspicion of possible effects of this on human health resulted in a significant reduction of DDT production and use in the 1970s.

Today, DDT is still authorized for selected use in public health, such as indoor residual application or mosquito net treatment in tropical countries.[5,6]

Apart from these selected uses in vector-borne disease control, DDT was substituted, from the end of the 1960s, by organophosphorous compounds (OPs), characterized by a highly effective insecticidal activity (cholinesterase inhibition) and by low or absent bioaccumulation and biomagnification characteristics. At the very start of their use, cases of acute poisonings and fatalities attributable to the high toxicity of these compounds were reported. Research thereafter focused on the development of less toxic but equally effective, or more specifically targeted chemicals. This objective was at least partially met with the synthesis of OP compounds that were easily metabolized by carboxylesterase, which is very well represented in mammals, but poorly represented in insects, or the less toxic cholinesterase inhibitors, such as the carbamates. In 1978, fenvalerate, the first representative of pyrethroids, a chemical class derived from natural pyrethrum, was synthesized. Due to their effective insecticidal activity and low toxicity to mammals, pyrethroids are the most commonly used group of insecticides today.

The examples and the history described above indicate that the major challenge has been the production of highly selective molecules toxic to their target species, but at the same time characterized by low toxicity to non-target species, including humans. The presence of biological activity in products deliberately spread into the environment requires specific risk assessment and management. Tests carried out before a new pesticide is released on to the market (pre-marketing phase) and after its release (post-marketing phase) include an assessment of any unacceptable risk to human or non-target species, and the environment. A safe pesticide management programme is achieved through action at international, national and local level. At the highest strategic level, international agencies and organizations such as the FAO (Food and Agriculture Organization of the United Nations), WHO (World Health Organization), EU (European Union) and OECD (Organisation for Economic Co-operation and Development), produce directives and guidelines for adoption at a national and local level within the existing legislation of a country. The process includes consideration of best practices, health surveillance and training of operators.

CLASSIFICATION OF PESTICIDES

The basis for classifying pesticides can be structural (by chemical formula) or functional (by mode of action). Data

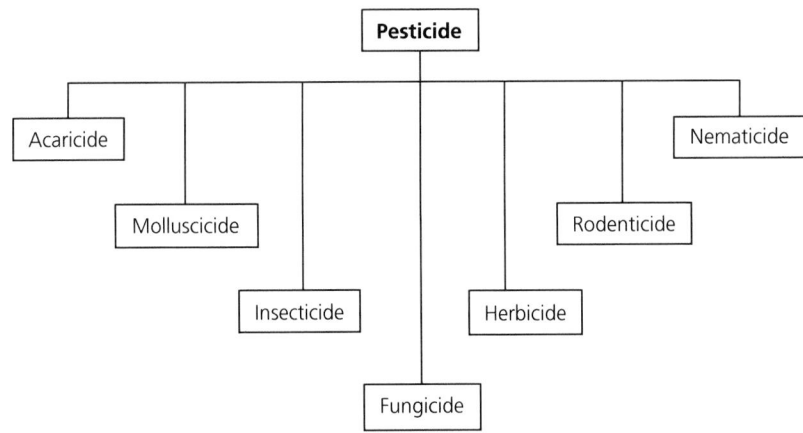

Figure 43.1 Classification by target organism.

on lethal dose 50 per cent (LD_{50}) can also be used to rank pesticides by toxicity, although there are species differences in terms of pathophysiological responses. The World Health Organization recommends the use of a specific pesticide classification system by member states, international agencies and regional bodies;[7] this uses a range of toxicity based on the LD_{50} for the rat model. An LD_{50} of 5 mg/kg, for an orally dosed solid, is classed extremely hazardous, whereas an LD_{50} of more than 500 mg/kg is classed slightly hazardous.

Classification by target organism

The simplest primary classification is illustrated in Figure 43.1.

Classification by mode of action

An alternative classification is by mode of action. A table that identifies the system or organ affected, with subcategories indicating the principal biochemical effect (mode of biochemical action) may be of use in dealing with clinical cases (see Table 43.1). In a case of poisoning, if the pesticide is known, then the major systems or organs affected can be considered and monitored. If the pesticide is unknown, but pesticide poisoning is suspected or on the list of differential diagnosis, then system or organ damage will help identify possible candidate chemical classes which can then be associated with the potential exposure or job, e.g. backpack spraying of an organophosphorus compound.

THE MECHANISMS FOR PESTICIDE TOXICITY

The mechanisms of toxicity for specific classes of pesticides can be discussed according to approximate order of toxicity.

Insecticides

Most insecticides with toxicity relevant to humans affect the nervous system. The major groups are as shown in Table 43.2.

Although mammals and insects share much in common with regards to their respective nervous systems, there are some very important differences which affect the toxicity of insecticides, for example:

- Insects have non-myelinated nerve fibres.
- Cholinergic (acetylcholine) transmission in insects only occurs in the central nervous system (CNS). In mammals, it occurs in the CNS and many peripheral nerves.
- Carboxylesterase activity is significantly less represented in insects than in mammals.
- Neuromuscular junctions in mammals are cholinergic (in insects, they are glutaminergic if excitatory and GABA-ergic if inhibitory).

The mechanism of neurotoxicity of insecticides is demonstrated in Figure 43.2, which indicates the site of action and biochemical mechanism of neurological disturbance.

The anticholinesterase class of insecticides exert their effect by mimicking the naturally occurring and widely distributed neurotransmitter acetylcholine (ACh). ACh is essential for opening ligand-binding sodium channels and requires two ACh molecules per channel. Within the post-synaptic membrane in junctional clefts, the enzyme acetylcholinesterase is present and this breaks down the ACh to non-active acetic acid and choline. The enzyme is therefore temporarily acetylated (Figure 43.3).

The neurotransmitter binding and cleavage into inactive choline and acetic acid is extremely rapid and one molecule of enzyme will hydrolyze 300 000 molecules of acetylcholine every minute. If an organophosphate is absorbed and finds the active site, then its similarity to ACh will allow it to bind to the esteratic site of the enzyme and phosphorylate (rather than acetylate) the enzyme and the esteratic bond is relatively stable to hydrolysis (Figure 43.4). This is therefore almost a permanent bond with one molecule of enzyme able to hydrolyze only 0.008 molecules of organophosphate per minute.

Carbamates have a similar pathophysiological action as organophosphates, but they compete with the acetylcholine for the enzyme surface and if successful, carbamylation

Table 43.1 The system or organ affected, with subcategories indicating the principal biochemical effect.

System/organ affected	Principal biochemical effect	Chemical class	Example of pesticides
Nervous system	Acetylcholinesterase inhibition	Organophosphorus (I)	Chlorpyrifos, pirimiphos-methyl, monocrotophos
		Carbamate (I)	Aldicarb, carbofuran
	GABA (gamma amino butyric acid) receptor antagonist	Phenylpyrazole (I)	Fipronil
		Cyclodiene (I)	Dieldrin
		Avermectin (I)	Abamectin
	Sodium channel opening enhanced	Pyrethroid (I)	Permethrin, deltamethrin
		Organochlorine (I)	DDT
	Nicotinic receptor agonist	Neonicotinoid (I)	Imidacloprid, thiacloprid
Blood	Methaemoglobin formation	Chloroacetamide (H)	Propanil
		Chloroaniline/urea (H)	Chlorotoluron
		Benzoylurea (I)	Diflubenzuron
		Diacylhydrazine (I)	Tebufenozide
	Coagulation inhibition (Anti-vitamin K)	Coumarin (R)	Warfarin
		Coumarin (2nd generation) (R)	Difenacoum
Kidneys	NADPH depletion, increased reactive oxygen	Bipyridylium (H)	Diquat, paraquat
Lung	NADPH depletion, increased reactive oxygen	Bipyridylium (H)	Paraquat
Electron transport	Uncoupling of oxidative phosphorylation	Dinitrophenol (F)	Dinoseb, dinocap
	Photosystem II inhibition	Chloroaniline/urea (H)	Chlorotoluron
	Mitochondrial complex III inhibition	Naphthalenedione	Acequinocyl
	Mitochondrial complex I inhibition	Pyridazinone (I and A)	Pyridaben
		—	Rotenone
Hormonal	Steroid hormone synthesis	Azole (F)	Fenbuconazole, tebuconazole
		Morpholine	Tridemorph
	Thyroid hormone disruption	Alkylenebis-(dithiocarbamates) (F)	Maneb, thiram, propineb
	Iodine uptake inhibition	Triazole (H)	Amitrole
	Androgen receptor binding	Dicarboximide (F)	Vinclozolin, procymidone
Cell division	Disruption of tubulin polymerization	Benzimidazole (F)	Carbendazim, benomyl
Immune system	Lymphocyte depletion	Organometallic (R and F)	Tributyltin
Non-specific toxicity	Macromolecular binding	Halogenated fumigants	Methyl bromide, sulfuryl fluoride dichlormethane
		Inorganic phosphide (fumigant)	Phosphine
Liver/red cells	Protoporphyrinogen oxidase/haem synthesis inhibition	Acyl triazolinone (H)	Sulfentrazone

After and with permission of Ian C Dewhurst, Chemicals Regulation Directorate (HSE), UK.

occurs. This relationship between enzyme and carbamate substrate is one of electrochemical alignment rather than chemical binding and competitive reversal may occur when the normal substrate ACh is in excess.

The action of anticholinesterase compounds is to allow the normal neurotransmitter, acetylcholine, to accumulate at the active site and cause excessive stimulation of the post-synaptic cells. In the normal course of events, ACh is

Table 43.2 Examples of insecticides.

Class	Subclass	Example
Anticholinesterase	Organophosphates (OPs)	Chlorpyrifos
		Diazinon
		Dichlorvos
		Malathion
	Carbamates	Aldicarb
		Carbaryl
Organochlorines (OCs)		DDT
		Aldrin
		Dieldrin
		Endosulfan
		Lidane (γ-HCH)
Pyrethrins and synthetic pyrethroids		Pyrethrum
		Permethrin
		Cypermethrin
		Tetramethrin
Chemicals that disrupt insect growth	Ecdysis agonists	Tebufenozide
	Chitin synthesis inhibitors	Difubenzurion
	Juvenile hormone analogues	Cyromazine
Natural compounds other than pyrethroids		Nicotine
		Totenone
		Abumectin

rapidly destroyed soon after it has been released from the synaptic cleft and this is usually accomplished by the strategic localization of acetylcholinesterase (AChE) in the post-synaptic and pre-synaptic membranes of the neuromuscular junctions. Failure to destroy ACh causes hyperactivity and then depression of activity at the autonomic ganglia, somatic muscles and some CNS neurones.

Organochlorine (OC) insecticides also have specific and well-documented neurotoxicological effects on the nervous system. The primary effects appear to be repetitive discharge of neurones, hyper-responsiveness and irritability, with the nerve membrane remaining in a potentially depolarized state and extremely sensitive. (This will lead to tremors and even convulsions as the physical signs in the affected species.) The mechanisms postulated[8] at the level of the neuronal membrane affect the permeability of potassium ions, reducing potassium transport across the membrane. The organochlorine DDT also alters the porosity of sodium channels and causes them to close more slowly, interfering with repolarization. In addition, DDT inhibits the enzyme ATPase (which is also critical to repolarization) and interferes with calcium transport (Figure 43.5).

Synthetic pyrethroids also have a number of neurotoxicological actions that are somewhat similar to the organochlorines and affect the gating kinetics of sodium channels. The inward flow of sodium ions (producing the action potential in cells where the channels are normally closed at the resting potential) are affected. Pyrethroids affect both activation (opening) and inactivation (closing) of the channel resulting in a hyperexcitable state as a consequence of a prolonged negative after-potential and therefore producing abnormal repetitive discharges (Figure 43.6).

There is also evidence that pyrethroids affect calcium channels and voltage-sensitive calcium-independent chloride channels,[9] and this would also contribute to the excitability. Sodium and calcium channels are common in both insects and mammals and the difference in toxicity between the species to synthetic pyrethroids is directly related to the slightly different stereochemistry between mammalian and insect ion channels (mammalian ion channels are far less sensitive). Mammals also possess specific enzyme systems that can rapidly metabolize and detoxify the synthetic pyrethroids, rendering them harmless.

Herbicides

Herbicides are substances that are designed and selected to kill plants with different degrees of specificity. As a general rule, the greater the specificity, the lower the mammalian toxicity.

The main groups in approximate order of toxicity and specificity are listed in Table 43.3.

SODIUM CHLORATE

Sodium chlorate is a non-selective herbicide and has been used as a desiccant. Ingestion causes acute gastrointestinal symptoms, methaemoglobinaemia and intravascular haemolysis.[10]

BIPYRIDYL HERBICIDES

Bipyridyl herbicides are non-selective and have a toxicological mechanism of action involving cyclic reduction-oxidation reactions producing reactive oxygen species, the depletion of NADPH and the production of lipid peroxidation. Paraquat and diquat, are examples of bipyridyl herbicides and have similar mechanisms for toxicity, although paraquat is more widely used than diquat.

Paraquat is one of the most specific pulmonary toxicants known and it is a highly polar compound, poorly absorbed by the gastrointestinal tract. Because of a unique amine/polyamine transport system in the alveolar cells, pulmonary tissue acquires high concentrations of paraquat which, in turn, undergoes a NADPH-dependent reduction to a free radical that reacts with molecular oxygen to regenerate the paraquat cation and the superoxide anion which is converted into hydrogen peroxide by the enzyme superoxide dismutase. Both O_2 and H_2O free radicals can damage the alveolar cell membrane by attacking polyunsaturated lipids. When ingested, concentrated paraquat can cause either rapid death from multisystem failure and cardiovascular shock or delayed death from progressive pulmonary fibrosis (see

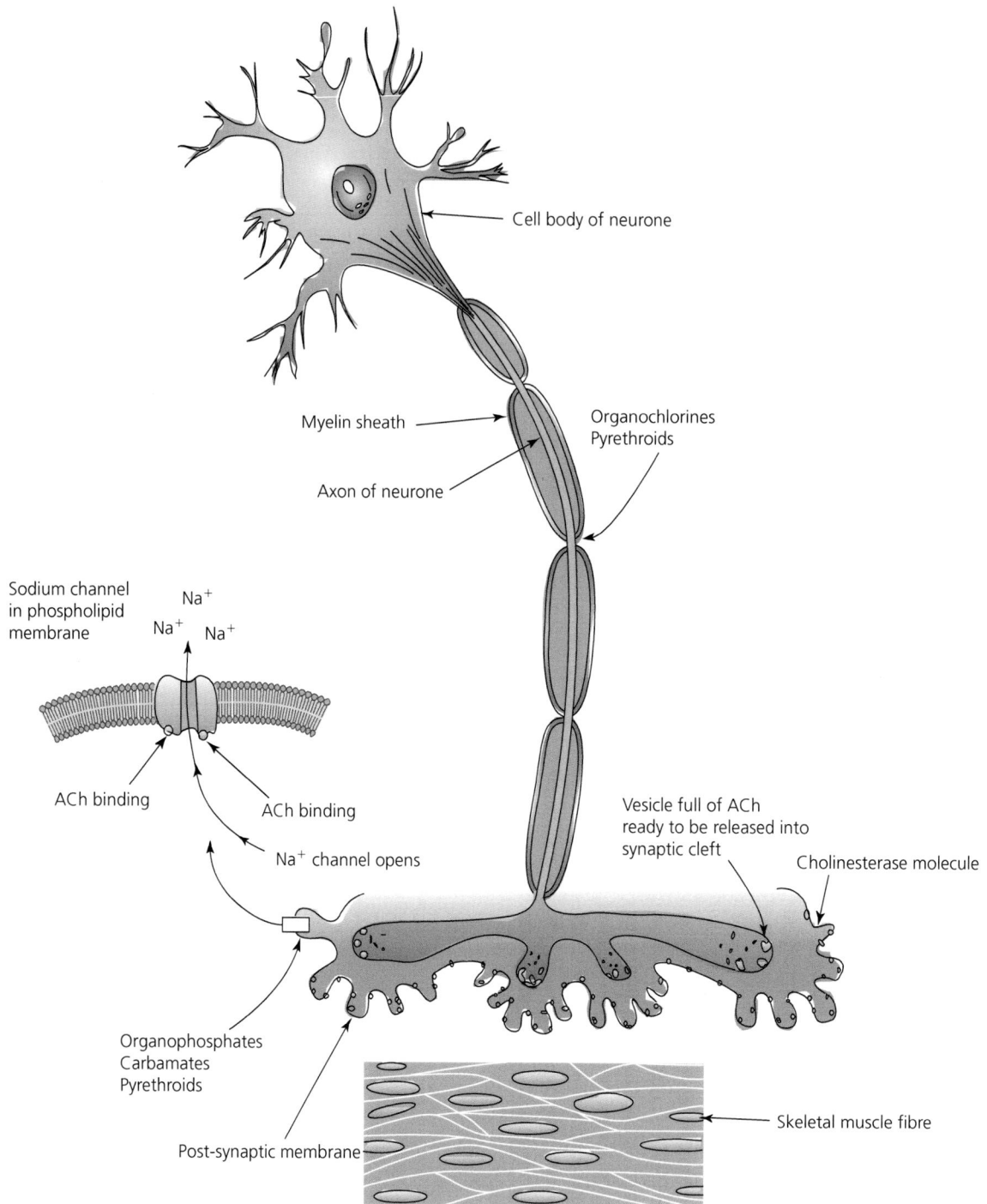

Figure 43.2 Typical motor neurone and site of action of neurotoxic insecticides.

under Acute effects, p. 403, and The management of acute pesticide poisoning, p. 409).

Diquat ingestion does not usually cause pulmonary fibrosis, but can produce early onset acute renal failure, although toxic effects are rarely reported.[11]

CHLOROPHENOXY COMPOUNDS

The organic chlorophenoxy acid herbicides are more selective as they are chemical analogues of auxins, a plant growth hormone. There is no equivalent hormone in animals. Chlorophenoxy acids have both agricultural and domestic uses. A number of compounds are included in this group, most notably 2,4-dichlorophenoxyacetic acid (2,4-D), 4-chloro-2-methylphenoxyacetic acid (MCPA), 2,4,5-trichlorophenoxyacetic acid (2,4,5-T) and mecoprop (MCPP). Chlorophenoxy herbicides are used widely for the control of broadleaved weeds. They exhibit a variety of mechanisms of toxicity including dose-dependent cell membrane damage, disruption of acetyl coenzyme A metabolism and an

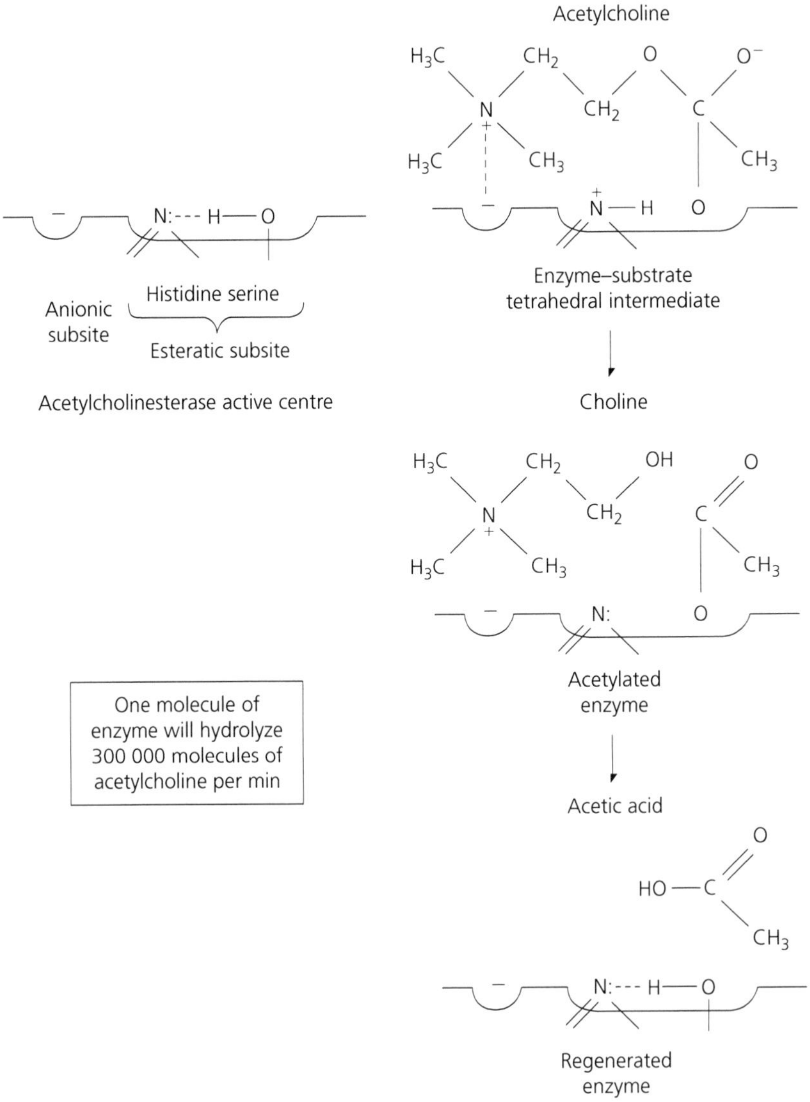

Figure 43.3 Under normal circumstances, acetycholine, a chemical neurotransmitter, is broken down by the enzyme acetylcholinesterase. Accumulation of acetylcholine is thus prevented. Reproduced with permission from Brown I. Agriculture (pesticides). In: Sadhra SS, Rampal KG (eds). *Occupational health: Risk assessment and management.* Oxford: Blackwell Science, 1999: 361–8.

effect related to their degree of chlorination (uncoupling oxidative phosphorylation). Details are given under Acute effects, p. 403.

Epidemiological studies suggest that an association exists between the manufacture and application of phenoxy herbicides, non-Hodgkin's lymphomas and soft tissue sarcomas. However, many of the studies have been confounded by an absence of quantitative data on exposure, multiple exposures to other substances and possible contamination of the phenoxy acids with other chemicals during manufacturing, especially highly carcinogenic and teratogenic dioxins (see under Cancer, p. 409).

OTHER HERBICIDES

Substituted anilines, ureas and thioureas are not of high toxicity, but may cause methaemoglobinaemia and interfere with red blood cell survival. Nitriles, such as ioxynil, act by inhibiting or uncoupling oxidative phosphorylation, but are not a major toxic risk to humans. Triazines and triazoles, and the non-cholinesterase inhibiting herbicide organophosphates, e.g. glyphosate, are highly plant specific and of low toxicity to humans.

Fungicides

These are a mixed group of substances that do not easily fit into a toxicological or chemical classification. They are in general of low to moderate acute toxicity to mammals and can vary from simple organic compounds, such as sulphur and copper sulphate, to complex metal-containing derivatives of organic chemicals, such as thiocarbamic acid. Acute toxicity varies from greater than 10 000 mg/kg (oral LD_{50} in the rat) for substances, such as vinclozolin (a dicarboximide), to around 400 mg/kg for some dithiocarbamates and chlorinated alkenes, and then down to 150 mg/kg for some fungicides with cholinesterase inhibitory effects, such as pyrazophos. This gives a relative toxicity of less than ethyl

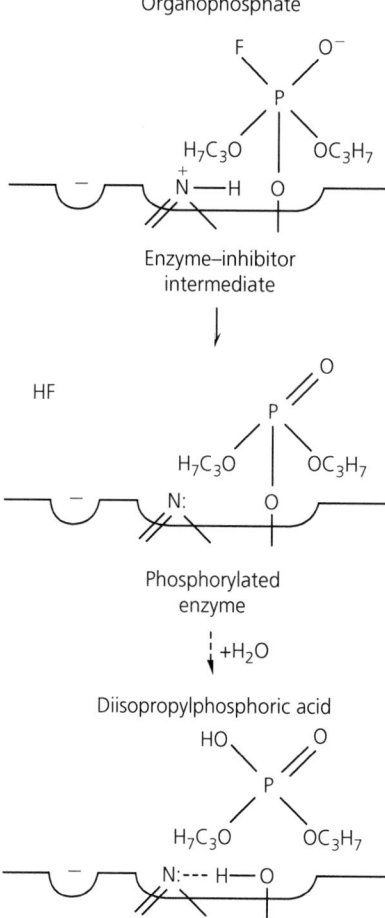

Figure 43.4 Organophosphate insecticides can phosphorylate the active site on the acetylcholinesterase enzyme, preventing it from breaking down acetylcholine. Reproduced with permission from Brown I. Agriculture (pesticides). In: Sadhra SS, Rampal KG (eds). *Occupational health: Risk assessment and management.* Oxford: Blackwell Science, 1999: 361–8.

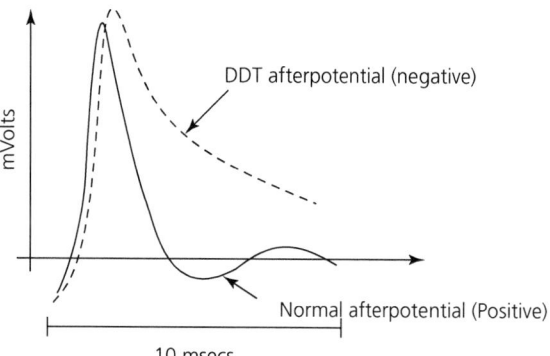

Figure 43.5 A recording of the depolarization and repolarization of a normal (untreated) neurone (—) and a DDT-treated neurone (---). Reproduced with permission from Ecobichon DJ. Toxic effects of pesticides. In: Klaassen CD (ed.). *Casarett and Doull's Toxicology. The basic science of poisons,* 6th edn. New York: McGraw-Hill, 2001: 763–843.

alcohol at best, down to the toxicity of phenobarbitone at worst.

The toxicological mechanisms have some common characteristics and many act upon the cellular or other supporting structures of the fungus. Others are barrier protectors on the plant cuticular surface or systemically toxic to the developing fungus. The low toxicity of fungicides may appear contradictory to their cytotoxic and mutagenic nature and, although not usually acutely poisonous, almost 90 per cent of all agricultural fungicides are carcinogenic in animal models and are considered to account for more than 50 per cent of the total estimated dietary carcinogenic risk. The withdrawal of more actively toxic fungicides, such as the organomercurials and organotins has considerably improved their safety profile.

Rodenticides and molluscicides

Anticoagulant rodenticides are widely and commonly used, and resistance has led to the introduction of the 'superwarfarins' which have a much longer duration of action. Their mechanism of toxicity is to inhibit the synthesis of blood clotting factors VII, IX and X, which are dependent on vitamin K.

Molluscicides kill slugs and snails and the most commonly used is metaldehyde. Its toxicity is due to its metabolism to acetaldehyde, but human poisoning is rare, unless significant quantities are ingested (more than 50 mg/kg).

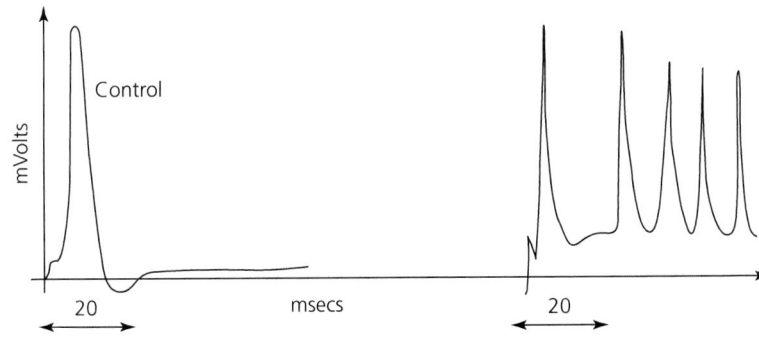

Figure 43.6 The effects of deltamethrin on muscle action potentials compared with the normal control action potentials. Reproduced with permission from Ray DE. Toxicology of pyrethrins and synthetic pyrethroids. In: Marrs TC, Ballantyne B (eds). *Pesticide toxicology and international regulation.* Chichester: Wiley, 2004: 129–58.

Table 43.3 The main groups of herbicides in approximate order of toxicity and specificity.

Class	Subclass	Example
Inorganic		Sodium chlorate
Bipyridyl derivatives		Paraquat
		Diquat
Organic acids	Chlorophenoxy compounds	2,4-D
		2,45-T
	Other organic acids	Haloxyfop
		Dicamba
Substituted anilines		Alachlor
		Propachlor
		Propanil
Ureas and thiomens		Diuron
		Linuron
Nitriles		Ioxynil
		Bromoxynil
Triazines and triazoles		Atrazine
		Amitrole
Organophosphates (non-cholinesterase inhibitor)		Glyphosate

The arrow indicates increasing toxicity.

EPIDEMIOLOGY AND INCIDENCE OF PESTICIDE POISONING

Pesticide poisoning is one of the most common causes of chemical poisoning. Acute poisoning can cause a range of symptoms in adults and children, depending on the type and quantity of pesticide, and can result in death, either rapidly or delayed, depending upon the characteristics of the formulation. Individuals can be exposed to pesticides while working, via food, soil, water or air, or by directly ingesting pesticide products. Pesticides are known to cause millions of acute poisoning cases per year. It has been estimated that 1–3 per cent of agricultural workers in the world suffer in their lifetime from at least one acute pesticide poisoning episode. Among acute intoxications worldwide, no less than one million require hospitalization with deaths amounting to an estimated 300 000 cases annually.[12] Safe storage promotion projects have been identified as a priority in the prevention of serious accidental pesticide poisoning, since poor storage of pesticides and bad management of used containers is an important determinant of risk.

Epidemiological surveillance is an important tool to monitor acute pesticide-related illness and to identify associated risk factors. Some attempts to monitor pesticide-related illness have been undertaken across the globe. In the United States, the National Institute for Occupational Safety and Health (NIOSH), Centre for Disease Control and Prevention (CDC), through the Sentinel Event Notification System for Occupational Risks (SENSOR) programme has provided technical and financial support for state-based surveillance of acute occupational pesticide-related illness and injury since 1987.[13] According to data generated by SENSOR, workers employed in agriculture have been found to have a greater incidence rate of acute occupational pesticide-related illness when compared to non-agricultural workers. Most of the cases (69.7 per cent) were of low severity. Severity was moderate in 29.6 per cent of the cases and high in 0.4 per cent. Insecticides were found to be the causative agent in 49 per cent of all cases.

CLINICAL EFFECTS OF PESTICIDE TOXICITY

Acute effects

Acute effects are described as any effect on the human organism in which symptoms develop rapidly and often subside after the exposure stops, and can be divided into local and systemic. In some cases, acute effects may arise following the storage in the body of large amounts of slowly metabolized compounds. Local acute effects consist mainly of dermal or mucosal injuries, from mild irritation to severe ulceration. Local acute effects are the result of both toxicological properties of the compound and physical/chemical properties of the formulation used and usually consist of damage to the body barriers, such as skin and respiratory tract, the eyes or gastric mucosa. Irritation, corrosion and ulcerative lesions are examples of such effects. Systemic effects consist of organ or system impairment following the absorption of an effective dose.

Insecticides can easily affect non-target organisms since they are often non-selective and the target sites and toxicity mechanisms may be similar in all species (see under The mechanisms for pesticide toxicity, p. 397). The target organ of the majority of chemical insecticides presently used is the nervous tissue. Since a certain analogy can be found in the organization and function of the central and peripheral nervous system between insects and humans, insecticides can elicit (following adequate exposure in terms of dose and duration), similar effects in the two species. Generally, insecticides interfere with the membrane transportation of sodium, potassium, calcium or chloride ions.[11]

Organochlorine insecticides exert their toxicity on the intact reflex arc consisting of a peripheral, afferent (sensory) neurone, inter-neurones and a peripheral, efferent (motor) neurone which in turn innervates a muscle. DDT is known to interfere with potassium, sodium and calcium transport across the neuronal membrane, leading to repetitive discharges in neurones and, consequently, to repetitive tremors, seizures and electrical activity triggered by tactile and auditory stimuli (see Figure 43.5). The clinical picture following organochlorine acute intoxication is characterized by tremors, motor seizures and respiratory failure. Organochlorine pesticides and their metabolites can be measured in blood samples by gas-liquid chromatography within a few days of exposure.

Anticholinesterase insecticides comprise the esters of phosphoric or phosphorothioic acid and those of carbamic acid (carbamates), and share a common mechanism of toxic action: the inhibition of the nervous tissue acetylcholinesterase (AChE), the enzyme responsible for the destruction of the neurotransmitter acetylcholine (see Figures 43.3 and 43.4). This inhibition leads to the accumulation of free ACh at the endings of all cholinergic nerves which results in a prolonged stimulation of electrical activity at:

- muscarinic receptors of the parasympathetic autonomic nervous system, with consequent increased secretions, bronchoconstriction, miosis, gastrointestinal cramps, diarrhoea, micturition and bradycardia;
- nicotinic junctions between nerves and muscles, with tachycardia, hypertension, muscle fasciculation, tremors, muscle weakness and flaccid paralysis;
- the central nervous system, with restlessness, emotional liability, ataxia, lethargy, mental confusion, memory loss, convulsions and coma.

Increased pulmonary secretions and respiratory failure are the usual causes of death from organophosphorus poisoning and recovery depends on regeneration of the enzyme within the critical tissues. The phosphorylation of AChE is irreversible in the case of the esters of phosphoric or phosphorothioic acid (organophosphorus compounds) and temporary for the derivatives of carbamates, leading to a wide ranging clinical picture in terms of seriousness and signs of the illness and the risk to life. The carbamyl–acetylcholinesterase combination dissociates more readily than the phosphoryl–acetylcholinesterase complex produced by organophosphorus compounds. Thus, carbamate poisoning tends to be of shorter duration and less serious. Most clinical manifestations of acute organophosphorus poisoning are resolved within days or weeks, although some symptoms, especially those of neuropsychological nature, can persist for months or longer.[11,14]

A second phase of organophosphorus insecticide poisoning is termed the 'intermediate syndrome', a paralytic condition consisting of neurological signs which appear 24–96 hours after the acute cholinergic crisis. Major effects are muscle weakness primarily affecting muscles innervated by cranial nerves, as well as those of the limbs. This is a life-threatening condition due to the unresponsiveness of the respiratory depression to atropine or oximes.[15] A third phase termed 'delayed neuropathy' (also termed 'organophosphorus pesticide-induced delayed polyneuropathy') is caused by some, but not all OPs, and is characterized by initial flaccidity (second motor neurone syndrome), followed in some cases by spasticity, hypertonicity, hyperreflexia and clonus indicative of a damage to the pyramidal tract. At a pathological level, the delayed neuropathy is accompanied by a Wallerian 'dying-back' degeneration of large diameter axons. Biochemical studies have demonstrated an inhibition of the neuropathic target esterase, a neuronal non-specific carboxylesterase, which is involved in the lipid metabolism of neurones.[16,17] The time scale for the acute and more chronic effects is shown in Figure 43.7, and greater detail is given about the 'chronic syndrome' and 'dippers' flu' under Chronic and long-term effects, p. 406.

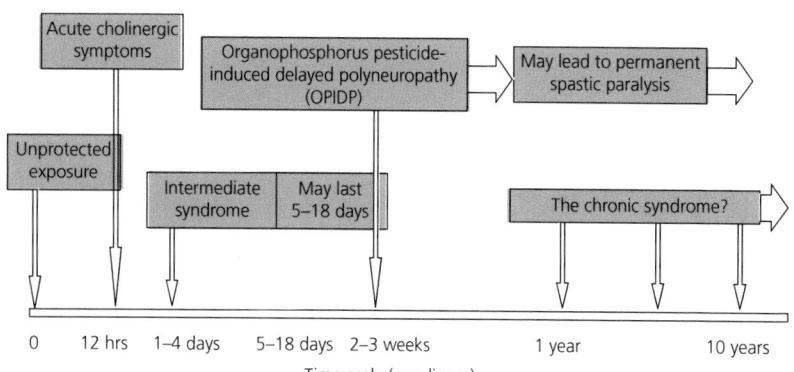

Figure 43.7 The spectrum of human response to organophosphorus chemicals.

Pyrethroids represent a group of widely used pesticides, obtained from chemical synthesis, but similar to the natural pyrethrum, a complex chemical mixture found in some species of chrysanthemum flowers, while the compounds obtained through extraction from a vegetable matrix are called pyrethrins. Pyrethroids and pyrethrins are similar from a toxicological point of view; in particular, they impair ion transport through the membrane of nerve axons, causing a rapid uncoordinated hyperactivity and then muscular paralysis in the insect, through an effect on sodium channels (see Figure 43.6). Systemic non-target species toxicity is limited because of low dermal and gastrointestinal absorption and their rapid degradation by mammalian liver enzymes and urinary excretion. Therefore, they usually do not cause any severe acute effect in humans, even after relatively high exposure. The main symptom observed is skin paraesthesia involving the face, hands or arms (without inflammatory signs), caused by the contact of the active ingredient with dermal nerve endings and consequent hyperstimulation. A further sign of exposure is the so-called 'upper respiratory tract sensory irritation', similar in mechanism of action to paraesthesia, but involving the mucosa.[18,19]

HERBICIDES

Chlorophenoxy herbicides are largely excreted unchanged in urine. They have long plasma half-lives of up to 220 hours in humans. The acute toxicity of the phenoxy acids is moderate to low and large doses are required to produce major toxic effects, which include alterations in consciousness, muscle fasciculation, vomiting and convulsions, all of which may be associated with a metabolic acidosis.

After acute exposure to lethal doses of paraquat, mortality is delayed by at least two days, although may take much longer. Damage is initially to the alveolar epithelial cells and progresses to the loss of large areas of alveolar epithelium followed by oedema, inflammatory infiltration and fibrosis which rapidly leads to death due to anoxia.

Paraquat is by far the most toxic bipyridyl and is a non-specific herbicide that has caused worldwide accidental and suicidal deaths since its introduction as a pesticide in 1962. Once absorbed, paraquat accumulates in the lung and kidney and it is these two organs that are the most susceptible to injury. The major toxicological concern is the acute localized effects, particularly in the lung and more specifically the affect on type 1 and type 2 alveolar epithelial cells and Clara cells. This specific toxicity is due to at least three biochemical mechanisms involving redox recycling, the formation of free radicals and eventually cell death. Poisoning can take place by ingestion, inhalation or dermal exposure. Following ingestion, an early clinical feature is vomiting, accompanied by abdominal pain, diarrhoea and, occasionally, gastrointestinal haemorrhage. Gastrointestinal fluid loss can lead to severe hypotension with cardiogenic shock and multiorgan failure. Hypotension can also result from direct myocardial toxicity, demonstrated by ECG changes such as T-wave flattening or inversion and QT interval prolongation. Neurotoxic features include coma, hypertonia, hyper-reflexia, ataxia, nystagmus, miosis, hallucinations, convulsions, fasciculation and paralysis. Respiratory failure can develop because of hypoventilation, usually in association with central nervous system depression, or because of myopathic symptoms including respiratory muscle weakness. Clinical signs include loss of tendon reflexes and myotonia, together with increased creatine kinase activity. Other clinical features are metabolic acidosis, rhabdomyolysis, renal failure, increased aminotransferase activity, pyrexia and hyperventilation. Dermal or inhalation exposure to 2,4-dichlorophenoxyacetic acid occasionally leads to systemic features, but no fatalities have ever been reported. Substantial dermal exposure has been reported to cause mild gastrointestinal irritation after a latent period followed by a progressive mixed sensory-motor peripheral neuropathy.[11,20]

FUNGICIDES

Pentachlorophenol (PCP), a very toxic, but nowadays rarely used fungicide, is readily absorbed by ingestion and inhalation in humans, but is less well absorbed by dermal contact. Its systemic distribution is limited, its metabolism extensive and it is slowly excreted. Severe exposure by any route may result in an acute and occasionally fatal illness caused by the uncoupling of oxidative phosphorylation. Tachycardia, tachypnoea, sweating, altered consciousness, hyperthermia and convulsions are the most notable features. Pulmonary oedema, intravascular haemolysis, pancreatitis, jaundice and acute renal failure have been reported. Survivors often display dermal irritation and exfoliation, irritation of the upper respiratory tract and possible impairment of autonomic function and circulation.[21] Apart from the 'historical example' of PCP poisoning, modern fungicides are, as a general rule, less toxic than insecticides and their acute toxicity to human beings is non-specific.

RODENTICIDES

Rodenticides comprise a diverse range of chemical structures with a variety of mechanisms of action. Although most rodenticides are formulated in baits that are unpalatable to humans, several rodenticide intoxications are registered each year. Among rodenticides, anticoagulants derived from coumadin are listed. Their toxicity is exerted through the antagonism of vitamin K in the synthesis of clotting factors (factors II, VII, IX and X). The emergence of warfarin-resistant strains of rats led to the introduction of a new group of anticoagulant rodenticides variously referred to as 'superwarfarins', which are very long acting. This group includes the second-generation 4-hydroxycoumarins: brodifacoum, bromadiolone, difenacoum, flocoumafen, and the indanedione derivatives chlorphacinone and diphacinone. Over 95 per cent of all rodenticides used in United States consist of superwarfarin, and brodifacoum is the most commonly used substance. Since the introduction of superwarfarins, a number of cases of ingestion resulting in coagulopathy have been reported, usually with minor outcomes, rapidly resolved and with no residual disability. Moderate outcomes (defined as more pronounced signs and symptoms of exposure with some form of treatment required), but no residual disability present or major outcomes (life-threatening event, resultant disability or death) have been reported. This is especially so with a prolonged coagulopathy due to the superwarfarin brodifacoum. The anticoagulant effect appears from eight to 12 hours after the ingestion, according to the half-lives of the various clotting factors. Following consumption over a period of days, bleeding of the gingival membranes and nose occurs, with haematomas at the knee and elbow joints. Gastrointestinal bleeding with spontaneous haemoperitoneum, haematuria and cerebrovascular accidents can also occur. Patients may remain anticoagulated for several days (warfarin) or days, weeks or months (longer-acting anticoagulants), after ingestion of large quantities.[11,22,23]

Chronic and long-term effects

The term 'chronic toxic effects', usually means effects as a consequence of prolonged exposure to toxic substances, at doses lower than those able to cause acute effects, or effects characterized by a prolonged latency, after exposure periods not necessarily prolonged, such as the appearance of tumours ('long-term effects'). A typical property of chronic effects is their slow development over time, and their persistence after the end of the exposure. Long-term pesticide exposure might affect farmers, professional pesticide applicators, and, to a lesser extent, the general population, exposed to pesticide residues via the environment, food and water consumption.

The causal attribution of such effects is complicated because of temporal considerations. For chronic and long-term effects, the identification of subjects who might have been chronically exposed to pesticides at the workplace is relatively easy, but the identification of the compound and source of exposure is less easy, because of the time elapsed since exposure and the exposure of agricultural workers to several different chemical substances over their working lifetime. Therefore, the identification of a single substance, or group of substances, to which the effects might be attributed, is difficult with poor historical exposure data and because most people are exposed to low doses of pesticide mixtures where delayed health effects are difficult to link to specific past exposures. Exposure assessment is therefore a crucial process in studying these associations, but the collection of historical exposure data is a complicated and often uncertain task.

The chronic and long-term effects that have been variably attributed to pesticide exposure are carcinogenesis, neurotoxicity (including behavioural impairment), immunotoxicity, reproductive effects and endocrine disruption. A summary of the existing evidence for these health outcomes is provided in the following paragraphs.

As a general rule, the epidemiological evidence suggests that agricultural workers experience a lower overall mortality rate with respect to the general population with a lower incidence of some specific causes of death, such as respiratory, cardiovascular diseases and tumours.[24–27] These findings are reasonably attributable to a healthier lifestyle and to the lower tobacco consumption of this employment sector.[27] However, pesticide exposure may also be associated with specific diseases. In particular, some pesticides may cause allergic or irritant dermatitis and, in some cases, the same compound may cause both of these problems.[28] The effects might also be attributable to co-formulants, instead of the active ingredients themselves, e.g. the solvents often present in the plant protection product. Irritant effects may also affect the respiratory tract and eye mucous membrane, which can be avoided by the use of personal protective equipment. The liver may be a target of the toxic effects of pesticides, but severe damage is now mainly a historical finding, with liver cirrhosis described in workers exposed to arsenical compounds in France in the 1940s and 1950s, or metabolic disturbances, such as diabetes observed in subjects heavily exposed to organochlorine compounds, such as DDT, hexachlorobenzene and lindane.[29] Inorganic metallic compounds and some solvents used as co-formulants may also affect the kidney. The respiratory tract may suffer non-specific irritant effects due to chronic exposure to some pesticides, and more unusually vineyard workers exposed to a mixture of calcium hydride and copper sulphate (Bordeaux mixture) develop an uncommon pulmonary granulomatosis also known as 'vineyard sprayer's lung'.[30] The reproductive system may be a target of pesticide effects and a historical example is represented by the cases of reduction in spermatocyte count, up to complete azoospermia, observed in workers exposed to the nematocide, dibromochloropropane (DBCP) which led to its ban in the United States.[31] Ethylene dibromide can also affect fertility by reducing semen quality (decreased sperm count, increase of percentage of morphologic abnormalities).[32,33] The effect is usually reversible after 12 to 18 months following the end of the exposure, but in the most severe cases permanent sterility has been observed. More recently, concerns have been focused on less direct effects, such as an alteration in the rate of male to female births, possibly as a consequence of a disturbance to the endocrine system.

THE IMMUNE SYSTEM

There is evidence that pesticides may cause direct immunotoxicity in exposed workers. Pesticides may affect the immune system by a variety of mechanisms of action, causing structural and functional alterations possibly resulting in decreased immunity, as well as an increase in immune response.[34] The immunotoxicological effects of xenobiotics include histopathological changes in immune tissues and organs, cellular pathology, altered maturation of immunocompetent cells, changes in B- and T-cell subpopulations, in addition to functional alterations of immunocompetent cells.[35] Chemical immunotoxicity can be modulated by several factors, including nutritional status, concurrent pathological conditions, biotransformation and activity of resulting metabolites, physical and emotional stress, and oxidative stress.[36]

While some pesticides show effects on the immune system in the experimental model, the evidence of human immunotoxicity in environmental or occupational exposure to pesticides is weaker. This topic, though, is very relevant for occupational health practice, because direct immune function suppression might be associated with an increase of infection rates and cancer, while an enhancement of the immune response might bring about disease states related to autoimmunity and allergy.[34] Current epidemiological evidence in western countries indicates that the prevalence of diseases associated with alterations of the immune response (such as asthma, certain autoimmune diseases and cancers) are increasing. Some researchers have queried whether such an observation could be attributed to improved diagnosis alone,[37] and there is also concern that this trend could be at least partially attributable to new or modified patterns of exposure to chemicals, including pesticides.[38] In some studies, allergic contact dermatitis has been reported, as well as a possible immunomodulatory activity (increase in the immune response) observed in exposed agricultural workers.[35] However, apart from some specific chemicals used in the past, such as some chlorinated compounds,[39] studies conducted on different groups of pesticide-exposed workers show only minor changes in some cell populations or in the blood concentration of mediators, without any sign of overt disease. Even though some doubt remains on the significance of these changes, it is evident that direct pesticide immunotoxicity in low-dose chronic exposure conditions, if present at all, is very low or undetectable.

THE NERVOUS SYSTEM

Apart from the well-described, pesticide-induced acute neurological effects (insecticides, especially OPs and carbamates), a small body of evidence is available suggesting that chronic exposure to some neurotoxic compounds may be responsible for the development of neurological disorders, affecting the central and/or peripheral nervous system (parkinsonism, neurobehavioural changes, suicidal ideation or behaviour). In particular, some studies conducted on (pesticide) exposed workers have shown increased prevalence of neurological symptoms and changes in neurobehavioural performance, reflecting cognitive and psychomotor dysfunction.[40,41] Most of the studies available suffer major limitations due to the different methodologies applied by the researchers, and to the possibility of bias related to significant differences in education between the exposed and the control population. There is good evidence that neurobehavioural impairment can be the consequence of a severe acute poisoning, with brain injury, but this may not be a specific toxic effect as similar impairments have been observed in subjects with evidence of other types of brain injury, including traumatic events and carbon monoxide poisoning.[40] Studies conducted on subjects chronically exposed to OPs, but never acutely poisoned, do not provide evidence of neurological impairment, but data do suggest that neurobehavioural impairment can be observed in workers heavily exposed to OPs such as, for example, sheep dippers.[40] Major limitations for the interpretation of the existing data are demonstrated by the difficulties in the comparison of the single studies, the limited knowledge of exposure levels, and the absence of a study protocol validated and accepted by most of the researchers. In conclusion, the only fully described effect on the peripheral nervous system is the OP-induced 'delayed neuropathy', which is a sequelae of acute poisoning, rather than a long-term or chronic effect (see under Acute effects, p. 403). As for other pesticides, some limited data suggest that chronic exposure to DDT and fumigants might be associated with a change in neurobehavioural functioning and increase in psychiatric symptoms, but this is inconclusive.[41]

Greater detail on the organophosphate-induced 'chronic syndrome' and 'dippers' flu' is given below.

The chronic syndrome and sheep dippers' flu

The clinical effects of acute exposure to OPs has been thoroughly investigated and documented with thousands of animal studies and reports of human poisoning. The pathophysiology of these acute effects is well understood. The possibility of more long-term effects, where there are no measurable cholinergic signs is less well understood and remains controversial. An extensive review of the literature was undertaken in 1997 and 1998 by the European Centre of Ecotoxicology and Toxicity of Chemicals.[42,43] This review investigates published work and other studies on the long-term effects of OP exposure in humans, discriminating between the chronic effects of acute exposure or repeated acute exposure with the dose being large enough to produce clinical signs and symptoms and the effects of chronic low level, apparently asymptomatic exposure. The report concludes the evidence at that time (1998) for chronic effects arising from low level exposure to be insufficient. The report goes on to state that there is no pharmacokinetic evidence for cumulative effects of chronic exposure to OPs at levels which are not acutely toxic and sensitivity even starts to decrease because of the development of tolerance. The authors also state that there is insufficient evidence in the epidemiological literature for the description of a 'chronic syndrome' resulting from chronic, apparently asymptomatic OP exposure. The task force did recommend that further epidemiological studies should be undertaken. A further report was published in November 1998 by the Royal College of Physicians and Royal College of Psychiatrists.[44] This was the result of the findings of a working party on OP sheep dip exposure with a widely drawn membership to hear evidence from sufferers, from those representing them, and from experts in the field. They concluded that the symptoms and distress were quite genuine and in some cases very long-standing. The report goes on to suggest that OP-exposed populations have shown subtle cognitive changes, perhaps suggesting that OPs may underlie some of the symptoms or perhaps that there are co-morbidities, such as severe anxiety or depression, that have been intuitively attributed by the sufferers to OP exposure. The report does though, make the point that the severity of the symptoms and the consequent disturbance to family life and work, make it essential to provide an adequate level of clinical care for those who experience symptoms following OP sheep dip exposure and existing clinical services do not appear to provide satisfactory management of the cases in the UK. The report recommended that the exposed patient with symptoms required particularly sympathetic handling with the symptoms and signs treated seriously and at face value. They also suggested that over-investigation is not recommended, as many of the patients have been found not to have abnormalities on specialized testing. More recently (2007), an extensive questionnaire-based survey on acute symptoms following work with pesticides was undertaken by Solomon et al.[45] They analysed 10 765 responders in three rural areas of England and Wales. They were particularly interested in the occurrence of flu-like symptoms following the use of sheep dip, although the study did not specify the nature of the chemical in the dipping solutions. They concluded that flu-like symptoms did not cluster unusually among the users of sheep dip and that acute symptoms were common following work with pesticides, but in many cases the illness may have arisen through psychological rather than toxic mechanisms. There is still considerable ongoing work on the aetiology and susceptibility of individuals to 'dippers' flu', but the present evidence does not appear to support this reported disorder as a specific syndrome and its relationship to organophosphate chemical exposure remains uncertain.

Evidence describing long-term neuropsychological or neuropsychiatric effects in humans following low-dose chronic exposure appears contradictory and relatively recent expert reviews conclude that the evidence does not support the existence of clinically significant neuropsychological effects, neuropsychiatric abnormalities or peripheral nerve dysfunction.[43,45]

Despite a 2004 summary of their 1998 report and consideration of more recent concerns about OPs (www.opin.info/rcp.php), the joint report of the Royal College of Physicians and Psychiatrists, recommend an open-minded, eclectic and pragmatic approach to the management of OP-related illness. This would include establishing a therapeutic alliance with the patient and agreeing specific treatment and management goals. Cognitive-behavioural therapy has been found to be useful and specific symptoms, such as depression, fatigue, sleep disorders and suicidal thoughts, should be managed vigorously in the usual way. They also state that consideration should be given to setting up specialist centres in appropriate areas to complement existing clinical services.

Perhaps, most importantly, two themes for research have emerged from the working party's original deliberations:

1. epidemiological studies aimed at developing a means of quantifying OP sheep dip exposure and relating this to clinical symptoms;
2. prospective trials to assess the efficacy of treatment.

In the United Kingdom, a number of government expert scientific advisory committees are again reassessing the evidence and will, in due course, make further recommendations.

Other neurological disorders

The 30–35 studies exploring the relationship between Parkinson's disease and pesticide exposures[40] are hardly comparable with different criteria used even for the definition of parkinsonism, and they show major limitations in the assessment of the levels of exposure. The available data suggest that the relationship between pesticide exposure and Parkinson's disease is therefore weak and there is no evidence of the development of a peripheral neuropathy without a previous history of severe, possibly life-threatening, OP poisoning.

THE ENDOCRINE SYSTEM

Few human data studies are available suggesting a possible effect of some pesticides on the endocrine system. Some organochlorinated compounds, such as DDT (and its metabolites), chlordecone, dicofol, methoxychlor, endosulfan and lindane[46] exert oestrogenic activity, while fungicides, such as vinclozolin and iprodione, may act as anti-androgens.[47] Some triazine herbicides, such as atrazine, may also interfere with oestrogens via indirect pathways.[48] Menstrual abnormalities, prolonged time-to-pregnancy and miscarriage have been described in some studies of pesticide-exposed women, but firm conclusions could not be drawn because of potential bias, uncertainty on exposure levels, concurrent exposure to a complex mixture of chemicals and other risk factors for miscarriage, such as heavy workload and high temperatures.[49–51] Due to the vulnerability of mother and fetus during pregnancy, endocrine disruption might potentially alter fetal and neonatal development, with the highest risks during prenatal and early post-natal development. In some studies, pesticide exposure has been associated with defects, such as cleft lip and palate, limb defects, cardiovascular malformations, spina bifida, hydrocephaly, cryptorchidism and hypospadias.[52]

Pentachlorophenol, a rarely used wood preservative, binds to human thyroid binding protein and may directly reduce the thyroxine uptake (T_4) into the brain.[53] Ethylene bisdithiocarbamate fungicides exert, at high doses, an inhibitory effect on thyroid hormone synthesis, and other currently used pesticides, including dicofol and bromoxynil, have, at least in the experimental model, effects on thyroxine binding, as does the restricted dinoseb.[53] Due to their short environmental persistence and low acute toxicity, ethylenebisdithiocarbamate (EBDCs) fungicides are largely used worldwide.[54] As a consequence, these compounds are a potential source of fungicide exposure for many agricultural workers. While the low acute toxicity of EBDCs is well known, data on possible effects due to prolonged, low-dose exposure are lacking. In the case of very high exposure to EBDCs, a goitrogenic effect has been observed, attributable to the main metabolite of these compounds, ethylenethiourea (ETU). ETU exerts its effect by the inhibition of the iodine peroxidase enzyme, with an impairment of the synthesis of thyroid hormones, and a consequent feedback activation of thyroid stimulation hormone (TSH) and a goitrogenic effect.

One of the possible outcomes of endocrine disturbance may be cancer, especially in organs strongly dependent on hormonal control (see under Cancer).

CANCER

In the context that the risk of cancer is lower than predicted in agricultural workers, some studies have shown an increased risk of certain specific malignancies, in particular leukaemia, myeloma, non-Hodgkin's lymphomas (NHL), lip, stomach, skin, brain and prostate tumours.[27] In some cases, the observed excesses might, at least in theory, be attributed to quite specific risk factors, for example, skin and lip tumours and exposure to ultraviolet radiation, or endocrine-mediated tumours and exposure, mainly during fetal life, to endocrine disruptors.[55] The epidemiology of cancer in agricultural workers is complex and a clear picture of the risk in relation to agricultural exposure is still unavailable.[56] Apart from the problem of multiple exposures, a further confounding factor is the concurrent exposure of agricultural workers to different non-pesticide risk factors, e.g. zoonotic viruses, solvents, oils and fuels, dusts, paints and welding fumes.[27]

The mechanisms by which pesticides could contribute to cancer causation vary, and one pesticide may operate by more than one mechanism. These include genotoxic effects (producing direct changes in DNA), promotion, causing fixation and proliferation of abnormal clones, immunotoxic effects, disturbing the body's normal cancer surveillance mechanisms, and epigenetic effects, causing enhancement or inhibition of specific genes involved in cell proliferation or apoptosis.

In respect of data available on specific compounds, some studies have linked phenoxy acid herbicides, in particular 2,4-D, with NHL.[57-62] Although phenoxy herbicides and their contaminants, mainly dioxins, are the most consistently NHL-associated chemicals, some investigators have raised carcinogenic and NHL concerns about other pesticides, including lindane (used also in some head and body lice treatments),[63] carbaryl, chlordane, DDT, diazinon, dichlorvos, malathion, nicotine and toxaphene.[64] Chlorophenols have also been associated with thyroid cancer.[65]

Organochlorine exposure has been linked with a variety of gastrointestinal and pancreatic malignancies.[66,67] The pesticides involved are DDT, chlordane, heptachlor, endrin, aldrin and dieldrin, which are no longer used in developed countries. However, exposure to these compounds may still occur because of their environmental persistence and, in some cases, illegal use. Some studies demonstrate small but significant correlations between prostate cancer and specific jobs involving pesticide exposure.[68]

The fungicide ethylenebisdithiocarbamate, the main metabolite of which is ethylenethiourea, has also been suspected of possible carcinogenic activity (thyroid neoplasm) but it is now known that the tumours observed in the experimental model (rat) are attributable to a specific metabolic mediated susceptibility of these animals and the existence of a carcinogenic risk to humans, under the usual conditions of exposure, has been excluded.[69]

Despite the enormous amount of variable work undertaken, the results of positive studies are often contradicted by negative studies, and significant limits and confounders affect the interpretation of the results. It is therefore reasonable to conclude that, apart from the well-known historical carcinogens, e.g. arsenic, there is not at present a convincing body of evidence to show that repeated exposure to pesticides at the workplace causes cancer in humans.

Pesticide carcinogenicity is usually fully evaluated in the experimental model before the formal registration of a compound, and compounds shown to be carcinogenic in animal models do not enter the market. However, the compounds that have been in use for some considerable time may not have been subject to such thorough testing. The International Agency for Research on Cancer (IARC) has evaluated more than 60 active pesticide substances and only a few of them are still in use today (ethylene dibromide in group 1A (carcinogenic in humans) and amitrole and dichlorvos in class 2B (possibly carcinogenic in humans)). The use of the most toxic and carcinogenic compounds (for example, arsenical derivatives) has been forbidden in many countries for many years. Therefore, the present risk is significantly reduced, but due to the long latency period for most occupational cancers, a comprehensive personal history together with accurate exposure data remain of paramount importance for the diagnosis and reporting of suspected tumours and malignancies caused by exposure to pesticides.

THE MANAGEMENT OF ACUTE PESTICIDE POISONING

The general principles of management

Most pesticide-related diseases have a presentation that is similar to other common medical conditions and display non-specific symptoms and physical signs. Diagnosis of mild poisoning can be difficult and this results in significant worldwide under-reporting. Only the suspicion of a possible poisoning in relation to the patient's specific signs and symptoms and the accurate recording of the personal history and exposure data, can lead to the correct diagnosis. It is very important to obtain further information on the suspected product from the pesticide label or the manufacturer's material safety data sheet.

In the case of suspected pesticide intoxication, some general rules need to be followed. The management of acute poisoning consists largely of appropriate decontamination, supportive measures including the administration of oxygen, respiratory assistance, removal of secretions from the respiratory tract, maintenance of fluid balance and general symptomatic care. Intravenous fluids to rehydrate the patient and ensuring an adequate urine output will be part of supportive care in most cases. Skin decontamination should be performed through showering the patient with soap and water, while avoiding direct contact with contaminated clothing and biological fluids by using personal protective equipment. The airways must be maintained and in the case of respiratory depression cuffed endotracheal intubation should be performed.

Once vital functions have been supported, therapy should address reducing the potential absorbed dose through gastric lavage which may be considered when the patient presents within one hour from contamination through ingestion. Activated charcoal administered orally (or through an orogastric tube if the patient has a depressed level of consciousness) is an effective absorbent for many poisons. Ipecacuana syrup, an emetic agent, is no longer recommended for routine use, being contraindicated in patients with diminished airway protective reflexes and in the case of ingestion of a corrosive substance.

In addition to general decontamination, specific pharmacological agents to control symptoms may be needed. In case of seizures, lorazepam or phenobarbitone are the drugs of choice. Moreover and when available, highly specific antidotal therapy may need to be used, but general supportive measures will remain the keystone of therapy.

It is very important, during first aid activities, to collect and store biological samples from the subject (vomit, urine, blood and faeces) and to continue collection before the diagnosis is made. In some cases, the diagnosis can be confirmed by the detection in the biological sample of the toxic active ingredient or its metabolites.[70]

The treatment of pesticide poisoning

INSECTICIDE POISONING

Organophosphate poisoning

General principles of treatment

Any suspected case of organophosphorus pesticide intoxication must be considered a serious medical emergency and the patient should be hospitalized as soon as possible.

Symptoms usually develop within 12 hours and in severe poisoning symptoms occur within four to six hours. However, this may be delayed in highly fat soluble organophosphates, such as fenthion. Blood samples should be taken in order to measure plasma pseudocholinesterase or preferably red blood cell acetylcholinesterase levels. In any remote rural area, it is strongly recommended that health personnel have available specific kits that are able to provide a quick and reliable estimate of the levels of cholinesterase inhibition based on a few drops of blood collected from a finger of the patient (the so-called 'paper test'). The severity of the clinical picture is directly proportional to the level of enzyme inhibition. Symptoms may arise when 50 per cent of cholinesterase activity is inhibited, with the most life-threatening situation occurring at 90 per cent or more enzyme inhibition. An excellent guide is provided by the Health and Safety Executive Laboratories in the United Kingdom and this can be found in the Appendix.

In addition to support of vital functions, specific therapeutic pharmacological agents should be used. Intravenous, intramuscular or endotracheal atropine sulphate is used to counter the effects of excessive concentrations of acetylcholine at the muscarinic nerve endings in target organs. Atropinization should be maintained through repeated doses according to clinical status and AChE levels. The administration of an oxime, usually pralidoxime chloride (2-PAM chloride), a highly specific antidote, is effective in reactivation of acetylcholinesterase when administered within 48 hours. However, pralidoxime is far less effective if used later when the phosphorylation of the enzyme is strengthened by the loss of one organophosphate alkyl group, a phenomenon known as 'ageing'.

Blood pressure should also be monitored during treatment because of the occasional occurrence of a hypertensive crisis. Favourable prognostic signs are the reversal of muscarinic symptoms and signs and the improvement of respiratory function and blood oxygenation. In organophosphate poisoning, treatment with activated charcoal is of little benefit because of the rapid absorption of the pesticide into the bloodstream. Management of a moderate to severe poisoning case (50–90 per cent cholinesterase inhibition), is best undertaken in an intensive care unit as mortality from severe poisoning is around 10 per cent and prompt skilled management will improve outcomes.[71]

Specific clinical detail

The effects of organophosphates on human physiology are complex, but inhibitions of esterases, particularly acetylcholinesterase is the most clinically important and leads to a collection of symptoms known as the 'acute cholinergic crisis'. This will be a mixture of muscarinic and nicotinic receptor responses, initially stimulation and then blockade. The balance depends upon the particular organophosphate and its absorption and activation characteristics, but muscarinic responses are essentially 'secretory and excretory' and are a mixture of diarrhoea, bronchorrhoea, urinary frequency, emesis, lacrimation and salivation, together with meiosis, bradycardia, bronchoconstriction, hypertension and possibly cardiac arrhythmia. These can be treated symptomatically and may not be life-threatening; although very severe bronchorrhoea can occur with some organophosphates, such as chlorpyrifos. Nicotinic responses are primarily neuromuscular, initially with fasciculation and then muscle weakness that may progress to paralysis and life-threatening respiratory failure. Mydriasis, tachycardia and hypertension may also paradoxically occur depending upon the balance of muscarinic to nicotinic responses.

Central nervous system responses always accompany this constellation of symptoms and signs and can be quite non-specific, for example anxiety, but severe poisoning will cause altered levels of consciousness and convulsions and will contribute to the respiratory distress. Respiratory embarrassment and even failure may reoccur after the acute cholinergic crisis and this is known as the 'intermediate syndrome'. This occurs some 24–96 hours after the primary symptoms and the patient may well be starting to recover. A useful early sign of the intermediate syndrome is weakness of the neck flexors and cranial nerve palsies[72] and this 'secondary' or type 2 paralysis usually lasts from five to 18 days and recovers spontaneously if the patient is supported. The cause is postulated to be later dysfunction of the nicotinic receptors situated at the neuromuscular junction.

The use of antidotes in acute organophosphate poisoning

Antidotes in the treatment of any poisoning are the exception rather than the rule and decontamination and support of vital functions remain the cornerstone of preliminary clinical responsibilities. Organophosphate poisoning is, however, exceptional and there are three broad classes that are used as specific antidotes:

1. **Muscarinic antagonists**. Atropine is the most commonly used agent and the dose is carefully titrated to reverse the muscarinic effects. This will reduce bronchorrhoea and increase the heart rate (which is a good measure of atropinization and should be kept at more than 80 beats per minute). The dose is much larger than that used in other therapeutic indications and in adults may be 1–3 mg initially by an intravenous route (0.02 mg/kg in children). Atropine will have no effect on the neuromuscular junction or on muscle weakness and therefore breathing will still be compromised.
2. **Oximes**. These are administered as an infusion and will facilitate dephosphorylation of the acetylcholinesterase enzyme, thereby restoring the catalytic site. This is only possible before 'ageing' of the enzyme–organophosphate complex and therefore early use is recommended in a confirmed case and the infusion should be continued until recovery. With praladoxime chloride, (2-PAM chloride), a loading dose of 30 mg/kg is given intravenously over 20 minutes followed by an infusion 8 mg/kg per hour.
3. **Benzodiazepines**. These agents will control some of the central nervous system effects, especially agitation and seizures. Most benzodiazepines are suitable and should be administered by an intravenous route. Diazepam is the most commonly given, at a starting dose of 0.05–0.03 mg/kg.

For greater practical detail on managing organophosphate poisoning, the authors strongly recommend the clinical review by Roberts and Aaron[73] published in the *British Medical Journal* in March 2007. This has a particularly useful 'decision tree' which compares the treatment of minor toxicity with major toxicity.

Carbamate poisoning

Carbamates very rarely cause life-threatening events, even with attempted suicide. In occupational poisoning, symptomatic treatment and fluid balance support is usually all that is required to manage the patient. A prompt differential diagnosis from OP poisoning is essential since symptoms are similar, but the use of pralidoxime is not recommended. Early management of the more severe cases relies on the early stabilization of the patient and the titrated administration of atropine to treat muscarinic symptoms. Assisted ventilation may rarely be required.[11]

Organochlorine poisoning

Treatment involves supportive care and avoiding exogenous sympathomimetic agents, since organochlorine pesticides are toxic to the central nervous system and sensitize the myocardium to catecholamines. Apart from decontamination and general supportive measures, diazepam and phenobarbitone are used to control irritability and seizures.[11]

Pyrethrum and pyrethroid poisoning

Apart from the allergic reactions observed as a consequence of exposure to natural pyrethrum compounds contaminated by allergens (such as resins), acute occupational or intentional poisoning from these compounds are only very seldom observed and, never so severe as to become a life-threatening event.[11]

HERBICIDE POISONING

Paraquat and diquat (bipyridyl compounds)

Paraquat is poorly absorbed from the gastrointestinal tract and the skin, and if its absorption can be prevented death may be avoided. Speed of interventional therapeutic action is therefore very important. Treatments have therefore focused on the prevent of absorption, removal of the chemical from the bloodstream by haemodialysis or haemoperfusion, prevention of its accumulation in the lung, the use of free-radical scavengers and the prevention of lung fibrosis.[11] In practice, only the prevention of absorption by emesis or purgation of the gastrointestinal tract has been found to be effective. To avoid accidental ingestion, the manufacturers have added a blue pigment, a stenching compound and an emetic substance to the formulation and this has been effective in reducing morbidity and mortality.

A dose of 20–30 mg/kg of paraquat can cause mild poisoning, while 40–50 mg/kg can cause delayed development of pulmonary fibrosis, which can be lethal. Higher doses usually cause death within a few days due to pulmonary oedema and renal and hepatic failure. Levels can be monitored by measuring the unchanged chemical in the urine.

The similar herbicide diquat is different toxicologically and does not accumulate in the lungs. On chronic exposure, the target organs for toxicity are the gastrointestinal tract, the kidney and in particular the eye. Diquat has been found to cause cataracts in mammals by a free-radical mechanism. Acute clinical symptoms include nausea, vomiting and diarrhoea, ulceration of the mouth and oesophagus, decline in renal function and neurological effects. There have been very few cases of human intoxication with diquat and the treatment remains the prevention of absorption and enhancing elimination, as with paraquat.[74]

Chlorate

Poisoning following ingestion of chlorate salts is characterized by methaemoglobinaemia (MetHb), haemolysis, disseminated intravascular coagulation and renal failure. The clinical features include nausea, vomiting, diarrhoea, cyanosis and dyspnoea. Very few data are available regarding the pathophysiology and specific effective treatment of sodium chlorate poisoning. Chlorate salts, which are powerful oxidizing agents, induce the formation of methaemoglobin from the oxidation of the ferrous ion in haemoglobin to the ferric state. Methylene blue, an effective reducing agent, is unfortunately unable to 'reduce' methaemoglobin from chlorate salts because of the concomitant denaturation of glucose-6-phosphate dehydrogenase caused by the chlorate *per se*. In severe poisonings, haemodialysis is recommended.[10]

Chlorophenoxy herbicides

In the absence of a specific antidote for chlorophenoxy herbicides, urinary alkalinization is the treatment of choice in promoting elimination. Alkalinization increases urinary flow and will dilute the concentration of chlorophenoxy herbicide in the glomerular filtrate which also decreases the rate of passive reabsorption (often termed 'forced diuresis').[75]

Glyphosate-containing herbicides

The mechanisms of toxicity of glyphosate formulations are complicated since it has at least five different salts and commercial formulations contain a number of different surfactants. Human poisoning usually follows exposure to a variable mixture where the toxicity of the surfactant polyoxyethyleneamine (POEA) contributes more to the toxicity than glyphosate alone. Accidental ingestion of glyphosate formulations is generally associated with only mild, transient, gastrointestinal effects, although there is a reasonable correlation between the amount ingested and the likelihood of serious systemic sequelae or death. Advancing age is associated with a less favourable prognosis and corrosion of the gastrointestinal tract has been observed. Renal and hepatic impairment are also frequent findings in significantly large absorbed doses and usually reflect reduced organ perfusion. Respiratory distress, impaired consciousness, pulmonary oedema with infiltration shown on the chest radiograph, shock, arrythmias, renal failure (requiring haemodialysis), metabolic acidosis and hyperkalaemia may all occur in severe cases. Bradycardia and ventricular arrhythmias are often present in the preterminal phase. Management is symptomatic and supportive.[11]

Triazine herbicides

Severe poisonings have rarely been observed and overexposure has resulted mainly from accidental or suicidal ingestion. In these cases, administration of activated charcoal is recommended.

RODENTICIDES

With aluminium phosphide poisoning, no antidote is available and many patients die despite intensive care and supportive measures are all that can be offered.[76] Some studies suggest a beneficial effect of magnesium sulphate, but available data are not sufficiently robust to recommend this treatment in standard treatment protocols.

In anticoagulant rodenticide poisoning, the international normalized ratio (INR) should be measured 36–48 hours post-exposure. If the INR is normal at this time, no further action is required. If active bleeding occurs, prothrombin complex concentrate, recombinant activated factor VII or fresh frozen plasma and phytomenadione i.v. should be given.

MOLLUSCICIDES

Although some cases of acute metaldehyde poisoning have been reported, the occurrence of severe poisonings is very uncommon. Supportive measures are all that is required (correction of acid-base balance, ventilatory support, correction of haemodynamic instability and anticonvulsant therapy, when appropriate).[77]

THE MONITORING OF EXPOSURE

Operator exposure

Risk assessment for exposure to pesticides in occupational settings starts with the definition of the hazard, as for any other chemical. Labelling the pesticide provides useful information about intrinsic toxicity and possible effects due to acute and chronic exposure. The next concern is operator exposure which has to be defined in both qualitative and quantitative terms, so that it can be compared with the acceptable operator exposure level, when available, or with any other appropriate occupational exposure limit (OEL).

Several factors can affect pesticide exposure in agricultural settings. With the same applied dose, wide ranges of pesticide exposure levels can be measured depending on weather conditions, machinery, personal protection equipment and operators' tasks and skills. In addition, since agricultural activities are performed outdoors and with typical seasonal variability, exposure levels show a significant variability over time. It is therefore often difficult to perform representative environmental monitoring. Thus, more than in any other occupational setting, exposure assessment has to be tailored to the worker.

As a general rule, exposure to pesticides in agriculture – especially in open field crops – is almost exclusively dermal. Dermal exposure occurs in part from direct physical contact with the pesticide and in part from cross-contamination of surfaces and work instruments. Respiratory exposure is minimal and does not significantly affect the overall operator's contamination.[78]

Operator exposure can be estimated by the measurement of the total amount of pesticide that can be found on patches applied on the surface of various parts of the body. The US Environmental Protection Agency (EPA) sets out in detail how dermal exposure assessment is to be performed.[79] Personal air sampling and environmental monitoring can also be applied when inhalation can contribute to the overall exposure, such as in greenhouse work and in pesticide production factories. Pesticide exposure can be significantly reduced through the prudent use of personal protection equipment (PPE). Due to the previously described characteristics of agricultural work, dermal protection is in general more important than respiratory protection. Overalls and gloves are essential personal protection devices, taking into account the covered body surface (see Table 43.4) and the relative importance of different body areas in dermal contamination. Also, the wearing of protective boots has been shown to significantly reduce dermal exposure.[80]

There is a continuity of exposure to the human population from manufacturing of the active product to possible

Table 43.4 Percentage of body surface of different body regions.

Body region	Surface area (% of total)
Head	5.6
Neck	1.2
Upper arms	9.70
Forearms	6.70
Hands	6.90
Chest, back, shoulders	22.80
Hips	9.10
Thighs	18.00
Calves	13.50
Feet	6.40
Total	100

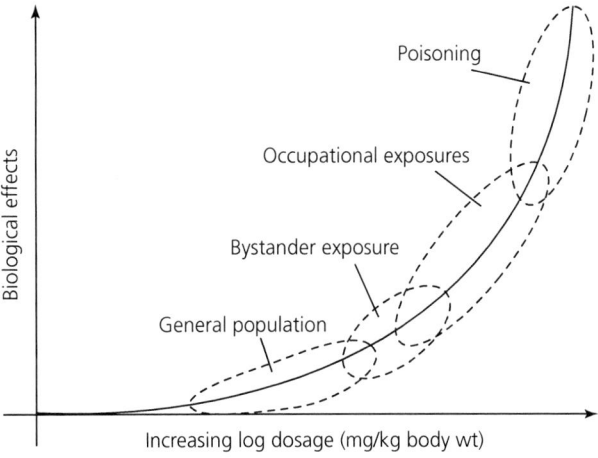

Figure 43.8 Biological effect on a human population increases exponentially if plotted against the log of the dosage in milligrams per kilogram of body weight. Reproduced with permission from Ecobichon DJ. Toxic effects of pesticides. In: Klaassen CD (ed.). *Casarett and Doull's Toxicology. The basic science of poisons*, 6th edn. New York: McGraw-Hill, 2001: 763–810.

residues in the treated crop or environment where spraying or distribution has taken place. The biological effect on a human population increases in an exponential fashion if plotted against the log of the dosage in milligrams per kilogram of body weight and can be illustrated as shown in Figure 43.8.

Acute symptomatic poisoning may occur at dosage levels hundreds if not thousands of times greater than exposure to the general population in food, air and water, but occupational exposure is on the upward slope and can end in an acute poisoning if poor systems of work practice are adopted (e.g. failure of enclosure of process, poor separation of employees and inadequate personal protective equipment).

Pesticide use in agriculture runs through three major phases: mixing and loading, application and re-entry. Pesticide exposure during mixing and loading contributes to less than 10 per cent of the total exposure.[81] A more practical approach to workplace exposure is illustrated in Figure 43.9, which follows the manufactured pesticide from the reaction vessel of the manufacturing plant to the end user and end usage, where some residual contamination may remain. This pathway history of the active ingredient pesticide is divided into distinct stages.

Exposure to the active product on the manufacturing plant must always be a safety consideration as the finished product will need to be tested and then dispatched to storage, usually in a holding tank (see stage (1)). It is rare for chemical processes to be completely contained, and worker exposure can occur during product sampling, maintenance, during decanting to bulk storage and packaging into containers for onward distribution (see stages (2) and (3)). Once the concentrate is bottled and packaged, exposure is minimized until the concentrate bottle or container is

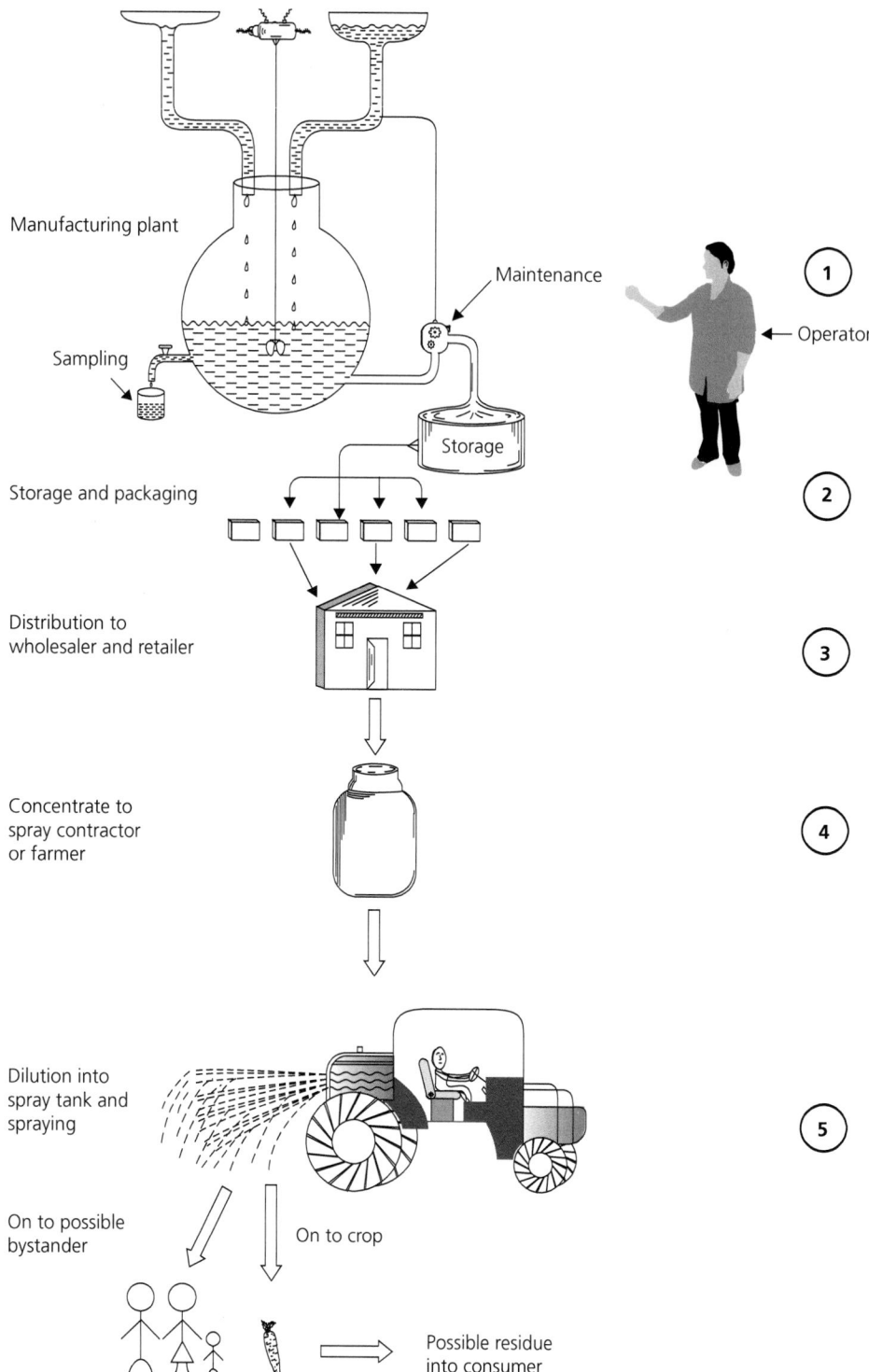

Figure 43.9 From manufacturing to crop treatment.

opened and decanted into a spray tank for dilution and distribution to the target crop or other environment (see stages (4) and (5)). A thorough review of organophosphate contamination risk in agricultural workers by the Committee on Toxicity of Chemicals in Food, Consumer Products and the Environment[82] demonstrated that potential exposure was greatest at the concentrate to dilution stage because of splashing and inadequate personal protective equipment and they suggested better pouring and dilution techniques with improved concentrate containers to facilitate this. Sole reliance on following the manufacturer's instructions and correct PPE may not always give adequate protection. Studies undertaken on manufacturing plants synthesizing the organophosphorus compound chlorpyrifos[83] revealed statistically significant depressions of the enzyme cholinesterase in apparently well-protected employees.

The total operator's exposure during application of a pesticide on to the crop can be higher than during mixing, loading and re-entry, with the most important determinant of a worker's contamination being the application technique.[84] Backpack sprayers have higher exposure potential compared to tractor applicators.[78] During tractor application, the use of an air-conditioned closed tractor can reduce exposure to negligible levels. Re-entry consists of all manual and/or mechanical activities performed on the crop after pesticide application. In re-entry activities, the skin is the major route of operator exposure and shows a linear correlation with the dislodgeable foliar residue (DFR), which is the amount of pesticide deposited on crop surfaces that is also available for operator contamination.[85,86] The occurrence of symptoms has been used to monitor exposure to backpack sprayers in some developing countries. This is far from safe or sensible and effectively adds to the pesticide poisoning burden in these countries.[87]

Biological monitoring, intended as the measurement of the dose that has been absorbed in the subject, is potentially the most useful tool for monitoring pesticide exposure of agricultural workers. The route of exposure for most farm workers is dermal and most pesticides in current use are metabolized rapidly, with the metabolites eliminated in urine. Urinary levels of pesticides or their metabolites can be performed with the aim of monitoring the exposure level indirectly.

Biological monitoring has several limitations, such as the difficult choice of the sampling time due to the variability (over time) of the exposure levels, the lack of biological exposure limits or reference values (for most of the compounds used) and poor knowledge of the toxicokinetics of most pesticides in humans. A single exposure is very time dependent, while repeated exposure measurements are more representative of the average with approximation to a steady state for blood or urinary level metabolites. Blood levels are usually more specific as the parent chemical is measured instead of the metabolite, but these are much more time dependent. Collection of 24-hour urine samples are inconvenient with poor compliance by exposed workers. Spot urine samples are more acceptable, but as the urine volume varies, correction factors must be used, the most common being micrograms of pesticide (or metabolite) per gram of creatinine.

Urinary measurements are specific if the parent compound is excreted in the urine unchanged, for example (2,4-dichlorophenoxy)acetic acid and glyphosate. Most organophosphates can be found unchanged in the blood for only very short periods of time and are then rapidly metabolized, often to an even more active intermediate. They may then be subsequently broken down to a specific leaving group and non-specific alkyl phosphates, which are found in the urine, usually well within 24 hours. These are useful tools for assessing exposure, especially at low doses, but this may not be as useful as measuring the biological effect of these chemicals (which is the inhibition of acetylcholinesterase), but this measurement in itself may well be complicated by inter- and intraindividual variability. However, cholinesterase inhibition remains the major clinically important measurement in a suspected case of significant exposure and possible OP poisoning.

Health surveillance is not merely the diagnosis of occupational disease or acute toxic effects. It should be carried out even when exposure is below permitted levels and to monitor the exposure and the safety of the work activity, including the effectiveness of personal protective equipment.

Health surveillance of pesticide workers include:

- a pre-employment medical examination to detect allergies or medical conditions which can be exacerbated by pesticide exposure, and to establish a baseline for comparison in any further evaluation of the worker;
- periodic medical examinations aimed at detecting any early specific adverse health effects attributable to the pesticide exposure;
- a medical examination after prolonged or repeated sickness absence to detect any significant change in health status which may compromise the ability to continue the assigned job, and to ensure that any illness is not pesticide related.

Biological effect monitoring should be considered especially when determination of a specific marker of biological effect is available, such as cholinesterase activity in plasma or red blood cells in pesticide manufacturers or applicators (see Appendix). Other parameters that have been considered as possibilities for biological effect monitoring include cytogenic analysis of lymphocyte micronuclei and semen quality. Presently, these remain as research procedures which have not been field tested for practicality or applicability. Liver and renal function tests may be indicated depending on the compounds used and the estimated levels of exposure, but abnormal liver function tests often lack specificity.

For determination of inhibition of cholinesterase levels in workers exposed to organophosphates and carbamates, venous blood is taken from the employee at regular intervals after potential exposure. For acute exposures, the samples are best taken immediately after exposure. Sampling towards the end of the day avoids the 'diurnal variation' effect. During collection of venous blood samples, precautions should be taken to avoid contamination of the blood by exposure to cholinesterases in the air or on the skin of the donor or sampler. Cholinesterases are also unstable when kept at room temperature for long periods and samples should therefore be stored on ice or frozen prior to analysis.

Levels of red blood cell acetylcholinesterase, plasma cholinesterase or both can be measured. The greater the inhibition of the cholinesterase levels, the greater the extent of absorption of the pesticide. If activity is reduced to 30 per cent or more of the pre-exposure level, the test should be checked immediately, and removal of the individual from further exposure considered. Cholinesterase levels are very variable in the population, and the variability in a single individual can be by as much as ± 16 per cent with a coefficient of variation between 7.6 and 11.3 per cent.[86–89] It may be possible to determine normal variation of cholinesterase levels in personnel involved in the manufacture of organophosphate pesticides before they are asked to work with the ingredients or final product. However, it is difficult to implement a system to establish the normal variation in cholinesterase levels for any individual pesticide applicator before he/she is assigned to using organophosphate pesticides. This is especially so for pesticide applicators in developing countries where laboratory and technical support is lacking or limited. In such situations, the emphasis should be on adequate training, safe systems of work, and care in the preparation, use and disposal of pesticides.

THE IMPORTANCE OF TRAINING FOR PESTICIDE OPERATORS

Since pesticides are known to be harmful for human and environmental health when misused, their use in the field should only be undertaken by authorized and trained operators. Operator training and education activities are of paramount importance for the prevention of pesticide exposure, and knowledge of the determinants of pesticide contamination can significantly reduce operator exposure. For example, knowledge and observation of 're-entry intervals' (time which must elapse after pesticide application and before the worker can safely enter and handle the crop without personal protective equipment) are critical in reducing workers' pesticide exposure. Good training of agricultural workers is also necessary to avoid risk of contamination to the environment, as well as of the food commodities produced.[89,90]

In many countries, programmes aimed at improving the operator's safety and skills about pesticide use and application are available. Some authoritative written documents addressed to agricultural workers have been produced, such as the booklet entitled 'Preventing health risks from the use of pesticides in agriculture'.[91] These give advice on how health risks can be reduced. Also, the private sector provides communication and instruction tools for the safe use of pesticides. The European Crop Protection Association (ECPA) has launched the 'Safe Use Initiative' aimed at reduction of potential exposure through innovative application techniques, recommendation of the best available specific PPE and improvement of hygiene practices. Acute toxicity information should always be available on product labels which are designed to inform users of the potential hazards associated with the use of a pesticide in a given formulation.

Based on the above considerations, it is evident that training and education represent a fundamental tool in preventing pesticide exposure risk for workers, the general population and the environment. In rural populations, the main providers of health education and training are the local healthcare practitioners, and it is therefore essential that they have adequate training on pesticide risk control.

CONCLUSIONS

The world market and registration of pesticides is very dynamic, and the oldest and most toxic substances are being eliminated or restricted. This will give a new generation of pesticides, probably safer, but toxicologically less well understood. It is essential that the occupational physician keeps properly up to date with this changing situation.

Key points

- Pesticide poisoning is one of the most common causes of chemical poisoning in the world. It has been estimated that 1–3 per cent of all agricultural workers, in their lifetime, suffer at least one acute pesticide poisoning incident. There are also 300 000 pesticide-related deaths every year.
- Pesticides are commonly classified by consideration of their target organism, but may also be described by their mode of action and this usually gives an indication of their structural chemistry and specific toxicity.
- Pesticides and agrochemicals are used throughout the world with the highest use rates in tropical countries. Around ten manufacturing companies produce 90 per cent of the 1000 or so active ingredients. Before an active ingredient can be marketed, it undergoes intensive regulatory testing in respect to its safety, efficacy and environmental impact.
- Insecticides are generally more acutely toxic than herbicides or fungicides and most affect the nervous system of the target species and possibly also humans.
- The more specific and targeted the active chemical is, the less likely it will be toxic to humans.
- Chronic and long-term pesticide affects have been extensively researched and this has been specifically investigated in relation to the immune system, the nervous system, the endocrine system and the development of cancer.
- General supportive measures remain the keystone of treatment in acute pesticide poisoning.
- Acute insecticide poisoning is usually neurological in nature and will often involve an organophosphorus chemical, a carbamate, or more rarely an organochlorine or synthetic pyrethroid.
- Acute herbicide poisoning is rare, except in the case of highly non-specific herbicides, such as paraquat and sodium chlorate.
- Exposure to the acute active chemical of the pesticide is potentially greatest at the

> manufacturing plant and thereafter declines exponentially to exceedingly low doses in food, water and the environment.
> - Biological and biological effect monitoring of pesticide users is very complex and usually undertaken during field trials of the chemical before formal registration for commercial use. Correct study design is essential for the generation of valid results.

APPENDIX. RECOMMENDED BIOLOGICAL EFFECT MONITORING STRATEGY FOR OCCUPATIONAL EXPOSURE TO ORGANOPHOSPHATES (OPS)[92]

- For routine monitoring, baseline activities of both plasma and erythrocyte enzymes should be established before each exposure season begins, or at least 60 days after the last exposure, then followed by monitoring of the plasma and erythrocyte enzymes at intervals which reflect work activities and likely risk of exposure. Multiple subclinical exposures can lead to cumulative depression of the blood enzymes.
- In cases of acute or suspected poisoning, both plasma and erythrocyte enzymes should be measured. An acute exposure will be obvious in the blood enzymes, if the blood sample is taken within three days of exposure. Detection of subclinical exposures may need the collection of a baseline post-exposure (60 days) and delay between exposure and venepuncture will limit the ability to detect exposure.
- To some extent, after OP inhibition, both blood enzymes undergo spontaneous reactivation to normal or 'ageing' to an inactive enzyme where activity is only replaced by new enzyme synthesis. The rates of spontaneous reactivation and ageing depend on the OP and enzyme. Aged plasma enzyme is replaced with a half-life of six to 12 days compared with the erythrocyte enzyme half-life of about 32 days. Thus, the erythrocyte enzyme may be depressed longer than the plasma enzyme. However, in our experience most OPs preferentially inhibit the plasma enzyme. Thus, the delay between exposure and venepuncture may alter the pattern of inhibition in the two blood enzymes.
- Ideally there should be little delay between exposure and venepuncture so as to minimize the recovery of enzyme activities. It is preferable to keep a blood sample for a couple of days under refrigeration after venepuncture close to the exposure period, rather than delaying venepuncture until the laboratory can receive the sample by post the next day.
- It is important that serial analyses should be performed by an established method in the same laboratory and subject to stringent quality control procedures.

Interpretation of results

With the analytical precision attained in the Health and Safety Laboratory, significant absorption of OPs is indicated if the percentage drop between successive estimations is:

- plasma >15 per cent;
- erythrocyte >12 per cent.

REFERENCES

1. Scialabba NE-H, Hattam C (eds). Organic agriculture, environment and food security. Rome: Environment and Natural Resources Service Sustainable Development Department FAO, 2002.
2. Smith AE, Secoy DM. Forerunners of pesticides in classical Greece and Rome. *Journal of Agricultural and Food Chemistry*. 1975; **23**: 1050–5.
3. Smith AE, Secoy DM. A compendium of inorganic substances used in European pest control before 1850. *Journal of Agricultural and Food Chemistry*. 1976; **24**: 1180–6.
4. World Health Organization. International Programme on Chemical Safety Environmental Health Criteria. DDT and its derivatives. Geneva: WHO, 1979.
5. World Health Organization, Regional Office of Europe. Joint WHO/Convention Task Force on the Health Aspects of Air Pollution. Health risks of POPs from long-range transboundary air pollution. Copenhagen: WHO, 2003.
6. United Nations Environment Program. Stockholm Convention on Persistent Organic Pollutants. Geneva: Stockholm Convention Secretariat, 2001.
7. International Programme on Chemical Safety. The WHO recommended classification of pesticides by hazard and guidelines to classification. Geneva: IPCS, 2005.
8. Matsumura F. *Toxicology of insecticides*. New York: Plenum Press, 1985: 122–8.
9. Forshaw PJ, Ray DE. A voltage dependent chloride channel in NIE 115 neuroblastoma cells is activated by protein-kinase-C and also by the pyrethroid deltamethrin. *Journal of Physiology*. 1993; **467**: 252.
10. Proudfoot A. *Pesticide poisoning: Notes for the guidance of medical practitioners*. London: The Stationery Office, 1996.
11. Ecobichon DJ. Toxic effects of pesticides. In: Klaassen CD (ed.). *Casarett and Doull's Toxicology. The basic science of poisons*, 6th edn. New York: McGraw-Hill, 2001: 763–810.
12. United Nations Environment Programme – Chemicals. Childhood pesticide poisoning: Information for advocacy and action. Geneva: UNEP, 2004.
13. Calvert GM, Plate DK, Das R *et al.* Acute occupational pesticide-related illness in the US, 1998–1999: Surveillance findings from the SENSOR Pesticides Program. *American Journal of Industrial Medicine*. 2004; **45**: 14–23.

14. Roldan-Tapia L, Nieto-Escamez FA, del Aguila EM *et al.* Neuropsychological sequelae from acute poisoning and long-term exposure to carbamate and organophosphate pesticides. *Neurotoxicology and Teratology.* 2006; **28**: 694–703.
15. Karalliedde L, Baker D, Marrs TC. Organophosphate-induced intermediate syndrome: Aetiology and relationships with myopathy. *Toxicological Reviews.* 2006; **25**: 1–14.
16. Glynn P. Neuropathy target esterase. *Biochemical Journal.* 1999; **344**: 625–31.
17. Glynn P. Neural development and neurodegeneration: Two faces of neuropathy target esterase. *Progress in Neurobiology.* 2000; **61**: 61–74.
18. World Health Organization. Communicable diseases. Control, prevention and eradication. WHO Pesticide Evaluation Scheme (WHOPES) and Protection of the Human Environment Programme on Chemical Safety (IPCS). Safety of pyrethroids for public health use. Geneva: WHO, 2005.
19. Reigart JR, Roberts JR. Pesticides, and toxic substances. In: *Recognition and management of pesticide poisonings*, 5th edn. US Environmental Protection Agency/Office of Prevention. EPA Document No. EPA 735-R-98-003, 1999: 68–9.
20. Bradberry SM, Watt BE, Proudfoot AT, Vale JA. Mechanisms of toxicity. Clinical features and management of acute chlorophenoxy herbicide poisonings: A review. *Clinical Toxicology.* 2000; **38**: 111–22.
21. Proudfoot AT. Pentachlorophenol poisoning. *Toxicological Reviews.* 2003; **22**: 3–11.
22. Nelson AT, Hartzell JD, More K, Durning SJ. Ingestion of superwarfarin leading to coagulopathy: A case report and review of the literature. *Medscape General Medicine.* 2006; **8**: 41.
23. Chua JD, Friedenberg WR. Superwarfarin poisoning. *Archives of Internal Medicine.* 1998; **158**: 1929–32.
24. Blair A, Malker H, Cantor KP *et al.* Cancer among farmers: A review. *Scandinavian Journal of Work, Environment and Health.* 1985; **11**: 397–407.
25. Blair A, Hoar-Zahm S, Pearce N *et al.* Clues to cancer aetiology from studies of farmers. *Scandinavian Journal of Work, Environment and Health.* 1992; **18**: 209–15.
26. Acquavella J, Olsen G, Cole P *et al.* Cancer among farmers: A meta-analysis. *Annals of Epidemiology.* 1998; **8**: 64–74.
27. Alavanja MCR, Dale P, Sandler DP *et al.* Cancer incidence in the Agricultural Health Study. *Scandinavian Journal of Work, Environment and Health.* 2005; **31** (Suppl. 1): 39–45.
28. Moretto A. Occupational aspects of pesticide toxicity in humans. In: Marrs T, Ballantyne B (eds). *Pesticide toxicology and international regulation*, 431. London: Wiley, 2002.
29. Lee DH, Lee IK, Song K *et al.* A strong dose–response relation between serum concentrations of persistent organic pollutants and diabetes: Results from the National Health and Examination Survey 1999–2002. *Diabetes Care.* 2006; **29**: 1638–44.
30. Eckert H, Jerochin S. Lung changes induced by copper sulfate. An experimental contribution to the so-called 'vineyard sprayer's lung'. *Zeitschrift für Erkrankungen der Atmungsorgane.* 1982; **158**: 270–6.
31. Milby TH, Whorton D. Epidemiological assessment of occupationally related, chemically induced sperm count suppression. *Journal of Occupational Medicine.* 1980; **22**: 77–82.
32. Ratcliffe JM, Schrader SM, Steenland K *et al.* Semen quality in papaya workers with long term exposure to ethylene dibromide. *British Journal of Industrial Medicine.* 1987; **44**: 317–26.
33. Schrader SM, Ratcliffe JM, Turner TW, Hornung RW. The use of new field methods of semen analysis in the study of occupational hazards to reproduction: The example of ethylene dibromide. *Journal of Occupational Medicine.* 1987; **29**: 963–6.
34. Colosio C, Birindelli S, Corsini E *et al.* Low level exposure to chemicals and immune system. *Toxicology and Applied Pharmacology.* 2005; **207** (Suppl. 2): 320–8.
35. Colosio C, Barcellini W, Maroni M *et al.* Immunomodulatory effects of occupational exposure to mancozeb. *Archives of Environmental Health.* 1996; **51**: 445–1.
36. Banerjee BD. The influence of various factors in immune toxicity assessment of pesticide chemicals. *Toxicology Letters.* 1999; **107**: 21–31.
37. Luster MI, Rosenthal GJ. Chemical agents and the immune response. *Environmental Health Perspectives.* 1993; **100**: 219–26.
38. Corsini E, Liesivuori J, Vergieva T *et al.* Effects of pesticide exposure on the human immune system. *Human Experimental Toxicology.* 2008; **27**: 671–80.
39. Salazar KD, Ustyugova IV, Brundage KM *et al.* A review of the immunotoxicity of the pesticide 3,4-dichloropropionanalide. *Journal of Toxicology and Environmental Health. Part B, Critical Reviews.* 2008; **11**: 630–45.
40. Colosio C, Tiramani M, Maroni M. Neurobehavioral effects of pesticides: State of the art. *Neurotoxicology.* 2003; **24**: 577–91.
41. Colosio C, Tiramani M, Brambilla G *et al.* Neurobehavioural effects of pesticides with special focus on organophosphorus compounds: Which is the real size of the problem? *Neurotoxicology.* 2009; **30**: 1155–61.
42. Brown I, Classen W, Ivens IA *et al.* Organophosphorus pesticides and long-term health effects. *Neurotoxicology.* 1997; **18**: 875–6.
43. Brown I, Classen W, Ivens IA *et al.* Organophosphorus pesticides and long term health effects. ECETOC Technical Report, 75. Brussels: European Centre for Ecotoxicology and Toxicology of Chemicals, 1998.
44. Royal College of Physicians and Royal College of Psychiatrists. Organophosphate sheep dip: Clinical aspects of long-term low-dose exposure. Report of a Joint Working Party. London: Royal College of Physicians and Royal College of Psychiatrists, 1998.
45. Solomon C, Poole J, Palmer KT *et al.* Acute symptoms following work with pesticides. *Occupational Medicine.* 2007; **57**: 505–11.
46. Bason CW, Colborn T. US application and distribution of pesticides and industrial chemicals capable of disrupting endocrine and immune systems. *Environmental Toxicology and Occupational Medicine.* 1998; **7**: 147–56.

47. Gray LE Jr, Ostby J, Monosson E, Kelce WR. Environmental antiandrogens: Low doses of the fungicide vinclozolin alter sexual differentiation of the male rat. *Toxicology and Industrial Health.* 1999; **15**: 48-64.
48. Van den Berg KJ. Interaction of chlorinated phenols with thyroxine binding sites of human transthyretin, albumin, and thyroid binding globulin. *Chemico-Biological Interactions.* 1990; **76**: 63-75.
49. Goulet L, Theriault G. Stillbirth and chemical exposure of pregnant workers. *Scandinavian Journal of Work, Environment and Health.* 1991; **17**: 25-31.
50. Rupa DS, Reddy PP, Reddi OS. Reproductive performance in a population exposed to pesticides in cotton fields in India. *Environmental Research.* 1991; **55**: 123-28.
51. Munger R, Isacson P, Hu S et al. Intrauterine growth retardation in Iowa communites with herbicide contaminated drinking water supplies. *Environmental Health Perspectives.* 1997; **105**: 308-14.
52. Arbuckel TE, Sever LE. Pesticide exposures and fetal death: A review of the epidemiologic literature. *Critical Reviews in Toxicology.* 1998; **28**: 229-70.
53. Van den Berg KJ, van Raaij AGM, Bragt PC, Notten WRF. Interactions of halogenated industrial chemicals with transthyretin and effects on thyroid hormone levels *in vivo. Archives of Toxicology.* 1991; **65**: 15-19.
54. Maroni M, Colosio C, Ferioli A, Fait A. Biological monitoring of pesticide exposure: A review. *Toxicology.* 2000; **143**: 1-123.
55. Birnbaum LS, Fenton SE. Cancer and developmental exposure to endocrine disruptors. *Environmental Health Perspectives.* 2003; **111**: 389-94.
56. Alexander BH, Bloemen L, Allen RH. Sessions on the epidemiology of agricultural exposure and cancer. *Scandinavian Journal of Work, Environment and Health.* 2005; **31** (Suppl. 1): 5-7.
57. Keller-Byrne JE, Khuder SA, Schaub EA, McAfee O. A meta-analysis of non-Hodgkin's lymphoma among farmers in the central United States. *American Journal of Industrial Medicine.* 1997; **31**: 442-44.
58. Morrison HI, Wilkins K, Semenciw R et al. Herbicides and cancer. *Journal of the National Cancer Institute.* 1992; **84**: 1866-74.
59. Persson B, Fredriksson M, Olsen K et al. Some occupational exposures as risk factors for malignant lymphomas. *Cancer.* 1993; **72**: 1773-8.
60. Zahm SH. Mortality study of pesticide applicators and other employees of a lawn care service company. *Journal of Occupational and Environmental Medicine.* 1997; **39**: 1055-67.
61. Blair A, Cantor KP, Zahm SH. Non-Hodgkin's lymphoma and agricultural use of the insecticide lindane. *American Journal of Industrial Medicine.* 1998; **33**: 82-7.
62. Hardell L, Eriksson M. A case-control study of non-Hodgkin's lymphoma and exposure to pesticides. *Cancer.* 1999; **85**: 1353-60.
63. Blair A, Cantor KP, Zahm SH. Non-Hodgkin's lymphoma and agricultural use of the insecticide lindane. *American Journal of Industrial Medicine.* 1998; **33**: 82-7.
64. Hardell L, Eriksson M. A case-control study of non-Hodgkin's lymphoma and exposure to pesticides. *Cancer.* 1999; **85**: 1353-60.
65. Grimalt JO, Sunyer J, Moreno V et al. Risk excess of soft-tissue sarcoma and thyroid cancer in a community exposed to airborne organochlorinated compound mixtures with a high hexachlorobenzene content. *International Journal of Cancer.* 1994; **56**: 200-3.
66. Wiklund K, Dich J. Cancer risks among male farmers in Sweden. *European Journal of Cancer Prevention.* 1995; **4**: 81-90.
67. Kauppinen T, Partanen T, Degerth R, Ojajarvi A. Pancreatic cancer and occupational exposures. *Epidemiology.* 1995; **6**: 498-502.
68. Van Der Gulden JW, Vogelzang PF. Farmers at risk for prostate cancer. *British Journal of Urology.* 1996; **77**: 6-14.
69. International Agency for Research on Cancer. Some thyrotropic agents. IARC Monographs on the Evaluation of Carcinogenic Risk to Humans. Geneva: IARC, 2001.
70. Reigart JR, Roberts JR (eds). General principles in the management of acute pesticide poisoning. In: *Recognition and management of pesticide poisonings,* 5th edn. Washington DC: US Environmental Protection Agency, 1999: 10-15.
71. Eddlestone M. Patterns and problems of deliberate self-poisoning in the developing world. *Quarterly Journal of Medicine.* 2000; **93**: 715-31.
72. Karalliedde L, Baker D, Marrs TC. Organophosphate-induced intermediate syndrome: Aetiology and relationships with myopathy. *Toxicological Reviews.* 2006; **25**: 1-14.
73. Roberts DM, Aaron CK. Managing acute organophosphorus pesticide poisoning. A clinical review. *British Medical Journal.* 2007; **334**: 629-34.
74. Jones GM, Vale JA. Mechanisms of toxicity, clinical features, and management of diquat poisoning: A review. *Journal of Toxicology. Clinical Toxicology.* 2000; **38**: 123-8.
75. Roberts DM, Buckley NA. Urinary alkalinisation for acute chlorophenoxy herbicide poisoning. *Cochrane Database of Systematic Reviews.* 2007; (**1**): CD005488.
76. Watt BE, Proudfoot AT, Bradberry SM, Vale JA. Anticoagulant rodenticides. *Toxicological Reviews.* 2005; **24**: 259-69.
77. Bleakley C, Ferrie E, Collum N, Burke L. Self-poisoning with metaldehyde. *Emergency Medicine Journal.* 2008; **25**: 381-2.
78. Blanco LE, Aragon A, Lundberg I et al. Determinants of dermal exposure among Nicaraguan subsistence farmers during pesticide application with backpack sprayers. *Annals of Occupational Hygiene.* 2005; **49**: 17-24.
79. US Environmental Protection Agency. Occupational and residential exposure test guidelines. OPPTS 875.2400 Dermal exposure. Washington DC: EPA, 1997.
80. Martinez Vidal JL, Egea Gonzalez FJ, Garrido Frenich A et al. Assessment of relevant factors and relationships concerning human dermal exposure to pesticides in greenhouse applications. *Pest Management Science.* 2002; **58**: 784-90.
81. Capri E, Alberici R, Glass CR et al. Potential operator exposure to procymidone in greenhouses. *Journal of Agricultural and Food Chemistry.* 1999; **47**: 4443-9.

82. Food Standards Agency. Minutes of the Committee on Toxicity of Chemicals in Food, Consumer Products and the Environment, September 4, 2007. London: The Food Standards Agency, 2007.
83. Brown I. The measurement and assessment of plasma and erythrocyte cholinesterase following potential low dose exposure to the organophosphate chlorpyrifos. Proceedings of the 24th Congress of the International Commission on Occupational Health, Nice, 1993 (Abstr.).
84. Brouwer DH, Brouwer R, De Mik G *et al.* Pesticides in the cultivation of carnations in greenhouses. Part I, Exposure and concomitant health risk. *American Industrial Hygiene Association Journal.* 1992; **53**: 575-81.
85. Brouwer R, Brouwer DH, Tijssen SC, van Hemmen JJ. Pesticides in the cultivation of carnations in greenhouses. Part II, Relationship between foliar residues and exposures. *American Industrial Hygiene Association Journal.* 1992; **53**: 582-7.
86. Samuel O, St Laurent L, Dumas P *et al.* Pesticides en milieu serricole. Caractérisation de l'exposition des travailleurs et évaluation des délais de réentrée. Rapport 315. Montreal: Institut de Recherche Robert-Sauvé en Santé et en Sécurité du Travail, 2002.
87. Koh D, Jeyaratnam J. Pesticide hazards in the developing countries. *Science of the Total Environment.* 1996; **188**: 78-85.
88. Dosemeci M, Alavanja MC, Rowland AS *et al.* A quantitative approach for estimating exposure to pesticides in the Agricultural Health Study. *Annals of Occupational Hygiene.* 2002; **46**: 245-60.
89. Mekonnen Y, Agonafir T. Pesticide sprayers' knowledge, attitude and practice of pesticide use on agricultural farms of Ethiopia. *Occupational Medicine.* 2002; **52**: 311-15.
90. Ngowi AVF, Maeda DN, Partanen TJ. Knowledge, attitudes and practices (KAP) among agricultural extension workers concerning the reduction of the adverse impact of pesticides in agricultural areas in Tanzania. *La Medicina del Lavoro.* 2002; **93**: 338-46.
91. International Centre for Pesticide Safety. Preventing health risks from the use of pesticides in agriculture. Protecting Workers' Health Series No. 1. Geneva: World Health Organization – Occupational and Environmental Health, 2001.
92. Nutley BP, Cocker J. Biological monitoring of workers occupationally exposed to organophosphate pesticides. *Pesticide Science.* 1993; **38**: 315-22.

44

Welding

GRANT McMILLAN

Introduction	421	Adverse health effects of employment as a welder	429
Principal welding processes	422	Adverse effects on reproduction	435
Source, nature and variation of emissions	423	Health surveillance	435
Sampling and analysis	427	Inhalation fevers	436
Control of workplace exposures in welding	428	References	438

INTRODUCTION

'Welding' is a generic term for any of the processes of joining materials at areas or points softened or liquefied by the application of heat derived in a variety of ways. Welding metal is the most ubiquitous of the industrial processes and welders are among the last craftsmen in industrialized and industrializing economies. Several sources of heat are used. These include friction, electron beams, lasers, ultrasound and combustion of fuel gases, but by far the most common source is an electric arc struck between two electrical conductors. Further consideration of the health and safety hazards of welding here will be limited almost entirely to arc welding processes.

Estimates suggest that well over three million workers worldwide use welding to some extent in their work. Welders and the many other individuals who work with them, or in their vicinity, may be exposed to emissions that pose a wide range of potential health hazards. With such large numbers of workers involved, a sound knowledge of welding processes and their emissions is important for controlling the hazards to health.

There is also economic pressure to improve the reality and perception of health and safety in the welding industry. Increasing global demand for these skilled workers is not being met. Recruiting is down and, after years of training, retention of qualified welders working through to normal retirement age is poor. International opinion-formers in the industry believe this is due in large part to the perception that welding is 'dirty and dangerous'. They are seeking to change that view. They recognize that this means accepting that welding and allied processes and the workplaces wherein these are used may indeed be damaging to health unless health and safety professionals are on hand to assess and ensure the many associated risks of harm are controlled.

Over the last decade, specific concerns for the occupational health and safety of welders and related workers have resurfaced yet again. This has been prompted by legislation, research findings, impending legislation on protection from electromagnetic fields and, from the United States, a catalyst for research provided by litigation over assertions that inhaled manganese compounds in fume from very commonly used welding and related processes may exert significant irreversible neurotoxic effects on exposed workers.

The industry's desire to shake off the 'dirty and dangerous' mantle has helped to prevent these new developments totally overshadowing and diverting attention from the need for more to be done about long-recognized hazards and their effects. These include wholly avoidable deaths at work; the damage done daily to hundreds of thousands of workers by 'minor' but painful injury accidents related to welding processes; respiratory diseases and the long-term toll of largely avoidable wear and tear of the musculoskeletal system which is one of the main causes of 'medical wastage'.

In the area of respiratory diseases, the spotlight has widened to highlight not only continuing uncertainty about causal links with chronic obstructive pulmonary disease (COPD), and chronic bronchitis and emphysema (CBE), and the long-standing apparent excess risk welders have for lung cancer, but also to include the hypothesis that inhaling welding fume may facilitate pneumonic infections.

Making health and safety of welders a naturally integrated part of education, training and good practice at all levels of the workforce and from project conception through to completion, and beyond to maintenance and repair, must be at the heart of moves to make welding less 'dirty and dangerous'. There is an urgent need to conclude research to clarify the situation regarding hazards such as manganese; for more pro-active measures to recognize, evaluate and control exposure to welding fumes without significant loss of productivity; and to make improvements to the ergonomics of the processes and workplaces. Welders need to be better trained, motivated and equipped to exercise their responsibility to contribute to protecting their own health and that of fellow workers by using their skills, knowledge and common sense to better effect, for example, to reduce exposure to potentially harmful materials by using the ventilation which is provided and keeping their head out of the plume of fume.

PRINCIPAL WELDING PROCESSES

A basic understanding of the principal welding processes is necessary to understand and appreciate the source and nature of the emissions and the potential which exists to control them. The main welding and allied processes are arc welding, resistance welding, gas welding, forge welding, brazing and soldering. Prime among these in terms of usage is arc welding, the main topic in this chapter, probably followed by resistance welding. Much information and technical details on these and the range of joining and related processes such as hardfacing, arc air gouging and burning are available at 'Job Knowledge' and other sections within the technical information area of the website of TWI World Centre for Material Joining Technology.[1]

Arc welding processes

In arc welding processes, in general terms, the great heat generated by an electric arc struck between the workpiece and an electrode held in a machine or by a manual welder in a handpiece melts abutting edges of the metal to be joined sufficiently for these to contribute molten metal to a common weld pool which, when cool, forms a solid joint. When the workpiece cannot contribute sufficient metal to the pool, metal may be added from a filler wire held in the arc. Alternatively, the filler wire may also conduct the electricity and act as the electrode which is the source of the arc. It is then called a 'consumable electrode'.

The wire may have a coating or core comprising a mixture of materials which together have properties to facilitate welding and improve the quality of the weld. It is usual for a gas shield to be formed over and around the arc and weld pool creating a bubble-like stable and reproducible micro-environment restricting access of oxygen and other gases, thus minimizing oxidation and other inclusions which could weaken the weld. This shield may be produced by combustion of components of the core or coating of the filler metal wire or be provided directly as a flow of inert or active gas, such as argon or carbon dioxide, respectively.

In manual metal arc (MMA) welding (Figure 44.1), the arc is struck between the workpiece and a consumable electrode in a holder held by the welder. The wire of the electrode is short to allow it to be controlled and is usually coated with a mixture of chemicals and alloying metals. In addition to forming a shield of combustion gases over the arc and weld pool this may contribute to the properties of the weld. It forms a temporary 'slag' over the weld bead to reduce oxidation and slow cooling. Slag is chipped off once the weld has cooled. This is a common source of foreign body eye injuries.

In tungsten inert gas (TIG) welding (Figure 44.2), the arc is formed between the workpiece and a contoured non-consumable electrode in the form of a conical spike of tungsten alloy in a pen-type holder. This may contain thorium (see under Radiation, p. 423). The electrode tip must be kept correctly contoured by periodic grinding at intervals of up to several weeks depending on use. Metal may be added from a filler wire fed into the weld pool by the operator independently of the electrode, resulting in both

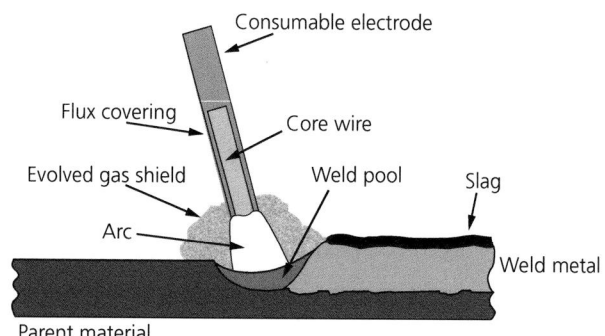

Figure 44.1 Schematic diagram of manual metal arc welding.

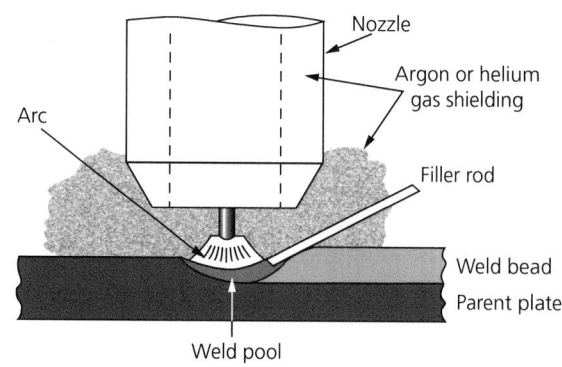

Figure 44.2 Schematic diagram of tungsten inert gas welding.

hands being used. The arc and weld pool are shrouded in inert (and thereby asphyxiant) shielding gas, such as argon and/or helium.

In metal inert gas (MIG) and metal active gas (MAG) welding, the electrode is a continuous consumable small diameter bare wire fed at a constant speed on to the parent metal of the workpiece. This wire is melted in its own arc to contribute directly to the weld pool. The wire may contain a flux in its core (flux core arc welding). The weld pool, tip of the electrode and arc are shrouded in a shield of piped inert and/or active gas. As the operator does not have to be concerned with controlling the arc length, this process is much favoured by amateur welders.

New processes

Although these arc welding processes are generally cheap and reliable, limitations in all of them have become evident.[2] Improvements and new technologies are required. Whether it is an established welding process which is being optimized or a new process being introduced, it is necessary to include an assessment of its impact on the health and safety of welders, and others, in the multidisciplinary development process of proving its suitability for purpose. New processes, such as laser and laser-hybrid processing, electron beam welding, magnetic pulse welding and friction stir welding, have been developed and are being or have been introduced with advantage to productivity and the health of workers.

Of the new technologies mentioned, friction stir welding (FSW) is of particular interest for improved occupational health because it welds in the solid phase – there is no melting and so no fume, and no arc so no ozone. Put simply, in friction stir welding, a wear-resistant, specially shaped tool is rotated at a very high speed and slowly plunged under a downward force by a machine into the joint line between the parts to be joined. These have to be clamped together so that the abutting faces cannot be forced apart. As it rotates, the tool heats the material by friction to about 70–85 per cent of its melting temperature so that it softens sufficiently for the rotating tool to traverse the joint line softening as the material goes. Its contoured shape ensures that, as it passes, it leaves material trailing behind it which forms into a solid phase bond between the two pieces. FSW is now well established worldwide especially for the welding of aluminium. Work is in hand to greatly extend its application.

SOURCE, NATURE AND VARIATION OF EMISSIONS

The emissions from arc welding processes comprise ultraviolet and infrared radiation, visible light, an often biologically active mixture of particles termed 'welding fume' and a mixture of gases derived from the process and the action of the arc on ambient air. The formation and emission rates and the composition of each and all of these pollutants may vary within and between welding processes. This can be troublesome when sampling and when prescribing control solutions, but can be turned to advantage to select, use and perhaps modify processes to ensure the maximum reduction of the risk of harm being caused by their emissions.

Variations in emissions within a process are influenced by many factors including the materials to be welded, those in the filler wire or other consumable, electrical parameters, shield gas and the individual welder's skill and self-protection measures,[3] the latter being a most powerful influence which can be reinforced by good education, training and motivation.

The air in the welding operator's breathing zone may also contain compounds originating from the surrounding workplace atmosphere, rather than the welding process, as was observed in a recent UK Health and Safety Executive investigation in which samples taken for analysis from three different arc welding techniques frequently contained commonly used solvents, such as acetone, cyclohexane and dichloromethane.[4] These and other materials may originate from surface coatings and contaminants or from other processes, such as degreasing, being carried out in the workplace.

Radiation

Arc welding is one of the most intense artificial sources of optical radiation. Each type of welding emits a different and continually changing spectrum and intensity.[5] For most processes ultraviolet (UV) (A, B and mainly C) and, to a much less extent, infrared radiation (IR), are the components of health and safety concern.

UV radiation is a known carcinogen. Excessive exposure to solar radiation increases risks of cancer of the lip, basal cell, and squamous cell carcinoma of the skin and cutaneous melanoma, particularly in fair skin populations. The short distance between the arc and the welders' and, sometimes, other workers' skin and eyes is likely to be insufficient to absorb much of the potentially damaging UVB and UVC, so they will be at significantly increased risk of eye and skin damage, including malignancy, if they have inadequate protection.

The possible health hazard of electromagnetic fields (EMF) is one of the most recent subjects of special interest in the health of welders. There is no clear-cut evidence of harm being caused to humans by this radiation other than occasional cases of local heating of the eye and male gonads. There is, however, a high level of suspicion that as-yet-undetected harm results from EMFs. It is anticipated that employers will be required to assess and measure levels of EMFs to which workers are exposed; where these levels exceed 'action values', to assess whether exposure limits are exceeded; to ensure that these limits are not exceeded; to erect warning signs when EMF exposure levels may cause exposure limits to be exceeded; and to provide appropriate information and training.

Arc welders are among those groups who may be exposed to the highest intensities of fields.[1] Although arc welding uses relatively low voltages, it requires high current. This flows through welding electrical equipment and cables. If that equipment is close to the welder and/or the welding cables are wrapped over or in direct contact with the body, as is often observed, then the welder may be exposed to relatively high intensities of field compared to other occupations. Much can be done to reduce the arc welder's exposure and relatively simple steps can have a tremendous benefit. Expert advice can be obtained from a reputable source, such as the national health and safety regulatory body or from an international[1] or the within-country national centre of welding expertise.

Ionizing radiation may be introduced into the welding scenario through ancillary processes, such as non-destructive testing radiography and, now unnecessarily, by the continued use of thoriated tungsten electrodes in TIG welding and, to a lesser extent, in plasma cutting. Tungsten is used because it can withstand very high temperatures with minimal melting or erosion. Performance is further improved by alloying the tungsten with small quantities of oxides of other metals. One such additive is thorium oxide which is radioactive, emitting mainly alpha particles. The main source of danger is in the ingestible and respirable dust produced during periodic grinding of the electrodes to maintain the necessary sharp point – but there is also a small external radioactive hazard.

Thorium-free tungsten electrodes incorporating alternative and only marginally radioactive additives, such as cerium, lanthanum, yttrium and zirconium oxides are available. These are technically acceptable in most welding situations and should be used, either as the only modification to the process or with equipment that eliminates the need for thoriated electrodes for arc starting. When this is not possible, strict precautions must be taken to minimize exposure to thorium-containing dust at all stages from receipt and storage of the electrodes through welding and grinding to cleaning and disposal of waste.

Particle emissions

Welding fume particles are derived from evaporation, condensation, oxidation, decomposition and combustion of materials involved in the joining process. The fume composition is largely (up to 95 per cent) determined by the composition of the filler metal and, when present, its flux core or coating. Usually less than 10 per cent of the particulate emissions derive from the metal being welded.

Twenty-first century technologies in imaging and analysing particles have provided an overall picture of welding fume previously unattainable.[6] When particles are characterized by size distribution, morphology, structure and chemical composition, it emerges that they can be classified into two main groups. The first of these comprises fractionated mixed metal oxide particles formed from metal vaporized in the high temperature of the arc, often oxidized following reactions with oxygen in the ambient air. These are present as individual irregular particles, individual spherical particles, and chains and aggregates formed by condensation of particles. They reflect the composition of the electrode with the more volatile constituents predominating. Many of the particles have a core-shell structure which suggests that surface composition can be quite different from the bulk composition.[6]

The second group of particles is termed 'spatter'. These are coarse, unfractionated particles of electrode, usually larger than respirable, but providing a secondary source of smaller respirable oxide particles as the hot metal spatter reacts with oxygen in the air, often explosively.

The size of the particles is critically important in assessing the bioavailability of their constituents as the lung is the principal potential route of entry. An important characteristic is the particle diameter (aerodynamic diameter for particles $>0.1\,\mu m$, diffusion equivalent diameter for particles $<0.1\,\mu m$). The size variation of welding fume particles is quite large.[6,7] It has long been known that many are in the respirable range. Whereas it had been estimated that some 50 per cent of the fume inhaled reached the lower respiratory tract and 35 per cent to the alveolar level, with most then being exhaled,[8] more recently it has been found that a substantial proportion comprises submicron/ultrafine/nanoparticles.[9–11] This may change our understanding and appreciation of the power of welding fume particles to initiate and promote inflammatory processes and systemic oxidative stress deriving from the soluble transition metals and, perhaps, to greatly facilitate the transfer of metals to various organs, such as manganese to the brain.[12]

An indication of the range of metallic oxides which may be present in the fume from several processes is given in Table 44.1 which was developed in discussion with fellow experts meeting under the aegis of the International Institute of Welding. In this context a principal component is of some occupational hygiene significance, while the key component has the greatest occupational hygiene significance and therefore requires the most stringent control measures to ensure that a welder is not exposed to an excessive level of the substance concerned.

While, as remarked earlier, emissions vary within and between processes, in general terms, of the most commonly used arc processes TIG welding gives the least fume followed by MIG/MAG and MMA, then flux cored welding which gives the most.

Although the metal compounds found in fume are considered in Section two, Metals, three (chromium, nickel and manganese) merit brief mention here solely in regard to their presence in welding fume. Further information on these substances in welding is available in separate publications.[13–15]

Table 44.1 Principal[a] and key[b] components of fumes from commonly encountered arc welding processes.

Type of process	Type of consumable	Typical principal components	Other possible principal components	Typical key component
MMA (SMAW)	Unalloyed and low alloy steel	Fe, Mn, Cr, Cr(VI), Ni, Cu	F	Mn, Cr, Cr(VI)
	High alloy steel	Cr, Cr(VI), Fe, Mn, Ni	F	Cr(VI), Ni
	Aluminium	Al, Cu, Mg, Mn, Zn	Be, Cl, F	Al, Mn or Zn
	Cast iron	Ni, Cu, Fe, Mn	Ba, F	Ni or Cu
	Hardfacing	Co, Cr, Cr(VI), Fe, Ni, Mn	V	Co, Cr, Cr(VI) Ni or Mn
	Work hardening	Fe, Mn, Cr		Mn
	Nickel-based	Co, Cr, Cr(VI), Mn, Ni	Fe	Cr, Cr(VI) or Ni
	Copper-based	Cu, Ni		Cu or Ni
MIG/MAG (GMAW) and GTAW	Unalloyed and low alloy steel	Fe, Mn, Cr, Cr(VI), Ni, Cu		Mn, Cr, Cr(VI)
	High alloy steel	Cr, Cr(VI), Fe, Mn, Ni		Cr, Cr(VI) or Ni
	Aluminium alloys	Al, Cu, Mg, Mn, Zn	Be	Al, Mn or Zn
	Nickel-based	Co, Cr, Cr(VI), Mn, Ni	Fe	Cr, Cr(VI) or Ni
	Copper-based	Cu, Ni		Cu or Ni
Gas-shielded FCAW	Unalloyed and low alloy steel	Fe, Mn, Cr, Cr(VI), Ni, Cu	F	Mn, Cr, Cr(VI)
	High alloy steel	Cr, Cr(VI), Fe, Mn, Ni	F	Cr(VI) or Ni
	Hardfacing	Co, Cr, Cr(VI), Fe, Ni, Mn	V	Co, Cr, Cr(VI) Ni or Mn
	Nickel-based	Co, Cr, Cr(VI), Mn, Ni	Fe	Cr, Cr(VI) or Ni
Self-shielded FCAW	Unalloyed and low alloy steel	Fe, Mn, Cr, Cr(VI), Ni, Cu, Al	Ba, F	Mn
	High alloy steel	Cr, Cr(VI), Fe, Mn, Ni, Al	Ba, F	Cr(VI) or Ni
	Hardfacing	Co, Cr, Cr(VI), Fe, Ni, Mn, Al	V	Co, Cr, Cr(VI) Ni or Mn

[a]A principal component is a component that is of occupational hygiene significance.
[b]A key component is the component that has the greatest occupational hygiene significance and therefore requires the most stringent control measures to ensure that a welder is not exposed to an excessive level of the substance concerned, i.e. it is the component whose limit value is exceeded at the lowest welding fume concentration.
FCAW, flux-coated arc welding; GMAW, gas metal arc welding; GTAW, gas tungsten arc welding; MAG, metal active gas welding; MIG, metal inert gas welding; MMA, manual metal arc welding; SMAW, shielded metal arc welding.

Trivalent and hexavalent chromium compounds are found in fume from welding on or with materials that contain chromium or chromates. These include high chromium nickel alloys and low alloy steels, high alloy flux covered wires, chromate paints and coatings, and chromium plating. Chromium is typically not added intentionally to mild steel or mild steel welding consumables but, because of the nature of steel making and the use of scrap metal, it is not unusual to find low levels.

Fume from welding stainless steel is rich in hexavalent chromium and trivalent chromium compounds, the amounts varying within and between processes. Hexavalent chromium compounds are a cause of occupational asthma (see under Occupational asthma, p. 434). Some hexavalent chromium compounds are known to be carcinogenic to the respiratory system by inhalation in a range of industrial processes other than welding, e.g. chrome plating and in the production of chromates, chromate pigments and ferrochromium. Dose–response relationships have been established for hexavalent chromium and cancer and the possibility of a threshold effect has been suggested. There is coincident exposure in most circumstances to trivalent chromium compounds. The International Agency for Research on Cancer (IARC) has found there to be inadequate evidence for classification regarding the carcinogenicity of trivalent chromium for humans,[16] nor has metallic chromium been found to be carcinogenic in humans.

When compounds containing hexavalent chromium are present in welding fume they can be absorbed and excreted. The extent to which retention, reduction and excretion of hexavalent chromium compounds and their solubility act as an important determinant of carcinogenic potential is uncertain.

IARC has classified nickel compounds as carcinogenic to man.[16] Evidence suggests that, in highly nickel-polluted environments, the risk appears to be stronger for water-soluble compounds of chromium rather than those which are water-insoluble. Nickel is found in welding fumes almost exclusively as nickel oxide and only when welding with pure nickel or nickel alloy filler material. The choice of welding process has a strong influence on the emission rate. The carcinogen nickel carbonyl has not been found in welding fume.

Manganese compounds have been proven to be occupational neurotoxins in a range of activities other than welding. Manganese is an essential component of steel. There is no suitable substitute. Compounds containing manganese, in complexes with iron and other oxides, are present in fume particles from steel welding and allied processes.

In recent years, it has been asserted by a few authors in the scientific literature, and during litigation in the United States, that occupational exposure to manganese compounds in fume from welding of steel causes or promotes the onset of Parkinson's disease and/or parkinsonism/ manganism in welders and those around them at work. These assertions have been vigorously contested.

Clinical manganism and Parkinson's disease are two separate diseases, which, with care and thorough investigation, can be differentiated from one another.[15] Follow-on studies have not supported the conclusion that welders are or have been at any greater risk of developing Parkinson's disease at all or at an earlier age than others of similar background in other occupations in their community. Whereas vast numbers of workers worldwide use arc welding to join metal, the literature contains reports of very few, if any, who have developed clinical manganism as a result of exposure to welding fume. The risk may be slightly greater in allied processes, such as thermal cutting and gouging or hardfacing in which fume emission levels are inherently higher, but again there have been very few cases. Furthermore, there is no convincing evidence that exposure to manganese-containing fume during employment as a welder can result in an increased risk of developing neurobehavioural deficiencies and loss of fine control of movements. There is, however, insufficient evidence to the contrary to dismiss the possibility with absolute certainty.

Gaseous emissions

Gaseous emissions comprise those formed in the arc and by the action of the arc on the ambient air, plus any shielding gases remaining after they have performed their role, and gases released from combustion or heating of surface coatings. The number of variables affecting workplace exposures means that a wide range of exposures is possible. Exposures of individual welders may come from general workshop levels rather than their own work.

The principal gases formed are ozone, oxides of nitrogen (NO_x) and carbon monoxide – each considered in detail in Chapter 8, Gases. The arc plays a key role in their formation. When arcing is not continuous, for example in manual processes, formation and emission of these gases peaks during and diminishes or is absent between arcing, so welders may be exposed for repeated short periods to concentrations very much higher than those indicated by an averaging sampling and measuring technique.[3]

It has been said that exposure to ozone is currently a major occupational hygiene problem with almost all gas-shielded arc welding processes and that, in recent years, the increasing use of aluminium and stainless steels, along with raised productivity, has increased the likelihood of unacceptable welder exposure.[17] This appears to be related more to achieving control down to at least within national occupational exposure limits, many of which have been reduced in recent years, than to there being evidence in the literature of exposures to ozone in workplaces causing ill health in welders – as this has not been found.

There is, however, no doubt that ozone is an irritant to mucous membranes, can cause acute discomfort to the eyes and upper respiratory tract, readily penetrates to small airways and alveoli and, even with brief exposures, if concentrations are sufficient, will cause a disabling inflammatory response with pulmonary oedema. The possibility of there being as-yet-undetected harm occurring in welders cannot be ignored – and so exposure to ozone must be minimized to at least within the national standards.

The generation of ozone is due to photodissociation of molecular oxygen in the ambient air around the welding process under the influence of direct or reflected UV radiation emitted from the arc. The gas forms in two distinct regions: approximately half within a 10–15 cm radius of the arc by the action of UV in the 130–175 nm range and the remainder in relatively low concentrations further from the arc, up to a metre, due to UV of wavelengths 175–240 nm. It decomposes when subjected to higher wavelengths. Usually, the ozone reaches the breathing zone in a few seconds after the arcing starts and the concentration returns to the background level almost within the same time after arcing has ended.[17]

Ozone concentration is affected by the number of welders at work (as several together can build up significant concentrations during welding in an inadequately ventilated space), the welder's care and skill, and any of the large number of other variables which influence the rate of formation and decomposition of the gas produced by each operator. These include the magnitude of the UV in the critical ranges for production – and beyond for decomposition of the gas once formed; the presence of fume particles, dust or other gases; the composition of the filler wire; the welding process and its parameters; and, often most complex and variable, the shielding gas. Together these, and the need for specialized equipment based on chemiluminescence, make measuring welders' exposure problematic.[17]

All else being equal, ozone concentration is greatest in processes with low fume emission and vice versa as it reverts to oxygen in contact with particles.

Process selection is a powerful influence on ozone exposure. For example, there tends to be a very fierce arc in TIG welding and so a great deal of ultraviolet radiation and much ozone are produced, particularly when welding on aluminium and stainless steel. Process modification may be useful in reducing ozone levels, at least experimentally, as small changes to the process and its parameters can have disproportionate effects.[18,19]

Oxides of nitrogen or nitrous gases (nitrogen monoxide, dioxide and peroxide) are generated as byproducts in most arc welding, cutting and heating processes as a result of heating the air in the arc or flame region. Emission rates during arc welding are very low compared to allied processes especially plasma cutting and oxyacetylene processes.[20] The rate of formation of nitric oxide is initially slower than that of ozone as the rapid production of the former is partly dependent on the air achieving a high temperature, whereas ozone production peaks in a fraction of a second after the arc is struck and UV is emitted.[3]

The first stage in the formation of these NO_x is oxidation of atmospheric nitrogen to nitrogen monoxide, a gas of very low toxicity. This occurs in contact with the very hot gas emanating from the arc and weld pool. Between 75 and 97 per cent of the oxides of nitrogen emitted may be nitrogen monoxide. Its rates of formation and emission peak during arcing as the temperature goes above 500–1000°C. They then fall, sometimes dramatically, as the NO is diluted by the ambient air and cools to its temperature whereupon it oxidizes, at rates dependent on concentration and temperature, to the biologically more active gases, nitrogen dioxide and peroxide, which have the potential to cause harm.

The ratio of nitrogen monoxide and dioxide can change if ozone or other oxidants are present in the air. In gas-shielded arc welding, because of ozone formation by the UV of the arc, almost all of the total oxides of nitrogen generated is nitrogen dioxide.[20]

The very low emission rates during arc welding compared to processes, such as plasma cutting or oxyacetylene burning where much higher rates may be encountered, may be of practical importance for occupational physicians and epidemiologists when seeking to select samples of workers for research studies as mixing those with superficially similar jobs may result in mixing those with notably different potential exposures to these gases, e.g. arc welders (low NO_x) and flame burners (higher NO_x).

Carbon monoxide is generated by thermal decomposition of carbon dioxide in metal active gas welding shielded by that gas and by the incomplete combustion of flux materials containing carbonates and/or cellulose in all or almost all processes. The amounts of carbon monoxide generated by fluxed arc welding processes are small and, generally, the risk of overexposure is low.

SHIELDING GASES

Shielding gases used in processes such as TIG, MIG/MAG and flux-cored arc welding (FCAW) may be inert, such as argon, helium or nitrogen, or active argon-based mixtures containing carbon dioxide, oxygen or both. Helium may be added to argon/carbon dioxide mixtures to improve productivity. Carbon dioxide may be used on its own. None of the gases can be seen and none has a smell[21] – although a method for odorization was described two decades ago.[22] Their presence in hazardous concentrations is difficult to detect without prior knowledge or measuring equipment. The main hazard arising from shielding gases is asphyxiation (see under Asphyxia, p. 432).

INFLUENCE OF COATINGS AND CONTAMINANTS ON EMISSIONS

The composition and amount of fumes and gases produced may be influenced significantly in complexity and potential to cause harm when the metal to be welded has a surface coating applied, e.g. by galvanizing, electroplating, painting on primer, thermal coating, or is contaminated by materials such as oil, degreasers or the products/byproducts of manufacturing processes, e.g. lead, manganese.

It is becoming increasingly common, particularly with resistance welding in the auto and white goods industries, to weld through or close to organic materials, such as shop primers, other coatings, adhesives, etc. This can generate a wide range of degradation products. Their composition may be difficult to predict even if knowledge of the composition of the product is available.[23]

Chlorinated hydrocarbons, such as trichloroethylene, may still be found in use for degreasing. These may present as vapour particles in the ambient air having passed from an adjacent tank or remain on metal parts which have just been cleaned but have not yet dried. The radiation from welding arcs may cause chlorinated hydrocarbons to decompose in the air or on the parts. The very toxic gas phosgene may be formed.

In many cases, the risk assessment will indicate that it would be best for the surface coatings and contaminants to be removed before welding. An exception may be made when the coating is classified as 'weld-through' and sufficient is known about it to conduct and act upon a properly informed risk assessment. With these coatings, fume composition and thus the risk of harm may be dependent on welding method as some processes produce more volatile organic compounds and less particulate than others when used on metal coated with the same primer.[4]

SAMPLING AND ANALYSIS

Air samples should be collected and analysed by qualified people using approved standardized methods and devices. The dynamism of the fume and the variation in gas emissions can present challenges to meaningful sampling. When assessing exposure, it is best to collect the fume in the breathing zone behind the welder's helmet – although this may not be possible with modern close-fitting helmets. If there is a national or international standard for sampling, this should be followed. Even with care, standardized methods and long experience, it can prove difficult to get reproducible results.

The content of the fume measured in the breathing zone may include significant contributions from neighbourhood activities, such as grinding and, as mentioned earlier, degreasing,[4] indicating the wider than perhaps expected range of exposure the workers may be experiencing. There are so many variables at work that often it will be imprudent to extrapolate results obtained in one situation, or even from one welder,[3] to another.

CONTROL OF WORKPLACE EXPOSURES IN WELDING

The hazards associated with welding and its allied processes are largely the same all round the world, yet the standards set for precautions to be taken to control the risks of harm vary greatly between countries.[24] Local enquiries must be made to determine the minimum levels to be achieved.

The multiplicity of situations in which welding and allied processes are used, the variations between and within them, and in legislation in many countries, make it obligatory for measures for control of workplace exposures to be selected following risk assessment of all relevant aspects of the individual work situation – including when this is off-site, e.g. at the customer's premises.[25,26]

Accurate risk assessment of exposure to welding emissions can be a difficult task. The assessment must consider not only the operators, but also the people working in the vicinity of welders. It should include the workers involved in the processes in discussions from the outset if at all possible. Guidance on assessment is available.[23,25,26] Means have been suggested to remove the requirement for expensive analysis of every fume sample.[23] The extent and method of health surveillance required must be included. This is considered under Health surveillance, p. 435.

The basic traditional occupational hygiene hierarchical approach must be taken to achieve adequate control of exposure:[27–30]

- prevent emission by selection/substitution of process; improve working practices by modification of process, process parameters or consumables to lower fume and gas emission rates or toxicity of the constituents;
- prevent exposure by natural ventilation and/or engineering controls, including isolation or segregation, control of pollutants at the source by local exhaust ventilation; and finally,
- prevent exposure by wearing respiratory protection equipment (RPE).

It is not appropriate to go directly to or rely solely on personal respiratory protection equipment. Although much guidance is available,[1,31] specialist advice may be required at any or every stage.

Selection of the process at the outset should include consideration of health risks alongside technical suitability, product quality, productivity and cost. In the last 25 years, technological improvements designed primarily to give better welds and improve productivity have also provided opportunities to reduce emissions. For example, enhanced control of power sources has allowed finer control of electrical parameters giving the potential to reduce emissions

sensitive to such changes. Process automation should be considered as this may greatly improve the possibilities for control of welding exposures in the welding environment.

Selection, substitution and process modification require knowledge of emissions of alternative processes and the effect of selected process parameters (such as weld speed, current and voltage), shielding gas or other consumables to allow meaningful comparisons to be made. In practice, process or parameter substitution or modification may be limited to situations where the product quality and overall production costs (including the cost of control measures) are not significantly adversely affected by the proposed changes. Experience has shown that opportunities for substitution lie in the selection of consumables using fume data provided by suppliers. It is important to ensure that hazards are not removed only to be replaced by others of equal or greater concern.

Isolation or segregation is often appropriate for automatic or semi-automatic processes, perhaps using remote control and/or an enclosure closely surrounding the source. It should be applied to the full range of manual processes in both stationary and non-stationary workplaces by reducing the number of people who are in the area of emissions to an absolute minimum and separating them from others by exclusion instructions and screens.

Local extraction ventilation (LEV) is usually required for welding and often provides the necessary control. It should be designed to capture the particulate fume and gases at source before these enter the breathing zone of the operator. It may be fixed, flexible or portable, or integrated in the welding equipment and should introduce air movement sufficient to capture and transport the pollutants away from the breathing zones of welders and those working with them. General ventilation is usually required as a supplement to LEV to supply fresh air and dilute pollutants. Guidance is available for self-help.[1,25,27,28] It may be prudent to seek specialist advice on the design and selection of extraction and general ventilation systems in all but the most straightforward situations.

Use of personal respiratory protection equipment is essential where previous steps cannot provide sufficient protection against exposure to fumes and gases. There are two aspects to be considered: (1) the selection and care of a suitable device and (2) the human aspects of achieving the expected level of respiratory protection. Both can present challenges.

The requirement may be met by filtering or air-fed respirators or helmets.[1,29–31] These should be fitted and supplied to the individual welder. All apparatus used should be marked with the appropriate nationally-used protection classification and quality scheme logo. Filters must protect against gases, as well as fumes – or alternative arrangements made for removal of gases. This should have been achieved by arrangements for ventilation. There must be adequate support arrangements (including education and training, cleaning and maintenance) and for supervision over such matters as length of use of filters.

ADVERSE HEALTH EFFECTS OF EMPLOYMENT AS A WELDER

Sudden deaths

Though fortunately rare, welders and allied workers are killed in the course of their work by electrocution, explosion or fire, and, as discussed below, asphyxia or acute chemical exposures. It would be hard to argue that these deaths were not entirely avoidable had a safe system of work based on sound risk assessment been followed. Much excellent guidance and direction are available from national and other health and safety agencies to assist in avoiding these and other potentially fatal hazards and how appropriate safe systems of work should be designed and operated.[1,31]

Other injury accidents

The Health and Safety Executive estimates that there are over 1000 work-related accidents to welders reported in the United Kingdom each year with around 300 classified as major accidents, such as fractures and amputations.[31] The three most common types of reported accidents to welders in the UK are related to handling, slips and trips, and being hit by a moving or falling object – which may be a foreign body heading for the eye!

BURNS AND OTHER NON-MALIGNANT SKIN LESIONS

Welders suffer a high incidence of burns and other skin lesions from hot metal, UV and IR radiation burns of unprotected areas of skin. UVR and IR radiation from electric arc welding processes commonly cause 'ray burn' (erythema) and, ultimately, persistent pigmentation in unprotected areas of skin, neck and chest exposed at the V-opening of an unbuttoned shirt or overall, the wrists due to stretching overhead, forehead and the fronts of the ankles in welders who squat to weld and allow their trousers to ride up.[32,33] The back of the ears may be affected by reflected radiation, e.g. when welding within an aluminium container.

Almost all welders have been burned by sparks, spatter and droplets of molten metal or slag and bear the scars of these repeated injuries. The occupational stigmata of ray burn and multiple small burn scars found on many welders can cause difficulties in 'blinding' controlled studies as it is so easy to distinguish the welders from others. Rarely, such burns occur inside the ear. These are particularly painful and may give rise to serious complications including perforation of the tympanic membrane with deafness and facial paralysis and unusually high rates of residual and recurring perforations.[34–37]

High velocity metal projectiles causing deep penetrating injuries with residual foreign body material may be emitted during spot or resistance welding, probably due to poor cleaning and maintenance of the equipment.[38,39]

Arc welding has been reported as affecting the exposed skin in other ways, including siderosis[40] and contact dermatitis due to chromium and nickel.[41] Atopic dermatitis has been exacerbated by UVC radiation from the arc[42] and the much rarer photodermatitis has been reported in a resistance welder.[43]

MALIGNANT SKIN LESIONS

Exposure to UVR, whether solar or of artificial origin, carries potential risks to human health. It is a known carcinogen. Excess exposure to solar radiation increases the risk of cancer of the lip, basal cell and squamous cell carcinoma of the skin and cutaneous melanoma, particularly in fair skin populations. Artificial UVR from welding torches may also contribute to the burden of disease from UVR.[44] It is possible that welders are at greater risk of developing these skin cancers than the general population, but there is a dearth of case reports or well-designed studies of that question.

The first of only two case–control studies found no excess of skin tumours in the welders[45] but, as has been remarked,[46] the welders examined were all well protected (so the dose level may have been unusually low) and young so the length of their exposure was relatively short compared to long-serving career welders and, moreover, they may not have had time to develop skin cancers as a response. The second case–control study found no persuasive evidence of occupational risk factors for melanoma.[47]

Reports have been published of basal cell carcinoma occurring after frequent episodes of cutaneous erythema and peeling induced by welding,[48] a group of five welders with non-melanoma skin cancer,[49] a welder with five squamous cell carcinomas on his hands[46] and a woman who had presented with numerous squamous cell carcinomas on her hands and commented that she had frequently experienced 'sunburn' on her hands after assisting her son with his welding business.[50] Interestingly, in regard to this last case, a case–control study of uveal melanoma has shown an increased risk associated with 'welding burn'.[51]

EYES

Welders normally require stereoscopic vision with good acuity to strike the arc and produce high quality joints. Their eyes should be especially precious to them, yet the eye is the part of the body most commonly injured by welding and related processes in industrial settings. It has been reported from the United States that, as a group, they sustain a higher number of eye injuries than most other types of workers[52] and that eye injuries account for 25 per cent of insurance compensation claims by welders.[53] In a survey of consumer product-related eye injury trauma treated in emergency rooms in hospitals across the United States in the period 1998–2000, welding equipment was estimated to be the product most commonly associated with eye injuries,[54] perhaps reflecting the increasing availability and unprotected use of that equipment by DIY amateurs, in addition to professional workers.

Foreign body eye injuries relate, in the main, to spatter during welding and to associated processes, such as chipping slag from the formed weld, or grinding metal in preparation for welding or after the joint has been made. The foreign body 'missile' may be set in flight by the actions of the injured welder or someone working closely adjacent. The particles may be carried on the wind or fall into the eye from the hair or skin or a protective goggle as it is moved from its perch on the welder's brow to cover his eyes; the process is completed by the welder rubbing his eye.

The high risk of injury makes it essential for the welder and those working around him to wear well-fitting goggles or spectacles with side pieces all the time in the workplace – including when the protection of the helmet or handheld shield is added before the arc is struck.

When a patient has a history of a known intraocular or periorbital foreign body or of occupational exposure to potential metallic ocular injury, as do welders, grinders and metalworkers, it is necessary to screen them with plain radiography before they have a magnetic resonance (MR) scan to ensure the latter is not undertaken during the continued presence of intraorbital metallic foreign bodies.[55]

Despite the periodic welding flashes from the arc, when the appropriate protection is worn, the UV radiation exposure levels reaching the eye are below those needed to cause permanent damage to the corneal endothelium and long-lasting eye damage is reported only very occasionally.[56,57] In contrast, the acute injury 'arc eye' is frequently recorded as the most commonly occurring eye injury of welders.

In that injury, the UV rays from the arc irritate the superficial corneal epithelium of the inadequately protected eyes provoking an inflammatory response which includes oedema, congestion of the conjunctiva and stippling of the corneal epithelium (superficial punctuate keratitis (SPK)), the latter characterized by small pinpoint defects in the superficial corneal epithelium which stain with fluorescein. If SPK is severe, it may be followed by total epithelial desquamation with conjunctival chemosis, lacrimation and blepharospasm. Re-epithelization occurs within 36–72 hours and long-term sequelae are rare.[58]

This is the classical 'arc eye'. It may occur in the welder who is actually producing the harmful emissions. It is often said to occur more commonly in neighbouring welders, other workers and in onlookers who are in the UV radiation area, but are not wearing appropriate eye protection. A recent report showed that whereas 85 per cent of cases received their overexposure from welding, only 3.8 per cent were professional welders with the remainder other occupations with occasional use of welding.[59]

Typically, arc eye is characterized by increasingly intense eye pain, photophobia, a feeling of grittiness, excess lacrimation and reduced visual acuity beginning some 4–12 hours after the exposure, by which time the damaged epithelial cells have sequestered. Symptoms usually resolve spontaneously within 48 hours of exposure.

Although the history may appear to make the diagnosis obvious, care must be taken to examine the eye carefully under local anaesthetic, such as proparacaine 0.5 per cent[58] to exclude trauma (including foreign body), conjunctivitis, corneal ulceration and ulcerative keratitis, and iritis and uveitis. The cornea must be stained with fluorescein to demonstrate the characteristic lesions. A full clinical record should be kept and this should include a note recording that other diagnoses, especially foreign body injury, were positively excluded.

As a first aid measure, some relief may be gained by flushing the eyes for several minutes with water or saline solution. Medical treatment involves administering a short-acting cycloplegic drug,[58,60] such as 1 per cent cyclopentolate or 2 per cent homatropine to relieve the pain of reflex ciliary spasm, a single drop being all that is usually necessary. It is essential to check for glaucoma as these drugs may induce acute glaucoma – though the risk may be small. The use of topical antibiotics in the absence of infection remains controversial but, as a secondary infection is a rare but devastating consequence of a corneal abrasion, their use has been said to be 'a very reasonable course of action' in that situation.[60] An eye patch is not recommended as routine treatment, but may give relief in those with large corneal abrasions.[60] These patients and others with extensive damage should be seen by an ophthalmic specialist without delay.

Patients should not leave the medical facility after treatment until the effects of the local anaesthetic have worn off and must be advised not to drive while the cycloplegic agent is still acting (it is usually safe after about 8–12 hours). They should be told to return if symptoms persist without steady diminution or are unresolved in 48 hours. They should not be given local anaesthetic to reapply as this introduces risks of further injury and may delay healing.

Retinal injuries attributed to radiation in the visible and near-infrared spectrum emitted by a range of arc welding processes have been reported in the literature under several titles,[61–72] but are all the same basic pathology. The radiation penetrates the eye to be absorbed by the retina and rarely causes clinically apparent photochemical or thermal damage. This may be permanent and sight-threatening. It has been reported that the prescription anti-psychotic medication fluphenazine may render workers particularly susceptible to retinal photic damage.[71]

Early diagnosis of the maculopathy may be difficult because it can be masked in the first few days by 'arc eye'. Multifocal electroretinography (ERG)[73] and automatic perimetry have been shown to be useful tools for the detection and quantification of the functional defects.[66] In most cases, retinal injuries heal spontaneously without loss of vision, but severe burns of the macula may lead to permanent complete or partial loss of central vision. They need to be seen by an ophthalmologist without delay.

After a controlled study of a group of welders,[68] it was concluded that the usual protective measures prescribed in professional welding to guard against radiation from the arc are sufficient to prevent an occupational risk of maculopathy and that its occurrence seems to be rather the result of a sequel of occupational accidents and neglect of safety regulations.

Ocular melanoma is the most common primary malignancy of the eye. A rare disease, it usually develops in the uveal tract, most commonly in the choroid which underlies the retina. Diagnosis tends to be late as it is quite literally 'out of sight'. It tends to metastasize before diagnosis, often to the liver, and this makes it a usually fatal disease. The first large case–control study seeking occupational links with melanoma found no persuasive evidence in their data or the scientific literature to link this neoplasm with welding – or any other occupation.[47] At about the same time, a large and more focused case–control study for intraocular melanoma found a significantly increased risk for occupations with welding exposure.[74] This view found some support from a study in France where the investigators considered that they had demonstrated an elevated risk of ocular melanoma in welders, increasing with job duration, and suggested that exposure to ultraviolet light was the likely causal agent.[75] A study in Australia found the risk of choroid and ciliary melanomas increased with increasing duration of welding exposure, although the trend was not significant overall.[76] A meta-analysis soon followed showing that there was evidence implicating welding as a possible risk factor for ocular melanoma.[77] The most recent and largest case–control study covering nine European countries found an excess risk for welders in only one, France.[78]

Accounts of contact lenses adhering to the cornea following exposure to UV and IR radiation from welding circulate periodically. None has been substantiated and there is no evidence to support the contention that welders should not wear contact lenses. Welders may do so, provided they observe the normal rules for their care and limitation on wear.

HEARING

The high sound pressure levels which can be found as background in some welding shops and are emitted by some welding and cutting processes may cause noise-induced hearing loss.[79] That injury may be seriously disabling to a welder as they use their hearing to detect changes in the sound of the welding arc which reflect what is going on at the weld.

PROTECTION OF SKIN, EYES AND HEARING

Care must be taken to protect the skin, eyes and hearing of arc welders and those working with them. Those within 2–3 metres of the arc should wear spark-, fire- and UV-proof protective clothing, without cuffs or pockets that catch sparks. This should be worn closed at the neck and be of a size which allows all exposed skin to be covered, even when the wearer is stretching or squatting.[32,33]

A broad-spectrum high factor, e.g. 50, sunscreen could be a useful adjunct affording extra protection against UVA and UVB in solar radiation should the welder be working outside, but reliance should not be placed on such a preparation to protect against the high intensity of UVC from arc welding as they are usually formulated to be effective between the wavelengths of 297 to 400 nm – with UVC being those wavelengths below 270 nm.

Welders should also wear fire-resistant gauntlet gloves, a helmet or handheld shield and suitable footwear. The headgear should be chosen to give protection from direct and reflected UV[80] and incorporate a filter selected to counter the expected emissions. The welding helmet filter may be 'passive' (constantly dark), in which case the helmet or shield will have to be lifted repeatedly to allow the worker to see the workpiece, or 'auto-darkening' with a light or other sensor to trigger lenses to automatically darken to the correct level of protection. Footwear must have insulating rubber soles which will not melt if hot spatter or metal splashes are stood upon. The uppers must also be impervious to these hot materials. Ankle boots with anti-crush toecaps are advised for all processes. Shoes with protective toecaps may be adequate for use with TIG.

Appropriate hearing protection should be added when working in a noise hazard area. Other additional protection may be needed in particular situations, e.g. a flame-retardant hood, cape with sleeves, chaps and leggings, bib and waist apron, and spats. Comfortable clothing and equipment is more likely to be used, so modern lighter-weight materials should be used whenever possible, provided these give adequate protection.

Because much time at risk is spent with the welding helmet raised or shield discarded, welders should also wear protective goggles or eyewear to guard against non-radiation hazards and arc radiation from neighbouring workers.

Prevention of arc eye requires more than eyewear alone and should follow the full gambit of risk assessment and control from elimination or substitution of the process through to improved personal protection. For example, MIG produces more UV than MMA and TIG. UV radiation also varies within the same process and with the metal being welded. Factors which increase UV emission such as arc energy, arc duration, electrical current and using argon as the shielding gas offer an opportunity to reduce the risks by process modification. Welders working on aluminium, and those in their vicinity, are at the greatest risk of heavy exposure to UV radiation and need the greatest protection, including from reflected rays.

Those in the vicinity of, but not involved in, the welding processes, and this includes passers-by in the street, should be protected from emitted radiation by containing it within the work area by strategically placed screens or curtains. These should absorb the radiation rather than reflect it back at the welder and those working with him/her.

MUSCULOSKELETAL SYSTEM

Manual welding involves a combination of high muscular strain, high precision demands and static muscle loads for the whole body, and especially for the arms and shoulders. Irrespective of position, the high precision demands of the work require postural stabilization, particularly of the hand and arm, which means that the stabilizing muscles of the shoulder are active to a high degree for as long as welding continues.[81,82]

Steps should be taken to minimize the physical stresses welders may experience should they have to lift, carry or manoeuvre heavy workpieces and welding or ventilation equipment; negotiate difficult worksite access or egress; work in confined spaces, such as in pipes or the double bottoms of ships, or in uncomfortable positions such as kneeling, leaning over the workpiece or straining to reach the weld line, always supporting the weight of the gun (electrode holder) and the cables connecting it to the welding unit. The welding gun plus cable may weigh between 1 and 7 kg or more, depending on the process being used.[82]

Musculoskeletal wear and tear injuries and disorders sustained by shipyard welders can render a significant proportion of them incapable of or motivated against work in the full range of normal tasks at the workplace or until the prescribed retirement age.[83,84] Welders were found to have a significantly higher prevalence of musculoskeletal pain than the rate in the general population in Sweden.[85] In the United Kingdom, the rate for those in the welding trade diagnosed with work-related musculoskeletal disorders by specialists in recent years was about twice that of all skilled trades taken together. All this information invites the conclusion that the stresses of manual welding are causing undue wear and tear to the welders' musculoskeletal system. There is evidence of particularly increased risk for shoulder pain and to a lesser extent for disorders in the neck, hand, lower back and lower extremities.[86–88]

Welders have been found in different studies to have significantly higher rates of problems in the shoulder and neck than controls. In one, almost a fifth of welders were affected[87] and it began at an earlier age than in workers in other arduous trades.[88] Much of the shoulder pain is due to inflammatory reactions in the rotator cuff, mainly tendonitis – a condition found ten times more often in those who commonly worked above shoulder level than in the overall study.[89] The supraspinatus muscle in the shoulder is particularly overloaded when the welder is working at or above shoulder level.[90–94]

Development of neck pain may be influenced by the individual welder's posture and static muscle load and in some cases by the dynamic biomechanical loading of the helmet/visor.[93] This is most likely if that equipment is heavy, not fully adjustable and has to be nodded down each time the welder arcs and both his hands are occupied.

Experience suggests that there can be early benefits if priority is given to correcting the intensity of work, the weight of the equipment and workpiece to be handled and the strain induced by the working position. Designing hazards out of the workplace from project conception to completion should proceed in parallel, in consultation with workers, and with improvements being made without delay. Automation should be sought and introduced wherever practicable.

In the workshop, physical strains would be reduced by providing welding tables and workholders which allow welders to set their preferred working height and angle. They may then optimize the hand position between waist and shoulder – without requiring twisted or bent postures – without involving any heavy lifting during adjustment and to choose whether they stand or sit.[94] The risk of shoulder strain should be reduced by designing out the need for overhead welding as far as possible and providing tool and arm support by suspension devices to reduce muscle loading.[92] Returning to neck pain, advantage should be gained by adjusting the welders' work so that less stressful postures can be adopted and equipping them with a lightweight, automatic darkening visor with adjustments for height and angle.

RESPIRATORY SYSTEM

Adverse effects on the respiratory system which have been related to employment as a welder include asphyxia; metal fume fever; perforation of the nasal septum; increased pulmonary infections in terms of severity, duration and frequency; parenchymal diseases such as siderosis; chronic bronchitis and emphysema; chronic obstructive pulmonary disease; occupational asthma; and an apparent increase in the risk of developing lung cancer.

A cause–effect relationship is seldom a matter of contention for the more acute effects of exposure to emissions from welding processes on the respiratory system. In contrast, the possibility and nature of chronic effects of exposure have long been the subjects of research studies with, in general, inconsistent or inconclusive results. This may be due to the absence of such a causal link, the variety of exposures (and thus effects) welders may experience, and/or deficiencies in the study designs. The latter may include healthy worker and survivor population effects operating within the study populations, i.e. workers who become welders or remain in that occupation over the long term may be healthier than the employed population in general.

ASPHYXIA

Asphyxia is a fortunately rare, but sometimes fatal, work-related acute condition suffered by welders through working in inadequately ventilated confined spaces, where the oxygen has been displaced by inert shielding gas or depleted by combustion or, reportedly, rusting of ferrous structures.

Shielding gases are supplied at a flow rate of some 15 L/min. The inert portion passes unchanged from the area of the arc into the workplace. They may leak from connections in supply pipes. Argon is heavier than air so tends to collect in low areas displacing oxygen-bearing air. Inhaling such a gas mixture, which contains little or no oxygen, can cause rapid loss of consciousness. A classic scenario is the welder welding with a gas-shielded process in a confined space with inadequate ventilation and, as he bends down, e.g. to retrieve a dropped object, his head enters the deadly concentration of argon, he loses consciousness, he falls into the gas – and asphyxiates. A Safe System of Work devised before the welding task is begun with inert gases in confined spaces, and followed during the work, should avert the risk of such tragedies. Workers should not enter an atmosphere that contains less than 18 per cent oxygen.

Foolish measures to counter the perceived risks of asphyxia by 'freshening the air' in hot ill-ventilated spaces with oxygen provided as a fuel gas have led to ferocious fires with loss of life in the 'oxygen-enriched' workplace. There is merit in reducing the risk of undetected accumulation of oxygen supplied as a fuel gas or of inert shield gas by odorizing them.[22]

NASAL SEPTUM PERFORATION

This is a rarely reported finding in welders. Once trauma, diseases and other conditions that cause this lesion have been excluded then, provided the welders have been welding stainless steel or other chromium-containing alloys, the perforation may be due to chronic exposure to low concentrations of hexavalent chromium from the fume directly or carried from the process by the contaminated hand.[95,96]

Metal fume fever

Metal fume fever[97–103] is one of the most common acute harmful effects of exposure to welding fume. It is usually an unpleasant, but short-lived, self-limiting flu-like toxic illness beginning some hours after welding has ceased. It may mimic other more serious diseases[104] and has been associated with development of symptoms of welding-related asthma[105] and other serious long-lasting health consequences.[106] It may well be that other effects remain to be identified, particularly in those who have had repeated attacks. Metal fume fever and other 'inhalation fevers' are discussed in more detail under Inhalation fevers, p. 436.

Great care must be taken to consider a diagnosis of pneumonitis during the initial assessment and observation.[107,108] Lest they actually have as-yet undeveloped and undetected chemical pneumonitis – which can progress to serious and even fatal consequences – before sending them home to recover, it is essential to warn workers thought to have metal fume fever to seek further medical assistance without delay if they develop worsening respiratory symptoms. Be especially cautious when cadmium is or may be involved. If this is the case, initial and monitoring investigations should include measuring urinary cadmium concentration and seeking evidence of renal damage.

Pneumonitis and adult respiratory distress syndrome

Rarely, freshly formed oxides of metals, notably zinc or cadmium, produced by welding on coated or plated metal[107,109,110] or using allied processes, such as flame cutting,[111,112] brazing with cadmium-containing solder[113] or metal spraying with an arc process,[114] cause chemical pneumonitis or adult respiratory distress syndrome. These conditions may have a fatal outcome due to respiratory failure. Survivors may be left with persistent pulmonary function abnormalities.[107] In the initial stages, these conditions may mimic metal fume fever. Sufficient investigation to allow an accurate differential diagnosis to be made is essential. It is better to err well on the side of caution, should there be any doubt.

Lobar pneumonia

National statistics of occupational mortality for England and Wales over two,[115] then three,[116] decades suggested that welders have an excess risk of dying from pneumonia attributable to exposure to metal fumes – and that this was not pneumonitis, but rather an excess of pneumococcal and unspecified pneumonia. There was no excess in men over retirement age adding weight to the conclusion that this was a work-related effect. It was suggested that metal components of welding fume, or possibly ozone or oxides of nitrogen, might reversibly increase the susceptibility of the lung to pneumonic infection[116] and, after case–control studies, that this may be attributable specifically to ferrous, and possibly other metal, fumes.[117]

Animal studies first showed that pre-exposure to fumes from MMA welding of stainless steel might result in suppression in immune response and an increase in susceptibility to infection[118] and more recently have demonstrated that short exposure to these fumes caused significant lung damage and suppressed lung defence mechanisms to bacterial infections.[119] Investigations on experienced welders, fresh from exposure at the workplace where they had received a high iron challenge from welding, found a 'noteworthy' absence of an inflammatory response.[120] The conclusion was drawn that chronic exposure to metal fume blunts responsiveness to inhaled particulate matter by an as-yet-undefined mechanism.

Chronic obstructive pulmonary disease

It might be expected from the nature of the mixture of fumes and gases arising from welding processes that, given sufficient time and concentration of exposure, the respiratory system would be irritated sufficiently for there to be a work-related excess risk of COPD and emphysema. This hypothesis has been investigated in many studies – though less so in recent years.

Although excess prevalence of both these diseases and/or adverse changes in lung function has been demonstrated in some studies, this has not been the case in all of them. There is insufficient consistent and statistically convincing evidence of a causal relationship between prolonged exposure to the concentrations of fumes and gases from arc welding processes found in industry and the development of COPD for these to be considered occupational diseases of welders. That said, for the purposes of risk assessments, worker protection and health surveillance, but not for purposes of legislation or litigation, the prudent occupational healthcare worker or employer will not wait for such evidence, but rather will act as if the link had been established – as logic demands that it must be there – and seek out those who may be susceptible and need special protection or are being affected adversely.

To clarify the situation, there is a need for epidemiological studies of sufficiently large cohorts of workers engaged only in welding, preferably mainly 'new starts',[121] and appropriate controls in sufficient numbers to give the required level of statistical power, thoroughly and appropriately assessed at the baseline and thereafter over, perhaps, a decade or two, and with concurrent records of work processes and measurement of exposures.

Occupational asthma

Asthma is characterized by variable airflow limitation and airway hyper-responsiveness. Once sensitized, exposure to very small concentrations of the causative agent will cause a reaction. The long-term effects can be significant in terms of employability. Symptoms include wheezing, coughing, chest tightness and/or shortness of breath. These can come on immediately after exposure or be delayed for several hours. Other associated conditions are rhinitis and/or conjunctivitis.

The incidence of occupational asthma appears to be generally low in welders.[122,123] Most cases are attributed to exposure to hexavalent chromium in fume emitted from welding on stainless steel. There may be no apparent difference in prevalence in surveyed employed welders working on stainless steel compared to those welding mild steel,[124] but this may be due to a survivor effect in the stainless steel welders studied as in most cases it is impossible for the patient to return to and continue with welding work after a diagnosis of occupational asthma.[125]

Employers should assess their workplace for known asthma agents, the risk of exposure, minimize exposure, inform their employees of the findings and precautions and conduct health surveillance, as under Health surveillance, p. 435.

Siderosis

Siderosis is a radiologically apparent pulmonary nodulation exhibited by varying proportions of arc welders of ferrous materials as a result of inhaling and retaining in their lungs a proportion of the iron oxide from the welding fume. It is seen more often after 15 years' exposure, the prevalence then increasing over time. Reports of siderosis being a fibrotic condition are unusual given the huge number of welders exposed to iron compounds in fume. With one exception, such proposals have arisen from individual case reports or small series, some with gross overexposure. The fact that iron clears from the lungs and radiological nodulation regresses after ferrous welding has ceased support the alternative conclusion which may be drawn safely from the many studies undertaken that siderosis alone is a benign condition without related fibrosis or pulmonary dysfunction.

Parenchymal fibrosis

There is, however, no doubt that siderosis and parenchymal fibrosis may coexist in the lungs of welders. Materials in their mixed exposure to which the fibrosis has been attributed include oxides of nitrogen, zinc, silica, hexavalent chromium, nickel compounds, aluminium and asbestos.

Aluminium and asbestos merit further attention as the first is becoming increasingly used and the second is a well-proven cause of parenchymal fibrosis in certain groups of arc welders.

ALUMINIUM

This metal merits attention because it is becoming increasingly used and welded. Emissions from refining aluminium, manufacture of certain abrasives with and the use of aluminium-containing powders are causally associated with specific chronic respiratory diseases. Increased activity of the small airways[126] and reduced expiratory flow through the airways[127] have been noted in aluminium welders. In contrast, the existence of interstitial lung disease caused by exposure to aluminium in general, let alone from aluminium welding, has been the subject of unresolved controversy. There are a very few published individual clinical cases.[128,129] Additionally, two cases of pulmonary granulomatous reactions,[130,131] one of desquamative interstitial pneumonia,[132] and one of severe non-reversible obstructive lung disease[133] have been reported in men employed as welders of aluminium. In each, alternative explanations are offered. No epidemiological evidence has been found in support of the hypothesis of there being a causal relationship between aluminium welding and development of chronic interstitial pulmonary disease. A well-designed and implemented cross-sectional controlled survey of clinical findings and lung function tests, albeit limited by small sample size, published in 1985, did not detect any evidence of pulmonary fibrosis in the study group of 64 aluminium welders.[134] The welders had a higher prevalence of chronic bronchitis than their controls and it is reported that these respiratory symptoms were related to ozone concentrations.

ASBESTOS

Parenchymal fibrosis due to asbestos is found in arc welders, especially those who were employed in shipbuilding or repair yards, locomotive works and similar workplaces, where there was heavy use of crocidolite and amosite – and no adequate protection from exposure. Historically, in such places, they worked among the asbestos during lagging, broke into it to gain access to metal on which to weld, were exposed during delagging and, probably of least importance, used it for their protection – tearing sheets to size, thus maximizing dust emission! They had high and sustained exposures to airborne fibres and have been shown to be affected by the whole range of asbestos-related diseases, including mesothelioma.[135]

Lung cancer

Welding fume has been classified as 'possibly carcinogenic to humans'.[16] National statistics and international epidemiological studies have shown that employment as an arc welder is associated with a sustained higher risk of developing lung cancer than is found in the general population.[16,136–138]

Welding fume from some welding processes contains compounds which are proven carcinogens in other work processes, e.g. hexavalent chromium. The evidence to link the increased risk of lung cancer to these substances or even to processes is not sufficiently strong or consistent to draw firm conclusions regarding specific processes or materials,[138] or even to differentiate between them.[137]

Surveys have shown that, on average, the proportion of welders who smoke or have smoked is likely to be higher than in the general working population.[136] As tobacco smoke is a known lung carcinogen, it must be a strong candidate for at least contributing to causation, but it is also thought likely that the work environment contributes to the excess risk of lung cancer.[13]

A history of working in asbestos-contaminated environments may be an important occupational factor in the excess risk of lung cancer in welders, especially those who smoke or smoked, as people who have been exposed to both asbestos and tobacco have the highest risk for lung cancer.[139] This risk reduces over time since they stopped smoking, emphasizing the importance of smoking prevention and smoking cessation programmes.[139]

Action is needed to control recognized risk factors, such as smoking (by assisting welders to cease), ending all exposure to asbestos (paying particular attention to developing countries[140]), and reducing exposure to the fume and gas emissions from welding processes to at least the nationally defined occupation limits.

ADVERSE EFFECTS ON REPRODUCTION

Investigation of reproductive dysfunction requires wide-ranging evaluation and enquiry, including defining occupation and exposures to environmental and industrial toxins.[141,142] Welders' reproductive health has attracted much research interest, more than most occupations, perhaps because they may be exposed to a combination of agents which have been linked in other circumstances to reproductive dysfunction, such as ionizing radiation, heat, lead, cadmium, chromium, copper and organic solvents. It has been said that the evidence for welding having an adverse effect on male reproduction is strongly supported in well-designed epidemiological studies.[143]

There can be no doubt that several studies present evidence that being a welder carries risks of adverse effects on sperm quality,[144–147] fertility[148] and rate of spontaneous abortion.[149,150] A minority have presented contrary conclusions on some of these matters.[151–153] Also, no adverse effect on the probability of implantation nor increased risk of spontaneous abortion in *in vitro* fertilization (IVF) have been demonstrated.[154,155] Statistically significant associations have been described between spina bifida and paternal exposure to welding fumes and UV.[156] The only reproductive disorder which has been associated with maternal employment as a welder is a possible association with low birthweight, but, importantly, this finding did not survive adjustment for key confounding variables.[157]

Should a welder suggest that his reproductive health is being compromised by his work as a welder, and the quality or quantity of his semen is shown to be subnormal, the several factors mentioned as possible 'causes' should be checked. He should stop smoking. Steps should be taken to reduce his exposure to fumes and/or excessive radiant heat.

HEALTH SURVEILLANCE

Welders should be under a health surveillance programme designed primarily to detect especially susceptible or sensitized workers with regard to occupational asthma, and, to a lesser but probably still worthwhile extent, to monitor and seek to prevent the development of COPD. It also offers opportunities for education and to encourage self-referral for non-respiratory conditions. It has been recommended or prescribed from time to time in regulations and guidance, but the methods to be adopted are rarely defined clearly other than that they are to be in line with the outcome of the risk assessment. An exception is the abundance of good guidance available to help when exposure includes an agent or agents known to cause occupational asthma.

The necessity and design of such health surveillance of welders should be determined after a formal risk assessment has been completed. Surveillance should be undertaken by appropriately trained healthcare workers.[158] Other personnel may be used for monitoring specific aspects or possible effects. Personal records must be kept. These should allow easy analysis of group health. A basic scheme would start with a baseline assessment for each worker, initially before they started work, with the programme being rolled out to encompass all welders and others identified by the risk assessment. This would include an occupational history and record of current work circumstances (place, process, exposures, protection, etc.); completion of a standardized, previously validated, respiratory questionnaire enquiring about work-related upper and lower respiratory symptoms including pre-existing sensitization to substances they might be exposed to in their (new) job; and standardized assessment of lung function (peak expiratory flow and/or FEV_1 and FVC). There should then be periodic review at intervals determined by the risk assessment and the health of the individual worker and an annual formal expert review of absence said to be due to ill health or injury. The workers should be given information, advice and education about the risk, how it should be controlled, recognizing and reporting symptoms, and stopping smoking tobacco. To this may be added an interview on return from absence and special tests, such as audiometry and biological monitoring, as indicated by the risk assessment.

INHALATION FEVERS

Inhalation fevers are related to many occupations other than welding, but are discussed here because the most common is metal fume fever – and welding is the activity most frequently associated with that disorder.

The term 'inhalation fever' collectively describes a group of acute, non-allergic, usually benign and, importantly, self-limiting flu-like illnesses, some with colourful names, which may follow shortly after exposure to any one of a disparate range of inhalable occupational and environmental pollutants. The attack rate is usually higher in those with the highest exposure. Unlike allergic response disorders, there is no discrimination between those with and without previous exposure. Putative pollutants may be grouped, in order of overall population incidence, as metal fumes; pyrolysis products of polymers, principally polytetrafluoroethylene; and bioaerosols. Each of these groups is considered separately below.

There is often a latent period between exposure and the onset of clinical features of an inhalation fever, so the worker may have left the workplace when the illness first becomes apparent. Features may include undulating low-grade – but sometimes high – fever, chills and difficulty keeping warm, shivering, muscle aches and joint pains, headache, malaise and nausea – even vomiting, thirst, chest pain and difficulty breathing and/or breathlessness – the latter ringing alarm bells.

Diagnosis depends largely on pinpointing the cause by way of an appropriately focused and analysed occupational and environmental history – and excluding more serious illness. Physical examination of the chest may be unremarkable or reveal rales and rhonchi. Pulmonary function is commonly unaffected. Although there is likely to be an inflammatory lung infiltrate of polymorphonuclear leukocytes, the chest radiograph should be clear. There is a peripheral blood leukocytosis.

Management of the uncomplicated case of inhalation fever is conservative and supportive. It is usual for the disorder to resolve within two to three days. Of course, the best management is by prevention – seeking to anticipate and control the exposure before cases result, and protecting others who may be at risk of exposure to the damaging pollutant by investigating occupational and environmental sites from which cases arose.

Inhalation fevers may closely mimic or, by their similarities, mask another lung disorder which may be progressive, potentially fatal and result from exposure to pollutants which arise in similar circumstances. It is vital to differentiate specifically between inhalation fever and much more serious conditions. The principal differential diagnosis relevant to inhalation fever includes acute lung injury, infection, hypersensitivity pneumonitis and other immunologic responses.

An alternative diagnosis is likely if improvement does not begin early in the course of the illness and is not completed within two to five days, if at any stage respiratory function is compromised, and/or if infiltrates or other changes are apparent on the chest radiograph. While in inhalation fever occasionally there may be transient acute impairment with reduced lung volume and transfer factor and rarely an asthma-like response, these features should be treated with special suspicion.

Before sending those thought to have an inhalation fever home to recover, it is prudent to consider these alternative diagnoses – and record that this process has been completed and why the decision has been made. Be especially cautious when cadmium is or may be involved. If this is the case, the patient should be kept under observation and initial and monitoring investigations should include measuring urinary cadmium concentration and seeking evidence of renal damage. If the patient is sent or left at home, it is essential to warn them to seek further medical assistance without delay if they develop worsening respiratory symptoms. If recovery does not occur as expected, the diagnosis must be reviewed and the possibility of pneumonitis reconsidered.

The pathogenesis of inhalation fever has yet to be elucidated. The symptoms cannot be engendered by ingestion or intravenous injection of the causative agent, only by inhalation. It is, however, apparent that the lung is not only the sole entry portal and principal target organ, but also the source of whatever substance or substances the inhaled pollutant stimulates to initiate the typical adverse pulmonary and systemic clinically apparent responses.

Research indicates the likelihood of pro-inflammatory cytokines playing a pivotal role.

Metal fume fever

Metal fume fever is one of the few ancient occupational diseases still encountered in modern industrial practice in developed countries. Caused by inhaling freshly formed fumes, and perhaps very finely divided dusts, of some metal oxides, most commonly zinc oxide, it is the most frequently encountered of the inhalation fevers and rejoices in a wide range of names including 'Monday morning fever', 'Monday ague' and 'welder's shakes'. Sometimes, quite moderate concentrations of the pollutant can provoke an attack, especially if the exposure time is prolonged over the work period. Clinical features typical of an inhalation fever (see under Inhalation fever, p. 436) tend to begin some hours after exposure began and often after work has ceased. Symptoms include thirst, chills, muscle aches, shivering and fever, headache and nausea.

If asked, the affected worker will often admit to welding or being in the vicinity of welding on zinc-containing material, galvanized metal being most commonly involved, but the oxides of several other metals have been implicated. These include magnesium, copper, cadmium, chromium, antimony and iron, but the evidence for these is sparse.

A worker with straightforward metal fume fever requires only conservative and supportive treatment while he recovers over one to three days (five days at most). Rarely, he or she will develop pneumonitis when the concentration of fumes has been unusually high or when the situation is complicated by specific acute metal toxic damage, e.g. due to cadmium. As previously mentioned, it is vital to seek to exclude this initially and to advise the patient of this risk, how to recognize that all is not well and to seek further medical aid promptly.

Some welders believe that an attack of metal fume fever early in the working week confers temporary immunity or resistance. There is no scientific evidence for this view, and it may be that the affected welder is more cautious about minimizing his exposure in the days following such an unpleasant illness!

In common with all inhalation fevers, the pathology of metal fume fever is poorly understood. It may mimic other more serious diseases and has been associated with development of symptoms of welding-related asthma and other serious long-lasting health consequences. It may well be that other effects remain to be identified, particularly in those who have had repeated attacks. It has been concluded in a prospective study that it could be a predictor for the development of respiratory symptoms, but not functional abnormalities, in welders.[159]

Treatment is conservative and supportive. Before sending those thought to have metal fume fever home to recover, it is prudent to consider the diagnosis lest they actually have as-yet-undeveloped and undetected chemical pneumonitis – which can progress to serious and even fatal consequences (see under Polymer fever). If the decision is made to send them home, it is essential to warn them to seek further medical assistance without delay if they develop worsening respiratory symptoms. Be especially cautious when cadmium is, or may be, involved. If this is the case, on referral of the individual to hospital, initial and monitoring investigations should also include measuring urinary cadmium concentration and seeking evidence of renal damage.

For completeness, it should be noted that inhalation of zinc chloride, as distinct from zinc oxide, while not precipitating an 'inhalation fever' can cause serious lung injury. Exposures can occur through the use of zinc chloride-containing smoke bombs in military or police training exercises. It is important not to confuse the effects of these two different exposures.

Polymer fever

First described in 1951, this fever has the general clinical characteristics of an inhalation fever. It may occur within eight hours or so of the inhalation of pyrolysis products of fluorocarbon polymers or copolymers, the most commonly reported being polytetrafluoroethylene (PTFE) or Teflon®), exposed to temperatures between 250/300 and 750°C. Under normal usage, Teflon is among the most inert non-toxic and non-inflammable substances, but if it is heated in excess of 750–800°C, it will decompose to form hydrogen fluoride, tetrafluoroethylene, hexafluoropropylene and octofluoroiso-butylene. Other common pyrolysis products include organic fluorides, carbonyl fluoride and perfluoropropane, depending upon the fluorocarbon polymer and the temperature and humidity at which it is burnt.

Outbreaks of polymer fever have been described in workers in an aircraft repair shop and in factories moulding or extruding PTFE, welding on PTFE-coated metal, testing electronic equipment, using mould release sprays and shoe sprays containing fluoropolymers, and in the manufacture of synthetic fabrics, plastics and chemicals, paint and rubber stamps.

Cigarettes rolled or smoked at the workplace and contaminated with particles of polymer may be a source of the fever, pyrolysis products being inhaled with the smoke. A no-smoking rule should be enforced and employees instructed to wash their hands before rolling or smoking cigarettes in permitted areas. Smoking immediately after using a waterproofing spray is thought to have caused an acute respiratory illness in a young man in Japan.[160]

Higher temperature breakdown of PTFE and related polymers produces highly irritant fumes that can cause acute lung injury, rather than inhalation fever. Severe, acute non-cardiogenic pulmonary oedema has been reported after such exposures, e.g. after overheating a Teflon-coated cooking pan.[161] This may have been the situation in a reported case of a syndrome resembling polymer fever, but with chest radiographs consistent with pneumonitis, occurring in the patient shortly after the inhalation of pyrolysed hair spray.[162] It appears that pyrolysis is not always necessary as four cases of toxic pneumonitis with chronic alveolar changes due to direct inhalation of industrial fluorocarbon used as a waterproofing spray for horse rugs has been reported.[163]

Bioaerosols

Inhalation fever may be a response to exposure to a range of bioaerosols, including mouldy organic dust (hay, grain, silage, wood and bark in trimming at sawmills and used as garden mulch); dust from flax, cotton, kapok or hemp; or mould or bacteria-contaminated water mists from humidifiers, air conditioning systems, showers and even jet bath tubs.

Organisms causing inhalation fever may also cause more serious pulmonary and systemic illness. *Legionella pneumophila* contaminating the water in these situations causes the inhalation fever called Pontiac fever and may also cause the more serious Legionnaires' disease (Legionella pneumonia). In contrast to the latter, in Pontiac fever the attack rate is high, the incubation period short at between five and 66 hours, and the illness is benign and self-limiting with resolution in one to five days. Cytophaga, an endotoxin-producing bacteria, was shown to be the cause of both humidifier fever and hypersensitivity pneumonitis in a nylon-producing plant.[164] This further emphasizes the importance and challenge of thorough differential diagnosis in cases of inhalation fever.

Key points

- The work of the welder is widely perceived by those in the occupation, often justifiably, as 'dirty and dangerous'.
- Adverse health effects of most concern include eye, skin and musculoskeletal injuries, acute and chronic respiratory disease, and malignancies of the skin and lung. Occupational injuries are common.
- It is essential to control the risk of exposure to a wide range of potentially harmful particle, gas and radiation emissions, which may vary between and within welding processes.
- A wide range of control and protection measures is available, but their implementation can be a challenging task. Good education and training gives a high return on investment.
- Welders generally warrant pre-employment and periodic health surveillance.
- Metal fume fever is the most common inhalation fever and is most prevalent in welders.

REFERENCES

1. TWI World Centre for Material Joining Technology. Available from: www.twi.co.uk.
2. Kristensen JK. Trends and developments within welding and allied processes. Houdremont Lecture. *Welding in the World.* 2002; **46**: 1–22.
3. Evans MJ, Ingle J, Molyneux MK, Swain J. An occupational hygiene study of a controlled welding task using a general purpose rutile electrode. *Annals of Occupational Hygiene.* 1979; **22**: 1–17.
4. Health and Safety Executive. Analysis of weld-through primers arc welding tests. Report HSL/2007/15. Bootle: HSE, 2007.
5. Tenkate TD. Optical radiation hazards of welding arcs. *Reviews on Environmental Health.* 1998; **13**: 131–46.
6. Sowards JW. Method for sampling and characterizing arc welding fume particles. *Welding in the World.* 2006; **50**: 9–10.
7. Hewett P. The particle size distribution, density and specific surface area of welding fumes from SMAW and GMAW mild and stainless steel consumables. *American Industrial Hygiene Association Journal.* 1995; **56**: 128–35.
8. Hewett P. Estimation of regional deposition and exposure for fumes from SMAW and GMAW mild and stainless steel consumables. *American Industrial Hygiene Association Journal.* 1995; **56**: 136–42.
9. Speigel-Ciobanua VE. The formation of ultrafine particles during welding and allied processes. BIA report 7/2003. BIA Workshop on Ultrafine Aerosols at Workplaces. August 21–22, 2002. St Augustin: BIA, 2002: 151–61, report in German. Available from: www.hvbg.de/d/bia/pub/rep/rep04/bia0703.html.
10. Stephenson D, Seshadri G, Veranth JM, Workplace exposure to submicron particle mass and number concentrations from manual arc welding of carbon steel. *American Industrial Hygiene Association Journal.* 2003; **64**: 516–21.
11. Hovde CA, Raynor PC. Effects of voltage and wire speed on fume characteristics. *Journal of Occupational and Environmental Hygiene.* 2007; **4**: 903–12.
12. Donaldson K, Tran L, Jimenez LA et al. Combustion-derived nanoparticles: A review of their toxicology following inhalation exposure. *Particle and Fibre Toxicology.* 2005; **2**: 10.
13. McMillan GHG. *Lung cancer and electric arc welding.* The Chromium File No. 12. Paris: International Chromium Association, March, 2005.
14. Fiore SR. Reducing exposure to hexavalent chromium in welding fumes. *Welding Journal.* 2006; **August**: 38–42.
15. McMillan GHG. Is electric arc welding linked to manganism or Parkinson's disease. *Toxicological Reviews.* 2005; **24**: 237–57.
16. International Agency for Research on Cancer. Chromium, nickel and welding. IARC Monograph on the Evaluation of Carcinogenic Risks to Humans. Lyon: IARC, 1990, Report No. 49.
17. Engström B. Exposure measurements of ozone in welding. In: Proceedings of International Conference Health and Safety

in Welding and Allied Processes, Copenhagen, Denmark, May 9-11, 2005.
18. Dennis JH, Mortazavi S, French MJ et al. The effects of welding parameters on ultraviolet light emissions, ozone and CrVI formation in MIG welding. *Annals of Occupational Hygiene*. 1997; **41**: 95-104.
19. Dennis JH, French MJ, Hewitt PJ et al. Control of occupational exposure to hexavalent chromium and ozone in tubular wire arc welding processes by use of a secondary shield gas. *Annals of Occupational Hygiene*. 2002; **46**: 43-8.
20. Hansen EB, Thernøe J. Oxides of nitrogen in welding, cutting and oxy-acetylene heating processes – A review of emission rates, exposure levels and control measures. In: Proceedings of International Conference Health and Safety in Welding and Allied Processes, Copenhagen, Denmark, May 9-11, 2005.
21. Health and Safety Executive. Asphyxiation hazards in welding and allied processes. Bootle: HSE, Information document HSE 288/6(REV).
22. Cain WS, Leaderer BP, Cannon L et al. Odorisation of inert gas for occupational safety: Psychophysical considerations. *American Industrial Hygiene Association Journal*. 1987; **48**: 47-55.
23. Carter GJ. Assessing exposure and fume control requirements during arc welding of steel. *Welding and Cutting*. 2004; **3**: 364-71.
24. McMillan GHG. Concerns for the health and safety of welders in 2005. *Welding in the World*. 2006; **50**: 38-44.
25. Health and Safety Executive. Control of fume arising from electric arc welding of stainless steel. Bootle: HSE, Information document HSE 668/29.
26. Semple S. Assessing occupational and environmental exposure. *Occupational Medicine*. 2005; **55**: 419-24.
27. Hansen EB. Measures for control of workplace exposures in welding and cutting. In: Proceedings of International Conference Health and Safety in Welding and Allied Processes, Copenhagen, Denmark, May 9-11, 2005.
28. Health and Safety Executive. Leaflet WL1, Workshop ventilation. Bootle: HSE.
29. Health and Safety Executive. Leaflet WL6. RPE used with forced ventilation. Bootle: HSE.
30. Balieu E. Fundamental aspects in selection and use of respiratory protective devices during welding and cutting processes. In: Proceedings of International Conference Health and Safety in Welding and Allied Processes, Copenhagen, Denmark, May 9-11, 2005.
31. Health and Safety Executive. Welding home page. Last accessed: November 3, 2007. Available from: www.hse.gov.uk/welding/index.htm.
32. Tenkate TD, Collins MJ. Personal ultraviolet radiation exposure of workers in a welding environment. *Journal of the American Industrial Hygiene Association*. 1997; **58**: 33-8.
33. McMillan GHG. Protection of dockyard welders. *The Safety Practitioner*. 1983; **May**: 8-16.
34. Stage J, Vinding T. Metal spark perforation of the tympanic membrane with deafness and facial paralysis. *Journal of Laryngology and Otology*. 1986; **100**: 699-700.
35. Fisher EW, Gardiner Q. Tympanic membrane injury in welders. *Journal of the Society of Occupational Medicine*. 1991; **41**: 86-8.
36. Mertens J, Bubmann M, Reker U. Welding spark injuries of the ear. *Laryngorhinotologie*. 1991; **70**: 405-8.
37. Panosian MD, Dutcher PQ. Transtympanic facial nerve injury in welders. *Occupational Medicine*. 1994; **44**: 99-101.
38. Giddins GE, Wilson Macdonald J. Spot welding injuries of the hand. *Journal of Hand Surgery*. 1994; **19**: 165-7.
39. Shanahan EM, Hanley SD. Soft tissue injury in resistance welding. *Occupational Medicine*. 1995; **45**: 137-40.
40. Jirasek L. Occupational exogenous siderosis of the skin. *Contact Dermatitis*. 1979; **58**: 334.
41. Weiler KJ. Nickel contact eczema caused by electric welding. *Dermatosen in Beruf und Umwelt*. 1979; **27**: 142.
42. Elsner P, Hassam S. Occupational UVC-induced atopic dermatitis in a welder. *Contact Dermatitis*. 1996; **35**: 180-1.
43. Shehade SA, Roberts PJ, Diffey BL, Foulds IS. Photodermatitis due to spot welding. *British Journal of Dermatology*. 1987; **1**: 117-19.
44. Gallagher RP, Lee TK. Adverse effects of ultraviolet radiation: A brief review. *Progress in Biophysics and Molecular Biology*. 2006; **92**: 119-31.
45. Emmett EA, Buncher CR, Suskind RB, Rowe KW Jr. Skin and eye diseases among arc welders and those exposed to welding operations. *Journal of Occupational Medicine*. 1981; **23**: 85-90.
46. Dixon AJ, Dixon BF. Ultraviolet radiation from welding and possible risk of skin and ocular malignancy. *Medical Journal of Australia*. 2004; **181**: 155-7.
47. Fritschi L, Siemiatycki J. Melanoma and occupation: Results of a case-control study. *Occupational and Environmental Medicine*. 1996; **53**: 168-73.
48. Donoughue AM, Sinclair MJ. Basal cell carcinoma after frequent episodes of cutaneous erythema and peeling induced by welding. *Occupational and Environmental Medicine*. 1999; **56**: 646.
49. Currie CL, Monk BE. Welding and non-melanoma skin cancer. *Clinical and Experimental Dermatology*. 2000; **25**: 28-9.
50. Dixon A. Arc welding and the risk of cancer. *Australian Family Physician*. 2007; **36**: 255-6.
51. Holly EA, Aston DA, Char DH et al. Uveal melanoma in relation to ultraviolet light exposure and host factors. *Cancer Research*. 1990; **50**: 5773-7.
52. Harris PM. Nonfatal occupational injuries involving the eyes, 2002. Washington, DC: Bureau of Labor Statistics, US Department of Labour. Compensation and Working Conditions Online. Last accessed October 26, 2007. Available from: www.bls.gov/opub/cwc/sh20040624ar01p1.htm.
53. Lombardi DA, Pannala R, Sorock GS et al. Welding related occupational eye injuries: A narrative analysis. *Injury Prevention*. 2005; **11**: 174-9.
54. McGwin G Jr, Hall TA, Seale J et al. Consumer product-related eye injury in the United States, 1998-2002. *Journal of Safety Research*. 2006; **37**: 501-6.

55. Murphy KJ, Brunberg JA. Orbital plain films as a prerequisite for MR imaging: Is a known history of injury a sufficient screening criterion? *American Journal of Roentgenology.* 1996; **167**: 1053-5.
56. Doughty MJ, Oblak E. A clinical assessment of the anterior eye in arc welders. *Clinical and Experimental Optometry.* 2005; **88**: 387-95.
57. Oblak E, Doughty MJ. Chronic exposure to the ultraviolet radiation levels from arc welding does not result in obvious damage to the human corneal endothelium. *Photochemical and Photobiological Sciences.* 2002; **1**: 857-64.
58. Brozen R. Ultraviolet keratitis. Available from: www.emedicine.com/EMERG/topic759.htm.
59. Yen YL, Lin HL, Lin HJ et al. Photokeratoconjunctivitis caused by different light sources. *American Journal of Emergency Medicine.* 2004; **22**: 511-15.
60. Khaw PT, Shah P, Elkington AR. ABC of eyes: Injury to the eye (authors' reply). *British Medical Journal.* 2004; **328**: 644.
61. Turut P, Isorni MC, Sicard C, Malthieu D. Macular photoinjury caused by a welding arc on an eye with an implant. *Bulletin des Sociétés d'Ophtalmologie de France.* 1986; **86**: 857-9.
62. Cellini M, Profazio V, Fantaguzzi P et al. Photic maculopathy by arc welding. A case report. *International Ophthalmology.* 1987; **10**: 157-9.
63. Brittain GP. Retinal burns caused by exposure to MIG-welding arcs: Report of two cases. *British Journal of Ophthalmology.* 1988; **72**: 570-75.
64. Garcia A, Wiegand W. Retinitis photoelectrica durch Elektroschweissen. *Klinische Monatsblätter für Augenheilkunde.* 1989; **195**: 187-9 (in German).
65. Fich M, Dahl H, Fledelius H et al. Maculopathy caused by welding arcs. A report of three cases. *Acta Ophthalmologica.* 1993; **71**: 402-4.
66. Denk PO, Profazio V, Fantaguzzi P et al. Phototoxische Makulopathie nach Lichtbogenschweissen: Stellenwert des multifokalen ERG [Phototoxic maculopathy after arc welding: value of multifocal ERG]. *Klinische Monatsblätter für Augenheilkunde.* 1997; **211**: 207-10 (in German).
67. Magnavita N. Photoretinitis: An underersimated occupational injury? *Occupational Medicine.* 2002; **52**: 223-5.
68. Maier R, Heilig P, Winker R et al. Welders' maculopathy? *International Archives of Occupational and Environmental Health.* 2005; **78**: 681-5.
69. Choi SW, Chun KI, Lee SJ, Rah SH. A case of photic retinal injury associated with exposure to plasma arc welding. *Korean Journal of Ophthalmology.* 2006; **20**: 250-3.
70. Kim EA, Kim BG, Yi CH et al. Macular degeneration in an arc welder. *Industrial Health.* 2007; **45**: 371-3.
71. Power WJ, Travers SP, Mooney DJ. Welding arc maculopathy and fluphenazine. *British Journal of Ophthalmology.* 1992; **76**: 255.
72. Vicuna-Kojchen J, Amer R, Chowers I. Reversible structural disruption of the outer retina in acute welding maculopathy. *Eye.* 2007; **21**: 127-9.
73. National Horizon Scanning Centre. New and emerging technology briefing. Multifocal electroretinography for the diagnosis of eye disorders. Birmingham, UK: University of Birmingham, July 2002.
74. Holly EA, Aston DA, Ahn DK, Smith AH. Intraocular melanoma linked to occupations and chemical exposures. *Epidemiology.* 1996; **7**: 55-61.
75. Guénel P, Lafirest L, Cyr D et al. Occupational risk factors, ultraviolet radiation, and ocular melanoma: A case-control study in France. *Cancer Causes and Control.* 2001; **12**: 451-9.
76. Vajdic CM, Kricker A, Giblin M et al. Artificial ultraviolet radiation and ocular melanoma in Australia. *International Journal of Cancer.* 2004; **112**: 896-900.
77. Shah CP, Weis E, Lajous M et al. Intermittent and chronic ultraviolet light exposure and uveal melanoma: A meta-analysis. *Ophthalmology.* 2005; **112**: 1599-607.
78. Lutz J-M, Cree I, Sabroe S et al. Occupational risks for uveal melanoma results from a case-control study in nine European countries. *Cancer Causes and Control.* 2005; **16**: 437-47.
79. Rodgers L. Hearing conservation in fabrication shops. *Welding Metal Fabric.* 1993; **May/June**: 417-22.
80. Tenkate TD, Collins MJ. Angles of entry of ultraviolet radiation into welding helmets. *American Industrial Hygiene Association Journal.* 1997; **58**: 54-6.
81. Sporrong H, Palmerus G, Kadefors R, Herbert P. The effect of light manual precision work on shoulder muscles – an EMG analysis. *Journal of Electromyography and Kinesiology.* 1998; **8**: 177-84.
82. Kadefors R. Static workload in the extreme. A review of musculoskeletal disorders in manual welders, and an evaluation model for welding work. *Zeitschrift für Arbeitswissenschaft.* 2005; **59**: 361-6.
83. McMillan GHG, Molyneux MK. The health of welders in naval dockyards: The work situation and sickness absence patterns. *Journal of the Society of Occupational Medicine.* 1981; **31**: 43-60.
84. Wanders SP, Zielhuis GA, Vreuls HJH, Zielhuis RL. Medical wastage in shipyard welders: A forty-year historical cohort study. *International Archives of Occupational and Environmental Health.* 1992; **64**: 281-91.
85. Report of the Health Risk Study Group to the Swedish Commission of Working Conditions. A survey of jobs posing special risks to health. Stockholm: Ministry of Labour, 1990.
86. Torell G, Sandén Å, Järvholm B. Musculoskeletal disorders in shipyard workers. *Journal of the Society of Occupational Medicine.* 1988; **38**: 109-13.
87. Herberts P, Kadefors R. A study of painful shoulder in welders. *Acta Orthopaedica Scandinavica.* 1976; **44**: 381-7.
88. Herberts P, Kadefors R, Anderson G, Petersén I. Shoulder pain in industry: An epidemiological study on welders. *Acta Orthopaedica Scandinavica.* 1981; **52**: 299-306.
89. Hageberg M, Wegman DH. Prevalence rates and odds ratios of shoulder-neck diseases in different occupational groups. *British Journal of Industrial Medicine.* 1987; **44**: 602-10.

90. Kadefors R, Petersén I, Herberts P. Muscular reaction to welding work: An electromyographic investigation. *Ergonomics.* 1976; **19**: 543–58.
91. Herberts P, Kadefors R, Högfors C, Sigholm G. Shoulder pain and heavy manual labor. *Clinical Orthopaedics.* 1984; **191**: 166–78.
92. Jarvholm U, Palmerud G, Kadefors R, Herberts P. The effect of arm support on supraspinatus muscle load during simulated assembly work and welding. *Ergonomics.* 1991; **34**: 57–66.
93. Eklund J, Gunnarsson K. Loadings on the neck when welding with vizors. Book of abstracts, PREMUS-92, *Arbete och Hälsa.* 1992; **17**: 78–9 (also available as International Institute of Welding Document VIII-1674-93).
94. Van der Veen F. Productivity or quality of work as the decisive factor in marketing ergonomics. Design considerations for a new ergonomic welding table. *Ergonomics.* 1990; **33**: 407–11.
95. Jindrichova J. Chromium-induced injuries in electric welders. *Zeitschrift für die gesamte Hygiene und ihre Grenzgebiete.* 1978; **24**: 86–8.
96. Lee CR, Yoo CI, Lee J, Kanq SK. Nasal septum perforation of welders. *Industrial Health.* 2002; **40**: 286–9.
97. Mueller EJ. Metal fume fever – a review. *Journal of Emergency Medicine.* 1985; **2**: 271–4.
98. McMillan GHG. Metal fume fever. *Occupational Health* 1986; **May**: 148–9.
99. Van Pee D, Vandenplas O, Gillet JB. Metal fume fever. *European Journal of Emergency Medicine.* 1998; **5**: 465–6.
100. Ebran B, Quieffin J, Beduneau G, Guyonnaud CD. Radiological evidence of lung involvement in metal fume fever. *Revue de Pneumologie Clinique.* 2000; **56**: 361–4.
101. Fuortes L, Schenck D. Marked elevation of urinary zinc levels and pleural friction rub in metal fume fever. *Veterinary and Human Toxicology.* 2000; **42**: 164–5.
102. Kelleher P, Pacheco K, Newman LS. Inorganic dust pneumonias: The metal-related parenchymal disorders. *Environmental Health Perspectives.* 2000; **108** (Suppl. 4): 685–96.
103. Kaye P, Young H, O'Sullivan I. Metal fume fever: A case report and review of the literature. *Emergency Medical Journal.* 2002; **19**: 268–9.
104. Hassaballa HA, Lateef OB, Bell J et al. Metal fume fever presenting as aseptic meningitis with pericarditis, pleurisy and pneumonitis. *Occupational Medicine.* 2005; **55**: 638–41.
105. El-Zeim M, Infante-Rivard C, Malo JL, Gautrin D. Is metal fume fever a determinant of welding related respiratory symptoms and/or increased bronchial responsiveness? A longitudinal study. *Occupational and Environmental Medicine.* 2005; **62**: 688–94.
106. Dube D, Puruckherr M, Byrd RP Jr, Roy TM. Reactive airways dysfunction syndrome following metal fume fever. *Tennessee Medicine.* 2002; **95**: 236–8.
107. Barnhart S, Rosenstock L. Cadmium chemical pneumonitis. *Chest.* 1984; **86**: 789–91.
108. Ando Y, Shibata E, Tsuchiyama F, Sakai S. Elevated urinary cadmium concentrations in a patient with acute cadmium poisoning. *Scandinavian Journal of Work and Environmental Health.* 1996; **22**: 150–3.
109. Patwardhan JR, Finckh ES. Fatal cadmium fume pneumonitis. *Medical Journal of Australia.* 1976; **1**: 962–6.
110. Taniguchi H, Suzuku K, Fujisaka S et al. Diffuse alveolar damage after inhalation of zinc oxide fumes. *Nihon Kokyuki Gakkai Zasshi.* 2003; **41**: 447–50 (in Japanese).
111. Fernández MA, Sanz P, Palomar M et al. Fatal chemical pneumonitis due to cadmium fumes. *Occupational Medicine.* 1996; **46**: 372–4.
112. Barbee JY Jr, Prince TS. Acute respiratory distress syndrome in a welder exposed to metal fumes. *Southern Medical Journal.* 1999; **92**: 510–12.
113. Seidal K, Jörgensen N, Elinder CG et al. Fatal cadmium-induced pneumonitis. *Scandinavian Journal of Work and Environmental Health.* 1993; **19**: 429–31.
114. Rendall REG, Phillips JI, Renton KA. Death following exposure to fine particulate nickel from a metal arc process. *Annals of Occupational Hygiene.* 1994; **38**: 921–30.
115. McMillan GHG, Pethybridge RJ. The health of welders in naval dockyards: Proportional mortality study of welders and two control groups. Appendix, An appraisal of the use of data in the Registrar General's Decennial Supplement on Occupational Mortality. *Journal of the Society of Occupational Medicine.* 1983; **33**: 75–84.
116. Coggon D, Inskip H, Winter P, Pannet B. Lobar pneumonia: An occupational disease in welders. *Lancet.* 1994; **344**: 4–5.
117. Palmer KT, Poole J, Ayres JG et al. Exposure to metal fume and infectious pneumonia. *American Journal of Epidemiology.* 2003; **157**: 227–33.
118. Antonini JM, Taylor MD, Millechia L et al. Suppression in lung defense responses after bacterial infection in rats pretreated with different welding fumes. *Toxicology and Applied Pharmacology.* 2004; **200**: 206–18.
119. Antonini JM, Stone S, Roberts JR et al. Effect of short-term stainless steel welding fume inhalation exposure on lung inflammation, injury and defense responses in rats. *Toxicology and Applied Pharmacology.* 2007; **223**: 234–45.
120. Palmer KT, McNeill Love RM et al. Inflammatory responses to the occupational inhalation of metal fume. *European Respiratory Journal.* 2006; **27**: 366–73.
121. El-Zein M, Malo JL, Infante-Rivard C, Gautrin D. Incidence of probable occupational asthma and changes in airway calibre and responsiveness in apprentice welders. *European Respiratory Journal.* 2003; **22**: 513–18.
122. Beach JR, Dennis JH, Avery AJ et al. An epidemiologic investigation of asthma in welders. *American Journal of Respiratory and Critical Care Medicine.* 1996; **154**: 1394–400.
123. McDonald JC, Chen Y, Zekveld C, Cherry NM. Incidence by occupation and industry of acute work related respiratory disease in the UK, 1992–2001. *Occupational and Environmental Medicine.* 2005; **62**: 836–42.
124. Wang ZP, Larsson K, Malmberg P et al. Asthma, lung function and bronchial responsiveness in welders. *American Journal of Industrial Medicine.* 1994; **26**: 741–54.

125. Hannu T, Piipari R, Tuppurainen M et al. Occupational asthma caused by stainless steel welding fumes: A clinical study. *European Respiratory Journal*. 2007; **29**: 85-90.
126. Nielsen J, Dahlqvist M, Welinder H et al. Small airways function in aluminium and stainless steel welders. *International Archives of Occupational and Environmental Health*. 1993; **65**: 101-5.
127. Fishwick D, Bradshaw L, Slater T et al. Respiratory symptoms and lung function changes in welders: Are they associated with workplace exposures? *New Zealand Medical Journal*. 2004; **117**: U872.
128. Vallyathan V, Bergeron WN, Robichaux PA, Craighead JE. Pulmonary fibrosis in an aluminium arc welder. *Chest*. 1982; **81**: 372-4.
129. Hull MJ, Abraham JL. Aluminum welding fume-induced pneumoconiosis. *Human Pathology*. 2002; **33**: 819-25.
130. De Vuyst P, Dumortier P, Schandené L et al. Sarcoid-like granulomatosis induced by aluminium dusts. *American Reviews of Respiratory Diseases*. 1987; **135**: 493-7.
131. Fireman E, Goshen M, Ganor E et al. Induced sputum as an additional tool in the identification of metal-induced sarcoid-like reaction. *Sarcoidosis, Vasculitis, and Diffuse Lung Diseases*. 2004; **21**: 152-6.
132. Herbert MJ, Sterling G, Abrahma J, Corrin B. Desquamative interstitial pneumonia in an aluminium welder. *Human Pathology*. 1982; **13**: 694-9.
133. Balkissoon R. A 26 year old welder with severe non-reversible obstructive lung disease. *Chronic Obstructive Pulmonary Disease*. 2006; **3**: 63-7.
134. Sjøgren B, Ulfvarson U. Respiratory symptoms and pulmonary function among welders working with aluminum, stainless steel and railroad tracks. *Scandinavian Journal of Work and Environmental Health*. 1985; **11**: 27-32.
135. McMillan GHG. The health of welders in naval dockyards. The risk of asbestos-related diseases occurring in welders. *Journal of Occupational Medicine*. 1983; **25**: 727-30.
136. Steenland K. Ten-year update on mortality among mild steel welders. *Scandinavian Journal of Work and Environmental Health*. 2002; **28**: 163-7.
137. Ambroise D, Wild P, Moulin JJ. Update of a meta-analysis on lung cancer and welding. *Scandinavian Journal of Work and Environmental Health*. 2006; **32**: 22-31.
138. Sørensen AR, Thulstrup AM, Hansen J et al. Risk of lung cancer according to mild steel and stainless steel welding. *Scandinavian Journal of Work and Environmental Health*. 2007; **33**: 379-86.
139. Reid A, de Klerk NH, Ambrosini GL et al. The risk of lung cancer with increasing time since ceasing exposure to asbestos and quitting smoking. *Occupational and Environmental Medicine*. 2006; **63**: 509-12.
140. Joshi TK, Gupta RK. Asbestos in developing countries. Magnitude of risk and its practical implications. *International Journal of Occupational Medicine and Environmental Health*. 2004; **17**: 179-85.
141. Sheiner EK, Sheiner E, Hammel RD et al. Effect of occupational exposures on male fertility: Literature review. *Industrial Health*. 2003; **41**: 55-62.
142. Burdorf A, Figà-Talamanca I, Jensen TK, Thulstrup AM. Effects of occupational exposure on the reproductive system: Core evidence and practical implications. *Occupational Medicine*. 2006; **56**: 516-20.
143. Jensen TK, Bonde JP, Joffe M. The influence of occupational exposure on male reproductive function. *Occupational Medicine*. 2006; **56**: 544-53.
144. Bonde JP. Semen quality and sex hormones among mild steel and stainless steel welders: A cross sectional study. *British Journal of Industrial Medicine*. 1990; **47**: 508-14.
145. Bonde JP. Semen quality in welders before and three weeks after non-exposure. *British Journal of Industrial Medicine*. 1990; **47**: 515-18.
146. Bonde JP. Semen quality in welders exposed to radiant heat. *British Journal of Industrial Medicine*. 1992; **49**: 1055-6.
147. Danadevi K, Rozati R, Reddy R, Paramjit G. Semen quality of Indian welders occupationally exposed to nickel and chromium. *Reproductive Toxicology*. 2003; **17**: 451-6.
148. Bonde JP, Hansen KS, Levine RJ. Fertility among Danish male welders. *Scandinavian Journal of Work and Environmental Health*. 1990; **16**: 315-22.
149. Kolstad HA, Bonde JP, Hjollund NH et al. Menstrual cycle pattern and fertility: A prospective follow-up study of pregnancy and early embryonal loss in 295 couples who were planning their first pregnancy. *Fertility and Sterility*. 1999; **71**: 490-6.
150. Hjollund NHI, Bonde JPE, Jensen TK et al. Male-mediated spontaneous abortion among spouses of stainless steel welders. *Scandinavian Journal of Work and Environmental Health*. 2000; **26**: 187-92.
151. Bonde JP, Ernst E. Sex hormones and semen quality in welders exposed to hexavalent chromium. *Human and Experimental Toxicology*. 1992; **11**: 259-63.
152. Hjollund NHI, Bonde JPE, Jensen TK et al. Semen quality and sex hormones with reference to metal welding. *Reproductive Toxicology*. 1998; **12**: 91-5.
153. Hjollund NHI, Bonde JPE, Jensen TK et al. A follow-up study of male exposure to welding and time to pregnancy. *Reproductive Toxicology*. 1998; **12**: 29-37.
154. Tielemans E, van Kooij R, Looman C et al. Paternal occupational exposures and embryo implantation rates after IVF. *Fertility and Sterility*. 2000; **74**: 690-5.
155. Hjollund NH, Bonde JP, Ernst E et al. Spontaneous abortion in IVF couples – a role of male welding exposure. *Human Reproduction*. 2005; **20**: 1793-7.
156. Blatter BM, Hermens R, Bakker M et al. Paternal occupational exposure around conception and spina bifida in offspring. *American Journal of Industrial Medicine*. 1997; **32**: 283-91.
157. Farrow A, Shea KM, Little RE et al. Birthweight of term infants and maternal occupation in a prospective cohort of pregnant women. *Occupational and Environmental Medicine*. 1998; **55**: 18-23.
158. McMillan GHG. Welders' health examinations. *Journal of the Society of Occupational Medicine*. 1979; **29**: 87-92.
159. El-Zein M, Infante-Rivard C, Malo JL, Gautrin D. Is metal fume fever a determinant of welding related respiratory

symptoms and/or increased bronchial responsiveness? A longitudinal study. *Occupational and Environmental Medicine.* 2005; **62**: 688–94.
160. Kobayashi K, Tachikawaka S, Horiquchi T *et al.* A couple suffering acute respiratory illness due to waterproofing spray exposure. *Nihon Kokuyi Gakkai Zasshi.* 2006; **44**: 647–52.
161. Son M, Maruyama E, Shindo Y *et al.* Case of polymer fever with interstitial pneumonia caused by inhalation of polytetrafluorethylene (Teflon). *Chudoku Kenkyu.* 2006; **19**: 279–82 (in Japanese, English abstract).
162. Delgado JH, Waksman JC. Polymer fume fever-like syndrome due to hairspray inhalation. *Veterinary and Human Toxicology.* 2004; **46**: 266–7.
163. Wallace GM, Brown PH. Horse rug lung: Pneumonitis due to fluorocarbon inhalation. *Occupational and Environmental Medicine.* 2005; **62**: 414–16.
164. Nordness ME, Zacharisen MC, Schlueter DP, Fink JN. Occupational lung disease related to cytophaga endotoxin exposure in a nylon plant. *Journal of Occupational Medicine.* 2003; **45**: 385–92.

45

The semiconductor industry

DAVID KOH AND JUDY SNG

Introduction	444
Semiconductor materials	444
Semiconductor devices	445
Work processes in semiconductor manufacturing	445
Hazards in semiconductor manufacturing	447
Health issues in the semiconductor industry	449
Impact on the environment	451
Conclusion	451
References	452

INTRODUCTION

The semiconductor industry has developed rapidly over the past few decades and is expected to continue expanding. In 1965, Gordon E Moore, cofounder of Intel (currently the world's largest silicon supplier), predicted that the number of transistors on a chip would double every two years.[1] This has come to be known as 'Moore's Law', which reflects the increasing complexity and performance of the devices and rapid progress of the industry. The sales volume of the electronics industry could comprise about 10 per cent of the gross world product if current growth trends continue. The electronics industry is heavily dependent on the semiconductor industry, thus both can be expected to grow together.[2] According to the Semiconductor Industry Association, worldwide semiconductor sales totalled US$232.7 billion in the first 11 months of 2008.[3]

A July 2007 press release from the Semiconductor Industry Association stated that in the United States, the chip industry employs a domestic workforce of 232 000 people.[4] In 2001, in the United Kingdom, about 10 000 people were employed directly within the semiconductor industry, and 5000 within the supply base, and a further 30 000 engineers were involved in research and development for the industry.[5]

In its early days, semiconductor manufacturing was mostly located in California (Silicon Valley) and Texas. However, since the 1960s, the industry has spread to many other countries such as Taiwan, Japan, Korea, Singapore, China and India. Taiwan alone is responsible for 70 per cent of total worldwide production of CD-ROM (compact disc read-only memory) devices, as well as 50 per cent of world production of light-emitting diodes with integrated circuit products. In a 2004 evaluation, more than 30 000 people were employed in Taiwan's semiconductor industry in 350 companies located in the Hsinchu science-based industrial park.[6] In 2006, in India, the semiconductor and embedded design industry generated a revenue of approximately US$4.6 billion and employed almost 102 000 people. By 2015, this is projected to increase to a revenue of US$43 billion and a workforce of 780 000.[4]

The industry is now growing most rapidly in the Asia Pacific region. Previously, this rapid growth was mainly due to demand from countries in the west resulting in a move of their manufacturing bases to Asia. Today, growth in production in this region is mainly a result of increasing domestic demand.[7]

SEMICONDUCTOR MATERIALS

At the heart of the industry is the unique electrical property of substances that are neither conductors nor insulators. A semiconductor is a material whose conductivity is normally between that of a metal and an insulator. In addition, altering temperature or chemical composition can change the conductivity of a semiconductor material.[8]

There are essentially three classes of semiconductor materials:

1. Elemental semiconductors, such as silicon and germanium
2. Compound semiconductors, such as gallium arsenide and indium phosphide
3. Alloy semiconductors, such as silicon germanium and aluminium gallium arsenide.

Silicon is currently still the most widely used material. Gallium arsenide and aluminium gallium arsenide have been used in recent years in the development of quantum-effect semiconductor devices.[9]

SEMICONDUCTOR DEVICES

The term 'semiconductor device' usually refers to an integrated circuit (IC or chip). This is a tiny electronic circuit that is created on the surface of a semiconductor substrate, such as a wafer of silicon. The world's first integrated chip was demonstrated by Texas Instruments in 1958.[10]

Integrated chips are now used in many home and office items, including personal computers, mobile phones and household appliances, such as washing machines and televisions. Diodes and transistors are also semiconductor devices. These are frequently seen in applications such as light emitting diodes (LEDs) and laser diodes which are used in digital video devices (DVDs) and compact disc read-only memory devices (CD ROMs).[11]

WORK PROCESSES IN SEMICONDUCTOR MANUFACTURING

In semiconductor device fabrication, electronic circuits are built on to a wafer of pure semiconductor material in a series of intricate processes. It takes several weeks to complete the entire manufacturing process from raw materials to packaged chips.

There is a high degree of automation in semiconductor fabrication factories and much of the work processes are enclosed and take place in clean rooms. In a typical semiconductor manufacturing clean room, the humidity is kept low and the air is recirculated through high efficiency particulate absolute filtration units to ensure a dust-free environment (Figure 45.1). These measures are for the protection of the highly sensitive products, where a single speck of dust or spot of condensation could cause profound damage and malfunction. In such an environment, workers are also required to wear special protective gowns, caps, facemasks and boots to prevent them from unintentionally contaminating the materials.

Briefly, the manufacturing process comprises front end processing, which involves production of wafers from pure silicon ingots and fabrication of integrated circuits on to the wafers, and back end processing, which involves assembly and testing, of the finished products (Figure 45.2). The work processes vary widely depending on the desired final product.

Front end processing

SILICON WAFER PRODUCTION

Sand is used to obtain purified polycrystalline silicon which is then melted. A pure silicon crystal ingot is grown

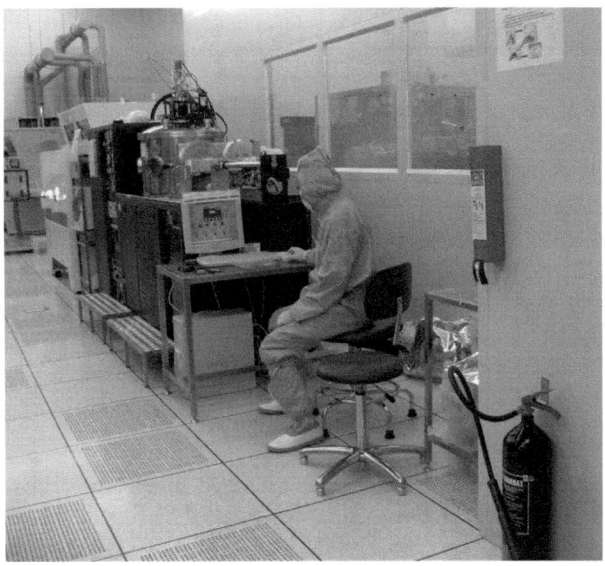

Figure 45.1 Typical clean room attire and set up. Note also the fire safety equipment in the foreground.

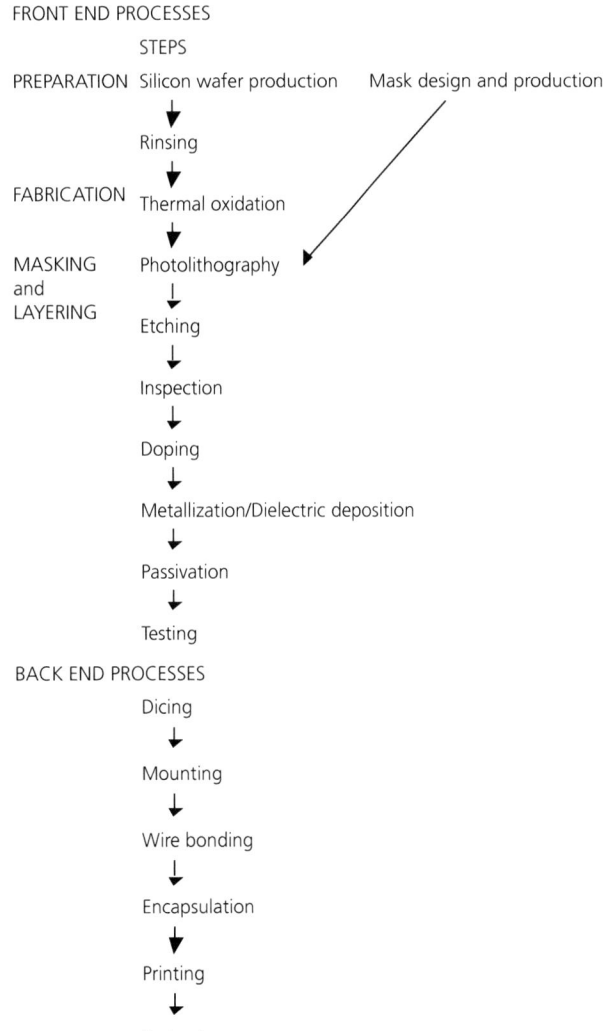

Figure 45.2 Manufacturing process for semiconductors.

from a 'seed' – a small piece of pure silicon placed in the molten silicon bath. The seed is gradually drawn up from the bath to form the ingot.

The ingot is sliced into thin wafers by a diamond blade, ground smooth and chemically polished. These wafers are the base for the manufacture of integrated circuits. Some companies list another step known as epitaxy, in which another 0.5–20 micron-thin layer of ultrapure silicon is grown over the wafer to enhance subsequent processes and overall performance of the wafer. The techniques for epitaxy vary from chemical vapour deposition to the newer molecular beam epitaxy.

PRODUCTION OF MASKS

The required patterns for the integrated circuits are drawn on to chromium-plated quartz glass plates to form reticles or stencil-like instruments. The chromium plating is removed by lasers or electron beams to form a negative image of the pattern. This plate will subsequently be used as a mask or stencil in photolithography to imprint the patterns on to the silicon chips.

FABRICATION

This is a key step in any semiconductor manufacturing, and takes from 1.5 to more than 4 weeks to complete, all within the highly controlled clean room environment.

The wafers are rinsed with deionized water and chemicals (such as diluted hydrochloric/hydrofluoric acid) and then exposed to high temperature and oxygen concentration to induce thermal oxidation – the growth of a uniformly thin insulating film of silicon dioxide on the surface.

Next, the wafers are coated with photoresist – a light-sensitive polymer film which becomes soluble when exposed to ultraviolet light (Figure 45.3).

In a process known as photolithography, ultraviolet light is passed through a patterned glass mask (a stencil) on to the wafer. Thus the pattern is transferred from the glass mask to the wafer. The exposed areas of photoresist become softened by the ultraviolet light and are subsequently washed away with a solvent. The areas of exposed silicon dioxide are etched away with chemicals such as hydrofluoric acid (wet etching) or plasma etching/reactive ion etching (dry etching). The rest of the photoresist is then removed and the wafers are visually inspected for accuracy of image transfer before being transferred to the next step.

Doping or ion implantation is the next process, where impurities (dopants) are introduced into the exposed areas of the wafer to alter the electrical conductivity of the silicon. Arsenic, boron, antimony and phosphorus are some commonly used dopants.

The above steps are repeated many times to achieve multiple differently patterned layers on the wafer.[12,13]

Atoms of metal (usually aluminium or copper) are deposited into windows created in the wafer, interconnecting the individual devices. This process is known as 'metallization'. Dielectric films (insulators) are also inserted to separate the components. The circuit is then coated with another protective insulating layer (passivation).

Hundreds of microprocessors are created on one wafer. Every wafer is inspected both macroscopically and with the use of a microscope for scratches and defective patterns. Every single microprocessor is also tested to ensure it is functioning properly. Defective chips are marked for automatic rejection.

At the back end processing factory, a diamond saw cuts the wafer, separating the individual microprocessors (dicing). The chips are mounted on lead frames ('lead' as in 'leader', not the metal Pb) and connected to the frame by wire bonding. Either gold, aluminium or copper is used to connect the chip to the package. The chips are then inspected again before being encapsulated in resin for protection.

The substances used in the manufacturing process are presented in Table 45.1. This is by no means an exhaustive list, but serves to illustrate the large number of chemicals involved.

Recent advances

New techniques and substrates are frequently being tried and introduced in the race to find more precise techniques to produce smaller and faster devices. As a result, the work processes in the semiconductor industry are continually changing. The implications of the substrates and equipment used in new work processes remain to be seen with time.

Shorter wavelength light produced using krypton fluoride or argon fluoride is gradually replacing ultraviolet light for more accurate transcription of miniaturized circuit patterns.[14]

Laser beams are also increasingly being used for more precise dicing of the wafers at the start of back end processing.

An interesting new development is the flexible thin film transistor which can be applied in novel ways, such as paper-like roll-up displays and conformable x-ray

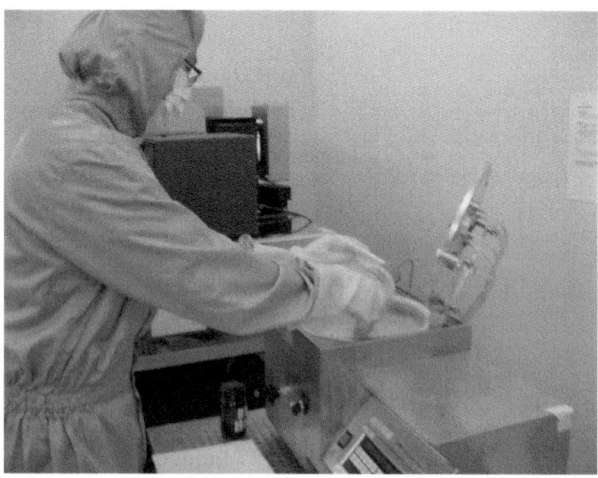

Figure 45.3 Cleaning the photoresist spin-coater in a research laboratory.

Table 45.1 Materials used in semiconductor manufacturing.

Substance		Use(s)
Semiconductors and metals	Aluminium	Integrated circuit metallization, conductor between components
	Boron	Dopant
	Copper	Lead frame component, metallization
	Germanium	Semiconductor substrate, often as compound or alloy
	Gold	Interconnecting wires between integrated circuit to lead frame
	Silicon	Semiconductor substrate
	Silver	In assembly, packaging
Acids	Hydrofluoric acid	Etching of silicon dioxide
	Hydrochloric acid	Etching
	Sulphuric acid	Stripping plastic and organic material
	Nitric acid	Etching, plastic package decapsulation
	Phosphoric acid	Removal of aluminium and silicon nitride
	Chromic acid	Cleaning and etching
Alkalis	Ammonium hydroxide	In etching processes
	Potassium hydroxide	As above
	Sodium hydroxide	As above
Amines and amides	Trimethylamine	Photoresist coating and stripping
	Triethylamine	
	Dimethylacetamide	
Organic solvents	Acetone	Solvents are mainly used for cleaning, rinsing and drying
	Ethylene glycol	
	Isopropyl alcohol	Ethylene glycol is used in etching
	Methyl alcohol	
	Methyl ethyl ketone	
	Xylene	
Oxidizers	Hydrogen peroxide	Cleaning and etching
	Oxygen	Thermal oxidation, plasma etching
Gases	Arsine	Source of arsenic for doping
	Ammonia	Source of nitrogen; wafer cleaning and polishing
	Boron trifluoride	Doping
	Chlorine	Etching
	Diborane	Doping agent and source of boron
	Nitrogen trifluoride	Cleaning of chemical vapour deposition reactors
	Ozone	Chemical vapour deposition, oxide growth, photoresist removal
	Phosphine	Source of phosphorus for doping
	Silane	
	Tungsten hexafluoride	

Adapted from www.siliconfareast.com/semicon_matls.htm.

imagers.[15] The use of dip-pen nanolithography in semiconductor manufacture processes is also being explored for use in the fabrication of multilayered metal-semiconductor nanostructures.[16]

HAZARDS IN SEMICONDUCTOR MANUFACTURING

Chemical hazards

Numerous chemicals are used in semiconductor wafer fabrication, many of which present either safety, corrosion or health hazards. Two issues arise from this. First, multiple concurrent chemical exposures from daily operations and maintenance work are likely to cause health issues that are very different from those resulting from single chemical exposure. There are few data on this issue. Second, possible health effects of other chemicals which might be overlooked (such as byproducts from the reactions between various process chemicals, as well as chemicals used for maintenance and cleaning) need to be considered.

Fortunately, most of these chemicals are used within contained systems in the high-tech environment of semiconductor factories, and thus typically exposure to employees would be minimal. Many companies have sophisticated engineering control measures to ensure that workers are protected from exposure during normal production runs. Common engineering control measures used include maintaining the processes under reduced pressure, purging of chambers with inert gas before products are removed by workers and monitored process exhaust systems.

However, when maintenance work needs to be performed, some of the engineering controls may need to be either bypassed or shut down. It is then that the possibility of workers coming into contact with the hazardous chemicals is higher. This would be less likely during routine scheduled maintenance work and more likely when the maintenance work is unscheduled, such as in the event of system malfunction. Additional exposure prevention measures need to be preplanned and communicated to the relevant workers.[17]

Hydrofluoric and hydrochloric acid are used in wet etching and to rinse the silicon wafers prior to thermal oxidation. Both are highly corrosive mineral acids which can cause severe chemical burns. Hydrogen fluoride can also cause hypocalcaemia, hypomagnesaemia and death if systemic absorption occurs.[18] Chromic acid used in etching and cleaning can ignite on contact with alcohol. The International Agency for Research on Cancer (IARC) has also designated chromic acid as a confirmed human carcinogen.[19]

Some etching processes also involve the use of strong alkalis such as sodium hydroxide and potassium hydroxide.

Arsine, phosphine and diborane gases used in doping are flammable or potentially explosive. These gases also carry a health risk: arsine is a potent haemolytic agent, while phosphine reacts with moisture to form phosphoric acid which can cause acute respiratory irritation. Gas detectors for toxic materials are commonly found in clean rooms. (Figure 45.4).

The thermal oxidation of pure silicon wafers requires high concentrations of oxygen coupled with high temperatures of about 1000°C. There is a potential fire and explosion hazard if any reactive or combustible material is accidentally included in the chamber.[20]

Some of the metals used to generate dopant atoms, as well as alloy and compound semiconductors, are health hazards. Inorganic arsenic causes hyperkeratosis, peripheral neuropathy and anaemia, and has been classified by the IARC as a confirmed human carcinogen. Antimony causes both acute effects of respiratory and mucous membrane irritation, as well as chronic effects of pneumoconiosis, pustular dermatitis and nasal septum perforation.[21] Antimony is a suspected human carcinogen.

Many organic solvents are used in semiconductor manufacturing to clean, rinse or dry the chips. The commonly encountered ones are isopropyl alcohol, n-butyl acetate, xylene, acetone, methanol, methoxy ethanol, petroleum distillates, trichloroethane, methylene chloride, tetrachloroethylene, ethylene glycol and methyl ethyl ketone.

Ethylene glycol ether used in photolithography has been linked to prolonged menstrual cycles[22] and prolonged time to pregnancy.[23] Although the use of ethyl and methyl glycol ethers appears to have been phased out since 1992 in the United States,[24] they may still be used in factories

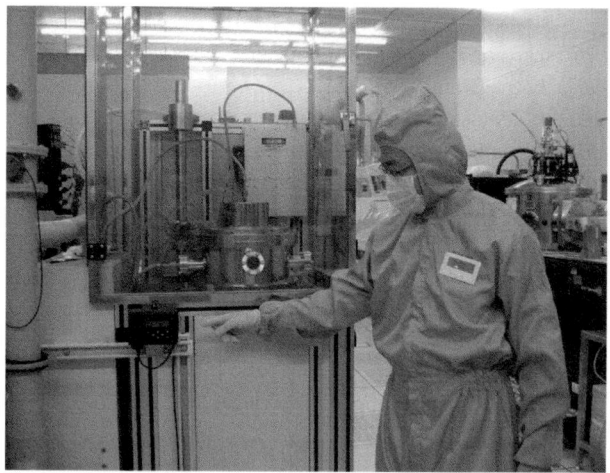

Figure 45.4 Toxic gas detector in a clean room.

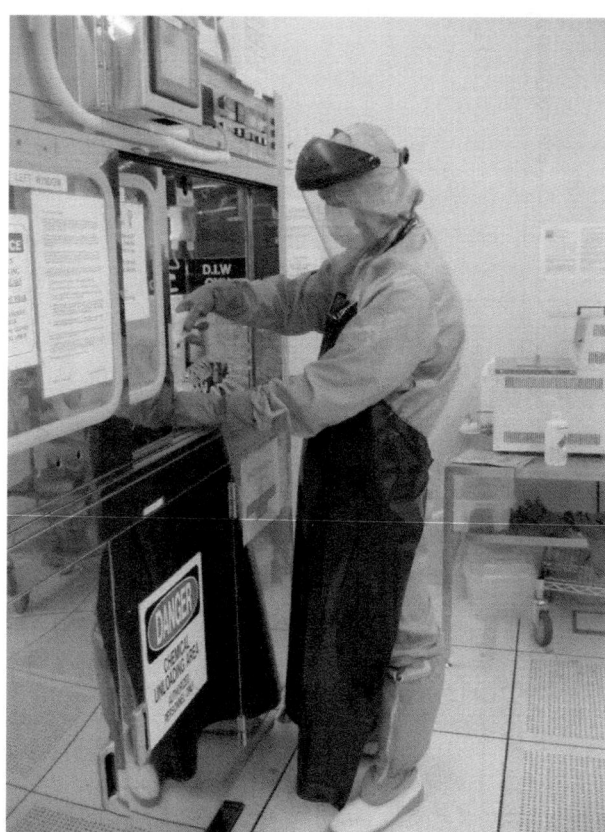

Figure 45.5 Laboratory officer using the solvent bench in a clean room in a research facility.

in other countries, and can still be found on the waste inventories of some semiconductor manufacturing companies (Figure 45.5).

Physical hazards

Ionizing and non-ionizing radiation are used for testing, quality control inspection and curing. Ionizing radiation (such as x-rays) is used in ion-transfer processes and in quality-control inspection of wafers. Non-ionizing radiation like ultraviolet light, infrared light or microwave is used in photolithography to harden the photoresist layer and to transfer the required patterns from the mask to the wafer. Shorter wavelength light or 'extreme ultraviolet light' is used if even greater precision is required.

Some workers may be exposed to high noise levels, although it is not usually considered to be a major issue within semiconductor factories. Vertical laminar flow hoods and ceilings normally create a background noise level of about 75–78 dBA in clean rooms. Core building areas which house the equipment for running the factory operations (for example, air-conditioner compressors, chillers or boilers) are usually the noisiest areas of the factory – often at about 85 to >95 dBA. The main group of workers at risk of noise exposure here would be the maintenance personnel. However, the total duration of work in the core building areas may not be sufficient to cause noise-induced hearing loss.[25]

The relative humidity level in clean rooms needs to be kept low to protect the components from corrosion. The levels are generally kept at or below 40–50 per cent relative humidity. Low humidity has been linked to skin disorders, such as physical irritant contact dermatitis.[26,27] Relative humidity of less than 35–40 per cent can induce pruritus and skin changes related to xerosis, especially in susceptible individuals.[28] Workers exposed to relative humidity of 2.5 per cent in an ultradry clean room of a high-tech device-developing laboratory had significantly higher prevalence of skin complaints, such as itch, dryness, rash and pain.[29]

Psychosocial

Shift work is common in the semiconductor industry, as most factories run continuously. Rotating shifts are a well-documented source of psychosocial stress. Monotonous and repetitive work at a fast and unvarying pace also contributes to psychosocial stress in the semiconductor industry.

This industry also has sizeable numbers of non-production workers. Sales and marketing staff are usually required to travel frequently, and are often under high stress levels due to intense competition between companies to promote their products.

Research and development engineers in the semiconductor industry are also under pressure to design smaller and faster chips with wider capacities and applications, within tight time lines.

Ergonomic

An increasing degree of automation may find ergonomic problems progressively being phased out. However, while automation reduces the physical strain on workers, they are often still required to lift the wafer cassettes in and out of the machines and monitor the running of multiple machines. The Semiconductor Health Study indicated a dose–response relationship between the numbers of hours spent on fabrication work and distal upper extremity pain.[30] A study conducted in 2004 on 906 female semiconductor workers from different factories in Malaysia found that 80.5 per cent of the workers had experienced pain in the past year in at least one part of the body, including the neck, shoulders, back, upper and lower limbs. The Malaysian factories studied dealt mostly with back end processing.[31]

Workers who are required to inspect the chips visually with the use of microscopes at various stages of the manufacturing process may be subject to visual fatigue and other ergonomic problems, such as prolonged or repeated neck flexion. However, much of this work can and has been automated.

Administrative and research and development staff may be subject to the ergonomic issues of office workers from prolonged work at the computer terminal.

Biological

Although biological hazards are not routinely encountered in semiconductor manufacturing work processes, the recycling of air in clean rooms may aid the spread of communicable diseases, such as upper respiratory tract infections.

The risk cannot be overlooked, especially with the experience of the severe acute respiratory syndrome (SARS) epidemic and concerns with influenza outbreaks and pandemics. During the 2003 SARS crisis in Singapore, a worker in an electronics company was diagnosed to have SARS. This resulted in a temporary shut down of the entire electronics line, as all 305 workers on the same shift as the infected worker had to be quarantined.[32]

An outbreak of conjunctivitis in a microelectronics factory resulted in a temporary plant shut down after safety glasses and routine hand-washing instructions failed to curb the spread of the infection. A total of 145 workers had been affected by that time, and the mode of disease transmission was believed to have been via the sharing of microscopes among workers.[33]

HEALTH ISSUES IN THE SEMICONDUCTOR INDUSTRY

Cancer incidence

Workers in semiconductor manufacturing facilities are exposed to known and suspected carcinogens. Commonly cited are arsenic and its compounds, antimony and ionizing radiation. These have all been linked with lung cancer occurrence. In addition, some researchers have suggested that prolonged night shift work increases the risk of breast cancer in women.[34] As previously mentioned, night shift is common in the semiconductor industry, especially among female line workers.

A study conducted in two major semiconductor companies in Taiwan found that the workers were exposed to high levels of arsenic, as well as to gallium and indium. The arsenic level in inhalable air for operators ranged from 5.26 to 106.12 $\mu g/m^3$. This was above the permissible exposure limit set by the United States Occupational Safety and Health Administration (OSHA). The levels for gallium and indium were between 0.34 to 101.26 $\mu g/m^3$ and 0.14 to 100.62 $\mu g/m^3$, respectively. Mirroring these results were the high metal levels in the urine of exposed workers, with a mean level of 39.35 $\mu g/L$ of urinary arsenic, 10.15 $\mu g/L$ of gallium and 6.98 $\mu g/L$ of indium. Cancer risk was calculated by the US EPA Carcinogen Assessment Group's multistage model to predict dose-specific cancer risk associated with inhalation of inorganic arsenic. The workers were found to have a cancer risk higher than the allowable risk-based US EPA's acceptable risk limits.[4]

In a large retrospective study of over 100 000 staff working in IBM factories, the mortality rates and causes of death were noted. No conclusive evidence of causal association between work and increased mortality from any form of cancer was found, although there was some suggestion of increased rates of central nervous system cancer in process equipment maintenance workers in one plant and prostate cancer among facilities/plant engineers and laboratory workers in another plant.[35]

A retrospective study was conducted based on 4388 workers in a Scottish semiconductor manufacturing facility. Fifty per cent of the male workers and 79 per cent of the female workers were recorded to have been involved in fabrication work in this factory. Although total cancer registrations were close to expected levels for both males and females, the authors identified increased rates of cancers of the respiratory tract, stomach and breast in females, and mortality from cancer of the brain among males. In females, the standardized registration ratio (SRR) for malignant neoplasms of the trachea, bronchus and lung was 273, for malignant neoplasms of the stomach the SRR was 438 and the SRR for breast malignancies was 134. (The SRRs were calculated for specific types of malignant neoplasms and adjusted for deprivation using Carstairs index.) For males, the main finding was a standardized mortality ratio (unadjusted) of brain cancer of 401.[36]

Another retrospective study published in 2005 that focused on 1807 workers from a semiconductor factory in the United Kingdom found significantly elevated standardized registration ratios for malignant melanoma (SRR, 217) and rectal cancer (SRR, 199) in males and females, and pancreatic cancer (SRR, 226) in females. Detailed work history was not analysed in this study.[37] A case–control study conducted in 1993 found increased risk of cutaneous melanoma (odds ratio, 2.03) in individuals who had previously worked in the electronics industry.[38]

The current data on cancer experience among workers in the semiconductor industry is patchy and inconclusive. Other studies are currently ongoing in an attempt to establish more clearly the relationship between occupational exposures and cancer incidence.

Reproductive problems

The association between semiconductor work and reproductive disorders remains a controversy. The main reason for this is the inherent difficulty of obtaining sufficient sample sizes of pregnancy-related epidemiological studies. In a United States retrospective cohort study, the spontaneous abortion rate of 904 female workers with eligible pregnancies was studied. The risk of spontaneous abortions was slightly higher in fabrication-area workers (adjusted risk ratio, 1.43) compared with non-fabrication workers. Further analysis of specific work exposures showed a dose–response association of spontaneous abortions with photoresist and developer solvents. The main constituent of these would be ethylene-based glycol ethers.[39] A later study that was conducted by the Health and Safety Executive in the United Kingdom found no evidence of increased risk of spontaneous abortion among female workers in the British semiconductor industry who were also exposed to ethylene glycol ethers. This was a nested case–control study that was based on a retrospective cohort of 2203 females. From these, 116 were selected as cases or controls. The adjusted odds ratio for spontaneous abortions was 0.58 for fabrication workers.[40]

In Taiwan, 292 pregnancies from 173 female workers from a wafer manufacturing company were studied and the relative fecundability as reflected by the fecundability ratio (FR) was calculated. The waiting time to pregnancy was prolonged (FR, 0.77) among female workers in the photolithography area compared to non-fabrication workers. In addition, among fabrication workers, those who worked in areas where they were potentially exposed to ethylene glycol ethers had longer time to pregnancy (FR, 0.59) compared to those who were not likely to be exposed.[23]

Another Taiwan-based study of 606 female workers compared workers in the fabrication areas with those working in non-fabrication areas. Fabrication workers had a 2.0 odds ratio for long menstrual cycles (defined as cycles that were more than 35 days long) compared to workers in non-fabrication areas. Fabrication workers in the photolithography areas, who were likely to be exposed to ethylene glycols and isopropyl alcohol had the highest odds of long cycles (5.0, compared to non-fabrication workers).[22] However, this is in contrast to other earlier studies that found shortened menstrual cycles in relation to ethylene glycol ether exposure, underscoring the need for further, more conclusive evidence.[41]

Male fertility was also assessed during the Semiconductor Health Study in 1990 to 1991, comparing men working in fabrication rooms with those in non-fabrication areas. Men who worked in the furnace, thin-film or ion implantation areas of fabrication sections were more likely to report previous difficulty conceiving (defined as needing one or more years to achieve conception; relative risk, 1.79) and to have lower past fertility (adjusted fertility ratio, 0.79). However, contraception data were not collected in this study.[42]

Decreased white cell counts

Male fabrication workers in a Taiwan semiconductor plant who were involved in photolithography and implantation work were found to have significantly lower white cell counts than male office workers in the same company. The office workers had a mean white cell count of $7350/mm^3$, while male workers in photolithography and implantation areas had mean counts of 5870 and $6190/mm^3$, respectively. The prevalence of leukopenia, defined for the purpose of the study as a white cell count of $5 \times 10^3/mm^3$ or less, was also significantly higher in male photolithography workers (30 per cent) compared to male office workers (5.6 per cent). The authors suggested the risk of intermittent short-term peak exposures to glycol ethers, ionizing radiation, arsenic and other toxins in these male workers to be the possible cause of lower white cell counts.

Female workers in the photolithography section had marginally elevated liver enzyme levels. The fabrication processes in this company were automated and workers had no direct contact with the chemicals under normal working circumstances. Previous studies had also found the estimated exposure concentrations of solvents to be below the permissible exposure limit. The control systems within the plant were found to be in good order, with careful attention paid to the prevention of toxic chemical leaks.

Thus, the finding of a biological effect on the workers, despite maintaining seemingly adequate environmental control, suggests that adverse health effects may occur at levels below the permissible exposure limit.[43]

Genotoxicity

In a 1991 German study, the genotoxic effect of exposure to chemicals including boron compounds was assessed by looking for the formation of micronuclei in lymphocytes. Twenty workers who had contact with open plasma etching processes had significantly higher mean frequency of micronuclei (9.2 micronuclei per 500 billion cells) than a control group of 21 workers who were not exposed (5.7 micronuclei per 500 billion cells). This was despite the fact that environmental levels of boron trifluoride and boron trichloride were under the detection rate. Urinary boron fluoride measurements also did not indicate significant chemical exposure. A second survey was conducted in 2004, 12 years after the implementation of numerous control measures. The levels of micronuclei in exposed workers had decreased to 3.2 per 500 billion cells. The conclusion drawn by the authors was that the workers could have been exposed to intermediate products formed by a variety of chemicals during the plasma etching process. These intermediate products were not individually identifiable, but had the potential to cause genotoxicity.[44]

IMPACT ON THE ENVIRONMENT

There has been concern about the discharge into the environment of toxic and persistent waste material by semiconductor manufacturing facilities. In early 2002, the Silicon Valley in the United States had more than 150 polluted groundwater sites.[45]

In a 2004 Taiwan survey, groundwater from around the semiconductor industrial park was tested for arsenic, gallium and indium levels. The average arsenic concentration in the well water samples was 34.19 μg/L. This far exceeds the level set by the Environment Protection Agency for drinking water of 10 μg/L. Average gallium and indium levels in the water were 19.34 and 9.25 μg/L respectively.[5] Gallium, arsenic, indium and thallium were also found in high concentrations in the kidney, liver and lung tissues of squirrels captured from a county adjacent to Taiwan's main semiconductor industry site. Squirrels of the same species that were captured from Japan had much lower levels of the elements tested. In particular, renal thallium concentrations were two to three times higher in the Taiwanese squirrels compared to the Japanese specimens.[46]

On the positive side, the industry has been able to find environmentally safer alternatives to the ozone-depleting chlorofluorocarbons (CFCs). In the 1970s to early 1980s, CFCs were being used in massive amounts in the Silicon Valley and in Japan as they were thought to be safer than trichloroethylene. When it was realized that CFCs were damaging the ozone, the semiconductor industry moved to develop alternatives. By the end of 1992, many electronics companies worldwide had stopped using CFCs.[47]

CONCLUSION

The semiconductor industry is large and rapidly growing in many aspects. The industry employs millions of people worldwide, and is an important driving force behind the economies of many countries. Cutting-edge research and development is a cornerstone of the industry, designing smaller yet faster and more complex products within a short time and finding more efficient ways to manufacture them.

The work processes within the industry are diverse, varying from country to country, and depending on consumer demand. Many hazardous chemicals and agents are used, albeit within enclosed and automated processes. The potential for exposure still exists, and occupational health personnel need to be aware of this and understand the unique work experiences of each set of workers under their care.

Key points

- In many countries, the semiconductor industry is an important employment sector.
- Work processes within the industry and resultant worker exposures vary greatly.
- While many highly toxic substances, such as arsine and hydrofluoric acid, are used, most processes in this high-tech industry are enclosed and automated.
- Work processes and materials used are continually changing as research and development progresses towards greater precision, smaller and more powerful devices, that consume less energy.
- Occupational health problems associated with semiconductor work are dermatitis, and issues related to shift work and work-related musculoskeletal disorders. Currently, there are insufficient data on cancer risk in semiconductor workers.

REFERENCES

1. Moore GE. Cramming more components on to integrated circuits. *Electronics*. 1965; **38**: 8, cited September 30, 2007. Available from: www.intel.com/technology/mooreslaw/index.htm.
2. Sze SM. *Semiconductor devices: Physics and technology*, 2nd edn. New York: John Wiley & Sons, 2002.
3. Semiconductor Industry Association. Semiconductor sales slow in November. Updated January 2, 2008; cited January 8, 2008. Available from: www.sia-online.org/cs/papers_publications/press_release_detail?pressrelease.id=1524.
4. India Semiconductor Association. Media kit. Cited September 26, 2007. Available from: www.isaonline.org/documents/mediakit.pdf.
5. Dyson CM. A learning network for the semiconductor industry. *International Journal of Electrical Engineering Education*. 2001; **38**: 290–304.
6. Chen HW. Exposure and health risk of gallium, indium, and arsenic from semiconductor manufacturing industry workers. *Bulletin of Environmental Contamination and Toxicology*. 2007; **78**: 113–17.
7. World Semiconductor Trade Statistics. WSTS Projects 2.3 percent global semiconductor growth in 2007. Updated May 30, 2007; cited August 1, 2007. Available from http://www.wsts.org/plain/content/view/full/553.
8. McNaught AD, Wilkinson A. *International Union of Pure and Applied Chemistry (IUPAC) compendium of chemical terminology*. Cambridge: Royal Society of Chemistry. Available from: www.iupac.org/goldbook/S05591.pdf.
9. Considine GD (ed.). Semiconductors. In: *Van Nostrand's scientific encyclopaedia*, 9th edn. New York: John Wiley and Sons, 2002: 3132.
10. Semiconductor Industry Association. SIA and semiconductor industry history. Cited July 28, 2007. Available from: www.sia-online.org/abt_history.cfm.
11. Van Zeghbroeck B. *Principles of semiconductor devices*, University of Colorado, 2004, cited July 28, 2007. Available from: ece-www.colorado.edu/~bart/book/.
12. Semiconductor Industry Association. Media resources: How is a semiconductor chip made? Cited August 2, 2007. Available from: www.sia-online.org/pre_resources_FAQ_Made.cfm.
13. Intel. Inside the Intel manufacturing process: How chips are made. Cited August 2, 2007. Available from: www.intel.com/education/makingchips/.
14. NEC Electronics Corporation. Advanced exposure techniques. Cited September 8, 2007. Available from: www.necel.com/v_factory/en/index.html.
15. Sun Y, Aun JH, Rogers JA. Printable semiconductors for flexible electronics. In: *McGraw-Hill yearbook of science and technology*. New York: McGraw-Hill, 2007: 192–7.
16. Clifton K, Shen F, Mirkin CA. Dip-pen nanolithography. In: *McGraw-Hill yearbook of science and technology*. New York: McGraw-Hill, 2006: 95–7.
17. Semiconductor Industry Association. Exploring opportunities to further minimise potential equipment-related exposures. SIA WHI Final Report, 2004.
18. Klaassen CD (ed.). *Casarett and Doull's toxicology: The basic science of poisons*. New York: McGraw-Hill, 1996: 534.
19. World Health Organization. International Agency for Research on Cancer. IARC monographs on the evaluation of carcinogenic risks to humans, vol. 49. Chromium, nickel and welding. Summary of data reported and evaluation. Last accessed June 2009. Available from: http://monographs.iarc.fr/ENG/Monographs/vol49/volume49.pdf.
20. Bretherick L. *Handbook of reactive chemical hazards*, 4th edn. Boston, MA: Butterworth-Heinemann, 1990.
21. Lewis R. Metals. In: LaDou J (ed.). *Current occupational and environmental medicine*. New York: McGraw-Hill, 2007: 413.
22. Hsieh GY, Wang JD, Cheng TJ, Chen PC. Prolonged menstrual cycles in female workers exposed to ethylene glycol ethers in the semiconductor manufacturing industry. *Occupational and Environmental Medicine*. 2005; **62**: 510–16.
23. Chen PC, Hsieah GY, Wang JD, Chang TJ. Prolonged time to pregnancy in female workers exposed to ethylene glycol ethers in semiconductor manufacturing. *Epidemiology*. 2002; **13**: 191–6.
24. Herrick RF, Stewart JH, Blicharz D et al. Exposure assessment for retrospective follow-up studies of semiconductor- and storage device-manufacturing workers. *Journal of Occupational and Environmental Medicine*. 2005; **47**: 983–95.
25. Williams ME, Baldwin DG. *Semiconductor industrial hygiene handbook: Monitoring, ventilation, equipment and ergonomics*. New Jersey: Noyes Publications, 1995, 92.

26. Koh D. Occupational dermatitis – What's new? Electronics industry. *Clinics in Dermatology.* 1997; **15**: 579–86.
27. Morris-Jones R, Robertson SJ, Ross JS et al. Contact dermatitis and allergy: Dermatitis caused by physical irritants. *British Journal of Dermatology.* 2002; **147**: 270–5.
28. White IR, Rycroft RJ. Low humidity occupational dermatosis – an epidemic. *Contact Dermatitis.* 1982; **8**: 287–90.
29. Sato M, Fukayo S, Yano E. Adverse environmental health effects of ultra-low relative humidity indoor air. *Journal of Occupational Health.* 2003; **45**: 133–6.
30. Pocekay D, McCurdy SA, Samuels SJ, Hammond SK. A cross-sectional study of musculoskeletal symptoms and risk factors in semiconductor workers. *American Journal of Industrial Medicine.* 1995; **28**: 861–71.
31. Chee HL, Rampal KG. Work-related musculoskeletal problems among women workers in the semiconductor industry in Peninsular Malaysia. *International Journal of Occupational and Environmental Health.* 2004; **10**: 63–71.
32. Prime Minister Lee Hsien Loong's 2003 May day rally speech. Cited September 25, 2007. Available from: http://app.mfa.gov.sg/pr/read_content.asp? View,1881.
33. Doyle L, Gallagher K, Heath BS, Patterson WB. An outbreak of infectious conjunctivitis spread by microscopes. *Journal of Occupational Medicine.* 1989; **31**: 758–62.
34. Schernhammer ES, Kroenke CH, Laden F, Hankinson SE. Night work and risk of breast cancer. *Epidemiology.* 2006; **17**: 108–11.
35. Beall C, Bender TJ, Cheng H. Mortality among semiconductor and storage device-manufacturing workers. *Journal of Occupational and Environmental Medicine.* 2005; **47**: 996–1014.
36. McElvenny DM, Darnton AJ, Hodgson JT et al. Investigation of cancer incidence and mortality at a Scottish semiconductor manufacturing facility. *Occupational Medicine (Lond).* 2003; **53**: 419–30.
37. Nichols L, Sorahan T. Cancer incidence and cancer mortality in a cohort of UK semiconductor workers, 1970–2002. *Occupational Medicine (Lond).* 2005; **55**: 625–30.
38. Nelemans PJ, Scholte R, Groenendal H et al. Melanoma and occupation: Results of a case-control study in The Netherlands. *British Journal of Industrial Medicine.* 1993; **50**: 642–6.
39. Schenker MB, Gold EB, Beaumont JJ, Eskenazi B. Association of spontaneous abortion and other reproductive effects with work in the semiconductor industry. *American Journal of Industrial Medicine.* 1995; **28**: 639–59.
40. Elliott RC, Jones JR, McElvenny DM. Spontaneous abortion in the British semiconductor industry: An HSE investigation. *American Journal of Industrial Medicine.* 1999; **36**: 557–72.
41. Cordier S, Multigner L. Occupational exposure to glycol ethers and ovarian function: Commentary on the paper by Hsieh et al. *Occupational and Environmental Medicine.* 2005; **62**: 507–8.
42. Samuels SJ, McCurdy SA, Pocekay D, Hammond SK. Fertility history of currently employed male semiconductor workers. *American Journal of Industrial Medicine.* 1995; **28**: 873–82.
43. Luo JCJ, Hsieh LL, Chang MJW, Hsu KH. Decreased white blood cell counts in semiconductor manufacturing workers in Taiwan. *Occupational and Environmental Medicine.* 2002; **59**: 44–8.
44. Winker R, Roos G, Pilger A, Rüdiger HW. Effect of occupational safety measures on micronucleus frequency in semiconductor workers. *International Archives of Occupational and Environmental Health.* 2008; **81**: 423–8.
45. Dooley EE. EHPnet – Silicon Valley toxics coalition. *Environmental Health Perspectives.* 2002; **110**: 4.
46. Suzuki Y, Watanabe I, Oshida T et al. Accumulation of trace elements used in semiconductor industry in Formosan squirrel, as a bio-indicator of their exposure, living in Taiwan. *Chemosphere.* 2007; **68**: 1270–9.
47. Perry TS. Cleaning up. *IEEE Spectrum.* 1993; February: 20–6.

PART THREE

DISEASES ASSOCIATED WITH PHYSICAL AGENTS

Section One: Noise	457
Section Two: Vibration	487
Section Three: Heat and cold	523
Section Four: Barometric pressure	545
Section Five: Radiation	621

SECTION ONE

Noise

---

46 Sound, noise and the ear 459
Richard T Ramsden and Shakeel R Saeed

46

Sound, noise and the ear

RICHARD T RAMSDEN AND SHAKEEL R SAEED

Introduction	459
The physics of sound	459
Anatomy and physiology of the ear	461
Occupational noise-induced hearing loss	464
Acoustic trauma and blast trauma	469
Assessment of hearing disability	470
Age-associated hearing loss	471
Hearing conservation programmes	471
Management	475
Non-organic (or exaggerated, or functional) hearing loss	476
Electric response audiometry (evoked response audiometry)	477
Occupational noise-induced tinnitus	480
Occupational noise-induced vertigo	480
Infrasound and ultrasound	480
Systemic effects of noise pollution	481
References	482

INTRODUCTION

There has been an awareness for several centuries that exposure to high levels of sound may be detrimental to an individual's hearing. The objectives of this chapter are to review the response of the ear to normal and hazardous sound levels, examine the issues of assessment and management of patients presenting with possible noise-induced afflictions of the ear, and discuss the legal provisions available for such individuals.

THE PHYSICS OF SOUND

The application of a mechanical force to an elastic medium, such as air, results in the displacement of the particles or molecules that constitute that medium. The energy in the displacing force effectively overcomes the mass or inertia of the molecules. This displacement is resisted by a force that tends to return the molecule or particle to its resting position, that is the elasticity. In effect, the displacing force sets up an oscillation or vibration in that medium, which is essentially sound. This oscillation would continue indefinitely if it were not for the frictional resistance that is also inherent to any vibrating system. As a result of this frictional resistance, the energy in the initial displacing force is dissipated as heat and the vibration ceases. The transfer of kinetic energy between vibrating molecules, however, leads to a propagation of the sound through the medium. This generates alternating areas of condensation (with a rise in ambient pressure) and rarefaction (with a fall in ambient pressure) within the medium (Figure 46.1). There is no net movement of the medium as such, but rather the movement of changes in pressure in the medium, which is a sound wave and takes the form of a sine wave when the pressure changes are plotted against time. A sound wave thus has two fundamental properties: its intensity (amplitude of the peak of the wave form), correlating subjectively with loudness, and its frequency, which has the subjective correlate of pitch.[1]

Sound wave intensity

By definition, the intensity of a sound wave is its power per unit area (expressed in watts per metre squared) and depends on the peak pressure of the sound wave and the peak velocity of the air molecules. The peak pressure and peak velocity are proportional to each other, the constant of proportionality being the impedance of the medium through which the wave is being propagated. The ambient pressure of a sound wave depends on the point on the sinusoid wave form at which it is measured and therefore the relationship between the intensity and the peak pressure will also vary in this manner. In order to overcome this during quantification, the average or root mean square (RMS) value of the pressure is calculated from pressure measurements at points along the waveform. This allows the intensity of the sound to be calculated from the RMS pressure for a medium with a known impedance. Unlike intensity, sound pressure can be readily measured with a

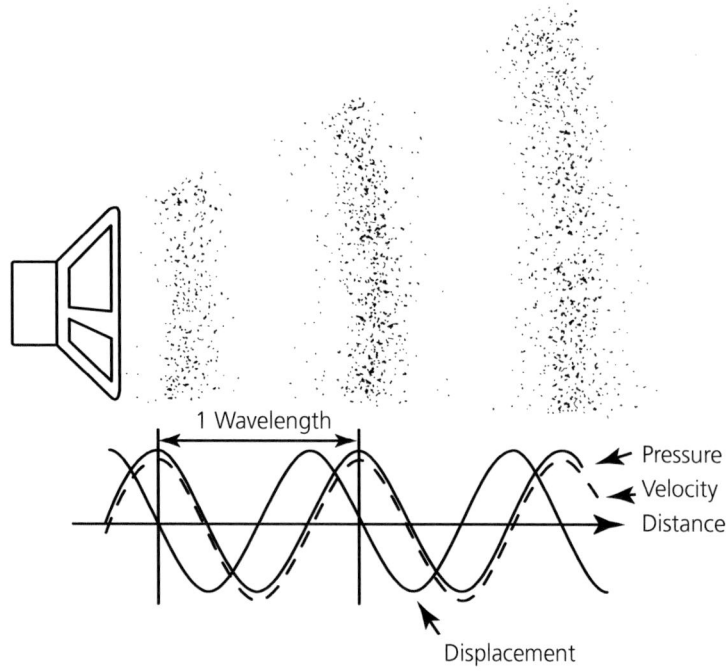

Figure 46.1 A sound wave generated by alternating areas of condensation and rarefaction of the medium through which it travels. Reproduced with permission from Ref. 1.

microphone and is expressed in newtons per square metre (N/m^2) (pascals (Pa)). The auditory system, however, is sensitive to a vast range of sound pressures: 2×10^{-5} N/m^2 for the threshold of hearing to around 1×10^8 N/m^2 next to a jet aircraft at take off. With such a wide numerical range, the impracticalities of quantification and calculation are obvious. Second, the ear does not respond in a linear manner to linear changes in sound pressure. In fact, the ear perceives changes in intensity more closely to logarithmic changes in power or sound pressure. The use of the logarithm of the ratio of the measured pressure to a reference pressure or ratios of intensity or indeed power overcomes the two difficulties cited.

Logarithms to the base 10 of these ratios are termed 'bels' after Alexander Graham Bell, as the scale was first used in telephony. In practical terms, one-tenth of a bel or decibel (dB) is more convenient for the sizes of the numbers involved. Thus:

$$\text{Sound pressure level in bels (SPL)} = \frac{\log_{10} \text{ RMS measured sound pressure}}{\text{Reference sound pressure}}$$

$$\text{Sound pressure level in dB (SPL)} = \frac{10\log_{10} \text{ RMS measured sound pressure}}{\text{Reference sound pressure}}$$

To express the sound intensity which varies as the square of the pressure:

$$\text{Intensity (dB SPL)} = \frac{20\log_{10} \text{ RMS measured sound pressure}}{\text{Reference sound pressure}}$$

Using this decibel scale for measuring sound pressure levels (SPL), the reference sound pressure is 2×10^{-5} N/m^2 (20 µPa), 0 dB SPL corresponds to the threshold of hearing and 130 dB SPL the threshold of pain. Audiometrically, however, the reference pressure is frequency dependent as the threshold sensitivity of the human ear is frequency dependent (see Sound wave frequency, p. 461). These reference pressures have been defined by the International Standards Organization (ISO 389: 1991)[2] and are the same as those of the British Standards Institution (BS 2497: 1992).[3] Using these reference pressures, an audiometric sound level of say 30 dB is written as 30 dB hearing level (HL) and if this corresponds to the threshold of hearing of an individual's ear then the threshold is said to be 30 dB HTL (hearing threshold level) for that ear.[4] Conveniently, the minimum detectable change in intensity is 1 dB SPL and an increase of 10 dB SPL gives a subjective sensation of doubling the loudness of a sound, although the intensity of the sound has increased ten-fold.

Table 46.1 shows the internationally agreed reference levels for the calculation of decibels of sound with respect to power, sound pressure and intensity. One other relevant consideration relating to sound intensity is the effect of distance from the sound source. For a theoretical point sound source in a homogenous medium, the intensity of the sound is a function of the power per unit area. Since the area increases as the square of the distance from the source, the intensity is inversely proportional to the square of the distance from the source of the sound. In reality, the presence of physical obstructions with the resultant reflection, diffraction and absorption effects tend to confound this relationship.

Table 46.1 The internationally agreed reference levels for the calculation of decibels of sound.

Scale	Abbreviation	Reference quantity
Power level	PWL	1.0 pW (10−12 W)
Intensity level	IL	10−12 W/m²
Pressure level	SPL	20 μPa (20 × 10^{-6} N/m²)

Sound wave frequency

The number of complete cycles of a sound wave per second is its frequency, expressed in hertz (Hz). At sea level with an ambient temperature of 15°C, the velocity of sound waves is 330 m/s in free air. Therefore, a sound wave with a frequency of 330 Hz has a wavelength of 1 m and as the frequency increases, the wavelength decreases. The human ear in a child or young adult has a frequency perception range between 20 Hz and 20 kHz. The high frequency sensitivity diminishes with age such that few adults over the age of 30 years can detect sound with a frequency greater than 16 kHz.

The frequency of a sound broadly correlates with the subjective sensation of pitch. The threshold of human hearing, however, varies with frequency with maximum sensitivity between 2 and 3 kHz which encompasses the important speech sounds. This necessitates the use of a correction factor or weighting when measuring sound pressure levels or hearing thresholds and several such weighting curves exist. Of these, the 'A' weighting scale (low and extremely high frequencies weighted less heavily) is commonly utilized as it best correlates with measured and perceived sound. A statement of a sound pressure level should also, therefore, indicate the weighting utilized by means of a suffix, e.g. 30 dB (A) SPL.

As with sound intensities, the ear subjectively responds to incremental changes in frequency ratios, rather than in a linear manner. Hence, doubling the frequency of a tone produces a perceived change in pitch of one octave. Conventionally therefore, tuning fork tests and audiometric testing is undertaken in multiples of 256 Hz (middle C) though among musicians, middle C corresponds to a frequency of 261 Hz. Everyday sounds, of course, are more complex than those of a simple sinusoid (sine wave). Analysis of a complex waveform by breaking it down into its component sinusoids (Fourier analysis) allows the relative contribution of the components to be determined by frequency and relative amplitude. Periodic sounds (waveforms in the same time interval) are shown to have components that are multiples of the fundamental frequency or harmonics. These in part give a musical note, for example, its particular timbre. For non-periodic sounds, such as the spoken voice, analysis shows that rather than discrete component frequencies, there is a continuous range of frequencies or spectrum.

Noise

The preceding discussion examines sound in terms of its physical properties. Physically, noise is a complex sound whose characteristics are not easily amenable to analysis and has little or no measurable periodicity. Physiologically, noise is an uninformative signal with variable intensity. Psychologically, any sound that is unpleasant, noxious or unwanted is noise irrespective of its waveform.[5] Noise may be classified as continuous (steady-state or fluctuant) or intermittent (impulse or impact). Impulse noise, such as the noise generated from a gun blast, is characterized by its short duration and shock-front pressure waveform. Impact noise, such as in pile driving, is characterized by little or no shock-front, but considerable reverberant sound. The characteristics of intermittent noise merge into those of continuous noise if the former is repeated very rapidly.

ANATOMY AND PHYSIOLOGY OF THE EAR

Structurally and functionally, the human ear is divided into three parts, namely the outer ear, middle ear and inner ear (Figure 46.2). Together with the central connections of the ear in the brain, each part plays a role in the process of hearing and therefore merits further consideration.

The outer ear

The outer or external ear comprises the auricle (pinna) and the external auditory canal. Collectively, these serve to modify incoming sound in two specific ways. First, the combination of the auricle behaving as an ear trumpet, concentrating sound from a large area to the smaller area of the external canal and the natural resonances of the external canal itself serves to increase the sound pressure level at the tympanic membrane by about 10 dB over a frequency range of 2–7 kHz.[1] Second, based on the above phenomenon and the fact that a proportion of incident sound is reflected off the head in a manner dependent on the direction of the sound, the outer ear provides some information about sound localization.

The middle ear

Embryologically derived from the outer and middle ear, the tympanic membrane (drumhead) constitutes the major component of the lateral or outer wall of the tympanic cavity. Within this cavity are the three ossicles, the malleus, incus and stapes, linking the drumhead to the inner ear. The middle ear cavity communicates with the pharynx at the back of the nose by the Eustachian tube and with the mastoid air cells by the aditus ad antrum. The fundamental function of the middle ear is mechanically to couple acoustic energy to the cochlea. To do this effectively, the middle ear has to match the impedance of air to

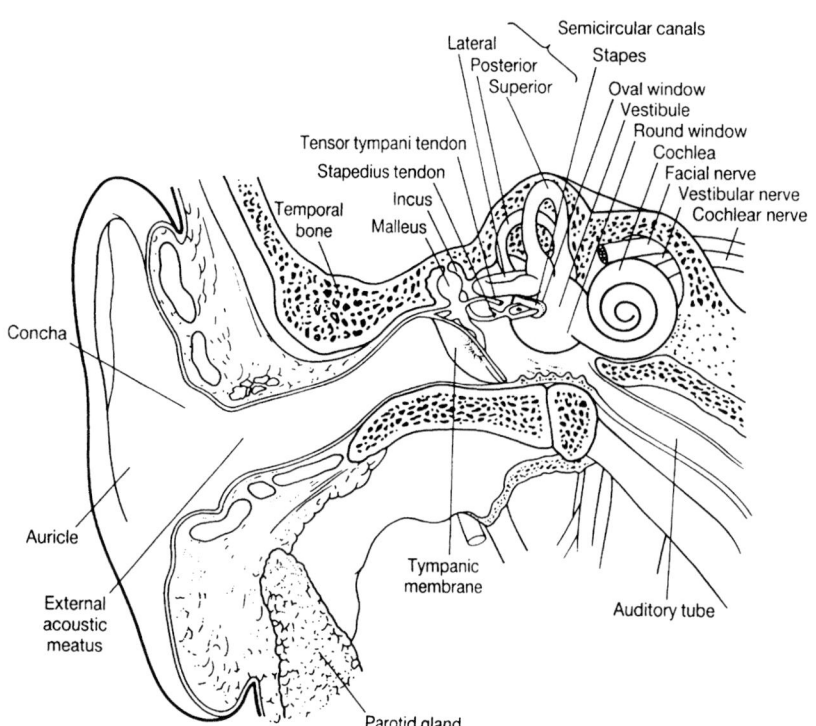

Figure 46.2 The external, middle and inner ears. Reproduced with permission from Ref. 104.

the considerably higher impedance of the inner ear fluids, that is, function as an acoustic sound pressure transformer. The effect of this, in combination with the effects of the outer ear already described means that up to 50 per cent of the incident sound energy is transmitted to the inner ear as opposed to the expected 1 per cent in the absence of the transformer.[6] This is achieved by two mechanisms. The leverage of the malleus and incus about their axis of rotation gives a ×1.3 mechanical gain. The difference in the functional surface area between the drumhead and the stapes footplate which sits in the oval window gives rise to a 14-fold hydraulic effect.[7] Combining the two provides an increase in pressure at the oval window by a factor of around 18.

The second consideration is that the cochlear fluids, like any fluid, are incompressible. The ossicular chain preferentially directs acoustic energy to the stapedial end of the cochlear compartment. The other end of this compartment is closed by the round window membrane which is able to deform in response to the pressure change in the cochlear fluids. Relative to the oval window, the incident acoustic energy at the round window is very small due to the effect of the ossicular chain and the presence of air (via the Eustachian tube) in the middle ear cavity (Figure 46.3).

The inner ear

The inner ear consists of two parts: the osseous labyrinth and the corresponding membranous labyrinth which lies within it. Descriptively, the labyrinth comprises the semicircular canals and vestibule which house the sensory end

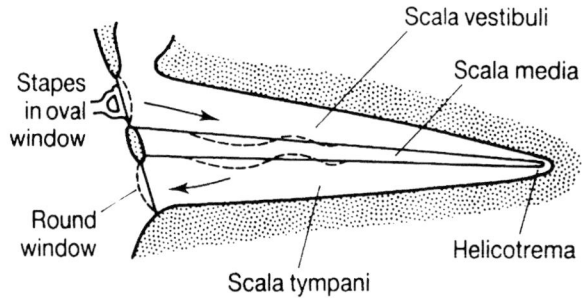

Figure 46.3 Schematic diagram of an unrolled cochlea showing the transmission of vibrations from the oval window to the round window. Reproduced with permission from Ref. 105.

organs of balance and the cochlea within which is the hearing organ (Figure 46.4). Lying in the medial wall of the middle ear, the cochlea is shaped like a snail's shell with two and three-quarter turns, 5 mm in height and 9 mm across the base.[8] The central bony axis of the cochlea (modiolus) has a spiral bony lamina projecting from it along its length which is completed by the basilar membrane. On this lies the cochlear duct (membraneous labyrinth) effectively dividing the cochlear lumen into three compartments, the scala vestibuli (in continuity with the vestibule, containing perilymph), the scala tympani (in continuity at the apex of the cochlea with the scala vestibuli and closed by the round window membrane) and the scala media (containing endolymph), within which is the organ of Corti (Figure 46.5). The organ of Corti is a specialized area of the lining of the cochlear duct that runs the whole length of the cochlear spiral and is around 35 mm long.[9]

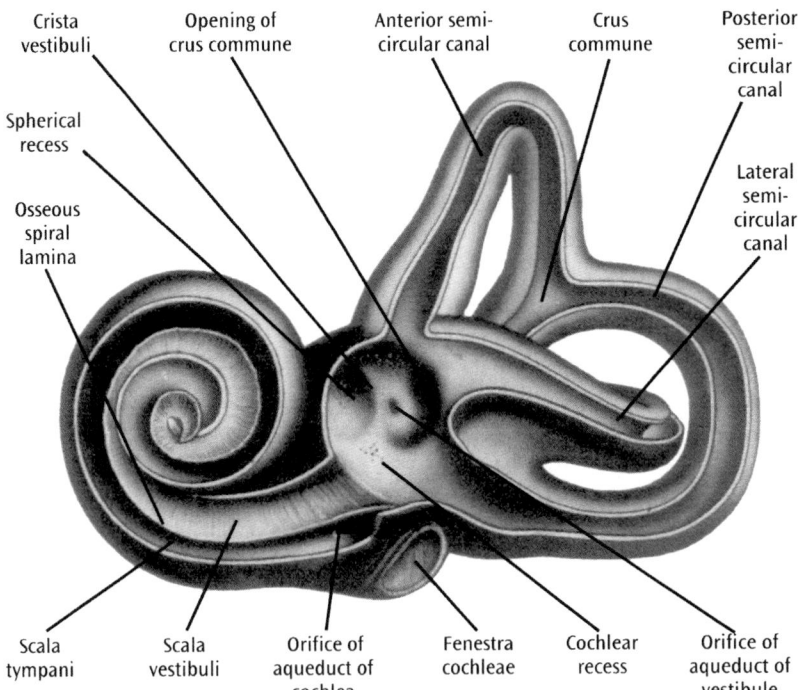

Figure 46.4 The interior of the osseous labyrinth showing the cochlea, vestibule and the semicircular canals. Reproduced with permission from Ref. 8.

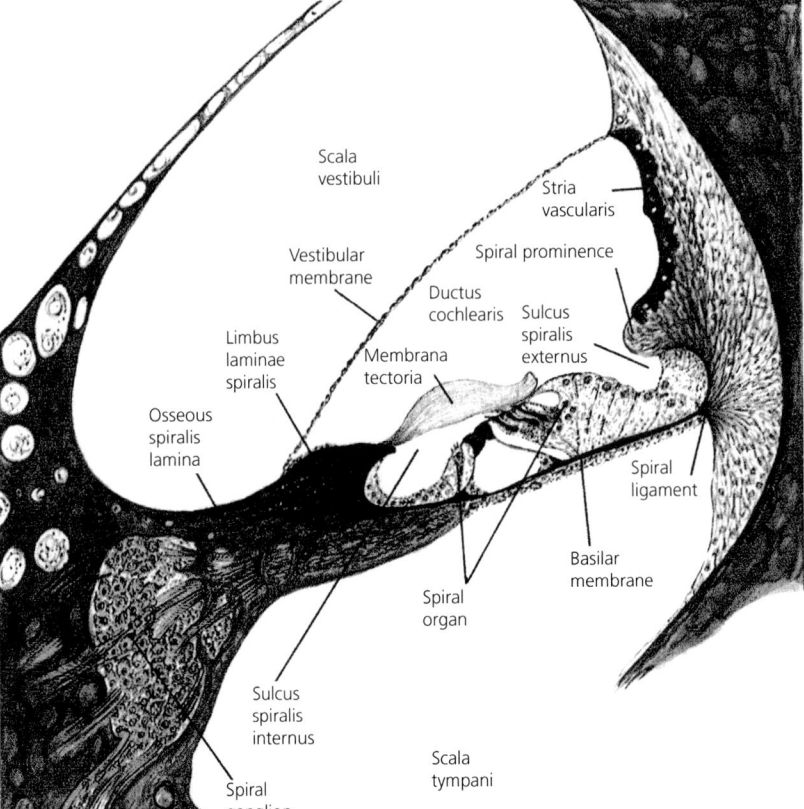

Figure 46.5 Section through the cochlea showing the organ of Corti. Mallory's stain. Reproduced with permission from Ref. 8. See website (www.hodderplus.com/hunters) for colour plate.

The sensory cells of the organ of Corti are arranged in one inner row and three to five outer rows. Microfilaments (stereocilia) from the sensory cell surface have given rise to the descriptive term sensory hair cells (Figure 46.6). This represents the interface where mechanical energy is converted to electrical energy: the organ of Corti is thus a specialized transducer. From the sensory cells, afferent nerve fibres pass together as the cochlear nerve to the brainstem and ultimately to the auditory cortex of the brain.

The incident mechanical energy at the oval window sets up a series of waves in the perilymph of the scala vestibuli which in turn distort the membranes of the cochlear duct.

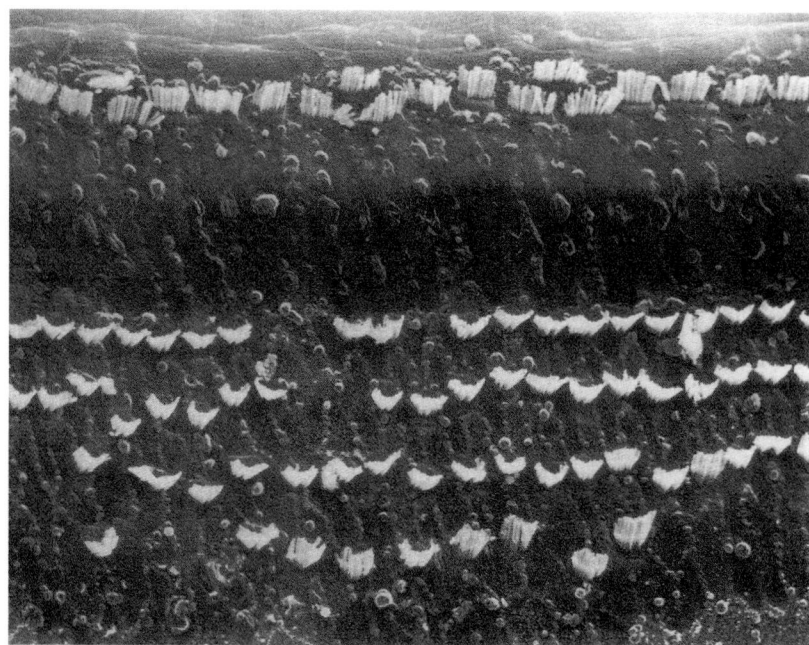

Figure 46.6 Scanning electron micrograph of part of the human organ of Corti. There is a single row of inner hair cells and several rows of outer hair cells. Reproduced with permission from Ref. 106.

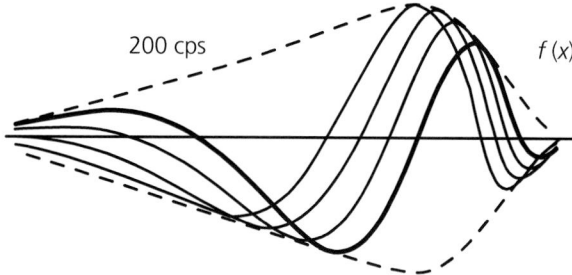

Figure 46.7 The cochlear travelling wave according to Békésy. The solid lines depict displacement at four successive instants and the dotted lines show the static envelope. Reproduced with permission from Ref. 1.

In the 1940s, Békésy introduced the concept of the travelling wave (Figure 46.7) following a series of experiments in which he observed the movements of cadaveric basilar membranes in response to high intensity sounds at different frequencies.[7,10] The travelling waves for higher frequencies peaked at the basal end of the cochlear, while the lower frequencies produced a peaked wave towards the apex. He correctly concluded that the basilar membrane had the property of frequency selectivity. More recent work has shown that the mechanical response of the basilar membrane (by way of tuning or frequency-threshold curves) and indeed the tuning curves for hair cells and the auditory neurons is very narrow.[11,12] There is thus a sharp band pass frequency for a given point on the basilar membrane, the hair cells in the organ of Corti at that point and the auditory neurons from those sensory cells.[13] The auditory system thus exhibits sensitivity and frequency selectivity, probably as an active as well as passive mechanical process in the basilar membrane.[1] The deflection of the basilar membrane results in deflection of the stereocilia of the sensory cells in the organ of Corti. Depending on the relative movements of the stereocilia, ion channels in the sensory cell membrane are either opened or closed.[14] The resultant movement of potassium and calcium ions from the endolymph into the hair cells and change in their relative electrical potentials leads to the release of neurotransmitters in the synapses at the base of the hair cells giving rise to action potentials in the auditory nerve fibres. This then completes the process of transduction as the inner hair cells are in contact with 95 per cent of the afferent fibres of the auditory nerve.

OCCUPATIONAL NOISE-INDUCED HEARING LOSS

Historical aspects

One of the earliest descriptions of the adverse effects of noise on hearing was by Francis Lord Bacon in 1627.[15] He wrote, 'A very great sound, near hand, hath strucken many deaf.' He relates his own experience of what was a temporary threshold shift, '… myself, standing near one that lured (whistled loudly to call back a falcon) loud and shrill, had suddenly an offence, as if somewhat had broken or been dislocated in my ear; and immediately after a loud ringing (not an ordinary singing or hissing, but far louder and differing) so I feared some deafness. But after some half quarter of an hour it vanished'.

Nearly a century later, a report by Ramazzini recognized the relationship between copper hammering and hearing impairment[16] and in 1782, Admiral Lord Rodney was deafened for two weeks following the firing of 80 broadsides from his ship HMS Formidable.[17] In 1831, Fosbroke accurately described noise-induced hearing loss in blacksmiths and coined the phrase 'blacksmith's deafness'.[18] It was the arrival of the Industrial Age, however, that led to a more widespread recognition of the deleterious effects of intense or prolonged noise on hearing: Roosa and Holt in the United States of America, Bezold in Germany and Barr in Great Britain.[5]

The work of Thomas Barr merits further consideration. He undertook field studies comparing the hearing in 100 boilermakers, 100 ironmoulders and 100 postmen.[19] He wrote, 'It is familiarly known that boilermakers and others who work in very noisy surroundings are extremely liable to dullness of hearing. In Glasgow, we would have little difficulty in finding hundreds whose sense of hearing has thus been damaged, by the noisy character of their work. We have therefore in our city ample materials at hand for investigation on this subject'. Barr found that 75 per cent of the boilermakers had difficulty in hearing at church or at a public meeting compared with 12 per cent of the ironmoulders and 8 per cent of the postmen. Four years later, in 1890, the pathology of noise-induced hearing loss was described by Habermann. Partial loss of the organ of Corti with destruction of the hair cells, particularly in the basal turn was noted.[20]

Following the introduction of audiometry, Fowler in 1929 observed the characteristic 4-kHz dips and the first systematic audiometric studies were reported in 1939 by Bunch and by Larsen.[21–23] The technological advancements seen after the Second World War were paralleled by ever-increasing noise levels in the workplace. While loss of earnings due to hearing loss caused by acute trauma at work was compensatable from the early part of the last century, it is only in the last 35 years that the legislative bodies of developed countries have recognized occupational noise-induced hearing loss, put into place mechanisms to confer responsibility on the manufacturing industries and compensate those individuals deemed to suffer this disorder.

Epidemiology

Occupational noise-induced hearing loss is considered one of the most common occupational disorders in industrial countries. Apparently, between 1 and 4 per cent of the population are exposed to harmful or potentially harmful noise levels and the presence or effectiveness of hearing conservation programmes will dictate the proportion of these individuals who do not have a noise-induced hearing deficit.[4] The paucity of hard data on hearing impairment in the adult population prompted the Medical Research Council to fund a multicentre epidemiological study which was carried out in the 1980s. This rigorous study (UK National Study of Hearing) found that 12 per cent of adults in the United Kingdom had a sensorineural hearing defect. Around one-third of these was accounted for by age and 5 per cent by noise.[24] This would imply that around 1 in 200 of the adult population has noise-related sensorineural hearing impairment. Putting aside principal factors, such as the level and nature of noise exposure, its duration and hearing conservation programmes, adjunctive factors are also recognized. Variations in individual susceptibility are now considered to be multifactorial, but nonetheless a real entity.[25] The evidence for differences in susceptibility between men and women or between dark- and fair-skinned individuals is conflicting.[25,26] Indeed, a recent pilot study showed that in view of their ambivalence to their disorder, women with noise-induced hearing loss are less likely to be reported than men in studies examining noise-induced hearing loss.[27] With regard to children, a study that screened over 14 000 Swedish schoolchildren found a greater than 20-dB, 4-kHz dip in 2.3 per cent with nearly two-thirds having an identifiable noise exposure factor, such as firearms and crackers.[28] Perhaps the greatest area of concern, however, is that while developed countries are slowly bringing noise under control, the developing nations are witnessing an ever increasing level of urban and industrial noise.

Effects of sound stimulation and hazardous noise

ADAPTATION (PERSTIMULATORY FATIGUE)

This is an immediate physiological phenomenon that occurs when a sound is presented to the ear. For sound pressure levels up to 80 dB, the greatest elevation in threshold occurs at the same frequency of the stimulating tone. There follows an exponential recovery which occurs within 1 second. Electrophysiological animal studies have shown that adaptation correlates with a reduction in auditory nerve action potentials.[29] For higher stimulating sound intensities, true temporary threshold shift sets in though the intensity of stimulation required varies from individual to individual and depends on the frequency of the stimulating tone.

TEMPORARY THRESHOLD SHIFT (POST-STIMULATORY FATIGUE)

The magnitude of a temporary threshold shift is proportional to the intensity and duration of the stimulus and the recovery, unlike adaptation is slow. Recovery usually occurs within 16 hours, but may take several days with higher intensities. The risk of developing permanent threshold shift has been studied by Mills and is complex.[30] Interactions between the level, nature and number of noise exposures, their duration and frequency and the susceptibility of the individual are all factors (Figure 46.8). Classically, there is a high frequency rise in threshold with a characteristic notch at 4 kHz (Figure 46.9), though the notch may centre at 3 or 6 kHz. This is often accompanied by tinnitus and after a short rest period, the rise in threshold recovers. With repeated exposure, there is a tendency to acquire resistance to the auditory effects in that the degree of temporary threshold shift lessens[31] though at

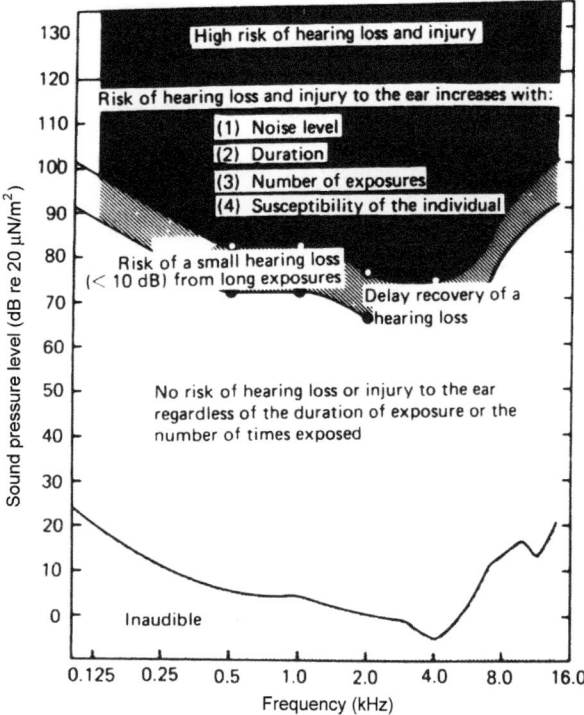

Figure 46.8 Most of the range of human audibility categorized with respect to the risk of hearing loss and injury. Reproduced with permission from Ref. 5.

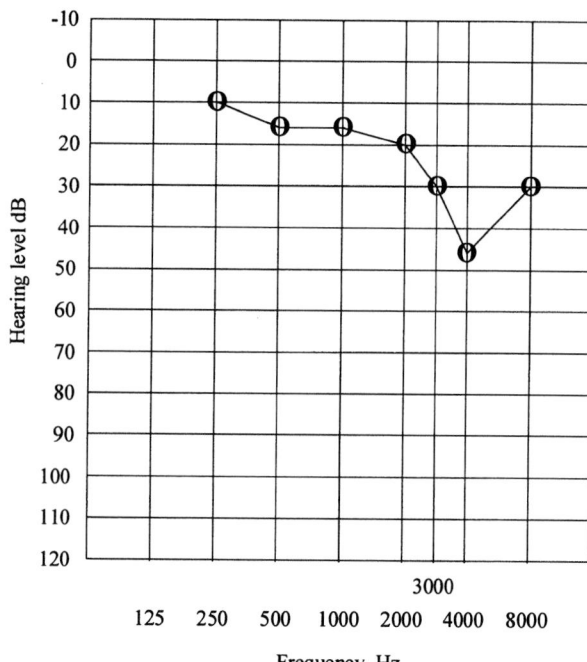

Figure 46.9 Pure tone audiogram, right ear, showing the typical 4-kHz notch after excessive noise exposure.

some arbitrary point, continued exposure leads to a permanent threshold shift.

PERMANENT THRESHOLD SHIFT

This is characterized by irreversible audiometric effects and pathological changes in the cochlea. The 4-kHz notch tends to deepen but also insidiously widens, encompassing adjacent high frequencies (Figure 46.10). Once the audiometric changes encroach upon the speech frequencies (2 and 3 kHz in particular), the affected individual becomes aware of the diminished acuity in his or her hearing. Speech discrimination with background noise becomes difficult and the associated tinnitus (which is highly variable in character) may become intrusive. The rate of progression again depends on the noise parameters cited previously and on individual susceptibility. Generally, progression at 4 kHz is initially rapid, but slows down after 10–12 years. Progression to involve the lower frequencies is associated with a flattening of the audiogram in the highest frequencies (Figure 46.11) such that the characteristic notched audiogram is not a prerequisite for a diagnosis of occupational noise-induced hearing loss. At this stage, the impaired speech discrimination in noise is accompanied by the complaint of sound generally being too quiet.[5]

With the progression of time, the increasing effects of ageing on auditory function come into play and this aspect assumes importance in the evaluation process of those being assessed with possible occupational noise-induced hearing loss (see below).

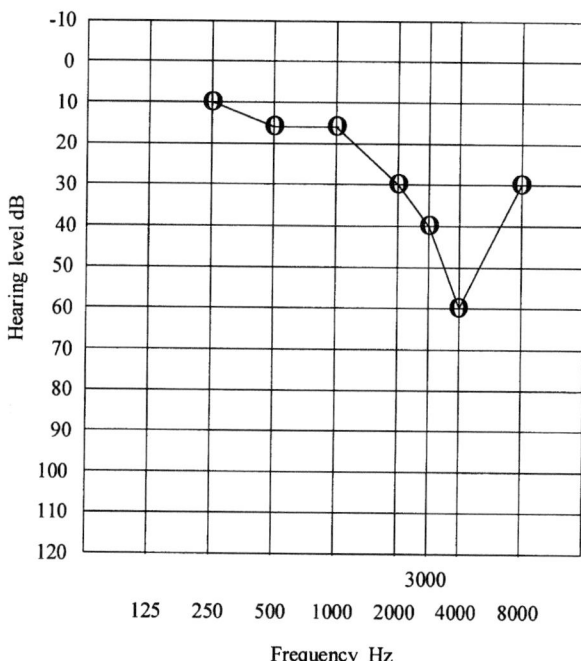

Figure 46.10 Pure tone audiogram, right ear, showing a deepening of the 4-kHz notch and involvement of adjacent frequencies.

Pathology

As mentioned previously, the correlation of occupational noise-induced hearing loss with cochlear pathology was first described by Habermann in 1890. He reported that it

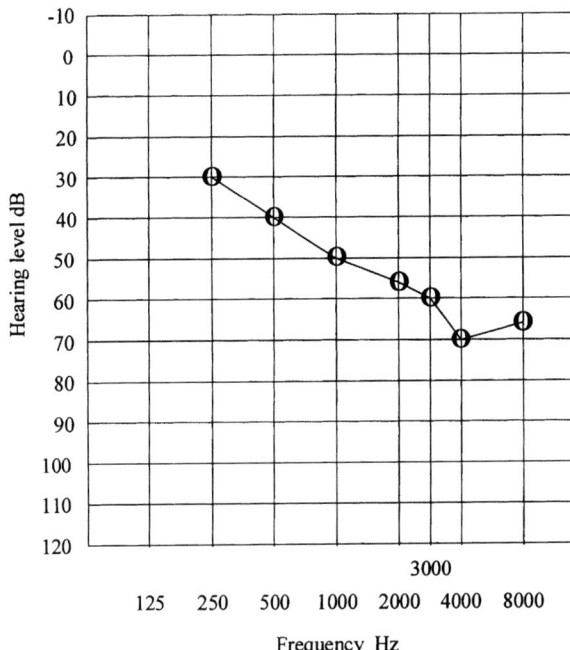

Figure 46.11 Pure tone audiogram, right ear, showing a rise in the thresholds across the mid and high frequencies after protracted exposure to noise.

was the organ of Corti, particularly the sensory hair cells and occasionally the spiral ganglion cells of the auditory nerve fibres that were affected.[20] Studies by Igarashi and colleagues[32] and Bredberg[33] showed that the site of predilection in the organ of Corti was 11 mm and 10.5–14 mm, respectively, from the beginning of the basal turn of the cochlea. This corresponds to an area that is responsive to sound frequencies around 4 kHz.

The work of Békésy in the 1940s not surprisingly led to attempts to tie in his mechanical travelling wave theories with pathological changes in the cochlea. If the maximal excursion of the basilar membrane in response to a travelling wave is in its central relatively unsupported part, then the shearing stress is exerted maximally at this point and would explain why the supporting cells of the inner hair cells and the first row of the outer hair cells are the structures that sustain most injury.[34] As the limitations of the Békésy model were realized and technological advances, such as electron microscopy, became available, the ultrastructure and function of the hair cells themselves has become the focus of attention.

Progressive degrees of stereocilial damage and hair cell death correlate with temporary and permanent threshold shifts (Figure 46.12).[35,36] The sensitivity of the afferent inner hair cells depends in part on the function of the efferent outer hair cells[37] and it is postulated that dysfunction of the latter has an adverse effect on the function of the former. The time-honoured belief that the pathological site correlated with the threshold shift has also been challenged as there is a variation in the distribution of the hair cell loss and loss of cochlear sensitivity, related perhaps to the response of the middle ear muscles to different types of hazardous sound stimulation.[38] In addition to these mechanical factors, metabolic and vascular factors have been postulated.[39]

It is becoming increasingly apparent that the damage to the cochlea caused by excessive noise is the result of cellular injury from reactive oxygen species (ROS). ROS are ions or small molecules that include oxygen ions, free radicals (hydroxyl radical OH, peroxynitrite radical ONOO) and peroxides (e.g. hydrogen peroxide, H_2O_2) and are produced in the mitochondria. They are a natural product of oxygen metabolism and have an important role in cell signalling. They may, however, be produced in excess in response to stress and are then capable of causing serious damage to cell structures, a condition known as 'oxidative stress'. They have a role in programmed cell death (aptoptosis), and also have some beneficial effects in the induction of host defence genes. The damaging effects of ROS include damage to DNA, oxidation of fatty acids and amino acids and inactivation of enzyme systems. Normally, there are enzyme systems that protect the cell from damage from ROS, such as superoxide dismutase, catalases, glutathione peroxidases. In addition, antioxidants, such as ascorbic acid (vitamin C) and tocopherol (vitamin E), have a major role in scavenging free radicals.

The cochlea is metabolically highly active and produces ROS which are in normal circumstances neutralized by endogenous antioxidant mechanisms. There is evidence that oxidative stress can be responsible for cochlear impairment as a result of an accumulation of harmful free radicals. Noise exposure is the most common cause of this stress, but similar mechanisms are at play in cochlear injury from ototoxic medication. One factor which seems to play a significant part in causing these metabolic changes is the role of reduced cochlear blood flow following stimulation with loud noise.

There is a body of animal work to support the ROS theory. During acoustic overstimulation, there is a change in cochlear homeostasis with an increase in the uptake of glucose and an increase in the perilymphatic oxygenation. Superoxide anions and hydroxyl radicals build up in the scala media after excessive exposure to noise.[40] Ohlemiller et al.[41] demostrated a two-fold increase in hydroxyl radical in the cochlea after a one hour exposure to broadband noise of 112 dB. The process of lipid peroxidation consists of a series of reactions through which free radicals and ROS can break down lipid molecules, such as cell membranes. There is evidence of increased lipid peroxidation after noise exposure.[42,43] Noise-induced changes in the sensory cells of the cochlea may also be mediated through the Src-protein tyrosine kinase (PTK) signalling cascade.[44] It is clear that there is much laboratory animal work being done and many points in the homeostatic pathway are being identified at which injury from noise may occur. It is interesting that the changes in the cochlea are not all immediate and that there is a significant late formation of free radical as late as seven to ten days following noise exposure.[45]

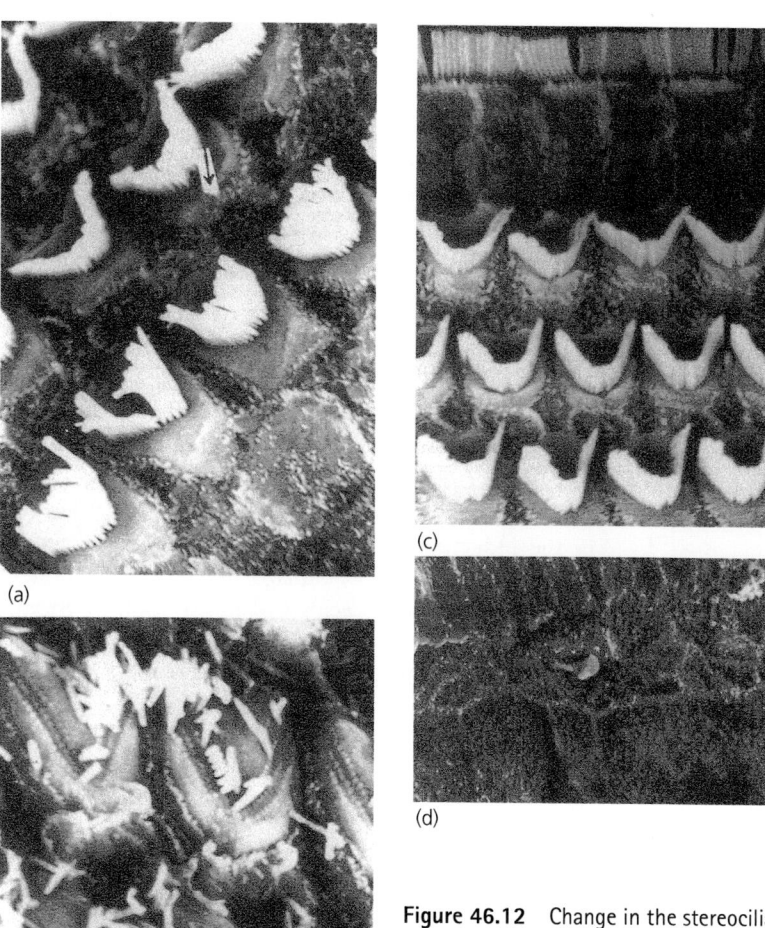

Figure 46.12 Change in the stereocilia of guinea pigs. (a) Exposure to 110 dB for 30 min; half an hour after exposure, there is swelling of the cuticular plate (arrow) ×2800. (b) Exposure to 110 dB for 30 min; 80 days after exposure, 9.5 mm from the round window. The inner and outer hair cells appear normal as was the hearing threshold (×1900). (c) Exposure to 120 dB for 150 min; half an hour after exposure, there is total loss of the stereocilia on the outer hair cells (×4300). (d) Exposure to 120 dB for 150 min; 80 days after exposure, 9 mm from the round window. The surface is devoid of both sterocilia and hair cells, correlating with a 30–35 dB permanent threshold shift at 2 and 4 kHz. Reproduced with permission from Ref. 5.

The effects of middle ear disease

The widely held belief that a conductive hearing loss due to middle ear disease serves to protect the inner ear from hazardous noise is open to debate as the literature is somewhat conflicting. Alberti and colleagues[46] studied a group of individuals with otosclerosis and presumed occupational noise-induced hearing loss and found that there was no difference in the bone conduction threshold curves between the operated and non-operated ear, even though the individuals concerned had continued to work in a noisy environment after their surgery. Similarly, Simpson and O'Reilly[47] could not demonstrate a protective effect on the inner ear in a worker with chronic middle ear disease. In contrast, a study by McShane and colleagues[48] examined the hearing in workers with unilateral unoperated otosclerosis and demonstrated a small protective effect (around 4 dB) in the affected ear at 4 kHz.

Hinchcliffe has discussed the reasons for such disparate findings and reduces them to two main factors.[4] First, the two most common causes of adult conductive hearing loss, otosclerosis and chronic inflammatory middle ear disease, may be associated with sensorineural hearing loss – the former as cochlear otosclerosis and the latter as a complication of the disease. The pathological status of the middle ear in terms of extent, nature and activity also has a bearing on inner ear function. Ossicular fixation (whether due to otosclerosis or otherwise) alters the middle ear resonance and may give rise to the 2-kHz Carhart notch in the bone conduction threshold. Second, the temporal relationship between the onset of the conductive hearing loss and noise exposure is also relevant. Clearly, the interaction between middle ear disease and inner ear function is complex and one cannot draw the intuitive conclusion that a conductive hearing loss acts as some form of hearing protective device.

Diagnosis of occupational noise-induced hearing loss

The process of establishing a diagnosis of occupational noise-induced hearing loss should be no different from the process of reaching a diagnosis when faced with any other clinical problem. The fundamental principles of taking a comprehensive and pertinent history, conducting a thorough examination and undertaking appropriate investigations are just as applicable. However, certain factors cloud this process and as a result the diagnosis is usually circumstantial.[5] When faced with an individual with hearing loss and a history of occupational noise exposure, the clinician has to make a decision as to whether the former is a result of the latter. This gives rise to the first problem. Of the 12 per cent of adults found to have a sensorineural hearing loss in the Medical Research Council study cited earlier under Epidemiology (p. 465), only 40 per cent of these could be accounted for by the effects of age or noise exposure.[24] Some of the remaining 60 per cent were no doubt due to the myriad of less common or rare disorders (in population terms) that cause a sensorineural hearing loss, but a significant proportion were idiopathic (cause unknown). If the diagnostic process is one of exclusion of known causes, Williams has put forward the argument that attempting to exclude that which cannot be identified defies logic.[49] However, appraisal by an appropriately trained clinician remains paramount as there is no reason why the prevalence of other otological disorders should be any different in the individual with noise-induced deafness than in the general population. The Department of Health and Social Security publication 'Occupational deafness' states that apart from the characteristic audiometric changes, there are no signs or symptoms specific to noise-induced deafness.[50] This implies that the diagnosis of occupational noise-induced hearing loss is an audiometric one. However, the characteristic audiogram with its 4-kHz notch is not a pathognomonic feature of noise-induced deafness. The notch may lie between 3 and 6 kHz (a notch centred at 6 kHz is considered to be an artefact), and with progression over time the notch may widen and be lost as the thresholds at the higher frequencies rise. Additionally, noise exposure is not the only cause of a 4-kHz notch and the hearing loss may not necessarily be symmetrical.[51]

The history must include not only audiovestibular symptoms, but also details of previous and intercurrent focal and systemic disorders that may affect the ear. This includes the administration of potentially ototoxic drugs. The history of noise exposure, whether occupational, military or otherwise, can be difficult to construct in temporal terms as individuals may have difficulty in recalling past events and employment accurately. Increasing recognition of non-syndromic familial sensorineural deafness and the familial nature of otosclerosis and some cases of Menière's disease underline the importance of obtaining a good family history. Autoimmune deafness may be associated with systemic symptoms and these should be enquired about. The examination of the ear, nose and throat must be complete. Much information regarding the health of the external and middle ear can be gleaned from pneumatic otoscopy and if the clinician is in any doubt, microscopic examination of the ear should be readily available, if nothing else, to clear the external meatus of wax that precludes a view of the drumhead. Aside from the audiometric evaluation, additional investigations are dictated by the clinical assessment and include haematological, serological and relevant immunological laboratory tests, in addition to radiology if indicated. Evaluation of the historical, clinical and investigative evidence usually allows, if present, the causal relationship between hearing loss and noise exposure to be established, but as there is currently no single clinical or investigative feature unique to noise-induced hearing loss, the diagnosis remains one of clinical probability and audiometric compatibility.

ACOUSTIC TRAUMA AND BLAST TRAUMA

The preceding discussion has primarily focused on the auditory effects of prolonged exposure to hazardous noise. The term 'acoustic trauma' describes permanent hearing loss following brief exposure to a single very loud noise. This encompasses, for example, the effects of gunfire, but also includes the effects of industrial impulse noise associated with drop forging and riveting. Gunfire noise in particular has the potential to be extremely hazardous. Peak sound pressure levels of 160 dB for hand-held weapons to 190 dB for field weapons have been recorded and therefore permanent injury to the inner ear may arise from the first exposure.[5] It is worth bearing in mind that with rifle fire, the forward ear (left ear in a right-handed individual) is closer to the muzzle, thereby bearing the greater brunt of the acoustic trauma than the opposite ear and this is often discernible audiometrically. Second, occupational noise-induced hearing loss and acoustic trauma may coexist in the same individual.

Blast trauma (otic blast injury) is due to the effects of an explosion such as a bomb blast, but may also be a component of the acoustic trauma from large calibre weapons. It is characterized by a greater severity and may be associated with damage to the tympanic membrane and the middle ear structures.[52] The shock wave from an explosion is longer than that of hazardous sound and consists of a short (5 ms) positive pressure followed by a longer (30 ms) negative pressure. Clinically, there may be a history of bleeding from the ear following the injury and examination shows a spectrum of tympanic membrane changes ranging from hyperaemia to frank perforation of the pars tensa which may be 'clean' or ragged. It is the initial positive pressure that perforates the drumhead and the subsequent negative pressure that leads to the characteristic everted edges of the perforation. The resultant deafness and tinnitus is immediate and severe but recovery, though incomplete for the higher pitches, is not uncommon and over three-quarters of drumhead perforations heal spontaneously.[52]

ASSESSMENT OF HEARING DISABILITY

Impairment, disability and handicap

These consequences of disease are differentiated by the World Health Organization.[53]

- **Impairment** relates to a loss or impairment of the structure or function of an organ or system. Within the auditory system, there are a number of impairments of function which could be measured. The one which has most relevance for the assessment of hearing disability is the alteration in the pure tone threshold.
- **Disability** is an index of the loss of an individual's functional performance as a consequence of impairment to the diseased organ or system. It thus represents a disturbance at the level of the individual. Hearing disability has been described as the restriction or lack of ability to perceive everyday sounds in the manner that is considered normal for healthy young people.[54]
- **Handicap** encompasses the disadvantages experienced by an individual as a consequence of impairments and disabilities. It thus reflects interactions between the individual and his social and working environment. Hearing handicap is the disadvantage to an individual resulting from a hearing impairment or disability, that limits or prevents the fulfilment of a role that is normal for that individual. Disability and handicap are thus seen to be multifaceted. A given degree of hearing impairment could represent a much greater handicap for a professional musician than for a sculptor for example. The complex picture of disability and handicap that may result from occupational noise-induced hearing loss has been painted by Hetu et al.[55]

In 1981, a working party of members of the British Association of Otolaryngologists (BAOL) and the British Society of Audiologists (BSA) was set up to address the problem of assessment of hearing disability for the purpose of compensation. Up to then, there was a plethora of conflicting recommendations, from a number of different sources. The results of the working party's deliberations were published in the so-called 'Blue Book' of 1983.[56] Because of some misgivings about its conclusions, a new group called the Inter-Society Working Group was established in 1986 with a wider membership including representatives of the British Association of Audiological Physicians (BAAP), and the British Association of Audiological Scientists (BAAS).

The results of this group's efforts are published in 'Guidelines for medicolegal practice', although the BAAP did not sign up to the final document because of problems on the definition of disability and on agreeing the scale of degrees of disablement. The group considered every aspect of hearing disability and its assessment. They stated that, 'hearing disability assessment should provide an accurate quantitative assessment of the actual disability suffered by the individual, appropriately weighted according to the way he uses his auditory facilities and the extent to which difficulties in hearing interfere with those activities'. The authors recognize, however, that the ideal is impossible to attain in an easily measurable, scientific and quantitative way because of the subjective nature of disability and handicap and the great variability between individuals. They identify instead a typical (median or average) individual and relate disability to that notional individual, and they recognize that such a concept may underestimate disability in some people and overestimate it in others. They also recognize the need to identify an audiometric surrogate (i.e. a measure of impairment) as a means of quantifying disability.

Several studies have been carried out to identify the audiometric descriptors which best relate with disability including those by Atherley and Noble,[57] Lutman et al.[58] and the Medical Research Council's National Study of Hearing from the early 1980s. These studies, by and large, looked at the different patterns on pure tone audiometry which were the best predictors of disability. It was concluded that the three-frequency average of 1, 2 and 3 kHz was the best predictor. Errors were introduced by the inclusion of 0.5 Hz and 6 kHz.[59] It may seem strange that 4 kHz is excluded from this formula, when one considers that this is the frequency most likely to be affected by occupational noise; however, the notches at 4 kHz may be narrow but quite deep, so that there is a danger of obtaining an inflated average hearing threshold measurement which does not truly reflect the degree of disability. Furthermore, it is convenient not to include 4 kHz in the estimate because of the difficulty in obtaining accurate bone conduction thresholds above 3 kHz. Finally, the three-frequency average coincides with the UK statutory hearing loss criteria, even though the fence values of the latter may be subject to some criticism.

Fence values

The low fence is that notional point on the continuum of elevation of the hearing threshold level at which disability is deemed to commence. It has never been satisfactorily identified, and indeed cannot be seen as anything other than an artifice erected for administrative convenience, with little relevance to the individual case. Robinson et al.[60] identified a 30 dB hearing threshold level averaged over 1, 2 and 3 kHz as the threshold of disability, and this coincides with British Standard BS 5330 (1976).[61] A low fence as high as 50 dB HL (1, 2, 3 kHz average) is employed in the UK statutory compensation scheme. Even the much lower value of 26 dB (0.5, 1, 2 kHz) that prevailed under the American Academy of Otolaryngology and Ophthalmology (AAOO) scheme underestimated the disability of those individuals who began life with hearing that was 'normal'. The high fence is that point in the continuum of elevation of hearing threshold level at which disability is deemed to be total. High fence values have been judged to be any level from 70 dB upwards, and are just as arbitrary as low fence values.

AGE-ASSOCIATED HEARING LOSS

Ageing is associated with a progressive loss of auditory function, a condition which has been described in the past as 'presbyacusis'. It is recognized that most of the impairment arises as a result of progressive cochlear dysfunction with loss of hair cells from the organ of Corti, affecting the higher frequencies first, but advancing through the cochlea to affect eventually the whole frequency range to some extent. Other structures may also undergo degenerative change, for example the auditory nerve and the central auditory pathways. There may also be a central loss of cognitive function. It is clearly important to be able to make some allowance for the effects of 'natural' ageing on the hearing of those middle-aged and elderly individuals who have also been exposed to the harmful effects of noise during their working lives.

Data on this subject are available from many sources. International Standard ISO 7029 (1984)[62] gives values of age-associated hearing loss as deviations relative to the median thresholds of young otologically normal subjects. The data are available for sex, for the age range 20–70 years, for frequencies ranging from 125 Hz to 8 kHz, and for percentiles of the population from the 5th to the 95th. They are available in table form for ease of reference so that allowance can be made in the individual case for the effects of ageing.[63]

The International Standard ISO 1999 (1990)[64] 'Determination of occupational noise exposure and estimation of noise-induced hearing impairment' assumes a direct additive effect between noise and age effects, although that is not true at profound levels of deafness. A word of caution is necessary, however. Burns and Robinson[65] and Robinson[66] have drawn attention to the complicated interrelationship of occupational noise-induced hearing loss and ageing. The former tends to produce an elevation in threshold which is initially rapid, but slows down with subsequent exposure. Age-related hearing loss takes a progressively accelerating course with time. Thus, the contribution of occupational noise-induced hearing loss to the total sensorineural hearing loss decreases with age, and by the age of 80 it would make virtually no difference what the noise had been.[49]

HEARING CONSERVATION PROGRAMMES

There are several areas in which employers may help to minimize the risks to the hearing of employees from the harmful effects of industrial noise:

- noise measurement and reduction;
- provision of personal ear protection;
- audiometric testing;
- education.

Noise measurement: the relationship of hearing loss to noise exposure

With the development of accurate methods of measuring both the sound stimulus and the hearing level, more precise determination of the relationship between hearing loss and noise exposure has become possible. Burns and Robinson[59] reduced the number of significant parameters to two: the noise level and the duration of exposure. Daily personal noise exposure (L_{EPd}) can be determined by wearing a personal sound dosimeter over a given period. A more accurate picture may, however, be established from the measured values of A-weighted sound pressure levels and the duration of exposure at work using a Noise Exposure Ready Reckoner as recommended in the 2005 Health and Safety Executive document 'Controlling Noise at Work'.[68] This employs a noise exposure points system relating average sound pressure levels (L_{Aeq} dB) with duration of noise exposure in hours. It is a simple way of working out the daily personal noise exposure especially in situations where the noise exposure is variable throughout the day, for example, if an employee spends part of a day in a very noisy environment and part of the day in a less noisy activity (Table 46.2). In the noise exposure points scheme, the upper exposure action value is 100 points (equivalent to an L_{EPd} of 85 dB) and the lower exposure action is 32 points (equivalent to an L_{EPd} of 80 dB) (Table 46.3). For a worked example of this scheme, the reader is referred to the original document. The 'first action level' of 80 dB is the level at which ear protectors should be available on demand. The 'second action level' of 85 dB is the level at which the use of ear protectors is mandatory. These values have each been reduced by 5 dB since the previous 1989 document.[67] A similar scoring system can be used to work out weekly exposure and is of particular value if there is significant variation in noise exposure from day to day during the working week.

There are also occasions when one wants to establish the L_{EPd} caused by repeated 'single event' noise produced for example by impact or cartridge-operated tools. Peak pressure meters provide rapid information and are easy to use. If the reading exceeds 125 dBA, more accurate measurements should be made. An integrating sound level meter (BS 6693: IEC 804) is the most convenient instrument for general use. It calculates the equivalent continuous sound pressure level

Table 46.2 Noise level and duration of exposure are combined to give 'noise exposure points'.

Sound pressure level, L_{AEq} (dB)	Duration of exposure (hours)							
	$\frac{1}{4}$	$\frac{1}{2}$	1	2	4	8	10	12
105	320	625	1250					
100	100	200	400	800				
97	50	100	200	400	800			
95	32	65	125	250	500	1000		
94	25	50	100	200	400	800		
93	20	40	80	160	320	630		
92	16	32	65	125	250	500	625	
91	12	25	50	100	200	400	500	600
90	10	20	40	80	160	320	400	470
89	8	16	32	65	130	250	310	380
88	6	12	25	50	100	200	250	300
87	5	10	20	40	80	160	200	240
86	4	8	16	32	65	130	160	190
85		6	12	25	50	100	125	150
84		5	10	20	40	80	100	120
83		4	8	16	32	65	80	95
82			6	12	25	50	65	75
81			5	10	20	40	50	60
80			4	8	16	32	40	48
79				6	13	25	32	38
78				5	10	20	25	30
75					5	10	13	15

Reproduced with permission from Ref. 67.

according to the equal energy principle. A peak sound pressure level of 140 dB is defined as the 'peak action level'. At this level, the use of ear protectors is mandatory.

It is clearly the responsibility of employers to ensure that all measurement equipment is accurately and regularly calibrated.

Employers in the music and entertainment industries were given an additional period of two years to comply with the 2005 regulations, while continuing to comply with the 1989 regulations.[67,68]

Noise reduction

This can be helped, *inter alia*, by the enclosure of noisy machines, the use of mufflers, damping, silencers and anti-vibration mountings, the treatment of reflective surfaces with absorbing materials, the limitation of the use of noisy equipment to times when it is actually required, and the distancing of workers from the areas of maximum noise. There are many more suggestions for the reduction of noise in the workplace in the consultative document 'Prevention of damage to hearing from noise at work' published by the Health and Safety Commission in 1987.[69] The publication 'Sound solutions' published by the Health and Safety Executive in 1995 provides employers with many examples of techniques to reduce noise in the workplace.[70]

ACTIVE NOISE CONTROL

The principles of active noise control (or active cancellation) have been known for 60 years, but the techniques remain rather experimental. One sound is cancelled by the introduction of a second sound of equal amplitude but reversed phase, derived electronically from the first sound. There are considerable difficulties in designing and commissioning these systems, but the technique does show considerable promise in the reduction of low frequency noise where control by passive measures can be difficult. Commercial interest in the technique is increasing.

EAR PROTECTION

Ear protection provides a system of attenuation of the incoming sound and thus minimizes the sound arriving at the tympanic membrane. Various types of protector are available.[71,72]

Ear muffs

Ear muffs (Figure 46.13) fit over the ears and are sealed to the side of the head by soft cushion seals filled with soft plastic foam or a viscous fluid. They are usually held in position by means of a headband, but may alternatively be attached to a safely helmet. Attenuation may be 'frequency selective', protecting some frequencies more than others,

Table 46.3 Total daily exposure points converted to a daily personal exposure. Note the first and second action levels at 80 and 85 dB.

Total exposure points	Noise exposure $L_{EP,d}$ (dB)
3200	100
1600	97
1000	95
800	94
630	93
500	92
400	91
320	90
250	89
200	88
160	87
130	86
100	85
80	84
65	83
50	82
40	81
32	80
25	79
20	78
16	77

Reproduced with permission from Ref. 67.

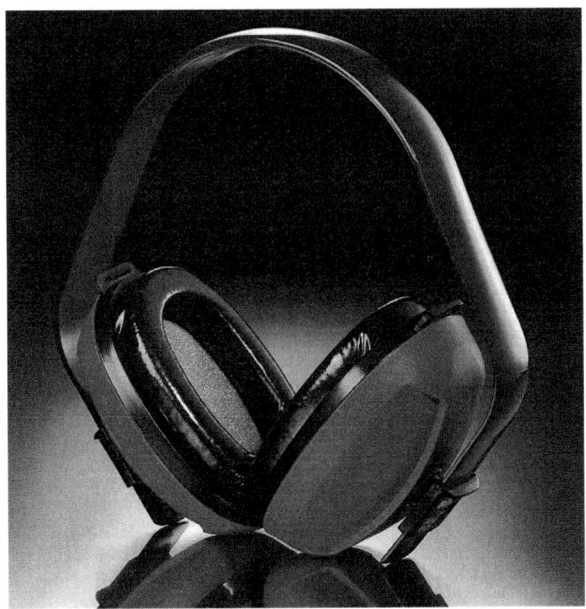

Figure 46.13 Sound-excluding ear muffs.

particularly the higher frequencies rather than the speech frequencies. 'Amplitude selective' devices are designed to provide attenuation that increases with sound level. Such a device usually has a small hole which acts as a mechanical filter, allowing low sound pressures to pass but offering more resistance at high pressures. 'Active devices' incorporate electronic circuitry which limits the transmission of sound at high intensity, and are of value when workers are exposed to short bursts of high intensity sound or impulsive sounds. 'Anti-noise' devices incorporate circuitry which cancels out incident noise especially at low frequency. These devices are still largely experimental. Many of the newer muffs incorporate an inbuilt communication system.

While ear muffs usually provide an effective level of attenuation, their value may be limited by any effect which decreases the efficiency of the seal, for example spectacle frames, goggles, beards and long hair, or scarves worn under the muffs. Furthermore, wear and tear may decrease the efficiency of the seal. It should also be emphasized that if protection is removed in noisy areas, even for a short period, the amount of protection will be severely limited. For example if a protector with an 'assumed protection' of 20 dB(A) is removed for 30 minutes per day the actual reduction in noise dose received by the wearer will be only 12 dB(A).

Ear plugs

Ear plugs are generally thought to be less efficient attenuators of sound than muffs, but have the advantage that they are easy to use. They may be disposable or permanent. Disposable plugs are made of a compressible or conformable material and fit most people without individual fitting. They are readily available commercially, but have a finite 'life expectancy' after which their effectiveness decreases. Permanent and custom moulded plugs have a longer survival, and are usually comfortable if made by an experienced technician. One of the main disadvantages of plugs is the increased propensity to otitis externa, although this too can occur with muffs.

Dual protection with the use of both muffs and ear plugs may be indicated when the noise levels are extremely high (e.g. when LEPd exceeds about 115 dBA).

Noise-excluding helmets

At extremely high levels of sound (e.g. in tunnelling), the protection offered by muffs and plugs, either alone or in combination, may be insufficient. Sound may still reach the ears through the nose, mouth, eye sockets and the skull itself. Experimental studies with helmets to protect the whole skull are at present under evaluation.

The attenuation provided by a protector should comply with British Standard BS 510866 (ISO 4869),[73,74] and the basic design features should comply with BS 6344.[75] The 'assumed protection' of a device will vary with frequency and most will attenuate higher frequency sound better than low frequency sound. The 'assumed protected level' of noise exposure is obtained by subtracting the assumed protection of the device at each octave band frequency from the sound pressure level at each frequency. Conversion should then be made to A-weighted sound levels (dBA). All this sounds complicated. Attempts to simplify the rating of devices by using a 'single number' rating which does involve frequency analysis, tends to sacrifice accuracy in the cause of simplicity. It is important that ear protection zones be identified within which use of ear protectors are advisable or mandatory.

Measurement of hearing: Audiometry in the workplace

Measurement of hearing using electroacoustic devices is generally referred to as audiometry. Pure tone audiometry records the threshold for each ear separately, at a series of test frequencies at octave intervals covering the frequencies most commonly encountered in everyday life and in particular in everyday speech. The frequencies usually tested in the clinical setting are 125 Hz, 250 Hz, 500 Hz, 1 kHz, 2 kHz, 4 kHz and 8 kHz. In the medicolegal and compensation fields, 3 kHz is always tested, and 6 kHz may be. Air and bone conduction thresholds are measured to establish the presence or absence of a conductive component of the overall hearing loss. Bone conduction thresholds are inaccurate above 3 kHz. Audiometry may be carried out by an audiometrician (manual audiometry) or using a self-recording audiometer.

Hinchcliffe has pointed out the possible shortcomings of manual audiometry.[4] Two different audiometricians might obtain significantly different thresholds at 3 and 4 kHz on the same patient on the same day. Test–retest reliability on the same patient by the same audiometrician may yield differences of up to 25 dB. Self-recording audiometry eliminates the variability due to the audiometrician. By utilizing a combination of continuous and pulsed test tones, there is a greater likelihood of picking up a spurious (non-organic) hearing loss. A permanent record is obtained without the need for transcription with the risk of errors. Sweep frequencies are used because this technique may pick up notches at intervals not tested on fixed frequency audiometry. Thus, the preferred technique is sweep frequency self-recording audiometry using both continuous and pulsed tones. An audiometry programme ideally should consist of a pre-employment test followed by tests at regular intervals. Important side issues include the calibration of equipment, the acoustic requirements of the test area, instructions to the subject and the format and storing of records. These are all covered in detail in the discussion document, 'Audiometry in industry', published by the Health and Safety Executive.[76] Electric response audiometry is an objective method of assessing hearing thresholds which has no place in the routine evaluation of hearing loss, but has a role in the medicolegal arena. It is described under Electric response audiometry (evoked response audiometry, p. 477).

Information and education

Workers at risk of occupational noise-induced hearing loss need to be educated about the harmful effects of noise and the importance of hearing conservation measures. They need to understand the importance of wearing properly fitting and appropriate ear protectors. The attitude that it is somehow 'macho' not to wear ear protectors must be changed. Workers should recognize and report the first symptoms of deafness, such as temporary threshold shift and tinnitus. Warning signs should be attached to machines or displayed in all areas likely to cause workers to receive a daily personal noise exposure of 90 dBA or a peak pressure of 200 Pa (the levels at which the use of ear protectors becomes mandatory). Oral explanations, individual counselling and lectures, as well as leaflets, posters, films and videos may all be employed. Education must be extended to management so that their responsibilities are clearly defined, and managers exposed to potentially damaging sound levels must themselves be seen to be conscientious in their observation of safety measures.

LEGAL DUTIES OF EMPLOYERS

The general obligations of employers in the United Kingdom to safeguard the health of their employees (including hearing) were laid out under the Health and Safety at Work Act of 1974. Specific requirements with regard to hearing were covered by the Noise at Work Regulations 1989, which came into force on January 1, 1990. These have been superseded by the Control of Noise at Work Regulations 2005 which were enforceable from April 6, 2006. The reader is referred to 'Noise at work: Guidance for employers on the Control of Noise at Work Regulations 2005' published by the Health and Safety Executive for full details,[67] but certain salient points can be highlighted here.

- **Regulation 5.1.** An employer who carries out work which is liable to expose any employees to noise at or above a lower exposure action value shall make a suitable and sufficient assessment of the risk from that noise to the health and safety of those employees, and the risk assessment shall identify the measures which need to be taken to meet the requirements of these regulations.
- **Regulation 6.1.** The employer shall ensure that risk from exposure of his employees to noise is either eliminated at source or, where this is not reasonably practicable, reduced to a low a level as is reasonably practicable.
- **Regulation 7.1.** Without prejudice to the provisions of regulation 6, an employer who carries out work which is likely to expose any employees to noise at or above the lower exposure action value shall make personal hearing protectors available on request to any employee who is so exposed.
- **Regulation 7.2.** Without prejudice to the provisions of regulation 6, if an employer is unable by other means to reduce the levels of noise to which an employee is likely to be exposed to below an upper exposure action value, he shall provide personal hearing protectors to any employee who is so exposed.
- **Regulation 8.1.** The employer shall (a) ensure so far as is practicable that anything provided by him in compliance with his duties under these regulations to or

for the benefit of an employee, other than personal hearing protectors provided under regulation 7.1 is fully and properly used, and (b) ensure that anything provided by him in compliance with his duties under these regulations is maintained in an efficient state, in efficient working order and in good repair.
- **Regulation 9.1.** If the risk assessment indicates that there is a risk to the health of his employees who are, or liable to be, exposed to noise, the employer shall ensure that such employees are placed under suitable health surveillance, which shall include testing of hearing.
- **Regulation 9.2.** The employer shall ensure that a health record in respect of his employees who undergo health surveillance in accordance with paragraph 9.1 is made and maintained and that the record or a copy thereof is kept in a suitable form.

In addition, the regulations define the responsibilities of the employer in the provision of ear protection zones, in the maintenance and use of equipment and the provision of information, instruction and training to employees. The employees' obligations under the regulations are also emphasized. The document also deals with the legal obligations of designers, manufacturers, importers and suppliers of plant and machinery for use at work to provide noise information and control the noise emission of machinery.

MANAGEMENT

With the exception of the transient phenomenon of temporary threshold shift, the hearing loss caused by noise exposure is permanent and is due to the loss of or damage to the organ of Corti and neuronal structures in the inner ear. There is, as yet, no medical or surgical treatment that can reverse the damage to these structures. Management of occupational noise-induced hearing loss is therefore based on prevention of further damage, suitable amplification with hearing aids, and the provision where indicated of other assistive devices. It is generally felt that the process of injury to the inner ear ceases when the subject is removed from, or protected from, his noisy working environment, but subjects should be warned of further possible damage from other sources, such as recreational noise exposure.

These effects on the inner ear are, as has been previously stated, most marked in the high frequencies commencing at 4 kHz, but spreading downwards across the frequency range. The early effects, therefore, are most marked for the high frequency components of speech, the consonants, the sibilants and fricatives. It is these elements which convey most of the meaning in speech. Neuronal damage causes a further loss of speech discrimination which may not be correctable by simple amplification. In addition, there are other psychoacoustic deficits which may come into play and for which hearing aids cannot compensate, such as impaired frequency discrimination, frequency selectivity or temporal acuity. Furthermore, the phenomenon of recruitment, a feature of cochlear deafness, may limit the usefulness of amplification. This is characterized by a disproportionately great increase in the perceived loudness for a small increase in the actual sound pressure level. This is a major factor in causing distortion with hearing aids, and may limit their use. The ability to discriminate speech in the presence of background noise is lost early in the evolution of sensorineural deafness, and involves factors other than a simple elevation of the hearing threshold. It is not restored by fitting a hearing aid and it remains one of the main grievances of hearing aid users who find it impossible to converse with one individual in a noisy environment, such as a bar, cocktail party, or if the television or a stereo system is on.

Despite these shortcomings it is, however, clear that individuals with noise-induced hearing impairment can derive appreciable benefit from hearing aids provided that careful attention is given to the type of aid and the design and engineering of the ear mould.

Different hearing aids have different frequency responses. Some preferentially amplify the higher frequencies and this would intuitively seem a sensible type of device for a subject with a high frequency hearing loss. The prescription of an aid with a customized frequency response for an individual hearing loss is beguiling and has commanded much attention in recent years. It is, nevertheless, a much more challenging problem than the prescription of spectacles for a simple refractive error, for reasons mentioned earlier in this section. Different hearing aids have different gain or amplification (i.e. some are stronger than others), and again it is clearly important to have the appropriate aid for the severity of the deafness. Hearing aids, like car engines, have a point or a range at which they function best. If one attempts to get more performance from an underpowered aid, there is a marked fall off in the efficiency of the device. It is better to get a stronger aid and have it working at its most efficient level. Compression aids incorporating automatic gain control, attempt to overcome the problem of the loud sound which exceeds the discomfort level of the listener.

Systems which address the problems of understanding speech in the presence of background noise have been developed and in the UK are at present only available in the private health sector, where they cost considerably over £1000.

The other factor of considerable importance is the design and fitting of the hearing aid mould. The aid must fit comfortably in the ear, but must be secure enough to prevent acoustic feedback problems – the whistling that one often associates with hearing aids is usually the result of a poorly fitting mould or an underpowered aid with the volume setting too high. The effect of occlusion of the ear canal may be to cause otitis externa in susceptible individuals. Some wearers develop an allergic reaction in the skin of the meatus to the mould material. Hypoallergenic alternatives are available to overcome such problems.

The physical properties of the mould have an effect on the acoustic output of the aid and modifications to the mould may influence the performance of the device. Venting entails the creation of a second hole next to the existing sound tube. This has a considerable effect in increasing the low frequency responses of the aid. It also incidentally may decrease the tendency to otitis externa by decreasing the greenhouse effect within the ear canal. Funnelling of the outlet tube where the sound leaves the mould may increase the high frequency response. Acoustic filters can be introduced into the tube. These may alter the shape of the frequency response curve. All of these facilities are available in the United Kingdom on the standard ear level hearing aids. The National Health Service does not, at present, provide small in-the-ear aids.

In addition to hearing aids, there are other assistive devices or environmental aids that can be used with or independent of conventional hearing aids[70] including amplifying devices, alerting and alarm systems, telephone modifications and speech-to-text transcription. They are not necessarily expensive and may provide significant personal benefit. They include induction loop systems, television listening aids, tactile and visual devices activated by sound stimuli (door bells, fire alarms, alarm clocks, telephone). Inductive coupling between coils in the handpiece and the hearing aid greatly helps telephone conversation. Text telephones using a computer link, or a relay service via an operator may help the very deaf. Speech-to-text transcription, such as Palantype, is a major help at public meetings, but is expensive and the system operators are relatively few. A simple overview of the devices available is given by Martin.[77]

Cochlear implantation

The cochlear implant is an electric device inserted into the inner ear of certain profoundly deaf individuals to take the place of a severely damaged organ of Corti and convey to the brain a processed sequence of electric stimuli which the brain perceives as sound. Cochlear implants have now reached such a level of sophistication that the best implantees can converse almost effortlessly even over the telephone. To 'qualify' for an implant, a subject must have a degree of deafness that cannot be aided with any conventional hearing aid. Pure occupational-induced hearing loss very rarely if ever produces deafness of that degree of severity, and with the present selection criteria for implantation, cochlear implantation is not a treatment option for such individuals. There are indications, however, that selection criteria may become less strict in the future.

Antioxidant treatment: a possibility for the future

With the new insights outlined earlier in this chapter into the cellular events that result in noise-induced deafness comes the possibility of prevention and treatment of the condition. Glutathione has been shown to limit noise-induced hearing loss in the guinea pig both on auditory evoked brainstem response audiometry and on histological studies of cochlear hair cell loss.[78] Kopke et al.[79] looked at three strategies for enhancing the cochlea's intrinsic stress defences in a chinchilla model. Acetyl-L-carnitine is an endogenous mitochondrial membrane compound that helps maintain mitochondrial function in the face of oxidative stress. Carbamathione is a glutamate antagonist. Glutathione levels are reduced in the noise damaged cochlea. Kopke and co-workers administered acetyl-L-carmine, carbamathione and a glutathione repletion drug D-methionine to three groups of chinchillas and demonstrated protection from cochlear damage by showing significant reduction in hearing threshold elevation and significant reduction in cochlear hair cell loss at postmortem examination. The same team[80] demonstrated a strong protective effect on the chinchilla model of the antioxidants acetyl-L-carnitine (ALCAR) and N-L-acetyl cysteine (NAC). Hight et al.[81] administered a combination of two antioxidants, glutathione monoethylester and R-PIA, to chinchillas subsequently exposed to impulse (145 dB SPL) or continuous (105 dB, 4 kHz) noise and demonstrated a significant protection from both. They also demonstrated raised glutathione levels in the perilymph. Other workers have looked at the effect of magnesium administration on the susceptibility to damaging noise levels in the guinea pig[82] and found that there was a protective effect if the magnesium was administered immediately after noise exposure. The magnitude of the effect lessened with the length of time that elapsed from the noise exposure and the administration of the drug. It seems that there may be a synergistic effect between magnesium and free radical scavengers, such as vitamins A, C and E in reducing noise trauma.[83]

How these animal observations relate to the protection of the ear from noise in human beings in an industrial environment is not yet clear, but they are a very encouraging pointer to future developments in the field. Human trials have not yet commenced, but the animal results would suggest that they cannot be far off, assuming safety factors have been addressed. Early clinical trials with the antioxidant N-acetylcysteine (NAC) are anticipated.[84]

Another phenomenon to attract increasing interest is that of 'cochlear toughening'. A sound of sufficient mid-intensity produces a temporary threshold shift (TTS) following exposure. If the same exposure is repeated on a daily basis the TTS gets progressively less compared with the original shift. The cochlea has become conditioned by the so-called toughening exposures.[85] Again it is not yet clear if and how this observation can be put to practical use in humans.

NON-ORGANIC (OR EXAGGERATED, OR FUNCTIONAL) HEARING LOSS

In the medicolegal context, with the attendant lure of financial gain from compensation, the doctor assessing an industrial deafness case has to be constantly aware of the possibility of exaggeration of a hearing loss. Experienced clinicians and audiometricians may develop a finely honed sixth sense, based on the inappropriate or pantomimic behaviour of an individual subject. There may be a clear discrepancy between the perceived hearing of the subject in interview, and the volunteered thresholds on pure tone audiometry. Further discrepancies may exist between the pure tone thresholds and the score on speech audiometry. There may be test–retest unreliability on audiometry, and there may be a lack of agreement between pure tone thresholds obtained with ascending and descending stimulus intensity. Sweep frequency audiometry may reveal a pattern suggestive of non-organic hearing loss. Suspicion may be heightened if the threshold for the stapedial reflex (acoustic reflex) is found to be close to, or better than, the volunteered pure tone threshold. Sometimes, these contradictions can be ironed out and the true threshold established by the employment of low cunning on the part of the tester. Not infrequently, however, one may have to turn to electric response audiometry for verification.

ELECTRIC RESPONSE AUDIOMETRY (EVOKED RESPONSE AUDIOMETRY)

Electric response audiometry (ERA) provides a method of objectively estimating the auditory thresholds, by the recording of the electrical events which occur in the auditory pathways following the exposure of the ear to an acoustic stimulus. The stimuli used are either broadband clicks containing a wide spectrum of frequencies, or more frequency-specific stimuli, such as filtered clicks or tone bursts. A single such stimulus will give rise to electrical potential changes in a series of neural structures from the cochlea to the auditory cortex. These events have a characteristic form and latency depending upon which part of the auditory pathway is being studied.

The cochlea and eighth nerve give rise to near field potentials of very short (or no) latency, such as the cochlear microphonic (CM), the summating potential (SP) and the eighth nerve action potential (AP). The components of the auditory brainstem response (ABR or BSER) have a latency of up to 7–8 ms, and arise from structures in the lower to mid brainstem. The middle latency response (MLR) takes origin higher in the brainstem and at higher subcortical levels. The slow vertex response (SVR), recorded on cortical ERA (CERA) is thought to take origin from the highest levels in the auditory pathways and naturally has the longest latency (50–300 ms).

Most of these responses are recorded through simple disc electrodes located on the skin of the scalp and are thus non-invasive. The exception is the recording of cochlear potentials by the process of electrocochleography (ECochG, ECoG), which entails the siting of a recording electrode deep in the ear canal on the surface of the ear drum, or sometimes from the medial wall of the middle ear by means of a transtympanic needle electrode. The potentials recorded are of very low voltage and are difficult to differentiate from random background electrical activity. They have to be extracted by the process of 'time domain averaging' of the responses to a series of stimuli, then amplified for display on a visual display/computer unit where they can be studied, manipulated and stored for future recall. The better the signal-to-noise ratio of the response the fewer stimulus repetitions will be required to produce a reliable recording. Near field responses, such as ECochG, therefore, require fewer stimuli that far field responses, such as the ABR. A greater number of stimuli are needed to produce a response as the threshold is approached.

Electric response audiometry is employed in the neuro-otological diagnosis of certain disease states. For example, ECochG, yields typical patterns in Menière's disease. The ABR frequently demonstrates latency abnormalities in tumours of the cerebellopontine angle or brainstem of which vestibular schwannoma is the most common example. The other main use for ERA is to help establish the true hearing threshold when it is difficult to obtain reliable thresholds using conventional techniques. In addition to its role in the case of suspected non-organic hearing loss, it is used to test very young children, or children or adults with multiple handicaps who are unable to cooperate in the performance of standard hearing tests. The great advantage of the technique is that the patient cannot influence the generation of the potentials.

There are, however, certain disadvantages with ERA, some of which are common to all techniques, and some of which are specific to the individual test. Subjectivity on the part of the tester remains, in that it is not always easy, when tracing an ever-decreasing response to a stimulus of decreasing intensity, to determine at exactly what point the response disappears (the end point). Thus, the threshold estimation is not always as precise as one might wish. All ERA techniques tend to give more accurate information about high frequency thresholds than about thresholds at frequencies below 1 kHz. In the industrial deafness case, this is not always such a problem as in pure clinical work, because most of the desired information is in the higher frequencies anyway. One misconception about ERA needs to be corrected. It is not a better test of hearing than conventional hearing tests. The best estimate of hearing is a standard pure tone audiogram carried out on a willing and cooperative subject; ERA is used when that ability or willingness are absent. The preferred technique in the evaluation of a subject suspected of exaggerated hearing loss is CERA, but two other techniques (ABR and ECochG) are occasionally employed and will also be described.

Auditory brainstem response

The ABR comprises a series of five potentials (N1–N5) which occur in the first 7–8 ms after acoustic stimulation.

The generators of these potentials are still the subject of debate, but have been suggested to be:

- N1, cochlear nerve/nucleus;
- N2, cochlear nucleus;
- N3, superior olivary complex;
- N4, lateral lemniscus;
- N5, inferior colliculus.

Of these, the largest component and the one most usually employed in the estimation of hearing threshold is N5 (Figure 46.14). Stimuli are presented initially at a moderately high intensity, say 70 dB, and if an N5 response is observed, the stimulus intensity is decreased stepwise. As threshold is approached, the latency of the N5 response increases and the amplitude decreases, until it is no longer recordable. In a subject with normal hearing, the N5 response can usually be recorded down to stimulus intensities of 25–30 dB. The reason it cannot be recorded at lower intensities is largely due to the small voltage of the response and distance of the recording scalp electrodes from the generators in the brainstem. Most workers in this field would state that if responses are recordable down to 25–30 dB, the hearing is likely to be close to normal.

The advantages of ABR are that in the hands of an experienced audiologist, it produces clear and reproducible waveforms, is non-invasive and carries no risk to the subject. It is also unaffected by general anaesthesia, which is of value in the assessment of the young and unco-operative. There are certain disadvantages. It is quite time-consuming because as the threshold is approached many hundred stimuli may be required to produce a good response, and in order to demonstrate reproducibility, the test may have to be repeated several times. The information it yields is greatest in the high frequencies, although as stated above this may be less of a problem in the industrial deafness case.

Electrocochleography

The most important component of the ECochG is the eighth nerve action potential. The signal–noise ratio is much more favourable than with ABR, so large and reliable responses can be obtained after very few stimuli, even at quite low stimulus intensities, at which the response again decreases in amplitude and increases in latency. Threshold estimation is usually more accurate than with ABR (probably to within 10–15 dB), but as with ABR the higher frequency responses are more reliable than the low. The main disadvantage is the fact that the recording electrode has to be sited in the ear. An ear canal electrode may be satisfactory, but the best responses are obtained from a transtympanic electrode which has to be passed through the tympanic membrane to lie on the cochlea. This is performed under topical anaesthesia using EMLA® (eutectic mixture of local anaesthetics) cream, and the tiny perforation created nearly always heals rapidly. Nevertheless, the invasiveness of the technique means that it is not the technique of first choice, although there are occasions when its reliability might be desirable.

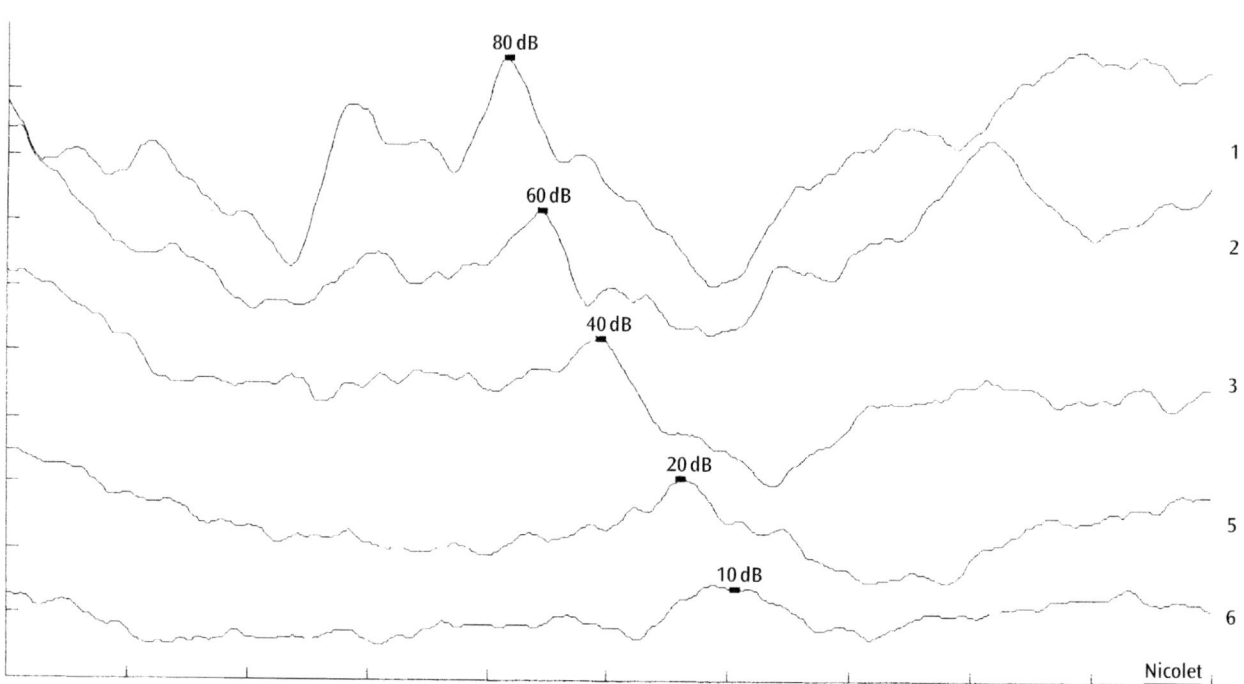

Figure 46.14 Auditory brainstem response. The stimulus intensity is marked on wave N5. Note that the latency of the N5 response increases and the amplitude decreases as the hearing threshold is approached.

Cortical evoked response audiometry

CERA records a response, the slow vertex response (SVR) which occurs between 50 and 250 ms after the delivery of sound to the ear (Figure 46.15). This long latency suggests that it is not a primary response. It is best recorded from scalp electrodes placed at the vertex.[86] The precise generators of the response are unclear, but it is known to arise from cortical structures. It thus has the theoretical advantage over ABR and ECochG of getting closer to recording 'hearing' than the other techniques which record events lower in the auditory pathway. The components of the waveform are two vertex positive waves and one vertex negative wave (the P1, N1, P2 complex).

Although frontal lesions do not affect the waveform, extensive temporoparietal lesions may eliminate the N1 component, but not P1. The SVR is influenced by general anaesthesia and to a lesser extent by sedation, so it is of little value in children. It is also influenced by EEG alpha activity, so is best tested with the subject's eyes open. In about 5 per cent of subjects, high levels of alpha activity make it very difficult to obtain an accurate SVR threshold.[87] In such a situation, ABR or ECochG might be preferred. The test is carried out with the subject reclining, perhaps reading. The scalp electrodes are non-invasive. In most cases, an audiogram at 500 Hz, 1 kHz, 2 kHz and 3 kHz can be obtained in an hour. In adults, it is usually accurate to about 10 dB of the true threshold[88] and furthermore its frequency specificity is better than that of ABR and ECochG. It is the technique of choice for verification of the pure tone audiogram in cases of suspected NOHL. If the pure tone threshold and the SVR threshold agree to within 10 dB, the behaviour threshold is confirmed. If the pure tone threshold exceeds the SVR threshold by 15 dB or more, exaggerated hearing loss should be strongly suspected.

Otoacoustic emissions: the possible use as a predictor of noise-induced hearing loss

Otoacoustic emissions (OAE) are sounds that are produced by the outer hair cells of normal ears. They are an epiphenomenon that seem to be the result of non-linearities in the way that the cochlea functions in reponse to acoustic stimulation. Spontaneous otoacoustic emissions (SOAEs) occur in about 40–50 per cent of normally hearing people. Transient otoacoustic emissions (TOAE) are the most useful clinically. These are low intensity sounds that are produced instantaneously by the cochlea in response to an acoustic stimulus. They are transmitted through the middle ear to the outer ear canal where they can be recorded using a small hand-held probe that delivers the test tone and records the response. TOAEs usually arise in frequency bands where hearing is normal so are fairly frequency-specific responses. They are very sensitive to changes in the cochlear hair cells. The technique is the basis for the newborn hearing screening programme. In general, the presence of a TOAE is a good indication that the hearing in that frequency band is within 30 dB HL of normal. The question arises as to whether the test or a modification of it could have any value in detecting preclinical changes in the hearing in individuals exposed to

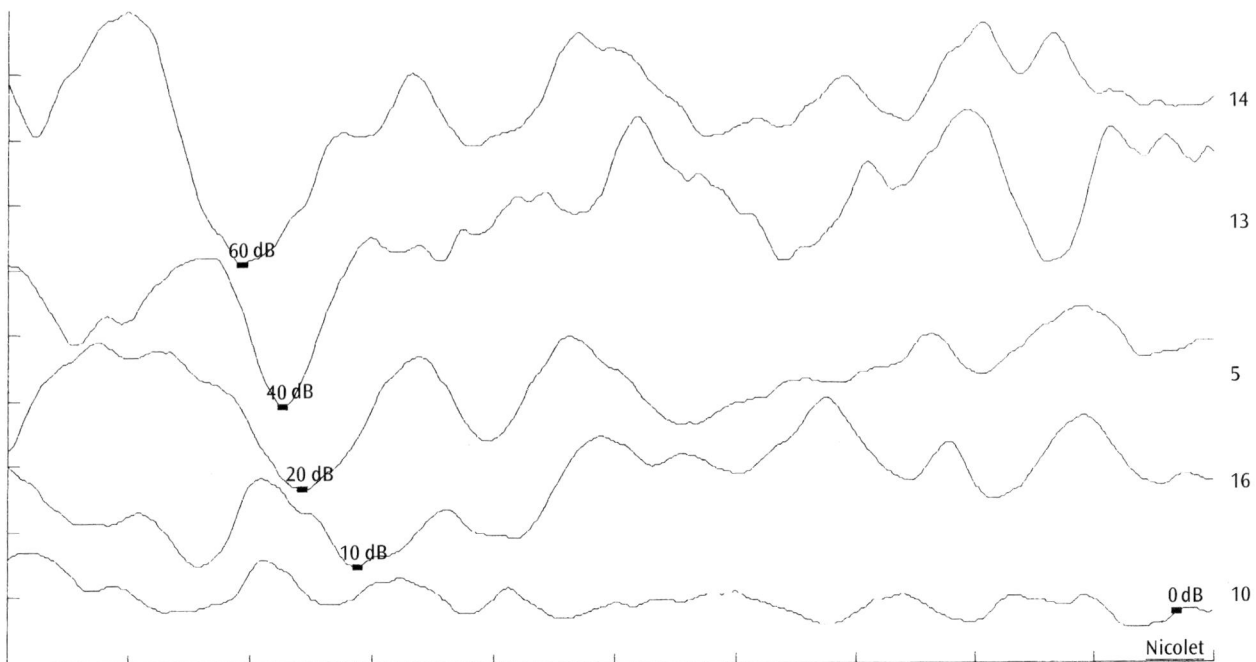

Figure 46.15 Cortical evoked response audiometry showing the slow vertex response. The vertex negative N1 wave is marked with the stimulus intensity.

noise – in other words, does the OAE change before the pure tone audiogram (PTA) threshold. A study from the Naval Submarine Medical Research Laboratory in Connecticut looked at just this issue in 338 volunteers working on aircraft carriers. While the average amplitude of the TOAE decreased significantly, the PTA average did not change. The best predictor was the TOAE amplitude in the 4-kHz half octave frequency band. The authors conclude that OAE may have predictive value for noise-induced hearing loss risk.[89] Another study looked at 135 ship engine room workers and concluded that, although TOAE changes after one year showed a high sensitivity (88 per cent) in predicting noise-induced hearing loss (NIHL) after two years of exposure, the test was a very poor screening tool because of the very low specificity (33 per cent) with an unacceptable false-positive rate.[90] The case for adoption of the technique for screening workers with noise exposure has not therefore yet been made, but it does seem likely that the test can be improved in the future using mathematical modifications of the technique, such as Volterra Slice techniques.[91]

OCCUPATIONAL NOISE-INDUCED TINNITUS

Many individuals have experience of the tinnitus that occurs after exposure to loud music, such as that of a rock concert or discotheque. This temporary tinnitus may be short-lived or last for days, depending on the duration and intensity of the exposure and may be associated with a measurable temporary threshold shift.[92] Similarly, tinnitus is reported often to accompany industrial noise exposure and while initially it is temporary, over a period of years it may become permanent in as many as 60 per cent, particularly in those exposed to impact noise.[93,94] There is some debate, however, regarding the importance of tinnitus in the assessment of occupational noise-induced hearing loss: Hinchcliffe and King suggest that tinnitus is often a symptom of those seeking compensation.[95] In contrast, a study of 647 individuals with occupational noise-induced hearing loss, showed a prevalence of tinnitus in 23.3 per cent, nearly one-third of whom felt that the tinnitus was intrusive to the point of having an effect on daily activities.[96] The issue is complicated further by the observation that solicitors advertising their services to potential claimants may do so with provocative statements linking noise exposure at work with tinnitus. The debate then is not so much as to whether tinnitus and occupational noise-induced hearing loss go hand in hand, but the weight that should be attributed to the tinnitus component during the evaluation of a claimant.

OCCUPATIONAL NOISE-INDUCED VERTIGO

Temporary vestibular disturbance in response to loud noises is referred to as the Tullio phenomenon. In a state of health, high sound intensities are required to evoke this response. In various otological disorders, however, lesser sound levels may have a similar effect in certain individuals. Firm evidence that occupational noise-induced vertigo is a real entity is lacking. However, three more recent studies merit consideration. Shupak and colleagues[97] demonstrated a reduced vestibulo-ocular reflex and reduced caloric response of the inner ear in 22 individuals with occupational noise-induced hearing loss compared with 21 controls, although all those evaluated were subclinical in terms of vestibular complaints. Manabe and colleagues[98] evaluated 36 patients with occupational noise-induced hearing loss cases, half of whom complained of vertigo. In the symptomatic group, a reduced caloric response was also shown, as were electrophysiological changes suggestive of endolymphatic hydrops. Histopathological evidence of endolymphatic hydrops in two patients with late onset vertigo and noise-induced hearing loss was provided by Kemink and Graham.[99] Thus, there is some evidence to substantiate a link between acoustic trauma and delayed endolymphatic hydrops, but further investigation into this aspect of hazardous noise exposure is required.

INFRASOUND AND ULTRASOUND

Evidence that excessive sound above or below the normal human auditory range may have an adverse effect on inner ear function remains scant.

Infrasound (conventionally sound below 20 Hz) is commonly felt as vibration rather than heard and is a component of natural phenomena such as earthquakes and thunder.[100] Heavy industrial machinery, high speed car travel with open windows and ship's engine rooms are potential sources of infrasound. More specifically, Pyykkö and colleagues[101] examined 203 lumberjacks over a six-year period, compared the hearing in those with and without vibration-induced white finger syndrome and found a statistically significant difference in thresholds at 4 kHz in those with the syndrome than those without. They postulated that the higher thresholds in the lumberjacks with vibration-induced white finger was due to reflex sympathetic vasoconstriction in cochlear blood vessels in response to vasospasm of the hands rather than a direct mechanical effect on the cochlea (see Chapter 47, Hand–arm vibration syndrome, p. 489).

The auditory effects of ultrasound (sound above 20 kHz) have been reviewed by Acton.[102] These include a full feeling in the ear, tinnitus and headaches. Utilizing low frequency ultrasound (10–28 kHz) in guinea pigs, Ishida and colleagues[103] noted auditory electrophysiological effects, including alteration in the cochlear microphonic and increased thresholds. Currently, the adverse auditory effects of hazardous levels of both infrasound and ultrasound in humans remain to be defined.

SYSTEMIC EFFECTS OF NOISE POLLUTION

Recently, the World Health Organization Noise Environment Burden of Disease (BoD) Working Group has identified environmental noise (as distinct from occupational noise) as a stressor in the evolution of cardiovascular disease.[107] In addition, there is increasing concern about the burden of sleep disturbance, of annoyance, of hearing impairment, of tinnitus and of cognitive impairment from environmental noise. It has been estimated[107] that the severe annoyance due to noise from traffic, trains and aircraft may account for approximately 3 per cent of coronary heart disease deaths in Europe each year (or about 210 000 deaths). Chronic noise exposure has been incriminated in elevation of systolic blood pressure in workers in the metal manufacturing industry, and in shipyard workers.[108,109] Risk tends to be associated with night-time noise exposure and the noise threshold for cardiovascular disease has been stated to be a night-time exposure of 50 dBA. The mechanism is thought to be the high levels of stress hormones, such as cortisol, adrenaline and noradrenaline, released into the circulation at times of stress at a subcortical level in the amygdala. This mechanism may be active during sleep and there are several reports in the literature that indicate that exposure to traffic noise and aircraft noise during sleep may cause autonomic changes, leading to hypertension and myocardial infarction.[110,111] It has been suggested[112] that the neuroendocrine changes associated with noise stress may modify immune function. Willich et al.[113] reported that the risk of myocardial infarction from chronic noise burden appears more closely associated with sound levels than with subjective annoyance.

As a means of further assessing the noise-related disease burden, the WHO Working Group have devised disability adjusted life years (DALY). These allow one to quantify the amount to which life expectancy is reduced by premature death or disease-related disability. It was estimated that in 2002, Europeans lost 880 000 DALYs to coronary heart disease related to road traffic noise. The group also recognized the possible interaction between traffic noise and air pollution in the increased BoD. Outdoor air pollution represents approximately 2 per cent of cardiopulmonary disease mortality, and it is not clear whether the impact of noise on ischaemic heart disease is independent, additive or synergistic to the impact of outdoor air pollution.

It is also suggested that sleep disturbance caused by environmental noise (noise-induced insomnia) can be a contributory factor to loss of performance and predispose to accidents at home, at work and when driving. The deleterious effects of noise on cognitive function are also under scrutiny. There are four components of cognitive impairment (reading, recall, recognition and attention) which appear to show a consistent relationship with noise exposure. It must be emphasized, however, that there are immense difficulties in acquiring robust data to establish a causal relationship. There are uncertainties in quantifying noise exposure, in separating the effects of noise from other variables, and in agreeing and in quantifying outcome measures. Pooling of data for meta-analysis is fraught with hazard because of differences in the assessment of exposure and outcome.[114]

In 2004, the World Health Organization published a guide for occupational health professionals aimed at the provision of a tool for carrying out detailed disease burden estimates of the hearing loss from occupational noise.[115] In Europe, environmental noise is becoming a major health concern for policy-makers. The European Directive related to the assessment and management of environmental noise (Directive 2002/49/EC) addresses the action plans to reduce harmful effects of noise exposure.[116]

The summary policy implications of these initiatives are:

- Estimates of the incidence of occupation-related NIHL in a given country or study population will provide quantitative information on the importance of the problem and help motivate interventions to reduce the risks and impact on health.
- While incurable and irreversible, NIHL is nevertheless preventable and it is essential that preventative programmes are implemented.
- Hearing conservation programmes should be integrated into the overall hazard prevention and control programme for the workplace.

On this basis, the WHO publication stipulates that such programmes require political will and decision-making, high-level management and workforce commitment, adequate human and financial resources, technical knowledge and experience, communication and monitoring mechanisms and continuous programme improvement. The WHO also recognizes the importance of local sociocultural aspects and financial climate, and that in developing countries a large proportion of the population works in the informal sector – a group that represents a major challenge in terms of occupational hazard prevention.

In an attempt to provide a common basis for tackling the environmental noise problem across the European Union (EU), the European Parliament and Council have adopted Directive 2002/49/EC of June 25, 2002 which encompasses the following environment policy directives:

1. Monitoring the environmental problem through member states drawing up strategic noise maps for major roads, railways and airports.
2. Informing and consulting the public about noise exposure and measures considered to address it.
3. Addressing local issues whereby competent authorities will need to devise action plans to reduce environmental noise.
4. Developing a long-term EU strategy to reduce the number of affected individuals.

The deadlines relating to the implementation of this Directive spanned from 2004 to July 2009, by which time the member states should have set up a database of information on strategic noise maps at which point the Commission must submit a report on the implementation of the Directive to the European Parliament and Council.

> **Key points**
>
> - Industrial noise exposure remains a significant cause of hearing impairment, disability and handicap in the Western world, and a major cause in developing coutries.
> - Permanent threshold elevation cannot yet be treated medically or surgically. Management is with hearing aids. The condition is best prevented.
> - In the future, there may be therapeutic possibilities in the use of antioxidants in protecting the ear from the damaging effects of noise.
> - Legislation places strict requirements on employers to reduce sound levels in the workplace and to provide adequate hearing protection at levels of noise defined by statute.
> - Evidence is emerging that environmental noise pollution can have serious long-term effects on health in general, particularly heart disease.

REFERENCES

1. Pickles JO. Physiology of hearing. In: Kerr AG (ed.). *Scott-Brown's Otolaryngology*, vol 1. Oxford: Butterworth-Heinemann, 1997: 2/1–34.
2. International Standards Organization. ISO 389. Acoustics – Standard reference zero for the calibration of pure-tone air conduction audiometers, 3rd edn. Geneva: ISO, 1991.
3. British Standards Institution. BS 2497. Specification for standard reference zero for the calibration of pure-tone air conduction audiometers. London: BSI, 1992.
4. Hinchcliffe R. Sound, infrasound and ultrasound. In: Raffle PAB, Adams PH, Baxter PJ, Lee WR (eds). *Hunter's Diseases of occupations*, 8th edn. London: Arnold, 1994: 271–94.
5. Alberti PW. Noise and the ear. In: Kerr AG (ed.). *Scott Brown's Otolaryngology*, vol 2. Oxford: Butterworth-Heinemann, 1997: 11/1–34.
6. Rosowski JJ, Carney LH, Peake WT. The radiation impedance of the external ear of the cat: Measurements and applications. *Journal of the Acoustical Society of America*. 1990; **84**: 1697–708.
7. Ludman H. Physiology of hearing and balance In: Ludman H (ed.). *Mawson's Diseases of the ear*. London: Edward Arnold, 1988: 74–101.
8. Williams PL, Warwick R (eds). Auditory and vestibular apparatus. In: *Gray's Anatomy*. Edinburgh: Churchill Livingstone, 1996: 1367–97.
9. Ulehlova L, Voldrich L, Janisch R. Correlative of sensory cell density and cochlear length in humans. *Hearing Research*. 1987; **28**: 147–51.
10. Békésy G von. The variation of phase along the basilar membrane with sinusoidal variations. *Journal of the Acoustical Society of America*. 1947; **19**: 452.
11. Sellick PM, Patuzzi R, Johnstone BM. Measurement of basilar membrane motion in the guinea pig using the Mossbauer technique. *Journal of the Acoustical Society of America*. 1982; **72**: 131–41.
12. Robles L, Ruggero MA, Rich NC. Basilar membrane mechanics at the base of the chinchilla cochlea. I. Input–output functions, tuning curves and response phases. *Journal of the Acoustical Society of America*. 1986; **80**: 1364–74.
13. Cody AR, Russell IJ. Acoustically induced hearing loss: Intracellular studies in the guinea pig cochlea. *Hearing Research*. 1988; **35**: 59–70.
14. Pickles JO, Corey DP. Mechanoelectrical transduction by hair cells. *Trends in Neuroscience*. 1992; **15**: 254–9.
15. Bacon FL. *Sylva sylvarum: Or a natural history*. London: W Rawley, 1627.
16. Ramazzini B. In: Wright WC (ed.). *Diseases of workers*. Translated from the Latin *De Morbis Artificum*. New York: Hafner, 1964: 438–9.
17. Ludman H. Inner ear trauma. In: Ludman H (ed.). *Mawson's Diseases of the ear*. London: Edward Arnold, 1988: 593–604.
18. Fosbroke J. Practical observations on the pathology and treatment of deafness II. *Lancet*. 1831; **VI**: 644–8.
19. Barr T. Enquiry into the effects of loud sound upon the hearing of boiler makers and others who work amid noisy surroundings. *Transactions of the Philosophical Society of Glasgow*. 1866; **17**: 223–9.
20. Habermann J. Über die Schwerhörigkeit des Kesselschmiede. *Archiv für Ohrenheilkunde*. 1890; **30**: 1–25.
21. Fowler EP. Limited lesions of basilar membrane. *Transactions of the American Society of Ophthalmologic and Otolaryngologic Allergy*. 1929; **19**: 182.
22. Bunch CC. Traumatic deafness. In: Fowler EP (ed.). *Nelson loose leaf medicine of the ear*. New York: Thos Nelson, 1939: 349–67.
23. Larsen B. Investigations of professional deafness in shipyard and machine factory labourers. *Acta Otolaryngologica Supplementum*. 1939; **36**: 3–255.
24. Browning GG, Davis AC. Clinical characterisation of the hearing of the adult British population. *Advances in Otorhinolaryngology*. 1983; **31**: 219–23.
25. Henderson D, Subramaniam M, Boettcher FA. Individual susceptibility to noise induced hearing loss: An old topic revisited. *Ear and Hearing*. 1993; **14**: 153–68.
26. Barrenäs ML, Lindgren F. The influence of eye colour on susceptibility to TTS in humans. *British Journal of Audiology*. 1991; **25**: 303–7.
27. Hallberg LR, Jansson G. Women with noise-induced hearing-loss: An invisible group? *British Journal of Audiology*. 1996; **30**: 340–5.
28. Rytzner B, Rytzner C. School children and noise. The 4 kHz dip-tone screening in 14391 school children. *Scandinavian Audiology*. 1981; **10**: 213–16.

29. Botte MC, Monikheim S. Psychoacoustic characterization of two types of auditory fatigue. In: Dancer AL, Henderson D, Salvi RJ, Hamerick RP (eds). *Noise-induced hearing loss*. St Louis: Mosby Year Book, 1992: 259–68.
30. Mills JH. Effects of noise on auditory sensitivity, psychophysical tuning curves and suppression. In: Hamernik RP, Henderson D, Salvi R (eds). *New perspectives on noise-induced hearing loss*. New York: Raven Press, 1982: 249–63.
31. Ryan AF, Bennett TM, Woolf NK, Axelsson A. Protection from noise induced hearing loss by prior exposure to a non-traumatic stimulus: Role of the middle ear muscles. *Hearing Research*. 1994; **72**: 23–8.
32. Igarashi M, Schuknecht HF, Myers EN. Cochlear pathology in humans with stimulation deafness. *Journal of Laryngology and Otology*. 1964; **78**: 115–23.
33. Bredberg G. The human cochlea during development and ageing. *Journal of Laryngology and Otology*. 1967; **81**: 739–58.
34. Beagley HA. Acoustic trauma in the guinea pig. II. Electron microscopy including the morphology of cell functions in the organ of Corti. *Acta Otolaryngologica*. 1965; **60**: 479–95.
35. Liberman MC. Chronic ultrastructural changes in acoustic trauma: Serial section reconstruction of stereocilia and cuticular plates. *Hearing Research*. 1987; **26**: 25–88.
36. Goa WY, Ding DL, Zheng XY et al. A comparison of changes in the stereocilia between temporary and permanent hearing losses in acoustic trauma. *Hearing Research*. 1992; **62**: 27–41.
37. Reuter G, Gitter AH, Thurm U, Zenner HP. High frequency radial movements of the reticular lamina induced by outer hair cell mobility. *Hearing Research*. 1992; **60**: 236–46.
38. Saunders JC, Cohen YE, Szymko YM. The structural and functional consequences of acoustic injury in the cochlea and peripheral auditory system: A five year update. *Journal of the Acoustical Society of America*. 1991; **90**: 136–46.
39. Saunders JC, Dear SP, Schneider ME. The anatomical consequences of acoustic injury: A review and tutorial. *Journal of the Acoustical Society of America*. 1985; **78**: 833–60.
40. Yamane H, Nakai Y, Takayama M et al. The emergence of free radicals after acoustic trauma and strial blood flow. *Acta Otolaryngologica Supplementum*. 1995; **519**: 87–92.
41. Ohlemiller KK, Wright JS, Duggan LL. Early elevation of cochlear reactive oxygen species following noise exposure. *Audiology and Neurotology*. 1999; **4**: 229–36.
42. Henderson D, Bielefeld EC, Harris KC, Hu BH. The role of oxidative stress in noise induced hearing loss. *Ear and Hearing*. 2006; **27**: 1–19.
43. Ohinata Y, Miller JM, Altschuler RA, Schacht J. Intense noise induces formation of vasoactive lipid peroxidase products in the cochlea. *Brain Research*. 2000; **878**: 163–73.
44. Harris KC, Hu B, Hangauer D, Henderson D. Prevention of noise induced hearing loss with Src-PTK inhibitors. *Hearing Research*. 2005; **208**: 14–25.
45. Le Prell CG, Yamashita D, Minami SB et al. Mechanisms of noise induced hearing loss indicate multiple methods of prevention. *Hearing Research*. 2007; **226**: 22–43.
46. Alberti PW, Hyde ML, Symons FM, Miller RB. The effect of prolonged exposure to industrial noise on otosclerosis. *Laryngoscope*. 1980; **90**: 407–13.
47. Simpson DC, O'Reilly BF. The protective effect of a conductive hearing loss in workers exposed to industrial noise. *Clinical Otolaryngology*. 1991; **16**: 274–7.
48. McShane DP, Hyde ML, Finkelstein DM, Alberti PW. Unilateral otosclerosis in noise-induced hearing loss. *Clinical Otolaryngology*. 1991; **16**: 70–5.
49. Williams RG. The diagnosis of noise-induced hearing loss. *Journal of Audiological Medicine*. 1996; **6**: 45–58.
50. Department of Health and Social Security. Occupational deafness. London: HMSO, 1973.
51. Alberti PW, Symons F, Hyde ML. The significances of asymmetrical hearing thresholds. *Archives of Otolaryngology*. 1979; **87**: 255–63.
52. Kerr AG, Byrne JET. Concussive effects of bomb blast on the ear. *Journal of Laryngology and Otology*. 1975; **89**: 131–43.
53. World Health Organization. International classifications, disabilities and handicaps. Geneva: WHO, 1980: 27, 73.
54. King PF, Coles RRA, Lutman ME, Robinson DW. *Assessment of hearing disability guidelines for medicolegal practice*. London: Whurr Publishers, 1992.
55. Hetu R, Riverin L, Getty Lalande N, St-Cyr C. Quantitative analysis of the handicap associated with occupational hearing loss. *British Journal of Audiology*. 1988; **22**: 251–64.
56. British Association of Otolaryngologists and British Society of Audiology. Method for assessment of hearing disability. London: BAO and BSA, 1983.
57. Atherley GRC, Noble WG. Clinical picture of occupational hearing loss obtained with the hearing measurement scale. In: Robinson DW (ed.). *Occupational hearing loss*. London: Academic Press, 1971: 193–206.
58. Lutman ME, Brown EJ, Coles RRA. Self reported disability and handicap in the population in relation to pure tone threshold, age, sex and type of hearing loss. *British Journal of Audiology*. 1987; **21**: 45–58.
59. Robinson DW. Relation between hearing threshold level and its component parts. *British Journal of Audiology*. 1991; **25**: 93–103.
60. Robinson DW, Wilkins PA, Thyer NJ, Lawes JF. Auditory impairment and the onset of disability and handicap in noise-induced hearing loss. ISVR technical report No. 126. Southampton: University of Southampton, 1984.
61. British Standards Institution. BS 5330. Method of estimating the risk of hearing handicap due to noise exposure. London: BSI, 1976.
62. International Standards Organization. ISO 7029. Acoustics – Threshold of hearing by air conduction as a function of age and sex for otologically normal persons. Geneva: ISO, 1989.
63. Shipton MS. Tables relating pure-tone audiometry threshold to age. National Physics Laboratory Report 94. Teddington: National Physics Laboratory, 1979.
64. International Standards Organization. ISO 1999. Acoustics – Determination of occupational noise exposure

65. Burns W, Robinson DW. *Hearing and noise in industry*. London: HMSO, 1970.
66. Robinson DW. Impairment and disability in noise-induced hearing loss. In: *Advances in audiology*, vol 5. Basel: Karger, 1988: 71–81.
67. Health and Safety Executive. Controlling noise at work, L108. Sudbury: HSE Books, 2005.
68. Health and Safety Executive. Noise at work. The noise at work regulations. Guidance on regulations. Sudbury: HSE Books, 1989.
69. Health and Safety Commission. Prevention of damage to hearing from noise at work. Draft proposals for regulations and guidance. Consultative document. London: HMSO, 1987.
70. Health and Safety Executive. Sound solutions. techniques to reduce noise at work. Sudbury: HSE Books, 1995.
71. Health and Safety Executive. Noise at work. Noise assessment, information and control. Noise guides 3–8. Sudbury: HSE Books, 1990.
72. Alberti PW (ed.). *Personal hearing protection in industry*. New York: Raven Press, 1982.
73. British Standards Institution. BS 5108. Sound attenuation of hearing protectors. London: BSI, 1991.
74. International Standards Organization. ISO 4869. Acoustics – Hearing protectors. Geneva: ISO, 1989, 1990.
75. British Standards Institution. BS 6344. Industrial hearing protectors. London: BSI, 1988, 1989.
76. Health and Safety Executive. Audiometry in industry. Discussion document. London: HMSO, 1978.
77. Martin M. In: Ballantyne J, Martin MC, Martin A (eds). *Deafness*. London: Whurr Publishers, 1993: 270–9.
78. Ohinata Y, Yamasoba T, Schacht J, Miller JM. Glutathione limits noise induced hearing loss. *Hearing Research*. 2000; **146**: 28–34.
79. Kopke RD, Coleman JK, Liu J et al. Candidates thesis: Enhancing intrinsic cochlear stress defenses to reduce noise induced hearing loss. *Laryngoscope*. 2002; **112**: 1515–32.
80. Kopke R Bielefeld E, Liu J et al. Prevention of impulse noise hearing loss with antioxidants. *Acta Otolaryngologica*. 2005; **125**: 235–43.
81. Hight NG, McFadden SL, Henderson D et al. Noise-induced hearing loss in chinchillas pretreated with glutathione monoethylester and R-PIA. *Hearing Research*. 2003; **179**: 21–32.
82. Scheibe F, Haupt H, Ising H, Cherny L. Therapeutic effect of parenteral magnesium on noise induced hearing loss in the guinea pig. *Magnesium Research*. 2002; **15**: 27–36.
83. Le Prell CG, Hughes LF, Miller JM. Free radical scavengers vitamins A, C and E plus magnesium reduce noise trauma. *Free Radical Biological Medicine*. 2007; **42**: 1454–63.
84. Kopke RD, Jackson RL, Coleman JK et al. NAC for noise: From the bench top to the clinic. *Hearing Research*. 2007; **226**: 114–25.
85. Hamernik RP, Qiu W, Davis B. Cochlear toughening, protection, and potentiation of noise-induced trauma by non-Gaussian noise. *Journal of the Acoustic Society of America*. 2003; **113**: 969–76.
86. Davis H, Zerlin S. Acoustic relations of the human vertex potential. *Journal of the Acoustical Society of America*. 1966; **39**: 109–16.
87. Hyde M, Alberti P, Matsumoto N, Yao-Li L. Auditory evoked potentials in the audiometric assessment of compensation and medicolegal patients. *Annals of Otology, Rhinology and Laryngology*. 1986; **95**: 514–19.
88. Lutman ME. Diagnostic audiometry. In: Kerr AG (ed.). *Scott-Brown's Otolaryngology*, vol 2. Oxford: Butterworth-Heinemann, 1997: 12/22–23.
89. Lapsley Miller JA, Marshall L, Heller LM, Hughes LM. Low level otoacoustic emissions may predict susceptibility to noise-induced hearing loss. *Journal of the Acoustic Society of America*. 2006; **120**: 280–96.
90. Shupak A, Tal D, Sharozi Z et al. Otoacoustic emissions in early noise induced hearing loss. *Otology and Neurotology*. 2007; **28**: 745–52.
91. de Boer J, Thornton AR. Volterra slice otoacoustic emissions recorded using maximum length sequences from patients with sensorineural hearing loss. *Hearing Research*. 2006; **219**: 121–36.
92. Coles RRA. Tinnitus. In: Kerr AG (ed.). *Scott-Brown's Otolaryngology*, vol. 2. Oxford: Butterworth-Heinemann, 1997: 18/1–34.
93. McShane DP, Hyde ML, Alberti PW. Tinnitus prevalence in industrial hearing loss compensation claimants. *Clinical Otolaryngology*. 1988; **13**: 323–30.
94. Axelsson A, Barrenås ML. Tinnitus in noise-induced hearing loss. In: Dancer AL, Henderson D, Salvi RJ, Hamerick RP (eds). *Noise-induced hearing loss*. St Louis: Mosby Year Book, 1992: 269–76.
95. Hinchcliffe R, King PF. Medicolegal aspects of tinnitus. I, II, III. *Journal of Audiological Medicine*. 1992; **1**: 38–58, 59–79, 127–47.
96. Phoon WH, Lee HS, Chia SE. Tinnitus in noise-exposed workers. *Occupational Medicine*. 1993; **43**: 35–8.
97. Shupak A, Bar-El E, Podoshin L et al. Vestibular findings associated with chronic noise induced hearing impairment. *Acta Otolaryngologica*. 1994; **114**: 579–85.
98. Manabe Y, Kurokawa T, Saito T, Saito H. Vestibular dysfunction in noise-induced hearing loss. *Acta Otolaryngologica Supplementum*. 1995; **519**: 262–4.
99. Kemink JL, Graham MD. Hearing loss with delayed onset of vertigo. *American Journal of Otology*. 1985; **6**: 344–8.
100. Westin JB. Infrasound. A short review of effects on man. *Aviation, Space, and Environmental Medicine*. 1975; **46**: 1135–43.
101. Pyykkö I, Starck J, Farkkila M et al. Hand–arm vibration in the aetiology of hearing loss in lumberjacks. *British Journal of Industrial Medicine*. 1981; **38**: 281–9.
102. Acton WI. Exposure to industrial ultrasound: Hazards, appraisal and control. *Journal of the Society of Occupational Medicine*. 1983; **33**: 107–13.
103. Ishida A, Matsui T, Yamamura K. The effects of low-frequency ultrasound on the inner ear: An electrophysiological study

using the guinea pig cochlea. *European Archives of Oto-Rhino-Laryngology*. 1993; **250**: 22-6.
104. Kessel RG, Kardon RH. *Tissues and organs: A text-atlas of scanning electron microscopy*. San Francisco: Freeman, 1979.
105. Pickles JO. *An introduction to the physiology of hearing*. New York: Academic Press, 1982.
106. Wright A. Anatomy and ultrastructure of the human ear. In: Kerr AG (ed.). *Scott-Brown's Otolaryngology*, vol. I. Oxford: Butterworth-Heinemann, 1997.
107. Babisch W. Quantifying burden of disease from environmental noise. Second technical meeting report. Bern: World Health Organization, 2005.
108. Lee JH, Kang W, Yaang SR *et al*. Cohort study for the effect of chronic noise exposure on blood pressure among male workers in Busan, Korea. *American Journal of Industrial Medicine*. 2009; **52**: 509-17.
109. Wu TN, Ko YC, Chang PY. Study of noise exposure and high blood pressure in shipyard workers. *American Journal of Industrial Medicine*. 1987; **12**: 431-8.
110. Jarup L, Babisch W, Houthuijs D *et al*. HYENA study team. Hypertension and exposure to noise near airports. *Environment Health Perspectives*. 2008; **116**: 329-33.
111. Leon Blum G, Berglind N, Nordling E, Rosenlund M. Road traffic noise and hypertension. *Occupational and Environmental Medicine*. 2007; **64**: 122-6.
112. Prasher D. Is there evidence that environmental noise is immunotoxic? *Noise and Health*. 2009; **11**: 151-5.
113. Willich SN, Wegscheider K, Stallmann M, Keil T. Noise burden and the risk of myocardial infarction. *European Heart Journal*. 2006; **27**: 276-82.
114. Babisch W, Kamp I. Exposure response relationship of the association between aircraft noise and the risk of hypertension. *Noise and Health*. 2009; **11**: 161-8.
115. Concha-Barrientos M, Campbell-Lendrum D, Steenland K. *Occupational noise: Assessing the burden of disease from work-related hearing impairment at national and local levels*. WHO Environmental Burden of Disease Series, No. 9. Geneva: World Health Organization, 2004.
116. Directive 2002/49/EC of the European Parliament and the Council of 25 June 2002 relating to the assessment and management of environmental noise – Declaration by the Commission in the Conciliation Committee on the directive relating to the assessment and management of environmental noise.

SECTION TWO

Vibration

47	Hand-arm vibration syndrome *Ian J Lawson, Frank Burke, Kenneth L McGeoch, Tohr Nilsson and George Proud*	489
48	Whole body vibration *Massimo Bovenzi and Keith Palmer*	513

47

Hand–arm vibration syndrome

IAN J LAWSON, FRANK BURKE, KENNETH L McGEOCH, TOHR NILSSON AND GEORGE PROUD

Introduction	489	Hand–arm vibration and muscle weakness	500
Classification	490	Hand–arm vibration and bone and joint disorders	502
Pathophysiology	490	Diagnosis and tertiary case assessment	502
Clinical features	494	Diagnosis	505
Vascular clinical features	495	Workplace health surveillance	505
Carpal tunnel syndrome	497	Management of cases	506
Dupuytren's disease	499	References	507

INTRODUCTION

The prolonged use of vibrating tools and equipment can lead to a number of pathological effects primarily in the peripheral neurological, vascular and musculoskeletal systems. The resulting symptom complex is now internationally known as the hand–arm vibration syndrome or HAVS.[1] The relative importance of the two main components, vascular (a Raynaud's phenomenon) and sensorineural (a peripheral neuropathy), has shifted since the condition was first recognized at the beginning of the last century. In Alice Hamilton's biography,[2] in a chapter entitled 'Dead fingers', she described the presentation in limestone cutters working in Bedford, Indiana in 1918:

> The men call the condition 'dead fingers' and it is a good name, for the fingers do look like those of a corpse, a yellowish-greyish white and shrunken. There is a clear line of demarcation between the dead part and the normal part.

These early reports did not reach a conclusion as to the cause of this condition, but presumed cold and tight gripping of tools to be responsible. It was the work of Seyring on vibration exposure in iron foundry workers in 1931 which made it clear that vibration transmitted to the hand–arm system was the underlying cause of the condition, and cold the trigger to the attacks of vasospasm.[3]

Towards the end of the twentieth century it became generally accepted that disability associated with the syndrome resulted from the effect of vibration on the peripheral nervous system rather than the visible presentation of whiteness. Presciently in Hamilton's original work she reported, 'they could not tell a dime from a nickel without looking at it'. Epidemiological evidence suggesting that the sensorineural and vascular components could develop independently emerged at a landmark workshop in Stockholm in 1986, and led to a new classification system, the Stockholm Workshop Scale (SWS).[4,5] The legacy term vibration white finger (VWF), which neatly encapsulates the cause and presentation, now tends to be confined to legal circles in the United Kingdom. A series of multiparty litigation cases in the early part of the twenty-first century in the United Kingdom, led to the examination of large volumes of claimants under standardized conditions.[6] Systematic reviews and international workshops have attempted to standardize the clinical assessment, testing and management of the syndrome.[7–9] However, the use of specialized tests remains confined to a limited number of centres of excellence in most countries.

An acceptance that the sensorineural component of the syndrome causes disability has been slow to receive recognition. It was only in 2004 in the United Kingdom, that the Industrial Injuries Advisory Council recommended the assessment of isolated sensorineural symptoms for the purposes of industrial injuries disability benefit. This led to amended regulations in 2007.

Exposure to hand–arm vibration (HAV) from hand-held vibrating tools and equipment is common, particularly in construction and engineering. The number of workers exposed to HAV varies significantly between countries. A national survey estimated that approximately 4.9 million workers are exposed in the United Kingdom alone.[10] An estimated 350 000 workers are regularly exposed in Sweden, 6.7 million in Germany, and 1.5 million in the United States.[11] A European Working Conditions Survey 2005 (EWCS) suggested usage was five times more common in men. Sources of HAV that can lead to HAVS are numerous and varied, including both electrically and pneumatically powered percussive and rotary tools, such as fettling tools, impact wrenches, needle guns, hammer drills, chipping hammers, nibblers, hand-held polishers, sanders, grinders, pedestal grinders, rock drills, road breakers, tampers, chain saws, brush saws, strimmers and concrete scabblers.[12] Foundry workers, construction workers, metal workers, miners and forestry workers are at greatest risk.[13]

Prevalence studies in HAVS have mostly considered finger blanching and may be confounded by differences in climate. One prevalence study in the United Kingdom reported 670 000 men and 104 000 women with episodes of finger blanching in response to cold.[14] These types of study have been mostly from developed countries, but other regions are now adding to the literature.[15]

The occupational health professional needs to have some understanding of vibration measurement and its implications when assessing individual cases. Vibration is an oscillatory motion that can be represented by a simple harmonic sine wave with the properties of displacement, a velocity and acceleration. In practice, the wave is a complex, of differing frequencies and acceleration. Vibration can move in three orthogonal directions (x, y and z axes) and it is the vector sum that is normally calculated (ISO 5349).[16] The measurement of interest, in terms of a biological effect, is the magnitude of vibration or 'A(8)' which incorporates intensity, duration and direction.[17]

The daily exposure to vibration of a person is ascertained using the formula:

$$A(8) = a_{hw} \sqrt{T/T_o}$$

where a_{hw} is the vibration magnitude, in metres per second squared (m/s^2); T is the duration of exposure to the vibration magnitude a_{hw} and T_o is the reference duration of eight hours (28 800 seconds).

A frequency weighting up to 16 Hz is factored into calculations to take account of the supposedly more damaging lower frequencies suggested by laboratory studies.[18] The validity of this frequency weighting and whether damaging frequencies extending from 6.3 to 5000 Hz should be adopted by unweighted measurement continues to cause controversy.[19]

Inaccuracy in both measurement of vibration and assessment of clinical effects has meant that a robust dose–response model has been elusive. The most frequently cited is in ISO 5349. This model bases the prediction of vascular symptom prevalence on groups of workers who use tools with vibration predominantly above the 30–50 Hz range such as grinders, rock drills and chain saws. Other factors thought to affect the severity of an individual's condition include temporal exposure patterns, intermittency of exposure, direction of vibration transmitted to the hand, including push and other ergonomic factors that may ultimately affect the transmission of vibration into the hand–arm system. Recent studies suggest that even low level vibration may lead to HAVS.[20] Individual susceptibility, particularly those with pre-existing Raynaud's phenomenon, peripheral neuropathy and nerve entrapment, also plays a part.[9]

An understanding of the relationship between the onset of symptoms and first exposure can be assisted by a general understanding of the group prevalences at given vibration magnitudes. It was accepted at an international workshop that the first onset of finger blanching in relation to exposure (the latent interval) might range from a few months after the start of vibration exposure to approximately one year after vibration exposure ceased[7] and can be 20 years or more. In turn, reversibility depends on age of the subject, the severity of symptoms, duration of exposure to vibration and the type of vibration tool used.[7]

CLASSIFICATION

The vascular and sensorineural components of HAVS are graded separately in the SWS (see Table 47.1). The scale is a clinical grading and not a disability scale. It has, however, been used to make recommendations on employability.[21] Limitations in definitions used in the scale has led to suggested modifications (see Table 47.3).[22]

It has been difficult to carry out powerful prospective studies because of the diminishing levels of manufacturing, and from younger employees more readily choosing to seek job alternatives.[23]

PATHOPHYSIOLOGY

There is uncertainty as to the exact pathogenesis of hand–arm vibration syndrome. The vascular and neurological components of the hand–arm vibration syndrome may, however, share a common pathogenesis. Vasospasm may be initiated by nerve fibre dysfunction in the vessel wall, or conversely numbness and tingling may be due to damage to the intraneural vessels. In addition, nerve injury, carpal tunnel syndrome and Dupuytren's contracture can all be associated with vascular dysfunction.

Table 47.1 The Stockholm Workshop Scale for the classification of the hand–arm vibration syndrome.

Stage	Grade	Description
Vascular component		
0		No attacks
1V	Mild	Occasional attacks affecting only the tips of one or more fingers
2V	Moderate	Occasional attacks affecting distal and middle (rarely also proximal) phalanges of one or more fingers
3V	Severe	Frequent attacks affecting all phalanges of most fingers
4V	Very severe	As in stage 3, with trophic changes in the fingertips
Sensorineural component		
0SN		Vibration-exposed, but no symptoms
1SN		Intermittent numbness with or without tingling
2SN		Intermittent or persistent numbness, reduced sensory perception
3SN		Intermittent or persistent numbness, reduced tactile discrimination and/or manipulative dexterity

Note. The staging is made separately for each hand. The grade of the disorder is indicated by the stage and number of affected fingers on both hands, e.g. stage/hand/number of digits.

Normal physiology of the skin

The skin regulates body temperature, stores blood and provides protection from uncontrollable fluid loss and sepsis. Cutaneous sensation allows an awareness of the environment. Sweating and the adjustment of blood flow are part of the homeostatic regulation of body temperature. Thermoreceptors in the skin provide local temperature control and neurons in the pre-optic area of the anterior hypothalamus contribute to central control.[24] Local skin temperature reflexes help prevent excessive heat exchange from locally cooled or heated portions of the body. These reflexes are weak in comparison with hypothalamic control. Moderate cooling or a brief exposure to severe cold leads to constriction of arterioles (resistance vessels) and venules (capacitance vessels) and arteriovenous anastomoses (AVA). The radial and ulnar arteries divide into the deep and superficial palmar arches. The ulnar artery is the main arterial input to the superficial palmar arch usually receiving a branch from the radial artery, but which may be small. The digital arteries, one of which lies on each side of the finger, are derived from the superficial palmar arch for the little, ring and middle fingers. The radial artery supplies the deep palmar arch and this produces the digital arteries to the thumbs and the index fingers. The deep arch also gives anastomotic arteries to the digital arteries from the superficial arch. The digital arteries may anastomose with each other in the digits, more especially at their tips. Acting together, the digital arteries are effectively end arteries: in digital arterial vasospasm the blood supply is effectively cut off and the finger skin becomes diffusely white. Acute injury to both digital arteries may result in loss of the digit unless microvascular repair can be carried out.

The arterial blood supply anatomy can be variable and the relative contribution of radial and ulnar arteries may be different from one person to another. An absent ulnar pulse reflects no more than an innocuous variant from the normal: it does not necessarily reflect pathology.

The cutaneous circulation is controlled by sympathetic vasoconstrictors and vasodilator nerves.[25] Sympathetic vasoconstrictor and vasodilator nerves innervate all areas of hairy skin (non-glabrous), whereas hairless (glabrous skin) is innervated by sympathetic vasoconstrictor nerves only. In glabrous skin, arteriovenous anastomoses are numerous and opening and closing of AVA can cause substantial change in blood flow.[25] Secondary Raynaud's phenomenon related to functional changes in blood flow would be expected more often to present in glabrous skin, for the second to the fifth digits and in relation to cold. In practice, the phenomenon is often circumferential.

Cutaneous sensation entails a variety of modalities including tactile (touch, pressure, vibration), thermal (heat and cold) and pain sensations carried through the peripheral nerves for interpretation in the central nervous system.

Pathogenesis of neurosensory dysfunction

Manifestations of neurosensory dysfunction can include reduced or absent sensibility, symptoms of pain or dysaesthesia and changed perception of cold (cold sensitivity). Disturbances of central nervous integration may be implied by reduced hand coordination and manual dexterity. Investigations on the sympathetic and parasympathetic autonomic activity have demonstrated an altered balance, with increased sympathetic drive in vibration-exposed subjects.[26] It is postulated that neurosensory pathogenesis may occur at multiple levels. These include changes to sensory receptors, compression or changes in nerve fibres and intrinsic muscles, and to the somatosensory and motor cortex.[27]

Takeuchi et al.[28] analysed finger biopsies from 30 patients with vibration-induced white fingers, and conducted electron microscopy biopsies from three additional patients with VWF.[29] The impairment of large myelinated fibres has been documented in both morphologic studies and nerve conduction studies. Histological assessments of patients with VWF revealed an increase in the thickness of the perineurium, and a decrease in the number of myelinated nerve fibres and thick lamellar fibrosis of the perineurium.[28,29] The nerve fibres were often reduced in size with an increase of collagen with fibroblasts in the endoneurium. The impairment arising from small diameter nerve fibres (A-delta and C-fibres) is documented in disturbed thermal perception studies. Ultrastructural studies using different neural markers for small diameter nerve fibres showed a significant reduction of epidermal nerve density (END) over the forearm among vibration-exposed subjects.[30]

Sensory and motor dysfunction could also be due to changes in cortical somatotopic mapping of the hand in the brain.[31] Here, Lundborg et al. conducted an fMRI study to compare the somatotopic cortical representation of the hands of workers exposed to vibration with controls. Cortical activation did not differ significantly between patients and controls, thus favouring a peripheral mechanism. The findings did show some shift in cortical activation suggesting a possible cortical remodelling.

Several different experimental animal models have been used to study vibration-induced neuropathology. Most studies have been conducted on rats. Early experiments often used the paws and assessed the results with light microscopy, while more recent studies use a rat-tail model,[32] and electron microscopy with immunostaining. Long-time exposure of a rat limb induces swelling (intraneural oedema) and permanent damage to the sciatic nerve.[33] Ultrastructural changes (such as detachment of myelin sheath from the axolemma at the nodes of Ranvier, axonal loss, and constriction of the axon) increase with the dose of vibration.[34] Axonal damage is seen both in myelinated and non-myelinated axons. Non-myelinated axons have also been found to be oedematous.[35] Rat tails exposed to vibration also exhibit elevated nitrotyrosine immunoreactivity indicative of free-radical damage.[36] Short-term vibration exposures have been associated with disrupted axoplasmic transport, and the experimental results indicate a cumulative effect.[37] Vibration and cold generate similar percentages of myelinated axons with disrupted myelin. Cold with and without vibration caused intraneural oedema, whereas vibration alone did not.[38]

Pathogenesis of vibration-induced Raynaud's phenomenon

Raynaud's phenomenon (RP) denotes an exaggerated vasospastic response to cooling. The aetiology of the phenomenon can be either primary (idiopathic) or secondary, where secondary RP relates to a number of different conditions, including vibration exposure. The phenomenon may be triggered or modified by emotion and stressors. The pathogenesis varies between the underlying conditions. From physical principles (Poiseuille's law) alone, three general mechanisms can be identified that influence peripheral microcirculation:

1. perfusion pressure
2. the luminal radius of the digital artery
3. blood viscosity.

Abnormalities in all three mechanisms have been described among vibration-exposed subjects. The vascular dysfunction may be due to functional or structural abnormalities or both.[39,40] Some dysfunction is better understood, while others are speculative.[41] The pathogensis of Raynaud's phenomenon either primary or secondary remains uncertain.

PERFUSION PRESSURE ABNORMALITIES

Both sympathetic vasoconstrictor and vasodilator systems in the skin participate in blood pressure regulation via the baroreflex. A decrease in perfusion pressure can be caused by systemic hypotension or by a proximal arterial obstruction. Raynaud's phenomenon has been associated with obstructive vascular disorders, such as cervical ribs[40] and thromboses. Subjects with entrapment in the carpal tunnel exhibit increased prevalence of RP.[42] Thenar- and hypothenar hammer syndrome are disorders with reduced blood flow and may appear similar in their manifestation to RP. The baseline cutaneous blood flow of healthy females is lower than that in males and may in part explain the higher prevalence of RP in women.

DYSREGULATION AND ABNORMALITIES OF THE LUMINAL RADIUS

The regulation of the luminal radius is balanced by vasoconstrictors and vasodilators. The neural vasoconstrictor system is tonically active in thermoneutral environments. Sympathetic vasoconstrictor nerves release norepinephrine, which interact with postsynaptic a_1- and a_2-receptors on cutaneous arterioles and arteriovenous anastomoses. Noradrenergic vasoconstrictor nerves also release neuropeptide-y and adenosine triphosphate. Cold augments smooth muscle α_2-adrenoreceptor function. Adrenoreceptor (AR) dysfunction among VWF cases causes weakened α_1-receptor-mediated response and predominance of α_2-receptor function. Cold-induced vasoconstriction is usually a protective response to prevent heat loss and is mediated by a reflex increase in sympathetic nerve activity. The α_2-adrenoreceptors comprise three subtypes and only the α_{2C} AR seems to be sensitive to cold. Results from rat-tail models indicate that vibration can augment sympathetic vasoconstriction by selectively increasing α_2 AR reactivity.[43] Cooling activates α_{2C} AR.

Intraneural swelling occurred in the rat model when the skin temperature was below 15°C.[44]

In addition to the neural regulation, there are endothelium-produced vasoconstrictors and vasodilators. The most potent vasoconstrictor is endothelin-1. Patients with VWF seem to exhibit lower endothelin-1 levels than primary RP[45] in response to cold provocation tests, but more advanced cases of VWF show an exaggerated response compared to normal subjects.[46] Cutaneous injection of endothelin-1 results in a large area with vasospasm, but a reduced vasodilator response which indicates a local axon-reflex deficit,[47] with abnormality in unmyelinated 'C-fibres' and thinly myelinated A-delta fibres.

Nerves supplying blood vessels produce several vasodilatory substances. Temperature increase normally causes vasodilation by stimulating local release of neuropeptides from sensory nerves, such as calcitonin gene-related peptide (CGRP), substance P (SP) and neurokinin-A (NKA). It also stimulates release of endothelin-related nitric oxide (NO).

Immunohistochemical studies have shown a reduction in the number of sensory-motor nerves containing the vasodilator CGRP in finger skin biopsies of patients with hand–arm vibration syndrome. There was also a reduction in the pan-neuronal marker protein gene product 9.5, suggesting that the CGRP depletion might be a consequence of damage with neuronal loss.[48]

Biopsies from patients with VWF reveal thickening of the muscular layers of the artery walls, with hypertrophy of individual muscle cells without intimal fibrosis.[28,29]

INTRAVASCULAR DYSFUNCTION

Changes in leukocytes, erythrocytes and the intima have been reported in long-term exposure to vibration.[41] Where reduced blood viscosity has been found, it has been interpreted as a compensatory mechanism in reaction to tissue ischaemia.

Pathogenesis of carpal tunnel syndrome

Recent studies have demonstrated neuropathies proximal to the hand among vibration-exposed workers[49] or at multifocal levels.[50] Structural changes found just proximal to the wrist may be involved in the development of carpal tunnel syndrome in vibration-exposed workers.[51] Histological findings in the wrist of post-mortem specimens showed synovial membrane hyperplasia, endothelial reduplication and increased epineural density inside the carpal tunnel. The findings are interpreted as steps in the pathogenetic path based mainly on pressure produced by forces and displacement of tendons.[52] This mechanical factor in the aetiogenesis of carpal tunnel syndrome (CTS) has later been modified and extended by supporters of an additional vascular pathogenesis for CTS. The pathophysiology of the microcirculation and the subsequent neuropathy varies with the various stages of the CTS lesion.[27] In the early stages, there is evidence for oedema formation and vascular insufficiency manifested as nocturnal paraesthesias, while in the advanced stage, there is severe injury with severe nerve fibre lesions of neuropractic and axonotometic type. Evidence from meta-analysis of studies on CTS and work supports and extends previous conclusions that there is a relation to vibration and to certain hand activities.[53]

Pathogenesis of Dupuytren's disease

Dupuytren's disease (DD) is characterized by thickening, nodule formation and contracture of the palmar fascia, resulting in flexion deformity of the fingers. Heredity, alcohol abuse, epilepsy, diabetes and smoking have been associated with DD.[54] When reviewing studies focusing on the relation between intensive manual work, trauma, vibration exposure and the development of DD, Liss and Stock[55] concluded that there was good support for an association between vibration and DD. However, a recent study including almost 100 000 subjects failed to show this association.[56] Biomolecular advancements at gene and cellular level have brought new insights to the pathogenesis of DD. Studies of gene expression using DNA microarray technology[54] revealed that several genes were upregulated, while at the same time others were downregulated in tissue samples of DD. Contractile myofibroblasts are involved in contracture deformity. Histologically, the cords of DD consist of a dense collageneous matrix with fibroblasts. The cause of myelofibroblast profileration on the cellular level in DD is unknown. One hypothesis is that reduced peripheral blood flow causes ischaemia and the generation of free radicals, which damage the surrounding tissue and cause fibroblast proliferation.[54] Initially, in the pathogenesis, there is a proliferative stage characterized by an increase in myelofibroblasts. In the subsequent involutional stage, the microvessels within this tissue are considerably narrowed. It has been suggested that the pathogenesis of DD is a result of vessel narrowing causing local hypoxia and chronic ischaemia, activating the xanthine oxidase pathway, releasing free radicals that stimulate fibroblasts to proliferate.[57]

Pathogenesis of vibration-associated muscular disease

Reduction of neuromuscular function and strength may occur following long-term exposure to work with vibrating machines.[58] Farkkila and co-workers reported loss of extrinsic hand muscle strength among lumberjacks with hand–arm vibration syndrome. More recent studies have confirmed reduction in both extrinsic and intrinsic hand muscle strength.[59] The results of Necking et al. demonstrate thenar muscle strength loss in subjects with long-term exposure to hand-held vibrating machines. The morphological assessments demonstrated centrally located myonuclei with fibre type grouping, angulated muscle fibres, ring fibres, regenerating fibres and fibrosis. The observed muscle necrosis, fibrosis and the structural disorganization were all interpreted as suggestive of direct muscle damage, whereas the angulated fibres and fibre type grouping suggests muscle denervation and reinnervation.[59] These findings are in accordance with those observed in short-term vibration in animal models.[60] Several theories regarding the pathogenesis have been suggested, including vibration, tonic vibration reflex with continuous elevation of muscle tone, blood flow reduction, and mechanical and metabolic changes. The evidence suggests that working with vibrating machines may cause both damage to the muscle units within the contractile muscle fibres and nerves.

CLINICAL FEATURES

Sensorineural hand–arm vibration syndrome

In the natural history of the condition, neurological (sensorineural) symptoms tend to occur first. Most surveys record them as twice as common as vascular symptoms and generally causing greater disability. The latent period for sensorineural symptoms varies from a few months to many years.

SIGNS AND SYMPTOMS

Use of vibratory tools causes transient paraesthesia in the fingers of most users. This usually passes off within 20 minutes. Often, the first abnormal symptoms are an extension of this time. Tingling or numbness usually starts at the fingertips, but can affect all, or the whole, of the fingers. With continuing exposure, these symptoms may become persistent lasting for hours or even all day. Although aggravated by coldness, the tingling and numbness can occur in a warm environment, causing considerable distress. The sensory loss causes workers to describe their fingers as feeling thick or 'like bananas' in many instances.

There is a loss of feeling, of temperature appreciation and of pain sensation. In severe cases, workers can experience clumsiness and loss of manual dexterity, with poor finger coordination causing inability to do fine work.

Assessing a case of suspected neurological HAVS requires details of vibration exposure, past medical history and a clinical history of date of onset of symptoms, site of paraesthesia, time of occurrence and duration of symptoms. Nocturnal symptoms may occur, but are less frequent than in cases of carpal tunnel syndrome.

Before reaching a diagnosis of sensorineural HAVS, all other causes of peripheral neuropathy must be considered (see under Diagnosis, p. 505).

There are no visible signs of neurological damage. This makes the use of tests all the more important before advice can be given to the worker on the severity of the condition and implications of further exposure to vibration.

As there is no gold standard to diagnose sensorineural HAVS, and no single test with sufficient specificity or sensitivity, researchers have recommended the use of a battery of tests.[21,61]

The appreciation of touch, vibration, temperature, joint position and motion are transmitted by nociceptors, thermoreceptors, mechanoreceptors and nerve fibres. Tests have been designed to detect abnormalities in these receptors and transmission pathways. Their main value is in assessing the severity of sensory loss.

Simple tests, such as cotton wool and moving two-point aesthesiometry, can demonstrate a loss of sensation, but are limited by inter-observer error, and generally will only pick up the later stages of sensory loss. These clinical findings have no normative data available for comparison. Semmes–Weinstein monofilaments have been used to grade such loss and are considered a better validated example of these types of test.[62]

Other psychophysical or quantitative sensorineural tests (QST) with a sound anatomical and physiological basis have been developed. As all these tests have a subjective input, they are not truly objective and are often referred to as 'standardized tests'.

These tests derive from the work on mechanoreceptors by Mountcastle.[63] Vibration stimulates mechanoreceptors, end organs and nerve fibres. The superficial Meissner corpuscles or fast adapting 1 (FA1) respond to frequencies between 5 and 60 Hz, while the deep Pacinian corpuscles or fast adapting 11 (FA11) react to frequencies between 50 and 400 Hz. These signals are transmitted by the large myelinated A-alpha and A-beta fibres.

There are also cold and warm receptors in the fingertips. Messages from the cold receptors are transmitted by small myelinated A-delta fibres, while those from warm receptors use unmyelinated C fibres.

The vibrotactile threshold test (VTT)[64,65] and thermal aesthesiometry test (TA)[66] have had their integrity investigated.[67–69] These tests must be performed in a temperature-controlled environment. As they are psychophysical tests, a random element should be built in to eliminate any deliberate exaggeration. In both tests, the flexor surface of the distal phalanx of the index and little fingers is tested to assess the median and ulnar innervation. The VTT requires a constant downward pressure of 1 Newton. Thresholds are generally measured at 31.5 Hz (Meissner corpuscles) and 125 Hz (Pacinian corpuscles), although some equipment includes a broader range of frequencies.

Change of the temperature in TA is 1°C per second. The 'pulse method' should be used.[70] The zone in which change in temperature cannot be felt is known as the temperature neutral zone (TNZ), and is calculated by subtracting the cold threshold from the warm threshold.

A test, such as the Purdue pegboard test (PPT), may demonstrate loss of dexterity against age-related normative data.[71,72] As an isolated test, it is of little discriminatory value.

Table 47.2 Scoring system for the standardized tests.

Scoring system			
Vibrotactile threshold (VTT) index and fifth finger			
At 31.5 Hz	$<0.3\,\text{ms}^2 = 0$	$\geqslant 0.3\,\text{ms}^2 - <0.4\,\text{ms}^2 = 1$	$\geqslant 0.4\,\text{ms}^2 = 2$
At 125 Hz	$<0.7\,\text{ms}^2 = 0$	$\geqslant 0.7\,\text{ms}^2 - <1.0\,\text{ms}^2 = 1$	$\geqslant 1.0\,\text{ms}^2 = 2$
Thermal aesthesiometry (TA) (1°/sec index and fifth finger)			
Temperature neutral zone (TNZ)	$<21°C = 0$	$\geqslant 21°C - <27°C = 2$	$\geqslant 27°C = 4$

As the mechanism and proportion of damage is unclear, the VTT and TA should be given equal weighting. A scoring system can be used to record the extent of this damage (see Table 47.2).[69]

The first attempt to grade the stages of vibration damage was the Taylor/Pelmear classification in 1967. Unfortunately, the only neurological category was the earliest stage 0N (numbness) or 0T (tingling). Once the importance of the neurological damage was recognized this neurological grading became inadequate and was replaced by the sensorineural component of SWS (see Table 47.1).[4]

A very large contract examining more than 100 000 miners with the use of VTT and TA gave the opportunity to recommend refinements to the sensorineural staging of the SWS.[6] As tingling was thought to be as important as numbness, the wording 'with or without tingling' was changed to 'numbness and/or tingling'.

Stage 2SN was thought to cover a very wide range of neurological damage from patients with relatively minor handicap to those with severe sensory loss, but without a dexterity problem in a warm environment. For this reason, the combined VTT and TA score was used to divide this stage into 2SN early and 2SN late (see Table 47.3).

True 3SN cases have severe persistent neurological damage. For a grading of stage 3SN, there had to be a loss of dexterity in a warm environment, VTT and TA score of equal to or greater than 9, and an abnormal Purdue pegboard test. As the maximum single test score per hand was 8, a score of $\geqslant 9$ was required to show evidence of damage in both tests. When these criteria were met, 10 was added to the combined VTT and TA score.

In the United Kingdom, the use of these tests, scoring system and modified sensorineural staging has been accepted by the Health and Safety Executive in their Guidance on Health Surveillance for Occupational Health Professionals 2005.[22]

VASCULAR CLINICAL FEATURES

The vascular component is one of arterial vasospasm, and the clinical features are indistinguishable from Raynaud's phenomenon. Raynaud's phenomenon is a very common condition in the community manifested by cold-induced

Table 47.3 Modification of Stockholm Workshop Scale for classification of the sensorineural component of hand–arm vibration syndrome staging.

Stage	Criteria
0SN	Vibration exposure, but no symptoms
1SN	Intermittent numbness and/or tingling with a sensorineural score of $\geqslant 3 - <6$
2SN (early)	Intermittent or persistent numbness and/or tingling, reduced sensory perception with a score of $\geqslant 6 - <9$
2SN (late)	As 2SN (early), but with a score of $\geqslant 9 - \leqslant 16$
3SN	Intermittent or persistent numbness and/or tingling, reduced manipulative dexterity and a SN score of $\geqslant 19$

episodic attacks of digital arterial vasospasm, causing 'whiteness' of the affected parts of the fingers. It is more common in colder climates. Overall, it affects up to about 15 per cent of the community with a female preponderance of approximately 3:1 compared with males. In temperate European countries, a prevalence of about 5 per cent for males and 30 per cent for females would be expected. In warm countries, fewer manifestations of Raynaud's phenomenon have been reported.

Raynaud's description in 1862 included a variety of conditions, but as time has passed, the condition has become much more clearly described and primary and secondary Raynaud's conditions are now recognized.

Primary Raynaud's phenomenon is otherwise known as Raynaud's disease. This condition affects younger people, mostly under the age of 40 years, and usually females. Individuals suffer episodic attacks of whiteness of the fingers and/or toes occurring in response to cold. Fingertips are affected first and, as the condition progresses, the entire fingers are affected in late cases. Although some or all of the digits can be affected, the extent of the blanching is usually variable from attack to attack and is diffuse.

The extensive use of vibrating powered tools in industrial processes is responsible for most cases of secondary Raynaud's phenomenon. However, there are other well-recognized diseases (many under the heading of collagen vascular disorder, for example, systemic sclerosis and CREST syndrome). These are all associated with digital artery vasospasm occurring in response to cold. In these conditions, the symptoms can come on at any age and may be rapidly progressive leading to ischaemia of the fingers and toes necessitating amputation. Investigations will normally show antibodies in the blood enabling the diagnosis to be made, and although these may be absent initially, they frequently emerge with time and it may be some years after first presentation of the disease that they become detectable. Severe Raynaud's disease is often said to be an autoimmune secondary Raynaud's phenomenon without the antibodies, yet being identifiable. It is rare for Raynaud's disease or Raynaud's phenomenon secondary to vibration to be as severe in its effect as secondary Raynaud's phenomenon arising in association with autoimmune vascular disease. A systematic review found evidence that vascular symptoms could occur in the lower limbs in those diagnosed with HAVS, providing symptoms were apparent in the hands.[9]

Vibration-induced Raynaud's phenomenon is graded on the Stockholm scale according to the severity of the symptoms and the extent of the blanching. In stages 0, 1, 2 and 3, there is a transition from vibration exposed, but no blanching to extensive blanching affecting all of the fingers in their entirety. A stage 4 category is reserved for those individuals who have trophic or ischaemic changes evident in the fingers: while it is true that some vibration-exposed workers will show trophic changes in the fingertips, it is the experience of the authors that all of these cases have another reason for the trophic change to be present. Almost certainly, stage 4 HAVS does not exist and if a case is seen in which stage 4 seems a likely diagnosis, full blood investigations for autoimmune vascular disease should be instigated, and repeated if the results are initially negative.

The onset of HAVS is dependent on two factors. The first is the susceptibility of the individual using vibrating tools to the harmful effects of vibration, and the second is the vibration dose received: higher dose leads to an earlier onset. Some individuals develop symptoms early in their careers, yet others may never develop symptoms or have the onset of symptoms delayed for many years.

The first symptom or sign of digital arterial vasospasm is the onset of blanching affecting the tips of one or more digits and occurring in response to cold. Gradually, the extent of the blanching increases until the full length of each finger may be affected. The thumbs tend to be spared, but they can be affected particularly in more severe cases of HAVS, or when the thumb is particularly exposed to vibration. The blanching of the fingers may just extend on to the most distal aspect of the palms. The blanching is circumferential and sometimes obliquely so, affecting the territory of one digital artery, but not both.

A typical attack lasts for between 20 and 30 minutes, although it can last longer for up to an hour or so. Longer-duration attacks are highly unusual and a regularly experienced 'attack' lasting more than two hours is more likely to be a description of a natural physiological response to the cold. Recovery can be hastened by warming of the hands, although this may be painful. True digital artery vasospasm is accompanied by numbness in the fingers due to the transient ischaemia of the digital nerves. The area of blanching is normally sharply demarcated from the surrounding normal skin.

In the recovery phase, the circulation is restored to the digit from the base towards the tip, and there is usually a reactive hyperaemia, reflecting the acidosis or acidaemia that will have developed in the digit during the period of ischaemia. The finger often appears a prominent red colour as recovery proceeds, with ultimately a normal pink hue being resumed. Many individuals describe this phase as being one of hot aches, and a comparison is often made with the sensation in the hands remembered from childhood after playing in the snow. In some people, the red discolouration does not occur, but a cyanotic colour is present instead. In addition, some people give a description of arterial vasospasm without whiteness, only cyanosis of the fingers. This is likely to be compatible with a diagnosis of HAVS.

Blotchiness of the fingers may be a complaint. This is not normally considered to be Raynaud's phenomenon, which causes a uniform blanching. Mottling is a common normal skin appearance.

Another common complaint is of cold fingers or cold sensitivity. In isolation, this is not Raynaud's phenomenon, nor does it necessarily reflect any underlying vascular pathology, although some consider it to be to a presymptomatic phase.

Some individuals describe a whiteness of the skin that is simply a normal appearance or a physiological response to cold. Some drug therapy is associated with the potential side effect of cold extremities (for example β-blocker therapy). These drugs do not *per se* cause Raynaud's phenomenon, although if an individual suffers from cold extremities when taking them, they may be more likely to suffer an attack of arterial vasospasm.

Eliasson and colleagues[73] reviewed the effects of β-blockers and concluded that when propranolol was used (propranolol is one of the earlier non-cardioselective agents) that around 3 per cent of patients experienced troublesome vasospastic phenomena of the periphery. The symptoms occurred within two months of starting the treatment and usually affected the extremities of all four limbs. At about the same time, Marshall and colleagues[74] published higher figures for the development of Raynaud's phenomenon, although the diagnosis was based only on the results of a questionnaire. Fifty-nine per cent of patients on propranolol had Raynaud's phenomenon compared with 35 per cent on atenolol. Overall, patient numbers were small; however, this study is important for it found that all patients with Raynaud's phenomenon attributable to β-blockers had developed it in both the hands and feet simultaneously.

These factors relating to the vasospastic phenomena of HAVS are probably of greater importance in the litigation arena than in the occupational health environment. It is suggested below that the management of the individual exposed to vibration, who has arterial vasospastic symptoms and signs, is based on the presence of the Raynaud's phenomenon, and not on whether β-blockers or other factors might be causing the symptoms.

People affected by HAVS present in either the occupational health setting or in the medicolegal arena. In the former, the symptoms may be under-reported, for there may be a genuine concern about continuing employment, but in the latter the symptoms may be exaggerated to try and increase the financial compensation. Much time and effort has been expended in trying to identify a test that might be useful in this respect (e.g. cold water provocation). Attempts to do this are confounded by the fugitive nature of the disease itself. There currently is no objective assessment of a sufficiently high sensitivity, specificity and positive predictive value to enable decisions to be made at an individual level regarding the presence, absence or severity of the disease.

While vibration causes the underlying disease to be present, it is cold which provokes an attack of arterial vasospasm. The affected person knows the circumstances that might lead to an attack occurring, but whether an attack will occur in those circumstances cannot be predicted. The attacks tend to be random. There are a number of variables that can confound the application of these tests. These include core body temperature, recent smoking and alcohol intake, recent vibration exposure, anxiety, drug therapies and the state of the arterial tree.

The nature of Raynaud's phenomenon means the response to cold in any individual varies from day to day. The sufferer knows the circumstances which may provoke an attack of blanching and also knows that an attack may or may not occur under those circumstances. The response is unpredictable. Despite these caveats, a number of these tests have been studied. These have included uncontrolled cold provocation tests, in which the worker's hands are plunged into ice or iced water for a variable period of time. The response is observed without any criteria having been established against which the results of the challenge can be assessed. These unpleasant and potentially dangerous tests are of no value and should be abandoned.[75]

In an attempt to produce an objective test to evaluate the vascular component of HAVS, some researchers have produced a test of controlled finger cooling with measurement of rewarming times of the digits.[76] Comparing the results with known normative data might allow for an objective assessment to be made. In this situation, 'objective' means that the test cannot be manipulated either by the observer or the subject. The test involves cooling the fingers for a defined time and then measuring, by means of thermocouples, the rewarming time. The application of this test on over 40 000 miners was assessed in the UK miners' compensation scheme established by the Department of Trade and Industry.[6,77] The results showed that the test employed was of little or no value in assessing these miners. The Health and Safety Laboratory of the HSE reported similar findings.[78] An alternative to measurement of finger skin temperature using a thermocouple is to use a thermographic measurement of the digital rewarming, but the principle remains the same.

Other techniques have included the measurement of finger systolic blood pressure after controlled cooling of the fingers.[79] This test is technically difficult to perform in the field setting, but is suited to an occupational health laboratory. However, considerable overlap of results has been documented in a study of dockyard workers with and without symptoms of HAVS.[80] Some researchers have suggested that the sensitivity and specificity of these tests might be improved after body cooling. Others suggest that a cooling test, with measurement of changes in the recovery phase, does offer a test of high sensitivity, specificity and positive predictive value.[81] Despite this, the Faculty of Occupational Medicine evidence review[9] concluded 'no current vascular test has been shown to accurately stage the extent of an abnormality in an individual as defined by the Stockholm Workshop Scale'.

There is no test or process which will enable a decision to be taken with absolute certainty as to whether Raynaud's phenomenon is secondary to vibration or is simply due to Raynaud's disease. The main potential causes, when considering the differential diagnosis, are presented in Table 47.4 (see under Diagnosis, p. 505).

CARPAL TUNNEL SYNDROME

Carpal tunnel syndrome (pressure on the median nerve at the wrist) has a high prevalence in the adult community. Episodes of intermittent mild numbness in the median innervated fingers will not necessarily take a person to their primary care physician for investigation or treatment. Two studies in the 1990s sought to identify the prevalence of carpal tunnel syndrome in the community by patient questionnaire and nerve conduction studies. De-Krom et al.[82] identified a prevalence of 3.4 per cent of adult females with known carpal tunnel syndrome, but an additional 5.8 per cent of females where the diagnosis had been previously undetected. The figures for men range from 0.6 to 8 per cent depending on the criteria used. Ferry et al.[83] felt the prevalence estimate lay between 7 and 18 per cent of the adult population (and was similar for male and female populations).

Patients complain of pain and paraesthesia in the distribution of the median nerve, with numbness in the fingers especially at night, and aggravation of symptoms when using the hand. There may be wasting of abductor pollicis brevis in long-standing cases. Provocation tests may be useful in diagnosing carpal tunnel syndrome; Phalen's test increases the pressure on the median nerve, as the wrist is moved from neutral dorsipalmar flexion to maximum

Table 47.4 Differential diagnosis of hand–arm vibration syndrome.

	Diagnosis
Hand conditions	Arteritis
	Drugs
	Carpal tunnel syndrome
Regional problems	Thoracic outlet syndrome (including cervical rib)
	Atherosclerotic vascular disease
Systemic disease	Primary Raynaud's phenomenon
	Connective tissue disorders, including CREST syndrome, rheumatoid arthritis and systemic lupus erythematosus
	Diabetes mellitus
	Hypothyroidism
	Chronic micro-embolism – from valvular heart disease and atheroma
	Polycythaemia
Neurological disease	Any peripheral neuropathy
	Cervical spondylosis
	Multiple sclerosis
Blood-borne factors	Malignant disease including multiple myeloma
	Cryoglobulinaemia and cold agglutinins
	Raised plasma viscosity
Drugs and chemicals	Beta-adrenergic blockers, ergot, some anti-cancer drugs, PVC exposure
	Metronidazole, anti-epileptic drugs, chronic alcohol excess, cyclosporine, anti-depressants – all cause neurological complications
	(The list of drugs is only indicative of some agents causing problems. Always check the side effects of drugs especially when the worker is on long-term medication)

CREST, calcinosis, Raynaud phenomenon, oesophageal dysmotility, sclerodactyly and telangiectasia.
This list is not a complete list, but it does cover some of the more common potential causes of doubt in the diagnosis. Inclusion here does not necessarily mean the second pathology or the presence of drugs is the cause of symptoms. Only a very small number of people on β-blocker therapy will develop Raynaud's-like symptoms; only a very small number of diabetic patients will have a peripheral neuropathy.

passive flexion. The test is considered diagnostic if the onset of paraesthesia occurs within 60 seconds of flexing the wrists. Tinel's sign may be demonstrated by gently percussing over the median nerve just proximal to the flexor retinaculum. A positive test produces paraesthesia in the fingers in the median nerve distribution.

Advice on workplace or home task modification may be very helpful in controlling symptoms of mild to moderate carpal tunnel syndrome. This may take the form of avoiding end range posture of joints during the working process by adjustments of working height, and the use of appropriately designed tools with suitably sized handles. Repetitive and forceful activities should, if possible, be shared through the entire working day, to minimize the prospect of difficulties. An ergonomic programme outlined by Eversman[84] reduced a workforce incidence of carpal tunnel syndrome by 60 per cent. Nerve and tendon gliding exercises have been shown to be of benefit in reducing the need for carpal tunnel decompression.[85,86] Wrist splints can also be extremely helpful in the earliest stages of the disease. The volume of the carpal tunnel is maximal in the neutral flexion extension range and the wrist splint should be applied in this position for maximal benefit.[87]

Harrington et al.[88] considered the surveillance criteria for carpal tunnel syndrome to be pain or paraesthesia or sensory loss in the median nerve distribution and one of the following, Tinel's test positive, Phalen's test positive, nocturnal exacerbation of symptoms, motor loss with wasting of abductor pollicis brevis or abnormal nerve conduction studies. Additional features that might aid the diagnosis included no signs or symptoms in the little finger or dorsum of the hand, no other cause apparent or a successful outcome following steroid injection or surgery. Carpal tunnel syndrome presenting in its classical form is readily diagnosed on history and examination alone. However, the diagnosis of carpal tunnel syndrome in the presence of neurosensory impairment arising from hand–arm vibration syndrome is more complex.

Carpal tunnel syndrome in workers exposed to vibration

A variety of papers have identified a high prevalence of carpal tunnel syndrome in vibration-exposed workers (Table 47.5). The studies mentioned are composed of relatively small numbers of workers. Stromberg et al.[95] reviewed 100 vibration-exposed workers and noted that 48 per cent had isolated neurosensory symptoms, 20 per cent isolated vasospastic problems and 32 per cent combined neurosensory and vascular problems. Twenty-two per cent of the cases were also considered to have carpal tunnel syndrome. The Industrial Injuries Advisory Council[96] in the United Kingdom has accepted carpal tunnel syndrome as a prescribed industrial disease, having reviewed the evidence and concluded a doubling of relative risk in vibration-exposed workers. The council did not consider there was sufficient evidence to offer an opinion on qualifying exposure, but would expect the symptoms to begin during employment when hand-held vibrating tools were used.

The relationship between carpal tunnel syndrome and hand–arm vibration is unclear. If there is an association, its pathological process is not known. Those exposed to vibration commonly use their hands for high force, high repetition activities, which Silverstein et al.[97] consider a potent cause of higher prevalence of carpal tunnel syndrome. Lundborg et al.[98] believe that vibration creates oedema

Table 47.5 Papers advising of an association between hand–arm vibration syndrome and carpal tunnel syndrome.

Author	No. vibration-exposed workers in study	Number with carpal tunnel syndrome (%)
Chatterjee et al.[89]	16	7 (44)
Lukas[90]	137	44 (32)
Boyle et al.[91]	19	12 (63)
Farkkila et al.[92]	79	20 (26)
Koskimies et al.[93]	125	25 (31)
Bovenzi et al.[94]	65	25 (38)
Stromberg et al.[95]	100	22 (22)

within the nerve and swelling of the synovial linings, creating increased pressure within the carpal tunnel. Stromberg, a co-worker, took biopsies of the posterior interosseous nerve in vibration-exposed workers and controls.[99] The posterior interosseous nerve lies on the dorsal surface of the wrist. There was evidence of myelin breakdown and intraneural fibrosis in those exposed to vibration, confirming that vibration damage can occur to nerves at wrist level.

The diagnosis of carpal tunnel syndrome in vibration-exposed workers with neurosensory impairment is difficult. Tinel's and Phalen's tests are helpful in classical cases of carpal tunnel syndrome,[100] but the specificity and sensitivity of these tests has not been evaluated in a vibration-exposed group. Stromberg et al.[101] assessed the value of nerve conduction studies and concluded that they did not discriminate between carpal tunnel syndrome and vibration-induced neurosensory impairment. Numbness and tingling in the median innervated fingers that wakes a patient at night, or is present on awakening in the morning, may be the most helpful clinical sign, confirming a diagnosis of carpal tunnel syndrome in vibration-exposed workers. Burke et al.[102] reported the assessments of 26 000 miners seeking compensation for hand–arm vibration syndrome. The doctors assessing the claimants observed 38 per cent to have nocturnal awakening, 15 per cent had a positive Tinel's test and 20 per cent a positive Phalen's test. The doctors assessing the claimants considered 15 per cent of the claimants to have carpal tunnel syndrome.

Carpal tunnel decompression in patients not exposed to vibration produces a very satisfactory outcome in most cases.[103] Decompression in vibration-exposed workers is effective at relieving night pain and intermittent numbness within the median nerve distribution.[104] Hagberg et al.[105] considered carpal tunnel decompression slightly less effective in vibration-exposed patients, but the majority still had a satisfactory outcome from surgery.

In conclusion, the Industrial Injuries Advisory Council considers there is a doubling of risk of carpal tunnel syndrome in vibration-exposed workers. However, the prevalence of carpal tunnel syndrome in the community is high, with many patients not seeking treatment for their complaints. Vibration exposure may be an aetiological risk factor for carpal tunnel syndrome, or alternatively a risk factor for provocation of symptoms of carpal tunnel syndrome. However, the relationship between carpal tunnel syndrome and hand–arm vibration remains uncertain.[106]

DUPUYTREN'S DISEASE

Dupuytren's disease commonly affects mature males in Northern Europe. The prevalence there varies between countries, with Gudmundsson et al.[107] noting very considerable variations in prevalence between communities in the United Kingdom, Norway, Sweden and Iceland.

The prevalence of Dupuytren's disease rises steeply with age. Hueston[108] noted 4 per cent prevalence in working male Australians if they were under the age of 40 years, but a 30 per cent prevalence in those older than 60 years. A genetic predisposition is noted in most cases, with a particularly high prevalence observed in diabetics.[109] An increased prevalence has also been noted in those with a high consumption of alcohol,[110] and in those who smoke tobacco.[111]

The condition manifests itself with the development of thickening in the palmar fascia, producing nodules, bands and pits. The ulnar border of the hand is most commonly involved, extending into the ring and little fingers, but all digits may be affected, including the thumb and first web space. Those with a strong Dupuytren diathesis will have deposits of Dupuytren tissue on the dorsal surface of the proximal interphalangeal (PIP) joint (Garrods pads), and there may be involvement of the plantar fascia (Ledderhose disease) or the penis (Peyronie's disease). Nodules may be tender at the outset, but the discomfort usually settles as the nodules mature, with shortening that can produce contracture to the metacarpophalangeal (MP) and PIP joints, particularly to the ulnar border of the hand. The distal interphalangeal joints are rarely involved in primary unoperated cases. Excision of the foreshortened fascia in the palm or fingers is effective at releasing contractures, but recurrence is common, particularly in younger patients.

The effect of heavy manual work on the prevalence of Dupuytren's disease has been debated for many years. Dupuytren[112] considered there was an association between manual work and the condition which bears his name. Hueston[113] was not supportive of an association. Mikkelsen[114] did consider there was a relationship and postulated that heavy manual work gives rise to rupture of the fibres in the palmar fascia initiating an unregulated fibrotic response creating nodules and contractures.

The subject was reviewed in 2004 by Khan et al.,[115] who compared the incidence of Dupuytren's disease across social classes in England and Wales, using data from the National Morbidity Survey. They reviewed the incidence rates of first ever consultations for Dupuytren's disease with general practitioners in a 500 000 population. They reviewed the prevalence of attendances with Dupuytren's disease combining skilled manual, partly skilled manual and unskilled manual workers as a group and compared them with a group of professional, managerial and technical and skilled non-manual workers. Accumulative standardized incidence of Dupuytren's disease rose in a similar way with increasing age until normal retirement age (65 years), but a divergence then occurred between the manual and non-manual groups. The non-manual group were found to have a higher incidence than manual workers. Their findings are in conflict with those of Mikklesen,[114] who found a higher incidence in retired manual workers in an epidemiological study involving 16 000 citizens of a small Norwegian town. Khan et al.[115] concluded that manual occupations were not associated with an increased incidence of Dupuytren's disease. Ross[116] reviewing the available literature considered that most authors believed there was no association between occupation and the risk of developing Dupuytren's disease.

The effect of a single traumatic event on the development of Dupuytren's disease has been investigated. Stewart et al.[117] studied patients who had sustained a Colles fracture and observed that 11 per cent of the 235 patients developed features of Dupuytren's disease between three and six months from injury. Contractures were mild and were not progressive when reassessed at a later date.

Dupuytren's disease in vibration-exposed workers

Some studies of vibration-exposed workers have revealed an increased prevalence of Dupuytren's disease. Liss and Stock[55] reviewed the literature and felt that there were three papers which offered reasonable evidence of an association.

Cocco et al.[118] matched 180 cases of Dupuytren's disease against controls with age matching ± five years. They found a statistically significant increase in the risk of Dupuytren's contracture in vibration-exposed workers, and there appeared to be a dose-response relationship. Bovenzi et al.[119] reviewed 570 quarry workers who had been exposed to vibration, using stone workers as controls. They considered the odds ratio for developing Dupuytren's contracture was 2.6, although no dose response was identified. Thomas and Clarke[120] identified a prevalence of Dupuytren's disease of almost 20 per cent in vibration-exposed workers (double the prevalence in the controls). They found no correlation between the Taylor Pelmear stagings for hand-arm vibration and the prevalence of Dupuytren's disease. The sample size of the three studies is relatively small and age matching relatively loose.

However, age does have a major effect on the prevalence of Dupuytren's disease. A review of over 97 000 miners seeking compensation for hand-arm vibration syndrome, revealed a Dupuytren's disease prevalence of 1.7 per cent in claimants in the 35–39 year age group.[56] The prevalence in 80–84 year olds was 19.6 per cent. Age was found to be the prime determinant of the prevalence of Dupuytren's disease in this study. An accurate assessment of vibration exposure throughout previous employment cannot usually be obtained, and employees who may overestimate time spent holding the vibrating tool (the 'anger time' or 'trigger time') by as much as a factor of four.[121] However, the vibration exposure in years (in all industries) was known for this large group of miners. There was no statistically significant correlation between the years of exposure to vibration and the prevalence of Dupuytren's disease (controlling for age). Stockholm vascular and neurosensory grading and thermal aesthesiometry and vibrotactile threshold scores (when corrected for age) were found not to be predictors of Dupuytren's disease. This study does not support Liss and Stock's view that there is an association between vibration exposure and the development of Dupuytren's disease.

The prime determinant for the prevalence of Dupuytren's disease is age, and any study of a possible association between Dupuytren's disease and occupation must be tightly controlled for age. On the available evidence, Dupuytren's disease is unlikely to occur more frequently in manual workers and is probably not more common in vibration-exposed workers.

HAND–ARM VIBRATION AND MUSCLE WEAKNESS

Normative data for grip are available from the United States[122,123] and in the United Kingdom.[124] All three studies used a Jamar dynamometer on the second grip setting, with a mean of three grips in standard positioning. Mathiowetz et al. obtained values from 310 males,[122] Hanten et al. 533 males[123] and Gilbertson and Barber-Lomax 130 males.[124] The Hanten series, and Gilbertson and Barber-Lomax are broadly supportive of Mathiowetz's male grip normative values. Grip reaches a maximum in the late 20s and early 30s and halves in old age. Males are noted to be almost 50 per cent stronger than females in comparable age bands. There was a slight preponderance to the right hand being stronger than the left, and minimal difference in the power of grip between dominant and non-dominant hands. Seven per cent of Mathiowetz's males and 11 per cent of Hanten's study were left-handed. Bohannon[125] reviewed ten studies and concluded that in all but one study, strength was greater to the dominant right hand. For dominant left-handers the results were equivocal.

Patients suffering from HAVS are frequently noted to suffer from weakness of grip.[68] Farkkila et al.[126] noted muscle forces to be significantly diminished among workers reporting numbness in the hands. Weakness was not found in forestry workers who had been exposed to less than 5000 hours of sawing. Farkkila et al.[58] explored the matter further, reassessing grip after a two-year interval. Lumberjacks with HAVS (described as white finger) lost 21 per cent of grip over the two years, while lumberjacks not suffering from HAVS only lost 5 per cent of grip. The numbers in the study are small. The HAVS group comprised 11 subjects with a mean age of 45 ± 8 years. The mean age of the 44 subjects considered to have normal grip and no HAVS was 39 (±10) years. Mirbod et al.[127] performed a similar study over a four-year interval. Fifty-three grinders were assessed for grip over a four-year interval. None were considered to have HAVS at the first assessment, two at the second assessment. The average diminution of grip was 7.4 per cent over the four-year interval. The mean age rose from 42.3 years (range, 37–59) to 46.3 years (range, 41–63).

Sorensson and Burstrom[128] assessed the translation of vibration to different parts of the arms (knuckle, wrist and elbow). They confirm that energy transmission decreases with increasing distance from the source. There is progressive dampening more proximally in the limb. If vibration causes nerve or muscle injury, the parts most at risk would be the intrinsic muscles of the hand, rather than the long flexor and extensor muscles of the forearm. Necking et al.[129] explored the effects of vibration on the intrinsic and extrinsic muscles of the arm in 81 workers exposed to vibration and 45 controls. They noted a 7 per cent reduction in extrinsic muscle power in vibration-exposed patients and a 19 per cent reduction in intrinsic muscle power compared to controls. Their study supports the view that the principle cause of weakness of grip in vibration-exposed workers relates to intrinsic muscle dysfunction in the hand rather than the forearm, where energy transmission is less.

Intrinsic muscle mass may be considered relatively small compared with the forearm muscles, but the intrinsic contribution to grip is significant. Kozin et al.[130] explored the contribution of extrinsic and intrinsic muscles to grip in 21 volunteers, who were subjected to low median and low ulnar nerve blocks. A low nerve block to the ulnar intrinsics reduced grip by 38 per cent and a low nerve block to the median innervated intrinsics reduced grip by 32 per cent. Blocks to both median and ulnar innervated intrinsics reduced grip from pre-injection levels by 49 per cent.

A series of studies from Malmo in Sweden have indicated that chronic vibration exposure can damage nerves at the level of the wrist. Stromberg et al.[131] biopsied the posterior interosseous nerve at the level of the wrist in ten patients who had been chronically exposed to vibration. A variety of pathological changes to the nerve was noted (including myelin breakdown and intraneural fibrosis). These features were not found in a similar number of cadaver controls that had not been exposed to vibration.

Necking and co-workers[60] in the same research institute, explored the short-term effects of vibration exposure to the hind paws of rats (five hours daily for two days). Exposure was noted to expand muscle fibres, and nuclei took on a more central position within the fibre. In a more recent study, the same group biopsied abductor pollicis brevis in 20 patients known to be suffering from HAVS.[132] A variety of abnormalities were noted (centrally located myonuclei, angulated muscle fibres, ring fibres, regenerating fibres and fibrosis). Most of these changes are indicative of direct muscle injury, but angulated fibres were considered to likely arise from muscle denervation and re-innervation, suggesting not only direct muscle damage, but additional injury to the motor nerve fibres.

In a separate study, Necking observed reduced index abduction power in patients suffering from hand–arm vibration syndrome.[59]

Grip strength assessments in 97 581 miners seeking compensation for hand–arm vibration syndrome revealed weakness of grip in two-thirds of cases.[133] Figure 47.1 compares the miner's grip, by age band, to UK and US normative values. The effect of vibration exposure on grip was not dose-related and was small when corrected for age (Figure 47.2). The Stockholm neurological and vascular stagings had little correlation with grip, except those with a 3SN rating. Thermal aesthesiometry and vibrotactile threshold staging also had little correlation with grip, when corrected for age. The claimants' low grip values in all age bands, when compared to normative data were not explained. An early vibration effect on grip during the first five years of exposure was not identified.

Workers exposed to the use of vibrating tools frequently complain of weakness of grip and research studies have shown that vibration can cause damage to the small muscles of the hand and the nerves that supply them. The onset

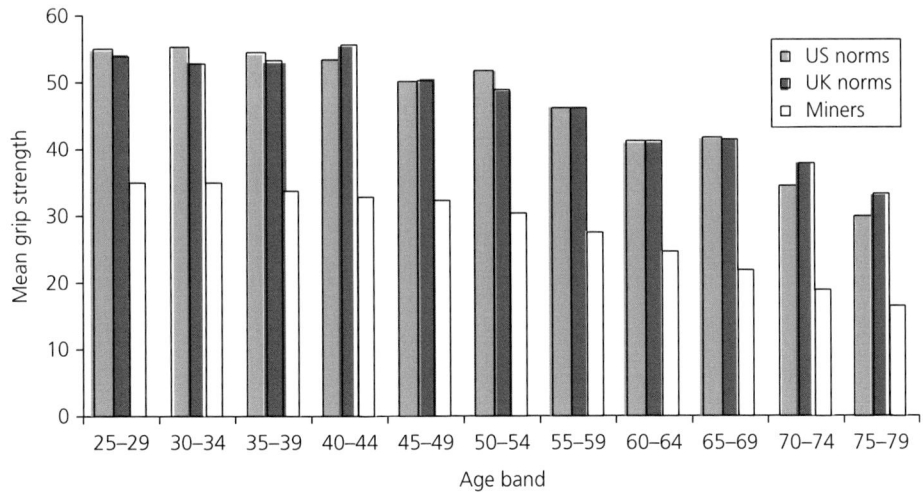

Figure 47.1 Mean grip by age band: The miners compared to United Kingdom and United States normative data.

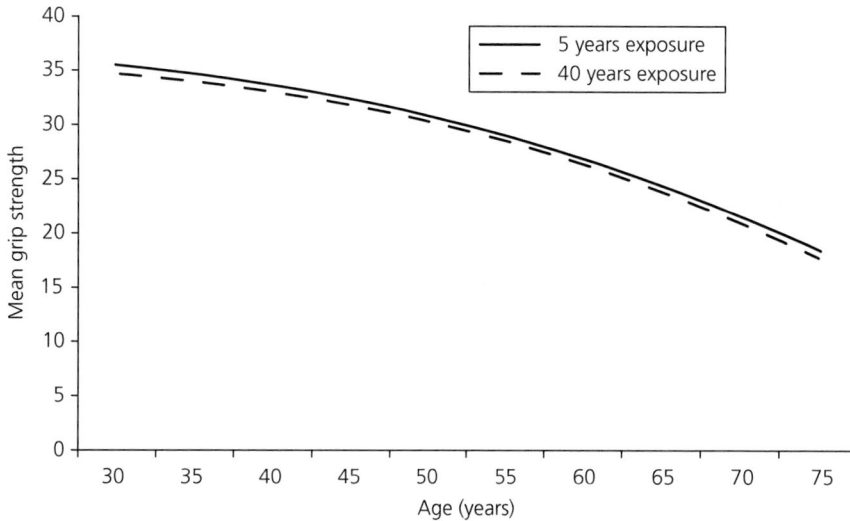

Figure 47.2 The effect of vibration exposure of five and 40 years on mean grip right hand by age band (line of best fit).

of weakness requires further investigation to identify any possible dose response. This will allow development of guidelines for working practice. All studies concerning grip strength need to be tightly controlled for age.

HAND–ARM VIBRATION AND BONE AND JOINT DISORDERS

Gemne and Saraste[134] reported a low frequency of bone and joint disorders with the use of percussive tools. These disorders take the form of bone cysts or osteoarthritis to elbow or wrist. Other authors have found cysts to be present in the carpal bones as frequently in controls as in those exposed to vibration. Local attitudes are to an extent moulded by variations in national compensation schemes. Most countries do not consider that the available evidence justifies compensation for bone and joint disorders routinely.

DIAGNOSIS AND TERTIARY CASE ASSESSMENT

Examination models for the diagnostic work up of subjects with possible injury from work with vibrating tools and equipment vary with the purpose of the assessment. These models range from questions about symptoms, signs, the possible association between exposure and injury; to questions on fitness for work, disability; through to the evaluation for medicolegal assessment and workers' compensation. In those instances where the purpose of the clinical examination is to confirm a possible association between vibration exposure at work and injury, the assessment may include the following aspects:

- evaluation and judgement of symptoms and signs, and grading of severity;
- exposure assessments that include both vibration and ergonomic aspects;
- excluding other potential differential diagnoses.

Scientific reviews on the diagnosis of HAVS are collected in the supplementary issues of the *International Archives of Occupational and Environmental Medicine*[135] which report the First International Workshop on Diagnosis of Injuries 2000 and from the corresponding second workshop held in Göteborg, 2006.[136] The Faculty of Occupational Medicine has reviewed the evidence on clinical testing and management of individuals exposed to hand–arm vibration.[9] A number of textbooks,[137] websites (for example, www.humanvibration.com) and articles present guidance in the diagnostic process for investigating subjects with suspected HAVS.

The level of diagnostic precision required is determined by the outcome required. Screening in the workplace for disease needs to be simple and easy to carry out, yet alert the professional to the possible presence of disease. When disease is suspected more sophisticated diagnosis will be required especially when outcomes may be expensive, such as workers' compensation claims or when deciding on ongoing fitness for work, or in terms of future harm occurring to the individual. The clinical picture of severe cases presenting to a tertiary care setting will be different from those manifesting early signs in a surveillance setting.

Neurological symptoms are usually the first manifestation of HAVS. Finger blanching, although visible, is almost invariably the second symptom or sign. Sensory symptoms can be classified as positive (paraesthesia, dysaesthesiae or pain), negative (motor or sensory loss) or provocable. Symptom disturbance in early cases of HAVS usually presents with tingling or numbness. Symptoms following immediately after vibration exposure (temporary threshold shift) are physiologically normal if they disappear within 20 minutes. Workers may refer to a reduced ability to withstand cold and damp conditions (cold sensitivity). For some susceptible individuals, symptoms may result in early incapacity and reduced workability, while others just have discomfort. Some cases may present with nothing more than a loss of sensitivity in the fingertips. As the condition progresses, more severe symptoms including a reduction in finger precision, manual dexterity, grip force or an increase in extent and frequency of finger blanching lead to a progressive reduction in hand function and resistance to cold.

In the occupational health setting, the medical interview is currently widely accepted as the best available method of diagnosing 'white fingers' (Raynaud's phenomenon). The medical interview should include information on symptoms, distribution, time and duration of blanching. The course, pattern and symptom distribution should ideally be specified pictorially on an upper limb or hand manikin or diagram. Identification of 'white fingers' by comparison with a standardized colour chart has long since been advocated.[138] The medical history should entail assessment of other diseases, injuries or medication that might be related to neuropathy[139,140] or those related to Raynaud's phenomenon,[141] such as autoimmune diseases, endocrine disorders, blood and vessel abnormalities, malignant diseases and infections (see Table 47.4).

Several drugs used to treat hypertension, asthma and cancer are also vasoactive. Medications such as beta-blockers (see under Vascular clinical features, p. 495), ergotamine, clonidine, metysergide, bleomycin, vinblastine, lithium and methylamphetamine may be relevant.[140] Enquire about potentially relevant occupational exposures – rarely specific organic solvents and heavy metals can cause neuropathy[139,140] and chemicals, such as arsenic, vinyl chloride and lead, are likely to influence the occurrence of Raynaud's phenomenon.[141] Exposure to stress and tobacco consumption may add to the interpretation of the medical history.

A history of exposure to a significant degree of vibration is required when diagnosing a presentation of Raynaud's phenomenon as VWF, or a sensory neuropathy as a vibration-associated neuropathy. An understanding of the level of vibration magnitude and its limitations is an essential stage in reaching a diagnosis. Mean frequency, intensity level, trigger times and overall duration are all important. The amount of vibration transmitted to the hand is modified by ergonomic factors such as grip and push forces and if possible an inspection of the job may provide valuable information especially where symptoms are asymmetric. Work organization and work technique may influence the amount of exposure indirectly.

Physical examination

Guided by a differential diagnosis from the history, a careful examination should be performed. Both upper and lower extremities should be examined in order to exclude possible signs of neuropathy, upper limb pain or other systemic disease. (This examination will assist in interpreting abnormal findings in subsequent quantitative sensory threshold (QST) and electrodiagnostic testing.) The examiner inspects the appearance of the distal parts of the hands and fingers for signs such as as scarring, callosities, trophic changes, nail abnormality or Dupuytren's contacture.

Tinel's and Phalen's tests should be performed if carpal tunnel syndrome is suspected. Grip strength can be assessed by Jamar dynamometer and dexterity by Purdue pegboard test and compared to age-related normative data. These along with Semmes–Weinstein monofilaments can be used for assessment in an office environment.

The assessment should include an assessment of upper limb circulation, including blood pressure in each arm, auscultation of the major vessels at the base of the neck and upper arm for bruits indicating possible presence of atheromatous disease and thoracic outlet syndrome (TOS). Roos test and Adson's manoeuvre can be useful if TOS is suspected by symptoms presenting on shoulder abduction. These clinical tests for TOS are of low discriminatory value.

Allen's test assesses the patency of the radial and ulnar arteries supplying the hands. It has always been of doubtful significance for it cannot distinguish between the normal, abnormal and simple anatomical variations that are of no clinical relevance. However, an 8-mHz hand-held Doppler probe is a more informative method for assessing arterial patency in the hands. The Doppler wave-form or laser Doppler may show evidence of conditions such as occlusive vascular disease and hypothenar hammer syndrome. Capillary recirculation time (Lewis–Prusik test) is of very limited diagnostic use.

If, after history and examination, there is no or low suspicion of an underlying disease, then there is no need for further specialized testing. If there is a suspicion that the patient has secondary RP, then further evaluation is needed.[140] The musculoskeletal examination should follow standard clinical orthopaedic examination,[142] specifically looking for signs of carpal tunnel syndrome, Dupuytren's contracture and osteoarthritis (Figure 47.3).

Laboratory tests

BLOOD TESTS

For subjects with a suspected neuropathy, blood tests will include blood count, sedimentation rate, blood glucose determination, serum protein electrophoresis, thyroid studies and vitamin B_{12} level. Although where a peripheral neuropathy exists it is unlikely that blood tests will reveal an unknown pathology.[139]

If secondary RP is suspected, blood tests should also include renal and liver function, rheumatoid factor, cold agglutinins, complement (C3 and C4) and ANA (if positive, tests for antitopoisomerase I and anticentromere antibodies are indicated). Although country-specific medical custom will determine who carries out these tests, it is recommended that they are performed in the tertiary specialist setting.

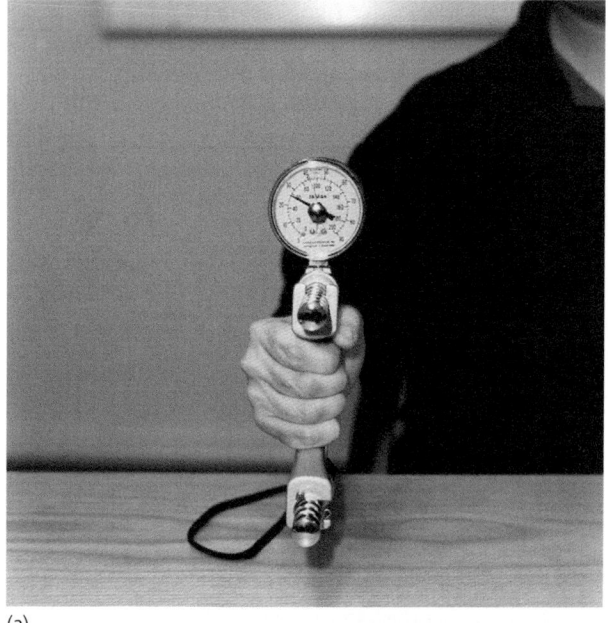
(a)

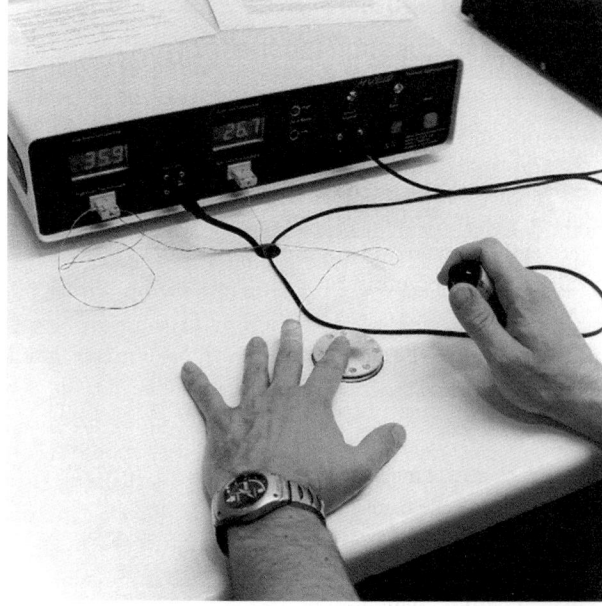
(d)

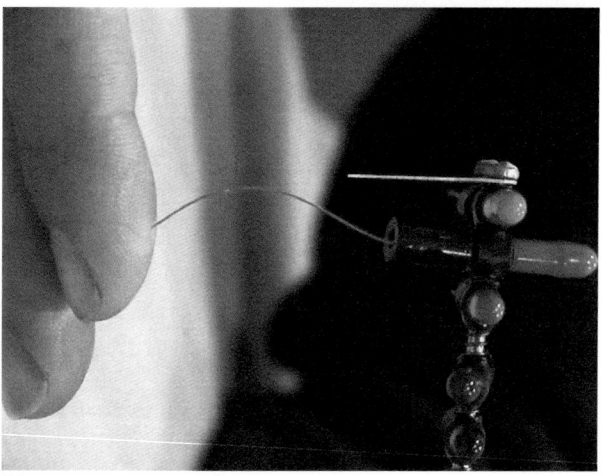
(b)

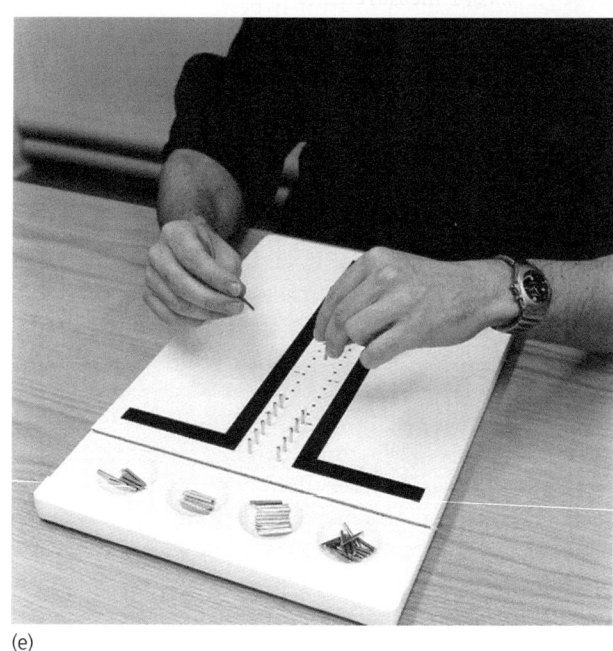
(e)

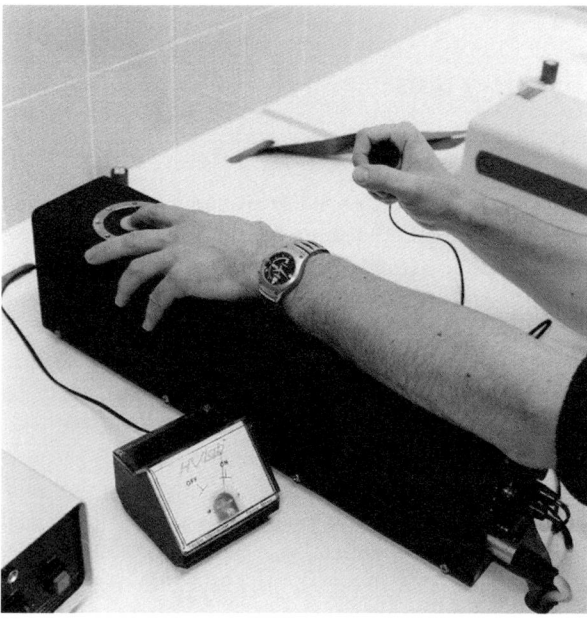
(c)

Figure 47.3 Equipment for the physical examination of subjects exposed to hand–arm vibration. *Motor function*: (a) Jamar grip test. *Sensory function*: (b) monofilaments, (c) vibrotactile thresholds, (d) thermal thresholds. *Dexterity*: (e) Purdue pegboard.

FINGER SYSTOLIC BLOOD PRESSURE

Raynaud's phenomenon can often be diagnosed on the basis of a medical interview, a questionnaire and by identification of white fingers on a colour chart. In some countries, medicolegal demands are for objective support despite ongoing uncertainty about sensitivity and specificity (see under Vascular clinical features, p. 495). This may justify finger systolic blood pressure measurement (comparing distal systolic blood pressure before and after cooling).

QUANTITATIVE SENSORY TESTING

QST provides modality-specific assessment of altered perception thresholds for both large (vibration perception threshold) and small (thermal perception thresholds) fibres. Vibrotactile threshold and thermal thresholds assist in staging severity (see under Sensorineural hand–arm vibration syndrome, p. 494). It should be remembered that upper extremity pain might influence the results from subsequent QST measurements.[143]

ELECTRODIAGNOSTIC TESTING

Electrodiagnostics are useful in cases where there is clinical uncertainty about whether weakness is neurogenic or myogenic, whether the neuropathy is axonal or demyelinating, or where the clinical localization of a nerve lesion is difficult.[144]

BIOPSY

Nerve and skin biopsies should never be performed in the occupational health setting and are rarely ever indicated in the specialist laboratory because of the risk of causing secondary injury or neuroma. However, biopsies have been performed to categorize injury in patients with symptoms that suggest involvement primarily of small fibres.[145] Symptoms of small fibre sensory neuropathy may entail paraesthesia, altered thermal sensation and pain.

RADIOGRAPHY AND MAGNETIC RESONANCE IMAGING

If osteoarthritis is suspected, radiographics are helpful to illustrate the severity and degree of the disorder, more rarely magnetic resonance imaging will reveal cases of nerve entrapment.

DIAGNOSIS

There is currently no established algorithm that unambiguously identifies the specific diagnosis of HAVS. A history of increase of tingling and/or numbness suggests possible sensorineural abnormalities requiring further investigation. A clinical description comprising cold-induced whitening of the skin of the distal phalanges, with a clear demarcation from the normal proximal skin, constitutes a minimum criterion for the diagnosis of Raynaud's phenomenon. For RP to be diagnosed as being secondary to vibration, then the exposure to hand–arm vibration must precede the appearance of the vasospastic episodes. Other probable cause of the Raynaud's phenomenon must also be excluded. To be active, these episodes of finger blanching have to have occurred within the last two years (when exposed to cold).

Staging is carried out in accordance with the Stockholm Workshop Scale (Table 47.1) with grading made separately for vascular and sensorineural components and for each hand.

The diagnosis of carpal tunnel syndrome rests on clinical and electrodiagnostic findings.

The diagnosis of HAVS rests largely on symptoms, signs and test results that rule out other conditions that might form a differential diagnosis, leaving vibration, on the balance of probability, as the cause.

WORKPLACE HEALTH SURVEILLANCE

Workplace health surveillance is primarily for the detection of adverse health effects at an early stage. It can also be used as a means of identifying and protecting susceptible individuals at increased risk from the effects of hand–arm vibration. In addition, it can provide feedback on the adequacy of risk assessment, and as a check on the effectiveness of control measures that have been introduced, and also to prevent the progression of HAVS to the more severe and disabling stages.[22] At the outset, it is critical to ensure that the company or industry concerned agrees a comprehensive policy, including identification, assessment, case management, information, instruction and training, and exposure control.[146] Full discussion with employee representatives and company legal advisers is essential.[147] A programme of health surveillance can only be introduced when these policies have been agreed. Decisions should be agreed on continuing exposure to vibration and at what point cessation of exposure or redeployment should be considered. The policy should include details of how risk assessments should be carried out and whether these should include vibration magnitude measurement and the level of health surveillance required. This may range from the use of a self-administered questionnaire to a fully validated questionnaire administered by a suitably trained occupational health professional. In Europe, the Physical Agents Vibration Directive mandates that health surveillance should be provided.[17] In effect, this means those who are:

- likely to be regularly exposed above the action level of 2.5 m/s (A8); or
- likely to be exposed occasionally above the action value and where the risk assessment identifies that the frequency and severity of exposure may pose a risk to health; or
- have a diagnosis of HAVS (even when exposed below the action value).

The application of this directive in six European countries has been reviewed and several countries, such as Italy, Sweden and Germany, have adopted local guidelines with differing approaches.[11]

The Control of Vibration at Work Regulations 2005 implemented in July 2005 in the United Kingdom describes a five-step tiered approach to health surveillance.[22] This includes a pre-employment or pre-placement baseline check by a qualified person, and annual review by either a qualified person or a responsible person. A positive result is referred to tier 3 for health assessment by a qualified person, normally a suitably trained occupational health nurse. A tentative diagnosis of HAVS should lead to referral to tier 4 which involves a formal diagnosis carried out by a suitably trained doctor qualified in occupational health, who can advise on fitness for work. An optional tier 5 involves referral to a specialist centre for standardized vascular and sensorineural tests.

MANAGEMENT OF CASES

Management of individual cases

The approach to managing individual cases of HAVS is limited by our understanding of the natural history and prognosis of the condition. Objective evidence of reversibility in HAVS is weak. Reversibility is greater for vascular symptoms than sensorineural symptoms, but unlikely in those with stage 3 symptoms.[148]

Regardless of the stage the condition has reached, there are a number of generic recommendations that may reduce the chance of progression. These include reduction in exposure and advice on maintaining general body warmth, avoiding cold damp conditions and specifically smoking cessation.[149,150] In practice, the progression in an individual case very much depends on intangible variables including whether the employer has a policy, individual susceptibility and inadequate exposure–response models.[146]

The Physical Agents Vibration Directive exposure action value (EAV) for the introduction of health surveillance effectively accepts a likely prevalence of 10 per cent finger blanching after nine years of exposure.[17] The apparently pragmatic recommendation to reduce exposure may not be practicable for the employee's patterns of work. The effective vibration dose can depend on intermittency of exposure, the magnitude and direction of applied grip forces and adopted body postures. Vibration magnitudes from the same tools can vary greatly depending on the background tool maintenance programmes.

International Organization for Standardization dose–response models suggest no observed effect levels at exposures of less than 1 m/s^2, although this cannot be regarded as a 'safe level' (ISO 5349, Annex C 2001).[16] The latent interval can vary from six months to 20 or more years between first exposure and onset of vascular symptoms. Some workers are peculiarly resistant to the effects of vibration.

Accepting differing national regulatory frameworks, it would seem reasonable that HAVS cases diagnosed at stage 1 on the SWS should be allowed to continue with exposure, unless there has been a particularly short latent interval or rapid progression of symptoms. Stage 1 cases should be reviewed annually with recommendations for reduction in exposure along with a review of control measures to reduce exposure as far as possible and ideally not exceed an $A(8)$ value of 1.0 m/s^2.

For later stages, consensus statements and evidence reviews have recommended exposure cessation that prevents the development of either stage 3 vascular or stage 3 sensorineural on the Stockholm Workshop Scale.[21,151] At the onset of stage 2, there should be closer monitoring, say six monthly, and a similar review of exposure and control measures. Follow up of existing cases after cessation of exposure should continue until they are free of symptoms. A more recent recommendation from the Health and Safety Executive (HSE) in the United Kingdom is to prevent HAVS stage 3 developing, as this represents a more severe form of disease with associated loss of function and disability.[22] The National Institute of Occupational Safety and Health recommends the removal from exposure at neurosensory or vascular Stockholm stage 2 or above.[19] Stage 2, however, ranges from minimal neurosensory symptoms, through to imminent functional disability. Lawson and McGeoch divided stage 2 into an early and late stage.[6] The progression to late stage 2 then becomes a stronger criterion for recommending cessation of exposure. The ultimate decision for removing an employee from exposure is between the employer and the employee. The employer's duty of care needs to be offset by the rights of the employee to have an informed acceptance of risk. The tipping point in favour of the employer's duty of care to accept a recommendation of removal from exposure is at late stage 2. Terms 'intermittent', 'persistent' and 'constant' have been suggested as a way of separating '2 early' from '2 late' in a sceening environment.[22] The HSE subsequently went on to recommend that an employee will only be declared unfit when the disease has reached 'a late stage 2'. They qualify this for older employees, closer to retirement, who fully understand the ongoing risks. They may continue work with limited exposure and regular surveillance.

In many respects, the ideal management of someone affected by HAVS is to remove them from vibration exposure altogether. Continuing exposure is a compromise between the ideal and the practical. Medically, however, it makes little sense to continue to expose someone to a physical agent which has already caused harm. From follow-up studies, once established sensorineural-only HAVS shows no sign of reversibility or regression, so preventive measures should be the main focus.

Treatment of the individual with HAVS

There is no active drug treatment for the neurological symptoms. The treatment of the vascular phenomena is the same as the treatment of Raynaud's disease. In general, measures are aimed at the prevention of the signs and symptoms. The worker should specifically keep the hands warm, as well as the body. Simply wearing gloves is not enough if the body is cold. Working in a warm environment is the ideal, but often not feasible. Drug treatment is often of little benefit and the side effects of medication usually preclude its use. Alpha-adrenergic blockers will cause vasodilatation, but are associated with tachycardia, hypotension and a stuffy nose.

Calcium-channel blockers, such as nifedipine, may be used with some success, but the beneficial effects are often not sustained in the long term with side effects such as hypotension, tachycardia and flushing.

Other agents, such as endothelin receptor antagonists, have been tried in the management of severe Raynaud's phenomenon (for example, systemic sclerosis). These have no part in the management of Raynaud's phenomenon in the vibration exposed. Similarly, interventions, such as cervicodorsal sympathectomy, are not indicated.

Key points

- The diagnosis of the vascular component of hand–arm vibration syndrome, a secondary Raynaud's phenomenon, relies on a description of diffuse, circumferential, well-defined finger blanching that occurs in response to cold. Cold-water provocation testing does not assist either diagnosis or staging severity.
- The diagnosis of the sensorineural component of HAVS relies on the presence of appropriate peripheral symptoms. Selective psychophysical tests can assist in staging severity.
- Identification of nocturnal paraesthesia (not involving the little finger) facilitates the diagnosis of carpal tunnel syndrome from the sensorineural component of HAVS.
- There is no association between the development of Dupuytren's disease and exposure to the use of vibrating tools.
- In managing an individual case, advice on continuing exposure to hand–arm vibration should aim to avoid anyone progressing past late stage 2.

REFERENCES

1. Gemne G, Taylor W. Foreward: Hand–arm vibration and the central autonomic nervous system. In: Gemne G, Taylor W (eds). Special Volume. *Journal of Low Frequency Noise, Vibration and Active Control.* 1983; **11**.
2. Hamilton A. Chapter XII, Dead fingers. In: *Exploring the dangerous trades. The Autobiography of Alice Hamilton, M.D.* Beverley Farms, MA: OEM Press, 1995: 200–7.
3. Seyring M. Maladies from work with compressed air drills. *Bulletin of Hygiene.* 1931; **6**: 25.
4. Brammer AJ, Taylor W, Lundborg G. Sensorineural stages of the hand–arm vibration syndrome. *Scandinavian Journal of Work and Environmental Health.* 1987; **13**: 279–83.
5. Gemne G, Pyykkö I, Taylor W, Pelmear PL. The Stockholm Workshop scale for the classification of cold-induced Raynaud's phenomenon in the hand–arm vibration syndrome (revision of the Taylor Pelmear scale). *Scandinavian Journal of Work and Environmental Health.* 1987; **13**: 275–8.
6. Lawson IJ, McGeoch KL. HAVS assessment process for a large volume of medico-legal compensation cases. *Occupational Medicine.* 2003; **53**: 302–8.
7. Gemne G, Brammer AJ, Hagberg M *et al.* (eds). Proceedings of the Stockholm Workshop 94. Hand–arm vibration syndrome: Diagnostics and quantitative relationships to exposure. Goteborg: Arbete och Hälsa, 1995: 5.
8. Gemne G (ed.). Report from a panel discussion on the clinical management of suspected cases of hand–arm vibration syndrome (HAVS). 9th International Conference on Hand-Arm Vibration, Nancy, France, June 5–8, 2001, 90–106.
9. Mason H, Poole K. *Clinical testing and management of individuals exposed to hand-transmitted vibration: An evidence review.* London: Faculty of Occupational Medicine of the Royal College of Physicians, 2004: 1–206.
10. Health and Safety Executive. Regulatory impact assessment of the draft Control of Vibration at Work Regulations 2005 as they relate to hand–arm vibration. Sudbury: HSE Books, 2004.
11. Bovenzi M, Peretti A, Nataletti P, Moschioni G (eds). Workshop: Application of 2002/44/EC Directive in Europe. Proceedings of the 11th International Conference on Hand-Arm Vibration, Bologna, Italy 2007.
12. Griffin MJ. *Handbook of human vibration.* London: Academic Press, 1990.
13. Palmer KT, Griffin MJ, Syddall H *et al.* Risk of hand–arm vibration syndrome according to occupational and sources of exposure to hand-transmitted vibration: A national survey. *American Journal of Industrial Medicine.* 2001; **39**: 389–96.
14. Palmer KT, Coggon DN, Bednell HE *et al.* Hand-transmitted vibration: Occupational exposures and their health effects in Great Britain. Health and Safety Executive contract report 232/1999.

15. Phillips IJ, Heyns S, Nelson G. Hand-arm vibration syndrome in the South African mining industry. In: Bovenzi M, Peretti A, Nataletti P, Moschioni G (eds). Proceedings of the 11th International Conference on Hand-Arm Vibration, Bologna, Italy, 2007.
16. International Organization for Standardization. ISO 5349-1. Mechanical vibration – Measurement and evaluation of human exposure to hand-transmitted vibration. Part 1: General requirements. Geneva: ISO, 2001.
17. Council Directive 2002/44/EC of 6 July 2002 on the minimum health and safety requirements regarding the risks arising from physical agents (vibration). Last accessed September 2009. Available from: http://eur-lex.europa.eu/LexUriServ/LexUriServ.do?uri=OJ:L:2002:177:0013:0019:EN:PDF.
18. Miwa T. Evaluation methods for vibration effects. Part 4: Measurement of vibration greatness for whole body and hand in vertical and horizontal vibration. *Health*. 1968; **6**: 1–10.
19. National Institute for Occupational Safety and Health. Criteria for a recommended standard. Occupational exposure to hand-arm vibration. Cincinnati, OH: NIOSH, 1989.
20. Burström L, Hagberg M, Lundström R, Nilsson T. Relationship between hand-arm vibration exposure and onset time for symptoms in a heavy engineering production workshop. *Scandinavian Journal of Work and Environmental Health*. 2006; **32**: 198–203.
21. Health and Safety Executive. Hand-arm vibration, HS(G)88. Bootle: HSE, 1994.
22. Hand-arm vibration. The control of vibration at work regulations 2005. Guidance on regulations, L140. Bootle: HSE, 2005.
23. Cherniack M, Brammer AJ, Lundstrom R et al. Prospective studies of vibration exposed cohorts: Hand-Arm Vibration International Consortium (HAVIC). Proceedings of the First American Conference in Human Vibration, June 2006. Cincinnati, OH: NIOSH.
24. Guyton A, Hall J. *Textbook of medical physiology*, 11th edn. Philadelphia: Elsevier Saunders, 2006: 1–1067.
25. Charkoudian N. Skin blood flow in adult human thermoregulation: How it works, when it does not, and why. *Mayo Clinic Proceedings*. 2003; **78**: 603–12.
26. Takahashi S, Iwamoto M, Yoshimura M et al. Factors influencing autonomic nervous function during cold-water immersion test in patients with hand-arm vibration syndrome. *International Archives of Occupational and Environmental Health*. 2003; **76**: 249–52.
27. Lundborg G. *Nerve injury and repair. Regeneration, reconstruction and cortical remodeling*, 2nd edn. Philadelphia: Elsevier Churchill Livingstone, 2004: 1–248.
28. Takeuchi T, Futatsuka M, Imanishi H, Yamada S. Pathological changes observed in the finger biopsy of patients with vibration-induced white finger. *Scandinavian Journal of Work and Environmental Health*. 1986; **12**: 280–3.
29. Takeuchi T, Takeya M, Imanishi H. Ultrastructural changes in peripheral nerves of the fingers of three vibration-exposed persons with Raynaud's phenomenon. *Scandinavian Journal of Work and Environmental Health*. 1988; **14**: 31–5.
30. Liang HW, Hsieh ST, Cheng TJ et al. Reduced epidermal nerve density among hand-transmitted vibration-exposed workers. *Journal of Occupational and Environmental Medicine*. 2006; **48**: 549–55.
31. Lundborg G, Rosen B, Knutsson L et al. Hand-arm vibration syndrome (HAVS): Is there a central nervous component? An fMRI study. *Journal of Hand Surgery*. 2002; **27**: 514–19.
32. Curry BD, Bain JL, Yan JG et al. Vibration injury damages arterial endothelial cells. *Muscle and Nerve*. 2002; **25**: 527–34.
33. Lundborg G, Dahlin LB, Danielsen N et al. Intraneural edema following exposure to vibration. *Scandinavian Journal of Work and Environmental Health*. 1987; **13**: 326–9.
34. Chang KY, Ho ST, Yu HS. Vibration induced neurophysiological and electron microscopical changes in rat peripheral nerves. *Occupational and Environmental Medicine*. 1994; **51**: 130–5.
35. Matloub HS, Yan JG, Kolachalam RB et al. Neuropathological changes in vibration injury: An experimental study. *Microsurgery*. 2005; **25**: 71–5.
36. Govindaraju SR, Curry BD, Bain JL, Riley DA. Comparison of continuous and intermittent vibration effects on rat-tail artery and nerve. *Muscle and Nerve*. 2006; **34**: 197–204.
37. Yan JG, Matloub HS, Sanger JR et al. Vibration-induced disruption of retrograde axoplasmic transport in peripheral nerve. *Muscle and Nerve*. 2005; **32**: 521–6.
38. Govindaraju SR, Curry BD, Bain JL, Riley DA. Effects of temperature on vibration-induced damage in nerves and arteries. *Muscle and Nerve*. 2006; **33**: 415–23.
39. Herrick AL. Pathogenesis of Raynaud's phenomenon. *Rheumatology*. 2005; **44**: 587–96.
40. Turton EP, Kent PJ, Kester RC. The aetiology of Raynaud's phenomenon. *Cardiovascular Surgery*. 1998; **6**: 431–40.
41. Stoyneva Z, Lyapina M, Tzvetkov D, Vodenicharov E. Current pathophysiological views on vibration-induced Raynaud's phenomenon. *Cardiovascular Research*. 2003; **57**: 615–24.
42. Chung MS, Gong HS, Baek GH. Prevalence of Raynaud's phenomenon in patients with idiopathic carpal tunnel syndrome. *Journal of Bone and Joint Surgery. British volume*. 1999; **81**: 1017–19.
43. Krajnak K, Dong RG, Flavahan S et al. Acute vibration increases alpha2C-adrenergic smooth muscle constriction and alters thermosensitivity of cutaneous arteries. *Journal of Applied Physiology*. 2006; **100**: 1230–7.
44. Krajnak K, Waugh S, Wirth O, Kashon ML. Acute vibration reduces A-beta nerve fiber sensitivity and alters gene expression in the ventral tail nerves of rats. *Muscle and Nerve*. 2007; **36**: 197–205.
45. Nakamura H, Matsuzaki I, Hatta K et al. Blood endothelin-1 and cold-induced vasodilation in patients with primary Raynauld's phenomenon and workers with vibration-induced white finger. *International Angiology*. 2003; **22**: 243–9.

46. Palmer KT, Mason H. Serum endothelin concentrations in workers exposed to vibration. *Occupational and Environmental Medicine*. 1996; **53**: 118–24.
47. Dowd PM, Goldsmith PC, Chopra S et al. Cutaneous responses to endothelin-1 and histamine in patients with vibration white finger. *Journal of Investigational Dermatology*. 1998; **110**: 127–31.
48. Goldsmith PC, Molina FA, Bunker CB et al. Cutaneous nerve fibre depletion in vibration white finger. *Journal of the Royal Society of Medicine*. 1994; **87**: 377–81.
49. Lander L, Lou W, House R. Nerve conduction studies and current perception thresholds in workers assessed for hand-arm vibration syndrome. *Occupational Medicine*. 2007; **57**: 284–9.
50. Hirata M, Sakakibara H. Sensory nerve conduction velocities of median, ulnar and radial nerves in patients with vibration syndrome. *International Archives of Occupational and Environmental Health*. 2007; **80**: 273–80.
51. Strömberg T, Dahlin LB, Brun A, Lundborg G. Structural nerve changes at wrist level in workers exposed to vibration. *Occupational and Environmental Medicine*. 1997; **54**: 307–11.
52. Armstrong TJ, Castelli WA, Evans FG, Diaz-Perez R. Some histological changes in carpal tunnel contents and their biomechanical implications. *Occupational Medicine*. 1984; **26**: 197–201.
53. Palmer KT, Harris EC, Coggon D. Carpal tunnel syndrome and its relation to occupation: A systematic literature review. *Occupational Medicine*. 2007; **57**: 57–66.
54. Shaw RB Jr, Chong AK, Zhang A et al. Dupuytren's disease: History, diagnosis, and treatment. *Plastic and Reconstructive Surgery*. 2007; **120**: 44e–54e.
55. Liss GM, Stock SR. Can Dupuytren's contracture be work-related? Review of the evidence. *American Journal of Industrial Medicine*. 1996; **29**: 521.
56. Burke FD, Proud G, Lawson IJ et al. An assessment of the effects to vibration, smoking, alcohol and diabetes on the prevalence of Dupuytren's disease in 97,537 miners. *Journal of Hand Surgery*. 2007; **32E**: 400–6.
57. Hart MG, Hooper G. Clinical associations of Dupuytren's disease. *Postgraduate Medical Journal*. 2005; **81**: 425–8.
58. Farkkila M, Aatola S, Starck J et al. Hand-grip force in lumberjacks: Two-year follow-up. *International Archives of Occupational and Environmental Health*. 1986; **58**: 203–8.
59. Necking LE, Friden J, Lundborg G. Reduced muscle strength in abduction of the index finger: An important clinical sign in hand-arm vibration syndrome. *Scandinavian Journal of Plastic and Reconstructive Surgery and Hand Surgery*. 2003; **37**: 365–70.
60. Necking LE, Lundstrom R, Lundborg G et al. Skeletal muscle changes after short term vibration. *Scandinavian Journal of Plastic and Reconstructive Surgery and Hand Surgery*. 1996; **30**: 99–103.
61. Pelmear PL, Wong L, Dembek B. Laboratory tests for the evaluation of hand-arm vibration syndrome. Proceedings of 6th International Conference on Hand-Arm Vibration, Bonn, 1992: 817–26.
62. Bell JA. Sensibility evaluation. In: Hunter JM, Schneider LH, Macken EJ, Callahan AD (eds). *Rehabilitation of the hand*. St Louis: Mosby, 1978: 399–406.
63. Mountcastle VB. Central nervous mechanisms in mechanoreceptive disorders. *American Physiological Society*. 1984; **1**: 789–878.
64. Harada N, Griffin MJ. Factors influencing vibration thresholds used to assess occupational exposures to hand transmitted vibration. *British Journal of Industrial Medicine*. 1991; **48**: 185–92.
65. Hayward R, Griffin MJ. Measures of vibrotactile sensitivity in persons exposed to hand transmitted vibration. *Scandinavian Journal of Environmental Health*. 1986; **12**: 423–7.
66. Ekenvall L, Nilsson BY, Gustavson P. Temperature and vibration thresholds in vibration syndrome. *British Journal of Industrial Medicine*. 1986; **43**: 825–9.
67. Lawson IJ. Review of objective tests for hand-arm vibration syndrome. *Occupational Medicine*. 1997; **1**: 15–20.
68. McGeoch KL, Gilmour WH. Cross sectional study of a workforce exposed to hand-arm vibration with objective tests and the Stockholm workshop scales. *Occupational and Environmental Medicine*. 2000; **1**: 35–42.
69. McGeoch KL, Lawson IJ, Burke F et al. Use of sensorineural tests in a large volume of medico-legal compensation claims for HAVS. *Occupational and Environmental Medicine*. 2004; **54**: 528–34.
70. Swerup C, Nilsson BY. Dependence of thermal thresholds in man on the rate of temperature change. *Acta Physiologica Scandinavica*. 1987; **131**: 623–4.
71. Reddon JR, Gill DM, Gauk SE, Maer MD. Purdue pegboard: Test-retest estimates. *Perceptual and Motor Skills*. 1988; **66**: 503–6.
72. Tiffin J, Asher EJ. The Purdue pegboard norms and studies of reliability and validity. *Journal of Applied Psychology*. 1948; **32**: 234–47.
73. Eliasson K, Lins LE, Sundqvist K. Vaso-spastic phenomena in patients treated with beta-adrenoceptor blocking agents. *Acta Medica Scandinavica*. 1979; **628**: 39–46.
74. Marshall AJ, Roberts CJC, Barritt DW. Raynaud's phenomenon as side effect of beta-blockers in hypertensions. *British Medical Journal*. 1976; **1**: 1498–9.
75. Welsh CL. In: Proud G, Hodgson C, Lees T (eds). *Hand-arm vibration syndrome*. HHSC Handbook 24. Leeds: H and H Scientific, 1999: 18–33.
76. Griffin MJ, Lindsell CJ. Cold provocation test for the diagnosis of vibration induced white finger: Standardisation and repeatability. Institute of Sound and Vibration Research Contract Research Report (for Health and Safety Executive). 1998; **173**: 1–44.
77. Proud G, Burke F, Lawson IJ et al. Cold provocation testing and hand-arm vibration syndrome – an audit of the results of the Department of Trade and Industry scheme for the evaluation of miners. *British Journal of Surgery*. 2003; **90**: 1076–9.
78. Mason H, Poole K, Saxton J. A critique of a UK standardised test of finger re-warming after cold provocation in the

diagnosis and staging of hand–arm vibration syndrome. *Occupational Medicine*. 2003; **53**: 325–30.
79. Bovenzi M. Finger systoloic blood pressure indices for the diagnosis of vibration-induced white finger. *International Archives of Occupational and Environmental Health*. 2002; **75**: 20–8.
80. Lindsell CJ, Griffin MJ. Thermal thresholds, vibrotactile thresholds and finger systolic blood pressures in dockyard workers exposed to hand-transmitted vibration. *International Archives of Occupational and Environmental Health*. 1999; **72**: 377–86.
81. Coughlin PA, Chetter IC, Kent PJ, Kester RC. The analysis of sensitivity, specificity, positive predictive value and negative predictive value of cold provocation thermography in the objective diagnosis of the hand–arm vibration syndrome. *Occupational Medicine*. 2001; **51**: 75–80.
82. De-Krom MC, Knipschild PG, Kester AD et al. Carpal tunnel syndrome prevalence in the general population. *Journal of Clinical Epidemiology*. 1992; **45**: 373–6.
83. Ferry S, Prichard T, Keenan J et al. Estimating the prevalence of delayed median nerve conduction in the general population. *British Journal of Rheumatology*. 1998; **37**: 630–5.
84. Eversman WW. Reduction of cumulative trauma disorders by a comprehensive ergonomic programme in a major commercial bakery. *American Society for Surgery of the Hand, News*. 1990; **9**: 1–8.
85. Totten PA, Hunter JM. Therapeutic techniques to enhance nerve gliding in thoracic outlet syndrome and carpal tunnel syndrome. *Hand Clinics*. 1991; **3**: 505–20.
86. Rozmaryn LM, Dovelle S, Rothman ER et al. Nerve and tendons gliding exercises and the conservative management of carpal tunnel syndrome. *Journal of Hand Therapy*. 1998; **11**: 171–9.
87. Gelberman RG, Hergenroeder PT, Hargens AR et al. The carpal tunnel syndrome. A study of carpal canal pressures. *Journal of Bone and Joint Surgery*. 1981; **63A**: 380–3.
88. Harrington JM, Carter JT, Birrell L, Gompertz D. Surveillance case definitions for work related upper limb pain syndromes. *Occupational and Environmental Medicine*. 1998; **55**: 264–71.
89. Chatterjee DS, Barwick DD, Petrie A. Exploratory electromyography in the study of vibration induced white finger in rock drillers. *British Journal of Industrial Medicine*. 1982; **39**: 89–97.
90. Lukas E. Peripheral nervous system and hand-arm vibration exposure. In: Brammer AJ, Taylor W (eds). *Vibration effects on the hand and arm in industry*. New York: John Wiley, 1982: 29–43.
91. Boyle JC, Smith MJ, Burke FD. Vibration white finger. *Journal of Hand Surgery*. 1988; **13B**: 171–5.
92. Farkkila M, Pyykkö I, Janhi V et al. Forestry workers exposed to vibration: A neurological study. *British Journal of Industrial Medicine*. 1988; **45**: 188–92.
93. Koskimies K, Farkkila M, Pykkö I et al. Carpal tunnel syndrome in vibration disease. *British Journal of Industrial Medicine*. 1990; **47**: 411–16.
94. Bovenzi M, Zadini A, Franzinelli A, Borgogni F. Occupational musculoskeletal disorders in the neck and upper limbs of forestry workers exposed to vibration. *Ergonomics*. 1991; **34**: 547–62.
95. Stromberg T, Dahlin LB, Lundborg G. Hand problems in 100 vibration-exposed symptomatic male workers. *Journal of Hand Surgery*. 1996; **21B**: 315–19.
96. Industrial Injuries Advisory Council. Work-related upper limb disorders. Report by the Industrial Injuries Advisory Council, DSS Cm 1936. London: HMSO, 1992.
97. Silverstein BA, Fine LJ, Armstrong TJ. Occupational factors and carpal tunnel syndrome. *American Journal of Industrial Medicine*. 1987; **11**: 343–58.
98. Lundborg G, Dahlin LB, Danielsen N et al. Intraneural oedema following exposure to vibration. *Scandinavian Journal of Work, Environment and Health*. 1987; **13**: 326–9.
99. Stromberg T, Dahlin LB, Lundborg G. Structural nerve changes at the wrist level in workers exposed to vibration. *Occupational and Environmental Medicine*. 1997; **54**: 307–11.
100. Szabo RM, Slater RR Jr, Fraver TB et al. The value of diagnostic testing in carpal tunnel syndrome. *Journal of Hand Surgery*. 1999; **24**: 704–14.
101. Stromberg T, Dahlin LB, Rosen I, Lundborg G. Neurophysiological findings in vibration exposed male workers. *Journal of Hand Surgery*. 1999; **24B**: 203–9.
102. Burke FD, Lawson IJ, McGeoch KL et al. Carpal tunnel syndrome in association with hand–arm vibration syndrome: A review of claimants seeking compensation in the mining industry. *Journal of Hand Surgery*. 2005; **30B**: 199–203.
103. Burke FD, Dias JJ, Webster H. Median nerve compression syndrome at the wrist. In: Hunter J, Schneider LH, Makin EJ (eds). *Tendon and nerve surgery in the hand – a third decade*. St Louis: Mosby, 1997: 145–8.
104. Savage R, Burke FD, Smith NJ, Hopper I. Carpal tunnel syndrome in association with vibration white finger. *Journal of Hand Surgery*. 1990; **15B**: 100–3.
105. Hagberg M, Nystrom A, Zetterland B. Recovery from symptoms after carpal tunnel syndrome surgery in males in relation to vibration exposure. *Journal of Hand Surgery*. 1991; **16A**: 66–71.
106. Lozano Calderon S, Anthony S, Ring D. The quality and strength of evidence for etiology: Example of carpal tunnel syndrome. *Journal of Hand Surgery*. 2008; **33A**: 525–38.
107. Gudmundsson KG, Arngrimsson R, Sigfusson N et al. Epidemiology of Dupuytren's disease. *Journal of Clinical Epidemiology*. 2000; **53**: 291–6.
108. Hueston JT. The incidence of Dupuytren's contracture. *Medical Journal of Australia*. 1960; **2**: 999–1002.
109. Leclercq C. Associated conditions in Dupuytren's disease. In: Tubiana R, Leclercq C, Hurst LC et al. (eds). *Dupuytren's disease*. London: Martin Dunitz, 2000: 108.
110. Su CK, Patek AJ. Dupuytren's contracture: Its association with alcoholism and cirrhosis. *Archives of Internal Medicine*. 1970; **126**: 278–81.
111. An HS, Southworth SR, Jackson WT, Russ B. Cigarette smoking and Dupuytren's contracture of the hand. *Journal of Hand Surgery*. 1988; **13A**: 872–974.

112. Dupuytren M le Baron. Leçon Oraies de Clinique chirurgicale faites ál'Hôtel Dieu de Paris. Paris: Germer Baillière, 1832.
113. Hueston JT. *Dupuytren's contracture*. Edinburgh: E&S Livingstone, 1963.
114. Mikkelsen OA. Dupuytren's disease: The influence of occupation and previous hand injuries. *Hand*. 1978; **10**: 1-8.
115. Khan AA, Rider OJ, Jayadev CU et al. The role of manual occupation in the aetiology of Dupuytren's disease in men in England and Wales. *Journal of Hand Surgery*. 2004; **29B**: 12-14.
116. Ross DC. Epidemiology of Dupuytren's disease. *Hand Clinics*. 1999; **15**: 53-62.
117. Stewart HD, Innes AR, Burke FD. Hand complications of Colles fracture. *Journal of Hand Surgery*. 1985; **10B**: 103-7.
118. Cocco PL, Frau P, Rapello M, Casula D. Occupational exposure to vibration and Dupuytren's disease: A case controlled study. *La Medicina del Lavaro*. 1987; **78**: 386-92.
119. Bovenzi M, Cerri S, Merseberger A et al. Hand-arm vibration syndrome and dose response relation for vibration induced white finger amongst quarry drillers and stone carvers. *Occupational and Environmental Medicine*. 1994; **51**: 603-11.
120. Thomas PR, Clarke D. Vibration white finger and Dupuytren's contracture: Are they related? *Journal of the Society of Occupational Medicine*. 1992; **42**: 155-8.
121. Gerhardsson L, Balogh I, Hambert PA et al. Vascular and nerve damage in workers exposed to vibrating tools. The importance of objective measurements of exposure time. *Applied Ergonomics*. 2005; **36**: 55-60.
122. Mathiowetz V, Kashman N, Volland G et al. Grip and pinch strength: Normative data for adults. *Archives of Physical Medicine and Rehabilitation*. 1985; **66**: 69-74.
123. Hanten WP, Chen WY, Austin AA et al. Maximum grip strength in normal subjects from 20-64 years of age. *Journal of Hand Therapy*. 1999; **12**: 193-200.
124. Gilbertson L, Barber-Lomax S. Power and pinch grip strength recorded using the hand held Jamar dynamometer and the B&L hydraulic pinch gauge. British normative data for adults. *British Journal of Occupational Therapy*. 1994; **57**: 483-8.
125. Bohannon RW. Grip strength: A summary of studies comparing dominant and non-dominant limb measurements. *Perceptual and Motor Skills*. 2003; **96**: 728-30.
126. Farkkila MA, Pyykkö I, Starck JP, Korhonen OS. Hand grip force and muscle fatigue in the aetiology of vibration syndrome. In: Bramer AJ, Taylor W (eds). *Vibration effects on the hand arm in industry*. London: John Wiley, 1983: 45-50.
127. Mirbod SM, Akbar-Khanzadeh F, Onozuka M et al. A four year follow-up study on subjective symptoms and functional capacities in workers using hand held grinders. *Industrial Health*. 1999; **37**: 415-25.
128. Sorensson A, Burstrom L. Transmission of vibration energy to different parts of the human hand-arm system. *International Archives of Occupational and Environmental Health*. 1977; **70**: 199-204.
129. Necking LE, Lundborg G, Friden J. Hand muscle weakness in long term vibration exposure. *Journal of Hand Surgery*. 2002; **27B**: 520-5.
130. Kozin SH, Porter S, Clark P, Thoder JJ. The contribution of intrinsic muscles to grip and pinch strength. *Journal of Hand Surgery*. 1999; **24A**: 64-72.
131. Stromberg T, Dahlin LB, Brun A, Lundborg G. Structural nerve changes at wrist level in workers exposed to vibration. *Occupational and Environmental Medicine*. 1997; **54**: 307-11.
132. Necking LE, Lundstrom R, Lundborg G et al. Hand muscle pathology after long term vibration exposure. *Journal of Hand Surgery*. 2004; **29B**: 431-7.
133. Lawson IJ, Burke FD, Proud G et al. Grip strength in miners with hand-arm vibration syndrome. Paper presented at Diagnosis of injuries caused by hand-transmitted vibration – 2nd International Workshop, Göteborg, Sweden, September 2006.
134. Gemne G, Saraste H. Bone and joint pathology in workers using hand-held vibratory tools: An overview. *Scandinavian Journal of Work and Environmental Health*. 1987; **13**: 290-300.
135. Griffin MJ, Bovenzi M. The diagnosis of disorders caused by hand-transmitted vibration: Southampton Workshop 2000. *International Archives of Occupational and Environmental Health*. 2002; **75**: 1-5.
136. Bovenzi, Griffin MJ, Hagberg M. New understanding of the diagnosis of injuries caused by hand-transmitted vibration. *International Archives of Environmental Health*. 2008; **81**: 505.
137. Pelmear PL, Wasserman DE. *Hand-arm vibration. A comprehensive guide for occupational health professionals*, 2nd edn. Beverly Farms: OEM Press, 1998.
138. O'Keeffe ST, Tsapatsaris NP, Beetham WP Jr. Color chart assisted diagnosis of Raynaud's phenomenon in an unselected hospital employee population. *Journal of Rheumatology*. 1992; **19**: 1415-17.
139. Asbury A. Approach to the patient with peripheral neuropathy. In: Kasper DL, Braunwald E, Hauser S et al. (eds). *Harrison's Principles of internal medicine*. New York: McGraw-Hill, 2005: 2500-10.
140. Willison HJ, Winer JB. Clinical evaluation and investigation of neuropathy. *Journal of Neurology, Neurosurgery, and Psychiatry*. 2003; **74** (Suppl. 2): 113-18.
141. Block JA, Sequerira W. Raynaud's phenomenon. *Lancet*. 2001; **357**: 2042-8.
142. McRae R. *Clinical orthopedic examination*, 5th edn. London: Churchill Livingston, 2004.
143. Leffler AS, Hansson P, Kosek E. Somatosensory perception in patients suffering from long-term trapezius myalgia at the site overlying the most painful part of the muscle and in an area of pain referral. *European Journal of Pain*. 2003; **7**: 267-76.
144. Nilsson T. Neurological diagnosis: Aspects of bedside and electrocardiagnostic examinations in relation to hand-arm vibration syndrome. *International Archives of Occupational and Environmental Health*. 2002; **75**: 55-67.

145. Lauria G, Lombardi R. Skin biopsy: A new tool for diagnosing peripheral neuropathy. *British Medical Journal.* 2007; **334**: 1159-62.
146. Lawson IJ, McGeoch KL. How likely is it that Stockholm stage 1 of the hand arm vibration syndrome will progress to stages 2 and 3? *Occupational Medicine.* 1999; **49**: 401-2.
147. Lawson IJ. Vibration. In: Sadhra SS, Rampal KK (eds). *Occupational health risk assessment and management.* Oxford: Blackwell Science, 1999: 379-89.
148. Ogasawara C, Sakakibara H. Longitudinal study on factors related to the course of vibration-induced white finger. *International Archives of Occupational and Environmental Health.* 1997; **69**: 180-4.
149. Cherniack M, Clive J, Seidner A. Vibration exposure, smoking, and vascular dysfunction. *Occupational and Environmental Medicine.* 2000; **57**: 341-7.
150. Petersen R, Andersen M, Mikkelsen S *et al.* Prognosis of vibration induced white finger: A follow up study. *Occupational and Environmental Medicine.* 1995; **52**: 110-15.
151. Faculty of Occupational Medicine of the Royal College of Physicians. Hand transmitted vibration: Clinical effects and pathophysiology. London: Royal College of Physicians, 1993.

48

Whole body vibration

MASSIMO BOVENZI AND KEITH PALMER

Introduction	513	Factors affecting exposures and control measures	519
Common sources of exposure	514	Health surveillance	520
Health effects	514	References	520
Control standards	519		

INTRODUCTION

The nature of whole body vibration and its assessment

Mechanical vibration arises from a wide variety of processes and operations performed in manufacturing industry, mining, construction, transport and haulage, forestry and agriculture, and the public utilities. Whole body vibration (WBV) occurs when the human body is supported on a surface that is vibrating.

Vibration is an oscillatory motion characterized in terms of the frequency of the oscillatory cycle, its magnitude and its direction.[1] The magnitude of vibration can be quantified by its displacement (m), its velocity (ms^{-1}) or its acceleration (ms^{-2}). However, it is usually expressed in terms of an average measure of the motion's acceleration (to give the root mean square (rms) value in ms^{-2} rms) so that a complex time-varying pattern is not unduly influenced by a few unrepresentative peaks. The rms magnitude can be related to the energy imparted and hence to the injury potential.

The frequency of vibration is expressed in cycles per second (Hertz, (Hz)). Biodynamic investigations have shown that the response of the human body to vibration is frequency dependent.[1] The adverse health effects of WBV seem to be related mainly to exposures in the low frequency range (from 0.5 to 80 Hz), although frequencies below 0.5 Hz can cause motion sickness. Thus, to account for differences of response, current standards for exposure evaluation recommend weighting the frequencies of measured vibration according to the assumed deleterious effects of each frequency.[2,3] Frequency weightings are applied to measurements taken in three orthogonal directions (x-, y- and z-axes) at the interfaces between the body and the vibration.

The evaluation of exposure is based on the vibration total value (a_v),[2] a quantity defined as the square root of the sum of the squares of the frequency-weighted acceleration values (a_w) determined on the three orthogonal axes x, y, z. For a seated or standing worker, the a_v for whole body vibration is calculated as $a_v = (k_x^2 a_{wx}^2 + k_y^2 a_{wy}^2 + k_z^2 a_{wz}^2)^{1/2}$, where $k = 1.4$ for x- and y-axes and $k = 1$ for z-axis.

The health effects of WBV may also be influenced by shocks or vibration peaks. To allow for this, international standard ISO 2631-1 recommends the fourth power vibration dose as the basis for averaging, rather than the second power of the acceleration time history (i.e. rms).[2] The fourth power vibration dose value (VDV) is expressed in the unusual units of metres per second to the power of 1.75 (i.e. ms$^{-1.75}$).

According to European Directive 2002/44/EC,[4] the assessment of exposure to WBV 'is based on the calculation of daily exposure $A(8)$ expressed as continuous equivalent acceleration over an eight-hour period, calculated as the highest (rms) value, or the highest vibration dose value (VDV) of the frequency-weighted accelerations, determined on three orthogonal axes (1.4a_{wx}, 1.4a_{wy}, a_{wz})' in accordance with the international standard ISO 2631-1.[2]

EU Directive 2002/44/EC establishes daily exposure action values and daily exposure limit values for WBV, above which administrative, technical and medical measures have to be implemented (as described below).

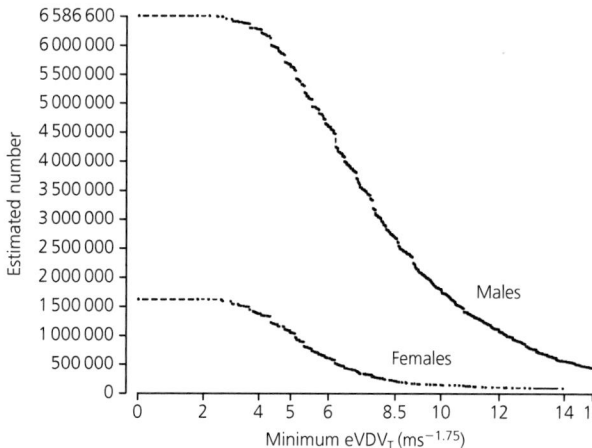

Figure 48.1 Minimum estimated numbers of men and women in Great Britain whose daily equivalent estimated vibration dose (eVDV) from all occupational sources in the past week exceeded the values indicated. Reproduced with permission from BMJ Publishing Group.[5]

COMMON SOURCES OF EXPOSURE

Exposure to WBV arises in workers who operate tractors, excavators, bulldozers, forklift trucks, armoured vehicles, buses, lorries and many other vehicles and machines.

Such exposures are common in the working population. Palmer et al.[5] conducted a national survey of exposures in the United Kingdom in 1998 and estimated that 7.2 million men and 1.8 million women were exposed to WBV at work in a one-week period. The most common sources of occupational exposure to WBV as estimated by the survey were cars, vans, forklift trucks, lorries, tractors, buses and loaders. In another large UK community survey, 7 per cent of respondents reported having been drivers of trucks, tractors, diggers and other industrial vehicles;[6] while in a third UK survey of self-reported working conditions in 1995, 12 per cent of men (95 per cent CI, 9–14) and 1 per cent of women (95 per cent CI, 0.5–2) reported their job sometimes involving sitting or standing on a vibrating machine or vehicle, the exposure prevalence being highest in farming, fishing and forestry, and in road transport.[7] A recent European survey on working conditions from the same period estimated that 24 per cent of respondents were exposed to mechanical vibration for at least a quarter of the time in EU workplaces, with craft workers, machine operators, agricultural workers and members of the armed forces having notable exposures to WBV.[8] Elsewhere, it has been estimated that 4–7 per cent of all employees in the United States, Canada and some European countries are exposed to potentially harmful WBV.[9]

Vibration doses arising from such sources vary, depending not only on the driving time but also on factors intrinsic to the vehicle (e.g. wear, tear, design of vehicle, seating and suspension) and specific to the driving situation (e.g. road surface and road speed). In the British National Survey of Vibration,[5] a population-based investigation, the estimated VDV exceeded a proposed British Standard action level of 15 ms$^{-1.75}$ in more than 374 000 men and 9000 women (Figure 48.1). Occupations in which the estimated exposures most often exceeded 15 ms$^{-1.75}$ included forklift truck and mechanical truck drivers, farm owners and managers, farm workers and drivers of road goods vehicles (Figure 48.2). The highest estimated median occupational eVDVs were found in forklift truck drivers, drivers of road goods vehicles, bus and coach drivers, and technical and wholesale sales representatives, among whom a greater contribution to total dose was received from occupational exposures than from non-occupational ones; but in many other occupations the reverse applied. Leisure time and commuting exposures are also very common.

Other measurements of vibration magnitude (vibration total value (or vector sum) of the frequency-weighted rms accelerations) have been made in industrial surveys covering specific vehicles, with reported values varying from 0.25 to 0.67 ms^{-2} in cranes, 0.36 to 0.56 ms^{-2} in buses, 0.35 to 1.45 ms^{-2} in tractors, and 0.79 to 1.04 ms^{-2} in forklift trucks and freight-container tractors.[10]

HEALTH EFFECTS

The best-recognized health effect of WBV relates to the outcome of low-back pain (LBP).[11–41] LBP is a symptom rather than a diagnosis, and consequently case definitions of outcome in research studies have varied in relation to anatomical distribution symptoms and in relation to their frequency, intensity and impact in terms of disability, medical consultation and sickness absence. Other common research end points have included radiating leg pain and sciatica. Some investigators have focused on lumbar disc degeneration, as assessed by imaging or presumed on clinical grounds (although degeneration is common in the absence of symptoms and only weakly correlated with LBP[41]). In addition, a few have studied surgically confirmed symptomatic prolapsed intervertebral disc.[11,12]

Other suggested effects of WBV include neck–shoulder pain or cervical disc degeneration, autonomic disturbance, disorders of balance and digestion, and effects on menstruation and perhaps labour.[1,9,34] However, evidence in many of these areas is very weak and we focus this account on back pain.

Back disorders and WBV: Epidemiological evidence

The effects of WBV on the low back have been the focus of many studies, variously set in the workplace,[13–30] in hospitals[11,12] and in the general community.[31–33] Findings have also been summarized and discussed in several detailed reviews.[1,10,34–40]

In general, these support the idea of a causal association between WBV and back problems defined in a range of ways.

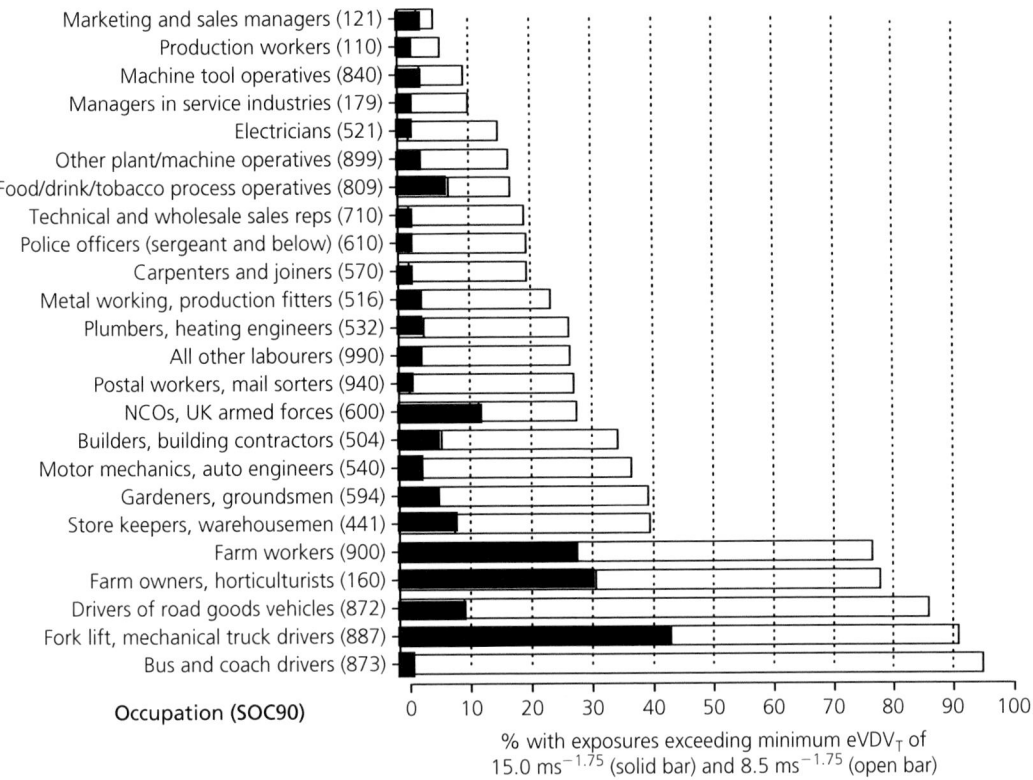

Figure 48.2 Occupations in which significant exposures to whole body vibration most commonly arose in the past week among employed men. Reproduced with permission from BMJ Publishing Group.[5]

Thus, for example, a systematic review by the US National Institute for Occupational Safety and Health (NIOSH) described evidence on the association with LBP as 'strong' (15 of 19 studies positive),[37] while a review by Bovenzi and Hulshof[10] reached similar conclusions and offers a model of the generally available evidence. In a systematic search using several databases and a broad definition of outcome, these authors retrieved 45 articles. The quality of each study was evaluated in terms of methodology and the care taken in assessing vibration exposure and health effects; then a meta-analysis was conducted to combine the results of independent studies of sufficient quality. Altogether, 17 articles reporting the occurrence of back disorders in 22 WBV-exposed occupational groups, met the inclusion criteria. Most of these studies were cross-sectional in design (13 occupational groups), but in four groups longitudinal data were available. The main reasons for exclusion of studies were insufficient quantitative information on exposures to WBV, lack of control information and a failure to consider important confounders. Typically, the qualifying studies focused on crane operators, bus drivers, tractor drivers and forklift truck drivers with administrative or manual workers as controls. Vibration measurements on the vehicles were performed according to ISO 2631-1, and vibration total value or vector sum of the frequency-weighted rms acceleration ranged from 0.25 to 1.45 ms^{-2}. Outcome assessment focused mostly on symptoms reported at medical interview or in response to the standardized Nordic questionnaire on musculoskeletal symptoms, but medical records and radiological investigations were sometimes also available.

Table 48.1 presents meta-analyses for four outcomes where results could be combined[10] – 12-month and acute LBP, sciatic pain and herniated disc – all based on self-reports in the original cross-sectional surveys. It may be seen that summary prevalence odds ratios (POR) are raised for all outcomes and by up to two-fold. A recent further meta-analysis, carried out by the first author, of cross-sectional studies published between 1986 and 2006, confirms previous findings, with a summary POR of 2.4 (95 per cent CI, 2.0–2.8) for 12-month LBP in 16 driver groups (Figure 48.3). On the basis of such evidence, WBV is considered one of the best-established risk factors for LBP.

However, longitudinal data are still relatively sparse and cross-sectional studies suffer some well-known limitations. These include the potential for affected workers to be selected out of exposure (healthy worker effect), with underestimation of risks, or (less likely) the selection of workers with back pain into driving jobs as an alternative to, say, heavy manual work, with overestimation of risks. Cross-sectional studies are also limited by inaccuracies in the assessment of prior exposures. In addition, a problem of interpretation arises in that prevalence depends not only on incidence but also on duration, and could be higher through prolongation of, rather than initiation of, symptoms. Thus, to strengthen the evidence base and to define safe working limits of exposure, interest has focused on

Table 48.1 Meta-analysis of several cross-sectional surveys of back problems and whole body vibration (1986–97).[10]

Occupation group	Prevalence OR (95% CI)			
	Low back pain, past year	Acute low back pain	Sciatic pain, past year	Self-reported herniated lumbar disc
Forklift truck drivers[14,22]	1.7 (0.9–3.1)	1.7 (0.7–4.2)	2.7 (0.6–1.2)	0.8 (0.2–2.6)
	7.3 (2.5–22)	2.8 (1.3–6.3)	1.0 (0.5–2.2)	
	1.6 (1.0–2.6)			
Tractor drivers[19,26]	2.0 (1.2–3.4)	1.0 (0.5–1.9)	1.6 (0.9–3.0)	2.1 (0.8–5.6)
	2.4 (1.6–3.7)	3.0 (1.8–5.0)	3.9 (1.8–8.7)	1.8 (0.7–4.7)
Wheel loaders[17]	1.3 (0.5–3.2)	0.5 (0.2–1.5)	1.0 (0.3–3.1)	
Bus drivers[24]	3.0 (1.8–5.1)	1.9 (1.2–3.3)	1.9 (1.2–3.3)	1.3 (0.6–3.0)
Crane operators[20]	3.3 (1.5–7.1)			
Straddle-carrier drivers[20]	2.5 (1.2–5.4)			
Subway train operators[21]			3.9 (1.7–8.6)	
Summary prevalence OR (95% CI)	2.3 (1.8–2.9)	1.7 (1.1–2.7)	2.0 (1.3–2.9)	1.5 (0.9–2.4)

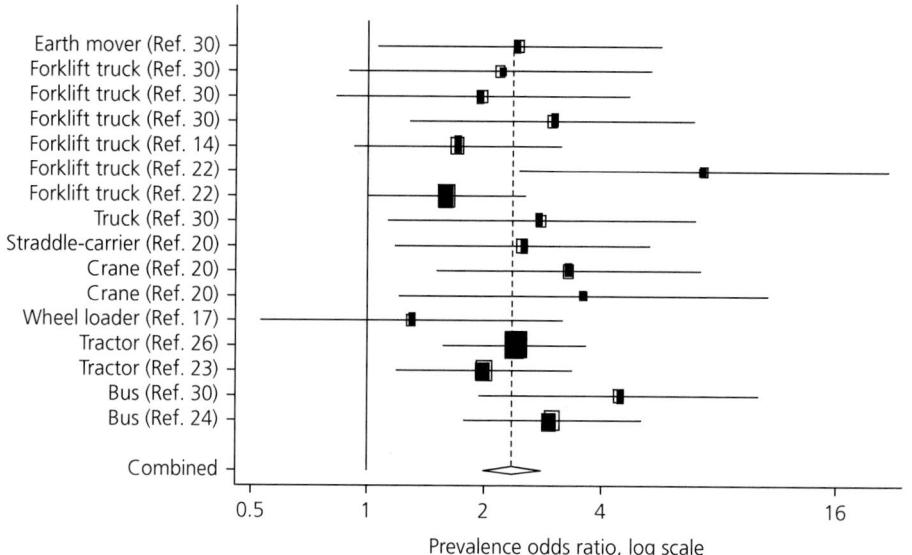

Figure 48.3 Prevalence odds ratios (POR) and 95 per cent confidence intervals (CI) for 12-month low-back pain in 16 driving occupations with exposure to whole body vibration compared to control groups. The POR of each study is adjusted for several confounders (individual characteristics, ergonomic risk factors and/or psychosocial variables). The area of each box is inversely proportional to the estimated variance in the study. Random effects estimation of the combined POR and 95 per cent CI is shown.

longitudinal studies and on evidence on exposure–response relations.

Current information in these areas comes largely from a series of studies commissioned by the Dutch Ministry of Social Services and Employment, in the 1980s. Retrospective cohort studies in crane operators,[15,16] tractor drivers[19] and other transportation workers examined risks for prolonged sick leave and disability pensioning, as demonstrated by social insurance and medical records. Findings were supplemented with in-fill cross-sectional surveys in other exposure groups.[17,18,22,23] A complex picture emerged. In one survey, a relation was found between intervertebral disc disorder and working for more than five years as a crane operator: the age-adjusted risk ratio for disability pension was raised almost three-fold and increased with years of driving experience,[15] while age-adjusted rates of prolonged sickness absence ($\geq$28 days) were also somewhat higher.[16] However, prolonged sickness absence was somewhat less common for non-specific LBP and back disorders overall.[16] Similarly, in tractor drivers, an increasing trend of sick leave with increasing dose was found for disc complaints, but not for non-specific LBP[19] – using a Cox model, estimated RRs were 2.47 and 0.94, respectively, for a dose increase of five years m^2/s^4.

In the cross-sectional surveys, there tended to be excesses of back complaints, but a less clear picture according to dose and disorder. In a small study involving drivers

Table 48.2 Effects of cumulative vibration exposure and postural load on chronic low-back pain in a population of 1155 tractor drivers and 220 controls unexposed to whole body vibration.

Cumulative vibration exposure (years m^{2}s^{-4})^a	OR (95% CI)	Postural load (grade)	OR (95% CI)
0 ($n = 220$)	1.0	Mild ($n = 96$)	1.0
<15 ($n = 335$)	1.48 (0.87–2.50)	Moderate ($n = 231$)	1.20 (0.60–2.40)
15–30 ($n = 374$)	1.90 (1.13–3.20)	Hard ($n = 450$)	1.61 (0.82–3.16)
>30 ($n = 446$)	2.00 (1.17–3.40)	Very hard ($n = 598$)	2.30 (1.17–4.54)

Odds ratios (OR) and 95% confidence intervals (95% CI) were estimated by multivariate logistic regression.[26]
ORs adjusted for age, body mass index, smoking, education, sporting activity, car driving, marital status, mental stress, climatic conditions and previous back trauma.
^{a}Cumulative vibration exposure was estimated as, $\sum a_{vi}^2 t_i$ where a_{vi} is the vibration total value (or vector sum) of the frequency-weighted rms accelerations of tractor i and t_i is the number of full-time working years driven on tractor i (year m^{2}s^{-4}).

of wheel loaders,[17] for example, back pain was somewhat less common in those from the low exposure band and somewhat more common in those from the high band, but in lift-truck and freight-container tractor drivers, back pain lasting several weeks was marginally less common in the high exposure group.[19] Back pain was more common than in non-driver referents, but within the exposed group was more common at younger ages, related largely to dose within the short term (the five years preceding back pain onset). In a cross-sectional survey of helicopter pilots,[18] much higher odds ratios were reported than in other surveys involving higher levels of exposure to WBV. LBP and lumbago were more prevalent in pilots from the least and most exposed bands, defined by dose and cumulative duration of flying (a U-shaped relationship), whereas these outcomes increased with hours of daily flight time, as did back pain lasting more than two weeks. Prevalence of sciatica showed a monotonic relationship to estimated vibration dose, but peaked with intermediate durations of lifetime and daily flight time.

Such differences may reflect real differences in the risks of different outcomes (e.g. LBP versus prolapsed disc) in relation to different metrics of exposure (e.g. short versus long term). However, they may also reflect a combination of measurement errors, selection effects and uncontrolled confounding. The high rates of back pain in helicopter pilots, for example, have been attributed partly to the cramped space of cockpits as a source of transient discomfort.[18] Other potential confounders common among professional drivers include heavy lifting (e.g. loading and unloading of delivery vehicles by hand), and twisting with a non-neutral trunk position (e.g. looking behind when manoeuvring a forklift truck).

In a growing number of surveys, special effort has been made to control for confounding by known causes of back disorders. A cross-sectional study of tractor drivers by Bovenzi and Betta[26] provides one example. In an epidemiological survey of 1155 tractor drivers and 220 controls unexposed to WBV, cumulative vibration exposure and postural load were found to be independently associated with chronic LBP, defined as daily experience of LBP or several episodes of LBP lasting more than 30 days in the previous 12 months (Table 48.2). A significant trend was found with higher levels of both vibration dose and postural load, such that tractor drivers with high exposure to both factors had a more than three-fold elevated risk of chronic LBP relative to subjects who scored low on these counts (Table 48.3). The analysis also took account of other risk factors for LBP such as age, body mass index, smoking, sporting activity, mental health and previous back trauma.

However, even with great care in execution, a problem exists in disentangling the separate risks of sitting and WBV. Intradiscal pressure is higher when sitting, and so prolonged sitting is a biologically plausible confounder, especially given that both exposures are almost always present together. Estimates of dose often incorporate an allowance for time as well as vibration magnitude, so

Table 48.3 Odds ratios^a for the combined effect of cumulative vibration exposure and postural load on the occurrence of chronic low-back pain in tractor drivers.[26]

Cumulative vibration exposure (years m^{2}s^{-4})^b	Postural load (grade)			
	Mild	Moderate	Hard	Very hard
5	1.29	1.79	2.50	3.48
10	1.41	1.96	2.73	3.79
20	1.55	2.15	2.99	4.16
30	1.63	2.27	3.16	4.39
40	1.70	2.36	3.29	4.58

^{a}With reference to controls exposed to mild postural load and unexposed to vibration.
^{b}Cumulative vibration exposure was estimated as in Table 48.2. Odds ratios were adjusted for age, body mass index, smoking, education, sport activity, car driving, marital status, mental stress, climatic conditions and previous back trauma.

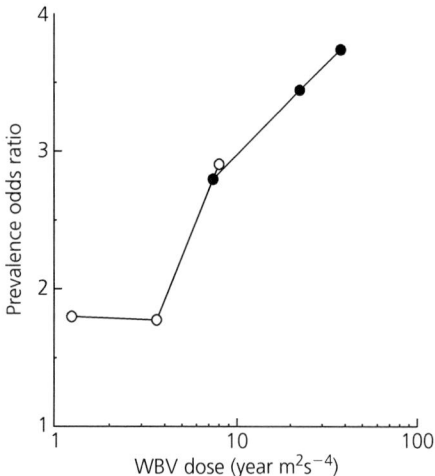

Figure 48.4 Prevalence odds ratio for low-back pain among tractor drivers as a function of lifetime cumulative whole body vibration (WBV) dose estimated as $\sum a_{vi}^2 t_i$, where a_{vi} is the vibration total value (or vector sum) of the frequency-weighted rms accelerations of tractor i and t_i is the number of full-time working years driven on tractor i (year m^{2}s^{-4}). Based on data from Refs 23 and 26.

dose–response patterns do not necessarily implicate vibration or exonerate sitting,[38] while higher vibration magnitudes themselves may be correlated with sitting (as the vehicles that generate such exposures tend to be operated by professional drivers). The ideal study design might compare drivers with people who sit equally long in blue-collar jobs that do not involve driving, or might take as a focus a controlled intervention to reduce vibration magnitude without reducing driving time. Some surveys have used office workers as controls,[24,26] but intervention studies have rarely been reported.[42] Driving of vehicles with relatively low vibration magnitudes has been linked with an excess of prolapsed intervertebral disc[11,12] and new onset simple LBP,[25] pointing to a possible role for posture rather than WBV; but, on the other hand, sitting in the absence of vibration (work in other sedentary occupations) does not seem to carry a very high or consistent risk of LBP.[38,43]

Vibration dose is a composite of vibration magnitude and time. Thus, in principle, the relative importance of sitting time and vibration could be assessed in exposed populations receiving doses held to be equivalent, but in which these subcomponents vary (high sitting time–low vibration versus low sitting time–high vibration). Few data of this kind are available at present. However, some studies offer risk estimates by cumulative vibration dose, vibration magnitude and duration of exposure separately,[23,26] and these seem to suggest that duration of exposure (driving years) is associated with LBP disorders more than vibration magnitude alone (ms^{-2}). In another recent survey,[30] LBP, high pain intensity in the lower back and disability from LBP (based on the Roland–Morris scale) were all significantly associated with total driving hours, but not with $A(8)$.

Assuming that the health effect arises from WBV, and taking risk estimates from careful cross-sectional investigations, some elements of an exposure–response relationship may be tentatively offered. Thus, for example, two large epidemiological studies of tractor drivers[23,26] used the same methods to measure WBV in the workplace and to assess cumulative vibration dose according to the equal energy principle. The two tractor driver groups differed with respect to mean duration of exposure (10 versus 21 years) and vibration magnitude (0.7 versus 1.1 ms^{-2} rms). LBP symptoms were collected with a similar questionnaire and the influence of a wide range of potential confounders, including postural load, was taken into account in the study design and data analysis. Figure 48.4 displays the estimated prevalence odds ratio for LBP as a function of the lifetime cumulative WBV dose, and suggests a trend of increasing risk with increasing exposure to WBV.

As may be judged from the foregoing discussion, a number of uncertainties in the knowledge base prompt continuing research interest in the field. Recently, these have encouraged a European research consortium (VIBRISKS) to mount several cross-European prospective cohort studies, the pooled analyses from which are awaited (see www.vibrisks.soton.ac.uk).

We summarize current epidemiological knowledge as follows:

- Consistent associations have been shown between various measures of LBP and professional driving in many cross-sectional and a small number of longitudinal and case–control studies. In keeping with this consistency, meta-analyses support a relationship.
- Such a pattern is unlikely to be due to chance. If attributable to confounding, then the most plausible confounder is sitting. However, most authorities assume the association is causal.
- Some evidence exists of an exposure–response pattern, but there is a substantial agreement that firm conclusions on the relationship between WBV exposure and LBP disorders cannot be drawn from available epidemiological data.

Pathophysiological mechanisms

While research continues apace, the role of WBV in the pathogenesis of LBP remains uncertain. A popular working hypothesis is that vibration causes mechanical overloading which leads to premature degeneration of the lumbar spine.[1,34,44,45] Biodynamic and physiological experiments suggest the possibility of several interacting mechanisms, e.g. muscle fatigue, reduced disc height and bending of the spine jointly leading to high strain on the vertebral column. Direct mechanical effect – fatigue failure and impaired nutrition of the disc[1,34,44,45] – may ensue.

However, mechanical injury to the spine appears to be neither a necessary nor sufficient cause of LBP in general (pain can occur in the absence of demonstrable pathology, disc changes are common even in people without LBP,[41] and symptoms come and go without a change in imaging status), and the same may be true of LBP associated with professional driving. Symptoms can arise from local soft tissue injury, or be moderated, reinforced or perpetuated by higher level inputs from the central nervous system.[46] Reflecting this, experience of LBP is common across all jobs and influenced importantly by psychological factors, including illness beliefs and mental health. Nociception, pain, suffering, pain behaviour and disability are only partially correlated.[47]

Local injury may be an initiating event, but a question arises as to whether high peak of exposures matter most (acute injury) or long-term steady exposures with insufficient recovery (chronic wear and tear). Some epidemiological studies have found a greater risk of back symptoms and referred pain with more years of driving, but this does not necessarily favour a long time course of pathogenesis – more time could simply give more opportunity for acute injury – and other studies have reported raised risks within quite short intervals of driving (e.g. in a study by Boshuizen et al.,[23] ORs were raised by five-fold for frequent or long-lasting LBP or prolapsed disc in tractor drivers with as little as 0–5 years of exposure) and at young ages.[19]

Animal experiments have demonstrated that excessive mechanical overload can result in structural injury and degeneration of the tissues of bones and joints.[48] Repeated impact loading can lead to cumulative microdamage and metabolic changes in bone and cartilage of the rabbit tibia;[49] and there is evidence that heavy vibration loads and repetitive mechanical shocks can cause stress damage in porcine intervertebral discs.[50] Animal experiments, however, have seldom been undertaken to explore mechanisms and the impact of different controlled patterns of vibration exposure.[51]

CONTROL STANDARDS

Reflecting current uncertainty, the distinction between shocks and steady continuous exposures is glossed over in current control standards. Table 48.4 sets out exposure standards for WBV according to the European Directive 2002/44/EC,[4] defined in terms of an exposure action value (EAV) – the daily amount above which employers must act to control exposure, and an exposure limit value (ELV) – the maximum amount an employee may be exposed to on any given day. (Regulations in member countries permit a transitional period until July 2010 for work equipment in use before July 2007.) EAVs and ELVs are expressed either in terms of $A(8)$ (rms), an averaging method, or VDV, a dose measure that accumulates exposures in accord with a fourth power time dependency. However, as Griffin[52] points out, these methods are not equivalent and show 'a large internal inconsistency … for short duration exposures to WBV'. Specifically, high short-term peaks (shocks) can be offset under the averaging method by periods of low vibration, whereas this does not reduce VDV. Griffin suggests that the Directive does rule out 'extraordinarily high' vibration of short duration if assessed by the rms method – severe enough to be intolerable to those exposed to vibration.[52] He suggests it would be prudent to base actions on qualitative guidance, to reduce risks to a minimum, rather than relying on this quantitative guidance.

Uncertainty is compounded because the thresholds chosen are not rooted in a clear understanding of the exposure–response relationship.

Table 48.4 Daily exposure action values and daily exposure limit values for whole body vibration (WBV) according to the European Directive 2002/44/EC on mechanical vibration.[4]

	$A(8)$ (rms)	VDV
Daily exposure action value	$0.5\,\mathrm{ms}^{-2}$	$9.1\,\mathrm{ms}^{-1.75}$
Daily exposure limit value	$1.15\,\mathrm{ms}^{-2}$	$21\,\mathrm{ms}^{-1.75}$

$A(8)$ is the daily vibration exposure value normalized to an eight-hour reference period and VDV is the Vibration Dose Value (see text for definitions).

FACTORS AFFECTING EXPOSURES AND CONTROL MEASURES

In addition to the magnitude, duration and pattern of WBV, several other factors may relate to the injury potential, including individual susceptibility to injury, the dynamic response of the human body (mechanical impedance, vibration transmissibility, absorbed energy), body posture and health status. Dose may be related to the design of the vehicle, the cabin seating, the suspension, the road conditions, the road speed and ultimately the behaviour and training of the driver.

Consistent with these notions, Article 4 of Directive 2002/44/EC[4] requires the employer to assess and, if necessary, measure the levels of WBV to which workers are exposed, giving particular attention to such items as:

a. *the level, type and duration of exposure, including any exposure to intermittent vibration or repeated shocks;*
b. *the Exposure Limit Values and the Exposure Action Values laid down in Article 3 of the Directive;*
c. *workers specially sensitive to risks;*
d. *any indirect effects on worker safety resulting from interactions between mechanical vibration and the workplace or other work equipment;*
e. *information provided by the manufacturers of work equipment in accordance with the relevant Community Directives;*
f. *the existence of replacement equipment designed to reduce the levels of exposure to mechanical vibration;*
g. *the extension of exposure to WBV beyond normal working hours under the employer's responsibility;*

h. specific working conditions such as low temperatures;
i. and appropriate information obtained from health surveillance, including published information.

Where exposures exceed the EAV, employers must eliminate or reduce risks as far as reasonably practicable and exposures should not exceed the ELV (Article 5).

The prevention of ill health and injury requires administrative, technical and medical responses, many of which are specified in or supported by the Directive. Administrative measures include adequate information and advice to employers and employees (Articles 6 and 7), organizational changes in the work, and training to instruct the operators of vibrating machinery in safe and correct work practices. Work schedules should be arranged to include rest periods.

Technical measures include the choice of vehicles with the lowest vibration and best ergonomic designs. An EC Directive concerning the safety of machinery [89/392/EEC] obliges manufacturers to state whether the frequency-weighted acceleration of WBV exceeds $0.5\,\mathrm{ms}^{-2}$ rms, to facilitate informed choice.

Within the United Kingdom, where the Directive is implemented as the Control of Vibration at Work Regulations 2005, the Health and Safety Executive[53] advises on several preventive precautions: drivers should adjust their seating, avoid rough, poor or uneven surfaces, and moderate their speed to suit road conditions; vehicle suspensions should be maintained as should site roadways, 'safer systems of work' should be encouraged with sufficient rest breaks and care should be taken in the choice of seating.

HEALTH SURVEILLANCE

The Directive also requires health surveillance, assuming a reasonable likelihood of health problems arising, a valid means of detection and sensible options for response. According to article 8, para 1: *'health surveillance, the results of which are taken into account in the application of preventive measures at a specific workplace, shall be intended to prevent and diagnose rapidly any disorder linked with exposure to mechanical vibration. Such surveillance shall be appropriate where:*

- *the exposure of workers to vibration is such that a link can be established between that exposure and an identifiable illness or harmful effects on health;*
- *it is probable that the illness or the effects occur in a worker's particular working conditions;*
- *there are tested techniques for the detection of the illness or the harmful effects on health.*

In any event, workers exposed to mechanical vibration in excess of the values stated in Article 3(1)(b) and (2)(b) [the daily Exposure Action Values] shall be entitled to appropriate health surveillance.'

Implementation is problematic however, in that LBP is so common in the general population as to be expected in many workers, drivers and non-drivers alike, while there are differing views on the added value of physician's examination over screening questionnaires (the HSE recommends a simple system of health monitoring for workers at greater risk).[53] Surveillance implies pre-employment and regular periodic inquiry, but back pain episodes may come and go in-between inquiries, and the immediate management of cases will mostly be dictated by severity of symptoms and incapacity in the acute phase, extremes of which normally lead to consultation independent of regular inquiry. Thus, the main virtues of health monitoring may lie in identifying extremes of unacceptable exposure, in ensuring systematic coverage, and in gaining a group level impression of the success in controlling health problems. Where surveillance is undertaken, it should be managed by certified occupational health personnel.

Key points

- Whole body vibration is a very common component of the working environment, especially when account is taken of the many professional drivers with low-level exposures in delivery and transport duties.
- Substantial industrial exposures are less common, but many workers still approach the exposure standards set in European legislation and many contribute additionally to total dose during leisure-time travels and commuting.
- Exposure to WBV is generally thought to be a cause of work-related back pain and a great deal of epidemiological evidence supports this, while not excluding a role for other concurrent risk factors, such as posture and prolonged sitting.
- Knowledge of the exposure–response relation is incomplete and the current control standards are to an important extent arbitrary.
- In spite of this uncertainty, many practical steps can be taken to mitigate risks of ill health which can be supported, to a greater or lesser extent, as sensible occupational health and safety practice.
- Control by engineering means is preferable to measures aimed at changing behaviour. Both, however, offer scope for intervention.

REFERENCES

1. Griffin MJ. *Handbook of human vibration.* London: Academic Press, 1990.
2. International Organization for Standardization. *Guide for the evaluation of human exposure to whole body vibration – Part 1: General requirements.* ISO 2631-1. Geneva: ISO, 1997.

3. International Organization for Standardization. *Measurement and evaluation of human exposure to hand-transmitted vibration – Part 1: General guidelines.* ISO 5349-1. Geneva: ISO, 2001.
4. Directive 2002/44/EC of the European Parliament and of The Council of 25 June 2002 *on the minimum health and safety requirements regarding the exposure of workers to the risks arising from physical agents (vibration) (sixteenth individual Directive within the meaning of Article 16(1) of Directive 89/391/EEC).* Official Journal of the European Communities, L 177/13, 6.7.2002.
5. Palmer KT, Griffin MJ, Bendall H *et al.* Prevalence and pattern of occupational exposure to whole-body vibration in Great Britain: Findings from a national survey. *Occupational and Environmental Medicine.* 2000; **57**: 229–36.
6. Walsh K, Cruddas M, Coggon D. Interaction of height and mechanical loading of the spine in the development of low-back pain. *Scandinavian Journal of Work, Environment and Health.* 1991; **17**: 420–4.
7. Jones JR, Hodgson JT, Osman J. *Self-reported working conditions in 1995.* London: HMSO, 1997.
8. Parent-Thirion A, Fernández Macías E, Hurley J, Vermeylen G. Fourth European Working Conditions Survey. Dublin: European Foundation for the Improvement of Living and Working Conditions, 2007.
9. Comité Européen de Normalisation. Mechanical vibration – guide to the health effects of vibration on the human body. CEN Technical Report 12349. Brussels: 1996.
10. Bovenzi M, Hulshof CTJ. An updated review of epidemiologic studies on the relationship between exposure to whole-body vibration and low back pain (1986–1997). *International Archives of Occupational and Environmental Health.* 1999; **72**: 351–65.
11. Kelsey JL, Hardy RL. Driving of motor vehicles as a risk factor for acute herniated lumbar intervertebral disc. *American Journal of Epidemiology.* 1975; **102**: 63–73.
12. Kelsey JL, Githens PB, O'Conner T *et al.* Acute prolapsed lumbar intervertebral disc: An epidemiological study with special reference to driving automobiles and cigarette smoking. *Spine* 1984; **9**: 608–13.
13. Backman AL. Health survey of professional drivers. *Scandinavian Journal of Work, Environment and Health.* 1983; **9**: 30–5.
14. Brendstrup T, Biering-Sørensen F. Effect of fork-lift truck driving on low-back trouble. *Scandinavian Journal of Work, Environment and Health.* 1987; **13**: 442–52.
15. Bongers PM, Boshuizen HC, Hulshof CTJ, Koemeester AP. Back disorders in crane operators exposed to whole-body vibration. *International Archives of Occupational and Environmental Health.* 1988; **60**: 129–37.
16. Bongers PM, Boshuizen HC, Hulshof CTJ, Koemeester AP. Long-term sickness absence due to back disorders in crane operators exposed to whole-body vibration. *International Archives of Occupational and Environmental Health.* 1988; **61**: 59–64.
17. Bongers PM, Boshuizen HC, Hulshof CTJ. Self-reported back pain in drivers of wheel-loaders. Academisch Proefschrift, Universiteit van Amsterdam, 1990, 205–20.
18. Bongers PM, Hulshof CTJ, Dijkstra L *et al.* Back pain and exposure to whole body vibration in helicopter pilots. *Ergonomics.* 1990; **33**: 1007–26.
19. Boshuizen HC, Boshuizen HC, Bongers PM, Hulshof CTJ. 1990. Long-term sick leave and disability pensioning due to back disorders of tractor drivers exposed to whole-body vibration. *International Archives of Occupational and Environmental Health.* 1990; **62**: 117–22.
20. Burdorf A, Zondervan H. An epidemiological study of low-back pain in crane operators. *Ergonomics.* 1990; **33**: 981–7.
21. Johanning E. Back disorders and health problems among subway train operators exposed to whole-body vibration. *Scandinavian Journal of Work, Environment and Health.* 1991; **17**: 414–19.
22. Boshuizen HC, Bongers PM, Hulshof CTJ. Self-reported back pain in forklift truck and freight-container drivers exposed to whole-body vibration. *Spine.* 1992; **17**: 59–65.
23. Boshuizen HC, Bongers PM, Hulshof CTJ. Self-reported back pain in tractor drivers exposed to whole-body vibration. *International Archives of Occupational and Environmental Health.* 1990; **62**: 109–15.
24. Bovenzi M, Zadini A. Self-reported low back symptoms in urban bus drivers exposed to whole-body vibration. *Spine.* 1992; **17**: 1048–59.
25. Pietri F, Leclerc A, Boitel L *et al.* Low-back pain in commercial drivers. *Scandinavian Journal of Work, Environment and Health.* 1992; **18**: 52–8.
26. Bovenzi M, Betta A. Low-back disorders in agricultural tractor drivers exposed to whole-body vibration and postural stress. *Applied Ergonomics.* 1994; **25**: 231–41.
27. Magnusson ML, Pope MH, Wilder DG, Areskoug B. Are occupational drivers at an increased risk for developing musculoskeletal disorders? *Spine.* 1996; **21**: 710–17.
28. Schwarze S, Notbohm G, Dupuis H, Hartung E. Dose–response relationships between whole-body vibration and lumbar disk disease – a field study on 388 drivers of different vehicles. *Journal of Sound and Vibration.* 1998; **215**: 613–28.
29. Kumar A, Varghese M, Mohan D *et al.* Effect of whole-body vibration on the low back. A study of tractor-driving farmers in north India. *Spine.* 1999; **24**: 2506–15.
30. Bovenzi M, Rui F, Negro C *et al.* An epidemiological survey of low back pain in professional drivers. *Journal of Sound and Vibration.* 2006; **298**: 514–39.
31. Liira JP, Shannon HS, Chambers LW, Haines TA. Long-term back problems and physical work exposures in the 1990 Ontario Health Survey. *American Journal of Public Health.* 1996; **86**: 382–7.
32. Xu Y, Bach E, Orhede E. Work environment and low back pain: the influence of occupational activities. *Occupational and Environmental Medicine.* 1997; **54**: 741–5.
33. Palmer KT, Griffin MJ, Syddall HE *et al.* The relative importance of whole-body vibration and occupational lifting

33. as risk factors for low-back pain. *Occupational and Environmental Medicine.* 2003; **60**: 715–21.
34. Dupuis H, Zerlett G. *The effects of whole-body vibration.* Berlin: Springer-Verlag, 1986.
35. Hulshof CTJ, Veldhuijzen van Zanten OBA. Whole-body vibration and low back pain – a review of epidemiologic studies. *International Archives of Occupational and Environmental Health.* 1987; **59**: 205–20.
36. Kuorinka I, Forcier L (eds). *Work-related musculoskeletal disorders (WMSDs): A reference book for prevention.* London: Taylor & Francis, 1995.
37. National Institute for Occupational Health and Safety. Musculoskeletal disorders and workplace factors. A critical review of epidemiologic evidence for work-related musculoskeletal disorders of the neck, upper extremity, and low back. Cincinnati, OH: US Department of Health and Human Sciences/NIOSH, 1997 (publication no. 97-141).
38. Burdorf A, Sorock G. Positive and negative evidence on risk factors for back disorders. *Scandinavian Journal of Work, Environment and Health.* 1997; **23**: 243–56.
39. Bovenzi M, Hulsof CTJ. An updated review of epidemiologic studies on the relationship between exposure to whole-body vibration and low back pain. *Journal of Sound and Vibration.* 1998; **215**: 595–612.
40. Ling S, Leboeuf-Yde C. Whole-body vibration and low back pain: A systematic, critical review of the epidemiological literature 1992–1999. *International Archives of Occupational and Environmental Health.* 2000; **73**: 290–7.
41. Lawrence JS. Disc degeneration – its frequency and relationship to symptoms. *Annals of Rheumatic Diseases.* 1969; **28**: 121–38.
42. Hulshof CTJ, Verbeek JHAM, Braam ITJ et al. Evaluation of an occupational health intervention program on whole body vibration in forklift truck drivers: A controlled trial. *Occupational and Environmental Medicine.* 2006; **63**: 461–8.
43. Hartvigsen J, Leboeuf-Yde C, Lings S, Corder EH. Is sitting-while-at-work associated with low back pain? A systematic, critical literature review. *Scandinavian Journal of Public Health.* 2000; **28**: 230–9.
44. Bongers P, Boshuizen H. Back disorders and whole-body vibration at work. PhD Thesis. Amsterdam: University of Amsterdam, 1990.
45. Wilder DG. The biomechanics of vibration and low back pain. *American Journal of Industrial Medicine.* 1993; **23**: 577–88.
46. Melzack R, Wall P. Pain mechanisms: A new theory. *Science.* 1965; **50**: 971–9.
47. Waddell G. *The back pain revolution.* Edinburgh: Churchill Livingstone, 1998.
48. Waters T, Rauche C, Genaidy A, Rashed T. A new framework for evaluating potential risk of back disorders due to whole body vibration and repeated mechanical shock. *Ergonomics.* 2007; **50**: 379–95.
49. Radin E, Martin R, Burr D et al. Effects of mechanical loading on tissues of the rabbit knee. *Journal of Orthopaedic Research.* 1984; **2**: 221–34.
50. Tsai K, Lin R, Chang G. Rate-related fatigue injury of vertebral disc under axial cyclic loading in a porcine body – disc-body unit. *Clinical Biomechanics.* 1998; **13**: S32–S39.
51. Seidel H. Selected health risks caused by long-term, whole-body vibration. *American Journal of Industrial Medicine.* 1993; **23**: 589–604.
52. Griffin MJ. Maximum health and safety requirements for workers exposed to hand-transmitted vibration and whole-body vibration in the European Union: A review. *Occupational and Environmental Medicine.* 2004; **61**: 387–97.
53. Health and Safety Executive. Vibration at work. Last accessed July 27, 2007. Available from: www.hse.gov.uk/vibration/index.htm.

SECTION THREE

Heat and cold

49 Heat and cold 525
E Howard N Oakley

49

Heat and cold

E HOWARD N OAKLEY

Introduction	525
Physical and physiological principles	526
Cold stress	528
Heat stress	534
Principles of the reduction of thermal strain	538
References	543

INTRODUCTION

Humans live and work in the widest range of thermal environments of any single species, and the strategies they have developed to support relatively normal activities in the face of extreme heat and cold have been crucial to the survival and success of the species.

Historically, techniques for surviving thermal challenges have extended and supported the underlying physiological responses by changing behaviour and the establishment of a favourable local microclimate within clothing. Nomadic hunter-gatherers and traders in hot, arid lands have developed activity patterns that minimize exposure to heat stress, wearing loose garments that isolate the skin from high solar radiation load, and move cooler air around an internal microclimate as the clothing moves. Others living in very cold areas have herded and hunted animals to supply the fur that humans lack, then fashioned those skins into layered garments to maintain a near-tropical microclimate at the skin.

Shelters have developed from small and temporary structures permitting the hands to be exposed for manual tasks and exclusion of wind and precipitation to allow a limited range of other activities, to massive fixed structures consuming huge amounts of power to condition the internal environment regardless of external conditions. However, many workers continue to spend much of their working day outdoors, away from the comfort of shelters. Others are involved in processes such as the filleting and preparation of fish that have to be performed in cold and wet conditions, or at the opposite extreme with molten metals at very high temperatures.

The twentieth century saw substantial improvements in mechanical handling that have reduced the number of workers who have to operate plant in extreme heat or cold. The frozen food industry, for example, has moved from largely manual handling within stores to highly mechanized warehouses in which products can be even better preserved by reducing atmospheric oxygen levels. There are still workers who need to enter modern cold stores, but they are mainly maintenance engineers who may have to carry out prolonged tasks that require tactile sensation and dexterity: great challenges in temperatures below $-30°C$ and at an equivalent altitude to half-way up Mont Blanc.

The future is increasingly uncertain, perhaps even bleak. Despite innovative efforts to reduce the carbon footprint of conditioned buildings, it is much less efficient to chill or heat the entire working environment than it is to cool or insulate the individual worker. With rising average temperatures, many buildings in previously temperate climates will prove costly and inefficient to chill during hotter summers. The only option may be for office and other workers to have to cope with hotter, and less comfortable, conditions for much of the year. Rising sea levels and more frequent heavy precipitation will increase the risks of flooding, particularly in densely populated coastal areas. Rescue workers who seldom had to cope with floods are more likely to have to work in floodwater, with its thermal and other challenges.

So far from being problems afflicting less industrialized societies, heat and cold are likely to become increasingly important as employment patterns and climate change in the future.

Throughout this chapter, careful distinction will be made between the terms 'stress' and 'strain'. In accordance with their engineering origins, these will be used rigorously: 'stress' is the force applied to an object (in a thermal context, the thermal load to which the body is subjected), while 'strain' is the response within that object to the applied stress (thermally, the physiological and behavioural responses that result from thermal load). The usefulness of this distinction should not be underestimated: for example, the measurement of stress is useful in predicting the safe exposure for groups, while measurement of strain can assess how well a given individual is coping with a certain stress, and thus whether or not that person should be withdrawn or treated.

This chapter reviews the fundamental factors in human heat exchange, describes the reactions to thermal stress and their adverse consequences, and outlines approaches to the modification of both stress and strain. Although coverage includes discussion of local cold injury, such as frostbite, thermal burns are omitted in deference to authoritative accounts elsewhere.

PHYSICAL AND PHYSIOLOGICAL PRINCIPLES

Overall, the human body is subject to the law of conservation of energy, succinctly expressed in the equation:

$$M + (R + C + K - E) = S$$

where M is the heat generated by metabolism (always positive); R is the net radiant heat exchange with the environment (negative for loss from the body); C is the convective heat exchange with the surrounding fluid (negative for loss); K is the conductive heat exchange with any contacting solid (negative for loss); E is the evaporative heat loss resulting from the evaporation of liquid from the body or its clothing (almost always positive for a loss from the body, or zero); and S is the heat stored (positive) or lost

---

Box 49.1 Examples of thermal balance

1. Sedentary, in balance. In sedentary work, M will be approximately 100 W. For $S = 0$, thermal equilibrium, most of that 100 W will be lost in C, with a small loss in E as a result of 'insensible perspiration'.

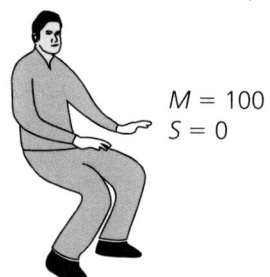

$M = 100$
$S = 0$

2. Exercising, in balance. When M rises to 250 W or more, thermal equilibrium can only be maintained by overt sweating to increase E substantially, to 200 W or more, as C will not increase much. This requires the effective evaporation of upwards of 300 mL of sweat per hour, comfortably within human capability.

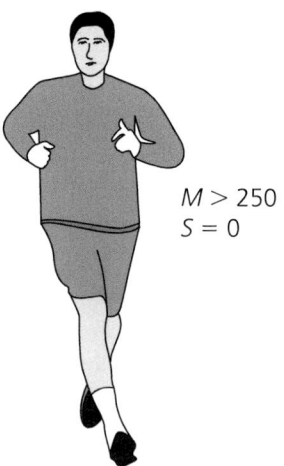

$M > 250$
$S = 0$

3. Exercising in occlusive clothing. Workers who are required to perform physical work inside occlusive clothing can find that R, C, K and E all fall close to 0 W, so that all the heat that they generate, perhaps 200 W or more, will be stored at S. This results in a rapid rise in body temperature, perhaps as high as 10°C per hour, and rapid onset of heat illness.

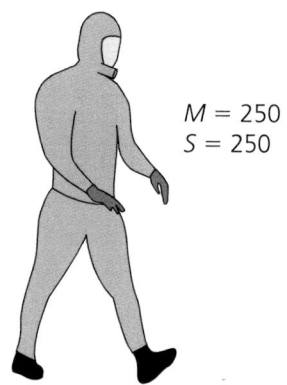

$M = 250$
$S = 250$

4. Cooling when wearing wet clothing. Inadequate protective clothing can result in excessive evaporative loss too. With a sedentary M of about 100 W, someone whose clothing is soaked might evaporate as much as a litre of water every hour, which would make E become about 700 W. S then becomes very negative and their body cools in spite of shivering attempting to increase M. They will become hypothermic unless their evaporative loss is stopped, perhaps by surrounding them with a plastic bag to act as a water vapour barrier.

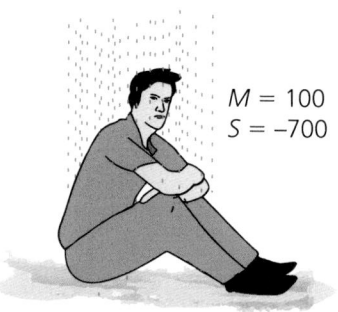

$M = 100$
$S = -700$

(negative) by the body, and thus reflected in a change in mean body temperature.

Basal metabolic heat generation remains relatively constant in health, but is diminished in hypothermia, endocrine disorders such as hypothyroidism, certain drug intoxications, and other disorders. It rises following a meal (the 'specific dynamic effect'), and in some endocrine and other disorders. However, the greatest variation in metabolism is seen in the additional heat generation resulting from physical activity. Depending on the intensity of that activity, total metabolic heat production can vary from less than 80 W when asleep, to over 500 W during short-duration intense exercise by a trained athlete.

The four modes of heat exchange (R, C, K and E defined above) are each governed by physical laws that, in theory at least, allow their precise computation. In practice though, information is seldom sufficiently complete, and more empirical relationships have to be used. Most popular are lumped equations analogous to Ohm's law:

$$q = t/h$$

where q is the heat flux by that route, t is the thermal differential driving that mode of heat exchange, typically the difference between the surface and ambient temperatures, but notably the difference between fourth powers of temperatures in the case of radiant heat transfer (R), and h is the coefficient of resistance to that mode of heat exchange.

Although empirical, such equations are valuable in demonstrating the crucial importance of temperature gradients in determining the direction and size of heat flows. Heat cannot flow against a temperature gradient.

The magnitude of each mode of heat exchange is thus set by a combination of environmental conditions, including ambient radiation, air movement, temperature and water content, together with skin temperature and clothing worn. For example, some industrial environments impose a high radiant heat load (R) from hot machinery, molten metals and flame; this can be usefully attenuated by garments coated with an outer metallized reflective layer. However, this may in turn render the garments impermeable to water vapour transfer, resulting in evaporative heat loss (E) falling to zero. Another major factor that affects thermal resistance is the difference in physical properties of fluids: convective exchange with water is much greater than that with air.

A common error in the application of physics to human thermoregulation is to assume that the body can be treated as a single inert and undifferentiated entity. Regulatory mechanisms respond to central (or 'core') temperatures quite differently from those in the periphery. When someone who is hyperthermic immerses their hands in cold water, peripheral vasodilatation is maintained and they can lose substantial amounts of heat into the water; euthermic or hypothermic subjects will not only vasoconstrict on (cold) hand immersion, but may not be able to vasodilate even if the hands are immersed in warm water.

Should heat production not match heat loss, heat will either be gained or lost from the body, according to the sign of S defined above, and it is this which results in a change in body temperature. The over-simplistic single-element model of the body then fails to show the change in internal thermal gradients that occurs. If excessive heat is being lost from the skin, the peripheries will cool first and there will be little effect on the 'core' other than its shrinking in effective volume; this strategy of 'sacrificing' the homeostasis of the peripheries in order to preserve the core environment is important in paving the way for local cold injury. Insufficient heat loss and a rising 'core' temperature tends to externalize the core by reducing thermal gradients with the peripheries, and increasing the volume of the body at core temperature.

Responses to cold

The primary physiological responses to cold exposure are peripheral vasoconstriction, piloerection, and the increase in metabolic heat production by shivering. Skin temperature falls first, a result of local cooling without a corresponding increase in the delivery of heat to the skin by the flow of blood. This fall in skin temperature stimulates peripheral cold receptors and leads to both locally mediated and centrally regulated vasoconstriction, which in turn allows a further fall in skin temperature. If the rest of the body is sufficiently warm, cyclical cold vasodilatation ('cold induced vasodilatation' or the 'hunting reaction') may ensue, with skin temperatures falling below 12°C, rising with the vasodilatation, and then falling again. The mechanism responsible for this phenomenon remains controversial, but extensive experimentation has shown that it is very variable between and within individuals, and absent if the rest of the body is cold.[1] Sustained peripheral vasoconstriction may be accompanied by fluid shifts resulting in a reduction in plasma volume. Shivering first appears as short bursts in a few groups of muscles, becoming continuous and generalized as a rectal temperature of about 35°C is reached. Further cooling or exhaustion results in shivering gradually tailing off, until it is replaced by generalized rigidity and finally the flaccidity of imminent death.

Responses to heat

Under heat stress, changes in blood flow to the periphery are again the earliest response, followed by an increase in evaporative heat loss by sweating. The normally low nutrient skin capillary flow is augmented by the opening of arteriovenous anastomoses in the skin, which allow high rates of heat transfer from the deeper body to its surface without altering capillary exchange. This increases skin temperature, driving higher rates of heat loss as long as the ambient temperature is lower than that of the skin. When this temperature difference becomes too small to support adequate heat loss or is actually reversed, the only significant means by which the body can lose heat is by the evaporation of sweat, which also makes high demands on peripheral blood flow.

These responses conflict with the requirement to perfuse working muscle during exercise, which may of course be the cause of the thermal stress. Fluid loss in sweat also threatens plasma volume, which is in turn essential to the maintenance of peripheral vasodilatation and sweating. A further problem is that thermally effective sweating requires evaporation from the skin (or, less effectively, the outermost layers of clothing); sweat which drips from the body makes no contribution to the loss of heat, while remaining a drain on fluid reserves. Failure of evaporation in humid conditions, with little air movement or impermeable clothing, explains many cases of heat illness in relatively moderate dry bulb temperatures.

COLD STRESS

Assessment of cold stress

The dominant components of cold stress are the temperature and nature (air or water) of the fluid surrounding the body. Wind speed, and to a lesser extent water movement, can also be important. A simple thermometer and a wind speed indicator are the main measuring instruments needed. Anemometers need not be complex: one of the cup type is best for outside use, whilst vane and hot wire systems are preferred in enclosed spaces. Inexpensive hand-held anemometers are popular in outdoor leisure activities and generally sufficiently accurate for these purposes. However, they often present derived measures such as 'wind chill equivalent temperature' that should be treated with suspicion. The measurement of radiant heat exchange is more difficult to measure accurately, although it is generally small except under a clear night sky.

Evaporative loss is even harder to assess and is small in cold-dry systems. However, if the clothing is wet, evaporative losses alone can exceed 700 W, exceeding the total of other modes of heat loss; simple techniques such as repeated weighing to estimate water loss can then only give a crude overestimate. Although convective losses in water are much greater than in air of the same temperature, partial immersion presents a particularly complex situation. Subtle differences in behaviour and conditions can result in large changes in heat loss, as the body switches from convective cooling in water, through evaporative cooling of wet surfaces in air, to dry convective cooling. The delayed evaporative cooling of sweat-soaked garments after exercise is also difficult to quantify, but of potentially great significance in those working hard in cold conditions.

Siple and Passell[2] were the first to attempt to incorporate dry bulb air temperature and wind speed into a single figure, now commonly referred to as 'wind chill equivalent temperature' (Table 49.1). Models for this vary and none is

> **Box 49.2 Some occupations with recognized thermal challenges**
>
> - Cold
>   - farmers, forestry workers and all other outdoor workers in temperate winter and colder conditions;
>   - construction and ground workers;
>   - delivery drivers and postal delivery workers;
>   - fishery workers, including fish farmers;
>   - food processors in chilled environments, including fish filleters;
>   - divers;
>   - cold store workers, now including maintenance engineers within cold stores;
>   - emergency service personnel working outdoors in all weathers;
>   - military personnel.
> - Heat
>   - foundry and hot metal workers;
>   - miners;
>   - welders and fabricators;
>   - firefighters;
>   - chemical and other hot process workers;
>   - radiation, decontamination and other workers required to wear occlusive clothing;
>   - aircrew wearing occlusive clothing in hot climates;
>   - athletes training or competing in warm or hot climates;
>   - military personnel.

universally applicable, despite considerable efforts to improve on the original work by Steadman and others in North America; for example, the cooling effect of wind depends greatly on whether the individual is wearing windproof clothing. Another crucial factor is that windchill to freeze fingers is acting over very different physical dimensions to that chilling clothed bodies, and it is not possible to derive a single index capable of expressing such disparate risks. However, these models usually give a useful first approximation of cold stress.

Assessment of cold strain

Any fall in core temperature below 35°C, the accepted threshold for hypothermia, is the best guide to a serious degree of general cold strain. Rectal measurement, at least 10 cm and preferably 15 cm beyond the anal sphincter, is the most reliable in cold conditions, though tympanic, oesophageal, gastric, vaginal, deep arterial and deep venous sites can each be used in different circumstances; detailed discussion is given in ISO 9886.[3] All require careful calibration of probes and measures to prevent the transmission of infections, such as HIV. Oral temperature is never reliable in

Table 49.1 Wind chill equivalent temperatures (°C)

Wind speed				Dry bulb air temperature (°C)							
Beaufort	miles/h	kt	m/s	−1	−7	−12	−18	−23	−29	−34	−40
0	0	0	0	−1	−7	−12	−18	−23	−29	−34	−40
2	4	3	2	−3	−9	−15	−21	−26	−32	−38	−44
3	9	8	4	−9	−16	−23	−30	−36	−43	−50	−57
4	13	12	6	−14	−21	−29	−36	−43	−50	−58	−65
4	17	15	8	−16	−24	−32	−40	−47	−55	−63	−71
5	22	19	10	−18	−26	−34	−42	−51	−59	−67	−76
6	26	23	12	−19	−28	−36	−44	−53	−61	−70	−79
6	35	31	16	−21	−30	−38	−46	−55	−64	−73	−82
										Wind chill equivalent temperature (°C)	

Derived from the work of Siple and Passell,[2] applicable to naked exposed fingers. The equivalent temperature indicated in the main body of the table for a given combination of wind speed (at the left) and dry bulb temperature (at the top) is claimed to be that at which there is an equal rate of heat loss, given a wind speed of 0 m/s. For example, at a wind speed of 15 kt and a dry bulb air temperature of −12°C, the wind chill equivalent temperature is indicated to be −32°C, i.e. the risk of cold injury is the same as that for a wind speed of 0 kt and a dry bulb temperature of −32°C.

the cold, as it is depressed by cold saliva, and infrared tympanic techniques are likely to be dangerously misleading.[4]

Skin temperatures can give warning of lesser degrees of general cold strain, and are necessary measures of local cold strain, particularly when there is a risk of cold injury. Techniques are based on thermistors or thermocouples, or infrared emission measurement systems for uncovered skin. Repeated efforts have been made to estimate core temperature from measurements of skin temperature taken under insulation. In cold environments at least, these are doomed to failure because of the great variation in subcutaneous insulation and local skin blood flow. Electromyography (EMG) and oxygen uptake can be used to assess shivering and total metabolic heat production, although these are of limited value outside the laboratory.

Adaptation and habituation

Repeated brief exposures to cold produce clear reductions in both the vasoconstrictor and metabolic responses to cold stress. A course of just eight repeated cold (15°C for 40 minutes) immersions has been shown to attenuate the initial hyperventilation and tachycardia found during the initial responses to cold immersion.[5] Adaptation of more sustained responses has been seen to be more variable and difficult to demonstrate, although they may play a part in the physiology peculiar to long-distance sea swimmers,[6] and in the reduced response to cold by aboriginal peoples in Australia and Ama divers. It may be that this 'hypothermic' adaptation has an advantage in increasing comfort during cold exposure, in particular permitting sleep, though it could be hazardous in cold exposure of longer duration. Many other attempts to demonstrate central adaptation or acclimatization to prolonged cold have failed to provide clear or consistent effects. The signal exception to this is earlier and more marked cold vasodilatation, which may be a result of reduced vasoconstriction, described in occupational groups subjected to repeated peripheral cold exposure, such as fish filleters.[7]

Freezing cold injury

Local freezing of tissues, the most rapid and dramatic form of cold injury, may occur when people are exposed to temperatures below 0°C without adequate protection or opportunities to return to warm environments when the extremities become chilled.

The areas most commonly affected include fingers and toes, followed by nose, cheeks and ears, and occasionally the male genitalia. The last can occur in association with excessive consumption of alcohol or drugs of abuse, or as a result of running without windproof underwear.[8] Such injuries may be associated with hypothermia, in which case the potentially life-threatening condition must be treated first, or with local or general trauma.[9] Although most commonly seen in wartime and the military, freezing cold injury is also seen in those undertaking winter sports and in outdoor workers in cold climes, sometimes when the air temperature is not particularly low.[10] Cases can occur in those working in cold stores and other processing plants. Those who now appear most vulnerable are maintenance engineers, who may need to work with limited hand protection, and lubricants may contaminate their clothing and reduce the effectiveness of its insulation. The damage is mainly caused by high concentrations of electrolytes left in tissue fluids when most of the water turns to ice. While frozen, the skin is white and hard; on thawing, there is first hyperaemia and then, in severe cases, pallor and a woody feel to the skin as local blood vessels become occluded by red cells.

FROSTNIP

'Frostnip' is popularly used to describe mild freezing cold injury in which the superficial tissues (that are the only layer affected) recover completely within 30 minutes of starting rewarming; such recovery must include the return of normal sensation. Classically, it involves any combination of the loss of peripheral sensation and the slight freezing of superficial tissues. Typically, one or more finger or toe tips are blanched, the skin is leathery to the touch, but not of wooden feel (which usually indicates deeper freezing) and anaesthetic. The immediate and diagnostic treatment is to rewarm the affected periphery against the warm skin of an understanding colleague; hands and feet may conveniently be placed in an axilla or groin, whilst portions of the nose, cheeks or ears are best rewarmed by firm contact with a hand or fur patch on the back of a mitten. Rubbing, massage and direct heat should be avoided. Provided that recovery is complete within the 30-minute period, no further treatment is necessary. However, those who have not returned to normal should then be treated for superficial frostbite.[11] Thereby hangs the dilemma in that this diagnosis is dependent on the outcome to field treatment; an adverse outcome has serious consequences in terms of further management. Anyone who suffers recurrent episodes of frostnip should be suspected of having a more significant problem and withdrawn from further cold exposure.

SUPERFICIAL FROSTBITE

More severe freezing injury that would not recover so rapidly is usually termed 'frostbite'. If confined to the skin and most peripheral layers of tissue, it can usefully be qualified as being 'superficial'. Initial appearances may be indistinguishable from frostnip, but in the hours and days following thawing, gross discoloration may occur, with haemorrhagic patches and blisters with fluid varying from clear serous exudate to the frankly haemorrhagic. Later still, small and superficial areas of dry gangrene may develop, with skin peeling and nail loss.

The standard treatment for superficial frostbite remains conservative. Rapid rewarming in a stirred waterbath at 38–41°C should be prolonged and thorough, with good analgesic cover.[12] Care must be taken to ensure that patches do not remain partially defrosted on removal from the waterbath. For some, rewarming is an exquisitely painful process that may even merit titration with intravenous morphine, but non-narcotic analgesics normally suffice. Although objective evidence of other beneficial effects is still needed, moderate quantities of alcohol can reduce the requirement for analgesia and improve general well-being, and a twice daily 'tot' is recommended. Infection must be prevented with liberal use of topical anti-bacterials, such as those based on chlorhexidine gluconate, preferably in combination with twice daily 'whirlpool' baths at 40°C. Tetanus prophylaxis is also required in most cases, although systemic antibiotics are normally only considered when there is active infection or deeper tissues are involved. Unfortunately, those with substantial areas of necrotic tissue are at risk of developing antibiotic-resistant hospital infections: the advice of a specialist in infection control is recommended at an early stage in management.

Blisters should not be burst or aspirated because of the risk of infection, unless a high standard of asepsis can be maintained. Their resolution will be aided by the elevation of the injured part, which should be kept comfortably warm, but not too hot. Early physiotherapy to restore functional movement is very important, particularly when hands are affected, as is the restraining of overenthusiastic surgeons; in the absence of any other threat to the injured tissues, surgery should be avoided for at least four and preferably six months. Careful conservative management will normally result in the loss of much less tissue than might originally be expected from appearances in the first few weeks after injury. One decisive factor is the avoidance of premature or incomplete rewarming. In spite of the diagnostic definition of frostnip, rewarming should never be attempted until it is certain that further freezing cannot occur and that the affected part will not be used or further damaged. For this reason, rewarming is generally best avoided in remote areas, unless the casualty can be evacuated by stretcher and in guaranteed warmth.

An almost complete lack of good clinical trials of adjuvant drugs makes it impossible to recommend pharmacological intervention. Different groups have advocated colloidal infusions, various vasodilators, even derivatives of snake venoms. To date, the only addition to the conservative regimen that might hold promise is the use of aloe vera-derived inhibitors of thromboxane, but few are licensed and evidence remains scant.[12]

DEEP AND COMPLICATED FROSTBITE

Freezing of muscles and other deeper tissues, including their blood vessels, is much rarer and more serious. Almost unseen in ordinary working situations, it is mainly a product of wartime and occasionally in mountaineering accidents. Whole limbs may freeze solid and victims are invariably hypothermic. Rapid rewarming should only be attempted in hospital under full biochemical control, as massive release of potassium from damaged cells can otherwise cause sudden death. Surgical decompression of tissue spaces may be needed before rewarming, to limit the rise of tissue pressures which results from the volume expansion accompanying the melting of ice crystals. The amount of tissue likely to be dead or dying demands the utmost care in preventing tetanus, gas gangrene and resistant infections.[13] Even so, proper conservative management may result in the salvage of much of the limb.[14]

Cyclical freezing, thawing and refreezing is even more destructive of cells, and can result in the very worst end result. Early and radical amputation, at two to three months following injury, may be preferred in these cases, as it might in established infections.[12]

LONG-TERM SEQUELAE OF FREEZING COLD INJURY

Military campaigns and civil disaster, such as an earthquake in winter, may leave swathes of the population recovering from the acute effects of freezing cold injury. Although often not as severe as the long-term consequences of non-freezing cold injury, those resulting from freezing injuries may be just as frequent.[11,15] Reviews of veterans as long as 45 years after their original injuries reveal many suffering from chronic problems as a result.

The most common sequelae include cold sensitization (which is more usually associated with non-freezing cold injury, see below), chronic pain, residual neurological defects that rarely may involve loss of proprioception rather than touch, joint pain and stiffness, hyperhidrosis, skin and nail abnormalities. Radiographic examination may reveal characteristic appearances of 'frostbite arthritis', but long-term changes in gait may be more commonly responsible for overuse injuries in more proximal joints, particularly in the lower limb. Although hyperhidrosis may lead to chronic fungal infection, the skin is often dry and scaly, and may crack painfully; topical application of lanolin cream, or preparations intended for the care of cows' udders, can alleviate this. Fungal infections of the nails may respond little to treatment and, together with disturbances of nail growth, can result in thickening and frank onychogryphosis, making a high standard of podiatry essential if mobility is to be maintained.

More unusual sequelae include recurrent ulceration and breakdown of old scars, which may in turn lead to an increased risk of local skin cancers. It is not clear whether this is specifically related to the frostbite or is common to other causes of recurrent ulceration. Although rare, complete local loss of proprioception is a neurological abnormality that is characteristic of old cold injury. In the hands, this can make dressing very hard, while in the feet it may threaten mobility.

Non-freezing cold injury

Longer exposures to less severe temperatures, particularly when coupled with other conditions liable to cause circulatory stasis, can result in injuries that appear generally mild in comparison with frostbite. A wide variety of terms have been applied to non-freezing cold injury (NFCI) since it was first described in the eighteenth century, including trench foot, immersion foot, shelter limb and Flanders foot, depending on the circumstances in which the variant was described. It often coexists with freezing injury, but in spite of its apparent innocence during the acute phase, NFCI frequently results in more severe long-term sequelae. In common with freezing injuries, NFCI is overtly more frequent in certain ethnic groups, most notably Africans and Caribbeans, even when their antecedents migrated to colder areas, such as northern Europe. However, most recent studies in the British army[16] have shown that previously reported relative incidences of up to five times those of Caucasian groups, found with freezing injuries, may be underestimates: African and Caribbean groups were found to have a relative incidence of NFCI of 30 compared to Caucasians, and they appeared to suffer more severe injuries too.

The great majority of cases of NFCI affect the feet alone, although recent series in the UK claim that a quarter of cases are found to have suffered NFCI of the hands as well as the feet. Apart from military personnel in cold wet climates, the main groups affected by classical NFCI are survivors in the water, in liferafts, or during flooding. Immersion of a hand for as little as 45 minutes in water at 0°C may produce mild NFCI, but three hours are needed to result in overt injury. Because seawater freezes at a temperature below 0°C (normally around $-1.9°C$), tissues immersed in very cold seawater may sustain freezing rather than non-freezing injury. Although circumstantial evidence points to dependence on a function of duration of exposure and low temperature, variation between individuals may obscure this. In the same person, the same injury might result from a short period at a low temperature, or a longer period exposed to a milder temperature. There also appear to be relationships with other similar conditions: long immersion in luke-warm water results in 'paddy foot', which is clinically indistinguishable from NFCI. The pathogenesis of these conditions remains obscure; factors that have been proposed include the direct effect of cooling on nerves, prolonged ischaemia during cold exposure and the liberation of reactive oxygen compounds during reperfusion. Some or all of these may be important in the evolution of vibration injuries, complex regional pain syndromes (formerly known as reflex sympathetic dystrophy) and other similar syndromes.[12]

PRESENTATION AND MANAGEMENT

Clinical appearances have been divided into four stages:

1. Injury: in which the foot is very cold, ischaemic and numb.
2. Rewarming: in which the foot becomes mottled blue-pink and exquisitely painful.
3. Hyperaemia: in which the pulses are full and bounding, but there is slow capillary refill, there is marked swelling, some degree of anaesthesia and paraesthesia, and severe pain (primarily nocturnal).
4. Recovery: in which the foot gradually returns towards normal, with residual sequelae including cold sensitization.

Stage 1 is seen throughout the period in which the injury is actually occurring, ranging from minutes to days in duration. It is therefore usually only witnessed by the patient, who may provide the diagnostic description of numbness or other sensory impairment. Stage 2 is seen fleetingly during rewarming, typically lasting just a few minutes. The great majority of cases present in stage 3, which lasts for several days or weeks. Stage 4 may then supervene for months, years, possibly lifelong.

Although NFCI is best managed using similar conservative principles to those for freezing injury, it has been established that rapid rewarming in a waterbath exacerbates both damage and pain. Slow (or 'passive') rewarming is therefore preferred. The management of early pain can be fraught: bedclothes should be cradled over the feet at night and conventional analgesics are invariably ineffective. Although it has never undergone formal trialling, and in most countries is beyond the normal licensed indications, the standard approach is to give a single daily dose of amitriptyline (25–150 mg) in the evening, much as is used for the treatment of other types of neuropathic pain. Morphine does not affect the pain but the patient no longer cares about the discomfort, while regional analgesia is highly effective but short-lived.[12] Patients who do not obtain good relief from amitriptyline alone can be tried on a combination of 10-mg amitriptyline at night together with pregabalin, the latter prescribed in accordance with the recommendations of a current formulary. Achieving good early pain relief is very important if chronic pain is to be avoided, and the involvement of a specialist in pain management may be valuable. However, experience with sympathetic blocks or sympathectomy is generally very discouraging and they should normally be avoided.

Late consequences are common and may last for life, even after subclinical NFCI. Most prominent is a prolonged vasoconstrictive response to further cold exposure; when a patient complains of this as a symptom, it is termed 'cold sensitivity', but assumes a diagnosis of 'cold sensitization' when supported by physical findings. A cold stimulus as innocuous as a 2-minute immersion in water at 15°C may precipitate a cold, vasoconstricted foot for four or more hours afterwards. This predisposes to further injury and is a prime reason for following up those who have sustained NFCI and investigating those claiming cold sensitivity.

The cause of cold sensitization remains ill understood. It was originally supposed that it resulted from a sympathetic denervation supersensitivity, but most recent assessment of other sympathetic nerve function in sensitized feet has shown this not to be the case. The cause may lie in a vascular endothelial abnormality (and NFCI is known to result in endothelial injury) or the devascularization which is known to arise when local blood flow is chronically reduced. No effective treatment is known, although exposure to heat may be ameliorative. This can be accomplished by living in a tropical country for some years, or possibly by bathing the affected parts in water at 40°C for at least 30 minutes every day; again trials are needed. Severe cases may enjoy slow and slight benefit from sustained release nifedipine, but it is hard to achieve therapeutic benefit without troubling side effects. Other long-term sequelae are common and include those mentioned for freezing cold injury above.[12] Because of the risk of long-term alteration in gait and resulting overuse injury, early and expert assessment of gait should be considered in those who have sustained NFCI of the feet.

Hypothermia on land

Taken across the working population as a whole, hypothermia is comparatively rare without immersion, and as a cause of death it is quite unusual. Even in social groups deemed to be at particular risk, notably the very young and very old in poorer circumstances, hypothermia is considerably less common than is usually portrayed. In those of working age, cases tend to occur in clusters when groups involved in military or leisure activities are exposed to particularly harsh conditions, frequently in association with inadequate planning and preparation.

On land, its onset is usually gradual, over a period of hours, when heat loss is greatly increased by evaporation from precipitation, previous immersion or accumulated sweat, but heat production is falling due to physical exhaustion. In many cases, victims have been maintaining thermal balance by hard physical exertion and then start to tire; as their fatigue causes them to reduce the rate of work, heat loss starts to exceed heat production and core temperature falls. Inadequate replenishment of energy and fluid, insufficient physical fitness, and previous alcohol intake (which can produce sustained hypoglycaemia)[17] are all common predisposing factors.

Detailed clinical descriptions of hypothermia and its management are given elsewhere.[18] In the field, actions should be directed at reducing further heat loss and evacuating the casualty. Although the risks associated with rough handling are thought to be lower on land than following immersion, evacuation should be careful and considered rather than rushed. Those providing assistance should not neglect the risk of others in the party succumbing to hypothermia: it may be necessary for them to be placed in shelter, or for their evacuation after that of the immediate casualties. Issues relating to rewarming are discussed below.

Immersion hypothermia and 'cold shock'

Immersion poses more threats beyond hypothermia alone. Many of those who die in the water do so because of drowning, although even then this simple diagnosis obscures a complex causal sequence. Golden and Hervey[19] have divided up the hazards of cold immersion into four phases according to the time since entry into the water.

Sudden immersion in cold water produces dramatic physiological responses that have been reviewed by Tipton.[20] In the great majority of adults, any tendency to the potentially protective effects of the 'diving response' is usually overwhelmed by an inspiratory gasp followed by hyperventilation, tachycardia and peripheral vasoconstriction. If trapped in a ditched helicopter, flooding building or capsized vessel, useful breath-hold time diminishes almost to zero, making underwater escape almost impossible; underwater breathing apparatus (particularly if not based on pressurized gas, with its concomitant risk of arterial gas embolism) can be invaluable in enabling successful escape. Hyperventilation not only makes the inhalation of water, thus primary drowning, more likely, but its effects on blood chemistry can be disabling. Cardiovascular responses may be dramatic, such as the sudden onset of lethal cardiac arrhythmia, and combine to produce a sharp rise in blood pressure, which may be sufficient to burst arterial aneurysms.

Those who survive the first 2–3 minutes of cold water immersion and thus suffer 'cold shock', may drown in the ensuing 10–15 minutes, apparently failing to swim even though they may be close to safety. Such 'swimming failure' is largely independent of warm water swimming ability and appears related to the direct cooling of peripheral nerves (making muscular control harder), failure to synchronize breathing with swim-stroke and other subtle effects. It is only when the casualty has been immersed for more than about 20 minutes that immersion hypothermia becomes a serious threat, and even then it may lead to disablement and thus drowning long before core temperatures reach lethal levels below about 28°C.

Divers have been claimed to be prone to two forms of hypothermia that may occur with minimal physiological responses. One may affect saturation divers who are dependent on careful control of breathing gas temperature and their hot water suits to maintain thermal balance.[21] If their inspired gas is slightly too cool, large amounts of heat could be lost from the core, while skin temperatures are held high. In the absence of stimulus to the peripheral cold receptors, the body may make little or no physiological response to the falling core temperature. The other form of insidious hypothermia may affect slightly underdressed free-swimming divers in water temperatures between about 20 and 25°C. Although cold enough to result in falling core temperature, such water may not elicit any sensation of cold, and once again peripheral vasoconstriction and shivering may not occur. These conditions remain controversial, and extensive review of thermal aspects of diving is sceptical of their occurrence in real life.[22]

The hazards of immersion do not stop when rescue starts. As high as 20 per cent of all those conscious, but thought to be hypothermic at the time of rescue, die during the following minutes. Golden et al.[23] have reviewed the causes, which are related to the mode of rescue and subsequent treatment. Because the ailing circulation receives substantial hydrostatic support during immersion, during which the margin for cardiac compensation is being eroded, vertical modes of recovery can result in sudden loss of venous return and complete circulatory collapse. The adoption of horizontal modes of rescue, such as double rescue strops, can reduce this risk, provided that they do not compromise the chances of successful recovery.

Another risk following rescue is that of rewarming collapse, which appears to be the result of peripheral vasodilatation during rewarming. For this reason, casualties should not be left unattended nor rewarmed in an upright position, for example a shower. Hot baths are often the method of choice for those who are cold, but not clinically hypothermic. Aggressive or active rewarming techniques should be avoided unless they are applied in sophisticated medical facilities, such as intensive therapy units; they may hasten complex and life-threatening problems during rewarming, and good evidence that they improve outcome is still lacking. Another pitfall is the decision to start external cardiac massage (ECM) should it be thought that cardiac output is insufficient in the hypothermic. Because this is likely to precipitate ventricular fibrillation (if still alive), and the cold heart cannot be defibrillated, starting ECM commits the first-aider to maintaining it – effectively – until the casualty is delivered to a place of definitive care. If this will only take 30 minutes, ECM may prove life-saving; if evacuation could take many hours or even days, it is probably wisest to avoid starting ECM for this reason.

Those who have inhaled insufficient water to cause primary drowning may exhibit signs of adult respiratory distress during the first one to three days after immersion; this is secondary drowning and requires immediate aggressive intensive therapy. All those who have become immersed and could have aspirated water, and thus could be at risk of secondary drowning, should be cautioned of the unlikely chance of the condition, and the need to seek medical aid as a matter of urgency.

The ideal protection from cold immersion is an integrated survival system, consisting of personal protective equipment to provide appropriate buoyancy and thermal protection, if necessary with underwater escape supported by a breathing system.[24] Those who may need to hold their breath to permit escape to the surface can have their initial responses attenuated by cold habituation, for example a daily cold shower,[5] or even psychological skills training.[25] It would appear that surfers, kayakers and others who submerge themselves out of choice have already learned their own techniques for coping with cold shock, including habituation and breath-hold training.

For longer-term survival, as when abandoning a ship in the ocean, dry-shod entry into a seaworthy and thermally effective liferaft should be the goal.

The prediction of survival during immersion is very important in determining how long search and rescue efforts should be maintained. As immersion incidents commonly happen when sea and weather conditions are most threatening to those engaged in searching, accurate prediction not only determines the cost of expensive assets such as helicopters, but also the risk to which the rescuers are exposed. National coastguard manuals include aids for the prediction of survival during immersion, and these should improve considerably in the coming years with the ongoing analysis of a large survey of immersion incidents in UK waters.[26] Traditional approaches to survival prediction generally work best in colder water temperatures, below 20°C. In warmer waters, in particular, there are many survivors' accounts of very long periods of complete or partial immersion that imply that several days could be the norm. However, the strong currents associated with movement of floodwater, and rough seas encountered during shipwrecks, appear much less forgiving, with high death tolls. There is an urgent need for objective study of this area.

The effect of cold on performance

Although opinion and anecdote invariably assert the deleterious effects of cold on a wide range of aspects of human performance,[27] objective assessments are less frequent and not as clear-cut.[28] There are many methodological problems to be overcome before the body of scientific evidence can be considered to be substantial enough either to confirm opinion or to modify it. The presence of large variations between individuals and differences between performances of the same individual on different occasions, have been of particular hindrance. Broadly speaking, cold has been described as impairing three different aspects of performance: sensory, motor and higher brain function. The first two are commonly combined in measures of dexterity, which are reduced either by cooling, or by the protective clothing worn to prevent cooling. Where studies have been able to show significant effects on dexterity, they are usually related to both local and central cooling.[29] In actual occupational settings, impairment of performance is commonly a result of many factors. The combination of cold, physical exertion and protective clothing can be particularly dangerous, as rest periods may result in rapid and severe peripheral cooling,[30] while the metabolic cost of submaximal work increases and maximal aerobic performance falls.

Observations that accident rates increase during cold periods of the year[27] are too crude to permit conclusions to be drawn about the influence of moderate cold on higher mental functions. However, a particularly disturbing study by Coleshaw et al.[31] demonstrated that even slight levels of body cooling (above those diagnosed as hypothermia) can have dramatic effects on simple measures of mental function, such as memory registration and the speed of reasoning.

HEAT STRESS

Assessment of heat stress

Because of the greater capacity for warm air to contain water vapour and the importance of evaporative heat loss in higher temperatures, the simple dry measures made in cold environments are insufficient to assess warmer conditions quantitatively. The one exception to this is when personnel are clad almost entirely in impermeable clothing, as they might be when working in toxic or radioactive environments, for instance. Then the exclusion of evaporative heat transfer permits simplification of the measurements detailed below.

Most measures of heat stress therefore attempt to combine weighted values of dry bulb temperature with some estimate of humidity, together with radiant heat load and sometimes other variables. Although different indices come into vogue at different times and for different purposes, that with perhaps the best all-round record is the wet bulb globe temperature (WBGT) index, which also has the advantage of being simple to compute and easily measured with compact instruments. More detailed work may require a psychrometric chart on which the relationship between air temperature, moisture content and relative humidity is shown. Body heat production is again important, and can be measured in the field by expired gas analysis using a portable respiratory system, or more crudely estimated from activity levels against standard scales. Methods for doing this are given in ISO 8996.[32]

WET BULB GLOBE TEMPERATURE INDEX

ISO 7243[33] prescribes a standard method for the estimation of heat stress using three temperature measurements: those of a standard dry bulb, a wet bulb and one inside a blackened globe of 150-mm diameter. The three temperatures are combined into the WBGT index using the following equation:

$$WBGT = 0.7T_{wet\ bulb} + 0.2T_{globe} + 0.1T_{dry\ bulb}$$

Under this ISO standard, it is permissible to ignore the dry bulb temperature if there is little difference between it and that of the globe (e.g. indoors with little radiant heat load), in which case the equation becomes:

$$Indoor\ WBGT = 0.7T_{wet\ bulb} + 0.3T_{globe}$$

The standard provides a set of reference index values for five levels of metabolic rate for both acclimatized and unacclimatized people, which may be of value in assessing the relative stress. For example, on a warm summer's day in a temperate climate the dry bulb temperature may rise as high as 34°C. When the relative humidity remains low, at 40 per cent, the wet bulb will remain low at 24°C. In full shade, the globe temperature should be close to that of the dry bulb, giving a WBGT index of 27, the threshold for sustaining moderate exercise in acclimatized individuals. If the air is wetter, with a higher relative humidity, the wet bulb will be higher, hence the WBGT index will exceed that threshold and make it impossible to exercise for long. In the full radiant heat load of the sun, the globe temperature will soar, with similar effects on WBGT index and exercise.

Related indices can be derived for environments in which formal measurement of the WBGT index are not possible. For example, Nunneley and Stribley[34] developed a 'fighter index of thermal stress' (FITS) for the cockpit of aircraft at low altitude, but using measurements taken at ground level on clear days:

$$FITS = 0.83T_{psychrometric\ wet\ bulb} + 0.35T_{dry\ bulb} + 5.08$$

Unfortunately, none of the temperatures used to derive the WBGT index is routinely measured in standard

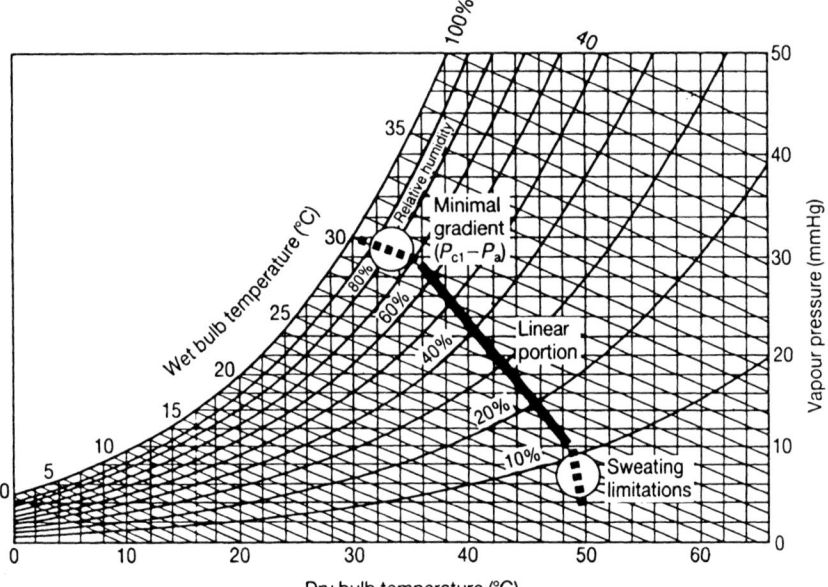

Figure 49.1 A psychrometric chart. The grid is laid over a graph of water vapour pressure against dry bulb air temperature. On this, curves of equal percentage relative to humidity are superimposed, as are lines of equal wet bulb temperature. Thus, the graph may be entered using any pair of dry bulb air temperature, water vapour pressure, relative humidity or wet bulb temperature. For a given garment assembly and work rate, it is possible to plot a straight line which determines the upper limit of the exposure envelope, marked as the 'linear portion' in this figure. Those conditions to the left of and below this line are acceptable. However, there are two additional linear segments which are also shown: at higher relative humidities, the small vapour pressure gradient from clothing to ambient limits tolerance, whilst at low relative humidities sweating endurance is limited and thus restricts the envelope.

meteorological practice, nor can normal meteorological forecast variables be substituted into the WBGT equation. However, work has been undertaken to permit estimation of the three input temperatures from normal forecast variables, and it is likely that some meteorological centres will produce WBGT forecasts in the future. It remains to be seen whether this becomes commonplace as average temperatures rise.

PSYCHROMETRIC CHARTS

In many situations, radiant heat loads are fairly small in comparison to the heat exchange by convection and evaporation. The psychrometric chart (ironically derived from the Greek *psychron* meaning cold), reproduced in Figure 49.1, is a clear graphical way of understanding the effect of changing humidity and temperatures alone. Use of the chart requires a measurement of the water content of the air (e.g. by some form of psychrometer capable of yielding relative or absolute humidity values) and the dry bulb temperature. Limits may be defined on the chart appropriate to a given group of individuals for specified activities and clothing, thus allowing the user to make recommendations as to how their physiological requirements may be met. The chart may also be used to understand the relative effects of lowering air temperature and humidity when trying to control an environment.

OTHER INDICES

Although the WBGT index is simple to measure quite accurately, it is only indirectly linked with heat strain. In most circumstances, operators prefer to employ measures that can give a more direct assessment of heat strain, and to this end many alternatives have been proposed. These have been compared by Parsons[35] and more formally in ISO 11399.[36] A potentially very attractive approach to the assessment of heat stress is to attempt to relate it to the amount of evaporative heat loss required for thermal balance; this was originally incorporated into a 'predicted 4-hour sweat rate' (P4SR), but has more recently evolved into the required sweat rate and 'predicted heat strain', as defined in ISO 7933.[37] Measurement essentially consists of a semi-empirical solution of the equation of heat balance, to arrive at an estimate of the sweat rate required for the maintenance of thermal equilibrium. It is thus considerably more complex than the WBGT index and more suited to experimental investigations rather than routine monitoring. The latest studies have confirmed its efficacy in predicting averages and limits to exposure,[38] although modifications have been required to the calculation of the evaporative efficiency of sweating.[39]

More moderate thermal stress may need to be assessed by more complex methods than the simple WBGT index, as the transfer of heat by each physical mode is usually more sensitive to subtle changes. Detailed accounts of the 'predicted mean vote' (PMV) and predicted percentage of dissatisfied (PPD) indices are given in ISO 7730,[40] based on measurements of air temperature, mean radiant temperature, humidity, air velocity, metabolic rate and clothing insulation. Indeed, in any situation in which clothed individuals are being assessed, reference will need to be made to the estimation of the thermal insulation and resistance to evaporative heat loss imposed by clothing; ISO 9920[41] provides a sound practical basis for this.

Assessment of heat strain

The principal measurement of heat strain, like that of cold, is core body temperature. However, core temperature can rise rapidly in the heat and the fact that rectal temperature changes later and more slowly than other sites makes it less suitable for safety purposes. Accordingly, it is more common to estimate deep body temperature in the heat from a tympanic membrane or auditory canal reading; this has the added advantage that this site should usually be a good indicator of the temperature of the brain, which is not only the central temperature controller, but is also one of the more critical organs in heat illness. Unfortunately, the otherwise convenient infrared tympanic membrane thermometers that have become so popular in general clinical practice are again a potential source of error, and should not be trusted: a thermistor or thermocouple needs to be placed just short of the tympanic membrane, and the auditory meatus occluded and carefully insulated if the temperature recorded is to be a reliable estimate of core temperature.

Three other variables are commonly recorded in heat studies: heart rate is the simplest of all to measure, loss of body mass due to sweating is also very easily determined, whilst skin temperatures are sometimes of value if judiciously interpreted.

Heart rate is well correlated with heat strain, provided that changes due to exercise are taken into consideration. It is often used, in conjunction with aural temperature, in establishing criteria for the withdrawal of people exposed to heat loads. The simple estimate of body weight loss is a useful measure of fluid loss in laboratory conditions. Skin temperatures can prove misleading, as they fall if there is good evaporation from the skin, but climb close to core if evaporation is limited or absent. These methods are described in ISO 9886.[3]

Acclimatization

Temperate residents cannot perform as well under heat stress as those used to living in the tropics. Careful studies during the middle of the twentieth century demonstrated that unacclimatized temperate residents show significant acclimatization after only two weeks of exposure to heat.[42] This can be produced by prolonged exposure to an environmental heat load (e.g. by living in the tropics or working in hot conditions) or by repeatedly raising the body temperature by undertaking sustained physical exercise, or by a combination of both. Pure fitness training produces similar changes to heat acclimatization and so improves tolerance to heat stress.

During the first week of acclimatization, the ability of the body to sweat is increased, so that thermal sweating occurs more rapidly under heat stress, and the amount of sweat produced is increased. Cardiovascular changes sustain peripheral vasodilatation and the blood flow required by active sweat glands. Salt is retained by the kidneys and salt content of the sweat declines, so that increased sweating does not result in severe hyponatraemia. Consequently, some individuals may need to increase dietary salt intake slightly during the first week of acclimatization, but seldom after that. It should be noted that required water intake may actually be increased in those who are acclimatized: popular belief that those conditioned to living in the tropics are also able to do without water, or even worse to substitute alcohol, is completely erroneous.

The process of acclimatization continues more gradually over the remainder of the first three months or so spent in the tropics, at the end of which the temperate-born individual is almost physiologically indistinct from those who have spent their entire lives under a heat stress. However, behavioural adaptation, in which dress and habits are changed to those most appropriate in the heat, may never occur.

De-acclimatization can occur surprisingly rapidly, after just a few days of withdrawal from heat stress. Those who spend a period working in air-conditioned comfort, or who return to more temperate climates for a holiday, therefore need to undergo supervised re-acclimatization on their return to heat exposure. This introduces a dilemma in choosing optimal living and working conditions in hot climates: while many find it more comfortable and sleep better in conditioned accommodation, more constant exposure to heat stress will maintain a better level of acclimatization.

Immediate consequences of heat strain

The continuing popularity of prolonged physical exercise in temperate climates, such as marathons and triathlons in the populous countries of the northern hemisphere, reinforces the need to move away from the traditional classification of heat illness. The latter, evolved during British Imperial days, endeavoured to distinguish acute, subacute and chronic disorders involving overheating, and water and electrolyte losses in a complex and probably misleading terminology. Setting aside a few discrete disorders, such as prickly heat and salt and water deficiencies, true heat illness can be spread along a continuum from heat exhaustion to heat stroke.[43] At the one extreme, this consists of little change in body temperature and overt hyperventilation, and at the other, a core temperature in excess of 41°C, absence of sweating and complete circulatory collapse. Patients can move rapidly from minor heat exhaustion to life-threatening heat stroke; so no matter how mild the symptoms may appear to be, anyone suffering from a heat illness should be considered to be in incipient heat stroke and thus in imminent danger of death.

HEAT EXHAUSTION

Heat exhaustion is typified by the moderately well-trained athlete competing in a marathon during the warmer months in a temperate country. It may also be seen in military personnel during fitness training in similar conditions and in groups of manual workers with moderate environmental heat loads. The first sign of impending heat exhaustion is usually hyperventilation, in someone who appears ill at ease with the exercise that they are performing.[43]

Classic signs and symptoms from the disturbance of the body's acid–base balance and the calcium–phosphate ratio in the blood follow, with dizziness, nausea, paraesthesiae in the peripheries and around the mouth, progressing to confusion, collapse, vomiting and even seizures. Core temperature at this stage is below 40°C, and usually between 37° and 39°C. Early cases respond rapidly to rest in a recumbent position, rebreathing from a paper bag to restore end-tidal CO_2 levels and simple cooling. Fluids may also be beneficial and should always be given by appropriate means. If these patients are allowed or even encouraged to continue exercising, they may rapidly develop frank heat stroke.

HEAT STROKE

Those working in very hot surroundings, particularly when evaporative cooling is ineffective due to high humidity, may undergo a rapid rise in core temperature, to the point at which thermoregulation fails.[44] The classic victim of heat stroke has stopped sweating and is dry to the touch. They may still maintain peripheral circulation and thus be red, or may have undergone circulatory collapse, in which case their skin colour is not diagnostic. They are very hot, semiconscious or comatose, and prone to convulsions, cardiac and respiratory arrest. The onset of this dramatic illness may have been very rapid, although many will have shown evidence of earlier heat exhaustion.

Cooling is best achieved in the field by stripping the patient in the shade, drenching with tepid water and fanning if there is little natural wind. Cold water or ice is less useful in adults because of the intense vasoconstriction which it can precipitate, which limits heat transfer from the core to the skin; however, there are recent claims that ice-water baths may still produce the most rapid fall in core temperature even in adults, as they do in infants with their much greater surface area to volume ratio. Alternating litres of isotonic dextrose and saline intravenously are the best means of fluid administration, but cannot be a substitute for immediate and effective cooling. The precise quantity given may be based on an estimate of fluid loss, but in unconscious cases it is probably best to give the first litre over 15 minutes or less, thereafter reducing the rate of infusion according to clinical indications and the perceived risk of hypervolaemia leading to pulmonary oedema. Such fluids should not be warmed, but neither should they be cooled below 15°C. Elevation of the legs to assist venous return, administration of oxygen and possibly sedatives, are of value. However, vasodilators and platelet inhibitors, such as aspirin, should be avoided. Rapid but careful evacuation to an intensive care unit is essential, where urinary output, blood biochemistry and direct measurement of the central venous pressure can be monitored closely. Cooling is normally discontinued when the rectal or aural temperature has reached 38°C, lest it overshoot. A useful if empirical guide to prognosis is the area under a curve of core temperature against time, during which core temperature exceeds 39°C: the greater the duration and elevation above that temperature, the poorer the likely outcome.

Unfortunately, the outcome of true heat stroke is not good. If core temperature rises to around 45°C, irreversible heat denaturation of proteins causes multiple organ failure or disseminated intravascular coagulation. If this is not immediately fatal, renal dialysis may be necessary during recovery. Heat illness, associated with exercise, can produce subacute rhabdomyolysis (necrosis of muscle) that can in turn lead to late renal failure. Follow up of military personnel who made complete recoveries from an initial episode of heat illness have suggested that subsequent episodes are more common than among those who have not suffered heat illness.[45] However, numbers were small and further work is merited. At least two national armed forces have now introduced work-in-heat testing of those who have suffered an episode of heat illness during military training. Although experience is limited and the optimal test protocol remains controversial, these have enabled the identification of individuals with metabolic disorders related to malignant hyperthermia, cases of anhidrosis and other conditions that predispose to further heat illness.

HYPONATRAEMIA

For much of the nineteenth and twentieth centuries, an important task in preventing heat illness among athletes, service personnel and workers in hot environments has been to encourage the replacement of body fluid lost by sweating with sufficient quantities of aqueous fluid. For a surprisingly long period in history, athletes and others consumed very little in the way of fluid, and the drinks used were often physiologically unsuitable, such as beer or even spirits. In the early decades of professional cycle racing, for instance, some competitors consumed at least a bottle of brandy a day when taking part in arduous stage races, while foundry workers were at one time notorious for drinking many pints of beer during their working day. Recent years have seen a dramatic change, in which fluids are thrust at athletes in particular in considerable quantities, to the point where many are now at risk of becoming hyponatraemic, which can cause collapse, death and severe neurological disturbances in those who survive.[46]

The aim of drinking during exposure to heat stress should be to replace fluid and electrolyte losses in sweat. Even when acclimatized and fit, few humans are capable of losing more than 2 litres an hour in sweat, so drinking should never exceed that rate. Over a typical extended working day, a ceiling of 10–12 litres of fluid intake is advisable. Most western diets provide ample daily sodium intake, but it is common for meals to be lightened or skipped when exercising in the heat. If a normal diet of three meals per day is not maintained, careful consideration needs to be given to supplementation with fluids containing electrolytes so that proper balance can be maintained. This is potentially very complex, and the margins for error can be narrow: injudicious consumption of sports gels and fluids can be as dangerous as inadequate intake of salt. It is far simpler to maintain a normal diet and balanced fluid intake.

OTHER CONDITIONS

Classic salt depletion, due to salt loss in sweat while on a low salt diet, with adequate water intake, is now rarely seen. The classic accompaniment of cramp (e.g. miner's cramp) only occurs in association with hard exercise and is now very unusual. Plasma sodium only falls in more severe cases, with milder cases showing a fall in extracellular fluid volume with normal plasma sodium. In the worst cases, vigorous treatment with oral or intravenous saline may be required. Subacute and other variants of this condition, sometimes attributed to different combinations of water and electrolyte depletion and 'disacclimatization', are similarly uncommon. They are best treated by cooling, rest, rehydration and the restoration of a normal diet. Those whose appetite has been suppressed and who have overindulged in alcohol, should recover quickly in this way. The blind administration of salt, even with the copious quantities of fluid that are required, is potentially dangerous and should be avoided.

One possible danger is that of hyperkalaemia; many young people often rehydrate following exercise in the heat using some form of orange juice, or a 'sports rehydration' fluid, which may be high in potassium. They should be advised to ensure that their rehydration fluid is well diluted with water.

Perhaps the most common of the 'mild' heat disorders is prickly heat or miliaria rubra, which results from blocking of the orifices of sweat glands. Because of the blockage, the glands rupture their ducts, raising a weal within an erythematous area, which is intensely itchy. Removal from the heat both abolishes sweating and prevents the body overheating as a result of its impaired ability to sweat. Other less well-understood conditions which may appear during heat stress include a transient ankle oedema (which may result from the thermal attenuation of the veno-arteriolar reflex) and mild muscular cramps. Some individuals experience dizziness and fainting that may have a common aetiology.

The effect of heat on performance

Reconciling the subjective and objective is no easier for the possible effects of heat than were noted above for cold. Ramsey[47] has reviewed more than 150 studies that attempted to find differences in 'perceptual motor performance' in the heat and commented on the remarkable lack of objective evidence of dominant effects. It appears that there is no significant detectable impairment in the performance of the great majority of tasks until the level of heat stress reaches a WBGT index of approximately 30°C. This is broadly in accordance with the criteria originally laid down by NIOSH in their original recommended exposure limit (REL).[48] Paradoxically, when revised 14 years later, NIOSH omitted this REL because of lack of supporting evidence.[49]

A few studies cast interesting and potentially different light on the area. There is much stronger support for adverse effects in circumstances in which core temperature has risen; when core temperature is 38°C or greater, a prominent effect is an increase in irritability independent of the rise in subjective discomfort.[50] Critics of studies which have used more artificial and perhaps oversimplified measures of performance may find some comfort in the work of Wyon et al.,[51] who examined the effect of moderate heat stress on driving performance. While they observed a heat-related increase in overt driving errors, it was found to occur only in women.

Perhaps the most useful tool (beyond tenuous attempts to relate accident statistics to heat stress or strain) in the practical examination of performance effects is the expression of subjective judgement scales. ISO 10551[52] lays down a standard approach to these, which allows inclusion of comfort, acceptability and tolerance in the assessment of thermal environments.

PRINCIPLES OF THE REDUCTION OF THERMAL STRAIN

Given that there are many industrial processes and situations that could lead to injury or illness resulting from cold or heat, and the potential consequences of such injuries or illnesses, the importance of prevention cannot be overemphasized. In addition to specific remarks in previous sections, the following provides general principles to form the basis of systematic plans for prevention. There are already a number of good examples of codes of practice that illustrate how preventive measures can be implemented.[53–57]

The worker

Working in particularly cold or hot environments makes many demands of the individual. The body and mind may be taken to the limits, something that is often viewed as an attraction for those who voluntarily expose themselves to thermal extremes in their leisure-time pursuits.

Any condition that impairs the physiological mechanisms responsible for compensating for heat or cold stress risks the safety of the individual and thus is contraindicated in workers exposed. Margins for such compensation generally decline with age, although experience in coping behaviourally increases with maturity, and the very young may be limited on both counts. The additional metabolic and cardiovascular demands of pregnancy make exposure to heat stress inadvisable for women during those times. Any form of concurrent illness, especially if febrile, increases risks whether the worker is exposed to heat or cold. The consumption of alcohol or drugs of abuse, even in small quantities, or of most medications, can compromise some or all of the physiological mechanisms; in the case of medication, it needs to be ascertained from recognized pharmacological authorities that the treatment in question is not likely to do this. On the other hand, general physical fitness of a cardiorespiratory or endurance nature is usually a great benefit.

If called upon to assess the fitness of an individual to undergo thermal stress, detailed knowledge of the environment, activities and clothing to be worn are essential. For those undertaking work in the cold, obesity is actually highly undesirable, as it impairs the mobility of someone required to wear already bulky protective clothing, and increases the likelihood of their being subject to heat stress when wearing that clothing. The level of physical fitness required is at least that of a person undertaking the same activity in more comfortable temperatures, while carrying the whole protective clothing ensemble.

Sedentary work in the heat, particularly following acclimatization, is not normally too physically demanding. However, those who have to wear restrictive protective clothing, breathing apparatus, and then have to perform arduous physical work, need to be physically very fit. For example, in both laboratory and field studies of firemen,[58] it is more usual that their ability to carry out work is limited by physical exhaustion than by dangerous elevation of body temperature; factors of particular importance include the duration of work and the use of breathing apparatus. In the face of these demands, firemen should have good pulmonary and cardiovascular function, and significant pathology such as myocardial ischaemia or lung disease should contraindicate further exposure. Formal tests of physical fitness, such as step tests and even the measurement of maximal oxygen uptake, are only guides in the overall assessment of individuals. In all cases, the examining doctor should ask the question as to whether the person presenting for examination is capable of undertaking the specific tasks in the given environment in reasonable safety, and not whether they have achieved an arbitrary standard in an artificial test.

Good progressive training, coupled with conditioning or acclimatization, is very valuable in preparing the individual for work in stressful environments. In the case of heat, every effort should be made to allow personnel to acclimatize before they are required to carry out any exercise in the heat.

Once they do start, the period for which they work should be carefully controlled according to the heat stress and strain, making due allowance for accidents and emergencies which might happen. For example, firefighting teams wearing breathing apparatus are limited in duration by the air supply which they carry with them; this supply should not encourage them to stay so long in the full heat of the fire that they suffer from heat illness, but at the same time it must allow for delays in withdrawing once their anticipated working time is over. The total number of teams should allow for a reasonable number of entries to be made, with adequate cooling and rest periods in between. In some cases, three teams will be needed to provide these breaks, but each team may then be limited in the number of entries that it can make. It should be borne in mind that, in these circumstances, cooling down takes longer than heating up.

In environments in which all other methods have failed and personnel are required to work hard physically, the only solution may be to plan that they undertake only brief periods of work, interspersed with rest periods in which they may cool. Although many factors have to be taken into consideration, guideline WBGT indices above which this may be required are 29–33°C for the sedentary, 24–28°C for those working moderately hard, and 20–26°C for those performing heavy exercise. Those who have acclimatized to the heat can generally tolerate higher temperatures for longer periods (provided that they are both kept well hydrated and are able to sweat effectively), and at higher work rates increased air movement may also reduce heat stress at a given WBGT index. In extremely hot environments, such as coke ovens, it may be necessary to restrict exposure to a very short period, which must be strictly enforced.

Although there is little physiological advantage to progressive training in the cold, it is psychologically and behaviourally of great benefit. Circumstantial evidence suggests that the experienced individual develops many small but very effective techniques for minimizing their cold stress, such as an ability to don and doff clothing quickly and with minimum cooling. The naive person in a cold environment can quickly run into trouble, particularly when things start going wrong or there is an accident or emergency. On the other hand, those who have had adverse effects, such as previous cold injury or any other evidence of cold intolerance, should be prevented from further cold exposure. This includes a small number of people with conditions which predispose to local cold injury, including those with vibration white finger, any form of Raynaud's disease, impaired circulation, skin grafts or other cold sensitivity (whether resulting in excessive vasoconstriction or allergic responses as in cold urticaria). Similarly, those with a history of previous heat illness should only be re-exposed under careful supervision, as further episodes are likely, and anyone with a skin disorder should avoid heat stress, as most will impair thermally effective sweating.

Care also needs to be taken in considering the nature of work to be performed, with regard to the effects of its impairment. In spite of the equivocal results from experimental

> **Box 49.3 The office worker**
>
> Traditionally, legislative requirements for sedentary workers, particularly those in offices, have set a minimum temperature for their environment, but no maximum. It is not hard to arrive at a reasonable minimum temperature based on acceptable dress and the need to keep hands warm enough to undertake typical tasks. However, healthy sedentary workers are physiologically capable of dissipating their metabolic heat output over a wide range of thermal environments. Whether or not an employer deems it acceptable for office workers to have to sweat 2 litres or more over the course of their working day, as long as they maintain adequate hydration and are fit and healthy (and preferably acclimatized to the heat), they should thermoregulate and there should be no danger to their health.
>
> In climates with seasonal differences in environmental heat stress, office environments can follow those changes, to exploit seasonal acclimatization in workers. In the winter, the tendency to wear warmer clothing can be used to lower office temperatures by a couple of degrees below their annual average. Once warmer summer temperatures have become established, office temperatures can be allowed to rise a couple of degrees above annual average. Allowing approximately two weeks lag in these changes of office environment should suffice to allow for changes in clothing and acclimatization.
>
> Careful consideration also needs to be taken of the effects on human performance, social interaction and psychology. In times of austerity, workers have been motivated to try to press on even when wearing multiple layers of heavy clothing and gloves, but current social attitudes would not tolerate that now. Those working under mental rather than physical pressure may deliver their best when their thermal expectations are met, or at least they perceive that they are. Uneven heating or cooling is as likely to result in discomfort and complaints as more uniform discomfort. Consideration must also be given to those whose health is not perfect, or are pregnant, growing old, or have a disability; it is usually necessary to reduce the potential thermal stress posed by an environment to ensure sufficient margin of comfort for those individuals.

> **Box 49.4 Disabilities and thermal stress**
>
> Although other types of disability may have subtle thermal implications, the most prominent considerations need to be given to those with generally impaired mobility, and disabilities that specifically impair thermoregulation.
>
> Mobility impairment usually results in lower average metabolic rates and lower peripheral perfusion, making individuals more susceptible to whole body and peripheral cooling when they are exposed to cold environments with the same thermal protection provided to more mobile workers. This requires consideration in workplace assessment, potentially the provision of more efficient personal protective equipment and shortened periods of exposure to compensate.
>
> The most common disabilities that result in dramatic alteration in thermoregulation are spinal injuries. From the approximate level of the injury distally, normal peripheral vasoconstriction and vasodilatation may be impaired or completely absent. Deprived of these fundamental defences against thermal stress, those with spinal injuries can quickly cool or heat up in environments that others may find perfectly comfortable. Assessment may need consultation with their neurologist to establish the nature of an individual's problems, followed by thorough planning of the workplace to accommodate their needs. Contingency plans may also be needed to protect them in the event of failure of environmental conditioning.

work discussed above, those operating plant and machinery, in particular vehicle drivers, should only ever be permitted to be exposed to very mild heat or cold stress. An extreme example of this is in aircrew, in whom even very subtle psychological impairment resulting from thermal stress may have disastrous consequences. Careful consideration should always be given to the potential role of thermal stress and its consequences in the investigation of all incidents and accidents.

Traditionally, it has been assumed that those exposed to challenging thermal environments will be fully fit and healthy and have no form of disability, but this is increasingly inaccurate, as endurance sports become popular among even severely disabled athletes, and a greater proportion of the disabled population expects to pursue a full range of working and leisure activities. Detailed understanding of the sometimes severe thermoregulatory problems in certain types of spinal injury, for example, can help tackle the problems that individuals may face, but there are no general solutions. Even in those working in the relative shelter of conditioned office environments, achieving thermal comfort needs careful attention to the individual.[59]

Personal protective equipment

Hot or cold working environments are often those in which there are more serious thermal hazards (e.g. in the steel industry or firefighting) or other serious threats (e.g. chemical or radioactive contamination) and personal protective equipment (PPE) is frequently required to counter the thermal and other hazards.

The use of PPE in the heat is a more serious problem, as almost all PPE adds to the heat stress. Garments that are worn necessarily increase the resistance to heat loss from the body and may, of course, abolish all effective evaporative

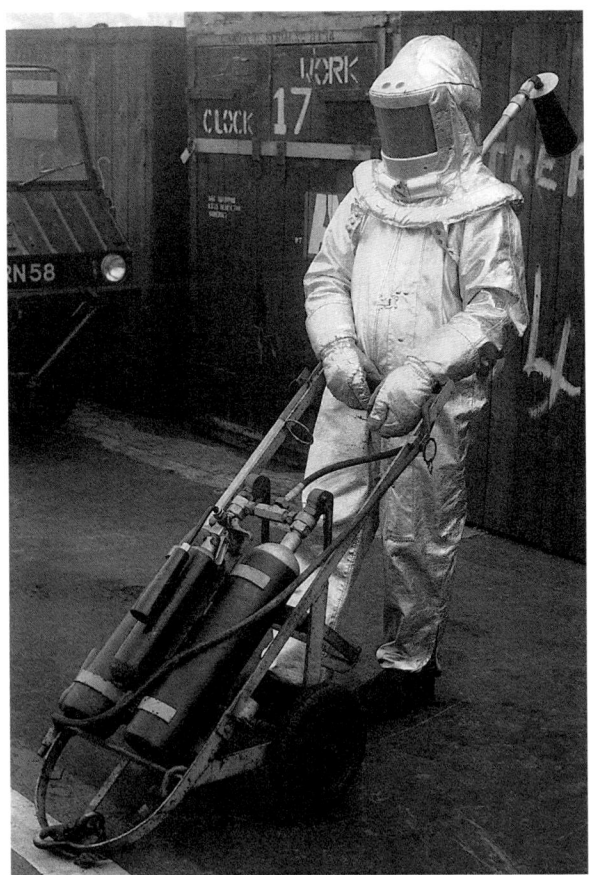

Figure 49.2 Specialist clothing for firefighters may include metallized garments which reflect the high radiant heat load. Below the reflective surface is a thick insulative layer to minimize heat gain by the body, which forms an almost complete barrier to heat loss from the body, even when worn in cold conditions (Crown copyright).

transfer; equipment that is carried increases the amount of work performed for a given task, and thus it increases the metabolic heat generated. In some cases, workers who require to wear effective PPE to protect them from a high radiant heat load, flame and contact burns, such as firefighters, find that this PPE imposes considerable heat stress on them (Figure 49.2). Apart from the impaired performance which results, there is the real risk that workers will not use the PPE completely or correctly, in an effort to increase their comfort, and there is the constant danger that their discomfort will detract from performance in an emergency, resulting in an accident.

There are no easy solutions to these problems. Active cooling systems still require substantial chilling plants and power, and may not always work with the body; a liquid-conditioned garment, for example, may be cooled with water so cold that it induces vasoconstriction in the skin and thus slows cooling, or with tepid water which must have a very high flow rate to remove sufficient heat. Workers who need to be mobile can often only carry the cooling plant with them, which may make matters still worse. A promising approach currently introduced into some industries is the use of regional cooling, for example periodic immersion of the hands in cold water, which does not result in vasoconstriction but may lead to substantial heat loss.[60] Phase-change packs, consisting of crystalline gels that freeze at a physiologically valuable temperature, sealed in plastic bags, appear promising, but packs need to be replenished periodically, and are heavy and bulky.

Another useful advance is in the availability of vapour-permeable materials, such as Goretex® which can sometimes replace impermeable protective layers, yet allowing evaporative cooling to occur through them. Garments using vapour-permeable materials are becoming very popular in many circumstances, for example in affording firemen a water-impermeable and chemical-resistant layer. However, consideration still needs to be given to the essential function of the garment, as failure to achieve that cannot be excused by the improvement of thermal comfort.

Selecting protective clothing for cold environments is also fraught with difficulty. The amount of thermal insulation provided by clothing is approximately proportional to its thickness (actually, it is more accurate to refer to the thickness of air trapped within), so the greater the insulation, the more cumbersome the garments. As the body sweats, so water may condense within these layers and reduce insulation. This is worst if the individual overdresses when working, leading to extensive wetting of their clothing, and then stops to rest; they may then become cold surprisingly rapidly. Workers who enter very cold environments only intermittently, such as those in cold stores, should always doff their protective clothing as soon as they return to warmer conditions, or they will quickly start to saturate the garments with sweat. Water may also mist or ice up eye protection, causing the wearer to remove it (Figure 49.3).

The most intractable problems in PPE for cold conditions are in protecting the hands and feet. Any form of glove reduces manual dexterity, while trying to work without in even cool conditions is just as deleterious to performance.[61] As temperatures fall below 0°C, gloves cannot provide sufficient insulation to keep the fingers warm, and mittens must be worn, very severely impairing work requiring tactile sensation and dexterity. Some of those working in cold conditions have additional protective requirements of their handwear, such as those preparing meat in cold rooms. Although metallic elements may be incorporated into their gloves, to reduce the risk of injury from knives and other cutting equipment, it must be remembered that metal is also an excellent conductor of heat and will reduce the thermal protection of such clothing. The situation with regard to the protection of the feet has been reviewed by Oakley,[62] albeit in a military setting, but the same considerations are needed when choosing footwear for workers (see Figure 49.4).

Using tables of thermal insulation and evaporative resistance for garments such as those in ISO 9920,[41] and the required values for the environment and physical

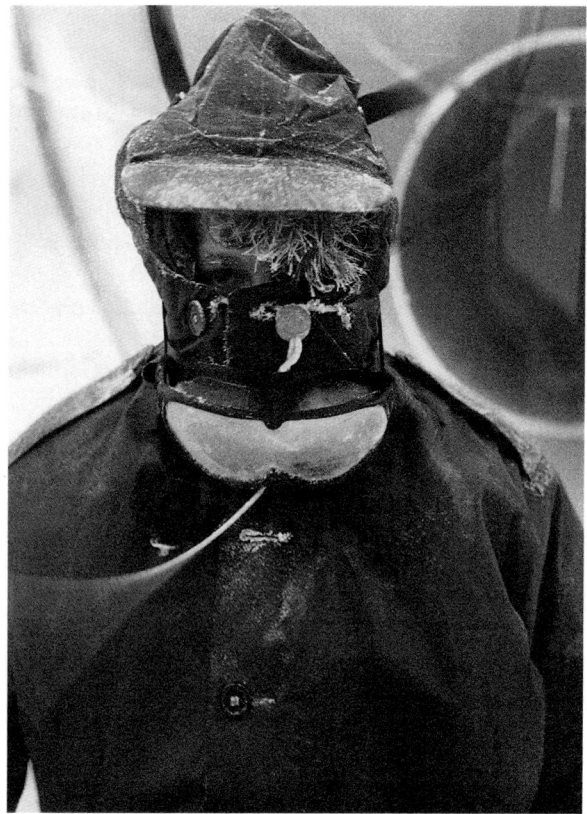

Figure 49.3 This worker in an experimental refrigerated wind tunnel requires good facial protection, but he has had to remove his goggles because of icing (Crown copyright).

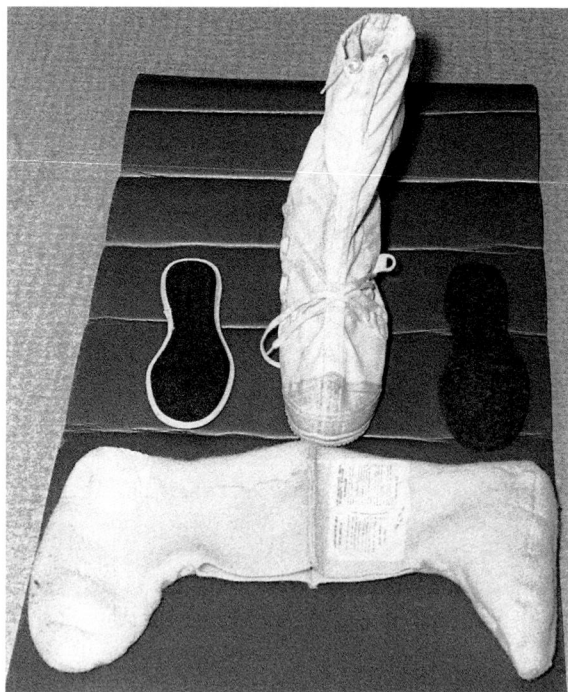

Figure 49.4 A complete mukluk assembly, consisting of a canvas outer boot, insulative insoles and a double felt inner boot, which has been used successfully in temperatures below −40°C (Crown copyright).

activity (e.g. IREQ, the calculated clothing 'Insulation REQuired'),[63] it is possible to make provisional choices as to suitable clothing ensembles. However, careful trials and experience in use are required before firm decisions can be made, owing to the extreme complexity of the situation. For example, the efficacy of closures such as zips and cuffs may be critical in a cold environment, and those with physical limitations or disabilities may need bespoke tailoring of clothing to allow it to be donned and doffed readily. Although aided by national and international standards, the selection of PPE remains a difficult task, which requires detailed knowledge, possibly careful trials, and is often only a rough compromise.

Control of the environment

In an ideal world, of course, all working environments would be thermally neutral, and all the preceding material irrelevant. While it is often impossible to achieve this, most situations are capable of improvement to the extent that the untenable may become at least temporarily acceptable, or the uncomfortable become not unpleasant. A range of standards for different occupational settings has been offered by the leading national and international standards organizations.[49,64–66]

Careful application of the equation of heat balance given at the start of this chapter can be of great value. For example, if ambient air temperature and humidity cannot be controlled, then forced ventilation can increase cooling markedly; thus, in enclosed machinery spaces, a very effective way of providing 'cooling off stances' is to force ventilate air into a number of places. Then, workers can stand in a draft to cool down intermittently and significantly extend their effective working time in the compartment. The provision of shade for those working exposed to the sun and the wetting of surfaces and even clothing in dry heat, are other examples. However, such an approach in a cold storage facility is much more difficult to implement, as deliberately warming several areas would add greatly to the problem of refrigerating the rest. A parallel in cold environments might be to heat small shelters in a cold and windy outdoor setting, allowing workers as much time as possible within them, out of the high wind chill.

The involvement of a good heating and refrigeration engineer can also save much wasted effort. Simple physical facts, such as the rising of warmed air, can be harnessed and turned to advantage, rather than negating that which is being attempted; expert advice at the earliest stage can anticipate such problems. Indeed, the appalling environments often found in working places that have no real intrinsically severe thermal problems (modern electronic share-dealing rooms, for example) usually arise because this has been neglected. For while heat and cold may be among man's oldest environmental enemies, there is a wealth of new and old technology available to control them.

> **Key points**
>
> - Illness and injury arising from hot or cold exposures remain relatively common in some occupations.
> - Local cold injury may be non-freezing, leading to cold sensitivity and pain in peripheries that have undergone only modest cold exposure.
> - Cold immersion can result in rapid death long before the onset of hypothermia; life jackets and protective clothing are key prevention.
> - Heat illness is a life-threatening emergency that can largely be prevented by acclimatization and wise exposure policies, and is often exacerbated by the wearing of personal protective equipment.
> - Cooling the hot and warming the cold remain therapeutic challenges.

REFERENCES

1. Daanen HAM, van der Struijs NR. Resistance index of frostbite as a predictor of cold injury in Arctic operations. *Aviation, Space, and Environmental Medicine.* 2005; **76**: 1119–22.
2. Siple PA, Passell CP. Dry atmospheric cooling in sub-freezing temperatures. *Proceedings of the American Philosophical Society.* 1945; **89**: 177–99.
3. ISO 9886. Ergonomics – evaluation of thermal strain by physiological measurements. Geneva: International Organization for Standardization, 2004.
4. Frim J, Ducharme MB. Physical properties of several infrared tympanic thermometers. Proceedings of the Sixth International Conference on Environmental Ergonomics, Montebello, Canada, September 1994.
5. Golden FStC, Tipton MJ. Human adaptation to repeated cold water immersions. *Journal of Physiology.* 1988; **396**: 349–69.
6. Golden FStC, Hampton IFG, Smith DJ. Lean long distance swimmers. *Journal of the Royal Navy Medical Service.* 1980; **66**: 26–30.
7. LeBlanc J. *Man in the cold.* Springfield, IL: Thomas, 1975.
8. Hershkowitz M. Penile frostbite, an unforeseen hazard of jogging. *New England Journal of Medicine.* 1977; **296**: 178.
9. Andrews RP. Cold injury complicating trauma in the subfreezing environment. *Military Medicine.* 1987; **152**: 42–4.
10. Miller CW. Diseases of sprout pickers. *Occupational Health and Safety.* 1983; **35**: 120–1.
11. Riddell DI. Is frostnip important? *Journal of the Royal Navy Medical Service.* 1984; **70**: 140–2.
12. Francis TJR, Oakley EHN. Cold injury. In: Tooke JE, Lowe GDO (eds). *A textbook of vascular medicine.* London: Edward Arnold, 1996: 353–70.
13. Killian H. *Cold and frost injuries.* Berlin: Springer-Verlag, 1981.
14. Mills WJ. Comment and recapitulation. *Alaska Medicine.* 1993; **35**: 69–87.
15. Oakley EHN. The long-term sequelae of cold injury among 'The Chosin Few'. Unpublished MOD Reports.
16. Burgess JE. 'Retrospective analysis of the ethnic origins of male British Army soldiers with peripheral cold weather injury'. MSc thesis, University of Surrey, 2007.
17. Haight JSJ, Keatinge WR. Failure of thermoregulation in the cold during hypoglycaemia induced by exercise and alcohol. *Journal of Physiology.* 1973; **229**: 87–97.
18. Maclean D, Emslie-Smith D. *Accidental hypothermia.* Oxford: Blackwell Scientific Publications, 1977.
19. Golden FStC, Hervey GR. The 'after-drop' and death after rescue from immersion in cold water. In: Adam JA (ed.). *Hypothermia ashore and afloat.* Aberdeen: Aberdeen University Press, 1981.
20. Tipton MJ. The initial response to cold-water immersion in man. *Clinical Science.* 1989; **77**: 581–8.
21. Keatinge WR, Hayward MG, McIver NKI. Hypothermia during saturation diving in the North Sea. *British Medical Journal.* 1980; **280**: 91.
22. Mekjavic IB, Tipton MJ, Eiken O. Thermal considerations in diving. In: Brubakk AO, Neuman TS (eds). *Bennett and Elliott's physiology and medicine of diving,* 5th edn. Amsterdam: Saunders, 2003: 115–52.
23. Golden FStC, Hervey GR, Tipton MJ. Circum-rescue collapse: Collapse, sometimes fatal, associated with rescue of immersion victims. *Journal of the Royal Navy Medical Service.* 1991; **77**: 139–49.
24. Tipton MJ. The concept of an 'integrated survival system' for protection against the responses associated with immersion in cold water. *Journal of the Royal Navy Medical Service.* 1993; **79**: 11–14.
25. Barwood MJ, Dalzell J, Datta AK et al. Breath-hold performance during cold water immersion: Effects of psychological skills training. *Aviation, Space, and Environmental Medicine.* 2006; **77**: 1136–42.
26. Oakley EHN. The prediction of survival during cold immersion: Results from the UK National Immersion Incident Survey. Unpublished MOD reports.
27. O'Neill R. Work in winter. *Occupational Health Review.* 1995; Jan/Feb: 10–13.
28. Enander A. Performance and sensory aspects of work in cold environments: A review. *Ergonomics.* 1984; **27**: 365–78.
29. Tanaka M, Tochihara Y, Yamazaki S et al. Thermal reaction and manual performance during cold exposure while wearing cold-protective clothing. *Ergonomics.* 1983; **26**: 141–9.
30. Rissanen S, Rintamäki H. Thermal responses and physiological strain in men wearing permeable and semipermeable protective clothing in the cold. *Ergonomics.* 1997; **40**: 141–50.
31. Coleshaw SRK, van Someren RNM, Wolff AH et al. Impaired memory registration and speed of reasoning caused by low body temperature. *Journal of Applied Physiology.* 1983; **55**: 27–31.
32. ISO 8996. Ergonomics of the thermal environment – determination of metabolic rate. Geneva: International Organization for Standardization, 2004.

33. ISO 7243. Hot environments – estimation of the heat stress on working man, based on the WBGT-index (wet bulb globe temperature). Geneva: International Organization for Standardization, 1989.
34. Nunneley SA, Stribley RF. Fighter index of thermal stress (FITS): Guidance for hot-weather aircraft operations. *Aviation, Space, and Environmental Medicine*. 1979; **50**: 639–42.
35. Parsons KC. International heat stress standards: A review. *Ergonomics* 1995; **38**: 6–22.
36. ISO 11399. Ergonomics of the thermal environment – principles and application of the relevant international standards. Geneva: International Organization for Standardization, 1995.
37. ISO 7933. Ergonomics of the thermal environment – analytical determination and interpretation of thermal stress using calculation of the predicted heat strain. Geneva: International Organization for Standardization, 2004.
38. Peters H. Testing climate indices in the field. *Ergonomics*. 1995; **38**: 86–100.
39. Mairiaux P, Malchaire J. Comparison and validation of heat stress indices in experimental studies. *Ergonomics*. 1995; **38**: 58–72.
40. ISO 7730. Ergonomics of the thermal environment – analytical determination and interpretation of thermal comfort using calculation of the PMV and PPD indices and local thermal comfort criteria. Geneva: International Organization for Standardization, 2005.
41. ISO 9920. Ergonomics of the thermal environment – estimation of the thermal insulation and evaporative resistance of a clothing ensemble. Geneva: International Organization for Standardization, 1995.
42. Clark RP, Edholm OG. *Man and his thermal environment*. London: Edward Arnold, 1985.
43. Oakley EHN. Heat exhaustion. *Journal of World Accident, Emergency and Disaster Medicine*. 1987; **3**: 28–30.
44. Khogali M, Hales JRS (eds). *Heat stroke and temperature regulation*. Sydney: Academic Press, 1983.
45. Phinney LT, Gardner JW, Kark JA, Wenger CB. Long-term follow-up after exertional heat illness during recruit training. *Medicine and Science in Sports and Exercise*. 2001; **33**: 1443–8.
46. Speedy DB, Noakes TD, Schneider C. Exercise associated hyponatremia: A review. *Emergency Medicine*. 2001; **13**: 17–27.
47. Ramsey JD. Task performance in heat: A review. *Ergonomics*. 1995; **38**: 154–65.
48. NIOSH. Criteria for a recommended standard – occupational exposure to hot environments. HSM 72-10269. Washington DC: National Institute for Occupational Safety and Health, 1972.
49. NIOSH. Criteria for a recommended standard – occupational exposure to hot environments. Revised criteria 1986. DDHS (NIOSH) 86-113. Washington DC: National Institute for Occupational Safety and Health, 1986.
50. Holland RL, Sayers JA, Keatinge WR et al. Effects of raised body temperature on reasoning, memory and mood. *Journal of Applied Physiology*. 1985; **59**: 1823–7.
51. Wyon DP, Wyon I, Norin F. Effects of moderate heat stress on driver vigilance in a moving vehicle. *Ergonomics*. 1996; **39**: 61–75.
52. ISO 10551. Ergonomics of the thermal environment – assessment of the influence of the thermal environment using subjective judgement scales. Geneva: International Organization for Standardization, 1995.
53. RFIC. Guidance on work in cold indoor environments. Bracknell: Refrigerated Food Industry Confederation, undated.
54. BSI. Draft British Standard: Ergonomics of the thermal environment – code of practice for the design and evaluation of working practices for cold indoor environments. London: BSI Standards, 1996.
55. Griefahn B. Arbeit in mässiger Kälte. Report no. Fb 716. Dortmund: Bundesanstalt für Arbeitsschutz, 1995.
56. Malchaire J, Mairiaux P. Strategy of analysis and interpretation of thermal working conditions. *Annals of Occupational Hygiene*. 1991; **35**: 261–72.
57. American College of Sports Medicine. Prevention of cold injuries during exercise. *Medicine and Science in Sports and Exercise*. 2006; **38**: 2012–29.
58. Smith DL, Petruzzello SJ, Kramer JM, Misner JE. The effects of different thermal environments on the physiological and psychological responses of firefighters to a training drill. *Ergonomics*. 1997; **40**: 500–10.
59. Parsons KC. The effects of gender, acclimation state, the opportunity to adjust clothing and physical disability on requirements for thermal comfort. *Energy and Buildings*. 2002; **34**: 593–9.
60. Allsopp AJ, Poole KA. The effect of hand immersion on body temperature when wearing impermeable clothing. *Journal of the Royal Navy Medical Service*. 1991; **77**: 51–7.
61. Provins KA, Clarke RSJ. The effect of cold on manual performance. *Journal of Occupational Medicine*. 1960; **2**: 169–76.
62. Oakley EHN. The design and function of military footwear: a review following experiences in the South Atlantic. *Ergonomics*. 1984; **27**: 631–7.
63. ISO/DIS 11079. Ergonomics of the thermal environment – determination and interpretation of cold stress when using required clothing insulation (IREQ) and local cooling effects. Geneva: International Organization for Standardization, 2005.
64. ASHRAE/ANSI. Standard 55-81: Thermal environmental conditions for human occupancy. Atlanta, GA: American Society of Heating, Refrigerating, and Air-Conditioning Engineers, 1981.
65. ASHRAE. Standard 62-1989: Ventilation for acceptable indoor air quality. Atlanta, GA: American Society of Heating, Refrigerating, and Air-Conditioning Engineers, 1989.
66. COST. Indoor air quality and its impact on man. Brussels: Commission of European Community, Working Group 6: Ventilation Requirements, 1990.

SECTION FOUR

Barometric pressure

50	Diving and work at increased pressure *Stephen Watt and Andrew Colvin*	547
51	Working at high altitude *Peter JG Forster*	570
52	Flying and spaceflight *Mike Gibson, David Gradwell and Alyson Calder*	591

50

Diving and work at increased pressure

STEPHEN WATT AND ANDREW COLVIN

Overview of the need for diving and tunnelling and the hazards	547	Diving tasks	556
		Current hazards and risks	559
The increased pressure environment	547	Long-term health effects	561
Physics of the pressure environment	548	Tunnelling tasks	562
Pressure-related physiology and pathophysiology	549	Decompression illness in compressed air work	564
Decompression sickness	551	Legal framework	565
Bone necrosis	553	Assessment of fitness for work at pressure	565
Loss of consciousness	555	References	567

OVERVIEW OF THE NEED FOR DIVING AND TUNNELLING AND THE HAZARDS

The history of mankind is inextricably linked with the sea. The sea and inland lakes and waterways have been vital as sources of food and for exploration and travel. As a result, numerous food stuffs and items of value have been sought from beneath the sea surface throughout the history of man. These driving forces, enhanced by military requirements, have resulted in enormous efforts to explore the subsea environment for profit, military advantage, scientific research and for pleasure. The history of diving begins with simple breath-hold diving as is still practised for gathering pearls and by recreational snorkellers, and moves through the development of breathing apparatus to modern saturation diving methods. Practical solutions have been found for many of the problems encountered in exploration of the subsea environment which now allow man to conduct a wide range of work activities underwater. However, the underwater environment remains alien to man and is always hazardous.

Within the last 200 years, the technological advances have also been applied in civil engineering situations where excavation beneath a water table results in ingress of water. By enclosing the excavation and applying increased pressure, the ingress of water can be prevented allowing continued excavation in a dry environment. These enclosures are called 'caissons' and have been extensively used in the building of bridge piers, tunnels and other civil engineering works. Workers in caissons do not dive, but do share exposure to increased pressure with divers, and hence many of the same problems and hazards. In the last 20 years, due to increasing health concerns, several of the techniques previously developed in military and commercial diving are now used within tunnelling operations involving compressed air work.

This chapter deals with the occupational health issues of both diving and compressed air work.

THE INCREASED PRESSURE ENVIRONMENT

On the surface of the Earth at sea level, we live in an air environment where the air pressure results from the mass of the air in the atmosphere above and the effect of the Earth's gravitational field. On ascent to altitude on mountains or in aircraft, the mass of air above is less and hence the pressure is also lower. On descent underwater, the environmental pressure results from both the mass of air above and the mass of water. Since water is many times denser than air, there is a very rapid increase in pressure with progressive descent underwater and pressure changes occur when compressed air is used in engineering works. This change in pressure is the most critical environmental factor in both diving and compressed air work.

Pressure can be measured in many alternative units which are in everyday use. The pressure on the Earth's

Table 50.1 Equivalent units of pressure.

Unit	Abbreviation	Value
Standard atmosphere absolute	ata	1
Bar (bar)	bar	1
Torr	torr	760
Millimetres of mercury	mmHg	760
Kilopascal	kPa	100
Pounds per square inch	psi	14.7
Kilogram force per sq centimetre	Kgf.cm^{-2}	1.033
Feet of seawater	fsw	33
Metres of seawater	msw	10

surface at sea level has been defined as 1 bar (=1000 millibar). (Fluctuations in pressure reported in millibar form an important measurement in weather forecasting.) One standard atmosphere absolute (ata) is almost equivalent to 1 bar. Other measures in regular use are torr and millimetres of mercury (mmHg), pounds per square inch (psi), kilogram force per square centimetre (Kgf.cm^{-2}), meters of seawater (msw), feet of seawater (fsw) and pascals (Pa). Many of these will be familiar in everyday medical or scientific use. Table 50.1 provides equivalent values. Pressure is most usefully measured in absolute terms where zero equals an absolute vacuum, but is often measured relative to surface air pressure (called gauge pressure) which introduces confusion in physical calculations. Although scientifically it is most appropriate to use SI units (Pa), the units in most common use in the diving and compressed air industry have been retained in this chapter. Care should be taken when comparing different pressure units to avoid mistakes and confusion, particularly where pressure is measured either as absolute or total pressure or gauge pressure (where the pressure above ambient is recorded).

Gases are compressible, so become denser as pressure increases. As a result on ascent to altitude, air density reduces with ascent and so the pressure reduction is not linear with height. Water is not compressible and hence underwater the pressure rises linearly with depth by 1 atmosphere for every 10 m additional depth. The absolute pressure underwater in ata can simply be calculated from the water depth in meters divided by 10 and adding 1 for surface air pressure. Hence, pressure at 50 m depth is $50/10 + 1 = 6$ ata. In compressed air work, 1 bar (gauge) is equivalent to 2 bar absolute pressure (i.e. 1 bar atmospheric pressure + 1 bar gauge pressure).

Both divers and compressed air workers operate in an environment where the ambient pressure is raised. Historically, compressed air work has rarely involved pressures above 3–4 ata, but in recent years the development of tunnel boring machines used in modern tunnel excavation has led to much higher pressures being required. Diving is regularly undertaken at pressures of up to 35 ata and the world record exceeds 70 ata.

Divers and compressed air workers also share other environmental problems. Both commonly require to use compression chambers and hence work in an enclosed space and while divers inevitably require breathing apparatus, compressed air workers may also need to use breathing apparatus for breathing alternative gases or protection in potentially contaminated environments.

PHYSICS OF THE PRESSURE ENVIRONMENT

The physical properties of the environment are defined by the gas laws. The following are of critical importance in understanding the pressure environment.

Boyle's law states that for a fixed mass of gas at constant temperature the volume is inversely proportional to the absolute pressure. Hence, if pressure is doubled, the volume is halved.

Charles' law states that for a fixed mass of gas at constant pressure, the volume is proportional to the absolute temperature.

Dalton's law states that 'in a mixture of gases, the pressure exerted by each of the constituent gases is the same as it would exert if it alone occupied the same volume'. The pressure exerted by each constituent is called a partial pressure. The total pressure in a gas mixture is the sum of the partial pressures of the constituents, and these partial pressures can be calculated from the total pressure and the fractional concentrations of the constituents. Hence, in air at sea level where oxygen forms 20.9 per cent of the gas mixture, the partial pressure of oxygen is 20.9 per cent of 1 ata or 760 mmHg, i.e. 0.209 ata, 159 mmHg.

Henry's law states that 'at constant temperature, the amount of gas which dissolves in a liquid with which it is in contact is proportional to the partial pressure of that gas'. Hence, while the amount or mass of gas which dissolves in a liquid is also dependent on that gas's solubility, an increase in partial pressure of the gas will increase the amount that goes into solution.

The effects of these laws can be seen in Table 50.2.

The constituent gases of the diver's breathing mixture have important pathophysiological effects. Oxygen is critical to metabolic processes and a reduced partial pressure of oxygen will result in hypoxaemia. However, the increase in oxygen partial pressure may also be toxic. Oxygen toxicity is more likely with increasing pO_2 and with duration of exposure. The lung may be affected with prolonged exposure to a pO_2 above 0.6 ata[1-3] and, in the central nervous system (CNS), prolonged exposure often manifests as convulsions with relatively short duration exposure to pO_2 above 1.6 ata.[4] CNS toxicity is enhanced by exertion,[4,5] so a diver at rest in a chamber can tolerate a pO_2 of 2.8 ata which would result in convulsions if the diver was active in the water. Oxygen tolerance can be extended if exposure is intermittent.[6] Nitrogen which is normally an inert component of the air we breath has narcotic and anaesthetic effects[7] at high partial pressures, which limits the depth at which air can be used as a breathing mixture and represents a distinct safety hazard. The narcotic effects begin to be noticeable at a depth of about 30 msw (pN_2 approximately

Table 50.2 Some implications of breathing air at increased pressure.

Depth (msw)	Pressure (ata)	Volume (L)	Density (g/L)	MVV (L/min)	pN2 (ata)	pO2 (ata)
0	1	8	1.2	200	0.8	0.2
10	2	4	2.4		1.6	0.4
20	3	2.66	3.6		2.4	0.6
30	4	2	4.8	100	3.2	0.8
40	5	1.66	6.0		4.0	1.0
50	6	1.33	7.2	80	4.8	1.2
70	8	1	9.6		6.4	1.6
160	17	0.47	20.4		13.6	3.4

Volume column shows the lung volume changes during a breath-hold dive from total lung capacity at the surface. MVV (maximum voluntary ventilation) shows the restriction of ventilation imposed by increasing gas density. pO_2 column shows how an inspired partial pressure of 1 ata can be achieved either by breathing 100% oxygen on the surface or by breathing air at a depth of 40 msw.

3 ata) and increase as the pressure goes up. Nitrogen narcosis and gas density issues become an important safety issue deeper than 30 msw and an important contributor to accidents or errors. Breathing air is considered to be a medical contraindication for routine commercial diving applications at depths greater than 50 m. In practice, this is the reason the Royal Navy prohibit air diving for military purposes at depths greater than 50 m and in the Health and Safety Executive (HSE)-approved compressed air tables breathing air is limited to a 3.45 bar (gauge) maximum pressure in the United Kingdom.[8] At higher pressures, the nitrogen requires to be replaced either partially or completely by an alternative 'inert' gas usually helium. Helium has the advantages of having no narcotic effect and being very light, so also overcomes some of the respiratory problems caused by gas density. However, it diffuses very easily, has high thermal conductivity, and so introduces significant thermal control problems and produces speech distortion which affects vocal communications. Other gases may also be encountered. Argon is used as a shielding gas in welding operations. It is breathable but more narcotic than nitrogen and hence a hazard. Hydrogen has been used in some experimental deep dives for its minimal density. It has high thermal conductivity and introduces the potential for explosive gas mixtures.

PRESSURE-RELATED PHYSIOLOGY AND PATHOPHYSIOLOGY

Barotrauma

MIDDLE EAR BAROTRAUMA

The most immediately recognized effect of change in environmental pressure is the result on the middle ear cavity. The Eustachian tube is normally closed and hence the middle ear cavity is a closed gas space with one flexible side, the tympanic membrane. The body tissues behave like a fluid and transmit pressure so any change in environmental pressure is transmitted to gas-containing spaces in the body. An increase in pressure results in a reduction in middle ear gas volume and causes movement of the tympanic membrane. This is readily sensed and can cause pain if the membrane is stretched enough. If the diver opens the Eustachian tube, air at ambient pressure passes up into the middle ear and the tympanic membrane moves back to the normal position. As a diver descends in the water or a tunneller is compressed in a gas environment, this action of 'equalizing' ear pressures is required recurrently until the diver reaches stable depth. If equalization is not performed, the differential pressure across the Eustachian tube may effectively prevent the diver from opening the tube and result in pain and trauma to the tympanic membrane or inner ear organs. The tympanic membrane may be bruised and haemorrhagic or may rupture, an event, which although painful, equalizes pressure. In most cases, middle ear barotrauma resolves within two weeks with complete healing of the ear drum. It is important to ensure Eustachian function has returned to normal before returning to diving or other pressure exposure. However, the transmitted pressure effects may also damage the organ of Corti and produce a permanent hearing loss. Vigorous attempts to equalize pressure by holding the nose and doing a valsalva manoeuvre increase intracerebral pressure and hence the pressure difference across the round window. Rupture of this membrane results in leak of endolymph into the middle ear and a gradual onset of vertigo, nausea and hearing loss. This is an emergency and requires urgent otological assessment.

SINUS BAROTRAUMA

Other gas-containing spaces in the body may also cause problems. Sinus cavities should normally communicate with the nasal airways and hence not behave as closed spaces. However, minor inflammatory change in the nasal mucosa may readily close sinus ostia and so prevent free gas movement. These spaces are of fixed volume in bony cavities so cannot change volume. In the event of the gas content reducing in volume interstitial fluid and blood is effectively sucked into the mucosa, a process which can generate some pain. On subsequent ascent, the trapped gas expands again and may force mucous and blood out of the ostia into the nasal cavity. Although the presentation can be dramatic, the injury is usually minor and resolves spontaneously. Persistent inflammatory change in the sinus mucosa may result in persistent obstruction of the ostia and long-term inability to dive. Rarely, the acute event may result in local nerve injury to the fifth or seventh cranial nerves.

PULMONARY BAROTRAUMA

The lungs are the largest gas-containing space in the body. In normal breathing, the lungs communicate freely with the upper airways and mouth so changes in volume of gas in the lungs can be easily compensated for during normal breathing. Should the diver either stop breathing, hold their breath or change depth rapidly, gas volume may change enough to injure the lung. Compression of the lung (squeeze) is extremely rare in normal diving or compressed air work, but a common issue in extreme breath-hold diving. Overexpansion of the lung (burst lung) is a much more important problem in diving with potentially fatal results. If during a rapid ascent, the diver does not exhale adequately, the lung will expand beyond normal volume and may rupture allowing gas to escape through the interstitial tissue of the lung. This gas may track to the pleural cavity causing pneumothorax often with tension, or into the mediastinum, or it may rupture into the pulmonary venous system and pass directly into the left heart and result in arterial gas embolism. Rarely, gas may track through the retroperitoneal space and cause pneumoperitoneum. Both tension pneumothorax and gas embolism may be rapidly fatal. Pneumothorax presents in a similar manner to spontaneous pneumothorax in other situations with chest pain and breathlessness and is treated in the same way. Pneumomediastinum often presents slowly after the dive, often several hours later with crepitus over the anterior chest and neck, discomfort in the neck and hoarse voice (Figure 50.1).

There is no specific treatment available, but breathing 100 per cent oxygen accelerates the removal of air from the tissues. Arterial gas embolism usually presents with an acute cerebral event, convulsion, loss of consciousness, sudden blindness or hemiplegia and is usually almost immediately following surfacing from a dive. Treatment is required rapidly and includes administration of 100 per cent oxygen and therapeutic recompression using an appropriate treatment procedure.

The pathogenesis of these disorders is incompletely understood. Arterial gas embolism occurs when the lung ruptures as a result of pulmonary barotrauma and gas is released into the pulmonary venous system. Relatively low transpulmonary pressure can rupture the lung, but many external factors may provide support to the thorax and lung, allowing the lung to sustain higher pressures.[9,10] When gas escapes into the pulmonary venous system, its main target organ is the brain. Gas enters the cerebral circulation and, although some will pass through, it triggers circulatory change with local hyperaemia and an increase in cerebral blood volume, systemic hypertension, a loss of cerebral autoregulation and rapid development of cerebral oedema.[11,12] The latter is almost certainly related to the injury to vascular endothelium. In those who survive the acute injury, the progress of the illness may be significantly affected by the presence of inert gas already dissolved in brain tissue. Dissolved gas may enhance the volume of gas involved exacerbating the pathological impact. Hence, an episode of arterial gas embolism occurring in the presence of a significant dissolved gas load may have a worse prognosis than one occurring without. Much

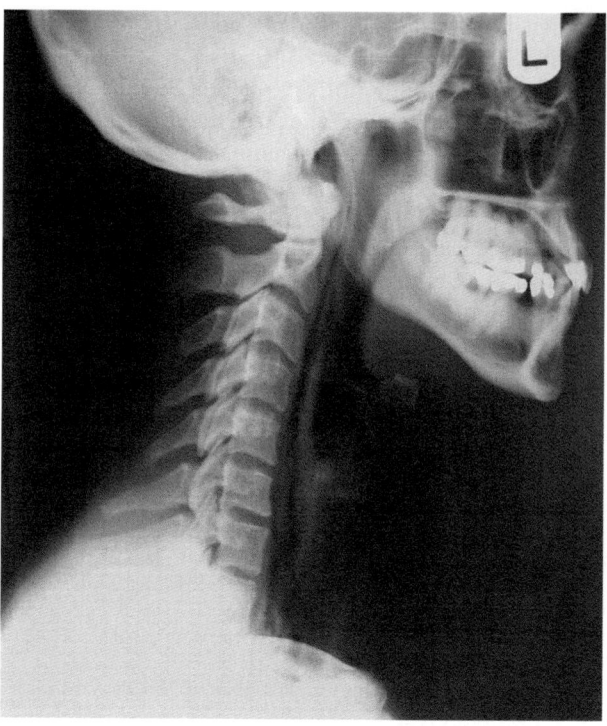

Figure 50.1 Lateral radiograph of a diver's neck showing extensive air in deep tissues, confirming the diagnosis of pneumomediastinum. The diver had presented with a sore throat after an uneventful air dive.

of the clinical information concerning prognosis is derived from submarine escape training where dissolved gas load is minimal and hence may not reflect outcomes after an incident occurring during other diving activity.

> During ascent from an air dive at 47 msw with planned surface decompression, a diver was raised rapidly from a 10 msw stop to the surface. During the surface interval he became confused and subsequently lost consciousness. He was therefore compressed to 18 msw rather than the planned 12 msw, where he regained consciousness but had persisting neurological abnormalities with right arm weakness, poor balance and visual disturbance. These abnormalities persisted despite further recompression treatment, but resolved slowly over a period of several months after the incident.

The risk of sudden change in pressure is much less in compressed air work where the working chamber pressure and compression and decompression rates are controlled by a pressure lock operator. However, there remains a risk of explosive decompression resulting from engineering or equipment failure.

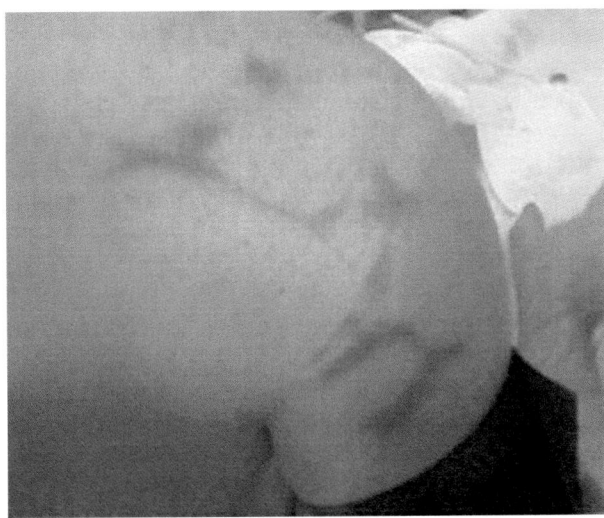

Figure 50.2 Appearance of a diver's arm following an air dive. He reported the presence of a rash. The characteristic linear bruises and the series of radial lines marking the site of his suit dump valve are typical. For colour image, see www.hodderplus.com/hunters.

BAROTRAUMA TO OTHER ORGANS

The bowel usually contains gas, but is distensible and ultimately open ended. Hence while gas movement may be recognized by the diver or tunneller, it is rarely pathological. A small number of cases of gastrointestinal barotrauma have been reported, but mostly associated with explosive uncontrolled ascent.

Gas spaces around the body are also affected. The gas space between a diver's breathing mask and face is affected by pressure change. A diver's mask includes the nose, allowing the diver to exhale through the nose to equalize pressure. Without this action, the diver's periorbital soft tissues are effectively sucked into the mask space producing oedema and haemorrhage. This results in a dramatic appearance, but is not a serious injury.

Divers wearing a dry suit have an enclosed gas space around them which will reduce in volume during descent. Eventually, the suit will be compressed around the diver and folds in the suit material may trap subcutaneous tissues of the diver and result in linear bruising (suit squeeze) which may be painful (Figure 50.2).

Many modern suits now have a gas injection system allowing the diver to introduce additional gas and release the pressure. This provides more comfort, but introduces an additional hazard due to buoyancy effects.

DECOMPRESSION SICKNESS

Decompression sickness is a spectrum of clinical syndromes which result from the effects of the formation of excessive amounts of gas microbubbles in the tissues and bloodstream, during or after a decompression, from gas which had previously been dissolved in body tissues according to Henry's law.[13]

When a diver or compressed air worker is exposed to increased environmental pressure and breathes a gas mixture containing an inert gas (e.g. nitrogen or helium), body tissues are exposed to an increase in partial pressure of that gas. As a result, additional gas dissolves. Some gas may diffuse through the skin directly into subcutaneous tissues, but the majority of the gas will dissolve initially in the pulmonary blood flow and be distributed gradually to all body tissues. This process of solution, distribution and diffusion is gradual and will take six to eight hours at a constant pressure until complete equilibrium in all body tissues is established. At this point, the diver is said to be saturated with the inert gas at that particular pressure. On return to the surface, the partial pressure of the gas reduces and so the tissues become effectively supersaturated with gas which is then released from solution. On slow ascent, this excess gas will mostly be transferred through the circulation to the lungs and exhaled. However, the difference in partial pressure between the diver's tissues and the environment may be sufficient to cause gas to come out of solution and form bubbles. Bubbles are not inert and the bubble surface is capable of triggering a reaction in tissues and in blood involving the coagulation system and an inflammatory process.[14]

Bubbles can be identified in both tissues and the circulation using ultrasound methods[15] and it is recognized that some bubble formation is commonly seen after apparently safe dives or compressed air exposures and not associated with any ill effects.[16] It appears most likely that a pathological outcome is triggered by a critical volume of gas bubbles, in particular tissues or perhaps a critical rate of formation. These critical factors may be different in different tissues and vary between individuals.

Recognized risk factors for clinical episodes of decompression sickness fall into two major categories: (1) pressure exposure-related factors, such as the depth (pressure) and duration of the exposure, previous exposures over the preceding hours and days; and (2) the ascent/decompression rate, decompression methodology and individual diver's predisposing clinical factors, such as intracardiac shunt[17,18] or personal susceptibility.[19] Many cases in divers are provoked by incautious ascent, omitting appropriate decompression stops or by rapid and uncontrolled ascent as a result of loss of buoyancy control. In civil engineering or tunnelling operations, the incidence of decompression illness is significantly higher than in commercial diving. This may reflect longer exposures often approaching or reaching saturation levels repeated daily with relatively inadequate decompression procedures.

Symptoms of decompression sickness are very variable, but fall into several main categories.[20]

Neurological

Neurological symptoms include paraesthesiae of any area, sensory loss, focal weakness and disturbance of balance.[21] More pronounced spinal cord involvement may cause marked weakness and paraplegia or even tetraplegia and be associated with sphincter disturbance. Low back pain or pain in a girdle distribution is often a precursor of spinal cord symptoms. Vestibular symptoms (staggers) of nausea, vertigo and loss of balance may occur either with or without other neurological symptoms. Disturbance of cerebral function is less common, but well documented, and may include behavioural change or even loss of consciousness. Although the ultimate prognosis for neurological disease is usually for considerable recovery,[22,23] this is the main cause of permanent disability resulting from decompression illness.[24]

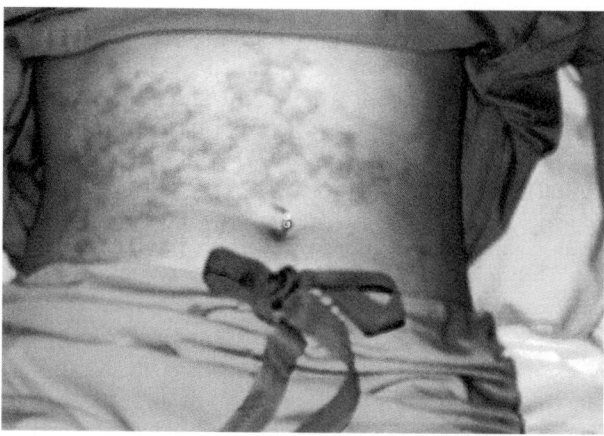

Figure 50.3 Appearance of a diver's torso following a deep air dive. The diver reported the presence of a rash. The widespread patchy rash, which is erythematous but may also have petechial areas, is characteristic of cutaneous decompression sickness. It is most commonly seen on the trunk and proximal limbs. For colour image, see www.hodderplus.com/hunters.

> A commercial diver with 12 years' experience of civil engineering diving at depths to a maximum of 22 msw obtained work in oil field diving which involved dives to 45 msw. In the course of three months, he developed three episodes of illness after uneventful diving, the first involving mainly gastrointestinal symptoms which resolved spontaneously, the second involved minor neurological features which resolved on recompression and the third obvious lower limb weakness which also responded rapidly to recompression treatment. Investigation following recovery demonstrated the presence of patent foramen ovale which was subsequently closed by percutaneous catheter technique. He has subsequently been able to return to normal diving activity with no further episodes.

Limb pain

Limb pain (bends) symptoms most commonly affect larger joints, typically the shoulder, elbow wrist and knee, but can affect any joint. Joint pain varies from being a mild ache (niggle) to severe and incapacitating pain, tends to be constant and unaffected by movement of the joint. Limb pain not localized to a joint sometimes occurs and may be due to oedema and swelling of a muscle. This is historically the most common presentation in compressed air workers often affecting the knees and typically presenting 4–12 hours after exposure.

Cutaneous

Cutaneous symptoms, include itching which is probably due to gas diffusing through the skin, urticaria and a more persistent rash, called cutis marmorata which comprises a patchy rash of erythematous and petechial lesions interspersed with normal skin spread over variable areas but usually over the trunk or proximal limbs (Figure 50.3). It is usually painless and not itchy and hence not observed until the diver removes their suit. This rash is often associated with more serious neurological manifestations of the illness which may be concurrent or follow later. Localized areas of oedema of the skin may occur which are probably due to local lymphatic obstruction.

Constitutional

Many patients also report constitutional symptoms of tiredness, nausea, feeling cold or weak. These symptoms are most likely a result of hypovolaemia resulting from loss of fluid through damaged capillary endothelium into interstitial tissues and often improve rapidly with rehydration and therapeutic recompression.

Pulmonary

Pulmonary involvement (chokes) results from massive bubble load in the venous circulation and obstruction of the pulmonary circulation. This results in cough, breathlessness and haemoptysis. The resulting high pulmonary arterial pressure results in intrapulmonary shunting and passage of bubbles to the arterial circulation and severe neurological symptoms usually follow. Individuals with significant pulmonary involvement are critically ill and there is a high mortality.

The underlying pathology results from the formation of gas within tissues from molecules previously dissolved in tissues and hence the mechanisms relate to the appearance of microbubbles. These may occur in many tissues, but have been most commonly identified in the bloodstream using Doppler methodology.[25] Microbubbles in tissue may migrate into the vascular bed. It is recognized that some gas microbubbles occur commonly after symptom-free decompressions, so it appears that the onset of disease may relate to a threshold which may be volume, number or rate of appearance.[26] It is clear that the passage of microbubbles results in damage to the endothelium which results in fluid leak into interstitial tissues.[27] This is important within the cerebral circulation resulting in cerebral oedema, but also results in significant haemoconcentration. Correction of haemoconcentration with large volumes of intravenous fluid often results in peripheral oedema and pleural effusion. Within the bloodstream, microbubbles trigger the coagulation cascade and stimulate platelet aggregation, and activate the complement system contributing to haemoconcentration.[28]

These effects are well established; however, how these effects relate to specific organ-related symptoms is less clear. There is evidence that pulmonary symptoms are associated with the venous vascular bubble load. Increasing obstruction to the pulmonary capillary bed results in hypoxia and increasing pulmonary arterial pressure[29,30] with symptoms of breathlessness, haemoptysis and chest tightness. Endothelial leak results in the development of pulmonary oedema.

As pulmonary arterial pressure rises, bubbles begin to appear in the arterial circulation. This is associated with the development of neurological manifestation, particularly of spinal cord origin. Whether spinal cord injury occurs primarily as a result of arterial bubble embolization or as a result of bubble formation *in situ* or a combination of both or other mechanisms is uncertain. The close association between spinal cord injury and right to left intracardiac shunt supports the theory that bubble embolization plays a role.[31,32] Conversely, animal experimental work has demonstrated that autochonous (*in situ*) bubble formation can occur.[33,34] The end result is the appearance of punctuate haemorrhagic lesions scattered in spinal cord tissue most obvious in white matter associated with axonal swelling and subsequent myelin degeneration.[35]

Other symptoms of decompression sickness are also difficult to explain in terms of pathogenesis. The characteristic musculoskeletal pain symptom has been explained on the basis of gas present within the joint, within soft tissues around the joint, within marrow cavities of adjacent bone and as referred pain of neurological origin. Constitutional symptoms have been explained on the basis of the proinflammatory processes associated with decompression sickness, but might readily be explained by the hypovolaemia. The classical cutaneous manifestation of cutis marmorata shows evidence of an acute vasculitis on biopsy, but its origin may relate to embolization of cutaneous vessels or the direct transcutaneous migration of gas. The close association of this rash with right to left intracardiac shunt suggests embolization is more relevant. Vestibular decompression illness may result from gas formation from endolymph with subsequent damage to the semicircular canal sensor cells.

Symptoms may develop at any time after the commencement of the ascent phase of a dive, but are most common in divers in the first one to two hours following surfacing. Over 90 per cent of cases present within 24 hours of completion of the last exposure in both divers and tunellers. However, the pattern is complicated by travel involving ascent to altitude after exposure either by road or in commercial aircraft. Such altitude exposure may provoke symptoms during a period of 24–48 hours following exposure that may prove to be slow to resolve even with appropriate hyperbaric oxygen therapy.

Immediate first aid treatment includes administration of 100 per cent oxygen and rehydration by the most effective means available. Patients presenting with decompression illness should receive specialist assessment and transfer to a recompression unit for further treatment with intravenous fluids and recompression. Those patients with severe neurological illness or paraplegia may also require the expertise of a specialist spinal injury unit in their continuing management.

A 32-year-old compressed air diver made an emergency rapid ascent from a 12 minute dive to a depth of 30 msw. This was followed immediately by an impairment of consciousness and hemiparesis which resolved spontaneously within minutes. Some 20 minutes later, he noticed woolliness in his feet which progressed into classic paraplegia. He was evacuated by air to a chamber, where some 24 hours later he was recompressed but with little response. While in the chamber, a surgeon conducted a laparotomy 'because of paralytic ileus' and after decompression the wound dehisced. The patient emerged still paraplegic, but six months later was able to walk with two sticks.

Comment

It may be speculated that after a relatively short dive with little nitrogen gas load, the rapid ascent resulted in pulmonary barotrauma and cerebral gas embolism. Although these symptoms resolved spontaneously, either the pulmonary injury, or diffuse endothelial injury interfered with normal nitrogen elimination and resulted in neurological decompression illness. Severe neurological illness does not always respond to recompression therapy and the delay in recompression may have contributed to the lack of response. Paralytic ileus is common after severe spinal injury and may complicate the decompression phase of treatment. Surgical intervention in a chamber is best avoided.

BONE NECROSIS

Both divers and compressed air workers are at risk of developing dysbaric osteonecrosis.[36] This is a form of aseptic bone necrosis which occurs as a long-term health effect (Figure 50.4). It may occur after a single pressure exposure, but is more likely after deeper and longer pressure exposures and it is more likely to occur in individuals with a history of acute decompression illness. It is discussed in detail below.

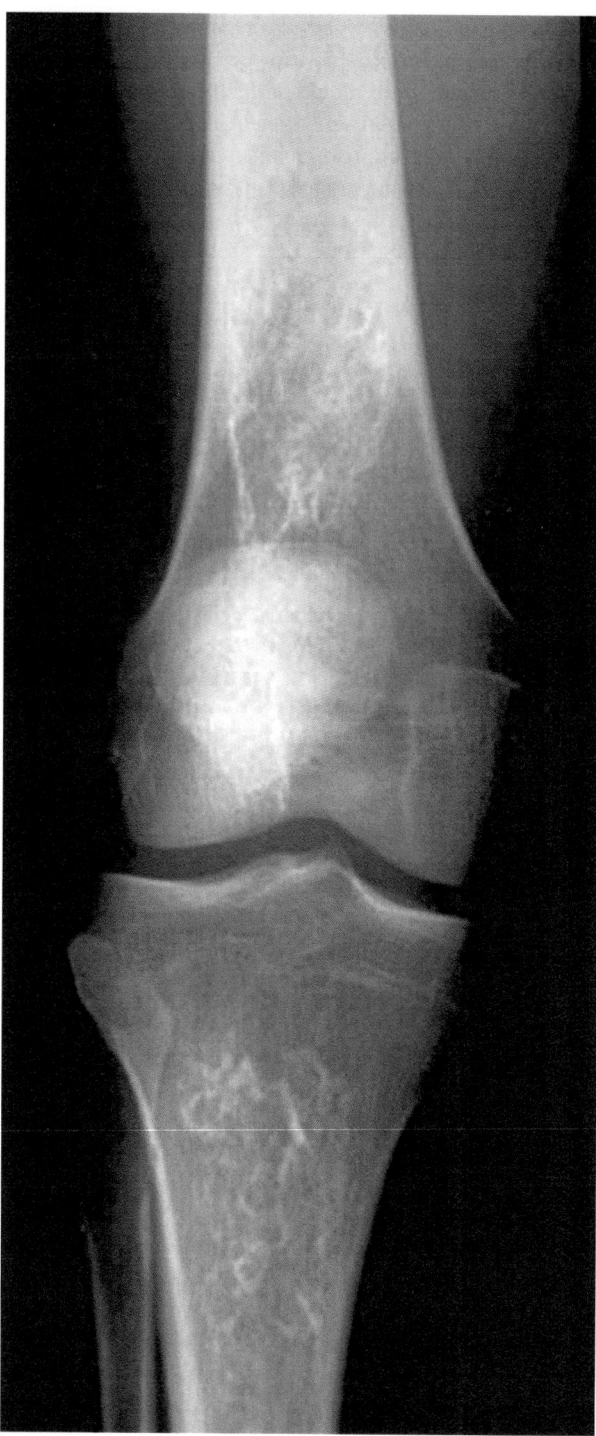

Figure 50.4 Radiograph of an experienced diver's knee joint, showing irregular sclerotic areas in the lower femoral and upper tibial shafts typical of dysbaric osteonecrosis.

Immersion-related physiology and pathology

IMMERSION

When the human body is placed upright in water, the water pressure difference between the feet and the head forces fluid to move upwards. As a result, a number of physiological changes occur. The normal distribution of blood volume is affected with blood from the lower limb extremity moving upwards and mainly being accommodated within the chest. This results in an increase in pulmonary blood volume and a rise in right atrial pressure. The former results in a small reduction in vital capacity impeding ventilation and the latter results in production of atrial naturetic hormone and a resultant diuresis. The pressure difference between the centre of the chest and the mouth introduces a resistance to breathing, as drawing air down into the chest against the pressure gradient increases the work of inspiration. Conversely, the work of expiration is aided. These changes disappear when the body is horizontal, for example when the diver is swimming and are reversed when the diver is head down. The changes may combine with gas density effects to result in a significant impairment of ventilatory capacity during exercise and a degree of carbon dioxide retention. This becomes important in some diving situations where it may enhance oxygen toxicity, particularly in nitrox diving or closed circuit oxygen breathing military divers.

Rarely, immersion may result in the development of acute pulmonary oedema.[37,38] This results in the dive being aborted, but is likely to reoccur with future dives and with increasing severity. It is most common in individuals with a history of mild hypertension.

BUOYANCY

The human body is almost neutrally buoyant, but buoyancy varies with the volume of gas in the lungs so breathing in allows the body to float, whereas breathing out allows it to sink. Most diving is carried out wearing thermal protective suits which contain gas within enclosed spaces to provide insulation. In neoprene suits, air is contained within the foam bubbles of the suit and in membrane dry suits gas is contained in the space between the diver's body and the suit. The gas or air contained within the suits is affected by pressure, so the volume shrinks as the diver descends. While on the surface, the suit increases buoyancy substantially as a result of the gas contained and the diver needs to carry additional weight in the form of lead to counteract this effect in order to get submerged. However, once submerged, the increasing pressure reduces the volume of air within the suit and the added buoyancy of the suit is progressively lost with depth. Hence, the diver who adjusted weight for neutral buoyancy on the surface becomes negatively buoyant at depth. This problem is solved by a buoyancy compensation device which may be either an air-filled jacket or suit in which the volume contained can be adjusted by the diver. This requires use of the diver's air supply to fill the device and use of valves to exhaust or dump the excess gas as the diver ascends. Such devices expand and rapidly provide positive buoyancy on ascent and hence careful control is required to maintain overall stable depth. Their failure or incautious use have been the cause of numerous episodes of rapid uncontrolled ascent.

CARDIOVASCULAR

Apart from fluid shifts which raise right atrial pressure, immersion of the face in water, particularly when it is cold provokes the diving reflex manifest by vagal stimulation and bradycardia. This is not a potent effect, but may be part of the mechanism which results in the rare development of arrhythmias in some divers and the development of immersion-induced pulmonary oedema.

THERMAL

The water in which divers immerse themselves is commonly cold so rapid loss of body heat is an important physiological challenge. Divers with more subcutaneous fat are better protected, but in almost all situations some form of thermal protection is required. A basic neoprene wetsuit traps a thin layer of water between suit and the diver's skin which is heated by the diver's body heat. The suit restricts water movement and provides some insulation, thereby reducing heat loss. Drysuits enclose the diver in a watertight suit which traps a layer of air or gas within the suit, which acts as insulation. The suit membrane is often thin. Fibre pile or other insulated clothing worn inside the suit provides a medium to hold and trap the insulating gas. Drysuits provide better protection than wet-suits, but have buoyancy problems and still do not really allow comfortable long dives. Flooded hot water suits are commonly used. These are essentially a baggy wetsuit with an internal pipe network. Hot water is pumped down to the diver and perfuses the suit. Multiple perforations in the suit pipe network provide a constant supply of hot water to the whole body in a fairly even distribution. Although the diver is wet, body heat can be well maintained for long periods in the coldest water environments. Unfortunately, these suits do not provide any protection from other hazards, e.g. chemical. In these circumstances, a liquid heated membrane suit can be used. These are a drysuit containing a network of thin-walled tubing in the suit material wall, which can be heated with a supply of hot water to maintain the temperature of the suit environment.

A diver's thermal comfort can be important in the control of decompression illness. Cold and poorly perfused peripheral tissues take up and release dissolved gas less readily. A diver who takes up inert gas while warm during a dive, but becomes cold during the following decompression may have a higher inert gas load at the end of the dive and hence an increased risk of decompression sickness.

Water has very high thermal conductivity compared to air. This is why garments and suits which trap a layer of air provide insulation for a person in either a cold environment or water. Unfortunately, helium also has high thermal conductivity, so when the air used for insulation purposes is replaced with helium–oxygen mixtures, there is a substantial loss of insulation effect.

WETNESS

Divers' skin is exposed to water or damp conditions during much of their work. In wet or flooded suits, the diver is wet throughout the period in the water. Drysuits are totally enclosed waterproof enclosures and if the physical work rate is high, there is very high humidity as a result of sweating. Saturation diving environments using heliox as the breathing gas require to be maintained at 28–32°C to maintain thermal balance. Keeping the humidity level under control generates significant problems, so divers may be exposed to high humidity for periods of weeks at a time with potential effects on the skin.[39]

LOSS OF CONSCIOUSNESS

Disturbance of consciousness or incapacitation while in the water prevents the diver from maintaining those actions essential to preserve life while underwater and hence may prove fatal. The ultimate cause of many diving fatalities is drowning, although this commonly results from an initial event which might be a preceding illness, injury or equipment failure. A detailed investigation of diving incidents, which should include assessment of equipment in use, is crucial in understanding how the incident occurred and hence how further events may be prevented in the future.

The causes of loss of consciousness fall into several categories:

- The presence of a gas phase within the body either from a cerebral gas embolism or decompression sickness may cause loss of consciousness either immediately after ascent or during the first few hours.
- The toxic effects of normal air constituents at pressure may result in loss of consciousness from nitrogen narcosis, but only at high pressures (pN_2 greater than 6 ata) or from cerebral oxygen toxicity, where the pO_2 exceeds 1.5 ata. The latter may occur when breathing an oxygen-enriched gas mixture (pure oxygen or nitrox) at shallow depth or a heliox or trimix mixture at deeper depths.
- Hypoxia can occur when breathing a gas mixture with a low pO_2 which can occur as a result of an error in dive planning or on ascent when breathing a gas which had adequate pO_2 at depth, but as pressure falls on ascent the pO_2 falls. This may occur when making an emergency ascent after losing an air supply. Hypoxia also results in loss of consciousness when it occurs as a result of drowning, aspiration of vomit or breathing a gas supply contaminated with carbon monoxide.
- Hypercapnia can occur when ventilation is restricted by gas density, for example when breathing air at depths below 40 msw. The high pO_2 of air at that depth prevents hypoxia and allows a diver to undertake high levels of physical exertion. The high metabolic rate

associated with exertion results in high CO_2 production which cannot be excreted normally because of limited ventilatory ability resulting in acute CO_2 narcosis.
- Hypothermia can occur rapidly as a result of inadequate suit heating or when breathing cold heliox at depth.
- Hyperthermia may also occur rapidly in a heliox environment when the breathing gas or chamber environment is too high.

> An air diver attempted a survey dive using a diving helmet at a depth of 45 msw. On arrival on the sea bed, he found his umbilical snagged, was unable to move, struggled and called for assistance before becoming unconscious. He was recovered by the standby diver who found him motionless and apnoeic. During recovery, spontaneous breathing commenced at a depth of 12 msw and he recovered consciousness at the surface, but complained of headache. He was immediately recompressed to manage omitted decompression and because the cause of the episode was uncertain. All symptoms resolved rapidly during recompression and he remained entirely well.
>
> **Comment**
>
> High workload when struggling and an element of panic while breathing dense air at 5.5 ata resulted in hypoventilation and acute carbon dioxide retention, leading to a period of anaesthesia. The high partial pressure of oxygen prevented severe hypoxaemia and the reduction of ambient pressure during ascent reduced gas density and alveolar pCO_2 allowing rapid recovery with only residual headache.

DIVING TASKS

Diving methodology

Modern commercial diving may involve a number of different diving methods.

Breath-hold diving is only in use for commercial purposes in traditional pearl diving communities. However, breath-hold dives may be undertaken as part of work activity, for example in helicopter underwater escape training (Figure 50.5).

Self-contained underwater breathing apparatus (SCUBA) allows a diver to carry a compressed breathing gas supply and hence be entirely independent in the water. This is most extensively used by recreational divers. The diver carries a cylinder of compressed gas with a regulator which reduces the pressure to a few ata above the diver's actual environmental pressure. The regulator supplies a demand valve which is usually attached to a mouthpiece held by the diver's teeth. The demand valve provides a supply of breathing gas as the diver inhales at the diver's ambient pressure. In the event of emergency, help can only be obtained from the immediate vicinity and hence divers dive with a buddy. Complete independence which is attractive to sport divers represents a

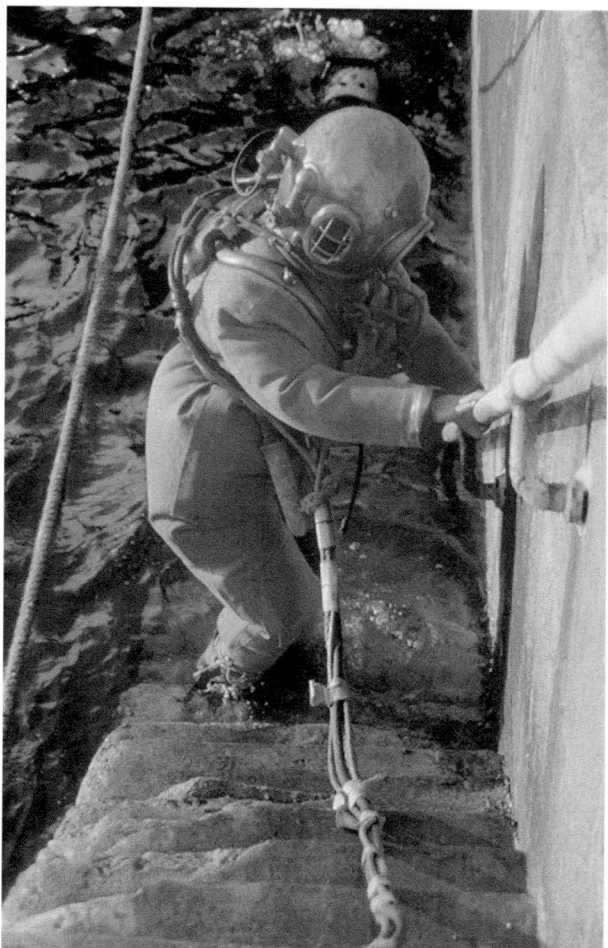

Figure 50.5 Diver entering water wearing 'standard dress' – a totally enclosed suit and rigid brass helmet supplied with compressed air from the surface.

hazard in most working diving environments, but the technique is still used in a limited range of applications including some scientific (marine science), media diving, police (search and rescue) and sea food harvesting, but has very restricted application elsewhere. More complex versions of SCUBA, such as closed or open circuit rebreather devices, have limited military or recreational applications.

Surface-supplied diving (SSD) provides a breathing gas supply from the surface by hose or umbilical. The diver normally wears a helmet and breathes through an oronasal mask, rather than a mouthpiece (Figure 50.6).

These two factors allow communications, so the umbilical also contains electric cables for communications and commonly a hot water supply and a depth/pressure monitor (pneumofathometer). The communication link allows the supervisor to listen to the diver's breathing pattern and talk with the diver and as the umbilical is attached to the diver's harness, it provides a means by which the diver can be recovered. No buddy diver is required, but a standby diver is available on the surface to follow the diver's umbilical to provide rapid support if necessary. Wearing a helmet, rather than using a mouthpiece, provides much greater security in the event of any incident involving loss

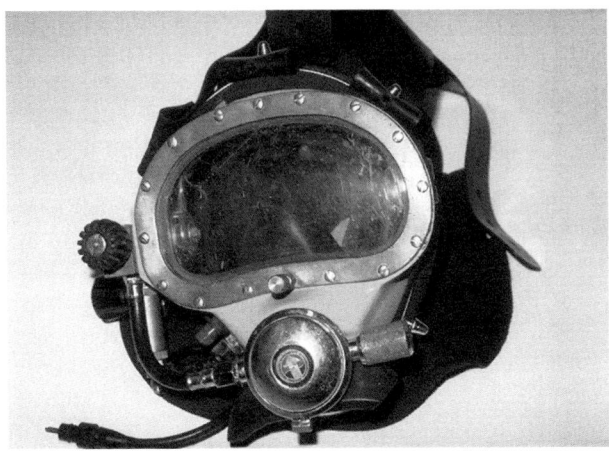

Figure 50.6 Commonly used commercial divers 'band mask' helmet comprising a rigid faceplate attached to a soft neoprene hood held on to the diver's head by a number of rubber straps (spider) attached to posts around the faceplate. The demand valve which supplies breathing gas to an oronasal mask within the helmet is clearly seen below the faceplate. For colour image, see www.hodderplus.com/hunters.

of consciousness or self-control or vomiting. This is the most common method used for air diving in oilfield work, inshore commercial diving and is increasingly being used in police and rescue diving activity. The risks associated with this method increase with the distance from safety (surface) and are widely regarded as unacceptable with an umbilical greater than 50 m in length.

In many commercial diving operations, getting the diver safely into and out of the water is a significant difficulty. A wet bell is essentially a transport device or lift which lowers divers from a surface structure down to the sea surface and on down further to the working dive depth. Although the divers are just standing on an open platform in the water it is possible to have a small air-filled space in the upper part of the structure which provides an opportunity to sort any helmet or breathing apparatus problems without necessarily returning to the surface. The bell, whose depth is controlled from the surface, also allows divers to make decompression stops during the ascent at accurate depths and times.

A closed diving bell is a pressure vessel with a hatchway and trunk in the floor which has doors on both inside and outside. Divers can travel from the surface to depth in the closed bell with pressure maintained at 1 ata with the external door closed. Pressurization of the bell can be delayed until the bell is in the appropriate position and the diver is ready to leave. At this point, the bell is pressurized to a depth equal to the position of the bell so that the door can be opened to allow the diver to exit to perform the task. On returning to the bell, the bell can be raised with the door open until bell depth reaches a decompression stop. At this point, the inside door is closed and while the bell pressure is maintained for the purposes of following the decompression plan, the bell can be lifted out of the water. The bell may then be locked on to a chamber allowing the divers to transfer to complete their decompression in a comfortable environment. Deep bell dives in which the diver completes the dive breathing heliox and then completes a decompression returning to the surface, have in the past been extensively used in oilfield diving. The risk of decompression sickness is high and problems resulting from oxygen toxicity from the high ppO_2 mixtures used to accelerate decompression are frequent. In most areas, the method has been replaced with saturation techniques.

The use of a chamber on the surface and a closed diving bell is the basis of a saturation diving system. To avoid long decompression periods after every dive, divers are 'stored' at increased ambient pressure in pressure chambers on the surface. They can then transfer to a diving bell and then into the water to conduct work without any significant change in pressure. This allows divers to work in the water for prolonged periods over a period of three weeks or more. However, there is then a need for a prolonged decompression which may last several days to retrieve the divers from storage to the surface. The very low risk of decompression illness and the absence of significant time restriction on divers' working time in the water, together with the more effective work time/decompression time ratio has made this the preferred method for most oilfield diving, other than shallow inspection work. The benefits compensate for the considerable increase in cost of plant and manpower and the method is being increasingly used for shallower work.

Decompression planning

Procedures which permit divers or compressed air workers to return to the surface following exposure to increased pressure without the development of decompression illness are critical to safe diving and compressed air work. The mathematics of decompression planning are a complex mixture of limited experimental data, empirical observation and theoretical calculation. The resulting algorithms provide valuable reduction in risk, but do not offer complete control. The risk of decompression illness is best controlled in saturation diving, where complete saturation is certain and one single final decompression is made using an appropriate slow decompression following many hours of underwater work. In all other (surface-orientated) diving, the extent of a diver's gas uptake is always an estimate and not surprisingly the incidence of decompression illness is much higher. The risk of decompression illness is also greater for longer and deeper dives. The gradual evolution of decompression algorithms continues to reduce the risk, but this appears unlikely ever to be completely eliminated due to variations in working activities and both inter- and intraindividual characteristics. Despite the undoubted benefits of scientific and theoretical calculations in developing decompression schedules, the best predictor of the safety of a diving or compressed air decompression procedure is the practical experience of it gained in actual commercial or military operations.

Decompression procedures or tables

The practical application of decompression algorithms at the dive site can be achieved either by the use of tables[40] or by the use of a portable computer device. Decompression tables comprise a list of procedures defining the ascent profile required following dives of varying depth and duration. Typically, if a dive is planned to a depth of, for example 32 msw, the dive supervisor would select a table for the next deeper depth which might be 35 msw. There will already be an approximate estimate of the time required for the dive, so in the course of the dive the supervisor would have available 35-msw tables for time intervals around the estimate. In the course of the dive, the supervisor would ensure that the planned depth was not exceeded and after the work is complete, would note the time at which the ascent is started. The duration of the dive from leaving the surface to commencement of ascent is called 'bottom time'. The supervisor selects the table time which is the next longer than the actual bottom time and then directs the diver to make stops during the ascent at depths and for times defined by the table procedure.

Recreational divers plan their dive in advance and then stick to the plan since their access to table data during a dive is limited to what can be recalled from memory or written on a waterproof slate. Not surprisingly, a hand- or wrist-held computer, which accurately measures depths and time and can then compute the required decompression profile while the diver is in the water, overcomes many practical difficulties and is an attractive option.

Diving tables are produced and published by various organizations including navies,[40] recreational diving organizations,[41] commercial diving contractors and others. The efficacy of decompression tables is somewhat variable, but in general continues to improve and as a result the incidence of decompression illness is falling. Diving tables are a critical component of a commercial diving contractor's equipment and a legal requirement in some countries.

Despite gradual improvements, there remain considerable differences between tables in the decompression requirement for the same dive. This highlights the fact that decompression table procedures reduce risk, but do not eliminate it. Individuals also differ in susceptibility to decompression illness when exposed to identical pressure exposure, working activity and conditions. Intraindividual variations must also occur to explain why individuals sometimes develop acute decompression illness, for no obvious reason, after many years of similar previous uneventful exposures. These factors have confounded the further development of decompression procedures and the study of associated risk factors.

Computers

The dive computer has revolutionized the conduct of recreational diving and their use is widespread. Currently, they have only limited application in commercial diving and are not used in compressed air operations. The ability to measure depth and duration of the dive accurately without the need to rely on the diver reading a watch and a depth gauge underwater represents a major advance and the opportunity to eliminate many calculation errors made in table selection. The computer can then accurately apply the decompression algorithm and provide a guide to the decompression profile required. However, in the use of tables, there was a consistent methodology to apply safety margins to the algorithm by using a deeper depth than actually dived, a longer bottom time and using the deepest depth reached as the depth of the dive rather than an average. The computer enables an absolute calculation of depth time profile to calculate gas uptake and then applies the algorithm. Effectively, this means that the algorithm is operated close to its limits at all times, whereas when using tables there would commonly be additional inbuilt safety allowances.

Computers are so widely used that direct comparison of table use versus computer use is now impossible. Computers inevitably permit more time in the water than would tables and hence are attractive to recreational divers. The ease with which a diver can conduct a decompression dive has contributed to the increasing depth of recreational diving. It is important that divers fully understand the background and limitations of diving computers and use them in a knowledgeable and sensible manner.

Mixed gas methods

As dive depth gets deeper, an increasing number of problems occur. First, when breathing compressed air, nitrogen narcosis becomes increasingly important at pressures above 4 ata and a major safety risk. Replacing the nitrogen with helium overcomes the narcotic effect and also some of the respiratory limitation resulting from increased breathing gas density. The elevated partial pressure of oxygen in compressed air may result in cerebral oxygen toxicity when the partial pressure exceeds 1.5 ata, i.e. at 65 msw, particularly where gas density results in some CO_2 retention.

These problems can be overcome by using a mixture of helium and oxygen (heliox) at depth. The oxygen content is reduced to ensure that the partial pressure of oxygen at the dive depth is not toxic and narcosis is eliminated. An important disadvantage is that the high rate of diffusion of helium contributes to a rapid uptake during the dive so that the diver approaches saturation more rapidly. As a result, decompression times for surface-orientated diving with heliox are longer than with air. Since decompression times get exponentially longer as the dive depth and duration increase, this becomes an important limitation on the use of heliox for surface-orientated diving. To enhance decompression rate, oxygen-enriched breathing gas mixtures and 100 per cent oxygen are used during the decompression; however, the potential for development of oxygen toxicity limits the extent of oxygen use.

Although deep heliox dives can be conducted using an umbilical from the surface, this technique presents high risk and the use of a closed bell is more appropriate.

Recreational deep divers, attracted to surface-orientated techniques as a result of cost and logistical factors, usually take a different approach to commercial divers, replacing some but not all of the nitrogen with helium to produce a 'trimix' in which the oxygen partial pressure is controlled, and narcosis controlled but not eliminated, while not suffering all the decompression disadvantage of using heliox.

Saturation diving

In deep diving, where safety demands the use of a closed diving bell, the number of personnel required to support the operation is large, the amount of time a diver can spend working on the seabed is very limited and a large component of time is taken up with the decompression. Deep surface-orientated dives carry a high risk of decompression illness. The logical solution to all these issues is saturation diving. A team of divers is 'stored' in a pressure chamber at a pressure which is very close to the depth at which work is required. Each small diving team comprising a standby diver and one or two working divers is transported by closed bell from the storage chamber to the worksite. The small pressure difference between the bell and the water at the worksite is equalized and the diver(s) can leave the bell to work. At the end of their shift they return to the bell which is then closed and sealed and the divers return to the storage chamber. Because there have been only very small pressure changes, there is no time limitation on the duration of the dive and no requirement for a staged decompression at this point. Another shift of divers can continue the work immediately. In this way, divers can work on the seabed for more than 20 in every 24 hours.

The divers become 'saturated' or equilibrated with the gas at the pressure they are stored at over a period of six hours. Once equilibrated, no more inert gas can dissolve in body tissues and hence the decompression time required is no longer after four weeks than after approximately six hours. At the completion of the work, decompressing the divers to the surface may take five to six days or even longer, but the system allows a much more effective use of divers' time and of plant and equipment and at the same time dramatically reduces the risk of decompression illness. At depths exceeding 150 msw, divers compressed rapidly may experience a complex neurological effect known as high pressure neurological syndrome,[42,43] characterized by tremor, incoordination and episodes of microsleep. In operational diving, this is readily avoided by appropriate compression profiles, but is a potential cause of poor diver performance and hence accidents during very deep saturation dives. It may also generate problems when additional support workers, for example medical staff, are compressed rapidly in an emergency situation.

Saturation diving has completely revolutionized subsea engineering. Large numbers of ships have been purpose-built to conduct saturation diving and subsea intervention and the associated technology is being applied to diving tasks in progressively shallower water.

While the saturation method largely protects divers from decompression illness,[44] the mode of work introduces a wide range of different medical problems. Perhaps most important of these is the isolation of the divers who cannot be returned to the surface in less than their decompression time, usually several days. This presents difficulties in the management of illness or injury. Although the concept of transporting an injured diver in a portable pressure chamber to a hospital-based hyperbaric facility has been explored, it is always simpler to transport a medical team and equipment to the dive vessel and provide care on site. Medical staff who attend a diver in saturation are likely to require the same prolonged decompression.

Dive planning

The methodology selected for an underwater diving project depends on a number of factors which include water depth, duration of work activity, cost, available equipment and personnel, and acceptable risk. For example, a single dive to a depth of 40 msw for a task lasting a few minutes might be safely conducted by a single surface-orientated air dive involving no decompression stops. A substantial work programme requiring many hours of work at a depth of 30 msw could be conducted by an air diving operation, but would require numerous dives which would all need to be of reasonable duration (30–40 minutes) and hence would involve decompression procedures. There would therefore be a significant risk of one or more episodes of decompression illness. The same work programme might be more rapidly achieved using saturation methodology in which a smaller number of divers could complete the work in shifts, all working for six hours at a time with a very low risk of decompression illness. It would, however, require expensive equipment and trained personnel, so would represent a more costly option.

CURRENT HAZARDS AND RISKS

Divers are exposed to a wide range of hazards. These may be considered under two major headings, environmental and related to the work activity. It is important to remember that diving is simply a method of getting workers to the workplace and while diving itself carries significant inherent hazards, there remain significant hazards of the work activity itself, many of which are shared by workers on the surface (Figure 50.7). Some of these hazards are modified by the underwater environment and may be difficult to

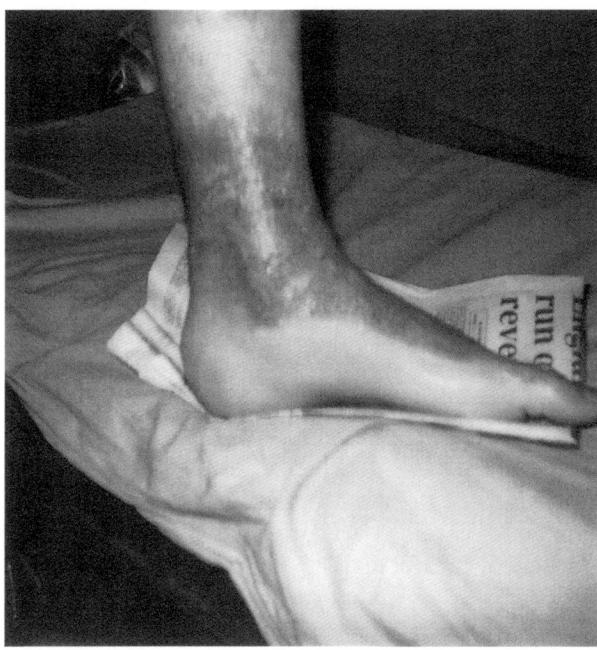

Figure 50.7 Extensive chemical dermatitis affecting the ankle and foot of an oilfield diver who had been working on the sea bed contaminated with drilling mud. For colour image, see www.hodderplus.com/hunters.

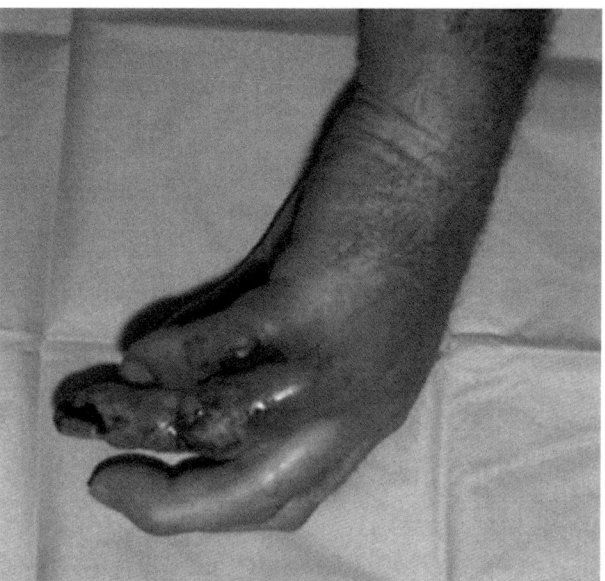

Figure 50.8 The hand of a diver whose fingers had been sucked into a valve as a result of pressure difference during a mechanical engineering task on the sea bed. Pressure differences between the ambient pressure at which the diver is working and gas spaces in mechanical components have caused major injury and fatalities. For colour image, see www.hodderplus.com/hunters.

assess and control. Some of these issues have been overshadowed by diving hazards and require further attention.

Environmental (dive-related) hazards include pressure-related illness (barotrauma and decompression sickness), drowning, breathing gas toxicity, noise, infection, thermal illness and marine animal attack. Work activity may result in direct trauma, noise exposure, chemical and vibration exposure.

Commercial diving has a reputation as a hazardous occupation, but there are large differences in risks between different sectors of the commercial diving industry. For example, scientific divers and police diving teams have very low incident rates, whereas oilfield commercial diving has much higher rates (Figure 50.8). This difference is mainly explained by the nature of the work environment and the type of work undertaken. Incident rates have fallen substantially over the course of the last 20 years, but diving remains a hazardous employment. Comparison with other groups of workers is difficult because of the pattern of divers' work. For example, an air diver might undertake 200 dives in a year, but spend between 50 and 600 hours in the water, whereas an onshore construction worker might expect to be at work for 2000 hours in a year. A saturation diver might spend 120 days at pressure (almost 3000 hours), but be in the water for less than 600 hours.

Incident control

Safety management in the diving industry is complex. Improved decompression procedures and restrictions on divers' pressure exposure have greatly reduced the incidence of decompression illness. Major improvements in equipment preventing catastrophic failure and control of the use of hazardous techniques, e.g. oxygen burning and high pressure water jetting have contributed to lower accident rates. The introduction of a risk assessment method to every task has also had a contribution, but is highly dependent on the expertise within the dive team to identify potential problems. Much of the risk control is managed by the diving supervisor who has responsibility for all aspects of a diving operation from the operational planning to the handling of problems occurring in the course of a dive.

In diving operations, even a trivial problem may result in a catastrophic outcome, so the severity of outcome is commonly greater than in comparable situations in other industries. In this situation, the efficiency with which potential hazards are identified and brought to the attention of the diving team is critical. In the United Kingdom, the speed with which hazardous incidents have been investigated and the conclusions and recommendations passed on to the industry, both by the Diving Inspectorate (both Department of the Environment and the Health and Safety Executive) and contractors, has been a major contribution to reduction in accident rate and the UK Offshore standards are regarded as a world leader in diving safety.

Management of incidents

Despite improvement in risk control, the environment in which diving operations are conducted is always hazardous and contingency planning for the management of incidents remains an important part of diving operation planning.

In the event of an incident resulting in illness or injury, the most immediate assistance is provided by other members of the dive team and hence appropriate first aid training of divers is important. Divers may be subject to the normal range of accidents which occur in working environments and in addition are at risk of specific diving-related illness. The immediate first aid management of the decompression illnesses, near drowning, hypoxia and carbon monoxide poisoning or contaminated gas supply includes oxygen administration and all divers should have this expertise and be familiar with the oxygen equipment available.

Most cases of decompression illness are treated with fluid replacement and recompression.[45] Divers presenting with symptoms on the surface are most commonly treated with an oxygen breathing procedure, such as Royal Navy Table 62 (United States Navy Table 6), in which the individual is compressed in a chamber to a depth equivalent of 18 msw and given 100 per cent oxygen to breath for periods of 20 minutes interspersed with breathing air for five minutes. After three to five periods of oxygen breathing, the pressure is reduced slowly to 9 msw and further periods of oxygen breathing lasting an hour are continued before a final decompression to the surface. A substantial proportion of cases resolve during this primary procedure, but others require further hyperbaric oxygen treatments before the condition has either resolved or reached a stable state. A variety of more complex procedures may be applied in specific situations based upon individual clinical assessment.[46–48]

Immediate access to specialist diving medical expertise is critical to ensure that continued care follows appropriate lines, and evacuation to an appropriate medical and/or hyperbaric facility occurs when necessary. This is particularly important when a recompression facility is available at the dive site where the opportunity exists for recompression treatment to be given without any direct medical assessment. In the past, a number of inappropriate and unsupervised recompression procedures conducted without adequate clinical support or medical advice have led to tragic outcomes.

Where medical care at a more advanced level than immediate first aid is required at the dive site, for example if a recompression facility is available or if the dive site is remote either geographically or because the affected diver is saturated in a storage living chamber, then it is appropriate for at least a proportion of the diving team to have more advanced first aid training. This is commonly called 'diver medic training' and involves a two-week training course which covers more medical procedures, such as venous cannulation and intravenous fluid administration, drug administration, advanced resuscitation, urinary catheterization, vital sign recording, aspects of neurological examination and wound care.

In the event of serious incident, there must be a contingency plan for evacuation of the diver to medical care or the provision of medical care at the dive site. In evacuation, the possible risk of decompression sickness in the period after the dive and the possibility of provocation during evacuation by air needs to be considered, but in most circumstances the risks associated with delay in receiving medical treatment are greater.

Outcome of incidents

Most incidents require careful investigation to ensure that the cause is fully understood and particularly that the sequence of events leading up to injury or the presentation of illness is fully established. This may be critical in establishing a diagnosis. For example, the onset of symptoms at stable depth before any decompression has taken place effectively excludes decompression illness as a cause of that symptom.

After illness or injury, reassessment of medical fitness to dive should be carried out by a doctor with diving medical knowledge and with complete information about the prognosis and the impact of any disability.

LONG-TERM HEALTH EFFECTS

Divers are at risk of acute diving-related illness, such as decompression sickness and barotrauma, as well as other work-related injury. Incomplete recovery from these events may leave the diver with a significant residual deficit or disability which will never recover.[20]

In addition, divers are at risk of health effects which result in the presentation of symptoms with a substantial delay after any pressure exposure and without a history of acute decompression illness or other overt symptomatology.

Dysbaric osteonecrosis is the best example of this phenomenon.[36] This is a form of aseptic bone necrosis which is associated with previous experience of decompression. Although the precise pathogenic mechanism remains unclear, it is assumed that decompression involving the release of inert gas from solution in body tissues is the underlying precipitant. The mechanism may involve microbubble emboli causing infarction in end arteries within bone[49] or pressure change within bone marrow.[50] The lesions which may occur in many bones are painless. The end result is areas of dead bone which usually remain asymptomatic for many years. The radiological classification of dysbaric osteonecrosis affecting divers and compressed air workers was established by the Medical Research Council Decompression Sickness Panel in the 1960s and has been widely used internationally ever since.[51] Two distinct types of lesion are defined. 'B' lesions are found in the shafts of long bones, particularly the femur, tibia and humerus. 'A' (juxta-articular) lesions occur adjacent to articular surfaces of large joints, particularly the shoulder and hip. Lesions are almost entirely painless and those in long bone shafts cause no symptoms and can be regarded as of no clinical significance. Over the course of years, some lesions adjacent to articular surfaces may result in a gradual collapse of the articular surface followed by the development of secondary osteoarthritis. Symptoms of joint pain and stiffness develop at this late stage and may require joint replacement due to severe disability. The prevalence of dysbaric osteonecrosis in different working populations appears to relate closely to the efficacy of the decompression tables or algorithm used. Although the prevalence in the UK commercial diving population was considered to represent a significant potential risk to the diving population as deep saturation diving developed,[52] this has not proved to be the case and the incidence of new cases in commercial (or military) diving appears to be very low. It is however, not possible to be certain because routine radiological screening is no longer considered to be acceptable from a radiation hazard aspect, and magnetic resonance imaging (MRI), which is the alternative screening method, has not yet been widely applied because of cost implications.

The reported incidence of dysbaric osteonecrosis in compressed air work projects in the past has reached as high as 25 per cent in the mid-1900s with a wide variation between different projects. The incidence rates appear to have reduced with improved safety and decompression procedures over many years. However, because of the latency before the appearance of radiological abnormality and even longer period before onset of symptoms, accurate incidence rates are difficult to establish. Cases of disability resulting from dysbaric osteonecrosis still present through the courts representing a significant ongoing work-related morbidity for previous compressed air workers. The risk remains significant particularly considering the relatively small number of exposures when compared to the commercial diving industry. Unfortunately, any beneficial effect on dysbaric osteonecrosis in compressed air workers from the use of oxygen decompression techniques has not yet been proven due to the lack of accurate data.

Neurological

There have been many suggestions that divers are at risk of long-term neurological injury as a result of diving in the absence of a history of acute decompression illness resulting in permanent disability.[53,54] Several reports have indicated that divers are more likely to complain of memory difficulties and possibly concentration problems. However, no distinct symptomatic pattern of illness or pathology has emerged. Many studies have been complicated by the absence of an appropriate control population and by failure to adjust for other factors, such as accidents, head injury and alcohol consumption, all of which influence neurological outcome. The issue has become a significant problem in Norway, where a significant proportion of divers who worked offshore in the 1970s and 1980s have claimed to be incapacitated as a result of diving work. There may, however, be significant psychosocial compounding factors, including the overall sickness absence rates, cultural factors, compensation and medicolegal issues as UK divers working at the same time and often at the same worksites do not appear to have similar problems.

Pulmonary

Divers have been demonstrated to have larger lungs than the normal population[55] and this has been associated with abnormalities in the expiratory flow pattern consistent with small airway obstruction.[56] However, although some of these changes appear to progress in the early part of a diver's career,[57] no specific pathological outcome has yet been identified.

Recent studies

A number of recent reports have addressed the concerns about development of long-term health effects in the commercial diving population. Some uncontrolled studies from Norway[58,59] have suggested that long-term disability due to unspecified neurological deficit is common in a population with experience of diving within the offshore oil industry. However, a large questionnaire survey of commercial divers in the United Kingdom,[60] compared to the offshore non-diving population revealed no major difference in health status, although divers did report more symptoms, particularly of forgetfulness and loss of concentration. More detailed evaluation of symptomatic divers showed only small differences in formal tests of memory,[61] which appeared to be related to work in the offshore oil industry, rather than any particular diving technique, suggesting that other factors associated with work in the industry, for example chemical exposure may be relevant.

TUNNELLING TASKS

Tunnelling or caisson work is part of civil engineering activity. Working at pressure becomes a requirement where excavation occurs beneath the level of the water table and where the ground is sufficiently porous to allow water to be forced into the tunnel or caisson as a result of the groundwater pressure. Hence, while it is possible to tunnel through solid impervious rock below water level without risk of flooding, tunnelling through softer water-permeable ground readily results in a water-filled tunnel with the risk of collapse of the (water-saturated) tunnel apex or face. In this situation, to allow work to progress, the open end of the tunnel is closed off with a pressure tight structure and the tunnel is pressurized to a pressure adequate to prevent water ingress and stabilize the tunnel face. A pressure chamber or lock is built into the tunnel enclosure to allow workers to transfer from the surface to the pressurized environment without loss of pressure in the tunnel. This enables the tunnel construction to continue with work conducted in a dry environment.

In the past, much of the work conducted at pressure was manual excavation using hand-held pneumatic tools to progress the tunnel. Tunnelling, therefore, required many man hours of hard manual work in compressed air and the relatively large tunnel labour force (sometimes hundreds of men on large projects) consisted mostly of labourers who worked on a daily shift system with five or six days' exposure, sometimes during a project which could last several years. Although some small projects still require this activity, most tunnels are now constructed mechanically using a sophisticated tunnel boring machine (TBM) which lines the tunnel as it is constructed and hence the only human work requiring a pressurized environment is maintenance work conducted at the front face of the machine, such as blade or tool changing (often called 'interventions') or technical or geological inspections (Figure 50.9). As a result, the number of man hours required at pressure and the number of workers exposed, is greatly reduced in comparison to historical projects. The type of work is often now of a more technical nature rather than simple manual activity, but may still be physically demanding, in very confined spaces under extreme conditions of temperature and humid or wet conditions. TBM interventions or inspections are usually conducted on a periodic basis during the project with the pressure exposure varying from 0.5 to 2 hours (for single inspections) to interventions with shift lengths of two to ten hours (subject to the maximum working pressure and conditions) and daily exposures for two to six days.

TBMs require short intense periods of compressed air interventions, sometimes at high pressures (4–8 ata), but use a relatively small compressed air workforce (typically 30–60 personnel). The number of workers per shift depends on the tunnel diameter and other factors, but usually only three to five men will work under pressure at any one time on a rotating 24-hour shift basis for the duration of the intervention. As the TBM progression is effectively halted until the intervention is completed, it is an operational priority to maximize working time under pressure and to minimize the risk of decompression sickness (since this removes the worker from the compressed air workforce for the duration of that intervention).

Most UK tunnel projects using compressed air in the past have been at relatively low pressure (often below 2 ata and rarely above 4 ata, but exposures tended to be long (six to eight hours)). However, increasing health concerns in the late 1980s and early 1990s led to much shorter pressure exposures being adopted by contractors following recommendations from their medical advisers, especially where working pressure exceeded 2 ata and this was eventually prescribed by HSE in the 1996 regulations. Working pressures greater than 3 ata restrict shift duration and the limit of current air tables is set at 4.45 ata as a result of physiological factors and safety issues. This has led to the need for the development and implementation of safer decompression techniques that give longer working time at higher pressures (4 ata or greater) and with reduced risk of decompression sickness or dysbaric osteonecrosis. Inevitably, this means the application of diving technologies in the civil engineering context, which includes the use of mixed gas and saturation techniques, in addition to oxygen decompression.

Like divers, tunnel workers may also require a gradual return to surface pressure to prevent the onset of decompression illness. The decompression or ascent is conducted in a pressure lock so can be very accurately controlled. Whole shifts will compress together and decompress at the end of the working shift.

Decompression procedures for tunnelling in the past have been quite different from diving procedures and appeared to permit much more rapid decompression from a given pressure exposure. The incidence of decompression illness has often been quite high and dysbaric osteonecrosis

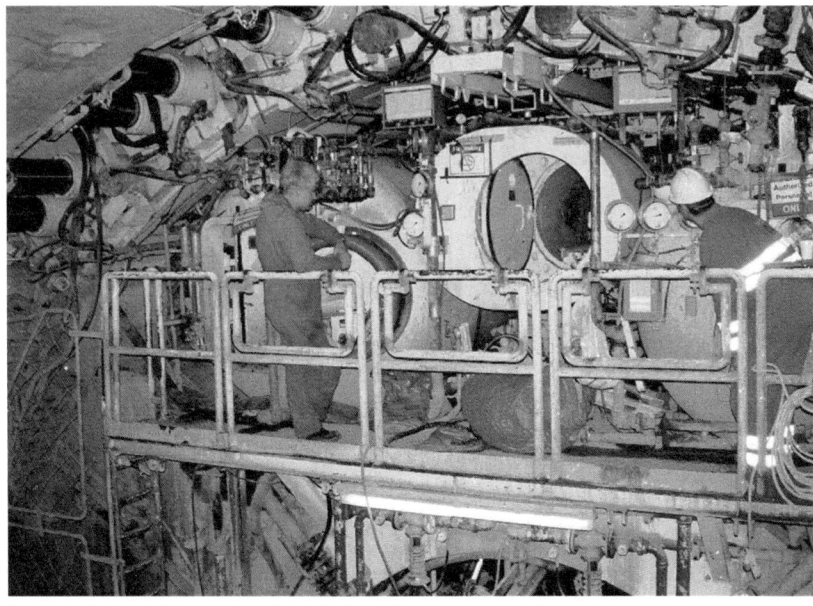

Figure 50.9 A modern tunnel boring machine for a tunnel in excess of 10-m diameter. The operators are in front of three pressure locks used by compressed air workers and equipment used to access the front face of the machine. Hydraulic rams which push the machine forward from the tunnel lining are clearly seen at the top right. For colour image, see www.hodderplus.com/hunters.

a more frequent result than in divers, often appearing many years after the pressure exposure.

Civil engineering projects requiring work at pressure are intermittent and relatively rare. As a result, the workforce only occasionally takes part in pressure-related activities while doing a wide range of other work usually within the construction industry. Long-term health surveillance has been difficult in this situation as most compressed air workers are not in long-term employment with any given contractor and thus health screening has usually only been managed on a project-specific basis when the need arises.

The development of TBMs has also led to a different type of workforce being involved. Due to the skills required and the technical complexity of the projects, there is now always a minority of workers with previous compressed air or pressure exposure experience and the health and safety culture is mainly derived from the construction industry. This has implications for the induction training, lock supervision and site management of the pressure systems with significant differences from the management approaches employed with commercial offshore divers who will work under pressure usually as a long-term career choice. Where mixed gas or saturation techniques are required in civil engineering projects, the selection and training of the workforce (who will optimally require a mixture of tunnelling and diving experience within teams) will always require careful consideration.

Tunnel and caisson environments have other significant safety issues. They are enclosed spaces and require appropriate ventilation. Carbon dioxide retention may be a contributory factor in decompression illness. It is critical to ensure that the environment is not contaminated by toxic chemicals, particularly carbon monoxide, and that all possible sources of ignition are controlled to avoid fire. Fire in a pressurized tunnel burns more intensely for a given flame size, spreads more vigorously and is harder to extinguish than at atmospheric pressure and all of these effects are magnified by oxygen enrichment. Hence, the fire risk depends on both pressure and percentage of oxygen in the environment and it remains a major safety consideration in compressed air work. Oxygen decompression techniques were effectively delayed in the United Kingdom within the civil engineering industry, until the Health and Safety Executive had fully assessed the possible increase in safety risk from fire compared to the reduction in risk of decompression sickness from breathing oxygen during decompression.

While it is possible to ensure that the structure constructed to enclose the tunnel is sound and adequate to withstand the applied pressure, it is equally important to ensure that the surrounding ground cover and tunnel wall itself is secure. While tunnelling under a river for example, if the depth of ground between the bed of the river and the upper part of the tunnel wall is too thin, then the tunnel may blow out with rapid loss of pressure and flooding of the tunnel. Good management of any compressed air project therefore requires effective and regular communications between management, engineering, hyperbaric and medical staff at all times.

DECOMPRESSION ILLNESS IN COMPRESSED AIR WORK

Historically, decompression sickness was common among tunnel workers and many factors contributed. Long exposure times associated with hard manual work activity, ineffective decompression procedures, inadequate tunnel ventilation and avoidance or incorrect application of the decompression procedure have all contributed. Limb pain has been a more common presentation than any other, although sensory neurological or other clinical manifestations are not uncommon. Severe neurological decompression illness occurs rarely. As decompression is always conducted in a chamber lock which is usually of a significant size, very rapid ascent is virtually unknown and hence pulmonary barotrauma is very rare. In the recent past, considerable effort has been directed at improving the decompression procedures without substantially prolonging overall working hours and this has been achieved by the use of oxygen breathing during decompression for pressures up to 3.45 bar (gauge). While this is a major advantage in terms of decompression safety, there remain some concerns about the safety aspects of using compressed oxygen in some situations, particularly where a lock on a tunnel boring machine may be at the closed end of a tunnel several kilometres long. In practice, this has implications for the competency of hyperbaric technical staff (lock attendants), training and supervision of the workforce and strict management and fire prevention procedures which must be fully implemented on site.

The risk of decompression illness requires the development of a contingency plan which covers surveillance of workers during the at-risk period after pressure exposure, and the provision of a recompression facility with appropriate medical support sufficient to manage a patient with severe neurological decompression illness.

Treatment of decompression illness in compressed air work projects

The treatment of decompression illness arising during tunnelling operations is now identical to that used in the management of diving illness. In the past, recompression procedures using air alone were extensively used with several therapeutic and practical disadvantages, but now that the use of oxygen at the worksite has been accepted, the use of oxygen treatment tables has become normal practice. Therapeutic recompression is carried out using on-site chambers operated by medical lock attendants under the clinical supervision of the contract medical adviser or by referral to the nearest appropriate hyperbaric facility if the compressed air worker is remote from site.

LEGAL FRAMEWORK

Diving

In the United Kingdom, commercial diving is conducted under the Diving at Work Regulations (1997)[62] issued under the Health and Safety at Work Act (1974).[63] In addition to the general provisions of the HSW Act, the Diving at Work Regulations place duties on the diving contractor, diving supervisor and diver which aim to support the overall safety of the operation. The regulations also define the requirement for the medical assessment of divers and the necessary contingency plans required for diving operations. Approved codes of practice[64] are published for different sectors of the diving industry (offshore commercial diving, inland/inshore commercial diving, scientific and archaeological, media, recreational and police) which provide specific interpretation and explanation of how the regulations impact on the different sectors of the industry.

In other countries, various different government authorities have responsibility for the regulation of commercial diving, some having a regulatory system based on a similar model to the UK system. In others, diving is completely unregulated. Within Europe, the European Diving Technology Committee attempts to coordinate standards for diving practice, including standards for medical assessment among member countries of the EU.

However, even within the EU, the regulatory bodies vary. In Norway, the Norwegian Petroleum Directorate regulates oilfield diving, but the Directorate of Labour Inspection regulates inshore diving. In the Netherlands, the State Supervisor of Mines is responsible for all diving activity, while in Denmark, the Danish Marine Authority is responsible. In the United States, the Occupational Safety and Health Administration (OSHA) regulates all diving.

Further complications arise because in various countries police or rescue diving activity is regulated separately and scientific diving may fall within or outwith regulation.

Work in compressed air

In the United Kingdom, tunnelling and caisson work is conducted under the Work in Compressed Air Regulations (1996),[8] which are currently under revision. The 1996 regulations were a major advance from the previous Work in Compressed Air Special Regulations of 1958. The new regulations formalized much of the contemporary industry guidance (contained in BS6164 and CIRIA 44 publications) and advances in compressed air practice and reflected good modern management of pressure systems similar to the standards of the UK offshore commercial diving industry.

The 1996 regulations accepted the need for oxygen breathing during on-site hyperbaric treatments of decompression sickness, but fell short of requiring routine oxygen decompression (breathing 100 per cent oxygen during decompression) in the tunnel locks due to fire safety concerns. The statutory requirement for oxygen decompression at pressures above 1 bar (gauge) finally took place in 2001 when an addendum to the HSE guidance on the 1996 regulations was issued which also permitted the use of mixed gas or saturation techniques, if required, subject to specific HSE approval.[65]

The framework of the compressed air regulations is similar to the diving regulations, but some significant differences are of interest because they reflect the different work environments in which diving and compressed air work takes place and the medical historical background. For example, decompression schedules are prescribed in the compressed air regulations or associated guidance. Specific HSE application for alternative decompression procedures in civil engineering projects is necessary from contractors with the full justification for the alternative procedure including the theoretical derivation, any laboratory evaluations and reference to practical operational experience within the UK or overseas. The diving regulations provide a right for a diver to appeal against a medical decision of unfitness. The work in compressed air regulations do not provide this right, but include a specific section relating to abuse of alcohol. Diving contractors are required to keep records of pressure exposure for two years, whereas compressed air contractors must keep records for 40 years. The compressed air regulations have a requirement for each project to have a contract medical adviser with a specific role of the professional supervision of all the occupational health aspects of working in compressed air. This includes the selection of the most appropriate decompression schedules, the planning and pattern of compressed air work, emergency medical response (including hyperbaric treatments), in addition to clinical examinations of medical fitness for work.

ASSESSMENT OF FITNESS FOR WORK AT PRESSURE

Both diving and work in compressed air involve exposure to increased pressure and hence the medical requirements are similar for both activities. The UK regulations for both work activities require that a medical assessment be conducted by a medical practitioner with appropriate knowledge and expertise and that the individual's fitness be documented or 'certified'.

The medical supervision of pressure workers involves a pre-employment assessment, periodic reassessment and aspects of health surveillance.

For divers, medical assessments are conducted by 'approved medical examiners of divers', doctors recognized by the Health and Safety Executive according to HSE guidance.[66] Their principal role is to ensure that divers are safe to be working in the water and not a risk to either themselves or other members of the dive team. Health surveillance for occupational health effects is a secondary function. In most countries, medical assessment is required on an annual basis.

The health assessment is fairly extensive. It covers general fitness issues, including the physical ability to undertake the work activity necessary and specific areas which are relevant to working at pressure. These include ear, nose and throat assessment to exclude an increased risk of barotrauma, pulmonary assessment both from the point of view of risk of barotrauma and the physical capacity to work while breathing gas of increased density,[67] cardiovascular assessment to cover risk of sudden incapacitation, increased risk of decompression illness resulting from intracardiac shunt or impaired peripheral vascular perfusion, neurological assessment to exclude risk of sudden incapacitation and to identify pre-existing neurological abnormality which might cause confusion in subsequent diagnosis of decompression illness. Skin disease can be important, as divers often remain wet for prolonged periods on a regular basis. Psychological suitability to work as a diver is a difficult area. Ability to cope with life-threatening emergencies in a challenging environment calmly and efficiently is a valuable asset for a diver, but is difficult to assess. In practice, the diver population is heavily self-selected and individuals who find that the environment induces anxiety or panic are unlikely to pursue a career. However, a change in mental response to the environment, as a result of an accident or other non-work-related life event, is not uncommon.

Where a diver is considered to be unfit, it is important that they fully understand the rationale behind the decision and the practical limitations of any disability. This may require a supervised test dive to demonstrate to all parties the practical effects and safety implications of a disability.

The assessment requires a number of investigations including lung function, vision testing, audiometry, electrocardiograph and assessment of exercise capacity. Measurement of exercise capacity is helpful for a number of reasons. It acts as a useful adjunct to lung function testing, as a crude screening test for ischaemic heart disease and as a guide to the individual's ability to cope with the physical aspects of the work which are mainly activities carried out on the surface. It also encourages divers to maintain physical fitness by doing regular exercise which provides some protection against decompression illness. However, the actual physical work rate conducted by divers while in the water is in most circumstances relatively low because divers are weightless in the water and other factors, such as restriction of ventilatory capacity by dense breathing gas and immersion, impairs exercise ability.

> A saturation diver reported recurrent episodes of wheeze, cough and breathlessness which came on during the course of repeated saturation dives, but which resolved within a few days after surfacing. On the surface, he remained well. Challenge tests revealed the cause to be exposure to a disinfectant agent used for cleaning the chamber (panacide). Changing to an alternative disinfectant agent allowed him to continue saturation diving uneventfully.

Tunnelling

Medical assessment of compressed air workers is conducted by a doctor approved for compressed air work and appointed to the project by the HSE. Workers are required to be assessed before and at intervals throughout (the periodicity related to the pressure and working conditions), and at the end of the project. The principal role of appointed doctors is to ensure that workers are safe to be employed in the compressed air environment and work role and not a risk to either themselves or other members of the team. Health surveillance for occupational health effects is a secondary, but important, function as exposure to respiratory and skin irritants is quite common and prevention often relies on the use of personal protective equipment.

The clinical assessment follows similar requirements to those for divers in the areas of physical fitness, barotrauma and risk of decompression illness. However, since the work is conducted in a dry environment, without the risk of sudden pressure changes or drowning in most cases, some aspects of the assessment are less critical to safety. The risk of dysbaric osteonecrosis remains higher than in diving, and health surveillance for this is problematic. In the past, routine practice was to include a limited skeletal survey radiological assessment before and after a project. In most cases, it proved impossible to continue surveillance longer as the workforce was mobile and since the radiological abnormalities may appear only some years after the last pressure exposure, this was unsatisfactory. Today, the radiation dose associated with this system is unacceptable. Osteonecrosis is readily detectable by MRI, with a high degree of sensitivity and specificity,[68] but there is limited experience using MRI for long-term health surveillance in asymptomatic working populations of either tunnel workers or commercial divers.[69] It remains possible that lesions detected at an early stage by MRI may resolve spontaneously and not necessarily develop into long-term pathological lesions associated with radiological abnormality. It seems likely, however, that greater experience will be obtained with MRI as a screening method for dysbaric osteonecrosis in compressed air workers, despite the increased costs, once the known health risks and current working practices and future trends (increased pressure associated with TBM interventions) are taken into account. Using MRI assessment of the heads of both radii and femurs or as part of a planned skeletal survey appears to be the most clinically appropriate methodology and, where MRI detects an abnormality, a radiograph should be obtained at least until greater familiarity with the new screening technique is gained. This approach will reduce the radiation dose required substantially, while providing the potential benefit of a more sensitive screening method and further information about the natural history of early lesions detected by MRI.

Compressed air workers in the UK and overseas have benefited considerably from a forum specifically devoted to their health and welfare. The Medical Research Council formed its Decompression Sickness Panel in the early 1950s. Members consisted of civil engineers, occupational physicians and hyperbaric or technical experts practising in the field of compressed air work. This panel issued advice to industry and the Health and Safety Executive and was replaced in 1986 by the Compressed Air Working Group (CAWG). The CAWG continues to hold regular meetings and issue guidance under the sponsorship of the British Tunnelling Society. The work of the HSE, which has conducted a long-term programme of research into both the safety and health aspects of work in the tunnelling hyperbaric environment in recent years, has helped make a major contribution internationally to improving health and safety in compressed air workers and underpins much of the current stringent legislation in the United Kingdom.

Key points

- Diving and tunnelling as occupations are simply a means of commuting to the workplace. Risks relate both to the environmental exposure and to the work task being undertaken.
- Decompression illness may vary from trivial, often unrecognized, symptoms to a serious and sometimes fatal illness. Fit divers with serious decompression illness are often misdiagnosed because they do not look unwell.
- Any new symptoms presenting within 24 hours of a pressure exposure may be decompression illness and appropriate advice should be sought.
- Saturation diving methodology has almost completely eliminated decompression illness.
- There are long-term health effects. The incidence of dysbaric osteonecrosis which can result in disabling arthritic change relates to the safety of decompression procedures used. Other health effects reported in divers are mainly related to lifestyle issues and trauma.

REFERENCES

1. Bruce Davis W, Rennard SJ, Bitterman PB, Crystal RG. Early reversible changes in human alveolar structures induced by hyperoxia. *New England Journal of Medicine.* 1983; **309**: 878-83.
2. Fisher AB, Hyde RW, Puy RJM *et al.* Effect of oxygen at 2 atmospheres on the pulmonary mechanics of normal man. *Journal of Applied Physiology.* 1967; **24**: 529-36.
3. Clark JM, Jackson RM, Lambertson CJ *et al.* Pulmonary function in man after breathing oxygen at 3.0 ata for 3.5 hr. *Journal of Applied Physiology.* 1991; **71**: 878-85.
4. Donald KW. Oxygen poisoning in man I and II. *British Medical Journal.* 1947; **1**: 667-72, 712-17.
5. Butler FK, Thalmann ED. Central nervous system toxicity in closed-circuit scuba divers. In: Bachrach AJ, Matzen MM (eds). Proceedings of the VIII Symposium of Underwater Physiology. Bethesda, MD: Undersea Medical Society, 1984: 15-30.
6. Lance-Hendricks P, Hall DA, Hunter WL, Haley PJ. Extension of pulmonary O_2 tolerance in man at 2ATA by intermittent O_2 exposure. *Journal of Applied Physiology.* 1977; **42**: 593-9.
7. Brauer R, Way RO. Relative narcotic potencies of hydrogen, helium, nitrogen and their mixtures. *Journal of Applied Physiology.* 1970; **29**: 23-31.
8. Statutory Instrument No. 1656. The work in compressed air regulations. London: HMSO, 1996.
9. Malhotra MS, Wright HC. The effects of raised intrapulmonary pressure on the lungs of fresh unchilled cadavers. *Journal of Pathology and Bacteriology.* 1961; **82**: 198-202.
10. Schaefer KE, McNulty WP, Carey C, Liebow AA. Mechanisms in development of interstitial emphysema and air embolism on decompression from depth. *Journal of Applied Physiology.* 1958; **13**: 15-29.
11. Johannsen BB. Cerebral air embolism and the blood brain barrier in the rat. *Acta Neurologica Scandinavica.* 1980; **62**: 201-9.
12. Van Hulst RA, Lameris TW, Hasna D *et al.* Effects of cerebral air embolism on brain metabolism in pigs. *Acta Neurologica Scandinavica.* 2003; **107**: 1-7.
13. Bert P. *La pression barometrique. Recherches dephysiologie experimentale.* Paris: Masson, 1898.
14. Francis TJR, Gorman DF. Pathogenesis of the decompression disorders. In: Bennett PB, Elliott DH (eds). *The physiology of medicine and diving*, 4th edn. London: WB Saunders, 1993.
15. Smith KH, Spencer MP. Doppler indices of decompression sickness: Their evaluation and use. *Aerospace Medicine.* 1970; **41**: 1396-400.
16. Ikeda T, Okamoto Y, Hashimoto A. Bubble formation and decompression sickness on direct ascent from shallow air saturation diving. *Aviation Space and Environmental Medicine.* 1993; **64**: 121-5.
17. Wilmshurst PT, Ellis BG, Jenkins BS. Paradoxical gas embolism in a scuba diver with an atrial septal defect. *British Medical Journal.* 1986; **293**: 1277.
18. Bove AA. Risk of decompression sickness with patent foramen ovale. *Undersea and Hyperbaric Medicine.* 1998; **25**: 175-8.
19. Wilmshurst P, Davidson C, O'Connell G, Byrne C. Role of cardiorespiratory abnormalities, smoking and dive characteristics in the manifestations of neurological decompression illness. *Clinical Science.* 1994; **86**: 297-303.
20. Elliott DH, Moon RE. Manifestations of the decompression disorders. In: Bennett PB, Elliott DH (eds). *The physiology and medicine of diving*, 4th edn. London: WB Saunders, 1993.
21. Rozsahegyi I, Roth B. Participation of the central nervous system in decompression. *Industrial Medicine and Surgery.* 1966; **35**: 101-10.

22. Blick G. Notes on diver's paralysis. *British Medical Journal.* 1909; **2**: 1796-8.
23. Palmer AC, Calder IM, McCallum RI, Mastaglia FL. Spinal cord degeneration in a case of 'recovered' spinal decompression sickness. *British Medical Journal.* 1981; **283**: 888.
24. Rozsahegyi I. Late consequences of neurological forms of decompression sickness. *British Medical Journal.* 1959; **16**: 311-17.
25. Smith KH, Spencer MP. Doppler indices of decompression sickness: Their evaluation and use. *Aerospace Medicine.* 1970; **41**: 1396-400.
26. Eatock BC. Correspondence between intravascular bubbles and symptoms of decompression sickness. *Undersea Biomedical Research.* 1984; **11**: 326-9.
27. Nossum V, Koteng S, Brubakk AO. Endothelial damage by bubbles in the pulmonary artery of the pig. *Undersea Hyperbaric Medicine.* 1999; **26**: 1-8.
28. Boussuges A, Succo E, Juhan-Vague I, Sainty JM. Activation of coagulation in decompression illness. *Aviation, Space and Environmental Medicine.* 1998; **69**: 129-32.
29. Butler BD, Hills BA. Transpulmonary passage of venous air emboli. *Journal of Applied Physiology.* 1985; **59**: 543-7.
30. Butler BD, Katz J. Vascular pressures and passage of gas emboli through the pulmonary circulation. *Undersea Biomedical Research.* 1988; **15**: 203-9.
31. Wilmshurst PT, Byrne JC, Webb-Peploe MM. Relation between interatrial shunts and decompression sickness in divers. *Lancet.* 1989; **2**: 1302-6.
32. Torti SR, Billinger M, Schwerzmann M et al. Risk of decompression illness among 230 divers in relation to the presence and size of patent foramen ovale. *European Heart Journal.* 2004; **25**: 1014-20.
33. Sykes JJW, Yaffe LJ. Light and electron microscopic alterations in spinal cord myelin sheaths after decompression sickness. *Undersea Biomedical Research.* 1985; **12**: 251-8.
34. Francis TJR, Pezeshkpour GH, Dutka AJ et al. Is there a role for the autochonous bubble in the pathogenesis of spinal cord decompression sickness? *Journal of Neuropathology and Experimental Neurology.* 1988; **47**: 475-87.
35. Dick EJ, Broome JR, Hayward IJ. Acute neurologic decompression sickness in pigs: Lesions of the spinal cord and brain. *Laboratory Animal Science.* 1997; **47**: 50-7.
36. Elliott DH, Harrison JAB. Bone necrosis: An occupational hazard for divers. *Journal of the Royal Naval Medical Service.* 1970; **56**: 140-61.
37. Wilmshurst P, Nuri M, Crowther A, Webb-Peploe MM. Cold-induced pulmonary oedema in scuba divers and swimmers and subsequent development of hypertension. *Lancet.* 1989; **I**: 62-5.
38. Hampson NB, Dunford RG. Pulmonary edema of scuba divers. *Undersea and Hyperbaric Medicine.* 1997; **24**: 29-33.
39. Ahlen C, Iverson OJ, Risberg J et al. Diver's hand: A skin disorder common in occupational saturation diving. *Occupational and Environmental Medicine.* 1998; **12**: 315-19.
40. US Navy Naval Sea Systems Command. US Navy Diving Manual, rev 6. Washington, DC: NAVSEA, 2008.
41. British Sub Aqua Club. BSAC 88 diving tables. Ellesmere Port: British Sub Aqua Club, 1988.
42. Halsey MJ. Effects of high pressure on the central nervous system. *Physiological Reviews.* 1982; **62**: 1341-77.
43. Logie RH, Baddeley AD. Cognitive performance during simulated deep sea diving. *Ergonomics.* 1985; **28**: 731-46.
44. Jacobsen G, Jacobsen JE, Peterson RE et al. Decompression sickness from saturation diving: A case control study of some diving exposure characteristics. *Undersea and Hyperbaric Medicine.* 1997; **24**: 73-80.
45. US Navy Naval Sea Systems Command. Diving medicine and recompression chamber operations, Chapter 5. In: US Navy Diving Manual, rev 6. Washington, DC: NAVSEA.
46. Miller JN, Fagraeus L, Bennett PB et al. Nitrogen-oxygen saturation therapy in serious cases of compressed-air decompression sickness. *Lancet.* 1978; **ii**: 169-71.
47. Hyldegaard O, Kerem D, Melamed Y. Effect of combined recompression and air, oxygen or heliox breathing on air bubbles in rat tissues. *Journal of Applied Physiology.* 2001; **90**: 1639-47.
48. Kol S, Adir Y, Gordon CR, Melamed Y. Oxy-helium treatment of severe spinal decompression sickness after air diving. *Undersea and Hyperbaric Medicine.* 1993; **20**: 147-54.
49. Kahlstrom SC, Burton CC, Phemister DB. Aseptic necrosis of bone. 1. Infarction of bones in caisson disease resulting in encapsulated and calcified areas in diaphyses and in arthritis deformans. *Surgery, Gynecology and Obstetrics.* 1939; **68**: 129-46.
50. Harrelson JM, Hills BA. Changes in bone marrow pressure in response to hyperbaric exposure. *Aerospace Medicine.* 1970; **41**: 1018-21.
51. Medical Research Council. Decompression Sickness Panel Report. Bone lesions in compressed air workers with special reference to men who worked on the Clyde Tunnels 1958-1963. *Journal of Bone and Joint Surgery.* 1966; **48**: 207-35.
52. Aseptic bone necrosis in commercial divers – a report from the Decompression Sickness Central Registry and Radiological Panel. *Lancet.* 1981; **ii**: 384-8.
53. Todnem K, Nyland H, Kambestad BK, Arli JA. Influence of occupational diving upon the nervous system: An epidemiological study. *British Journal of Industrial Medicine.* 1990; 47: 708-14.
54. Todnem K, Nyland H, Skeidsvoll H et al. Neurological long term consequences of deep diving. *British Journal of Industrial Medicine.* 1991; **48**: 258-6.
55. Crosbie WA, Reed JW, Clarke MC. Functional characteristics of the large lungs found in divers. *Journal of Applied Physiology.* 1979; **46**: 639-45.
56. Thorsen E, Segedal K, Kambestad BK, Gulsvik A. Diver's lung function: Small airways disease. *British Journal of Industrial Medicine.* 1990; **47**: 519-23.
57. Skogstad M, Thorsen E, Haldorsen T. Lung function over the first 3 years of a professional diving career. *Occupational and Environmental Medicine.* 2000; **57**: 390-5.

58. Irgens A, Gronning M, Troland K et al. Reduced health-related quality of life in former North Sea divers is associated with decompression sickness. *Occupational Medicine*. 2007; **57**: 349–54.
59. Troland K, Gronning M, Skeidsvall H et al. The Haukeland University Hospital prospective study of Norwegian occupational divers – CNS effects of diving. *Undersea and Hyperbaric Medicine*. 2006; **33**: 666.
60. Ross J, Macdiarmid J, Osman L et al. A questionnaire study of health effects in United Kingdom male professional divers and offshore oil industry workers. *Occupational Medicine*. 2007; **57**: 754–61.
61. Taylor CL, Macdiarmid JI, Ross JAS et al. Objective neuropsychological test performance of professional divers reporting a subjective complaint of 'forgetfulness or loss of concentration'. *Scandinavian Journal of Work, Environment and Health*. 2006; **32**: 310–17.
62. Statutory Instrument No. 2776. The Diving at Work Regulations 1997. London: HMSO, 1997.
63. Health and Safety at Work Act. London: HMSO, 1974.
64. Health and Safety Executive. Commercial diving project: Inland/inshore. The Diving at Work Regulations 1997. Approved Code of Practice. Bootle: HSE, 1998.
65. Health and Safety Executive. Guidance on oxygen decompression and the use of breathing mixtures other than compressed natural air in the working chamber. Addendum to 'A guide to the Work in Compressed Air Regulations 1996'. Bootle: HSE, 1996.
66. Health and Safety Commission. Medical examination and assessment of divers, MA1. UK: Health and Safety Commission, 2008.
67. Godden D, Currie G, Denison D et al. British Thoracic Society Guidelines on respiratory aspects of fitness for diving. *Thorax*. 2003; **58**: 3–13.
68. Koo KH, Kim R, Kim YS et al. Risk period for developing osteonecrosis of the femoral head in patients on steroid treatment. *Clinical Rheumatology*. 2002; **21**: 299–303.
69. Bolte H, Koch A, Tetzlaff K et al. Detection of dysbaric osteonecrosis in military divers using magnetic resonance imaging. *European Radiology*. 2005; **15**: 368–75.

51

Working at high altitude

PETER JG FORSTER

High altitude illness	570	Anaesthesia at high altitude	581
At-risk groups	578	Altitude sickness	581
Sleep at high altitude	580	References	587

HIGH ALTITUDE ILLNESS

The journals of intrepid mountaineers give clear testimony to the discomforts and perils of life at high altitude. In 1879, on Chimborazo in Ecuador, Edward Whymper, conqueror of the Matterhorn in 1865 and the foremost mountaineer of his time, suffered intense headache which 'rendered us almost frantic or crazy' and an 'indescribable feeling of illness which pervaded the whole body ... and we were preoccupied by the paramount necessity of obtaining air'.[1] Whymper succeeded in reaching the summit of Chimborazo (6290 m). However, Edward Fitzgerald failed to achieve his personal ambition of the first ascent of Aconcagua (6980 m), the highest mountain in the western hemisphere, because, as he records in his book published in 1899: 'I got up, and tried once more to go but I was only able to advance from two to three steps at a time and then to stop, panting for breath, my struggles alternating with violent fits of nausea.'[2]

The discomfort experienced by mountaineers on ascent to high altitude is compounded by the additional hardships of exertion, fatigue, exposure, low temperature, gastrointestinal upsets, alteration in diet and dehydration. Fitzgerald's discomfort was intensified by a diet which on Christmas morning 1896, camping cold and hungry at 4900 m, consisted of 'some tins of Irish Stew ... melting the great white frozen lumps of grease slowly in our mouths, and then swallowing them'. In 1913, TH Ravenhill, medical officer to a mining district in the Chilean Andes, described the features of altitude sickness affecting miners transported by rail from Antofagasta, a seaport on the Pacific Ocean, to mines situated above 4600 m. The miners in Ravenhill's study were subject to the effects of altitude without other complicating influences. Based on his clinical observations, Ravenhill identified three types of altitude sickness: normal puna (acute mountain sickness), cardiac puna (high altitude pulmonary oedema) and nervous puna (high altitude cerebral oedema).[3] It is tribute to Ravenhill's astute clinical acumen and observational skills that his classification of the 'benign' (acute mountain sickness) and 'malignant' (high altitude pulmonary oedema, high altitude cerebral oedema) forms of altitude sickness remains in use in the modern era.

Acute mountain sickness is a self-limiting condition characterized by headache, sleep disturbance, anorexia, nausea, vomiting and cerebral symptoms, such as profound fatigue, dizziness, irritability, lack of concentration and confusion. Physical signs include periorbital and peripheral oedema and manifestations of normal physiological response to high altitude exposure, such as shortness of breath on exertion and tachycardia. Acute mountain sickness (AMS) affects unacclimatized visitors at elevations above 2500 m. Symptoms become manifest after a period of approximately six hours at high altitude and reach their maximum severity at 24–48 hours. Symptoms subside gradually after two or three days' acclimatization. If the condition is ignored and ascent to greater altitude is attempted, AMS may progress to potentially fatal high altitude cerebral oedema (HACO) or high altitude pulmonary oedema (HAPO).[4]

The incidence of AMS in sea-level residents ascending to altitudes greater than 3000 m has been estimated from large population studies of trekkers and soldiers on single ascents. Hackett and Rennie[5] reported an incidence of 43 per cent in 200 hikers reaching Pheriche (4243 m) on the trail to Mount Everest. One-third of the hikers were symptom free. Of the thousands of climbers making the rapid ascent to the summit of Mount Rainier (4392 m) every year, 50–75 per cent suffer from AMS.[6] Of over 250 hikers walking the Mount Everest base camp trek from Namche Bazaar (3440 m) to a final altitude of over 5500 m, 57 per cent developed AMS; concomitant symptoms of respiratory and gastrointestinal infection were common (87 per cent of the study group) and were more prevalent in AMS sufferers.[7] Singh et al.[8] reported an 8.3 per cent incidence of severe AMS in thousands of soldiers transported from sea level to above 3500 m. These published studies have involved young, physically fit and, predominantly, male subjects. In a general population of visitors (age range 16–87 years, one-third female) to modest elevations (1900–3000 m) in the Rocky Mountains of Colorado, 25 per cent suffered AMS) within the first 12 hours of arrival.[9] Males and females are affected equally by altitude sickness: the young suffer more than the old. As a rough guide a rule of thirds applies: moderate to severe symptoms of AMS occur in one-third of sea-level residents at high altitude, mild symptoms in one-third and one-third are symptom free.[10]

A study of sea-level residents transported rapidly to high altitude, similar to the experience of the Andean miners in Ravenhill's paper, was conducted in 1980 on personnel manning astronomical observatories at the summit of Mauna Kea (4200 m, 13 796 ft), on the island of Hawaii.[11,12] In 1980, four major telescopes were situated at the summit which because of the dry atmosphere, absence of pollution and ready access, was the pre-eminent site for terrestrial infrared and submillimeter astronomy (Figures 51.1–51.3). At the summit, barometric pressure is 625 mbars (62.5 kPa, 475 mmHg) and the ambient partial pressure of oxygen is 60 per cent of the sea-level value.

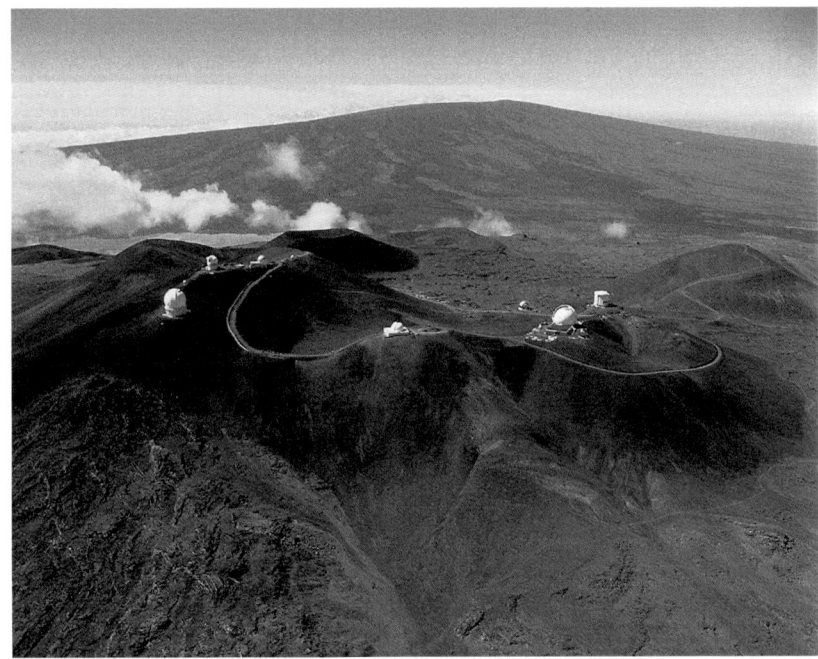

Figure 51.1 Mauna Kea Observatory, Hawaii 1989. Reproduced with permission of UK ATC, Royal Observatory, Edinburgh, UK.

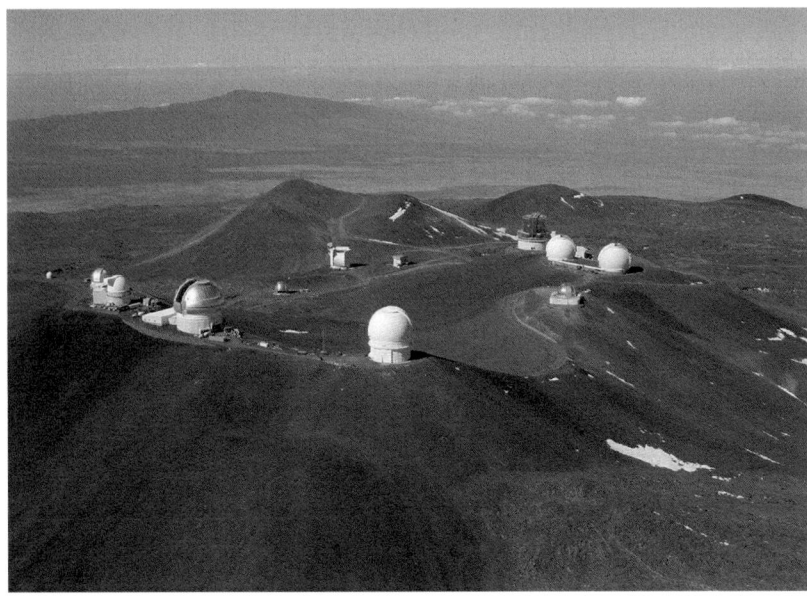

Figure 51.2 Mauna Kea Observatory 1998. Reproduced with permission of Richard Wainscoat, Institute for Astronomy, University of Hawaii (www.ifa.hawaii.edu).

The partial pressure of oxygen in inspired air is 12.6 kPa (95 mmHg) compared with 20 kPa (150 mmHg) at sea level and 7.6 kPa (57 mmHg) in alveolar air, compared with 14 kPa (105 mmHg) at sea level. Telescope personnel make frequent ascents by four-wheel drive vehicle from sea level to the summit with minimal provision for acclimatization above 3000 m. They remain on the mountain for five day shifts working at the telescopes and sleeping in dormitories at 3000 m. On Mauna Kea, 80 per cent of the shift workers were affected by altitude sickness symptoms on the first day. Headache and breathlessness were the most common and troublesome complaints. Other common symptoms were insomnia, lethargy, poor concentration and impairment of memory.

After five days on the mountain, 60 per cent of workers were free of symptoms, while the remainder continued to experience minimal symptoms of exertional dyspnoea, headache and insomnia. There was no difference in the incidence of AMS in shift workers who worked at the summit following a four-day sojourn at sea level compared to a 30-day rest period at sea level; acclimatization to altitude achieved during five days above 3000 m appeared to be lost within days of return to sea level. Telescope personnel who commuted to the summit for a single day did not suffer from severe AMS symptoms. However, commuters were only at an advantage if the duration of the visit to the summit was limited to less than six hours, the period of time that elapses usually between arrival at high altitude and the development of AMS: symptoms of headache, poor concentration, lethargy and dyspnoea were developing as commuters descended after five hours. The disadvantage of the commuter's work schedule was that commuters did not acclimatize.

A 2007 study on Mauna Kea used the Lake Louise AMS Questionnaire (Appendix 51.1) to survey AMS amongst telescope shift workers and day visitors.[13] Using this standardized self-report symptom assessment, which was not available in 1980, AMS was detected in 69 per cent of shift workers. Over 65 per cent of the telescope staff reported headache with 13 per cent suffering incapacitating headache. Difficulties with sleeping were common (70 per cent), as were nausea and lethargy. The majority of workers (70 per cent) were aware that symptoms reduced their level of activity.

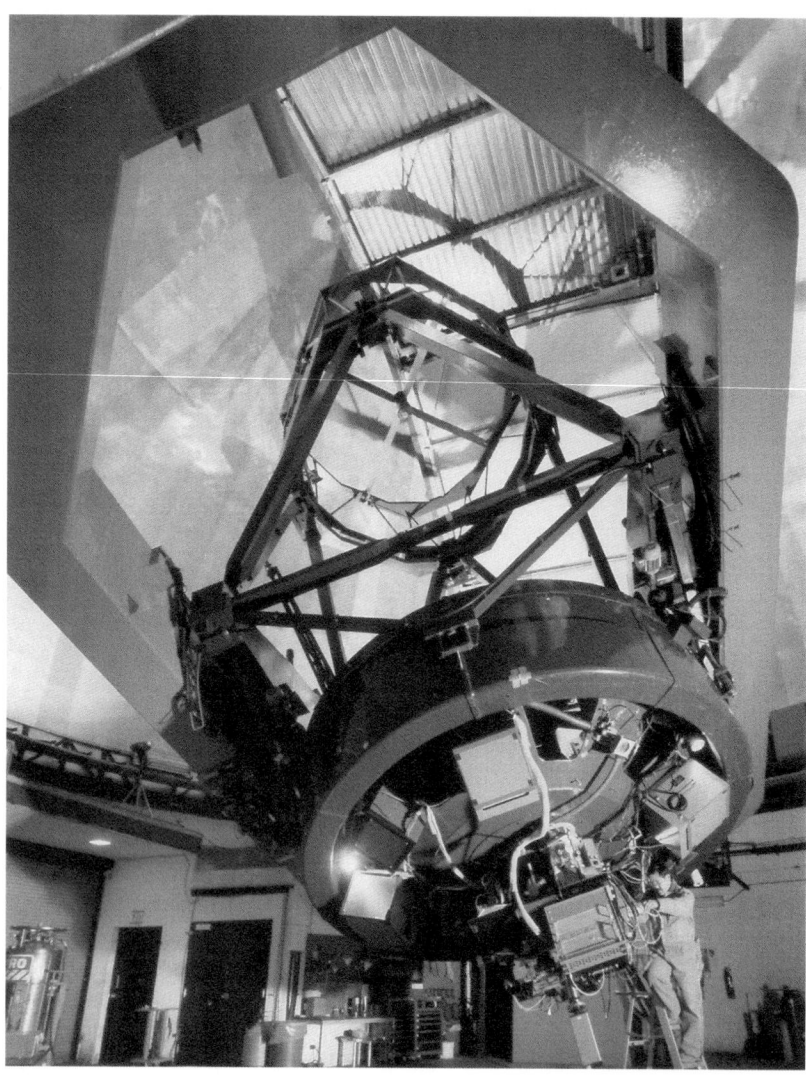

Figure 51.3 Technician working on the 3.8-m UK infrared telescope (UKIRT) on Mauna Kea. Reproduced with permission of UK ATC, Royal Observatory, Edinburgh, UK.

High altitude pulmonary oedema (HAPO) is a non-cardiogenic form of pulmonary oedema. Pulmonary hypertension is the principal pathological process causing leakage of oedema fluid from intravascular space into the alveolar bed in association with an exaggerated pulmonary vasoconstrictive response to hypoxia and exercise, which is distributed unevenly throughout the lung vasculature. In addition, abnormal endothelial synthesis of vasoactive substances disturbs the balance between vasodilators (e.g. nitric oxide) and vasoconstrictors (e.g. endothelin-1).[14] HAPO may follow viral respiratory infections in children[15] and HAPO victims may exhibit infective and inflammatory signs: low-grade pyrexia, peripheral leukocytosis and raised ESR. However, examination of bronchoalveolar lavage fluid collected from climbers within hours of arrival at 4559 m has shown no increase in inflammatory markers or neutrophils.[16] Hence, inflammation is thought to be a secondary response to extravasation of fluid into alveoli rather than a primary pathological process in HAPO.[4]

The signs of HAPO are marked breathlessness at rest, a rapid respiratory rate (>30 breaths/min) and a dry cough, which as the condition worsens may be productive of white, frothy or blood-streaked sputum. The victim appears deeply cyanotic and may complain of chest discomfort. Extensive bilateral crepitations (rales) are heard on auscultation. In extreme cases, gurgling sounds from the lungs may be audible to the victim and his companions without the use of a stethescope. Signs of cardiac failure are not evident, although tachycardia (pulse rate >120 beats/min) and a low systemic blood pressure are frequently present. Cardiac murmurs are not a feature of HAPO. However, the second heart sound is accentuated and sometimes palpable, reflecting elevation of pulmonary artery pressure. An erroneous diagnosis of bronchopneumonia may be suggested by the presence of low-grade pyrexia and moderate leukocytosis, but respiratory infection may coexist with HAPO.

Arterial blood gas measurements confirm severe hypoxaemia with low arterial partial pressure of oxygen (PaO_2) and decreased arterial carbon dioxide tension ($PaCO_2$) from hyperventilation resulting in respiratory alkalosis. Prominence of the pulmonary arteries and patchy infiltrates seen in chest radiographs in early disease progress to homogenous bilateral infiltration in severe cases. Right ventricular overload pattern (right axis deviation, right bundle block and right ventricular strain) is present on electrocardiograph tracings. Echocardiography may demonstrate incompetence of the tricuspid valve. Cardiac catheterization studies performed on HAPO victims before treatment or descent show a high pulmonary arterial pressure and low or normal pulmonary artery wedge pressure.[17] Descent to low altitude and administration of oxygen lowers pulmonary artery pressure, clears radiographic pulmonary infiltrates and relieves symptoms within one to two days. The development of HAPO is related to the speed of ascent, the altitude achieved, the exertion involved and the susceptibility of the individual.

An incidence of HAPO has been reported as high as 15.5 per cent in thousands of lowland troops flown up to the Himalayas.[18] Seven cases of HAPO were encountered amongst 278 unacclimatized hikers at 4243 m in Nepal, an incidence of 2.5 per cent.[19] At the Regina Margherita hut (4559 m) in the Alps Valais, 4 per cent of climbers were diagnosed as suffering from HAPO as indicated by pulmonary crepitations on auscultation.[20] On Mauna Kea, one case of HAPO was diagnosed in 41 shift workers during a two-year study (Table 51.1). Calculated in terms of the 2000 ascents per annum to a single telescope, this low incidence of HAPO may reflect the lack of physical exertion involved in ascent to 4200 m. However, in contrast to the low incidence of HAPO reported in earlier studies, a 2002 prospective study of 262 climbers to Monte Rosa (4559 m) found clinical and radiographic evidence of interstitial oedema in 40 subjects (15 per cent) without HAPO-related symptoms. Using airway closing volume as a proxy for interstitial water, 74 per cent of the healthy climbers had subclinical pulmonary oedema without clinical or radiographic evidence. The researchers concluded that 'even at modest altitudes and rates of ascent, with heavy but not extreme exertion, the healthy lung is on the edge of failure in terms of fluid balance'. Hypoxia was proposed as the putative agent rather than exercise.[21,22]

Individuals with an over-exaggerated pulmonary vasoconstrictive response to hypoxia and exertion or abnormalities of cardiopulmonary circulation leading to increased pulmonary artery pressure (e.g. unilateral absent pulmonary arteries, primary pulmonary hypertension) are at increased risk of HAPO.[23-25] Although it is not possible to predict who will suffer from HAPO on a particular ascent, individuals who have suffered a previous episode have a risk of recurrence of 60 per cent on reascent to over 4500 m.[26] A genetic predisposition to HAPO may be linked to up- or downregulation of the genes that control synthesis of the vasodilator nitric oxide and the vasoconstrictor endothelin-1. Other studies of genetic predisposition to HAPO have included investigations of polymorphisms in angiotensin-converting enzyme genes, HLA haplotypes and the amiloride-sensitive epithelial sodium channel which has a key role in clearance of fluid and sodium from the alveolar space.[27]

Failure to descend or to treat HAPO effectively may result in a fatal outcome within a few hours of onset; the mortality rate is quoted in the range 4-11 per cent. In a review of 166 reported cases of HAPO, untreated victims had a mortality rate of 44 per cent compared to a 3 per cent mortality in subjects who were treated by descent and oxygen administration.[28] Half of HAPO sufferers who die have coexistent HACO evident at post-mortem.[29]

Cerebral oedema (HACO) presents typically with intense headache, profound lethargy, ataxia, impaired coordination, confusion, disorientation and hallucinations. Convulsions and focal features, such as cranial nerve palsies and visual field loss, may occur. Cerebral oedema occurs in people exhibiting 'benign' AMS: the progression

Table 51.1 Medical emergencies at United Kingdom Infrared Telescope (UKIRT) on Mauna Kea.

Case	Patient	Symptoms	Treatment	Outcome
Case 1: High altitude pulmonary oedema	Male, aged 29 years	Progressive dyspnoea, tachypnoea, cyanosis; occurred at rest camp (3000 m) following third night shift at summit	Immediate descent and oxygen administration (6 L/min)	Clinical examination at sea level – symptoms and signs of HAPO resolved; chest radiograph normal; subsequent work at summit without recurrence of HAPO
Case 2: High altitude cerebral oedema	Male, age 30 years	Slurred speech, frontal headache with neck stiffness, temporary loss of peripheral vision, impaired coordination, ataxic gait; symptoms presented on first day at summit	Descent and oxygen	Complete resolution of signs and symptoms at sea level; no subsequent work at telescope
Case 3: Acute mountain sickness	Male, aged 30 year	Headache, nausea, lethargy, poor concentration, impaired memory, cyanosis, periodic respiration: no focal central nervous system signs. Symptoms present on first day of work at summit of every shift, necessitating descent. Subject attempted, unsuccessfully, to ameliorate symptoms by gradual staging of ascent	Acetazolamide prophylaxis (dose 500 mg to 1.5 g/day); minimal reduction in AMS symptoms. Adverse effects – paraesthesia, diuresis	Exemption from work at high altitude
Case 4: Migraine headache	Male, age 29 years	History of classical migraine. Eighth day on mountain – symptoms of expressive dysphasia, loss of right peripheral visual field, numbness right arm; nausea: no headache	Descent, anti-emetic for nausea	Neurological symptoms resolved at sea level, EEG, isotope brain scan – normal
Case 5: Bronchopneumonia	Male, aged 34 years	Cough productive of purulent sputum, dyspnoea at rest, fever, anorexia, ataxic gait – following flu-like illness	Descent under supervision by colleague (patient exhibited marked loss of insight), antibiotics, bed rest	Uneventful return to summit after 4 days
Case 6: Bronchopneumonia	Male, aged 30 years	Two episodes on consecutive visits to Mauna Kea, cough productive of purulent sputum, severe dyspnoea, central cyanosis	Descent to sea level, antibiotics, bronchodilators, bed rest	Completed work schedule at observatory after 3 days sojourn at sea level; following second episode, persistent dyspnoea; astronomical research aborted, returned home; subsequent examination by respiratory physician – no underlying chest disease
Case 7: Perforation of ear drum	Male, aged 55 years	Contracted coryza at sea level, developed right otitis media on Mauna Kea. Impaired hearing, 'pressure in right ear', discharge from ear	Remained on mountain, antibiotics, decongestant	Healing of perforation

Assuming a complement of three day staff and three night observers, approximately 2000 'man-days' were worked each year at the UKIRT facility during the two-year period of study. An average working day constituted nine hours at the summit.

to HACO is indicated by deterioration in existing AMS, despite treatment and no further ascent, or the appearance of neurological signs, such as ataxia on walking (poor heel to toe walking) or sitting (truncal ataxia), cranial nerve palsies and visual field loss.[30] Convulsions may occur. Features of HAPO may coexist and complicate diagnosis and management of HACO. Papilloedema develops in over 50 per cent of HACO victims. Retinal vein engorgement and retinal haemorrhage are of minor prognostic significance in HACO as these fundoscopic abnormalities are not uncommon in asymptomatic subjects at high altitude. Rapid deterioration in conscious level leading to death has been widely reported.[31] Investigations off the mountain show raised cerebrospinal fluid pressure on lumbar puncture and increased signal in white matter reflecting oedema of the corpus callosum on T-2 and diffusion-weighted magnetic resonance imaging (MRI).[29] Post-mortem examination reveals extensive cerebral oedema, intracerebral haemorrhages and thrombosis in cerebral veins and dural sinuses.[32,33]

Current thinking is that HACO is due to vasogenic oedema related to disruption of the blood–brain barrier with extravasation of fluid into the interstitial space rather than cytotoxic oedema related to cell death due to increased intracellular osmolarity.[4] Damage to the blood–brain barrier may be 'mechanical' induced by impairment of cerebral vascular autoregulation or 'chemical' related to release of mediators of barrier permeability, such as bradykinin and hydroxyl-free radicals. Cerebral hypoxia is exacerbated by exercise which reduces oxygenation further.[34] If swelling of the brain is commonplace in all people on ascent and AMS is a mild form and precursor of HACO, the 'tightfit' hypothesis proposes that susceptible individuals have less cranial capacity to accommodate the swollen brain. Capacity would depend on the ratio of cranial cerebrospinal fluid to brain volume which varies between individuals and could explain variability of response to high altitude exposure.[29] Perhaps people aged over 50 years are more tolerant of high altitude because of a degree of cerebral atrophy.[35]

Cerebral oedema occurs usually in unacclimatized people above 3000-m elevation, although cases of HACO in well acclimatized climbers at extreme altitudes (>7000 m) have been documented. Typically, HACO appears as a progression of AMS developing over 24–36 hours: the risk factors for both conditions are the same. HACO is less common than HAPO. In a study of 278 trekkers in the Himalayas, five cases were diagnosed at 4243 m, an incidence of 1.8 per cent (compared to 2.5 per cent for HAPO).[12] Singh et al.[18] described 24 cases of 'severe' neurological abnormality amongst 1925 AMS victims at altitudes between 3350 and 5486 m.[18] A single episode of HACO occurred during the Mauna Kea study (Table 51.1).

Physical fitness offers no protection against altitude sickness. Ravenhill[3] records in his 1913 paper: 'There is, in my experience, no type of man whom one may say that he will, or will not, suffer from puna (altitude sickness). Most of the cases I have instanced were men to all appearances perfectly sound. Young, strong and healthy men may be completely overcome: stout, plethoric individuals of the chronic bronchitic type may not even have a headache.' Edward Whymper, a proud man, could not hide his irritation with one of his fellow travellers: 'strange to relate Mr Perring did not appear to be affected at all. Except for him, we should have faired badly … yet at sea level, in the normal course of things he was a rather debilitated man and was distinctly less robust than ourselves. He could scarely walk on a flat road without desiring to sit down.'

Cognitive and psychomotor function at high altitude

In a series of papers published in the late 1930s, RA McFarland reported several studies from the Andes of the effects of high altitude on psycho-physiological performance. Comparing sudden ascent to 5000 m in unpressurized airplanes while flying over the Andes with slower ascent to 4700 m by road or rail, he observed that the performance of mental tests of complex reactions (e.g. mental arithmetic, writing) were more impaired than motor and sensory tests and that there was a 'close interdependence between the partial pressure of oxygen in the internal environment of the organism and the functional capacity of the central nervous system': the rate of ascent was an important variable.[36] In a second paper, sensory (auditory threshold, visual after images) and motor functions (reaction times, hand–eye coordination) showed significant deterioration only above 5330 m; acclimatization lessened deterioration.[37] In the third paper, memory, speed of word recognition and mental flexibility were not significantly affected until an altitude of above 4700 m was achieved. The research subjects noted 'that the effort of mind needed to carry out a task was greater than the loss of capacity to do it'.[38] In his fourth paper, McFarland reported that Andean sulphur miners working at 5330 m had slower reaction times and blunted auditory sensitivity than age- and race-matched workmen at sea level.[39]

Impairment of higher cerebral functions has been reported at lower altitudes than the threshold altitude of 4700 m in McFarland's studies. Psychomotor efficiency (eye–hand coordination test) was compromised in accuracy and speed in a group of Indian soldiers over a period of ten months at 4000-m altitude. Although accuracy recovered over the next 13 months, presumably due to acclimatization, recovery of speed of performance did not return to sea-level values, while the subjects remained at high altitude.[40] Psychomotor and information processing tests were not impaired in Mauna Kea telescope staff at 4200 m. Numerate memory was impaired on the first summit day, but corrected by the fifth day.

Elite climbers who had reached summits over 8000 m without supplementary oxygen were found to have residual cognitive impairment in short-term memory, cognitive flexibility and ability to concentrate two to six months after the last of repeated exposures to extreme altitude. The three most severely affected individuals exhibited EEG abnormalities.[41] In a group of young fit mountaineers using supplemental oxygen to climb Everest (altitude 8850 m, 29 029 ft: barometric pressure 337 mbars, 33.7 kPa, 253 mmHg), transient mild deterioration in learning, memory and expression of verbal material was detected within three days of descent to Kathmandu, but had recovered by one year. Reduction in motor speed (finger tapping test) characterized by rapid muscle fatigue persisted for a year.[42] In a study of mountaineers before and 1–30 days after ascent to altitudes above 5488 m and altitude chamber 'ascent' to 8848 m, neuropsychological testing revealed a decline in visual and verbal long-term memory expression.[43] However, in an earlier study, Clark et al.[44] found no evidence of cerebral impairment as judged by neurophysiological tests performed before and 16–221 days after climbs ranging from 5335 to 8848 m in the Himalayas.

Magnetic resonance imaging of the brains of nine climbers before and after a 7500-m climb without supplementary oxygen showed cortical atrophy (high signal areas) in five before the expedition with new areas of cortical atrophy in two of the group. Both had suffered severe neurological symptoms during the climb.[45] In a more extensive study, MRI abnormalities were present in 61 per cent (13/21) of climbers who had ascended to altitudes over 8000 m, but in only 14 per cent (1/7) of Himalayan sherpas with similar high-altitude exposure. Although no relationship was found between the MRI changes and the number of climbs or the duration of exposure to high altitude, these studies confirm the risk to the brain of hypoxia at extreme altitude with over half of sea-level native climbers affected and relative sparing of high altitude natives.[46]

Female gender

At high altitude, females are equally likely to suffer from AMS as men. Peripheral oedema is more common in females, but the incidence of HAPO is lower. There are no data regarding difference in the incidence of HACO between the genders.[47] Acclimatization is similar as is exercise performance at high altitude.[48] Although females have an increased ventilatory response to hypoxia which is assumed to be due to the protective effect of the respiratory stimulant hormone progesterone, this does not appear to confer benefit in terms of ventilatory acclimatization.[49] Females lose less weight at high altitude than males possibly because they recover from hypoxia-induced anorexia more quickly.

Women are advised to confine their ascents to modest altitudes (<2500 m) during early pregnancy because of the possible risk of hypoxia to fetal development. During the first trimester, prophylaxis with the carbonic anhydrase inhibitor acetazolamide is contraindicated because of the known teratogenic properties of sulphonamide drugs. Recommendations for pregnant women going to high altitude, including who should not go high, based on a comprehensive review of the literature has been published in an International Mountaineering and Climbing Federation consensus paper.[47]

Combined oestrogen and progestogen oral contraceptives (COCP) can be taken to control the menstrual cycle in wilderness conditions, but there is a theoretical risk of increased thrombotic episodes due to dehydration and an increase in haematocrit occurring at high altitude. Synthetic progestogen formulations may be more suitable for stabilizing the menstrual cycle and for use as contraceptives due to the theoretical reduction in risk of thrombosis. However, different preparations have different characteristics and advantages (see Table 51.2). Newer progestogen-only pills containing desogestrel (75 µg) may have advantages over conventional COCPs by inhibiting ovulation as do COCPs without the increased thrombotic risk. Alternatives to oral preparations include the progestogen-releasing (levonorgestrel) intrauterine system or etonorgestrel implants. To establish effectiveness for the individual female, these formulations should be tried for a minimum of three months, ideally six months, before travel.

Children

Children are susceptible to the adverse effects of altitude and suffer AMS, HAPO and HACO.[50] Most studies have shown a similar incidence of AMS in children and adults. Children living at high altitude are more susceptible than adults to 're-entry HAPO' when they return home after a sojourn at lower altitude.

The inherent risks to children travelling to high altitude demand special attention in the planning for and management of altitude-related illness and subsequent specialist follow up.[51]

Lake Louise acute mountain sickness scoring system

To aid diagnosis and to assess the severity of altitude sickness, the Lake Louise acute mountain sickness scoring system was developed at consensus meetings held in Lake Louise, Canada in 1991 and 1993.[52] The scoring system was formulated initially to allow standardization of diagnosis and severity of illness for research studies. Nevertheless, the simple and short self-reporting questionnaire of five key symptoms has sufficient sensitivity and specificity for use by non-medical trekkers and mountaineers for the detection of altitude sickness in themselves and their companions (Appendix 51.1).

The Lake Louise score can be confounded by extraneous factors (e.g. concomitant illness) leading to over-diagnosis of altitude sickness, hence the score should be calculated in the context of a recent gain in altitude.

Table 51.2 Contraception and menstrual cycle control for women at high altitude.

	Administration	Licensed contraceptive	Increase theoretical risk of thrombosis	Time to stabilize treatment (months)	Cycle control
Combined oral contraceptive pill (COCP)	Daily oral pill to be taken within 12-hour window	Yes, may be reduced if on antibiotics	Yes	3 months	Good, no period if taken continually, but in this case risk of breakthrough bleeding
Progesterone only pill (POP)	Daily oral pill to be taken within 3-hour window	Yes, may be difficult to take on time	No	3 months	Variable
Desogestrel (POP)	Daily oral pill to be taken within 12-hour window	Yes	No	3 months	Generally good, variable
Levonorgestrel IUDs	Intrauterine system lasts for 5 years	Yes	No	6–9 months	Generally good after 6 months, may well result in little or no period
Etonogestrel implant	Subdermal implant lasts for 3 years	Yes	No	3 months	Variable, may try desogestrel POP first to establish efficacy and side-effect profile
Medroxyprogesterone acetate injection	Intramuscular injection lasts for 12 weeks	Yes	No	4 months	Variable but if suits, generally excellent, may result in no period
Medroxyprogesterone acetate orally 30 mg daily	Oral daily medication	No	No	2 months	Generally good, may have no bleeding but risk of breakthrough bleeding
Norethisterone 5 mg tds days 5–26	Oral three times daily medication	No	No	3 months	Good, will have a period, should be fairly light

Reproduced with permission of Dr Jane Preston, Consultant Obstetrician and Gynaecologist, James Paget University Hospital, Gorleston, Great Yarmouth, UK.

A clinical assessment score involving change in mental status, ataxia (heel–toe walking test) and the presence of peripheral oedema, as well as an overall functional score can be added to the Lake Louise self-assessment score for research purposes. The Lake Louise scoring system is not suitable for the detection of altitude sickness in preverbal children (i.e. under the age of three years). A modified scoring system (Children's Lake Louise Score) has been developed for this purpose.[53]

Susceptibility to altitude sickness

Susceptibility to altitude sickness varies greatly between individuals; however, in general, individuals respond consistently on each ascent. On Mauna Kea, mean arterial oxygen tension (PaO_2) recorded in the study group ranged from 4.4 kPa (33 mmHg) to 7.6 kPa (57 mmHg) at the summit. The worker with the highest PaO_2 during the first ascent (7.0 kPa, 52.5 mmHg) recorded the highest PaO_2 on a subsequent ascent (7.6 kPa, 57 mmHg). Similarly, one subject recorded the lowest PaO_2 (4.4 kPa, 33 mmHg: 5.1 kPa, 38 mmHg) on both ascents.[54] The reproducibility of individual response to high altitude exposure implies that the surest means of predicting an individual's performance at high altitude is their response on previous ascents. Inevitably, anomalies do occur: the healthy 29-year-old male astronomer who suffered from HAPO on Mauna Kea worked for two years before the episode of HAPO, and three years subsequently, without incident.

Predisposition to AMS may be related to individual sensitivity of hypoxic drive.[55] Subjects with a low ventilatory response to hypoxia are liable to develop AMS.[56] The magnitude of the increase in pulmonary arterial pressure in response to hypoxia is a further risk factor. The search for a genetic marker for AMS predisposition is wide-ranging and on-going.

Rapid ascent by sea-level residents to high altitude

As previously stated, there is a time delay of several hours on arrival at high altitude before the development of AMS; nevertheless, 'high altitude novice' sea-level residents report unpleasant symptoms on immediate arrival at high altitude before the onset of 'classical AMS'. Tourists visiting mountain tops report impaired mental and physical performance. Businessmen on tight schedules feel so unwell on reaching La Paz (3600 m) that their presentations are poor and multimillion dollar contracts are lost.[57]

In the 2007 survey of AMS on Mauna Kea, day visitors to the summit by vehicle were invited to complete a self-report assessment Lake Louise Symptom Score (LLSS) on descent. The majority were at the summit for less than two hours. Despite the lack of exertion on ascent, 60 day visitors (30 per cent) suffered AMS defined as a LLSS of 3 or greater. Headache was recorded in all sufferers, mental status changes in 17 per cent and shortness of breath in 29 per cent.[13] The authors of this study observed that to differentiate symptoms induced directly by hypoxia from those caused by changes in vascular permeability, which are involved in the pathogenesis of AMS,[58] would be difficult. Nevertheless, the time scale of the onset of symptoms indicates that these novice visitors to high altitude experienced either AMS of unusually rapid onset or a different condition altogether.

Illness at high altitude which is not high altitude illness

A personal account by a senior physician and experienced researcher emphasizes that not all sickness at high altitude is high altitude sickness. At Pheriche (4243 m) on the path to the Everest base camp, his dyspnoea, chest discomfort ('a severe weight on my chest – like a dead yak') and tachycardia were due to atrial flutter with 2:1 block and left ventricular failure and 'not real AMS'.[59]

The number of confounding conditions which can mimic or confuse the diagnosis of altitude sickness is legion. Neurological conditions reported include subarachnoid haemorrhage, transient global ischaemia, transient ischaemic attacks and strokes, convulsions, migraine and isolated sixth nerve palsies. Ophthalmic diagnoses, such as radial keratotomy and retinal haemorrhages, need to be recognized. Pulmonary embolism and respiratory infection, so often a mimic of HAPO, occur at high altitude and may be hypoxia-related. Miscellaneous problems may be linked to alcohol and recreational drug use, exhaustion, hypothermia, dehydration and carbon monoxide poisoning occurring in snow holes and tents. The authors of a comprehensive review of acute medical problems in the Himalayas outside the setting of acute altitude sickness recommend 'in most instances and when the diagnosis is uncertain it is best to descend'.[60]

AT-RISK GROUPS

Ischaemic heart disease

On the first day of work on the summit of Mauna Kea, mean PaO_2 was 5.6 kPa (42 mmHg) measured in 27 subjects on 40 ascents. Hypoxaemia induces increased sympathetic stimulation. As pulse rate increases, so does cardiac work and systemic blood pressure. The increase in cardiac work can be expressed in terms of the 'double product', i.e. the product of heart rate and systolic blood pressure. Among the Hawaiian telescope workers, the mean sea level 'double product' was 8925 units (mean resting pulse rate 75 beats/minute × mean systolic blood pressure 119 mmHg). At 4200 m, the 'double product' rose to 10 285 units, an increase in cardiac work of approximately 15 per cent.

By five days, sympathetic activity had fallen and the 'double product' stood at 9840 units. This indicates that the period of greatest risk for exacerbation or precipitation of ischaemic heart disease is the first three days at high altitude: the threat to coronary patient diminishes by five to seven days. Modest increases in cardiac output at high altitude will have little deleterious effect on people with controlled ischaemic heart disease and these people can work safely at high altitude. However, subjects experiencing angina or exertional dyspnoea at sea level may suffer a worsening of symptoms shortly after arrival at high altitude when cardiac output is highest. Common-sense advice should include recommendations for a slower than usual ascent profile with additional rest days at intermediate altitudes, limitation of physical activity to less than the level that precipitates symptoms at sea level and control of blood pressure.[61] People whose level of activity is severely curtailed by ischaemic symptoms at sea level are likely to suffer a marked deterioration at high altitude and must be cautioned against ascent. For such people who decide to ascend, facilities for rapid retreat down the mountain are mandatory taking precedence over other precautions, e.g. provision of oxygen or medical supervision.

In a population study, Shlim and Houston[62] surveyed reports of illness in 148 000 trekkers in Nepal during a three-year period. In the 23 fatalities, the cause of death were trauma (11), 'illness' (8) and AMS (3); no cardiac deaths were reported. Hultgren[63] reports that in the 25 years of his experience, the Chief Medical Officer at La Oroya (altitude 3750 m) never witnessed a myocardial infarction in a known sufferer from ischaemic heart disease among the hundreds of visitors who ascend each year from Lima, near sea level, to La Oroya.

Hypertension

There is no consistent change in blood pressure reported in normotensive sea-level residents at high altitude. On Mauna Kea, systolic pressure rose after two days at high altitude (mean 124 versus mean 118 mmHg at sea level) and returned to baseline levels on return to sea level. Diastolic pressure rose on arrival at 3000 m, remained elevated during five days on the mountain and fell on descent. No adverse effects related to elevation in systemic pressure occurred (Table 51.3). Hypertensive individuals demonstrate both increases and decreases in blood pressure at altitude.[48] Controlled hypertensive subjects can be reassured regarding ascent and advised to continue their prescribed antihypertensive medication.

Table 51.3 Effect of repeated exposure to high altitude (4200 m) on subjects with pre-existing medical conditions.

Case	Patient	Symptoms	Treatment
Case A: Bronchial asthma	Male, aged 32 years	Exercise-induced asthma since childhood; modest severity – no regular medication, bronchodilator by inhalation as required. No asthmatic attacks on mountain during 2.5 year work programme; single attack of bronchospasm at 3000 m precipitated by cardiac exercise test – self-limiting, no medication required	
Case B: Mitral valve prolapse and paroxysmal supraventricular tachycardia	Male, aged 34 years	Single episode of tachycardia during 3 years work on Mauna Kea; episode curtailed by carotid massage performed by subject	
Case C: Paroxysmal atrial tachycardia	Male, aged 40 years	No episodes of tachycardia on mountain; cardiac stress test (3000 m) normal	Self-treatment with β-blocker drug (oxyprenolol 80 mg)
Case D: Wolff–Parkinson–White syndrome (pre-excitation syndrome)	Male, aged 26 years	No episodes on Mauna Kea. Normal cardiac stress test (3000 m)	
Case E: Essential hypertension	Male, aged 45 years	Moderate increase in blood pressure on each ascent to 4200 m; no deterioration in blood pressure control during 3 years of supervision	Salt-restricted diet; diuretic (hydrochlorthiazide); β-blocker (propranolol 80 mg three times daily)
Case F: Crohn's disease	Male, aged 29 years	No deterioration in bowel condition during 2 years at Mauna Kea telescopes	Diet, sulphasalazine; corticosteroid (oral and rectal administration)

Respiratory disorders

CHRONIC OBSTRUCTIVE PULMONARY DISEASE

Sea-level dwellers rendered hypoxic by chronic lung disease will suffer a further reduction in PaO_2 at high altitude. Graham and Houston[64] accompanied eight patients with chronic obstructive airways disease (COAD), who had an average resting PaO_2 of 8.8 kPa (66 mmHg) at sea level, to an altitude of 1920 m. Within three hours of ascent, resting PaO_2 fell to 6.9 kPa (52 mmHg). Six minutes on a treadmill produced severe arterial hypoxaemia (mean PaO_2 6.2 kPa (46.5 mmHg) compared to 8.4 kPa (63 mmHg) at sea level). Despite levels of PaO_2 which would qualify as respiratory failure in COAD patients at sea level, none of the study patients came to harm and altitude sickness symptoms were trivial. In this study, tolerance of modest high altitude by COAD patients was facilitated by the exclusion criteria of coexistent disease (cor pulmonale, hypertension, angina) or elevated $PaCO_2$. Many COAD patients will be afflicted by these complications and the results of this study must be interpreted with caution. Other factors may compromise high altitude tolerance in chronic lung disease patients. Smokers experience more profound arterial hypoxia than non-smokers at high altitude.[65] Obese individuals are more prone to sleep apnoea at high altitude[66] and during periods of apnoea PaO_2 falls precipitously. Marked nocturnal arterial desaturation contributes to the exaggeration of altitude sickness symptoms present on morning waking.

ASTHMA

Bronchial airway narrowing in asthmatics can be provoked by stimuli, such as exercise and inhalation of cold air. Nevertheless, exposure to mountain air relatively free of air pollutants (tobacco smoke, petrol fumes) and exogenous allergens (house dust mites) is of benefit to asthmatics and treatment clinics have flourished in the alpine regions at altitudes as high as 3200 m in the Northern Tien-Shan mountains in Kyrgyzstan. Asthmatics with well-controlled disease may be encouraged to go to high altitude. Pre-treatment with acetazolamide protects against AMS symptoms and lessens arterial desaturation during sleep.[67] Asthmatics who self-monitor by serial peak flow measurements should be aware that the decrease in air density at high altitude results in under-reading by meters.[68] Readings taken with a mini-Wright meter can be corrected by adding 6.6 per cent for every 100 mmHg reduction in barometric pressure.[50] Overall PEF increases at high altitude, while FVC falls. Neither of these changes in pulmonary function measurements correlate with AMS.[69]

Diabetes mellitus

Hypoxia *per se* does not appear to have a deleterious effect on glucose metabolism and diabetic control. However, the inevitable increase in exercise during an ascent will consume carbohydrate stores and altitude-related nausea and vomiting will reduce carbohydrate intake leading to a reduction in insulin requirements. Hypoglycaemia may develop if insulin dosage is not adjusted accordingly. In wilderness conditions, intercurrent illness and vomiting associated with altitude sickness may predispose the diabetic to ketoacidosis. The respiratory alkalosis of hyperventilation at high altitude may complicate the clinical presentation of a metabolic acidosis. Furthermore, the prescription of a carbonic anhydrase inhibitor, such as acetazolamide as prophylaxis against AMS (see below under Prevention), may exacerbate metabolic acidosis. A climber with diabetes must be prepared to monitor their glycaemic control even more assiduously than usual. This necessity is compromised by under-reading of glucose meters at high altitude and low temperature. People with diabetes and their climbing companions must be well versed in the recognition and treatment of hyperglycaemia and hypoglycaemia.

On Kilimanjaro (5700 m), a group of type I diabetics were not more prone to AMS than their non-diabetic companions, although the diabetic climbers attained Gillman's Point (5700 m), whilst the non-diabetic others reached Uhuru Peak (5900 m).[70]

Haemoglobinopathies

Sickle cell anaemia, the homozygous form of the disease with HbS accounting for more than 90 per cent of haemoglobin, carries a high childhood mortality and considerable morbidity for adult survivors. People with the heterozygote sickle cell trait (HbA 60 per cent; HbS 40 per cent) are usually symptom-free at sea level and, with normal respiratory function, are unlikely to be at risk at altitudes up to 2000 m. Above this altitude, there is a risk of splenic and renal infarction and hence workers should be screened for the sickle cell trait before they are employed to work at high altitude. Avoidance of dehydration, caution in the event of infection and awareness of the significance of unexplained abdominal pain or haematuria will afford some protection to individuals with haemoglobinopathies who wish to venture to high places.[71] Treatment of a sickling crisis at high altitude is descent, in addition to the administration of oxygen and fluids and the prescription of analgesia.

SLEEP AT HIGH ALTITUDE

Periodic breathing (Cheyne–Stokes respiration) occurs during sleep at high altitude and periods of apnoea interspersed with rapid respiration cause frequent arousals during the night.[72] Insomnia is a common complaint. At relatively modest altitudes below 1400 m, sleep duration is reduced and the sleep efficiency index (ratio of total sleep time to the time in bed) falls. Above 4000 m, sleep duration and efficiency deteriorate further; sleep onset latency is increased and rapid eye movement (REM) sleep is decreased.[73] Disruption of the normal respiratory rhythm produces marked hypoxaemia during sleep. Sleep quality can be improved and sleep hypoxaemia alleviated by acetazolamide.[74] The use of hypnotic drugs by climbers at extreme altitude is not recommended because of the accompanying depression of ventilation which exacerbates nocturnal hypoxia. Nevertheless, the prescription of a short-acting benzodiazepine at low doses (e.g. 10-mg temazepam) in conjunction with acetazolamide reduces sleep onset latency and increases sleep efficiency at 4000 m to values comparable to sea level.[73]

ANAESTHESIA AT HIGH ALTITUDE

In a review of anaesthesia at high altitude, Stoneham[75] advises that the greater the altitude the greater the risks of anaesthesia and the less the likelihood of available anaesthetic expertise. At all altitudes, general anaesthesia will cause an increase in the alveolar to arterial gradient with physiological shunting. In addition, anaesthetic agents act as respiratory depressants and abolish peripheral chemoreceptor hypoxic drive upon which hyperventilation and survival at high altitude depend. At altitudes of 2000 m (e.g. Denver, Colorado) general anaesthesia should provide no particular problems. At altitudes above 3500 m (e.g. La Paz, Bolivia), the anaesthetic gas mixture should be oxygen enriched: close attention must be given to avoid post-operative hypoxia. At altitudes above 4000 m, general anaesthesia should be avoided unless life saving. Every attempt must be made to evacuate to a lower altitude.

Oxygen enrichment at high altitude

The pre-eminence of Mauna Kea as the highest terrestrial observatory in full-time operation has been superseded by the establishment of telescopes on the Chajnantor plateau in Northern Chile (5050 m, 16 470 ft). At this site, the California Institution of Technology has been operating a cosmic background imager (CBI) since 1999.

At 5050-m elevation, the barometric pressure is 551 mbars (55.1 kPa, 419 mmHg) and the partial pressure of oxygen in inspired air is 10.3 kPa (78 mmHg), only 52 per cent of sea-level values. These figures compare with a barometric pressure of 625 mbars (475 mmHg) and partial pressure of inspired oxygen of 12.6 kPa (95 mmHg) at the Mauna Kea summit. The CBI workers are exposed to approximately 10 per cent less oxygen than their Mauna Kea colleagues. To reduce the deleterious effects of hypoxia at over 5000 m, the atmosphere in the CBI control room and laboratory is enriched with oxygen to 27 per cent using oxygen concentrators.[76,77] Enrichment of oxygen to 27 per cent reduces the equivalent altitude (i.e. the altitude at which the moist inspired PO_2, when a subject is breathing ambient air, is the same as the inspired PO_2 in the oxygen-enriched environment) to 3200 m. Between altitudes of 3000 and 6000 m, each 1 per cent of oxygen enrichment results in a reduction of equivalent altitude of about 300 m.[48]

Oxygen enrichment was first used at the El Tambo mine in Northern Chile (4200 m) where 16 dormitory rooms were supplied with 24–26 per cent oxygen from a liquid oxygen source. Sleep quality was enhanced. The miners improved in the performance of psychometric tests assessing ability to concentrate, short-term memory, visual perception, attention span and auditory and topographical memory.[78] Oxygen enrichment technology has developed with the introduction of oxygen concentrators and can be implemented without an increase in fire risk at high altitude.[79] In a study at White Mountain (3800 m), Luks et al.[80] confirmed that oxygen enrichment enhanced sleep, but cognitive function improvement did not occur after one night of breathing oxygen-enriched air in this environment. In a 1972 paper, McFarland reported that cognitive function was only minimally impaired at this altitude.[81] However, at a simulated 5000-m altitude, oxygen enrichment improved motor function (hand–eye coordination) and response times, although not cognitive function. Undoubtedly, oxygen enrichment does increases the sense of well-being in workers at high altitude and over the seven years of operation, oxygen enrichment has shown benefit.[82] At Chajnantor, construction of the multinational Atacama large millimeter array (ALMA) started in 2003 and will be completed in 2012: it will become operational in 2010. ALMA is a single instrument composed of 66 high-precision antennas which can be moved across the altiplano desert over distances up to 15 km. In living and enclosed work areas (e.g. main control room, electronics and computing areas, engineering offices and antenna receiver cabins), the atmosphere will be oxygen enriched to 27 per cent.

In a 1984 review of high altitude medicine and physiology, Cudaback[83] concluded that the detrimental effect of hypoxia on performance and health at 4000-m high telescopes was sufficiently severe to warrant intervention. Considering the options of oxygen enrichment of enclosed air spaces, raising inside ambient barometric pressure or administration of medication, he concluded that oxygen enrichment was the answer. However, none of the 13 Mauna Kea observatories in operation employ oxygen enrichment, although the capability exists at two telescopes and neither is this provision available at the dormitory and living facilities at 3000 m. The opinion and experience of Mauna Kea staff was that the evidence of the need for oxygen enrichment at 4000-m altitude was not convincing.

ALTITUDE SICKNESS

Prevention

Wise mountaineers who wish to avoid the debilitating effects of high altitude respect the maxims 'climb high, sleep low' and 'hasten slowly'. These precepts are of particular relevance for people with a previous history of altitude sickness. A slow ascent of only 300 m/day above 3000 m altitude is recommended.[84,85] Staging the climb so that a rest day and two consecutive nights are spent at the same altitude every third day (or every 1000 m) facilitates acclimatization. By following these cautious guidelines, the majority of sea-level residents ascend safely, but some will develop altitude sickness above 3000 m. Common sense must prevail: an attempt to climb higher while in the throes of an attack of altitude sickness is foolhardy. Victims of altitude sickness must descend; a descent of 500 m may be sufficient to relieve AMS. Alternatively, AMS sufferers should remain at a safe moderate altitude (below 3000 m) until their condition improves. General measures to ease discomfort include avoidance of strenuous exercise on arrival at high altitude, maintenance of an adequate fluid intake and abstinence from alcohol and tobacco. Cold exposure and lack of sleep aggravate the discomforts of a hypoxic environment. Infection is associated with a higher incidence of AMS and markedly increases the misery of altitude sickness; climbers with infections should ascend at a slower rare or preferably remain at an intermediate altitude.[7]

People whose work or leisure schedules do not allow gradual ascent can be offered prophylactic treatment with acetazolamide and this is a wise precaution if they have a previous history of altitude sickness. Acetazolamide and methazolamide inhibit the enzyme carbonic anhydrase which regulates CO_2 transport out of cells. Inhibition of the enzyme in the renal tubule promotes renal excretion of bicarbonate and conserves hydrogen ion (H^+). The increased arterial H^+ concentration counteracts the respiratory alkalosis caused by hyperventilation in the low oxygen environment of high altitude. Respiratory alkalosis produces a negative feedback on central respiratory drive: carbonic anhydrase inhibition removes this negative feedback, thus enhancing respiratory activity and increasing oxygen uptake (Figure 51.4). Prophylactic treatment with acetazolamide raises arterial H^+ concentration and PaO_2 and ameliorates AMS symptoms.[86–89] Prescriptions of acetazolamide (500 mg/day, sustained release tablet or a dose of >125 mg twice a day[90]) should be given for 24 to 48 hours before ascent and continued for two days at high altitude. The period of time needed for acclimatization will depend upon the speed of ascent, the altitude achieved and the individual's unique physiology. Adverse effects of carbonic anhydrase inhibitors include limb and perioral paraesthesia which diminish over time and an alteration of the taste of carbonated drinks. Mountaineers recognize that individuals resistant to altitude sickness urinate profusely on reaching altitude – the 'Hohendiuresis' of the alpine climber. Although acetazolamide is a diuretic, the diuretic effect is short-lived and its efficacy in altitude sickness is not due to this property. Frusemide, a potent loop diuretic, has been advocated for the prevention of AMS;[8] however, there is a danger of aggravating fluid depletion in climbers who are dehydrated by hyperventilation, intense physical activity and the twin scourges of vomiting and diarrhoea. Hypercoagulability of the blood and sequestration of platelets provoke pulmonary thrombosis at high altitude. The dehydrating effect of a powerful diuretic may aggravate this thrombotic tendency.

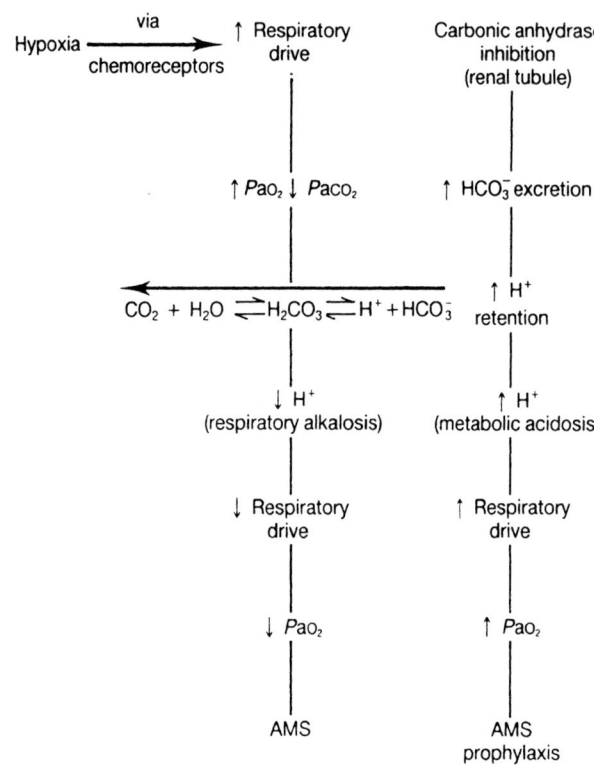

Figure 51.4 Mode of action of carbonic anhydrase inhibition in prophylaxis of acute mountain sickness (AMS).

Dexamethasone, a potent synthetic glucocorticoid with some mineralocorticoid activity, has been demonstrated to reduce AMS symptoms when given prior to simulated ascent to high altitude (4570 m)[91] and during rapid ascent of Mount Rainier.[92] In the latter study, dexamethasone was administered at a 4-mg dose every eight hours for 24 hours before ascent. The potentially serious adverse effects of corticosteroids limit the duration of prophylactic treatment. Dexamethasone has no effect upon oxygen consumption or carbon dioxide transport. Reduction of cerebral oedema of vasogenic origin may be the action whereby dexamethasone is effective as AMS prophylaxis.

Theophylline, a phosphodiesterase inhibitor and potent bronchodilator used in the treatment of obstructive airways disease has a range of pharmacological properties advantageous to the AMS victim, including suppression of capillary permeability in lung and brain, decrease in pulmonary artery pressure and stimulation of central respiratory drive. A decompression chamber study (simulated altitude 4500 m) and a mountain study (3454 m) showed that slow-release theophylline (375 mg bid or 250 mg bid for subjects <70 kg) taken three days before ascent reduced AMS (Lake Louise symptom score) and raised arterial oxygen saturation. These benefits were short lived.[93]

An alternative remedy for AMS prophylaxis is ginkgo biloba. This herbal extract is reputed to have anti-oxidant and anti-hypoxic properties which led to its use in patients with cerebral and peripheral vascular disease. Ginkgo biloba is reputed to stabilize the cerebral blood–brain barrier, hence the rationale for its use in AMS. A study in the Himalayas of 44 mountaineers ascending to 5200 m showed a significant reduction in AMS with none of the gingko-treated group (five days of 120-mg gingko) suffering from AMS compared to 41 per cent of placebo group.[94] In a study on Mauna Kea, with subjects following an ascent profile similar to that of shift workers in the 1980 study, gingko (60 mg tds) taken one day before ascent reduced the severity of AMS in the treated group, but there was no significant reduction in incidence of AMS. This study was discontinued early because of the unexpected and unexplained incidence of severe AMS with 42 per cent (11/26) of subjects needing evacuation from the summit. No difference in oxygen saturation was found between the treatment and placebo groups.[95] The case for gingko prophylaxis requires further study; however, with few adverse effects (occasional headaches) and available without prescription, gingko will appeal to those unable or reluctant to take acetazolamide or dexamethasone as AMS prophylaxis.

Chemoprophylaxis for HAPO is an important therapeutic intervention because of the recurrent nature of the condition. The calcium channel blocker nifedipine is effective as a slow-release preparation at a dose of 20 mg every eight hours and has been demonstrated to prevent HAPO after rapid ascent to 4559 m. Individuals with a history of HAPO who wish to climb should consider nifedipine prophylaxis.[26] However, nifedipine is not recommended as prophylaxis or treatment of AMS or HACO.[96] HAPO-susceptible individuals have an impairment of sodium-dependent alveolar fluid clearance. The beta-sympathetic agonist salmeterol facilitates clearance of alveolar fluid by stimulating trans-epithelial sodium transport via effects on the amiloride-sensitive channel and Na^+/K^+-ATPase pump. Prophylactic inhalation of salmeterol (125 μg by pressurized metered-dose inhaler connected to a spacer every 12 hours), administered on the morning of a day-long ascent to 4559 m, decreased the incidence of HAPO by over 50 per cent in a group of HAPO-susceptible mountaineers.[97] Manipulation of pulmonary vasoactive mediators is another possible HAPO chemoprophylactic avenue to explore. The phosphodiesterase-V inhibitor sildenafil is a potent vasodilator of both peripheral and pulmonary vessels. Combined with red wine, a known antioxidant and endothelin-1 suppressor, sildenafil may, in the words of one reviewer, 'lead to an enthusiastic number of subjects going to high altitude for more than just the enjoyment of the view'.[27]

Treatment

Acute mountain sickness of moderate severity – without respiratory distress or neurological dysfunction – may be managed at intermediate altitudes between 3000 and 4000 m, particularly if the victim is able to sleep at a lower altitude. Exercise induces sodium and water retention, decreases oxygen saturation and increases pulmonary artery pressure, thus aggravating the pathological processes leading to altitude sickness: rest is an important component of treatment for all grades of severity of AMS.[98] In difficult circumstances, the need for rest may be outweighed by the need for exertion to descend. Abstinence from alcohol, adequate fluid intake and frequent small meals of carbohydrate content are recommended. Non-steroid anti-inflammatory drugs (e.g. ibuprofen) have been proven effective in relieving high altitude headache in a placebo-controlled double-blind trial.[99] The association of nausea, vomiting and visual disturbance with debilitating headache has led to the supposition that AMS could share a similar pathophysiological mechanism to classical migraine.[100] However, selective stimulation of 5-hydroxytriptamine receptors by sumatriptan (100-mg dose), a rapid and comprehensive treatment for migraine, was not efficacious for high altitude headache.[101] To ease nausea and vomiting, anti-emetics (e.g. prochlorperazine 10-mg oral, or intramuscular injection three times a day) may be administered. To aid sleep short-acting sedatives (e.g. temazepam) should be used at the lowest effective dose for the shortest time possible. The use of carbonic anhydrase inhibitor drugs for the treatment of AMS has been established in several studies. In a double-blind, placebo-controlled trial on Mt McKinley (4200 m), low-dose acetazolamide (250 mg) was prescribed at diagnosis and eight hours later. Symptoms were relieved, arterial oxygenation improved and pulmonary gas exchange was stabilized.[102] High-dose acetazolamide (1.0–1.5 g) and methazolamide (400–500 mg) were studied on three separate expeditions at between 3200 and 5486 m: as in the low-dose study, AMS symptoms and arterial oxygenation improved significantly.[103] High-dose acetazolamide was associated with more adverse effects and a quarter of subjects suffered headache. This is sufficient reason to favour the lower-dose treatment regime.

The treatment for severe AMS, HAPO and HACO is immediate descent to the lowest altitude feasible and administration of oxygen. All other therapeutic measures are of secondary importance. The consequences of delayed descent may be fatal pulmonary and cerebral disease.[104] Once HAPO or HACO are established, oxygen therapy may not be beneficial even at the recommended flow rate of 6–8 L/min; the failure of supplementary oxygen to be invariably effective is because hypoxia, the initiating insult, triggers increased capillary permeability causing oedema of the lungs and brain which can only be reversed by retreat from a hypoxic and hypobaric environment. In addition to descent and oxygen, dexamethasone is administered in severe AMS (4 mg every six hours for 24 hours) and HACO at a dose of 8 mg initially followed by 4 mg every six hours by mouth, i.m. or i.v. injection.[105] Nifedipine, a calcium channel blocker, reverses hypoxic pulmonary hypertension and lowers pulmonary artery pressure in HAPO victims.

Oxygenation improves and the clinical manifestations of HAPO are relieved.[106] Nifedipine is prescribed at a dose of 10 mg sublingually and 20 mg slow release capsule stat followed by 20-mg slow release capsule every six hours until descent for established HAPO. HAPO is not caused by cardiac failure and the use of frusemide may worsen the condition of a hypotensive, shocked HAPO victim.

In remote high altitude regions of the world, many miles from medical attention, the sick climber suspected of HACO and HAPO can be administered dexamethasone (8 mg stat followed by 4 mg six-hourly for 24 hours) and nifedipine (20 mg tablet six-hourly for 24 hours) simultaneously to allow for repatriation to a lower altitude. Carrying these medications for use in an emergency has been recommended by physicians experienced in high altitude medicine. It must be emphasized that such treatment should neither exceed 24 hours nor be a substitute for descent.[107]

The practical problems of transporting cylinders to high altitude limit the availability of oxygen in an emergency. Simulated descent in a portable fabric hypobaric chamber (Gamow bag®, Certec bag®, portable altitude chamber) is a popular alternative. The Gamow bag (weight 6.6 kg, including foot pump) is inflated to an inside pressure of 103 mmHg above ambient atmospheric pressure. At this inflation pressure, a patient inside the chamber experiences a simulated descent;[108] for example, at 4500 m (ambient atmospheric pressure 433 mmHg), a treated subject experiences a pressure of 536 mmHg equivalent to an altitude of 2780 m, a 'descent' of 1720 m. Hyperbaric treatment alleviates symptoms and PaO_2 rises for the duration of treatment in the chamber, but falls within minutes of return to the outside atmospheric pressure.[109,110] Symptom relief is greater and quicker with pressurization treatment than with oral dexamethasone (8 mg initially, 4 mg after six hours), but the benefits of corticosteroids are of greater duration: both treatments can be administered together to AMS patients.[111] It is possible to place an oxygen cylinder in the bag for use by the victim. The inevitable build up of exhaled carbon dioxide in the bag, despite venting by foot pump action, has a measurable beneficial effect in increasing peripheral and cerebral oxygenation possibly by stimulation of the respiratory centre or dilatation of cerebral vasculature.[112] Hyperbaric treatment is not to be recommended as a substitute for descent, but may obviate the need for storing large quantities of oxygen at high altitude work stations. Other novel methods to improve gas exchange and oxygenation include the use of a portable continuous positive airways pressure in HAPO[113] and the addition of 3 per cent carbon dioxide to inhaled air in AMS.[114]

Safe working at high altitude

Assessed against the parameters of the quality of astronomical research and safety of the work force, the Mauna Kea Observatory has been an outstanding success. A visible sign of this success is shown in Figures 51.1 and 51.2: between 1989 and 1998 the number of telescopes increased from six major telescopes with one under construction to 11 telescopes sited at the summit.

According to management staff at Mauna Kea, in a 2007 survey of AMS, there had not been any reported deaths or permanent morbidity related to HAPO or HACO on the mountain.[13] Remote observation technology has advanced since the early days; nevertheless, in 1999 staffing requirements at one telescope (United Kingdom Infra Red Telescope, UKIRT) still necessitated 2000 man-days per annum. Overall, 30 000 man-days per annum are spent at the major telescopes on Mauna Kea. There has been a single cardiac death at the summit among the telescope personnel. A 37-year-old smoker and diabetic suffered a myocardial infarction after staying at the summit all night and working through the days. Post-mortem examination revealed extensive coronary disease. Following this fatality, revised health screening protocols were established (Table 51.4). All UKIRT personnel undergo a medical evaluation at sea level which includes physical examination, a comprehensive range of blood tests, resting ECG and treadmill stress test, chest x-ray and pulmonary function tests. Recommendations are that medical evaluations should be repeated annually for individuals above age 40 years, every two years between ages 30 and 39 years and every three years for those younger than age 30 years. In the late 1990s, a 40-year-old construction worker suffered a fatal cardiopulmonary arrest at the summit: construction company employees were not required to undergo a rigorous screening programme.[115] The confidence of the workforce – technical, scientific and managerial – in operating the telescopes on Mauna Kea has been greatly facilitated by ease of descent from the mountain and ready access to high quality medical care in the event of an emergency. Within two hours of leaving the summit by road, a victim of HAPO or HACO could be undergoing MRI or computed tomography (CT) scanning at sea level. Provision of sleeping and living facilities at a mid-level station (Onazaku Center, Hale Pohaku, 3000 m) affords protection and comfort for the staff.

Education of the workforce is essential. The initial trepidation of the telescope staff at the prospect of working in a hypoxic and hypobaric environment has been supplanted by knowledge of the consequences of altitude exposure, and the awareness that problems can be predicted and coping strategies developed. The converse 'machismo' attitude of denial of the hazards of altitude has been replaced by respect for the mountain site and acceptance that people react to altitude exposure in an individual manner irrespective of age, fitness, gender or 'toughness'. Information cards describing the serious symptoms requiring immediate evacuation from the summit are displayed at the telescope. Bottled oxygen is available on site. Experience has established clear directives for the workforce. No individual is allowed at the summit alone and sufficient unlocked vehicles must always be available at the telescope: the so-called 'two man, two vehicle' rule. No one sleeps at the telescope. No alcohol is permitted on the mountain. Staff

Table 51.4 Prevention and management of altitude sickness.

Prevention/ treatment	Treatment	
Prevention	Gradual ascent. Above 3000 m ascend 300 m per day	
	Staging ascent. Two days stay at intermediate altitude (i.e. 3000 m): rest day and 2 consecutive nights at same altitude every 3rd day (or 1000 m ascent)	
	Avoid excessive exertion	
	Consider prophylaxis. AMS: acetazolamide 500 mg sustained-release or 250 mg twice daily 2 days before ascent and 2 days at high altitude	
	dexamethasone: 4 mg every 8 hours for 24 hours before ascent (for subjects intolerant or refractory to acetazolamide)	
	HAPO: nifedipine 20 mg slow release every 8 hours	
Treatment	Mild AMS	'If in doubt, go down'
		Rest: no further ascent, avoid exertion
		Analgesia for headache
		Anti-emetics for nausea, vomiting
	Moderate/severe AMS	Descend 500 m or more, sleep at lower altitude
		Rest
		Adequate fluid intake and small frequent meals
		Ibuprofen or paracetamol for headaches, anti-emetics for nausea
		Acetazolamide: 250 mg twice daily or 500 mg sustained release
		Dexamethasone: 4 mg every 6 hours for severe AMS if descent is not possible
		Antibiotics for infection (if suspected)
	High altitude cerebral oedema	Immediate descent or evacuation
		Dexamethasone: 8 mg stat (oral, i.m. or i.v. route), then 4 mg every 6 hours
		Oxygen (2–4 L/min)
		Hyperbaric pressurization (if descent not possible)
	High altitude pulmonary oedema	Immediate descent or evacuation
		Oxygen 4–6 L/min (then 2–4 L/min if improvement)
		Nifedipine: 10 mg oral/sublingual with 20 mg stat, then 20 mg slow release every 6 hours
		Hyperbaric pressurization (if descent not possible)
		Dexamethasone: as above if neurological features indicate HACO

are only allowed to drive on the mountain road after having experienced three return trips as a passenger. It is clearly understood that a staff member is the responsible officer at the summit and has the authority to close the facility if hazard threatens. Many of these measures have been adopted at the Chajnantor site to complement the two elements underpinning safe operation at the site – the establishment of an operations support base at a modest altitude (2400 m) and oxygen enrichment of the air inside the buildings at 5000 m.[116]

Over several decades of scientific endeavour on Mauna Kea, the calibre of astronomical research produced has demonstrated that high altitude is not detrimental to high performance. Men endure high altitude for reasons more prosaic than gazing at the stars. At the Aucanquilcha sulphur mines in the Chilean Andes, native miners live and sleep at 5330 m and each day ascend to the mines at 5950 m. Miners refuse to inhabit the camp erected at the mine because of difficulty with sleep at the higher elevation; nevertheless, the top camp is occupied by a gang of caretakers. Each Sunday, the caretakers descend to the comfort of 4220 m to play football.[117] However, at the international level, there is controversy that adaptation to life at high altitude may confer unfair advantage to high altitude natives over sea-level opponents when playing 'the beautiful game' in thinner air. In May 2007, football's international governing body (FIFA) banned World Cup-qualifying matches from being played at more than 2750 m elevation because of 'possible distortion of competition' to the delight of the Brazilians (Rio de Janiero, sea level) and the outrage of the Bolivians (La Paz, 3600 m). Under pressure from the Bolivian president Evo Morales, who enlisted the support of Diego Maradona in a campaign against 'football apartheid' and the South American Football Confederation, FIFA relented and awarded a special dispensation for Bolivia to host World Cup-qualifying games in La Paz.[118]

On May 23, 2007, medical researchers sampled femoral arterial blood at the 'Balcony' (8400 m) on their descent from the summit of Everest (8850 m). PaO_2 was in the range of 2.55–3.93 kPa. One of the key objectives of the Caudwell Xtreme Everest expedition was to investigate how humans could survive in environmental hypoxia, when at sea level artificial ventilation would be required to preserve life. It is hoped that the experiments will extend knowledge which will aid the care of critically ill patients in whom hypoxia is a fundamental problem.[119]

'Because it is there', answered George Mallory, reputedly, when asked why he wanted to climb Everest. Mallory and Andrew Irvine died in the attempt. And yet men and women still climb and die on the mountain: some alone and cold, some overwhelmed by avalanche, ice falls or falling rocks, some in the depths of crevices, and some stumbling exhausted and incapacitated by high altitude illness.[120] Humans, ascending mountains for many different reasons as well as science and commerce, can find there an unforgiving world.

Box 51.1 Useful sources of information

- Birmingham Medical Research Expeditionary Society: www.bmres.org.uk/
- CIWEC Clinic, Travel Medicine Centre, Kathmandu, Nepal: www.ciwec-clinic.com/
- Diabetes at high altitude: www.idea2000.org/
- International Society for Mountain Medicine: www.ismmed.org/
- Medex: Travel at high altitude: www.medex.org.uk/
- Wilderness Medical Society: www.wms.org/

Key points

- Altitude sickness affects unacclimatized sea-level residents ascending to altitudes above 2500 m.
- The clinical diseases associated with high altitude sickness are 'benign' acute mountain sickness (AMS) which is usually self-limiting and resolves after two to three days and 'malignant' high altitude cerebral oedema (HACO) and high altitude pulmonary oedema (HAPO), both of which are potentially fatal.
- Altitude sickness is avoided by slow, staged ascent ('hasten slowly') allowing acclimatization, sleeping at the lowest possible altitude ('climb high, sleep low') and avoidance of strenuous exertion.
- The essential treatment for severe AMS, HACO and HAPO is immediate descent to lower altitude. All other treatments (e.g. drugs, oxygen administration) are adjuncts to descent.
- Experience derived from decades of work at high altitude mines and astronomical observatories have shown that working at high altitude is possible, safe and effective if appropriate working practices are established and if the means for descent is always available.

Appendix 51.1 Calculating the Lake Louise Acute Mountain Sickness (AMS) score.[121]

Add up the responses to each of the questions of the self-report score (questions 1–5).
A diagnosis of AMS is based on a recent rise in altitude, the presence of a headache and at least one other symptom and a total score of at least 3.
AMS = Altitude Gain AND Headache AND at least one other symptom AND a total score of 3 or more.

Self-Report Questionnaire:		
	1. Headache	0. No headache
		1. Mild headache
		2. Moderate headache
		3. Severe headache, incapacitating
	2. Gastrointestinal symptoms	0. No gastrointestinal symptoms
		1. Poor appetite or nausea
		2. Moderate nausea or vomiting
		3. Severe nausea and vomiting, incapacitating
	3. Fatigue and/or weakness	0. Not tired or weak
		1. Mild fatigue/weakness
		2. Moderate fatigue/weakness
		3. Severe fatigue/weakness, incapacitating
	4. Dizziness/ lightheadedness	0. Not dizzy
		1. Mild dizziness
		2. Moderate dizziness
		3. Severe dizziness, incapacitating
	5. Difficulty sleeping	0. Slept as well as usual
		1. Did not sleep as well as usual
		2. Woke many times, poor nights sleep
		3. Could not sleep at all

Additional Lake Louise Scoring: The Self-Report Score above (questions 1–5) stands alone and this is recommended for non-medical mountain travellers. Additional observations are sometimes used by researchers. The Clinical Assessment score (questions 6–8) can be added to the Self-Report Score, in which case, in the context of a recent rise in altitude, a score of 5 or more would be taken as AMS (AMS = altitude rise AND headache AND at least one other symptom (from questions 1–5) AND a total score of 5 or more (questions 1–8)

Clinical Assessment:		
	6. Change in mental status	0. No change in mental status
		1. Lethargy/lassitude
		2. Disorientated/confused
		3. Stupor/semi-conscious

(Continued)

Appendix 51.1 (*Continued*)

	7. Ataxia (heel-toe-walking)	0. No ataxia
		1. Manoeuvres to maintain balance
		2. Steps off line
		3. Falls down
		4. Can't stand
	8. Peripheral oedema	0. No peripheral oedema
		1. Peripheral oedema in one location
		2. Peripheral oedema in two or more locations
Functional score:	Overall, if you had any symptoms, how did they affect your activity?	0. No reduction in activity
		1. Mild reduction in activity
		2. Moderate reduction in activity
		3. Severe reduction in activity (e.g. bed rest)

Reproduced with permission of Dr Paul Richards, Honorary Lecturer in Travel Medicine, University College, London, UK.

REFERENCES

1. Whymper E. *Travels amongst the Great Andes of the Equator.* London: John Murray, 1892.
2. Fitzgerald EA. *The highest Andes. A record of the first ascent of Aconcagua and Tupungatoin Argentina and the exploration of the surrounding valleys.* London: Methuen & Co, 1899.
3. Ravenhill TH. Some experiences of mountain sickness in the Andes. *Journal of Tropical Medicine and Hygiene.* 1913; **16**: 313–20.
4. Basynat B, Murdoch DR. High-altitude illness. *Lancet.* 2003; **361**: 1967–74.
5. Hackett PH, Rennie D. Rales, peripheral edema, retinal haemorrhage and acute mountain sickness. *American Journal of Medicine.* 1979; **67**: 214–18.
6. Roach RC, Larson EB, Hornbein TF *et al.* Acute mountain sickness, antacids and ventilation during rapid, active ascent of Mount Rainier. *Aviation, Space and Environmental Medicine.* 1983; **54**: 397–401.
7. Murdoch DR. Symptoms of infection and altitude illness among hikers in the Mount Everest region of Nepal. *Aviation, Space and Environmental Medicine.* 1995; **66**: 148–51.
8. Singh I, Khanna PK, Srivastava MC *et al.* Acute mountain sickness. *New England Journal of Medicine.* 1969; **280**: 175–84.
9. Honigman B, Theis MK, Koziol-McLain J *et al.* Acute mountain sickness in a general tourist population at moderate altitudes. *Annals of Internal Medicine.* 1993; **118**: 587–92.
10. Wright AD. Medicine at high altitude. *Clinical Medicine.* 2006; **6**: 604–8.
11. Forster PJG. *Work at high altitude: A clinical and physiological study at the United Kingdom Infrared Telescope, Mauna Kea, Hawaii.* Edinburgh: Royal Observatory, 1983.
12. Heath D, Williams DR. *High altitude medicine and pathology.* Oxford: Oxford University Press, 1995.
13. Onapa J, Haley A, Yeow ME. Survey of acute mountain sickness on Mauna Kea. *High Altitude Medicine and Biology.* 2007; **8**: 200–5.
14. Schoene RB. Unravelling the mechanism of high altitude pulmonary edema. *High Altitude Medicine and Biology.* 2004; **5**: 125–35.
15. Durmowicz AG, Noordeweir E, Nicholas R *et al.* Inflammatory processes may predispose children to high-altitude pulmonary edema. *Journal of Pediatrics.* 1997; **130**: 838–40.
16. Swenson ER, Maggiorini M, Mongovin S *et al.* Pathogenesis of high altitude pulmonary edema: Inflammation is not an etiologic factor. *Journal of American Medical Association.* 2002; **287**: 2228–35.
17. Hultgren HN. High altitude pulmonary edema: Current concepts. *Annual Review of Medicine.* 1996; **47**: 267–84.
18. Singh I, Kapila CC, Khanna PK *et al.* High altitude pulmonary oedema. *Lancet.* 1965; **I**: 229–34.
19. Hackett PH, Rennie D, Levine HD. The incidence, importance and prophylaxis of acute mountain sickness. *Lancet.* 1976; **2**: 1149–54.
20. Maggiorini M, Buhler M, Waiter M, Oelz O. Prevalence of acute mountain sickness in the Swiss Alps. *British Medical Journal.* 1990; **301**: 853–5.
21. Cremona G, Asnaghi R, Baderna P *et al.* Pulmonary extravascular fluid accumulation in recreational climbers. *Lancet.* 2002; **359**: 303–9.
22. Sonna LS. Pulmonary oedema at moderately high altitudes. *Lancet.* 2002; **359**: 276–7.
23. Hackett PH, Roach RC. High altitude illness. *New England Journal of Medicine.* 2001; **345**: 107–114.
24. Hackett PH, Creagh CE, Grover RF *et al.* High altitude pulmonary edema in persons without the right pulmonary artery. *New England Journal of Medicine.* 1980; **302**: 1070–3.
25. Naeije R, De Backer D, Vachiery JL, De Vuyst P. High-altitude pulmonary edema with primary pulmonary hypertension. *Chest.* 1996; **110**: 286–9.
26. Bartsch P, Maggiorini M, Ritter M *et al.* Prevention of high-altitude pulmonary oedema by nifedipine. *New England Journal of Medicine.* 1991; **325**: 1284–9.
27. Schoene RB. Unraveling the mechanism of high altitude pulmonary edema. *High Altitude Medicine and Biology.* 2004; **2**: 125–35.
28. Richalet JP. High altitude pulmonary oedema: Still a place for controversy. *Thorax.* 1995; **50**: 923–9.
29. Hackett PH, Roach RC. High altitude cerebral oedema. *High Altitude Medicine and Biology.* 2004; **5**: 136–46.
30. Milledge JS. High altitude. In: Harries M, Williams C, Standish WD, Micheli L (eds). *Oxford textbook of sports medicine.* Oxford: Oxford University Press, 1996: 217–30.

31. Houston CS, Dickinson J. Cerebral form of high altitude illness. *Lancet.* 1975; **2**: 758–61.
32. Dickinson J, Heath D, Gosney J, Williams D. Altitude related deaths in seven trekkers in the Himalayas. *Thorax.* 1983; **38**: 646–56.
33. Rennie D. High altitude oedema – cerebral and pulmonary. In: Clarke C, Ward M, Williams E (eds). *Mountain medicine and physiology.* London: Alpine Club, 1975: 85–98.
34. Imray CHE, Myers SD, Pattinson KTS *et al.* Effect of exercise on cerebral perfusion in humans at high altitude. *Journal of Applied Physiology.* 2005; **99**: 699–706.
35. Roach RC, Houston CS, Honigman B *et al.* How well do older persons tolerate moderate altitude? *Western Journal of Medicine.* 1995; **162**: 32–6.
36. McFarland RA. Psycho-physiological studies at high altitude in the Andes. I. The effects of rapid ascents by aeroplane and train. *Comparative Psychology.* 1937; **23**: 191–225.
37. McFarland RA. Psycho-physiological studies at high altitude in the Andes. II. Sensory and motor responses during acclimatisation. *Comparative Psychology.* 1937; **23**: 227–58.
38. McFarland RA. Psycho-physiological studies at high altitude in the Andes. III. Mental and psychosomatic responses during gradual adaptation. *Comparative Psychology.* 1938; **24**: 147–88.
39. McFarland RA. Psycho-physiological studies at high altitude in the Andes. IV. Sensory and circulatory responses of the Andean residents at 17500 feet. *Comparative Psychology.* 1938; **24**: 189–220.
40. Sharma VM, Malhotra MS, Baskaran AS. Variations in psychomotor efficiency during prolonged stay at high altitude. *Ergonomics.* 1975; **18**: 511–16.
41. Regard M, Oelz O, Brugger P *et al.* Persistent cognitive impairment in climbers after repeated exposure to extreme altitude. *Neurology.* 1989; **39**: 210–13.
42. Townes BD, Hornbein TF, Schoene RB *et al.* Human cerebral function at extreme altitudes. In: West JB, Lahiri S (eds). *High altitude and man.* Bethesda, MD: American Physiological Society, 1984: 31–6.
43. Hornbein TM, Townes BD, Schoene RB *et al.* The cost to the central nervous system of climbing to high altitude. *New England Journal of Medicine.* 1989; **321**: 1714–19.
44. Clark CF, Heaton RK, Wiens AN. Neuropsychological functioning after prolonged high altitude exposure in mountaineering. *Aviation, Space and Environmental Medicine.* 1983; **54**: 202–7.
45. Garrido E, Segura R, Capdevila A *et al.* New evidence from magnetic resonance imaging of brain changes after climbs to extreme altitude. *European Journal of Applied Physiology.* 1995; **70**: 477–81.
46. Garrido E, Segura R, Capadevila A *et al.* Are Himalayan sherpas better protected against brain damage associated with extreme altitude climbs? *Clinical Science.* 1996; **90**: 81–5.
47. Jean D, Leal C, Kriemler S *et al.* Medical recommendations for women going to high altitude. *High Altitude Medicine and Biology.* 2005; **6**: 22–31.
48. Ward MP, Milledge JS, West JB. *High altitude medicine and physiology.* London: Arnold, 2000.
49. Hultgren HN. High altitude medical problems. *Western Journal of Medicine.* 1979; **131**: 8–23.
50. Pollard AJ, Murdoch DR. *The high altitude medicine handbook.* Oxford: Radcliffe Medical Press, 2003.
51. Yaron M, Niermeyer S. Travel to high altitude with young children: An approach for clinicians. *High Altitude Medicine and Biology.* 2008; **9**: 265–9.
52. Roach RC, Bartsch P, Hackett PH and the Lake Louise AMS Scoring Consensus Committee. The Lake Louise acute mountain sickness scoring system. In: Sutton JR, Houston CS, Coates G (eds). *Hypoxia and molecular medicine.* Burlington, VT: Queen City Printers, 1993.
53. Yaron M, Niermeyer S, Lindgren K *et al.* The diagnosis of acute mountain sickness in pre-verbal children. *Archives of Pediatric Adolescent Medicine.* 1998; **152**: 683–7.
54. Forster PJG. Reproducibility of individual response to high altitude exposure. *British Medical Journal.* 1984; **2**: 1269.
55. Lakshminarayan S, Pierson DJ. Recurrent high altitude pulmonary oedema with blunted chemosensitivity. *American Review of Respiratory Diseases.* 1975; **111**: 869–72.
56. Milledge JS. Acute mountain sickness. *Thorax.* 1983; **38**: 641–5.
57. Medex. Travel at high altitude. Last accessed July 2009. Available from: www.medex.org.uk.
58. Lewis DM, Bradwell AR, Shore AC *et al.* Capillary filtration coefficient and urinary albumin leak at altitude. *European Journal of Clinical Investigation.* 1997; **27**: 64–8.
59. Harvey TC. Om Mani Padme Hum. *Lancet.* 1993; **342**: 363.
60. Basnyat B, Cumbo TA, Edelman R. Acute medical problems in the Himalayas outside the setting of altitude sickness. *High Altitude Medicine and Biology.* 2000; **1**: 167–74.
61. Alexander JK. Coronary problems associated with altitude and air travel. *Cardiology Clinics.* 1995; **13**: 271–8.
62. Shlim D, Houston R. Helicopter rescues and deaths among trekkers in Nepal. *Journal of the American Medical Association.* 1989; **261**: 1017–19.
63. Hultgren HN. Coronary heart disease and trekking. *Journal of Wilderness Medicine.* 1990; **1**: 154–61.
64. Graham WGB, Houston CS. Short term adaptation to moderate altitude. Patients with chronic obstructive pulmonary disease. *Journal of the American Medical Association.* 1978; **240**: 1491–4.
65. Brewer GJ, Eaton JW, Grover RF, Weil JV. Cigarette smoking as a cause of hypoxemia in man at altitude. *Chest.* 1971; **59**: 30S–31S.
66. Rennie D, Wilson R. Who should not go high. In: Sutton JR, Jones NL, Houston CS (eds). *Hypoxia: Man at altitude.* New York: Thieme-Stratton Inc, 1982: 186–90.
67. Mirrakhlmov M, Brimkulov N, Cieslicki J *et al.* Effects of acetazolamide on overnight oxygenation and acute mountain sickness in patients with asthma. *European Respiratory Journal.* 1993; **6**: 536–40.

68. Forster PJG, Parker RW. Peak expiratory flow rate at high altitude. *Lancet.* 1983; **ii**: 100.
69. Pollard AJ, Mason NP, Barry PW *et al.* Effect of altitude on spirometric parameters and the performance of peak flow meters. *Thorax.* 1996; **51**: 175-8.
70. Moore K, Vizzard C, Coleman C *et al.* Extreme altitude mountaineering and type 1 diabetes: The Diabetes Federation of Ireland Kilimanjaro Expedition. *Diabetes Medicine.* 2001; **18**: 749-55.
71. Winslow RM. Notes on sickle cell disease. In: Sutton JR, Jones NL, Houston CS (eds). *Hypoxia: Man at altitude.* New York: Thieme-Stratton Inc, 1982: 179-81.
72. Weil JV. Sleep at high altitude. *High Altitude Medicine and Biology.* 2004; **5**: 180-9.
73. Nicholson AN, Smith PA, Stone BM *et al.* Altitude insomnia: Studies during an expedition to the Himalayas. *Sleep.* 1988; **11**: 354-61.
74. Sutton R, Houston CS, Mansell AL *et al.* Effect of acetazolamide on hypoxemia during sleep at high altitude. *New England Journal of Medicine.* 1979; **310**: 1329-31.
75. Stoneham MD. Anaesthesia and resuscitation at altitude. *European Journal of Anaesthesiology.* 1995; **12**: 249-57.
76. West JB, Readhead A. Working at high altitude: Medical problems, misconceptions, and solutions. *The Observatory.* 2004; **124**: 1-14.
77. West JB. Oxygen enrichment of room air to relieve the hypoxia of high altitude. *Respiration Physiology.* 1995; **99**: 225-32.
78. Napier PJ, West JB. Medical and physiological considerations for a high altitude MMA site. *MMA Memo.* 1996; **162**: 1-18. Available from: www.mma.nrao.edu.
79. West JB. Fire hazard in oxygen-enriched atmospheres at low barometric pressures. *Aviation, Space and Environmental Medicine.* 1997; **68**: 159-62.
80. Luks AM, van Melick H, Batarse RR *et al.* Room oxygen enrichment improves sleep and subsequent day-time performance at high altitude. *Respiration Physiology.* 1998; **113**: 247-58.
81. McFarland RA. Psychophysiological implications of life at high altitude and including the role of oxygen in the process of aging. In: Yousef MK, Horvath SM, Bullard RW (eds). *Physiological adaptations: Desert and mountain.* New York: Academic Press, 1972: 157-81.
82. Gerard AG, McElroy MK, Taylor MJ *et al.* Six percent oxygen enrichment of room air at simulated 5000m altitude improves neuropsychological function. *High Altitude Medicine and Biology.* 2000; **1**: 51-61.
83. Cudaback DM. Four km altitude effects on performance and health. *Publications of the Astronomical Society of the Pacific.* 1984; **96**: 463-77.
84. Johnson TS, Rock PB. Acute mountain sickness. *New England Journal of Medicine.* 1988; **319**: 841-5.
85. Pollard AJ. Altitude induced illness. *British Medical Journal.* 1992; **304**: 1324-5.
86. Forwand SA, Landowne M, Follansee JN, Hansen JE. Effect of acetazolamide on acute mountain sickness. *New England Journal of Medicine.* 1968; **279**: 839-45.
87. Birmingham Medical Research Expeditionary Society Mountain Sickness Study Group. Acetazolamide in control of acute mountain sickness. *Lancet.* 1981; **1**: 180-3.
88. Wright AD, Bradwell AR, Fletcher RF *et al.* Methazolamide and acetazolamide in acute mountain sickness. *Aviation, Space and Environmental Medicine.* 1983; **54**: 619-21.
89. Larson EB, Roach RC, Schoene RB, Hornbein TF. Acute mountain sickness and acetazolamide: Clinical efficacy and effect on ventilation. *Journal of the American Medical Association.* 1982; **248**: 328-32.
90. Basnyat B, Gertsch JH, Holck PS. Acetazolamide 125mg bd is not significantly different from 375mg bd in the prevention of acute mountain sickness. *High Altitude Medicine and Biology.* 2006; 7: 17-27.
91. Johnson ST, Rock PB, Fulco CS *et al.* Prevention of acute mountain sickness by dexamethasone. *New England Journal of Medicine.* 1984; **310**: 683-6.
92. Ellsworth AJ, Larson EB, Strickland D. A randomised trial of dexamethasone and acetazolamide for acute mountain sickness prophylaxis. *American Journal of Medicine.* 1987; **83**: 1024-30.
93. Fischer I, Lang SM, Steiner U *et al.* Theophylline improves acute mountain sickness. *European Respiratory Journal.* 2000; **15**: 123-7.
94. Roncin JP, Schwartz F, D'Arbigny P. EGb in control of acute mountain sickness and vascular reactivity to cold exposure. *Aviation Space and Environmental Medicine.* 1996; **67**: 445-52.
95. Gertsch JH, Todd BS, Mor J, Onopa J. Gingko biloba for the prevention of severe acute mountain sickness (AMS) starting one day before rapid ascent. *High Altitude Medicine and Physiology.* 2002; **3**: 29-37.
96. Hohenhaus E, Niroomand F, Goerre S *et al.* Nifedipine does not prevent acute mountain sickness. *American Journal of Respiratory and Critical Care Medicine.* 1994; **150**: 857-60.
97. Sartori C, Allemann Y, Duplain H *et al.* Salmeterol for the prevention of high-altitude pulmonary edema. *New England Journal of Medicine.* 2002; **346**: 1631-6.
98. Bartsch P. Treatment of high altitude diseases without drugs. *International Journal of Sports Medicine.* 1992; **1**: 71-4.
99. Broome JR, Stoneham MD, Beeley JM *et al.* High altitude headache: Treatment with ibuprofen. *Aviation, Space and Environmental Medicine.* 1994; **65**: 19-20.
100. Bartsch P, Maggi S, Kleger GR *et al.* Sumatriptan for high altitude headache. *Lancet.* 1994; **344**: 1445.
101. Burtscher M, Likar R, Nachbauer W *et al.* Ibuprofen versus sumatriptan for high altitude headache. *Lancet.* 1995; **346**: 255-6.
102. Grissom CK, Roach RC, Sarnquist FH, Hackett PH. Acetazolamide in the treatment of acute mountain sickness: Clinical efficacy and effect on gas exchange. *Annals of Internal Medicine.* 1992; **116**: 461-5.
103. Wright AD, Winterborn MH, Forster PJG *et al.* Carbonic anhydrase inhibition in the immediate therapy of acute mountain sickness. *Wilderness Medicine.* 1994; **5**: 49-55.

104. Sutherland AI. Why are so many people dying on Everest? *British Medical Journal.* 2006; **333**: 452.
105. Ferrazzini G, Maggiorini M, Kriemler S *et al.* Successful treatment of acute mountain sickness with dexamethasone. *British Medical Journal.* 1987; **294**: 1380–2.
106. Oelz O, Maggiorini M, Ritter M *et al.* Nifedipine for high altitude pulmonary oedema. *Lancet.* 1989; **2**: 1241–4.
107. Clark C. Diamox, dexamethasone and nifedipine at high altitude. UIAA Mountain Medicine Centre information sheet 3.2002. Available from: www.thebmc.co.uk.
108. Gamow RI, Geer GD, Kasic JF, Smith HM. Methods of gas balance control to be used with a portable hyperbaric chamber in the treatment of high altitude illness. *Journal of Wilderness Medicine.* 1990; **1**: 165–80.
109. Forster PJG, Bradwell AR, Winterborn MJ *et al.* Alleviation of hypoxia at high altitude: A comparison between oxygen, oxygen and carbon dioxide inhalation and hyperbaric compression. *Clinical Science.* 1990; **79**: 1P.
110. Bartsch P, Merki B, Hofstetter D *et al.* Treatment of acute mountain sickness by simulated descent: A randomised controlled trial. *British Medical Journal.* 1993; **306**: 1098–101.
111. Keller HR, Maggiorini M, Bartsch P, Oelz O. Simulated descent versus dexamethasone in the treatment of acute mountain sickness. *British Medical Journal.* 1995; **310**: 1232–5.
112. Imray CHE, Clarke T, Forster PJG *et al.* Carbon dioxide contributes to the beneficial effect of pressurization in a portable hyperbaric chamber at high altitude. *Clinical Science.* 2001; **100**: 151–7.
113. Davis PR, Kippax J, Shaw GM *et al.* A novel continuous positive airways pressure device for use at high altitude. *High Altitude Medicine and Biology.* 2002; **3**: 101 (Abstr.).
114. Harvey TC, Raichle ME, Winterborn MH *et al.* Effect of carbon dioxide in acute mountain sickness: A rediscovery. *Lancet.* 1988; **ii**: 639–41.
115. Forster P. Chronic intermittent exposure to high altitude: The view from Mauna Kea. *International Society of Mountain Medicine Newsletter.* 2000; **10**: 3–5.
116. Napier PJ, West JB. High-altitude medical and operations problems and solutions for the Millimeter Array. MMA Memo 1998. NRAO. Available from: www.mma.nrao.edu/library/napier/napier.html.
117. West JB. *High life: A history of high-altitude physiology and medicine.* New York: Oxford University Press, 1998.
118. Carroll R. FIFA suspends ban on high-altitude football. *The Guardian.* May 29, 2008.
119. Grocott MPW, Martin DS, Levett DZH *et al.* Arterial blood gases and oxygen content in climbers on Mount Everest. *New England Journal of Medicine.* 2009; **360**: 140–8.
120. Firth PG, Zheng H, Windsor JS *et al.* Mortality on Mount Everest, 1921–2006. *British Medical Journal.* 2008; **337**: 1430–3.
121. Richards P. Lake Louise Acute Mountain Sickness (AMS) score. Available from: www.abdn.ac.uk/~src248/peru/documents/ams_scoring.doc.

52

Flying and spaceflight

MIKE GIBSON, DAVID GRADWELL AND ALYSON CALDER

Flying	591	Spaceflight	607
Introduction	591	Background	607
Pressure change	592	The space environment	608
Gravitational stress	595	Pre-launch and launch	608
Advanced life support systems	596	The spacecraft environment	608
Extremes of temperature	597	Extra-vehicular activity	609
Noise and vibration	598	Re-entry	609
Vision	599	Space physiology and pathophysiology	609
Spatial disorientation	601	Astronaut selection	611
Air sickness	602	Medical emergencies in space	611
Fatigue and jet lag	603	Research and ground-based analogues	613
Food and drink	604	The future of spaceflight	613
Exposure to chemicals	604	References	613
Aircraft accidents	604	Further reading	620
Fitness for flight	605		

FLYING

INTRODUCTION

Flying can be an exciting occupation or hobby, providing exposure to unfamiliar environmental and physiological stressors. Although over 200 years have passed since the first manned balloon flight by Pilâtre de Rozier, François Laurent and the Marquis d'Arlandes, most of the understanding of the effects of the aviation environment on the human body has come since 1900. In the first 70 years of aviation, when mankind progressed from Kitty Hawk to the moon, aircraft flew ever higher, ever faster. Since then, development has tended to be limited to improvements in noise reduction, range and payload by environmental and economic considerations.

In 1909, there was one fatality for every 1500 miles flown. By 1912, the safety of aircraft had developed to the extent that the mileage flown for each fatality had risen 100-fold.[1] Even in the first half of the First World War, accidents accounted for some 25 per cent of all pilot fatalities, more than attributed to enemy action. Flying is now safer than road travel. Every day, 1.7 million passengers board aircraft in the United States.[2] At any one time, over half a million passengers are airborne in some part of the world and over 2 billion people fly every year. Civilian aircrew live longer than the general population of England and Wales and their patterns of death do not appear to be attributable to their occupation.[3]

Although flying has become so much safer since the pioneering days, the risks of exposure to an unforgiving environment cannot be ignored. Physiologically, man has evolved to live at ground level, at normal gravity ($+1\,G_z$), within strict temperature limits and with certain limitations to his special senses and his psychology. Adaptation and acclimatization can increase the physiological range to an extent, while training can improve performance. However, flying is usually an acute exposure, so physiological adaptations have a limited role to play. Protection from the environment, by means of engineering solutions, can increase the operating range of the human, but it also has limitations. The potential for failure of that protection necessitates the provision of back-up systems or a restriction in the operating envelope of the aircraft. Thus, human tolerances have increasingly set the limits to which aircraft can be engineered.

People work in the air in a variety of capacities. Military aviators fly in aircraft ranging from helicopters to high speed, single-seat jets. Crews of military transport aircraft may face additional challenges that do not affect crews of commercial aircraft. Civilian flight in small aircraft can range from recreational flight to instructional duties to crop spraying. Many people, of course, fly just as passengers and many need to be fit for work on arrival at their destination, but some also work while they are flying. This chapter outlines the stresses and hazards of flight, describes the ways of overcoming them and considers fitness for flight, both for professional aviators and passengers.

PRESSURE CHANGE

As altitude increases, pressure decreases exponentially. For fliers, this gives rise to four potential problems: gas expansion, hypoxia, decompression sickness and rapid decompression (Figure 52.1).

Gas expansion

As ambient pressure decreases, volume increases in accordance with Boyle's law. Where the gas in the human body is enclosed, this may cause problems. Gas is enclosed in the body after surgery. Thus, 30 mL of intracranial air would expand by 30 per cent at a cabin altitude of 8000 ft, resulting in a rise of intracranial pressure from 10 to 21 mmHg or from 20 to 31.8 mmHg.[4] Therefore, it is unwise to fly within ten days of laparotomy (unless a drainage tube is left in place), within three weeks of craniotomy or air contrast x-ray studies of the spine, or within two weeks of thoracotomy or pneumothorax unless a Heimlich valve or similar device is in place. In addition, penetrating injury of the eyeball can produce subluxation of the lens on ascent to altitude and a case of sudden blindness has been reported caused by expansion of an air bubble introduced during retinopexy.[5] Patients with these conditions may be flown, but only if the cabin pressure of the aircraft is held at the ambient pressure of the departure airfield. Similarly, a small gas bubble beneath a badly filled tooth can cause excruciating pain on ascent (aerodontalgia) which usually improves on descent,[6] although occasional dental fracture may occur.[7]

Where the gas is incompletely enclosed, there is less of a problem. The gut normally contains between 100 and 200 mL of gas at ground level in the stomach and large bowel. The rise in intra-abdominal pressure limits the volume increase. The usual symptom is of abdominal fullness or bloating and is reduced by eructation or passing flatus. The problem can be limited by avoiding dietary items which predispose to flatulence, such as fizzy drinks or certain vegetables. Gas in the middle ear also has an outlet to ambient air. On ascent, the gas expands easily along the Eustachian tube and the ears 'pop' automatically. On descent, however, the increased pressure in the pharynx causes the Eustachian tube to act as a flap valve. The resulting pressure differential causes the eardrum to be inverted, causing pain (which is often severe) and deafness. In severe cases, vertigo and nausea may occur. Rarely, facial palsy may result.[8] The way to equalize pressures is to yawn, swallow or waggle the jaw if the pressure change is gradual, or to perform a Valsalva manoeuvre (holding the nose and straining against a closed glottis) or Frenzel manoeuvre (holding the nose and raising the pressure in the nasopharynx without increasing intrathoracic pressure) if the change is rapid. Topical decongestants before or during flight may be effective. There is no evidence that earplugs which claim to equalize pressure are effective.[9] Future

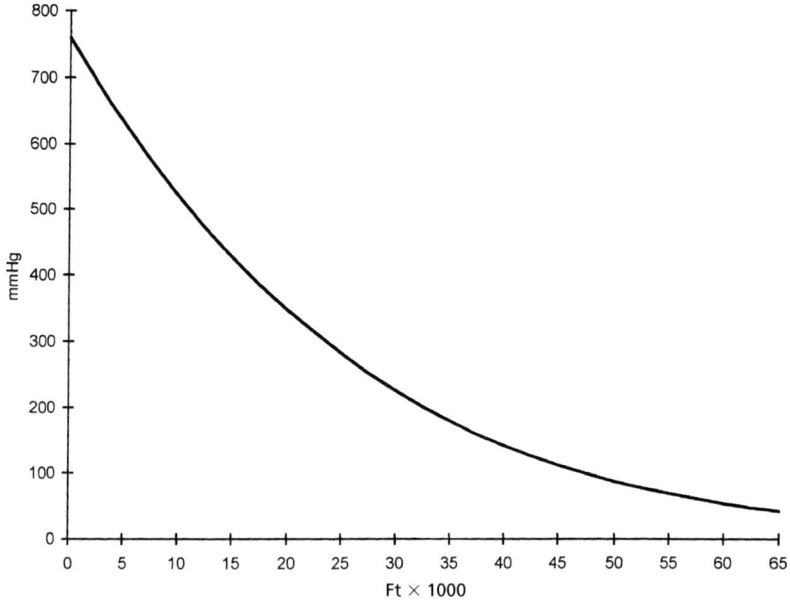

Figure 52.1 Relationship of barometric pressure to altitude.

developments may include the use of surfactants which play a role in maintaining patency of the Eustachian tube.[10] If descent is continued without the pressure equalizing, there is haemorrhage into the drum and it may perforate with subsequent relief from pain. Colds and upper respiratory tract infections predispose to this inability to 'clear the ears'. Since ear pain, deafness and vertigo are flight safety hazards, aircrew with these conditions should not fly until they can clear their ears. Inability to clear the ears during flight can, if possible, be helped by a re-ascent to altitude and a more gradual descent. Otitic barotrauma usually clears spontaneously in two to three weeks.

The frontal and paranasal sinuses usually vent to ambient easily on ascent and equally easily repressurize on descent. Again, infection may interfere with this, causing pain. Nasal polyps or deviated nasal septum can also predispose to sinus barotrauma. Topical decongestants before or during flight may help. Symptomatic treatment may be required on the ground for a few days afterwards.

Finally, at an altitude of 63 000 ft, the total ambient pressure is 47 mmHg. This is also the pressure exerted by water vapour at body temperature. At this altitude (known as the Armstrong Line), body tissues begin to vaporize. Small pockets of gas appear beneath the skin within 2–3 seconds, there is gas evolution within the abdominal cavity in 10 seconds and in the heart in about 20 seconds. Although man can recover from brief exposures, it is better to protect an individual at risk by means of a pressure cabin or pressure suit.

Hypoxia

At all altitudes, the fractional concentration of oxygen in the air remains at 21 per cent. However, as pressure falls on ascent to altitude, the partial pressure exerted by that oxygen also falls, in accordance with Dalton's law of partial pressures. Up to an altitude of about 10 000 feet, the amount of oxygen available to the body remains almost the same because of the shape of the oxygen–haemoglobin dissociation curve. However, the oxygen saturation can fall below 90 per cent even in commercial pressurized aircraft[11] and this may have detrimental effects on some patients. Although it is unlikely to affect the occurrence of acute mountain sickness, it may contribute to increased reporting of discomfort in passengers in medium duration flights.[12]

The most common causes of hypoxia in flight are ascent to altitude without supplementary oxygen, failure of personal breathing equipment to provide an adequate supply of oxygen and decompression of the cabin at high altitude. Human failure to turn on the supply, check hoses are connected or to ensure the mask seals to the face properly, plays a significant role in hypoxia in military aircrew.

The symptoms of hypoxia are insidious and include euphoria, loss of insight, impairment of cognitive functions, reduction of visual acuity (including colour vision), inco-ordination, cyanosis, hyperventilation and, eventually, loss of consciousness and death. The gradual onset explains those cases where loss of cabin pressure has led to all on board becoming unconscious, the aircraft then flying on automatic pilot until it crashed when fuel was exhausted. A survey of helicopter crew showed most had experienced symptoms suggestive of hypoxia at an average altitude of just over 8000 ft. The most common signs were difficulty with calculations, delayed reaction time and confusion; non-pilots were more affected than pilots.[13] It is widely quoted in the literature that mild hypoxia (8000 ft) impairs the learning of a novel task,[14] but later research failed to confirm this.[15] Smokers may take longer to detect hypoxia than non-smokers.[16] Tolerance to hypoxia is reduced by exercise, exposure to cold, the presence of illness and after taking alcohol.

The insidious nature of the symptoms of hypoxia has led many military air forces to adopt a training regime in decompression chambers to allow aviators a greater chance of spotting hypoxia in themselves. In one survey of military aircrew, 76 per cent of cases of hypoxia were recognized by the aviator involved.[17] The symptoms of hypoxia are very difficult to distinguish from those of hyperventilation. Any symptoms in flight which could be either, must be treated as hypoxia until proved otherwise. On acute exposure to high altitude, either from failure of a pressure cabin or of the oxygen supply, the oxygen stored in the tissues allows a 'time of useful consciousness' before capability is lost. This time ranges from about 4 minutes at 25 000 ft to about 20 seconds at 40 000 ft and 10–15 seconds at 52 000 ft. Impairment of performance occurs sooner (45 seconds at 25 000 ft, 12–15 seconds at 40 000 ft).

Hypoxia can be prevented by ensuring that the aircraft does not fly above 10 000 ft, by providing supplemental oxygen to breathe or by pressurizing the aircraft to maintain a cabin pressure of equivalent to an altitude below 10 000 ft. The alveolar oxygen tension (P_AO_2) at sea level can be maintained up to 33 000 ft by breathing 100 per cent oxygen and the 10 000 ft equivalent can be maintained up to 40 000 ft. However, there are two disadvantages to providing 100 per cent oxygen. First, if the aircraft has an aerobatic capability, the gravitational forces may occlude small airways in the lung leading to absorption of all the oxygen distal to the occlusion. The localized pulmonary collapse is called 'acceleration atelectasis'. Second, a similar problem may occur in the middle ear after landing, causing pain (oxygen ear). The usual solution is to provide oxygen/air mix sufficient to allow a ground level P_AO_2 (103 mmHg) until 33 000 ft when 100 per cent oxygen is supplied. The P_AO_2 then falls to a 10 000 ft equivalent at 40 000 ft.

Above this altitude, oxygen has to be provided under pressure to maintain adequate oxygenation (pressure breathing). In military aircraft, pressure breathing is usually applied through an oronasal mask. The barometric pressure at 40 000 ft is 141 mmHg. The aim of pressure breathing is to maintain that absolute pressure delivered to the lungs. Thus the breathing pressure will be (141-ambient pressure) mmHg. Breathing pressures up to 70 mmHg will protect against hypoxia at altitudes up to 56 000 ft. However, there are disadvantages. Pressure breathing gives rise to physiological problems. The increased work of expiration, which is usually passive, produces discomfort, as does the distension of cheeks, mouth and respiratory passages. The nasolachrymal duct can be forced open causing severe blepharospasm and the Eustachian duct can also be forced open causing ear pain. Blood return to the heart is compromised. Peripheral pooling of the blood and the passage of fluid from the circulation into the tissues reduce effective blood volume, leading to reduced tolerance to gravitational stresses and syncope. The likelihood of syncope during pressure breathing is increased in the presence of hypoxia, hypocapnia, heat stress, anxiety, infection or after alcohol. The effects of pressure breathing can be minimized by providing counterpressure to bladders in a sleeved or sleeveless partial pressure jacket and to the anti-G trousers. An alternative in military aviation is to use a full pressure suit with either a full or a partial pressure helmet, but these have the significant disadvantages of reduced mobility and increased heat load. One significant flight safety hazard remains. It is very difficult to talk when pressure breathing. Sudden loss of cabin pressure in a multicrew aircraft flying above 40 000 ft will lead to the requirement to read through check lists. Practice is vital.

Decompression sickness

Decompression sickness (DCS) during diving activities is dealt with fully in Chapter 50, Diving and work at increased pressure. It is commonly believed that altitude DCS does not occur below 18 000 ft. However, bubbles in the circulation have been recorded at altitudes down to 13 000 ft. Bubbles do not form at low altitude unless the individual has been diving in the preceding 24 hours. The rate of symptoms of DCS is related to the final altitude and the time spent at altitude. Other predisposing factors are known susceptibility, exercise at altitude,[18] age, body build, general health and previous exposure to altitude within the preceding 24 hours. Female gender *per se* does not appear to be a risk factor,[19] although women may be more at risk during the first week of their cycle than mid-cycle.[20] Flying after diving is particularly dangerous.[21] At least 12 hours should be spent at ground level after diving; this time should be doubled if the dive lasted more than four hours and redoubled if the subsequent flight is to be at a cabin altitude above 8000 ft.

The symptoms in one series of over 400 cases arising from decompression chamber experience ranged from joint pains (the bends, 83 per cent, with the knee accounting for 70 per cent), respiratory effects (the chokes, 2.7 per cent), skin symptoms (formication or the creeps, 2.2 per cent), paraesthesia (10.8 per cent) to neurological manifestations (0.5 per cent).[22] Visual symptoms include blurred vision, loss of vision, scintillation and scotoma. Neurological symptoms and collapse can occur after return to ground level (one study demonstrated a 45 per cent incidence of symptoms at altitude, with 24 per cent in the first hour after return to ground level and 21 per cent between one and six hours).[23]

The incidence of DCS in those individuals exposed to an altitude of 25 000 ft or less is low. The U-2, however, had an altitude ceiling of >73 500 ft for more than 15 hours unrefuelled, at a cabin altitude of 29 500 ft. Despite precautions, more than 75 per cent of U-2 pilots experienced symptoms of DCS, and 13 per cent had, at some stage, to alter the flight profile or abort the mission.[24]

Treatment[25] depends on the severity and resolution of the symptoms. If the symptoms clear on descent and neurological examination is normal, the patient should ideally breathe 100 per cent oxygen for two hours and undergo aggressive oral rehydration. The patient should be observed for 24 hours. If pain or cutaneous symptoms persist after descent, in addition to 100 per cent oxygen and oral rehydration, the patient should be exposed to treatment in a hyperbaric chamber. In Scotland, advice may be obtained from Aberdeen Royal Infirmary (Tel. 0845 4566000, asking for the diving doctor on call). For the rest of the United Kingdom, guidance is obtained from the Duty Diving Medical Officer at the Institute of Naval Medicine (Tel. 07831 151523). If the symptoms are not relieved within 10 minutes of compression on Royal Navy Treatment Table 61 (equivalent to US Navy Treatment Table 5), subsequent decompression should follow RN Treatment Table 62 (USN Table 6).[26] Travel to the chamber should be by road. If air travel is absolutely necessary, then either a cabin altitude of sea level or an absolute aircraft altitude of 1000 ft should be maintained. The patient should be supine, intubated if necessary, or in the lateral decubitus position. Intravenous fluids should be either normal saline or Ringer's solution (i.e. isotonic), 1 litre in the first hour and then ~1.5 mL/kg per hour. Avoid solutions (oral or intravenous) containing glucose. If there are spinal cord symptoms, there may be benefit in giving a bolus of 30 mg/kg of methylprednisolone and then 5.4 mg/kg per hour for 23 hours. It is important to control the body temperature of the patient. On recovery from mild DCS without central nervous system (CNS) complications, the pilot can return to flying within 72 hours if there are no symptoms and examination is normal.

Prevention is based on three factors: (1) selection of individuals who are not susceptible to DCS by testing them in a decompression chamber; (2) limiting exposure to altitude by use of pressurized aircraft; and (3) denitrogenation by breathing 100 per cent oxygen before take-off. Prebreathing schedules are a mixture of experience and pragmatism. Pre-oxygenation for 30 minutes will protect against short exposure to 48 000 ft as long as total time above 25 000 ft is less than 10 minutes. Exposure to 40 000 ft for 3 hours requires 3 hours of pre-oxygenation at ground level. U-2 pilots prebreathe for 60 minutes. Exercise while denitrogenating can reduce the time that prebreathing is necessary while retaining the same level of protection, although this effect may be limited.[27]

Rapid decompression

The respiratory passages can easily cope with the expansion of gas in the lung on rapid decompression (except that air embolus may occur if the breath is held). The effects of rapid decompression depend on the altitude at which the aircraft is flying, the pressure differential of the cabin, the volume of the aircraft and the size and location of the defect in the pressure cabin. Hypoxia, exposure to cold and, eventually, DCS may all occur. The initial problem for aircrew in a rapid decompression is that the flow of air can raise dust and debris; visibility may also be restricted by the condensation of water vapour that occurs. Provided P_AO_2 remains above 30 mmHg, there will be no expected decrement in the aircrew's performance. The transient cabin altitude can be lower than outside because of the Venturi effect or it may be higher because of a ram air effect. The airblast can even suck passengers out of a window. Because of the physics, the risk is only to those immediately next to the defect. The time of rapid decompression can be as little as 0.005 seconds for loss of a canopy in a military aircraft to 30 seconds if a window is lost in a large passenger aircraft. The incidence is low: $2–3/10^5$ flying hours for military aircraft and 30–40 a year worldwide for commercial aircraft.

Low differential pressure cabins, such as in military aircraft, require the aircrew to use oxygen equipment throughout. Provided it can give 100 per cent oxygen at 33 000 ft and pressure breathing above 40 000 ft, hypoxia is unlikely following rapid decompression. In civilian, high pressure differential aircraft, there is little risk of hypoxia in the crew provided they can don oxygen equipment delivering 100 per cent oxygen within 5 seconds of cabin altitude exceeding 10 000 ft. The crew will then make an emergency descent to at least 10 000 feet. In Concorde, the protection was provided by designing the aircraft so that, even if a window were lost at 65 000 ft, the cabin altitude would not exceed 36 000 ft provided emergency descent was started within 30 seconds.[28] Sufficient oxygen is carried on all commercial aircraft for passengers' P_AO_2 to be maintained above 50 mmHg in the event of a rapid decompression, although it is unlikely that they will all be able to use the drop-down masks successfully.

As already noted, although seemingly less dramatic, slow decompression may occur. Unless prompt action is taken in response to warning signals, there may be a risk to the aircraft and its occupants.

GRAVITATIONAL STRESS

The most common long duration accelerations experienced in flying are radial accelerations – those produced by change of direction of motion without change of speed. Acceleration is conventionally described by a three-axis system (Figure 52.2). The acceleration of most interest in military aviation is $+/-G_z$. Current agile aircraft can easily achieve $+9.5\,G_z$ at onset rates of over 10 G/s. In these circumstances, the limiting factor on the performance of the aircraft is the physiology of the aircrew.

Effects of $+G_z$

The effects of acceleration are exacerbated by heat stress, hypoglycaemia, ingestion of alcohol, hyperventilation and intercurrent infection. Even at $+2\,G_z$, there is noticeable difficulty in moving the limbs and and the face sags. At levels greater than $+3\,G_z$, it is impossible to escape unaided from an aircraft. Movement becomes more difficult as $+G_z$ rises and raising the head once it is flexed becomes impossible at $+8\,G_z$ even without a helmet. Head movement generally at high G_z is difficult, particularly with the

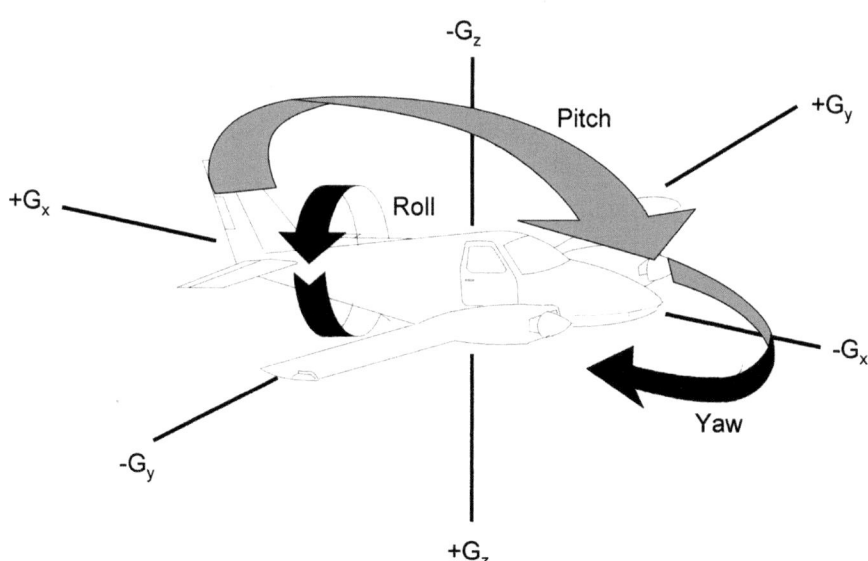

Figure 52.2 G axes and vectors of motion in aviation.

new generation of helmets which carry helmet-mounted sights and displays or, when required, night vision goggles. Exposure to high G flight causes a temporary diminution in height of up to almost 5 mm due to spinal compression[29] and musculoskeletal symptoms,[30] fatigue,[31] cervical disc bulges[32] and premature cervical spine degeneration[33] have been reported.

Acceleration in the G_z axis has a hydrostatic effect on the circulation. The mean arterial pressure at the level of the heart is 100 mmHg at both +1 and +4 G_z. At eye level, some 30 cm vertically above the heart, the respective pressures are 100 mmHg minus the hydrostatic pressure exerted by the column of blood (22 mmHg at +1 G_z and 88 mmHg at +4 G_z), i.e. 78 and 12 mmHg. Similarly, the corresponding pressures in the posterior tibial artery, some 80 cm below the heart in the sitting individual, can be calculated to be 157 and 324 mmHg.

The blood pressure changes at head level affect vision, cerebral blood flow, cerebral oxygenation and the level of consciousness. Eyeball pressure is 20 mmHg. Thus, the blood pressure at head level has to be above that for retinal perfusion to occur. Application of G results in constriction of the pupils which may help to maintain vision.[34] In the relaxed individual, peripheral vision starts to deteriorate at about +3 G_z (grey-out) and totally disappears near +4 G_z. The symptom takes a few seconds to develop because of retinal oxygen stores and, at sustained, low rates of +G_z will often fade in a few seconds because of adaptive changes in the circulation. At +5 to +6 G_z, consciousness is lost (G-induced loss of consciousness, known as G-LOC) but at higher rates of +G_z, consciousness can be lost before visual symptoms arise. The incidence of G-LOC is lower than would be predicted because of various physiological mechanisms which tend to maintain regional cerebral perfusion. In one survey, 21 per cent of aircrew reported that they had experienced black-out and 20.1 per cent reported G-LOC.[35] Not all aircrew who experience G-LOC in centrifuge training remember the episode, so the incidence may be much higher than reported. The US Air Force lost 29 aircraft in crashes attributed to G-LOC in one 20-year period.[36] There is no evidence that relaxed +G_z tolerance and endurance on simulated air combat manoeuvring (SACM) are any different in females than males.[37,38] In this respect, the shorter stature (and hence smaller heart–eye vertical distance) of females may compensate for lack of physical strength.

Below the heart, the effects of +G_z produce pooling of blood in the periphery, transudation of fluid from the blood to the tissues and rupture of unsupported skin capillaries to produce petechiae. The pooling and loss of blood volume eventually produce intense peripheral vasodilatation and bradycardia, leading to syncope. In addition to the effects described above, rupture of the diaphragm[39] and acute inguinal hernia[40] in response to +G_z and/or the effects of straining against G have been reported.

Negative acceleration (−G_z) is experienced in outside loops and spins and in inverted flight. Tolerance is much lower than for positive G_z. The general effects include heaviness of the limbs, fullness and pressure in the head (which can produce severe headache), congestion of the air passages which can cause difficulty in breathing, bradycardia, epistaxis, eye discomfort, subconjunctival haemorrhages and petechiae in unsupported skin. The transition from −G_z to +G_z (sometimes called the 'push–pull') can reduce tolerance to +G_z,[41] which is worsened by the duration of the preceding −G_z.[42]

Protection against +G_z

The major ways of increasing tolerance to +G_z are by use of an Anti-G Straining Manoeuvre (AGSM), anti-G suits, posture, positive pressure breathing (PPB) and training, or by various combinations of these. The commonly used AGSMs, which all include isometric muscle tensing, are the M-1 manoeuvre (exhaling forcibly against a partially closed glottis with a rapid inspiration every 4–5 seconds), the L-1 manoeuvre (periods of raised intrathoracic pressure with a closed glottis separated by short inspiratory and expiratory gasps) and the Qigong manoeuvre (rapid panting with tensed muscles).[43] Training in a centrifuge can help to maximize the effectiveness of the AGSM.[44]

Without an anti-G suit, increasing G_z lowers the diaphragm, increasing the functional residual capacity. Inflation of the abdominal bladder of the anti-G suit reverses this. The closing volume of the lung increases linearly with +G_z, and use of an anti-G suit, by raising the diaphragm, increases the number of non-ventilated alveoli in the base of the lung. Thus there is a change to the ventilation/perfusion ratio from the apex to the base of the lung, with the apex tending to be ventilated, but underperfused, and the base tending to be perfused, but underventilated. This is of particular importance when air enriched with oxygen is breathed, for it assists in the development of acceleration atelectasis. The increased respiratory work of anti-G straining manoeuvres produces respiratory fatigue that may contribute to the degree of overall tolerance to prolonged +G_z.[45]

ADVANCED LIFE SUPPORT SYSTEMS

In the most modern generation of combat fast jet aircraft, the requirements to provide protection against exposure to altitude and high acceleration have driven the development of advanced life support systems. Commonly, the requirement for protection against hypoxia is addressed by the provision of a continuous supply of oxygen derived from compressed air taken from the compressor stages of the aircraft's engines and passed through a two or three bed molecular sieve oxygen concentrator (MSOC). Such systems cannot produce 100 per cent oxygen, since argon is also concentrated, but do remove the requirement to replenish the main oxygen supply between sorties. A back-up supply of

100 per cent oxygen is therefore required to cope with high altitude decompressions and ejection.

Above 40 000 feet, there remains a requirement to provide positive pressure breathing for altitude protection (PBA) in the event of a decompression, but this can be combined in a common system with pressure breathing for G protection (PBG). Counter-pressure layers can be incorporated in the life preserver, whose main function is to provide buoyancy, allied with inflation of the anti-G trousers to provide lower body counter-pressure. Inflation of the counter-pressure layer of the upper garment, to the same pressure as oxygen is delivered to the mask, prevents over-distension of the chest and relieves the fatigue of breathing against pressurized gas. Inflation of the lower garment improves venous return and reduces the likelihood of pressure breathing-induced syncope. In the most advanced systems, the lower garment inflation pressure is 1.5–2 times the breathing pressure, as this has been found to enhance the circulatory support provided.

Modern anti-G trousers cover a greater part of the body surface than traditional (so-called skeletal) anti-G trousers and are often termed full coverage anti-G trousers (FCAGTs). Such garments are mechanically more efficient and provide enhanced G protection, as well as reducing the fatigue associated with 'pulling G'. When combined with PBG, there is a very substantial improvement in G protection, commonly allowing a 'relaxed' exposure to up to 9 Gz with little or no requirement for physical straining to retain full vision and reduce the risk of loss of consciousness (Figure 52.3).

Such systems carry the additional burdens of increased resistance to movement and greater thermal load because of the additional layers and greater coverage of the body with impermeable materials. In addition, some advanced anti-G systems are associated with an incidence of arm pain, where the vasculature is unprotected by counter-pressure.

EXTREMES OF TEMPERATURE

Details on heat and cold can be found in Chapter 49, Heat and cold. This chapter will highlight those aspects relevant to flying.

Cold

Exposure to extreme cold may occur when operating at high altitude, on the ground in very cold countries and following accidents in isolated locations. At very low cockpit temperatures, simple oxygen systems run the risk of the expiratory valve freezing open because of the accumulation of condensed and frozen water vapour from the expirate. This may lead to hypoxia because the resistance of inspiring through an open expiratory valve is less than that of cracking open an inspiratory valve. Most military oxygen systems overcome the problem by design of the expiratory valve, by the use of safety pressure in the mask above certain altitudes (which would lead to continuous flow being sensed and shown on the flow indicator if there was a leakage) and by the use of cockpit heating.

Heat

There are several ways in which a flier may become hot in the aircraft. First, thermal radiation from the sun becomes

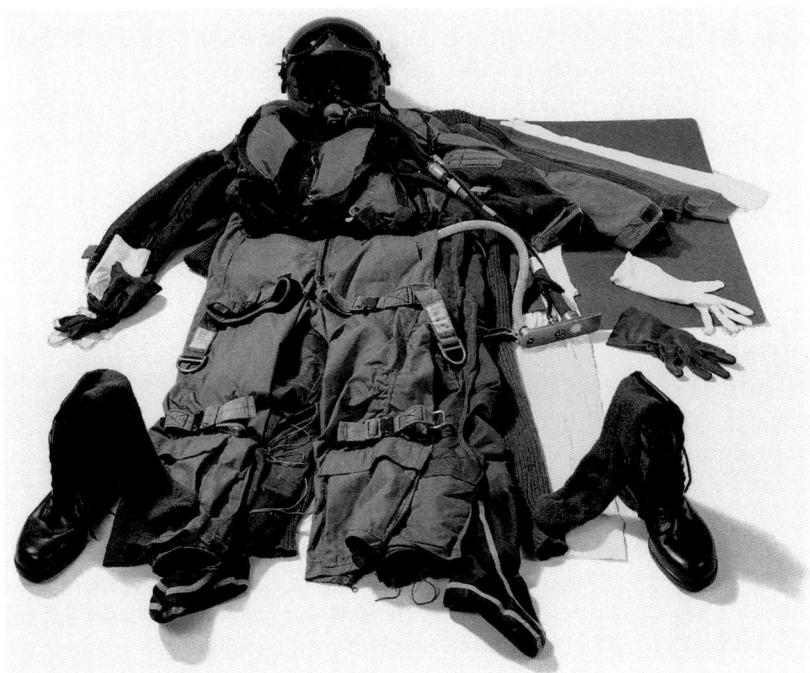

Figure 52.3 Example of aircrew clothing and equipment available for one aircraft type.

trapped in the cockpit rather like a greenhouse. In small aircraft, the large relative size of the cockpit transparency exacerbates the problem. Surface temperatures of seats can exceed 60°C. Second, electrical components, of which there are many in military aircraft, consume power inefficiently, radiating heat to the aircrew. Third, aerodynamic heating of the aircraft exterior can conduct heat into the cockpit. Temperatures above 110°C have been recorded on the skin of aircraft flying at high speed and low level. Finally, individuals produce heat from their own metabolism. These sources of heat would not be an embarrassment to the aircrew if they were able to dissipate the heat load. Unfortunately, particularly in military aviation, the clothing worn interferes with heat loss by being bulky and insulating and also by incorporating materials impermeable to water vapour, thus preventing sweat evaporation. Moreover, the specialized flying ensemble of military aviators is multilayered, increasing the work required to move while wearing it. Certainly, deep body temperatures of above 38°C have been measured in aircrew at cockpit temperatures below a wet bulb globe temperature (WBGT) index of 30°C. Laboratory simulations of aircrew wearing ensembles including nuclear, biological and chemical (NBC) protection, in cockpit temperatures previously measured in flight suggest that sortie length may be limited in the heat[46] or performance affected.[47]

There are two main approaches to solving the problem of heat in the cockpit: cabin and personal conditioning systems. The former are frequently not as effective as they could be, occasionally even being de-rated to reduce cockpit noise. Furthermore, the aircrew are insulated from the cooling air by their flying clothing. Personal conditioning systems do have the advantage that the cooling fluid is circulated where is it most required – next to the skin. However, cool air systems cannot be used in potential NBC conditions and liquid systems, whilst physiologically effective, are not yet in widespread use. Both systems require the aircrew to wear yet another layer of clothing.

NOISE AND VIBRATION

Noise

Noise is covered in Chapter 46, Sound, noise and the ear. The human tolerance to noise is exceeded in many aircraft with the risks of interference with performance of the flying task, fatigue, degradation of communication and hearing damage. Noise in flight arises from the aircraft power source, subsidiary noise from equipment, flow of air over aircraft surfaces and weapon firing. Sonic booms do not affect the occupants since the aircraft leaves the sonic boom behind. The noise profile will differ between aircraft types, seat positions and profiles flown. Cabin noise levels up to 120 dB have been measured in fixed wing aircraft when flying at 480 knots at 250 ft,[48] with the highest peaks being in the 0.5–4.0-kHz range. Even motor gliders can reach a cockpit noise level of 117 dBA at start up with levels of 92–99.5 dBA in the cruise.[49] Noise in helicopters is related to the rotors (at about 20 Hz) and the gearbox and transmission chains (from 400–600 Hz). In propeller-driven aircraft, the noise is primarily related to the number of propeller blades and the speed of rotation. In passenger jet aircraft, the major contributors are aerodynamic noise and noise from the conditioning systems; the noise in a window seat may be as much as 6 dB higher than in the centre of the aircraft.

Protection is obtained by careful engineering of the aerodynamic properties of the aircraft and (less frequently) of the cabin conditioning system. In military aircraft, an important degree of protection is afforded by the aircrew helmet. Attenuation is generally low at low frequencies but attenuation of 30 dB at 500 Hz to 50 dB at 4 kHz can be achieved. Careful attention to fitting can maximize the attenuation of perceived noise at the ear. In addition, active noise reduction (ANR, a mechanism of destructive interference by sampling the noise field, inverting the phase and then reintroducing it to the headset to cancel the original noise) can produce a further benefit of up to 10 dB. Passengers in noisy aircraft will benefit from the use of earplugs. Even with protection, workers on the ground and in the air may be at risk of hearing loss[50,51] and thickening of the mitral valve with a higher incidence of prolapse than the general population.[52]

Vibration

Vibration is considered in detail in Chapter 48, Whole body vibration. This chapter will address only those aspects relevant to flying. Complex structures, such as human bodies and aircraft, can vibrate in one or more of the six geometric degrees of freedom (three rotational: yaw, pitch and roll; three translational: heave, surge and sway). In flying, the sources of vibration are the power unit and the air through which the aircraft is travelling.

In helicopters, vibration is generally related to the rotor rate and to the number of rotor blades. The former is generally four revolutions per second, which gives rise to vibration within the helicopter of 4 Hz. The rotor rate multiplied by the number of blades gives the blade pass frequency which can give vibrations generally in the region of 8–20 Hz. Further vibration is generated at higher harmonics of the blade pass rate and also at levels related to the tail rotor. Vibration is usually similar in intensity in each of the x, y and z axes and is worse on transition to the hover.

In fixed-wing aircraft, the vibration from the engines is usually at a higher frequency than in helicopters. A single-stage turbine usually produces vibration at about 130 Hz, while a dual stage one produces 230 Hz. In propeller-driven aircraft, the blade pass frequency is about 100 Hz, although desynchronized propellers may give beating at lower frequencies. In fixed-wing aircraft, the most noticeable turbulence is caused by the atmosphere, for example during cloud penetration, during low level flight or in 'clear air turbulence'. In military aircraft, the firing of weapons can also give rise to vibration.

The effects of vibration in the aviator can range from imperceptible to inconvenient to unpleasant. The body is least tolerant of vibration between 4 and 8 Hz. The main symptoms limiting tolerance in the laboratory are precordial and abdominal pain. However, in flying, the most important effect for the pilot is on vision. The instrument panel and the pilot's eyes are usually vibrating out of phase. This results in degraded visual acuity. This is often exacerbated when helmet-mounted display systems are in use, particularly at frequencies of 4–6 Hz.[53] Outside the aircraft, the image is stable in space and at optical infinity, with other aircraft unlikely to be moving so fast that they exceed the angular velocity limitations of the pursuit reflex. In addition, vibration can also give rise to illusions of motion and to symptoms of motion sickness. At normal levels of vibration in flight, there are no great effects on the cardiovascular system, although there may be an increase in metabolic rate reflecting an increase in muscular activity required to maintain posture. Vibration can cause hyperventilation. A fall in P_aCO_2 to less than 25 mmHg has been recorded after 2 minutes of vibration at 9.5 Hz with an acceleration-amplitude of 1 G_z.[54] This is sufficient to reduce cerebral blood flow by 35 per cent.[55] Vibration has also been implicated in orthopaedic problems in helicopter aircrew, although seating, posture and ergonomic factors undoubtedly play a part.

Protection can be afforded against vibration by careful engineering of the aircraft, the use of dynamic vibration absorbers and by vibration isolation of the aircrew seat or of stretcher mounts and the use of seat cushions.[56] Finally, if the source of vibration is turbulent air, the effects may be minimized by routing away from it, changing cruising altitude and by ensuring passengers remain in their seats with seat belts fastened.

Casualties from military operations tend to be evacuated by helicopter before definitive surgery is conducted away from the front line. Vibration of unstabilized fractures can cause severe pain and may contribute to complications. Casualties evacuated by helicopter must be given adequate analgesia and their fractures adequately stabilized.

VISION

The importance of vision in aviation was first recognized during the First World War.[57] Despite the increase of equipment to increase flight safety, vision is still important in collision avoidance and target identification. Intact colour vision is more than ever necessary in the 'glass cockpit' where displays and warnings are presented in a wider variety of hues than ever before. Aircrew need to be protected from insults such as glare, lasers and chemicals with the addition in military aircraft of birdstrike, blast, explosive devices and nuclear flash. Visual illusions are covered below under Types of illusion, p. 601.

When there are no visual clues, the eye tends to focus at a point 1–2 m away. This functional short sight, called 'empty field myopia', can reduce the chances of a pilot seeing another aircraft, since objects at infinity are blurred. This is an important cause of road accidents in fog. Pilots should be trained to look at their wing tips from time to time to relax their accommodation. If a pilot looks at the instruments and then outside again, the gaze can be distracted for 2.5 seconds or more and the requirement to refocus frequently from infinity to near vision can be fatiguing. It was for these reasons that the first head-up display (HUD) – where the instrument image is focused at infinity on a glass screen in front of the pilot – was developed for the Beaufighter in the Second World War.[58]

It can take up to 5 seconds from the time an image first falls on the pilot's retina for an aircraft to change course. During this time, the aircraft can cover almost a mile if travelling at 500 knots. However, if two aircraft are on a collision course, they will remain on a constant bearing from each other, thus denying the pilots the stimulus of a moving object in the visual field.[59] Objects are more easily seen in the peripheral visual fields, especially if they are moving. Tracking is optimal up to 30° per second, but visual acuity is halved at 40° per second. Pilots must therefore be trained to maintain a good lookout at all times.

Eye protection

In civil flight and military transport aircraft, protection from glare is given by sunglasses. Sunglasses and visors should have a transmittance of 10–15 per cent. In addition to increasing visual acuity in bright sunlight, they also protect the eye from the effects of UV light.

Military fast jet aircrew usually wear helmets whose polycarbonate visors (one clear, one tinted) afford protection against glare, birdstrike and blast. Ideally, the cockpit transparency should be tough enough to withstand birdstrike, but this often conflicts with the need for rapid escape in an emergency. About 95 per cent of birdstrikes occur below 750 ft[60] and therefore are more commonly suffered during take off, landings and high speed, low-level flight. The clear visor can also protect against lead spatter from canopy fragmentation devices used to clear the ejection path. Although lead spatter usually causes superficial damage only, cases of ocular penetration have occurred. Visors also form an integral part of the overall protection against windblast during the ejection sequence. Design of the ensemble of helmet, visor and mask is important so that they remain on the head during ejection. Current RAF systems provide adequate protection up to 650 knots and aircrew are advised to have at least one visor selected down at all stages of flight.

The fireball from a nuclear explosion can cause direct and indirect flash blindness and may even cause a retinal burn. The problem is worse at night when, theoretically, a pilot could be effectively blind for as long as a minute after exposure. Various protective devices have been proposed, ranging from an eyepatch which could be raised after exposure to complex electro-optical devices.

Lasers, on the other hand, are more likely to pose a problem. Damage can range from transient stress temporary conditions (e.g. acute keratitis) to permanent damage, such as cataract, corneal opacity or retinal burning. The international aviation community is attempting to minimize the problem by legislation controlling the use of such devices near airfields. In military flying, lasers are used for target designation and thus may be deliberately aimed at aircraft. Protection is best provided by distance, but visor coatings designed to protect against specific wavelengths may be necessary. These have the diasadvantages that they only protect against specific threats, they produce a blending of surface colours and loss of terrain features, a reduction in depth perception and difficulties with warning lights and displays, maps and weapons displays.

Spectacles and contact lenses

The clinical indications for visual correction and visual standards are covered below. Approximately 27 per cent of pilots, 51 per cent of navigators and 40 per cent of other aircrew in the US Air Force need to wear glasses. Over 12 per cent need bifocals.[61] More then half of civilian pilots need lenses to correct defective vision in order to satisfy licensing requirements.[62] Evidence suggests that there is no difference in civil accident rates or in US naval carrier landing accidents in pilots who wear visual correction.[63] One survey has reported that glasses cause more flight safety incidents in military aviation than contact lenses.[64] Generally speaking, contact lenses are the preferred option for visual correction for aircrew.

Both soft (SCL) and hard contact lenses (HCL) have been used in flight. High water content SCL are preferred in the low humidity of aircraft cockpits, but HCL are still required in some conditions such as keratoconus. Rigid, gas-permeable lenses may offer advantages for this group in the future. Daily, disposable contact lenses are convenient and give rise to fewer problems for aviators with simple myopia. The major difficulties quoted in flight are foreign body incursion and movement off-centre. In both of these, the incidence is greater for HCL than SCL.[65] The greatest difficulty experienced in the Gulf War related to resupply problems with replacement lenses.[66] Some US Air Force aircrew have lost SCL or HCL during ejection, but the overall experience is small.

Overall, sunglasses and visors should give as wide a field of vision as possible. The optical quality should be high and it may be necessary to incorporate anti-scratch and anti-reflection coatings. Corrective flying spectacles must be capable of integration with the rest of the aircrew equipment without impairment of hearing protection or interference with the seal of an oxygen mask. They must be comfortable, resistant to fogging, minimize internal reflections and not move under conditions of vibration or G. Tinted spectacles should not be worn with tinted visors (see below). Photochromatic lenses are not yet sufficiently reactive to respond quickly enough on entering a cloud layer from high sunlight. Many military aircrew have reported losing a lens from their spectacles in flight and thus it seems sensible to carry a spare pair. In the RAF, most spectacles and helmets are retained on the head during ejection. In the US Air Force, on the other hand, sorties are flown higher with clear visors up and up to 80 per cent lost their eyewear.[67]

Eye surgery

As laser techniques have evolved, radial keratotomy (RK) has declined as a surgical method of correcting myopia. Photorefractive keratotomy (PRK) usually produces visual stability in three to six months. Laser *in-situ* keratomileusis (LASIK) produces a more predictable and safer method of correcting higher levels of myopia than PRK. The results are good for both PRK and LASIK. About 85 per cent of such patients achieve 6/6 or better.[68] The eye often becomes dry and requires lubricants for up to six months after operation and some patients experience night vision problems, such as haloes or starbursts around light sources. Recertification for military flying depends on the outcome and the type of procedure. For civilian flying, the Civil Aviation Authority (CAA) will consider class 1 certification three months after LASIK and six months after PRK as long as certain criteria are met.

The use of intraocular lenses is compatible with both military and civil flying once vision has stabilized. In one reported case, the implanted lens remained stable during ejection when the imposed acceleration reached an estimated $+14\,G_z$ for 200 ms.[69]

Night vision

During the Second World War, interceptors had to pick up their targets before they themselves were spotted, bomb-aimers needed to be able to place their bombs accurately despite the attentions of searchlights and tracer and pilots had to be capable of judging their landings correctly on darkened airfields. In the Second World War, much emphasis was given to dark adaptation of aircrew before take-off.

The introduction of night vision goggles (NVG) has changed things, but has introduced new problems. Some accidents have been directly linked to the use of NVG. In effect, NVG present an isochromatic view of the world limited in contrast and detail. Visual acuity, as well as visual fields, are degraded. For example, switching from forward-looking infrared (FLIR) to NVG gave a 4-second visual loss, a two-fold reduction in visual acuity and a three-fold reduction in contrast sensitivity.[70] The cockpit lighting needs to be compatible with the use of such devices and set carefully.[71] Careful fitting and training are required. In one study, training improved visual acuity from 6/15 to 6/12.[72]

SPATIAL DISORIENTATION

Spatial disorientation (SD) occurs when a pilot does not sense correctly the position relative to the ground, motion or attitude of himself or his aircraft. The broader term 'situational awareness' (SA) is taken to include a tactical appreciation of the position of other aircraft, as well as a sense of geographical location. SD is caused by inadequate or erroneous cues to the brain and by central processing errors, such as errors of perception or coning of attention.

SD is a significant cause of aircraft accidents. The majority of accidents occur in poor visibility when the pilot may not be aware that his interpretation of aircraft attitude is incorrect. However, some occur in good conditions when visual cues are misinterpreted. The type of incident where the pilot is aware that there is a mismatch between his aircraft instruments and what his brain is telling him is less likely to lead to an accident if appropriate training is given. Spatial disorientation is more likely at times of high workload, when undergoing treatment with certain drugs or with upper respiratory tract infections. It is also more prevalent in poor weather, at night, at high altitude and during flight over sea or featureless terrain. Certain flight manoeuvres contribute, such as prolonged linear acceleration or deceleration and prolonged angular motion, particularly when combined with head movement. Transfer to instrument meteorological conditions (IMC) when landing in helicopters, when the downwash from the rotor kicks up dust or snow, is also a potent cause of SD. Subthreshold changes in attitude are unlikely to be detected and thus can also lead to SD.

Types of illusion

The illusions may be caused by false information from the otoliths and kinaesthetic receptors during sustained acceleration (somatogravic illusions) and on moving the head in an atypical force environment (G excess illusions) or from the semicircular canals on recovery from prolonged rotation (somatogyral illusions) and on moving the head during rotation (cross-coupled or Coriolis illusions).

Man is habituated to expect any sustained acceleration to be due to gravity. When a sustained acceleration is applied, the resultant combined acceleration is interpreted as the vertical. For example, when an aircraft accelerates on take-off, the resultant acceleration from the rearward inertial force and downwards gravity is between the two; the pilot senses this resultant force and mentally orientates it so that it is vertical. He thus senses that the aircraft nose is high and tends to want to push the stick forwards. A brief G_x acceleration of 5 G for 2–3 seconds, such as in a catapult launch from an aircraft carrier, gives an apparent nose-up attitude of 5° for a minute or more. There is little time to overcome this particular illusion on take-off. If the pilot pushes the stick forward, he introduces a radial acceleration that will make matters worse. When performed at high altitude, pilots approaching the vertical in a bunt manoeuvre have reported feeling as if the aircraft was flipped on its back. Similarly, a pilot in a flat turn will feel as if he is rolled out of the turn and a pilot in a banked turn may feel himself to be level. Head movement during these manoeuvres can induce further illusions.

When external visual clues are inadequate, for example at night, the apparent movement of light sources in the external environment may be interpreted as a change in attitude of the aircraft. For example, during linear acceleration, the backward rotation of the resultant force vector may make a bright star appear to move upwards. This may be interpreted as a nose-down change in the aircraft attitude.

One of the most common illusions is 'the leans'. If a pilot is in a gentle turn to the right, at a rate below that which would stimulate the otoliths, he could feel that the wings are level. If he then rolls wings level abruptly, he can feel that he is banking to the left. Even though this can be recognized as level flight on the instruments, there is a distinct temptation to lean to align the body with the perceived vertical.

In the same way that the otoliths can misinterpret linear accelerations, so can the semicircular canals misinterpret angular accelerations in yaw, pitch and roll. At constant angular speed, the body's sensors will only give the correct information during the first 8 seconds of the manoeuvre.[73] During recovery from a prolonged spin, not only is there a somatogyral illusion that the aircraft is turning in the opposite direction, but vision may also be degraded by the nystagmus induced by the spin; this will make reading of instruments difficult at a critical time. In reduced light conditions, oculogyric illusions may occur with an illusory perception of movement of an isolated light. Responses during banking may be complicated by the optokinetic cervical reflex where pilots tend to move their heads to keep a constant horizon rather than keep them in line with the vertical axis of the aircraft.[74]

Movement of the head during angular accelerations can produce quite compelling sensations of movement by cross-coupled or Coriolis forces. For example, a head movement in roll from 45° left to 45° right while rotating at a steady speed about the z body axis will produce a strong sense of pitching forward. In highly manoeuvrable aircraft, there is a potential for cross-coupling illusions independent of pilot head motion.[75]

Imbalance between middle ear pressure on ascent or descent can also cause vertigo which, although usually lasting only seconds, can last some minutes. It is more common when there is a respiratory tract infection. The flicker of propellers or rotor blades have also caused vertigo and nausea, but the more usual presentation is irritation.

Occasionally, pilots in single-seat aircraft at high altitude report a feeling of detachment, isolation or remoteness from the aircraft. Some even describe it as an 'out of body' experience, watching themselves controlling the aircraft. A similar 'break-off phenomenon' has been described in helicopters flying at lower altitudes, but in conditions of limited visual cues.

Another form of misinterpretation is caused by the error of expectancy. When flying in cloud, the cloud is brighter in the direction of the sun. The brain interprets this direction as 'up' and stimulates the pilot to 'lean on the sun'. Another example of expectancy is when lights on fishing boats at night are interpreted as stars, which are expected to be above the aircraft; the pilot then inverts the aeroplane. Other errors can occur when interpreting heights of mountains or trees, in misinterpreting a short runway as a longer one seen from a greater height or in assuming a sloping cloudbank to be the horizon.

Incidence

Spatial disorientation is surprisingly common. In one survey, 92 per cent of respondents had experienced the leans, 82 per cent had lost the horizon because of atmospheric conditions, 79 per cent reported misleading altitude cues, 75 per cent had experienced a sloping horizon and 66 per cent reported SD arising from distraction. Helicopter pilots using NVG reported more SD than fast jet pilots.[76] Similar estimates are not available for general aviation pilots, although confidential reporting for commercial flights gives a much lower incidence.

Protection

There are some aircraft factors that can help to reduce SD. The instruments should be reliable and able to be read clearly and unambiguously by day and night. The instruments should be able to cope with the manoeuvres flown by the aircraft and the conditions in which it will operate. A head-up display will also help. The instruments should be laid out so that they can be read without undue head movement.

Aircrew factors include rejection for licensing of those likely to be affected by SD, for example those with Ménière's disease. Aircrew should not fly while suffering from upper respiratory tract infections or acute labyrinthitis, nor should they fly while taking medications whose potential side effects include nausea, vertigo or sensory disturbance. Alcohol has been shown to compromise a pilot's ability to detect angular acceleration and this may continue even after blood alcohol level reaches zero.[77]

Training in the air, as well as on the ground, plays a major part in preventing SD. Instrument flying must be continually practised. In military aviation, spatial disorientation familiarization devices can give valuable experience on the ground of the various illusions.

AIR SICKNESS

Air sickness is a normal response to flying in the unadapted individual. The incidence is related to the intensity of the motion stimulus, the frequency spectrum of the motion and the time of exposure. The condition reduces tolerance to acceleration[78] and may have significant effects on flight safety. It is most commonly experienced during flying training, when the quietness and withdrawal it produces may be misinterpreted as disinterest or inaptitude by the instructor. Severe air sickness in a trained aviator is uncommon unless the stimulus is unduly provocative, for example during flights to study hurricanes. Commercial flying as a passenger does not induce much air sickness, but paratroopers or special forces, who may be flown tactically in more adverse weather, may be particularly affected. Their performance on the ground immediately after landing may suffer.

Some people may not be affected at all, some may experience minor inconvenience, while others will be prostrated. In addition to individual susceptibility, there is a gradual decrease in susceptibility with increasing age from 12 years onwards. Females are more susceptible than males[79] and there appear to be ethnic differences.[80]

Symptoms

The condition does not differ essentially from any of the other forms of motion sickness and presents commonly as nausea, vomiting, pallor and cold sweating. The first symptom is usually epigastric awareness which progresses to nausea. Cold sweating with facial pallor then occur. There is then a crescendo of symptoms (the avalanche phenomenon) with increased salivation, lightheadedness, yawning, and often depression and apathy. Vomiting then follows, which often temporarily improves the symptoms. The feelings of lethargy and drowsiness can last for some hours after landing.

Prevention and treatment

The best treatment is adaptation, particularly for aircrew who should not fly while taking drugs for air sickness. Flying training should introduce exposure to the more adventurous flight manoeuvres gradually. Return to flying after a period away should follow the same principle. The distraction of flying the aircraft or other demanding mental activity rather than being a passenger often keeps the symptoms at bay. However, reading does not help because of the risk of introducing anomalous visual cues. Passengers generally can reduce their incidence by closing their eyes and limiting movement of the head.

About 5 per cent of military aircrew do not manage to adapt by normal means. However, desensitization to strong vestibular stimuli has proven to be transferable to aircraft motion.[81] In the RAF, about 85 per cent of those affected have been salvaged by a programme of increasing exposure to cross-coupled stimuli on the ground before a similarly progressive exposure to aerobatic flight in a dual controlled aircraft.[82] Later work has suggested that it is the number of challenges rather than the severity of malaise achieved that is the important factor determining habituation.[83]

The number of remedies available is large and none can completely prevent everyone from experiencing air sickness in all conditions. One of the most effective drugs is L-hyoscine hydrobromide (L-scopalamine hydrobromide in the United States; Kwells®). In conditions where 10 per cent of the population would be airsick, 0.4 mg of the drug can increase protection so that only 2 per cent suffer symptoms. In more severe conditions, when 50 per cent of those exposed would be sick without prophylactic treatment, 1.0 mg of the drug can provide protection for all but 8 per cent.[84] Unfortunately, most of the drugs used have side effects unacceptable for use by aircrew.[85] Hyoscine can cause blurred vision, dry mouth, sedation, dizziness and significant performance decrements. Promethazine (Phenergan®, Avomine®) 25 mg can also impair psychomotor performance, while dimenhydrinate (Dramamine®, Gravol®) is a central depressant. For short-term protection in passengers, oral L-hyoscine hydrobromide (0.3–0.6 mg) is the drug of choice. For longer benefit, transdermal administration of hyoscine by patch may be useful if placed at least six hours before protection is needed. Antihistaminic drugs, such as cinnarizine (Stugeron®) give protection for six hours, while related drugs, for example, promethazine can give protection for 12 hours. One study found that a combination of 25-mg promethazine and 200-mg caffeine (to counteract the sedative effect of the promethazine) was most helpful.[86] Other proposed prophylactics, such as wristbands, which claim to work by pressure on the acupoints, have not proved effective.[87] Although the severity of symptoms can be reduced by the use of stroboscopic illumination or shutter glasses with a frequency of 4 Hz (to reduce retinal slip),[88] such devices are not yet practicable in aviation.

FATIGUE AND JET LAG

Chapter 91 (Shift work and extended hours of work) addresses the subject of shift work and extended hours of work. For crews of both short-haul and long-haul flights, sleep deprivation occurs because of the work schedules.[89] For the short-haul pilot, the adaptation to encroachment of duty hours on sleep is mainly by prolongation of sleep periods. Rapid and large time zone changes, coupled with sleep disturbance related to overnight flights, are particularly important in flying. Jet lag adds to the acute fatigue for the crews of long-haul, transmeridian flights. Older people tend to be more affected than younger individuals.

Time zone changes may lead to lethargy, loss of appetite, a general feeling of malaise and disruption to the normal pattern and quality of sleep. Until rhythms are resynchronized, the nadir of psychomotor performance no longer coincides with sleep. After flights westward, when the normal sleep onset is delayed, individuals tend to fall asleep quickly and sleep more deeply. Sleep later in the night is more disturbed. By the third night, the sleep pattern is more adapted to the new time zone and this is reflected in daytime alertness and general well-being. Eastward flights impose an advanced sleep onset time. If sleep during the flight and during daytime at the destination is avoided, the first night's sleep may be good. However, once the immediate effects of sleep loss are overcome, the sleep pattern does not adapt to local time for several days. Sleep quality is reduced and there are more night-time awakenings.

Protection

Airline scheduling is largely governed by commercial factors. In an ideal world, an overnight, eastwards flight, after a period of desynchronization caused by the flight west, would be timed to arrive when alertness and performance would be high. However, this is not always possible and flight safety is maintained by imposing statutory flight time limitations. For aircrew required to work overnight, an anticipatory sleep of about four hours in the afternoon or evening will improve overnight performance. Light visor treatment for jet lag may accelerate circadian re-entrainment, but the effect is modest and unaccompanied by subjective improvement in symptoms.[90] An alertness device based on wrist inactivity may be useful in preventing long-haul pilots from falling asleep in the cockpit, but does not obviate the need for sensible rostering.[91]

For the statesman or businessman, there are two ways of limiting the effects of time zone changes. One is to time the trip so that adaptation to the local time zone is complete by the time important business is transacted and to allow adequate time for recovery on return. Another is to travel by supersonic aircraft (if and when these are available again), conduct the business and then return by supersonic aircraft; adaptation to a new time zone is therefore unnecessary. For those who have neither the time nor the money to adopt these techniques, napping when necessary and the use of hypnotics may be the only answer.

Hypnotics have been used for some years to impose sleep at unusual times or in unusual conditions. A rapidly absorbed drug with a short half-life, such as temezepam 10–20 mg has been found to have an acceptable margin of safety when used sparingly. It was used successfully in the Falklands campaign[92] and in the Gulf War. Psychostimulants have not been used by the RAF since the Second World War, but dextroamphetamine (5 mg every two to four hours) has been used extensively and effectively by the US Air Force[93] and 20 mg doses of caffeine every hour have been reported to be useful after sleep deprivation.[94] More recently, attention has been focused on the use of melatonin, which has been reported to prevent jet lag symptoms in east and west transmeridian flight.[95] A dose of 10 mg can advance bed and rise times by two to three hours and maintain sleep duration between seven and eight hours compared to placebo, and produces fewer performance errors on awakening than placebo.[96] In general terms, all use of such drugs requires medical oversight.[97]

FOOD AND DRINK

Food

Food has been recognized as an important factor in flight safety from the earliest days of flying.[98] First, gastrointestinal upsets are the most common cause of in-flight incapacitation.[99] For this reason, flightdeck crew must select different menu items for meals both in-flight and when down the route. In addition, it is sensible, for obvious reasons, for the flightdeck crew to stagger their times of eating when in flight. Second, hypoglycaemia can reduce tolerance to $+G_z$ and has been cited as a significant finding in more than 50 per cent of incidents of unconsciousness in the air.[100] This has led to a requirement to eat sensibly before flying and to provide in-flight rations during long flights.

Drink

The cabin air of all aircraft is dry, as is the breathing mixture provided by military aircraft oxygen systems. This, combined with fluid shifts in the body caused by sitting for long periods, produces dehydration.[101] In turn, dehydration can affect tolerance to $+G_z$ and to heat load and may contribute to an increased risk of deep venous thrombosis.[102] An adequate fluid intake on long flights is therefore important.

However, alcohol in large quantities is not sensible. Not only does alcohol itself contribute to dehydration, but it also affects performance, tolerance to $+G_z$, incidence of DCS and can potentiate SD. Most airlines and military air forces impose a 'bottle to throttle' time for aircrew. The usual time allowance, of 8 to 12 hours, could be considered insufficiently stringent bearing in mind its continuing contribution to accident rates.[103,104] Alcohol plays a significant role in cases of passenger misconduct in flight.[105]

EXPOSURE TO CHEMICALS

Ordinarily, the aviator should not be exposed to noxious chemicals. However, there are four main circumstances in which exposure may occur: toxic fumes in the cockpit, fire, aircraft crash and deliberate release, for example crop spraying[106] or when attacked by chemical warfare agents. In an incident, gas chromatography of blood samples taken as soon as possible after landing may identify the chemicals concerned. Protection against toxic fumes in the cockpit is given by use of an oxygen system with 100 per cent oxygen selected, thereby avoiding inhalation of air from the cockpit environment. Exposure of crop sprayers to chemicals may require skin decontamination and systemic treatment. Protection of aircrew against chemical warfare agents is provided by deployment of detection devices, a robust reporting system, training, protective clothing including respirators which maintain a positive internal pressure to prevent inward leaks, decontamination schedules, filtered air in accommodation for briefing and rest and, finally, medical treatment if required. Pyridostigmine 30 mg every eight hours may be given as pre-exposure treatment against nerve agents.

The aviation worker is also exposed to jet fuel fumes. Chronic exposure can affect neurocognitive functioning in refuelling workers.[107] The effect is greater at the end of the working day and in smokers, who smoke downwind of the site. From time to time, claims are made about exposure to other chemicals in the normal cabin environment. To date, no evidence has been found of exposure to toxic substances at levels that would be expected to cause acute or cumulative embarrassment.

AIRCRAFT ACCIDENTS

Not all accidents involving aircraft require flight. The airfield and the hangar both entail significant working hazards. Ground crew accidents have occurred at the rate of 0.47 per 10^6 aircraft departures, approximately 25 per cent of which were fatal.[108] Over 40 per cent of incidents were caused by a vehicle collision with the aircraft, 34 per cent by individuals coming into contact with moving aircraft parts and 11 per cent from jet blast or fires. Procedures for working airside need to be carefully devised and strictly applied. Medical standards are required, particularly for vision and hearing, and frequent airfield safety training is essential.

In addition, not all injuries in flight relate to crashes. Injuries caused by turbulence amount to 1.9 injuries per 10^6 flying hours with fractures of the ankle being the most common.[109] Not surprisingly, cabin staff are most at risk. Most injuries to passengers occur when the 'fasten seat belts' sign is not illuminated, allowing them to move around the cabin. Thus, most injuries occur in the cruise.

Aircraft crashes are, fortunately, relatively rare events. Commercial flying is the safest form of mass transport. Military flying, when conducted at high speed and low level, is inherently more dangerous, but the risks are reduced by meticulous planning and training. Crashes can occur following engineering or design failure; home-built aircraft accounted for 3 per cent of the hours flown in the United States in 1993, but for 10 per cent of the crashes.[110] The majority of accidents is caused by human factors which may include physiological or psychological causes. SD was a major contributing factor in 20 per cent of one series of military aircraft crashes.[111] Adverse weather is a recurring theme in aircraft accidents and may be associated with greater pilot workload increasing the risk of pilot error.[112]

The most common pilot errors in an analysis of American civil crashes over a period of 14 years were mishandling of the aircraft, inattention and poor decision making.[113] However, there is no evidence of an increase in pilot error with increasing age of the pilot up to the early 60s.[114] The majority of crashes occur in the vicinity of an airfield, being related to take-off or landing. Many crashes occur during training; in one series of civilian crashes, an instructor was present for 50 per cent of crashes following stalls and 32 per cent of those resulting from fuel mismanagement.[115]

Aircraft have notoriously been used for acts of terorism but are also used as a method of committing ordinary suicide,[116] accounting for between 0.72 and 2.4 per cent of all accidents.[117] Such pilots have tended to be younger than those involved in other accidents; 24 per cent had used alcohol and 14 per cent illicit drugs. Other factors involved were domestic and social issues (46 per cent), legal problems (40 per cent) and pre-existing psychiatric disorder (38 per cent).[118]

Most accidents involve ground impact. Injury can result from sudden deceleration, crushing loads on the fuselage, break up of the floor structure or by fire. Protection from mechanical forces is given by restraint harnesses and, in military aircraft, energy-attenuating seating. The more efficient the restraint in the seat, the higher is the likelihood of survival. In one study of fire in 134 fatal civil aircraft accidents, 360 individuals had insignificant antemortem injury, but carboxyhaemoglobin levels >20 per cent, enough to impair chances of escape.[119] Almost 60 per cent of fires start during the impact sequence, with another 17 per cent occurring after the aircraft has come to rest. Rescue is then hampered by terrain, bad weather and the dark.[120] Smoke hoods for passengers have been developed but are not in use by the airlines.[121]

Many military aircraft have ejection seats which can allow the aviator to be on a fully deployed parachute within 3 seconds of initiating ejection. The risks are of not initiating ejection soon enough, of back injury as a result of the forces of ejection, of collision with canopy or canopy fragments, windblast and flail injuries and landing injury. The design of the seat, the use of miniature detonating cord (MDC) to fragment the canopy to clear the escape path and use of leg and arm restraint can minimize the risks. Although more modern aircraft are associated with a lower risk of injury from ejection,[122] there will always be injuries caused by ejection outside the design specifications of the ejection seat. However, injury can occur from anticipated, in-envelope, ejection forces alone, with anterior wedge fractures of the thoracolumbar region being the most common. The risk is greater with taller and heavier aircrew.[123] After ejection, a full spinal radiographic screen from C1 to the sacrum should be carried out. Even with a negative screen, a Technetium-99 bone scan will often demonstrate 'hot spots' indicative of fresh bony injury. Treatment is by total bed rest for three weeks in hospital followed by gradual mobilization. Resumption of flying on ejection seats is possible after three months.

Escape from helicopters offers different challenges. Up to half of military helicopter accidents involve ditching in water.[124] The problems of escape include physical restriction from equipment or trapped air, limited air supply, poor underwater visibility, exit design and fear. The solutions include comprehensive training in a crash simulator, better design of exits and hatches, more streamlined personal equipment, underwater lighting and breathing aids. The death rate in helicopter crashes on land is reduced by using the shoulder restraint harness.[125]

At a crash, the first priority is to save life. The next priority is to preserve evidence. Fire and crash sites are controlled by incident commanders who restrict access depending on risk. The risks to accident investigators can range from bugs to bears, encompassing explosive, chemical, biological, terrain, meteorological and psychological hazards. The chemicals involved at a crash site include aviation fuels, hydraulic fluid, metals (such as cadmium, beryllium, chromium, mercury and their salts), plastic resins and surface coatings and products of combustion. Unexploded ordnance, for example ejection seat cartridges when ejection was not initiated, may also be present.

FITNESS FOR FLIGHT

The formation of the Special Royal Flying Corps Medical Board in 1916 significantly improved the proportion of candidates who passed flying training.[126] Nowadays, it can cost over £1 million to train a military fast jet pilot. The aircraft flown can cost over 100 times that figure. Moreover, medical factors frequently feature in accident reports. One study cited medical factors as causing or contributing to 4.7 per cent of fatal accidents.[103] Aviation medicine policy must therefore balance the risks to individual health, flying safety and mission completion against conservation of resources, flying experience and training costs. Civilian aviation authorities have set a goal of one fatal accident in multicrew aircraft in each 10^7 flying hours.[127] If the medical contribution to this is an arbitrary 10 per cent, then incapacitation in flight should cause an accident no more than once in every 10^8 flying hours. This is attainable if the risk to an individual pilot of incapacitation is <1 per cent a year,[128] although there has been recent discussion about the logic of reducing this to 2 per cent.[129] The actual figure for the United States Air Force over a ten-year period was 1.9 in 10^7 flying hours.[130] Although some doubt has been expressed regarding the predictive value of periodic aircrew medical examination,[131] one retrospective study showed that there were no important risk factors that could have been detected at such examinations in a series of military aircraft crashes.[132] The only blood test that has shown any value is a blood lipid profile which should be carried out on initial examination and repeated at age 40.[133]

It is a generally accepted principle that not only should aircrew be protected against the rigours of the aviation environment, but also that the general public should be protected from accidents caused by aircrew illness. This is achieved by agreeing to medical standards which are the minimum compatible with professional flying. Aircrew are then selected for training who meet those standards. They are required to be not abnormally susceptible to the stresses of flying, either by disease or by unusual physiological response. Once the aircrew are trained, they are regularly examined to ensure that they continue to meet medical standards. Military aircrew are subject to the standards imposed by their parent armed force. Civilian aircrew in the United Kingdom are subject to licensing by the CAA. The frequency and content of the examination depends on the age of the pilot, the type of flying envisaged and the existence of risk factors. For many years, the upper age limit for captaincy of civilian passenger aircraft was set at 60 years. Experience reduces, but does not eliminate, age-related decline. However, the Aerospace Medical Association has concluded that there is insufficient evidence to support restriction of pilot certification based on age alone.[134]

To allow any aircrew to fly with particular medical conditions, the following criteria must be satisfied:

- There must be minimal risk of sudden incapacitation.
- There must be minimal risk of subtle performance decrement.
- The condition must have resolved or be stable and be expected to remain so under the stresses of the aviation environment.
- If there is a risk of progression or recurrence, the symptoms and signs must be easily detectable and must not pose a risk to the safety of the individual or others.

In addition, for professional aircrew, the condition must not need exotic tests, regular invasive procedures or frequent absences to monitor for stability or progression. Finally, for military aircrew, the condition must be compatible with performance of sustained flying operations in austere environments worldwide.[135] The role of the doctor dealing with aircrew must be clearly understood. Most aviators regard doctors as only marginally better than the angel of death because of the risk of being grounded. The medical officer must work to obtain and hold the trust of the aircrew and make it clear that his main aim is to maintain their flying status – but that he also has a responsibility to the employer and the general public as one of the guardians of flight safety. The three most common conditions seen by the United States Navy requiring a decision on fitness for flying are allergic rhinitis, obesity and decreased visual acuity.[136] In one series in a European airline, the rate of grounding was $9.2/10^3$ crew members a year. Ear, nose and throat disorders accounted for 30.1 per cent, musculoskeletal disorders for 21.3 per cent and psychiatric conditions for 12.5 per cent.[137] The rate of disqualification on medical grounds in the United States Air Force declined from 4.1 per cent a year in 1984 to 0.18 per cent by 1999, largely as a result of the use of clinical management groups to provide an evidence base, new therapies and effective preventive medicine efforts.[138] In the final analysis, the decision on whether or not to return an aviator to flying rests with the appropriate national authorities, civil or military.

Miscellaneous conditions caused or affected by flight

Backache is one of the most common conditions reported by aircrew and this is related to the relatively poor ergonomics often found in aircraft. Helicopter pilots have a greater incidence of prolapsed intervertebral disc,[139] osteoarthritis of the spine[140] and backache than controls.[141] Over half of Sea King helicopter crew reported backache in the previous two years, sufficient to interfere with performance, and this incidence increased with the total numbers of hours flown.[142] In addition, almost all flight attendants report musculoskeletal symptoms in one year, particularly in the lower back.[143] Active female flight attendants report more menstrual irregularity than former flight attendants.[144] In addition, an increased incidence of skin cancer has been reported in civilian airline pilots;[145] this may be related to behavioural factors but some influence of exposure to cosmic radiation could be implicated.[146] An elevated risk of brain cancer and carcinoma of the prostate for male pilots and of breast cancer for female flight attendants compared to the ground-based population has been described, but both occupational and non-occupational risk factors may have contributed.[147]

Most airlines are now smoke-free. The withdrawal of nicotine from an addicted smoker may cause decrements in psychomotor performance. Aircrew who try to stop smoking should ideally be grounded for one to two weeks. Nicotine replacement therapies, such as patches or gum, may be allowed but systemic drugs such as buproprion (Zyban®) should not be permitted when on flying status.[148]

Most aircrew who have had a hip replacement may be able to return to civilian flying. The risk for military aircrew would be expected to be greatest during the ejection sequence,[149] but some methods of ingress to and egress from cramped cockpits may predispose to dislocation and vibration may contribute to loosening of the prosthesis.

Use of therapeutic drugs

The use of therapeutic agents, whether by self-medication or prescribed, may be particularly dangerous in aviation. Most have side effects, some of which may be hazardous in aviation. Particular care should be taken with over-the-counter medication and unlicensed, herbal remedies. The key questions that have to be asked are:

- Does the condition for which the drug is being taken necessitate grounding in its own right?
- What monitoring of the condition is required?
- What are the potential side effects relevant to aviation?
- Does the patient have any untoward reaction to the drug on the ground?

The use of statins to reduce cholesterol levels has been found to be aeromedically safe provided side effects are minimal.[150] Hypertensive patients undergoing treatment with selected anti-hypertensive agents may be returned to flying duty once their blood pressure is within limits, provided there are no untoward side effects and other risk factors are under control. In the end, the final decision on medication and flying rests with the relevant licensing authority.

Fitness for flight as a passenger

Passengers fly with all sorts of medical conditions every day and survive. However, with some conditions there is a degree of risk. The doctor asked to advise a patient must bear in mind the inactivity of a long flight, the relative hypoxia, the low humidity, the hassle, the ready availability of alcohol and the time zone changes. These may all impact on the timing of medications, particularly relevant to insulin-dependent diabetics. The swelling of legs may cause circulatory embarrassment to patients in plaster of Paris leg casts. Susceptible passengers may be at increased risk of deep vein thrombosis.[102] Risk factors are:[151]

- Low: Age over 40, active inflammation, minor surgery in last three days. These passengers should be given information about mobilization and hydration. Support tights or non-elasticated long socks may be helpful.
- Medium: Varicose veins, uncontrolled heart failure, heart attack in the last six weeks, the taking of either hormone replacement therapy (HRT) or the oral contraceptive pill, polycythaemia, paraplegia, injury to the lower limb in the last six weeks, pregnancy or six weeks post-natal. These passengers should follow the advice above and use graduated compression stockings. The doctor may advise the use of aspirin if there are no contraindications.
- High: previous stroke or pulmonary embolus, major surgery within the last six weeks, malignancy, family history of pulmonary embolus. The advice for the above two groups should be followed, but the doctor may recommend the use of low molecular weight heparin instead of aspirin.

Airlines expect that passengers with known medical conditions will need to be medically cleared before flight, either by their own or an airline doctor. One survey found one request for medical clearance for almost every 11 000 passengers.[152] Almost one-quarter of requests were for musculoskeletal disorders or fractures, with psychiatric patients accounting for 17.6 per cent. Three-quarters required either a qualified escort or travel companion. Wheelchairs were needed by 30 per cent, in-flight oxygen by 28 per cent and stretchers by 27 per cent. When such patients are accepted as passengers, on-board oxygen, special diets or individual embarking, debarking or transfer arrangements may be made available. Kerbside check-in of baggage may be recommended. The airlines reserve the right not to accept infectious patients, patients who would be expected to deteriorate in flight or those whose conditions would be offensive to fellow travellers. Carriage of unstable patients is a skilled business which should only be undertaken by specially trained operators.

Transmission of disease

Worldwide flight exposes aircrew and passengers, as well as ground personnel, to a variety of disease vectors. For example, transmission of *Mycoplasma tuberculosis* from one crew member to another on a single flight has been reported.[153] Communicable disease can enter the country by an infected person, infected vector or by infected material. International Health Regulations exist to detect, reduce and eliminate sources of infection, improve sanitation around airports and prevent the dissemination of vectors. Despite disinfection, cases of malaria have occurred in non-travellers living in the vicinity of airports in non-malarious countries. The regulations provide for notification of disease, health organization at airports, procedures at and between airports, documentation and disinfection. In the United Kingdom, the Public Health (Aircraft) Regulations 1979 cover cholera, plague, yellow fever, the viral haemorrhagic fevers and rabies.

It should be remembered that aircrew travel and therefore need to be immunized.[154] The number of mandatory immunizations is small, but there are additional ones that may be recommended. Aircrew should not fly immediately after immunization because of the risk of side effects. Some malaria prophylaxis, for example mefloquine, should not be taken by aircrew for the same reason. Chloroquine (300 mg weekly, despite an occasional, temporary effect on visual accommodation) and proguanil (200 mg daily) have been overtaken as the mainstay of malaria prophylaxis for aircrew by malarone. Other drugs, such as doxycycline, may be given in areas of chloroquine resistance. The main actions to be taken are avoidance involving use of mosquito nets, sprays, long-sleeved and long-legged clothing. For aircrew staying overnight in malarial areas in air-conditioned hotels in urban or semi-urban areas, and transferring there in air-conditioned cars, the risks are very low, provided al fresco dining or safari trips are eschewed.[155]

SPACEFLIGHT

BACKGROUND

'Never before has medicine been called upon to certify that an individual will be healthy enough to perform for three years following the examination'.[156] On July 21, 1969, Neil Armstrong became the first man to walk on the moon. It is only a matter of time before some nation or group of nations will return to the moon and then go on to explore Mars. Such plans depend on political will and support. When this happens, the success of the mission will depend upon the health of the crew.

Over 500 people have flown in space since Yuri Gagarin became the first in 1961. Space travel has changed greatly over the intervening decades and is set to progress dramatically in our lifetime. The space shuttle programme is drawing to a close and plans are being made to return to the moon and on to Mars. Space travel will become more available to paying 'space tourists'. Man will be spending longer in space and at greater distances from Earth. Maintaining astronaut health is vital to the success of future missions. Space medicine studies the effects of microgravity on the human body and develops strategies for dealing with medical conditions and emergencies in space. This section summarizes the most important issues affecting the health of astronauts.

THE SPACE ENVIRONMENT

The space environment is inhospitable. Space starts at 63 000 feet above sea level (Armstrong's Line) and has a barometric pressure of less than 1 mmHg. Temperatures range from +1500°C to −130°C. Astronauts experience microgravity since spacecraft are in a state of freefall. Objects retain their mass, but have no weight.

Space radiation poses a serious threat to astronaut health since there is little protection from Earth's atmosphere or magnetic field. Three main sources of space radiation exist: galactic cosmic radiation (very high energy electrons, protons and heavy atom nuclei), solar radiation (mainly x-rays and high energy electrons and protons) and trapped radiation in the van Allen belts (energetic protons and electrons). Solar particle storms generate potentially lethal fluxes of radiation approximately every 11 years, so future exploration class spacecraft will require a 'storm shelter' to protect crews. Spacecraft may not protect the crew from background cosmic radiation, which has the highest energy and so is the most penetrating and potentially damaging. When solar activity is at a minimum, astronauts are exposed to a dose equivalent of 0.78 mSv/day on the international space station (ISS).[157] Career limits for low-Earth orbit astronauts are 1500 mSV for males and 900 mSv for females aged 45. Annual limits for astronauts en route to Mars are yet to be determined, but astronauts are likely to be exposed to several sieverts during a three-year Mars mission.[158]

Effects of radiation on the body are covered in Chapter 53, Ionizing radiations. Chronic effects relevant to space are the increased risk of carcinogenesis, CNS damage and cataract formation.[159] Acute radiation sickness (ARS) from solar particle events would cause nausea, gastrointestinal upset, pancytopenia, seizures and even death. Drugs, such as amifostine, may be used to scavenge radiation-induced free radicals and protect tissues from ionizing radiation damage.[160]

PRE-LAUNCH AND LAUNCH

Safety of both astronauts and ground crew is of paramount importance to the on-site flight and occupational physicians. In 1967, a ground test of the Apollo 1 spacecraft killed three astronauts when the pressurized 100 per cent oxygen atmosphere caught fire from a spark from an electrical cable. Cabin atmosphere composition was changed as a result. Launch of the spacecraft is a dangerous time with high levels of vibration and noise. Risk of fire, explosion and toxins on the launch pad are posed by the large quantities of pressurized highly explosive propellants present. Gravitational pull reaches 3 G on the shuttle and 4 G on the Russian Soyuz capsule. In 1986, the space shuttle Challenger disintegrated shortly after launch killing all seven astronauts on board.

THE SPACECRAFT ENVIRONMENT

The spacecraft is a pressurized vehicle which provides atmospheric control, waste management and shielding against micrometeorites and some radiation. The international space station is maintained at 1 atm, 80 per cent nitrogen and 20 per cent oxygen.[161] CO_2 is actively removed using lithium hydroxide filters to keep levels below 0.01 per cent. Charcoal in the mixture removes odours. Toxicology, water quality, microbiology and radiation levels of the spacecraft environment are regularly monitored. Noise levels on the international space station are 75 dB mainly generated by the environmental control system, avionics and experiments. This may affect hearing, concentration and sleep.

Toxic chemical exposure is a potential hazard. Chemicals, such as freon, from cooling loops are toxic in small quantities if the leak enters the spacecraft, the airlock or crystallizes on extra-vehicular activity (EVA) suits. Chemicals used for orientation control systems, such as hydrazine and nitrogen tetroxide, can immediately irritate the respiratory tract and eyes or be absorbed through the skin. More long-term effects include kidney failure, hepatic failure and respiratory arrest.

Analysis of the space shuttle atmosphere detected benzene, acetaldehyde and dimethyl sulphides[162] at levels below the maximum allowable concentration limits. Dichloromethane and formaldehyde have also been detected and are potentially toxic.[163] Toxic contamination of the spacecraft occurred in 1975 when nitrogen tetroxide was released into the Apollo craft as it undocked from Soyuz. Three astronauts developed pneumonitis as a result; one lost consciousness briefly as they were putting on the oxygen masks.[164]

Damage to the spacecraft's protective shell could lead to decompression sickness. Astronauts had a 'near miss' in 1997 when the unmanned Progress module collided with and punctured the Spektr module of the MIR space station causing it to lose pressure. Fire in a spacecraft is even more dangerous than on Earth since it behaves differently and more unpredictably. Oxygen canisters caught fire on MIR releasing smoke and particles (Ewald, personal communication).

EXTRA-VEHICULAR ACTIVITY

The first EVA was performed by Alexei Leonov in 1965. EVAs are necessary for repair, construction and maintenance of the international space station and Earth satellites. The spacesuit contains its own life support system. The spacesuit atmosphere is 100 per cent oxygen at a pressure 30 per cent of that in the spacecraft (26–40 kPa compared to 101.3 kPa).[165] This lower pressure in the suit allows it to be more flexible. Astronauts 'pre-breathe' 100 per cent oxygen before initial depressurization to prevent decompression sickness. Russian and American pre-breathing protocols differ, the Russian one being shorter which may be useful in emergency situations.[166,167]

Basic medical checks (blood pressure, heart rate, temperature) are recorded before EVA permission is granted. During EVA electrocardiogram, respiratory rate, heart rate, temperature, spacesuit pressure, radiation exposure, and spacesuit F_iCO_2 are measured.[166] A liquid cooling garment is used for thermoregulation and hydration is maintained using a drink bag with straw inside the spacesuit.

EVAs are very arduous and metabolic use is high. At the peak of activities, astronauts' heart rates have risen to above 170 with a respiratory rate over 40.[166] Blunt or penetrating trauma may be caused because of the momentum of the large masses often moved during EVAs. Should the astronaut need medical help, he would need to be moved into the airlock before removal of the EVA suit. In extreme situations, if the suit becomes disrupted during EVA, the astronaut's ambient pressure would quickly drop to zero and result in hypoxia and ebullism causing the astronaut to lose consciousness in 15 seconds.

RE-ENTRY

During re-entry, gravitational pull depends upon the trajectory (1.5 G in the shuttle and 3–4 G in the Russian Soyuz). An emergency return in Soyuz may reach 8 G. Increased G forces may put the astronaut's already deconditioned cardiovascular systems under extra stress. Vladimir Komarov died in 1967 on impact when the parachutes on his returning Soyuz capsule failed to deploy properly. In 1971, three cosmonauts died on return from Salyut 1 following a sudden depressurization of their Soyuz capsule. More recently, Space Shuttle Columbia disintegrated on re-entry in 2003 as a result of failure of a heat shield tile damaged during launch. During re-entry, the temperature of the heat shield can rise to 3000°C.

SPACE PHYSIOLOGY AND PATHOPHYSIOLOGY

Because humans evolved in a 1-G environment, our physiology is significantly altered in microgravity. Many of these physiological changes are similar to those occurring in old age. Some of the changes can be regarded as pathophysiological and return to 1 G can be problematic. Space physiology research requires a balance between regarding astronauts as research subjects and patients in their own right.

Space motion sickness

Space motion sickness (SMS) affects up to 70 per cent of Shuttle astronauts.[168] As spacecraft size has grown, the incidence of SMS has risen. Symptoms of SMS are similar to motion sickness and include drowsiness, nausea, vomiting (often with little warning), stomach fullness, loss of appetite, facial flushing, dizziness, headache, inability to concentrate and sweating.[168,169] SMS also includes the 'sopite syndrome' of fatigue, mood and personality changes and lack of initiative.[170] These symptoms start within a few hours of weightlessness and recover after 72–96 hours. Symptoms like this affect astronaut productivity and EVAs are not routinely recommended during the first three days of spaceflight. Forty-seven per cent of medication used on board the international space station is for the treatment of space motion sickness.[171,172]

There are several hypotheses regarding the aetiology of SMS, including sensory conflict, otolith asymmetry and otolith tilt–translation reinterpretation. Astronauts recover due to neuronal plasticity and remodelling of the CNS, but suffer from similar symptoms on return to Earth ('mal de débarquement'). Manual control of a returning space vehicle when the pilot is experiencing such symptoms may be hazardous.

Cardiovascular system and orthostatic intolerance

The lack of gravitational pull results in blood shift into the thorax and head. Activity in carotid and aortic baroreceptors increases and activates mechanisms to decrease the central blood volume (BV). It was initially thought that BV decreases due to diuresis, but astronauts' urine volumes do not increase and total body water remains constant.[161] Fluid is thought to move from the intravascular space to the interstitial space. These changes happen within a matter of days. Decrease in thirst compounds the relative dehydration.[173] Red cell mass decreases creating a 'space anaemia'.[174] This follows decreased erythropoietin levels rather than increased destruction (the number of reticulocytes falls).[175,176] This is a response to the decreased plasma volume so haematocrit is normal in microgravity but falls on Earth when plasma volume recovers.

These changes in fluid distribution are appropriate for the microgravity environment, but can be problematic on return to Earth. Two-thirds of astronauts suffer from orthostatic intolerance (OI) on return to Earth with longer flights being associated with higher incidence.[177] This causes symptoms of pre-syncope and syncope which could be dangerous if astronauts had to egress the capsule in an emergency. The aetiology of post-flight OI is multifactorial, including decreased central blood volume, decreased inability to increase peripheral vascular resistance, cardiac atrophy, baroreflex dysfunction and increased venous compliance. Left ventricular mass falls by an average of 14 per cent after just ten days in space.[178] Stroke volume falls significantly post-flight.[179] As a result, VO_{2max} measured in astronauts in space for 9 and 14 days decreases by an average of 22 per cent post-flight.[180] This means that astronauts' endurance is reduced in flight, which may be of particular importance during an EVA.

Several countermeasures are used to counteract the cardiovascular deconditioning seen in astronauts, none with complete success. These include fluid loading before re-entry, medication (e.g. midodrine[181]), anti-G suits inflated to 1 psi during re-entry, exercise and lower body negative pressure. Astronauts may re-enter the atmosphere in the recumbent position to try to minimize the $+G_z$ load on re-entry. It is uncertain how a reduced gravitational field, such as occurs on Mars (0.38 G) and the moon (0.18 G) will affect the incidence of OI.

Whether exposure to microgravity increases the risk of cardiac arrhythmias or not is still disputed. The QT interval is increased in space[182] and an episode of asymptomatic ventricular tachycardia has been recorded,[183] the significance of which has yet to be ascertained. Although debated, the NASA Bioastronautics Roadmap recognizes arrhythmia as a potential risk during spaceflight.[184]

Musculoskeletal

Muscle atrophy increases with time spent in microgravity, the greatest reduction being seen during the first month in space. This atrophy occurs since use of postural and lower limb muscles decreases in microgravity. Losses of muscle mass, force, power and increased fatiguability have been reported.[185] Following an eight-day mission, a reduction in postural muscle size up to 11 per cent was recorded.[186] Countermeasures include exercise and the elasticized Russian 'penguin' suit, which provides resistance exercise. However, these countermeasures do not completely prevent muscle atrophy. Backache is commonly thought to be related to lengthening of the vertebral column.[187]

Decreased mechanical loading in microgravity leads to bone mineral density (BMD) loss of weight-bearing bones at an average rate of 1–2 per cent per month[186] and up to 3–5 per cent per month in some bones.[188] The extent to which osteoclast activity increases and osteoblast activity decreases is yet to be ascertained. Unlike disuse osteoporosis during bed rest on Earth, rate of bone loss in microgravity does not appear to plateau. On return to Earth, the rate of recovery is slower than the rate at which it was lost[189] and the extent to which bone fully recovers is debatable.[190] A three-year Mars mission could potentially result in losing 50 per cent of BMD at some skeletal sites if untreated. Such losses of BMD would increase the risk of fractures during long-term spaceflights.

Several countermeasures have been tried, but none found to be completely effective. Bisphosphonates, resistive exercise and artificial gravity may work synergistically to combat osteoporosis.[191]

Renal/urinary

Urinary calcium and phosphate levels increase as a result of the decreased BMD.[192] This increases the risk of renal calculi which are expected in 0–5 per cent of astronauts. Other reasons for the increased risk of renal stones are decreased urine output, dehydration, decreased urine pH, magnesium and citrate. These factors increase urinary super-saturation of renal stone-forming salts. Hypercalciuria may affect sodium and water balance. There was one incidence of calculi in flight which would have caused early evacuation of the astronaut, but the stone was passed spontaneously. Eleven US astronauts have had 14 calculi after flights of over a fortnight. There have been four cases of urinary retention requiring catheterization on the Shuttle. Ten per cent of astronauts flying on the Shuttle between 1981 and 1998 (89 missions, 438 males, 69 females) suffered from genito-urinary symptoms during flight. Good hydration and potassium citrate may be a useful countermeasure to this problem.[191]

Immunology

The immune system is suppressed by microgravity which may increase the risk of infection, reactivation of latent viruses (e.g. Epstein–Barr,[193] varicella zoster[194]) and may alter wound healing, regulation of autoimmune disease and tumour growth.[195] Cell-mediated immunity is decreased during spaceflight.[196] *Escherichia coli* and *Staphylococcus aureus* have been found to have increased resistance to some antibiotics in space.[197] Rates of microbial mutation increase in space and there is reduced diversity of the body's normal microflora.

Respiratory effects

The apicobasal gradients in lung perfusion and ventilation diminish in microgravity. Lung vital capacity decreases initially by 8–10 per cent because of engorgement of the pulmonary circulation.[198,199] This normalizes to pre-flight values after nine days. Membrane diffusion capacity improves with the increased thoracic blood volume. Respiratory changes in microgravity are not regarded as detrimental.

Psychological aspects

The psychological stresses of being in space are just as important as the physiological challenges. The mental and psychological health of astronauts is vital to the success of the mission and coping strategies for being in such a remote environment are required. The unique dynamics of mixed sex, race and multicultural groups are important. Behavioural, cultural and social differences are all important. Problems which have occurred during spaceflight to date include stress, anxiety, altered concentration, depressed mood, malaise and fatigue. Sleep disturbance is common: on average, astronauts get six hours sleep a night.[200] The potential for dysfunctional relationships between crew members and ground staff is possible. Careful crew testing, selection and training may decrease the likelihood of this occurring.

ASTRONAUT SELECTION

Selecting healthy astronauts aims to minimize medical and behavioural problems in space. Physical requirements differ depending on whether the astronauts are to become pilots, commanders, mission specialists or payload specialists. Pilots and mission specialists must pass a NASA class I or II space physical, respectively (similar to a military or civilian class I or II flight medicals). Selection criteria for astronauts and cosmonauts differ. Commercial spaceflight participants ('space tourists') have a different set of selection criteria, likely to be less stringent than typical current astronaut selection. Psychological testing is as important as fitness testing. Future crews will need to be cross-trained and multi-skilled, perhaps in several specialities, e.g. doctor and geologist (Cockrell, personal communication).

MEDICAL EMERGENCIES IN SPACE

To date, more astronauts have died as a result of equipment failure than from medical problems. However, medical emergencies can occur in space and they would have a major impact on mission success.[201] Medical events occurred on 1867 occasions in 508 astronauts on shuttle flights STS-1 to STS-89 between 1981 and 1998. 498 astronauts reported medical symptoms other than SMS, including general malaise, respiratory events, digestive symptoms and injuries.[202] The potential conditions which may occur are very varied. In descending order of frequency, the conditions which occurred were anorexia, space motion sickness, fatigue, insomnia, dehydration, dermatitis, back pain, upper respiratory infection, conjunctivitis, subungal haemorrhage, urinary tract infection, arrhythmia, headache, muscle strain, diarrhoea, constipation, barotitis, decompression sickness (limb pains mainly) and chemical pneumonitis.[200] The median age of astronauts is increasing which may increase the likelihood of medical problems occurring.[203]

Several medical evacuations from space have been necessary as a result of septic prostatitis, urinary retention, possible appendicitis and supraventricular tachycardia.[204] Toothache in space has been reported and is potentially debilitating.[205]

Not every mission flies a medical doctor, but each mission has a designated medical officer. Crew medical officers (CMO) receive at most 40–60 hours of training. They refresh their training using one hour of computer training per month. Non-CMO crew receive 17 hours of medical training. In close Earth orbit, astronauts can take guidance from flight surgeons in Mission Control. However, signals take approximately 20 minutes to travel to Mars and back, so exploration-class crews will need to become more medically autonomous.

Equipment is limited because it costs €20 000 (US$28 000) to launch 1 kg into space. Storage space and power are restricted.[161] However, medical capabilities are similar to those available on board a submarine or Antarctic mission. Capabilities for basic first aid, treating minor medical problems, performing a physical examination, wound closure, inject medications, minor dentistry, advanced life support (drugs and defibrillator with pacing capabilities), maintaining an airway, ventilation and patient monitoring are present. Monitoring includes electrocardiogram, blood pressure, $P_{ET}CO_2$, pulse oximetry (Christgen, personal communication).

Administration of intravenous fluids requires a pump due to bubbles forming in intravenous bags in microgravity. The problem of inadequate supplies of intravenous fluids for treatment of haemorrhage, for example, may be solved by onboard production of sterile intravenous fluids using reverse osmosis and other ultrafiltration methods (Scarpa, personal communication). Hypotension in such a situation could be exacerbated by pre-existing low blood volume and increased gravitational forces during emergency re-entry (e.g. 8 G during an emergency Soyuz trajectory).

Making a diagnosis in microgravity

Physical examination must be adapted for the unique environment and physiological changes of microgravity – the 'microgravity examination technique'. There are, for example, decreased bowel sounds, distended jugular veins, altered posture, hyper-reflexia and the diaphragm is elevated by two intercostal spaces. Using a stethoscope may be difficult in the noisy spacecraft environment. The crew medical restraint kit allows astronauts to be examined more easily.

Ultrasound is the only imaging modality presently flown in space.[206] Ultrasound sensitivity and specificity are likely to be no different in microgravity than on Earth. It can be used for obtaining images of a great variety of systems including abdominal, urinary pathology, echocardiography, sinus or dental infection, ocular trauma, musculoskeletal injury.[207] Ultrasound has reliably diagnosed pneumothorax in anaesthetized pigs in microgravity[208] and could also be used to diagnose haemothorax.[209] Endotracheal tube position could be checked using ultrasound to rule out oesophageal positioning and endobronchial intubation. Ocular ultrasound has been performed in space under the real-time guidance of doctors on the ground.[210] Musculoskeletal ultrasound of the shoulder has been performed successfully on the international space station.[211] These images can be relayed to physicians back on Earth for interpretation, although transmission delays require acute medical problems on an exploration mission be diagnosed initially by a well-trained, on-board clinician. On-board computer training may help astronauts retain and improve their diagnostic skills.[207]

Surgery in space

It has been predicted that one medical event requiring anaesthesia and/or surgery will occur every three to four years of spaceflight.[212] As missions increase in length and leave Earth's orbit, space crews will require the capability to perform surgery on board the spacecraft since return to Earth may not be possible or timely. Alternative approaches to surgical conditions may be required. For example, non-operative treatment of appendicitis has been shown to be effective in remote environments[213] as has prophylactic appendicectomy. Protection of the surgical field from the surrounding air will be needed in microgravity. There are more antibiotic-resistant bacteria in space, so sterile techniques are paramount.

Surgery in a microgravity environment has been shown to be possible, although conditions are clearly different. The surgeon's tactile sensation and proprioception are altered.[214] Laparotomies on rabbits were carried out by Russian research teams on board parabolic flights in the 1960s.[215] Rats have been operated on in a neutral buoyancy tank, during which a variety of surgical techniques were practised, including nephrectomy, small bowel resection and splenectomy.[214] Tissue planes separate more easily and comments have been made on improved visualization during laparotomy (Campbell M, personal communication). Bleeding behaves differently in microgravity. Arterial bleeding forms droplets and streamers, while venous bleeding stays close to the wound because of surface tension.[214] Surgical instruments float and so attachment aids (e.g. Velcro, magnets) are necessary for safety and ease of use.

Anaesthesia in space

In order to perform surgery, anaesthesia is required. In microgravity, the anaesthetist faces logistical challenges and altered physiological norms. There is no liquid–gas interface in microgravity and so anaesthetic vaporizers would not function.[203] Total intravenous anaesthesia may be the most practical technique since regional blockade is likely to be limited by the skills available. Pharmacodynamics and pharmacokinetics may be altered, e.g. neuromuscular junction physiology is affected by muscular atrophy. The changed acetylcholine receptor function may preclude use of depolarizing muscle relaxants to avoid theoretical hyperkalaemia.

The best way of securing an airway is likely to be the laryngeal mask airway (LMA). Intubating LMA and endotracheal tubes are flown (Christgen and Williams, personal communications). Tracheal intubation may be difficult because of facial oedema and the need to tether both the patient and the intubator. Gastric motility is decreased in microgravity so the risk of aspiration during general anaesthesia increases.

Anaesthesia could be altered on return from microgravity. Two rhesus monkeys who flew 14 days in space on the Bion 11 mission experienced significant complications, one dying, after anaesthesia to obtain biopsies.

Adult life support

Should chest compressions be required in microgravity, a modified technique will be required to maintain contact between the patient and provider.[204] Studies on mannikins and pigs during microgravity on parabolic flights have demonstrated that successful chest compressions

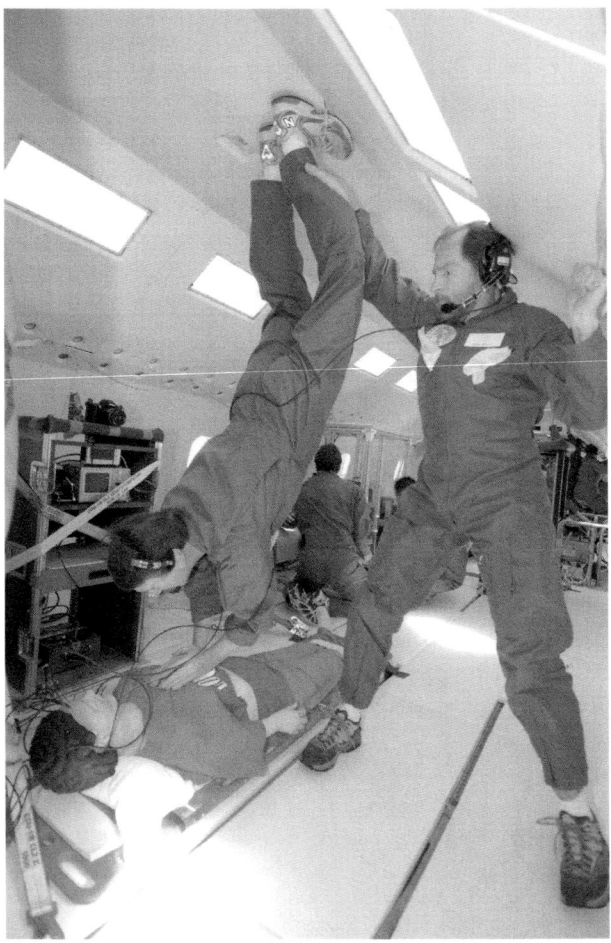

Figure 52.4 Demonstration of vertical inverted chest compressions in microgravity. Image courtesy of NASA.

are possible in this environment. Several methods of performing chest compressions have been devised: the Evetts–Russomano method, reverse Heimlich (bear hug), vertical-inverted (hand stand (Figure 52.4)) and conventional 1-G method with patient and provider restrained.[216] Performing chest compressions in a hypogravity environment, such as the moon or Mars, will require use of upper body strength rather than simple body weight.[217]

RESEARCH AND GROUND-BASED ANALOGUES

Studies into health in microgravity have been limited by small sample sizes and expense. To address this, space researchers use ground-based analogues to microgravity to carry out research relevant to microgravity. Such analogues include head-down bed rest, head-out water immersion and head-out dry immersion. Parabolic flights on aircraft nicknamed 'the vomit comet' produce brief periods of microgravity (approximately 20–30 seconds) up to 40 times each flight. Analogue environments (e.g. Antarctica, submarines) can be useful in trying to predict the sort of conditions which may occur as a result of long-term spaceflight since such explorers live in cramped isolated conditions.

THE FUTURE OF SPACEFLIGHT

Commercial spaceflight

In 2004, history was made when the Ansari X prize was won by the first private spaceship to go into space. Commercial space passengers may be older than the average astronaut and more likely to have chronic medical problems. Standards for such paying space participants are less rigorous than those of career astronauts. This has already been seen when a recent 57-year-old space participant visited the international space station despite a history of moderately severe bullous emphysema, previous spontaneous pneumothorax, a lung parenchymal mass, renal cyst and ventricular and atrial ectopy. He underwent thorascopic pleurodesis pre-flight to prevent pneumothorax recurrence.[218] The Space Passenger Task Force of the Aerospace Medical Association has issued some general medical guidelines for space passengers.[219]

Artificial gravity

Artificial gravity may be used in future long-term, exploration missions to counteract some of the physiological changes occurring in microgravity. This can be achieved by rotating future spacecraft or flying on-board, short-arm centrifuges. Artificial gravity is different from terrestrial gravity because of gravity gradients, Coriolis forces and cross-coupled angular accelerations.

> **Key points**
>
> - Flying and spaceflight expose the human to a variety of stresses which can destabilize the physiological equilibrium, degrade performance and can pose a risk to flight safety.
> - These stresses, and the resulting physiological strains, can be ameliorated by selection against predetermined medical standards, training, protective equipment, suitable exposure planning, development of techniques and protocols, appropriate engineering design and, occasionally, suitable medication.
> - If financial considerations are ignored, human, rather than engineering, factors will continue to limit the future development of flight and space exploration.

REFERENCES

1. Dépagniat MR. *Les martyrs de l'aviation*. Paris: E Bassett, 1912. Cited in Holden HCL, Lessons accidents have taught. *Aeronautical Journal*. 1914; **XVIII**: 204–11.
2. DeHart RL. Health issues of air travel. *Annual Review of Public Health*. 2003; **24**: 133–51.
3. Irvine D, Davies DM. British airways flightdeck mortality study, 1950–1992. *Aviation, Space, and Environmental Medicine*. 1999; **70**: 548–55.
4. Andersson N, Grip H, Lindvall P et al. Air transport of patients with intracranial air: Computer model of pressure effects. *Aviation, Space, and Environmental Medicine*. 2003; **74**: 138–44.
5. Polk JD, Rugaber C, Kohn G et al. Central retinal artery occlusion by proxy: A cause for sudden blindness in an airline passenger. *Aviation, Space, and Environmental Medicine*. 2002; **73**: 385–7.
6. Harvey W. Some aspects of dentistry in relation to aviation. *Proceedings of the Royal Society of Medicine*. 1944; **37**: 465–74.
7. Zadik Y, Einy S, Pokroy R et al. Dental fractures on exposure to high altitude. *Aviation, Space, and Environmental Medicine*. 2006; **77**: 654–7.
8. Grossman A, Ulanovski D, Barenboim E et al. Facial palsy aboard a commercial aircraft. *Aviation, Space, and Environmental Medicine*. 2004; **75**: 1075–6.
9. Klokker M, Vesterhauge S, Jansen EC. Pressure equalling earplugs do not prevent barotrauma on descent from 8000 ft cabin altitude. *Aviation, Space, and Environmental Medicine*. 2005; **76**: 1079–82.
10. Fen L-N, Chen W-X, Cong R, Gou L. Therapeutic effects of Eustachian tube surfactant in barotitis media in guinea pigs. *Aviation, Space, and Environmental Medicine*. 2003; **74**: 707–10.

11. Muhm JM. Predicted arterial oxygenation at commercial aircraft cabin altitudes. *Aviation, Space, and Environmental Medicine.* 2004; **75**: 905–12.
12. Muhm JM, Rock PB, McMullin DL et al. Effect of aircraft-cabin altitude on passenger discomfort. *New England Journal of Medicine.* 2007; **357**: 18–27.
13. Smith A. Hypoxia symptoms reported during helicopter operations below 10,000 ft: A retrospective survey. *Aviation, Space, and Environmental Medicine.* 2005; **76**: 794–8.
14. Denison DM, Ledwith F, Poulton EC. Complex reaction times at simulated cabin altitudes of 5,000 feet and 8,000 feet. *Aerospace Medicine.* 1966; **37**: 1010–13.
15. Paul MA, Fraser WD. Performance during mild acute hypoxia. *Aviation, Space, and Environmental Medicine.* 1994; **65**: 891–9.
16. Tomoda M, Yoneda I. Effect of smoking habit on the symptoms of hypoxia. *Aviation, Space, and Environmental Medicine.* 1996; **67**: 711 (Abstr.).
17. Cable GG. In-flight hypoxia incidents in military aircraft: Causes and implications for training. *Aviation, Space, and Environmental Medicine.* 2003; **74**: 169–72.
18. Webb JT, Krause M, Pilmanis AA et al. The effect of exposure to 35,000 ft on incidence of altitude decompression sickness. *Aviation, Space, and Environmental Medicine.* 2001; **71**: 509–12.
19. Webb JT, Kannan N, Pilmanis A. Gender not a factor for altitude decompression sickness risk. *Aviation, Space, and Environmental Medicine.* 2003; **74**: 2–10.
20. Lee V, St Leger Dowse M, Edge C et al. Decompression sickness in women: A possible relationship with the menstrual cycle. *Aviation, Space, and Environmental Medicine.* 2003; **74**: 1177–82.
21. Freiberger JJ, Denoble PJ, Pieper CF et al. The relative risk of decompression sickness during and after air travel following diving. *Aviation, Space, and Environmental Medicine.* 2002; **73**: 980–4.
22. Ryles MT, Pilmanis AA. The initial signs and symptoms of altitude decompression sickness. *Aviation, Space, and Environmental Medicine.* 1996; **67**: 983–9.
23. Fitzpatrick DT. Visual manifestations of neurologic decompression sickness. *Aviation, Space, and Environmental Medicine.* 1994; **65**: 736–8.
24. Bendrick GA, Ainsclough MJ, Pilmanis AA, Bisson RU. Prevalence of decompression sickness among U-2 pilots. *Aviation, Space, and Environmental Medicine.* 1996; **67**: 199–206.
25. Moon RE, Sheffield PJ. Guidelines for treatment of decompression illness. *Aviation, Space, and Environmental Medicine.* 1997; **68**: 234–43.
26. Risdall J. Clinical management of decompression illness. In: Rainford DJ, Gradwell DP (eds). *Ernsting's Aviation medicine.* London: Hodder Arnold, 2006: 761–2.
27. Webb JT, Pilmanis AA, Fischer MD, Kannan N. Enhancement of preoxygenation for decompression sickness prevention: Effect of exercise duration. *Aviation, Space, and Environmental Medicine.* 2002; **73**: 1161–6.
28. Preston FS. Medical aspects of supersonic travel. *Aerospace Medicine.* 1975; **46**: 1074–8.
29. Hämäläinen O, Vanharanta H, Hupli M et al. Spinal shrinkage due to +Gz forces. *Aviation, Space, and Environmental Medicine.* 1996; **67**: 659–61.
30. Green NDC. Acute soft tissue neck injury from unexpected acceleration. *Aviation, Space, and Environmental Medicine.* 2003; **74**: 1085–90.
31. Oksa J, Hämäläinen O, Rissanen S et al. Muscle fatigue caused by repeated aerial combat maneuvering exercises. *Aviation, Space, and Environmental Medicine.* 1999; **70**: 556–60.
32. Hämäläinen O, Visuri T, Kuronen P, Vanharanta H. Cervical disk bulges in fighter pilots. *Aviation, Space, and Environmental Medicine.* 1994; **65**: 144–6.
33. Petrén-Mallmin M, Linder J. Cervical spine degeneration in fighter pilots and controls: A 5 yr follow-up study. *Aviation, Space, and Environmental Medicine.* 2001; **72**: 443–6.
34. Cheung B, Hofer K. Acceleration effects on pupil size with control of mental and environmental factors. *Aviation, Space, and Environmental Medicine.* 2003; **74**: 669–74.
35. Green NDC, Ford SA. G-induced loss of consciousness: Retrospective survey results from 2259 military aircrew. *Aviation, Space, and Environmental Medicine.* 2006; **77**: 619–23.
36. Lyons T, Davenport C, Copley CB et al. Preventing G-induced loss of consciousness: 20 years of operational experience. *Aviation, Space, and Environmental Medicine.* 2004; **75**: 150–3.
37. Navathe PD, Gomez G, Krishnamurthy A. Relaxed acceleration tolerance in female pilot trainees. *Aviation, Space, and Environmental Medicine.* 2003; **74**: 29–36.
38. Doolet JW, Hearon CM, Shaffstall RM, Fischer MD. Accommodation of females in the high-G environment: The USAF female acceleration tolerance enhancement (FATE) project. *Aviation, Space, and Environmental Medicine.* 2001; **72**: 739–46.
39. Manigas PA, di Julio MA, Dronen SC. Diaphragmatic rupture during G-maneuvers in a J-3 jet trainer. *Aviation, Space, and Environmental Medicine.* 1983; **54**: 1037–9.
40. Snyder QC, Kearney PJ. High +Gz induced acute inguinal herniation in an F-16 aircrew member: Case report and review. *Aviation, Space, and Environmental Medicine.* 2002; **73**: 68–72.
41. Prior ARJ, Adcock TR, McCarthy GW. In-flight arterial blood pressure changes during −Gz to +Gz manoeuvring. *Aviation, Space, and Environmental Medicine.* 1993; **64**: 428 (Abstr.).
42. Banks RD, Grissett JD, Saunders PL, Mateczun AJ. The effect of varying time at −Gz on subsequent +Gz physiological tolerance (Push-Pull effect). *Aviation, Space, and Environmental Medicine.* 1995; **66**: 723–7.
43. Guo H-Z, Zhang S-X, Jing B-S. The characteristics and theoretical basis of the Qigong maneuver. *Aviation, Space, and Environmental Medicine.* 1991; **62**: 1059–62.

44. Balldin UI, Werchan PM, French J, Self B. Endurance and performance during multiple intense high +Gz exposures with anti-G protection. *Aviation, Space, and Environmental Medicine.* 2003; **74**: 303–8.
45. Bain B, Jacobs I, Buick F. Respiratory fatigue during simulated air combat maneuvering (SACM). *Aviation, Space, and Environmental Medicine.* 1997; **68**: 118–25.
46. Belyavin AJ, Gibson TM, Anton DJ, Truswell P. Prediction of body temperatures during exercise in flying clothing. *Aviation, Space, and Environmental Medicine.* 1979; **50**: 911–16.
47. Gibson TM, Allan JR, Lawson CJ, Green RG. Effect of induced changes of deep body temperature on performance in a flight simulator. *Aviation, Space, and Environmental Medicine.* 1980; **51**: 356–60.
48. Rood GM, James SH. Noise. In: Rainford DJ, Gradwell DP (eds). *Ernsting's Aviation medicine*. London: Hodder Arnold, 2006: 404.
49. Steuben U. Hearing loss from cockpit noise in motor gliders. *Aviation, Space, and Environmental Medicine.* 2001; **72**: 827–30.
50. Raynal M, Kossowski M, Job A. Hearing in military pilots: One-time audiometry in pilots of fighters, transports, and helicopters. *Aviation, Space, and Environmental Medicine.* 2006; **77**: 57–61.
51. Abel SM. Hearing loss in military aviation and other trades: investigation of prevalence and risk factors. *Aviation, Space, and Environmental Medicine.* 2005; **76**: 1128–35.
52. Marciniak W, Rodriguez E, Olszowska K *et al.* Echocardiographic evaluation in 485 aeronautical workers exposed to different noise environments. *Aviation, Space, and Environmental Medicine.* 1999; **70**: A46–A53.
53. Wells MJ, Griffin MJ. Benefits of helmet-mounted display image stabilisation under whole-body vibration. *Aviation, Space, and Environmental Medicine.* 1984; **55**: 13–18.
54. Ernsting J. Respiratory effects of whole body vibration. Flying Personnel Research Committee Report No. 1164, 1961.
55. Gibson TM. Hyperventilation in aircrew – a review. *Aviation, Space, and Environmental Medicine.* 1979; **50**: 725–33.
56. Smith SD. Seat vibration in military propellor aircraft: Characterization, exposure assessment, and mitigation. *Aviation, Space, and Environmental Medicine.* 2006; **77**: 32–40.
57. Wells HV. Some aeroplane injuries and diseases, with notes on the aviation service. *Journal of the Royal Naval Medical Service.* 1916; **ii**: 65–71.
58. Gibson TM, Harrison MH. *Into thin air.* London: Hale, 1984: 201.
59. Morris CC. Midair collisions: Limitations of the see-and-avoid concept in civil aviation. *Aviation, Space, and Environmental Medicine.* 2005; **76**: 357–65.
60. Wright P, Scott RAH. Optics and vision. In: Rainford DJ, Gradwell DP (eds). *Ernsting's Aviation medicine*. London: Hodder Arnold, 2006: 289.
61. Miller RE, Kent JF, Green RP. Prescribing spectacles for aviators: USAF experience. *Aviation, Space, and Environmental Medicine.* 1992; **63**: 80–5.
62. Nakagawara VB, Montgomery RW, Wood KJ. Aviation accidents and incidents associated with the use of ophthalmic devices by civilian airmen. *Aviation, Space, and Environmental Medicine.* 2002; **73**: 1109–13.
63. Still DL, Temme LA. Eyeglass use by US Navy jet pilots: Effects on night carrier landing performance. *Aviation, Space, and Environmental Medicine.* 1992; **63**: 273–5.
64. Partner AM, Scott RAH, Shaw P, Coker WJ. Contact lenses and corrective flying spectacles in military aircrew – implications for flight safety. *Aviation, Space, and Environmental Medicine.* 2005; **76**: 661–5.
65. Dennis RJ, Tredici TJ, Ivan DJ, Jackson WG Jr. The USAF aircrew medical contact lens study group: Operational problems. *Aviation, Space, and Environmental Medicine.* 1996; **67**: 303–7.
66. Moore RJ, Green RP. A survey of US Air Force flyers regarding their use of extended wear contact lenses. *Aviation, Space, and Environmental Medicine.* 1994; **65**: 1025–31.
67. O'Connell SR, Markovits AS. The fate of eyewear in aircraft ejections. *Aviation, Space, and Environmental Medicine.* 1995; **66**: 104–7.
68. Scott RAF, Wright P. Opthalmology. In: Rainford DJ, Gradwell DP (eds). *Ernsting's Aviation medicine*. London: Hodder Arnold, 2006: 701.
69. Smith P, Ivan D, LoRusso F *et al.* Intraocular lens and corneal status following aircraft ejection by a USAF aviator. *Aviation, Space, and Environmental Medicine.* 2002; **73**: 1230–4.
70. Rabin J, Wiley R. Switching from forward-looking infrared to night vision goggles: Transitory effects on visual resolution. *Aviation, Space, and Environmental Medicine.* 1994; **65**: 327–9.
71. Howard CM, Riegler JT, Martin JJ. Light adaptation: Night vision goggle effect on cockpit instrument reading time. *Aviation, Space, and Environmental Medicine.* 2001; **72**: 529–33.
72. DeVilbiss CA, Antonio JC, Fiedler GM. Night vision goggle (NVG) visual acuity under ideal conditions with various adjustment procedures. *Aviation, Space, and Environmental Medicine.* 1994; **65**: 705–9.
73. Wickens CD, Self BP, Small RL *et al.* Rotation rate and duration effects on the somatogyral illusion. *Aviation, Space, and Environmental Medicine.* 2006; **77**: 1244–51.
74. Merryman RFK, Cacioppo AJ. The optokinetic cervical reflex in pilots of high performance aircraft. *Aviation, Space, and Environmental Medicine.* 1997; **68**: 479–87.
75. Pancratz DJ, Bomar JB, Raddin JH. A new source for vestibular illusions in high agility aircraft. *Aviation, Space, and Environmental Medicine.* 1994; **65**: 1130–3.
76. Holmes SR, Bunting A, Brown DL *et al.* Survey of spatial disorientation in military pilots and navigators. *Aviation, Space, and Environmental Medicine.* 2003; **74**: 957–65.

77. Ross LE, Maghni WN. Effect of alcohol on the threshold for detecting angular acceleration. *Aviation, Space, and Environmental Medicine*. 1995; **66**: 635–40.
78. Eiken O, Tipton MJ, Kolegard R et al. Motion sickness decreases arterial pressure and therefore acceleration tolerance. *Aviation, Space, and Environmental Medicine*. 2005; **76**: 541–6.
79. Flanagan MB, May JG, Dobie TG. Sex differences in tolerance to visually-induced motion sickness. *Aviation, Space, and Environmental Medicine*. 2005; **76**: 642–6.
80. Klosterhalfen S, Kellermann S, Pan F et al. Effects of ethnicity and gender on motion sickness susceptibility. *Aviation, Space, and Environmental Medicine*. 2005; **76**: 1051–7.
81. Cheung B, Hofer K. Desensitisation to strong vestibular stimuli improves tolerance to simulated aircraft motion. *Aviation, Space, and Environmental Medicine*. 2005; **76**: 1099–104.
82. Bagshaw M, Stott JRR. The desensitisation of chronically motion sick aircrew in the Royal Air Force. *Aviation, Space, and Environmental Medicine*. 1985; **56**: 1144–51.
83. Golding JF, Stott JRR. Effect of sickness severity on habituation to repeated motion challenges in aircrew referred for airsickness treatment. *Aviation, Space, and Environmental Medicine*. 1995; **66**: 625–30.
84. Brand JJ, Perry WLM. Drugs used in motion sickness. *Pharmacological Reviews*. 1966; **18**: 895–924.
85. Shupak A, Gordon CR. Motion sickness: Advances in pathogenesis, prediction, prevention and treatment. *Aviation, Space, and Environmental Medicine*. 2006; **77**: 1213–23.
86. Estrada A, LeDuc PA, Curry IP et al. Airsickness prevention in helicopter passengers. *Aviation, Space, and Environmental Medicine*. 2007; **78**: 408–13.
87. Miller KE, Muth ER. Efficacy of acupressure and acustimulation bands for the prevention of motion sickness. *Aviation, Space, and Environmental Medicine*. 2004; **75**: 227–34.
88. Reschke MF, Somers JT, Ford G. Stroboscopic vision as a treatment for motion sickness: Strobe lighting vs. shutter glasses. *Aviation, Space, and Environmental Medicine*. 2006; **77**: 2–7.
89. Bourgeois-Bougrine S, Carbon P, Gounelle C et al. Perceived fatigue for short- and long-haul flights: A survey of 739 airline pilots. *Aviation, Space, and Environmental Medicine*. 2003; **73**: 1072–7.
90. Boulos Z, Macchi MM, Stürchler MP et al. Light visor treatment for jet lag after westward travel across six time zones. *Aviation, Space, and Environmental Medicine*. 2002; **73**: 953–63.
91. Wright N, Powell D, McGown A et al. Avoiding involuntary sleep during civil air operations: Validation of a wrist-worn alertness device. *Aviation, Space, and Environmental Medicine*. 2005; **76**: 847–56.
92. Baird JA, Coles PKL, Nicholson AN. Human factors and air operations in the South Atlantic campaign. *Journal of the Royal Society of Medicine*. 1983; **76**: 933–7.
93. Emonson D, Vanderbeek R. The use of amphetamine in US Air Force tactical operations during Desert Shield and Storm. *Aviation, Space, and Environmental Medicine*. 1995; **66**: 260–3.
94. Kamimori GH, Johnson D, Thorne D, Belenky G. Multiple caffeine doses maintain vigilance during early morning operations. *Aviation, Space, and Environmental Medicine*. 2005; **76**: 1046–70.
95. Petrie K, Conaglen JV, Thompson L, Chamberlain K. Effect of melatonin on jet lag after long haul flights. *British Medical Journal*. 1989; **298**: 705–7.
96. Comperatore CA, Lieberman HR, Kirby AW et al. Melatonin efficacy in aviation missions requiring rapid deployment and night operations. *Aviation, Space, and Environmental Medicine*. 1996; **67**: 520–4.
97. Caldwell JA, Caldwell JL. Fatigue in military aviation: an overview of US military-approved pharmacological countermeasures. *Aviation, Space, and Environmental Medicine*. 2005; **76** (Suppl.): C39–51.
98. Anderson HG. *The medical and surgical aspects of aviation*. London: Hodder & Stoughton, 1919: 147.
99. Buley LE. Incidence, causes and results of airline pilot incapacitation while on duty. *Aerospace Medicine*. 1969; **40**: 64–70.
100. Powell TJ, Carey TM, Brent HP, Taylor WGR. Episodes of unconsciousness in pilots during flight in 1956. *Journal of Aviation Medicine*. 1957; **28**: 374–86.
101. Carruthers M, Arguelles AE, Mosovich A. Man in transit: Biochemical and physiological changes during intercontinental flights. *Lancet*. 1976; **I**: 977–81.
102. Sahiar F, Mohler SR. Economy class syndrome. *Aviation, Space, and Environmental Medicine*. 1994; **65**: 957–60.
103. Cullen SA, Drysdale HC, Mayes RW. Role of medical factors in 1000 fatal aviation accidents: Case note study. *British Medical Journal*. 1997; **314**: 1592.
104. Chaturvedi AK, Kraft KJ, Canfield DV, Whinnery JE. Toxicological findings from 1587 civil aviation accident pilot fatalities, 1999–2003. *Aviation, Space, and Environmental Medicine*. 2005; **76**: 1145–50.
105. Pierson K, Power Y, Marcus A, Dahlberg A. Airline passenger misconduct: Management implications for physicians. *Aviation, Space, and Environmental Medicine*. 2007; **78**: 361–7.
106. Cable GG, Doherty S. Acute carbamate and organophosphate toxicity causing convulsions in an agricultural pilot: A case report. *Aviation, Space, and Environmental Medicine*. 1999; **70**: 68–72.
107. Tu RH, Mitchell CS, Kay GG, Risby TH. Human exposure to the jet fuel, JP-8. *Aviation, Space, and Environmental Medicine*. 2004; **75**: 49–59.
108. Grabowski JB, Baker SP, Li G. Ground crew injuries and fatalities in US commercial aviation, 1983–2004. *Aviation, Space, and Environmental Medicine*. 2005; **76**: 1007–11.
109. Tvaryanas AP. Epidemiology of turbulence-related injuries in airline cabin crew, 1992–2001. *Aviation, Space, and Environmental Medicine*. 2003; **74**: 970–6.

110. Hasselquist A, Baker SP. Homebuilt aircraft crashes. *Aviation, Space, and Environmental Medicine*. 1999; **70**: 543-7.
111. Cheung B, Money K, Wright H, Bateman W. Spatial disorientation-implicated accidents in Canadian Forces 1982-92. *Aviation, Space, and Environmental Medicine*. 1995; **66**: 579-85.
112. Li G, Baker SP, Grabowski JG, Rebok GW. Factors associated with pilot error in aviation crashes. *Aviation, Space, and Environmental Medicine*. 2001; **72**: 52-8.
113. Baker SP, Lamb MW, Grabowski JG *et al*. Characteristics of general aviation crashes involving mature male and female pilots. *Aviation, Space, and Environmental Medicine*. 2001; **72**: 447-52.
114. Li G, Baker SP, Lamb MW *et al*. Human factors in aviation crashes involving older pilots. *Aviation, Space, and Environmental Medicine*. 2000; **71**: 134-8.
115. Baker SP, Lamb MW, Li G, Dodd RS. Crashes of instructional flights. *Aviation, Space, and Environmental Medicine*. 1996; **67**: 105-10.
116. Ungs TJ. Suicide by use of aircraft in the United States. *Aviation, Space, and Environmental Medicine*. 1994; **65**: 953-6.
117. Cullen SA. Aviation suicide: A review of general aviation accidents in the UK, 1970-96. *Aviation, Space, and Environmental Medicine*. 1998; **69**: 696-8.
118. Bills CB, Grabowski JG, Li G. Suicide by aircraft: A comparative analysis. *Aviation, Space, and Environmental Medicine*. 2005; **76**: 715-19.
119. Chaturvedi AK, Sanders DC. Aircraft fires, smoke toxicity and survival. *Aviation, Space, and Environmental Medicine*. 1996; **67**: 275-8.
120. Li G, Baker SP, Dodd RS. The epidemiology of aircraft fire in commuter and air taxi crashes. *Aviation, Space, and Environmental Medicine*. 1996; **67**: 434-7.
121. Reader DC. Smoke hoods revisited. *Aviation, Space, and Environmental Medicine*. 1997; **68**: 617 (Abstr.).
122. Werner U. Ejection associated injuries within the German Air Force from 1991-1997. *Aviation, Space, and Environmental Medicine*. 1999; **70**: 1230-4.
123. Edwards M. Anthropometric measurements and ejection injuries. *Aviation, Space, and Environmental Medicine*. 1996; **67**: 673 (Abstr).
124. Higenbottam C, Redman P. Underwater escape from helicopters. *Defence Science Journal*. 1997; **2**: 161-6.
125. Krebs MB, Li G, Baker SP. Factors related to pilot survival in helicopter commuter and air taxi crashes. *Aviation, Space, and Environmental Medicine*. 1995; **66**: 99-103.
126. Gibson TM, Harrison MH. British aviation medicine to 1939. Royal Air Force Institute of Aviation Medicine Report R593, 1981.
127. Chaplin JC. In perspective – the safety of aircraft, pilots and their hearts. *European Heart Journal*. 1988; **9** (Suppl. G): 17-20.
128. Tunstall-Pedoe H. Risk of a coronary heart attack in the normal population and how it might be modified in fliers. *European Heart Journal*. 1988; **9** (Suppl. G): 13-15.
129. Mitchell SJ, Evans AD. Flight safety and medical incapacitation risk of airline pilots. *Aviation, Space, and Environmental Medicine*. 2004; **75**: 260-8.
130. McCormick TJ, Lyons TJ. Medical causes of in-flight incapacitation: USAF experience 1978-1987. *Aviation, Space, and Environmental Medicine*. 1991; **62**: 884-7.
131. McLoughlin DC, Jenkins DIT. Aircrew periodic medical examinations. *Occupational Medicine*. 2003; **53**: 11-14.
132. Weber F, Kron M. Medical risk factors in fatal military aviation crashes: A case control study. *Aviation, Space, and Environmental Medicine*. 2003; **74**: 560-3.
133. Curry IP. An analysis of routine blood testing of British Army pilots. *Aviation, Space, and Environmental Medicine*. 2003; **74**: 332-6.
134. Aerospace Medical Association Aviation Safety Committee, Civil Aviation Sub-Committee. The age 60 rule. *Aviation, Space, and Environmental Medicine*. 2004; **75**: 708-15.
135. Gibson TM, Giovanetti PM. Aeromedical risk management for aircrew. In: *The clinical basis for aeromedical decision making*. NATO AGARD Conference Proceedings. Neuilly-sur-Seine: AGARD. 1994; CP553: 1.1-1.8
136. Bailey DA, Gilleran LG, Merchant PG. Waivers for disqualifying medical conditions in US naval aviation personnel. *Aviation, Space, and Environmental Medicine*. 1995; **66**: 401-7.
137. Pombal R, Peixoto H, Lima M, Jorge A. Permanent medical disqualification in airline cabin crew: Causes in 136 cases, 1993-2002. *Aviation, Space, and Environmental Medicine*. 2005; **76**: 981-4.
138. McCrary BF, van Syoc DL. Permanent flying disqualifications of USAF pilots and navigators (1995-1999). *Aviation, Space, and Environmental Medicine*. 2002; **73**: 1117-21.
139. Mason KT, Harper JP, Shannon SG. Herniated nucleus pulposis: Rates and outcomes among US Army aviators. *Aviation, Space, and Environmental Medicine*. 1996; **67**: 338-40.
140. Aydog ST, Turbedar E, Demirel AH *et al*. Cervical and lumbar spinal changes diagnosed in four-view radiographs of 732 military pilots. *Aviation, Space, and Environmental Medicine*. 2004; **75**: 154-7.
141. Sheard SC, Pethybridge RJ, Wright JM, McMillan GHG. Back pain in aircrew – an initial survey. *Aviation, Space, and Environmental Medicine*. 1996; **67**: 474-7.
142. Hansen ØB, Wagstaff AS. Low back pain in Norwegian helicopter aircrew. *Aviation, Space, and Environmental Medicine*. 2001; **72**: 161-4.
143. Lee H, Wilbur J, Conrad KM, Mokadam D. Work-related musculoskeletal symptoms reported by female flight attendants on long-haul flights. *Aviation, Space, and Environmental Medicine*. 2006; **77**: 1283-7.
144. Lauria L, Ballard TJ, Caldora M *et al*. Reproductive disorders and pregnancy outcomes among female flight attendants. *Aviation, Space, and Environmental Medicine*. 2006; **77**: 533-9.
145. Hammar N, Linnersjö A, Alfredsson L *et al*. Cancer incidence in airline and military pilots in Sweden

1961–1996. *Aviation, Space, and Environmental Medicine.* 2002; **73**: 2–7.
146. Pukkala E, Aspholm R, Auvinen A *et al.* Cancer incidence among 10,211 airline pilots: A Nordic study. *Aviation, Space, and Environmental Medicine.* 2003; **74**: 699–706.
147. Ballard T, Lagorio S, de Angelis G, Verdeccia A. Cancer incidence and mortality in flight personnel: A meta-analysis. *Aviation, Space, and Environmental Medicine.* 2000; **71**: 216–24.
148. Grossman A, Landau D-A, Barenboim E, Golstein L. Smoking cessation therapy and the return of aviators to flying duty. *Aviation, Space, and Environmental Medicine.* 2005; **76**: 1064–7.
149. Tormes FR, Webster DE. Return to flight status following total hip replacement: A case report. *Aviation, Space, and Environmental Medicine.* 2002; **73**: 709–12.
150. Beigel R, Barenboim E, Sofer BA *et al.* Statin efficacy and safety for lipid modification in apparently healthy male aircrew. *Aviation, Space, and Environmental Medicine.* 2005; **76**: 857–60.
151. Air Transport Committee. Medical Guidelines for airline travel. *Aviation, Space, and Environmental Medicine.* 2003; **74** (Suppl.): A7–8.
152. Jorge A, Pombal R, Peixoto H, Lima M. Preflight medical clearance of ill and incapacitated passengers: 3-year retrospective study of experience with a European Airline. *Journal of Travel Medicine.* 2005; **12**: 306–11.
153. Driver CR, Valway SE, Morgan WM *et al.* Transmission of mycobacterium tuberculosis associated with air travel. *Journal of the American Medical Association.* 1994; **212**: 1031–5.
154. Siedenberg J, Perry IC, Stuben U. Tropical medicine and travel medicine. *Aviation, Space, and Environmental Medicine.* 2005; **76** (Suppl.): A1–A30.
155. Byrne NJ, Behrens RH. Airline crews' risk for malaria on layovers in urban sub-Saharan Africa: Risk assessment and appropriate prevention policy. *Journal of Travel Medicine.* 2004; **11**: 359–63.
156. Nicogossian A. Cited in Clement G. *Fundamentals of space medicine.* Dordrecht: Kluwer Academic Publishers, 2003.
157. NCRP. Radiation protection guidance for activities in low Earth orbit. NCRP Report No. 132. Bethesda, MD: National Council on Radiation Protection and Measurements, 2000.
158. Simonsen L, Wilson J, Kim M. Radiation exposure for human Mars exploration. *Health Physics.* 2000; **79**: 515–25.
159. Jones JA, McCarten M, Manuel K *et al.* Cataract formation mechanisms and risk in aviation and space crews. *Aviation, Space, and Environmental Medicine.* 2007; **78** (Suppl.): A56–A66.
160. Facorro G, Sarrasague MM, Torti H *et al.* Oxidative study of patients with total body irradiation; effects of amifostine treatment. *Bone Marrow Transplant.* 2004; **33**: 793–8.
161. Aubert EA, Beckers F, Verheyden B. Cardiovascular function and basics of physiology in microgravity. *Acta Cardiologica.* 2005; **60**: 129–51.
162. James JT, Limero TF, Leano HJ *et al.* Volatile organic contaminants found in the habitable environment of the space shuttle: STS-26 to STS-55. *Aviation, Space, and Environmental Medicine.* 1994; **65**: 851–7.
163. Pierson D, James J, Russo D *et al.* Environmental health. In: Sawin CF, Taylor GR, Smirg WL (eds). Extended Duration Orbiter Medical Project. Final report 1989–1995. NASA Special Publication SP-1999-534. Houston: National Aeronautics and Space Administration, 1999.
164. Dejournette R. Rocket propellant inhalation in the Apollo-Soyuz astronauts. *Radiology.* 1977; **125**: 21–4.
165. Hamilton DR. Cases in space medicine. *Aviation, Space, and Environmental Medicine.* 2004; **75**: 288–92.
166. Katuntsev VP, Osipov YY, Barer AS *et al.* The main results of EVA medical support on the Mir Space Station. *Acta Astronautica.* 2004; **54**: 577–83.
167. McBarron JM II. The US prebreathe protocol. *Acta Astronautica.* 1994; **32**: 75–8.
168. Davis JR, Vanderploeg JM, Santy PA *et al.* Space motion sickness during 24 flights of the space shuttle. *Aviation, Space, and Environmental Medicine.* 1988; **59**: 1185–9.
169. Reschke MF, Bloomberg JJ, Harm DL *et al.* Posture, locomotion, spatial orientation and motion sickness as a function of space flight. *Brain Research Reviews.* 1998; **28**: 102–7.
170. Lackner JR, DiZio P. Space motion sickness. *Experimental Brain Research.* 2006; **175**: 377–99.
171. Putcha L. Pharmacotherapeutics in space. *Journal of Gravitational Physiology.* 1999; **1**: 165–8.
172. Putcha L, Berens KL, Marshburn TH *et al.* Pharmaceutical use by US astronauts on space shuttle missions. *Aviation, Space, and Environmental Medicine.* 1999; **70**: 705–8.
173. Leach CS, Alfrey CP, Suki WN *et al.* Regulation of body fluid compartments during short-term space flight. *Journal of Applied Physiology.* 1996; **81**: 105–16.
174. Johnson PC, Driscoll TB, Fisher CL. Blood volume changes. In: Biomedical results from Skylab. NASA Special Publication SP-377. Washington DC: National Aeronautics and Space Administration, 1977.
175. Alfrey CP, Udden MM, Leach-Huntoon CS *et al.* Control of red blood cell mass in space flight. *Journal of Applied Physiology.* 1996; **81**: 98–104.
176. Gunga H, Kirsch K, Roecker L, Jelkmann W. Haemopoietic, thrombopoietic and vascular endothelial growth factor in space. *Lancet.* 1999; **353**: 470–1.
177. Buckey JC Jr, Lane LD, Levine BD *et al.* Orthostatic intolerance after spaceflight. *Journal of Applied Physiology.* 1996; **81**: 7–18.
178. Perhonen MA, Franco F, Lane LD *et al.* Cardiac atrophy after bed rest and spaceflight. *Journal of Applied Physiology.* 2001; **91**: 645–53.
179. Bungo MW, Charles JB, Johnson PC. Cardiovascular deconditioning during spaceflight and the use of saline as a countermeasure to orthostatic intolerance. *Aviation, Space, and Environmental Medicine.* 1985; **56**: 985–90.
180. Levine BD, Lane LD, Watenpaugh DE *et al.* Maximal exercise performance after adaptation to micogravity. *Journal of Applied Physiology.* 1996; **81**: 686–94.

181. Ramsdell CD, Mullen TJ, Sundby GH et al. Midodrine prevents orthostatic intolerance associated with simulated spaceflight. *Journal of Applied Physiology.* 2001; **90**: 2245-8.
182. D'Aunno DS, Dougherty AH, DeBlock HF, Meck JV. Effect of short- and long-duration spaceflight on QTc intervals in healthy astronauts. *American Journal of Cardiology.* 2003; **91**: 494-7.
183. Fritsch-Yelle JM, Whitson PA, Bondar RL, Brown TE. Subnormal norepinephrine release relates to presyncope in astronauts after spaceflight. *Journal of Applied Physiology.* 1996; **81**: 2134-41.
184. Bioastronautics Roadmap. A risk reduction strategy for human space exploration. February 2005. NASA SP-2004-6113.
185. Riley DA, Ellis S. Research on the adaptation of skeletal muscle to hypogravity: Past and future directions. *Advances in Space Research.* 1983; **3**: 191-7.
186. LeBlanc A, Rowe R, Schneider V et al. Regional blood loss after short duration space flight. *Aviation, Space, and Environmental Medicine.* 1995; **66**: 1151-4.
187. Wing PC, Tsand IK, Susak L et al. Back pain and spinal changes in microgravity. *Orthopedic Clinics of North America.* 1991; **22**: 255-62.
188. Vico L, Collet P, Guignandon A et al. Effects of long-term microgravity exposure on cancellous and cortical weight-bearing bones of cosmonauts. *Lancet.* 2000; **355**: 1607-11.
189. Bikle DD, Halloran BP, Morey-Holton E. Space flight and the skeleton: Lessons for the earthbound. *Endocrinologist.* 1997; **7**: 10-22.
190. LeBlanc A, Shackelford L, Schneider V. Future human bone research in space. *Bone.* 1998; **22**: 113S-116S.
191. Jones JA, Jennings R, Pietryzk R et al. Genitourinary issues during spaceflight: A review. *International Journal of Impotence Research.* 2005; **17**: S64-S67.
192. Lutwak L, Whedon GD, Lachance PA et al. Mineral, electrolyte and nitrogen balance studies of the Gemini-VII fourteen-day orbital space flight. *Journal of Clinical Endocrinology.* 1969; **19**: 1140-56.
193. Pierson DL, Stoew RD, Phillips TM et al. Epstein-Barr virus shedding by astronauts during spaceflight. *Brain Behaviour and Immunity.* 2005; **19**: 235-42.
194. Mehta SK, Cohrs RJ, Forghani B et al. Stress-induced subclinical reactivation of Varicella zoster virus in astronauts. *Journal of Medical Virology.* 2004; **72**: 174-9.
195. Harm DL, Jennings RT, Meck J et al. Gender issues related to spaceflight: A NASA perspective. *Journal of Applied Physiology.* 2001; **91**: 2374-83.
196. Taylor GR, Janney RP. *In vivo* testing confirms a blunting of the human cell-mediated immune mechanism during space flight. *Journal of Leukocyte Biology.* 1992; **51**: 129-32.
197. Lapchine L, Moatti G, Gassett G et al. Antibiotic activity in space. *Drugs under Experimental and Clinical Research.* 1986; **12**: 933-8.
198. Sawin CF, Nicogossian AE, Rummel JA et al. Pulmonary function evaluation during the Skylab and Apollo-Soyuz missions. *Aviation, Space, and Environmental Medicine.* 1976; **47**: 168-72.
199. Paiva M, Estenne M, Engel LA. Lung volumes, chest wall configuration and patterns of breathing in microgravity. *Journal of Applied Physiology.* 1989; **67**: 1542-50.
200. Clement, G. *Fundamentals of space medicine.* Dordrecht: Kluwer Academic Publishers, 2003.
201. Bilica RD, Simmons SC, Mathes KL et al. Perception of the medical risk of spaceflight. *Aviation, Space, and Environmental Medicine.* 1996; **67**: 467-73.
202. Bilica R. In-flight medical events for US astronauts during space shuttle program STS-1 through STS-89, April 1981-January 1998. Presentation to the Institute of Medicine Committee on Creating a Visions for Space Medicine During Travel Beyond Earth Orbit, February 22. Houston, TX: Johnson Space Center, 2000.
203. Agnew JW, Fibuch EE, Hubbard JD. Anesthesia during and after exposure to microgravity. *Aviation, Space, and Environmental Medicine.* 2004; **75**: 571-80.
204. Campbell MR, Billica RD, Johnston SL III, Muller MS. Performance of advanced trauma life support procedures in microgravity. *Aviation, Space, and Environmental Medicine.* 2002; **73**: 907-12.
205. Wheatcroft M. Effects of simulated Skylab missions on the oral health of astronauts. *Journal of the Greater Houston Dental Society.* 1989; **61**: 7.
206. Sargsyan AE, Hamilton DR, Jones JA et al. FAST at MACH 20: Clinical ultrasound aboard the international space station. *Journal of Trauma.* 2005; **58**: 35-9.
207. Foale CM, Kaleri AY, Sargsyan AE et al. Diagnostic instrumentation aboard ISS: Just-in-time training for non-physician crewmembers. *Aviation, Space, and Environmental Medicine.* 2005; **76**: 594-8.
208. Sargsyan AE, Hamilton DR, Nicolaou S et al. Ultrasound evaluation of the magnitude of pneumothorax: A new concept. *The American Surgeon.* 2001; **67**: 232-6.
209. Melton S, Beck G, Hamilton D et al. How to test a medical technology for space: Trauma sonography in microgravity. *McGill Journal of Medicine.* 2001; **6**: 66-73.
210. Chiao L, Sharipov S, Sargsyan AE et al. Ocular examination for trauma: Clinical ultrasound aboard the International Space Station. *Journal of Trauma.* 2005; **58**: 885-9.
211. Fincke EM, Padalka G, Lee D et al. Evaluation of shoulder integrity in space: First report of musculoskeletal US on the international space station. *Radiology.* 2005; **234**: 319-22.
212. Campbell MR. Surgical care in space. *Aviation, Space, and Environmental Medicine.* 1999; **70**: 181-4.
213. Campbell MR, Johnston SL, Marshburn T et al. Nonoperative treatment of suspected appendicitis in remote medical care environments: Implications for future spaceflight medical care. *Journal of the American College of Surgeons.* 2004; **198**: 822-30.
214. Satava RM. Surgery in space, phase I: Basic surgical principles in a simulated space environment. *Surgery.* 1988; **103**: 633-7.
215. Yaroshenko GL, Terentlyen VG, Mokov MD. Characteristics of surgical intervention under conditions of weightlessness. *Voenno-Meditsinski Zhurnal.* 1967; **10**: 69.

216. Jay GD, Lee P, Goldsmith H *et al.* CPR effectiveness in microgravity; comparison of three positions and a mechanical device. *Aviation, Space, and Environmental Medicine.* 2003; **74**: 1183–9.
217. Dalmarco G, Calder A, Falcao F *et al.* Evaluation of external cardiac massage performance during hypogravity simulation. *Engineering in Medicine and Biology.* 2006; (Suppl.): 2904–7.
218. Jennings RT, Murphy DMF, Ware DL *et al.* Medical qualifications of a commercial spaceflight participant: Not your average astronaut. *Aviation, Space, and Environmental Medicine.* 2006; **77**: 475–84.
219. Aerospace Medical Association Task Force on Space Travel. Medical guidelines for space passengers. *Aviation, Space, and Environmental Medicine.* 2001; **72**: 948–50.

FURTHER READING

Committee on Creating a Vision for Space Medicine During Travel Beyond Earth Orbit. Ball JR, Evans CH (eds). *Safe passage: Astronaut care for exploration missions.* Washington DC: National Academies Press, 2001.

Clement G. *Fundamentals of space medicine.* Dordrecht: Kluwer Academic, 2003.

Harding RM. *Survival in space.* London: Routledge, 1989.

Nicogossian AE, Huntoon CL, Pool SL (eds). *Space physiology and medicine*, 2nd edn. Philadelphia: Lea & Febiger, 1989.

Rainford DJ, Gradwell DP (eds). *Ernsting's Aviation medicine*, 4th edn. London: Hodder Arnold, 2006.

Rayman RB, Hastings JD, Kruyer WB *et al. Clinical aviation medicine*, 4th edn. New York: Professional Publishing Group, 2006.

SECTION FIVE

Radiation

53	Ionizing radiations *Chris Sharp and Fred A Mettler Jr*	623
54	Non-ionizing radiation and the eye *Michael E Boulton and David H Sliney*	644
55	Extremely low frequency electric and magnetic fields *Leeka Kheifets and Gabor Mezei*	663
56	Radiofrequency fields *Gabor Mezei and Leeka Kheifets*	675

53

Ionizing radiations

CHRIS SHARP AND FRED A METTLER JR

Introduction	623	Health surveillance	634
Ionizing radiations	623	Basic plan for the handling of casualties following a nuclear reactor accident	638
Dose quantities	624		
Natural background radiation	625	Accidents and radiation risk	640
Detection of radiation	625	Acknowledgements	641
Health effects of ionizing radiation	625	References	641
Medical aspects	634	Further reading on medical treatment of casualties	643

INTRODUCTION

On November 8, 1895, Wilhelm Roentgen was examining the effects of passing an electric current through a glass tube from which air had been evacuated, when he found that a sheet of photosensitive paper glowed when the current was switched on. He had discovered x-rays and by the turn of the last century radiographs were being used in many fields, in particular for diagnostic purposes. In 1896, Henri Becquerel discovered that certain types of substances, in particular radium, darkened photographic plates. He called this phenomenon 'radiation' and, with a student who worked with him, Madame Marie Curie, continued to investigate and experiment in this field. Due to a lack of knowledge of the harmful biological effects that radiation could produce, they adopted no precautions or gave no thought to the hazards. As a result, Madame Curie received very high doses of radiation and died of leukaemia, possibly due to her radiation exposure. Similarly, many radiologists received high doses of radiation to their hands resulting in erythema and subsequently many died of radiation-induced cancers.[1] Throughout the twentieth century, the use of radiation increased, so that now radiation sources and radioactive elements are found in wide and diverse environments, embracing, *inter alia*, nuclear medicine and therapy, non-destructive testing, nuclear power and smoke detectors.

Accident and emergency personnel, hospital specialists, occupational health and public health physicians are likely to become involved with radiation issues if the stringent statutory controls for radiation sources or equipments are bypassed or ignored. For example, the theft of a caesium-137 source in Goiânia, Brazil led to 50 people receiving significant exposure and four deaths.[2] Large areas of land and property were affected. There have been many accidents with irradiator sources using non-destructive testing or irradiation of foods and materials where individuals have received very high doses, often leading to death. In the Chernobyl nuclear power plant accident, 28 members of the workforce died of radiation-related injuries and the release of radioactivity led to widespread contamination of houses, land and foodstuffs.[3,4] These low probability events can lead to significant radiation exposures to both the workforce and the public and their clinical management would clearly involve hospital physicians, occupational and public health physicians, and general practitioners. Experience suggests that in all these scenarios both the individual employee's health outcome and the public's health concerns dominate the agenda and place a burden on health professionals. Coherent plans to deal with these events are essential.

IONIZING RADIATIONS

Atoms, radioactivity and radiation

All matter is made up of atoms. Each atom contains a nucleus around which electrons orbit. In the nucleus, there are protons and neutrons. All atoms of the same chemical element have an identical number of positively charged protons in the nucleus and negatively charged electrons on

Table 53.1 Properties of ionizing radiations.

Type	Range in air	Range in tissue	Hazard	Examples
Alpha (α)	Few cm	10s of μ	Internal	Plutonium
Beta (β)	Up to several metres	Few mm	External and internal	Caesium
Gamma (γ)	Many metres	Many cm	External and internal	Cobalt source
x-Rays	Many metres	Many cm	External	Hospitals
Neutrons	Many metres	Many cm	External	Reactors

Tables 53.1–53.10 created by, and reproduced with permission from National Radiological Protection Board, Chilton, UK. (now the Radiation Protection Division of the Health Protection Agency).

the orbits. So, an undisturbed atom is electrically neutral. The number of protons defines the atomic number of the element. The mass of the atom is determined by the number of protons and neutrons and the total number is called the mass number. The same element can have different numbers of neutrons and consequently different mass numbers. These variants of the elements are known as isotopes. Some of these isotopes are unstable and eventually transform into atoms of another element with the simultaneous emission of alpha (α)- or beta (β)-particles and accompanied usually by gamma (γ)-rays. This property of the unstable atom is called radioactivity; the change itself is called radioactive decay and the unstable atom is said to be a radionuclide. The time necessary to reach a stable form depends on the particular isotope and may take a few fractions of a second to several thousand years. The time for the activity to decay by one-half is termed the half-life ($t_{1/2}$). For example, sodium-23 (^{23}Na) is the stable form of sodium and ^{24}Na is a radioactive isotope with a $t_{1/2}$ of 15 hours. The latter decays emitting a β-particle to become ^{24}Mg, a stable isotope of magnesium. This activity is measured by the numbers of disintegrations per unit time. The unit by which radioactivity is measured is the becquerel (Bq) and 1 Bq equals one atomic disintegration per second; 60 Bq is the average amount of natural potassium-40 (^{40}K) in every kilogram of the average person. This means that about 15 million ^{40}K atoms disintegrate inside a person each hour.

What are ionizing radiations?

Ionizing radiation may be higher energy electromagnetic radiations (x-rays and γ-rays) or energetic subatomic particles such as α- and β-particles and neutrons. According to their energy, x-rays and γ-rays interact with matter and tissue and although the mechanisms may be different, they all produce positively and/or negatively charged ions, which then interact with the absorbing matter to produce physicochemical changes by adding or subtracting electrons. The energy of these electromagnetic radiations will also determine their penetration, higher energy photons penetrating further than low energy ones. When they do interact with tissues and cells, energy is deposited within the tissue.

The different radiations penetrate matter in different ways, the properties being determined by the size, charge and energy of each type; α-particles are stopped by a thin piece of paper or the dead layer of the skin, while β-particles can penetrate the hand but will be stopped by a thin sheet of aluminium; x- and γ-rays penetrate the body and an aluminium sheet, but are stopped by lead. Neutrons penetrate most materials, but may be stopped by thick polythene or concrete (hydrogenous materials); high energy neutrons have a high penetrance in tissue but low energy neutrons can be absorbed in the body because of the body's high water content (see Table 53.1). These overall properties of radiation affect the degree of cellular damage following exposure and the methods needed for protection.

In general α-particles do not constitute a significant hazard as an external source, but are hazardous when taken into the body. When incorporated, they can irradiate adjacent cells in, for example, the liver. Neutrons, because of their absence of electrical charge, produce ionization indirectly and tend to be more penetrating. Ionizing radiations have sufficient energy to break chemical bonds and ionize atoms and molecules, producing an ion pair. These ions are charged and capable of causing further ionization and energy deposition leading to physicochemical changes in cellular constituents.

DOSE QUANTITIES

Some of these changes may be of no biological consequence and others may be repaired, but there is a finite probability that damage may cause cell death or irreparable damage to vital cell constituents. The absorbed dose is a measure of the mean energy absorbed by unit mass of tissue, and the absorbed dose in grays (Gy) is equal to the deposition of one joule (J) of energy in 1 kilogram (kg) of tissue. Overall, the greater the dose, the greater the likelihood of a biological effect being seen. Energy is deposited along the path of ionizing radiation as it traverses tissues in the form of ionizations. The average deposition of energy per unit length is called the linear energy transfer (LET).

Charged particles tend to have higher LET values than x- or γ-rays. The International Commission on Radiological Protection (ICRP) has introduced a weighting factor related to LET to take into account these differences.[5] These radiation weighting factors (w_R) may range from 1 to 20 for different radiations. Thus photons, such as x- or γ-rays, are assigned a w_R of 1 (low LET) and α-particles 20 (high LET). Tissues are also assigned weighting factors (w_T) to differentiate the wide variation in tissue sensitivity to radiation, the lymphopoietic stem cells and gonadal germ cell cells being the most sensitive and bone being relatively insensitive. These radiation and tissue weighting factors are used to convert the absorbed dose in grays to an effective dose in sieverts (Sv). This system allows external and internal exposures to be combined into one dose – on the basis of equality of risk. Once a radionuclide is incorporated, it will continue to expose surrounding tissues until final decay or it is excreted. It is usual to calculate this committed effective dose following the ingestion or inhalation so that extra care can be taken to reduce future external exposures.

Submultiples of the sievert are commonly used, such as the millisievert (mSv), which is one-thousandth of a sievert; for example, the world average individual dose received due to exposure to natural background radiation is about 2.4 mSv per year compared with the occupational dose limit of 20 mSv average per year over defined periods of five years.[5] It is sometimes useful to have a measure of the total dose to groups of people or a population. The quantity used to express this total is the collective effective dose: it is obtained by summing the product of all the doses in a group and the number of people in the group and is usually expressed in person-sieverts. Throughout this chapter, these various dose quantities will be referred to as dose, except where further clarification is required.

NATURAL BACKGROUND RADIATION

Radiation of natural origin pervades the whole environment. Cosmic rays reach the earth from outer space, the earth itself is radioactive, and natural activity is present in our diet and in the air. Everybody is exposed to natural radiation to a greater or lesser extent, and for most people it is the major source of exposure.[6]

DETECTION OF RADIATION

Physical

Ionizing radiations cannot be directly detected by the human senses, but they can be detected and measured by a variety of means, such as photographic films, Geiger tubes and scintillation counters. There are also relatively new techniques using thermoluminescent materials and silicon diodes. Some of these techniques are used to measure individual doses on dosemeters (generally called film badges). Measurements made with such dosemeters can be interpreted to represent the energy deposited in the body or in a particular part of the body by the radiation concerned.

Biological

When a radionuclide is deposited in an internal organ, for instance via ingestion or inhalation, doses are generally calculated, because the activities are too small to be measured. The dose (or activity) can be assessed or measured by taking urine or blood samples and applying biokinetic models or be measured directly by special detection systems, e.g. whole body monitors. These systems are only available at special sites in the United Kingdom, such as British Nuclear Fuels, the Atomic Weapons Establishment, the Health Protection Agency, Sellafield Ltd or Harwell.

In an accident situation, estimating the whole body dose by changes in circulating absolute lymphocyte counts in the first 48 hours is possible and by cytogenetic assays for chromosome aberrations in cultured lymphocytes. These techniques use either dicentric counting or more recently fluorescence *in situ* hybridization (FISH) painting of chromosomes and measuring the translocation of genetic material. The threshold for whole body dose-validated chromosomal changes is around 1–200 mSv. More recently, electron paramagnetic spin resonance techniques have been developed using teeth or, in the case of cadavers, bone, which permits a retrospective assessment of the dose. The accurate range for this technique is from around 100 mGy to lethal doses. Another technique using post-subcapsular lens opacities also offers a possible way to assess historic doses; however, its accuracy is not yet proven.

HEALTH EFFECTS OF IONIZING RADIATION

Any organ or tissue may be affected, the degree varying with the dose and the radiosensitivity of the given organ or tissue. Distinguishing two types of effects is possible, somatic and hereditary. The somatic effects relate to the individual who is exposed, and may be early or late, and in the embryo or fetus may be teratogenic. The hereditary effects would occur in the offspring, through genetic damage to germ cells of the exposed individual.

Somatic effects

Somatic effects are classified as deterministic and stochastic. Deterministic effects are those for which the severity increases with the dose and for which a threshold exists. Stochastic effects are those whose probability of occurrence increases with the dose and whose severity is independent of the dose and without a threshold. With deterministic effects, cause and effect can be seen. However, due to the random nature of the interaction of radiation with matter, for stochastic effects the inference of cause can only be based on an increase in the probability of that effect. Where the dose is low (as is likely in occupational exposures), only stochastic effects might be seen. The severity of stochastic effects is not dose dependent as it is with deterministic effects. So an increase in a dose produces an increase in the probability of a stochastic effect.

DETERMINISTIC EFFECTS

Generally, dose–response relationships are sigmoid in shape and exhibit a threshold. For each deterministic effect, the two main parameters to consider are the threshold dose (ED_0), at which the given effect may appear, and its relative severity. These effects are characterized by the median dose, ED_{50}, at which 50 per cent of exposed individuals will exhibit the effect, and by the slope of the curve at the median. The dose–response relationships are generally quoted for acute exposure; protraction of exposure increases the median dose for the effect.[7,8]

Doses below which selected deterministic effects should not occur in a normally distributed population (ED_0) are given in Table 53.2. These levels take into account the individual variation and sensitivity rather than the average value. They are not complete and are for guidance only. The values should not be used in conditions of known radiosensitivity, e.g. ataxia telangiectasia.

Table 53.2 Approximate threshold levels of dose (ED_0) for deterministic effects (adult exposure).

Organ	Effect	ED_0 (threshold dose) (Gy)
Whole body	Early death	1.5
	Prodromal syndrome (e.g. vomiting)	0.5
Bone marrow	Early death	1.5
	Depression of haematopoiesis	0.5
Lung	Early death	6
	Pneumonitis	3–5
Skin	Prompt erythema, dry desquamation	>8
	Moist desquamation and necrosis	>15
Thyroid	Hypothyroidism	3
Lens of the eye	Detectable opacity	0.5–2
	Cataract with loss of vision	5
Testes	Temporary sterility	0.15
	Permanent sterility	3.5–6
Ovaries	Permanent sterility	2.5–6
Embryo or fetus	Teratogenesis	0.10

Haematopoietic system

The bone marrow is the main organ of concern since exposure to penetrating radiation at high dose rate can lead to death within a few weeks. This early mortality results from stem cell depletion in the marrow. The lymphocytes are the most sensitive indicators of injury to the bone marrow. Acute doses of 1–2 Gy reduce their concentration in blood to about 50 per cent of their normal level within about 48 hours. Neutrophils and platelets also show a dose-related decrease in concentrations and the levels can be used to predict the likelihood of survival and the necessity for treatment. People with bone marrow aplasia show an increased susceptibility to infection and frequently spontaneous bleeding (from thrombocytopenia) as a direct result of damage to the immune and haematopoietic systems. In severe cases of radiation injury, marrow aplasia is the likely cause of death.[6,9]

Because of the lack of quantitative human data, there has been considerable uncertainty about the dose–effect relationship for death due to irradiation of the bone marrow following acute or chronic radiation exposure. Extensive data have been published on the effects of whole-body irradiation in animals.[10] However, they cannot be used directly to predict dose–response relationships for man due to marked variation between species, but they do provide information on the likely shape of the dose–response relationship.

The median lethal dose for humans is not precisely known. Several estimates have been published ranging from 2.4 to 5.1 Gy bone marrow dose. The higher values of the estimates of the LD_{50} involved cases where significant supportive and therapeutic medical treatment was provided. With minimal medical treatment involving no more than basic first aid, a value for LD_{50} of 3 Gy has been adopted by United Nations Scientific Committee on the Effects of Atomic Radiations (UNSCEAR),[6] the National Radiological Protection Board (now part of the Health Protection Agency)[7] and the Nuclear Regulatory Commission, USA (NUREG).[11] For supportive medical treatment which includes procedures such as reverse isolation procedures, the use of antibiotics, white cell and platelet transfusions and intravenous feeding, NRPB7 and NUREG11 recommend a value for LD_{50} of 4.5 Gy. This is based partly on human and partly on animal data. Recent advances in rescuing depleted marrow with stem cell stimulating growth factors[12,13] would now be included in treatment. These offer hope that the LD_{50} will be raised, possibly to the point where death no longer depends on haematopoietic damage.

The lymphocyte count decreases within a few hours of irradiation and the platelet and granulocyte counts within a few days or weeks, while the erythrocyte count begins to decrease rather slowly only after a number of weeks. The exposed individual may die from infection or from haemorrhage. The consensus value for the median lethal dose within 60 days ($LD_{50/60}$) is estimated to range from 2.5 to

5 Gy, after homogeneous exposure. The slope of the dose–response curve is relatively steep, expressing a rapidly increasing probability of death for small increments of dose without medical treatment.

Gastrointestinal tract

There is considerable variation in response as the different parts of the gastrointestinal tract have markedly different radiosensitivity. The oesophagus and rectum are relatively radioresistant, while the stomach and small intestine are much more sensitive.[14] The small intestine is the most sensitive because of the rapidly proliferating mucosal cells of the mucosal epithelium in the crypts of Lieberkühn.[15] Single acute doses to the abdomen of around 6–16 Gy produces early onset of nausea, vomiting and diarrhoea, the symptoms occurring earlier and being prolonged broadly in proportion to the dose. These symptoms are thought to be caused by the release of 5-hydroxytryptamine (5-HT) into the bloodstream which stimulates the nausea/vomiting centres in the brain and other 5-HT receptors.[16] There is a concomitant increase in bowel motility which may be caused by bile salts and other substances acting on the damaged mucosa. Very few human data are available on this gastrointestinal syndrome. It is known, however, that cancer patients given whole body doses of 10 Gy or more (generally as a single dose delivered in about four hours, in conjunction with bone marrow transplantation) have survived the gastrointestinal syndrome.[17] Data obtained from studies in which x-rays were used to irradiate acutely the gastrointestinal tract of rats indicate an LD_{50} of about 15 Gy, an LD_{10} of 10 Gy and an LD_{90} of 20 Gy.

For gastrointestinal symptoms, the following figures are given as guidelines for adults; anorexia may be seen in 5 per cent of those at 0.4 Gy and 95 per cent at 3 Gy, nausea in 5 per cent at 0.5 Gy and 95 per cent at 4.5 Gy, vomiting in 5 per cent at 0.6 Gy and 100 per cent at 7 Gy, and diarrhoea in 5 per cent at 1 Gy and over 20 per cent at 8 Gy. If the time from exposure to onset of any of the above symptoms is less than one hour, the whole body dose is likely to be >3 Gy, if more than three hours <1 Gy and if they last for more than 24 hours, the dose is likely to be >6 Gy. The onset of symptoms within 30 minutes indicates an abdominal dose >3 Gy. These signs and symptoms are sometimes referred to as the acute radiation syndrome.

Lung

The lung can be exposed to external radiation from a beam or internal radiation after inhalation of radioactive materials. Radiation pneumonitis appears some weeks or months after exposure. It is a complex phenomenon, including oedema, cell death, cell desquamation, fibrin exudate in the alveoli, fibrous thickening of alveolar septa and proliferative changes in the blood vessels. The main effect is interstitial pneumonitis, followed by pulmonary fibrosis, resulting principally from the damage and response of the fine vasculature and the connective tissues. Development of the lesions is highly influenced by the volume of the organ irradiated and the dose. An acute exposure of both lungs shows a threshold at about 6–7 Gy, with an ED_{50} at about 9 Gy.[8]

Thyroid

The adult thyroid is not especially sensitive to radiation; however, it should always be considered if iodine isotopes are inhaled or ingested by some employees as it accumulates rapidly in the gland. The radiation-induced diseases include acute radiation thyroiditis and hypothyroidism. Total ablation of the thyroid requires high doses, about 1000 Gy delivered within a short period (two weeks).[8] Hypothyroidism is produced by much lower doses, with 50 per cent incidence at about 60 Gy for acute external exposure and 300 Gy for prolonged internal exposure. The childhood thyroid is more sensitive to radiation (see under Carcinogenesis, p. 629).

Skin

The skin is a relatively radioresistant organ, but is likely to be exposed in any type of accident. Skin responses depend upon various factors, such as size of the irradiated area, depth distribution of dose, duration of exposure and dose rate.[18] Radiation damage to the skin may be observed as erythema, moist desquamation and necrosis, with thresholds of 2, 12–20 and >18 Gy, respectively.[18] Moist desquamation often results in chronic changes, with hyperkeratosis and telangiectasia of the capillaries and of superficial and deep blood vessels. The chronic phase may lead to ulceration, atrophy and necrosis.

Protraction of exposures for 1–14 days will increase the threshold and ED_{50} values by a factor of about two compared with acute exposure.[8] As radiation burns involving large areas can precipitate the same systemic effects as thermal injury, overall management may be complicated especially where other body systems have been affected, e.g. bone marrow.

Eye

Experience has shown that radiation doses received by the lens may result in lenticular opacities or cataracts. There is currently a debate as to whether these changes are deterministic or stochastic. The eye may be exposed either after local irradiation – acute or protracted – or after whole body irradiation. The threshold level for detectable opacity is estimated to be less than 0.5 Gy.[19] Protraction does not increase the threshold so much as for some other organs. The cataract does not appear early after exposure; the latent period varies from six months to 35 years, with an average of three years.

Gonads

The germ cells of the reproductive system are highly radiosensitive. The threshold dose for transient sterility lasting for several weeks averages 0.15 Gy for men and about five to ten times higher for women.[8] Recovery time in men is dose dependent and may take many years. Doses of 2.5–6 Gy or more are required for permanent sterility in both men and women.

Embryo and fetus

The embryo and fetus should also be considered, as women in the workforce may become pregnant. The developmental effects of radiation in the embryo and fetus are strongly related to the gestational age at which the exposure occurs, i.e. whether it occurs during organogenesis.[20] The most serious health consequences of prenatal exposure are embryonic death, gross congenital malformation, growth retardation or severe mental retardation. For exposures at high dose rates, severe mental retardation has been shown for exposure occurring during the 8th–15th week and to a lesser degree during the 16th–25th week after conception. The threshold dose is estimated to be around 0.4 Gy between the 8th and 15th week and 0.1–0.2 Gy between the 16th and 25th, respectively.[21]

Central nervous system

The acute central nervous system effects are generally reached only when the whole body radiation dose exceeds about 50 Gy. The survival time is usually less than 48 hours.[8,22] Death is believed to be a function of several causes, including vascular damage, meningitis, myelitis and encephalitis. Fluid also infiltrates the brain causing marked oedema. However, any person who exhibits even mild symptoms of central nervous system syndrome would inevitably die from gastrointestinal or haematopoietic damage.

Effects of acute whole body radiation exposure

The effects which are likely to be seen following a homogenous whole body irradiation over a short period (minutes or hours) are shown in Table 53.3. Experience from several accidents has shown that most casualties have only part of their bodies exposed to the radiation. The non-uniform and heterogeneous nature of the exposure leads to variable signs and symptoms and the outcomes are different. Some high localized doses do not present with the classical prodromal signs of nausea and vomiting. This complicates the initial triage and subsequent therapy. For example, in patients with severe but partial bone marrow irradiation residual stem cells in unaffected bone marrow can reject bone marrow grafts causing host-versus-graft disease. This was one of the prime reasons why most of the transplantations at Chernobyl were unsuccessful.[4]

Effects of whole body chronic radiation exposure

In a chronic exposure (measured in days, weeks, months), the symptoms are usually more subtle. The usual feature is of general malaise, with influenza-type symptoms, fever and or diarrhoea and vomiting. Several cases have arisen where people have been exposed chronically to an industrial or a medical therapy radiation source, sometimes discarded or procured illegally. In one case (unpublished), where a radiation source had been taken into a house, it was only after an elderly member of the household died and others started to suffer from general malaise that radiation exposure was suspected. It has been reported that chronic radiation exposures have been implicated in life

Table 53.3 Expected signs and symptoms following whole body irradiation.

Dose	Signs/symptoms	
0–100 mSv	No signs or symptoms	Dose clinically undetectable
100–500 mSv	No signs or symptoms	Expected laboratory findings:
		Small decrease in lymphocyte count in blood (1–4 days)
		Increase in accuracy of chromosome dosimetry from limit of sensitivity
500 mSv–2 Sv	Nausea and vomiting probable, onset usually >2 h	Laboratory findings:
		Diagnostic changes in blood within days
		Accurate chromosome dosimetry
2–6 Sv	Nausea, vomiting and headache onset within 30 min to 2 h	Laboratory findings:
		Early diagnostic changes in blood
		Accurate chromosome dosimetry (*Note*: Lethal dose 50% without treatment ~3 Sv)
		Early diagnostic changes in blood
>6 Sv	Rapid onset nausea, vomiting, headache and pyrexia (within 30 min)	
>8 Sv	Chromosome dosimetry becoming saturated	
	Gastrointestinal syndrome – diarrhoea	
10 s of Sv	Rapid onset of apathy, prostration, convulsions and death	

shortening, accelerated ageing and premature atherosclerosis, but the evidence was inconclusive, when the data were critically reviewed by UNSCEAR in 2006. They concluded that while there was an increase in circulatory diseases at doses in excess of several grays, the evidence for an association in the range of 1–2 Gy comes only from the atomic bomb survivors and that at lower doses there was not sufficient evidence to establish a causal relationship. For other non-cancer diseases, there was even less evidence of a radiation dose–response relationship.[23] Chronic fatigue has also been reported in other accidents and is a characteristic seen in patients who have undergone radiotherapy.[24] Some researchers consider that a chronic radiation syndrome exists; however, the signs and symptoms are non-specific and do not present as a defined syndrome. In many places where these complaints have been reported, other environmental hazards exist, such as extensive environmental heavy metal contamination.

Effects of partial body exposure to radiation

In almost all partial body exposures, whether acute or chronic, the skin will be affected. Table 53.4 shows the severity of skin damage with increasing dose. The effects would only be seen in accident situations or where flagrant breaches of safety practices have occurred.[25] Depending on the type of exposure, deeper tissues may also be affected. Incidents where small sources have been carried in shirt pockets for short periods have given rise to exceptional doses (measured in hundreds of Gy) leading to serious necrotic lesions of the chest wall.

STOCHASTIC EFFECTS

Carcinogenesis

Following irradiation, a viable but modified somatic cell may retain its mitotic capacity and may result, after a prolonged and variable period, in the development of a malignancy. The cancers induced by radiation, with or without the contributions of other agents, are indistinguishable from those occurring 'spontaneously' or from other causes. Since the probability of cancer resulting from the radiation is related to dose, this type of effect of radiation can only be detected by statistical means in epidemiological studies carried out on exposed population groups. If the number of people in an irradiated group and the doses that they have received is known, and if the number of cancers eventually observed in the group exceeds the number that could be expected in an otherwise similar but non-irradiated group, the excess number of cancers may be attributed to radiation, and the risk of cancer per unit dose may be calculated, i.e. the risk factor. The probability of causation can be ascribed based on radioepidemiological tables (see below).

A major source of information on the risk of radiation-induced cancer following whole body irradiation is the follow-up studies of the survivors of the atomic bombing in Hiroshima and Nagasaki in Japan in 1945.[26,27] Data have also been obtained for a number of tissues from other exposed human population groups, for example, tuberculosis patients who had high x-ray doses during treatments,[28–32] and from people exposed to nuclear weapons fallout in the Marshall Islands.[33] Risk estimates have also been developed for cancers of some individual organs, based on information on the effects of incorporated radionuclides, in miners exposed to radon and its decay products,[34] from employees exposed to radium in the luminizing industry,[35] and from patients given the x-ray contrast medium thorotrast (thorium oxide).[36] Some of the available epidemiological data of second cancers, for example of the breast, in patients who have been irradiated for Hodgkin's disease[37] are far from ideal for calculating risk estimates because of the confounding influence of various chemotherapy and radiotherapy regimes. A further example is the significant increase in childhood thyroid cancer in Belarus, the Ukraine and the Russian Federation following the inhalation and ingestion of radio-iodines after the Chernobyl accident. It has proved difficult to reconstruct the thyroid doses and so the risk estimates are not yet robust. Furthermore, the accuracy of the dosimetry involved in many of the large epidemiological studies is also a potential source of error and needs careful evaluation. Recent risk estimates are based largely on the Japanese bomb survivor data,[26] and one drawback to the use of these data for risk estimates at low dose and dose rates, is the contribution from neutron exposure, although this forms only a small part of the total exposure. Estimates of the dose were revised in 2002[38] which has led to a revision downwards of about 8 per cent in the risk estimates.

Information of this nature has been reviewed in BEIR VII,[39] in ICRP 103[5] and in the 2006 report of UNSCEAR.[40] These reports assess the risks of radiation-induced cancer, based predominantly on data on the Life Span Study (LSS) of the atomic bomb survivors. Recent risk assessments have used data on cancer incidence in the A-bomb survivors,[27] as well as data on mortality in this population.[26] Where risk factors are not available from the LSS, they have been developed from the many other epidemiological studies.

Table 53.4 Effects of radiation on the skin.

Skin dose	Signs
0–100 mGy	Nil
100–400 mGy	Nil expected
400 mGy–4 Gy	Transient erythema expected within 3 days of exposure
4–8 Gy	As above followed by fixed erythema after variable latent period
	Temporary hair loss
8–15 Gy	Prompt erythema followed by vesication
	Permanent hair loss
>15 Gy	Severe vesication, tissue slough
	Very slow to heal
	Possible site of malignant change

The risks have increased partly as a result of new estimates of tissue doses received by the Japanese population, because more cancers have appeared in the longer period of follow up to 1990, and because different models have been used to predict the risk over a lifetime. However, there is uncertainty in how many cancers will arise in the future as almost half of the Japanese cohort were still alive in 1997.

The research on the atomic bomb survivors in Japan has shown that leukaemia appears first after whole body irradiation, with a latent period of two years and peaks at six to seven years. Solid tumours generally begin to appear after about ten years and their incidence continues to increase for several decades. No threshold is detectable and statistically significant increased risks exist at doses down to 150 mSv.[26] This is important for setting acceptable occupational dose limits (see under Occupational doses, p. 632).

However, as discussed earlier, the cancer risks derived from such exposed groups are influenced largely by exposures to high doses, which were delivered over a short period of time. In practice, most people are exposed occupationally to low doses of radiation received over relatively long periods. On the basis of available information, therefore, UNSCEAR[6] and ICRP[5] have assessed that the risk factors obtained directly from observations at high doses and high-dose rates should be reduced by at least a factor of two to give more realistic risk factors for low doses and dose rates. The risk factor or lifetime fatality probability coefficient from ICRP for a reference population of both sexes and of working age is 4.1×10^{-2}/Sv for the sum of all fatal malignancies, i.e. a dose of 1 Sv in a working lifetime results in a 4 per cent chance of a fatal cancer occurring.[5] More recent epidemiological studies involving lower dose exposures from the UK National Registry for Radiation Workers have shown that the leukaemia incidence trend with dose is consistent with the ICRP risk estimates.[41]

Probability of causation

The concept of the probability of causation (*PC*) has been developed to answer the question: if a person has been exposed to ionizing radiation and subsequently develops a cancer, what is the probability that the cancer was due to the earlier exposure? The US National Institutes of Health[42] used data on the Japanese atomic bomb survivors to compile tables on the probability of causation relating an individual's cancer to a prior radiation dose. This topic has also been reviewed by the International Atomic Energy Agency (IAEA).[43] In essence, the probability that a radiation dose to an organ of a person's body leads to the subsequent development of cancer can generally be calculated as:

$$PC = \frac{ERR}{(1+ERR)}$$

where *ERR* is the excess relative risk associated with the exposure, i.e. *ERR* is the relative increase in risk, with the value 1 subtracted. For example, an *ERR* of 1 represents a doubling of the risk, relative to that in the absence of exposure. This gives a probability of causation of

$$PC = 1/(1 + 1) = 0.5$$

i.e. a 50 per cent chance that the cancer was induced by radiation. The *ERR* can depend on a number of factors. Among them, the size of the radiation dose is very important. Generally, the *ERR* varies in direct proportion to the dose, although in some circumstances the trend in risk with dose is more complex. For example, data on the Japanese survivors indicate that the risk of leukaemia varies not as a simple linear function of dose, but according to both linear and quadratic functions of dose. As well as dose, *ERR* can be affected by factors such as sex, the age at which the exposure occurred, and the time between exposure and the development of the disease. For example, for leukaemia and for many solid cancers, data from the Japanese survivors and other studies indicate that the *ERR* is greater for exposure in childhood than in adulthood. Also, the *ERR* for leukaemia tends to be higher soon after exposure than at later times whereas – at least for exposures in adulthood – the *ERR* of solid cancers is fairly stable over time. The degree to which the dose was protracted may also need to be taken in calculating the *ERR*, since various animal studies have suggested that, for a given total dose, radiation risks may be higher if received acutely rather than over a prolonged period.

For a given exposure scenario, i.e. the size of the dose, the sex of the person exposed, the age of exposure, the time between exposure and the onset of disease, the degree of dose protraction, it is therefore possible using models such as those developed by the US BEIR VII Committee[39] to derive an estimate of the *ERR*. This can then be used, via the approach described above to estimate the *PC*. However, in instances where the dose is not known or where there are differing views about its magnitude, the calculation can be reversed to obtain the dose required to produce a given value for *PC*. For example, it was explained earlier than a 50 per cent probability of causation (i.e. a *PC* of 0.5) corresponds to an *ERR* of 1. For a given person and a likely time of exposure, it is then possible using a standard risk model to derive an estimate of the dose required to give such an *ERR*. This approach could be used to calculate the doses required to attain various values for the *PC* in individual employees who have cancer.

In the United Kingdom, the nuclear industry has set up a no-fault compensation scheme based on *PC* calculations, to avoid unnecessary litigation and allow the current scientific risk factors to be used in a generous manner for those claiming a radiation-induced cancer.

Hereditary effects

The other main late effect of radiation is the concept of hereditary damage and arises through irradiation of the germ cells. Ionizing radiation induces mutations which are frequently harmful in the germ cells or their precursors. The hereditary diseases that mutations may cause range from afflictions, such as colour blindness or minor disorders of metabolism (e.g. disorders of amino acid metabolism) to serious defects which may cause early death or severe mental retardation (e.g. Down's syndrome).

The study of genetic or hereditary effects caused by radiation is even more difficult than the study of cancer. However, no conclusive evidence for hereditary effects attributable to exposure to radiation has been found in human offspring.[6,44] Genetic and cytogenetic studies of the progeny born to the atomic bomb survivors in Japan have so far yielded no evidence of a statistically significant increase in severe hereditary defects.[45] Extensive studies made on experimental animals provide some information of the frequency with which genetic effects, including chromosome aberrations (numerical or structural) and mutations of genes (dominant and recessive), can be expected to occur. The research so far suggests that the doubling dose for all genetic effects is around 1–1.5 Gy.[46] ICRP estimates that for exposures at low dose rates, the radiation detriment due to hereditary effects is a few per cent of the corresponding detriment for cancer.[5]

Follow up of the atomic bomb survivors and their offspring has not yielded evidence for a statistically significant excess of malignancy in those children conceived after exposure;[47] a study in the UK suggested a link between paternal occupational exposure to radiation at the Sellafield nuclear reprocessing plant (West Cumbria, UK) and the incidence of leukaemia in the offspring.[48] However, this finding has generally not been confirmed in other studies and the UK Committee on the Medical Aspects of Radiation in the Environment (COMARE) has concluded that those excesses that have been reported may be associated with lifestyle factors, work practices or population mixing.[49]

BIOLOGICAL BASIS FOR RADIATION EFFECTS

It is generally accepted that for carcinogenesis, the cellular DNA of the genome is the critical molecule. Damage to this molecule leading to cancer can be mediated through direct ionization by the radiation or by its indirect action in the formation of free radicals in the fluid in close proximity to the genome. This indirect effect accounts for about two-thirds of the biological effect in the case of low LET radiation, but the direct effect predominates with high LET radiation. Evidence is building that there are fragile sites unusually prone to breakage and rearrangement in DNA, which could explain particular sensitivities.

In some medical conditions, such as ataxia telangiectasia and Li-Fraumeni syndrome, there exist genetic defects in cell repair mechanisms which produce an increase in individual sensitivity to ionizing radiation. At high doses, cell death will predominate leading to organ malfunction, whose severity is dependent on the dose.

FACTORS INFLUENCING RADIOSENSITIVITY AND MODIFICATION OF EFFECTS OF EXPOSURE

Susceptibility to the carcinogenic effects of radiation is summarized in BEIR VII,[39] and can be affected by a number of factors, such as genetic constitution, sex, age, physiological state, smoking habits, drugs and various other physical and chemical agents. The genetic basis of some diseases including increased cancer susceptibility is becoming clearer. For example, it has been shown that the full expression of ataxia telangiectasia, including enhanced cancer susceptibility, results from homozygous mutated genes on chromosome. In addition, the heterozygous carriers, who do not express the full-blown disease, are known to be subject to a higher cancer incidence, especially for breast cancer. This mutation is thought to act through inactivation of repair mechanisms.[50,51] The mechanisms through which these factors influence the radiosensitivity are, however, not fully understood. They depend on the particular type of cancer, the tissue at risk and the specific modifying factor under consideration.

Cancer rates are highly age dependent and, in general, increase exponentially in older age groups. The expression of radiogenic cancers varies with age in a similar way, so that the age-dependent increase in the excess risk of radiogenic cancer is conventionally expressed in terms of relative risk; that is, the increased risk tends to be proportional to the baseline risk in the same age interval. However, in some cases such as breast cancer, the change in the baseline cancer rate with age is more complicated. For lung cancer, the situation is also not simple. Smoking and prolonged exposure to inhaled α-particle emitters interact synergistically and this is then said to be a multiplicative effect.

For lung cancer and most other non-sex-specific solid cancers, it is unclear how a person's sex affects the risk of radiogenic cancer. In general, baseline rates for such cancer in males exceed those in females, possibly because of increased exposure to carcinogens and promoters in occupational activities and lifestyle factors, such as increased smoking and consumption of alcohol. While sex-specific excess rates of cancer can generally be modelled adequately as being proportional to the corresponding sex-specific baseline rates, in many cases an additive excess risk model fits the data equally, that is, the number of radiation-induced cancer per unit dose is nearly the same in both sexes.

For example, as it is known, the carcinogenic process includes the successive stages of initiation, promotion and progression. The promotion phase, appears to be particularly sensitive to cigarette smoking.

SOURCES AND MAGNITUDES OF HUMAN EXPOSURE

Cosmic radiation

Cosmic rays come mainly from our galaxy and some come from outside it. In addition, they may arise from the sun in bursts during solar flares. The numbers of cosmic rays entering the earth's atmosphere are also affected by the earth's magnetic field: more enter near the poles than at the equator. As they penetrate the atmosphere, they are gradually absorbed, so that the dose decreases as altitude decreases. The average annual dose from cosmic rays at ground level in the UK is about 0.3 mSv. The intensity of cosmic rays for a typical flying altitude is greater than on the ground and also varies with latitude.

Gamma rays from the earth

All materials in the earth's crust are radioactive. For example, uranium is dispersed throughout the soil and rock at various low concentrations around a few parts per million (ppm). Potassium-40 constitutes 120 ppm of the stable element, which in turn makes up 2.4 per cent by weight of the earth's crust. The γ-rays are emitted by the radionuclides in the earth and since building materials are extracted from the earth, they too are radioactive, and people are irradiated indoors as well as outdoors. Doses are affected by the geology of the area and the structure of the buildings, but the average dose from earth γ-rays in the United Kingdom is about 0.35 mSv in a year.

Radon

The average annual effective dose in the UK from radon decay products is estimated to be 1.3 mSv. There are pronounced variations about this mean, and in some dwellings the dose to the occupants was found to be more than two orders of magnitude higher (range 0.1–500 mSv). The indoor radon levels depend on the geology of the area and also building structures. Poorly ventilated properties or workplaces, e.g. mines, have higher levels (see Chapter 36, Uranium, p. 243). Radon-affected areas have been identified in Cornwall, Devon, Derbyshire, Northamptonshire and Somerset and in parts of Scotland and Northern Ireland. The UK action level for radon in homes is 200 Bq/m^3. A lifetime exposure in dwellings at this level would lead to a 50 per cent increase in fatal lung cancer. Among smokers and non-smokers combined, about 6 per cent of deaths in the UK are due to lung cancer. A lifetime exposure at the UK action level of 200 Bq/m^3 would increase the risk of fatal lung cancer from 6 to 9 per cent. Many other parts of the world have higher radon levels (e.g. Finland and Germany). A number of large pooled studies of residential radon exposure have validated the risk of residential radon.[52–54]

Activity in diet

Other radionuclides from the uranium and thorium series are present in air, food and water, in particular lead-210 and polonium-210 which irradiate the body internally. Potassium-40 is taken into the body in the diet and is the major source of internal irradiation apart from radon decay products. A number of radionuclides, such as carbon-14, are created in the atmosphere by cosmic rays, and these also contribute to internal irradiation. The average annual dose from these sources of internal radiation in the UK is estimated to be 0.25 mSv in a year.

Total doses

The total dose from radiation of natural origin is, on average, about 2.2 mSv in a year in the UK. Differences in average doses from one locality to another may exceed 10 mSv in a year, and differences in individual doses may exceed 100 mSv in a year owing to the existence of dwellings with particularly high concentrations of radon.

Occupational exposures

Radiation is used in electricity generation (nuclear power), general industry (primarily for process and quality control), and for diagnostic purposes in medicine, dentistry and veterinary practice. Furthermore, it is used as a research tool in colleges, universities and industry. All these processes result in occupational exposures to ionizing radiations and in the first years of the twenty-first century, the total numbers of people working with ionizing radiations in the UK was about 34 000 in the nuclear power industry, and about 115 000 in general industry, health, defence and research. Some employees receive increased exposure to natural sources of radiation, the most notable being underground miners to radon and aircrew exposed to elevated levels of cosmic rays. About 96 000 employees are exposed to elevated levels of natural radiation.

Occupational doses

Legal controls (see under Legislation, p. 634) require that the doses received by the more exposed employees are routinely assessed and records kept of their doses. These employees are often referred to as 'classified' persons. A significant proportion of the non-classified employees are also monitored, but the records for this group, who generally receive low doses anyway, are less comprehensive. Approximately every four years, the Radiation Proection Division of the Health Protection Agency, UK (formerly the National Radiological Protection Board) conducts a major review of the radiation exposure of the UK population, which along with public and medical exposure routes, also provides comprehensive data on all occupational exposure. The last such review was published in 2005 and related to data from 2001–2003.[55] It is these data that are primarily quoted below.

In the period, no nuclear power industry workers received annual doses in excess of the dose limit of 20 mSv in a year. Most employees, however, received doses that are a relatively small fraction of the limit. The average dose in the nuclear power industry was 0.4 mSv and the collective dose was 14.6 person-Sv. The measure of the collective dose allows the employer and the regulators to assess whether the total dose for a site has remained static or been reduced and acts as a method of assessing the amount of sharing of dose. Doses had decreased significantly from the previous survey. The averages and collective doses are around a third of that in the 1990s.

The equipment used in general industry is normally well shielded and doses to employees are generally very low. One major exception had been where radiographers in the construction and engineering industries are required to carry out their radiography *in situ* and appreciable doses, sometimes in excess of the limit, were received. Improvements in techniques and vigilance are being instituted to reduce these high doses. The average dose in industry as a whole was 0.4 mSv, but encouragingly that for industrial radiographers was the same. However, 0.67 per cent of radiographers were over 6 mSv and 0.04 per cent over 15 mSv. The doses to those who work in medicine, dentistry and veterinary practices are generally low. In many cases, monitoring is conducted more for the reassurance of staff than to fulfil statutory requirements. To establish exposures, a sample of 26 000 workers in the group were surveyed. Ninety-eight per cent had doses under 1 mSv and only 1.9 per cent over 6 mSv. The overall average was 0.14 mSv, slightly higher than previously, probably due to the increased use of interventional radiography – mainly due to increased exposures to radiologists.

In round terms, about 96 000 people in the UK are routinely monitored for occupational exposure to artificial sources of radiation. Their dose was 2.7 mSv on average in the latest survey. However, the figure disguises a wide range of exposures.

Occupational doses from natural radiation sources

The average annual dose to crew members of subsonic aircraft is currently estimated to be about 2.4 mSv. Higher dose rates were experienced by the crews of Concorde (now out of service) with the result that the annual doses were somewhat higher at ~3 mSv, at the hours typically flown. The introduction to service of long-range aircraft has increased the potential for higher doses for subsonic flight crews, with the possibility of doses up to 5–6 mSv per year for some personnel. However, when ICRP reviewed the most recent scientific information it came to the conclusion that the weighting factor for protons was too high and reduced this from 5 to 2. This would have the effect of reducing doses by around 50 per cent, in most aviation circumstances.[5]

The average radon daughter concentrations in non-coal mines, such as gypsum, tin and fluorspar mines, were generally high in the past. However, the size of the industry has dramatically reduced to under 6000 and the types of mines have changed leading to an average dose of about 0.7 mSv, a seven-fold decrease from the previous survey.

In some parts of the UK, radon concentrations in buildings, such as offices, schools and libraries, are much higher than the national average. Tentative analysis indicates some 5000 premises with levels above that at which the Ionizing Radiations Regulations 1999 apply.[56] The average dose was estimated to be 5.3 mSv with 10 per cent of the employees exceeding 20 mSv. More attention is being given to this area because of the significance of the doses.

In round terms, some 96 000 people are considered to be exposed to elevated levels of natural radiation at work.

MEDICAL EXPOSURES

On average, individual doses to medical personnel are of the order of 1 mSv/year with values usually somewhat higher for radiologists and those involved in interventional radiological procedures. In nuclear medicine, there is a need for protection against ingestion or inhalation during the production, analysis and administration of radiopharmaceutical preparations. In some cases, there can also be external exposure, as with technetium-99 m, which can deliver substantial doses at very high dose rates to the hands of the operator if no protection is provided. The average doses here are around 1.6 mSv per individual per year. Female nuclear medical technicians who are pregnant may be exposed above the special recommended dose limits if they continue their work for the duration of their pregnancy (see under Reassurance, p. 635).

Overall, workers in the UK had a collective exposure of 385 manSv, 3.8 per cent in the nuclear industry, 0.6 per cent in defence, 0.8 per cent in general industry, 2.7 per cent in health, 21 per cent in aviation, 0.01 per cent in mining and 70 per cent from radon in other places.

RADIATION PROTECTION

The main principles of radiation protection are set out and promulgated by the ICRP in Publication 103.[5] They can be summarized as follows:

1. No practice involving exposure to radiation should be adopted unless it produces at least sufficient benefit to the exposed individuals or to society to offset the radiation detriment it causes (termed 'justification of a practice').
2. In relation to any particular source of radiation within a practice, all reasonable steps should be taken to adjust the protection so as to maximize the net benefit, economic and social factors being taken into account (termed 'optimization of protection').
3. Finally, a limit should be applied to the dose (other than from medical exposures) received by any individual as the result of all the practices to which he is exposed (termed 'application of individual dose limits').

In simple terms, this framework is derived from three principles that apply to many human activities, and especially to medicine:

- The justification of a practice implies doing more good than harm.
- The optimization of protection implies maximizing the margin of good over harm.
- The use of dose limits implies an adequate standard of protection even for the most highly exposed individuals.

These three principles overall avoid the possibility of deterministic effects and minimize the risk of stochastic effects in normal operations.

Protection against external irradiation

The general principles deployed in the workplace to keep external doses as low as reasonably practicable are to keep exposures as short as possible, keep as far away from the source as possible and wherever possible place shielding between the source and the employee. This simple concept of time, distance and shielding is practised routinely in all clinical radiography departments with screens, lead aprons and special rooms for exposures.

Protection against external contamination

The use of protective clothing prevents contamination of the skin; however, loose contamination on such clothing will still irradiate the skin and so exposure times need to be strictly limited. Containment of contamination is essential wherever possible to prevent activities producing an inhalation hazard.

Protection against internal irradiation

The use of containment, such as with fume cupboards or glove boxes, is effective and is used at a level appropriate to the level of hazard. Work with α-emitting radionuclides presents a major hazard and these facilities require special detection systems for leaks to reduce the possibility of either inhalation or contamination of wounds.

LEGISLATION

In the UK, the use of ionizing radiations at work is governed by the Ionizing Radiations Regulations 1999 (IRR99).[56] The legislation was enacted in the UK to implement the EU Council Directive 96/29/Euratom.[57] The Directive and the regulations incorporate the guiding principles of the ICRP and the dose recommendations in its Publication No. 60.[58] Employees who are occupationally exposed to radiation and who are likely to receive 6 mSv in any one year are known as 'classified persons'. Those who are occasionally exposed to radiation by virtue of their employment and at levels below 6 mSv are known as 'non-classified persons'. The third category is the general public and the dose limitation placed upon this category takes into consideration radiation doses from natural background. Table 53.5 shows the annual dose limits in mSv for the foregoing three categories.

The regulations require exposures to be limited to no more than 100 mSv in any consecutive period of five years, i.e. effectively 20 mSv per year, and with a maximum in any single year of 50 mSv. This will equate to an annual risk of early death from radiation exposure at work of around 10^{-3} per annum. The dose limits take account of increased knowledge of the radiation risk factors and the present acceptability of risk for occupational exposures.

An investigation level has been set at 15 mSv whole body dose for any classified person and, if exceeded, a local investigation is undertaken to establish whether all steps are being taken to keep radiation exposures as low as reasonably practicable (ALARP).

Table 53.5 Current UK annual dose limits (mSv).[56]

Part of the body	Classified person	Non-classified person	General public
Whole body[a]	20	6	1
Any single organ or tissue	500	150	50
Hands, forearms, feet and ankles	500	150	50
Lens of the eye	150	50	15

[a]The dose limit in any three-month interval for female employees of reproductive capacity is 13 mSv to the abdomen, concurrent with a whole body dose limit of 20 mSv. Once a female employee has declared pregnancy, the employer must ensure the dose to the fetus is unlikely to exceed 1 mSv in the rest of the pregnancy. This is practically interpreted as an external dose limit of 2 mSv to the abdomen over the declared term of pregnancy.

MEDICAL ASPECTS

Classified persons are required to have health surveillance conducted by a doctor formally appointed by the Health and Safety Executive (HSE) under the IRR99.[56] In large organizations, this occupational health cover may include one or more occupational physicians, health physicists, occupational nurses, occupational hygienists and safety specialists, and the workers themselves. The routine health surveillance of people occupationally exposed to ionizing radiations is no different from that for other groups exposed to other hazards. However, the physician will require special training, especially where radioactive contamination is anticipated.

It is emphasized that the statutory dose limits are set at levels well below those at which deterministic effects will occur and so no changes will be detectable by clinical examination, routine blood examination or special examinations, such as cytogenetic studies. For this reason, routine medical examinations and investigations are not necessary. However, routine biological investigations, such as urine analyses, are sometimes performed for reassurance purposes.

HEALTH SURVEILLANCE

Employees should be medically examined prior to employment, and thereafter their medical fitness should be reviewed at periodic intervals (normally annually). The primary purpose of this medical surveillance is to assess the initial and continuing fitness of employees for their intended tasks. The nature of the periodic reviews will depend on the type of work that is undertaken. The frequency of examinations should normally be comparable with that of any other occupational health surveillance programme. Three situations may arise where special surveillance may be required:

1. Fitness for wearing respiratory protection devices;
2. Fitness for handling unsealed sources in the case of employees with skin diseases or skin damage;
3. Fitness of employees with psychiatric or psychological disorders.

Employees who wear respiratory protective equipment in the course of their radiation work, for example, inside contaminated confined spaces, need to be checked periodically to verify their lung function. Employees with skin diseases, such as psoriasis, may need to be excluded from work with unsealed radioactive materials, unless the levels of activity are low and appropriate precautions are taken, such as covering the affected parts of the body. However, there may be a need for periodic medical checks to ensure that unprotected areas have not become affected by the skin disease. In employees with psychiatric or psychological disorders, the primary concern is whether the employees could pose a danger to themselves or their colleagues, particularly in high radiation dose-rate areas and the handling of unsealed and portable sources.

There is no particular reason why employees who have previously been treated for malignant disease should be excluded from work with radiation if they are otherwise fit for the job. Any additional risk of radiation-related disease caused by future occupational exposure is likely to be small in comparison with the risks from the treatment with surgery, chemotherapeutic agents and/or radiotherapy. However, it may be necessary to restrict their employment in emergency teams where high doses in accident situations might be permissible, and essential when saving life.

Reassurance

Two types of employees may need special reassurance by the physician, sometimes supported by other medical specialists. These are:

- women who are, or may become pregnant;
- individual employees who have been or may have been exposed substantially in excess of the dose limits.

Once the physician or the management has been informed that a woman believes she is pregnant, arrangements may need to be made to change her conditions of work. The physician is often the best person to advise management on the need for any particular precautions or procedures to be adopted regarding the working conditions of pregnant women. The physician should also be able to inform the pregnant woman of the risks to her conceptus associated with her work and, in particular, reassure her on all the health issues. Pregnancy does not require a ban from working in designated areas or on handling radioactive sources, but does imply restriction where there is the potential for high-dose exposures. Separate dose limits apply to pregnant women.

In the case of accidental exposure or overexposure, the physician needs to liaise with the management and other safety specialists to ensure that all suitable arrangements for evaluating the scale of the exposure are undertaken. The medical aspects of the management of overexposed employees is dealt with below.

MEDICAL MANAGEMENT OF ACCIDENTALLY EXPOSED EMPLOYEES

As soon as an unexpected exposure is suspected, management should undertake an investigation to determine the dose to the employee. If a dose is established, an injury is sustained, or contamination occurs, then the appointed doctor or occupational health service should be informed.

External exposures

The majority of unexpected exposures are determined to be false alarms, such as the improper use of a dosemeter, and no further action is required. However, once the dose is deemed to have been received, the appointed doctor or occupational health service must be informed. The investigation should include the dose estimates from all types of available dosimetry. It is convenient to divide exposures into three categories of increasing doses.

Doses close to the dose limits

Normally, such doses do not require any special clinical investigations or therapy. The role of the occupational health personnel is to counsel the overexposed employee that the exposure is unlikely to produce adverse health effects.

Doses well above the dose limits

Where the exposure is significantly higher, but below the threshold for deterministic effects, the prime role of the occupational physician is to advise the employee of the risks. Then they need to determine whether biological dose indicators, such as lymphocyte counts and chromosome aberration assays, are needed to confirm the dose estimates. Normally, no further action is required other than counselling.

Doses at or above the threshold for deterministic effects

If the assessed external doses are around the threshold for deterministic effects, therapeutic action may need to be undertaken. In order to make this decision, the overexposed employee needs to be examined clinically and any abnormal findings or symptoms recorded. Haematological examination will need to be undertaken in order to monitor the clinical course of the overexposure. If the exposure is severe enough to lead to the acute radiation syndrome, early transfer to a designated hospital is essential.

The occupational physician should institute the initial investigations and treatment of the early symptoms. Immediate life-threatening injuries, such as fractures and burns, must be treated as a priority before transfer to a hospital.

The clinical management of such highly exposed individuals is dealt with below.

Internal exposures

Where the exposure is internal in origin (internal contamination), the employee should be removed temporarily from the workplace to prevent any further exposure, even when the dose is expected to be close to, but below, the dose limit. This action will allow more accurate dose estimates from sequential counting either of the body, an organ or body fluids.

High exposures may warrant interventional therapy to accelerate the excretion of radionuclides. Such therapeutic measures might include the administration of chelating agents to enhance the excretion of transuranic radionuclides, as for example in lead poisoning, forced diuresis for high doses from tritium intakes and pulmonary lavage for some inhaled plutonium compounds. For plutonium internal contamination intravenous administration of diethylene triamine pentoacetic acid (DTPA) will enhance excretion by chelation. Incidents involving radionuclides, such as plutonium, can only occur in specialist industries and they usually hold supplies of DTPA.

Medical procedures are not without risk and should only be undertaken when the expected benefit from saving the future dose from the incorporated radionuclide (committed dose) outweighs the risk of the intervention. Many of these therapeutic procedures would be undertaken only at a major hospital, for example lung lavage for a large inhalation of plutonium.

The occupational physician should be prepared to administer the first dose of chelating agents (such as DTPA for transuranic radionuclides) or give stable iodine (see under Additional aspects of treatment of internally contaminated casualties, p. 638) for radio-iodine uptake.

External contamination

Where an employee has been externally contaminated, decontamination, by simple washing, should be undertaken as quickly as possible. Significant skin contamination with β-emitting radionuclides can result in radiation burns if not treated quickly. It should be remembered that thermal burns could complicate skin decontamination and both may need to be treated simultaneously. The only justification for delay would be the immediate treatment of life-threatening physical injuries.

It is emphasized that a contaminated casualty will not represent a hazard to the physician or attending staff wearing standard medical dress, such as a gown, gloves and simple face mask.

Some radionuclides may be absorbed through the skin depending on their chemical form, and can lead to internal contamination. This is particularly true where skin contamination occurs with tritiated water and with some compounds of iodine and caesium.

Return to radiation work

Exposures which do not approach deterministic levels need not affect an employee's fitness for further radiation work. An employee should be advised by the physician on the level of the increased risk for stochastic effects. Where their own actions contributed to an overexposure, consideration should be given by management to retraining before return to work. Return to work after internal contamination may be delayed until an adequate dose assessment has been made.

Where there is partial body overexposure which produces deterministic effects, for example, in industrial radiography where the source is handled producing skin and deep tissue hand damage, the employee should be advised on the future risks involved not only in radiation work (e.g. the stochastic risks), but also on future manual work involving exposure to cold and other physical agents, such as chemicals.

Medical records of overexposures

The medical record should be as complete as possible. It should contain details of all examinations, treatment and advice. It will also require copies of any dose reconstruction or assessment performed by health physics staff.

MEDICAL ASPECTS OF A MAJOR RADIATION ACCIDENT

The overall medical role will involve those responsible for the management and treatment of casualties, the provision of public health information, advice on the health hazards of ionizing radiation and the application of any public health countermeasures.

Treatment of casualties

It is likely that most non-essential personnel would be evacuated from a nuclear site as soon as an emergency was declared and before any serious release or irradiations could occur and so an accident, for example to a nuclear reactor, should not result in many casualties. At the Chernobyl accident, however, there was no warning and there were many casualties.[4] Casualties can be considered under three headings.

Conventional injury

These could arise from events, such as fires or steam leaks, or follow incidents and panic.

External irradiation

Personnel bringing the plant under control or attempting to save life, and injured individuals immobilized close to the reactor or plant, could receive significant doses of whole body external radiation.

Contamination

Personnel exposed, either within the plant or in the open, to a radioactive cloud would become externally contaminated. In addition, the radioactive cloud, which could comprise fission products or actinides, could be swallowed and, without respiratory protection, inhaled with resultant internal contamination.

Radiation accident casualties, no matter what level their contamination, will not present a significant hazard to appropriately trained and equipped medical teams. Assessment of radiation exposure and contamination levels or actual decontamination procedures must never take precedence over life-saving medical procedures.

Externally irradiated casualties

Following a nuclear accident, individuals suspected of being exposed to high doses of external penetrating radiation should be managed according to Table 53.6.

CONTAMINATED CASUALTIES

External exposure to contamination

Patients exposed to high levels of contamination may suffer the effects of skin irradiation from the β- and γ-emitting isotopes. This was a significant problem at Chernobyl mainly in those who were watch keepers on duty and in the emergency personnel (fire-fighters).[4] Skin lesions were also a serious problem in people contaminated by caesium in Goiânia, Brazil.[2] Overall medical management requirements for contaminated casualties are shown in Table 53.7.

Internal exposure to contamination

Once in the body, the hazards depend on (1) the elements concerned, for example iodine to thyroid, radium and strontium to bone; (2) the chemical form, for example tritiated water absorbed more rapidly than tritium gas;

Table 53.6 Treatment of externally exposed casualties.

Type of exposure	Possible consequences	Treatment
Localized more often to hands	Localized erythema with possible development of blisters, ulceration and necrosis	Clinical observation and treatment Specialist advice may be sought
Total or partial body with minimal and delayed clinical signs	No clinical manifestation for 3 h or more following exposure Not life-threatening Minimal haematological changes	Clinical observation and symptomatic treatment Sequential haematological investigations
Total or partial body with early prodromal signs	Acute radiation syndrome of mild or severe degree dependent on dose	Start treatment as above Patient requires specialized treatment Full blood count and HLA typing are essential before transfer to a designated hospital, if feasible
Total or partial body with thermal, chemical or radiation burns and/or trauma	Possible severe combined injuries, life-threatening	Treat life-threatening conditions Carry out actions as above and early transfer to a designated hospital

HLA, human leukocyte antigen.

Table 53.7 Treatment of externally contaminated casualties.

Type of contamination	Possible consequences	Treatment
Low-level intact skin which can be cleaned promptly	Unlikely; possible mild radiation burns	Decontaminate skin and monitor
Low-level intact skin where cleaning is delayed	Possible radiation burns; possible percutaneous intake of radionuclides	Specialist advice may be sought
Low level with thermal, chemical or radiation burns and/or trauma	Possible internal contamination	Specialist advice should be sought
Extensive with associated wounds	Likely internal contamination	Specialist advice should be sought
Extensive with thermal, chemical or radiation burns and/or trauma	Possible severe combined injuries and internal contamination	First aid, plus treatment of life-threatening injuries; early transfer to a designated hospital

Table 53.8 Treatment of internally contaminated casualties.

Type of exposure	Possible consequences	Treatment
Inhalation and ingestion of radionuclides insignificant quantity (activity)	No immediate	Specialist advice must be sought
Inhalation and ingestion of radionuclides significant quantity (activity)	No immediate	Nasopharyngeal lavage important. Early transfer to a designated hospital is essential to enhance excretion of radionuclides
Absorption through damaged skin (see Table 53.7)	No immediate	Specialist advice should be sought
Major incorporation with or without external total, or partial body or localized irradiation, serious wounds and/or burns	Severe combined radiation injury	Treat life-threatening conditions and transfer to a designated hospital

Table 53.9 Examples of treatments for internal contamination.

Isotope	Treatment
Iodine	Administration of stable iodine
Tritium	Forced diuresis
Plutonium	Chelating agents, e.g. diethylene triamine pentaacetic acid (DTPA). May be given i.v. or as an aerosol inhalation
Caesium	Prussian blue given orally inhibits intestinal reabsorption

(3) the solubility, generally soluble substances are more hazardous than insoluble ones. Alpha emitters are the most hazardous isotopes when incorporated. Particle size is important in inhalation, smaller particles penetrating deeper into the lungs than larger ones and overall the stay time in body (effective half-life) which is determined by a combination of the radioactive decay or half-life ($t_{1/2}$ (physical) and the biological half-life ($t_{1/2}$ (biol)):

$$\text{Formula: } t_{\frac{1}{2}}(\text{effective}) + \frac{t_{\frac{1}{2}}(\text{biol}) \times t_{\frac{1}{2}}(\text{physical})}{t_{\frac{1}{2}}(\text{biol}) + t_{\frac{1}{2}}(\text{physical})}$$

The overall management aspects of treating internally contaminated patients are shown in Table 53.8. Examples for accelerating the decorporation of some isotopes in internally contaminated patients are shown in Table 53.9.

ADDITIONAL ASPECTS OF TREATMENT OF INTERNALLY CONTAMINATED CASUALTIES

Once radionuclides have been incorporated, the treatment principles are to reduce absorption and deposition in critical organs (e.g. thyroid for iodine and bone for plutonium) and enhance excretion. Administration of stable iodine, which is normally in the form of potassium iodate tablets, may block significant uptake of radio-iodine in the thyroid gland, but late administration does not enhance excretion. The normal dose of potassium iodate for an adult is 200 mg orally, but the blocking efficacy depends on early administration (ideally when an accident is threatened and before a release occurs) with approximately 50 per cent effectiveness if administered six hours after the exposure.[59,60]

KEY FACTORS FOR HOSPITAL STAFF AND FACILITIES

Protection of medical staff

All paramedical and medical staff involved in the handling and treatment of contaminated patients should wear simple protective clothing consisting of overalls, surgical rubber gloves, boots or overshoes (operating theatre dress) and a face mask or respirator. A simple gown and mask would be adequate if other clothing was not available.

Designated treatment areas

Treatment areas should be clearly demarcated from adjacent clean areas and have adequate space to allow an initial triage and resuscitation and then space for decontamination and treatment. Wherever possible, only decontaminated casualties should be allowed into the clean areas of the hospital. Monitoring of patients for radioactive contamination should take place at a suitable barrier between clean and dirty areas.

Areas designated to receive contaminated casualties must have an adequate water supply for decontamination and consideration should be given to control of ventilation systems to prevent spread of contamination.

BASIC PLAN FOR THE HANDLING OF CASUALTIES FOLLOWING A NUCLEAR REACTOR ACCIDENT

Reception centre

The plant operators and other personnel within the immediate vicinity will normally evacuate to a designated reception centre taking their casualties with them where possible in accordance with their detailed plans. These plans are usually required by the national legislation, such as the Ionizing Radiations Regulations in the UK[56] or recommended by the International Atomic Energy Agency. The initial medical triage should be undertaken by the most experienced medical staff member available, which could be a first-aider. This triage should identify any personnel requiring immediate despatch to a hospital without any radiation or contamination assessment.

Hospitals

Local plans to deal with accidents should include a designated hospital where radiation or contamination casualties should be taken. Where possible, these should be National Health Service providing assistance within the National Arrangements for Incidents involving Radioactivity (NAIR). This applies to Great Britain (England, Scotland and Wales) only. If the hospital designated to receive the radiation and contamination casualties is not the nearest accident and emergency unit, the local plan should also include the use of that unit to receive uncontaminated casualties. While the plan should include the transfer of radiation and contamination casualties to the specialized hospitals, it must also include instructions to direct casualties requiring immediate life-saving treatment to the nearest unit whatever the patient's radiation exposure status.

CLINICAL TREATMENT OF RADIATION INJURIES

Periodically, consensus treatment conferences on the treatment of radiation injuries have been held.[61] At the last held in Geneva in 2009,[62] it was agreed that four main medical effects determined the treatment, which interlink: sepsis, marrow aplasia, gastrointestinal injury and cutaneous injury. The consensus publication has an excellent summary for the treatment of radiation casualties. If conventional injuries are present, then the patient is deemed to have a combined injury and the prognosis is worse. The World Health Organization (WHO) has set up a worldwide Radiation Emergency Medical Preparedness Assistance Network (REMPAN). Physicians who need advice or assistance should contact WHO at Geneva, who can then suggest suitable therapies and arrange for the nearest REMPAN Centre to give direct advice.

CLINICAL CARE OF RADIATION CASUALTIES

General

- Experience from many accidents has shown that the heterogeneous nature of the exposures tends to confound both the clinical and pathological picture, so that estimating the scale of the radiation damage and exposure is difficult.
- The early treatment of conventional injuries is the main factor that determines survival in patients who have been accidentally irradiated.
- Casualties on admission can be classified into four treatment categories: mild, moderate, severe and lethal.
- Stating specific dose ranges for these categories is not possible, primarily because of the difficulty in converting an exposure to a meaningful tissue dose; however, equivalent whole body dose ranges would be <2, 2–5, 5–10 and >10 Gy, respectively.
- The most reliable prognostic guides for treatment in the early stage are the change in absolute lymphocyte counts and cytogenetics, levels of blood cells, which will give a good estimate of dose.
- The degree of radiation-induced marrow aplasia (reversible or irreversible) may not be known for days because of the uncontrolled nature of the exposure and the likelihood that it was non-uniform and heterogeneous.
- Assessment of the dose, while important, is secondary to the treatment.
- Reliable triage and good clinical care based on comprehensive biological data will ensure the best chance of recovery, provided some critical stem cells survive the radiation exposure (see Table 53.10).
- Professional help may be necessary to treat psychological problems accompanying radiation accidents.

Sepsis

- The suppression of bone marrow activity will reduce the resistance to bacterial and viral infections.
- For febrile neutropenic casualties blood, urine and faecal samples for cultures need to be taken on admission.
- Patients need to be started on broad-spectrum antimicrobials and these should be given until the patient is afebrile.
- Experience has shown that fungal lung infections can be the cause of late deaths, when all the other radiation effects have been stabilized.
- Early use of antifungal agents and gamma globulin for viral infections is essential.

Marrow aplasia

- Following a suspected high radiation exposure, initial patient assessment should be based on dosimetric testing (biological, physical), daily full blood counts, viral titres (e.g. cytomegalovirus, human immunodeficiency virus), human leukocyte antigen subtyping for possible bone marrow transplantation and the administration of haematopoietic growth factors (colony-stimulating factors, such as G or GM-CSF) (see Table 53.10).
- Particular care is needed if the patient has other injuries, such as pulmonary infections, burns or smoke inhalation.
- Subsequent supportive therapy might include platelet transfusions particularly if surgery is indicated for other injuries. Other treatments might include the use of thrombopoietic drugs.
- Bone marrow transplants should only be given if an autologous donor is available.

Gastrointestinal

- Vomiting should be controlled by use of effective anti-emetics, e.g. ondansetron. This relaxes the gut and reduces mechanical damage of lining of the small intestine. Anti-emetics also help to reduce fluid loss.
- Diarrhoea should be treated with fluids and electrolytes and efforts should be made to improve host defences by appropriate nutritional support.

Cutaneous

- Remove all clothing as soon as possible, bathe very gently in lukewarm water, use acetic acid or ion exchangers if surface contamination is thought to be soluble caesium, and only remove contamination mechanically from soles of feet or palms of hands.
- Later treatments might include use of topical creams, systemic acitretin and γ-interferon. These have been found to be helpful in treating the chronic skin damage seen in the Chernobyl firemen.

Combined injury

- Radiation injury is not immediately life-threatening and initial care should address the associated conventional injuries, for example, thermal burns and wounds.
- After stabilization, radioisotope decontamination should be performed before emergency surgery, definitive care and treatment of radiation injuries.
- Collection of biological samples during the resuscitation stages will supplement the initial data collected during triage.
- Ideally, definitive care should immediately follow resuscitation.
- Management of soft tissue wounds requires alternative ways to close wounds, for example, biological wound coverings and skin grafts.
- Surgical correction of life-threatening and other major injuries should be carried out as soon as possible (within 36–48 hours); elective procedures should be postponed until late in the convalescent period (45–60 days) following haematopoietic recovery.
- Treatment of thermal burns should include early excision of potentially septic tissue and closure of the wounds, preferably by skin grafting.
- Radiation burns and thermal burns should be treated differently, especially when using surgery, which should be delayed in the case of radiation burns (see Table 53.7).

ACCIDENTS AND RADIATION RISK

In any radiation accident, the workforce would take countermeasures to protect themselves. This would involve sheltering or considering evacuation. Similar actions may be necessary for the public. Workers and public would also be advised not to eat open foodstuffs. National authorities usually set the dosimetric criteria for taking these actions based on ICRP recommendations[63] in case of a nuclear power plant accident, where radio-iodines might be released and inhaled or ingested. Reducing doses to the thyroid can be effective by taking stable iodine tablets (see under Additional aspects of treatment of internally contaminated casualties, p. 638). Prophylactic iodine was issued to the workforce at Chernobyl and to most of the population in Poland immediately after that accident and no adverse side effects were reported.[64,65] The failure to implement adequate early countermeasures against iodine contamination in the former Soviet Union in the immediate aftermath of the Chernobyl accident has resulted in over a 100-fold increase in the incidence of childhood thyroid cancer in the affected republics.[66] The Chernobyl accident showed that accident contingency plans need to be exercised regularly and that the decontamination of casualties needs to be carried out as soon as possible.[4]

Ionizing radiation is a highly emotive subject and a radiation accident can cause widespread concern in a workplace. Individual perceptions of risk, knowledge of medical effects of radiation and the best methods of communicating these effects to people is important. The former Chief Medical Officer at the Department of Health in the UK, has made some tentative proposals on the language of risk.[67] Many facets of life affect perceptions, attitudes and behaviour. Changes in society also have affected attitudes and acceptability of different risks. Radiation risks from occupational exposures are low when compared with many other occupations or activities (Figure 53.1). Determining acceptable levels of risk is central to the process of setting occupational and public dose limits. However, if the degree of risk that society is prepared to accept changes, then the need for robust epidemiological and molecular biological studies to underpin the risk estimates and, *inter alia*, dose limits is emphasized.[68]

Table 53.10 Important laboratory samples to be taken.

Sample	
Blood, approximately 20–30 mL for the following analyses	Full blood count
	Cytogenetic analysis (24 h after exposure is optimum time)
	Biochemical analysis (serum amylase)
	Analysis for radionuclide content
Urine	Routine analysis
	Biochemical (creatinuria is a measure of tissue damage)
	Analysis for radionuclide content
Stools (for estimation of radionuclide contents)	

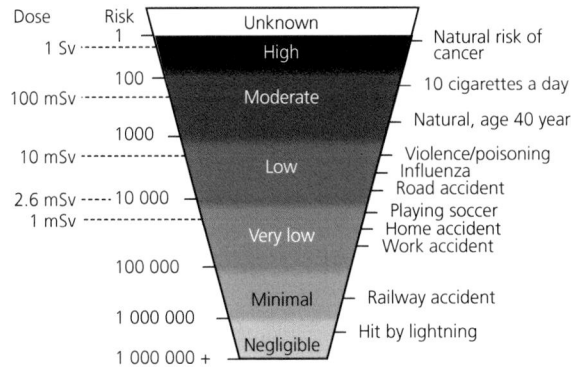

Figure 53.1 Risks – on the state of the public health (1995).

Key points

- Natural radiation and radioactivity are all around us and humans have evolved in that environment.
- The man-made use of radiation in medicine and industry, and for nuclear power has shown that high doses are lethal and early (deterministic) effects are visible and can be life-shortening.
- Latent (stochastic) effects particularly cancer are well documented and risk estimates, based on the study of occupationally and medically exposed cohorts, are reasonably robust.
- Legislation to control radiation exposures at work by defining dose limits is based on these risk estimates.
- Occupational exposures below the dose limits will prevent deterministic effects and reduce the risk of stochastic effects to an acceptable level, although all doses should be kept as low as reasonably practicable.
- The acceptability of risk by the public may change.

ACKNOWLEDGEMENTS

The authors thank Colin Muirhead for reviewing the epidemiology section of this chapter and making recommendations for changes. This chapter is updated from Harrison JR and Sharp C, Ionizing radiations, in Baxter PJ, Adams PH, Aw T-C, Harrington JM (eds). *Hunter's Diseases of Occupations*, 9th edn, London: Arnold, 2000: 725–37.

REFERENCES

1. Berry RJ. The radiologist as a guinea pig: Radiation hazards to man as demonstrated in early radiologists, and their patients. *Journal of the Royal Society of Medicine*. 1986; **79**: 506–9.
2. International Atomic Energy Agency. The radiological accident in Goiânia. Vienna: IAEA, 1988.
3. World Health Organization. Health effects of the Chernobyl accident and special health care programmes. Report of the UN Chernobyl Forum Expert Health Group. Geneva: WHO, 2006.
4. UNSCEAR. Sources, effects and risks of Ionising radiation. Report to the General Assembly. Annex on Health Effects of Radiation due to the Chernobyl Accident. New York: United Nations, 2008.
5. International Commission on Radiological Protection. 2007 Recommendations of the International Commission on Radiological Protection. Publication 103. *Annals of the ICRP*. 2007; **37**: 2–4.
6. UNSCEAR. Sources, effects and risks of Ionising radiation. Report to the General Assembly. Annex on Exposures of the Public and Workers from Different Sources of Radiation. New York: United Nations, 2008.
7. Edwards AA, Lloyd DC. Risk from deterministic effects of ionising radiation. *Documents of the National Radiation Protection Board*. 1996; **7**: 3.
8. Mettler FA, Upton AC. *Medical effects of ionizing radiation*, 3rd edn. Philadelphia: Saunders/Elsevier, 2008.
9. Scott BR, Hahn, FF. (1985). Early and continuing effects. In: Evans JS, Moeller JW, Cooper DW (eds). *Health effects models for nuclear power plant accident consequence analysis*. USNRC, NUREG/CR-4214 (SAND85-7185). Springfield, VA: NTIS.
10. Jones TD, Morris MD, Wells SM, Young RW. *Animal mortality resulting from uniform exposure to photon radiations: Calculated LD50s and a compilation of experimental data*. ORNL-6338. Oak Ridge, TN: Oak Ridge National Laboratory, 1986.
11. Evans JS, Abrahamson S, Bender MA et al. *Health effects models for nuclear power plant accident consequence analysis*. USNRC NUREG/CR-4214. Rev. 2, Part I, ITRI-141. Springfield, VA: NTIS, 1993.
12. Gusev IA, Guskova AK, Mettler FA. *Medical management of radiation accidents*, 2nd edn. Orlando, FL: CRC Press, 2001.
13. Fliedner TM, Chao NJ, Bader JL et al. Stem cells, multi-organ failure in radiation emergency medical preparedness: A US/European Consultation Workshop. *Stem Cells*. 2009; **27**: 1205–11.
14. Trott K, Hermann T. Radiation effects on abdominal organs. In: Scherer E, Streffer C, Trott K (eds). *Radiopathology of organs and tissues*. Berlin: Springer-Verlag, 1991.
15. Becciolini A. *Relative radiosensitivities of the small and large intestine*. Advances in Radiation Biology, 12. New York: Academic Press, 1987.
16. Andrews PLR, Davis CJ. The physiology of emesis induced by anti-cancer therapy. In: Reynolds DJM, Andrews PLR, Davis CJ (eds). *Serotonin and the scientific basis of anti-emetic therapy*. Oxford: Oxford Clinical Communications, 1995.
17. Thomas RL, Storb R, Clift RA. Bone marrow transplantation. *New England Journal of Medicine*. 1975; **292**: 832.

18. Balter S, Hopewell JW, Miller DL et al. Fluoroscopically guided interventional procedures: A review of radiation effects on patients' skin and hair. *Radiology.* 2010; **25**: 326–41.
19. Ainsbury EA, Bouffler S, Dorr W et al. Radiation cataractogenesis: A review of recent studies. *Radiation Research.* 2009; **172**: 109.
20. International Commission on Radiological Protection. Biological effects after prenatal irradiation (embryo and fetus). ICRP Publication No. 90. *Annals of the ICRP.* 2003; **33**: 1–2.
21. Otake M, Schull WJ, Yoshimaru H. A review of radiation-related brain damage in prenatally exposed atomic bomb survivors. Report TR4-89. Hiroshima: Radiation Effects Research Foundation, 1990.
22. Gutin PH, Leibel SA, Sheline GE. *Radiation injury to the central nervous system.* New York: Raven Press, 1991.
23. UNSCEAR. Ionizing radiation. Sources and biological effects: Annex B, Epidemiological evaluation of cardiovascular disease and other non-cancer diseases following radiation exposure. New York: United Nations, 2006.
24. Smets E, Garssen B, Schuster-Utterhoeve A et al. Fatigue in cancer patients: A review. *British Journal of Cancer.* 1993; **68**: 220–4.
25. Lloyd DC, Edwards AA, Fitzsimmons EJ et al. Death of a classified worker probably caused by overexposure to γ radiation. *Occupational and Environmental Medicine.* 1994; **51**: 713–18.
26. Preston DL, Shimizu Y, Pierce DA et al. Studies of the mortality of atomic bomb survivors. Report 13, Solid cancer and non-cancer disease mortality. Cancer: 1950–1997. *Radiation Research.* 2003; **160**: 381–407.
27. Preston DL, Ron E, Tokuoka S et al. Solid cancer incidence in atomic bomb survivors 1958–1998. *Radiation Research.* 2007; **168**: 1–64.
28. Miller AB, Howe GR, Sherman GJ et al. Mortality from breast cancer after irradiation during fluoroscopic examinations in patients being treated for tuberculosis. *New England Journal of Medicine.* 1989; **321**: 1285–9.
29. Davis F, Boice JD, Hubre Z et al. Cancer mortality in a radiation exposed cohort of Massachusetts tuberculosis patients. *Cancer Research.* 1989; **49**: 6130–6.
30. Boice JD, Engholm G, Kleinerman RA et al. Second cancer risk in patients treated for cancer of the cervix. *Radiation Research.* 1988; **116**: 3–55.
31. Darby SC, Doll R, Gill SK, Smith PG. Long-term mortality after a single treatment course with x-rays in patients treated for ankylosing spondylitis. *British Journal of Cancer.* 1987; **55**: 179–90.
32. Weiss HA, Darby SC, Doll R. Cancer mortality following x-ray treatment for ankylosing spondilitis. *International Journal of Cancer.* 1994; **59**: 327–38.
33. Conrad RA, Paglia D, Larsen P et al. Review of medical findings in a Marshallese population 26 years after accidental exposure to radioactive fallout. Report No. BNL 5161. Upton, NY: Brookhaven National Laboratory, 1980.
34. National Research Council, Committee on the Biological Effects of Ionizing Radiations. Health risks of radon and other internally deposited alpha-emitters (BEIR IV). Washington, DC: National Academic Press, 1988.
35. Baverstock K, Papworth D. The UK radium luminiser survey. In: Taylor DM, Mays CW, Gerber GB et al. (eds). *Risks from radium and thorotrast.* BIR Report 21. London: British Institute of Radiology, 1989.
36. dos Santos Silva I, Malveiro F, Jones ME et al. Mortality after radiological investigation with radioactive thorotrast: A follow-up study of up to 50 years in Portugal. *Radiation Research.* 2003; **159**: 521–34.
37. Bhatia S, Robison LL, Oberlin O et al. Breast cancer and other second neoplasms after childhood Hodgkin's disease. *New England Journal of Medicine.* 1996; **334**: 745–51.
38. Preston DL, Pierce DA, Shimizu Y et al. Effect of recent changes in atomic bomb survivor dosimetry on cancer mortality risk estimates. *Radiation Research.* 2004; **160**: 377–89.
39. National Research Council Committee on the Biological Effects of Ionizing Radiations. Health effects of exposure to low levels of ionizing radiation (BEIR VII). Washington, DC: National Academic Press, 2006.
40. UNSCEAR. Sources, effects and risks of Ionising radiation. Report to the General Assembly. Annex A Epidemiological studies of radiation and cancer. New York: United Nations, 2006.
41. Muirhead CR, O'Hajan JA, Haylock RG et al. Mortality and cancer incidence following occupational radiation exposure: Third analysis of the National Registry for Radiation Workers. *British Journal of Cancer.* 2009; **100**: 206–12.
42. Land CE, Gilbert E, Smith J et al. Report of the NCI-CDC Working Group to revise the 1985 NIH radioepidemiological tables. NIH Publication No. 03-5387. National Institutes of Health, US Department of Health and Human Services, 2003.
43. International Atomic Energy Agency. Methods for estimating the probability of cancer from occupational radiation exposure. IAEA-TECDOC-870. Vienna: IAEA, 1996.
44. UNSCEAR. Sources and effects of ionising radiation. Report to the General Assembly with annexes. New York: United Nations, 1977.
45. Neel JV, Schull WJ, Awa AA et al. The children of parents exposed to atomic bombs. Estimates of the genetic doubling dose of radiation in humans. *American Journal of Human Genetics.* 1990; **46**: 1053–72.
46. International Commission on Radiological Protection. Risk estimation for multifactorial diseases, Publication 83. *Annals of the ICRP.* 1999; **29**: 3–4.
47. Yoshimoto Y, Neel JV, Kato H et al. Malignant tumours during the first two decades in the offspring of atomic bomb survivors. *American Journal of Human Genetics.* 1990; **46**: 1041–52.
48. Gardner MJ, Snee MP, Hall AJ et al. Results of a case control study of leukaemia and lymphoma among young people near Sellafield nuclear plant in West Cumbria. *British Medical Journal.* 1990; **300**: 423–9.
49. COMARE Seventh Report. Parents occupationally exposed to radiation prior to conception of their children. A review of

the evidence concerning the incidence of cancer in their children. London: NRPB, 2002.
50. International Commisssion on Radiological Protection. Genetic susceptibility to cancer, Publication No. 79. *Annals of the ICRP.* 1998; **28**: 1–2.
51. Thacker J. Cellular radiosensitivity in ataxia telangiectasia. *International Journal of Radiation Biology.* 1994; **66**: 587–96.
52. Darby S, Hill D, Auvinen A et al. Radon in homes and risk of lung cancer: Collaborative analysis of individual data from 13 European case-control studies. *British Medical Journal.* 2005; **330**: 223.
53. Krewski D, Lubin JH, Zielinski JM et al. Residential radon and risk of lung cancer: A combined analysis of 7 North American case-control studies. *Epidemiology.* 2005; **16**: 137–45.
54. Lubin JH, Wang ZY, Boice JD et al. Risk of lung cancer and residential radon in China: Pooled results of two studies. *International Journal of Cancer.* 2004; **109**: 132–7.
55. Watson SJ, Jones AL, Oatway WB, Hughes JS. *Ionising radiation exposure of the UK population – 2005 review.* HPA-RPD-001. Oxford: HPA, 2005.
56. Ionising Radiations Regulations 1999. SI 3232. London: HMSO 1999.
57. Council Directive 96/29/Euratom. *Offical Journal of the European Communities.* 1996; **39**: 1–114.
58. International Commission on Radiological Protection. 1990 Recommendations of the International Commission on Radiological Protection, Publication No. 60. *Annals of the ICRP.* 1991; **21**: 1–3.
59. International Commission on Radiological Protection. Protecting people against radiation exposure in the event of a radiological attack. Publication No. 96. *Annals of the ICRP.* 2005; **35**: 1.
60. Kovari MD, Morrey ME. The effectiveness of iodine prophylaxis when delayed: Implications for emergency planning. *Journal of Radiological Protection.* 1994; **14**: 345–8.
61. Ricks RC, Berger ME, O'Hara FM (eds). The medical basis for radiation accident preparedness: Clinical care of victims. Proceedings of the Fourth International Conference, March 2001. Orlando, FL: Parthenon Publishing, 2001.
62. World Health Organization. International Atomic Energy Agency Conference. Medical management of acute radiation syndrome: First global consensus and evidence-based recommendations. Geneva: WHO, March 16–18, 2009.
63. International Commission on Radiological Protection. Protection of the public in situations of prolonged radiation exposure. Publication No. 82. *Annals of the ICRP.* 1999; **29**: 1–2.
64. Nauman J, Wolff J. Iodide prophylaxis in Poland after the Chernobyl reactor accident: Benefits and risks. *American Journal of Medicine.* 1993; **94**: 524–32.
65. Harrison JR, Paile W, Beaverstock KF. Public health implications of iodine prophylaxis in radiological emergencies. In: Proceedings of International Sympsium on Radiation and the Thyroid. Cambridge: World Science, 1999: 455–63.
66. Williams ED, Becker D, Dimidchik S et al. Effects on the thyroid in populations exposed to radiation as a result of the Chernobyl accident. In: International Atomic Energy Agency. International conference on one decade after Chernobyl: Summing up the consequences of the accident. Vienna: IAEA, 1996.
67. Calman KC. Cancer: Science and society and the communication of risk. *British Medical Journal.* 1996; **313**: 799–802.
68. Clarke RH. Managing radiation risks. *Journal of the Royal Society of Medicine.* 1997; **90**: 88–92.

FURTHER READING ON MEDICAL TREATMENT OF CASUALTIES

Fliedner TM, Friesewcke I, Beyer K (eds). *Manual on the acute radiation syndrome. Medical management of radiation accidents.* London: British Institute of Radiology, 2001.

Flynn DF, Goans RE. Nuclear terrorism: Triage and medical management of radiation and combined injury casualties. *Surgical Clinics of North America.* 2006; **86**: 601–36.

MacVittie TJ, Monroy R, Vigneulle RM et al. The relative biological effectiveness of mixed fission-neutron gamma radiation on the hematopoietic syndrome in the canine: Effect of therapy on survival. *Radiation Research.* 1991; **128**: 529–36.

Peter RU. Chronic cutaneous damage after accidental exposure to ionizing radiation: The Chernobyl experience. *Journal of the American Academy of Dermatology.* 1994; **30**: 719–23.

Powles R, Smith C, Milan S et al. Human recombinant GM-CSF in allogeneic bone-marrow transplantation for leukaemia. Double-blind, placebo-controlled trial. *Lancet.* 1991; **336**: 1417–20.

Thierry D, Gourmelon P, Parmentier C, Nenot JC. Haematopoietic growth factors in the treatment of therapeutic and accidental irradiation-induced bone marrow aplasia. *International Journal of Radiation Biology.* 1995; **67**: 103–17.

Wilson A. A meeting report (with extended abstracts): CEIR forum on the effects of cytokines on radiation responses. *International Journal of Radiation Biology.* 1993; **63**: 529–40.

54

Non-ionizing radiation and the eye

MICHAEL E BOULTON AND DAVID H SLINEY

Introduction	644
What is non-ionizing radiation?	644
Basic principles of vision	644
Basic mechanisms of light damage in tissues	648
Light absorption by ocular tissues	649
Ocular light damage	650
Acute light damage	650
Chronic light damage	654
Damage by infrared and microwaves	654
Photosensitization	655
Protection against light damage	656
Conclusions	659
References	659

INTRODUCTION

Visual deterioration, whether through disease or excessive exposure to non-ionizing radiation (generally referred to as light damage), is often severely debilitating. Any reduction of normal vision which affects our everyday functions can place a considerable socioeconomic burden on the family and government agencies. Light damage, though less common in recent years due to improved protective measures and health and safety at work, can still result as a complication of occupation. Anyone believed to have suffered occupational light damage should be referred to a doctor for a medical opinion.

WHAT IS NON-IONIZING RADIATION?

The electromagnetic radiation spectrum has been divided into a number of frequency regions. The most useful divisions are between ionizing (x-rays, gamma (γ) rays and cosmic rays) and non-ionizing radiation (ultraviolet (UV) radiation, visible, infrared radiation, radiofrequency waves).[1] The division between ionizing and non-ionizing radiation is generally considered to be at wavelengths around 1 nm in the far UV region. Non-ionizing radiation is that part of the electromagnetic spectrum which does not have sufficient energy to ionize matter, but can excite atoms by raising their outer electrons to higher orbitals, a process which may store energy, produce heat or cause chemical reactions (photochemistry). The wavelengths of non-ionizing radiation of major importance to the eye are grouped under the following headings:

Ultraviolet	100–400 nm (wavelength)
Visible	380–760 nm
Infrared	760 nm–1 mm
Microwave	1 mm–1 m

The natural, and major source, of these wavelengths is sunlight which has a broad emission ranging from far UV (200–280 nm) to far infrared (3000–10 000 nm). However, it should be noted that the eye is not normally exposed to the far UV component of the spectrum since this solar component is blocked by the atmosphere. In addition to sunlight, there is an ever-increasing amount of man-made candescent and incandescent sources which cover the full non-ionizing radiation spectrum. Details of the source and wavelength of non-ionizing radiation reaching the eye are given in Table 54.1.

BASIC PRINCIPLES OF VISION

Visual perception results from a series of optical and neural events; visible radiation arriving at the eye is focused by the cornea and lens creating a retinal image which is then converted by photoreceptors to nerve impulses which are conducted to the visual area of the cerebral cortex. The light pathway to the retina (consisting of cornea, aqueous, lens and vitreous) is almost completely transparent to all

Table 54.1 The pathophysiology of optical radiation and the eye.

Spectral domain		Wavelength (nm)	Sources		Absorbtion site		Nature of damage	
Physical	Biological		Lasers	Others	Tissue	Location		
Far ultraviolet	Ultraviolet C	200–280	Excimer	Sunlight Arc lamps Germicidal lamps Mercury lamps	Cornea	Epithelium	Photochemical	Photokeratitis Corneal opacity –
Far ultraviolet	Ultraviolet B	280–315	Excimer	Sunlight Sun lamps Welding arcs	Cornea	Epithelium	Photochemical	Photokeratitis Corneal opacity
		295–315			Lens Nucleus	Epithelium	Photochemical	Cataract
Near ultraviolet	Ultraviolet A	315–400	Excimer	Sunlight UV-A sun lamps Sunbeds	Lens	Epithelium Nucleus	Photochemical	Cataract –
Visible	Visible	380–780	Argon Dyes Helium-neon Krypton	Sunlight Incandescent lamps Fluorescent lamps Arc lamps	Retina	Pigment Epithelium Haemoglobin Macular pigment Visual cells	Thermomechanical Thermal Photochemical Thermal Thermal Photochemical	Visual loss Visual loss Visual loss Insidious visual loss Colour vision problems Accelerated ageing
Near infrared	Infrared A	780–1400	Gallium arsenide Neodymium YAG	Sunlight Arc lamps Electric fires Furnaces	Retina	Pigment epithelium	Thermal	Visual loss
					Iris Lens	Pigment epithelium Nucleus	Thermal	Cataract
Far infrared	Infrared B	1400–3000	Erbium	Sunlight Furnaces	Cornea	Epithelium	Thermal	Corneal opacity Aqueous flare
					Lens	Epithelium	Thermal	Cataract
Far infrared	Infrared C	3000–10000	Carbon dioxide	Furnaces	Cornea	Epithelium	Thermal	Cataract

Modified from Ref. 2.

wavelengths of visible light (although transmission characteristics do vary with age).[2] In considering the basic principle of vision, we will briefly describe the anatomy of the eye and phototransduction. A more comprehensive review of these areas can be acquired from a variety of general texts.[3–6]

Ocular anatomy

The eyeball is situated in the anterior part of the orbital cavity, towards the roof and to the temporal side. The eyeball is not completely spherical being made up of the segments of two spheres; the anterior segment, the transparent cornea, occupies about one-sixth of the whole surface, while the opaque posterior segment, the sclera, occupies the remainder of the exterior surface. Anatomy textbooks classically consider the eye to consist of three layers: (1) the fibrous tunic (cornea and sclera), (2) the vascular or uveal tunic (choroid, ciliary body and iris) and (3) the retina (neural retina and retinal pigment epithelium) (Figure 54.1a). Within lie the internal media, aqueous humor, lens and vitreous. Since this chapter concentrates on ocular light damage, the following description of ophthalmic anatomy will concentrate on those tissues which lie on the optic axis.

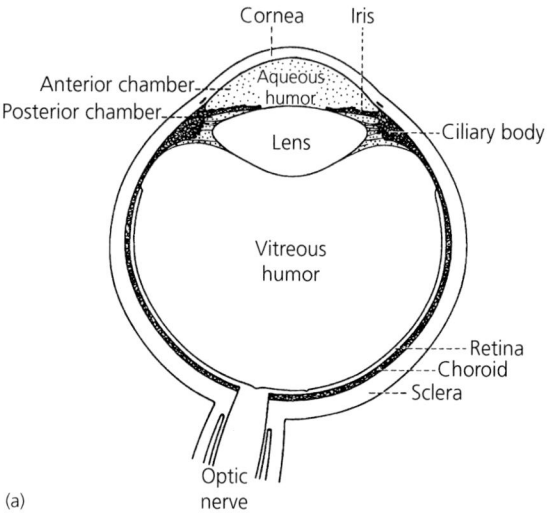

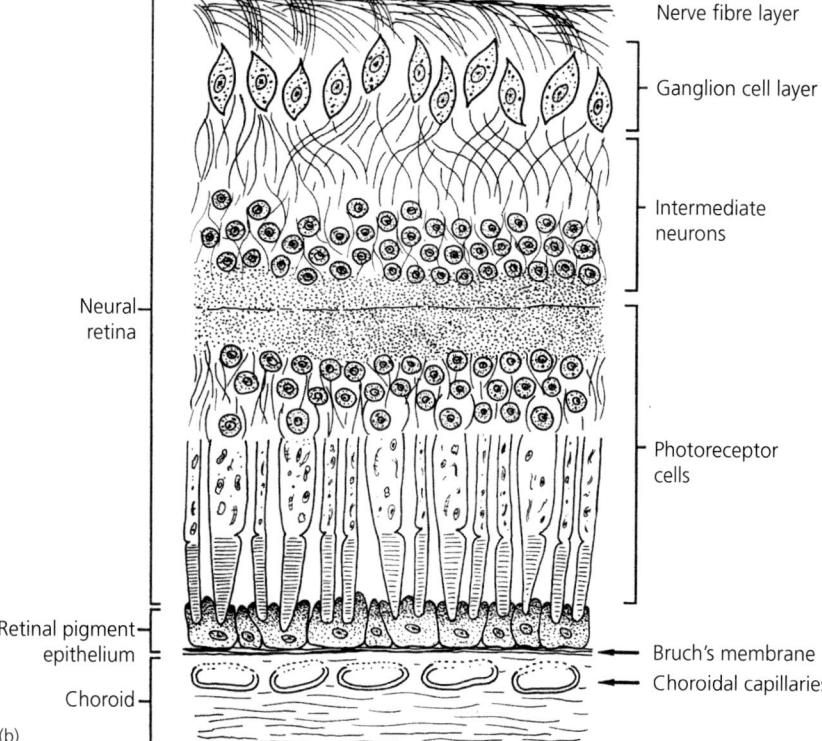

Figure 54.1 (a) Cross-section of an eyeball. (b) Cross-section of the retina.

CORNEA

Microscopically, the cornea consists of five distinct layers:

1. the epithelium
2. Bowman's layer
3. the stroma
4. Descemet's membrane
5. the endothelium.

The corneal epithelium

The corneal epithelium which is located at the front of the eyeball and is protected by the tear film, is a non-keratinized stratified epithelium five to six cells deep.

Bowman's layer

Bowman's layer is an acellular basement membrane consisting of interwoven collagen fibres which is located immediately beneath the epithelium. The membrane is about 10 μm thick and forms a strong attachment site for the basal cells of the epithelium.

The stroma

The stroma forms about 90 per cent of the corneal thickness. This transparent, avascular structure consists of between 200 and 250 flattened lamellae with each lamella consisting of collagen fibres lying parallel to one another and embedded in a glycosaminoglycan matrix. The lamellae are arranged in a definite pattern with collagen fibres in alternate layers, often being at right angles to one another. Interspersed between the flattened lamellae are stromal fibroblasts (often referred to as 'keratocytes'). The transparency of the cornea is dependent upon the thickness of the collagen fibres, their arrangement into parallel patterns and the constant separation between fibrils. Disease or trauma can cause the loss of the regular stromal structure culminating in corneal opacification.

Descemet's membrane

This is a thin elastic basement membrane (8–10 μm thick) located between the stroma and the corneal epithelium.

The corneal endothelium

The corneal endothelium is a monolayer of flattened polygonal endothelial cells whose major role is to control the normal hydration of the cornea.

The cornea is avascular, but is extensively innervated with nerve fibres derived from the ophthalmic division of the trigeminal nerve.

AQUEOUS

The aqueous is a colourless, transparent liquid whose composition includes protein, glucose, electrolytes and oxygen which is generated at the ciliary processes. The aqueous enters the anterior chamber via the pupil whence it supplies nutrients to the avascular cornea and lens and removes waste substances as it flows out of the anterior chamber into the canal of Schlemm.

LENS

The lens is a biconvex structure situated between the vitreous and the back of the iris. The lens is composed of three major parts:

1. an elastic capsule that envelops the entire lens;
2. the lens epithelium which is a monolayer of cuboidal cells which are attached to the posterior surface of the anterior capsule;
3. the lens fibres which constitute the majority of the lens and are high in the protein crystallin which provides the focusing power of the lens.

Opacification of the lens, usually resulting from the degeneration of the lens fibres, is referred to as cataract. The lens is held in position by radially arranged suspensory ligaments, termed 'zonules', which connect the ciliary processes and the lens capsule.

VITREOUS

The vitreous is a colourless, transparent gel which occupies the majority of the posterior chamber. It consists of 99 per cent water, collagen fibrils, hyaluronan, soluble proteins and salts.

RETINA

The retina extends from the vitreous base towards the optic nerve covering the whole of the eye cup. It functions to capture an ocular light image and to transduce it into a pattern of electrical signals for processing into a visual image in the brain. The retina can be divided into two layers:

1. the neural retina
2. the retinal pigment epithelium.

The neural retina

The neural retina contains three zones of neurons, named in the order which they conduct impulses, the photoreceptor cells, the intermediate neurons and the ganglion cells (Figure 54.1b). The photoreceptor cells are located in the outer retina adjacent to the retinal pigment epithelium. Two types of photoreceptor are present, rods (specialized for vision in dim light and do not recognize colour) and cones (specialized for colour vision and visual acuity). The photoreceptors consist of an inner and outer segment and it is the outer segment, abutting the retinal pigment epithelium which contains the light-sensitive pigment rhodopsin. The inner segments project into the inner retina where they synapse with inner retinal neurons which in turn synapse with the retinal ganglion cells. The ganglion axons exit through the optic nerve head and send nerve impulses to the visual cortex. In addition, the neural retina also contains supporting glial cells and the retinal vasculature.

The retinal pigment epithelium

The retinal pigment epithelium is a single layer of polarized hexano-cuboidal cells located beneath the neural retina and separated from the choroid by Bruch's membrane (Figure 54.1b). These cells contain melanin (an absorber of stray light), form the outer blood retinal barrier (controlling the supply of nutrients to the photoreceptors) and maintain the integrity of photoreceptor outer segments by ingesting the spent tips of photoreceptor outer segments.

At the posterior pole of the eye, approximately 3 mm lateral to the optic disc, is a shallow depression in the retina which forms the centre of the macula. The macula is an oval yellowish area approximately 5.5 mm in diameter. The yellowish colouration of the macula is caused by the macular pigment which principally consists of the carotenoid xanthophyll. The fovea is a depression in the centre of the macula and is about 1.5 mm in diameter. The floor of this depression, about 0.35 mm in diameter, is called the 'foveola'. The depressed area is formed by the nerve cells being displaced peripherally, leaving only densely packed photoreceptors in the centre. There are no blood vessels and no rod photoreceptor cells in the foveola, i.e. this is an all-cone region of the retina. The macula is anatomically adapted to permit light to have greater access to the photoreceptors than elsewhere in the retina and explains in part why this is the area of the most acute vision.

In addition to the ocular structures which lie on the optical axis, the eye is also made up of:

- the sclera – the outer, opaque, fibrous coat constituting the posterior 83 per cent of the outer surface of the eye;
- the iris – a contractile diaphragm which forms a central aperture, the pupil, which controls the amount of light entering the eye and impinging on the retina;
- the ciliary body – an annular portion of the uvea extending from the ora serrata to the root of the iris which provides the necessary muscular changes for accommodation and produces the aqueous fluid;
- the choroid – predominantly a vascular structure whose principal function is to nourish the retinal photoreceptors and pigment epithelium; this tissue contains melanocytes whose melanin granules absorb light and xenobiotics.

Phototransduction

Within picoseconds after an image is formed on the retina, photons are absorbed by the light-sensitive pigment rhodopsin, the chromophore is isomerized and the protein portion becomes activated.[7] The photoexcitation of rhodopsin triggers a rapid chain of molecular events within the photoreceptor outer segments which results in the closure of ion channels such that the receptor potential takes the form of a hyperpolarization and a decrease in the rate of neurotransmitter release. The generator potentials produced by the photoreceptor cells induce signals in both bipolar neurons and horizontal cells which are transmitted as a partially processed excitatory visual signal to the ganglion cells. The ganglion cell axons connect via the optic nerve and optic chiasma to the visual areas located in the occipital lobes of the cerebral cortex.

BASIC MECHANISMS OF LIGHT DAMAGE IN TISSUES

While optical radiation is essential for visual perception it can also, given the appropriate conditions, produce tissue damage.[8] Such damage, although generally considered detrimental to visual function, can be of considerable therapeutic value if used appropriately. Radiation damage is thought to occur via at least one of three fundamental processes:[9] mechanical (or ionization), thermal and photochemical (Figure 54.2). It should be noted that although this broad classification is used for simplicity, light damage often results from more than one of these processes through a continuum of photoinduced events.

Mechanical damage

Mechanical damage results from extremely short wavelength light exposures (nanosecond or less) at high irradiance levels causing sonic transients or shock waves that mechanically disrupt the tissue.[9] The injury may be due to ionization where electrons are stripped from the outer orbitals of atoms resulting in a plasma. In the eye, such mechanical damage is normally associated with radiation originating from Q-switched or mode-locked lasers.

Thermal damage

Thermal damage can occur if incident energy is trapped or absorbed in a substrate molecule resulting in a significant increase in temperature. A rise in temperature of 10°C or more in the retina is considered sufficient to cause coagulative tissue damage.[10] Such damage usually occurs

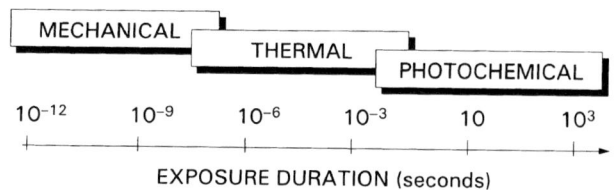

Figure 54.2 The mechanisms of light-induced retinal damage related to exposure duration. Modified from Ref. 9.

at longer wavelengths than for mechanical damage with exposure duration usually between 10^{-6} and 10^{-3} seconds and is dependent on the absorption of light by specific chromophores.[9] The retina contains a number of chromophores which readily absorb visible light, i.e. melanin, blood, xanthophyll and lipofuscin. Typical sources of thermal energy are xenon arc and laser photocoagulators, the extent of tissue damage being dependent on exposure time. The depth of penetration is dependent on wavelength, e.g. optical radiation from argon lasers (457–524 nm) is primarily absorbed at the retinal pigment epithelium, while that from the krypton red (around 650 nm) and diode lasers (790–830 nm) is absorbed by the choroid, as well as the retinal pigment epithelium.

Photochemical damage

This has been the most extensively studied form of light damage owing to its ability to cause damage under ambient conditions and its potential role in ocular pathologies (e.g. cataract and age-related macular degeneration). Photochemical damage is brought about by prolonged exposure (seconds to years) to the more energetic short wavelengths of light, such as blue and UV, which, when absorbed by a chromophore, lead to an electronic transition of the substrate to an excited state with a potential for causing tissue damage.[9]

Although photochemical damage is reported to occur in most ocular structures, it has been most studied in the lens and the retina.[11] The interactions of endogenous, as well as exogenous, biomolecules with UV radiation has demonstrated that the major UV absorbers in the lens are free or bound aromatic amino acids, as well as numerous age pigments and fluorophores.[11] Photochemical changes in the lens appear to be cumulative and certainly contribute to ageing changes and the development of cortical cataract.[12]

Retinal photochemical damage is currently classified as either type 1 or type 2 on the basis of animal studies.[9] Type 1 damage is caused by prolonged exposure (hours or days) to low irradiances, which at threshold result in damage to the retinal photoreceptors. The action spectra of type 1 damage corresponds reasonably with the absorption spectrum of the visual pigments thus supporting the view that these pigments are the prime chromophores responsible for the generation of type 1 damage.[13] By contrast type 2 damage is considered to originate in the retinal pigment epithelium and appears to correlate with relatively higher retinal irradiances than for type 1 damage delivered over shorter time spans (seconds to minutes).[14] However, current evidence suggests that prolonged exposure to low retinal irradiances can result in cumulative damage similar to that of type 2 (see Chronic light damage, p. 654). Ham and colleagues[15,16] measured the action spectrum of type 2 damage and reported that its sensitivity increased with decreasing wavelength, a feature which led to this type of damage being referred to as 'blue light damage'. Melanin in the retinal pigment epithelium has been proposed as the major chromophore, although more recent evidence suggest that the age-pigment lipofuscin which accumulates within retinal pigment epithelium cells with age may be the primary chromophore in man.[17]

LIGHT ABSORPTION BY OCULAR TISSUES

Visual perception results from a response to visible radiation (400–780 nm) reaching the retina. The light pathway to the retina is almost completely transparent to all wavelengths of visible light (although transmission characteristics do change with age). However, these 'transparent' tissues do have the ability to absorb varying amounts of non-ionizing radiation normally present in the environment.[2,11] Thus, the various structures of the eye can also be considered as a consecutive series of spectral filters with each component absorbing exclusive wavelengths and preventing/reducing the likelihood of retinal photodamage (Figure 54.3).[18] Table 54.1 provides details of spectral domain, wavelength, non-ionizing radiation sources, absorption site and type of light damage for different ocular tissues.

All non-ionizing radiation below approximately 295 nm is cut off by the cornea and does not reach the lens. The cornea is thus capable of absorbing the UV-C (100–280 nm) and the short wavelengths in the UV-B between 280 and 295 nm. It should be noted that the cornea is only exposed to UV-C from artificial non-ionizing radiation sources since this solar component is blocked by the atmosphere. The lens absorbs strongly in the long UV-B (300–315 nm) and the full UV-A (315–400 nm); appreciable irradiances of UV-B and UV-A reach the retina only in aphakic eyes. Both the cornea and the lens absorb in the infrared (1400–10 000 nm). Neither the aqueous nor the vitreous demonstrates any significant absorption of radiant energy

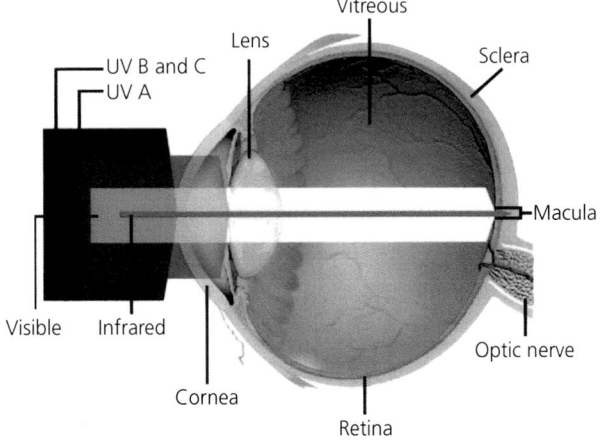

Figure 54.3 The penetration/absorption of ultraviolet, visible and infrared radiation by the different structures of the eye.

under non-pathological conditions. Thus, the light reaching the retina is the so-called 'visible component' of the electromagnetic spectrum (380–760 nm). The most obvious absorber in the retina is the visual pigment which has a broad band absorption across the whole of the visible spectrum. In addition, the retina contains a number of chromophores which readily absorb visible light:

- the broad band absorbers melanin and lipofuscin – absorption increases with decreasing wavelength and thus these chromophores have been implicated in blue light damage to the retina;
- haemoglobin which has absorption properties between 400 and 600 nm;
- macular pigment which strongly absorbs between 400 and 530 nm – this spectral absorption may protect the macula from potential blue light damage.

It should be noted that the absorption characteristics of different ocular tissues vary with age, e.g. the yellowing of the lens increases its absorptive characteristics between 300 and 400 nm with end absorptions extending to 500 nm.

A final point that should be emphasized is that the combined refractive powers of the cornea and lens can increase the light intensity reaching the fovea.

OCULAR LIGHT DAMAGE

Although light is essential for vision its absorption by various tissues can result in tissue damage (Figure 54.4). As discussed earlier, dependent on wavelength, irradiance energy and exposure duration, three different types of light damage can be identified: ionizing, thermal and photochemical. The damaging effect of non-ionizing radiation can be broadly divided into acute and chronic depending on the immediacy of the response, type of damage and the ability of the damaged tissue to recover.

ACUTE LIGHT DAMAGE

Ultraviolet damage most commonly occurs in the superficial structures of the eye and is caused by excessive exposure to UV light (e.g. photokeratitis, photoconjunctivitis).[19,20] There is usually a latent period of up to 12 hours following UV exposure before damage to ocular tissues becomes apparent. The adverse effects of UV are related to the duration, intensity of the exposure and the degree of penetration (i.e. UV-A will reach the lens, while the majority of UV-B is absorbed by the cornea). By contrast, light in the visible spectrum will usually affect the retina (e.g. solar retinopathy, welding arc maculopathy).[21] Infrared damage is discussed under Damage by infrared and microwaves, p. 654.

Photokeratitis and photoconjunctivitis

The acute damage to ocular tissues by exposure to excessive UV is well documented and usually affects the corneal (photokeratitis) and conjunctival (photoconjunctivitis) epithelia. This damage is photochemical and is most commonly caused by exposure to UV-A, B and/or C. The acute inflammatory reaction of the superficial part of the cornea (and conjunctiva) to UV was originally termed 'photophthalmia'. One of its forms (snowblindness, photokeratitis) was first described in 1722, although the condition became more common and better recognized after the introduction of the electric arc furnace and lighting in 1879. Epithelial damage is observed within 8–12 hours of exposure. The

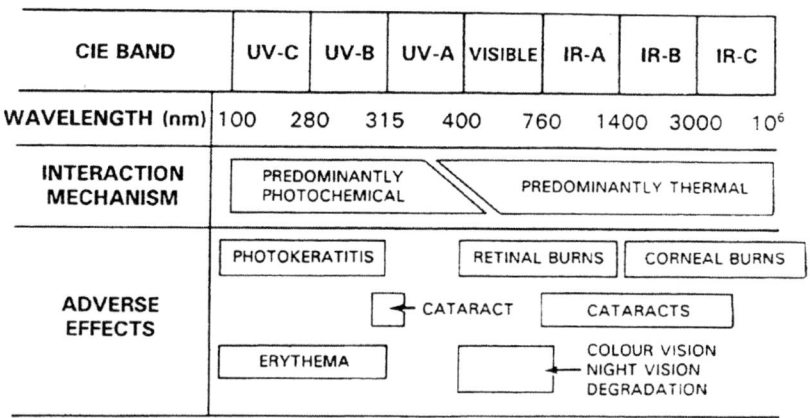

Figure 54.4 International Commission on Illumination (CIE) spectral bands with their corresponding effects. The direct biological effects of optical radiations are frequency dependent. In the visible and infrared (IR) regions, the interaction mechanism is primarily thermal. In the ultraviolet (UV) region, the interaction mechanism is predominantly photochemical, although thermal injury is also present. The biological effects for IR radiation are corneal burns and cataracts. The biological effects for visible radiation are retinal burns, cataracts and degradation of colour or night vision. The biological effects for UV radiation are photokeratitis, cataracts and erythema. UV-A and UV-B also cause skin cancer. Reproduced from Ref. 1.

photochemical changes induce a painful (foreign body sensation), red, photophobic profusely lacrimating eye with pronounced blepharism,[20,22] all manifestations of inflammatory keratoconjunctivitis (e.g. arc-eye, flash-eye, ophthalmia electra, snowblindness, exposure from sun lamp/sunbeds). Resolution takes between two and seven days, depending on the severity of the burn and the patient may be advised to lubricate the eye with antibiotic ointment (e.g. chloramphenicol) and take analgesics during the recovery period which involves the proliferation and migration of healthy epithelium to replace the damaged cells.

Despite the normal use of protective goggles, the most common industrial cause of damage is from welding arcs. It should be noted that damage can be cumulative; short exposures are additive within a period of 24 hours. Individuals receiving repeated exposure to UV radiation over extended periods (e.g. welders, those inhabiting snowy regions) can develop chronic blepharoconjunctivitis (with loss of elasticity of the conjunctiva and band degeneration of the cornea), as well as playing a role in the pathogenesis of pterygia, pinguecula and act as a trigger for recurrent corneal erosion.[23,24]

Ophthalmic instruments

Powerful light from ophthalmic instruments used for diagnostic and therapeutic purposes has been reported to cause iatrogenic phototoxicity in some patients.[25–27] To date, there have been no confirmed reports of occupational risk from the use of these instruments in either the clinic or operating theatre. However, there is a potential occupational risk from ophthalmic lasers.[28] This will be discussed in more detail (see Lasers, p. 652).

Solar retinopathy

Solar retinopathy is a well-recognized form of acute light damage caused by direct or indirect viewing of the sun.[20,21] Duke-Elder[29] reports that solar retinopathy has been recognized since the time of the ancient Greeks; Socrates advised that 'a solar eclipse should be only observed by looking at its reflection in water'. Galileo injured his eye while viewing the sun through his telescope. As detailed by De La Paz and D'Amico[21] the most common cause of solar retinopathy is the direct viewing of a solar eclipse, but photic retinopathy has also been described in association with direct sun gazing by sunbathers and patients with psychotic disorders, religious festivals, military personnel and the use of hallucinogenic drugs, such as lysergic acid diethylamide (LSD).

Retinal damage is considered to be photochemical since sunlight exposure is insufficient to raise the retinal temperature by 10°C provided macular choroidal blood flow is maintained.[30] The patient complains of blurred central vision immediately or soon after (usually within minutes) and the damage is usually, but not always, bilateral. The fundus presents initially with a yellow spot at the fovea which after several days changes to a reddish area with surrounding pigmentary change (Figure 54.5). There is a marked drop in visual acuity with a central scotoma. By two weeks, a red, well-circumscribed lamellar hole (100–200 μm diameter) often with a larger area of retinal pigment epithelium mottling is apparent. Visual acuity usually improves to near normal by six months, although a slight-to-moderate loss in visual acuity may persist in some individuals. A very small central red spot may remain throughout life. Oral corticosteroids have been advocated as a treatment for acute lesions with severe visual loss, but their efficacy remains unproven.

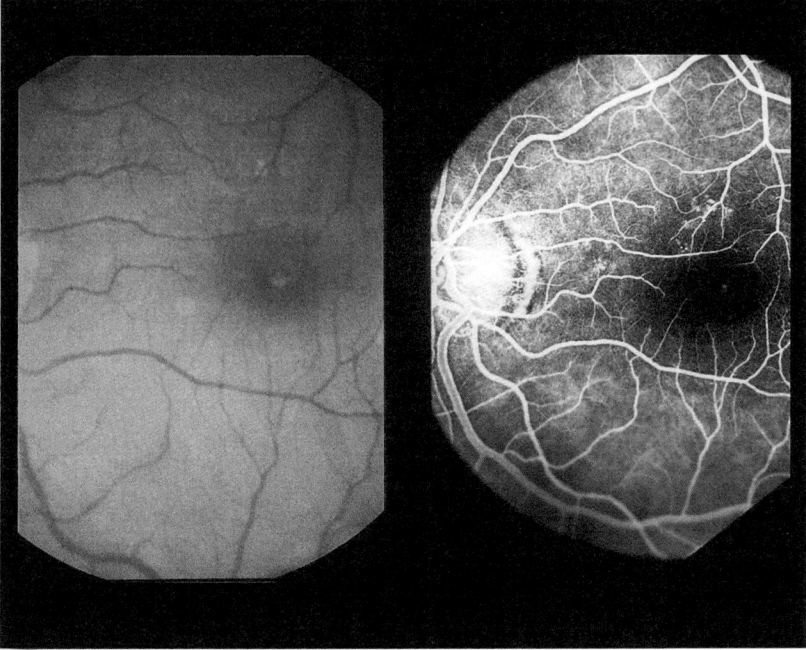

Figure 54.5 Photographs of solar retinopathy. The fundus photograph shows pigmentary disturbance at the fovea and the angiogram confirms a focal window defect in the pigment epithelium at the fovea. Image provided by Professor D McLeod, Manchester, UK.

Welding arc maculopathy

Photic retinopathy may occur, due to photochemical damage by the blue light component of the welding arc, to individuals welding without goggles. In general, patients present with a decrease in vision which occurs immediately or soon after the injury; fundus appearance and visual recovery resemble those described for solar retinopathy (see Chapter 44, Welding).[21,31]

Laser

Laser is an acronym for Light Amplification by the Stimulated Emission of Radiation. Lasers are sources of non-ionizing radiation that can operate in the UV, visible and infrared region of the electromagnetic spectrum. The light emitted has a unique combination of spatial coherence (i.e. all the waves are in step), monochromaticity (one colour or narrow wavelength range) and usually high collimation. Furthermore, the emission may be continuous wave or pulsed for either long or short (Q-switched) duration.

The known effects of acute light damage to ocular tissues are exploited in preventive ophthalmology. Optical breakdown damage from Q-switched or mode-locked lasers are important procedures in iridotomy and posterior capsulotomy. Photoreactive keratectomy is now a standard procedure in Europe for the correction of refractive error less than 4 dioptres, as well as becoming fashionable for the treatment of high myopia and is routinely undertaken using an Excimer laser emitting in the UV-C region of the spectrum.[32] Providing irradiance, exposure time, pulse rate and beam alignment are optimal, the operation is successful, however, poor quality control can result in corneal fibrosis and opacification.[33] Argon, krypton and diode lasers are routinely used in retinal scatter photocoagulation to induce the regression of subretinal and preretinal vessels in conditions such as proliferative diabetic retinopathy.

Lasers are commonly used both in the industrial (e.g. drilling, cutting, welding, communication) and military (e.g. rangefinders, tactical target designators, night vision) settings and there have been numerous reports of accidental exposure resulting in immediate loss of central vision. Depending on the type of laser, damage occurs by either a thermal or mechanical mechanism.[34,35] In the case of retinal damage, a gliotic scar develops and a paracentral or central scotoma may persist. Lasers are divided into four major classes depending on the potential safety hazard. These classes are defined by British Standard BS/EN/IEC 6082:2007 and ANSI Z136.1: 2007.

- Class 1 – non-hazardous lasers; (i) the output is so low the laser is inherently safe or (ii) the laser is part of a totally enclosed system. A class 1M laser product is safe to view without optical aids, but otherwise is potentially hazardous.
- Class 2 – low power visible continuous wave and pulsed lasers which, whether repetitively pulsed or continuous wave lasers, are not hazardous within the eye's aversion response (i.e. ≤0.25 second). Normally only procedural controls such as not directly pointing the laser at the eye are required. Class 2M laser products pose the same risk if viewed without optical aids, but otherwise are potentially hazardous to view with telescopes.
- Class 3 – divided into class 3R and class 3B. Class 3R – low to medium power lasers where the risk is minimal largely because of the extremely low probability of the pupil being large, of all the beam energy entering the eye and the eye accommodated to focus the beam to a minimal spot. Nevertheless, the eye may be exposed technically to levels up to five times the maximum permissible exposure (MPE). Hazard can be controlled by relatively simple procedures (e.g. use of beam stops and ensuring that beam paths are not at eye level). The only documented injuries from this type of laser have occurred from intentional direct-beam exposure. Class 3B – medium power lasers where the viewing beam either directly or by specular reflection is hazardous, but diffuse reflections are almost always safe. Hazard can be controlled by the use of beam enclosures, beam stops (ensuring that beam paths are not at eye level) and, if needed, laser eye protection.
- Class 4 – high power lasers which are not only a hazard from direct viewing and from specular reflections, but also from diffuse reflections. The direct beam may also be a skin and fire hazard. Their use requires extreme caution.

Most laser accident experience comes from careless use of lasers in the research laboratory, with fewer in industry and military applications.[1,36–42] A review of the accident data suggests that at least one type of laser is responsible for the majority of accidental injuries that result in a significant visual loss: the Q-switched neodymium: YAG (Nd:YAG) laser which emits invisible, near-infrared radiant energy at 1064 nm. Although a continuous wave (CW) laser causes thermal coagulation of tissue, a Q-switched laser having a pulse of only nanoseconds duration disrupts tissue by thermomechanical processes. A visible or near-infrared laser can be focused on the retina, resulting in a vitreous haemorrhage (Figure 54.6). Despite macular injuries[43] and an initially serious visual loss, the vision of many patients recovers surprisingly well.[44,45] Others may have severe vision loss. Corneal injuries resulting from exposure to reflected laser energy in the far-infrared account for surprisingly few reported laser accidents. The explanation for this accident statistic is not really clear. However, with the increasing use of lasers operating at many new wavelengths, the ophthalmologist may see more accidental injuries from lasers. Not all laser incidents result in injury, and temporary visual effects are now also of concern.[46]

As discussed, the eye is particularly vulnerable to injury in the retinal hazard region from 400 nm at the short-wavelength end of the visible spectrum to 1400 nm in the near-infrared part of the spectrum.[1,2,47,48] In this spectral

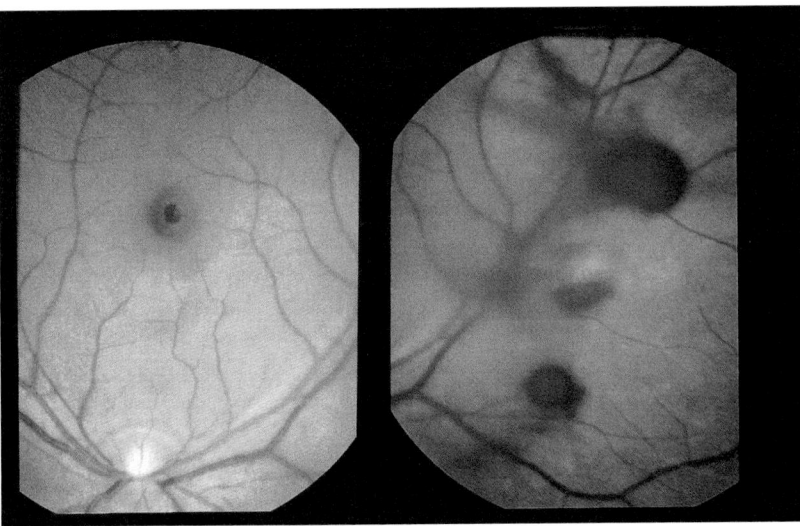

Figure 54.6 Photographs of an accidental laser lesion causing a macular hole, a cuff of surrounding subretinal haemorrhage and choroidal bleeding into the surrounding vitreous. Provided by Professor A Bird, Moorfields Eye Hospital, London, UK.

band, a collimated beam can be focused to a 15–20 μm diameter retinal spot (i.e. much smaller than the diameter of a human hair). Because of the great brightness of a laser, its radiant energy can be greatly concentrated when focused (e.g. upon the retina) compared with the rays from conventional light sources which are much less bright. The gain in beam irradiance from cornea to retina is approximately 100 000 times in the visible spectrum. Hence, a corneal beam irradiance of 1 W/cm^2 becomes 100 kW/cm^2 at the retina. Vision loss can vary from temporary afterimages to a permanent blind spot (scotoma) or even total loss of vision in an eye.[1,44,49]

Diffuse reflections of laser beams are normally safe to view, since the energy is dissipated upon reflection into all directions and the resulting image on the retina is that of an extended source. However, under special conditions, it is a realistic possibility to produce a hazardous diffuse reflection.[50] This can result from a diffuse reflection of a Q-switched (1–100 ns) laser in the retinal hazard region. Colour contrast sensitivity can be reduced in ophthalmologists using argon blue-green lasers for retinal photocoagulation.[28] After argon blue-green laser treatment sessions, sensitivity was reduced for colours lying along a tritan colour-confusion line for several hours. This acute effect was due to spectacular 'flashbacks' from the aiming beam off the surface of the contact lens. In addition, a correlation has been made between the number of years of laser experience and a chronic reduction in tritan colour sensitivity. Appropriate safety procedures have now been introduced following this finding.

Hand-held laser pointers (class 2 or class 3R) have engendered a considerable degree of concern in many quarters because of deliberate misuse by the public. Indeed, in some countries, only class 2 laser pointers are authorized for use by the general public. Claims in the media of individuals 'blinded' by a laser pointer are almost universally over-exaggerations and certainly related to being flash-blinded by the visually bright beam.[46]

Exposure limits

Occupational exposure limits have been promulgated by a number of organizations (see list of Health and Safety directives at end of chapter). In the United States, both the American Conference of Governmental Industrial Hygienists (ACGIH) and the American National Standards Institute (ANSI) have produced a comprehensive set of exposure limits which apply for pulse durations of 100 fs to 30 ks (eight hours) for wavelengths from 180 nm in the ultraviolet (UV) to 1 mm in the extreme infrared. These exposure limits are virtually identical, although exposure limits are termed 'threshold limit values' by ACGIH and maximum permissible exposure limits in the ANSI standard Z-136.1.[51] On the international scene, the International Commission on Non-ionizing Radiation Protection (ICNIRP) published guidelines for limits of human exposure to laser radiation in 1996. The basic resource used for the development of the laser exposure limits was the Environmental Health Criteria Document of the World Health Organization (1982). The International Electrotechnical Commission (IEC) and European guidelines (EU Optical Radiation Directive) are all based upon the ICNIRP, ACGIH and ANSI exposure limits. Although the complete listing of all laser exposure limits is beyond the scope of this text, Table 54.2 provides a brief summary of some of the most commonly used limits.

Screening tests

Although not obligatory, some employers undertake a pre-employment check of a potential employee's fundus appearance and visual acuity. This is largely for employer protection should an employee with a retinal lesion prior to working with a laser develop reduced vision and enter into litigation. Routine screening of employees is uncommon, particularly since small or subthreshold lesions are difficult

Table 54.2 Selected occupational exposure limits for some common lasers.

Type of laser	Wavelength	Exposure limit
Argon-fluoride	193 nm	3.0 mJ/cm² over 8 h
Xenon-chloride	308 nm	40 mJ/cm² over 8 h
Argon ion	488, 514.5 nm	3.2 mW/cm² for 0.1 s
		2.5 mW/cm² for 0.25 s
Helium-neon	632.8 nm	1.8 mW/cm² for 1.0 s
		1.0 mW/cm² for 10 s
Helium-neon	632.8 nm	100 µW/cm² for 8 h
Neodymium-YAG	1064 nm	5.0 µJ/cm² for 1 ns to 100 µs
		5 mW/cm² for 10 s
Erbium glass	1540 nm	1.0 J/cm² for 1 ns–10 s
Erbium: YAG	2940 nm	10 mJ/cm² for 1–100 ns
Hydrogen-fluoride	2.7–3.1 µm	10 mJ/cm² for 1–100 ns
Carbon dioxide	10.6 µm	100 mW/cm² for 10 s to 8 h, limited area
		10 mW/cm² for >10 s

Source: ACGIH EL.
Note: To convert exposure limits in mW/cm², multiply by exposure time in seconds, e.g. the He-Ne or Argon EL at 0.1 s is 0.32 mJ/cm².

to detect; an individual will be aware of a large retinal lesion due to visual loss.

CHRONIC LIGHT DAMAGE

Chronic light damage has been clearly demonstrated in animal models, but is difficult to prove in man; subclinical photodamage is believed to accumulate through a lifetime, eventually exceeding a threshold at which overt clinical damage is evident. However, to what extent such damage, particularly in the aged population, is primarily due to light exposure or other factors is open to debate. Furthermore, the major source of chronic light exposure has shifted dramatically over the last 50 years. Sunlight used to be the major non-ionizing radiation source; however, fluorescent lighting (and even lighting from light-emitting diodes (LEDs) is now a common feature both at home and in the workplace. Furthermore, computers are now commonplace. Thus, an increasing number of individuals are being exposed to non-ionizing radiation from visual display units in an environment of fluorescent lighting. Only time will tell if these changes in lighting sources will increase or reduce ophthalmic conditions attributable to chronic light exposure.

Sunlight

There are numerous epidemiological studies which have reported an association between chronic light exposure and cataract, pterygium, climatic droplet keratopathy and age-related macular degeneration.[20] The most detailed study of sun exposure and cataract was undertaken on 838 Chesapeake watermen in Maryland and a 60 per cent increase in risk of cortical cataract with a doubling of cumulative sun exposure was noted.[52] This observation was subsequently supported by the smaller study undertaken by Bochow and colleagues.[53] Other less detailed studies have reported that the risk for posterior subcapsular cataract is slightly increased in people with moderate and high light exposures.[12] Surprisingly, no association has yet been noted between light exposure and nuclear cataract. Studies organized by a group at Kanazawa, Japan, have pointed to a strong correlation of nuclear cataract and ambient lifetime ambient termperature; whereas – as in the other studies – cortical cataract was associated with UV exposure.[54,55] Severe cases of age-related macular degeneration have been shown to have received significantly greater exposures to either blue and/or full spectrum visible light over a 20-year period compared with controls especially in older subjects.[56] However, the role of light in the initiation and progression of early age-related macular degeneration remains a subject for debate.[57] Thus, high levels and chronic exposure of individuals to all or part of the visible light spectrum can manifest as ocular disease later in life.

Fluorescent lights

Many of the animal studies of light damage to the retina have employed fluorescent lamps, and this has given rise to concerns about human exposure to fluorescent lighting. It is important to recognize that the typical light exposure conditions for the test animals employed ring fluorescent lamps such that the animals (rats) could not look in any direction without seeing a bare fluorescent lamp. Under such conditions, where the luminance exceeded that of sunlight reflected from snow, retinal damage resulted after some days of exposure for 12 hours per day. Such conditions simply do not occur in human activity, where such a luminance would preclude seeing and result in almost continued 'bleaching' of the retinal pigment. It was necessary to dilate an animal's eyes in order to obtain this result in primates. There is no evidence of any detrimental effect in humans to date.

VISUAL DISPLAY UNITS

There is a large amount of literature on the viewing of visual display units and the suspected health hazards. Fundamentally, the research over the past two decades shows that while ergonomic (human-factor), refractive and visual comfort problems are real, there is no long-term adverse effect upon the visual system.[58,59]

DAMAGE BY INFRARED AND MICROWAVES

Infrared

Sources of infrared (IR) (which is normally invisible to the naked eye) include molten glass, furnaces, acetylene welding, the sun, various heating appliances, lasers (both commercial and opthalmic) and military weapons. IR-A damage is predominantly observed in the choroid, retina, iris and lens, while the longer wavelength IR-B and IR-C are absorbed by the cornea and lens but do not reach the retina (Table 54.1). Specific sources of IR-B and IR-C are the erbium and carbon dioxide lasers, respectively. Tissue damage is normally thermal, and in the case of the retina, largely irreversible.

Ocular damage from exposure to IR-A was common in workers involved with furnaces, molten glass or molten metals at temperatures over 1500°C. It was recognized as long ago as 1786 by Wenzel who observed that glass blowers had an increased incidence of cataract. Cataract formation appeared to be more common in the left eye probably due to the tendency for greater exposure to infrared on the left side as a result of common working practice.[60] It was calculated that the temperature of a human lens can increase by 9°C if the eye is exposed to molten glass at 1 foot (0.3048 m) distance for one minute.[61]

Infrared-induced cataract was 'prescribed' as an occupational disease in the United Kingdom in 1907 and the subsequent introduction of shields and goggles reduced the incidence of cataract in glass blowers dramatically, such that in 1908 some 20 per cent of workers had cataract while by 1945 only one case was reported in the United Kingdom in a whole year. Subsequently, the bulk of glass production and foundry work has been mechanized, leaving only a small number of workers, especially in craft centres, at risk. However, a significant problem will still exist in developing countries where mechanization and safety procedures are minimal.

Lens damage appears to be cumulative as a posterior cataract begins to develop after a decade or two of working near high intensity infrared sources. Cataract presents with a blurring of vision and associated lens opacities. Clinically, the infrared cataract starts as a cobweb-like opacity which increases in size and density and develops into a saucer-shaped posterior cataract.[62] The opacity will continue to grow and will ultimately form a complete opacity resembling a senile cataract. Treatment is by cataract extraction and intraocular lens implantation. Retinal damage often goes unnoticed since infrared is invisible and the retina has no pain receptors. However, pain may be experienced if the choroid is affected. Damage is thought to result from absorption of energy by melanin in the retinal pigment endothelium and choroidal melanocytes. This can result in a scotoma which, if at or near the fovea, can produce a profound loss of visual acuity. Examination may reveal localized areas of retinal oedema or patches of pigmentary disturbance, lesions often not appearing until 48 hours after exposure (fluorescein angiography can be used to identify burn areas not apparent by ophthalmoscopic examination). There is no recognized treatment for this condition.

Flash burns to the cornea may occur by the flashback of large artillery and by the flash of an atomic explosion. These burns which are a combination of infrared and ultraviolet are identical to those caused by other types of thermal exposure.[22] In most flash burns, the blink reflex protects the eyes from damage; however, in some instances the cornea is involved. The condition results in a painful eye which resolves within a few days. Treatment normally consists of topical antibiotics if epithelial defects and cycloplegia for discomfort. In more severe burns, there is corneal thinning, neovascularization and scarring.

Microwaves

Microwave radiation is the high-frequency end of the radiofrequency region of the electromagnetic spectrum with a wavelength range of 1 mm to 1 m. Sources of microwaves include household ovens, radar, satellite communication, insect control appliances and surgical diathermy apparatus. It is unlikely that domestic appliances will pose a risk to the individual, but military and civilian radar/communications workers may be at risk of exposure to dangerous levels of microwave radiation during service procedures near the antenna.[1] It has been hypothesized that in some tissues, especially the lens, repeated exposure causes cumulative damage and can manifest as cataract. However, evidence from chronic exposure animal and epidemiological studies have failed to confirm a direct correlation between microwave irradiation and cataract. Acute, accidental exposure of the eyes to microwave radiation may lead to skin burns, conjunctival infection and loss of corneal epithelium, as well as stromal oedema and opacification. Epithelial loss can be managed with topical antibiotics (e.g. chloramphenicol or fuscidic acid) and cycloplegia (e.g. cyclopentolate), while topical steroids (e.g. prednisolone acetate) may also be considered if stromal damage and inflammation occur (indicated by corneal oedema and opacification). Exposure limits vary from approximately 1 to 10 mW/cm^2 in different standards and with animal ocular injury thresholds being in the order of 100 mW/cm^2.[63,64] More recent studies by Kues et al.[65] suggest that short-pulse exposures at 2.45 GHz may produce effects at lower average power densities. Individuals usually recover within two weeks, although some stromal haze could persist for more than 12 months.

PHOTOSENSITIZATION

Photosensitizers, often given as drugs, can contribute to light-induced ocular damage.[8] Two groups of compounds, phenothiazides and psoralens, have been clearly identified as intraocular photosensitizing agents, capable of causing photochemical damage to the choroid, retina and lens in man, as well as experimental animals. 8-Methoxypsoralen (8-MOP) is a typical example of such a photosensitizer which is used in the photodynamic therapy of psoriasis and other skin diseases.[66] Interaction between 8-MOP and the lens or retina results in the photobinding of the dye to these tissues. The phototoxic side effects of psoralen plus UV-A therapy (PUV-A) in patients on oral 8-MOP were evaluated in a large prospective study over five years. No significant dose-dependent increase in the risk of cataract formation was found in the group of patients receiving PUV-A therapy and using protective glasses constantly for 24 hours after therapy to block out UV-A and hence prevent photobinding. Lens opacities have been reported to occur within months in patients who did not use eye protection for 24 hours after PUV-A treatment. However, photosensitizers such as verteporfin, have been used to abolish or regress pathological blood vessels associated with age-related macular degeneration. Verteporfin is a light-activated drug used in photodynamic therapy that preferentially locates to new blood vessels and when activated by light in the presence of oxygen, generates highly reactive, short-lived reactive oxygen radicals that cause endothelial cell damage.[67]

PROTECTION AGAINST LIGHT DAMAGE

The eye is well adapted to protect itself against acute optical radiation (ultraviolet, visible and infrared radiant energy) injury from ambient sunlight. It is protected by a natural aversion response to viewing bright light sources that normally protects against injury from viewing sources such as the sun, arc lamps and welding arcs, since this aversion limits the duration of exposure to a fraction of a second (about 0.25 s). However, sources rich in ultraviolet radiation without a strong visual stimulus can be particularly hazardous. One can force oneself to stare at the sun, a welding arc or a snow field and thereby suffer a temporary loss of vision, which in some cases may be permanent. In the industrial setting, when bright lights appear low in the field of view, the eye's protective mechanisms are less effective, and hazard precautions are particularly important.[68]

Safety standards

Safety standards for arc welding have long existed and specify eye protectors, curtains and barriers. Safety standards for lasers are also well developed worldwide; most following the general equipment and user guidance in IEC 60825-1-2007. Lasers are grouped into several hazard classes and so labelled by manufacturers; the user then follows certain specified control measures based upon the laser class. However, standards for lamp safety are actually more recent. In the United States, the Illuminating Engineering Society of North America (IESNA) issued photobiological safety standards for lamps and lighting systems for the first time in 1996 and lamp groups are placed in risk groups somewhat similar to laser hazard classes. Since then, this approach has been followed in the joint standard CIE-S009 of the International Commission on Illumination (the CIE) and in standard IEC-62471:2006 of the International Electrotechnical Commission (IEC).

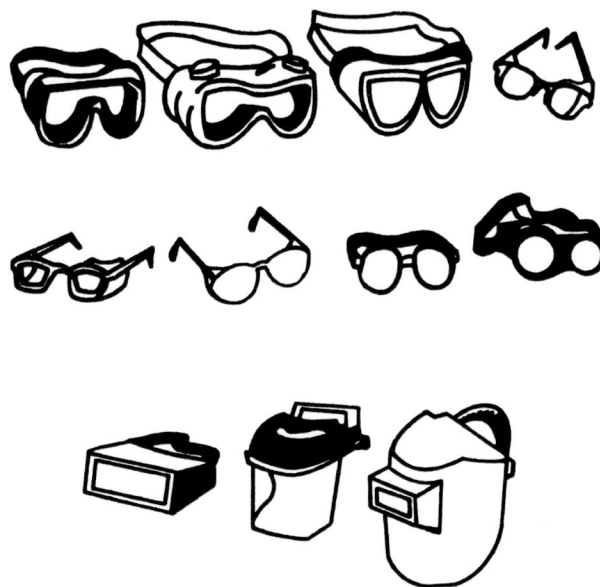

Figure 54.7 Eye protectors. Eye protection for optical radiation hazards are produced in a variety of configurations from spectacles with and without sideshields to goggles, face shields and welding helmets. The choice of protector is dependent on the specification of the optical hazard together with local and national health and safety directives.

Eye protector design and standards

The design of eye protectors for welding and other industrial optical sources (foundries, steel and glass manufacture, etc.) began at the beginning of this century with the development of Crooke's glass.[69] Eye protector standards which evolved later followed the general principle that since infrared and ultraviolet were not needed for vision, those spectral bands should be blocked as best as possible by the then currently available glass materials. Figure 54.7 illustrates the wide variety of design from spectacles to goggles and full-face welding helmets.

The empirical standards for eye protective equipment were tested in the 1970s and shown to have large safety factors for infrared and ultraviolet when the transmissions factors were tested against current occupational exposure limits, whereas the protection factors for blue light were just sufficient. Some standards' requirements were therefore adjusted. Table 54.3 summarizes recommended eye protectors for different types of optical sources.

Laser protective eyewear was developed after occupational exposure limits had been established, and specifications were drawn up to provide the optical densities (a logarithmic measure of attenuation factor) that would be needed as a function of wavelength and exposure duration for specific lasers. Although specific laser eye protector standards exist in Europe, guidelines for laser eye protection are provided in the American National Standard ANSIZ136.1 and ANSIZ136.7 in the US.[30,70]

Table 54.3 Selecting eye protection for intense optical radiation.

Type	Assessment	Protector type	Shade No.	Limitations	Not recommended
Welding electric arc	Shade based on visual comfort	Welding helmet	10–14	Protection from optical radiation directly related to filter lens density; select the darkest shade that permits adequate task performance	Protectors that do not provide protection from optical radiation
Welding gas	Shade based on visual comfort	Welding goggle or welding face shield	4–8	Face shield can be worn over the primary protector	
Cutting			3–6		
Torch brazing			3–4		
Torch soldering	Shade based on visual comfort	Spectacles or welding face shield	1, 3–5	Face shield can be worn over the primary protector	
Glare	Shade based on visual comfort	Spectacle frontal protection	1–4	Shaded or special purpose lenses, as suitable	
Laser specified	Optical density as maximum laser exposure divided by exposure limit	Laser protective goggle or spectacle	Optical density units used	Choose filter lens based on comfort, optimal visual performance	Uncomfortable goggles, users fail to wear
RF/microwave	Psychological	Goggles made but not recommended	NA	NA	Not effective

Adapted from Ref. 68. This table was published in *Opthalmology Clinics of North America*, **8**, Vinger P, Sliney D, Issues in ocular trauma. The prevention of sports and work related injury, 709–21, copyright Elsevier (1995).
NA, not applicable.

Human exposure limits

From knowledge of the optical parameters of the human eye and the radiance of a light source, it is possible to calculate irradiances (dose rates) at the retina. Exposure of the anterior structures of the human eye to ultraviolet radiation may also be of interest; and the relative position of the light source and the degree of lid closure can greatly affect the proper calculation of this ultraviolet exposure dose. For ultraviolet and short-wavelength light exposures, the spectral distribution of the light source is also important.

A number of national and international groups have recommended occupational exposure limits for optical radiation (i.e. ultraviolet, light and infrared radiant energy) (see list of Health and Safety directives at end of the chapter). Although most such groups have recommended exposure limits for UV and laser radiation, only one group has recommended exposure limits for visible radiation (i.e. light). This is the American Conference of Governmental Hygienists who, as previously mentioned, refer to its exposure limits as threshold limit values, and these are issued yearly, so there is an opportunity for a yearly revision. They are based in large part on ocular injury data from animal studies and from data from human retinal injuries resulting from viewing the sun and welding arcs. The threshold limit-values also have an underlying assumption that outdoor environmental exposures to visible radiant energy are normally not hazardous to the eye, except when fixating the sun or in very unusual environments such as snow fields and deserts.

Optical radiation safety evaluation

Since a comprehensive hazard evaluation requires complex measurements of spectral irradiance and radiance of the source, or very specialized instruments and calculations, this is rarely done by occupational hygienists and safety engineers. Instead, the eye protective equipment is mandated by safety regulations in hazardous environments. Research studies have evaluated a wide range of arcs, lasers and thermal sources in order to develop broad recommendations for practical, easier-to-apply safety standards.[30]

Protective filter materials

ULTRAVIOLET AND INFRARED PROTECTION

Almost all glass and plastic lens materials block ultraviolet radiation below 300 nm and infrared radiation at wavelengths greater than 3000 nm (3 μm), and for a few lasers and optical sources, ordinary impact-resistant clear safety eyewear will provide good protection (e.g. clear polycarbonate lenses effectively block the 10.6 μm CO_2 wavelength). However, absorbers such as metal oxides in glass or organic dyes in plastics, must be added to eliminate UV-A and UV-B up to about 380–400 nm, and infrared beyond 780 nm to 3 μm.[30,70] Depending upon the material, this may be easy, or very difficult or expensive, and the stability of the absorber may vary somewhat. Filters that meet ANSI Z87.1 must have the appropriate attenuation factors in each critical spectral band.

FOUNDRY AND GLASS INDUSTRY EYEWEAR

Spectacles and goggles designed for ocular protection against infrared radiation generally have a light greenish tint, although the tint may be darker if some comfort against visible radiation is desired. Such eye protectors should not be confused with the blue lenses used in the steel and foundry operations where the objective is to visually check the temperature of the melt; these blue spectacles do not provide protection, and should only be worn briefly.[69]

FIREFIGHTING

Firefighters may be exposed to intense near-infrared radiation, and apart from the crucially important head and face protection, infrared attenuating filters are frequently prescribed. Here, impact protection is also important.

ULTRAVIOLET RADIATION PROTECTION

A number of specialized UV lamps are used in industry for fluorescence detection and for photocuring of inks, plastic resins, dental polymers, etc. Although UV-A sources normally pose little real risk, these sources may either contain trace amounts of hazardous UV-B or pose a disability glare problem (from UV-A fluorescence of the crystallin lens); UV filter lenses with very high attenuation factors are widely available to protect against the entire UV spectrum with either glass or plastic lenses. A slight yellowish tint may be detectable if protection is afforded to 400 nm. Of paramount importance in these types of eyewear (and for industrial sunglasses) is peripheral protection. Side-shields or wrap-around designs are important to protect against the coroneo effect (focusing of temporal, oblique rays into the nasal equatorial area of the lens (where cortical cataract frequently originates).

LASER EYE PROTECTORS

The objective of laser eye protective filters is to transmit as much visible light for seeing while at the same time blocking the laser wavelength(s) of concern. The protective factor used for laser eyewear is termed optical density (OD). The OD is a logarithmic expression for attenuation factor, e.g. a protection factor of 1000 (10^3) is an OD of 3.0, and a protection factor of one million (10^6) is an OD of 6.0. Since most lasers emit powers or energies of the order of thousands to millions of times the maximum permissible exposure limit, optical densities of 4–6 are most typical. The ANSI standard Z136.1 *Safe use of lasers* provides detailed methods for determining the appropriate eyewear and ANSI standard Z136.7 *Testing and labelling of laser protective equipment* provides extensive technical detail. Although some eyewear vendors and laser safety promoters have argued for very robust filters of coated glass to withstand extremely high beam irradiances of many kilowatts per cm^2, this is overkill, and polycarbonate laser protective lenses are quite adequate (the skin will be severely charred at much lower irradiances). Polycarbonate has superior burn-through characteristics[70] compared with other plastics and is also superior to all other lens materials for industrial impact protection.

At present, prescription lenses in laser filter materials are only available on a limited basis for glass lenses, but there are a number of companies which supply cover goggles for laser protection. The Laser Institute of America in Orlando, FL is a useful source of information on laser safety and laser eye protectors.

Welding filters

Infrared and UV radiation filtration is readily achieved in glass filters with additives such as iron-oxide, but the visible attenuation determines the shade number, which is a logarithmic expression of attenuation. Normally a shade 3–4 is used for gas welding (goggles), and 10–14 for arc welding and plasma arc operations (helmet protection required). The rule of thumb is that if the welder finds the arc to view, adequate attenuation is provided against ocular hazards. Supervisors, welders' helpers and other people in the work area may require filters with a relatively low shade number (e.g. 3–4) to protect against welder's photokeratitis (arc-eye).[69] In recent years, a new type of welding filter, the autodarkening filter has appeared on the scene. Regardless of the type of filter, it should meet ANSI Z87.1 and Z-49.1 standards for fixed welding filters specified for the dark shade.

AUTODARKENING WELDING FILTERS

Autodarkening welding filters represent an important advance in the ability of welders to produce consistently high-quality welds more efficiently and ergonomically.[71] Considering the total welding process, the welder formerly had to lower and raise the helmet or filter each time an arc was started and quenched. The welder had to work blind just prior to striking the arc. Furthermore, the helmet is frequently lowered and raised with a sharp snap of the neck and head which can lead to neck strain or more serious injuries. Faced with this uncomfortable and cumbersome procedure, some welders frequently initiate the arc with a conventional helmet in the raised position – leading to 'welder's flash' (arc-eye or photokeratitis). Under normal ambient lighting conditions, a welder wearing a helmet fitted with an autodarkening filter can see well enough with the eye protection in place to perform tasks such as aligning and fixturing the parts to be welded, precisely positioning the welding equipment and striking the arc. Then, in the most typical helmet designs, light sensors detect the arc flash and direct an electronic drive unit to switch a liquid crystal filter from a light shade to a preselected dark shade. The aforementioned drawbacks of fixed shade filters are largely eliminated by autodarkening filters which explains the widespread popularity of these newer systems.

Questions have frequently been raised whether there are hidden safety problems with the new autodarkening filters. For example, can after-images (flash-blindness) result in impaired vision in the workplace? Do the new types of filters really offer equivalent or better protection than conventional fixed filters? The answer to the second question is Yes, but not all autodarkening filters are equivalent. Filter closure speeds and light and dark shade values vary, as does the weight of each unit. The temperature dependence of performance, variation of shade with electrical battery degradation, the 'resting state shade' and other technical factors vary depending upon each manufacturer's design. These are being addressed in new standards.

Since adequate filter attenuation is afforded by all systems, the single most important attribute specified by the manufacturers of autodarkening filters is the speed of filter switching. Current autodarkening filters vary in switching speed from 1/10th second (0.1 s) to faster than 1/10 000th second (100 µs). Buhr and Sutter[72] have indicated a means of specifying the maximum switching time, but their formulation varies relative to the time-course of switching. Switching speed is crucial, since it gives the best clue to the really important (but unspecified) measure of how much light will enter the eye when the arc is struck compared with when wearing a fixed filter of the same working shade number. If too much light enters the eye for each switching during the day, the accumulated light energy dose produces transient adaptation and complaints about eye strain, etc. Current products with switching speeds of the order of 10 ms or less will provide adequate protection against photoretinitis. However, the shortest switching time of the order of 30–100 µs (0.03–0.1 ms) has the advantage of reducing 'transient adaptation' effects.[71,73] Transient adaptation is the visual experience caused by sudden changes in one's light environment which may be accompanied by discomfort, glare and temporary loss of detailed vision.

Simple check tests are available to the welder short of extensive laboratory testing. Suggest to the welder to simply look at a page of detailed print through each autodarkening filter. This will give an indication of its optical quality. Next, try striking an arc while observing it through each filter being considered for purchase. Fortunately, one can rely on the fact that light levels which are comfortable to view will not be hazardous. The UV radiation and IR filtration should be checked in the manufacturer's specification sheet to make sure that the unnecessary bands are filtered out. A few repeated arc strikings should give the welder a sense of whether discomfort will be experienced from transient adaptation, although a one-day trial would be best.

The resting or failure state shade number of an autodarkening filter (e.g. if the battery fails) should provide 100 per cent protection of the welder's eyes for at least one to several seconds. Some manufacturers use a dark state as the 'off' position and others use an intermediate shade between the dark and the light shade states. In either case, the resting state transmittance for the filter should be appreciably lower than the light shade transmittance to preclude a retinal hazard. In any case, the device should provide a clear and obvious indicator to the user when the filter is switched off or when a system failure occurs. This will ensure that the welder is warned in advance when the filter is not switched on or is not operating properly before beginning to weld. Other features, such as battery life, performance under extreme temperature conditions, etc. may be of importance to certain users.

CONCLUSIONS

Although technical specifications can appear to be somewhat involved for eye protectors against optical radiation sources, safety standards exist which specify shade numbers, and these standards provide a conservative safety factor for the wearer. However, should damage occur the recipient should be immediately referred to a doctor for a medical opinion.

Key points

- Excessive non-ionizing radiation can damage the eye.
- Damage is usually to the cornea or retina and can result in visual deterioration.
- Users exposed to acute or chronic non-ionizing radiation should be aware of exposure limits, safety standards and the appropriate eye protection.

REFERENCES

1. DeFrank J, Bryan P, Hicks C, Sliney D. Nonionizing radiation. In: Zatjchuk R (ed.). *Textbook of military medicine*. Office of the Surgeon-General, Department of the Army, 1993: 539–80.
2. Marshall J. Radiation and the ageing eye. *Ophthalmic and Physiological Optics*. 1985; **5**: 241–63.

3. Hogan M, Alvarado J, Weddell J. *Histology of the human eye.* Philadelphia: WB Saunders, 1971.
4. Davson H. *Physiology of the eye.* London: Macmillan Academic, 1990.
5. Saude T. *Ocular anatomy and physiology.* Oxford: Blackwell Scientific, 1973.
6. Snell R, Lemp M. *Clinical anatomy of the eye.* Boston: Blackwell Scientific, 1989.
7. Berman E. *Biochemistry of the eye.* New York: Plenum Press, 1991.
8. Lerman S. Light-induced changes in ocular tissues. In: Miller D (ed.). *Clinical light damage to the eye.* New York: Springer Verlag, 1987: 183–215.
9. Mellerio J. Light effects on the retina. In: Albert D, Jakobiec F (eds). *Principles and practice of ophthalmology: Basic sciences.* Philadelphia: WB Saunders, 1994: 1326–45.
10. Mainster M, Sliney D, Belcher C, Buzney S. Laser photodistruptors, damage mechanisms, instrument design and safety. *Ophthalmology.* 1983; **90**: 937–44.
11. Dillon J. The photophysics and photobiology of the eye. *Journal of Photochemistry and Photobiology. B, Biology.* 1991; **10**: 23–40.
12. Hankinson S. The epidemiology of age-related cataract. In: Albert D, Jakobiec F (eds). *Principles and practice of ophthalmology: Basic sciences.* Philadelphia: WB Saunders, 1994: 1255–66.
13. Noell W, Walker V, Kang, Berman S. Retinal damage by light in rats. *Investigative Ophthalmology and Visual Science.* 1966; **5**: 450–73.
14. Marshall J. The ageing retina: Physiology or pathology. *Eye.* 1987; **1**: 292–5.
15. Ham W, Mueller H, Sliney D. Retinal sensitivity to damage from short wavelength light. *Nature.* 1976; **260**: 153–5.
16. Ham W. The photopathology and nature of the blue-light and near-UV retinal lesion produced by lasers and other optical sources. In: Wolbarsht M (ed.). *Laser applications in medicine and biology.* New York: Plenum Press, 1989: 191–246.
17. Rozanowska M, Jarvis-Evans J, Korytowski W et al. Blue light-induced reactivity of retinal age pigment. *Journal of Biological Chemistry.* 1995; **270**: 18825–30.
18. Wolbarsht M. The function of intraocular color filters. *Federation Proceedings.* 1976; **35**: 44–9.
19. Pitts D. The ocular effects of ultraviolet radiation. *American Journal of Optometry and Physiological Optics.* 1978; **55**: 19–35.
20. Roh S, Weiter J. Light damage of the eye. *Journal of the Florida Medical Association.* 1994; **81**: 248–51.
21. De La Paz M, D'Amico D. Photic retinopathy. In: Albert D, Jakobiec F (eds). *Principles and practice of ophthalmology: Basic sciences*, vol. 2. Philadelphia: WB Saunders, 1994: 1032–7.
22. Parrish CM, Chandler JW. Corneal trauma. In: Kaufmann H, Barron B, McDonald M, Waltman S (eds). *The cornea.* New York: Churchill Livingstone, 1988: 599–646.
23. Zuclich J. Cumulative effects of near-UV induced corneal damage. *Health Physics.* 1980; **38**: 833–8.
24. Mills B, Brown R, Saunders D. Non-ionising radiation and the eye. In: Raffle P, Adams P, Baxter P, Lee W (eds). *Hunter's Diseases of occupations*, 8th edn. London: Edward Arnold, 1994: 387–400.
25. Mainster M, Ham W, Delori F. Potential retinal hazards. Instrument and environmental light sources. *Ophthalmology.* 1983; **90**: 927–32.
26. Davidson P, Sternberg P. Potential retinal photoxicity. *American Journal of Ophthalmology.* 1993; **116**: 497–501.
27. Azzolini C, Brancato R, Venturi G et al. Updating on intraoperative light induced retinal injury. *International Ophthalmology.* 1994; **18**: 269–76.
28. Berninger TA, Canning C, Gunduz K et al. Using argon laser blue light reduces ophthalmologists' color contrast sensitivity. Argon blue and surgeons vision. *Archives of Ophthalmology.* 1989; **107**: 1453–8.
29. Duke-Elder S. Radiational injuries. In: *System of ophthalmology*, vol. 14, part 2. St Louis: CV Mosby, 1972: 888–912.
30. Sliney D, Wolbarsht M. *Safety with lasers and other optical sources.* New York: Plenum Press, 1980.
31. Naidoff M, Sliney D. Retinal injury from a welding arc. *American Journal of Ophthalmology.* 1974; **77**: 663–8.
32. McGhee C, Taylor H, Gartry D, Trokel S. *Excimer lasers in ophthalmology: Principles and practice.* London: Martin Dunitz, 1997.
33. McGhee C, Ellerton C. Complications of excimer laser photorefractive surgery. In: McGhee C, Taylor H, Gartry D, Trokel S (eds). *Excimer lasers in ophthalmology: Principles and practice.* London: Martin Dunitz, 1997: 379–402.
34. Sliney D. Interaction mechanisms of laser radiation with ocular tissues. In: Count LA, Duchene A, Courant D (eds). First International Symposium on Laser Biological Effects: Lasers et Normes de Protection. Fontenay-aux-Roses: Commissariat à l'Energie Atomique, Departement de Protection Sanitaire, 1988.
35. Hemstreet H, Bruce W, Altobelli K et al. Ocular hazards of picosecond and repetitive pulse argon laser exposures. First Annual Report, February 1973–February 1974. San Antonio, TX: USAF Contract for School of Aerospace Medicine. Technology Inc/Brooks AFB, 1974.
36. Boldrey E, Little H, Flocks M, Vassiliadis A. Retinal injury due to industrial laser burns. *Ophthalmology.* 1981; **88**: 101–7.
37. Gabel V, Birngruber R, Lorenz B, Lang G. Clinical observations of six cases of laser injury to the eye. *Health Physics.* 1989; **56**: 705–10.
38. Gibbons W, Allen R. Retinal damage from supra-threshold Q-switched laser exposure. *Health Physics.* 1978; **35**: 461–9.
39. Henkes H, Zuidema H. Accidental laser coagulation of the central fovea. *Ophthalmologica.* 1975; **171**: 15–25.
40. Liu H, Gao G, Wu D et al. Ocular injuries from accidental laser exposure. *Health Physics.* 1989; **56**: 711–6.
41. Rathkey A. Accidental laser burn of the macula. *Archives of Ophthalmology.* 1965; **74**: 346–8.

42. Wolfe C. Laser retinal injury. *Military Medicine.* 1985; **150**: 177–81.
43. Zweng H. Accidental Q-switched laser lesion of human macula. *Archives of Ophthalmology.* 1967; **78**: 596–9.
44. Hirsch D, Booth G, Schockett S, Sliney D. Recovery from pulsed-dye laser retinal injury. *Archives of Ophthalmology.* 1992; **110**: 1688–9.
45. Sliney D. Ocular injuries from laser accidents. In: *Proceedings of Laser-inflicted Eye Injuries: Epidemiology, Prevention and Treatment.* San Jose, CA, 1996: 25–33.
46. Mainster M, Sliney D, Marshall J et al. But is it really light damage? *Ophthalmology.* 1997; **104**: 179–80.
47. Ham W, Mueller H, Wolbarsht M, Sliney D. Evaluation of retinal exposures from repetitively pulsed and scanning lasers. *Health Physics.* 1988; **54**: 337–44.
48. Ham W, Ruffolo J, Mueller H, Guerry D. III: The nature of retinal radiation damage, dependence on wavelength, power level and exposure times. *Vision Research.* 1980; **20**: 1105–11.
49. Baleshevich L, Zhokov V, Kirillov YL, Preobrazhenskiy P. Some incidents of eye damage by laser radiation. *Vestnik Oftalmologii.* 1981; **1**: 60–1.
50. Curtin T, Boyden D. Reflected laser beam causing accidental burn of retina. *American Journal of Ophthalmology.* 1968; **65**: 188–9.
51. Wolbarsht M. Sliney D. Historical development of the ANSI Z136 laser safety standard. *Journal of Laser Applications.* 1991; **3**: 5–11.
52. Taylor H, West S, Rosenthal F et al. Effect of ultraviolet radiation on cataract formation. *New England Journal of Medicine.* 1988; **319**: 1429–33.
53. Bochow T, West S, Azar A et al. Ultraviolet light exposure and risk of posterior subcapsular cataract. *Archives of Ophthalmology.* 1989; **107**: 369–72.
54. Sasaki H, Jonasson F, Shui YB et al. High prevalence of nuclear cataract in the population of tropical and subtropical areas. *Developmental Ophthalmology.* 2002; **35**: 60–9.
55. Sasaki H, Kawakami Y, Ono M et al. Localization of cortical cataract in subjects of diverse races and latitude. *Investigative Ophthalmology and Visual Science.* 2003; **44**: 4210–14.
56. Taylor H, West S, Munoz B et al. The long-term effects of visible light on the eye. *Archives of Ophthalmology.* 1992; **110**: 99–104.
57. Mainster M, Boulton ME. Retinal light damage. In: Albert D, Miller J, Azar D, Blodi BA (eds). *Albert and Jacobiec's Principles and practice of ophthalmology*, 3rd edn. London: Elsevier, 2008: 2195–205.
58. Yeow P, Taylor S. Effects of long term visual display terminal usage on visual factors. *Optometry and Vision Science.* 1991; **68**: 930–41.
59. Jackson A, Barnett C, Stevens A et al. Vision screening, eye examination and risk assessment of display screen users in a large regional teaching hospital. *Ophthalmic and Physiological Optics.* 1997; **17**: 187–95.
60. Lydahl E, Glansholm A. Infrared radiation and cataract: Differences between the two eyes of glassworkers. *Archives of Ophthalmology.* 1985; **63**: 39–44.
61. Goldman H. Genesis of heat cataract. *Albrecht von Graefe's Archiv für Ophthalmologie.* 1933; **9**: 314–23.
62. Hanna C. Cataract of toxic ecology. In: Bellow J (ed.). *Cataract and abnormalities of the lens.* New York: Grune and Stratton, 1975: 217–24.
63. Lin R, Dischinger P, Conde J et al. Occupational exposure to electromagnetic fields and the occurrence of brain tumors. *Journal of Occupational Medicine.* 1985; **27**: 413–19.
64. Sliney D, Stuck B. Microwave exposure limits for the eye: Applying infrared laser-threshold. In: Klauenberg B (ed.). *Radiofrequency standards.* New York: Plenum Press, 1994: 79–87.
65. Kues HA. Microwave biological effects program review. Report JHU/APL, SR 90-2. Laurel, MD: Johns Hopkins University Applied Physics Laboratory, April 1990.
66. Andley U. Photoxidative stress. In: Albert D, Jakobiec F (eds). *Principles and practice of ophthalmology: Clinical practice*, vol. 2. Philadelphia: WB Saunders, 1994: 1032–7.
67. van den Bergh H. Photodynamic therapy of age-related macular degeneration: History and principles. *Seminars in Ophthalmology.* 2001; **16**: 181–200.
68. Vinger P, Sliney D. Issues in ocular trauma. The prevention of sports and work related injury. *Ophthalmology Clinics of North America.* 1995; **8**: 709–21.
69. Sliney D, Freasier B. The evaluation of optical radiation hazards. *Applied Optics.* 1973; **12**: 1–24.
70. Sliney D, Sparks D, Wood R. The protective characteristics of polycarbonate lenses against CO_2 laser radiation. *Journal of Laser Applications.* 1993; **5**: 49–52.
71. Sliney D. A safety managers guide to the new welding filters. *Welding Journal.* 1992; **71**: 45–7.
72. Buhr E, Sutter E. Dynamic filters for protective devices. In: Mueller G, Sliney D (eds). *Dosimetry of laser radiation in medicine and biology*, vol. IS–5. Bellingham, WA: SPIE, 1989: 101–7.
73. Eriksen P. Time resolved optical spectra from MIG welding are ignition. *American Industrial Hygiene Association Journal.* 1985; **46**: 101–4.

Health and Safety Directive references

American Conference of Governmental Industrial Hygienists. *Threshold limit values and biological exposure indices for 2009.* Cincinnati, OH: ACGIH, 2009.

American National Standards Institute. *Safety with welding and cutting and allied processes.* ANSI Z49.1. Miami, FL: ANSI, American Welding Society, 2005.

American National Standards Institute. *Safe use of lasers.* Z-1361-2007, Orlando, FL: ANSI, Laser Institute of America, 2007.

American National Standards Institute. *Occupational and educational eye and face protection devices.* ANSI Z87.1, Arlington, VA: ANSI, International Safety Equipment Association, 2009.

American National Standards Institute. *Testing and labelling of laser protective equipment.* ANSI Z136.7, Orlando, FL: ANSI, Laser Institute of America, 2008.

British Standards Institute. *Radiation safety of laser products and systems.* BS4803. London: BSI, 1984.

International Electrotechnical Commission. *Radiation safety and users guide.* IEC 60825-1:2007, also available as British Standards Institute BS EN 60825. Milton Keynes: BSI, 2007.

Duchene AS, Lakey JRA, Repacholi MH (eds). *IRPA Guidelines on protection against non-ionizing radiation.* New York: Macmillan, 1991.

Health Council of the Netherlands. *Optical radiation. Health based exposure limits for electromagnetic radiation in the wavelength range from 100 nanometer to 1 millimeter.* Rijswijk: Gezondheidsraad, 1993.

Illuminating Engineering Society of North America. *Photobiological safety of lamps and lighting systems.* ANSI RP27.1, ANSI RP27-2 and RP27.3. New York: IESNA, 2007.

International Electrotechnical Commission. *Radiation safety of laser products, equipment classification, and user's guide.* Document IEC 60825-1. Geneva: IEC, 2009.

International Commission on Non-Ionizing Radiation Protection (ICNIRP). Revision of the guidelines on limits of exposure to laser radiation of wavelengths between 400 m and 1.4 μm. *Health Physics.* 2000; **79**: 431–40.

International Commision on Non-Ionizing Radiation (ICNIRP). Guidelines on limits of exposure to broad-band incoherent optical radiation (0.38 to 3 μm). *Health Physics.* 1997; **73**: 539–54.

International Commision on Non-Ionizing Radiation (ICNIRP). Guidelines on limits of exposure to ultraviolet radiation of wavelengths between 180 nm and 400 nm (incoherent optical radiation). *Health Physics.* 2004; **87**: 171–86.

Prevention Blindness America. *Caution: Battery on board.* Schaumburg, IL: PBA, 1994.

Sliney DH, Mellerio J, Gabel V-P, Schulmeister K. What is the meaning of threshold in laser injury experimentation? Implications for human exposure limits. *Health Physics.* 2002; **82**: 335–47.

World Health Organization. *Lasers and optical radiation.* Environmental Health Criteria No. 23. Joint publication. Geneva: United Nations Environmental Program/The International Radiation Protection Association/WHO, 1982.

55

Extremely low frequency electric and magnetic fields

LEEKA KHEIFETS AND GABOR MEZEI

Nature of electric and magnetic fields	663	Magnetic resonance imaging	670
Occupational exposures	663	Conclusions	671
Acute effects in humans	664	References	671
Long-term health effects	664		

NATURE OF ELECTRIC AND MAGNETIC FIELDS

Electricity use has grown throughout the industrialized world since the first public power station began operation in London on January 12, 1882. Electricity is generated and usually transmitted as alternating current (ac) in the United States at 60 cycles per second, or 60 Hertz (Hz), and in Europe at 50 Hz.

Electricity is generally considered safe, but it is not completely without hazard. For example, in the United States each year there are about 1100 deaths attributed to electric shocks. Approximately three-quarters of these deaths occur from unsafe operation of electrical appliances in the home and the remainder are from accidents in the workplace.[1] However, the subject of clinical treatment of electric shocks and burns resulting from direct contact with electrical conductors is beyond the scope of this section, which considers health effects postulated from exposure to electric and magnetic fields associated with the delivery and use of electricity.

Electric and magnetic fields are ubiquitous in modern societies. The magnitude of electric fields, measured in kV/m, is directly proportional to line voltage, while magnetic fields, measured in tesla (T) or microtesla (μT), are determined by the magnitude of the electric current. These fields are found around every electrical conductor, motor and appliance. In office buildings, computers and copy machines are common sources of magnetic fields. Power distribution facilities and large motors used to drive building air conditioning systems can also contribute significantly to the magnetic field environment. In factories, high magnetic fields are encountered near large electric machines, electrical heating equipment and other high current-carrying devices.

Measurement of 50–60-Hz electromagnetic fields (EMF) is easily carried out with hand-held field meters. However, extreme variability of fields, both in space and time, make exposure assessment and the development of proper exposure surrogates of past exposures difficult. This is further complicated by the lack of knowledge regarding what aspects of exposure are biologically relevant and what might constitute a dose.

OCCUPATIONAL EXPOSURES

Occupational EMF exposures are considerably higher than non-occupational ones, which are usually in the 0.01–0.3 μT range (Figure 55.1). Occupational exposures have been studied most extensively in the electric utility industry. Average exposures have been found to be higher in electrical occupations than in other occupations, such as office work, ranging from 0.4–0.6 μT for electricians and electrical engineers to approximately 1.0 μT for power line workers. Welders have the highest average exposures at 3.7 μT. Average measurements or arithmetic means, however, can be strongly influenced by a few high measurements. Geometric means, which are not thus influenced, are much lower. Geometric means are 0.2–0.3 μT for electricians and electrical engineers, 0.4 μT for power line workers and 0.6 μT for welders.

Much less is known about exposures in non-electrical occupations. Few data, if any, are available for many jobs

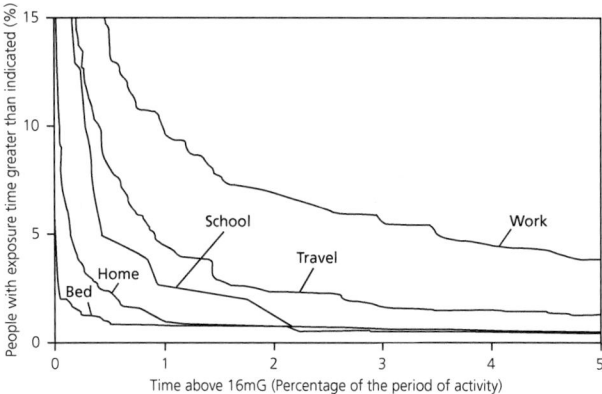

Figure 55.1 Length of time during different periods with field exceeding 16 mG estimates for the US population.

and industrial environments. Of note in the few surveys conducted are high exposures among railway engine drivers (about 4 μT) and seamstresses (about 3 μT). The best information on work exposures among the general population is available in a survey conducted by Zaffanella and Keaton.[2] The survey included 525 workers employed in a variety of occupations. The largest geometric mean (0.16 μT) for exposure to magnetic fields during work occurred in electrical occupations and in service occupations. Technical, sales and administrative support positions had a geometric mean of 0.11 μT; managerial and professional specialty occupations had 0.10 μT; and precision production, craft and repair occupations and operators, fabricators and labourers had a geometric mean 0.09 μT. At 0.05 μT, farming, forestry and fishing occupations had the lowest geometric mean. Work exposures were often significantly higher and more variable than other exposures; people spent significantly more time, for example, in fields exceeding 1.6 μT at work than at home. Nevertheless, average work exposures for the general population are low, with only 4 per cent exposed to magnetic fields above 0.5 μT.

ACUTE EFFECTS IN HUMANS

Electric fields can be detected as a slight tingling of the hair at field strengths of 5–10 kV/m. Electrical workers may also be affected by microshocks which can be experienced by a person touching a conducting object in an elevated electric field greater than about 2 kV/m. Imperceptible contact current flows into the person's body as long as it remains in contact with the conductor. Microshocks have been suggested as the source of certain effects in cells and tissues, such as chromosomal anomalies.[3] It should be noted, however, that there is no substantial evidence implicating microshocks as harmful beyond their nuisance effects (see under Neurobehavioural and neurodegenerative effects, p. 669).

There is evidence that certain animals and organisms (e.g. birds, bacteria) can detect and be guided by the Earth's static magnetic field and very low frequency ac fields (<10 Hz). Humans cannot sense time-varying magnetic fields of 50–60 Hz, except at very high field strengths (on the order of 3–5 mT). At this field strength, humans perceive visual flashes of light,[4] i.e. magnetophosphenes, which are transient and not thought to produce any permanent retinal lesions.[5] Extremely high fields may result in nerve stimulation.

In the past, exposures to ambient EMF have been thought to be without biologic effects. The first suggestion that exposures might be detrimental to health arose from studies conducted in the Soviet Union in the early 1960s.[6] These studies focused on utility workers, particularly substation employees. Studies of these employees found an excess of symptoms such as sleeplessness, headache and upper respiratory distress. Investigations of the general health of electrical workers in several western countries have failed to confirm these findings. Indeed, in evaluations of health between electrical workers[7] and comparison groups, no differences were found based on the response to a survey questionnaire of people in whom field measurements had been made.[8]

Some experimental studies suggest that electric and magnetic fields can, under certain exposure conditions, produce physiologic effects in human volunteers. Changes in heart rate, heart rate variability, cognitive function and evoked cerebral potentials were observed to be slightly affected by exposures to EMF.[9] These observations, however, were not confirmed unambiguously in later studies.[10]

LONG-TERM HEALTH EFFECTS

The first publication linking EMF to human cancer appeared in 1979.[11] The paper reported an association between childhood cancer and presumed residential exposure to EMF, originating from neighbourhood power lines. This observation spurred a number of epidemiologic studies which examined the effect of occupational exposure to EMF on cancer development. The focus of this chapter is on occupational epidemiologic studies of workers with potential exposure to EMF.

The health effects that have received the most attention are cancer, reproductive effects, neurobehavioural and neurodegenerative conditions and cardiovascular diseases.

Cancer

EPIDEMIOLOGIC STUDIES

The study of the hypothesized association of EMF exposure with human cancer has mostly followed these two lines of investigation: cancer among children whose exposure to EMF is residential in origin, and cancer among workers in broadly defined electrical occupations whose exposure to EMF presumably occurs at the workplace. Based on epidemiologic studies, childhood leukaemia risk appears to double at average residential exposure levels above 0.3–0.4 μT.[12,13] Studies of residential exposure in adults and biological effects from EMF are largely negative thus far. Detailed discussion of the studies of residential exposures is outside the scope of this chapter, for a review, see Ref. 28.

Occupational studies of EMF have employed several designs such as proportionate mortality, case–control and cohort analysis. The occupational groups studied included the following categories of workers: linemen, substation workers, welders, electricians, motion picture projectionists, electronic assemblers and electrical engineers. Unfortunately, the definition of electrical workers in these studies is broad, varies considerably among investigations and does not always reflect a high EMF exposure. More recent and better quality studies have assessed magnetic field exposures through job–exposure matrices (JEMs) populated with personal measurements of time-weighted average (TWA) magnetic fields. JEMs for electric utility workers[14,15] and for the general population[16,17] have been constructed from extensive full-shift measurements. These data are combined with activity records to calculate the TWA and other metrics, such as time above a threshold, that summarize a worker's exposure.

A major limitation of magnetic field JEMs is that occupation is not the main determinant of exposure. A person's occupational exposure depends on the performed job tasks, field sources encountered during work, the average strength of sources and the proportion of time spent at different locations relative to sources. Consequently, measured exposure varies widely among individuals within the same occupations.[18] Furthermore, JEMs based on contemporaneous measurements may not properly represent historical exposures.

Several improvements to JEMs have been tried. Miller developed a JEM that classifies exposure measurements by location as well as by job.[19] Renew et al.[20] assessed exposures of power station workers with a magnetic field model that takes account of the engineering design, layout and operational history for each power station. Results from this model were combined with data on the proportion of time spent in specific plant areas for each job and with occupational history to give individual exposure values. Good agreement was found between modelled and measured exposures. This approach had the added advantage of reconstructing historical exposures. While this approach is valuable for power plant occupations with fixed working locations, exposures for transmission and distribution workers are still best assessed by JEMs.

Elevated electric field exposures occur only where there are unshielded, high-voltage conductors and therefore do not normally occur in indoor facilities, such as power stations or factories. Moderate-to-high levels (0.1 to >1 kV/m) are found only near high-voltage transmission lines or exposed, energized busbars in substations. In these limited environments, adequate estimates of TWA electric field exposures can be obtained from spot measurements or computer modelling.[21]

A brief summary of the numerous studies investigating occupational EMF exposures and several cancers is presented below. Leukaemia and brain cancer, and, more recently, breast cancer have received the most attention, although many of the breast cancer studies focused on residential exposures. Also, occupational exposures to electric fields have re-emerged as an issue of potential importance.

Because of the large number of occupational studies of EMF and leukaemia and brain cancers, specific study references which have been included in meta-analyses are omitted below. Reference should be made to Kheifets et al.[22–24]

LEUKAEMIA

The risks of leukaemia associated with occupational exposure to magnetic fields are generally low. A meta-analysis of occupational epidemiologic studies suggested an excess of all leukaemias with a risk estimate of 1.18 (95 percent confidence interval (CI) 1.12–1.24),[22] with slightly higher risks for the various leukaemia subtypes. Although most studies reported a small elevation in risk, the apparent lack of a clear pattern of exposure to EMF substantially detracts from the hypothesis that magnetic fields in the work environment are responsible for it. These findings were not sensitive to assumptions, influence of individual studies, weighting schemes or modelling. Some evidence of publication bias was noted.[22] A pooled analysis of large cohort studies of electric utility workers showed similar weak but positive associations between occupational magnetic field exposure and adult leukaemia. More recent cohort studies of electric utility workers in the United Kingdom and Denmark showed no elevation in leukaemia risk in association with occupational magnetic field exposure (Figure 55.2).

A recent update to the previous meta-analyses on occupational EMF and adult leukaemia collected and evaluated all relevant 1993–2007 publications.[24] Combining the new and past studies leads to a small overall increase in risk of 17 per cent for all leukaemia with little indication of heterogeneity. A more detailed look indicates somewhat higher risk increases for specific leukaemia subtypes (an excess ranging from 15 to 37 per cent), but the excess is largely limited to the previous analysis with newer studies providing little indication of risk. Additionally, while in the past analysis the highest estimate was obtained for chronic lymphocytic leukaemia now the highest risk appears for acute lymphocytic leukaemia.

Improvements in study quality have not clarified the relationship between occupational EMF exposure and leukaemia. While recent studies represent substantial improvements over earlier research, each has unique limitations. The most recent studies do not point to strong biases or confounding in the earlier studies. However, so little is known of the risk factors for adult leukaemia that confounding from an as yet unidentified risk factor remains a possibility. Also, the lack of an exposure–response relationship and the inconsistencies in results from different studies makes it difficult to conclude that

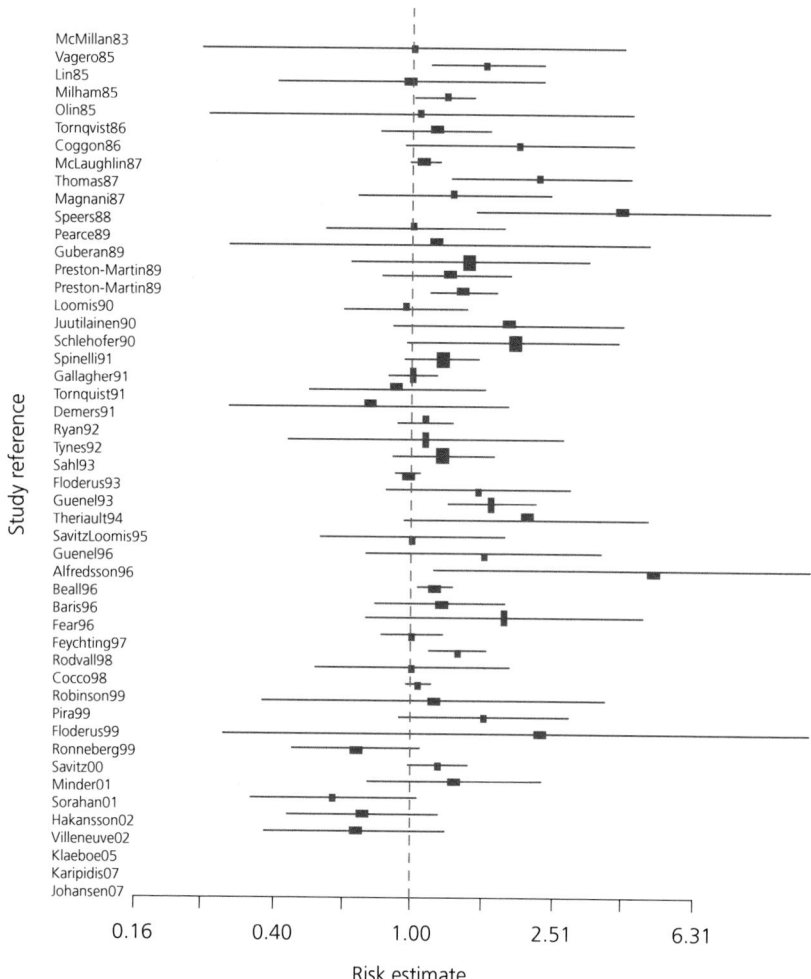

Figure 55.2 Leukaemia estimates with confidence intervals. For study details, see Refs 22–24.

occupational EMF exposure is a risk factor for adult leukaemia. Large increases in adult leukaemia risk in association with occupational EMF exposure, however, are unlikely based on the available results.

BRAIN CANCER

Similarly, there is a small but significant increase in brain cancer risk associated with estimates of potential workplace magnetic field exposure (relative risk (RR) = 1.21, CI 1.11–1.33).[23] While most studies reported a small elevation in risk, there was considerable heterogeneity in the results. Pooled risk estimates (based on inverse-variance weighted pooling) decreased over time. The findings of this meta-analysis were not affected by inclusion of unpublished data, influence of individual studies, weighting schemes or model specification. A pooled analysis of large utility cohort studies showed a weak-positive association between occupational exposure to EMF and adult brain cancer. More recent electric utility cohort studies from Denmark and the United Kingdom observed no increases in brain cancer risk. An update to the earlier meta-analysis for brain cancer[24] leads to an overall 14 per cent increase in risk for brain cancer and an 18 per cent increase for glioma, with some presence of heterogeneity.

While some studies reported a slight elevation in risk for adult brain tumours among people in electrical occupations, the lack of a dose–response relation in some studies and the lack of knowledge of other risk factors for brain tumours which could be confounding variables limit our ability to reach conclusions about the risks for adult brain cancer from occupational exposure to EMF. Similar to leukaemia, however, large increases in the risk of adult brain cancer in relation to occupational EMF exposure may be excluded on the available epidemiologic results (Figure 55.3) and previously observed risk patterns are not strengthened by new and better quality data.[24]

BREAST CANCER

Numerous studies have examined cancer in electrical occupations, with many considering breast cancer as one of the outcomes. These studies were motivated by a specific, biologically based hypothesis, which proposed that magnetic field exposure suppresses melatonin production at night and that reduced melatonin levels would result in an

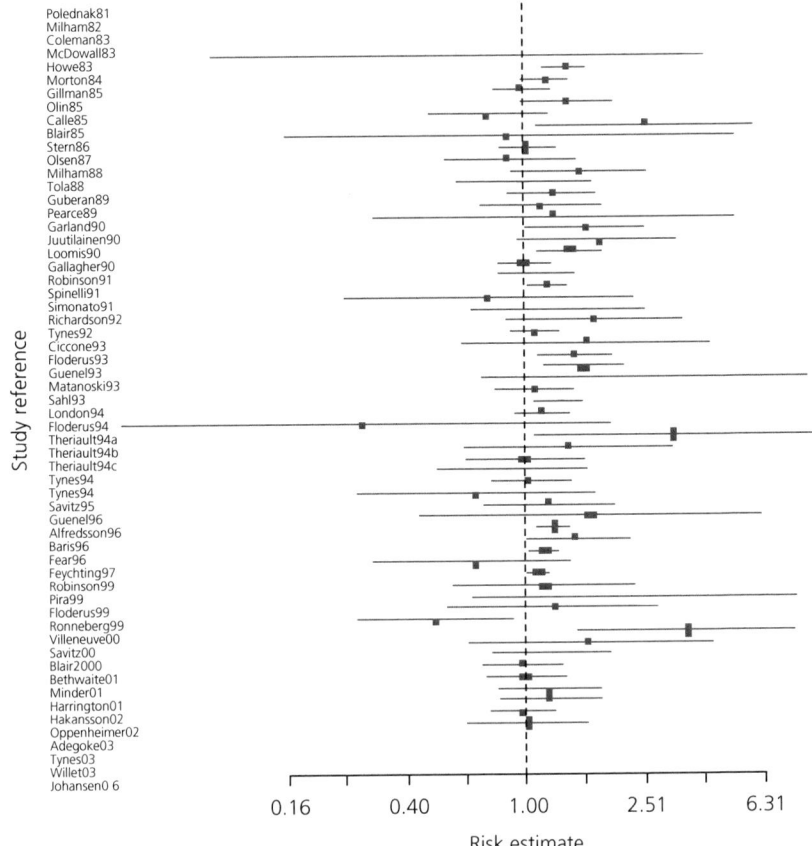

Figure 55.3 Brain estimates with confidence intervals. For study details, see Refs 22–24.

increased risk of breast cancer. Male breast cancer is very rare and most of the studies were not based on sufficiently large populations, so estimates of risk for male breast cancer were often not included in the tables of results unless an excess risk had been observed. This makes it difficult to evaluate the risk of male breast cancer. Although several reports were suggestive of a positive association, the more recent large studies of electrical workers[25–27] did not identify any excess of male breast cancer.

Few occupational studies of electrical workers included sufficient numbers of females to address the potential association of occupational EMF exposure and female breast cancer. Although some studies supported a possible association between EMF exposure and oestrogen receptor-positive breast cancer among premenopausal women, other studies did not. Most recently, a very large and well-designed occupational case–control study of Swedish women using a sophisticated female-occupation specific job–exposure matrix found no increase in breast cancer risk with exposure to magnetic fields. Available epidemiologic results, overall, do not provide support for an association between occupational exposure to EMF and breast cancer.

OTHER CANCERS

Sporadic reports of elevated risks for other cancers, such as malignant melanoma, non-Hodgkin's lymphoma, testicular cancer and prostate cancer,[28] have appeared in the literature but these have been inconsistent and none has been sufficiently strong to warrant further discussion here. Overall, epidemiologic results do not indicate that occupational EMF exposure may be a risk factor for these types of cancers.

ELECTRIC FIELDS

Magnetic, rather than electric, fields have been identified as the exposure of potential interest in most epidemiologic studies. In addition to the plethora of well-known difficulties in measuring magnetic field exposures today and extrapolating them to workers who held similar jobs in the past, measuring electric field exposure presents unique difficulties. Electric fields are perturbed by conducting objects, such as humans and their surroundings. The interaction of the subject with the field affects the reading of a field meter placed on the body. The field that is recorded by the instrument is therefore very dependent on where the device is worn, the posture of the subject and the relative location of sources of fields. This makes measurements of the electric fields difficult to perform and interpret, often yielding relative, as opposed to absolute, values of exposure for different individuals. Because most of the exposure assessments in the occupational environments have focused on magnetic, rather than on electric fields, little is known about the reliability and validity of electric field measurements. However, reanalyses of two cohorts of the Canada–France study[29–32] and of a study in Los Angeles County[33] considered electric field exposure (the original focus of these studies was magnetic fields).

In the first, Miller et al.[29] reported an association of all leukaemias and leukaemia subtypes (but not for brain cancer) with increasing electric field exposures. The primary effect occurred when both electric and magnetic field exposures were considered together. In contrast to these results, the second reanalysis[30] found no evidence of an increased risk of leukaemia and some evidence of an increased risk of brain tumours among utility workers exposed to electric fields. Finally, a limited reanalysis of data from Los Angeles County did not find an association between leukaemia and electric field exposures in a variety of occupations.[33] The two further analyses of the Ontario portion of the Canada–France electric utility worker study found an increased risk of leukaemia and non-Hodgkin's lymphoma with elevated exposures to electric fields.[31,32]

Due to the inconsistency of results and the special difficulties in assessing electric field exposure, there is currently little research studying possible associations between electric field exposure and cancer.

SUMMARY OF EPIDEMIOLOGIC RESEARCH

In summary, over 100 occupational studies have examined magnetic fields as a potential risk factor for a variety of cancers. A few of these studies also considered electric fields as a risk factor and one investigated the combination of electric and magnetic fields appearing together. These studies have varied widely in the design, types of study subjects, methods of exposure assessment, outcomes considered and quality.

Of the many cancers and exposures examined, a weak positive association exists between occupational exposure to magnetic field and leukaemia and brain tumours; the epidemiologic literature is consistent with either no association or a small association for these cancers. Based on epidemiologic results, overall, breast cancer is not likely to be related to magnetic field exposure.

The likelihood of positive findings due to chance alone is difficult to evaluate. Many of the studies were not specifically designed to test the EMF hypothesis, but rather were secondary analyses of existing data collected for other purposes. Biases are undoubtedly present in many or all of the epidemiologic studies. However, the magnitude and direction of biases in the studies of EMF are not well understood. These potential biases vary from study to study and over time some sources of bias have been largely eliminated, while others remain.

EMF exposure is an uncertain risk factor for the cancers studied based on the small to modest elevation in risk reported in some studies, general lack of a dose–response relationship, possible uncontrolled confounding, and inconsistencies among the studies in specific cancers and in exposures identified as most important. As the methodology of studies improved, the estimates of risk have become lower, making it unlikely that a large risk is being missed.

LABORATORY STUDIES

No biophysical mechanisms operating at low levels have been identified, in particular: effects below $5\,\mu T$ are implausible, at about $50\,\mu T$, no specific mechanism has been identified, but the basic problem of implausibility is removed. Above about $500\,\mu T$, there are established or likely effects from accepted mechanisms.[34]

As a whole, laboratory research does not support EMF exposure as a carcinogenic agent. Multiple studies have failed to show those cellular or tissue findings usually associated with the transformation of normal cells into neoplastic cells.[35] For example, with certain rare exceptions, EMF has not been shown to be mutagenic,[36] clastogenic or teratogenic, nor has any mechanism been established for weak to moderately strong fields.[37]

A review of animal models for carcinogenicity concluded that long-term continuous exposure to magnetic fields in the range of $2-5000\,\mu T$ is not likely to result in carcinogenesis in rats or mice.[38] Based on available evidence, a weak promoting effect of EMF under certain exposure conditions cannot be ruled out. Most of the studies addressing promotion and progression, however, were negative.

The absence of laboratory evidence of EMF as a cancer-initiating agent has led to some speculation and evaluation of EMF as synergetic with other agents. Juutilainen et al.[39] reviewed effects of such co-exposures in cell culture and short-term animal studies. The results of this analysis showed a high percentage of positive studies, suggesting that EMFs do interact with other physical and chemical exposures. All studies on apoptosis and embryotoxicity were positive while it was not the case for genotoxicity. Most of these studies on combined effects used magnetic fields of $100\,\mu T$ or higher.

Overall, the majority of animal and *in vitro* studies have found no evidence of genotoxic effects of extreme low frequency (ELF) magnetic fields at field strengths relevant to human exposure.

Reproductive effects

Reports of the effects of EMF on human reproductive outcomes, particularly in the occupational setting, are fewer than those of cancer. While there are a number of reports linking some forms of adverse reproductive outcome to occupational EMF exposure, overall, the body of evidence does not support an association between occupational exposure and reproductive outcomes, such as miscarriages or intrauterine growth retardation.[40] Among occupationally exposed populations, a variety of effects has been examined.

PREGNANCY OUTCOMES AND VIDEO DISPLAY UNIT USE

The potential influence of occupational EMF exposure on reproduction has been examined among women working with video display units (VDU). Initial concern was based on reports of several clusters of spontaneous abortions and congenital malformations among VDU operators.

Subsequently, several epidemiologic studies[41,42] provided very limited or no evidence of an association between VDU use and spontaneous abortion or other adverse pregnancy outcome. A study by Goldhaber et al.[43] offered some evidence that extensive work with VDUs had a detrimental effect on pregnancy outcome. However, the results of this study did not show consistent increases in risk with either extent of VDU use or particular job categories. Moreover, both recall and information biases could explain the study findings. With the exception of the study by Schnorr et al.,[42] all of these investigations did not involve any measurements of fields produced by VDUs. EMF exposures from VDUs in the Schnorr et al.[42] study were found to be similar to the exposures encountered in the home.

CONGENITAL MALFORMATIONS

Studies of congenital malformations among offspring of VDU operators have also been negative, although most of the studies were small and thus did not have the ability to detect small risks. Furthermore, laboratory studies and appropriate animal models employing VDU signals have not found adverse reproductive effects.

Only a small number of studies looked at paternal occupational exposure to magnetic fields and malformations among the offspring of males exposed to EMF. In 1983, Nordstrom et al.[44] used a written questionnaire to examine reproductive outcomes among Swedish workers employed in high voltage switching facilities. He reported an increase in a variety of malformations. Two more recent studies found no consistent pattern in the relationship between paternal exposure and congenital malformations. While some type of anomalies showed a positive association, others showed negative association with paternal occupational exposure.[45,46]

Animal studies of possible teratogenic effects of EMF exposure have been conducted with electric and magnetic fields separately at several intensity levels. They have generally been negative.[47–49]

PARENTAL EXPOSURE AND CANCER IN THE OFFSPRING

Childhood leukaemia

Early studies were concerned with childhood leukaemia as a possible consequence of parental exposure. No association was found in any of 24 studies conducted,[50] or in a secondary analysis[51] of a major childhood cancer study in Denver.[52] A 1991 investigation[53] reported an increased risk with maternal exposure to non-ionizing radiation, but not specifically EMF, during pregnancy. Paternal (but not maternal) exposure was associated with an increased risk of childhood leukaemia in one study[54] and for male offspring (but not female) in another one.[55] Thus, findings for childhood leukaemia and parental exposure do not show any consistency.

Brain tumours

Eight case–control studies examined the occurrence of childhood brain tumours or neuroblastoma among the children of fathers whose work presumably exposed them to EMF.[54–61] As in most occupational studies, exposure assessment was based on job title. Elevated relative risks (above 2.0) reported in two of the studies[56,67] were not confirmed in later studies. Selective reporting in earlier reports may account for the discrepancy. More recent analyses of childhood brain tumour studies[45,51,54,55,62,63] found no association.

In summary, there is little evidence to implicate occupational EMF exposure in the adverse pregnancy outcomes. However, because of methodological problems such as the potential for omission of early miscarriages, recall bias and the fact that the level of EMF exposure under study was not substantially different from the background level, additional studies designed to address these issues may be necessary to resolve this question definitively.

Neurobehavioural and neurodegenerative effects

A number of studies have focused on two categories of possible neurobehavioural effects in occupationally exposed populations: generalized neurasthenic effects and suicide. As a result of the early observations of Soviet scientists on depressive symptoms, several psychologists and industrial physicians conducted studies of such symptoms and found no effects.[8,9,64,65] Other investigators have examined suicide as a possible effect of EMF exposure and while some studies found an increased suicide risk, it has not been consistently confirmed in other occupational studies.[66–70]

Although the findings to date do not appear to produce a strong evidence of neurobehavioural effects in humans, there is some evidence of behavioural effects in animal studies. For example, learning ability in laboratory animals exposed to EMF was impaired.[71] Furthermore, some evidence that EMF might influence the secretion of melatonin suggests that both neurobehavioural and circadian effects in occupationally exposed human populations deserve further evaluation.

A series of studies investigated the potential relationship between occupational magnetic field exposure and neurodegenerative diseases, most notably Alzheimer's disease (AD)[72,73] and amyotrophic lateral sclerosis (ALS).[74] These investigators also suggested biological pathways that might be responsible for the association.[74,75]

In addition to the known difficulties of exposure assessment in epidemiologic studies of occupational magnetic field exposure, studies of neurodegenerative diseases are also hampered by difficulties of case ascertainment. Hospital-based studies in which cases and controls are typically identified through hospitals and clinics are more susceptible to selection bias, while population-based studies which mostly rely on death certificates for case identification are more likely to suffer from disease misclassification; death certificates are known to be incomplete for Alzheimer's disease in particular.

Some support for the hypothesis that exposure to power-frequency magnetic fields is related to Alzheimer's disease is mostly provided by hospital-based studies.[72,73,76] The results of population-based studies are less supportive and more inconsistent. For ALS, epidemiologic evidence appears to suggest that workers in electrical occupations may be at an increased risk. However, studies with measured fields showed less consistent association between ALS and magnetic fields than between ALS and self-reports of experiencing electric shocks. Further research on ALS which includes better exposure assessment, larger numbers and consideration of potential confounding due to electric shock and occupational exposures to solvents is needed.

Cardiovascular effects

The first epidemiologic study[77] specifically examining the association between occupational magnetic field exposure and cardiovascular diseases was motivated by a hypothesis suggesting that magnetic fields reduce heart rate variability which in turn results in acute cardiovascular events. In support of their hypothesis, Savitz et al.[77] found an increase in risk for death due to acute myocardial infarction and arrhythmia, but not due to chronic heart disease. The hypothesis was supported by the initial findings in a human volunteer study which showed an effect of magnetic field exposure on heart rate variability, and by several prospective cohort studies which suggested that reductions in some components of heart rate variability are associated with increased risk for heart disease, overall mortality rate in survivors of myocardial infarction and sudden cardiovascular death. Most of the epidemiologic studies with rigorous and varied designs which followed showed no effect. In a detailed review and analysis of the totality of evidence, Kheifets et al.[78] conclude that the weight of evidence speaks against an aetiologic relation between EMF exposure and cardiovascular disease. The potential for interference with implanted medical devices, such as pacemakers, needs to be considered in the case of very high electric and magnetic fields. All patients with pacemaker and defibrillators should be informed of the potential problems that could be associated with exposure to EMF. Interference of electric and magnetic fields is usually temporary and moving away from the source will alleviate the response. Advice to patients with these devices is to consult their cardiologist and the device manufacturers if concerned about potential EMF interference.

MAGNETIC RESONANCE IMAGING

Magnetic resonance imaging (MRI) is now widely used in clinical medicine and new applications with the potential fields of 10 T and higher are being developed. These imaging devices produce static, time-varying magnetic and radiofrequency fields. While the patient is exposed to all of these fields, technicians and other occupational personnel are exposed mostly to the static fields. Occupational exposure during construction and testing of these devices may result in exposure levels above 1 T. Field strengths very close to the machine during typical use may be as high as 10 mT. This field decreases to 1 mT at 3 m from the machine where a technician may stand for a few minutes. Farther away at the operating console, the technician is exposed to a considerably lower field level. The development of interventional magnetic resonance techniques will increasingly involve the exposure of staff involved in clinical procedures during real-time MRI scanning and at much higher levels. From the available scientific data and the magnitude of measured fields, it is unlikely that the health of operators is affected by their exposure to these magnetic fields, but studies capable of rigorously addressing this issue have not been conducted.[4,79] There are some contraindications for using MRI for individuals with metal implant and pacemakers[80] or who have had operations involving metal aneurysm slips or metal sutures. In addition, caution is indicated for patients who are pregnant and infants.

Exposure guidelines

Exposure standards are based on studies that provide information on the health effects of EMF, as well as the physical characteristics and the sources in use, the resulting levels of exposure and the people at risk. Exposure standards generally refer to maximum levels to which whole or partial body exposure is permitted from any number of sources. This type of standard normally incorporates safety factors and provides the basic guide for limiting personal exposure. There are two main international standards or guidelines: the International Commission on Non-Ionizing Radiation Protection (ICNIRP) and the Institute of Electrical and Electronic Engineers (IEEE).[81,82] Additionally, many national authorities have developed their own guidelines, which often adopt or modify ICNIRP guidelines. The European Union's directive to limit occupational exposure to EMF in its member countries, and which was based on ICNIRP guidelines, was introduced in 2004.[83] Its implementation, however, was recently delayed for four years[84] due to concerns that proposed guidelines for occupational MRI exposures are overly cautious and would prevent researchers and practising physicians from using the most recent generations of MRI technology.

Acute effects on the nervous systems form the basis of international guidelines. None of the guidelines consider potential long-term effects, such as cancer, to be sufficiently established to serve as a basis for standards. In particular, exposure limits are based on the acute effects on electrically excitable tissues, particularly those in the central nervous system (CNS). The current ICNIRP[81] limits for workers are 10 kV/m and 500 µT for 50 Hz and 8.3 kV/m and 420 µT for 60 Hz. The IEEE[82] exposure levels are 20 kV/m and 2710 µT at 60 Hz. The differences in the guidelines, derived independently by the IEEE and the ICNIRP, result from the use of different adverse reaction thresholds, different safety factors and different transition frequencies, i.e. those frequencies at which the standard function changes slope.

The occupationally exposed population consists of adults who are generally exposed under known conditions and are trained to be aware of potential risks and to take appropriate precautions. By contrast, the general public comprises individuals of all ages and of varying health status and may include particularly susceptible groups or individuals. Therefore, typically, exposure limits for the general public are lower by a factor of 5 than occupational exposure limits or exposures in the 'controlled environments', as they are referred to in some guidelines.

CONCLUSIONS

A large body of epidemiologic literature examined the potential health effects of residential and occupational magnetic field exposure. A number of national and international expert panels uniformly concluded that an association between residential exposure and childhood leukaemia development provides the strongest evidence. This relationship, however, cannot be considered causal since alternative explanations, such as bias, could not be excluded with certainty. Lack of a plausible biophysical mechanism and lack of evidence showing carcinogenic effects of magnetic fields in laboratory studies also weakens the argument for a causal effect. This uncertainty of the nature of the observed relationship is reflected in the classification of power-frequency magnetic field exposure as a possible human carcinogen (group 2B) by the International Agency for Research on Cancer and World Health Organization.[28,85]

Previous epidemiologic evidence also suggested an association between occupational magnetic field exposure or work in electrical occupations and adult leukaemia and cancer of the brain. However, the inadequate quality of exposure assessment, small elevations in risk, general lack of a dose–response relationship, possible uncontrolled confounding and inconsistencies among the studies in specific cancer types and exposures identified as the most important made the interpretation of the data difficult. Furthermore, more recent studies, presumably of better quality, have not strengthened this association – thus real risk increases for these and other cancers, including breast cancer, are unlikely. The data that are available do not meet the criteria of known occupational carcinogenic agents, i.e. EMF does not function either as a mutagen or a complete carcinogen.

An increase in risk of ALS among workers in electrical occupations should be investigated further. The evidence, however, remains weak, and it is unclear what aspects of the workplace exposure (magnetic fields, small electric shocks or some other confounders), if any, are responsible for the observed association. Risk increases in cardiovascular diseases in relation to occupational magnetic field exposure are unlikely in light of the current scientific literature.

Electricity use has grown throughout the industrialized world since the first public power station began operation. Today, the developing nations look to electricity as the means of providing jobs and improving lifestyle. Yet, concern over adverse health effects from electric and magnetic fields generated by electric power delivery and use has been a concern since the 1960s. Much has been learned from the many years of research on EMF and the many studies that have been published to date. It is clear that EMF do not pose a large public health or occupational hazard. The widespread use of electricity justifies research designed to resolve the remaining uncertainties.

> **Key points**
>
> - Exposures to extremely low frequency electric and magnetic fields (ELF, EMF) are widespread and highly variable in many work environments.
> - Acute effects on the nervous systems form the basis of international ELF guidelines. None of the guidelines consider potential long-term effects, such as cancer, to be sufficiently established to serve as a basis for standards – mainly due to a lack of generally accepted mechanism or replicated laboratory evidence below guideline limits.
> - Although a small risk increase for leukaemia and brain cancer from occupational exposures cannot be entirely excluded, the lack of a clear exposure–outcome pattern suggests that magnetic fields as presently measured are by themselves not responsible. No consistent indication of an association has been found for other cancers, including breast cancer.
> - The evidence speaks against an aetiologic role for EMF exposure in cardiovascular disease.
> - Among the major neurodegenerative disorders, amyotrophic lateral sclerosis (ALS) has been most strongly and consistently related to electrical occupations, thus warranting further investigation. Multi-country collaborative studies of ALS are needed to clarify this relationship.

REFERENCES

1. Baker SP, O'Neill B, Karpf RS. *The injury fact book*. Lexington, MA: DC Heath & Company, 1984: 149.
2. Zaffanella LE, Keaton GW. Survey of personal magnetic field exposure, phase II: 1000-person survey. Oak Ridge, TN: Lockheed Martin Energy Systems Inc., 1998.
3. Nordenson I, Hansson-Mild K, Nordstrom S *et al*. Clastogenic effects in human lymphocytes of power frequency electric fields: *In vivo* and *in vitro* studies. *Radiation and Environmental Biophysics*. 1984; **23**: 191–201.
4. World Health Organization. *Environmental health criteria 69*. Magnetic fields. UN Environmental Programme, International Labour Organisation. Geneva: WHO, 1987.

5. Silny J. The influence threshold of the time varying magnetic field in the human organism. In: Bernhardt JH (ed.). *Biological effects of static and extremely low frequency magnetic fields.* Munich: MMV Medizin-Verlag, 1986: 105–12.
6. Asanova TP, Rakov AI. The state of health of persons working in the electric field of outdoor 400 and 500 kV switchyards. Study in the USSR of medical effects of electric fields on electric power systems. 78 CH01020-7-PWR. New York: The Institute of Electrical and Electronics Engineers. *Gigiena Truda i Professionalnye Zabolevaniia.* 1978; **10**: 50–2 (in Russian).
7. Stopps GJ, Janischewskyj W. *Epidemiologic study of workers maintaining HV equipment and transmission lines in Ontario.* Montreal: Canadian Electrical Association, 1979.
8. Broadbent DE, Broadbent MPH, Male JC, Jones MRL. Health of workers exposed to electric fields. *British Journal of Industrial Medicine.* 1985; **42**: 75–84. Correction in *British Journal of Industrial Medicine.* 1985; **42**: 357.
9. Graham C, Cook MR, Cohen HD. Immunological and biochemical effects of 60 Hz electric and magnetic fields in humans. Final report. Kansas City, MO: Midwest Research Institute. DOE-FC01-84-CE76246; 1990 January 30. Prepared for the US Department of Energy, Office of Energy Storage and Distribution. Available from NTIS; Order No. DE90006671.
10. Graham C, Sastre A, Cook MR et al. Exposure to strong ELF magnetic fields does not alter cardiac autonomic control mechanisms. *Bioelectromagnetics.* 2000; **21**: 413–21.
11. Wertheimer N, Leeper E. Electrical wiring configurations and childhood cancer. *American Journal of Epidemiology.* 1979; **109**: 273–84.
12. Greenland S, Sheppard AR, Kaune WT et al. A pooled analysis of magnetic fields, wire codes, and childhood leukemia. Childhood Leukemia-EMF Study Group. *Epidemiology.* 2000; **11**: 624–34.
13. Ahlbom A, Day N, Feychting M et al. A pooled analysis of magnetic fields and childhood leukaemia. *British Journal of Cancer.* 2000; **83**: 692–8.
14. Sahl JD, Kelsh MA, Smith RW, Asseltine DA. Exposure to 60 Hz magnetic fields in the electric utility work environment. *Bioelectromagnetics.* 1994; **15**: 21–32.
15. Johansen C, Raaschou-Nielsen O, Skotte J et al. Validation of a job–exposure matrix for assessment of utility worker exposure to magnetic fields. *Applied Occupational and Environmental Hygiene.* 2002; **17**: 304–10.
16. Forssen UM, Mezei G, Nise G, Feychting M. Occupational magnetic field exposure among women in Stockholm County, Sweden. *Occupational and Environmental Medicine.* 2004; **61**: 594–602.
17. Bowman JD, Touchstone JA, Yost MG. A population-based job exposure matrix for power-frequency magnetic fields. *Journal of Occupational and Environmental Hygiene.* 2007; **4**: 715–28.
18. Kelsh MA, Kheifets L, Smith R. The impact of work environment, utility, and sampling design on occupational magnetic field exposure summaries. *AIHAJ: A Journal for the Science of Occupational and Environmental Health and Safety.* 2000; **61**: 174–82.
19. Miller RD, Neuberger JS, Gerald KB. Brain cancer and leukemia and exposure to power-frequency (50- to 60-Hz) electric and magnetic fields. *Epidemiologic Reviews.* 1997; **19**: 273–93.
20. Renew DC, Cook RF, Ball MC. A method for assessing occupational exposure to power-frequency magnetic fields for electricity generation and transmission workers. *Journal of Radiological Protection.* 2003; **23**: 279–303.
21. Bracken TD, Senior R, Tuominen M. Evaluating occupational 60-hertz electric-field exposures for guideline compliance. *Journal of Occupational and Environmental Hygiene.* 2004; **1**: 672–9.
22. Kheifets LI, Afifi AA, Buffler PA et al. Occupational electric and magnetic field exposure and leukemia: A meta-analysis. *Journal of Occupational and Environmental Medicine.* 1997; **39**: 1074–91.
23. Kheifets LI, Afifi AA, Buffler PA, Zhang ZW. Occupational electric and magnetic field exposure and brain cancer: A meta-analysis. *Journal of Occupational and Environmental Medicine.* 1995; **35**: 1327–41.
24. Kheifets L, Monroe J, Vergara X et al. Occupational EMF and leukemia and brain cancer: An update to two meta-analyses. *Journal of Occupational and Environmental Medicine.* 2008; **6**: 677–88.
25. Sahl JD, Kelsh MA, Greenland S. Cohort and nested case-control studies of hematopoietic cancers and brain cancer among electric utility workers. *Epidemiology.* 1993; **4**: 104–14.
26. Theriault G, Goldberg M, Miller AB et al. Cancer risks associated with occupational exposure to magnetic fields among electric utility workers in Ontario and Quebec, Canada, and France: 1970–1989. *American Journal of Epidemiology.* 1994; **139**: 550–72.
27. Savitz DA, Loomis DP. Magnetic field exposure in relation to leukemia and brain cancer mortality among electric utility workers. *American Journal of Epidemiology.* 1995; **141**: 123–34.
28. International Agency for Research on Cancer (IARC). IARC monographs on the evaluation of carcinogenic risks to humans, vol. 80. Non-ionizing radiation, part 1: Static and extremely low-frequency (ELF) electric and magnetic fields. Lyon: IARC Press, 2002.
29. Miller AB, To T, Agnew DA et al. Leukemia following occupational exposure to 60-Hz electric and magnetic fields among Ontario electric utility workers. *American Journal of Epidemiology.* 1996; **144**: 150–60.
30. Guenel P, Nicolau J, Imbernon E et al. Exposure to 50-Hz electric field and incidence of leukemia, brain tumors and other cancers among French electric utility workers. *American Journal of Epidemiology.* 1996; **144**: 1107–21.
31. Villeneuve PJ, Agnew DA, Miller AB et al. Leukemia in electric utility workers: The evaluation of alternative indices of exposure to 60 Hz electric and magnetic fields. *American Journal of Industrial Medicine.* 2000; **37**: 607–17.

32. Villeneuve PJ, Agnew DA, Miller AB, Corey PN. Non-Hodgkin's lymphoma among electric utility workers in Ontario: The evaluation of alternate indices of exposure to 60 Hz electric and magnetic fields. *Occupational and Environmental Medicine.* 2000; **57**: 249–57.
33. Kheifets LI, London SJ, Peters JM. Leukemia risk and occupational electric field exposure in Los Angeles County. *American Journal of Epidemiology.* 1997; **146**: 1–4.
34. Swanson J, Kheifets L. Biophysical mechanisms: A component in the weight of evidence for health effects of power-frequency electric and magnetic fields. *Radiation Research.* 2006; **165**: 470–8.
35. Kavet R. EMF and current cancer concepts. *Bioelectromagnetics.* 1996; **17**: 339–57.
36. Valberg PA, Kavet R, Rafferty CN. Can low-level 50/60-Hz electric and magnetic fields cause biological effects? *Radiation Research.* 1997; **148**: 2–21.
37. McCann J, Dietrich F, Rafferty C, Martin AO. A critical review of the genotoxic potential of electric and magnetic fields. *Mutation Research.* 1993; **297**: 61–95.
38. McCann J, Kavet R, Rafferty CN. Assessing the potential carcinogenic activity of magnetic fields using animal models. *Environmental Health Perspectives.* 2000; **108** (Suppl. 1): 79–100.
39. Juutilainen J, Kumlin T, Naarala J. Do extremely low frequency magnetic fields enhance the effects of environmental carcinogens? A meta-analysis of experimental studies. *International Journal of Radiation Biology.* 2006; **82**: 1–12.
40. Shaw GM. Adverse human reproductive outcomes and electromagnetic fields: A brief summary of the epidemiologic literature. *Bioelectromagnetics.* 2001; **5** (Suppl.): S5–S18.
41. Windham GC, Fenster L, Swan SH, Neutra RR. Use of video display terminals and the risk of spontaneous abortion. *American Journal of Industrial Medicine.* 1990; **18**: 675–88.
42. Schnorr TM, Grajewski BA, Hornung RW et al. Video display terminals and the risk of spontaneous abortion. *New England Journal of Medicine.* 1991; **324**: 727–33.
43. Goldhaber MK, Polen MR, Hiatt RA. The risk of miscarriage and birth defects among women who use visual display terminals during pregnancy. *American Journal of Industrial Medicine.* 1988; **13**: 695–706.
44. Nordstrom SB, Birke E, Gustavsson L. Reproductive hazards among workers at high voltage substations. *Bioelectromagnetics.* 1983; **4**: 91–101.
45. Törnqvist S. Paternal work in the power industry: Effects on children at delivery. *Journal of Occupational and Environmental Medicine.* 1998; **40**: 111–17.
46. Blaasaas KG, Tynes T, Irgens A, Lie RT. Risk of birth defects by parental occupational exposure to 50 Hz electromagnetic fields: A population-based study. *Occupational and Environmental Medicine.* 2002; **59**: 92–7.
47. Chernoff N, Rogers JM, Kavet R. A review of the literature on potential reproductive and developmental toxicity of electric and magnetic fields. *Toxicology.* 1992; **74**: 91–126.
48. Rommereim DN, Rommereim RL, Miller DL et al. Developmental toxicology evaluation of 60-Hz horizontal magnetic fields in rats. *Applied Occupational and Environmental Hygiene.* 1996; **11**: 307–12.
49. Juutilainen J. Developmental effects of electromagnetic fields. *Bioelectromagnetics.* 2005; (Suppl. 7): S107–S115.
50. Savitz DA, Chen JH. Parental occupation and childhood cancer: Review of epidemiologic studies. *Environmental Health Perspectives.* 1990; **88**: 325–37.
51. Feingold L, Savitz DA, John M. Use of a job–exposure matrix to evaluate parental occupation and childhood cancer. *Cancer Causes and Control.* 1991; **3**: 161–9.
52. Savitz DA, Wachtel H, Barnes FA et al. Case-control study of childhood cancer and exposure to 60-Hz magnetic fields. *American Journal of Epidemiology.* 1988; **128**: 21–38.
53. London SJ, Thomas DC, Bowman JD et al. Exposure to residential electric and magnetic fields and risk of childhood leukemia. *American Journal of Epidemiology.* 1991; **134**: 923–37 (erratum in *American Journal of Epidemiology.* 1993; **137**: 381).
54. Feychting M, Floderus B, Ahlbom A. Parental occupational exposure to magnetic fields and childhood cancer (Sweden). *Cancer Causes and Control.* 2000; **11**: 151–6.
55. Pearce MS, Hammal DM, Dorak MT et al. Paternal occupational exposure to electro-magnetic fields as a risk factor for cancer in children and young adults: A case-control study from the North of England. *Pediatric Blood and Cancer.* 2007; **49**: 280–6.
56. Spitz MR, Johnson CC. Neuroblastoma and paternal occupation. A case-control analysis. *American Journal of Epidemiology.* 1985; **121**: 924–9.
57. Nasca P, Baptiste M, MacCubbin P et al. An epidemiologic case-control study of central nervous system tumors in children and parental occupational exposures. *American Journal of Epidemiology.* 1988; **128**: 1256–65.
58. Wilkins JR, Koutras RA. Paternal occupation and brain cancer in offspring: A mortality-based case-control study. *American Journal of Industrial Medicine.* 1988; **14**: 299–318.
59. Johnson C, Spitz M. Childhood nervous system tumors: An assessment of risk associated with paternal occupations involving use, repair or manufacture of electrical and electronic equipment. *International Journal of Epidemiology.* 1989; **18**: 756–62.
60. Bunin GR, Ward E, Kramer S et al. Neuroblastoma and parental occupation. *American Journal of Epidemiology.* 1990; **131**: 776–80.
61. Wilkens JR, Hundley VD. Paternal occupational exposure to electromagnetic fields and neuroblastoma in offspring. *American Journal of Epidemiology.* 1990; **131**: 995–1007.
62. Preston-Martin S, Navidi W, Thomas D et al. Los Angeles study of residential magnetic fields and childhood brain tumors. *American Journal of Epidemiology.* 1996; **143**: 105–19.
63. Wilkins JR 3rd, Wellage LC. Brain tumor risk in offspring of men occupationally exposed to electric and magnetic fields.

64. Knave B, Gamberale F, Bergstrom S. A cross-sectional epidemiologic investigation of occupationally exposed workers in high-voltage substations. *Scandinavian Journal of Work and Environmental Health.* 1979; **5**: 115-25.
65. Baroncelli P, Battisti S, Chuccucci A *et al.* A health examination of railway high-voltage substation workers exposed to ELF electromagnetic fields. *American Journal of Industrial Medicine.* 1986; **10**: 45-55.
66. Baris D, Armstrong BG, Deadman J, Theriault G. A mortality study of electrical utility workers in Quebec. *Occupational and Environmental Medicine.* 1996; **53**: 25-31.
67. Kelsh MA, Sahl JD. Mortality among a cohort of electric utility workers, 1960-1991. *American Journal of Industrial Medicine.* 1997; **31**: 534-44.
68. van Wijngaarden E, Savitz DA, Kleckner RC *et al.* Exposure to electromagnetic fields and suicide among electric utility workers: A nested case-control study. *Occupational and Environmental Medicine.* 2000; **57**: 258-63.
69. van Wijngaarden E. Suicide mortality among electricians. *Occupational and Environmental Medicine.* 2002; **59**: 649.
70. Baris D, Armstrong B. Suicide among electric utility workers in England and Wales. *British Journal of Industrial Medicine.* 1990; **47**: 788-9.
71. Salzinger K, Frelmark S, McCullough M *et al.* Altered operant behavior of adult rats after perinatal exposure to a 60-Hz electromagnetic field. *Bioelectromagnetics.* 1990; **11**: 105-16.
72. Sobel E, Davanipour Z, Sulkava R *et al.* Occupations with exposure to electromagnetic fields: A possible risk factor for Alzheimer's disease. *American Journal of Epidemiology.* 1995; **142**: 515-24.
73. Sobel E, Dunn M, Davanipour Z *et al.* Elevated risk of Alzheimer's disease among workers with likely electromagnetic field exposure. *Neurology.* 1996; **47**: 1477-81.
74. Davanipour Z, Sobel E, Bowman JD *et al.* Amyotrophic lateral sclerosis and occupational exposure to electromagnetic fields. *Bioelectromagnetics.* 1997; **18**: 28-35.
75. Sobel E, Davanpour Z. Electromagnetic field exposure may cause increased production of amyloid beta and eventually lead to Alzheimer's disease. *Neurology.* 1996; **47**: 1594-600.
76. Davanipour Z, Tseng CC, Lee PJ, Sobel E. A case-control study of occupational magnetic field exposure and Alzheimer's disease: Results from the California Alzheimer's Disease Diagnosis and Treatment Centers. *BMC Neurology.* 2007; **7**: 13.
77. Savitz DA, Liao D, Sastre A *et al.* Magnetic field exposure and cardiovascular disease mortality among electric utility workers. *American Journal of Epidemiology.* 1999; **149**: 135-42.
78. Kheifets L, Ahlbom A, Feychting M *et al.* Extremely low-frequency magnetic fields and heart disease. *Scandinavian Journal of Work and Environmental Health.* 2007; **33**: 5-12.
79. Stuchly MA, Lecuyer DW. Survey of static magnetic fields around magnetic resonance imaging devices. *Health Physics.* 1987; **53**: 321-4.
80. National Institutes of Health. Magnetic resonance imaging. NIH Consensus Statement Online. 1987; **6**: 1-31.
81. International Commission on Non-Ionizing Radiation Protection. Guidelines for limiting exposure to time-varying electric, magnetic, and electromagnetic fields (up to 300 Ghz). *Health Physics.* 1998; **74**: 494-522.
82. Institute of Electrical and Electronics Engineers, Inc. IEEE standard for safety levels with respect to human exposure to electromagnetic fields, 0-3 kHz. IEEE Std C95.6 IEEE International Committee on Electromagnetic Safety on Non-Ionizing Radiation. 2002.
83. Directive 2004/40/EC of the European Parliament and of the Council. Official Journal of the European Union L 159, 30 April 2004.
84. Proposal for Amending Directive 2004/40/EC. Brussels, 26 October 2007. Available from: http://ec.europa.eu/employment_social/news/2007/oct/emf_en.pdf.
85. World Health Organization. Extremely low frequency fields. Magnetic fields. Environmental Health Criteria 238. Geneva: WHO, 2007.

Radiofrequency fields

GABOR MEZEI AND LEEKA KHEIFETS

Radiofrequency exposure	675	Conclusions	679
Acute effects	675	References	679
Chronic effects	676		

RADIOFREQUENCY EXPOSURE

Radiofrequency fields (RF) are a segment of the non-ionizing part of the electromagnetic spectrum. RF frequencies range from a few kHz to several hundreds of GHz. During the past few decades, we have witnessed tremendous advancement and proliferation of technologies using RF energy, and people in all societies are increasingly exposed to various sources and frequencies in the RF range. The public may be exposed to RF produced by AM and FM radio and television broadcast antennae, navigations systems, cordless telephones, wireless local area networks, and increasingly by mobile phone base stations and mobile phone handsets. Occupational exposures to RF may be experienced while operating and maintaining radio and television broadcasting and telecommunications systems. Additional significant sources of occupational RF exposures are dielectric heaters used for heating, sealing and melting vinyl and other materials and from military and civilian use of radar systems. In the medical field, exposures can occur from the use of magnetic resonance imaging (MRI), diathermy or electrosurgery. Workers in the electric utility industry may also be exposed to RF from antennae located on or near electric utility facilities. RF exposure in the far fields (at least several wavelengths away from the antenna) is typically measured as power density in W/m^2 or mW/cm^2. In near fields (close to the source of exposure relative to wavelength), exposure to RF is measured as electric and magnetic fields, in V/m and A/m, respectively. Since the actual amount of exposure a person receives from an RF field is also dependent on many factors, such as body size, grounding state of the person and frequency, uniformity and polarization of the field, in addition to field intensity, the internal exposure is typically expressed as specific absorption rate (SAR), in W/kg. Measurement of RF exposures of individuals and human populations appears to be even more complicated than that of extreme low frequency (ELF) due to potential distortions from other objects and bodies. In addition, communication technology is rapidly changing, which further complicates exposure assessment. Meters capable of capturing personal exposures have only recently been developed and are yet to be implemented in large-scale epidemiologic studies. In the RF studies, the lack of details about sources and exposures is still a major obstacle and extensive measurement studies within occupational groups are lacking.

ACUTE EFFECTS

Exposure to RF radiation induces heating in body tissues and imposes a heat load on the whole body, thus thermal mechanisms are accepted and prevention of excessive heating (above 1°C) serve as a basis for most international guidelines.[1,2] Exposure to very high intensity microwave beam can result in skin erythema and burns through tissue heating due to direct energy absorption. High RF may also interfere with pacemakers and other implanted medical devices. Direct contact with or very close proximity to an RF source, through an electric arc, may result in severe burns which tend to heal poorly. The lens of the human eye, due to lack of circulation and inefficient mechanisms to eliminate thermal energy, is known to be sensitive to heat. Therefore, heating due to high RF exposure could result in cataract. Observational studies in human populations, however, did not suggest that long-term, low-level RF exposure is associated with cataract development.[3,4] Many different effects at low RF energy, thought to be non-thermal in nature, have been reported in recent studies. Generally, it is thought that such interactions are unlikely to be biologically significant at the RF levels below guidance values, but much of the ongoing research focuses on the search for non-thermal mechanisms.

Exposure guidelines

RF exposure guidelines are currently based on avoiding the risk to health that results from localized rises in tissue temperature and from the physiological stress engendered by excessive whole-body heat loads. An SAR of at least 4 W/kg is required to result in an increase of 1°C in the tissue temperature. Present guidance on occupational exposure is based on restricting the RF-induced whole body SAR to less than 0.4 W/kg (a safety factor of 10); a heat-load sufficiently small that its contribution to other possible heat loads, generated from hard physical work and/or imposed by high ambient temperatures, can be neglected. Basic restrictions on localized SARs, averaged over any 10 g of contiguous tissue, are 10 W/kg in the head and trunk and 20 W/kg in the limbs. These are intended to restrict local tissue temperature rises to acceptable levels. Guidance on public exposure incorporates an additional safety factor of five, reducing the basic restrictions to 0.08 W/kg for the whole body and to 2 W/kg for localized exposures. Temperatures are derived from dosimetric calculation and thermal modelling. SARs are also related to external field values via dosimetric calculation.[1,2]

Of note are recent calculations indicating that for the frequencies in the GHz range far field waves, the whole body SAR is substantially larger for short subjects.[5,6]

Cognitive and neurobehavioural effects

Cognitive and neurobehavioural effects may result in occupational safety hazards if workers' judgement is impaired. Several studies examined potential cognitive effects of RF exposure from mobile phones in humans in laboratory settings. Earlier studies by Preece et al.[7] and Koivisto et al.[8] showed shortening reaction times in various cognitive tests but no impairment in overall accuracy. The effects were seen for analogue but not for digital phones. It was hypothesized that these effects were thermal effects due to local tissue heating. Later replication attempts, however, did not show consistent and statistically significant cognitive or neurobehavioural effects.[9–12] Nevertheless, electroencephalogram (EEG) changes, effects on regional cerebral blood flow and on sleep have been repeatedly reported in association with RF exposure from mobile phones in human laboratory studies.[13–17] The clinical significance of these EEG changes, however, are unclear. As human laboratory studies have been generally conducted at levels generally assumed to be too low to induce significant heating, if robust and replicable effects are identified this will have broad implications for our understanding of the plausibility of non-thermal RF effects in general.

CHRONIC EFFECTS

Cancer

EPIDEMIOLOGIC STUDIES

Several epidemiologic studies examined potential long-term effects, most notably cancer development, in association with RF exposure from various sources. Among cancer types, brain cancer and leukaemia were addressed most extensively in the literature. These epidemiologic studies are generally grouped into three categories based on the source of RF exposure: exposure from occupational sources, residential exposure from radio and television broadcast antennae, and exposure from use of hand-held mobile phones. Only the first type of epidemiologic studies investigated directly the potential health effects of occupational RF exposure and is the focus of this section. Additionally, mobile phone studies are also briefly discussed here because mobile phones produce relatively high exposures to the head and are increasingly part of many occupational environments.

Available case–control studies generally examine specific types of cancer and presumed occupational RF exposure in the general adult population, while cohort studies typically focus on well-defined groups of people exposed to a specific source through their work or hobby. All studies suffer from major methodological weaknesses. None of the studies included RF exposure measurements and exposure classification is often based on job title alone. In addition, no or only limited control for confounding has been made in these studies.

Occupational case–control studies

Two studies, conducted in the United States, showed a small increase in the risk of brain tumours in association with assumed occupational exposure to RF.[18,19] One of them investigated brain tumours among US Air Force personnel, and assessed exposure through job title and reports of exposure incidents above permissible limits.[18] Based on 230 cases and 920 controls, a small but statistically significant risk increase was observed (odds ratio 1.4, 95% confidence interval (CI) 1.0–1.9). The other study compared 435 deaths due to brain cancer to 386 deaths due to other causes identified through death certificates.[19] Exposure was assessed based on job titles ascertained through interviews with relatives of the deceased subjects. The study reported a risk increase for brain tumours with assumed occupational exposure with RF (odds ratio 1.6, 95% CI 1.0–2.4); the risk increase, however, was only seen with RF in electrical or electronics occupations and not with RF in other occupations. A third case–control study of occupational RF exposure and brain cancer, recently conducted in Germany included 366 glioma and 381 meningioma cases.[20] A slight, statistically not significant, increase in risk was observed for both glioma and meningioma. The odds ratios and 95% CI were 1.2 (0.7–2.2) and 1.4 (0.7–2.9), respectively. When the analyses were restricted to the exposure for more than ten years, the observed odds ratios further increased. Finally, in an Australian occupational epidemiologic study of RF exposure and glioma risk, exposure was estimated for 416 cases of glioma and 422 controls based on job titles linked to a job–exposure matrix (JEM) from a study in Finland.[21] No increased risks were observed for self-reported exposure, exposure based on expert assessment or exposure based on JEM.

Both male and female breast cancers were investigated in case–control epidemiologic studies. Demers et al.[22] compared potential exposure to occupational RF of 227 male breast cancer cases to that of 300 controls. Based on seven cases, the authors reported a three-fold but statistically not significant risk increase among radio and communications workers. A 1995 US case–control study compared possible exposure to RF based on job titles from death certificates of women who died of breast cancer to that of women who died of other causes.[23] The authors found no trend in breast cancer risk with either likelihood or level of occupational RF exposure.

Ocular melanoma was examined in two case–control occupational epidemiologic studies.[24,25] The first of these studies examined 221 cases of ocular melanoma and 447 controls, and obtained exposure information through interviews on a large number of chemical and physical agents.[24] The authors reported a roughly two-fold risk increase of ocular melanoma for subjects ever exposed to microwave or radar through their occupations (odds ratio 2.1, 95% CI 1.1–4.0). A German case–control study of 118 cases of ocular melanoma and 475 controls found a three-fold risk increase with occupational exposure to radio set or mobile phones, but no risk increase with occupational exposure to radar units.[25] The authors acknowledged that methodological limitations of the study may have contributed to the observed inconsistent pattern of associations.

A case–control study of testicular cancer relying on two methods for exposure assessment also reported inconsistent results; while with self-reported RF exposure, the risk appeared to increase three-fold, with RF exposure determined through job titles no risk increases were observed.[26]

A study of 694 cases of non-Hodgkin's lymphoma and the same number of controls in Australia investigated RF and other occupational exposures based on a Finnish JEM.[27] Based on very small numbers, the authors observed a three-fold, but statistically non-significant risk increase in the upper tertile of RF exposure (odds ratio 3.2, 95% CI 0.6–15.9).

Occupational cohort studies

Szmigielski et al. reported statistically significant risk increases with RF exposure for several cancer types of the haematopoietic and gastrointestinal systems and the brain among Polish military personnel based on information obtained from service records.[28,29] These observations, however, were later attributed to methodological limitations of the study rather than actual risk increases.[30]

Two studies that evaluated cancer mortality among US Navy personnel and veterans in relation to potential radar exposure showed no risk increases for cancer in general, or for leukaemia or brain cancer risks in particular.[31,32] Although a statistically significant risk increase was seen for non-lymphocytic leukaemia in one of the studies, it was only observed in one of the three highly exposed occupations in that study,[32] and was conflicting with the results from the other study.[31]

Milham examined mortality among about 67 000 registered amateur radio operators in California and Washington states.[33] Statistically significant increases were observed in acute myeloid leukaemia and cancers of other lymphatic tissue. Statistically decreased risks were also observed, however, for cancers of the respiratory tract and the pancreas.

Occurrence of cancer was investigated in a cohort of about 2600 Norwegian female radio and telegraph operators.[34] Statistically significant risk increases were observed for breast and uterine cancers; no other types of cancer showed elevated risks. This risk increase may also be explained by potential confounding by shift work. Shift work has recently been classified as a probable human carcinogen by the International Agency for Research on Cancer (IARC).[35]

Among operators of RF sealers in a small Italian manufacturing plant, a non-significant increase in cancer mortality and overall mortality was observed. The results, however, were based on very small numbers.[36]

An excess risk for melanoma and testicular cancer was also found among police officers in Ontario.[37] No information was available on radar use (potential source of RF exposure) in this study.

Researchers at McGill University in Montreal and Institut National de la Santé et de la Recherche Medicales in Paris examined cancer incidence in a cohort of about 170 000 workers at two electric utility companies in Quebec and France.[38] They assessed exposure to pulsed electromagnetic fields (PEMF) based on a JEM that was developed based on extensive full-shift measurements using meters calibrated to measure exposure in the 5–20-MHz range. Characteristics of detected fields are unclear because the meters used to measure them were very sensitive to fields at frequencies other than those originally intended by the manufacturer. The authors reported a statistically significant risk increase for lung cancer in the highest exposure category of PEMF. The apparent risk increase persisted even when adjustments were made for various potential confounding variables. Although adjustments were made for exposure to cigarette smoke, a potent lung carcinogen, they may have been incomplete because information on smoking was incomplete. Findings were not confirmed in several follow-up analyses of existing data.[39–41] Limitations of these follow-up analyses include suboptimal exposure assessment (as they had to use a JEM from the original work) and no information on smoking. Improved assessment of relevant exposures in the workplace, as well as better information on cigarette smoking, may clarify inconsistencies in these studies.

Cancer mortality of about 200 000 workers of a US wireless communication products company was examined over a 20-year period by Morgan et al.[42] Exposure to RF was assessed by a qualitative JEM. An expert panel categorized job titles into one of four categories (background, low, moderate, high). No excess risk was found for any type of cancers when the high exposure group was compared to either the background and low exposure groups, or the general population. The validity of the exposure assessment has not been assessed as no measurements were included.

Mobile phone studies

Most epidemiologic studies of mobile phone use examined tumours of the head and neck, mostly brain tumours and tumours of the acoustic nerve. Some of these studies relied on billing records from mobile phone companies to determine use and estimate exposure. This method is often constrained by limited access to billing records and is prone to exposure misclassification due to people sharing phones, using more than one phone, using company phones and switching carriers. Other studies assess exposure based on number and duration of calls, and duration of use in years as reported by study participants. Additionally, type of phone, urban/rural environment and use of hands-free devices can also be assessed in the interview-based studies. The main limitation of this exposure assessment method is the potential for recall bias, which might be particularly important for outcomes with impaired brain capacity. Both exposure assessment methods tend to be limited by lack of information on other factors greatly influencing RF exposure (e.g. signal strength, relative position of antenna, etc.). A novel exposure assessment method incorporating interviews, records and measurements is needed.

Most notable of the mobile phone epidemiologic studies is the ongoing Interphone study, which is a multinational population-based case–control study of mobile phone use and cancer of the brain (glioma and meningioma), the acoustic nerve and the parotid gland among adults in 13 countries.[43] Exposure is assessed by computer-assisted interviews of subjects using standardized structured questionnaires on aspects of mobile phone use, demographic characteristics and exposure to potential other risk factors, such as ionizing radiation and smoking. The study overall will include more than 2700 glioma cases, about 2400 meningioma cases, about 1100 cases of acoustic nerve tumour and about 100 cases of parotid gland tumour. The overall Interphone results are yet to be published. Combined results available from five countries suggest no overall association between regular mobile phone use and tumours of the brain and the acoustic nerve.[44,45] Subset analyses, however, suggest the possibility of a slight increase in the risk of glioma and, particularly, of acoustic nerve tumours among long-term users (more than ten years). The relatively small number of cases among long-term users, however, does not allow firm conclusions.

In summary, the currently available epidemiologic literature does not provide sufficiently convincing evidence to link RF exposure to brain cancer or other types of cancer. Due to severe limitations in RF exposure assessment and other methodological problems in most occupational RF and mobile phone use epidemiologic studies, the available epidemiologic evidence is also insufficient to rule out any potential effects. Most of the non-cancer outcomes are yet to be properly investigated.

LABORATORY STUDIES ON CARCINOGENICITY

Several two-year bioassays with rodents, such as Sprague–Dawley rats, Fischer rats and mice, were conducted to study the potential carcinogenic effect of long-term, daily RF exposure in typical mobile phone frequency ranges (0.8–1.6 GHz). The exposure systems in most cases were set up to achieve SAR levels of 1–2 W/kg in the brain and about a magnitude lower (0.1–0.4 W/kg) averaged over the whole body.[46–50] The results of these studies, overall, do not suggest that RF exposure, at these levels, are associated with increased incidence of brain tumours or other tumours.

Similar long-term exposure studies with rodents genetically susceptible to tumour development (e.g. transgenic mice) were also conducted to investigate the effect of RF exposures on cancer development. Although two initial studies showed increased development of lymphoma and mammary tumours,[51,52] these results were not reproduced in later replication studies.[50,53,54] Other rodent studies combined exposure to RF fields with known carcinogenic agents, such as ENU and DMBA.[46–48,55,56] These studies, overall, do not suggest that RF exposure modifies the effects of other carcinogenic agents.

Most genotoxicity studies in animals and cell cultures showed no effect when examining mutation, DNA and chromosome damage, or cytogenetic effects. Positive findings in individual studies could not be replicated independently, and most of these observations may be explained by thermal effects.

REPRODUCTIVE EFFECTS

A number of experimental studies examined possible teratogenic effects of RF exposure among various non-mammalian and mammalian species.[57] Teratogenicity was clearly demonstrated at RF exposure levels that result in maternal body temperature increases of 2°C or more. These exposure levels, however, are well above current guideline limit values. No consistent laboratory evidence is available to suggest non-thermal teratogenic effects at RF exposure levels below guideline values. This research area, however, has received much less attention.

Potential reproductive effects of occupational RF exposure were mostly investigated by epidemiologic studies conducted among physiotherapists using therapeutic microwave or shortwave diathermy.[58–63] The examined outcomes included delay in conception, miscarriage, stillbirth, preterm birth, birth defects and change in the offspring sex ratio. Although some of these studies showed increased risks for a few of the examined outcomes, no consistent pattern arose to implicate any specific type of adverse pregnancy outcomes.

Most experimental studies investigating effects of RF exposure on testicular function in rats found no adverse effects, or the decreased sperm parameters were attributed to the effect of hyperthermia.[64–69] Semen quality was also assessed in several studies among men exposed to RF mostly from military use of radar or microwaves.[70] Some indication of decreased sperm count and density was observed in some of these studies. Two recent cross-sectional studies conducted at infertility clinics showed inverse relationship between semen quality and self-described mobile phone use.[71,72] Limitations of exposure assessment, the highly selective study population and the cross-sectional design itself preclude any firm conclusions based on these results. Since spermatogenesis is known to be extremely sensitive to heat, some reduction in fertility as a result of low-level RF exposure cannot be ruled out.

CONCLUSIONS

No convincing evidence currently available suggests that occupational RF exposure below current exposure guideline limits results in increased risk of cancer or other adverse health effects. Due to severe limitations in study quality in most epidemiologic studies published to date, with particular deficiencies in exposure assessment, and due to poor current understanding of occupational and other RF exposures, potential adverse health effects cannot be ruled out, either, based on available scientific data.

Key points

- With the rapid advancement of communication technologies, exposure to radiofrequency fields (RF), has increased rapidly both in the general population and in occupational environments.
- Current RF exposure guideline limits are based on avoiding known acute health risks due to local tissue heating and whole body heat loads (thermal effects). No generally accepted mechanism or replicated laboratory evidence exist for non-thermal effects below established guideline limits.
- Current epidemiologic evidence does not point consistently to an increased risk of cancer or other adverse health effects. However, due to severe limitations of available epidemiologic studies and poor understanding of occupational and other RF exposures, potential adverse health effects cannot be ruled out based on available scientific data. Rigorous studies for a variety of outcomes are needed to close this gap.

REFERENCES

1. International Commission on Non-Ionizing Radiation Protection (ICNIRP). Guidelines for limiting exposure to time-varying electric, magnetic, and electromagnetic fields (up to 300 GHz). *Health Physics.* 1998; **74**: 494–522.
2. Institute of Electrical and Electronics Engineers, Inc. (IEEE). IEEE standard for safety levels with respect to human exposure to radio frequency electromagnetic fields, 3 kHz to 300 GHz. IEEE Std C95.1, IEEE International Committee on Electromagnetic Safety (SCC39), 2005.
3. Castren J, Lauteala L, Antere E *et al.* On the microwave exposure. *Acta Opthalmologica.* 1982; **60**: 647–54.
4. Elder JA. Ocular effects of radiofrequency energy. *Bioelectromagnetics.* 2003; **6** (Suppl.): S148–S161.
5. Hirata A, Kodera S, Wang J, Fujiwara O. Dominant factors influencing whole-body average SAR due to far-field exposure in whole-body resonance frequency and GHz regions. *Bioelectromagnetics.* 2007; **28**: 484–7.
6. Wang J, Fujiwara O, Kodera S, Watanabe S. FDTD calculation of whole-body average SAR in adult and child models for frequencies from 30 MHz to 3 GHz. *Physics in Medicine and Biology.* 2006; **51**: 4119–27.
7. Preece AW, Iwi G, Davies-Smith A *et al.* Effect of a 915-MHz simulated mobile phone signal on cognitive function in man. *International Journal of Radiation Biology.* 1999; **75**: 447–56.
8. Koivisto M, Revonsuo A, Krause C *et al.* Effects of 902 MHz electromagnetic field emitted by cellular telephones on response times in humans. *Neuroreport.* 2000; **11**: 413–15.
9. Russo R, Fox E, Cinel C *et al.* Does acute exposure to mobile phones affect human attention? *Bioelectromagnetics.* 2006; **27**: 215–20.
10. Keetley V, Wood AW, Spong J, Stough C. Neuropsychological sequelae of digital mobile phone exposure in humans. *Neuropsychologia.* 2006; **44**: 1843–8.
11. Preece AW, Goodfellow S, Wright MG *et al.* Effect of 902 MHz mobile phone transmission on cognitive function in children. *Bioelectromagnetics.* 2005; (Suppl. 7): S138–S143.
12. Haarala C, Bjornberg L, Ek M *et al.* Effects of a 902 MHz electromagnetic field emitted by mobile phones on human cognitive function: A replication study. *Bioelectromagnetics.* 2003; **24**: 283–8.
13. Hamblin DL, Croft RJ, Wood AW *et al.* The sensitivity of human event-related potentials and reaction time to mobile phone emitted electromagnetic fields. *Bioelectromagnetics.* 2006; **27**: 265–73.
14. Cook CM, Saucier DM, Thomas AW, Prato FS. Exposure to ELF magnetic and ELF-modulated radiofrequency fields: The time course of physiological and cognitive effects observed in recent studies (2001–2005). *Bioelectromagnetics.* 2006; **27**: 613–27.
15. Krause CM, Bjornberg CH, Pesonen M *et al.* Mobile phone effects on children's event-related oscillatory EEG during an auditory memory task. *International Journal of Radiation Biology.* 2006; **82**: 443–50.

16. Aalto S, Haarala C, Brück A et al. Mobile phone affects cerebral blood flow in humans. *Journal of Cerebral Blood Flow and Metabolism.* 2006; **26**: 885-90.
17. Hung CS, Anderson C, Horne JA, McEvoy P. Mobile phone 'talk-mode' signal delays EEG-determined sleep onset. *Neuroscience Letters.* 2007; **421**: 82-6.
18. Grayson JK. Radiation exposure, socioeconomic status, and brain tumor risk in the US Air Force: A nested case-control study. *American Journal of Epidemiology.* 1996; **143**: 480-6.
19. Thomas TL, Stolley PD, Stemhagen A et al. Brain tumor mortality risk among men with electrical and electronics jobs: A case-control study. *Journal of the National Cancer Institute.* 1987; **79**: 233-8.
20. Berg G, Spallek J, Schuz J et al. Occupational exposure to radio frequency/microwave radiation and the risk of brain tumors: Interphone study group, Germany. *American Journal of Epidemiology.* 2006; **164**: 538-48.
21. Karipidis KK, Benke G, Sim R et al. Occupational exposure to ionizing and non-ionizing radiation and risk of glioma. *Occupational Medicine.* 2007; **57**: 518-24.
22. Demers PA, Thomas DB, Rosenblatt KA et al. Occupational exposure to electromagnetic fields and breast cancer in men. *American Journal of Epidemiology.* 1991; **134**: 340-7.
23. Cantor KP, Stewart PA, Brinton LA, Dosemeci M. Occupational exposures and female breast cancer mortality in the United States. *Journal of Occupational and Environmental Medicine.* 1995; **37**: 336-48.
24. Holly EA, Aston DA, Ahn DK, Smith AH. Intraocular melanoma linked to occupations and chemical exposures. *Epidemiology.* 1996; **7**: 55-61.
25. Stang A, Anastassiou G, Ahrens W et al. The possible role of radiofrequency radiation in the development of uveal melanoma. *Epidemiology.* 2001; **12**: 7-12.
26. Hayes RB, Brown LM, Pottern LM et al. Occupation and risk for testicular cancer: A case-control study. *International Journal of Epidemiology.* 1990; **19**: 825-31.
27. Karipidis KK, Benke G, Sim R et al. Occupational exposure to ionizing and non-ionizing radiation and risk of non-Hodgkin lymphoma. *International Archives of Occupational and Environmental Health.* 2007; **80**: 663-70.
28. Szmigielski S. Cancer morbidity in subjects occupationally exposed to high frequency (radiofrequency and microwave) electromagnetic radiation. *Science of the Total Environment.* 1996; **180**: 9-17.
29. Szmigielski S, Sobiczewska E, Kubacki R. Carcinogenic potency of microwave radiation: Overview of the problem and results of epidemiological studies on Polish military personnel. *European Journal of Oncology.* 2001; **6**: 193-9.
30. Ahlbom A, Green A, Kheifets L et al. ICNIRP (International Commission on Non-Ionizing Radiation Protection) Standing Committee on Epidemiology. Epidemiology of health effects of radiofrequency exposure. *Environmental Health Perspectives.* 2004; **112**: 1741-54.
31. Garland FC, Shaw E, Gorham ED et al. Incidence of leukemia in occupations with potential electromagnetic field exposure in United States Navy personnel. *American Journal of Epidemiology.* 1990; **132**: 293-303.
32. Groves FD, Page WF, Gridley G et al. Cancer in Korean war navy technicians: Mortality survey after 40 years. *American Journal of Epidemiology.* 2002; **155**: 810-18.
33. Milham S Jr. Silent keys: Leukaemia mortality in amateur radio operators (letter). *Lancet.* 1985; **1**: 812.
34. Tynes T, Hannevik M, Andersen A et al. Incidence of breast cancer in Norwegian female radio and telegraph operators. *Cancer Causes and Control.* 1996; **7**: 197-204.
35. Straif K, Baan R, Grosse Y et al. on behalf of the WHO International Agency for Research on Cancer Monograph Working Group. Carcinogenicity of shift-work, painting, and fire-fighting. *Lancet Oncology.* 2007; **8**: 1065-6.
36. Lagorio S, Rossi S, Vecchia P et al. Mortality of plastic-ware workers exposed to radiofrequencies. *Bioelectromagnetics.* 1997; **18**: 418-21.
37. Finkelstein MM. Cancer incidence among Ontario police officers. *American Journal of Industrial Medicine.* 1998; **34**: 157-62.
38. Armstrong B, Theriault G, Guenel P et al. Association between exposure to pulsed electromagnetic fields and cancer in electric utility workers in Quebec, Canada, and France. *American Journal of Epidemiology.* 1994; **140**: 805-20.
39. Baris D, Armstrong BG, Deadman J, Thériault G. A mortality study of electrical utility workers in Québec. *Occupational and Environmental Medicine.* 1996; **53**: 25-31.
40. Kelsh MA, Sahl JD. Mortality among a cohort of electric utility workers, 1960-1991. *American Journal of Industrial Medicine.* 1997; **31**: 534-44.
41. Savitz DA, Dufort V, Armstrong B, Theriault G. Lung cancer in relation to employment in the electrical utility industry and exposure to magnetic fields. *Occupational and Environmental Medicine.* 1997; **54**: 396-402.
42. Morgan RW, Kelsh MA, Zhao K et al. Radiofrequency exposure and mortality from cancer of the brain and lymphatic/hematopoietic systems. *Epidemiology.* 2000; **11**: 118-27.
43. Cardis E, Richardson L, Deltour I et al. The Interphone study: Design, epidemiological methods, and description of the study population. *European Journal of Epidemiology.* 2007; **22**: 647-64.
44. Schoemaker MJ, Swerdlow AJ, Ahlbom A et al. Mobile phone use and risk of acoustic neuroma: Results of the Interphone case-control study in five North European countries. *British Journal of Cancer.* 2005; **93**: 842-8.
45. Lahkola A, Auvinen A, Raitanen J et al. Mobile phone use and risk of glioma in 5 North European countries. *International Journal of Cancer.* 2007; **120**: 1769-75.
46. Zook BC, Simmens SJ. The effects of 860 MHz radiofrequency radiation on the induction or promotion of brain tumors and other neoplasms in rats. *Radiation Research.* 2001; **155**: 572-83.
47. Adey WR, Byus CV, Cain CD et al. Spontaneous and nitrosourea-induced primary tumors of the central nervous system in Fischer 344 rats chronically exposed to 836 MHz modulated microwaves. *Radiation Research.* 1999; **152**: 293-302.

48. Adey WR, Byus CV, Cain CD et al. Spontaneous and nitrosourea-induced primary tumors of the central nervous system in Fischer 344 rats exposed to frequency-modulated microwave fields. *Cancer Research.* 2000; **60**: 1857–63.
49. Anderson LE, Sheen DM, Wilson BW et al. Two-year chronic bioassay study of rats exposed to a 1.6 GHz radiofrequency signal. *Radiation Research.* 2004; **162**: 201–10.
50. Utteridge TD, Gebski V, Finnie JW et al. Long-term exposure of E-mu-Pim1 transgenic mice to 898.4 MHz microwaves does not increase lymphoma incidence. *Radiation Research.* 2002; **158**: 357–64.
51. Repacholi MH, Basten A, Gebski V et al. Lymphomas in E-mu-Pim1 transgenic mice exposed to pulse 900 MHz electromagnetic fields. *Radiation Research.* 1997; **147**: 631–40.
52. Szmigielski S, Szudzinksi A, Pietraszek A et al. Accelerated development of spontaneous and benzopyrene-induced skin cancer in mice exposued to 2450-MHz microwave radiation. *Bioelectromagnetics.* 1982; **3**: 179–91.
53. Frei MR, Berger RE, Dusch SJ et al. Chronic exposure of cancer-prone mice to low-level 2450 MHz radiofrequency radiation. *Bioelectromagnetics.* 1998; **19**: 20–31.
54. Jauchem JR, Ryan KL, Frei MR et al. Repeated exposure of C3H/HeJ mice to ultra-wideband electromagnetic pulses: Lack of effects on mammary tumors. *Radiation Research.* 2001; **155**: 369–77.
55. Bartsch H, Bartsch C, Seebald E et al. Chronic exposure to a GSM-like signal (mobile phone) does not stimulate the development of DMBA-induced mammary tumors in rats: Results of three consecutive studies. *Radiation Research.* 2002; **157**: 183–90.
56. Verschaeve L, Heikkinen P, Verheyen G et al. Investigation of co-genotoxic effects of radiofrequency electromagnetic fields in vivo. *Radiation Research.* 2006; **165**: 598–607.
57. Heynick LN, Merritt JH. Radiofrequency fields and teratogenesis. *Bioelectromagnetics.* 2003; **6** (Suppl.): S174–S186.
58. Ouellet-Hellstrom R, Stewart WF. Miscarriages among female physical therapists who report using radio- and microwave-frequency electromagnetic radiation. *American Journal of Epidemiology.* 1993; **138**: 775–86.
59. Cromie JE, Robertson VJ, Best MO. Occupational health in physiotherapy: General health and reproductive outcomes. *Australian Journal of Physiotherapy.* 2002; **48**: 287–94.
60. Taskinen H, Kyyrönen P, Hemminki K. Effects of ultrasound, shortwaves, and physical exertion on pregnancy outcome in physiotherapists. *Journal of Epidemiology and Community Health.* 1990; **44**: 196–201.
61. Larsen AI, Olsen J, Svane O. Gender-specific reproductive outcome and exposure to high-frequency electromagnetic radiation among physiotherapists. *Scandinavian Journal of Work and Environmental Health.* 1991; **17**: 324–9.
62. Källén B, Malmquist G, Moritz U. Delivery outcome among physiotherapists in Sweden: Is non-ionizing radiation a fetal hazard? *Archives of Environmental Health.* 1982; **37**: 81–5.
63. Lerman Y, Jacubovich R, Green MS. Pregnancy outcome following exposure to shortwaves among female physiotherapists in Israel. *American Journal of Industrial Medicine.* 2001; **39**: 499–504.
64. Dasdag S, Akdag MZ, Aksen F et al. Whole body exposure of rats to microwaves emitted from a cell phone does not affect the testes. *Bioelectromagnetics.* 2003; **24**: 182–8.
65. Akdag MZ, Celik MS, Ketani A et al. Effect of chronic low-intensity microwave radiation on sperm count, sperm morphology, and testicular and epididymal tissues of rats. *Electromagnetic Biology and Medicine.* 1999; **18**: 133–45.
66. Dasdag S, Ketani MA, Akdag MZ et al. Whole-body microwave exposure emitted by cellular phones and testicular function of rats. *Urological Research.* 1999; **27**: 219–23.
67. Lebovitz RM, Johnson L, Samson WK. Effects of pulse-modulated microwave radiation and conventional heating on sperm production. *Journal of Applied Physiology.* 1987; **62**: 245–52.
68. Johnson L, Lebovitz RM, Samson WK. Germ cell degeneration in normal and microwave-irradiated rats: Potential sperm production rates at different developmental steps in spermatogenesis. *Anatomical Record.* 1984; **209**: 501–7.
69. Lebovitz RM, Johnson L. Testicular function of rats following exposure to microwave radiation. *Bioelectromagnetics.* 1983; **4**: 107–14.
70. Jauchem JR. Effects of low-level radio-frequency (3kHz to 300GHz) energy on human cardiovascular, reproductive, immune, and other systems: A review of the recent literature. *International Journal of Hygiene and Environmental Health.* 2008; **211**: 1–29.
71. Agarwal A, Deepinder F, Sharma RK et al. Effect of cell phone usage on semen analysis in men attending infertility clinic: An observational study. *Fertility and Sterility.* 2008; **89**: 124–8.
72. Fejes I, Závaczki Z, Szöllosi J et al. Is there a relationship between cell phone use and semen quality? *Archives of Andrology.* 2005; **51**: 385–93.

PART FOUR

DISEASES RELATED TO ERGONOMIC AND MECHANICAL FACTORS

Section One: The musculoskeletal system 685
Section Two: Back and spinal pain 713

SECTION ONE

The musculoskeletal system

57 Repeated movements and repeated trauma affecting the musculoskeletal system   687
    Cyrus Cooper and Keith Palmer

57

Repeated movements and repeated trauma affecting the musculoskeletal system

CYRUS COOPER AND KEITH PALMER

Introduction	687	Osteoarthritis	699
Shoulder problems	688	Risk factors for work-related musculoskeletal	
Neck problems	691	disorders and intervention studies	702
Elbow	692	Identifying work-related musculoskeletal disorders	705
Tenosynovitis and peritendinitis	693	Preventing and managing work-related musculoskeletal	
Carpal tunnel syndrome	694	disorders	706
Chronic upper limb pain	696	Acknowledgements	707
Dupuytren's contracture	698	References	707
Other soft tissue rheumatic conditions	699		

INTRODUCTION

Work-related musculoskeletal disorders (WMSDs) are considered an important source of occupational morbidity. Estimates of the size of the problem and its human and economic costs vary, depending on case definition and the source of the statistics. However, it is believed to represent the largest category of work-related illness in Britain today. The Health and Safety Executive (HSE) estimates[1] that in 2004/5 WMSDs affected a million people and cost society £5.7 billion in direct and indirect costs. Although back pain was the most common complaint (450 000 prevalent cases), disorders of the neck and upper limb were almost as common (375 000 cases).

WMSDs comprise a heterogeneous group of disorders – some well-defined, some ill-defined, whose natural history is for the most part poorly characterized. In some cases the debate concerns whether a recognized clinical entity is actually being described at all; in others it is the epithet 'work-related' that is contentious.[2]

Physicians are most likely to be concerned with the following questions:

1. Which upper limb and neck conditions may be caused or aggravated by work, and which conditions make work difficult to perform?
2. How can such cases be identified clinically and how should they be managed?
3. Who is most at risk? And how can the risk be assessed?
4. What can be done to prevent such problems, and how effective is the intervention likely to be?

Information exists on some of these questions, and this chapter will attempt a synthesis of the available information. However, it will help the reader in interpreting this information to possess some overview of the areas of difficulty and controversy.

The apparently simple question: 'Which musculoskeletal problems are known to be work-related?' has proved surprisingly difficult to answer. It is necessary first to state the problem more precisely, for example, to distinguish between exposures that *cause* a condition, and those that *aggravate* or accelerate it; and to identify unambiguously the end points of interest (discomfort or disability, accepted rheumatological and orthopaedic conditions or ill-defined regional pain disorders?). In assessing the individual complainant, the clinician would then need to consider several issues that bear on the likelihood of injury or complaint:

- the background level of the disorder and its natural history in unexposed populations (how unusual is its presentation?);

- factors personal to the worker (such as age, sex, the individual's anthropometrics and physical strength, medical history, mental health and threshold for complaint);
- factors particular to the working environment (e.g. job tasks and ergonomic stressors, workplace psychosocial conditions); and
- factors arising outside work (such as sport, housework and home craft activities).

He might turn to the epidemiologist for further guidance and would then find that these issues have been studied, to a greater or lesser extent, but that knowledge is incomplete and that its interpretation would be carefully qualified. For example, in general terms, there are data on the prevalence and incidence of complaints in the community, and how these vary by age and sex;[3-6] many studies describe associations between job title and musculoskeletal complaint,[7] and many others report a link in working groups between mental well-being and upper limb complaint.[8] However, the epidemiologist would point out that most surveys of WMSD have been cross-sectional in design, and may therefore have suffered from the problem of selection bias (for example, those worst affected may have selected themselves out of employment and escaped observation, leading to an underestimate of the problem); also that this study design does not permit the time sequence of events to be observed, and makes it harder to separate cause from effect. (For example, does the association between poor mental well-being and upper limb symptoms stem from a causal relationship, or do anxious and depressed workers simply complain more often than others about their aches and pains?) He would point out that some studies are of pain reports rather than specific diagnoses and that cross comparison is hindered because diagnostic criteria have varied, been ill-defined or not been applied in a uniform or standardized way; and he would say that it has proved difficult to grade the complex biomechanical workplace exposures that combine elements of force, frequency, repetition and movement and then vary them so thoroughly, so that in assessing causality there is scant information on dose–response relationships. The net result is that doctors entertain different views on the relation between work and particular symptom patterns presenting to them.

Two broad groups of musculoskeletal disorders that may be related to work will be considered in this chapter: neck/upper limb pain (Table 57.1) and osteoarthritis. We describe for each principal disorder in turn, its epidemiology, the evidence for its apparent association with work, its clinical presentation and its management. Later in the chapter we consider aspects of detection and prevention, as well as the current path on which research enquiries are headed.

Table 57.1 Upper limb and neck conditions that may be work related.[a]

	Condition
Shoulder	Shoulder tendinitis
	Rotator cuff tendinitis
	Bicipital tendinitis
	Shoulder capsulitis (frozen shoulder)
Neck	Cervical spondylosis
	Thoracic outlet syndrome
	Tension neck
Elbow	Lateral epicondylitis
	Medial epicondylitis
Wrist and forearms	Tenosynovitis of the wrist
	De Quervain's disease of the wrist
	Carpal tunnel syndrome
	Non-specific diffuse forearm pain (repetitive strain injury, RSI)

[a]Some authorities include ganglia, Dupuytren's contracture and trigger finger within the definition.

SHOULDER PROBLEMS

The glenohumeral joint has a greater range of movement than any other joint and this is permitted at the expense of stability. The glenoid fossa is shallow, the capsule is lax and there are no strong traversing ligaments. Stability, therefore, mainly depends on the muscles and tendons of the rotator cuff (supraspinatus, infraspinatus, teres minor and subscapularis), while the deltoid muscle provides a further mechanical support. The joint is protected superiorly by an arch formed by the coracoid process, the acromion and the coracoacromial ligament.

Epidemiology

Fraying and tearing of the rotator cuff tendons, thickening of the bursae and proliferative changes of the synovium are common age-related phenomena. They are often asymptomatic in life, but may be discovered at post-mortem. However, shoulder pain is also fairly common in community prevalence surveys. Bergenudd et al.[5] reported that 14 per cent of middle-aged men and women in a sample from Malmo, Sweden, had experienced shoulder pain lasting a day or more in the preceding month, and 3 per cent had taken sick leave because of it in the preceding year. A study of 15 268 Stockholm residents reported a point prevalence of shoulder pain of 20 per cent in subjects aged 40–74 years[9] and Dimberg et al.[4] found that 13.1 per cent of workers in an aeroengineering factory had current shoulder pain. Complaints become more common with age, although the Stockholm data suggest a peak around ages

Table 57.2 Occupational studies of shoulder tendinitis.

Cases	Controls	Study design	Relative risk	Source
Male shipyard workers and plate workers	Office workers	C	11–13	Herberts et al.[14]
Female packers	Female shop assistants	C	2.6	Luopajarvi et al.[15]
Male and female packers	Knitters	C	2.2	
Sewers	Knitters	C	2.4	McCormack et al.[3]
Board manufacturers	Knitters	C	2.1	
Garment workers	Health service workers	C	2.2	Punnett et al.[16]
Assembly workers	General population	C	3.4	Ohlsson et al.[17]
Female data entry workers	Other female office workers	C	0.54	Kuorinka and Koskinen et al.[18]
Male industrial workers with shoulder tendinitis	Age and workshop matched non-cases	CC	11[a]	Bjelle et al.[19]

[a]Relative risk for work with hands at or above shoulder level.
C, cross-sectional study; CC, case–control study.

55–60 years.[9] In the younger age group, there appears to be little difference in prevalence between the sexes, but in the 50s and thereafter men complain more commonly.[9]

Data on incidence derive principally from the National Morbidity Surveys in General Practice in England and Wales, a general practice-based surveillance system which collects details of consultations in participating practices over a one-year period. The 1981 survey indicated an annual incidence for all shoulder syndromes of 6.6 per 1000 practice-registered patients.[10] In the Stockholm survey, a subset of the cross-sectional respondents was interviewed and examined a year on, also providing incidence data: around 1–2.5 per cent had developed a painful shoulder, which included clinically verified restricted movement.[9] The peak annual incidence rate occurred in the fifth decade and there was little difference between the sexes.

Occupational studies

Injury appears to arise because of regular impingement of a relatively hypovascular area of the cuff against the acromioclavicular arch, an event that may be aggravated functionally through superior migration of the humeral head in abduction and elevation, or by an acromial spur or degenerative acromioclavicular joint. Studies of blood flow in the supraspinatus muscle[11,12] and muscle fatigue[13] confirm the importance of postural risk factors in the development of shoulder disorders. Occupational studies have therefore concentrated on working groups who elevate the shoulder repeatedly or for sustained periods at work, such as crop production workers, assembly line and other production workers.

Table 57.2 summarizes some of the older findings, based upon a comparison of occupational titles. Although risk estimates vary, most reports have concluded that there is good evidence of an association between overhead work and shoulder problems. In more recent investigations, exposure contrasts have been defined in terms of work activity, rather than the cruder measure of job title. A number of exposures (e.g. repetitive movements, vibration, high psychological demands) have been studied in this way. Van der Windt et al.,[20] in their systematic review, comment that in studies of good methodological quality associations were 'generally not strong'; while another review by National Institute for Occupational Safety and Health (NIOSH)[21] referred to 'evidence' (meaning some degree of support) for associations with repeated or sustained shoulder postures with greater than 60° of flexion or abduction, but 'insufficient evidence' in relation to vibration and forceful movements. Only recently have prospective studies been undertaken. However, in an Arthritis Research Campaign cohort study of new employees, lifting, carrying, pushing/pulling, monotonous employment and work with the hands above shoulder height were all found roughly to double risks of the relatively softer outcome of new onset shoulder pain during a two-year follow up.[22]

It should be noted that these studies have mainly investigated the occurrence of rotator cuff tendinitis (defined operationally as localized shoulder pain and tenderness over the humeral head[23]) or shoulder pain; the relation of other shoulder problems to work activity has not been examined in detail, although they may arise, coexist or become confused with tendinitis, and may certainly contribute to work incapacity when they occur. For this reason, they are described separately under Rotator cuff tendinitis, Calcific tendinitis, Bicipital tendinitis and Shoulder capsulitis (frozen shoulder).

Clinical aspects

ROTATOR CUFF TENDINITIS

Rotator cuff tendinitis (most commonly an inflammation of the supraspinatus tendon), tends to have an insidious onset, causing a dull shoulder aching or discomfort in the absence of a trauma history. Nocturnal pain is a prominent feature. Pain is felt over the deltoid region, and difficulty is encountered in reaching up, in dressing and in overhead work.

On examination, there may be tenderness over the humeral head and greater tuberosity, and the diagnosis is confirmed by reproducing the pain in resisted movement of the affected tendon. Supraspinatus tendinitis causes discomfort on abduction with a painful arc occurring between 70–120 degrees of abduction.

Chronic rotator cuff tears are often found at autopsy,[24,25] and in life these tend to be associated with falls on the outstretched hand, as well as overuse, and are noteworthy clinically because of weakness and muscle wasting, and because of the inability to maintain abduction (a positive 'drop off' sign).

Plain x-rays show evidence of calcification in the rotator cuff tendons in 8 per cent of the asymptomatic population over age 30 years,[26] and sometimes cystic and sclerotic changes at the greater tuberosity insertion. Ultrasound and magnetic resonance imaging (MRI) may be used to demonstrate rotator cuff tears, while arthrography will demonstrate full thickness tears.

CALCIFIC TENDINITIS

Calcific tendinitis often arises against a background of chronic shoulder pain on movement and arises at the site of rotator cuff injury and calcification, but it has a clinical pattern distinctive enough to be separately described. Pain is severe, localized to the deltoid area and quite abrupt in onset. Passive and active shoulder movements are greatly limited by pain, and there is extreme tenderness over the humeral head. X-rays reveal well-defined or fluffy calcium deposits in the affected tendon (usually the supraspinatus). The erythrocyte sedimentation rate (ESR) and white cell count are normal. Acute calcific tendinitis is a self-limited process, lasting one to two weeks. Sometimes it occurs spontaneously and not in apparent relation to injury.

BICIPITAL TENDINITIS

The long head of the biceps tendon tends to become inflamed as part of a more generalized shoulder problem (such as rotator cuff or adhesive capsulitis), rather than in primary overuse. However, it has occurred following weight lifting, and may well arise occupationally from prolonged repetitive carrying.

Pain occurs over the anterior shoulder, radiates into the biceps and is felt in overhead work and in shoulder extension, abduction and rotation. Tenderness is usually found over the tendon as it passes through the bicipital groove. In Yergason's test,[27] pain is provoked over the anterior inner shoulder in resisted active supination of the forearm with the elbow bent at 90°.

SHOULDER CAPSULITIS (FROZEN SHOULDER)

The primary form of this condition is characterized by global restriction of glenohumeral movement in all planes in the absence of significant underlying joint disease. It is believed to affect 2–3 per cent of the population[28] and onset nearly always occurs after the age of 40 years. Classically, there are three phases in the natural history of the condition, each lasting several months: a painful shoulder (phase 1) becomes painful and stiff (phase 2), and then profoundly stiff with slow natural resolution (phase 3). A minority of patients (7–15 per cent) have persistent functional difficulties afterwards.[29,30]

The onset is insidious, with pain in the deltoid area increasing gradually until sleep is disturbed. In the adhesive phase, there is equal restriction of active and passive glenohumeral movement in a capsular pattern (external rotation more than abduction, more than internal rotation). The aetiology of the condition is poorly understood and a particular relation with work has not been demonstrated thus far.

Management of shoulder problems

A Cochrane review by Green et al.,[31] in summarizing the evidence base on management of shoulder problems, found that certain physical therapies (exercise, laser therapy, ultrasound, pulsed electromagnetic field therapy) offered some benefit over placebo in certain disorders (e.g. rotator cuff disease, adhesive capsulitis, calcific tendonitis), but that more robust conclusions were undermined by small studies with weak statistical power and other methodological limitations. This information gap notwithstanding, a number of treatment options have gained currency in clinical practice.

The treatment of rotator cuff tendinitis is often difficult. Rest and modification of aggravating activities are necessary to prevent the problem becoming chronic. Initial treatment should be directed at reducing inflammation by means of physical therapy (for example, ultrasound) and a non-steroid anti-inflammatory agent. If symptoms fail to settle within three weeks, a subacromial injection of corticosteroid is useful. Once pain has eased and normal shoulder movements have been restored, a muscle-strengthening exercise programme should be instituted, concentrating on rotator cuff exercises. Failure to respond to a conservative programme within a year or so is a reasonable indication for surgical repair of the rotator cuff and release of acromial impingement.

Many therapies have been tried to modify the natural history of adhesive capsulitis of the shoulder joint. The mainstay of treatment remains intra-articular corticosteroid injection during the early phase when pain is the most prominent clinical complaint. During the phase of movement restriction without pain, it has been difficult to demonstrate the efficacy of any modality of treatment (including injection therapy, physiotherapy and anti-inflammatory drugs). Carefully directed corticosteroid injections also comprise the mainstay of treatment for a number of other shoulder problems, including acromioclavicular joint dysfunction, bicipital tendinitis and subacromial bursitis.

NECK PROBLEMS

Epidemiology

Neck pain is extremely common. According to studies from Finland and Canada, two-thirds of adults experience neck pain at some time;[6,32] in adults aged 25 years and over from the Netherlands the 12-month period prevalence was 31 per cent, with a point prevalence of 21 per cent and a prevalence of chronic symptoms (lasting more than three of the past 12 months) of 14 per cent;[33] a study from the UK estimated the prevalence of neck pain lasting greater than one week in the past four weeks in adulthood to be about 14 per cent;[34] and three studies from Sweden variously estimated a prevalence of chronic neck pain (more than three or more than six months) of 14–23 per cent.[35–37]

Prevalent neck pain, including chronic neck pain, is reported more often by older subjects, with a peak sometimes described in mid-life. Chronic neck pain, like back pain, is episodic and recurrent, with many individuals shifting their status over time. Thus, for example, in one study from Saskatchewan,[38] the 12-month cumulative incidence of new symptoms was 14.6 per cent among those free of neck pain at baseline, but disabling pain developed rarely, in only 0.6 per cent of the cohort. However, among subjects with neck pain initially, only a third enjoyed a complete resolution a year on, a further third reported persistence, almost 10 per cent experienced an aggravation of symptoms and a fifth had recurrent episodes of discomfort.

Pathogenesis of neck pain

The cervical spine is the most mobile and least stable section of the spine. Pain may arise from vertebrae, intervertebral discs, articulations or the complex system of ligaments and muscles. Unfortunately, although the International Association for the Study of Pain (IASP) recognizes some 60 sources of neck pain, the origin of symptoms is often unclear. Clinical and radiographic features are a weak guide to pathogenesis: tender points, restricted neck movement and degenerative changes on x-ray can be seen in the absence of neck pain.[39,40] In the general population, signs and symptoms correlate along a continuum with no distinct clustering suggestive of separate diagnostic entities.[40,41]

In the absence of clearer clinical pointers to pathogenesis, approaches to the classification of neck pain have varied. The diagnostic outcomes most often studied in occupational research are cervical spondylosis, cervical syndrome, tension neck syndrome and thoracic outlet syndrome, while the most popular classification schemes are those by Waris et al.,[42] Viikari-Juntura[43] and Ohlsson et al.[44]

Occupational studies

Neck complaints do appear to show an association with occupation, with lower incidence rates in office workers than in manual workers.[45] Four categories of neck problem have been particularly considered in surveys: cervical spondylosis, cervical syndrome, tension neck syndrome and thoracic outlet syndrome.

CERVICAL SPONDYLOSIS

This condition is characterized by degenerative changes in the intervertebral discs (particularly of the lower cervical spine) with the development of osteophytes and spurs. These changes are commonly accompanied by osteoarthritic change in the facet and neurocentral joints. The diagnosis of cervical spondylosis is often made on clinical grounds, but can be made with certainty only by the finding of typical changes on radiographs of the cervical spine. Cervical spondylosis is common from middle adult life and onwards, so that by the age of 65 years nearly everyone (90 per cent) will show radiographic evidence of the disease, irrespective of their occupational history. Some patients complain of stiffness, creaking and pain in the neck (which sometimes radiates to the occiput, shoulders and arms and is made worse by movement of the cervical spine), but many with similar radiographic evidence of disease do not. This lack of consistency between the symptoms and radiographic features of cervical spondylosis is a source of diagnostic difficulty. For these various reasons, surveys aimed at defining the extent and clinical significance of cervical spondylosis in different populations must be of limited value when based simply on the radiographic appearances of the cervical spine and/or symptom questionnaires. Radiographically verified cervical spondylosis has been found to occur significantly more commonly in meat carriers, dentists and miners than other groups.[23]

CERVICAL SYNDROME

Cervical syndrome is said to be present when pain in the neck coincides with symptom radiation along the distribution of a spinal nerve root. Some authorities also require limitation of neck movement and pain provoked by test manoeuvres before making the diagnosis. Although separately defined, this syndrome most probably arises from nerve root entrapment secondary to degenerative changes in the cervical spine. There have been relatively few studies of cervical syndrome in the occupational setting, and no compelling evidence of work-related risk.

TENSION NECK SYNDROME

Tension neck syndrome (TNS) is reported in Scandinavian and American studies of occupation, but is not described in standard textbooks of rheumatology and orthopaedics, and not widely recognized in the UK. However, it most closely corresponds to a regional pain disorder of the neck–shoulder area. It has been defined as a constant feeling of fatigue or stiffness in the neck associated with other subjective symptoms (such as neck pain or headache) and tender spots, palpable hardenings and neck muscle tightness.[23]

Such clinical patterns have been described in excess in assembly line workers,[46] data entry operators,[47] scissor makers,[18] lamp assemblers[48] and other groups, with reported risk ratios of 2.3 to 7.3. In keeping with this literature, a recent systematic review[49] found 'moderate' evidence that neck pain with palpation tenderness (TNS) and mixed neck–shoulder disorder (predominantly TNS) were causally related to repetition at the shoulder and neck flexion allied with repetition, but only limited evidence in relation to other factors, such as hand–wrist repetition and static loading in the absence of repetition. In the high quality Danish Project on Research and Intervention in Monotonous Work (PRIM) health study[50] – which involved pain-staking reconstruction of work tasks, videotape analysis of rates of repetition and proportion of time spent with the neck in various postures, and prospective blinded standardized assessment of outcome – strong exposure–response gradients were seen with the physical risk factors investigated, and odds ratios were raised by two- to three-fold in those whose jobs typically involved >15 versus 0 shoulder movements per minute or with the neck flexed >20° for at least two-thirds of the time.

Various mechanisms have been suggested for occupationally related TNS, including local muscle ischaemia, disturbed muscular microcirculation and sensitized pain receptors, but no specific pathological lesion has been identified. It seems plausible that tasks involving dynamic loading and tension of the shoulder and neck muscles produce such symptoms, but less clear whether they constitute a defined, discrete WMSD. (This may be a semantic point for occupational physicians who are interested in good ergonomic practice and worker comfort.)

THORACIC OUTLET SYNDROME

A constellation of neurological and vascular features ascribed to entrapment of the brachial nerve plexus and subclavian vessels by a cervical rib or congenital fibrous band. The frequency of this condition is highly contentious – some orthopaedic authors regard the syndrome as very rare in the general population, whereas others describe large panels of successfully treated patients.[51] A similar divergence of opinion exists in occupational medicine: some authorities have described high prevalences of the condition in assembly line workers (14–44 per cent),[52] cash register operators (32 per cent)[52] and plate workers (31 per cent),[53] but by contrast a UK expert workshop of occupational physicians, rheumatologists and orthopaedic surgeons considered it so rare as to obviate the need for consensus definition. This is in addition to the many sensory motor and vascular symptoms ascribed to thoracic outlet syndrome (TOS) which does not permit a ready description of established diagnostic criteria.

Management

The management of cervical pain syndromes is predominantly non-surgical. Acute exacerbations of neck pain are managed with a soft cervical collar, an eight-week course of combined analgesic and anti-inflammatory therapy and a physiotherapy programme. The physical therapy should include the use of heat pad, neck exercises, ultrasound/short-wave diathermy and massage. Traction and transcutaneous electrical nerve stimulation (TENS) are helpful in controlling brachial root irritation. Manipulative therapy and acupuncture may assist in selected resistant cases. The principal indication for structural imaging (MRI or computed tomography (CT)) is objective neurological deficit. If severe foraminal encroachment or myelopathy is discovered, surgical decompression may become necessary.

ELBOW

The elbow joint actually comprises a compound synovial joint with articulation between the ulnar notch and the trochlea of the humerus, and also between the radial head and the humeral capitellum. In consequence, a large variety of movements are possible, including flexion of 150°, pronation of 75–80° and supination of 85–90°. Apart from epicondylitis and olecranon bursitis, soft tissue problems of the elbow are uncommon.

Epidemiology

Epicondylitis is a pattern of pain at the origins of the extensors of the fingers and wrists on the lateral epicondyle (lateral epicondylitis), or at the origin of the flexors on the medial epicondyle of the humerus (medial epicondylitis). Lateral epicondylitis (tennis elbow) is about seven times more common than medial epicondylitis (golfers' elbow). The point prevalence of elbow pain has been reported at 11–13 per cent in aeroengineering workers[4] and textile workers[3] and in a population survey the period prevalence of elbow pain during the previous year was 7 per cent in 40–50 year olds and 14 per cent in those over 50 years.[54] However, clinically verified epicondylitis is less common: among the textile workers only 2 per cent had tender as well as painful elbows[3] and in a Swedish community survey that included clinical examination the prevalence in 31–74 year olds was

2.5 per cent.[9] Clinical epicondylitis reaches a peak prevalence and incidence in the fifth decade of life, and becomes increasingly less common after the age of 50 years.[9] It more commonly affects the dominant hand. Although 40–50 per cent of tennis players have the condition,[55] less than 5 per cent of cases arise from the sport.[56]

Aetiology

Lateral epicondylitis is believed to arise principally from overexertion of the finger and wrist extensors – in repeated hand dorsiflexion or in alternating forearm pronation and supination.[56] In those cases coming to clinical attention, there is often a history of unaccustomed, forceful, repetitive use.

However, the pathological lesion remains a point of debate, and there have been at least 25 suggested causes.[57] The most widely held theory is that macroscopic or microscopic tears occur between the common extensor tendon and the periosteum of the lateral humeral epicondyle,[58] and such tears have been identified in surgical procedures,[59] but not consistently enough to resolve the argument.[56]

Occupational studies

Over 20 epidemiological studies have examined workplace physical risk factors and their relation to epicondylitis. A major review by NIOSH[21] found 'insufficient' evidence for associations with repetition and postural factors when considered individually, and only weak evidence in relation to forceful work, but the evidence was considered 'strong' when these factors existed in combination. As examples of the evidence base, in three cross-sectional surveys comparing meat cutters, sausage makers and packers with workers in less strenuous jobs, Viikari-Juntura et al.[60] found that elbow symptoms were 1.6–1.8 times more common in the exposed groups, but the prevalence of clinically verified epicondylitis was identical (0.8 per cent). Dimberg et al. reported a higher prevalence in aircraft factory workers (7.4 per cent), but found no difference between white- and blue-collar workers.[4] McCormack et al. described a relative risk of 1.5 in packers and sewers compared with knitters,[3] a moderate excess of clinical epicondylitis has been described in a cross-sectional survey of public gas and water workers with long-term exposure to strenuous elbow work[61] and Luopajarvi et al. described a similar-sized effect when women packers were compared with non-cashier shop assistants,[15] but these differences are comparatively modest and the confidence intervals for the risk estimates were compatible with chance.

In 1997, when the review was written, just one cohort study had been published,[62] with strongly positive findings: an incidence rate 7–10 times higher in meat cutters and sausage makers (designated as jobs with high force and repetition) relative to other workers. Ten years on, the evidence base is scarcely more extensive, although one case–control and one cohort study point in the same direction. Haahr et al.[63] compared work exposures in 267 cases and 388 referents, recruited from Danish general practices and found associations with various activities performed for three-quarters or more of the time versus never/almost never – namely, arms lifted in front of the body (odds ratio (OR) 4.0 for women), hands bent or twisted (OR 7.4 for women, 3.2 for men), same movements of the arm (OR 3.7 for women) and work requiring precise movements (OR 5.2 for men). In France, where workers have routine statutory medicals, Leclerc et al.[64] reported that jobs that involved repetitive turning and screwing doubled the risks of incident epicondylitis after allowing for other factors.

Clinical aspects

The hallmark of lateral epicondylitis is slow onset pain and tenderness over the lateral epicondyle. The pain is reproduced by resisted dorsiflexion of the wrist with the elbow extended. Grip is impaired and this may limit working ability. In medial epicondylitis, the pain and tenderness (which are medially located) are often less prominent. Pain is reproduced over the medial epicondyle by resisted palmar flexion of the wrist. Investigations are generally unhelpful and unnecessary.

Management

Many treatments have been proposed, though not all have been validated. Placing the arm in a sling or plaster cast may help, but recovery often requires six weeks of immobility. A wrist splint (to prevent wrist dorsiflexion) sometimes provides symptomatic relief. Pulsed ultrasound has been shown to be efficacious,[65] while up to 90 per cent of subjects respond to local injection of corticosteroids. In resistant cases, surgery may be required as a last resort. After conservative treatment relapse is fairly common (18–50 per cent within six months[66,67]), especially in manual workers such as mechanics and builders.[68] In a case series of 88 workers visiting an occupational health department,[69] splint therapy combined with indomethacin was compared with cortisone therapy; neither duration of absence from work, nor recurrence rate differed between the treatment groups.

It is said that lateral epicondylitis resolves spontaneously in eight to twelve months,[57] but in one rheumatology clinic a majority of sufferers were still symptomatic at the one year stage.[68]

TENOSYNOVITIS AND PERITENDINITIS

There is some confusion in the literature about the appropriate terminology for this lesion. Some authors draw a distinction between inflammation of the tendon sheath of the wrist (tenosynovitis), the paratendon at the muscle–tendon junction rather further up the arm (peritendinitis), and the tendon itself (tendinitis), but such a distinction is not often drawn in the classification criteria adopted in occupational and community surveys. For this reason, we use the terms interchangeably in this account.

Epidemiology

In the US National Health Interview, 20 per 1000 adults reported that a doctor had told them they had 'tendinitis',[70] while in the UK Primary Care Study for 1981, the incidence of tenosynovitis, tendinitis, synovitis and bursitis combined was 10.9 per 1000 persons per year.[10] The incidence was more common in women than men at all ages, and peaked in middle age.

Occupational studies

There have been several cross-sectional surveys of hand–wrist tendinitis in the workplace. In a recent systematic review,[71] elevated relative risks (RRs) were found in four studies of assembly and packing – one in the shoe industry (prevalence ratio (PR) 3.7),[46] one in automobile workers (PR 2.5),[72] one of assembly line packers (PR 4.1)[15] and one of meat packers (RR 36).[62] In addition, two positive surveys were found of meat cutters. A longitudinal study by Kurppa et al.[62] found an incidence rate ratio of 13.9, while an odds ratio (OR) of 3.1 was reported in a smaller investigation by Roto et al.[73] The first of these studies also indicated a high RR (24.1) in women making sausages.[62] Finally, in a cross-sectional study that examined risks by physical activity, jobs that combined high force and high repetition carried a 29-fold greater risk of tendinitis than those lacking such features.[74]

Clinical aspects

The tendons most frequently involved are the radial extensors of the wrist and the long abductor and short extensor of the thumb. The flexor tendons are affected far less often.

TENOSYNOVITIS OF THE WRIST (DE QUERVAIN'S DISEASE)

Tenosynovitis of the wrist (De Quervain's disease) is characterized by pain on movement, localized to the tendon sheaths in the wrist and reproduced by resisted active movement. Pain is centred on the radial aspect of the wrist and thumb base, and particularly aggravated in grasping and employing the pinch grip. Typically symptoms appear following return to work after a long lay off, or following a change to unfamiliar work requiring new, rapid movements. For example, many cases occurred in the 1940s when people were required as part of the war effort to undertake unaccustomed work in factories and in agriculture.[75] Initially, a dull aching is experienced, but continuation of the work can give rise to severe pain. In the classical case, a sausage-shaped swelling is present on the radial side of the lower part of the dorsal surface of the forearm, proximal to the radial styloid process. The swelling, which is generally about 4 cm long, is tender and crepitus is often palpable and audible over it, sometimes extending up the forearm. Local redness and warmth may occur. In the less florid case, the diagnosis may be confused with osteoarthritis of the thumb base, but radiological assessment assists in this differential diagnosis.

The treatment consists of local heat, non-steroidal anti-inflammatory drugs (NSAIDs), and wrist and thumb immobilization by thermoplastic splinting. In patients with severe or persistent pain, one or more local corticosteroid injections can be helpful, giving complete and lasting relief in about 70 per cent of patients. Surgical decompression of the first extensor compartment (with or without tenosynovectomy) is indicated in those with persistent symptoms lasting longer than six months.

TRIGGER FINGER

Trigger finger is the result of tenosynovitis affecting the flexor tendons of the finger or thumb. The consequent fibrosis and constriction impair the tendon's motion at the first annular pulley, which overlies the metacarpophalangeal joint. The most common cause of trigger finger is said to be overuse of the hands in repetitive gripping activities. Management consists of modification of hand activity, local heat treatment, gentle exercises and NSAIDs as required. One or more corticosteroid injections to the affected flexor tendons cure the majority of patients. Surgical transection of the fibrous annular pulley is rarely required.

The evidence of benefit in these various treatments usually relates to short-term improvement, and there is clearly a need to demonstrate their longer-term benefit in controlled trials of adequate design. Such trials should reflect the occupational environment in which the pain syndrome developed and the effect of ergonomic interventions instituted during the trial period.

CARPAL TUNNEL SYNDROME

As it passes through the carpal tunnel into the wrist, the median nerve lies immediately beneath the palmaris longus tendon and anterior to the flexor tendons. Conditions that decrease the size of the carpal tunnel or increase the volume of structures contained within it, tend to compress the median nerve against the transverse ligament which bounds the tunnel's roof. Such circumstances can arise traumatically, congenitally or due to systemic or inflammatory effects (for example, diabetes mellitus, rheumatoid arthritis, acromegaly, hypothyroidism, pregnancy and tenosynovitis).

Table 57.3 Case-control studies of carpal tunnel syndrome and its relation to work activities.

Exposure		Odds ratio	Reference
Vibration	Use of vibrating tools	7.0	Cannon et al.[87]
	Exposure for more than 20 years	4.8	Wieslander et al.[88]
	Use of vibrating tools		Voog et al.[89]
	1–10 hours per week	3.2	
	More than 10 hours per week	14.0	
	Powered tools or machinery		Nordstrom et al.[90]
	2.5–5.5 hours per day	1.6	
	More than 6 hours per day	3.3	
Flexed wrist	1–7 hours per week	1.5	De Krom et al.[76]
	8–19 hours per week	3.0	
	20–40 hours per week	8.7	
Extended wrist	1–7 hours per week	1.4	
	8–19 hours per week	2.3	
	20–40 hours per week	5.4	
Repetitive wrist movements	1–20 years	1.5	Wieslander et al.[88]
	More than 20 years	4.6	
	3.5–6 hours per day	2.7	Nordstrom et al.[90]
	More than 6 hours per day	2.1	
	Keyboard typist	3.8	Voog et al.[89]

Epidemiology

The symptoms, signs and nerve conduction abnormalities of carpal tunnel syndrome (CTS), can arise separately, or in combination. Estimates of prevalence and incidence therefore vary according to the chosen case definition. In a large Dutch population survey that took as its definition sensory disturbance in the median nerve distribution occurring at least twice a week, generally waking the patient from sleep, and associated with neurophysiological abnormalities, the point prevalence was estimated at 0.6 per cent in men and 8 per cent in women.[76] Clinically diagnosed CTS occurred with a prevalence of 1.1 per cent in textile workers[3] and 2.1 per cent in other industrial workers.[74] The crude incidence rate is reported to be one per thousand person years in hospital diagnosed patients,[77,78] and around two per thousand person years in UK primary care (unpublished data from the Royal College of General Practitioners).

Obesity and short stature appear to be independent risk factors for CTS.[78,79] In case reports, pregnancy, the oral contraceptive pill, the menopause, hysterectomy and breast feeding have all been linked with the syndrome, although epidemiological evidence is contradictory. The condition is often bilateral and symptoms tend to be worse in the dominant hand.

Occupational studies

The relation between CTS and worker activities has been investigated repeatedly. For example, a review by Hagberg et al.[80] in 1992 identified 15 cross-sectional studies and six case–control studies that met high quality criteria for case ascertainment. In the cross-sectional studies, the prevalence of CTS between different occupational groups varied from 0.6 to 61 per cent. Particularly high prevalences and odds ratios were reported in grinders,[81] grocery store workers,[82] frozen food factory workers[83] and platers.[84] The authors concluded that repetitive and forceful gripping were major risk factors for occurrence of the syndrome. Silverstein et al.[85] classified the occupation of 652 workers from seven different industries according to the degree of force and repetition required, and found, compared with low force–low repetition jobs, that both high force and high frequency increased the risk moderately (odds ratios 1.8 and 2.7, respectively), but that the combination of high force and high frequency resulted in an odds ratio of more than 15.

The strongest associations in case–control studies have been with use of vibratory tools and with activities that frequently flex or extend the wrist (Table 57.3). The link with vibratory exposure has also been described in industry-specific surveys, notably among foresters[86] and is accepted for compensation purposes by the UK State Industrial Injuries Benefits Scheme. However, use of vibrating tools is often correlated with forceful repetitive work and it remains unclear whether the effect arises from the ergonomic aspects of vibratory tool use or from a more general effect of vibration on peripheral nerves.

A review by Palmer et al.,[91] in summarizing 38 other primary research reports (including those identified by Hagberg et al.[80]), also drew attention to the substantial body of evidence that highly repetitious flexion and extension of the wrist can more than double risks of CTS, and recently this association has been accepted for compensation purposes witin the terms of the UK State Industrial Injuries Benefits Scheme.

It should be remembered that case–control studies, like cross-sectional surveys, are susceptible to well-recognized biases. The association with a particular exposure may be spuriously inflated by recall bias, or by the effect of disease on work (if the decision to consult relates especially to difficulty in getting the job done). In CTS investigations, however, the studies have been in broad agreement. The more classically specific the case definition, the stronger the association with physical risk factors.[92] Furthermore, it can be demonstrated experimentally that extreme flexion and extreme extension of the wrist increase the pressure in the carpal tunnel sufficiently to impair blood perfusion of the median nerve, so that epidemiological and physiological investigations provide a coherent view of causation.

Clinical aspects

The history is typically one of gradual onset of numbness and tingling in the median nerve distribution of the hand. Strenuous use of the hand usually aggravates symptoms, although this may not become apparent until several hours after the activity. Night-time pain commonly disturbs sleep and patients often hang the affected hand over the side of the bed in an effort to gain relief. Many sufferers also complain of progressive weakness and clumsiness in their hands and tend to drop things.

Tinel's test (percussion over the flexor retinaculum reproducing parasthesiae over the median nerve distribution) is positive in about three-quarters of sufferers, and Phalen's test (sustained complete flexion of the wrist for 1 minute producing symptoms over the median nerve distribution) is positive in a similar proportion.[93] In one large case series, clinical impairment of sensation could be demonstrated over the median nerve in a quarter of cases, and thenar atrophy in a fifth.

The most important diagnostic test is nerve conduction. A slowed sensory nerve conduction velocity across the carpal tunnel and a prolonged distal motor latency support the diagnosis. Electrodiagnostic tests are often quoted as the gold standard, but even the most sensitive latency tests confirm no more than 90 per cent of 'classical' clinical cases.

Management

The specific treatment of carpal tunnel syndrome depends to a large degree on whether there is an identifiable cause of the entrapment. Conservative measures may suffice when symptoms are of short duration. Electromyographic determinations repeated over time may help the clinician determine the correct therapeutic approach. Other measures which are known to be of benefit include splinting, local corticosteroid injection, the use of anti-inflammatory drugs and, ultimately, surgical release.

CHRONIC UPPER LIMB PAIN

In describing upper limb disorders, different physicians have used a variety of terms in a variety of ways. For some, 'work-related upper limb disorders', 'cumulative trauma disorders' and 'repetitive strain disorders' are synonymous, and describe collectively the full range of recognized and ill-defined disorders arising (or appearing to arise) from frequent, forceful overuse of the upper limb at work. For others, repetitive strain injury (RSI) refers to a particular diagnosis made by exclusion, i.e. chronic upper limb pain ascribed to overuse at work, for which no clinical diagnosis can be made. Inevitably, confusion has ensued among doctors and especially in medical litigation.

The problem can be illustrated by reference to some topical cases that have attracted publicity. In 1981, an enquiry over upper limb complaints in an Inland Revenue office accepted that complaints, such as lateral epicondylitis and tenosynovitis, could sometimes arise from the use of the visual display unit (VDU). In December 1991, Judge Byre found in the High Court that two British Telecom keyboard operators had RSI that had been induced by the nature of the work (at least 10 000 depressions per hour with a bonus for higher totals) and long hours in constrained postures on defective seating (the complaints were diagnosed as tenosynovitis and epicondylitis). In 1994, a legal secretary received an award for tenosynovitis provoked by periods of intense typing. By contrast, in 1993 Judge Prosser, dismissed the complaints of a Reuters journalist, concluding that 'RSI did not exist'. Such a ruling plainly does not disprove the existence of well-established entities, like lateral epicondylitis and tenosynovitis, and the debate is really on two different fronts: (1) how often such specific complaints can arise from work activity and (2) whether there is a condition of chronic upper limb pain which presently defies clinical diagnosis, and which may be caused by work. Information on these questions has been tainted by studies that have drawn no distinction between potentially dissimilar clinical end points.

In this chapter we have attempted to draw a clearer distinction. The term RSI in the text that follows refers to chronic upper arm pain for which no diagnosis can be made and which has been ascribed to occupational overuse.

Epidemiology

It has proved difficult to define the epidemiology of a condition for which no clear definition and no validated or accepted diagnostic criteria exist. Routinely collected statistics tend to involve umbrella classifications that make it

Table 57.4 Incidence rates of compensated repetitive strain injury (RSI) by industry in Australia, 1985–86 (adapted from Gun[94]).

Industry	Male incidence[a]	Female incidence[a]
Manufacturing		
Food, beverages	4.5	7.4
Textiles, clothing, footwear	4.7	4.2
Public administration	3.9	4.8
Agriculture	3.1	1.7
Transport equipment	3.0	16.2
Basic metal manufacture	2.5	16.7
Finance, business services	0.2	3.0
Mining	0.5	1.5
Health services	0.3	1.2
All industries combined	1.4	2.6

[a]Per thousand person-years.

hard to disentangle information on non-specific upper limb pain. However, in Australia, the Bureau of Statistics separately codes compensation awards for injuries without explicit diagnosis ascribed to repetitive movement. Table 57.4 illustrates the variation in incidence rate of compensated RSI between men and women, and by industry.[94] Overall, RSI was more common in blue-collar workers than in clerical workers. For men, the highest rates occurred in the manufacture of textiles, clothing and footwear, food and beverages. In women, very high incidence rates occurred in parts of the manufacturing sector.

Sequential data over the period 1980–87 showed dramatic changes with time. The number of successful claims among women in 1984–85 was five times greater than in 1980–81, and that amongst men 50 per cent greater. Hocking[95] reported on the Australian RSI epidemic as it affected one large employer, the nationalized telephone operator Telecom Australia between 1981 and 1985. Nearly half of the 3976 reports within the company arose in telephonists, providing an incident rate of 343 cases per thousand keyboard workers over the five years, as compared with 284 per thousand in clerical workers, 116 per thousand in process workers and 34 per thousand in telegraphists. Women accounted for 83 per cent of all reports. Sixteen per cent of subjects had symptoms lasting longer than six months and the cost of the epidemic was estimated at more than $15 million dollars.

Of course, the decision to lodge a complaint or to compensate a claim, or even to pay attention to a symptom, can be heavily influenced by local awareness and health beliefs, fuelled by media publicity. It has been found, for example, that arm pain is far less commonly reported by Indian workers in Mumbai (who have a very low awareness of RSI) than in UK Asian workers doing essentially similar work,[96] and that arm pain is far more often attributed to work in surveys than can be explained by known physical risk factors from the workplace.[97] By the 1990s, the compensation rate in Australia had declined to a more normal level without any reduction in occupational physical demands. Similar transient epidemics have been seen in other countries and other time periods: in Japan, an epidemic of 'occupational cervicobrachial disorders' was reported between 1958 and 1982 and an epidemic of writer's cramp occurred among male clerks in the British Civil Service in 1830. In the Japanese outbreak, the workers who most frequently complained were typists and keyboard operators, punchcard operators and telephone operators (10–28 per cent of people claimed to be affected in some of the occupational groups[98]). As a result, the Japanese Ministry of Labour introduced guidelines that restricted working time at the keyboard to no more than five hours a day and the maximum number of key strokes to 40 000 per day, and this was followed by a fall in the frequency of complaints.[99] Another crop of upper limb complaints developed in the Inland Revenue Department of the British Civil Service in 1981.

The time variation in these various data sets suggests that psychosocial variables play an important part in the presentation and recognition of the condition, if not also in its development.

Clinical aspects

Miller et al.[100] have described a series of 200 consecutive patients referred for specialist opinion with suspected RSI in whom no other specific diagnosis could be made. In 75 per cent, the onset of pain was gradual, beginning as localized distal pain, but more diffusely spread by the time of clinic attendance. Nearly all of the patients described paraesthesiae and 73 per cent described subjective swelling of the limb. The dominant hand was more commonly affected, but bilateral disease was also common. Anxiety, irritation, mood change, fatigue and sleep disturbance were nearly always present. Clinical signs were generally absent, although most of the patients described tenderness at multiple sites.

In this respect, RSI has many similarities with fibromyalgia, a chronic musculoskeletal disorder of uncertain cause characterized by chronic widespread pain and multiple tender points. Fibromyalgia sufferers also tend to complain of fatigue, sleep disturbance, stiffness and paraesthesiae, and the clinical similarity between these two conditions has led to the suggestion that RSI is a fibromyalgia variant.[100,101] Fibromyalgia is fairly common, affecting around 1–2 per cent of the population,[102,103] 5–8 per cent of hospital attendees[104] and 14–20 per cent of patients referred to a rheumatology clinic.[105,106] The diagnostic criteria of the American College of Rheumatologists requires the pain of fibromyalgia to be present for at least three months in all four quadrants of the body and axial skeleton, with tenderness at 11 of 18 defined examination points.[107] The key point of clinical distinction is that fibromyalgia, pain and tender points occur in the trunk and lower limbs, as well as in the arm, shoulder and neck.

It has been suggested that RSI is a condition of pain amplification leading to abnormally low cutaneous pain threshold (allodynia), muscle stiffness and vasomotor changes. However, these ideas remain largely untested. Clinical and some epidemiological observations suggest that personality, emotional state, health beliefs, culture and psyche are important too, and pessimism about recovery is a poor prognostic indicator in arm pain sufferers, even when account is taken of case severity.[108]

No standard scheme exists to classify case severity in suspected cases of RSI, but the Australian Occupational Repetitive Strain Injuries Advisory Committee of the New South Wales Government of Industrial Relations proposed a three-stage clinical grading scale. The first stage was characterized by aching and tiredness occurring at work but settling overnight. In stage 2 disease, symptoms failed to settle overnight and disturbed sleep, a condition that could persist for several months. Finally, in stage 3 disease symptoms persisted at rest, prevented even light duties and were persistent over months or years. The relation between this proposed clinical grading scheme and the various specific and non-specific disorders that may be encountered in practice remains unclear.

Management

These aetiological components suggest and support a biopsychosocial approach to treatment. A structured rehabilitation programme including graduated exercises, behavioural approaches to pain control, analgesic medication and assistive devices, such as short-term splinting, may achieve dramatic benefits in the small number of severely affected patients. In this subgroup, there is otherwise a very low probability of returning to gainful employment.

DUPUYTREN'S CONTRACTURE

Dupuytren's contracture is a nodular proliferation of fibrous tissue of the palmar fascia which leads to contracture and permanent flexion of the fingers (especially the fourth and fifth fingers) of one or both hands.

Epidemiology

Dupuytren's contracture is a common condition. In northern Europe, for example, it affects about 10 per cent of men aged over 65 years. The condition is more common in men than women, and the prevalence increases with age.[109]

The condition is frequently bilateral. In a recent case–control study, the condition was found to be independently associated with cigarette smoking and alcohol consumption.[110] It is also known to be more common in patients with diabetes and epilepsy.

Occupational studies

The relation between Dupuytren's contracture and acute or cumulative traumatic injury is controversial. Case reports exist of Dupuytren's contracture arising soon after an acute injury to the hand, such as a penetrating wound, crush injury or fracture,[111] although epidemiological studies have not been conducted so far to investigate the association more formally. The relation between Dupuytren's contracture and chronic cumulative trauma has been reviewed recently by Liss and Stock.[112]

Bennett[113] observed a standardized morbidity ratio of 1.96 for Dupuytren's contracture among bagging and packing plant workers as compared with the expected age-adjusted prevalence from an earlier survey, and an odds ratio of 5.5 compared with workers from the local plant who did not undertake these activities. While Mikkelsen[114] reported a sex-adjusted odds ratio of 3.1 for heavy versus light manual work in a population-based sample from Norway. However, the literature is comparatively sparse.

The relation with use of vibrating tools has been investigated more extensively. Thomas and Clarke[115] observed that Dupuytren's contracture was twice as common in 500 men claiming vibration-induced white finger than in 150 controls admitted to hospital for elective surgery. An Italian case–control study[116] reported an odds ratio of 2.3 for exposure to vibration at work after adjustment for alcohol. In another Italian investigation, Bovenzi et al.[117] observed an increased frequency of Dupuytren's contracture among quarry drillers and stone carvers compared with stone workers who performed manual work but were not exposed to vibration (odds ratio 2.6, 95 per cent CI 1.1–6.2). Other researchers, by contrast, have failed to observe such an association.[112]

In summary, there is some evidence that Dupuytren's contracture may arise from occupational activities and this evidence is strongest for exposure to hand-transmitted vibration. The relation between Dupuytren's contracture and other manual work is uncertain at present.

OTHER SOFT TISSUE RHEUMATIC CONDITIONS

Two other categories of complaint that may be related to repetitive physical activity are recognized (prescribed) for state compensation under the UK Department for Work and Pensions (DWP)'s Industrial Injuries Disablement Benefits (IIDB) provisions:

- cramp of the hand or forearm 'due to repetitive movements';

- the 'beat' conditions – subcutaneous cellulitis of the hand (beat hand) and subcutaneous cellulitis or bursitis of the knee (beat knee) or elbow (beat elbow).

The epithet 'beat' has been removed in a recent revision of IIDB terminology. Carpal tunnel syndrome in vibrating tool users and tenosynovitis are also prescribed.

Writer's cramp, telegraphist's cramp, twister's cramp or craft palsy

This is said to be a condition of occupations that involve a great deal of handwriting, typing or other repetitive movement of the hand or arm. According to Department for Work and Pensions examiners' guidelines, it manifests as symptoms of spasm, tremor and pain in the hand or forearm (Focal dystonia) brought about by attempts to perform a familiar repetitive muscular action, and occurs in the absence of physical signs or detectable abnormalities on investigation. Many physicians would question whether such an entity exists as a defined disease. The time course and chronicity of disease is not clearly defined, and it would appear difficult in practice to distinguish this condition from transient occupational discomfort or chronic non-specific upper limb pain. Despite these uncertainties, around 120 new cases undergo assessment each year for prescription purposes.

The beat conditions

These are a more clearly recognized group of disorders. Repeated use of picks, shovels and hand tools in miners, quarrymen and labourers has sometimes been associated with a subcutaneous cellulitis of the hand with associated pain, tenderness, redness and swelling (beat hand) which may leave some residual disability. A sterile bursitis (beat knee) may sometimes arise in work that entails prolonged kneeling, such as coal mining, plumbing or carpet fitting. A similar disorder may arise at the elbow (beat elbow), although its association with occupational activity has been less clearly defined. It is assumed in each of these conditions that repeated physical trauma, friction and pressure are causal factors. It is not known how commonly these complaints occur, but nearly 200 new claims per year are assessed by DWP special medical boards in connection with them.

OSTEOARTHRITIS

Epidemiology and clinical features

Osteoarthritis (OA) is probably the most common joint disorder in the world. In western populations, radiographic evidence of OA occurs in the majority of people by the age of 65 years, and in about 80 per cent of those aged 75 years and over.[118] The disorder is second only to ischaemic heart disease as a cause of work-related disability in men over 50 years of age.

OA is defined as focal loss of articular cartilage with variable subchondral bone reaction. There is incomplete concordance between these pathological features and radiographic or clinical characteristics of the disorder. However, the difficulties encountered in using a pathological definition for epidemiological studies of OA have led to the widespread use of radiological and clinical markers. The radiographic features conventionally used to define the severity of OA include joint space narrowing, osteophyte, subchondral sclerosis, cyst formation and abnormalities of bony contour. These radiographic features can be incorporated in rating scales at the commonly affected joint sites (for example, the hand, knee and hip), permitting standardized grading of disease severity.[119] The two clinical sequelae of OA that are most relevant are joint pain and functional impairment.

The development of OA at any joint site depends upon a generalized predisposition to the condition, and biomechanical abnormalities that act at specific joints.[118,120] Individual risk factors that may be associated with a generalized susceptibility to the disorder include obesity, a family history and hypermobility. Those that reflect local biomechanical insults include trauma, abnormalities of joint shape and physical activity, including work.

Occupational studies

KNEE OSTEOARTHRITIS

The four major non-occupational risk factors for knee OA are obesity, knee injury, meniscectomy and the presence of Herberden's nodes.[121] Evidence has accumulated in recent years that risk is also increased by work that entails prolonged or repetitive knee bending, squatting, kneeling and load bearing with the knee flexed. These data fall into four categories: (1) comparisons of the prevalence of knee OA in different occupational groups, (2) assessment of the risk of knee OA in different occupations, (3) case–control studies in which general assessments of activity level in the workplace are compared in patients with knee OA and controls and (4) more detailed case–control studies in which a history of specific activities in the workplace is obtained.

Observational studies on the prevalence of symptomatic or radiographic knee OA in different occupational groups date back over 40 years (Figure 57.1). In 1952, Kellgren and Lawrence found that the prevalence of moderate to severe radiographic knee OA was almost six times greater among miners than clerical workers.[122] Later studies in dockers and civil servants,[123] painters and concrete workers[124] and shipyard workers and clerks,[125] all confirmed that the risk of knee OA is greater among men involved in heavy manual labour.

These observations have been extended by a register-based Swedish cohort study,[126] in which the risk of knee OA coming to arthroplasty in various occupational groups was compared with the baseline population risk. Men employed as firefighters, farmers and construction workers presented significantly more often for surgery. Among women, there was a significant excess among cleaners. The risk estimates for these occupations varied from 1.4 to 3.0. These observations agree with the findings of three case–control studies of knee OA in the United States,[127] the Netherlands[128] and Sweden.[129] When workplace activity was classified as heavy or light, the cases in all of these studies were between two and three times more likely to have been engaged in heavy activity occupations before the occurrence of knee OA. However, the risk estimates in all three studies failed to attain statistical significance.

Perhaps the most compelling evidence linking knee OA with occupational activity comes from two population-based surveys in the United States. In an analysis of cross-sectional data from the HANES I study,[130] radiographic OA of the knee at age 55–64 years was three times more common in people whose jobs were judged likely to entail knee bending. In a follow-up study of 1400 men and women from Framingham,[131] the risk of radiographic knee OA was highest in subjects whose earlier jobs were classified as both physically demanding and likely to involve bending of the knees.

In each of these studies, data on knee use in the workplace was obtained by extrapolation from job title rather than through direct questioning about workplace activity, but two British population-based case–control studies of knee OA examined specific occupational activities in some detail. Cases with symptomatic knee OA from a defined population in Bristol were compared with age- and sex-matched controls who had no evidence of knee pain or radiographic abnormality.[132] A lifetime occupational history was obtained, as well as details of specific workplace physical activities (kneeling, squatting, stair climbing, walking, standing, heavy lifting, sitting and driving). The risk of symptomatic knee OA (after adjustment for body mass index and the presence of Heberden's nodes) was significantly increased among men and women whose major previous occupation had entailed prolonged squatting (greater than 30 minutes daily), prolonged kneeling (greater than 30 minutes daily) and repeated stair climbing (greater than ten flights daily). There was no increase in risk associated with prolonged walking, standing, sitting or driving. Regular heavy lifting (25 kg daily) was not independently associated with an increase in risk, but subjects whose occupations involved heavy lifting and repeated knee flexion in combination had a substantial increase in risk (Figure 57.2). Jobs frequently reported by the cases as involving squatting or kneeling included teaching and nursing in women and steel erecting, electrical maintenance, roofing and other construction work in men. It was estimated from the data that around 5 per cent of all symptomatic knee OA might result from occupations involving repetitive knee use. Extrapolation from the Framingham study suggests an even greater attributable risk.

A second British case–control study by Coggon et al.[133] compared patients listed for surgical treatment of knee

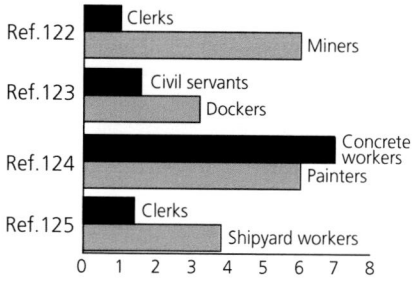

Figure 57.1 Observational studies examining the prevalence of radiographic knee osteoarthritis among various occupational groups.

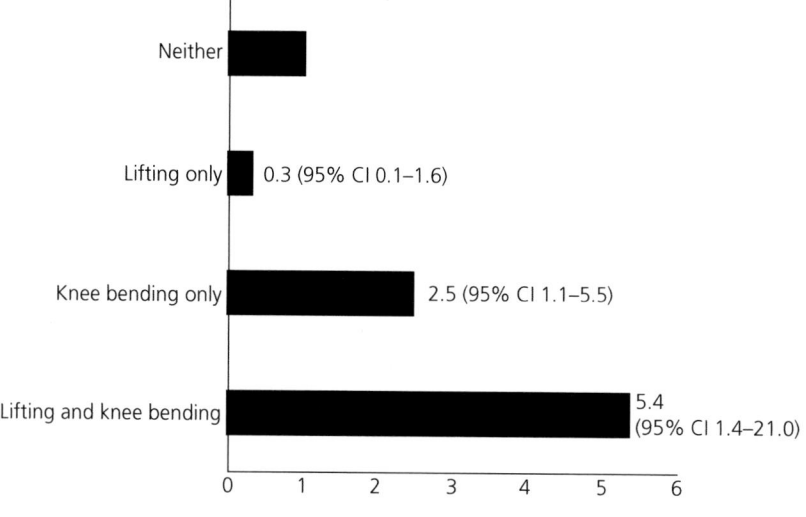

Figure 57.2 Risk of knee osteoarthritis according to occupations involving heavy lifting and repetitive knee flexion. Data derived from a population-based case–control study in Bristol.

Table 57.5 Medical management of patients with osteoarthritis of the knee or hip.

Therapy	
Non-pharmacological therapy	Patient education (self-management programmes (e.g. Arthritis Self-Help Course))
	Health professional social support (via telephone contact)
	Weight loss (if overweight)
	Physiotherapy
	Range of motion exercises
	Quadriceps strengthening exercises
	Assistive devices for ambulation
	Occupational therapy
	Joint protection and energy conservation
	Assistive devices for ADLs
	Aerobic exercise programmes
Pharmacological therapy	Intra-articular steroid injections
	Analgesics (e.g. paracetamol), topical analgesics (e.g. capsaicin) and topical anti-inflammatory creams, nonsteroidal anti-inflammatory drugs, opioid analgesics

ADL, activities of daily living.

osteoarthritis with age- and sex-matched controls from the same communities. After statistical adjustment for body weight, history of knee injury and the presence of markers of Heberden's nodes, risks were more than doubled in subjects kneeling or squatting at work for more than one hour per day over at least one year and raised 1.7-fold in those lifting weights of ≥25 kg more than ten times per week for at least a year. There was also an association with occupational climbing of ladders and stairs in men (odds ratio 2.3), but not in women. Even greater risks were reported from work that entailed both kneeling/squatting and heavy lifting (OR relative to neither activity 2.9 in men and 4.2 in women).

The balance of evidence thus favours occupational physical workload as a risk factor for knee OA, with risks being notably high in workers with non-occupational risk factors, such as morbid obesity.

HIP OSTEOARTHRITIS

The risk factor profile for hip OA is somewhat different from that for knee OA. There is a weaker association with obesity, hip injury and Heberden's nodes[118,120] and a greater influence from developmental disorders of the hip joint, such as congenital dislocation of the hip, slipped upper femoral epiphysis and Perthes' disease.

Data on the relationship between specific work activities, such as heavy lifting, and the risk of hip OA are not currently available. However, some studies have compared the occurrence of hip OA according to occupational title. Strong evidence has emerged that one such occupation – farming – is associated with high rates of the disorder.[134] Early studies from France, Norway and Sweden suggested that farmers had higher rates of total hip arthroplasty for OA than other occupational groups. In the large Swedish cohort study, which included 250 000 people in the blue-collar occupations,[126] the relative risk for hip arthroplasty among farmers was 3.8 (95 per cent CI, 2.9–3.9). However, farmers may seek treatment more often than other occupational groups, not because they have a higher incidence of the disorder, but because they are more handicapped by it when it occurs. This issue may be addressed by population-based radiographic studies comparing the prevalence of hip OA in farmers and other workers. In a British study[134] comparing men from a defined population aged 60–75 years who had ever been in farming with a group of controls who had spent their entire careers in clerical work, the prevalence of moderate/severe radiographic hip OA (defined as a minimal joint space <1.5 mm) was found to be 18 per cent in the former group, as compared with 2.4 per cent in the controls. This gave a summary odds ratio for hip OA among the farmers of 7.8 (95 per cent CI, 1.8–33.8), a risk estimate comparable with a Swedish study in which 15 000 agricultural workers were asked about previous hip radiography: 565 men and 151 women had had such examinations and the prevalence of hip OA in male farmers was increased more than ten-fold compared to the male population of similar age.

The evidence on farmers has proved sufficiently compelling for hip OA in farmers to be added to the list of prescribed diseases recognized for Industrial Injuries Disablement Benefit in the UK. However, the precise risk factors for hip OA in farmers have not been defined with certainty and it is not known whether an excess risk also exists in other heavy manual workers, such as construction workers and labourers. In a second British case–control study,[135] the risk of hip OA was found to be related to occupations that entailed regular heavy lifting (for example, the daily moving of weights greater than 25 kg by hand), prolonged standing and walking over rough ground, but the magnitude of risk associated with these exposures was much lower than that found in farmers, and further research is warranted.

Management

The goals of management in hip and knee osteoarthritis are to control pain, minimize disability and educate the patient about the disorder and its therapy. The medical modalities of management currently available are shown in Table 57.5 and can be divided into non-pharmacological and pharmacological components.

The role of exercise in knee and hip osteoarthritis has been widely reviewed. Three randomized control trials in patients with knee OA have demonstrated that strengthening of quadriceps musculature with isometric or isotonic exercises was associated with significant improvement in quadriceps strength, knee pain and function, when compared with controls. Recent data suggest that exercise regimens, particularly those incorporating hydrotherapy, have similar benefits at the hip.

Proper use of a stick (in the hand contralateral to the affected knee or hip) reduces loading forces on the limb and is associated with decreased pain and improved function. In addition, patients may benefit from shoe inserts to correct abnormal biomechanical problems arising from angular deformity at the knees. Although trial data are not available, the wearing of shock-absorbing shoes with insoles is believed to be of benefit. Finally, the use of lightweight knee braces may be helpful in patients with tibiofemoral disease, especially if complicated by lateral instability. Education also plays a central role.

Several studies have found that obesity is a major risk factor for the development and progression of knee OA, and in one study, weight loss was associated with lower odds of developing symptomatic disease. Overweight patients with OA of the lower limb joints, especially those being considered for arthroplasty, should be encouraged to participate in a comprehensive weight management programme, including dietary counselling and aerobic exercise.

Pain relief is the main indication for drug therapy in OA. No drugs are available presently that reverse the structural or biochemical abnormalities of the disorder, but chondroprotective agents have been studied in animal models of OA and may become available in the future for human use.

Traditionally, non-steroid anti-inflammatory drugs have been the agents of choice for pain relief. Recently, however, because of concerns about their possible deleterious effects on articular cartilage metabolism, questions about the role of synovial inflammation in natural disease progression and recognition of the greater risk of toxicity from prolonged therapy, the central role of these agents in the treatment of OA has been questioned. Randomized controlled clinical trials suggest that anti-inflammatory agents offer no advantage over paracetamol in simple pain relief, whereas the adverse effects of paracetamol are substantially less than for long-term NSAID use, so paracetamol should be the analgesic agent of first choice in OA. However, anti-inflammatory agents can be used in short courses among patients who have polyarticular disease with synovial inflammation.

In individuals with knee OA who do not respond to oral analgesics or who do not wish to take systemic therapy, topical analgesics or even capsaicin cream can be effective. Finally, patients who do not respond satisfactorily to these modalities may benefit from open or closed tidal knee irrigation with saline.

The response to surgical intervention in osteoarthritis of the hip and knee is dramatic. Pain is the most important single reason for surgery. When pain becomes intolerable or unmanageable by medical means, operative treatment should be considered. Other reasonable indications for surgery include progressive loss of movement, increasing deformity, complications such as sudden locking of the knee and progressive disability and dependency.

RISK FACTORS FOR WORK-RELATED MUSCULOSKELETAL DISORDERS AND INTERVENTION STUDIES

A basic hypothesis exists that WMSDs are caused or aggravated by forceful, repetitive and awkward movements with insufficient rest or recovery time. The evidence from case reports, workplace surveys and a mixed bag of formal epidemiological investigation points in this direction, although, as indicated earlier, evaluation is not straightforward.

A better gold standard might be high-quality blinded randomized control trials, to show that removal of a given exposure reduced the incidence of a given upper limb disorder in a target population. However, in practice some serious methodological challenges arise in mounting such trials – in blinding (where it may be possible to disguise the intervention from the clinician assessing outcome, but not from the participant), in randomization (which is most conveniently allocated at the factory, workshop or plant level), in standardized approach to diagnosis (a common omission), and in implementation (fear of litigation limits the number of employers willing to experiment, there being a bias towards solutions proposed on the basis of ergonomic theory and enforced by regulatory authorities). The evidence that has accrued so far is rather sparse.

However, three recent randomized trials in computer keyboard users suggest that the challenge is now being taken up. Gerr et al.[136] monitored the incidence of neck–shoulder complaints in workers randomized to receive an ergonomically adjusted workstation or the usual set-up. No important difference was found. By contrast, Aarås et al.[137] found a decrease in shoulder pain in parallel with a reduction in trapezius loading in a small group of female data workers, after instituting a training programme with more ergonomic information. Most recently, Rempel et al.[138] tested the provision of ergonomic training, a wide forearm support surface and a trackball input device in call-centre workers using computers extensively. Arm board support halved the incidence of neck–shoulder disorders and reduced weekly pain scores. Whether these findings can be taken as evidence in support of work causation is, of course, a matter of interpretation. However, cohort studies of arm pain and work activity are being undertaken in increasing numbers across Europe and the United States, including studies that include planned elements of intervention, so the evidence base on work causation is set to grow significantly.

In the meantime, a variety of physiological, biomechanical and ergonomic investigations underpin the causal hypotheses, so WMSDs have come to be described as repetition strain injuries or cumulative trauma or overuse disorders. The mechanisms of injury are unclear (and perhaps different for different outcomes), but it is generally felt that undesirable permutations of force, repetition, duration and posture contribute to disease onset.

Unfortunately, work factors of this kind are only too common in industry. High productivity targets and machine pacing encourage highly repetitive actions of short cycle time with limited opportunity for respite. Persistent static loading arises in jobs that involve prolonged standing, holding objects at arms' length and working above shoulder height for long periods. Work in confined spaces often requires awkward postures that load joints asymmetrically and require prolonged kneeling or squatting. Other common work circumstances include ill-considered workstation, tool and task design, and the manipulation of heavy loads, sometimes under adverse conditions (such as a slippery or uneven footing). Figure 57.3 illustrates some typical situations.

The different risk factors often coexist and in practice it is difficult to disentangle their effects. Thus, undesirable forces matter because of the load they impose on muscles and the torques they impose on joints, but the outcome probably depends upon the degree and direction of loading (posture), its duration and its frequency, muscle fatigue and recovery times. The effort of work can be minimized by 'good' postures that allow as many strong muscles to contribute as possible, or exaggerated by 'bad' ones, such as poor grip and ulnar or radial deviation of the wrist (which may reduce grip strength by up to 50 per cent) – hence force and posture are interrelated. In general, avoidance of prolonged static loading is desirable, as high intramuscular tensions interrupt the blood supply and enforce anaerobic metabolism, but the problem is heightened if high forces are required, the posture is awkward or effort needs to be maintained for any length of time. Work by Monod and Scherrer[139] and Rohmert[140] indicates that effort that exerts 50 per cent of the maximal force can last no more than a minute, while field studies suggest that loads of 15–20 per cent at maximum will induce painful fatigue if kept up for days or months.

There are reasons for considering some occupational groups such as typists to be at special risk from these factors. The static loading of the neck and trapezius muscles in VDU workers has been reported to be 20–30 per cent of the maximum voluntary contraction. Furthermore, the increasing use of a computer mouse encourages typists to spend more time with their wrist in ulnar deviation and with their shoulder externally rotated.

The concurrence of risk factors matters particularly as they may act synergistically. The study of carpal tunnel syndrome by Silverstein et al.[74] described under Carpal tunnel syndrome, p. 694, provides an example of synergistic interaction between force and repetition: when either was present the risk increased about two- to three-fold, but when present together the risk of CTS was raised many times over.

Approaches to risk assessment and risk reduction take their cue from the putative risk factors, attempting to measure or control some combination of unwanted forces, repetitions and work positions. Many assessment methods have been attempted, though none has achieved primacy. Some techniques are time consuming, expensive and research focused. Others have been advocated for use in the workplace in the assessment and planning of control measures.

Most elaborate are the video recording methods. These often employ pairs or panels of cameras providing alternative views of the work, with markers on the body (such as reflective spots or small lights) to provide measurement points. The results can be digitally encoded and analysed by computer, providing detailed spatial and temporal information on work postures and movements. Alternatively, workers have worn electronic pendulum potentiometers and flexible lightweight tubes containing strain gauge strips that allow reconstruction of postures and movements (again computerized analysis is possible).

Static work activity has been assessed by mapping the various joint angles (for example, using photographs or goniometers), while static workloads and muscle fatigue have been investigated using electromyography (EMG). A high correlation has been shown between EMG activity and muscular force (for both static and dynamic activities), and muscle fatigue can be detected as an increase in the amplitude of the low frequency range of EMG activity. For research purposes, needle electrodes have been lodged in particular muscles, but in workplaces the technique has been adapted so that records can be obtained from surface electrodes.

These various analytical approaches enable biomechanical measurements of force, posture, frequency and duration to be compared with known human capability and the outcomes of health investigations. They further allow comparison across jobs, so that those expected to carry higher risk can be identified.

However, they require special expertise and skills. In occupational practice, simpler more rapid assessment techniques are required, and a number of systems have been proposed. In one of the earliest, the Ovako Working Posture Analysing System (OSWAS) method,[141] postures were observed and recorded using a six-figure code during each stage of a representative task cycle. The first

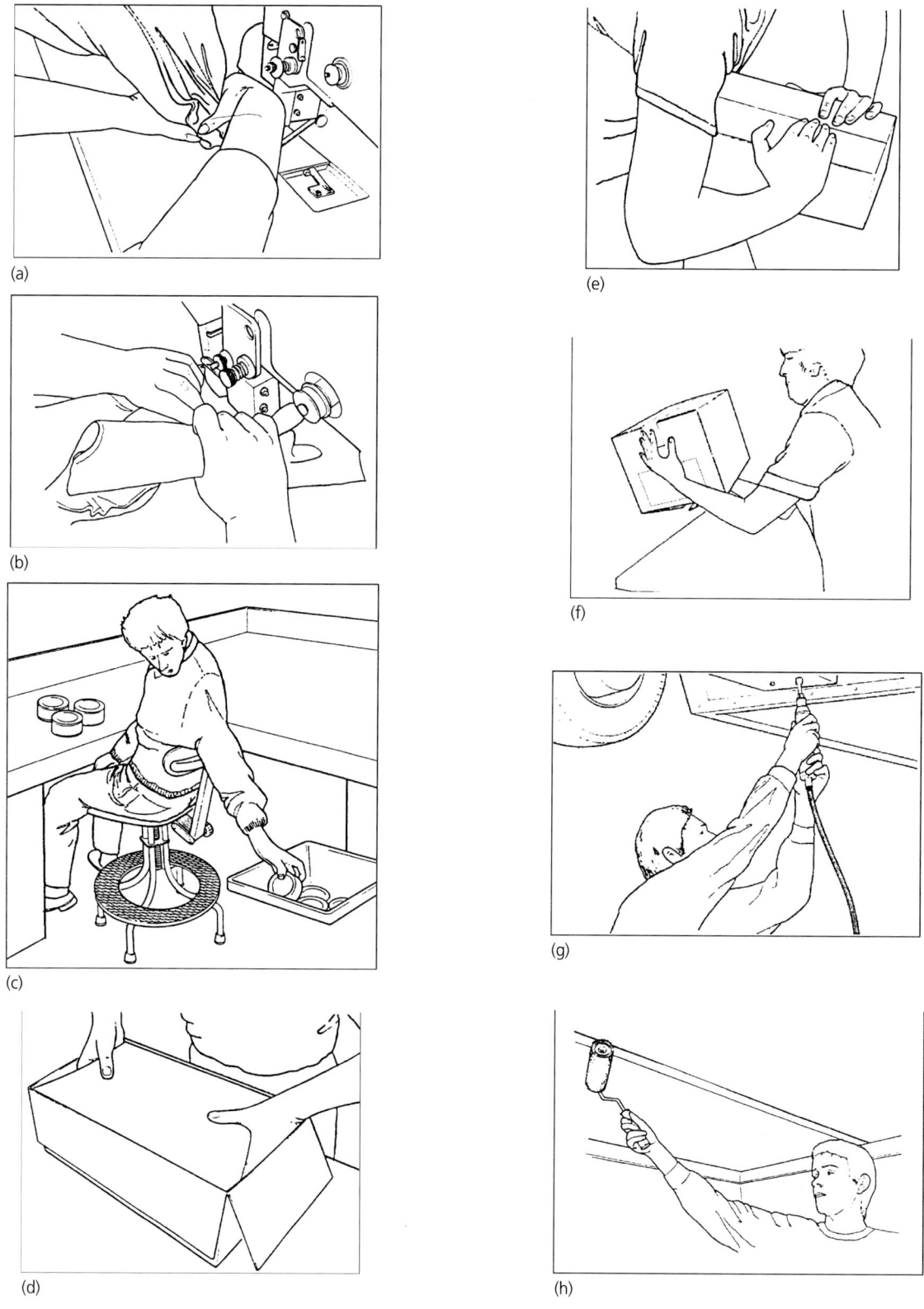

Figure 57.3 Examples of some ergonomic risk factors in the workplace. (a, b) Some tasks requiring high force levels to be applied. (c–h) Some examples of static or awkward posture. Material taken from HS(G) 60 – Work related upper limb disorders – a guide to prevention, Health and Safety Executive, ISBN 0717619783.[147] © Crown copyright material is reproduced with the permission of the Controller of HMSO and Queen's Printer for Scotland.

three digits represented a fairly crude description of trunk and limb postures. The fourth figure indicated the load or force employed, and the remainder were task designated. The procedure, which requires observer training and standardization, is to glance, look away and record it. For frequent activities the proportion of time in which particular postures are adopted and loads incurred can be estimated.

Other analogous scoring procedures exist for the upper limbs and neck, such as the Rapid Upper Limb Assessment (RULA) technique,[142] and these generally result in a risk score that is marked against advice on the urgency of corrective action. An alternative approach employs a risk factor checklist. Table 57.6 provides an example. In some cases, it has been suggested that the priority for remedial action should be determined by the number of risk factors identified: the situation is clearly more complicated than this, but in the absence of better information this provides a convenient means for assembling an action plan.

In some cases, these pragmatic tools have been tested empirically against levels of discomfort at work,[142] but at present there is no hard evidence concerning their predictive value for occurrence of WMSDs, and hence for the adequacy of the risk assessment produced. Nonetheless, they have evident attractions: they can be readily understood and applied, and facilitate attempts to prioritize remedial actions in an area where knowledge is far from complete.

IDENTIFYING WORK-RELATED MUSCULOSKELETAL DISORDERS

WMSDs arise in the context of a background incidence of musculoskeletal complaint, in workers who do not always seek medical advice. In some cases (as in hip and knee OA), they may present after retirement. Their multifactorial character and, for some disorders their transience, tend to impede detection. In clinical practice a high level of awareness is required if early recognition and intervention are to be achieved.

The starting point should be a knowledge of the occupations and tasks most likely to generate concern. Health professionals and safety managers should also be alert to the possibility of disease clustering. An 'outbreak' of apparently related symptoms in workers with a shared exposure suggests the need for wider investigation – for example, a health survey and a review of the work activity. The problem may be circumscribed, or bigger than first appreciated, and the process or materials may have changed, adding unrecognized risk to the job.

Many soft-tissue studies have used the Nordic questionnaire[143] as the basis of health enquiry. This simple self-completed questionnaire has been developed to standardize the data collected by the researchers, and has been validated to some extent. It allows an estimate of the

Table 57.6 Checklist for identifying work-related upper limb disorders.

	Checklist
1	Organizational factors
	Is operator training thorough enough?
	Is repetitive work arranged without a break or with compulsory overtime?
	Do bonus systems encourage the exceedance of good working practice?
2	Task and equipment design factors
	Applied forces
	Is excessive force being used?
	Are there static muscle loads?
	Are forces applied with the joints at or near extremes of their range of movement?
	Movements
	Are the same movements repeated frequently?
	Are they repeated rapidly?
	Do they include forceful twisting or rotation of the wrist, movement of the wrist from side to side, highly flexed fingers and wrist, or upper limb motions beyond a comfortable range?
	Postural factors
	Are the arms raised high or outstretched at the shoulder?
	Is the forearm held above the horizontal?
	Is the upper arm held away from the vertical?
	Do poor overall postures exist?
	Duration of effort
	Are tasks performed for long periods without relief?
	Are short bursts of energetic work included in longer periods of activity?
	Tool and equipment factors
	Are women using tools designed for men?
	Do the tools vibrate, without vibration dampening?
	Do the tools impose shock loading upon the user?
	Do the tools need to be held firmly to resist reaction torques?
	Do tools have a jerking action?
	Is considerable pressure required to hold/operate the tool?
	Are the handles too large/too small/too short/too slippery to be gripped easily?
	Do operators have to twist and turn to reach everyday items?
	Do the operator's gloves affect grip or dexterity?
3	Personal and anthropometric factors
	Do operators suffer from work or domestic stress?
	Are operators at one or other of the extremes of height/reach/strength of the working population?
4	Environmental factors
	Do levels of noise cause mental stress or interfere with communications?
	Do lighting levels encourage awkward postures?
	Do flickering lights and glare cause visual difficulties?
	Does protective clothing constrain posture and affect grip?

Material taken from HS(G) 60 – Work related upper limb disorders – a guide to prevention, Health and Safety Executive, ISBN 0717619783.[147]
© Crown copyright material is reproduced with the permission of the Controller of HMSO and Queen's Printer for Scotland.

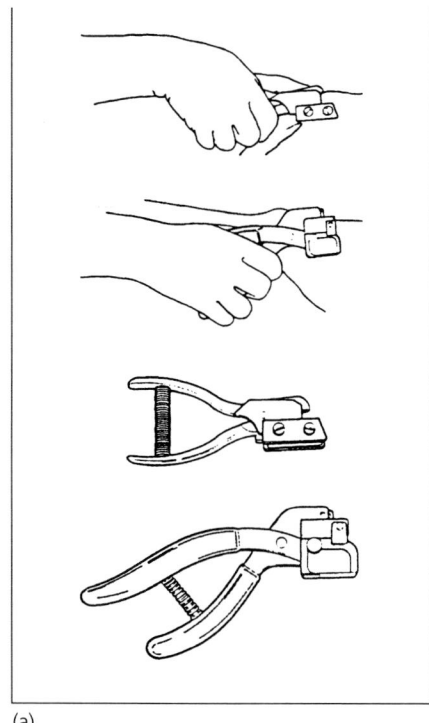
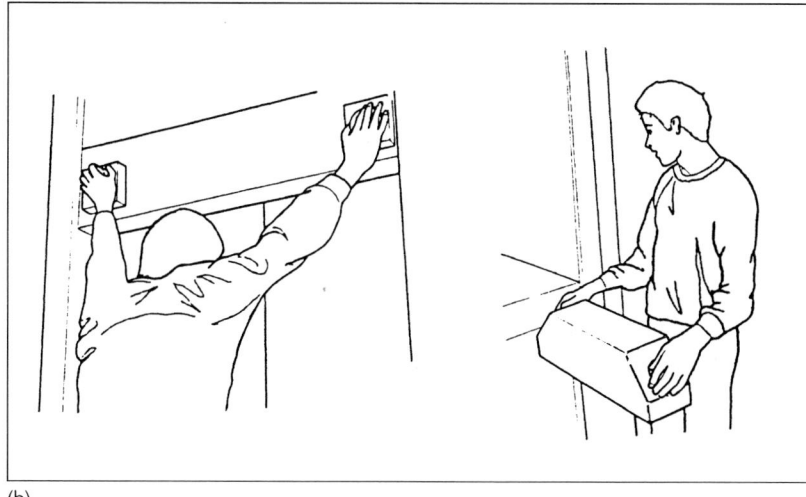

(a) (b)

Figure 57.4 Examples of some simple ergonomic solutions. (a) Redesigning the handles of a tool can lead to more comfortable hand positions and reduce the force required to do the job. (b) In this press operation repositioning of the control panel has eliminated the need for prolonged overhead work. Material taken from HS(G) 60 – Work related upper limb disorders – a guide to prevention, Health and Safety Executive, ISBN 0717619783.[147] © Crown copyright material is reproduced with the permission of the Controller of HMSO and Queen's Printer for Scotland.

one-week and one-year period prevalences of limb and neck complaint (such as pain and interference with work), but further assessment would be required before making a clinical diagnosis. Other questionnaires of similar scope have been developed for use in surveys and screening, and some authors have given advice on analysing and interpreting the findings.[144]

PREVENTING AND MANAGING WORK-RELATED MUSCULOSKELETAL DISORDERS

Success in the prevention of work-related musculoskeletal disorders depends upon an informed assessment of risk, a sharing of information between medical personnel and employees, and a package of risk reduction measures, underpinned by suitable management systems for monitoring and enforcement.

A similar approach will help the affected worker to return to work, and to avoid a recurrent problem.

Preventive measures may include:

1. Advice and training, to ensure a higher risk awareness and better working practices.
2. An induction period, to allow new employees to start work at a slower pace than the established workforce.
3. Job rotation or job enlargement, to provide respite from work that requires repetitive monotonous use of the same muscles and tendons.
4. Rest breaks. These are often advocated as an alternative to job rotation, although little information exists on their value or the length that the break should be.
5. A rehabilitation programme, to ease affected workers back into productive work.
6. Redeployment, in recalcitrant and recurrent cases.
7. Task optimization. Better design of tools and equipment, and a better work layout make the task easier to perform. Often only a little thought is required to reduce work effort and to avoid undesirable working postures. Figure 57.4 illustrates, for example, how one tool and one task were redesigned to eliminate undesirable wrist and shoulder postures. The HSE website provides further useful further guidelines (www.hse.gov.uk/msd/hsemsd.htm).

Work with visual display units in Great Britain now falls under the Health and Safety (Display Screen Equipment) Regulations 1992,[145] which are based on the premise that use of VDUs is associated with musculoskeletal effects, visual fatigue and mental stress that can be controlled by simple ergonomic principles. Detailed guidance has been provided on the appropriate design of screens, chairs, desks, document holders and foot rests for work stations in users, as well as the need for frequent rest breaks.[146]

Finally, for non-specific low-back pain, randomized trial evidence has shown that patients tend to fare better if encouraged to remain active within the limits of pain, rather than strictly resting and this begs the presently unanswered research question – whether the same might be true of those with diffuse non-specific arm pain.

> **Key points**
>
> - Work-related musculoskeletal disorders are common and may be disabling.
> - They belong to one of two broad clinical categories: either to one of a number of specific diseases or to one of a number of non-specific pain syndromes. Among the specific disorders, osteoarthritis of the hip and the knee are most important in the lower limb, while shoulder capsulitis and tendinitis, elbow epicondylitis, wrist tenosynovitis and carpal tunnel syndrome are important disorders of the upper limb. However, the relative contribution of specific and non-specific disorders to the overall burden of disease is not well described at present.
> - Two broad categories of risk factor are considered important in the causation of work-related musculoskeletal disorders: mechanical and psychosocial. In addition, personal vulnerability, health beliefs, mental health and pain perception may play an important part. The relative contribution of these factors is likewise poorly characterized and may perhaps differ between specific and non-specific disorders. Evidence exists for many health outcomes that adverse ergonomic factors pose a risk, but the role of psychosocial factors in the causation and presentation of disease is more problematic.
> - When assessing a patient with musculoskeletal complaints, the physician should always consider whether or not work may have caused or aggravated his condition, whether a rehabilitation programme could ease the patient's return to work, whether job modifications may be required, to mitigate against the risk of a recurrence and whether the risk posed by existing work circumstances has been adequately assessed and controlled.

ACKNOWLEDGEMENTS

A portion of this text appeared in *Topical Reviews. Reports on the Rheumatic Diseases* Series 5: *Work-related Disorders of the Upper Limb*. Chesterfield: Arthritis Research Campaign, 2006. We are grateful to the Arthritis Research Campaign for permission to reproduce the material.

REFERENCES

1. Health and Safety Commission. Health and safety statistics 2004/05. Available from: www.hse.gov.uk/statistics/overall/hssh0405.pdf.
2. Barton NJ, Hooper G, Noble J, Steel WM. Occupational causes of disorders in the upper limb. *British Medical Journal*. 1992; **304**: 309–11.
3. McCormack RR Jr, Inman RD, Wells A et al. Prevalence of tendinitis and related disorders of the upper extremity in a manufacturing workforce. *Journal of Rheumatology*. 1990; **17**: 958–64.
4. Dimberg L. The prevalence and causation of tennis elbow (lateral humeral epicondylitis) in a population of workers in an engineering industry. *Ergonomics*. 1987; **30**: 573–80.
5. Bergenudd H, Lindgarde F, Nilsson B, Petersson CJ. Shoulder pain in middle age. A study of prevalence and relation to occupational work load and psychosocial factors. *Clinical Orthopaedics*. 1988; **231**: 234–8.
6. Makela M, Heliovaara M, Sievers K et al. Prevalence, determinants, and consequences of chronic neck pain in Finland. *American Journal of Epidemiology*. 1991; **134**: 1356–67.
7. Hagberg M, Silverstein B, Wells R et al. *Work-related musculoskeletal disorders (WMSDs): A reference book for prevention*. London: Taylor & Francis, 1995.
8. Bongers PM, De Winter CR, Kompier MAJ, Hildebrandt VH. Psychosocial factors at work and musculoskeletal disease. *Scandinavian Journal of Work, Environment and Health*. 1993; **19**: 297–312.
9. Allander E. Prevalence, incidence and remission rates of some common rheumatic diseases or syndromes. *Scandinavian Journal of Rheumatology*. 1974; **3**: 145–53.
10. Royal College of General Practitioners. Third national morbidity survey in general practice 1980-1. Series MB5 No. 1. London: HMSO, 1986.
11. Jarvholm U, Styf J, Suurkula M, Herberts P. Intramuscular pressure and muscle blood flow in supraspinatus. *European Journal of Applied Physiology and Occupational Physiology*. 1988; **58**: 219–24.
12. Jarvholm U, Palmerud G, Karlsson D et al. Intramuscular pressure and electromyography in four shoulder muscles. *Journal of Orthopaedic Research*. 1991; **9**: 609–19.
13. Hagberg M. Electromyographic signs of shoulder muscular fatigue in two elevated arm positions. *American Journal of Physical Medicine*. 1981; **60**: 111–21.

14. Herberts P, Kadefors R, Hogfors C, Sigholm G. Shoulder pain and heavy manual labour. *Clinical Orthopaedics.* 1984; **191**: 166–78.
15. Luopajarvi T, Kuorinka I, Virolainen M, Holmberg M. Prevalence of tenosynovitis and other injuries of the upper extremities in repetitive work. *Scandinavian Journal of Work, Environment and Health.* 1979; **5** (Suppl. 3): 48–55.
16. Punnett L, Robins JM, Wegman DH, Keyserling WM. Soft tissue disorders in the upper limbs of female garment workers. *Scandinavian Journal of Work, Environment and Health.* 1985; **11**: 417–25.
17. Ohlsson K, Attewell R, Skerfving S. Self-reported symptoms in the neck and upper limbs of female assembly workers. Impact of length of employment, work pace, and selection. *Scandinavian Journal of Work, Environment and Health.* 1989; **15**: 75–80.
18. Kuorinka I, Koskinen P. Occupational rheumatic diseases and upper limb strain in manual jobs in a light mechanical industry. *Scandinavian Journal of Work, Environment and Health.* 1979; **5**: 39–47.
19. Bjelle A, Hagberg M, Michaelsson G. Clinical and ergonomic factors in prolonged shoulder pain among industrial workers. *Scandinavian Journal of Work, Environment and Health.* 1979; **5**: 205–10.
20. van der Windt DA, Thomas E, Pope DP et al. Occupational risk factors for shoulder pain: A systematic review. *Occupational and Environmental Medicine.* 2000; **57**: 433–42.
21. National Institute for Occupational Safety and Health. Musculoskeletal disorders (MSDs) and workplace factors: A critical review of epidemiologic evidence for work-related musculoskeletal disorders of the neck, upper extremity, and low back. Cincinnati, OH: US Department of Health and Human Services/NIOSH, publication No. 97-141, 1997.
22. Harkness EF, Macfarlane GJ, Nahit ES et al. Mechanical and psychosocial factors predict new onset shoulder pain: A prospective cohort study of newly employed workers. *Occupational and Environmental Medicine.* 2003; **60**: 850–7.
23. Hagberg M, Wegman DH. Prevalence rates and odds ratios of shoulder–neck diseases in different occupational groups. *British Journal of Industrial Medicine.* 1987; **44**: 602–10.
24. Hazlett JW. Tears of the rotator cuff. *Journal of Bone and Joint Surgery.* 1971; **53**: 772.
25. Nixon JE, DiStefano V. Ruptures of the rotator cuff. *Orthopedic Clinics of North America.* 1975; **6**: 423–47.
26. Boyle AC. Disorders of the shoulder joint. *British Medical Journal.* 1969; **3**: 283–5.
27. Yergason RM. Supination sign. *Journal of Bone and Joint Surgery.* 1931; **13**: 160.
28. Lundberg BJ. The frozen shoulder. *Acta Orthopaedica Scandinavica.* 1969; **119**: 1–59.
29. Reeves B. The natural history of the frozen shoulder syndrome. *Scandinavian Journal of Rheumatology.* 1976; **4**: 193–6.
30. Binder A, Bulgen DY, Hazleman BL, Roberts S. Frozen shoulder: A long-term prospective study. *Annals of the Rheumatic Diseases.* 1984; **43**: 361–4.
31. Green S, Buchbinder R, Hetrick S. Physiotherapy interventions for shoulder pain. *Cochrane Database of Systematic Reviews.* 2003; (**2**): CD004258.
32. Côté P, Cassidy JD, Carroll L. The factors associated with neck pain and its related disability in the Saskatchewan population. *Spine.* 2000; **25**: 1109–17.
33. Picavet HSJ, Schouten JSAG. Musculoskeletal pain in the Netherlands: Prevalences, consequences and risk groups, the DMC3-study. *Pain.* 2003; **102**: 167–78.
34. Urwin M, Symmons D, Alison T et al. Estimating the burden of musculoskeletal disorders in the community: The comparative prevalence of symptoms at different anatomical sites, and the relation to social deprivation. *Annals of the Rheumatic Diseases.* 1998; **57**: 649–55.
35. Andersson HI, Ejlertsson G, Leden I, Rosenberg C. Chronic pain in a geographically defined general population: Studies of differences in age, gender, social class, and pain localisation. *Clinical Journal of Pain.* 1993; **9**: 174–82.
36. Brattberg G, Thorslund M, Wikman A. The prevalence of pain in the general population. The results of a postal survey in a county of Sweden. *Pain.* 1989; **37**: 215–22.
37. Linton SJ, Hellsing AL, Halldeń K. A population-based study of spinal pain among 35–45-year-old individuals. *Spine.* 1998; **23**: 1457–63.
38. Côté P, Cassidy JD, Carroll LJ, Cristman B. The annual incidence and course of neck pain in the general population: A population-based cohort study. *Pain.* 2004; **112**: 267–73.
39. Levoska S. Manual palpation and pain threshold in female office employees with and without neck-shoulder symptoms. *Clinical Journal of Pain.* 1993; **9**: 236–41.
40. Reading I, Walker-Bone K, Palmer KT et al. Utility of restricted neck movement as a diagnostic criterion in case definition for neck disorders. *Scandinavian Journal of Work, Environment and Health.* 2005; **31**: 387–93.
41. Kaergaard A, Andersen JH, Rasmussen K, Mikkelsen S. Identification of neck–shoulder disorders in a one year follow-up study. Validation of a questionnaire-based method. *Pain.* 2000; **86**: 305–10.
42. Waris P, Kuorinka I, Kurppa K et al. Epidemiologic screening of occupational neck and upper limb disorders. *Scandinavian Journal of Work, Environment and Health.* 1979; **5**: 25–38.
43. Viikari-Juntura E. Neck and upper limb disorders among slaughterhouse workers: An epidemiologic and clinical study. *Scandinavian Journal of Work, Environment and Health.* 1983; **9**: 283–90.
44. Ohlsson K, Attewell RG, Johnsson B et al. An assessment of neck and upper extremity disorders by questionnaire and clinical examination. *Ergonomics.* 1994; **37**: 891–7.
45. Holt L. Frequency of symptoms for different age groups and professions. In: Hitsch C, Zotterman Y (eds). *Cervical pain.* New York: Pergamon Press, 1971: 17–20.
46. Amano M, Umeda G, Nakajima H, Yatsuki K. Characteristics of work actions of shoe manufacturing assembly line workers and a cross-sectional factor-control study on occupational cervicobrachial disorders. *Japanese Journal of Industrial Health.* 1988; **30**: 3–12.

47. Hunting W, Laubli TH, Grandjean E. Postural and visual loads at VDT workplaces. I. Constrained postures. *Ergonomics.* 1981; **24**: 917–31.
48. Onishi N, Namura H, Sakai K *et al.* Shoulder muscle tenderness and physical features of female industrial workers. *Journal of Human Ergology.* 1976; **5**: 87–102.
49. Palmer KT, Smedley J. The work-relatedness of chronic neck pain with physical findings: A systematic review. *Scandinavian Journal of Work, Environment and Health.* 2007; **33**: 165–91.
50. Andersen JH, Kaergaard A, Mikkelsen S *et al.* Risk factors in the onset of neck/shoulder pain in a prospective study of workers in industrial and service companies. *Occupational and Environmental Medicine.* 2003; **60**: 649–54.
51. Roos DB. Congenital anomalies associated with thoracic outlet syndrome. *American Journal of Surgery.* 1976; **132**: 771–8.
52. Sallstrom J, Schmidt H. Cervicobrachial disorders in certain occupations, with special reference to compression in the thoracic outlet. *American Journal of Industrial Medicine.* 1984; **6**: 45–52.
53. Toomingas A, Hagberg M, Jorulf L *et al.* Outcome of the abduction external rotation test among manual and office workers. *American Journal of Industrial Medicine.* 1991; **19**: 215–27.
54. Cunningham LS, Kelsey JL. Epidemiology of musculoskeletal impairments and associated disability. *American Journal of Public Health.* 1984; **74**: 574–9.
55. Gruchow HW, Pelletier BS. An epidemiologic study of tennis elbow. *American Journal of Sports Medicine.* 1979; **7**: 234–8.
56. Goldie I. Epicondylitis lateralis humeri: A pathogenetical study. *Acta Chirurgica Scandinavica.* 1964; **339** (Suppl.): 119.
57. Cyriax JH. The pathology and treatment of tennis elbow. *Journal of Bone and Joint Surgery.* 1936; **18**: 921–40.
58. Cyriax JH. *Textbook of orthopaedic medicine.* London: Baillière Tindall, 1982.
59. Coonrad RW, Hooper RW. Tennis elbow: Its course, natural history, conservative and surgical management. *Journal of Bone and Joint Surgery of America.* 1973; **55A**: 1177–82.
60. Viikari-Juntura E, Kurppa K, Kuosma E *et al.* Prevalence of epicondylitis and elbow pain in the meat-processing industry. *Scandinavian Journal of Work, Environment and Health.* 1991; **17**: 38–45.
61. Ritz BR. Humeral epicondylitis among gas- and water-work employees. *Scandinavian Journal of Work, Environment and Health.* 1997; **21**: 478–86.
62. Kurppa K, Viika RI, Juntura E *et al.* Incidence of tenosynovitis or peritendinitis and epicondylitis in a meat-processing factory. *Scandinavian Journal of Work, Environment and Health.* 1991; **17**: 32–7.
63. Haahr JP, Andersen JH. Physical and psychosocial risk factors for lateral epicondylitis: A population based case-referent study. *Occupational and Environmental Medicine.* 2003; **60**: 322–9.
64. Leclerc A, Landre MF, Chastang JF *et al.* Study Group on Repetitive Work. Upper-limb disorders in repetitive work. *Scandinavian Journal of Work, Environment and Health.* 2001; **27**: 268–78.
65. Binder A, Hodge G, Greenwood AM *et al.* Is therapeutic ultrasound effective in treating soft tissue lesions? *British Medical Journal.* 1985; **290**: 512–14.
66. Clarke AK, Woodland J. Comparison of two steroid preparations used to treat tennis elbow, using the hypospray. *Rheumatology and Rehabilitation.* 1975; **14**: 37–49.
67. Nevelos AB. The treatment of tennis elbow with triamcinolone acetonide. *Current Medical Research and Opinion.* 1980; **6**: 507–9.
68. Binder AI, Hazleman BL. Lateral humeral epicondylitis. A study of natural history and the effect of conservative therapy. *British Journal of Rheumatology.* 1983; **22**: 73–6.
69. Kivi P. The etiology and conservative treatment of humeral epicondylitis. *Scandinavian Journal of Rehabilitation Medicine.* 1982; **15**: 37–41.
70. Kramer JS, Yelin EH, Epstein WV. Social and economic impacts of four musculoskeletal conditions. *Arthritis and Rheumatism.* 1983; **26**: 901–7.
71. Palmer KT, Harris EC, Coggon D. Compensating occupationally-related tenosynovitis and epicondylitis: A literature review. *Occupational Medicine.* 2007; **57**: 67–74.
72. Bystrom S, Hall C, Welander T, Kilbom A. Clinical disorders and pressure-pain threshold of the forearm and hand among automobile assembly line workers. *Journal of Hand Surgery – British Volume.* 1995; **20**: 782–90.
73. Roto P, Kivi P. Prevalence of epicondylitis and tenosynovitis among meatcutters. *Scandinavian Journal of Work, Environment and Health.* 1984; **10**: 203–5.
74. Silverstein BA, Fine LJ, Armstrong TJ. Hand wrist cumulative trauma disorders in industry. *British Journal of Industrial Medicine.* 1986; **43**: 779–84.
75. Thompson AR, Plewes LW, Shaw EG. Peritendinitis crepitans and simple tenosynovitis: A clinical study of 544 cases in industry. *British Journal of Industrial Medicine.* 1951; **8**: 150–60.
76. de Krom MCTFM, Kester ADM, Knipschild PG, Spaans F. Risk factors for carpal tunnel syndrome. *American Journal of Epidemiology.* 1990; **132**: 1102–10.
77. Stevens JC, Sun S, Beard CM *et al.* Carpal tunnel syndrome in Rochester, Minnesota, 1961 to 1980. *Neurology.* 1988; **38**: 134–8.
78. Vessey MP, Villard Mackintosh L, Yeates D. Epidemiology of carpal tunnel syndrome in women of childbearing age. Findings in a large cohort study. *International Journal of Epidemiology.* 1990; **19**: 655–9.
79. de Krom MC, Knipschild PG, Kester AD *et al.* Carpal tunnel syndrome: Prevalence in the general population. *Journal of Clinical Epidemiology.* 1992; **45**: 373–6.
80. Hagberg M, Morgenstern H, Kelsh M. Impact of occupations and job tasks on the prevalence of carpal

tunnel syndrome. *Scandinavian Journal of Work, Environment and Health.* 1992; **18**: 337–45.
81. Nathan PA, Meadows KD, Doyle LS. Occupation as a risk factor for impaired sensory conduction of the median nerve at the carpal tunnel. *Journal of Hand Surgery – British Volume.* 1988; **13B**: 167–70.
82. Osorio AM, Ames R, Jones J. Carpal tunnel syndrome among grocery store workers. Field Investigation FI-86-005. Californian Occupational Health Program, California Department of Health Services: Berkeley, CA, 1989: 61.
83. Chiang HC, Chen SS, Yu HS, Ko YC. The occurrence of carpal tunnel syndrome in frozen food factory employees. *Kaohsiung Journal of Medical Sciences.* 1990; **6**: 73–80.
84. Nilsson T, Hagberg M, Burstrom L, Lundstrom R. Prevalence and odds ratios of numbness and carpal tunnel syndrome in different exposure categories of platers. In: Okada A, Dupuis WTH (eds). *Hand–arm vibration.* Kanozawa: Kyoei Press, 1990: 235–9.
85. Silverstein BA, Fine LJ, Armstrong TJ. Occupational factors and carpal tunnel syndrome. *American Journal of Industrial Medicine.* 1987; **11**: 343–58.
86. Bovenzi M, Zadini A, Franzinelli A, Borgogni F. Occupational musculoskeletal disorders in the neck and upper limbs of forestry workers exposed to hand-arm vibration. *Ergonomics.* 1991; **34**: 547–62.
87. Cannon LJ, Bernacki EJ, Walter SD. Personal and occupational factors associated with carpal tunnel syndrome. *Journal of Occupational Medicine.* 1981; **23**: 255–8.
88. Wieslander G, Norback D, Gothe CJ, Juhlin L. Carpal tunnel syndrome (CTS) and exposure to vibration, repetitive wrist movements, and heavy manual work: A case-referent study. *British Journal of Industrial Medicine.* 1989; **46**: 43–7.
89. Voog L, de Laval J, Ahlborg G, Holm Glad J. Compression of the median nerve at the wrist and work with vibrating tools. Report project 82-0545. Stockholm: Swedish Work Environment Fund, 1985.
90. Nordstrom DL, Vierkant RA, Layde PM, Smith MJ. Comparison of self-reported and expert-observed physical activities at work in a general population. *American Journal of Industrial Medicine.* 1998; **34**: 29–35.
91. Palmer KT, Harris EC, Coggon D. Carpal tunnel syndrome and its relation to occupation: A systematic literature review. *Occupational Medicine.* 2007; **57**: 57–66.
92. Reading I, Walker-Bone K, Palmer KT et al. Anatomic distribution of sensory symptoms in the hand and their relation to neck pain, psychosocial variables and occupational activities. *American Journal of Epidemiology.* 2003; **157**: 524–30.
93. Phalen GS. The carpal tunnel syndrome. *Journal of Bone and Joint Surgery.* 1966; **48A**: 211–8.
94. Gun RT. The incidence and distribution of RSI in South Australia 1980-81 to 1986-87. *Medical Journal of Australia.* 1990; **153**: 376–80.
95. Hocking B. Epidemiological aspects of 'repetition strain injury' in Telecom Australia. *Medical Journal of Australia.* 1987; **147**: 218–22.
96. Madan I, Reading I, Palmer KT, Coggon D. Cultural differences in musculoskeletal symptoms and disability. In: *Frontiers of occupational epidemiology.* 19th Symposium of Epidemiology in Occupational Health, Banff, Alberta, Canada, 9–12 October 2007, A210, p. 109.
97. Palmer KT, Reading I, Calnan M, Coggon D. How common is repetitive strain injury? *Occupational and Environmental Medicine.* 2008; **65**: 331–5.
98. Harris JE. Repetition strain injury. Proceedings of the Royal Australian College of Surgeons/Royal Australia College of Physicians Seminar Disability in the Workforce. RACS/RACP, 1984.
99. Ohara H, Aroyama H, Itani T. Health hazard among cash register operators and the effects of improved working conditions. *Journal of Human Ergology (Tokyo).* 1976; **5**: 31–40.
100. Miller MH, Topliss DJ. Chronic upper limb pain syndrome (repetitive strain injury) in the Australian workforce: A systematic cross-sectional rheumatological study of 229 patients. *Journal of Rheumatology.* 1988; **15**: 1705–12.
101. Wigley RD. Repetitive strain syndrome – fact not fiction. *New Zealand Medical Journal.* 1990; **103**: 75–6.
102. Hartz A, Kirchdoerfer E. Undetected fibrositis in primary care practice. *Journal of Family Practice.* 1987; **25**: 365–9.
103. Jacobsson L, Lindgarde F, Manthorpe R. The commonest rheumatic complaints of over six weeks' duration in a twelve-month period in a defined Swedish population. Prevalences and relationships. *Scandinavian Journal of Rheumatology.* 1989; **18**: 353–60.
104. Muller W. The fibrositis syndrome: Diagnosis, differential diagnosis and pathogenesis. *Scandinavian Journal of Rheumatology.* 1987; **16**: 40–53.
105. Yunus M, Masi AT, Calabro JJ et al. Primary fibromyalgia (fibrositis): Clinical study of 50 patients with matched normal controls. *Seminars in Arthritis and Rheumatism.* 1981; **11**: 151–71.
106. Wolfe F, Cathey MA. Prevalence of primary and secondary fibrositis. *Journal of Rheumatology.* 1983; **10**: 965–68.
107. Wolfe F, Smythe HA, Yunus MB et al. The American College of Rheumatology 1990 criteria for the classification of fibromyalgia. Report of the Multicenter Criteria Committee. *Arthritis and Rheumatism.* 1990; **33**: 160–72.
108. Palmer KT, Reading I, Linaker C et al. Population-based cohort study of incident and persistent arm pain: role of mental health, self-rated health and health beliefs. *Pain.* 2008; **136**: 30–7.
109. Early PF. Population studies in Dupuytren's contracture. *Journal of Bone and Joint Surgery.* 1962; **44B**: 602–13.
110. Burge P, Hoy G, Regan P, Milne R. Smoking, alcohol and the risk of Dupuytren's contracture. *Journal of Bone and Joint Surgery.* 1997; **79B**: 206–10.
111. Hueston JT. Dupuytren's contracture and specific hand injury. *Medical Journal of Australia.* 1960; **1**: 1084–5.
112. Liss GM, Stock SR. Can Dupuytren's contracture be work-related? Review of the evidence. *American Journal of Industrial Medicine.* 1996; **29**: 521–32.

113. Bennett B. Dupuytren's contracture in manual workers. *British Journal of Industrial Medicine.* 1982; **39**: 98–100.
114. Mikkelsen OA. Epidemiology of a Norwegian population. In: McFarlane RM, McGrouther DA, Flint MH (eds). *Dupuytren's disease: Biology and treatment.* New York: Churchill Livingstone, 1990: 191–200.
115. Thomas PR, Clarke D. Vibration white finger and Dupuytren's contracture: Are they related? *Journal of the Society of Occupational Medicine.* 1992; **42**: 155–8.
116. Cocco PL, Frau P, Rapallo M, Casula D. Occupational exposure to vibrations and Dupuytren's disease: A case-control study. *La Medicina del Lavoro.* 1987; **78**: 386–92.
117. Bovenzi M, Cerri S, Merseburger A *et al*. Hand-arm vibration syndrome and dose-response relation for vibration induced white finger among quarry drillers and stonecarvers. *Occupational and Environmental Medicine.* 1994; **51**: 603–11.
118. Cooper C. The epidemiology of osteoarthritis. In: Klipel J, Dieppe P (eds). *Rheumatology.* New York: Mosby, 1994: 7.3.1–7.3.4.
119. Spector TD, Cooper C. Radiographic assessment of osteoarthritis in population studies: Whither Kellgren and Lawrence? *Osteoarthritis and Cartilage.* 1993; **1**: 203–6.
120. Felson DT. Epidemiology of hip and knee osteoarthritis. *Epidemiological Reviews.* 1988; **10**: 1–28.
121. Cooper C, McAlindon T, Snow S *et al*. Mechanical and constitutional risk factors for symptomatic knee osteoarthritis: Differences between medial tibiofemoral and patellofemoral disease. *Journal of Rheumatology.* 1994; **21**: 307–13.
122. Kellgren JH, Lawrence JS. Rheumatism in miners: Part II, X-ray study. *British Journal of Industrial Medicine.* 1952; **9**: 197–207.
123. Partridge REH, Duthie JJR. Rheumatism in dockers and civil servants: A comparison of heavy manual and sedentary workers. *Annals of the Rheumatic Diseases.* 1968; **27**: 559–68.
124. Wickstrom G, Hanninen K, Mattsson T *et al*. Knee degeneration in concrete reinforcement workers. *British Journal of Industrial Medicine.* 1983; **40**: 216–19.
125. Lindberg H, Montgomery F. Heavy labour and the occurrence of gonarthrosis. *Clinical Orthopaedics.* 1987; **214**: 235–6.
126. Vingard E, Alfredsson L, Goldie I, Hogstedt C. Occupation and osteoarthrosis of the hip and knee: A register-based cohort study. *International Journal of Epidemiology.* 1991; **20**: 1025–31.
127. Kohatsu ND, Schurman DJ. Risk factors for the development of osteoarthrosis of the knee. *Clinical Orthopaedics.* 1990; **261**: 242–6.
128. Schouten JSAG, Van den Ouweland FA, Valkenburg HA. A 12 year follow up study in the general population on prognostic factors of cartilage loss in osteoarthritis of the knee. *Annals of the Rheumatic Diseases.* 1992; **51**: 932–7.
129. Bagge E, Bjelle A, Eden S, Svanborg A. Factors associated with radiographic osteoarthritis: Results from the population study 70-year-old people in Goteborg. *Journal of Rheumatology.* 1991; **18**: 1218–22.
130. Anderson JJ, Felson DT. Factors associated with osteoarthritis of the knee in the first national Health and Nutrition Examination Survey (HANES I). Evidence for an association with overweight, race, and physical demands of work. *American Journal of Epidemiology.* 1988; **128**: 179–89.
131. Felson DT, Hannan MT, Naimark A *et al*. Occupational physical demands, knee bending, and knee osteoarthritis: Results from the Framingham Study. *Journal of Rheumatology.* 1991; **18**: 1587–92.
132. Cooper C, McAlindon T, Coggon D *et al*. Occupational activity and osteoarthritis of the knee. *Annals of the Rheumatic Diseases.* 1994; **53**: 90–3.
133. Coggon D, Croft P, Kellingray S *et al*. Occupational physical activities and osteoarthritis of the knee. *Arthritis Rheumatism.* 2000; **43**: 1443–9.
134. Croft P, Coggon D, Cruddas M, Cooper C. Osteoarthritis of the hip: An occupational disease in farmers. *British Medical Journal.* 1992; **304**: 1269–72.
135. Croft P, Cooper C, Wickham C, Coggon D. Osteoarthritis of the hip and occupational activity. *Scandinavian Journal of Work, Environment and Health.* 1992; **18**: 59–63.
136. Gerr F, Marcus M, Monteilh C *et al*. A randomised controlled trial of postural interventions for prevention of musculoskeletal symptoms among computer users. *Occupational and Environmental Medicine.* 2005; **62**: 478–87.
137. Aarås A, Horgen G, Ro O *et al*. The effect of an ergonomic intervention on musculoskeletal, psychosocial and visual strain of VDT data entry work: the Norwegian part of the international study. *International Journal of Occupational Safety and Ergonomics.* 2005; **11**: 25–47.
138. Rempel D, Krause N, Goldberg R *et al*. A randomized controlled trial evaluating the effects of two workstation interventions on upper body pain and incident musculoskeletal disorders among computer operators. *Occupational and Environmental Medicine.* 2006; **63**: 300–6.
139. Monod H, Scherrer J. The work capacity of a synergic muscle group. *Ergonomics.* 1965; **8**: 329–38.
140. Rohmert W. Problems in determining rest allowances. *Applied Ergonomics.* 1973; **4**: 158–62.
141. Karhu O, Kansi P, Kuorinka I. Correcting working postures in industry: A practical method for analysis. *Applied Ergonomics.* 1977; **84**: 199–201.
142. McAtamney L, Corlett EN. RULA: A survey method for the investigation of work-related upper limb disorders. *Applied Ergonomics.* 1993; **24**: 91–9.
143. Kuorinka I, Jonsson B, Kilborn A *et al*. Standardised Nordic questionnaire for the analysis of musculoskeletal symptoms. *Applied Ergonomics.* 1987; **18**: 233–7.
144. Hagberg M, Silverstein B, Wells R *et al*. Health and risk factor surveillance for work related musculoskeletal

disorders. In: *Work-related musculoskeletal disorders (WMSDs): A reference book for prevention.* London: Taylor & Francis, 1995: 213–45.
145. Health and Safety (Display Screen Equipment) Regulations 1992. SI 1992/2792. London: HM Stationery Office, 1992.
146. Health and Safety Executive. Display Screen Equipment Work: Guidance on Regulations (L26). London: HM Stationery Office, 1992.
147. HMSO. Work-related Upper Limb Disorders: A Guide to Prevention. H5(G) 60. London: HMSO, 1990.

SECTION TWO

Back and spinal pain

58 Occupational back pain 715
    Jos H Verbeek and Frederieke Schaafsma

58

Occupational back pain

JOS H VERBEEK AND FREDERIEKE SCHAAFSMA

Introduction	715	Prevention of back pain at work	718
Historical treatment of occupational back pain	715	Clinical management and return to work	719
Prevalence of back pain	716	Conclusions	721
Causes of back pain at work	717	References	722

INTRODUCTION

Back pain is commonly defined as a symptom that originates from a malfunction of a structure in the back. Even though pain is often not felt in the back, the definition also includes pain radiating from the back into the buttocks and the legs because its cause is located in the back. In the majority of cases, the back pain is called non-specific because the cause of the pain cannot be located with current diagnostic methods. Because the pain is mostly felt in the lower part of the back, it is also termed 'low back pain', but there is no specific additional value of this adjective because pain higher in the back does not seem to be different from low back pain. Low back pain is reported four times more frequently than mid-back pain.[1]

In the majority of cases, back pain is a minor affliction only, but the impact on individuals and society is considerable, because in a minority of cases pain becomes chronic and results in long-lasting disability.[2] Back pain is limiting in activities where posture must be maintained for a long time (such as standing or sitting) and carrying out specific movements (such as lifting, bending or walking). In turn, the limitation of these activities leads to work disability and the restriction of participation in other important activities. In a small minority of patients, the pain and disability do not subside, leading to unemployment and loss of quality of life. The non-medical indirect costs of back pain that originate from work disability constitute a major proportion of all social security costs or general worker compensation. Chronic suffering and the economic consequences of lost productivity are the major drivers to improve the outcome of disability resulting from back pain.[3]

This chapter is based on our experience as occupational health physicians both in clinical practice and research. Our experiences are backed up by evidence from the scientific literature. Medline searches for systematic reviews of the specific aspects of back pain, such as aetiology, prognosis and treatment, have been carried out for the most up-to-date research.

HISTORICAL TREATMENT OF OCCUPATIONAL BACK PAIN

Research on back pain cannot be properly understood without some insight into its history. In 1996, Dempe gave an excellent overview of how social factors have influenced the concept of occupational back pain over the centuries.[4]

Throughout history, there have been descriptions of case reports involving back pain. There are no indications that the incidence of back pain has radically changed over time either in the distant or more recent past.

Views of back pain and theories as to its causes have changed according to prevailing medical opinion. Back pain has historically only occasionally been linked to occupational activities, such as sitting and other static postures. This was mentioned by Ramazzini in his classic work *De Morbis Artificum* in 1713. Throughout history, back pain has been attributed to rheumatism caused by the collection of rheumatic fluid and phlegm and aggravated by cold and draught.

Between 1850 and 1900, the concept of the 'irritable spine' was developed. The theory was formulated that pressure and constant movement could lead to all kinds of symptoms due to irritation of the spine. The irritable spine was then attributed to the discomfort and injuries endured by travelling by train when railways became more common around 1850. Many injuries occurred while travelling by train due to low safety measures, with resulting legal liability of railroad companies for compensation of passengers injured during collisions. This increased the epidemic of railway spine injuries. However, after thorough discussion in the medical literature, the railway spine sank into oblivion around 1900.

Rheumatism was debated as the cause of back pain through new medical discoveries and measurement techniques. For example, the availability of x-rays around 1900 made anatomical changes in the spine, such as disc and joint degeneration, visible and the German anatomist Schmorl related these findings to autopsy findings. The first operations for herniated intervertebral discs were performed in the 1930s by Mixter and Barr in the United States and these were very influential in research on back pain.[5] The now visibly ruptured disc led to an increasing belief that injury was the most important mechanism behind back pain.

Based on these medical developments, the injured back became the model for work-related back pain after the Second World War. The back injury was explained as an overload of the structures in the back. Measuring spinal load thus became an important aspect of research into occupational causes of back pain. Nachemson was one of the first to measure the pressure in the intervertebral disc directly.[6] He showed that the pressure was highest when sitting on a chair without a backrest. This led to increased interest in seating with a proper back support as a means to prevent back pain among workers.

The more recent introduction of magnetic resonance imaging techniques made it possible to view different structures in the back, such as vertebral endplate signal changes and their relation to low back pain. Even though there might be an association with low back pain, it is unclear what their role is in its development.[7]

Attention being paid to work as the cause of back pain coincided with improved social security in the twentieth century. This led to an exponential increase in the number of people on sick leave due to back pain and later to an increase in the number of people on disability benefit. During the 1970s and 1980s, the main strategy to counterbalance these increases was to improve working conditions. At the same time, the emphasis of working life in industrialized countries changed, at least for men, from heavy physical work in manufacturing industry to administrative work in the service sector.

Medical opinions on the treatment of back pain have changed over time. Until about 1990, the prevailing opinion was that rest was needed to cure the injured structures. One of the landmark studies on the management of back pain was published by the Quebec Task Force in 1987. The group was one of the first to perform a systematic review of the literature and to critically appraise its quality. They proposed a standard nomenclature for back pain diagnosis, diagnosing subgroups with acute, subacute or chronic pain, restricted diagnostic procedures and a non-inference policy for most cases of acute low back pain.[8] At about the same time, Waddell published an influential conceptual article in which he proposed to use a biopsychosocial model for the diagnosis and management of low back pain.[9]

Medical practice also changed as a result of the introduction of clinical practice guidelines based on research evidence from systematic reviews. The American Agency for Health Care Quality and Research produced one of its first guidelines on back pain in 1994. It contained many of the notions on back pain that we currently still use: such as diagnostic triage and continuing ordinary activities in spite of the back pain. To date, occupational medicine associations have made practice guidelines on the management of low back pain at work specifically for occupational health practitioners.[10–12]

The Cochrane Collaboration started its programme on reviewing the effects of healthcare interventions in 1992. Given the enormous amount of literature on back pain, systematic reviewing is needed to be able to transform this information into knowledge that can be used in practice. To date, the Cochrane Collaboration has produced 46 systematic reviews of prevention and treatment for back pain. The reviews are used as input for the development of practice guidelines.

The various drivers for change of management of low back pain have probably led to considerable changes in practice even though this is difficult to measure.[13] Waddell is one of the strongest advocates of these changes and sees this as 'the back pain revolution'.[14]

PREVALENCE OF BACK PAIN

Because back pain is a symptom, it is fairly easy to ask people about their back pain experience to shed light on the prevalence of back pain. However, different ways of phrasing questions about back pain experience lead to enormous differences in back pain prevalence. Both recall and the intermittent course of back pain lead to biased results. In addition, there is a gradual increase from no pain to severe and disabling pain. It has been agreed that asking about pain in the past four weeks, limitation of usual activities, radiation into the leg, the duration of the pain episode and a numerical pain rating scale probably give the best results for measuring back pain prevalence.[15]

Given the uncertainties surrounding back pain prevalence, the following figures give a rough indication of the situation.[16,17] The lifetime prevalence, meaning a positive answer to the question did you ever have back pain in your life, is around 70 per cent with variations between studies from 11 to 84 per cent. The one-year prevalence (Did you have back pain in the past 12 months?) lies around 50 per cent and varies from 31 to 65 per cent. The point prevalence (Do you have back pain now?) ranges from 12 to 33 per cent. The incidence of new episodes of back pain is estimated to be considerably lower, with population studies reporting an incidence of new episodes of 4 per cent.[18]

The prevalence of back pain increases from early adult life to the late 40s or early 50s and remains relatively constant thereafter, at least to the mid-60s. In those who continue to have back pain, it is more likely to be more frequent or more constant with increasing age.[19]

Worldwide, 37 per cent of low back pain is estimated to be attributable to occupational risk factors. This fraction varies among different regions in the world and is higher in areas with lower health status in general, mostly due to the high proportion of farmers.[20] Overall, the attributable risk fraction was higher for males than for females, largely because of men's higher participation in the labour force and in occupations with heavy lifting and whole body vibration.

CAUSES OF BACK PAIN AT WORK

Research on occupational back pain, especially epidemiological research, is fraught with difficulties. Both measuring the outcome and the exposure are difficult and easily subject to bias.[21] Over the past few years, many research groups have worked on obtaining consensus about which are the best measures to use and how to measure them.[22–26] Despite these efforts, there are still a considerable number of measurement options which makes comparison between studies difficult.

The measurement problems also relate to how the development of back pain is conceptualized. We suggest that the clinician should look at back pain as a process starting with pain and finally leading to disability and unemployment. Some people experience only one clearly limited episode of back pain, but for most new episodes occur or the pain becomes a diffuse chronic problem. For others again, these chronic problems lead to disability and loss of employment over time. At different phases of this process, work and other factors have a varying influence on back pain outcome. In the first phase of incident back pain, back pain is thought to be related to work through biomechanical overloading that damages structures in the back. In general, genetic and biological determinants probably play a major role. Which structures cause the pain is unclear and also the relation between overload, damage and back pain is unclear. Personal factors, such as an individual's beliefs about back pain, play a major role in reporting sick or becoming disabled.

There are a few older systematic reviews of epidemiological studies on work-related aetiology of back pain. The reviews differ considerably in the methodology used, but all come to more or less similar conclusions.

A NIOSH review of epidemiologic research on low back pain and occupational risk factors with 42 studies up to 1997 concluded that there was strong evidence for an association between lifting and forceful movements and back disorders. Thirteen of 18 studies found an association between these work factors and back pain. They also found evidence for an association between work-related awkward postures and back disorders, but not for an association between static work postures and back disorders.[27]

Burdorf and Sorock[28] gathered evidence on a relation between individual characteristics or exposure at work and back disorders from the literature. They used a simple vote-counting method to combine the results of 35 cross-sectional and cohort studies and did not stratify according to study type. They concluded that there is evidence for a relationship between exposure due to manual material handling, frequent bending and twisting, heavy physical load and whole body vibration. They found contradictory evidence for psychosocial factors. For individual characteristics, there was evidence for a relation with back pain for age, smoking and education, and no evidence for a relation for gender, height, weight, exercise and marital status.

In a methodologically better systematic review, Hoogendoorn et al.[29] used a rating system to assess the strength of the evidence for a relation between physical load at work and back pain. They based the rating on the methodological quality of 19 cohort and two case-referent studies which had looked into work-related factors. They found strong evidence for manual materials handling, bending and twisting, and whole body vibration as risk factors for back pain. The evidence was moderate for patient handling and heavy physical work, and no evidence was found for standing, walking or sitting.

Later, Lotters et al.[30] carried out a systematic review and meta-analysis partly based on similar material as Burdorf and Sorock's 1997 study.[28] The review included 40 studies, 35 cross-sectional and five cohort studies. They adjusted the risk estimates for possible confounders and were able to statistically combine the study results. The pooled OR was 1.5 (95 per cent confidence interval (CI) 1.3–1.7) for manual materials handling, 1.7 (95 per cent CI 1.4–2.0) for frequent bending or twisting, 1.4 (95 per cent CI 1.2–1.6) for whole body vibration, 1.3 (95 per cent CI 1.2–1.5) for job dissatisfaction. Since the proportion of people with back pain in the studies is around 30 per cent, the reported odds-ratios are overestimations of the real risk. Transforming the odds-ratios to risk ratios would yield, respectively, 1.3, 1.4, 1.2 and 1.2 for the risk factors mentioned above. This means that the prevalence of back pain of 30 per cent in a non-exposed population would increase to 39 per cent due to exposure to manual materials handling.

Biomechanics provides another important part of the evidence underpinning the relation between spinal loading and back pain.[31] Over the years, there has been considerable progress in measurement techniques that can predict the compression and shear forces on the lumbar intervertebral discs.[32,33] Co-contraction of trunk muscles has been identified as an important factor in spinal loading. It has also been observed that due to inappropriate muscle contraction, patients with low back pain exhibit a greater than necessary spinal loading that might maintain their back pain. Waddell very strongly argues that mechanical overloading leads to dysfunction which he defined as any disturbance of normal strength, endurance, flexibility, coordination or balance, but he also admits that there is little evidence to support his theory.[14]

Biomechanical modelling using a so-called linked segment model can be used to better understand the forces that are elicited by various work tasks and it can be used for preventive purposes. However, it is difficult to translate biomechanical findings to effective interventional strategies. For example, most of our knowledge about lifting techniques is derived from biomechanical models. However, training workers in lifting techniques to prevent back pain has so far led to disappointing results.[34]

Various other approaches to measure spinal load have been tried in the past. Spinal shrinkage has been postulated as a biomarker for spinal load. It is a precision measurement of body length that enables a measurement of the shrinkage of the spine due to water loss of the intervertebral discs during loading. However, it is unclear what the benefits are over biomechanical modelling.

The advances in research on cartilage structure and metabolism have induced a search for biomarkers that could be used as either markers for spinal loading or as markers for early damage. Even though there have been promising studies, the contribution to unravelling the causes of occupational back pain is still unclear.[35]

The evidence for psychosocial occupational risk factors for low back pain is more difficult to interpret. There are no objective criteria for psychosocial load and the evidence on this topic has been somewhat contradictory. A systematic review by Hoogendoorn et al.[36] published in 2000 found 13 studies, of which five were high quality studies that dealt with social support in the workplace. The authors concluded that there was strong evidence for a positive association between low social support and back pain based on four studies with risk estimates of 1.3 to 1.9. For job satisfaction, they also concluded that there was a positive association with back pain based on seven studies.

A systematic review published in 2001 of 21 studies concluded that there was evidence for a relation between the following six psychological risk factors and back pain: job satisfaction, monotonous work, work relations, work demands, stress and perceived ability to work. The strength of the relationships varied between the studies, but was consistent according to the authors.[37]

In a more recent systematic review of cohort studies, Hartvigsen et al.[38] concluded, based on 40 cohort studies of which ten were considered high quality, that there was no evidence for an association between back pain and perception of work, organizational aspects of work or social support at work.

Person-related factors, such as smoking and obesity, have been studied to find a possible relation with the risk for low back pain.[39,40] No clear evidence was found for a causal relation. A previous episode of low back pain is the most strong predictor for future sick listing because of low back pain.[41–43]

PREVENTION OF BACK PAIN AT WORK

Researchers have proposed various interventions to prevent occupational back pain.

Pre-employment strength testing and ergonomic job design together were seen as the most promising intervention methods in review articles in the 1980s and 1990s.[44,45] Snook[46] concluded that it appears possible to control back pain by reducing the probability of the initial episode, reducing the length of the disability, and reducing the chance of recurrence. Realization of these goals was deemed possible with a combination of job design, job placement and education/training. However, recent evaluation studies have shown disappointing results from these preventive interventions.

Exposure limits

If spinal loading at work is a main risk factor for back pain, then it makes sense to try to reduce spinal load by setting maximum permissible limits. The American National Institute of Occupational Safety and Health (NIOSH) has greatly contributed to this idea by developing a relatively simple risk assessment tool that can be used to assess a 'recommended weight limit'. The maximum recommended weight limit is 23 kg. The lifting conditions, such as distance of the load to the body and the degree of trunk rotation, have to be specified and entered into a formula which returns a recommended weight limit for these conditions.[47] Even though the tool covers a wide range of situations, there remain difficulties in applying it to all workplaces.[48,49] It is a serious drawback for its application that there are no studies that have evaluated the effectiveness of the NIOSH standard in reducing back pain due to lifting. Moreover, there are no exposure limits for bending and twisting.

Based on the risk for back disorders, exposure to whole body vibrations has been regulated in the EU. Exposure beyond an intensity of more than 0.25 m/s^2 is considered potentially dangerous and, beyond 0.50 m/s^2, it is required to take action to remediate the danger of exposure. The most frequently occurring whole body vibration in forklift trucks would be around 1.0 m/s^2. There are some studies that have evaluated the effectiveness of measures to reduce whole body vibration if the exposure were above the standard, but they could not show a decrease of exposure.[50]

Workplace improvements, participatory ergonomics

Ergonomics is commonly known as 'the scientific study of human work' or 'the application of scientific information concerning human beings to the design of objects, systems and environments'. Recently, participatory ergonomics has stressed the importance of a participatory approach to prevention and solution finding to increase effectiveness.[51] In a review of participatory ergonomic interventions, Cole et al.[52] found five studies of which two were randomized controlled trials. In these studies, they found limited evidence that participatory interventions decreased musculoskeletal symptoms with four studies reporting a decrease and one no effect. Effect size could be estimated only in one study and it was small. In a recently published study on the effectiveness of kitchen ergonomics, the intervention did not reduce physical work load nor musculoskeletal disorders.[53] In a partly overlapping review on workplace interventions for computer users, Van Eerd et al.[54] found four studies that showed no effect of workstation adjustments on musculoskeletal symptoms. In another four studies, ergonomics training yielded contradictory results on musculoskeletal outcomes. Even though ergonomic improvements may improve comfort and efficiency, they apparently contribute little to the prevention of back pain.

Pre-employment examinations

In general, researchers are sceptical about the possibilities of reducing health problems through pre-employment selection. The problem is that, at the individual level, it is difficult to tell who is at risk for the disease and who is not. The positive predictive value of tests is low which means that there will be a high number of applicants who will be rejected, but that would never have been afflicted with the occupational disease.[55] As part of an ongoing systematic review, we found three low-quality studies that evaluated pre-employment strength testing with contradictory results.[56]

Worker education and training

A recent Cochrane systematic review found six randomized controlled trials and five cohort studies that evaluated worker training and advice on manual material handling. The included studies all had follow-up times of at least one year and had varying degrees of training intensity and hands-on training. None of the studies showed that the intervention decreased the occurrence of back pain.[34] In their review on workplace interventions for computer users, Van Eerd et al.[54] found four studies on ergonomics training that yielded contradictory results on musculoskeletal outcomes.

Exercise

Exercise is believed to be beneficial for many disorders, including back pain. The following three mechanisms are held responsible for the preventative effect of exercise: (1) strengthening of the back muscles and increasing trunk flexibility, (2) increasing the blood supply to the spine muscles, joints and intervertebral discs and (3) improving mood and thereby altering the perception of pain. A review found six randomized controlled trials that evaluated the effectiveness of an exercise programme for various types of workers in 2001. Four out of five studies that compared exercise with no intervention found a significant reduction in back pain experience and reduced work absenteeism. One study reported inconsistent findings. The conclusion of this review was that there is consistent evidence that exercise may be effective in preventing back pain. One other study reported that exercises are more effective than training in back care, but this result was contradicted in another study.[57]

Reporting of occupational back pain to inform policy-making

Reporting of occupational diseases by physicians has been advocated as a useful instrument to inform policy-makers about preventive policy.[58] Many countries maintain a system through which physicians can report cases of occupational diseases often including occupational back pain. The quality of these systems varies and many do not provide guidelines for diagnosis of the diseases to be reported but rely entirely on the professional expertise of the reporting physicians. Moreover, there is little evidence that reporting of occupational diseases to national registries leads to actual policy changes.

Occupational back pain can best be defined as back pain that for a major part is caused by exposure at work. As a clinical disorder, occupational back pain cannot be distinguished from back pain in general by specific symptoms or signs, nor are there specific tests that can elicit these symptoms or signs. Dutch researchers have constructed a model to calculate the probability of work-relatedness. This three-step method calculates this probability on the basis of data on exposure to established risk factors in the work situation. The calculated probability of work-relatedness provides information that can be used to support professional assessment of the work situation and proposals for improving it in the interests of workers with non-specific low-back pain.[30]

The diagnosis of occupational back pain at the individual level can be at odds with the prevailing advice to continue ordinary activities as much as possible. If back pain is attributed to work, it will be difficult to return to the same job which caused the back pain in the first place. On the other hand, leaving a job because of back pain could easily lead to unemployment. A practical solution could be to discuss the pros and cons of continuing in the same job with the worker.

CLINICAL MANAGEMENT AND RETURN TO WORK

Many workers will experience back pain without occupational exposure, but there will still be a risk of long-term disability and unemployment. These risks are related to personal beliefs about the cause of back pain and the fear of reinjury. Proper management of back pain both within the work organization and by the attending physician probably decrease the risk of long-term disability.[59]

The management of back pain is the topic of clinical guidelines that have been developed in many countries and languages. In principle, the clinical management of occupational back pain is no different from management of back pain in general and the authors refer readers to those clinical guidelines. We will summarize the general principles of clinical management of back pain in the following paragraphs.

For any health professional, it is important to differentiate at an early stage between non-specific low back pain, radicular syndrome and specific low back pain. Based on the medical history and the physical examination, symptoms and signs for specific diseases can be detected. These signs and symptoms are called red flags because they potentially indicate serious disease. The absence of red flags excludes specific disease and thus leads to a diagnosis of non-specific back pain. The following red flags are mentioned in most clinical guidelines:

- back pain in workers less than 20 or more than 55 years old;
- constant progressive back pain;
- trauma;
- history of malignancy;
- prolonged use of corticosteroids;
- immunosuppression, drug use, HIV;
- general malaise or unexplained weight loss;
- neurological dysfunction (motor dysfunction, sensory abnormalities and/or miction disturbances);
- lumbar kyphosis and/or past history of lumbar lordosis;
- complaints that might relate to an infectious disease.

If one or more of these symptoms or signs are observed, further investigations should be carried out to exclude specific causes, such as a radicular syndrome due to a herniated disc, malignancy, osteoporotic vertebral fracture, vertebral canal stenosis, spondylitis ankylopoetica (Bechterew's disease) and or forms of spondylolisthesis.

In the history, it is also important to identify psychosocial factors, potential obstacles to recovery and to identify workplace factors (physical and psychosocial) that may be related to the back pain problem and return to work.[10,11,60–62]

People with non-specific back pain can generally be expected to recover, because most episodes settle uneventfully with or without formal health care. Most patients recover at least enough to return to most normal activities, even if with some persistent or recurrent symptoms. Waddell and Burton[63] state that only 1 per cent progress to long-term incapacity, but this is not backed up by evidence. The problem is not what makes these people develop long-term incapacity, but more so why do some people with a problem such as non-specific back pain not recover as expected.[63] Biopsychosocial factors, separately and in combination, can aggravate and perpetuate disability. Workplace factors, such as the attitude of the employer towards low back pain, attitudes of co-workers, communication at the workplace, rules and regulations around sickness absence management, and occupational health provision are examples of obstacles for recovery.

The following psychosocial factors have been listed by a group of experts as yellow flags for risk of chronicity:[63,64]

- dysfunctional attitudes, beliefs and expectations about pain and disability;
- inappropriate attitudes, beliefs and expectations about health care;
- uncertainty, anxiety, fear avoidance;
- depression, distress, low mood, negative emotions;
- passive or negative coping strategies (e.g. catastrophizing);
- lack of 'motivation' and readiness to change, failure to take personal responsibility for rehabilitation, awaiting a 'fix', lack of effort;
- illness behaviour.

The list should be interpreted with caution because not all of these factors are based on findings from rigorous research. Pincus et al. reported conflicting findings on the relation between fear-avoidance and both short- and long-term pain in a review of nine prospective cohort studies.[65] In another review of six cohort studies, she found psychological distress, depressed mood and somatization to be prognostic for chronic pain and to some extent also catastrophizing as a coping strategy.[66]

Prognosis

Assessment of prognosis is important because it is important information for workers and employers based on which they can adapt their personal circumstances or work. In addition, it will help the clinician to focus on those patients who need help most as they are at greatest risk of becoming a chronic patient. Most people will recover rapidly from an episode of acute low back pain and most of those absent from work with back pain also return to work within one month.[67] Further but smaller improvements occur up to three months, after which pain and disability levels remain almost constant. Pengel et al.'s[67] systematic review on prognosis of acute low back pain concluded that, although most people return to work within 12 months, low levels of pain and disability persist. From the studies included, it was not clear if these levels of long-term pain and disability reflect a small subgroup with high levels of pain and disability or a large subgroup with low levels of pain and disability. Nor is it clear whether chronic low levels of pain and disability are due to persistence of the original episode or to recurrences.

Steenstra et al. studied prognosis for duration of sick leave in patients absent from work because of low back pain. They found that the following factors were prognostic for longer sick leave: specific low back pain, higher disability levels, older age, female gender, more social dysfunction and more social isolation, heavier work and receiving higher compensation. A history of low back pain, job satisfaction, educational level, marital status, number of dependants, smoking, working more than eight-hour shifts, occupation, and size of industry or company did not influence duration of sick leave due to low back pain.[68]

Treatment interventions

EXERCISES

Exercise is widely used as therapy for back pain. A Cochrane review summarized the evidence of the effectiveness of exercise therapy based on 61 randomized controlled with 6390 participants for chronic back pain patients relative to comparisons at various follow-up periods. The pooled mean improvement in pain score was 7.3 points (95 per cent CI, 3.7–10.9) out of a maximum score of 100, 2.5 points (95 per cent CI, 1.0–3.9) for function out of a maximum score of 100 at earliest follow-up. In studies that included only patients presenting to healthcare providers, mean improvement was slightly better with 13.3 points (95 per cent CI, 5.5–21.1) for pain and 6.9 score points (95 per cent CI, 2.2–11.7) for function.

In patients with subacute low back pain in occupational settings, there is some evidence of effectiveness of a graded-activity exercise programme, although the evidence for other types of exercise therapy in other populations is inconsistent.

In patients with acute back pain, exercise did not have an effect different from other interventions.[69]

EDUCATION IN BACK CARE

Knowledge of back pain and how to prevent it are assumed to decrease the risk of back pain. Therefore, educational programmes try to increase knowledge on the causes of back pain, often in combination with exercises to improve function or physical fitness. A Cochrane review on back care education included 19 randomized controlled trials with 3584 patients. The authors reported that there is moderate evidence that education in back care provides better short- and intermediate-term effects on pain and functional status than other treatments for patients with recurrent and chronic back pain. There is moderate evidence suggesting that back schools for chronic back pain in an occupational setting, are more effective than other treatments and placebo or waiting list controls on pain, functional status and return to work during short- and intermediate-term follow up.[70]

BEHAVIOURAL TREATMENT PROGRAMMES

Behavioural treatment emphasizes the modification of behavioural processes assuming that pain and disability are not only influenced by somatic factors, but also by psychological and social factors. A Cochrane review showed that both combined respondent-cognitive therapy and progressive relaxation alone relieve pain more effectively than waiting list control in chronic patients. No significant differences could be detected between various types of cognitive-behavioural treatments, between treatments with the addition of behavioural components and the usual treatment programmes, such as physiotherapy, nor between behavioural treatment and exercises. Whether clinicians should refer patients with chronic low-back pain to behavioural treatment programmes or to active conservative treatment cannot be concluded from this review.[71]

MULTIMODAL TREATMENT PROGRAMMES

Multimodal treatment programmes are based on the biopsychosocial model of pain which suggests that physical, psychological and social factors play a role in decreasing pain and disability. A Cochrane review on multidisciplinary biopsychosocial rehabilitation showed that only intensive multidisciplinary biopsychosocial rehabilitation programmes with a functional restoration approach improve pain and function.[72] Functional restoration programmes refer to any intervention aimed at restoring a reasonable functional level for daily living.[73] The idea behind these programmes is that after a certain time, limitation of activities because of low back pain leads to lack of physical fitness, also called 'deconditioning syndrome'. This is associated with decreased lumbar spine mobility and back muscle strength and endurance, with psychosocial implications, such as increased anxiety and depression. A systematic review on functional restoration programmes showed different results in terms of return-to-work rates for controlled studies. Four studies conducted in the United States reported positive results with return-to-work rates of 80–90 per cent at 1 and 2 years' follow up. Two studies from Denmark reported better results for functional restoration programmes compared to control groups at four months and one year, but the positive effects disappeared after two and five years. Results on return-to-work improved when programmes incorporated the provision of suitable modified duties.[74]

Communication, cooperation and common agreed goals between the worker with back pain, the occupational health team, supervisors, management and primary healthcare professionals appears to be important for improvement in clinical and occupational health management outcomes. There is general consensus, but limited evidence, that workplace organizational and/or management strategies can reduce absenteeism and duration of work loss. Examples of such cultures and strategies are an organizational culture committed to health and safety, high stakeholder commitment to improve safety, providing optimum case management and encouraging and supporting early return to work.[11,19,75,76] A Cochrane review focusing on return to work outcomes and functional restoration programmes concluded that successful interventions incorporated:[77]

- a physical conditioning programme specifically designed to restore the individual's systemic, neurological, musculoskeletal or cardiorespiratory function;
- significant cognitive-behavioural components (e.g. correcting dysfunctional beliefs);
- a close association with the workplace, with work-related goals and outcomes.

CONCLUSIONS

Occupational back pain is a result of spinal loading at work due to lifting, twisting and bending, whole body vibration and psychosocial factors. The concept is not unequivocal due to a lack of evidence that exposure, physical damage and back pain are interrelated. Attribution of specific causes to back pain has changed considerably over time as a result of social and political factors. Back pain research is complicated due to the difficulty of measuring both exposure and outcome.

Preventative efforts to redesign workplaces, screen workers with limited physical capacities, train and educate workers in proper lifting techniques or the use of office ergonomics have not been shown to be effective in decreasing back pain outcomes.

Advising workers with back pain to continue ordinary activities has been shown to have beneficial effects on back pain-related disability. A simple clinical model of triage and advice will suffice for most workers with non-specific back pain. Workers with specific back pain should be referred to the appropriate medical specialist. Exercises are beneficial for workers with chronic back pain, but the effect size is only modest. The specific diagnosis and reporting of the work-relatedness of occupational back pain should be balanced against the potential increased risk of disability.

In spite of an immense body of scientific publications, the causes of occupational back pain are still not well understood. Improving the methodological quality of both primary research and systematic reviews will help. In addition, better collaboration between different disciplines will be beneficial. Better understanding of the causes of back pain and back pain-related disability are prerequisites for progress in the field.

Key points

- Back pain has a one-year prevalence of about 50 per cent and a yearly incidence of about 4 per cent.
- Factors at work, both physical and psychological, increase the risk of back pain by about 30 per cent. Occupational back pain is defined as back pain that is mainly caused by factors at work.
- Chronic pain and long-term disability occur probably only in a small percentage of back pain episodes and are the main drivers for better therapy and prevention.
- Clinical management of occupational back pain is similar to non-occupational back pain: triage and simple advice about maintaining normal activities suffice in the acute stage. In chronic pain patients, therapeutic exercises reduce pain levels by about 10 per cent and physical exercise is probably also helpful in preventing back pain.
- A work-directed approach involving patients and supervisors reduces the risk of disability and sick leave.
- Most preventive interventions, such as lifting advice and ergonomic improvements, do not lead to a reduction of back pain prevalence.
- Exercise after treatment might help in preventing recurrences of back pain.
- Better understanding of the mechanisms behind pain and disability is needed for progress in prevention and treatment.

REFERENCES

1. Niemelainen R, Videman T, Battie MC. Prevalence and characteristics of upper or mid-back pain in Finnish men. *Spine.* 2006; **31**: 1846–9.
2. Dunn KM, Croft PR. Epidemiology and natural history of low back pain. *Europa Medicophysica.* 2004; **40**: 9–13.
3. Dagenais S, Caro J, Haldeman S. A systematic review of low back pain cost of illness studies in the United States and internationally. *Spine Journal.* 2008; **8**: 8–20.
4. Dempe A. Back pain. In: Dembe AE (ed.). *Occupation and disease. How social factors affect the conception of work-related disorders*, 1st edn. New Haven/London: Yale University Press, 1996: 102–59.
5. Mixter WJ, Barr JS. Rupture of the intervertebral disc with involvement of the spinal canal. *New England Journal of Medicine.* 1934; **211**: 210–15.
6. Nachemson A. Lumbar intra-discal pressure. In: Jayson MIV (ed.). *The lumbar spine and back pain*, 3rd edn. Edinburgh: Churchill Livingstone, 1984: 191–203.
7. Jensen TS, Karppinen J, Sorensen JS et al. Vertebral endplate signal changes (Modic change): A systematic literature review of prevalence and association with non-specific low back pain. *European Spine Journal.* 2008; **17**: 1407–22.
8. Quebec Task Force. Scientific approach to the assessment and management of activity-related spinal disorders. A monograph for clinicians. Report of the Quebec Task Force on Spinal Disorders. *Spine.* 1987; **12** (7 Suppl.): S1–S59.
9. Waddell G. 1987 Volvo award in clinical sciences. A new clinical model for the treatment of low-back pain. *Spine.* 1987; **12**: 632–44.
10. NVAB. *Richtlijn, handelen van de bedrijfsarts bij rugklachten* (Practice guideline, occupational health management of back pain). Utrecht: Nederlanse Vereniging voor Arbeids en Bedrijfsgeneeskunde, 2009.
11. Carter JT, Birell LN. *Occupational health management guidelines for the management of low back pain at work; principal recommendations.* London: Faculty of Occupational Medicine, 2000.
12. Harris JS, Sinnott PL, Holland JP et al. Methodology to update the practice recommendations. In: American College of Occupational and Environmental Medicine's Occupational Medicine Practice Guidelines, 2nd edn. *Journal of Occupational and Environmental Medicine.* 2008; **50**: 282–95.

13. Steenstra IA, Verbeek JH, Prinsze FJ, Knol DL. Changes in the incidence of occupational disability as a result of back and neck pain in the Netherlands. *BMC Public Health.* 2006; **6**: 190.
14. Waddell G. *The back pain revolution.* Amsterdam: Elsevier Health Sciences, 2006.
15. Dionne CE, Dunn KM, Croft PR *et al.* A consensus approach toward the standardization of back pain definitions for use in prevalence studies. *Spine.* 2008; **33**: 95–103.
16. Walker BF. The prevalence of low back pain: A systematic review of the literature from 1966 to 1998. *Journal of Spinal Disorders.* 2000; **13**: 205–17.
17. Leboeuf-Yde C, Lauritsen JM. The prevalence of low back pain in the literature. A structured review of 26 Nordic studies from 1954 to 1993. *Spine.* 1995; **20**: 2112–18.
18. Waxman R, Tennant A, Helliwell P. A prospective follow-up study of low back pain in the community. *Spine.* 2000; **25**: 2085–90.
19. Snook SH. Work-related low back pain: secondary intervention. *Journal of Electromyography and Kinesiology.* 2004; **14**: 153–60.
20. Punnett L, Pruss-Utun A, Nelson DI *et al.* Estimating the global burden of low back pain attributable to combined occupational exposures. *American Journal of Industrial Medicine.* 2005; **48**: 459–69.
21. Punnett L, Wegman DH. Work-related musculoskeletal disorders: the epidemiologic evidence and the debate. *Journal of Electromyography and Kinesiology.* 2004; **14**: 13–23.
22. Deyo RA, Battie M, Beurskens AJ *et al.* Outcome measures for low back pain research. A proposal for standardized use. *Spine.* 1998; **23**: 2003–13.
23. de Vet HC, Heymans MW, Dunn KM *et al.* Episodes of low back pain: A proposal for uniform definitions to be used in research. *Spine.* 2002; **27**: 2409–16.
24. Ostelo RW, Deyo RA, Stratford P *et al.* Interpreting change scores for pain and functional status in low back pain: Towards international consensus regarding minimal important change. *Spine.* 2008; **33**: 90–4.
25. Griffith LE, Wells RP, Shannon HS *et al.* Developing common metrics of mechanical exposures across aetiological studies of low back pain in working populations for use in meta-analysis. *Occupational and Environmental Medicine.* 2008; **65**: 467–81.
26. Griffith LE, Hogg-Johnson S, Cole DC *et al.* Low-back pain definitions in occupational studies were categorized for a meta-analysis using Delphi consensus methods. *Journal of Clinical Epidemiology.* 2007; **60**: 625–33.
27. Bernard BP. *Musculoskeletal disorders and workplace factors. A critical review of epidemiologic evidence for work-related musculoskeletal disorders of the neck, upper extremity, and low back.* Cincinnati, OH: NIOSH, 1997.
28. Burdorf A, Sorock G. Positive and negative evidence of risk factors for back disorders. *Scandinavian Journal of Work and Environmental Health.* 1997; **23**: 243–56.
29. Hoogendoorn WE, van Poppel MN, Bongers PM *et al.* Physical load during work and leisure time as risk factors for back pain. *Scandinavian Journal of Work and Environmental Health.* 1999; **25**: 387–403.
30. Lotters F, Burdorf A, Kuiper J, Miedema H. Model for the work-relatedness of low-back pain. *Scandinavian Journal of Work and Environmental Health.* 2003; **29**: 431–40.
31. Chaffin DB, Andersson GBJ, Martin BJ. *Occupational biomechanics.* Chichester: John Wiley, 2006.
32. McGill SM. Linking latest knowledge of injury mechanisms and spine function to the prevention of low back disorders. *Journal of Electromyography and Kinesiology.* 2004; **14**: 43–7.
33. Marras WS. The future of research in understanding and controlling work-related low back disorders. *Ergonomics.* 2005; **48**: 464–77.
34. Martimo KP, Verbeek J, Karppinen J *et al.* Effect of training and lifting equipment for preventing back pain in lifting and handling: Systematic review. *British Medical Journal.* 2008; **336**: 429–31.
35. Kuiper JI, Verbeek JH, Frings-Dresen MH *et al.* Exploration of the use of biomarkers to monitor recovery after surgery for lumbar disc herniation: a prospective cohort study. *Journal of Spinal Disorders.* 2002; **15**: 398–403.
36. Hoogendoorn WE, van Poppel MN, Bongers PM *et al.* Systematic review of psychosocial factors at work and private life as risk factors for back pain. *Spine.* 2000; **25**: 2114–25.
37. Linton SJ. Occupational psychological factors increase the risk for back pain: A systematic review. *Journal of Occupational Rehabilitation.* 2001; **11**: 53–66.
38. Hartvigsen J, Lings S, Leboeuf-Yde C, Bakketeig L. Psychosocial factors at work in relation to low back pain and consequences of low back pain: A systematic, critical review of prospective cohort studies. *Occupational and Environmental Medicine.* 2004; **61**: e2.
39. Leboeuf-Yde C. Smoking and low back pain. A systematic literature review of 41 journal articles reporting 47 epidemiologic studies. *Spine.* 1999; **24**: 1463–70.
40. Leboeuf-Yde C. Body weight and low back pain. A systematic literature review of 56 journal articles reporting on 65 epidemiologic studies. *Spine.* 2000; **25**: 226–37.
41. Muller CF, Monrad T, Biering-Sorensen F *et al.* The influence of previous low back trouble, general health, and working conditions on future sick-listing because of low back trouble. A 15-year follow-up study of risk indicators for self-reported sick-listing caused by low back trouble. *Spine.* 1999; **24**: 1562–70.
42. Feyer AM, Herbison P, Williamson AM *et al.* The role of physical and psychological factors in occupational low back pain: a prospective cohort study. *Occupational and Environmental Medicine.* 2000; **57**: 116–20.
43. Van NA, Somville PR, Crombez G *et al.* The role of physical workload and pain related fear in the development of low back pain in young workers: Evidence from the BelCoBack Study; results after one year of follow up. *Occupational and Environmental Medicine.* 2006; **63**: 45–52.
44. Yu TS, Roht LH, Wise RA *et al.* Low-back pain in industry. An old problem revisited. *Journal of Occupational Medicine.* 1984; **26**: 517–24.
45. Garg A, Moore JS. Prevention strategies and the low back in industry. *Occupational Medicine.* 1992; **7**: 629–40.

46. Snook SH. Approaches to the control of back pain in industry: Job design, job placement and education/training. *Occupational Medicine*. 1988; **3**: 45–59.
47. Waters TR, Putz-Anderson V, Garg A, Fine LJ. Revised NIOSH equation for the design and evaluation of manual lifting tasks. *Ergonomics*. 1993; **36**: 749–76.
48. Dempsey PG. Usability of the revised NIOSH lifting equation. *Ergonomics*. 2002; **45**: 817–28.
49. Waters TR. When is it safe to manually lift a patient? *American Journal of Nursing*. 2007; **107**: 53–8.
50. Hulshof CT, Verbeek JH, Braam IT et al. Evaluation of an occupational health intervention programme on whole-body vibration in forklift truck drivers: a controlled trial. *Occupational and Environmental Medicine*. 2006; **63**: 461–8.
51. Buckle P. Ergonomics and musculoskeletal disorders: overview. *Occupational Medicine*. 2005; **55**: 164–7.
52. Cole D, Rivilis I, Van Eerd D et al. *Effectiveness of participatory ergonomic interventions. A systematic review*, vol. 2. Toronto: Institute for Work and Health, 2005.
53. Haukka E, Leino-Arjas P, Viikari-Juntura E et al. A randomised controlled trial on whether a participatory ergonomics intervention could prevent musculoskeletal disorders. *Occupational and Environmental Medicine*. 2008; **65**: 849–56.
54. Van Eerd D, Brewer S, Amick III BC et al. *Workplace interventions to prevent musculoskeletal and visual symptoms and disorders among computer users. A systematic review*. Toronto: Institute for Work and Health, 2006.
55. Sorgdrager B, Hulshof CT, van Dijk FJ. Evaluation of the effectiveness of pre-employment screening. *International Archives of Occupational and Environmental Health*. 2004; **77**: 271–6.
56. Mahmud N, Schonstein E, Lehtola M et al. Health examination for preventing occupational injuries and disease in workers. *Cochrane Database of Systematic Reviews*. 2009 (in press).
57. Linton SJ, van Tulder MW. Preventive interventions for back and neck pain problems: What is the evidence? *Spine*. 2001; **26**: 778–87.
58. Spreeuwers D, de Boer AG, Verbeek JH et al. Diagnosing and reporting of occupational diseases: A quality improvement study. *Occupational Medicine*. 2008; **58**: 115–21.
59. van Oostrom SH, Driessen MT, de Vet HC et al. Workplace interventions for preventing work disability. *Cochrane Database of Systematic Reviews*. 2009; (**2**): CD006955.
60. Staal JB, Hlobil H, van Tulder MW et al. Occupational health guidelines for the management of low back pain: An international comparison. *Occupational and Environmental Medicine*. 2003; **60**: 618–26.
61. Accident Compensation Corporation and National Health. *Active and working! Managing acute low back pain in the workplace*. Wellington, New Zealand: Accident Compensation Corporation and National Health, 2000.
62. Victorian Work Cover Authority. *Guidelines for the management of employees with compensable low back pain*. Melbourne: Victorian Work Cover Authority, 1996.
63. Waddell G, Burton AK. Concepts of rehabilitation for the management of low back pain. *Best Practice and Research. Clinical Rheumatology*. 2005; **19**: 655–70.
64. Kendall N, Linton SJ, Main C. *Guide to assessing psychosocial yellow flags in acute low back pain. Risk factors for long-term disability and work loss*. Wellington, New Zealand: Accident Rehabilitation and Compensation Insurance Corporation of New Zealand and the National Health Committee, 1997.
65. Pincus T, Vogel S, Burton AK et al. Fear avoidance and prognosis in back pain: A systematic review and synthesis of current evidence. *Arthritis and Rheumatism*. 2006; **54**: 3999–4010.
66. Pincus T, Burton AK, Vogel S, Field AP. A systematic review of psychological factors as predictors of chronicity/disability in prospective cohorts of low back pain. *Spine*. 2002; **27**: E109–E120.
67. Pengel LH, Herbert RD, Maher CG, Refshauge KM. Acute low back pain: Systematic review of its prognosis. *British Medical Journal*. 2003; **327**: 323.
68. Steenstra IA, Verbeek JH, Heymans MW, Bongers PM. Prognostic factors for duration of sick leave in patients sick listed with acute low back pain: A systematic review of the literature. *Occupational and Environmental Medicine*. 2005; **62**: 851–60.
69. Hayden JA, van Tulder MW, Malmivaara AV, Koes BW. Meta-analysis: Exercise therapy for nonspecific low back pain. *Annals of Internal Medicine*. 2005; **142**: 765–75.
70. Heymans MW, van Tulder MW, Esmail R et al. Back schools for non-specific low-back pain. *Cochrane Database of Systematic Reviews*. 2004; (**4**): CD000261.
71. Ostelo RW, van Tulder MW, Vlaeyen JW et al. Behavioural treatment for chronic low-back pain. *Cochrane Database of Systematic Reviews*. 2005; (**1**): CD002014.
72. Guzman J, Esmail R, Karjalainen K et al. WITHDRAWN: Multidisciplinary bio-psycho-social rehabilitation for chronic low-back pain. *Cochrane Database of Systematic Reviews*. 2006; (**2**): CD000963.
73. Bendix T, Bendix AF, Busch E, Jordan A. Functional restoration in chronic low back pain. *Scandinavian Journal of Medicine and Science in Sports*. 1996; **6**: 88–97.
74. Poiraudeau S, Rannou F, Revel M. Functional restoration programs for low back pain: A systematic review. *Annales de Réadaptation et de Médecine Physique*. 2007; **50**: 425–24.
75. Burton AK, Balague F, Cardon G et al. How to prevent low back pain. *Best Practice and Research. Clinical Rheumatology*. 2005; **19**: 541–55.
76. Anema JR, Steenstra IA, Urlings IJ et al. Participatory ergonomics as a return-to-work intervention: A future challenge? *American Journal of Industrial Medicine*. 2003; **44**: 273–81.
77. Schonstein E, Kenny DT, Keating J, Koes BW. Work conditioning, work hardening and functional restoration for workers with back and neck pain. *Cochrane Database of Systematic Reviews*. 2003; (**1**): CD001822.

PART FIVE

OCCUPATION AND TRANSMISSIBLE DISEASES

Section One: Occupational infections 727
Section Two: Bioterrorism and biotechnology 771

SECTION ONE

Occupational infections

59	Occupational infections *Julia Heptonstall and Anne Cockcroft*	729
60	Zoonoses *Alastair Miller and Julia Heptonstall*	750

59

Occupational infections

JULIA HEPTONSTALL AND ANNE COCKCROFT

Introduction	729	Infections associated with occupational travel	742
Healthcare workers and related occupations	729	Others	743
Laboratory research workers and animal handlers	741	References	744

INTRODUCTION

This chapter will consider in turn the main occupations at risk, and the infections associated with each occupation. The occupational groups considered here are:

- healthcare workers and people in related occupations;
- laboratory workers;
- people whose work involves frequent travel or living abroad;
- others.

Workers in almost any occupation may contract an infection as a result of their work, even if the occupation is not associated with a clearly recognized risk of infection, so the possibility that an infection may have been occupationally acquired should always be considered during the initial clinical assessment.

HEALTHCARE WORKERS AND RELATED OCCUPATIONS

Healthcare professionals, ancillary workers and staff in service laboratories have always been at risk of contracting infections from their patients. The spectrum of these infections has changed over time, as a result of changes in the pattern of infectious disease in the general population and advances in immunization and exposure prevention. However, with the exception of smallpox, none of the agents causing infections classically contracted by healthcare workers has been eradicated. A risk of infection, albeit small, remains, especially where lapses in exposure prevention occur. In developed countries, there are regulations covering the control of exposure to infectious agents at work; for example, in Europe there is the Biological Agents Directive, incorporated into the Control of Substances Hazardous to Health (COSHH) Regulations in the UK.[1]

Blood-borne viruses

The hepatitis viruses (particularly hepatitis B (HBV) and hepatitis C (HCV)) and the human immunodeficiency virus (HIV) are important causes of occupational infectious disease, especially in healthcare workers. The occupational hazard is increased because of the frequently long carrier phase when patients with undiagnosed infection are relatively well, but nevertheless able to transmit infection. One estimate of the global burden of occupational blood-borne virus infections suggests that 16 000 HCV, 66 000 HBV and 200–5000 HIV infections due to percutaneous exposure may have occurred in healthcare workers worldwide in the year 2000, with the fraction of infections attributable to occupational percutaneous exposure being 39, 37 and 4.4 per cent for HCV, HBV and HIV, respectively. More than 90 per cent of these infections occur in low-income countries, where the prevalence of infection tends to be higher, and where there are fewer resources for occupational health services, or exposure prevention and management.[2]

EVIDENCE OF RISK OF INFECTION IN HEALTHCARE WORKERS

Hepatitis B virus

Viral hepatitis is a prescribed industrial disease in the United Kingdom in people whose work activities expose them to frequent contact with blood and body fluids.[3] It is well recognized that hepatitis B can be transmitted via infected blood and other body fluids, either from those with acute infection or from individuals who have become virus carriers. Hepatitis B virus is usually transmitted by unprotected sexual intercourse, by sharing of blood-contaminated needles or injecting equipment between drug users, and by transmission from an infected mother to her child at or during delivery. It may also be transmitted by transfusion of infected blood, particularly in countries where the prevalence of infection is high and resources for transfusion services are small, and by accidental exposure to blood and other body fluids. It is the transmission by blood-exposure incidents that is particularly relevant to occupational risk.

Surveys undertaken before the hepatitis B vaccine became widely available show an excess of serological markers of hepatitis B infection in workers exposed to blood and body fluids. West[4] reviewed evidence from a number of seroprevalence studies in the United States and concluded that the overall risk to people employed in health-related fields was four times that of the general adult population; physicians and dentists were at five to ten times the risk of the general population; groups with over ten times the risk included surgeons, clinical workers in dialysis units and mental handicap units, and laboratory workers having frequent contact with blood samples. Later studies confirmed these findings.[5–8] Among 5813 Italian healthcare workers tested prior to hepatitis B immunization, 23 per cent had markers of past or present hepatitis B infection, including 2 per cent who were HBsAg positive.[9] A study from Stockholm of healthcare workers enrolling for hepatitis B immunization found a prevalence of hepatitis B markers of 4 per cent, not greater than in the general population, but related to age, duration of healthcare work and history of blood-exposure incidents.[10] In the United States, a survey of hospital-based surgeons showed a significant rate of hepatitis B infection; 17 per cent of 770 surgeons tested had markers of infection and 0.4 per cent were HBsAg positive.[11] Risk factors for infection were non-vaccination and surgical practice for ten years or more.

In the United Kingdom, in the 1970s and 1980s, there was an excess rate of acute hepatitis B among healthcare workers compared with the general population. In 1975–79, the average annual rate for men in the whole population was 4 per 100 000, while healthcare workers had rates of up to 36 per 100 000.[12] In 1980–84, the average annual rate in men in the general population was 6 per 100 000 and again up to 37 per 100 000 among healthcare workers.[13] However, cases of acute hepatitis B acquired occupationally in the United Kingdom are now rare.[14] This is likely to reflect the results of the campaign to ensure hepatitis B immunization of healthcare workers and pre-entry medical students; the few cases that did occur in the period of review were in people who had not had hepatitis B vaccine. A similar effect has been seen in the United States, where the reported incidence of acute hepatitis B in healthcare workers is now lower than that in the general population, the result of improvements in transfusion and dialysis safety, the implementation of standard ('universal') infection control precautions, and the use of hepatitis B vaccine.[15,16]

Even in countries where hepatitis B infection is endemic and the background seroprevalence is high, serosurveys provide evidence that there is an additional occupational risk among healthcare workers. Among 234 dentists in the Philippines, the prevalence of markers of hepatitis B infection was found to be 58 per cent, similar to the prevalence in the general population, but increasing with the number of years in dental practice.[17] In Japan, a seroprevalence study found that over a third of hospital workers had evidence of previous hepatitis B infection, about the same as that in a group of healthy controls, but that the seroprevalence among nurses and surgeons was significantly higher than in other staff or the controls.[18] A study in Cairo revealed a higher prevalence of hepatitis B infection markers among non-professional staff (60 per cent) than among doctors and nurses, presumably as a result of non-occupational infection in early life, but still found a relationship between infection markers and blood exposures and years of practice among the physicians.[19] A serosurvey of healthcare workers in Belize found that 29 per cent had markers of past hepatitis B infection and 1 per cent had detectable HBsAg. Prevalence of hepatitis B markers reached 57 per cent in workers from one ethnic group.[20] Similarly, a recent serosurvey of 167 surgeons working in hospitals in Lagos, Nigeria, found that 25 per cent were hepatitis B surface antigen positive, compared with 15 per cent of a control group of 193 administrative staff.[21]

Occupations allied to health care may also carry a risk of hepatitis B infection. A serosurvey of 133 embalmers[22] found that they had hepatitis B infection markers at about twice the rate of a blood donor comparison group and commonly gave a history of needlestick injuries at work. A Canadian study reported that 13 per cent of staff (and more than 20 per cent of specialized teachers) in a day school for mentally handicapped children had markers of hepatitis B infection.[23] Emergency medical workers, such as emergency ambulance staff and paramedics, have been reported to have an increased risk of hepatitis B infection.[24–26] However, other studies of groups of emergency workers and public-safety workers have not found an excess of hepatitis B infection markers. Morgan-Capner and Wallice[27] found no excess of hepatitis B markers among Lancashire ambulance personnel compared with blood donors; their subjects undertook both routine and emergency work. Studies of police officers,[28–30] prison officers[31] and firemen[32] have not documented an increased risk of hepatitis B infection.

Occupational hepatitis B infection has also been reported in professions unrelated to health care or the emergency services. Outbreaks of hepatitis B have been reported in butchers' shops[33,34] apparently spread from infected employees to colleagues as a result of frequent cuts sustained at work. Several studies have found an excess of hepatitis B infection among naval personnel and merchant seamen; this can be partly explained by work in a healthcare setting for some personnel, but appears to be related mainly to para-occupational factors, such as injecting drug use, unprotected sexual contact and tattooing performed in areas of high endemicity.[35–37]

Hepatitis C virus (HCV)

Seroconversion after occupational percutaneous exposure to HCV infected blood is well documented,[38] although most serosurveys of healthcare workers have indicated that the prevalence of hepatitis C antibodies is low. Abb found hepatitis C antibodies in eight of 738 healthcare workers (1 per cent), compared with much higher seroprevalences among certain patient groups.[39] In another study, although only 0.58 per cent of 1033 hospital employees had antibodies to hepatitis C, this prevalence was significantly greater than the 0.24 per cent of 2113 blood donor controls.[40]

Klein et al.[41] found antibodies to hepatitis C among 2 per cent of 456 dentists in New York compared with 0.1 per cent of 723 controls; among a small group of oral surgeons, the prevalence was 9 per cent. Dentists who had antibodies to hepatitis C reported more exposure incidents, and having treated more intravenous drug users in the previous month than did seronegative dentists. Among those dentists who had not been immunized against hepatitis B, 25 per cent had anti-HBs. Some 6 per cent of these had antibodies to hepatitis C, compared with only 2 per cent among those who were anti-HBs negative. This suggests a common mode of transmission for the two viruses, though with a lower risk for hepatitis C.

Later studies confirmed the low prevalence of hepatitis C antibodies among healthcare workers and investigated risk factors. In Argentina, a survey of 439 healthcare workers found antibodies to hepatitis C by enzyme immunoassay in 1.6 per cent.[42] In the Johns Hopkins Hospital in the United States, antibodies to hepatitis C were found in 0.7 per cent of 943 healthcare workers and 0.4 per cent of local blood donors.[43] Similarly, a study in a London teaching hospital among 1053 healthcare workers exposed to blood and body fluids found antibodies to hepatitis C in 0.28 per cent, no higher than reported in blood donors in the same area.[44] Another UK study, from Nottingham, reported similar findings, with antibodies to hepatitis C in 0.2 per cent of 1949 healthcare workers enrolled in a hepatitis B immunization programme.[45] Among 343 oral surgeons and 305 general dentists in the United States, 2 and 0.7 per cent, respectively, were found to have antibodies to hepatitis C.[46] Hepatitis C infection was more prevalent in those who were older, had more years of practice and had serological markers of hepatitis B infection; but hepatitis C infection was much less common than markers of previous hepatitis B infection (8 per cent in general dentists and 21 per cent in oral surgeons). In serosurveys at 16 Italian hospitals, 2 per cent of 3073 healthcare workers had antibodies to hepatitis C.[47] Infection was associated with previous acute hepatitis, blood transfusions, poor housekeeping and older age, but not with occupational risk factors.

The occupational risk of hepatitis C is lower than that of hepatitis B. In a study of hospital-based surgeons in the United States, 0.9 per cent of the 770 surgeons had antibodies to hepatitis C, compared with 17 per cent who had markers of hepatitis B infection[11] and in a study of 3411 orthopaedic surgeons in the United States, 13 per cent without non-occupational risk factors had markers of HBV infection and 1 per cent had HCV antibodies.[48] The prevalence of infection markers for both HBV and HCV was higher in older workers.

Human immunodeficiency virus (HIV)

In contrast to hepatitis B and C, the studies that have examined the seroprevalence of HIV among healthcare workers have found a low seroprevalence and no evidence of an excess related to occupation; most healthcare workers with HIV will have acquired it non-occupationally. For example, in a study of orthopaedic surgeons in the United States, none of the 3267 surgeons without non-occupational risk factors had antibodies to HIV.[49] In six urban areas of the United States, only two of 8519 healthcare workers who had donated blood were HIV positive; information was not available on non-occupational risks.[50]

TYPES OF EXPOSURE AND RISK OF TRANSMISSION IN THE HEALTHCARE SETTING

The most important means of transmission of blood-borne viruses in the occupational setting is by percutaneous exposure to infected blood, either by skin-penetrating injuries with blood-contaminated needles (needlestick injuries) or by cuts with scalpels or other sharp instruments contaminated with blood (sharps injuries). There is a lower risk of transmission associated with mucocutaneous exposure: blood contamination of eyes, mouth and broken skin. In addition, cases of hepatitis B, hepatitis C and HIV transmission by skin-penetrating bite have been reported. Blood-borne viruses do not cross intact skin, and faeco-oral transmission does not occur.

Blood exposure is particularly common in surgery. Lowenfels et al.[51] contacted surgeons in New York by letter or telephone and reported a median rate of puncture injuries of 4.2 per 1000 operating room hours, with 25 per cent of the surgeons having injury rates of nine or more per 1000 operating room hours. Hussain et al.[52] asked 18 surgeons in Saudi Arabia to record all accidental injuries during surgery and reported that sharps injuries occurred in 5.6 per cent of operations. An observational study of 1307 surgical procedures at San Francisco General Hospital revealed accidental blood exposures in 6.4 per cent of procedures and percutaneous exposure to blood in 1.7 per cent.[53] The risk of blood exposure was highest for procedures lasting more than three hours, when blood loss exceeded 300 mL, and for major vascular and gynaecological procedures. The lower rate of injuries in San Francisco was thought to reflect greater attention to safe practices because of the high rate of HIV infection among the patients.

However, in a later prospective observational study in four hospitals in the United States, sharps injuries were noted in 6.9 per cent of procedures[54] and injuries were recorded by operating theatre staff in Glasgow at a rate of 1.6 per cent per surgeon per operation, calculated to give 4.6 per cent per operation overall.[55] Williams[56] studied blood exposures in theatre staff during 6096 operations over a six-month period. Sharps injuries occurred in 1.6 per cent of operations. The risk was increased with long procedures, high blood loss, major operations, wound closure with staples and the main surgeon wearing corrective spectacles. It was concluded that wearing spectacles could be a surrogate for increased age and reduced manual dexterity or that the spectacles themselves could be obscuring the operative field.

Blood exposures other than sharps injuries are also common in surgical practice. These include glove tears and perforations,[57–59] and eye splashes with blood and other body fluids.[60–62] It has been reported that even minor suturing procedures undertaken in the Accident and Emergency Department are associated with one or more glove perforations in 11 per cent of cases.[63]

The risk of blood exposures is not confined to surgery. Albertoni et al.[64] found an overall rate of needlestick injuries over a one-year period of 29 per cent among 20 000 Italian healthcare workers interviewed in 1985; the rate was highest among surgeons (55 per cent) and nurses (35 per cent). Collins and Kennedy[65] have reviewed a number of studies of sharps injuries among groups of healthcare workers and compared the results in terms of needlestick injuries per 100 employee-years for different occupational groups. Nurses appear to suffer the highest number of injuries, even allowing for the number of nurses employed. A group of workers at particular risk are phlebotomists, who spend most of their working day using needles to gain access to veins.[66] Other groups at risk include domestic and portering staff, who get injured from improperly disposed needles and other sharp instruments, and laboratory staff.

Relatively few injuries in reported studies occur to doctors. Sharps injuries and other blood and body fluid exposures have also been found to be frequent among embalmers.[67]

Surveys of routinely reported incidents must be interpreted with caution because of the high rate of under-reporting, particularly among doctors. Some authors have attempted to quantify this under-reporting. Astbury and Baxter,[68] using questionnaire responses to estimate the incidence of sharps injuries and bites and scratches over the preceding year, found that only 5 per cent of injuries had been reported by staff to the hospital occupational health service. The low (45 per cent) response rate to their questionnaire may have biased their results. McGeer et al.[69] reported a less than 5 per cent reporting rate for sharps injuries among medical students, interns and residents in Toronto, but they asked respondents to recall incidents occurring over several previous years, which may have led to inaccuracies. A questionnaire study of 158 operating department staff at the Royal Free Hospital in London on reporting of needlesticks recorded 26 sharps injuries and 240 other blood-exposure incidents during the preceding month; only 15 per cent of the sharps injuries and none of the other blood exposures were reported to the occupational health department (or indeed to anywhere else).[70]

TRANSMISSION RISKS

The risk of transmission of HBV to a susceptible person following a single needlestick from a source who is HBeAg positive may be as high as 30 per cent. The risk of transmission when the source is HBsAg positive but HBeAg negative is much lower, with studies reporting rates of transmission of between 1 and 6 per cent (see Table 59.1 for a description of HBV serology).[71–74] The risk of hepatitis C transmission is around 2 per cent,[75–79] ranging from 0 to 10 per cent depending on the clinical status of the source patients and the tests used to identify infection in

Table 59.1 Serological markers of hepatitis B infection and immunity.

Clinical situation	Serological markers					
	HBsAg	Anti-HBc	Anti-HBc IgM	HBe Ag	Anti-HBe	Anti-HBs
Very early acute infection	+	−	−	+/−	−	−
Acute hepatitis B	+	+	+	+/−	−	−
Hepatitis B carrier: higher infectivity	+	+	−	+	−	−
Hepatitis B carrier: lower infectivity	+	+	−	−	+/−	−
Recent past HBV infection	−	+	+	−	+/−	+/−
Distant past HBV infection	−	+	−	−	+/−	+/−
Vaccine-induced immunity	−	−	−	−	−	+
True vaccine non-responder	−	(+)	−	−	−	−
False positive anti-HBc	−	+	−	−	−	−

HBsAg, hepatitis B surface antigen; anti-HBc, antibody to hepatitis B core antigen (anti-core antibody); anti-HBc IgM, IgM antibody to hepatitis B core antibody (anti-core IgM antibody); HBeAg, hepatitis B e antigen; anti-HBe, antibody to hepatitis B e antigen (anti-e antibody); anti-HBs, antibody to hepatitis B surface antigen (anti-surface antibody).
Anti-HBc IgM lasts three to six months after an acute HBV infection.

the workers, markedly lower than for hepatitis B. The overall risk of transmission of HIV after percutaneous exposure to infected blood has been extensively studied and is around 0.3 per cent.[80,81]

Some exposures may be of higher risk than others. A case–control study suggested that factors increasing the risk of HIV seroconversion after a percutaneous exposure to HIV-infected blood include: a 'deep' injury; the presence of visible blood on the instrument; procedures involving insertion of a device into an artery or vein; and exposure to a source patient who is terminally ill.[82] These are probably proxy measures for increased risks associated with exposure to a greater volume of blood and exposure to higher titres of HIV. Similarly, a recent European case–control study found that the risk of HCV seroconversion after percutaneous exposure increased with deep injuries and procedures involving placement of a hollow-bore needle in the source patient's vein or artery, and also suggested that the transmission risk increased with titre of virus in the source patient.[83]

By 2002 (the latest date for which aggregate data from published reports worldwide are available), there were 106 reported cases of documented HIV seroconversion after occupational exposure and a further 238 reported cases of possible occupationally acquired infection.[81] Most (87 per cent) of the documented seroconversions were reported from the United States or Europe; relatively few were reported from high-prevalence low-income countries, which have limited resources for occupational health and the enhanced surveillance needed to document seroconversion. Of the 57 documented seroconversions reported from the United States between 1991 and 2006, only three occurred after 1995, with the most recent in 1999.[84] This decline in incidence probably reflects a combination of factors: improved exposure prevention; improved post-exposure management; and the widespread use of highly active antiretroviral therapy for HIV infection, which, by reducing the numbers of HIV-infected people needing inpatient treatment for advanced HIV-related disease, reduced the overall transmission risks for healthcare workers.[85]

CLINICAL FEATURES IN INFECTED HEALTHCARE WORKERS AND RISK OF TRANSMISSION TO PATIENTS

The clinical features of infections with blood-borne viruses acquired occupationally by healthcare workers are essentially no different from the features of these infections acquired by any other means.

Hepatitis B

Acute icteric hepatitis, sometimes fulminant, can occur three to six months after occupational exposure to the virus in non-immune workers; though only around a third of adults who become infected will develop clinically significant symptoms. In clinically apparent hepatitis, a prodromal illness with fever, nausea, anorexia and abdominal discomfort precedes the development of jaundice and dark urine. In some cases of acute hepatitis B infection, the first symptom may be urticaria. Reports of acute infections acquired occupationally in the United Kingdom and other countries that have effective systems for ensuring that healthcare workers are vaccinated against hepatitis B are now rare.

Confirmation that a case of hepatitis is due to HBV infection requires serological testing. The serology of HBV infection is described in Table 59.1. This shows the pattern of hepatitis B markers found in different situations, including acute infection, natural immunity, the carrier state, and immunity as a result of vaccination.

During the acute infection, supportive treatment is usually all that is required. Severe cases should be managed in specialist units. Sexual partners and other family and close contacts should be investigated and offered vaccination if they are non-infected and non-immune.

Fewer than 10 per cent of adults with acute hepatitis B infection will fail to clear the virus and become carriers. The carrier state is indicated by *either* the presence of hepatitis B surface antigen (HBsAg) on two occasions at least six months apart *or* the finding of HBsAg in the absence of anti-core antibody of IgM type (anti-HBc IgM). Those carriers who remain positive for HBeAg have much greater infectivity than those who clear the HBeAg, but remain positive for HBsAg (see above). Treatment with antiviral drugs, such as alpha-interferon and other new agents, may sometimes be effective in helping to clear HBeAg or suppress viral replication. Long-term sequelae of chronic hepatitis B infection include chronic liver disease and hepatocellular carcinoma. Healthcare workers found to be infected with hepatitis B should be referred for specialist care.

Acutely or chronically infected healthcare workers who undertake exposure-prone procedures can transmit hepatitis B infection to their patients. An exposure-prone procedure is one where there is a risk that the patient's open tissues may be exposed to the blood of a healthcare worker, as in surgery, dentistry and midwifery during complicated or instrumental deliveries. The risk of transmission depends on the types of procedure being performed, the role of the worker and the infectivity of the worker. In outbreaks associated with HBeAg-positive surgeons, overall transmission rates have been around 5 per cent, but transmission rates of 20 per cent have been recorded in groups of patients undergoing longer and more complex procedures.[86] There is also evidence that some healthcare workers who are HBsAg positive but HBeAg negative can also transmit hepatitis B to patients during exposure-prone procedures, probably because of carriage of variants of hepatitis B virus, in which there is continuing viral replication, even though HBeAg is not detectable in the blood.[87]

Hepatitis C

It is now known that HCV is the cause of a large proportion of cases of what was formerly called 'non-A, non-B hepatitis'. Acute and even fulminant hepatitis can occur after occupational transmission of HCV but is rare. The majority of infections will be anicteric, and many will be asymptomatic, occupational transmission being indicated by a rise in liver enzymes or by the detection of HCV RNA or of antibody to HCV on testing. Treatment with antiviral drugs, especially if instituted early, may help to prevent the carrier state being established. In chronic HCV carriers, there is sometimes a fluctuating hepatitis with 'yo-yo' transaminases. Sequelae can be serious, including cirrhosis, chronic liver disease and hepatocellular carcinoma.

Healthcare workers infected with hepatitis C virus can transmit the infection to patients during exposure-prone procedures.[88–92] The transmission rate has not been quantified precisely, but, by analogy with the evidence on transmission to healthcare workers from needlestick exposures, it is likely to be substantially less than for hepatitis B (with HBeAg).

Human immunodeficiency virus

A seroconversion illness typically occurs about four to six weeks after the exposure. This is characterized by fever, generalized lymphadenopathy and a rash. Thereafter, the infection is asymptomatic until an HIV-related illness or full-blown AIDS occurs. The first AIDS illness in a young healthcare worker with undiagnosed HIV infection may be pneumonia due to *Pneumocystis jirovecii*. This may present with unexplained breathlessness on exertion or as failure of a chest infection to respond to the usual antibiotics. Immunocompromised people with AIDS can develop a variety of bacterial and fungal infections, sometimes with opportunistic organisms and parasitic infestations. Tuberculosis is a particular problem, especially in areas with a high prevalence in the population. There is a risk of infection with atypical mycobacteria or with multidrug-resistant *Mycobacterium tuberculosis*. Modern combination antiretroviral therapy for HIV infection and primary prophylaxis against opportunistic infections have greatly improved the prognosis of HIV infection in developed countries, prolonging survival and delaying the onset of AIDS in people infected with HIV. The prognosis remains very poor in countries where this effective but expensive treatment is not available. Anyone with HIV antibodies is considered to be infectious through sexual contact or contact with their blood, but infectivity is higher at times when the level of virus in the blood is higher, for example during seroconversion and in the late stages of AIDS.

The potential for HIV-infected healthcare workers to transmit to patients during exposure-prone procedures is a cause of great concern, given the very serious consequences of such an occurrence. There are three reports of transmission from a healthcare worker to patients: a dentist in Florida,[93] an orthopaedic surgeon in France[94] and a gynaecologist in Spain.[95] The estimated risk of transmission to patients is much lower than for either hepatitis B or hepatitis C.

MANAGEMENT OF INFECTED HEALTHCARE WORKERS

A healthcare worker may be found to have an infection with a blood-borne virus, either as a result of routine testing (see below), or by testing in relation to an illness or reported occupational exposure, or by testing during investigation of the source of infection in one or more infected patients.

In the United Kingdom, all healthcare workers who undertake exposure-prone procedures are required to demonstrate by testing of an identified validated blood sample that they are immune to hepatitis B as a result of immunization or that they are not hepatitis B infected (HBsAg positive). Hepatitis B-infected healthcare workers who are HBeAg positive, or who are HBeAg negative but have a hepatitis B virus DNA level (HBV DNA) of more than 10^5 genome equivalents per mL (geq/mL), may not perform exposure-prone procedures. Hepatitis B-infected healthcare workers who are HBeAg negative and have a baseline HBV DNA level of below 1000 geq/mL may practise unrestricted provided that their HBV DNA level is monitored annually, and remains below 10^3 geq/mL. HBeAg-negative healthcare workers whose baseline viral load is 10^3–10^5 geq/mL may, if on continuous oral antiviral treatment, and closely monitored by a consultant occupational health physician and a designated hepatologist, practise exposure-prone procedures, provided that their hepatitis B infection remains well controlled (i.e. HBV DNA level remains below 10^3 geq/mL).[96–98]

Healthcare workers in the United Kingdom who have hepatitis C (HCV) infection and who are HCV RNA positive must not perform exposure-prone procedures; successful antiviral treatment may permit a return to practice.[92] HIV-infected healthcare workers must not undertake exposure-prone procedures.[99] Recent guidance on health clearance in the United Kingdom recommends that all new and returning healthcare workers should routinely be offered hepatitis B vaccine (with post-vaccination testing of response) and testing for HCV and HIV infection. If the worker is to undertake exposure-prone procedures, the worker should be shown, by testing of an identified validated blood sample, to be non-infectious for HBV, HIV and HCV before the offer of appointment is confirmed.[98] The guidance also requires that healthcare workers who believe they might have been exposed to HIV or HCV (whether sexually, through injecting drug use or occupationally) promptly seek advice on whether they should be tested to confirm their status. National authorities in other European countries and the United States have made similar, though usually less prescriptive, recommendations. In the United Kingdom, recommendations on testing medical and dental students for blood-borne virus infections have recently been revised and are closely aligned to new health clearance guidance. They require post-admission testing of medical students, and pre-entry clearance of dental students, and set out the roles and responsibilities of the college, the occupational health service and the student. They also make it clear that being infected with a blood-borne virus is not, of itself, a barrier to medical school entry or to medical registration.[100]

It is recommended in the United Kingdom that, where there is evidence of HIV transmission from a healthcare worker to a patient, all patients on whom the worker has undertaken exposure-prone procedures should be contacted and offered testing to confirm that they have not acquired HIV infection from the healthcare worker. In the absence of evidence of transmission, the decision on whether to undertake a 'look-back exercise' should be considered on a case-by-case basis.[99] Recommendations on HCV are similar.[92]

More general issues about fitness to work may arise in HIV-infected healthcare workers and other people in jobs of high responsibility. These include concerns about their risk of acquiring infection if they become immunocompromised and about the effects of the neurological complications of HIV infection. The infection in most people, including healthcare workers, will have been acquired non-occupationally. The issues about HIV infection and fitness to work are considered in detail elsewhere.[101]

If a healthcare worker is found to be infected with a blood-borne virus, it is important to establish whether the infection is likely to be occupational, since they are eligible for certain benefits if this is the case. In the United Kingdom, since hepatitis B and hepatitis C are prescribed industrial diseases, all that is needed is to show that the person is infected and that their work involves (or has involved) exposure to potentially infected blood, whether in the clinical setting or the laboratory. HIV infection is not a prescribed industrial disease, but infected workers in the UK may be eligible for National Health Service Injuries Benefit if it can be shown that their infection is likely to be occupational in origin. For all blood-borne viruses, the most obvious way to demonstrate an occupational origin is to show seroconversion following an occupational exposure incident.

PREVENTION OF INFECTION WITH BLOOD-BORNE VIRUSES

Prevention rests mainly on reduction of the risk of exposure to blood or other infected body fluids. The most important risk is percutaneous exposure to blood, so reducing the use of sharp instruments, developing safer techniques and types of equipment, and making proper use of suitable containers and systems for disposal of used needles and sharp instruments are important.[102] Advances in the last decade include the widespread adoption of standard infection control precautions (formerly 'universal precautions'), the introduction of safety-engineered intravenous cannulae and phlebotomy devices, which have been shown to reduce needlestick injury rates,[103–105] and, in the United States, legislation that makes provision of safety-engineered devices to healthcare workers mandatory. Together, these have resulted in a decline in hollow-bore needle injury rates, most marked for the injuries that present the greatest risk.[85] In the United Kingdom, the Health and Social Care Act 2008 requires that NHS trusts consider making 'provision of medical devices that incorporate sharps protection mechanisms where there are clear indications that they will provide safe systems of working for healthcare workers' in order to demonstrate compliance, but it is not clear to what extent this requirement has been implemented.[106]

In the laboratory setting, the use of sharp instruments or equipment can be virtually eliminated. Suitable personal protective equipment (PPE) and safe laboratory practice prevents exposure of broken skin and the mucosae of the eyes and mouth.

However, not all occupational blood-exposure incidents are preventable and some will occur even where preventive measures have been well implemented. Other preventive strategies are available. For hepatitis B, the most infectious of the agents, there is fortunately an effective and safe vaccine. Immunization of all healthcare workers who may have contact with blood and body fluids is recommended. Vaccines against hepatitis C and HIV have not yet been developed.

Around 90 per cent of young, fit healthcare workers produce an adequate anti-HBs response to hepatitis B vaccine. Response rates are lower in males, smokers, older people and those who are immunosuppressed. Response rates are also lower when vaccine is given intradermally (rather than intramuscularly), or given intramuscularly into the gluteal muscles rather than the deltoid. True vaccine failure is rare.[107] Apparent non-responders (no or low level anti-HBs response) should be tested for evidence of HBV infection. True non-responders, with no evidence of previous HBV infection, should be informed they are not protected and strongly advised to report any occupational exposures to blood. Non-response to vaccine should not be considered a bar to employment as a healthcare worker in any capacity. Although a quarter of a century has passed since hepatitis B vaccine first became available, there are still reports of under-vaccination of healthcare workers at risk: a study of transplant surgeons in the United States in 2003 found that a fifth (70/311) of respondents were inadequately vaccinated, and that surgeons under-estimated the risks of having a percutaneous exposure while operating, and of becoming infected if exposed; the authors suggest that the most expedient way to ensure protection is to require documented evidence of vaccination and testing for all staff at risk.[108]

Once an exposure to infected blood has occurred, other measures can reduce the risk of infection in the worker. For hepatitis B, active immunization with the vaccine, using an accelerated course in those not previously immunized, is recommended. Passive protection may also be provided using hepatitis B immune globulin (HBIG). However, HBIG gives incomplete protection and should be given in conjunction with the first dose or booster dose of vaccine; in workers who have failed to respond to the vaccine, it is the only protection available. For hepatitis C, no effective post-exposure prophylaxis is available at present, but follow up to six months is recommended to check that transmission has not occurred.[92,109]

For HIV, recommendations about post-exposure prophylaxis (PEP) have recently been revised in the United Kingdom[110] and in the United States.[111] A retrospective case–control study suggests that the use of prophylactic zidovudine is associated with a reduced risk of HIV seroconversion after percutaneous (needlestick) exposure to HIV-infected blood.[82] By extrapolation from the effectiveness of combined antiretroviral therapy in established infection, and in preventing mother-to-child HIV transmission, current guidelines on PEP now recommend routine use of three antiretroviral drugs in the United Kingdom (or two, sometimes three in the United States) for four weeks after a significant occupational exposure to HIV. The recommended three drugs for PEP in the UK and USA are zidovudine, lamivudine and indinavir, with modification of this regime if the source patient is believed to have infection resistant to any of these drugs. The prophylaxis should be started as soon as possible after the exposure and preferably within one hour. The effectiveness of this regime in reducing the rate of seroconversion (in any case small) is unknown, and seroconversion despite prompt prophylaxis has been reported. A significant proportion of those given PEP will experience side effects, which may be severe enough to require time off work. Although higher adverse event rates are reported among those given a three-drug regime, the discontinuation rates for three-drug regimes are similar to those for two-drug regimes.[112]

Initiation of suitable post-exposure prophylaxis depends upon knowledge of the worker's immunity (for hepatitis B) and the source patient's infection status. Post-exposure testing of source patients for blood-borne virus infection is therefore important. Patients should be tested only with their consent and with appropriate pre-test discussion. If approached sensitively, few patients will refuse testing. If immediate testing is not feasible, or the patient refuses testing, but there is a strong suspicion of infection, for example with HIV, then PEP should be considered.

Healthcare workers who have been involved in blood-exposure incidents, especially when the source patient is known to be infected with a blood-borne virus, are understandably anxious and may become extremely anxious; post-traumatic stress syndrome has been reported.[113] They should have access to timely, sympathetic and knowledgeable advice from an experienced designated physician (the occupational physician often takes on this responsibility). Giving accurate information and providing immediate and ongoing support is an important, though not always recognized, part of the management of blood exposures at work.

Other workers may have occasional contact with blood or contaminated sharp instruments, for example emergency care workers, refuse workers, police and prison officers. These workers should be trained to take appropriate precautions to reduce the risk of exposure to blood (especially sharps injuries) and should know how to obtain immediate post-exposure care. The need to offer them routine pre-exposure hepatitis B immunization is less clear-cut, although this may be appropriate for selected subgroups. Arrangements should be made for them to have access to expert advice, and treatment if necessary, if they are involved in a blood-exposure incident.

Other viruses as occupational risks for healthcare workers

VIRAL HAEMORRHAGIC FEVERS

Viral haemorrhagic fevers, caused by a range of viruses (from the arenavirus, flavivirus, filovirus and bunyavirus families), are severe and potentially life-threatening diseases. They are endemic in Africa, parts of South America, and in rural Eastern Europe and the Middle East. Cases in the United Kingdom are very rare and virtually always imported, but laboratory-acquired infection has been reported.

The infections are transmitted to humans by mosquito bite (yellow fever, dengue, Rift valley fever, Chikungunya); tick bite (Omsk haemorrhagic fever, Kyanasur Forest disease, Crimean Congo haemorrhagic fever (CCHF)); or through contact with virus excreted by infected rodents or other animal reservoir (the arenaviruses, including Lassa virus; Hantaan virus); the geographic distribution of the viruses matches that of any animal reservoir. However, only four of these infections are known to be readily capable of spreading from person to person and thus present a potential risk of transmission to healthcare workers: Lassa fever, CCHF, Marburg disease and Ebola haemorrhagic fever. A newly described arenavirus, presumptively termed Lujo virus, may also fit into this category: a safari booking agent, who had a possible history of a recent tick bite and contact with horses, was transferred by air from Zambia to South Africa with an undiagnosed, but clearly severe, illness in early October 2008 and died soon afterwards. Three fatal secondary cases occurred in healthcare workers (a paramedic who accompanied the transfer, an intensive care nurse and the worker responsible for terminal cleaning of the index case's hospital room); a tertiary case (a nurse) survived; all had potential for exposure to the index case's blood or body fluids.[114]

CCHF was first recognized in the USSR in 1944, and the virus isolated from the patients was subsequently shown to be identical to that isolated in 1956 from a sick child in Zaire. The virus is now known to be widely spread in Africa, Central Asia, southern Europe and parts of the Middle East, though there appear to be geographical variations in virulence, the disease being more severe in Asia than in Africa.[115] Lassa fever was first described in 1969 after three missionary nurses working in Lassa in north eastern Nigeria became seriously ill with an unknown infection, from which two died. The third nurse, who had cared for the other two, was flown to North America for treatment, and a new arenavirus was isolated from her serum, and subsequently from similar cases in Nigeria, and named Lassa virus.

Marburg virus takes its name from an outbreak of haemorrhagic fever among laboratory workers in Marburg, Germany in 1967. Workers in laboratories in Frankfurt and Belgrade also became infected. All 25 with primary infections had been in contact with organs, blood or cell cultures from a batch of wild-caught African green monkeys from Uganda; six secondary cases occurred amongst those who had contact with infected patients' blood. Small numbers of cases have since occurred in South Africa, Zimbabwe, Kenya and Uganda; large outbreaks, amplified by nosocomial transmission, occurred in the Democratic Republic of the Congo (formerly Zaire) in 1998–2000, and in Uige province, Angola in 2004–2005. Ebola haemorrhagic fever was recognized in 1976, when outbreaks of a new haemorrhagic fever, with a high case fatality rate and considerable secondary spread through blood contact, occurred simultaneously in Zaire and in the Sudan. Five ebolavirus species have so far been recognized: *Zaire ebolavirus*, *Sudan ebolavirus*, *Reston ebolavirus*, *Cote d'Ivoire ebolavirus* and, most recently, in an outbreak in Uganda in 2007–2008, *Bundibugyo ebolavirus*.[116,117] Outbreaks have occurred in Gabon, Sudan, the Democratic Republic of the Congo, and the Republic of the Congo. *Cote d' Ivoire ebolavirus* was isolated from a zoologist working in the country who became accidentally infected while doing a post-mortem on a chimpanzee found dead in the wild. *Reston ebolavirus* was first isolated from batches of cynomolgus macaques imported to the United States and Italy from the Philippines, and has since also been isolated from domestic pigs in the Philippines. An animal caretaker in the Reston primate facility became viraemic after a virus-contaminated scalpel injury, and he and three other asymptomatic workers had serological evidence of infection. Antibody has also been detected in workers in primate-supply facilities in the Philippines and, more recently, in pig farmers, but human illness associated with this ebolavirus species has not been reported.[118]

The clinical illnesses are characterized by fever, haemorrhage and collapse, although serosurveys have suggested that subclinical and mild infections also occur. For Lassa fever, reported mortality rates range from 3 per cent (in a community outbreak) to 66 per cent (in hospitalized cases). Lassa fever tends to have a more insidious onset than Marburg or Ebola disease and can therefore be difficult to diagnose. The differential diagnosis of a fever in a patient who has been in rural West Africa within the previous three weeks includes Lassa fever, typhoid fever and malaria. In Lassa fever, there is usually fever and headache followed by pharyngitis, abdominal tenderness, sometimes with vomiting and diarrhoea, and evidence of pleural effusion. There may be little or no evidence of haemorrhage other than some bleeding of the gums. Severe haemorrhage is unusual in Lassa fever, but more common in Marburg or Ebola disease. Treatment is largely a question of providing intensive supportive care; antiviral drugs (specifically, ribavirin) reduce the mortality of Lassa fever, if started early, and may also be helpful in CCHF, but have not been shown to influence the course of either Marburg or Ebola disease.

The viral haemorrhagic fevers pose a significant risk of infection to healthcare workers caring for cases, laboratory workers handling specimens from them, and to research laboratory workers. The main risk in the healthcare setting is direct contact with infected blood (for example, by needlestick injury or contamination of broken skin or mucous membranes). In the ebolavirus epidemic in the Sudan in 1979, it was reported that staff providing direct clinical care for ill patients had a five times higher risk of contracting infection than staff with less physical contact with the patients, and there were no cases of infection in staff who entered the room but had no physical contact.[119] UK guidelines on management and control of viral haemorrhagic fevers[115] advise that patients returning from abroad with a fever should be categorized on the basis of a risk assessment that covers: area visited, clinical features and time of onset in relation to travel, household or occupational contact with known or suspected cases, or contact with potentially infected blood or body fluids. Any patient known or suspected to be suffering from a viral haemorrhagic fever, or in whom the diagnosis cannot immediately be excluded, should be urgently discussed with a senior infectious disease clinician working in a specially designated high security infectious disease unit. Nearly all suspected cases will in fact have malaria. The guidelines also cover the special precautions needed to obtain, transport and examine laboratory specimens from a patient with a suspected viral haemorrhagic fever and the management of patients' contacts. The first investigation should always be to confirm or refute a diagnosis of malaria. If there is doubt, empirical treatment for malaria should be instituted.

SARS CORONAVIRUS

In 2002, a new infection, severe acute respiratory syndrome (SARS) emerged in Guandong province, China. Rapid person-to-person spread of virus caused outbreaks in Hong Kong SAR, Vietnam, Singapore and Canada in 2003, with more than 8000 cases in more than 30 countries.[120] Transmission was amplified within hospitals, as early cases were cared for without effective routine infection control measures; 22 per cent of SARS cases in Hong Kong and nearly half (43 per cent) of SARS cases in Toronto and Singapore (41 per cent) occurred in healthcare workers. Further cases in Singapore, Taiwan and China in late 2003 and 2004 were associated with laboratory-acquired infections.[121,122] Overall, 20 per cent of hospitalized patients required mechanical ventilation and 15 per cent of hospitalized cases died. Mortality was greater in the elderly and in those with co-morbidity. The usual incubation period is three to five days (range, two to ten days). Clinical features include fever, chills, rigors, malaise and myalgia, sometimes accompanied by diarrhoea, followed two to four days later by a non-productive cough, dyspnoea and pneumonia, with progression to respiratory failure in severe cases.[123] However, there is a spectrum of disease, and many cases are mild and will not require hospital admission. Antiviral drugs (e.g. ribavirin) or other drugs, such as steroids, have not been shown to be effective; treatment is essentially supportive. Asymptomatic contacts are not infectious; cases are non-infectious from ten days after resolution of fever. SARS coronavirus, although a newly emergent virus, is transmitted from person to person in the same way as more common respiratory infections, mainly by respiratory droplet spread and direct contact, and the SARS epidemic was controlled by the efficient application of long-recognized public health control measures: rapid identification and early isolation of cases, and stringent adherence to infection control precautions.[124] In a study of almost 800 critical care workers who had cared for patients needing intubation during the outbreak in Toronto, factors identified as being predictive of the consistent use of recommended barrier precautions included caring for a patient identified as a definite SARS case and having had recent or interactive training in infection control.[125] Of 17 healthcare workers from six centres in Toronto, who acquired SARS after infection control measures had been implemented, 15 were well enough to be interviewed in depth about their infection control practice; results suggested that risk factors for infection included the performance of high-risk patient care procedures (e.g. intubation, nebulizer therapy), inconsistent use of personal protective equipment, fatigue and lack of adequate infection control training.[126]

One of the effects of SARS has been to provoke renewed interest in infection control and prevention of transmission of respiratory infections, which has led to development of the concepts of 'cough etiquette'.[127] Healthcare staff who will predictably undertake aerosol-generating procedures (intubation and related procedures including manual ventilation and suctioning, bronchoscopy, cardiopulmonary resuscitation) shown to be associated with an increased risk of respiratory pathogen transmission, for which the use of a respirator (e.g. FFP3 respirator) is required, and those (e.g. nebulization, non-invasive positive pressure ventilation) where evidence on transmission is less clear-cut, but where the use of a respirator may nevertheless be prudent, should be fit-tested by the occupational health service and trained in the use of the selected respirator, including fit-checking and safe removal and disposal. Such staff might include intensivists, emergency care clinicians, critical care response teams, chest physicians, respiratory therapists, surgeons and post-mortem room staff. Disposable respirators may not be suitable for all staff (e.g. those who have beards), but alternatives, including reusable powered respirators and helmets, are available.[128,129]

SARS coronavirus may re-emerge: the virus is probably zoonotic (SARS-like coronaviruses have been identified in Chinese horseshoe bats, which may be the natural reservoir; masked palm civets were likely the intermediate host in the 2002–2003 epidemic).[130] Occupational health clinicians have an important role to play in surveillance and should remain alert to cases of severe atypical respiratory illness in healthcare workers, particularly if there is more than one case within a short time span, and need also to be prepared to provide ongoing psychosocial support for workers involved, directly or indirectly in an outbreak, particularly if mortality is high or the outbreak prolonged.

VARICELLA ZOSTER

Varicella zoster virus (VZV) causes chickenpox (primary infection) and shingles (reactivation of previous infection). Healthcare workers who are susceptible to VZV are vulnerable to contracting the infection from patients. Chickenpox in adults tends to be more severe than in children, but the major concern is that healthcare workers who have chickenpox (who will have been particularly infectious in the 48 hours preceding the onset of the characteristic rash) may transmit the virus to susceptible patients. Any healthcare worker with chickenpox should remain off work until there are no new lesions and the existing lesions have crusted and dried; those with shingles are also infectious and should similarly remain off work. Recent UK guidance recommends that staff who will have direct patient contact (including ambulance staff, cleaners and receptionists) in hospitals or the community and who do not have a definite history of chickenpox should be tested to determine their immune status.[131,132] More than half of UK healthcare workers give a history of chickenpox in childhood and have antibodies as a result, and antibodies are also detectable in most of those without a history of chickenpox: about 10 per cent of adults will be seronegative (i.e. have no detectable antibody to VZV). UK guidance also recommends that healthcare workers who were born and raised overseas should be serologically tested regardless of their clinical history. Non-immune workers should receive varicella zoster vaccine (two doses of live attenuated vaccine four to eight weeks apart); routine post-vaccination testing is not advised. Varicella vaccine is contraindicated in pregnancy and in the immunosuppressed. At the time of vaccination, healthcare workers should be told that they may develop a rash in the month after vaccination and that if this occurs they should be assessed by the occupational health service. Those who develop a generalized rash that is papular or vesicular should avoid all patient contact until the lesions have crusted or resolved. Non-immune healthcare workers who have a significant exposure to VZV should be offered vaccine if there are no contraindications; work exclusion (from day 8 to day 21 post-exposure) or occupational health surveillance for fever and rash is also necessary. Post-exposure management of susceptible healthcare workers who are immunosuppressed or pregnant requires consideration of the use of zoster immune globulin.

CYTOMEGALOVIRUS

Cytomegalovirus is found in many body tissues including blood, urine, breast milk, saliva and vaginal fluid. It is not vaccine-preventable. However, provided even the most basic infection control procedures are followed, any risk of transmission to healthcare workers from their patients is extremely small. Indeed, several studies have failed to show any excess of cytomegalovirus in healthcare workers with clinical contact compared with others with no clinical contact.[133] The most important consequence of cytomegalovirus in immunocompetent females is its potential to cause fetal damage if acquired in pregnancy.

MEASLES, MUMPS AND RUBELLA

Measles is a highly transmissible acute viral illness, characterized by a prodromal illness (fever, conjunctivitis, coryza or cough) followed by the development of an erythematous maculopapular rash which spreads over the body from the head downwards over three to four days. Koplik spots may be seen on the mucous membranes of the mouth 24–48 hours before the rash appears. Complications include diarrhoea, pneumonia, convulsions, encephalitis and subacute sclerosing panencephalitis. In the United Kingdom, it is estimated that 1 in 5000 cases is fatal. The case fatality-rate is age-related; disease tends to be more severe in infants and in teenagers and adults than young children, and is also more severe in the chronically ill, under-nourished or immunosuppressed.

Rubella infection in children (German measles) is usually a mild, self-limiting illness characterized by fever and a morbilliform rash. In adults, however, infection is more severe, with rash, fever, debility and prominent symptoms in small joints. Maternal infection in the first 16 weeks of pregnancy, particularly if in the first trimester, causes severe fetal damage. Healthcare workers are unlikely to be at increased risk of rubella, especially since many countries now vaccinate infants as well as adolescents against rubella. However, healthcare workers have been the source of rubella outbreaks.

Mumps is an acute viral infection caused by a paramyxovirus, with an incubation period of around 16 days (range, 12–25 days). It is characterized by a short prodromal illness (fever, headache, myalgia, anorexia) followed by bilateral or unilateral parotid swelling. Asymptomatic infection is common, particularly in children. Meningism occurs in 15 per cent of cases; other complications include orchitis (25 per cent of post-pubertal men), oophoritis (5 per cent of post-pubertal women), pancreatitis (4 per cent) and sensorineural deafness. The virus is spread by droplet and airborne transmission. Non-immune healthcare workers who have an unprotected exposure to the virus must be excluded from work from the 12th to the 25th day after exposure.

Measles, mumps and rubella (MMR) vaccine prevents all three of these infections; vaccination of healthcare workers is particularly important because they may transmit infection to vulnerable groups. Self-reported immune status may be inaccurate. In the United Kingdom, satisfactory evidence of protection is documentation of receipt of two doses of MMR vaccine or serological evidence of immunity to measles and rubella.[132]

PARVOVIRUS

Parvovirus B19 infection (which is not vaccine preventable) produces a febrile illness with a transient macular rash which may be mistaken for rubella. In adults, particularly females, it can cause arthropathy which is usually self-limiting. It can cause complications in people with haemoglobinopathies and those who are immunosuppressed, and fetal damage. There is no specific treatment. Diagnosis is made serologically. Outbreaks in healthcare settings may necessitate ward closures to interrupt transmission.[134]

HERPETIC WHITLOW OR PARONYCHIA

These lesions on the fingers are due to direct contact with herpes simplex virus and used to be quite a common problem in healthcare workers. Diagnosis is by culture of virus from the lesions, electron microscopy or immunofluorescence. Contact with the mouth area, such as in mouth care or dentistry, with ungloved hands seems to be the major risk, and infection is therefore preventable by adherence to standard infection control precautions.[135]

Other infectious risks for healthcare workers

TUBERCULOSIS

The clinical features of pulmonary tuberculosis include fever, weight loss, cough, malaise, sweats and haemoptysis. The diagnosis should be considered in any healthcare worker who presents with such symptoms and no other apparent cause. Radiographs may be normal in early infection or show a rather diffuse bronchopneumonia, but in more advanced cases there may be the more typical upper lobe pneumonia with cavitation. Healthcare workers in the United Kingdom remain at increased risk of tuberculosis (TB), where although TB incidence rates have stabilized, they remain at higher levels than in the 1980s.[136]

Guidelines in the United Kingdom cover the health clearance of new and transferring National Health Service workers, protection of workers against infection (including the use of BCG (bacillus Calmette-Guérin)) and safe working practices (Figure 59.1).[98,100,132,137] BCG is recommended for healthcare workers, whatever their age, who will have contact with patients or clinical material and who are not tuberculin skin test positive as a result of previous BCG immunization. BCG should not be used in HIV-infected workers; workers should be individually risk-assessed for HIV before BCG is given. Healthcare workers from high TB incidence countries, or who have worked in high TB prevalence settings who have a positive tuberculin test (or a positive interferon gamma test) should be referred to a chest clinic. Healthcare workers from low TB incidence countries, such as the United Kingdom, who are tuberculin test (or interferon gamma test) positive and have not previously had BCG should have a medical assessment and a chest x-ray, but should also be referred to a chest clinic for consideration of treatment of disease or latent infection. Healthcare workers who are found to be HIV positive during employment should have medical and occupational assessments of TB risk, and may need to be offered redeployment to reduce exposure. Guidance is also given on the management of

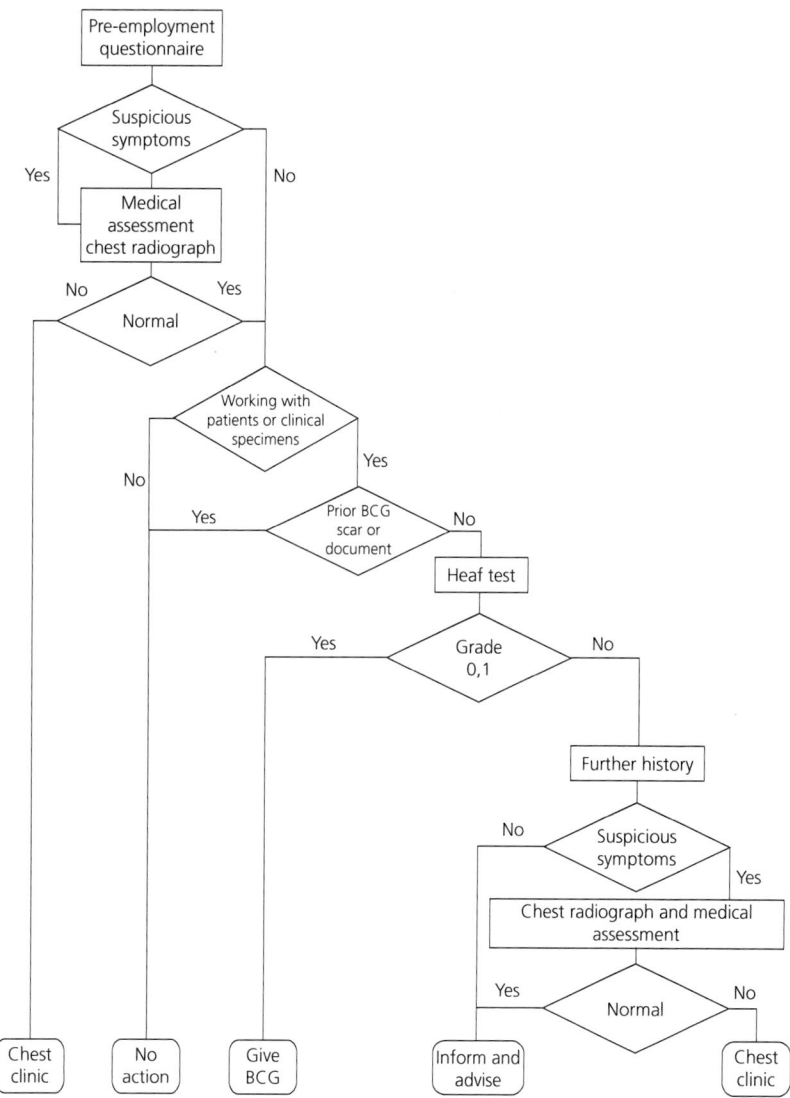

Figure 59.1 Screening of healthcare workers for tuberculosis. Reproduced with permission from Ref. 137.

healthcare workers who have a significant occupational exposure to TB, and of those who are infected with TB, regardless of source. Tuberculosis acquired through an occupation involving contact with sources of tuberculous material is a prescribed disease in the United Kingdom.

In the last 20 years, multidrug-resistant tuberculosis (MDR-TB) has become a problem. It remains uncommon in the United Kingdom, accounting for around 1 per cent of new isolates, but worldwide, about 20 per cent of isolates are multidrug resistant. MDR-TB strains are not more transmissible, or more virulent, but are considerably more difficult, and more costly, to treat. The more recently described extensively drug-resistant strains of *Mycobacterium tuberculosis*, which first emerged in South Africa against a background of high HIV prevalence, may not be treatable. Occupational transmission of MDR-TB to workers has been described.[138,139] HIV-infected workers and patients or those who are immunosuppressed for other reasons are at greater risk. In the United States, detailed guidelines for preventing transmission of *M. tuberculosis* in healthcare facilities were produced in response to several serious outbreaks of multidrug-resistant *M. tuberculosis* and, coupled with implementation of a national TB control strategy, have resulted in a reduction in TB incidence.[140] The guidelines, which were recently revised, include several levels of control: administrative controls to prevent exposing uninfected individuals to people who have infectious tuberculosis; then engineering controls to reduce spread of infectious droplet nuclei, such as local exhaust ventilation, air flow control and air filtration; and finally, the use of personal respiratory protective equipment in areas where there is still a risk of exposure to infection. The guidelines stress the need for early identification and treatment of patients with tuberculosis. Infection control guidelines for preventing the spread of tuberculosis in relation to HIV and multidrug-resistant tuberculosis have also been produced in the United Kingdom, designed to protect both patients and healthcare workers.[141,142]

SCABIES

This skin disease is caused by the mite *Sarcoptes scabei* and transmitted by close personal contact. The itchy rash characteristically presents on the finger webs, wrist and elbow flexures, and axillae but may sometimes present as a more widespread generalized dermatitis (Norwegian scabies). Linear burrows on the skin are present, but will not always be visible, particularly if hypersensitivity to mite antigen has developed. Nurses and other workers who provide physical care to patients are at risk. Cases are usually sporadic, but more extensive outbreaks have been described.[143] The use of gloves and gowns when handling patients who may have scabies is advisable. Treatment of the case and family members is with malathion or permethrin, which should be applied to the whole body from the neck down and left for 24 hours. Benzyl benzoate can also be used, but often causes irritation and may need to be applied on up to three consecutive days.

Occasionally, strains of mites from infected pets can also cause a highly pruritic papular urticarial rash. In this case, it is pet owners (and possibly veterinary surgeons) who are at risk, rather than healthcare workers.

STAPHYLOCOCCAL INFECTIONS

Healthcare workers can become colonized with meticillin-resistant *Staphylococcus aureus* (MRSA), carried in the nose, throat, axillae, perineum and on damaged skin. Such colonized workers pose a risk of transmitting to patients an infection which can be extremely difficult to treat and may be fatal in immunocompromised patients, including those who have undergone recent surgery. Even non-colonized healthcare workers can spread the infection between patients. Scrupulous attention to hand washing and to changing any barrier garments (gloves, aprons) between each patient is vital. Where a colonized worker has been detected as a result of an outbreak investigation, eradication of the organism may be attempted, but sometimes proves difficult to achieve. In rare cases, for example a cardiovascular surgeon or a nurse on the intensive care unit, failure to eradicate MRSA may, if there is evidence of continuing transmission to patients, mean that they require long-term redeployment.

In the United Kingdom, where reporting MRSA bacteraemia to the national surveillance system is a mandatory requirement, recent guidelines cover the prevention and management of MRSA in hospitals and other institutions.[144,145]

LABORATORY RESEARCH WORKERS AND ANIMAL HANDLERS

The infection risk to laboratory research workers will depend on the precise nature of the work in which they are engaged and the techniques applied. Risk assessments of individual processes are necessary under the COSHH (control of substances hazardous to health) regulations, and should result in the development, implementation and monitoring of safe standard operating procedures.

Workers should carry a medical contact card which gives details of their work and provides the name of the doctor who should be contacted if the worker develops an unexplained fever or other signs of infection. Workers seeking medical advice should tell the doctor about their work, as well as doctors asking their patients about their occupations.

Human immunodeficiency virus infection

At least three research laboratory workers worldwide have acquired HIV infection after exposure while working with concentrated HIV.[66,80] Workers should have the same access to post-exposure prophylaxis and care as described above for clinical healthcare workers.

Work with primates

Staff working with primates may be exposed to a number of infections, including herpes B virus, Marburg virus, *Reston ebolavirus*, monkeypox virus, rabies, tuberculosis, hepatitis A and enteric infections. Primates from reputable suppliers will, if wild caught, have been quarantined for six months and screened for these infections, although negative serological tests do not guarantee absence of infection. Primates for use in research which will involve human contact should, therefore, ideally have been bred in captivity and be herpes B virus seronegative. All primates should be regarded as potentially infective and handled with extreme care by trained staff. Suitable protective clothing should always be worn.

Infected animals shed herpes B virus from the oropharynx and genital tract; workers may acquire infection through bites or skin abrasions and subsequently develop a severe encephalomyelitis with a fatality rate of around 70 per cent. There is no evidence of asymptomatic infection in primate handlers. Guidelines have been published for the prevention and treatment of herpes B virus infections in exposed people. Wounds should be gently irrigated with soap and water or normal saline. Antibiotic prophylaxis against oropharyngeal bacteria (including anaerobes) should also be given for bites. Aciclovir may be given as prophylaxis after an exposure to a source known or potentially infected with herpes B virus, and should also be used to treat any worker with suspected infection.[146–148]

Work with vaccinia virus

A number of occupationally acquired infections with vaccinia virus have recently been reported in research workers; any worker who will be handling cultures or animals contaminated or infected with non-highly attenuated vaccinia virus or other orthopox viruses that infect humans should have vaccinia vaccine before any exposure.[149] If vaccine is contraindicated, redeployment may be necessary.

INFECTIONS ASSOCIATED WITH OCCUPATIONAL TRAVEL

The risk to travellers will depend on the countries visited, the proportion of time spent abroad, and working and living conditions while abroad. The most important hazard for occupational travellers is non-infectious: injury, particularly in road traffic accidents, is common and may often be fatal. There is good evidence that risk-taking behaviour abroad may differ from that at home; travellers should be counselled that unprotected sexual intercourse poses a clear risk of HIV and other infections and should be avoided.

Malaria

Malaria is a major infectious risk for travellers. Around 2000 cases are imported into the United Kingdom each year, of which rather more than half are due to *Plasmodium falciparum*, which is the most serious of the four species of malaria parasite which cause disease in man, and is potentially fatal. *P. vivax*, *P. ovale* and *P. malariae* are less likely to cause life-threatening illness. Most malaria infections will have been acquired through being bitten by an infected mosquito, but transfusion-acquired infection, transplacental transmission and acquisition through needlestick exposure to infected blood are also well recognized. Prevention requires risk recognition; travellers should be encouraged to take measures to avoid being bitten by mosquitoes (appropriate clothing, insect repellents (used directly on the skin or impregnated in wrist or ankle bands), insecticide-treated mosquito nets and insecticide sprays). They should comply with an appropriate chemoprophylactic regimen, but should understand that there is no chemoprophylactic regime which is 100 per cent effective. In choosing a regime, the risk of adverse reactions to any drug must be balanced against the risk of acquisition of disease.[150] Guidelines for the prevention of malaria in travellers from the United Kingdom have recently been revised,[151] and are regularly reviewed and updated. These contain up-to-date information about recommended chemoprophylaxis regimes by geographical area, and advice on the use of regimes for emergency self-treatment. The drugs most commonly used currently for prophylaxis include chloroquine, proguanil and mefloquine. Specialist advice should be sought on prophylaxis for people who will be sent on long-term postings, or who intend to live in a malaria-endemic area.

The incubation period for malaria varies depending on the species. Malaria due to *P. falciparum* usually presents either in the endemic area or within two months of leaving and typically 9–14 days after a bite from an infected mosquito. Malaria due to other species, particularly *P. vivax*, can take up to 12 months to present. Symptoms, especially in the early stages, are non-specific and include fever, headache, malaise and myalgia. The classically described fevers of specific periodicity associated with different species of malaria parasite are in practice rarely useful in diagnosis. It is important to have a high index of suspicion of malaria in anyone with an unexplained fever who has been in an endemic area. Particularly for falciparum malaria, sudden and catastrophic deterioration in clinical condition may occur; deaths can and do result. Complications of malaria include pulmonary oedema, coma, fits, hypoglycaemia, anaemia, renal failure and abortion.[152] Widespread haemolysis can lead to haemoglobinuria, so called 'black water fever'. Falciparum malaria should be treated as a medical emergency. The diagnosis of malaria is made by identification of the parasite in thick blood films; specialist help may be needed for interpretation. A single negative film does not exclude the diagnosis, particularly in a first episode of malaria when severe symptoms can occur with a low parasitaemia, and empirical treatment against *P. falciparum* may be appropriate.

The treatment regime depends on the known or suspected species of parasite and its likely sensitivities (depending on area of origin) as well as the severity of the clinical illness.[153] Expert advice should be sought about the appropriate treatment regime in each case. Chloroquine-resistant *P. falciparum* is now so widespread that choroquine should no longer be used for the treatment of falciparum malaria in the United Kingdom, although it remains the drug of choice for *P. malariae* and *P. ovale* and uncomplicated *P. vivax* infections. Additional treatment with primaquine is needed for infection with *P. vivax* and *P. ovale* to eradicate the hypnozoite stage of the parasite in the liver and prevent relapse. If this is not done, there is a risk of late relapse, which may occur years after the primary infection. Oral treatment can be used unless the patient is severely ill, confused or unconscious. Supportive care is an integral part of management and may include fluid replacement, management of fits, control of blood glucose, ventilation and renal dialysis.

Traveller's diarrhoea

In developed countries, *Campylobacter* sp. and salmonellae are the most common causes of infective diarrhoea. However, enterotoxin-producing strains of *Escherichia coli* (ETEC) are the most common cause of diarrhoea in travellers to less developed countries, where other infections which have a human, rather than an animal, reservoir are also more likely to be acquired. Diarrhoea caused by ETEC, shigellae and *Giardia lamblia*, although unlikely to be life threatening, may cause considerable morbidity, misery and loss of efficiency.

PREVENTION

In theory, travellers' diarrhoea is wholly preventable if simple precautions are followed faithfully. These include eating only thoroughly cooked food freshly prepared; washing and peeling all fruit; avoidance of salads, shellfish, unpasteurized milk or milk products, and tap water (including ice in drinks). In practice, it may be difficult to follow this advice to the letter, especially for those who have little control over catering arrangements (e.g. delegates at an international conference). Some clinicians would advocate antibiotic chemoprophylaxis, which has also been shown to reduce the incidence of travellers' diarrhoea. However, although this approach might perhaps be justifiable in people who are susceptible to infection or who suffer from inflammatory bowel disease, it cannot be generally endorsed, since it may increase susceptibility to infection with a resistant pathogen, will be ineffective against viral or parasitic causes of travellers' diarrhoea, and may engender a false sense of security. Bismuth subsalicylate has also been shown to reduce the incidence of traveller's diarrhoea and could be considered as an adjunct provided there are no contraindications.

MANAGEMENT

Most cases of travellers' diarrhoea occur while the traveller is abroad, are self-limiting (90 per cent resolve within a week) and are never investigated. Travellers can treat themselves effectively. They should be instructed on how to replace lost fluids using a suitable oral rehydration solution (proprietary packs are available). It is, of course, essential to make up the solution using clean water. Short-term use of a simple anti-diarrhoeal agent (such as loperamide) may be helpful in limiting symptoms, but should not be used by patients with fever or bloody diarrhoea, and has been associated with adverse events, including toxic megacolon and severe sepsis. Where fever persists for more than 48 hours, or diarrhoea is severe, self-treatment with short course antibiotic therapy could be started. Appropriate agents would be ciprofloxacin or other fluoroquinolone (doxycycline or trimethoprim are no longer recommended because of the high level of drug resistance); bismuth subsalicylate can also be used in treatment.

Travellers who have bloody diarrhoea should seek medical advice. Causes include *Entamoeba histolytica*, which may cause liver abscess, and is usually treated with metronidazole.[154]

Diarrhoeal symptoms that persist despite simple measures require further investigation, including stool microscopy and culture. Blood cultures are appropriate in febrile patients. Symptoms beginning more than a week after travel or which persist for more than ten days suggest the possibility of *Giardia lamblia* infection. This infection may become chronic and cause malabsorption. Diagnosis is usually by stool microscopy, but this may be negative in chronic cases. Treatment is with metronidazole or tinidazole.

Food handlers who have suffered traveller's diarrhoea following a trip abroad should consult their occupational health department before returning to work.

Hepatitis A

Hepatitis A virus (HAV) is transmitted by the faeco-oral route, through close contact with an infected person or through contaminated food (particularly bivalve molluscs) or water. Travel to countries of high or intermediate endemicity is a well-recognized risk for infection. Other potential occupational risks include directly handling the virus in the laboratory, direct contact with untreated sewage and direct contact with faeces of infected patients. In the United Kingdom, where the numbers of cases reported annually have been declining for a decade, recent outbreaks have occurred amongst men who have sex with men, injecting drug users and the homeless.[132] After an incubation period of two to six weeks, symptoms of fever, anorexia, nausea, abdominal pain, pale stools, dark urine and jaundice develop. Disease severity is age-related; 70–80 per cent of adults will develop jaundice, but young children are usually asymptomatic or have non-specific symptoms of viral illness. Viral excretion is at a maximum towards the end of the prodromal period, in the 48 hours before the onset of jaundice. Hepatitis A infection cannot be distinguished from other causes of viral hepatitis by clinical examination alone; diagnosis is made by testing for specific IgM antibody to HAV. The infection is usually self-limiting. There is no carrier state, but full recovery may take three to six months. Treatment is largely supportive. The mortality rate is below 0.1 per cent overall, but somewhat higher in those aged 45 years or over, and in those with pre-existing liver disease.

An inactivated hepatitis A vaccine is available, either as a monovalent vaccine or combined with either hepatitis B vaccine or typhoid vaccine. Passive prophylaxis, with human normal immunoglobulin (containing antibody to HAV) can provide immediate protection against infection for up to three months, but is no longer recommended for travellers, though it is still used, alone or in combination with vaccine, for post-exposure protection of contacts of a case and in outbreak control. Hepatitis A vaccine is recommended for those aged one year and over, travelling to countries of high or moderate endemicity for prolonged periods, and those who are posted to or will reside in, hepatitis A endemic countries. Vaccine may also be useful for those likely to make frequent short trips to endemic areas. Vaccine is also recommended for patients with chronic liver disease and for those with lifestyle risks for infection.

OTHERS

Sex workers

Sex workers are clearly at risk of a variety of sexually transmitted infections and, if their transactions involve sex for drugs rather than money, may also be at risk of infective conditions associated with injecting drug use, including hepatitis C, abscesses, endocarditis and severe clostridial infection. The risks of sexually transmitted infection may be reduced by the use of condoms, although this may be difficult to negotiate with clients.

Sex workers in the United Kingdom with local symptoms of a sexually transmitted infection will usually present to a genitourinary medicine clinic for treatment, where investigations for the full range of infections, including HIV, syphilis, gonorrhoea and hepatitis B should be undertaken. Those who present to other services may be less likely to disclose their occupation.

Sewage workers

There is evidence that sewage workers are at increased risk of enteric infections, including hepatitis A.[155,156] They are also at risk of leptospirosis (Weil's disease) (see Chapter 60, Zoonoses). The risks are mainly confined to those who come into contact with raw sewage[157] and can be reduced by the use of protective clothing. Hepatitis A immunization is recommended for higher risk subgroups, such as those with more frequent contact with raw sewage.

Archaeologists

Smallpox was officially declared to have been globally eradicated in 1980, but there is concern that viable virus could survive in corpses buried in permafrost or in cool dry crypts.[158] Other viruses, including strains of influenza from previous pandemics, may also be able to survive in similar circumstances. Expert advice about the risks and about protective equipment should be taken before corpses are exhumed.

Key points

- Many infections can be transmitted by occupational exposure, but a relatively small number pose a significant risk.
- Healthcare workers are at particular risk, but occupational infections also occur in a wide range of other occupational groups.
- Knowledge of the worker's occupation may provide a key clue to the diagnosis of an infection.
- Many occupational infections are preventable if measures to prevent or reduce exposure are implemented.
- Where a safe and effective vaccine is available, it should be offered to at-risk workers.

REFERENCES

1. Health and Safety Commission. Biological agents ACOP (control of biological agents): Control of substances hazardous to health regulations. London: Health and Safety Executive, 1994.
2. Prüss-Ustün A, Rapiti E, Hutin Y. Estimation of the global burden of disease attributable to contaminated sharps injuries among health-care workers. *American Journal of Industrial Medicine.* 2005; **48**: 482-90.
3. UK Benefits Agency. If you have an industrial disease: Industrial injuries disablement benefit (NI 2, August 1989, revised October 1991). London: HMSO, 1991.
4. West DJ. The risk of hepatitis B infection among health professionals in the United States: A review. *American Journal of Medical Science.* 1985; **287**: 26-33.
5. Iserson KV, Criss EA. Hepatitis B prevalence in emergency physicians. *Annals of Emergency Medicine.* 1985; **14**: 119-22.
6. McLean AA, Monahan GR, Finkelstein DM. Public health briefs: Prevalence of hepatitis B serologic markers in community hospital personnel. *American Journal of Public Health.* 1987; **77**: 998-9.
7. Hadler SC, Doto IL, Maynard JE et al. Occupational risk of hepatitis B infection in hospital workers. *Infection Control.* 1985; **6**: 24-31.
8. Reingold AL, Kane MA, Hightower AW. Failure of gloves and other protective devices to prevent transmission of hepatitis B virus to oral surgeons. *Journal of the American Medical Association.* 1988; **259**: 2558-60.
9. Petrosillo N, Puro V, Ippolito G and the Italian Study Group on Blood-Borne Occupational Risk in Dialysis. Prevalence of hepatitis C antibodies in health-care workers. *Lancet.* 1994; **344**: 255-6.
10. Struve J, Aronsson B, Frenning B et al. Prevalence of hepatitis B virus markers and exposure to occupational risks likely to be associated with acquisition of hepatitis B virus among healthcare workers in Stockholm. *Journal of Infection.* 1992; **24**: 147-56.
11. Panlilio AL, Shapiro CN, Schable CA et al. Serosurvey of human immunodeficiency virus, hepatitis B virus, and hepatitis C virus infection among hospital-based surgeons. *Journal of the American College of Surgeons.* 1995; **180**: 16-24.
12. Polakoff S, Tillett HE. Acute viral hepatitis B: Laboratory reports 1975-9. *British Medical Journal.* 1982; **284**: 1881-2.
13. Polakoff S. Acute viral hepatitis B: Laboratory reports 1980-4. *British Medical Journal.* 1986; **293**: 37-8.
14. Collins M, Heptonstall J. Occupational acquisition of acute hepatitis B infection by healthcare workers in England and Wales, 1985-93. *Communicable Disease Report. CDR Review.* 1994; **4**: R153-5.
15. Goldstein ST, Alter MJ, Williams IT et al. Incidence and risk factors for acute hepatitis B in the United States, 1982-1998: Implications for vaccination programs. *Journal of Infectious Diseases.* 2002; **185**: 713-19.
16. Mahoney FJ, Stewart K, Hu H et al. Progress toward the elimination of hepatitis B virus transmission among healthcare workers in the United States. *Archives of Internal Medicine.* 1997; **157**: 2601-5.
17. Lim DJ, Lingao A, Macasaet A. Sero-epidemiological study on hepatitis A and B virus infection among dentists in the Philippines. *International Dental Journal.* 1986; **36**: 215-18.

18. Kashiwagi S, Hayashi J, Ikematsu H *et al*. Prevalence of immunologic markers of hepatitis A and B infection in hospital personnel in Miyazaki Prefecture, Japan. *American Journal of Epidemiology*. 1985; **122**: 960–9.
19. Goldsmith RS, Zakaria S, Zakaria MS *et al*. Occupational exposure to hepatitis B virus in hospital personnel in Cairo, Egypt. *Acta Tropica*. 1989; **46**: 283–90.
20. Hakre S, Reyes L, Bryan JP, Cruess D. Prevalence of hepatitis B virus among healthcare workers in Belize, Central America. *American Journal of Tropical Medicine and Hygiene*. 1995; **53**: 118–22.
21. Belo AC. Prevalence of hepatitis B virus markers in surgeons in Lagos, Nigeria. *East African Medical Journal*. 2000; **77**: 283–5.
22. Turner SB, Kunches LM, Gordon KF *et al*. Public health briefs. Occupational exposure to human immunodeficiency virus (HIV) and hepatitis B virus among embalmers: A pilot seroprevalence study. *American Journal of Public Health*. 1989; **79**: 1425–6.
23. Remis RS, Rossignol MA, Kane MA. Hepatitis B infection in a day school for mentally retarded students: Transmission from students to staff. *American Journal of Public Health*. 1987; **77**: 1183–6.
24. Kunches LM, Craven DE, Werner BG, Jacobs LM. Hepatitis B exposure in emergency medical personnel: Prevalence of serologic markers and need for immunization. *American Journal of Medicine*. 1983; **75**: 269–72.
25. Pepe PE, Hollinger FB, Troisi CL, Heiberg D. Viral hepatitis risk in urban emergency medical services personnel. *Annals of Emergency Medicine*. 1986; **15**: 454–7.
26. Valenzuela TD, Hook EW, Copass MK, Corey L. Occupational exposure to hepatitis B in paramedics. *Archives of Internal Medicine*. 1985; **145**: 1976–7.
27. Morgan-Capner P, Wallice PDB. Hepatitis B markers in ambulance personnel in Lancashire. *Journal of the Society of Occupational Medicine*. 1990; **40**: 21–2.
28. Peterkin M, Crawford RJ. Hepatitis B vaccine for police forces? *Lancet*. 1986; **ii**: 1458–9.
29. Morgan-Capner P, Hudson P. Hepatitis B markers in Lancashire police officers. *Epidemiology and Infection*. 1988; **100**: 145–51.
30. Welch J, Tilzey AJ, Bertrand J *et al*. Risk to Metropolitan police officers from exposure to hepatitis B. *British Medical Journal*. 1988; **297**: 835–6.
31. Radvan GH, Hewson EG, Berenger S, Brookman DJ. The Newcastle hepatitis B outbreak: Observations on cause, management, and prevention. *Medical Journal of Australia*. 1986; **144**: 461–4.
32. Crosse BA, Teale C, Lees EM. Hepatitis B markers in West Yorkshire firemen. *Epidemiology and Infection*. 1989; **103**: 383–5.
33. Gerlich WH, Thomssen R. Outbreak of hepatitis B at a butcher's shop. *Deutsche Medizinische Wochenschrift*. 1982; **107**: 1627–30.
34. Mijch AM, Barnes R, Crowe SM *et al*. An outbreak of hepatitis B and D in butchers. *Scandinavian Journal of Infectious Diseases*. 1987; **19**: 179–84.
35. Dembert ML, A-Shaffer R, Baugh NL *et al*. Epidemiology of viral hepatitis among US navy and marine personnel, 1984–85. *American Journal of Public Health*. 1987; **77**: 1446–7.
36. Hyams KC, Palinkas LA, Burr RG. Viral hepatitis in the US navy, 1975–1984. *American Journal of Epidemiology*. 1989; **130**: 319–26.
37. Siebke JC, Wessel N, Kvandal P, Lie T. The prevalence of hepatitis A and B in Norwegian merchant seamen: A serological study. *Infection*. 1989; **17**: 77–80.
38. Cariani EA, Zonaro D, Primi E *et al*. Detection of HCV RNA and antibodies to HCV after needle stick injury. *Lancet*. 1991; **337**: 850.
39. Abb J. Prevalence of hepatitis C virus antibodies in hospital personnel. *International Journal of Medical Microbiology*. 1991; **274**: 543–7.
40. Jochen ABB. Occupationally acquired hepatitis C infection. *Lancet*. 1992; **339**: 304.
41. Klein RS, Freeman K, Taylor PE, Stevens CE. Occupational risk for hepatitis C virus infection among New York City dentists. *Lancet*. 1991; **338**: 1539–2.
42. Frider B, Sookoian S, Castano G *et al*. Prevalence of hepatitis C in healthcare workers investigated by 2nd generation enzyme-linked and line immunoassays. *Acta Gastroenterologica Latinoamericana*. 1994; **24**: 71–5.
43. Thomas DL, Factor SH, Kelen GD *et al*. Viral hepatitis in health care personnel at the Johns Hopkins Hospital. *Archives of Internal Medicine*. 1993; **153**: 1705–12.
44. Zuckerman J, Clewley G, Griffiths P, Cockcroft A. Prevalence of hepatitis C antibodies in clinical healthcare workers. *Lancet*. 1994; **343**: 1618–20.
45. Neal KR, Dornan J, Irving WL. Prevalence of hepatitis C antibodies among healthcare workers of two teaching hospitals: Who is at risk? *British Medical Journal*. 1997; **314**: 179–80.
46. Thomas DL, Gruninger SE, Siew C *et al*. Occupational risk of hepatitis C infections among general dentists and oral surgeons in North America. *American Journal of Medicine*. 1996; **100**: 41–5.
47. Puro V, Petrosillo N, Ippolito G *et al*. and the Italian Study Group on Occupational Risk of Bloodborne Infections. Occupational hepatitis C virus infection in Italian healthcare workers. *American Journal of Public Health*. 1995; **85**: 1272–5.
48. Shapiro CN, Tokars JI, Chamberland ME. Use of the hepatitis-B vaccine and infection with hepatitis B and C among orthopaedic surgeons. The American Academy of Orthopaedic Surgeons Serosurvey Study Committee. *Journal of Bone and Joint Surgery. American volume*. 1996; **78**: 1791–1800.
49. Tokars JI, Chamberland ME, Schable CA *et al*. A survey of occupational blood contact and HIV infection among orthopaedic surgeons. *Journal of the American Medical Association*. 1992; **268**: 489–94.
50. Chamberland ME, Petersen LR, Munn VP *et al*. Human immunodeficiency virus infection among healthcare

workers who donate blood. *Annals of Internal Medicine.* 1994; **121**: 269–73.
51. Lowenfels AB, Wormser GP, Jain R. Frequency of puncture injuries in surgeons and estimated risk of HIV infection. *Archives of Surgery.* 1989; **124**: 1284–16.
52. Hussain SA, Latif ABA, Choudhary AAAA. Risk to surgeons: A survey of accidental injuries during operations. *British Journal of Surgery.* 1988; **75**: 314–16.
53. Gerberding JL, Littell C, Tarkington A et al. Risk of exposure of surgical personnel to patients' blood during surgery at San Francisco General Hospital. *New England Journal of Medicine.* 1990; **322**: 1788–93.
54. Tokars J, Bell D, Marcus R et al. Percutaneous injuries during surgical procedures. Proceedings of the VII International Conference on AIDS, vol 2. Florence, Italy, 1991: 83.
55. Camilleri AE, Murray S, Imrie CW. Needlestick injuries in surgeons: What is the incidence? *Journal of the Royal College of Surgeons of Edinburgh.* 1991; **36**: 317–8.
56. Williams S. Variables associated with the risk of blood exposures in operating theatres. MD thesis, University of London, 1997.
57. Brough SJ, Hunt TM, Barrie WW. Surgical glove perforations. *British Journal of Surgery.* 1988; **75**: 317.
58. Camilleri AE, Murray S, Squair JL, Imrie CW. Epidemiology of sharps accidents in general surgery. *Journal of the Royal College of Surgeons of Edinburgh.* 1991; **36**: 314–16.
59. Wright JG, McGeer AJ, Chyatte D, Ransohoff DF. Mechanisms of glove tears and sharp injuries among surgical personnel. *Journal of the American Medical Association.* 1991; **266**: 1668–71.
60. Brearley S, Buist LJ. Blood splashes: An underestimated hazard to surgeons. *British Medical Journal.* 1989; **299**: 1315.
61. Porteous MJ, Le F. Operating practices of and precautions taken by orthopaedic surgeons to avoid infection with HIV and hepatitis B virus during surgery. *British Medical Journal.* 1990; **301**: 167–9.
62. Hinton AE, Herdman RC, Timms MS. Incidence and prevention of conjunctival contamination with blood during hazardous surgical procedures. *Annals of the Royal College of Surgeons of England.* 1991; **73**: 239–42.
63. Richmond PW, McCabe M, Davies JP, Thomas DM. Perforation of gloves in an accident and emergency department. *British Medical Journal.* 1992; **304**: 879–80.
64. Albertoni F, Ippolito G, Petrosillo N et al. Needlestick injury in hospital personnel: A multicenter survey from central Italy. *Infection Control and Hospital Epidemiology.* 1992; **13**: 540–4.
65. Collins CH, Kennedy DA. Microbiological hazards of occupational needlestick and 'sharps' injuries. *Journal of Applied Microbiology.* 1987; **62**: 385–402.
66. Metler R, Ciesielski C, Ward J, Marcus R. HIV seroconversions in clinical laboratory workers following occupational exposure, United States. VIIIth International Conference on AIDS, Amsterdam. July 1992: PoC 4147.
67. Beck-Sague CM, Jarvis WR, Fruehling JA et al. Universal precautions and mortuary practitioners: Influence on practices and risk of occupationally acquired infection. *Journal of Occupational Medicine.* 1991; **33**: 874–8.
68. Astbury C, Baxter PJ. Infection risks in hospital staff from blood: Hazardous injury rates and acceptance of hepatitis B immunization. *Journal of the Society of Occupational Medicine.* 1990; **40**: 92–3.
69. McGeer A, Sinor AE, Low DE. Epidemiology of needlestick injuries in house officers. *Journal of Infectious Diseases.* 1990; **162**: 961–4.
70. Williams S, Gooch C, Cockcroft A. Hepatitis B immunisation and blood exposure incidents amongst operating department staff. *British Journal of Surgery.* 1993; **80**: 714–16.
71. Hoofnagle JH, Seeff LB, Buskell Bales Z et al. Veterans Administration Study Group. Passive-active immunity from hepatitis B immunoglobulin. Re-analysis of a Veterans Administration Cooperative Study of needle-stick hepatitis. *Annals of Internal Medicine.* 1979; **91**: 813–18.
72. Grady GF, Lee VA, Prince AM et al. Hepatitis B immune globulin for accidental exposures among medical personnel: Final report of a multicenter controlled trial. *Journal of Infectious Diseases.* 1978; **138**: 625–38.
73. Werner BA, Grady GF. Accidental hepatitis B surface antigen positive inoculations. *Annals of Internal Medicine.* 1982; **97**: 367–9.
74. Reger A, Schiff ER. Clinical features of hepatitis. In: Thomas HC, Lemon SM, Zuckerman AJ (eds). *Viral hepatitis*, 3rd edn. Oxford: Blackwell Publishing, 2005: 33–49.
75. Kiyosawa K, Sodeyama T, Tanaka E et al. Hepatitis C in hospital employees with needlestick injuries. *Annals of Internal Medicine.* 1991; **115**: 367–9.
76. Mitsui T, Iwano K, Masuko K et al. Hepatitis C virus infection in medical personnel after needlestick accident. *Hepatology.* 1992; **16**: 1109–14.
77. Puro V, Petrosillo N, Ippolito G and the Italian Study Group on Occupational Risk of HIV and other Bloodborne Infections. Risk of hepatitis C seroconversion after occupational exposure in healthcare workers. *American Journal of Infection Control.* 1995; **23**: 273–7.
78. Hamid SS, Farooqui B, Rizvi Q et al. Risk of transmission and features of hepatitis C after needle stick injuries. *Infection Control and Hospital Epidemiology.* 1999; **20**: 63–4.
79. Henderson DK. Managing occupational risks for hepatitis C transmission in the health care setting. *Clinical Microbiology Reviews.* 2003; **16**: 546–68.
80. Ippolito G, Puro V, Heptonstall J et al. Occupational human immunodeficiency virus infection in health careworkers: Worldwide cases through September 1997. *Clinical Infectious Diseases.* 1999; **28**: 365–83.
81. UK Health Protection Agency Centre for Infections. Occupational transmission of HIV: Summary of published reports. March 2005 edition; data to December 2002. Last accessed June 19, 2009. Available from: www.hpa.org.uk/infections/topics_az/bbv/bbmenu.htm.

82. Cardo DM, Culver DH, Ciesielski CA et al. A case-control study of HIV seroconversion in healthcare workers after percutaneous exposure. *New England Journal of Medicine*. 1997; **337**: 1485–90.
83. Yazdanpanah Y, De Carli G, Migueres B et al. Risk factors for hepatitis C virus transmission to healthcare workers after occupational exposure: A European case-control study. *Clinical Infectious Diseases*. 2005; **41**: 1423–30.
84. Do AN, Ciesielski CA, Metler RP et al. Occupationally acquired human immunodeficiency virus (HIV) infection: National case surveillance data during 20 years of the HIV epidemic in the United States. *Infection Control and Hospital Epidemiology*. 2003; **24**: 86–96.
85. Jagger J. Caring for healthcare workers: A global perspective. *Infection Control and Hospital Epidemiology*. 2007; **28**: 1–4.
86. Heptonstall J. Outbreaks of hepatitis B virus infection associated with infected surgical staff. *Communicable Disease Report*. 1991; **1**: R81–R85.
87. The Incident Investigation Teams and others. Transmission of hepatitis B to patients from four infected surgeons without hepatitis B e antigen. *New England Journal of Medicine*. 1997; **336**: 178–84.
88. Esteban JI, Gomez J, Martell M et al. Transmission of hepatitis C virus by a cardiac surgeon. *New England Journal of Medicine*. 1996; **334**: 555–60.
89. Duckworth GJ, Heptonstall J, Aitken C for the Incident Control Team and others. Transmission of hepatitis C virus from a surgeon to a patient. *Communicable Disease and Public Health*. 1999; **2**: 188–92.
90. Ross RS, Viazov S, Roggendorf M. Phylogenic analysis indicates transmission of hepatitis C virus from an infected orthopaedic surgeon to a patient. *Journal of Medical Virology*. 2002; **66**: 461–7.
91. Ross RS, Viazov S, Thormahlen M et al. Risk of hepatitis C virus transmission from an infected gynecologist to patients: Results of a 7-year retrospective investigation. *Archives of Internal Medicine*. 2002; **162**: 805–10.
92. Department of Health. Implementing getting ahead of the curve: Action on bloodborne viruses. Hepatitis C-infected healthcare workers. London: Department of Health, 2002.
93. Ciesielski C, Marianos D, Ou C-Y et al. Transmission of human immunodeficiency virus in a dental practice. *Annals of Internal Medicine*. 1992; **116**: 798–805.
94. Lot F, Seguier JC, Fegueux S et al. Probable transmission of HIV from an orthopedic surgeon to a patient in France. *Annals of Internal Medicine*. 1999; **130**: 1–6.
95. Bosch X. Second case of doctor-to-patient HIV transmission. *Lancet Infectious Diseases*. 2003; **3**: 261.
96. Department of Health. Hepatitis B infected healthcare workers. Guidance on implementation of Health Service Circular 2000/020. London: Department of Health, 2000.
97. Department of Health. Hepatitis B infected healthcare workers and antiviral therapy. London: Department of Health, 2007.
98. Department of Health. Health clearance for tuberculosis, hepatitis B, hepatitis C, and HIV: New healthcare workers. London: Department of Health, 2007.
99. Department of Health. HIV infected healthcare workers: Guidance on management and patient notification. London: Department of Health, 2005.
100. The Medical Schools Council, the Council of Heads and Deans of Dental Schools, Association of UK University Hospitals, and the Higher Education Occupational Physicians Group. Medical and dental students: Health clearance for hepatitis B, hepatitis C, HIV and tuberculosis, February 2008. Last accessed June 22, 2009. Available from: www.chms.ac.uk/documents/BBVsGuidance Feb2008_000.pdf.
101. Cockroft A, Griffiths P. Acquired immune deficiency syndrome (AIDS). In: Cox RAF, Edwards FC, Palmer K (eds). *Fitness for work, the medical aspects*, 3rd edn. Oxford: Oxford University Press, 2000: 463–79.
102. UK Health Departments. Guidance for Clinical Healthcare workers: Protection against infection with blood-borne viruses. Recommendations of the Expert Advisory Group on AIDS and the Advisory Group on Hepatitis. London: UK Health Departments, 1998.
103. Lamontagne F, Abiteboul D, Lolom I et al. Role of safety-engineered devices in preventing needlestick injuries in 32 French hospitals. *Infection Control and Hospital Epidemiology*. 2007; **28**: 18–23.
104. Azar-Cavanagh M, Burdt P, Green-McKenzie J. Effect of the introduction of an engineered sharps injury prevention device on the percutaneous injury rate in healthcare workers. *Infection Control and Hospital Epidemiology*. 2007; **28**: 165–70.
105. Valls V, Lozano MS, Ya'nez R et al. Use of safety devices and the prevention of percutaneous injuries among healthcare workers. *Infection Control and Hospital Epidemiology*. 2007; **28**: 1352–60.
106. Department of Health. The Health and Social Care Act 2008. Code of practice for the NHS on the prevention and control of health care associated infection and related guidance. Department of Health, London, United Kingdom, January 2009. Last accessed June 23, 2009. Available from: www.dh.gov.uk/en/publicationsandstatistics/publications/publicationspolicyandguidance/DH_093762.
107. Boot HJ, van der Waaij LA, Schirm J et al. Acute hepatitis B in a health care worker: A case report of genuine vaccine failure. *Journal of Hepatology*. 2009; 50: 426–31.
108. Halpern SD, Asch DA, Shaked A et al. Inadequate hepatitis B vaccination and post-exposure evaluation among transplant surgeons. *Annals of Surgery*. 2006; **244**: 305–9.
109. Ramsey ME. Guidance on the investigation and management of occupational exposure to hepatitis C. *Communicable Disease and Public Health*. 1999; **2**: 258–62. Last accessed May 29, 2009. Available from: www.phls.co.uk/topics_az/hepatitis_c/HepCguidelines.pdf.
110. Department of Health. HIV post-exposure prophylaxis: Guidance from the UK Chief Medical Officers' Expert Advisory Group on AIDS. September 2008. London:

Department of Health, 2008. Last accessed June 24, 2009. Available from: www.dh.gov.uk/en/publications andstatistics/publications/publicationspolicyandguidance/DH_088185.
111. Centers for Disease Control and Prevention. Updated US public health service guidelines for the management of occupational exposures to HIV and recommendations for postexposure prophylaxis. *Morbidity and Mortality Weekly Reports.* 2005; **54**: RR-9.
112. Young T, Ahrens FJ, Kennedy GE *et al.* Antiretroviral post-exposure prophylaxis (PEP) for occupational HIV exposure. *Cochrane Database Systematic Reviews.* 2007; (1): CD002835.
113. Worthington MG, Ross JJ, Bergeron EK. Post traumatic stress disorder after occupational HIV exposure: Two cases and a literature review. *Infection Control and Hospital Epidemiology.* 2006; **27**: 215-17.
114. Briese T, Paweska JT, McMullan LK *et al.* Genetic detection and characterization of Lujo virus, a new hemorrhagic fever-associated arenavirus from southern Africa. *PLoS Pathogens.* 2009; last accessed June 24, 2009. Available from: www.plospathogens.org/article/info:doi/10.1371/journal.ppat.1000455. PMID: 19478873.
115. Advisory Committee on Dangerous Pathogens. Management and control of viral haemorrhagic fevers. London: HMSO, 1996.
116. Towner JS, Sealy TK, Khristova ML *et al.* Newly discovered ebola virus associated with hemorrhagic fever outbreak in Uganda. *PLoS Pathogens.* 2008; Last accessed June 24, 2009. Available from: www.plospathogens.org/article/info:doi/10.1371/journal.ppat.1000212.
117. Peters CJ. Marburg and Ebola-arming ourselves against the deadly filoviruses. *New England Journal of Medicine.* 2005; **352**: 2571-3.
118. World Health Organization. Ebola Reston found in domestic pigs in the Philippines. Available from: www.wpro.who.int/health_topics/ebola_reston/EbolaReston_FAQ.htm.
119. Baron RC, McCormick JB, Zubeir OA. Ebola virus dissemination in southern Sudan: Hospital dissemination and intrafamilial spread. *Bulletin of the World Health Organization.* 1983; **61**: 997.
120. World Health Organization. Summary of probable SARS cases with onset of illness from 1 November 2002 to 31 July 2003. Based on data as of 31 December 2003. Last accessed June 17, 2009. Available from: www.who.int/csr/sars/country/table2004_04_21/en/index.html.
121. Lim PL, Kurup A, Gopalakrishna G. Laboratory-acquired severe acute respiratory syndrome. *New England Journal of Medicine.* 2004; **350**: 1740-5.
122. World Health Organization. Severe acute respiratory syndrome (SARS) in Taiwan, China. December 17, 2003. Last accessed May 23, 2006. Available from: www.who.int/csr/don/2003_12_17/en/index.html.
123. Tsang K, Ho P, Ooi G *et al.* A cluster of cases of severe acute respiratory syndrome in Hong Kong. *New England Journal of Medicine.* 2003; **348**: 1977-85.
124. Svoboda T, Henry B, Shulman L *et al.* Public health measures to control the spread of severe acute respiratory syndrome during the outbreak in Toronto. *New England Journal of Medicine.* 2004; **350**: 2352-61.
125. Shigayeva A, Green K, Raboud JM *et al.* for the SARS Hospital Investigation Team. Factors associated with critical-care healthcare workers' adherence to recommended barrier precautions during the Toronto severe acute respiratory syndrome outbreak. *Infection Control and Hospital Epidemiology.* 2007; **28**: 1275-83.
126. Ofner-Agostini M, Gravel D, McDonald LC *et al.* Cluster of cases of severe acute respiratory syndrome among Toronto healthcare workers after implementation of infection control precautions: A case series. *Infection Control and Hospital Epidemiology.* 2006; **27**: 473-8.
127. Centers for Disease Control and Prevention. Respiratory hygiene/cough etiquette in healthcare settings. Last accessed May 23, 2009. Available from: www.cdc.gov/flu/professionals/infectioncontrol/resphygiene.htm.
128. World Health Organization. Infection prevention and control of epidemic- and pandemic-prone acute respiratory diseases in health care. WHO interim guidelines, June 2007. WHO/CDS/EPR/2007.6. Available from: www.who.int/csr/resources/publications/csrpublications/en/index7.html.
129. Department of Health. Pandemic influenza: Guidance for infection control in hospitals and primary care settings. November 2007. London: Department of Health, 2007.
130. Wang L-F, Shi Z, Zhang S *et al.* Review of bats and SARS. *Emerging Infectious Diseases.* 2006; 12: 1834-40. Last accessed June 24, 2009. Available from: www.cdc.gov/ncidod/EID/vol12no12/06-0401.htm.
131. Department of Health. Chickenpox (varicella) immunisation for healthcare workers PL/CMO/2003/8, PL/CNO/2003/9, PL/CDO/2003/1, PL/CPHO/2003/6. London: Department of Health. December 4, 2003.
132. Department of Health. Immunisation against infectious disease, 2006 edition. London: Department of Health, 2006. Available from: www.dh.gov.uk/en/Publichealth/Healthprotection/Immunisation/Greenbook/DH_4097254.
133. Geberding JL, Bryant-LeBlanc CE, Nelson K *et al.* Risk of transmitting the human immunodeficiency virus, cytomegalovirus, and hepatitis B virus to healthcare workers exposed to patients with AIDS and AIDS-related conditions. *Journal of Infectious Diseases.* 1987; **156**: 1-8.
134. Pillay D, Patou G, Hurt S *et al.* Parvovirus B19 outbreak in a children's ward. *Lancet.* 1992; **339**: 107-9.
135. Rosato FE, Rosato EF, Plotkin SA. Herpetic paronychia – An occupational hazard of medical personnel. *New England Journal of Medicine.* 1970; **283**: 804-5.
136. Meredith S, Watson JM, Citron KM *et al.* Are healthcare workers in England and Wales at increased risk of tuberculosis? *British Medical Journal.* 1996; **313**: 522-5.
137. Joint Tuberculosis Committee of the British Thoracic Society. Control and prevention of tuberculosis in the United Kingdom: Code of practice, 2000. *Thorax.* 2000; **55**: 887-901.

138. Beck-Sagu C, Dooley SW, Hutton MD et al. Outbreak of multidrug-resistant *Mycobacterium tuberculosis* infections in a hospital: Transmission to patients with HIV infection and staff. *Journal of the American Medical Association.* 1992; **268**: 1280–6.
139. Pearson ML, Jereb JA, Frieden TR et al. Nosocomial transmission of multidrug-resistant *Mycobacterium tuberculosis*: A risk to patients and healthcare workers. *Annals of Internal Medicine.* 1992; **117**: 257–8.
140. Centers for Disease Control and Prevention. Guidelines for preventing the transmission of *Mycobacterium tuberculosis* in health-care settings, 2005. *Morbidity and Mortality Weekly Reports.* 2005; **54**: 1–141.
141. The Interdepartmental Working Group on Tuberculosis. The prevention and control of tuberculosis in the United Kingdom: UK guidance on the prevention and control of transmission of 1. HIV-related tuberculosis 2. Drug-resistant, including multiple drug-resistant, tuberculosis. Department of Health, The Scottish Office, The Welsh Office, September 1998.
142. National Institute for Health and Clinical Excellence. Clinical diagnosis and management of tuberculosis, and measures for its prevention and control, 2006. Last accessed June 24, 2009. Available from: www.nice.org.uk/page.aspx?o=CG033&c=infections.
143. Barrett NJ, Morse DL. The resurgence of scabies. *Communicable Disease Report. CDR Review.* 1993; **3**: R32–34.
144. Gemmell CG, Edwards DI, Adam P et al. Guidelines for the prophylaxis and treatment of methicillin-resistant *Staphylococcus aureus* (MRSA) infections in the United Kingdom. *Journal of Antimicrobial Chemotherapy.* 2006; **57**: 589–608.
145. Coia E, Duckworth GJ, Edwards DI et al. Guidelines for the control and prevention of methicillin resistant *Staphylococcus aureus* (MRSA) in healthcare facilities. *Journal of Hospital Infection.* 2006; **66** (Suppl. 1): 1–44.
146. Holmes GP, Hilliard KJ, Kloutz KC et al. B virus (Herpes virus simiae) infection in humans: Epidemiologic investigations of a cluster. *Annals of Internal Medicine.* 1990; **112**: 833–9.
147. Holmes GP, Chapman LE, Stewart JA et al. Guidelines for the prevention and treatment of B-virus infections in exposed persons. The B virus Working Group. *Clinical Infectious Diseases.* 1995; **20**: 421–39.
148. Freifeld AG, Hilliard J, Southers J et al. A controlled seroprevalence survey or primate handlers for evidence of asymptomatic herpes B virus infection. *Journal of Infectious Diseases.* 1995; **171**: 1031–4.
149. Centers for Disease Control and Prevention. Laboratory-acquired vaccinia exposures and infections – USA 2005-2007. Morbidity and Mortality Weekly Report. 2008; **57**: 401–4.
150. Croft AMJ, Clayton TC, Gould MJ. Side effects of mefloquine prophylaxis for malaria: An independent randomised controlled trial. *Transactions of the Royal Society of Tropical Medicine and Hygiene.* 1997; **91**: 199–203.
151. Advisory Committee on Malaria Prevention in UK Travellers (ACMP). Guidelines for malaria prevention in travellers from the United Kingdom 2007. London: Health Protection Agency, 2007.
152. Warrell DA, Molyneux ME, Beales PF. Severe and complicated malaria. *Transactions of the Royal Society of Tropical Medicine and Hygiene.* 1990; **84** (Suppl. 2): 1–65.
153. Lalloo DG, Shingadia D, Pasvol G et al. (on behalf of the HPA Advisory Committee on Malaria Prevention in UK Travellers). UK malaria treatment guidelines. *Journal of Infection.* 2007; **54**: 111–21.
154. Knight R. Amoebiasis. In: Weatherall DJ, Ledingham JE, Warrel DA (eds). *Oxford textbook of medicine*, 3rd edn. Oxford: Oxford University Press, 1996: 825–35.
155. Chriske HW, Abdo R, Richrath R, Braumann S. Risk of hepatitis A infection among sewage workers. *Arbeitsmedizin, Sozialmedizin, Präventivmedizin.* 1990; **25**: 285–7.
156. Skinhoj P, Hollinger FB, Hovind-Hougen K et al. Infectious liver diseases in three groups of Copenhagen workers: Correlation of hepatitis A infection to sewage exposure. *Archives of Environmental Health.* 1981; **36**: 139–43.
157. Brugha R, Heptonstall J, Farrington P et al. Risk of hepatitis A infection in sewage workers. *Occupational and Environmental Medicine.* 1998; **55**: 567–9.
158. Baxter PJ, Brazier AM, Young SEJ. Is smallpox a hazard in church crypts. *British Journal of Industrial Medicine.* 1998; **45**: 359–60.

60

Zoonoses

ALASTAIR MILLER AND JULIA HEPTONSTALL

Introduction	750	Occupational zoonoses presenting with skin problems	762
Occupational zoonoses presenting as chest disease	751	Other important zoonotic infections	765
Occupational zoonoses presenting as fever	754	References	766
Occupational zoonoses presenting as gastrointestinal infection	759		

INTRODUCTION

The World Health Organization (WHO) defines zoonoses as diseases or infections that are transmitted naturally between vertebrate animals and man. Other authorities extend the definition to encompass infections that are transmitted only between human hosts by arthropod vectors, but this is a less common use of the term. In some circumstances, man is a dead-end host and in others he may transmit onwards to other animals or humans. A 2001 review concluded that 75 per cent of emerging pathogens and 61 per cent of all infectious organisms are zoonotic.[1]

Important recent examples include the emergence of novel influenza virus H1N1 in Mexico and the United States in 2009, with rapid evolution into a global pandemic, the severe acute respiratory syndrome (SARS) epidemic in 2002–2003, and the introduction of monkeypox into the United States from Africa in 2003.[2–4]

Zoonotic infections encompass the whole range of infective agents, including bacteria, rickettsia, viruses, fungi, protozoa and helminths. In addition to occupational exposure to zoonoses, humans can be infected by recreational exposure, keeping of pets, overseas travel, and ingestion of animal products. Many routes of infection are possible, including respiratory spread, gastrointestinal acquisition, percutaneous exposure by animal bite and spread by insect vector. Some zoonotic infections having initially been acquired from an animal source are then capable of human-to-human transmission and in these situations human health workers can be at risk through occupational exposure.

A large variety of occupational settings may expose man to the risks of infections transmitted from animals. Key areas are detailed in Table 60.1. Zoonotic infection may produce no disease, may produce organ damage with no initial symptoms or may present with any of the characteristic syndromes of clinical infection. There are usually no clinical features that specifically draw attention to the chance of its being an infection derived from animals and so clearly the history of animal exposure is critical and should be sought whenever an infection is diagnosed and its source is not immediately obvious. In this context, a detailed occupational history is vital. Characteristic clinical syndromes are illustrated in Table 60.2.

It is difficult to obtain accurate figures about the proportion of infections that are attributable to occupational exposure, but many countries have surveillance and notification systems that provide data on zoonotic infection in general. In Europe, data on zoonotic infections provided by member states to the European Centre for Disease Control are included in the centre's annual report.[5] In the United Kingdom, the Department of Environment, Food and Rural Affairs (DEFRA), in conjunction with the Health Protection Agency (HPA) and other agencies produces an annual report on the incidence of zoonotic infection.[6] A summary of the UK data for 2006 is shown in Table 60.3.

The risk to a worker of acquiring a zoonotic infection depends on the prevalence of the infection among the animals involved (which may be modified by specific control mechanisms), the infectivity and route of infection of the organism, and the steps taken to limit exposure. Measures to prevent or minimize exposure may include: provision of appropriate protective clothing, including masks and respirators (collectively known as personal protective

Table 60.1 Occupational settings for zoonotic exposure.

Contact with live animals	Contact with animal carcasses or byproducts	Laboratory exposure to infectious animal specimens	Environmental exposure
Veterinary workers	Abattoir workers, slaughtermen	Veterinary laboratory workers	Arable agricultural workers
Animal farmers	Butchers	Animal researchers	Forestry workers
Zoo workers	Meat inspectors	Medical laboratory workers	Sewage workers
Hunters, trappers	Workers with animal skin/hides/hair		Outdoor activity instructors/guides
Fishermen, fish farmers	Fishmongers, catering industry workers		
Animal trainers			
Animal sanctuary workers, cruelty inspectors			
Pet shop workers			

Table 60.2 Characteristic presenting clinical syndromes of zoonoses with examples.

Skin lesions	Fever	Diarrhoea (±fever)	Chest symptoms (±fever)	Miscellaneous (±fever)
Anthrax	Brucellosis	Salmonellosis	Q fever	Hepatitis E
Orf	Leptospirosis	Campylobacteriosis	Tuberculosis	Echinococcosis
Mycobacterium marinum	Viral haemorrhagic	Cryptosporidiosis	Psittacosis/ornithosis	
Erysipeloid	Tuberculosis	Yersiniosis	Tularaemia	
			Anthrax	
Animal ringworm	Rabies	*E. coli* O157/VTEC		

equipment (PPE)) accompanied by training to use it effectively; safe disposal of animal carcasses and waste products; environmental engineering (e.g. ventilation and/or filtration to reduce dust exposure, caging systems); standard good hygiene (e.g. hand washing), and pre-exposure vaccination (e.g. against rabies or anthrax) in some occupational groups.

OCCUPATIONAL ZOONOSES PRESENTING AS CHEST DISEASE

Anthrax

Anthrax is a bacterial infection caused by a Gram-positive spore-forming organism, *Bacillus anthracis*. The term 'anthrax' is derived from the Greek word for coal and refers to the black eschar that is characteristic of cutaneous anthrax. It is the vegetative bacilli that cause diseases in animals and man and when they are excreted in body fluids or when the host dies, then the bacilli will sporulate and spores may survive in the soil and remain viable for many years. They may even replicate in the soil.[7] After the Scottish island of Gruinard (Figure 60.1) was used for anthrax experiments during the Second World War, it remained quarantined for 48 years. Soil is contaminated in

Table 60.3 Zoonotic infections in England and Wales, 2006.[144]

Infection	Human cases	Comment
Campylobacter	46339	
Salmonella	14060	
Escherichia coli 0157	1002	
Cryptosporidia	3618	
Bovine tuberculosis	25	
Brucellosis	11	All acquired overseas
Anthrax	1	One fatality in Scotland

many areas of the world especially in Africa, the Middle East and Asia, but the concentration of spores is higher when infection in animal herds (principally herbivores, such as cattle, sheep and goats) is highest so annual vaccination of at-risk herds, coupled with case-finding and safe disposal of animal carcasses remains the mainstay of disease control.

Man becomes infected either by inoculation of spores through the skin to produce cutaneous anthrax, by inhalation of spores to give inhalational anthrax (historically, 'wool sorter's disease', caused by exposure to spore-contaminated fleeces) or by ingestion of contaminated meat containing viable vegetative bacilli to give gastrointestinal

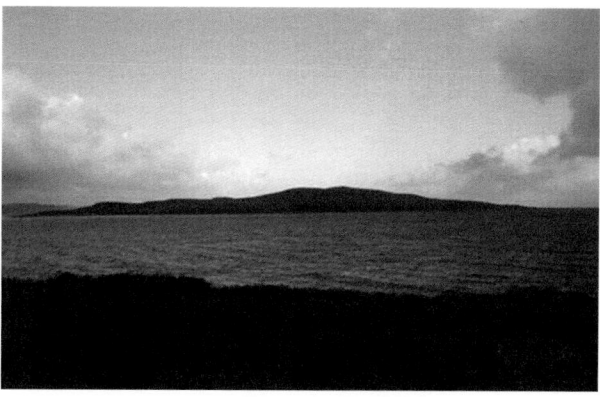

Figure 60.1 Gruinard Island, north west Scotland. Anthrax bombs were tested here during the Second World War and spores remained in the soil until the island was decontaminated in 1986. See website (www.hodderplus.com/hunters) for colour plate.

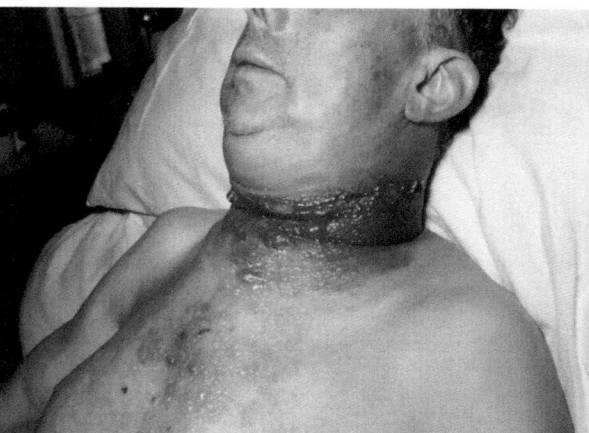

Figure 60.2 Acute cutaneous anthrax on the neck of a leather worker who carried animal hides, showing erythema, vesicles and oedema. The black eschar develops after a few days (AB Christie and Tropical and Infectious Disease Unit, Liverpool, UK). See website (www.hodderplus.com/hunters) for colour plate.

anthrax. Thus, anyone in close contact with animals and animal products may be at risk of infection.

Occupational exposure to anthrax can be divided into non-industrial exposure affecting farmers, butchers, slaughtermen and abattoir workers, and vets; and industrial exposure affecting those involved in processing animal hides, carcasses, or animal byproducts, e.g. bone meal, gelatin, bristles or hair (Figure 60.2). Recently, cases of inhalational anthrax have been reported in the United States and in the UK in drummers making, or using and handling drums made from imported, untreated, goatskin hides.[8]

Human anthrax is not a common problem in the west. Prior to the two recent 'drum-related' UK cases, there had been only 18 reported cases of human anthrax in England and Wales between 1981 and 2006 – all of these were cases of cutaneous disease. In the United States between 1980 and 2000, only seven cases of human anthrax were reported.[9] Anthrax has long been suggested as a favoured weapon of bioterrorism and in 2001, shortly after the attacks on the New York World Trade Center, 22 cases of suspected or confirmed anthrax occurred in the United States when anthrax spores were sent through the US mail.[10–12] There were 11 cutaneous cases and 11 inhalational cases, of which five were fatal (see Chapter 61, Bioterrorism). These were the first cases of inhalational anthrax in the United States since 1976.

Anthrax is essentially a disease caused by exotoxins. Three principal protein toxins are involved: protective factor, oedema factor and lethal factor. These toxins are elaborated by the vegetative bacilli and may disseminate around the host to cause cell and organ damage.

Cutaneous anthrax is the most common form of occupationally acquired anthrax. Spores are inoculated into the skin (minor cuts or abrasions are probably required for entry) by direct contact with infected animals or animal products. The usual incubation period is five to seven days, but a range of 1–19 days has been reported. The skin lesion (historically, known as 'malignant pustule') usually occurs on an exposed area of skin, and consists initially of a painless, often itchy, papule that rapidly evolves into the classical black eschar, and is associated with considerable surrounding oedema. There are frequently systemic manifestations as the toxins are released into the bloodstream, but the case–fatality rate is said to be very low if appropriate antibacterial agents are administered.

Inhalational anthrax is uncommon, and our understanding of the clinical presentation, disease process and outcome is derived from a relatively small number of cases: a recent systematic review of case reports published over the last century (1900–2005) identified 82 cases that were described in sufficient detail for inclusion in the analysis.[13] These included the cases from the 2001 US outbreak, but 74 cases from an outbreak in Sverdlovsk, Ukraine in 1979 that followed the inadvertent dissemination of anthrax spores from a military research facility were among the 178 cases excluded.[14] Inhalational anthrax occurs when spores are inhaled and are of an appropriate size (less than 5 μm) to enter the terminal bronchioles, from where they are carried by macrophages to the regional lymph nodes and germinate into vegetative bacilli. The release of toxin into the mediastinum leads to a haemorrhagic mediastinitis, rather than a pneumonia. The characteristic radiological appearances are of a widened mediastinum, but pleural effusions and consolidation can also be seen. Bacilli and toxins may disseminate via the bloodstream to produce features of general sepsis and anthrax meningitis is also frequent, and, being an indicator of late-stage, fulminant disease, is a poor prognostic sign.[13]

Gastrointestinal anthrax is rare in a western setting, but may occur more frequently in the developing world when contaminated meat is eaten and therefore is often reported as a point source outbreak. This is not usually an occupational issue. It may be either oropharyngeal or intestinal.

The former presents as oral ulceration, with oedema and membrane formation, so may be difficult to distinguish from diphtheria. The intestinal form may present as a generalized abdominal catastrophe and has a high mortality, particularly if presentation is late. Ascites may be a prominent feature.[10,15]

The differential diagnosis of anthrax is wide and depends on the clinical form. For cutaneous disease, this includes rickettsial infections, tularaemia, pseudomonal bacteraemia (ecthyma gangrenosum), orf, herpes virus infection, spider bites and other bacterial skin infections. In gastrointestinal anthrax, any severe abdominal pathology may be included in the differential diagnosis; inhalational anthrax can be confused with any severe chest infection. The diagnosis is established by culture of B. anthracis from appropriate clinical specimens. A polymerase chain reaction (PCR)-based test is also available. A high index of suspicion is required and diagnosis may be delayed unless other recent cases have been reported.

Treatment is with appropriate antibiotics. B. anthracis is sensitive to benzyl penicillin and this was traditionally the treatment of choice. Naturally occurring penicillin-resistant B. anthracis is extremely rare. However, because of concern about genetically manipulated resistance in organisms destined for deliberate release, and because beta-lactams do not penetrate so well into cells and tissues, the treatment of choice these days is usually ciprofloxacin, supplemented, in inhalational anthrax, with at least two of rifampicin, clindamycin and vancomycin. B. anthracis is not sensitive to cephalosporins. Prior to the 2001 cases in the United States, the mortality of inhalational anthrax was reported as being greater than 80 per cent, but with early combination antibiotic therapy, pleural fluid drainage, and modern intensive care the mortality in 2001 was less than 50 per cent. Presentation with fulminant late-stage disease and a requirement for intubation or tracheostomy were poor prognostic features.[13]

Prevention of occupationally acquired anthrax requires careful management and handling of animal products to minimize exposure to the infective spores. Hair, wool, hide and bone meal should be sterilized or disinfected before processing; in industrialized countries, importation of these products is tightly regulated. An inactivated vaccine is available, and recommended in the UK for selected workers at risk of exposure in higher-risk occupations, including veterinary medicine, research laboratory work, wool or hide-processing plants, and certain military settings.[16] Following a known exposure, post-exposure antibiotic prophylaxis may be offered. Ciprofloxacin and doxycycline are the two agents that are favoured. Antibiotics will be inactive against the spores and because of the long incubation period from acquisition of the spores to germination, post-exposure treatment is prolonged (up to 60 days was recommended in the 2001 outbreak in the United States). An alternative is to start a vaccination course and give antibiotics for 30 days until it is felt that the vaccine will be effective.

Chlamydophila infection (chlamydiosis, ornithosis, psittacosis)

The two most important zoonotic chlamydial infections are caused by *Chlamydophila psittaci* and *Chlamydophila abortus*. Both are found worldwide.

Chlamydophila psittaci infects a wide range of wild and caged birds, but human infection is usually the result of exposure to pet psittacine birds (e.g. parrots, parakeets, macaws, budgerigars) or to poultry. Infected birds may be asymptomatic, but nevertheless shed the organism in nasal discharges and faeces; infection in imported, quarantined birds may pass undetected. Chlamydophilae can survive in the environment for months. Human infection follows inhalation of the organism, usually during activities like cage cleaning, pet handling, or carcass evisceration or dressing.[17] Outbreaks have been described in poultry processors, pet shop workers, vets and veterinary medicine students, bird-fanciers, zoo and wildlife workers, and others (for example, customs officials exposed to birds at work may also be at risk).[18–23] Human infection is probably underdiagnosed. The incubation period ranges from one to four weeks; infection typically presents as an influenza-like illness with features of a community-acquired pneumonia, although milder and asymptomatic infections also occur. Diagnosis is made by serology on paired sera; PCR-based assays can be used to determine the infecting serovar, which may give a clue to the source. Clinical algorithms for the management of severe community-acquired pneumonia usually now include treatment with a macrolide (clarithromycin, azithromycin, erythromycin), which will treat the infection; doxycycline is an alternative.

Chlamydophila abortus is the most common cause of abortion and fetal loss in sheep (ovine enzootic abortion, enzootic abortion of ewes), and also causes abortion in goats and cattle. The organism is found in quantity in birthing fluids and placentae from infected animals; human infection is thought to occur by inhalation, and there may be a greater risk of transmission when birthing takes place in barns or lambing sheds rather than outdoors. However, infection after handling footwear and clothing contaminated during contact with infected animals has also been reported. Infection is a particular risk for pregnant women, as it may cause a severe febrile systemic illness, with multiorgan involvement, disseminated intravascular coagulation, and fetal death or premature delivery. Treatment (with a macrolide or, provided that the effects of tetracycline use in pregnancy have been considered, a tetracycline) of severe disease should not await confirmation of diagnosis, which is made serologically, or, if the test is available, by direct detection by PCR. Pregnant women should therefore avoid risk exposure (e.g. lambing, kidding, bottle-feeding young, milking, handling boots, clothing or other possibly contaminated objects), and should also avoid exposure to the live vaccine used to prevent infection in animals.[24,25]

Q fever

Q fever is a febrile illness caused by a Gram-negative coccobacillus, *Coxiella burnetii*. The disease was originally described following an outbreak of a febrile respiratory illness among workers in an abattoir in Queensland in 1935[26] and it has long been controversial whether the 'Q' stands for 'Query' or for Queensland. Q fever is a widespread zoonotic infection that can affect many mammals and birds. Domestic herbivores (cattle, sheep and goats) are the principal source of human infection; the main occupational groups at risk are agricultural workers, meat-processing workers, vets and research laboratory workers. Arthropods, such as ticks, can also be infected and may be responsible for maintaining the animal reservoir. Pet dogs, cats and rodents may also be infected. Animal infection is usually asymptomatic and chronic, but may cause abortion in sheep, goats and cattle. High concentrations of the organism are found in amniotic fluid, fetal membranes and the placenta, which may contain as much as 10^9 organisms/g. Birthing fluids may contaminate the surrounding environment, and, because the organism is relatively resistant to heat and to drying, it can survive in litter, bedding and dust for weeks. It can also be found in the milk, urine and faeces of infected animals, but inhalation of aerosolized organisms seems to be the major method of spread to humans. The infective dose is low: fewer than ten organisms may be sufficient to produce clinical disease. In a well-known outbreak in Switzerland, more than 400 people living along a road on which sheep descended from their mountain pastures became infected.[27,28] In Briançon, France, investigation of a community outbreak suggested airborne infection from exposure to a sheep slaughterhouse, where aerosols of contaminated dust were created by helicopters flying over from a nearby heliport.[29] More recently, extensive community outbreaks, associated with large-scale goat farming, have been reported from the Netherlands.[30] Other reported outbreaks have involved workers in a cosmetics supply factory that handled ovine products,[31] staff and patients of a psychiatric institution who worked on a goat farm,[32] veterinary high school students on a training course on a sheep farm,[33] workers in a cardboard manufacturing plant where a recent refurbishment might have exposed them to straw board dust,[34] and military or peace-keeping personnel deployed to Bosnia, Kosovo and Iraq.[35–37]

In man, many infections are asymptomatic (54 per cent in the Swiss outbreak[28]). The main features of clinically apparent infection are an acute pneumonic syndrome (one of the causes of the so-called 'atypical pneumonias'), a non-specific febrile illness or acute hepatitis. The incubation period following exposure is about two weeks (mean, 15 days; range, 2–41 days). The non-specific symptoms are usually self-limiting within one to three weeks as is the pneumonia, although this will often have been treated empirically with antibiotics before the diagnosis becomes apparent. Headache and myalgia are prominent features in the pneumonic and non-pneumonic forms of illness. The hepatitis can mimic acute viral hepatitis or become more chronic with the development of granulomata.

In addition to hepatitis, the major manifestation of chronic Q fever is endocarditis. This tends to occur in those who have previous heart valve damage, are pregnant, or are immune compromised.[38,39] Q fever endocarditis is often a delayed diagnosis and it is common for patients to have the more chronic features of endocarditis, such as finger clubbing and splenomegaly, together with features of immune complex activation.

There are no specific clinical features to aid in diagnosis and therefore there must be a high index of suspicion and requests for specific diagnostic testing. It is important to take a careful history about occupational or other exposure. Routine blood cultures are negative. There may be elevated inflammatory markers, white blood cell count is typically normal, but there may be thrombocytopenia and elevated liver transaminases.

The diagnosis is usually made by serological testing using immunofluorescence or complement fixation to detect antibodies to phase-1 and -2 antigens. Somewhat confusingly, antibodies to phase-2 antigens suggest acute Q fever (especially if there is an IgM response), whereas high titre antibody to phase-1 antigens suggests chronic infection.

Treatment of acute Q fever is usually with doxycycline.

In Australia, a Q fever vaccine has been licensed and used in a national programme targeted at abattoir workers and farmers, and an online register of workers' immune status has been developed. The number of cases of Q fever notified in Australia decreased by 50 per cent between 2002 and 2005.[40,41] Vaccine is contraindicated in those previously exposed to *C. burnetii* because severe local reactions may occur at the vaccination site, so pre-vaccination serology and skin testing are required. The vaccine is not commercially available elsewhere, but in other countries, vaccine for researchers working with live *C. burnetii* may be available under investigational new drug protocols. Guidelines on safety in laboratories and sheep research facilities cover risk reduction for workers and visitors; guidance has also been produced for farmers.[42–44]

OCCUPATIONAL ZOONOSES PRESENTING AS FEVER

Brucellosis

Brucellae are facultative intracellular Gram-negative coccobacilli that produce the clinical condition known as 'brucellosis'. There are at least eight named species, each closely associated with specific animal hosts, but *Brucella abortus*, *B. melitensis* and *B. suis* cause most human disease. *B. melitensis*, first isolated by Bruce in 1886, and soon after shown to be the cause of Malta fever, acquired by drinking unpasteurized milk from infected goats, is found also in sheep and camels, and has recently emerged as a problem in cattle in southern Europe. *B. abortus* was shown by Bang to cause abortion in cattle, and also occurs in buffalo, bison and elk. *B. suis* was first isolated from aborted pigs, and is also found in wild boars and hogs, and cattle; one serovar is host adapted to reindeer and caribou. The other species – *B. ovis* (found in sheep), *B. neotomae* (found only in desert wood rats), *B. canis* (dogs), *B. maris* (possibly three separate species, found in marine mammals) and *B. microti* (voles and red foxes) are either rarely (*B. canis*, *B. maris*) or never (*B. neotomae*) associated with human disease.[45–48]

Nearly all human cases of brucellosis are acquired directly or indirectly from animals, and disease incidence in humans reflects the prevalence of infection in local domestic animal herds. Infection is found worldwide, but is especially prevalent in the Mediterranean countries, the Middle East, South Asia, Africa and parts of Latin America. Humans acquire infection by direct contact with infected animals, or their birthing or abortion products (when the organism gains entry through cut or abraded skin, or conjunctivae or mucous membranes) or by inhalation of aerosolized animal material. Infection can also follow ingestion of raw milk or unpasteurized dairy products. Human-to-human spread by sexual contact has been described, but is uncommon.[49] Test and slaughter policies combined with vaccination programmes have led to the near eradication of *B. abortus* in cattle in the United States, United Kingdom and other industrialized countries, and this has been paralleled by a decline in the incidence of cases in humans. Programmes to control *B. melitensis* have been less effective. Many countries in Northern Europe are animal brucellosis free, although infections may occur in returning migrants occupationally exposed abroad, in travellers who have eaten unpasteurized dairy products, and in older or retired workers infected when animal disease was still prevalent.

Brucellosis is an occupational hazard for agricultural workers, veterinary workers, abattoir workers and meat packers, hunters and laboratory personnel. Although laboratory work on brucellae has long been recognized as hazardous, and work with the organisms requires biosafety level 3 containment, laboratory-acquired infection still occurs.[50] Cases are often attributable to open-bench exposure to cultures derived from patients in whom the diagnosis had not been suspected.

The clinical syndrome of brucellosis usually develops between two and four weeks after exposure. The onset may be acute or more insidious and the features can be divided into general systemic features and those features related to more specific sites of infection. The initial features are usually those of non-specific pyrexia of unknown origin – fever, malaise, sweats, headache, back pain and anorexia. Chronic brucellosis has been described as causing a depressive illness and cases of suicide in farmers have been attributed to this, but the evidence is not convincing.

Objective physical findings are not usually prominent. Rash is rarely apparent and apart from the fever, unimpressive lymphadenopathy has been described together with an enlarged liver and/or spleen.[48,51]

There is not thought to be any major distinction between the clinical syndromes produced by the different species. In a review of 530 cases of disease caused by *B. melitensis* approximately one-third developed a localized complication.[47] These may include bone and joint infection (especially sacroiliitis and/or spondylitis), aseptic meningitis, endocarditis (which is uncommon, but may account for much of the mortality from brucellosis), hepatic abscess (granulomatous hepatitis on liver biopsy when investigating pyrexia of unknown origin (PUO) is a common finding, but very non-specific) and epididymo-orchitis. Rarer complications include pneumonitis, uveitis, other abscesses (e.g. paraspinal, spleen, brain) and occasionally infection of prosthetic material.

Initial laboratory findings are non-specific and include evidence of an acute-phase response often accompanied by pancytopenia. Liver function tests may show a low-grade hepatitis. Various imaging modalities may be used to demonstrate abscess or other localized infection in areas that may then be accessible for biopsy or fine needle aspiration.

Diagnosis is achieved either by isolation of brucellae from blood cultures or by demonstrating a definitive serological response to brucella infection. It is important to consider the diagnosis on the basis of the clinical picture together with a detailed travel, occupational, recreational and dietary history. Cultures may be positive in up to 90 per cent of cases and the yield may be greater if bone marrow and liver biopsy (or other clinical material, e.g. from an abscess) samples are cultured in addition to blood.[52] It is essential that clinicians inform laboratory colleagues that a diagnosis of brucellosis is suspected: this not only ensures that the samples will be processed safely, but also ensures that they will be processed in a way that will provide the optimum diagnostic yield, by prolonging the period for which samples are incubated.

Serological testing usually uses the tube agglutination test or an ELISA technique. A single titre of antibody at a dilution greater than 1:160 in the context of a compatible clinical picture is regarded as diagnostic. Demonstration of a greater than four-fold change in titre over 4–12 weeks provides even stronger evidence of infection. The ELISA test is generally felt to have higher sensitivity and specificity than tube agglutination. Tests for antigen detection are in development.

Treatment of brucellosis with antibiotics improves symptoms, shortens the duration of illness and reduces risk of complications and relapse. Single-drug therapy has produced an unacceptably high level of relapse, so combination therapy with doxycycline and an aminoglycoside and/or rifampicin is recommended.[53] Most of the early aminoglycoside studies used streptomycin, whereas these days most clinicians would probably be more familiar and comfortable with gentamicin. Doxycycline should be given in a dose of 100 mg twice daily together with rifampicin

600–900 mg once daily for six weeks. Some clinicians may wish to add gentamicin at 5 mg/kg for the first one or two weeks of treatment. Monotherapy with any agent, and regimes based on cotrimoxazole or quinolones, are all felt to be inadequate.[53]

Hantavirus infection

Hantaviruses, RNA viruses that form a genus in the bunyavirus family, generally each have a single species of rodent (e.g. cotton rat, striped field mouse, deer mouse, bank vole) as their primary reservoir.[54] The viruses do not cause overt illness in the rodent hosts, but an infected animal excretes virus in urine, saliva and faeces. Hantaviruses cause two clinical syndromes: haemorrhagic fever with renal syndrome (HFRS) and hantavirus pulmonary syndrome (HPS). Infection is thought to be usually acquired by inhalation of dust containing virus-contaminated saliva or excreta; infection has also followed the bite of an infected rodent.

Four hantaviruses (Hantaan, Seoul, Puumala and Dobrava viruses) found largely in Europe and Asia, cause HFRS of varying severity. Hantaan virus infection (first described in the English language literature as Korean haemorrhagic fever, but occurring more widely in eastern Asia, in China and Russia) is the most severe, with a mortality rate of up to 15 per cent. By contrast, Puumala virus, which occurs throughout northwestern Europe, and is the cause of 'nephropathia epidemica', has a mortality rate of less than 1 per cent. Seoul virus occurs worldwide; infection after exposure to infected laboratory rats has been described.[55]

HPS occurs in North and South America. Hantaviruses were identified as the cause in 1993, when Sin Nombre virus was discovered during the investigation of an outbreak of adult respiratory distress syndrome with a high case fatality rate in the southwestern United States.[56,57] HPS is relatively uncommon in the United States, where fewer than 100 cases are reported annually; most are caused by Sin Nombre virus, although other hantaviruses (New York, Bayou, Monongahela and Black Creek Canal) are also known to cause disease.[55,58] HPS is more common in South America, where it has been caused by Andes, Oran, Lechiguanas and Juquitiba viruses; Andes virus is unusual in that it is the only hantavirus known to have been transmitted from person to person, and nosocomially.[59]

Hantavirus infection is diagnosed serologically; reference laboratory testing is usually required. Intravenous ribavirin is effective in the treatment of HFRS, but not useful in HPS, for which treatment is essentially supportive.

Guidelines on risk reduction highlight precautions that may limit the occupational risk (likely to be greatest for those whose work involves frequent handling of wild rodents, e.g. field biologists, mammologists, rodent operators), including the use of personal protective respiratory equipment.[60]

Henipavirus infections

Two highly pathogenic zoonotic paramyxoviruses, Hendra virus and Nipah virus, together form the genus henipavirus.

Both have pteropid bats ('flying foxes') as their natural reservoir, but both have a wide host range. Hendra virus (once named equine morbillivirus) was first recognized in Australia in 1994.[61,62] A horse trainer and a stablehand in Hendra, Brisbane developed severe influenza-like illness after exposure to horses that had developed a lethal respiratory infection. The trainer died; severe interstitial pneumonitis was found at post-mortem. At the same time, a trainer in Mackay, Queensland who had cared for two sick horses, and later helped with their necropsies, developed acute meningitis two weeks later, recovered, but a year later developed fatal encephalitis.[63] Since then, around a dozen clusters of infection have occurred in horses in eastern Australia, with a further four infections in humans (three veterinarians and a veterinary nurse), of which two (in 2008 and 2009, both in veterinarians) were fatal.[64] In the most recent outbreak, exposed workers were given post-exposure prophylaxis with intravenous ribavirin and oral chloroquine; full details have not yet been reported. The virus has not been detected outside Australia.

In 1997, Nipah virus emerged in Malaysia in pigs in Ipoh and subsequently spread to pigs farmed in villages in Negri Sembilan. An outbreak of severe acute encephalitis in pig farmers, and others who had close contact with pigs (e.g. pen cleaners, abattoir workers, vaccine sellers and pig cullers) followed in 1998–99.[61,65,66] Most had a febrile illness and acute encephalitis, but a pneumonic illness occurred in about a quarter of cases. Workers in an abattoir in Singapore exposed to infected pigs from Malaysia also became infected.[67] The infection has a high acute mortality rate (40 per cent in Malaysia), with neurological sequelae in survivors, some of whom develop relapsed encephalitis months or years after initial infection. More recently, clusters of Nipah virus infection have been reported from Bangladesh and India. In these incidents, risk factors for infection have variously included climbing trees, exposure to pigs, drinking date palm sap possibly contaminated by fruit bat urine or saliva, and exposure to an infected case. At least one outbreak was amplified by nosocomial transmission, and limited person-to-person spread by the respiratory route may be possible, but occupational risks have generally been less clear cut than in the outbreak in the Malay peninsula.[68]

Henipaviruses are categorized as hazard group 4 pathogens, and diagnosis and research work must therefore be undertaken only in BSL4/ABSL4 facilities.

Hepatitis E

Hepatitis E virus is a non-enveloped single-stranded RNA virus, which is usually transmitted by the faeco–oral route, causing fever and acute hepatitis, with anorexia, jaundice and hepatomegaly. Infection late in pregnancy may be especially severe, with fulminant hepatitis and a high (>20 per cent) mortality rate. In industrialized countries, infection is usually sporadic, but large epidemics, associated with contamination of water supplies, have occurred in developing countries. Swine and wild boar may act as an animal reservoir; viruses found in sporadic human cases in non-endemic areas have been found to be closely related to hepatitis E viruses detected in pigs. There are case reports of infection in butchers and slaughterhouse workers without a history of travel to an endemic area, and there is some evidence also from seroprevalence surveys of a possible occupational risk from work that involves exposure to swine.[69–72] Diagnosis is made serologically; infection is clinically indistinguishable from other causes of viral hepatitis. There is no carrier state, nor is there a specific treatment. A vaccine is not available; prevention of sporadic infection involves adoption of standard infection prevention measures, including good hand hygiene.

Leptospirosis

Leptospirosis is a zoonotic infection that can cause a variety of different clinical pictures in man ranging from asymptomatic infection to severe multiorgan disease with hepatorenal failure (Weil's disease). It has a worldwide distribution (except for the polar regions), but is particularly prevalent in the tropics. The taxonomy of leptospires (spirochaetes with hooked ends) is complex and still evolving. Historically, two phenotype-based species – *Leptospira interrogans* (containing pathogenic strains) and *L. bireflexa* (containing non-pathogenic strains) – were further subdivided on the basis of serological tests into more than 250 serovars, with antigenically related serovars grouped into a smaller number of serogroups. Each serovar has a defined host range, and the number of serovars present in any given geographical area tends to be restricted, particularly in temperate zones. Advances in molecular biology have led to a genotype-based classification, which recognizes at least 17 different species. For the moment, the two systems exist in parallel.[73]

Rodents and other small mammals are the most important animal reservoir. They become infected in infancy, develop a chronic renal infection and excrete leptospires in their urine throughout their life. Excreted organisms may remain viable in soil or water for weeks. Larger mammals, such as dogs, cattle and pigs, develop a symptomatic infection that may be fatal, or become chronically infected and shed leptospires into the environment. People who have direct contact with animals, water or soil are at greatest risk of occupationally acquired leptospirosis, which was first described in miners in the early twentieth century, although jaundice in rice-paddy workers has been recognized since ancient times in China. Infection is seasonal, with a peak in incidence in the rainy season in the tropics, and in the summer or autumn in countries with temperate climates. Infection rates may rise after heavy rainfall or flooding.[74]

Occupational risk groups include dairy and pig farmers, vets, abattoir workers, hunters and trappers, rodent control workers, sewage and canal workers, fish workers and fish farmers, sugar cane cutters and banana farmers, and the military. In a western setting, infection is also acquired by recreational exposure to water, and has been reported in canoeists, wild-swimmers, cavers, white-water rafters and triathletes, and in the UK, an increasing proportion of infections are reported in travellers exposed on adventure holidays abroad.[6]

Leptospires invade through mucous membranes, conjunctivae or microabraded or water-sodden skin; it is not known whether they can penetrate intact skin. They are disseminated via the bloodstream and are therefore widely distributed throughout the body where they produce a vasculitis, the exact mechanism of which remains obscure.

The clinical features are very variable. Many of those infected will have an asymptomatic seroconversion. Others may have a mild non-specific febrile illness and others may have one of the more easily appreciated syndromes. The average incubation period seems to be about ten days, although it is often difficult to establish exactly when exposure occurred and a range of incubation periods from two to 26 days has been reported. The majority of symptomatic cases present with sudden onset of fever, rigors, myalgia and headache. Nausea, vomiting, diarrhoea and cough are also common features. On examination, the most characteristic finding is conjunctival suffusion and muscle tenderness, but these probably only occur in a minority of cases. Less common physical findings include lymphadenopathy, hepatosplenomegaly, chest signs and a rash. Clinical features of meningitis may also be present. Although the illness is often described classically as 'biphasic', in practice such a pattern is rarely recognized. However, as the immune response appears the patient may deteriorate and develop one or more of the more specific syndromes associated with leptospiral infection. These include aseptic meningitis, Weil's disease (with the classic triadic presentation of jaundice), thrombocytopenia and renal failure (where, despite the jaundice, liver function is usually relatively well preserved), cardiac syndrome (with myocarditis leading to cardiac failure), and pulmonary syndrome. The pulmonary syndrome has been described particularly in South America, and may vary from mild respiratory symptoms and signs to severe pulmonary haemorrhage and adult respiratory distress syndrome. A recent review in Peru suggested that nearly 4 per cent of patients with serologically confirmed leptospirosis had severe pulmonary manifestations, but would not have been otherwise diagnosed if they had not been part of the study.[75]

The differential diagnosis during the non-specific febrile phase is wide and includes malaria, typhoid, influenza, rickettsial infection (especially scrub typhus) and arbovirus infection (including dengue fever). Routine laboratory investigations are similarly non-specific – the white cell count may be elevated or lowered (usual range 3000–25 000/mm^3) often with a left shift. About half the patients have elevations of liver transaminases (fairly mild) and creatinine kinase. The urine is often abnormal with proteinuria, white cells, casts and occasional microscopic haematuria. In Weil's disease, renal function deteriorates and the bilirubin may be very high. The chest x-ray may show non-specific shadowing. The platelet count may sometimes be reduced. The cerebrospinal fluid may show an elevated white cell count with neutrophils or lymphocytes, minimal to moderately elevated protein concentrations and normal glucose.

Because of the non-specific nature of the clinical picture and the laboratory findings, a high index of suspicion must be maintained if the diagnosis is not to be missed.

Leptospira can be seen by dark ground microscopy of blood or urine, but sensitivity and specificity are low and the technique is rarely used in practice. The organism can be cultured from blood (taken in the first ten days of the illness and before antibiotics have been administered) and from urine from the end of the first week and for some time afterwards, but culture requires special media, prolonged incubation, and is also relatively insensitive. Most patients have their infection identified serologically. The traditional gold standard test has been the microscopic agglutination test (MAT), which uses live organisms and can be technically demanding to perform. Therefore, most laboratories use a screening test first, such as an ELISA for IgM antibodies – these are usually detectable on day 5 of illness. PCR-based methods are in development, but are not yet in widespread use.

Leptospira are susceptible to many antibiotics *in vitro*, including penicillins, third-generation cephalosporins, macrolides and tetracyclines; intravenous penicillin has been used in the treatment of severe infection for decades. There is debate about the effectiveness of antibiotics if given any later than early in infection, doubt about whether mild disease needs to be treated, and few trials on which to base recommendations. Nevertheless, in endemic areas, where it is common for leptospirosis to be misdiagnosed as a rickettsial infection or vice versa, oral doxycycline 100 mg bid is a sensible option,[76] as it will treat both conditions empirically while serological diagnosis is awaited. If the patient is very unwell, then intravenous penicillin 1.2 g six-hourly or ceftriaxone 1 g once daily should be used. There are no trials on duration of therapy, but ten days is usually recommended.

Infection risks can be reduced by effective rodent control, avoidance of high risk exposure, and use of personal protective equipment (e.g. boots, goggles, rubber gloves, waterproof overalls, depending on the type of exposure expected) and standard veterinary infection control precautions when dealing with potentially infected animals.[77] A human vaccine has been used, but is not widely available. Animal vaccines are more widely used, but most do not prevent the excretion of leptospires. A study on chemoprophylaxis from 1984 showed significant benefit of weekly doxycycline 200 mg among American troops in the jungles of Panama.[78]

Streptococcus suis infection

Streptococcus suis is a porcine pathogen with a worldwide distribution, found wherever pigs are farmed. It causes septicaemia, meningitis, arthritis and meningitis in pigs; illness is more common when pigs are intensively farmed in suboptimal conditions. Human infection is associated with direct contact with sick or carrier pigs, and with eating undercooked pork products (particularly traditional foods, e.g. pig's blood), so there is an occupational risk for pig farmers (including 'backyard farmers'), abattoir workers, slaughterers, butchers and veterinarians. Wild boar hunters may also be at risk.[79,80]

Although more than 30 serotypes of *S. suis* have been recognized, human infection is usually caused by *S. suis* serotype 2. Infection is uncommon and sporadic in the United Kingdom and the United States, but the organism has recently been recognized as an important zoonotic pathogen in China and Southeast Asia.[81] In 2005, it caused an outbreak of streptococcal toxic shock syndrome (STSS) and meningitis that affected 204 people (with 38 deaths), mostly men who had slaughtered or eaten sick pigs; recent surveys suggest that *S. suis* is a common cause of acute bacterial meningitis in adults in Thailand, Vietnam and Hong Kong SAR.[82,83] The infection has a short incubation period (from a few hours to three days); cases present with clinical features of meningitis (fever, headache, neck stiffness, photophobia, nausea or vomiting) or septicaemia, and may in addition have signs of STSS, including purpura or a haemorrhagic rash. Septic arthritis and endocarditis may also occur. Diagnosis is made by culture of blood and cerebrospinal fluid (CSF); a PCR-based test is also available. The organism is sensitive to penicillins (although resistant strains have been reported), cephalosporins and vancomycin. Mortality rates (particularly in STSS) may be high; deafness is a common sequel of meningitis.

Prevention involves standard good hygiene (e.g. using appropriate PPE during slaughtering, hand hygiene) and ensuring that all pork products are thoroughly cooked before being eaten.

Toxoplasmosis

This is the clinical condition caused by infection with the intracellular protozoon parasite *Toxoplasma gondii*. Cats are the definitive host; humans, other mammals and birds serve as intermediate hosts. In sheep and goats, infection may cause abortion or fetal loss, with considerable economic costs. Humans become infected either by exposure to oocysts excreted from cats (e.g. by handling cat litter or through gardening), by handling raw meat, or eating undercooked meat derived from an infected intermediate host. Seroprevalence of infection increases with age (because of cumulative exposure), but is generally falling with increased standards of living. Overall, between 20 and 70 per cent of adults in the United States have serological evidence of previous exposure (and therefore have long-term subclinical infection).[84]

There may be an occupational risk for workers exposed to animals with clinical toxoplasmosis or to aborted lambs, kids, piglets and their placentas (e.g. farmers, shepherds, vets, animal shelter employees), and those who may be exposed to infected animal carcasses or raw meat (e.g. hunters, abattoir workers, meat packers, butchers, chefs and zoo workers). Infection might be acquired orally (by transfer of organisms on unwashed hands to the mouth), or through inoculation via damaged skin. Laboratory-acquired infections have been reported (including infection caused by needlestick injury while performing the Sabin Feldman dye test, which requires the use of live organisms), but a study of workers in a toxoplasma reference laboratory concluded that the risks to workers were low.[85] The live attenuated vaccine used to control infection in sheep may cause human infection if accidentally inoculated, and should not be administered by women of child-bearing age. In practice, most infections are probably acquired non-occupationally. However, an information sheet on preventing exposure in pregnant women during the lambing season is available.[86]

Most acute infections result in an asymptomatic seroconversion. A small proportion of immunocompetent adults develop a 'glandular fever-like syndrome' of malaise, fever, headache and lymphadenopathy. Atypical lymphocytes may be found in the peripheral blood and there may be a pharyngitis, although this is probably less prominent than with the infectious mononucleosis produced by Epstein–Barr virus (EBV) infection. Monospot or Paul Bunell testing is negative, as is IgM serology for EBV. The differential diagnosis includes cytomegalovirus (CMV), human herpes virus 6, lymphoma, HIV seroconversion illness and cat scratch disease. Toxoplasmosis is sometimes diagnosed histologically when lymph nodes are excised, but is more often diagnosed by tests for specific antibody. Acute toxoplasmosis is usually a benign self-limiting condition with no sequelae; no active treatment is needed. If a woman acquires toxoplasma infection during pregnancy, there is a significant risk of transmission to the unborn child, which can result in congenital toxoplasmosis and disability in the infant. Infection early in pregnancy is less likely to transmit to the fetus, but more likely to cause severe damage, whereas infection later in pregnancy is more likely to transmit to the fetus, but less likely to result in organ damage, although infants who have subclinical infection at birth may develop signs of disease much later. As most acute infections are asymptomatic, some countries (e.g. France) have serological screening programmes. Elsewhere, prevention is dependent on exposure reduction through education.[87]

The greatest concern about T. gondii infection is in patients who are immune compromised as a result of malignancy (especially myelo- or lymphoproliferative disease), iatrogenic immune suppression or by HIV. In these individuals, latent toxoplasma infection can reactivate, causing encephalitis, pneumonitis and chorioretinitis. Diagnosis of cerebral toxoplasma in an HIV-positive patient is made by diagnostic imaging (magnetic resonance imaging (MRI), plus possibly positron emission tomography (PET)). The majority of patients have positive serology for toxoplasma. Primary prophylaxis reduces the incidence of reactivation-associated disease; treatment of established disease is with pyrimethamine and sulphadiazine.

West Nile virus

West Nile virus is a flavivirus that is a pathogen for birds (the natural hosts), equines and humans. The virus was first identified in Uganda, and recognized as a cause of acute meningoencephalitis in Israel 20 years later. It is endemic in Africa and the Middle East, and since 1999 has emerged as a cause of meningoencephalitis throughout the United States, with spread to adjacent countries.[88–90] The majority of clinically apparent infections are mild, with fever, headache and occasionally a rash on the trunk. Neuroinvasive disease occurs in less than 1 per cent of infections, but mortality in hospitalized cases is significant; the risk of severe disease increases with age. Treatment is essentially supportive. Human infection is usually mosquito borne, but infection in laboratory workers after exposure via needlestick or aerosol while working with infected animal tissues or cell cultures has been reported.[91] A cluster of cases among turkey breeder farm workers in Wisconsin led to recommendations to include the use of insect repellents, alongside standard infection prevention measures that include good hand hygiene and use of personal protective equipment.[92] Infection in an alligator farm worker who had cared for sick alligators has also been reported.[93,94] Recommendations to prevent West Nile virus exposure in outdoor and field workers (likely to be primarily mosquito-borne) also emphasize the importance of insect repellents and protective clothing.[94,95] A vaccine has been developed for prevention of equine infection, but a vaccine for humans is not yet available.

OCCUPATIONAL ZOONOSES PRESENTING AS GASTROINTESTINAL INFECTION

Salmonellosis

The nomenclature of the salmonellae has recently been revised to accommodate advances in taxonomy. DNA hybridization studies showed that the 'one serotype, one species' concept – which, as the number of organisms distinguishable by serotyping increased, had led to an accumulation of over 2000 pathogenic species – was no longer tenable because the organisms had such closely related DNA. All clinically important salmonellae are now classified as a single species – *Salmonella enterica* – with serotypes (now grouped within one of six subspecies) referred to with a capital letter and in plain, rather than italic, type. For example, *Salmonella typhimurium* becomes *S. enterica* subsp. *enterica* ser Typhimurium, or is shortened to *S.* Typhimurium.[96,97]

Despite their microbiological similarities, there are major clinical and epidemiological distinctions between the so-called 'typhoidal' and 'non-typhoidal' salmonellae. The former group, which includes *S.* Typhi and *S.* Paratyphi, are exclusively human infections that are spread from person to person. Infection is acquired by the faeco–oral route, but the major manifestations (at least in the early stages) of infection are due to bacteraemia rather than luminal infection within the gastrointestinal tract. By contrast, the non-typhoidal salmonellae are mainly zoonoses and having been acquired via the faeco–oral route, their initial pathogenesis is within the gut to produce 'gastroenteritis', although they may go on to produce invasive disease, with bacteraemia and subsequent localized infection. Most infections are caused by ingestion of contaminated food or water, and are not occupationally acquired. Many cases are associated with overseas travel and several serotypes of salmonella can also be acquired from pet animals, including amphibians, and reptiles and the small rodents used to feed them.[98,99] The main occupational groups at risk are veterinary and agricultural workers, and laboratory workers. Infection of workers in a vaccine production plant has also been reported.[100] Food handlers may transmit infection; food safety and hygiene regulations cover employment and exclusion practices.[101,102]

Salmonellosis as a cause of gastrointestinal infection has been declining in the west since a peak in the mid-1990s.[5,6] *S.* Enteritidis and *S.* Typhimurium are the most frequently isolated serotypes. The former organism is a particular problem in the poultry and egg production industries, though rates of infection in breeder flocks have fallen in the last decade; the latter organism is found in dairy products, pork, turkey, beef and lamb. Monitoring farm premises for control purposes often reveals widespread environmental contamination, with reports of isolation of salmonellae from farm offices, tractor cabins, boots and animal pens post-disinfection.[6] Workers who are occupationally exposed to salmonellae may inadvertently contaminate their home environment. In New Zealand, where *S.* Brandenburg has emerged as a pathogen only in the last decade, a case–control study found that infection was significantly associated with occupational contact with sheep, or having a household member who had occupational contact with sheep.[103] In the United States, *S. enterica* was isolated from the contents of vacuum cleaner bags in 27 per cent (15/55) of households where one or more occupants had workplace exposure (in veterinary practice, a salmonella reference laboratory or on livestock farms), but not from households without such exposure.[104]

The gastrointestinal illness produced by infection with non-typhoidal salmonella is clinically indistinguishable from that caused by many other gastrointestinal pathogens. Diarrhoea is the main feature and this may be initially, or may become, bloody. It may often be associated with vomiting, abdominal pain and cramps, and sometimes with fever. The usual incubation period following ingestion of contaminated food or water is 12–72 hours (in contrast to typhoid where the incubation period is 10–14 days and the initial presentation is with fever, often accompanied by constipation). Approximately 5 per cent of patients with salmonella gastroenteritis will develop a salmonella bacteraemia; this is more likely with *S.* Typhimurium infection, especially if the organism is quinolone resistant.[105] Localized infection (e.g. of bones or joints) may then follow; more rarely endocarditis may occur.

Salmonellae have also been reported as a cause of pustular dermatitis (usually of the forearm), without gastrointestinal symptoms, in veterinarians who had delivered calves without adequate personal protective equipment.[106]

A recent Cochrane review found no clinical evidence of benefit in treating otherwise healthy adults (or children) with antibiotics for non-severe salmonella gastroenteritis, confirming previous reports that giving antibiotics increases the risk of adverse events and of prolonged stool carriage of salmonellae.[107] Antibiotics are recommended in those who are ill enough to require hospitalization, especially if they have high fever suggestive of invasive infection. Quinolones remain the first choice of treatment, although reports of resistance in typhoidal and non-typhoidal salmonellas mean that sensitivity should not be assumed. Third-generation cephalosporins (cefotaxime or ceftriaxone) or azithromycin are potential alternatives.

Campylobacteriosis

Campylobacters are colonizing organisms found in the gut of many vertebrates and were first shown to be human pathogens in the early 1970s. By the mid-1980s, they had become the most commonly identified bacterial cause of acute infectious intestinal disease in the United Kingdom.[6,108] Two species, *Campylobacter jejuni* (found in poultry and a broad range of farm animals) and *C. coli* (found in swine) are responsible for most human infections. Studies suggest that a high proportion of fresh chicken may be contaminated with campylobacter.

Campylobacter gastroenteritis is clinically indistinguishable from any other cause of gastroenteritis and presents with diarrhoea that is often bloody, associated with abdominal pain and nausea. Vomiting seems to be less common than with salmonella infection, and bacteraemia is less frequently identified, although it may be underestimated. The abdominal pain may be severe, may precede the diarrhoea and may mimic an acute abdomen. The role of antibiotics in the treatment of campylobacter is not clear. A meta-analysis suggested that antibiotic treatment shortened the duration of diarrhoea by 1.32 days.[109] Quinolones and erythromycin are effective treatments, but there is concern because of increasing resistance to quinolones (perhaps worsened by their use in veterinary medicine). In practice, most illness is self-limiting, and infection is often not diagnosed sufficiently early for antibiotic therapy to be beneficial. Guillain–Barré syndrome is a well-recognized complication.[108]

The greatest risk for campylobacter infection is eating undercooked poultry or food cross-contaminated by contact with poultry; infection is also associated with foreign travel. However, agricultural workers and those employed by the meat and poultry industries are at risk of campylobacter infections, as are veterinary staff. Outbreaks among workers on poultry (including turkey and pheasant) farms have been reported.[109,110] The risk of infection may be greater early in the course of employment: an explosive outbreak among workers in a poultry abattoir occurred when temporary student workers were employed to provide cover during the holiday season.[111,112] In the United States, a case–control study of sporadic *C. jejuni* infection estimated that 18 per cent of infections in rural areas were attributable to poultry husbandry, although poultry husbandry was not necessarily the primary occupation.[113] These infections are largely preventable, by good hand hygiene.

Enterohaemorrhagic *Escherichia coli* infection

In the United Kingdom, these organisms are called Vero cytotoxin-producing *E. coli* (VTEC), whereas in the United States they are called Shiga toxin-producing *E. coli* (STEC). These organisms are also known as enterohaemorrhagic *E. coli* (EHEC), and cause a characteristic, toxin-mediated, bloody diarrhoea, first recognized in 1982, when two outbreaks of haemorrhagic colitis were associated with eating hamburgers from a national restaurant chain.[114] There are a number of serotypes in the group: *E. coli* 0157: H7 is the most frequently identified in Europe and the United States; in Australia *E. coli* 0111: H- is more common. Their main 'natural' habitat is the gut of healthy cattle and other ruminants; carcasses become contaminated at slaughter. Outbreaks have been associated with inadequately cooked contaminated beef and exposure to other foodstuffs (including raw milk, cured sausages and cheese) or contaminated water.[115] Infection may also follow direct contact with live animals; risks extend to visitors to open farms and petting zoos. VTEC present occupational risks similar to those of campylobacter and salmonella, although the lower infective dose may make infection after direct exposure and transmission from person to person more likely.

The incubation period after ingestion of organisms is about three or four days, although a range from one to nine days has been reported. The spectrum of disease ranges from mild diarrhoea to severe haemorrhagic colitis, haemolytic uraemic syndrome (HUS), thrombotic thrombocytopenic purpura (TTP) and death.[116] The disease is more severe and mortality is higher in children and the elderly. There is usually the onset of abdominal cramps followed by diarrhoea that initially may be watery, but in the majority of cases becomes bloody at some stage in the illness. Fever is often absent, which may, in the absence of a known outbreak, lead attending clinicians to entertain diagnoses of non-infectious diarrhoea, such as ischaemic colitis or inflammatory bowel disease. A detailed occupational and food history is important; cases should be promptly reported to relevant public health authorities to enable rapid outbreak detection and control.

HUS is a syndrome of acute renal failure, microangiopathic haemolytic anaemia and thrombocytopenia. It can occur in between 5 and 10 per cent of those infected with *E. coli* 0157; young children are especially vulnerable. At least half of those diagnosed with HUS will need acute renal support and the long-term sequelae are not insubstantial – there is a 12 per cent risk of death or end-stage renal disease and a 25 per cent risk of other sequelae, such as hypertension, persistent proteinuria or some degree of chronic kidney disease.[117] If HUS does not develop then there are generally no renal sequelae from *E. coli* 0157 diarrhoea. TTP has similar underlying mechanisms, but is more likely to occur in the elderly, and to also affect the central nervous system to produce stroke syndromes or the colon to produce ischaemic colitis.

Treatment is essentially supportive; prompt, effective volume repletion may prevent the development of HUS. The effect of antibiotic therapy on the subsequent risk of developing HUS, TTP or other complications remains controversial, but most authorities advise against it on the grounds that no benefit of antibiotic treatment has been demonstrated and some studies have suggested that antibiotics induce the expression and release of toxin and may precipitate HUS.

Prevention of EHEC infection requires scrupulous attention to hygiene in handling of animal carcasses in abattoirs and butchers' premises, and to standard good practice in the catering industry, including adequately cooking meat. Patients admitted to hospital with bloody diarrhoea should be isolated and strict enteric precautions must be taken by all staff to minimize the risk of person-to-person transmission. There is specific guidance about avoiding risks of zoonotic infection at farms and petting zoos that have been opened to the public.[118]

Cryptosporidiosis

Cryptosporidia are coccidian protozoa that were first described in the stomach of mice in 1907. By the early 1970s, they were recognized as a cause of diarrhoea in cattle, but were not really thought of as a human pathogen until the 1980s, when it was recognized that they were the cause of a severe, intractable, diarrhoeal syndrome in patients with AIDS or other severe immune suppression. It is now realized that cryptosporidia can cause an unpleasant diarrhoeal illness even in the immune-competent. Although 16 species of cryptosporidia are now recognized, *C. hominis* (usually not zoonotic) and *C. parvum* (usually zoonotic) cause most human infections. Cattle farmers are at particular risk of cryptosporidia infection[119] and it is a risk to others on farm visits and open days.

Cryptosporidian oocysts are excreted by infected animals (especially calves and lambs) and may survive in the environment for some time. They are resistant to chlorination and have a low infective dose, so waterborne spread – either from drinking water or recreational or occupational use of water – is possible. The oocysts are infective at the time they are released, so person-to-person spread can occur. Cryptosporidia are found worldwide, although infection is probably underdiagnosed in developing countries.

The diarrhoea is usually watery and free of blood. It may be accompanied by nausea, anorexia and abdominal discomfort. Fever is uncommon. Infection is generally self-limiting and resolves within about two weeks. In AIDS patients, the diarrhoea generally improves as immune restoration takes place in response to antiretroviral drugs; nitazoxanide may be an effective specific therapy. Treatment is not indicated in the immune-competent.

In the developed world, prevention has focused on reducing the risk of cryptosporidial contamination of drinking water supplies, by fencing off reservoirs from animals and improvement of water treatment processes.

OCCUPATIONAL ZOONOSES PRESENTING WITH SKIN PROBLEMS

Lyme disease

Lyme disease is the most common tick-borne infection in the northern hemisphere. It was first formally described in 1977, after an outbreak of arthritis associated with a characteristic skin rash affected residents of the towns of Lyme and Old Lyme in southeast Connecticut over a five-year period.[120] Transmission by an arthropod vector was postulated, but it was not until 1982 that the causative organism was isolated both from humans and ticks.[121] The condition is caused by infection with organisms of the genus *Borrelia*. The main species responsible for Lyme disease is *Borrelia burgdorferi* sensu strictu, although in Europe the condition may be caused by two closely related organisms, *B. afzelii* and *B. garinii*. The bacterium is transmitted by hard ticks of the genus *Ixodes* (Figure 60.3). Forest rodents and small mammals, such as deer, are the usual animal hosts. Man is infected by the bite of an infected tick (usually the nymph stage). Lyme disease can theoretically occur wherever there is the pool of infected mammals and the appropriate hard ticks to maintain transmission. In practice, it is mainly reported from the United States and Europe. In the United States, more than 90 per cent of cases are reported from the northeastern states with just a few reports from the southwest. It occurs in the United Kingdom, but is more often reported from other European countries, particularly Austria, Germany, Slovenia and Sweden, usually from rural areas that have the requisite mammal and tick populations. The distribution of Lyme disease outside North America and Europe remains unclear: there is controversy about whether infection occurs in Australia, and few data for Africa, Asia or Latin America.

Occupational exposure may occur in forestry workers, agricultural workers, veterinarians and those employed in the leisure industry in endemic areas.

The clinical manifestations are conventionally divided into three stages: (1) early localized cutaneous involvement, (2) disseminated infection to heart, nervous system and joints and (3) persistent or late Lyme disease.[122] In most patients with Lyme disease (80 per cent), the initial indication of infection (stage I) is the characteristic skin rash known as erythema (chronicum) migrans (Figure 60.4).

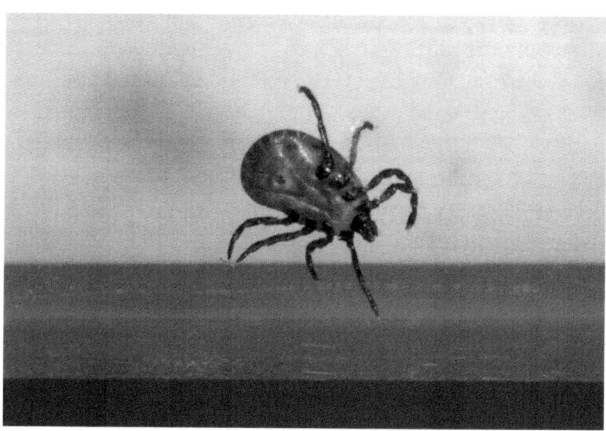

Figure 60.3 A hard tick. Vector for a number of zoonotic infections including Lyme disease. See website (www.hodderplus.com/hunters) for colour plate.

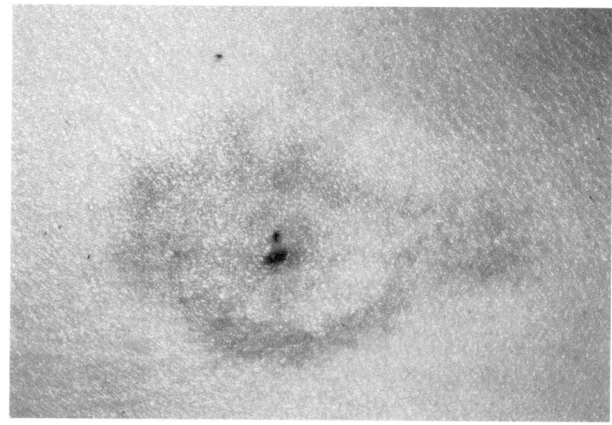

Figure 60.4 The classical rash of Lyme disease. See website (www.hodderplus.com/hunters) for colour plate.

This is a red lesion centred on the site of the tick bite. There is often some fading of the rash in the middle zone of the lesion so that the rash is said to resemble a 'bull's eye'. This usually appears any time between three and 30 days after the tick bite and may be accompanied by systemic features of general malaise, fever, arthralgia and headache. The rash fades slowly over a few weeks with or without treatment and may be the only manifestation of infection.

The early disseminated stage (stage II) is initially characterized by disseminated erythema migrans lesions and then later by neurological or cardiac involvement. The main neurological symptoms are isolated cranial nerve palsies (especially Bell's palsy), a lymphocytic meningitis, a radiculopathy and more controversially a form of encephalitis. These are described in about 15 per cent of patients with initial Lyme disease. Cardiac involvement is more rare and includes conduction disturbances or a myocarditis that can be severe and lead to long-term cardiac damage. Cardiac involvement occurs in about 5 per cent of untreated initial infections.

Late Lyme disease may develop months or years after initial infection especially if the initial episode was unrecognized or inadequately treated. It can affect up to 60 per cent of those initially infected. The most common manifestation is a chronic or intermittent arthritis that affects large joints, especially the knee. The arthritis may become established and chronic and may fail to improve even after long-term high-dose antibiotic therapy.[123]

Neurological late Lyme disease (sometimes known as chronic neuroborreliosis) can afflict up to 5 per cent of those initially infected.[124] This may present as sensory disturbances, radicular pain, and sometimes as muscular weakness. The pathology seems to be an axonal neuropathy with characteristic features on electromyography (EMG). A picture of encephalitis with cranial nerve involvement or cognitive impairment has also been described. Cerebrospinal fluid serology for B. burgdorferi antibody is commonly positive in those with late neuroborreliosis, but PCR testing is usually negative.

The diagnosis should be suspected on the basis of the clinical features and the history of potential exposure in an endemic area. If Lyme disease is suspected, serological tests for antibody to B. burgdorferi should be carried out; positive serology in the appropriate geographical and clinical setting is diagnostic. During the first few weeks of infection (even when erythema migrans is present) only 20–30 per cent of those infected have positive serology (usually IgM antibodies), but in the convalescent phase, several weeks later, up to 80 per cent have positive serology, even after antibiotic therapy. However, a significant proportion of those who are treated rapidly and appropriately never develop a serological response.[125] Antibody titres may fall slowly after antibiotic treatment and may persist for several years.

Evidence-based guidelines for the treatment of Lyme disease were published by the Infectious Diseases Society of America (IDSA) in 2006.[126] They recommend doxycycline 100 mg twice daily, amoxicillin 500 mg three times daily or oral cefuroxime axetil 500 mg twice daily for treatment of early disease, whether localized or disseminated (stages I and II), unless there is a suggestion of cardiac or neurological involvement. Macrolides are not recommended unless the three first-line drugs are inappropriate or unavailable for some other reason. For early Lyme disease with a suggestion of neurological or cardiac involvement, intravenous ceftriaxone 2 g once daily for two weeks is recommended (although oral treatment with first-line drugs is a possible strategy for cardiac problems). Late Lyme arthritis can be treated with first-line oral therapy, whereas late Lyme neurological involvement is an indication for four weeks of intravenous ceftriaxone (or cefotaxime).

A controversial area in the management of Lyme disease is whether the condition of 'chronic Lyme disease' really exists. Campaign groups in the United States and to a lesser extent in Europe believe that a variety of medically unexplained symptoms, such as those that make up the chronic fatigue syndrome, are caused by Lyme disease, even if there is no serological evidence of exposure to infection. The main medical and scientific view is that this condition does not exist and that long-term antibiotic therapy (longer than 30 days) should not be offered.[127,128] However, this view is vigorously disputed by campaign groups, and the area remains contentious.

Erysipeloid

Erysipeloid ('pork finger', 'whale finger', 'fish-handler's disease') is caused by the Gram-positive bacterium *Erysipelothrix rhusiopathiae*, which is widely distributed in nature and found in a wide range of vertebrates and invertebrates, including domestic swine (causing swine erysipelas), sheep, poultry, shellfish and fish (where it survives in mucoid exterior slime).[129,130] Most human infections are occupationally acquired, by direct contact with infected animals, fish or their products; minor trauma (e.g. puncture wounds from crab claws, fish hooks or bone spicules; cuts during autopsy or butchery) facilitates transmission. Infection usually presents five days to two weeks after exposure as an extremely painful, well demarcated, slightly raised cellulitis on the finger or hand, centred on the site of inoculation, which is characteristically violaceous at the spreading edge with central clearing. Fever is unusual. Less commonly, disseminated cutaneous infection, with bulla formation, occurs. *E. rhusiopathiae* is a rare cause of endocarditis (usually of a native aortic valve); around 40 per cent of cases have a recent history of an erysipeloid-like skin lesion, or a concurrent one.

Diagnosis requires culture (blood, needle aspirate or biopsy from the leading edge of the cellulitis); the organism is sometimes misidentified as a 'diphtheroid' or a lactobacillus. *E. rhusiopathiae* is sensitive to penicillins, cephalosporins and macrolides, but intrinsically resistant to vancomycin – important because the empirical treatment of severe sepsis in penicillin-allergic patients often relies on vancomycin to cover Gram-positive organisms. Although the localized skin infection will heal naturally within three to four weeks, healing is faster with antibiotic therapy.

Listeriosis

Although *Listeria monocytogenes*, the usual cause of listeriosis (septicaemia, meningitis, or, in pregnant women, abortion or congenital infection of the fetus) in humans, is a frequent cause of similar disease in animals, infection is usually sapronotic rather than zoonotic, and normally not associated with occupational exposure. However, cutaneous infection, presenting as pustular dermatitis, may occur in farmers and veterinarians one to four days after exposure to an infected animal (e.g. during delivery of an infected calf), usually affecting the forearm or hand.[131] Diagnosis is made by culture of the organism, which is usually sensitive to penicillins and macrolides.

Monkeypox

Monkeypox, an uncommon zoonotic orthopox viral infection that can mimic smallpox, occurs mainly in tropical central and west Africa. In 2003, a cluster of 47 confirmed and probable human cases occurred in the midwestern United States among people who had direct or close contact with sick pet prairie dogs, which had become infected when they were co-housed with wild-caught rodents imported as exotic pets from Ghana. Common clinical features included fever, headache, chills, lymphadenopathy (unusual in smallpox) and a vesiculopustular rash.[132] Occupational exposure was identified as a risk: cases included veterinarians and clinic staff, pet shop employees and animal distributors, as well as prairie dog owners.[132] Investigators noted that standard veterinary infection control precautions had not been universally implemented: although their use would not have prevented the outbreak, it might have limited transmission. Control measures included expansion of existing restrictions on the importation and sale of animal species likely to carry monkeypox virus.

Mycobacterium marinum

Mycobacterium marinum, the cause of 'fish tank finger' is a non-tuberculous mycobacterium that is widely distributed in aquatic environments and is also recognized as a pathogen of fish, including farmed food species and farmed tropical species (e.g. Siamese fighting fish). Cutaneous infection in humans follows exposure of cut or damaged skin while cleaning fish tanks or inoculation via a scratch or puncture wound (e.g. in fish filleters, boat builders). After an incubation period of several weeks, a reddish tender papule develops (usually on the hand or forearm, or other cooler, exposed area of the body) which may ulcerate, but eventually heals with scarring. Less often, multiple papules develop in a sporotrichoid distribution, or infection may involve deeper tissues, e.g. tendon or bone. Disseminated infection may occur in the immunosuppressed. Diagnosis is by histology and culture of the organism from a tissue biopsy. It is important to inform the laboratory of the suspected diagnosis, as the organism grows at a lower temperature than that routinely used for incubation. Treatment is usually with doxycycline, minocycline, clarithromycin or rifampicin with ethambutol; surgical debridement may also be required.[133] Strong, water-impermeable gloves, and covering cuts and lacerations with waterproof dressings will prevent exposure, but there may be a lack of awareness of the hazard amongst those at risk.[134]

Orf

Orf is a classic occupationally acquired zoonotic infection. It is caused by a DNA parapox virus that usually infects sheep and goats, and is sometimes called 'contagious pustular dermatitis'. It can also occur in cattle and reindeer. In ewes, pustular and scabby lesions develop on the teats and udder. Lambs then become infected when suckling, and develop lesions on the lips and nostrils, and inside the mouth. The occupationally at-risk population includes farm workers and shepherds (particularly after bottle-feeding lambs or after shearing), abattoir workers and slaughterers, veterinarians and others with frequent exposure to sheep and goats.

Orf infections in flocks are controlled by vaccination with a live, non-attenuated vaccine. Vaccinated sheep develop a mild form of orf, and recently vaccinated animals therefore also present a transmission risk to their handlers.[135] Infection may also follow needlestick exposure.

Three to five days after exposure, an erythematous, itchy, macule develops, usually on the finger, hand or forearm. This becomes papular, and then develops into a vesicle surrounded by erythema. The lesion may grow to about 2–3 cm in diameter and may progress to ulceration within two to three weeks (Figure 60.5). Complete healing generally takes place by four to six weeks. The lesions may be solitary or there may be several at the point of inoculation; infections in the immune-suppressed may be much more severe. The differential diagnosis includes erysipeloid, tularemia and cutaneous anthrax. If there is diagnostic doubt, then a skin biopsy will show characteristic histological features; a PCR-based test (of vesicle fluid, scab debris or tissue sections) is also available. There is no specific treatment. Secondary bacterial infection can be treated with standard antibiotics. There is anecdotal support for the use of cidofovir cream.[136] In practice, orf is

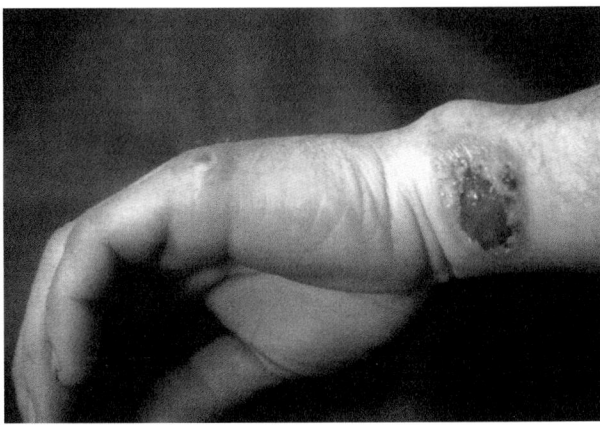

Figure 60.5 Orf on the hands of a sheep farmer. Note the presence of two lesions (AB Christie and Tropical and Infectious Disease Unit, Liverpool, UK). See website (www.hodderplus.com/hunters) for colour plate.

well recognized by the farming community, and usually self-diagnosed; treatment is rarely sought.[137,138] Infection does not lead to protective immunity and reinfection is not uncommon.

OTHER IMPORTANT ZOONOTIC INFECTIONS

Echinococcosis (hydatid disease, hydatidosis)

Echinococcosis is a parasitic infection caused by the larval stages of cestodes (tapeworms) of *Echinococcus granulosus* (which causes cystic echinococcosis (CE)) and *E. multilocularis* (which causes alveolar echinococcosis (AE)).[139] The adult *E. granulosus* tapeworm lives in the small intestine of dogs or other canids (e.g. dingoes); gravid tapeworm segments and eggs are excreted in the faeces. Sheep, cattle or other intermediate hosts ingest the eggs when grazing on contaminated pasture; the oncospheres released in the gastrointestinal tract then migrate to the liver, lungs or less often, other organs, where they slowly mature into a metacestode (hydatid cyst). The cycle is perpetuated when dogs eat, or are fed, infected meat or viscera. The parasite is found worldwide, particularly in Asia, Africa, Central and South America, and throughout the Mediterranean. In the United Kingdom, animal infection is most common in sheep-farming areas in Wales, Herefordshire and the Western Isles.[140] Control measures include voluntary, incentivized or mandatory dog worming, abattoir inspection, the prompt and correct disposal of animal carcasses, and education. Humans become infected through close contact with infected dogs, either by hand-to-mouth transfer of eggs after handling the animal or its faeces, or, less often, by exposure to contaminated food. Infection is often acquired in childhood, but adults, including shepherds and farmers who keep sheep (or other intermediate host, e.g. cattle, camels) and dogs are also at risk of infection.

E. multilocularis is found only in the northern hemisphere, with red foxes (including urban foxes), arctic foxes and dogs as definitive hosts, and small rodents as intermediate hosts. Again, man is an accidental intermediate host; possible routes for occupational infection include exposure to infected sled or hunting dogs, or foxes, or their faeces. Risk groups therefore include animal hunters and trappers, fur traders, and field and wildlife biologists.

Human infection is always asymptomatic initially, and may remain so. CE may be discovered by the incidental finding of a calcified cyst wall on radiographic or ultrasound examination, or may present with clinical features caused by the pressure effects of a mass lesion, or by the effect of spontaneous or traumatic cyst rupture. Most patients have a single cyst in a solitary organ, most often of the liver (60 per cent) or lungs (20 per cent); less often in brain, kidney, spleen, heart or bone. Pulmonary disease tends to present earlier than hepatic disease. Alveolar echinococcosis primarily affects the liver, and – since the metacestode has no capsule, but is multiloculate – more invasive than CE, though like CE, infections are initially asymptomatic and cyst growth may be very slow. Diagnosis of CE and AE is by serology (though false negatives are not uncommon) combined with imaging. Management requires specialist assessment: treatment options include surgical resection or PAIR (puncture, aspiration, injection of a scolicide, re-aspiration) combined with pre- and post-procedure anti-helminthic therapy (usually with albendazole), or long-term anti-helminthics alone.

Special safety precautions are recommended for laboratorians and for field workers at high risk of exposure to infective *Echinococcus* eggs, which are highly adapted for environmental survival and disinfectant resistant. Serological testing after a single, identified, one-off exposure may be appropriate, and regular testing of workers potentially exposed over longer periods is recommended.

Rabies and related lyssavirus infections

Rabies is an acute viral encephalitis caused by rabies virus genotype 1 (classical rabies), or, less often, by the related bat lyssaviruses (European bat lyssaviruses (EBLVs), the African bat lyssaviruses (Duvenhage and Mokola) and Australian bat lyssavirus) which cause a clinically indistinguishable disease.[141,142]

Infection usually follows exposure to saliva via a bite or scratch from an infected animal (most often a dog), but has also followed mucous membrane exposure. The viruses do not cross intact skin. The incubation period is usually 3–12 weeks, but may be as short as four days, or, rarely, longer than a year. Disease onset is insidious, with non-specific prodromal symptoms including fever, headache, sore throat and malaise, sometimes accompanied by itching, tingling or fasciculation at the site of the wound. These are followed by the development of signs of encephalitis, with hyperanxiety, aerophobia or hydrophobia, bizarre behaviour, seizures and signs of autonomic disturbance, or an ascending flaccid paralysis. Rabies is almost invariably fatal.

The World Health Organization estimates that between 40 000 and 70 000 human cases of classical rabies occur annually, mostly in developing countries, especially in South and South East Asia. Human infections caused by the other lyssaviruses are far less common: fewer than a dozen cases have been reported worldwide. These include a fatal case in an unvaccinated bat conservationist in Scotland in 2002.[143]

In the United Kingdom, pre-exposure prophylaxis with rabies vaccine is recommended for laboratory workers handling lyssaviruses (including those working in vaccine production), workers who will regularly be exposed to animals imported from rabies-enzootic areas, e.g. in primate holding facilities, quarantine centres, ports; state veterinary and technical staff, licensed and voluntary bat handlers; animal inspectors; veterinarians and zoologists who will be exposed to animals in enzootic areas, and healthcare workers who are about to provide care for a rabies case. Pre-exposure vaccine is also recommended for longer-term travellers to enzootic areas, and for short-term travellers whose activities may place them at risk, if access to post-exposure care is likely to be limited. In the UK, the Department of Health recommends that those who are working with live virus and others at high risk should be serologically tested at regular intervals, and reinforcing doses of vaccine given to maintain an antibody level above the recommended acceptable minimum.[16] Recommendations elsewhere are similar. Post-exposure vaccine, with or without rabies-specific immunoglobulin is given after a significant risk exposure; expert advice is available from national public health authorities.

Key points

- Seventy-five per cent of emerging pathogens and 61 per cent of all infectious organisms are zoonotic.
- No specific clinical features will suggest zoonotic origin for any particular infection. A detailed occupational history is essential to exclude zoonotic exposure in an occupational setting.
- Agricultural workers and veterinarians are at particular risk, but many other occupations may potentially expose workers to zoonotic infection.
- Most zoonotic infections will present with fever with or without skin lesions, chest symptoms or diarrhoea.
- The risk to a worker of acquiring a zoonotic infection depends on the prevalence of that infection among the animals involved, the infectivity and route of infection of the organism, and the steps taken to limit exposure.

REFERENCES

1. Taylor LH, Latham SM, Woolhouse ME. Risk factors for human disease emergence. *Philosophical Transactions of the Royal Society of London. Series B, Biological Sciences.* 2001; **356**: 983-9.
2. Chan M. World now at the start of 2009 influenza pandemic. Statement to the press by WHO Director-General, 11 June 2009. Last accessed October 2009. Available from: www.who.int/mediacentre/news/statements/2009/h1n1_pandemic_phase6_20090611/en/index.html.
3. World Health Organization. Summary of probable SARS cases with onset of illness from 1 November 2002 to 31 July 2003. Based on data as of December 31, 2003. Last accessed 20 October 2009. Available from: www.who.int/csr/sars/country/table2004_04_21/en/index.html.
4. Reed KD, Melski JW, Graham MB *et al.* The detection of monkeypox in humans in the Western Hemisphere. *New England Journal of Medicine.* 2004; **350**: 342-50.
5. European Centre for Disease Prevention and Control. Annual epidemiological report on communicable diseases in Europe 2008. Stockholm: European Centre for Disease Prevention and Control, 2008.
6. Department for Environment, Food and Rural Affairs. Zoonoses report, United Kingdom, 2007. London: DEFRA, 2008.
7. Titball RW, Turnbull PC, Hutson RA. The monitoring and detection of *Bacillus anthracis* in the environment. *Society for Applied Bacteriology Symposium Series.* 1991; **20**: 9S-18S.
8. Health Protection Agency. Anthrax and animal hide drums: Summary literature review and risk assessment. *Health Protection Report* 2008; **2**: 2. Last accessed October 20, 2009. Available from: www.hpa.org.uk/hpr/archives/2008/news4508.htm.
9. Hopkins RS, Jajosky RA, Hall PA *et al.* Summary of notifiable diseases – United States, 2003. *Morbidity and Mortality Weekly Report.* 2005; **52**: 1-85.
10. Inglesby TV, O'Toole T, Henderson DA *et al.* Anthrax as a biological weapon in bioterrorism: Guidelines for medical and public health. *Journal of the American Medical Association.* 2002; **287**: 2236-52.
11. Jernigan JA, Stephens DS, Ashford DA *et al.* Bioterrorism-related inhalational anthrax: The first 10 cases reported in the United States. *Emerging Infectious Diseases.* 2001; **7**: 933-44.
12. Jernigan DB, Raghunathan PL, Bell BP *et al.* Investigation of bioterrorism-related anthrax, United States, 2001: Epidemiologic findings. *Emerging Infectious Diseases.* 2002; **8**: 1019-28.
13. Holty J-EC, Bravata DM, Liu H *et al.* Systematic review: A century of inhalational anthrax cases from 1900 to 2005. *Annals of Internal Medicine.* 2006; **144**: 270-80.
14. Meselson M, Guillemin J, Hugh-Jones M *et al.* The Sverdlovsk anthrax outbreak of 1979. *Science.* 1994; **266**: 1202-8.
15. Kanafani ZA, Ghossain A, Sharara AI *et al.* Endemic gastrointestinal anthrax in 1960's Lebanon: Clinical

manifestations and surgical findings. *Emerging Infectious Diseases*. 2003; **9**: 520–4.
16. Department of Health. Immunisation against infectious disease, 2006. London: Department of Health, 2006. Last accessed October 20, 2009. Available from: www.dh.gov.uk/en/Publichealth/Healthprotection/Immunisation/Greenbook/dh_4097254.
17. Smith KA, Bradley KK, Stobierski MG, Tengelsen LA. Compendium of measures to control *Chlamydophila psittaci* (formerly *Chlamydia psittaci*) infection among humans (psittacosis) and pet birds, 2005. *Journal of the American Veterinary Medical Association*. 2005; **226**: 532–9.
18. Irons JV, Sullivan TD, Rowen J. Outbreak of psittacosis (ornithosis) from working with turkeys or chickens. *American Journal of Public Health*. 1951; **41**: 931–7.
19. Newman CP, Palmer SR, Kirby FD, Caul EO. A prolonged outbreak of ornithosis in duck processors. *Epidemiology and Infection*. 1992; **108**: 203–10.
20. Palmer SJ, Andrews BE, Major R. A common-source outbreak of ornithosis in veterinary surgeons. *Lancet* 1981; **2**: 798–9.
21. Heddema ER, van Hannen EJ, Duim B *et al*. An outbreak of psittacosis due to *Chlamydophila psittaci* genotype A in a veterinary teaching hospital. *Journal of Medical Microbiology*. 2006; **55**: 571–5.
22. Matsui T, Nakashima K, Ohyama T *et al*. An outbreak of psittacosis in a bird park in Japan. *Epidemiology and Infection*. 2008; **136**: 492–5.
23. De Schrijver K. A psittacosis outbreak in Belgian customs officers. *Euro Surveillance*. 1995; pii=173. Available from: www.eurosurveillance.org/ViewArticle.aspx?ArticleId=173.
24. Walder G, Hotzel H, Brezinka C *et al*. An unusual cause of sepsis during pregnancy: recognizing infection with *Chlamydophila abortus*. *Obstetrics and Gynecology*. 2005; **106**: 1215–17.
25. Meijer A, Brandenburg A, de Vries J *et al*. *Chlamydophila abortus* infection in a pregnant woman associated with indirect contact with infected goats. *European Journal of Clinical Microbiology and Infectious Diseases*. 2004; **23**: 487–90.
26. Derrick EH. 'Q' fever, a new fever entity: Clinical features, diagnosis and laboratory investigation. *Medical Journal of Australia*. 1937; **2**: 281–99.
27. Centers for Disease Control. Q fever outbreak – Switzerland. *Morbidity and Mortality Weekly Reports*. 1984; **33**: 355–61.
28. Dupuis G, Petite J, Peter O, Vouilloz M. An important outbreak of human Q fever in a Swiss Alpine valley. *International Journal of Epidemiology*. 1987; **2**: 282–7.
29. Armengaud A, Kessalis N, Desenclos JC *et al*. Urban outbreak of Q fever, Briancon, France, March to June 1996. *Euro Surveillance*. 1997; **2**: pii=137. Last accessed October 20, 2009. Available from: www.eurosurveillance.org/ViewArticle.aspx?ArticleId=137.
30. Schimmer B, Morray G, Dijkstra F *et al*. Large ongoing Q fever outbreak in the south of the Netherlands, 2008. *Euro Surveillance*. 2008; **13**: pii=18939. Last accessed October 20, 2009. Available from: www.eurosurveillance.org/ViewArticle.aspx?ArticleId=18939.
31. Wade AJ, Cheng AC, Athan E. Q fever outbreak at a consmetics supply factory. *Clinical Infectious Diseases*. 2006; **42**: e50–2.
32. Fishbein DB, Raoult D. A cluster of *Coxiella burnetii* infections associated with exposure to vaccinated goats and their unpasteurized dairy products. *American Journal of Tropical Medicine and Hygiene*. 1992; **47**: 35–40.
33. Grilc E, Socan M, Koren N *et al*. Outbreak of Q fever among a group of high school students in Slovenia, March–April 2007. *Euro Surveillance*. 2007; **12**: pii=3237. Available from: www.eurosurveillance.org/ViewArticle.aspx?ArticleId=3237.
34. van Woerden HC, Mason BW, Nehaul LK *et al*. Q fever outbreak in industrial setting. *Emerging Infectious Diseases*. 2004; **10**: 1282–9.
35. Faas A, Engeler A, Zimmermann A, Zöller L. Outbreak of Query fever among Argentinean special police unit officers during a United Nations mission in Prizren, South Kosovo. *Military Medicine*. 2007; **172**: 1103–6.
36. Splino M, Beran J, Chlíbek R. Q fever outbreak during the Czech Army deployment in Bosnia. *Military Medicine*. 2003; **168**: 840–2.
37. Faix DJ, Harrison DJ, Riddle MS *et al*. Q fever among US military in western Iraq, June–July 2005. *Clinical Infectious Diseases*. 2008; **46**: e65–8.
38. Maurin M, Raoult D. Q fever. *Clinical Microbiology Reviews*. 1999; **12**: 518–53.
39. Fenollar F, Fournier PE, Raoult D *et al*. Risks factors and prevention of Q fever endocarditis. *Clinical Infectious Diseases*. 2001; **33**: 312–16.
40. Gidding HF, Wallace C, Lawrence GL, McIntyre PB. Australia's national Q fever vaccination programme. *Vaccine*. 2009; **27**: 2037–41.
41. Meat and Livestock Australia. Australian Q fever register. Last accessed October 20, 2009. Available from: www.qfever.org/aboutregister.php.
42. World Health Organization. *Laboratory biosafety manual*, 3rd edn. Geneva: World Health Organization, 2004 (WHO/CDS/CSR/LYO/2004.11).
43. Office of Laboratory Security. Public Health Agency of Canada Guidelines for biomedical facilities using sheeps as research animals (December 2000). Health Canada, Office of Laboratory Security, 2006. Last accessed October 20, 2009. Available from: www.phac-aspc.gc.ca/ols-bsl/animres-eng.php.
44. Health Protection Agency. Q fever: Information for farmers. London: Health Protection Agency 2009. Last accessed October 20, 2009. Available from: www.hpa.org.uk/HPA/Topics/InfectiousDiseases/InfectionsAZ/1191942172161.
45. Foster JT, Okinaka RT, Svennson R *et al*. Real-time PCR assays of single-nulceotide polymorphisms defining the major *Brucella* clades. *Journal of Clinical Microbiology*. 2008; **46**: 296–301.
46. VanBressem M-F, Van Warebeck K, Raga JA *et al*. Serological evidence of *Brucella* species infection in odontocetes from the South Pacific and the Mediterranean. *Veterinary Record*. 2001; **148**: 657–61.
47. Corbel MJ. Brucellosis: An overview. *Emerging Infectious Diseases*. 1997; **3**: 213–19.

48. Young EJ. An overview of human brucellosis. *Clinical Infectious Diseases.* 1995; **21**: 283–9.
49. Rubin B, Band JD, Wong P et al. Person-to-person transmission of *Brucella melitensis. Lancet.* 1991; **1**: 14–15.
50. Robichaud S, Libman M, Behr M et al. Prevention of laboratory-acquired brucellosis. *Clinical Infectious Diseases.* 2004; **38**: 119–22.
51. Colmenero JD, Reguear JM, Martos F et al. Complications associated with *Brucella melitensis* infection: A study of 530 cases. *Medicine (Balt)* 1996; **75**: 195–211.
52. Yagupsky P. Detection of brucellae in blood cultures. *Journal of Clinical Microbiology.* 1999; **37**: 3437–42.
53. Skalsky K, Yahav D, Bishara J et al. Treatment of human brucellosis: Systematic review and meta-analysis of randomised controlled trials. *British Medical Journal.* 2008; **336**: 701.
54. Schmaljohn C, Hjelle B. Hantaviruses: A global disease problem. *Emerging Infectious Diseases.* 1997; **3**: 95–104.
55. Lloyd G, Bowen ETW, Jones N, Pendry A. HFRS outbreak associated with laboratory rats in UK. *Lancet.* 1984; **1**: 1175.
56. Ksiazek TG, Peters CJ, Rollin PE et al. Identification of a new North American hantavirus that causes pulmonary insufficiency. *American Journal of Tropical Medicine and Hygiene.* 1995; **52**: 1017–23.
57. Duchin JS, Koster FT, Peters CJ et al. Hantavirus pulmonary syndrome: A clinical description of 17 patients with a newly recognized disease. *New England Journal of Medicine.* 1994; **330**: 949–55.
58. Khan AS, Khabbaz RF, Armstrong LR et al. Hantavirus pulmonary syndrome: The first 100 US cases. *Journal of Infectious Diseases.* 1996; **173**: 1297–303.
59. Padula PJ, Edelstein A, Miguel SD et al. Hantavirus pulmonary syndrome outbreak in Argentina: Molecular evidence for person-to-person transmission of Andes virus. *Virology* 1998; **241**: 323–30.
60. Centers for Disease Control. Hantavirus pulmonary syndrome – United States: Updated recommendations for risk reduction. *Morbidity and Mortality Weekly Reports.* 2002; **51**: 1–12.
61. Eaton BT, Broder CC, Middleton D, Wang L-F. Hendra and Nipah viruses: Different and dangerous. *Nature Reviews. Microbiology.* 2006; **4**: 23–35.
62. Murray K, Selleck P, Hooper P et al. A morbillivirus that caused fatal disease in horses and humans. *Science.* 1995; **268**: 94–7.
63. O Sullivan JD, Allworth AM, Paterson DL et al. Fatal encephalitis due to a novel paramyxovirus transmitted from horses. *Lancet.* 1997; **349**: 93–5.
64. ProMED-mail. PRO/AH/EDH > Hendra virus, human, equine – Australia (04): (QL) fatal; ProMED 2009; 03 September; 20090903.3095. Last accessed October 20, 2009. Available from: www. promedmail.org.
65. Chua KB, Goh KJ, Wong KT et al. Fatal encephalitis due to Nipah virus among pig-farmers in Malaysia. *Lancet.* 1999; **354**: 1257–9.
66. Parashar UD, Sunn LM, Ong F et al. Case-control study of risk factors for human infection with a new zoonotic paramyxovirus, Nipah virus, during a 1998–1999 outbreak of severe encephalitis in Malaysia. *Journal of Infectious Diseases.* 2000; **181**: 1755–9.
67. Paton NI, Leo Y-S, Zaki SR et al. Outbreak of Nipah virus infection among abattoir workers in Singapore. *Lancet.* 1999; **354**: 1253–6.
68. Lo MK, Rota PA. The emergence of Nipah virus, a highly pathogenic paramyxovirus. *Journal of Clinical Virology.* 2008; **43**: 396–400.
69. Perez-Gracia MT, Mateos ML, Galiana C et al. Autochthonous hepatitis E infection in a slaughterhouse worker. *American Journal of Tropical Medicine and Hygiene.* 2007; **77**: 893–6.
70. Jary C. Hepatitis E and meat carcasses. *British Journal of General Practice.* 2005; **55**: 557–8.
71. Meng XJ, Wiseman B, Elvinger F et al. Prevalence of antibodies to hepatitis E virus in veterinarians working with swine and in normal blood donors in the United States and other countries. *Journal of Clinical Microbiology.* 2002; **40**: 117–22.
72. Galiana C, Fernandez-Barredo S, Garcia A et al. Occupational exposure to hepatitis E virus (HEV) in swine workers. *American Journal of Tropical Medicine and Hygiene.* 2008; **78**: 1012–15.
73. Levett PN. Leptospirosis. *Clinical Microbiology Reviews.* 2001; **14**: 296–326.
74. Gaynor K, Katz AR, Park SY et al. Leptospirosis on Oahu: An outbreak associated with flooding of a university campus. *American Journal of Tropical Medicine and Hygiene.* 2007; **76**: 882–6.
75. Segura ER, Ganoza CA, Camposi K et al. Clinical spectrum of pulmonary involvement in leptospirosis in a region of endemicity, with quantification of leptospiral burden. *Clinical Infectious Diseases.* 2005; **40**: 343–51.
76. Takafuji ET, Kirkpatrick JW, Miller RN et al. An efficacy trial of doxycycline chemoprophylaxis against leptospirosis. *New England Journal of Medicine.* 1984; **310**: 497–500.
77. Elchos BL, Scheftel JM, Cherry B et al. Compendium of veterinary standard precautions for zoonotic disease prevention in veterinary personnel. *Journal of the American Veterinary Medical Association.* 2008; **233**: 415–32.
78. McClain JB, Ballou WR, Harrison SM et al. Doxycycline therapy for leptospirosis. *Annals of Internal Medicine.* 1984; **100**: 696–8.
79. Arends JP, Zanen HC. Meningitis caused by *Streptococcus suis* in humans. *Reviews of Infectious Diseases.* 1988; **10**: 131–7.
80. Bensaid T, Bonnefoi-Kyriacou B, Dupel-Pottier C et al. *Streptococcus suis* meningitis following wild boar hunting. *La Presse Médicale.* 2003; **32**: 1077–8.
81. Lun Z-R, Wang Q-P, Chen X-G et al. *Streptococcus suis*: An emerging zoonotic pathogen. *Lancet Infectious Diseases.* 2007; **7**: 201–9.
82. Yu H, Jing H, Chen Z et al. Human *Streptococcus suis* outbreak, Sichuan, China. *Emerging Infectious Diseases.* 2006; **12**: 914–20.
83. Mai NT, Hoa NT, Nga TV et al. *Streptococcus suis* meningitis in adults in Vietnam. *Clinical Infectious Diseases.* 2008; **46**: 659–67.

84. Benson C, Kaplan J, Masur H et al. Treating opportunistic infections among HIV-infected adults and adolescents: Recommendations from CDC, the National Institutes of Health, and the HIV Medicine Association/Infectious Diseases Society of America. *Clinical Infectious Diseases.* 2005; **40**: S131.
85. Parker SL, Holliman RE. Toxoplasmosis and laboratory workers: A case control assessment of risk. *Medical Laboratory Sciences.* 1992; **49**: 103–6.
86. Thiebaut R, Leproust S, Chene G et al. Effectiveness of prenatal treatment for congenital toxoplasmosis: A meta-analysis of individual patients' data. *Lancet* 2007; **369**: 115–22.
87. Health Protection Agency. Infection risks during the lambing season. Last accessed October 20, 2009. Available from: www.hpa.org.uk/web/HPAweb&Page&HPAwebAutoListName/Page/1191942128199.
88. Nash D, Mostashari F, Fine A et al. The outbreak of West Nile virus infection in the New York City area in 1999. *New England Journal of Medicine.* 2001; **344**: 1807–14.
89. Weiss D, Carr D, Kellachan J et al. Clinical findings of West Nile virus infection in hospitalized patients, New York and New Jersey, 2000. *Emerging Infectious Diseases.* 2001; **7**: 654–7.
90. Campbell GL, Marfin AA, Lanciotti RS, Gubler DJ. West Nile virus. *Lancet Infectious Diseases.* 2002; **2**: 519–29.
91. Centers for Disease Control. Laboratory-acquired West Nile virus infections – United States, 2002. *Morbidity and Mortality Weekly Report.* 2002; **51**: 1133–5.
92. Centers for Disease Control. West Nile virus infection among turkey breeder farm workers – Wisconsin, 2002. *Morbidity and Mortality Weekly Reports.* 2003; **42**: 1017–19.
93. Idaho Department of Health and Welfare. West Nile virus found in bird in Gooding County (press release, August 26, 2004). Last accessed October 20, 2009. Available from: www.healthandwelfare.idaho.gov.
94. National Institute for Occupational Safety and Health. Recommendations for protecting outdoor workers from West Nile virus exposure. NIOSH publication No. 2005: 155. Atlanta, GA: NIOSH, September 2005.
95. National Institute for Occupational Safety and Health. Recommendations for protecting field, laboratory and clinical workers from West Nile virus exposure. NIOSH publication No. 2006: 115. Atlanta, GA: NIOSH, December 2005.
96. Tindall BJ, Grimont PAD, Garrity GM, Euzeby JP. Nomenclature and taxonomy of the genus Salmonella. *International Journal of Systematic and Evolutionary Microbiology.* 2005; **55**: 521–4.
97. Brenner FW, Villar RG, Angulo FJ et al. Salmonella nomenclature. *Journal of Clinical Microbiology.* 2000; **38**: 2465–7.
98. Woodward DL, Khakhria R, Johnson WM. Human salmonellosis associated with exotic pets. *Journal of Clinical Microbiology.* 1997; **37**: 2786–90.
99. Lee KM, McReynolds JL, Fuller CC et al. Investigation and characterisation of the frozen feeder rodent industry in Texas following a multi-state *Salmonella typhimurium* outbreak associated with frozen vacuum-packed rodents. *Zoonoses and Public Health.* 2008; **55**: 488–96.
100. Centers for Disease Control. Salmonella serotype enteritidis infections among workers producing poultry vaccine – Maine, November–December 2006. *Morbidity and Mortality Weekly Reports.* 2007; **56**: 877–9.
101. Kimura AC, Palumbo MS, Meyers H et al. A multi-state outbreak of *Salmonella* serotype Thompson infection from commercially distributed bread contaminated by an ill food handler. *Epidemiology and Infection.* 2005; **133**: 823–8.
102. Food Standards Agency. Food handlers: fitness to work. Regulatory guidance and best practice advice for food business operators. London: Food Standards Agency, 2008. Last accessed October 20, 2009. Available from: www.food.gov.uk.
103. Rice DH, Hancock DD, Roozen PM et al. Household contamination with *Salmonella enterica*. *Emerging Infectious Diseases.* 2003; **9**: 120–2.
104. Baker MG, Thornley CN, Lopez LD et al. A recurring salmonellosis epidemic in New Zealand linked to contact with sheep. *Epidemiology and Infection.* 2007; **135**: 76–83.
105. Helms M, Simonsen J, Molbak K. Quinolone resistance is associated with increased risk of invasive illness or death during infection with *Salmonella* serotype *Typhimurium*. *Journal of Infectious Diseases.* 2004; **190**: 1652–4.
106. Williams E. Veterinary surgeons as vectors of *Salmonella dublin*. *British Medical Journal.* 1980; **280**: 815–18.
107. Sirinavin S, Garner P. Antibiotics for treating salmonella gut infections. *Cochrane Database of Systematic Reviews.* 2000; (**2**): CD001167.
108. Moore JE, Corcoran D, Dooley JSG. Camplyobacter. *Veterinary Research.* 2005; **36**: 351–82.
109. Ternhag A, Asikainen T, Giesecke J et al. A meta-analysis on the effects of antibiotic treatment on duration of symptoms caused by infection with *Campylobacter* species. *Clinical Infectious Diseases.* 2007; **44**: 696–700.
110. Ellis A, Irwin R, Hockin J et al. Outbreak of *Campylobacter* infection among farm workers: An occupational hazard. *Canada Communicable Disease Report.* 1995; **21**: 153–6.
111. Heryford AG, Seys SA. Outbreak of occupational campylobacteriosis associated with a pheasant farm. *Journal of Agricultural Safety and Health.* 2004; **10**: 127–32.
112. Christenson B, Ringner A, Blucher C et al. An outbreak of *Campylobacter enteritis* among the staff of a poultry abattoir in Sweden. *Scandinavian Journal of Infectious Diseases.* 1982; **15**: 167–72.
113. Church-Potter R, Kaneene JB, Hall WN. Risk factors for sporadic *Campylobacter jejuni* infections in rural Michigan: A prospective case-control study. *American Journal of Public Health.* 2003; **93**: 2118–23.
114. Riley LW, Remis RS, Helgerson SD et al. Haemorrhagic colitis associated with a rare *Escherichia coli* serotype. *New England Journal of Medicine.* 1983; **308**: 681–5.
115. Waters JR, Sharp JC, Dev VJ. Infection caused by *Escherichia coli* O157:H7 in Alberta, Canada, and in

115. Scotland: a five-year review, 1987-1991. *Clinical Infectious Diseases.* 1994; **19**: 834-43.
116. Slutsker L, Ries AA, Greene KD et al. *Escherichia coli* O157:H7 diarrhea in the United States: Clinical and epidemiologic features. *Annals of Internal Medicine.* 1997; **126**: 505-13.
117. Garg AX, Suri RS, Barrowman N et al. Long term renal prognosis of diarrhoea-associated haemolytic-uraemic syndrome. *Journal of the American Medical Association.* 2003; **290**: 1360-70.
118. Health and Safety Executive. Agriculture information sheet number 23 (revised). Avoiding ill health at open farms: advice to farmers (with teachers' supplement). Last accessed October 20, 2009. Available from: www.hse.gov.uk/pubns/ais23.pdf.
119. Lengerich EJ, Addiss DG, Marx JJ et al. Increased exposure to cryptosporidia among dairy farmers in Wisconsin. *Journal of Infectious Diseases.* 1993; **167**: 1252-5.
120. Steere AC, Malawista SE, Snydman DR et al. Lyme arthritis: An epidemic of oligoarticular arthritis in children and adults in three Connecticut communities. *Arthritis and Rheumatism.* 1977; **20**: 7-17.
121. Burgdorfer W, Barbour AG, Hayes AF et al. Lyme disease – a tick borne spirochetosis? *Science.* 1982; **216**: 1317-9.
122. Steere AC. Lyme disease. *New England Journal of Medicine.* 2001; **345**: 115-25.
123. Steere AC, Levin RE, Molloy PJ et al. Treatment of Lyme arthritis. *Arthritis and Rheumatism.* 1994; **37**: 878-88.
124. Logigian EL, Kaplan RF, Steere AC. Chronic neurologic manifestations of Lyme disease. *New England Journal of Medicine.* 1990; **323**: 1438-44.
125. Dressler F, Whalen JA, Reinhardt BN, Steere AC. Western blotting in the serodiagnosis of Lyme disease. *Journal of Infectious Diseases.* 1993; **167**: 392-400.
126. Wormser GP, Dattwyler RJ, Shapiro ED. The clinical assessment, treatment, and prevention of Lyme disease, human granulocytic anaplasmosis, and babesiosis: Clinical Practice Guidelines by the Infectious Diseases Society of America. *Clinical Infectious Diseases.* 2006; **43**: 1089-134.
127. Feder HM, Johnson BJB, O'Connell S et al. A critical appraisal of chronic Lyme disease. *New England Journal of Medicine.* 2007; **357**: 1422-30.
128. Health Protection Agency. HPA statement on IDSA guidelines on Lyme disease diagnosis and treatment. May 21, 2009. Last accessed September 18, 2009. Available from: www.hpa.nhs.uk/web/HPAweb&HPAwebStandard/HPAweb_C/1213603246853.
129. Sheard K, Hicks DG. Skin lesions among fishermen at Houtman's Abrolhos, Western Australia, with an account of erysipeloid of Rosenbach. *Medical Journal of Australia.* 1949; **2**: 352-4.
130. Reboli AC, Farrar WE. *Erysipelothrix rhusiopathiae*: An occupational pathogen. *Clinical Microbiology Reviews.* 1989; **2**: 354-9.
131. McLaughlin J, Low JC. Primary cutaneous listeriosis in adults: An occupational disease of veterinarians and farmers. *Veterinary Record.* 1994; **135**: 615-17.
132. Croft DR, Sotir MJ, Williams CJ et al. Occupational risks during a monkeypox outbreak, Wisconsin, 2003. *Emerging Infectious Diseases.* 2007; **13**: 1150-7.
133. Aubry A, Chosidwa O, Caumes E et al. Sixty-three cases of *Mycobacterium marinum* infection: Clinical features, treatment, and antibiotic susceptibility of causative isolates. *Archives of Internal Medicine.* 2002; **162**: 1746-52.
134. Schmoor P, Descamps V, Bouscarat F et al. Tropical fish salesmen's knowledge and behavior concerning 'fish tank granuloma'. *Annales de Dermatologie et de Vénéréologie.* 2003; **130**: 425-7.
135. Centers for Disease Control. Orf virus infection in humans – New York, Illinois, California, and Tennessee, 2004-2005. *Morbidity and Mortality Weekly Report.* 2006; **55**: 65-8.
136. Geernick K, Lukito G, Snoeck R et al. A case of human orf in an immunocompromised patient treated successfully with cidofovir cream. *Journal of Medical Virology.* 2001; **64**: 543-9.
137. Buchan J. Characteristics of orf in a farming community in mid-Wales. *British Medical Journal.* 1996; **313**: 203-4. Last accessed September 18, 2009. Available from: www.bmj.com/cgi/content/full/313/7051/203.
138. Paiba GA, Thomas DR, Morgan KL et al. Orf (contagious pustular dermatitis) in farmworkers: Prevalence and risk in three areas of England. *Veterinary Record.* 1999; **145**: 7-11.
139. Eckert J, Gemmell MA, Meslin F-X, Pawlowski ZS (eds). *WHO/OIE manual on echinococcosis in humans and animals: A public health problem of global concern.* Paris: World Organization for Animal Health, 2001. Last accessed September 30, 2009. Available from: whqlibdoc.who.int/publications/2001/929044522X.pdf.
140. Buishi I, Walters T, Guildea Z et al. Re-emergence of canine echinococcosis infection, Wales. *Emerging Infectious Diseases.* 2005; **11**: 568-71.
141. Warrell MJ, Warrell DA. Rabies and other lyssaviruses. *Lancet.* 2004; **363**: 959-69.
142. Cliquet F, Picard-Meyer E. Rabies and rabies-related viruses: A modern perspective on an ancient disease. *Revue Scientifique et Technique (International Office of Epizootics).* 2004; **23**: 625-42.
143. Nathwani D, McIntyre PG, White K et al. Fatal human rabies caused by European bat lyssavirus type 2a infection in Scotland. *Clinical Infectious Diseases.* 2003; **37**: 598-601.
144. Department for Environment, Food and Rural Affairs. UK Zoonoses report 2006. Last updated July 20, 2009. Available from: www.defra.gov.uk/animalh/diseases/zoonoses/ncp.htm.

SECTION TWO

Bioterrorism and biotechnology

61 Bioterrorism 773
    Julia Heptonstall
62 Genetic modification and biotechnology 782
    David Roomes

61

Bioterrorism

JULIA HEPTONSTALL

Introduction	773	Emergency preparedness	778
Smallpox	774	References	779
Anthrax	774		

INTRODUCTION

The use of microorganisms with intent to cause harm or fear has a long history. Ancient Persian, Greek and Roman manuscripts describe the use of decaying bodies to contaminate water sources; the Tartars, laying siege to Caffa in 1346, catapulted the corpses of plague victims over the city walls, and during the French and Indian War (1754–67) the British forces attempted to spread smallpox amongst American Indians by distributing blankets from a smallpox hospital.[1,2] In the early twentieth century, interest in the hostile uses of pathogens developed in parallel with increasing understanding of the effects of specific pathogens and other technological advances, which included industrial-scale production of microorganisms. Although the Geneva Protocol of 1925 proscribed the use of biological weapons by signatory states, it does not prevent their possession or development, and many nations, including Canada, France, Great Britain, the United States and the former Soviet Union invested in bioweapons research.[3] These programmes, which were not without occupational risk (456 cases of laboratory-acquired infection occurred between 1942 and 1969 in workers at Fort Detrick, United States, including two fatal cases of anthrax and one fatal case of viral encephalitis[4]) had largely been terminated by the 1970s. The 1972 Biological Weapons Convention – which has over 140 nation-state signatories – prohibits the development, production or stockpiling of biological agents (or their toxins) in 'quantities that have no justification for prophylactic, protective or other peaceful purposes'.[3] However, in some states, notably the Russian Federation and Iraq, offensive bioweapons research continued until at least the early 1990s.[5] In 1979, the accidental release and airborne spread of anthrax spores from a research facility in Sverdlovsk caused more than 60 deaths from inhalational anthrax in the surrounding community, and in 1990, immediately before the Gulf War, concern about a possible threat resulted in the vaccination of more than 150 000 coalition military personnel against anthrax.[6,7] The revelation that Iraq had developed bioweapons, the deliberate release of sarin gas on the Tokyo subway by the Aum Shinrikyo sect in 1995, and fears that a sharp decline in financial support might have compromised biosecurity in laboratories in Russia and the former Soviet Union provided the impetus for a detailed review series that examined the potential use of specific pathogens as bioweapons and encouraged policy-makers and planners to ensure that health and other civilian services were adequately prepared to deal with the potential threat of bioterrorism.[8–11]

In the last 50 years, there have been only five reported incidents involving the intentional release of pathogens. Four involved gastrointestinal or foodborne pathogens (*Salmonella typhi*, *Salmonella enteritidis*, *Shigella dysenteriae* and *Ascaris suum*). In the largest of these incidents, over 700 people developed symptoms after eating from salad bars in two restaurants in Dalles, OR, in 1984, though the source of the outbreak was not recognized until late in 1985, when it was discovered that followers of Baghwan Shree Rajneesh had deliberately contaminated salads with cultures of *S. enteritidis*.[12–15] In 2001, however, the attacks on the World Trade Center and the Pentagon were followed, a month later, by an outbreak of anthrax caused by deliberate dissemination of anthrax spores via the US Postal Service.[16] These events stimulated a period of intense public health activity at international and national levels, focused initially on improving biosecurity and emergency preparedness for bioterrorism, but which now seek to ensure that preparedness planning for bioterrorist threats is integrated in a more rational, generic 'all-hazards' approach, with planning for infectious disease emergencies (including pandemic influenza), natural disasters and other public health emergencies.

The Centers for Disease Control (CDC) in the United States has combined the risk assessment concepts used to develop laboratory biosafety guidance (which assign pathogens to a risk category by considering the severity of human infection, transmission potential and the availability of effective treatment or prophylaxis) with assessments of ease of dissemination and estimates of the overall impact that any accidental or deliberate dissemination of the pathogen would have, and used the results to identify the pathogens for which preparedness is most essential. These 'category A agents' are: variola virus (smallpox), *Bacillus anthracis* (anthrax), *Yersinia pestis* (plague), *Clostridium botulinum* toxin (botulism), *Francisella tularensis* (tularaemia), filoviruses (Ebola and Marburg haemorrhagic fevers) and arenaviruses (Lassa fever). 'Category B agents' include *Burkholderia pseudomallei* (melioidosis), *Burkholderia mallei* (glanders), *Coxiella burnetii* (Q fever), and *Brucella abortus*, *B. suis* and *B. melitensis* (brucellosis), staphylococcal enterotoxin B, and Venezuelan equine encephalitis virus.[17] The global eradication of smallpox was certified in 1980, and infections caused by the other agents listed above are rare in industrialized countries, where few clinicians will have direct clinical experience of them. It is nevertheless essential that all clinicians maintain a working knowledge of their epidemiology, clinical features, differential diagnosis and initial investigation and management (Table 61.1). Extensive web-based and other training materials, including pathogen-specific guidelines, fact sheets, slide sets and decision-based algorithms for clinical management, have been developed since 2001, can be readily accessed through national authorities' websites and are particularly useful for self-directed learning when formal face-to-face training is not readily available.[18–20]

SMALLPOX

The last community-acquired case of smallpox – a severe infection with a case-fatality rate of around 30 per cent in susceptible people – occurred in Somalia in 1977. The last case of laboratory-acquired infection occurred in Birmingham, UK, in 1978.[21] Smallpox (variola) virus is now held only in two secure repositories, in Russia and the United States, and research work on the virus is strictly regulated. Routine smallpox vaccination programmes ceased around 30 years ago, although vaccination is still recommended for those who directly handle vaccinia (smallpox vaccine) virus cultures, infected dressings or other potentially infectious materials, recombinant vaccinia virus or other orthopox viruses (e.g. monkeypox), or handle animals infected or contaminated with any of these viruses.[22] In the pre-outbreak setting, vaccination is contraindicated in those who have atopic dermatitis, eczema or any other active or chronic skin condition involving the epidermis, are pregnant or immunosuppressed, or have a close contact who has any of these conditions. Adverse events after smallpox vaccination include inadvertent inoculation, generalized vaccinia, eczema vaccinatum, fetal vaccinia, progressive vaccinia and post-vaccinial encephalomyelitis.[23] In 2001, concerns about the possible bioterrorist use of smallpox led many industrialized countries to develop national smallpox preparedness plans, to stockpile vaccine supplies and to vaccinate selected military personnel and healthcare workers in 'smallpox response teams' – infectious disease clinicians, public health workers and first responders – who would be involved in the diagnosis and immediate management of any initial cases. In the most extensive programme, in the United States, 39 566 civilian volunteers had been vaccinated by June 2004; vaccination of military personnel is ongoing, but more than 1.4 million defence staff and contract workers had been vaccinated by June 2007.[24–26] Since so few clinicians were expected to have experience of smallpox vaccination, intense preparation and training were required: around 1.7 million people accessed the smallpox training materials provided on the CDC website, and the 318 people who attended central 'train the trainers' courses subsequently trained a further 15 349 people in disease recognition, differential diagnosis of fever rash-illness syndromes, pre-vaccination screening, vaccination technique (which requires multiple punctures with a bifurcated needle) and vaccination site care and follow up.[25] Adverse events mostly occurred at, or below, the frequency expected, perhaps because the civilian programme (though not the military programme) preferentially selected workers with a history of previous smallpox vaccination and because of the intensive education on deferring those at risk and on vaccine site care. Safety monitoring also confirmed an association between vaccination and myo/pericarditis, but did not confirm an association between vaccination and ischaemic cardiac events, though amended selection criteria for pre-event vaccination exclude people with a history of ischaemic heart disease, or three or more cardiac risk factors (including hypercholesterolaemia, smoking, diabetes and hypertension), or an immediate family member with onset of cardiac disease before the age of 50 years.[27–29]

ANTHRAX

Anthrax is a zoonosis, caused by *Bacillus anthracis*, which primarily affects sheep, cattle and goats. The organism has a spore form that is extremely well adapted for environmental survival and can persist in soil for decades: Gruinard Island, off the northwest coast of Scotland, was contaminated during experiments in the 1940s; spores remained detectable until the island was decontaminated in 1987.[30] Naturally acquired human infection follows contact with an infected animal, carcass or animal product (e.g. hide, wool, bone). The clinical features of infection depend on the route of exposure to the spores: contact with abraded skin (e.g. while butchering an animal or handling a hide) causes cutaneous anthrax; breathing the spores

Table 61.1 Potential bioterror agents: Clinical features and differential diagnoses.

Infection	Incubation period (median, range)	Clinical features	Differential diagnosis	Additional facts
Smallpox (Variola virus)	12 days (range 7–19 days)	Abrupt onset moderate fever, severe prostration Evolving rash (maculopapular > vesicular > pustular); begins on day 3 of illness Rash denser on face and extremities; all pocks on any one part of body at same stage of development Death can occur early, before rash develops	Febrile prodrome: influenza, malaria, meningitis Erythematous stage: measles, rubella, parvovirus B19 Papular stage: measles, chickenpox Later rash: chickenpox, monkeypox, drug rash, disseminated herpes simplex, hand foot and mouth disease, disseminated herpes zoster, contact dermatitis, erythema multiforme	Eradication certified 1980 Public health emergency: seek immediate public health advice Transmission usually airborne, but also occurs via contact with vesicle fluid, saliva, scabs or virus-contaminated fomites Airborne infection isolation essential Treatment is supportive; mortality rate in outbreaks 25–30% Tracing and post-exposure vaccination of contacts essential Asymptomatic, afebrile contacts are not infectious
Anthrax (Bacillus anthracis)	1–7 days (range 1–60 days)	Depend on route of exposure (contact, inhalation, ingestion) Cutaneous anthrax: fever, painless skin lesion evolves over 2–6 days to form black eschar, extensive local oedema, lymphadenopathy Pulmonary anthrax: fever, malaise, rapid onset sepsis, non-productive cough, dyspnoea, wide mediastinum on x-ray, haemorrhagic meningitis	Cutaneous: staphylococcal or streptococcal cellulitis, necrotizing soft tissue infection, orf, ecthyma gangrenosum, brown recluse spider bite, rickettsial pox, tularaemia Pulmonary: pneumonic plague (haemoptysis uncommon in anthrax), severe community-acquired pneumonia, tularaemia	Naturally acquired human anthrax is the result of contact with an infected animal, carcass or animal product; now rare in industrialized countries, but remains endemic elsewhere Occupational risks: working with animals or animal hides (e.g. drum-making), skins or hair, or working with the organism in the laboratory No person-to-person transmission: standard infection control precautions sufficient Cutaneous disease responds rapidly to antibiotic therapy; high mortality in pulmonary anthrax despite multidrug regimens
Plague (Yersinia pestis)	2–4 days (range 1–8 days)	Depend on route of exposure	Bubonic plague: staphylococcal/streptococcal adenitis, cat scratch disease, lymphogranuloma venereum, chancroid, strangulated inguinal hernia, tularaemia, syphilis, mycobacterial infection	Naturally acquired human disease is zoonotic, usually bubonic form, the result of a bite from an infected flea

(Continued)

Table 61.1 Continued

Infection	Incubation period (median, range)	Clinical features	Differential diagnosis	Additional facts
		Bubonic plague: fever; bubo – a swollen, very painful, tender lymph node (usually in the groin, axilla or on the neck); overlying skin is red and indurated, usually unilateral; hypotension, confusion	Pneumonic plague: severe community acquired pneumonia (*Streptococcus pneumoniae*, *Staphylococcus aureus*, etc.), hantavirus infection, anthrax (but haemoptysis uncommon), tularaemia, non-infective causes of haemoptysis	1500–3000 reported cases worldwide each year from Africa, Asia and Americas (including US)
		Pneumonic plague: fever, severe malaise; cough, increasing dyspnoea; watery, bloody sputum; chest pain; respiratory failure		Person-to-person transmission of pneumonic (but not bubonic or septicaemic) plague can occur: respiratory + standard infection control precautions required; post-exposure antibiotic prophylaxis for close contacts Occupational risks: laboratory work on organism; in endemic areas outside UK, animal trapping, hunting or skinning
Botulism (*Clostridium botulinum* toxins A–G)	1–3 days (range <1–8 days)	Symmetrical descending flaccid paralysis	Guillain–Barré syndrome	Toxins lethal, but inactivated by normal cooking of food and chlorination of water
		Alert, afebrile, with normal sensation	Myasthenia gravis	Toxin blocks acetylcholine release at neuromuscular junction
		Early prominent bilateral cranial nerve signs: facial weakness, ptosis, dysphonia, dysarthria, diplopia, dysphagia	Lambert–Eaton syndrome	Natural food-borne disease rare in UK, less so where home-canning common
		Respiratory failure, death	Organophosphates, belladonna, other toxins	Mortality reduced by early antitoxin administration (usually held by national public health authority) and good supportive care
			Stroke or CNS mass lesion	No person-to-person transmission: standard infection control precautions sufficient
			CNS viral infection, polio	
Tularaemia (*Francisella tularensis*)	3–5 days (range 1–14 days)	Depend on route of exposure: inhalation causes pneumonia; infection via bite or abraded skin causes ulcero/glandular disease; ingestion causes oropharyngeal disease; eye inoculation causes oculoglandular disease; all can disseminate, to sepsis syndrome	Differential diagnosis broad, initial symptoms non-specific and diagnosis easily missed:	Zoonosis, common in parts of rural Europe (not UK), Asia, Americas and Australasia, with small mammal reservoirs, e.g. rabbit, lemming, vole, muskrat

Disease	Incubation	Symptoms	Differential diagnosis	Comments
		Fever, malaise, headache, plus tender local lymphadenopathy ± painful ulcer/exudate at site of infection	Local disease: orf, anthrax, syphilis, herpes simplex infection, chancroid, staphylococcal/streptococcal infection, cat scratch disease, mycobacterial infection, rickettsial infection, sporotrichosis	Naturally acquired human disease follows exposure by: bite of infected vector (tick, mosquito, deerfly); handling infected animal or carcass; breathing infected aerosol (from infected animal or carcass, contaminated hay, lawn mowing); eating contaminated food or water
				Occupational risks: laboratory work; hunting, trapping, or farming
				Deliberate release most likely to be via aerosol, causing pneumonic tularaemia
				Very low risk of person-to-person spread: use standard precautions
		Pneumonia: fever, dry cough, pleuritic pain	Pneumonia: community-acquired pneumonia (bacterial or viral), Q fever, tuberculosis, lung abscess/empyema, anthrax, plague	Mortality low given appropriate antibiotic therapy (aminoglycoside or quinolone)
Viral haemorrhagic fever (including Marburg, Lassa, Congo Crimean haemorrhagic fever and Ebola viruses and others, e.g. dengue virus)	Disease-specific (range 1–21 days)	Febrile prodrome (fever, malaise, nausea, vomiting, myalgia, prostration) of up to seven days, followed by signs of vascular involvement	Malaria	All are zoonoses; distribution of natural disease is governed by the geographic distribution and ecology of the animal reservoir
		In second week of illness, cases either recover or deteriorate rapidly	Typhoid, shigellosis	Imported cases are rare in industrialized countries
		High mortality in outbreaks, particularly for filoviruses	Meningitis	High risk of person-to-person spread via percutaneous or mucocutaneous exposure to blood or infected body fluids; nosocomial amplification of outbreaks
			Leptospirosis	Occupational risk for: healthcare workers, laboratory workers
			Tularaemia, plague	Asymptomatic afebrile contacts are not infectious
			Other causes of DIC (including Gram-negative sepsis, leukaemia, lymphoma, liver failure	Ribavirin effective against Lassa virus and Congo Crimean haemorrhagic fever virus

CNS, central nervous system; DIC, disseminated intravascular coagulation.

causes pulmonary anthrax; eating undercooked spore-contaminated meat causes gastrointestinal anthrax. There are an estimated 2000–20 000 cases of human anthrax each year, largely in countries where animal infection is still endemic; human anthrax in industrialized countries is rare. Cutaneous infection accounts for 95 per cent of reported cases.[31]

The intentional dissemination of anthrax via the US Postal Service (USPS) in 2001, in envelopes containing *B. anthracis*-positive powder and addressed to prominent media or government figures, led to 22 cases of anthrax (11 pulmonary, 11 cutaneous) among residents in seven states in the eastern United States. These were the first cases of pulmonary anthrax in the USA since 1976; five (45 per cent) were fatal.[16,32–37] Cases occurred in two clusters, associated with at least two separate mailings of spore-containing envelopes. Most occurred in people who worked either at the USPS sites through which the contaminated mail passed (mail processor, three cases; mail worker, four cases; mail machine mechanic, one case) or at sites where the contaminated mail was received (government office or media company mail room worker, three cases; media company employee, six cases). Widespread contamination with anthrax spores was detected at these sites by environmental testing. Cases also included a seven-month-old infant, who was probably exposed while visiting one of the media companies, and four other people (a mail carrier, a book-keeper, a hospital storeroom worker and a retired elderly female) who were thought to have become infected after exposure to mail that had been cross-contaminated as it passed through the postal system.[38] It was not initially realized that anthrax spores could leak through sealed, intact envelopes, and lack of familiarity with the clinical signs of cutaneous anthrax (which should be included in the differential diagnosis of an unusual skin lesion, particularly if the lesion is relatively painless, but is accompanied by intense, extensive oedema) may have led to delays in diagnosis of the cases in the first cluster, many of which had already occurred before the index case of pulmonary anthrax was diagnosed in Florida by an alert clinician who had recently undergone bioterrorism preparedness training. Post-exposure antimicrobial prophylaxis (a 60-day course of ciprofloxacin, doxycycline or amoxicillin) was recommended for approximately 10 000 people assessed as being at risk of pulmonary anthrax; no cases of anthrax occurred in this group. In a follow-up study, over half of those (3032/5343; 57 per cent) who reported taking at least one dose of prophylaxis reported adverse events during treatment. Fewer than half (2712, 44 per cent) reported completing the 60-day course; reasons for stopping treatment reported by the 2631 who did not complete the course included: adverse events (43 per cent); low perceived risk of anthrax (25 per cent) and concerns about the effects of long-term antimicrobial use (7 per cent).[39,40]

Health and safety guidance for workers at sites where mail is handled or processed is designed to reduce the potential for inhalational or cutaneous exposure to anthrax spores, and emphasizes the importance of risk assessment-based selection of control measures. These include engineering controls (e.g. avoiding the use of compressed air to clean machinery and advice to use industrial vacuum cleaners fitted with HEPA filters to clean high-speed mail sorting machinery); administrative controls (developing strategies to limit the numbers of personnel and visitors exposed); housekeeping (e.g. using 'wet' dusting techniques in preference to 'dry' dusting) and the selection and use of appropriate personal protective equipment, which may include protective clothing, gloves and masks or respirators. All workers who process, handle or receive mail should be trained to recognize and manage a 'suspect package', and every worksite should have an emergency plan that describes the actions that should be taken if a suspect package incident or a potential exposure to *B. anthracis* occurs.[41,42] Pre-exposure vaccination is recommended for laboratory workers who will work directly with the organism or with high-risk specimens, and for occupational groups at risk of exposure to infected animals or their byproducts.[43]

EMERGENCY PREPAREDNESS

It is important that all clinicians remain open to the possibility that a deliberate release may occur – and that they may be the first to recognize it. Clinicians must be prepared to consult urgently with their local infectious disease specialist, clinical microbiologist or public health department on the basis of suspicion alone, and should keep a regularly updated list of relevant emergency contacts. Although the initial cases in any deliberate release are most likely to present to primary care or emergency medicine clinicians, occupational health clinicians are well placed to identify unusual or unexpected sickness absence, and should remain alert for changes in expected patterns and for the case that 'just doesn't fit'. Examples include an unusual number of cases of the same illness presenting in a short time-frame; an illness unusual for the time of year (influenza in summer); an illness unusual for the patient's age group (chicken pox in a middle-aged adult) or with an unusual clinical presentation (chicken pox rash concentrated on the extremities), or an illness, or report of a diagnosis of an illness acquired in an unusual place (e.g. tularaemia in a worker who has not travelled outside the United Kingdom).

As a result of the resurgence in biodefence-related research, and the recent expansion in the numbers of BSL3 and BSL4 (high and maximum containment) laboratories, more laboratory workers are working with category A and other high-risk pathogens than at any time in the last 50 years, increasing the risks of occupational exposure and occupationally acquired infection. Since 2000, there have been reports of occupationally acquired glanders (in a worker in a military research laboratory; the first case of glanders in the United States since 1945);[44,45] tularaemia (three cases, in research scientists working on vaccine development using an attenuated strain of *F. tularensis* that was subsequently found to have become contaminated with a virulent strain);[46] staphylococcal enterotoxin B-related illness (three cases, in workers in a military research laboratory between 1989 and 2002)[47] and Ebola haemorrhagic fever (a research scientist in a Russian laboratory who developed infection and died after a needlestick injury sustained while working with ebolavirus-infected guinea pigs in 2004;[48] in the same year a virologist in a military laboratory in the United States was isolated, but did not become infected, after scratch from a needle potentially contaminated with ebolavirus;[49] a similar incident occurred in Germany in 2009).[50] Laboratory workers in clinical laboratories may be exposed while working on diagnostic or surveillance-related samples (a case of cutaneous anthrax was reported in a laboratory worker in Texas who processed environmental samples associated with the 2001 anthrax outbreak),[51] or during laboratory proficiency testing. In 2007, a US laboratory participating in an exercise designed to test laboratory preparedness inadvertently processed a test sample containing *B. abortus* RB51 on the open bench, potentially exposing 24 laboratory workers to the organism, which, although attenuated, has been associated with human infection. Written information about safe processing had been provided with the test samples, but further investigation identified 916 potentially exposed workers in 254 of the 1316 laboratories involved in the exercise. Post-exposure prophylaxis was recommended for workers assessed as having had a high-risk exposure; no infections were identified.[52]

Guidelines on laboratory biosafety advise that laboratory workers should have access to expert occupational health advice, including, where appropriate, pre-exposure prophylaxis. An occupational history is an integral part of the initial management of any sick patient, and, if a laboratory or animal house worker presents with an unexplained febrile illness, further information should be sought urgently from the laboratory director about the agents to which the patient may have been exposed, regardless of whether the patient can recall a specific exposure. Workers in BSL3 or BSL4 laboratories require a pre-employment medical examination and should carry and use 'medical contact' cards.[53] Provision of occupational health care for workers in BSL-4 laboratories is highly specialized and presents special challenges and effective care provision requires close collaboration between the laboratory and the occupational health clinician.[54,55] Occupational infection may result from trivial or inapparent exposure, and since the initial signs and symptoms of laboratory-acquired infection may be non-specific, systems for monitoring and follow up of unexplained worker absence should be in place. Facilities working with, or storing, risk group 3 or risk group 4 pathogens should have a written contingency plan for dealing with accidents and other emergencies, based on a thorough biorisk assessment, and containing operational procedures for immediate incident management, decontamination, surveillance and emergency and clinical management of exposed people, with relevant contact details so that access to specialist medical advice can be rapidly obtained. Guidelines on the evaluation and management of exposures to potential bioterror agents have been published.[54] It is recommended that all procedures and protocols should be tested and practised through a programme of regular drills or exercises, thus improving emergency preparedness.

Preparedness for a bioterrorist incident – a 'low likelihood, high impact' event – should be integrated with major incident and business continuity planning; occupational health clinicians have key roles to play in such planning. All major events – whether accidents, natural disasters or outbreaks caused by newly emergent infections – and the fear and uncertainty associated with them – have profound psychosocial effects on individuals and communities. Provision of, and access to, psychosocial support for those involved, either directly, or indirectly, is essential.

Key points

- The risk of a bioterror event is small, but real.
- Integrated preparedness planning of emergency responses is essential.
- Occupational health clinicians have key roles to play in planning, surveillance, response and recovery.
- Know the main clinical features of illnesses caused by potential bioterror agents.
- Remain alert to the unusual and the unexpected – and be prepared to consult urgently with local public health clinicians on suspicion.

REFERENCES

1. Christopher GW, Cieslak TJ, Pavlin JA, Eitzen EM Jr. Biological warfare. A historical perspective. *Journal of the American Medical Association.* 1997; **278**: 412–17.
2. Wheelis M. Biological warfare at the 1346 Siege of Caffa. *Emerging Infectious Diseases.* 2002; **8**: 971–5.
3. World Health Organization. Public health response to biological weapons: WHO guidance (2004). Geneva: World Health Organization, 2004.
4. United States Army Medical Research Institute into Infectious Diseases. *Medical management of biological casualties*, 6th edn. Frederick, MD: USAMRIID, 2005.
5. Monterey Institute of International Studies. Chemical and biological weapons resource page. Chemical and biological weapons: Possession and programs past and present. Monterey, CA: Monterey Institute of International Studies, 2002. Last accessed April 6, 2009. Available from: http://cns.miis.edu/cbw/possess.htm.

6. Meselson M, Guillemin V, Hugh-Jones M et al. The Sverdlovsk anthrax outbreak of 1979. *Science.* 1994; **266**: 1202-8.
7. Department of Defense. Information paper: Vaccine use during the Gulf War. Department of Defense, December 2000. Last accessed April 5, 2009. Available from: www.gulflink.osd.mil/va/index.htm.
8. Zillinskas RA. Iraq's biological weapons: The past as future? *Journal of the American Medical Association.* 1997; **278**: 418-24.
9. Okumura T, Takasu N, Ishimatsu S et al. Report on 640 victims of the Tokyo subway sarin attack. *Annals of Emergency Medicine.* 1996; **28**: 129-35.
10. Henderson DA. Bioterrorism as a public health threat. *Emerging Infectious Diseases.* 1998; **4**: 488-92.
11. Henderson DA, Inglesby TV, O Toole T. *Bioterrorism: Guidelines for medical and public health management.* Chicago, IL: American Medical Association, 2002.
12. Anonymous. Deliberate spreading of typhoid in Japan. *Science Journal.* 1966; **2**: 11-12.
13. Torok TJ, Tauxe RV, Wise RP et al. A large community outbreak of salmonellosis caused by intentional contamination of restaurant salad bars. *Journal of the American Medical Association.* 1997; **278**: 389-95.
14. Kolavic SA, Kimura A, Simons SL et al. An outbreak of *Shigella dysenteriae* type 2 among laboratory workers due to intentional food contamination. *Journal of the American Medical Association.* 1997; **278**: 396-8.
15. Phills JA, Harrold AJ, Whiteman GV, Perelmutter L. Pulmonary infiltrates, asthma and eosinophilia due to *Ascaris suum* infestation in man. *New England Journal of Medicine.* 1972; **286**: 965-70.
16. Jernigan JA, Stephens DS, Ashford DA et al. Bioterrorism-related inhalational anthrax: The first 10 cases reported in the United States. *Emerging Infectious Diseases* 2001; **7**: 933-44.
17. Centers for Disease Control and Prevention. Biological and chemical terrorism: Strategic plan for preparedness and response. Recommendations of the CDC Strategic Planning Workgroup. *Morbidity and Mortality Weekly Reports.* 2000; **49**: 1-14.
18. Centers for Disease Control and Prevention. Emergency preparedness and response. Emergency A-Z. Last accessed April 5, 2009. Available from: www.bt.cdc.gov.
19. Heptonstall J, Gent N. *CBRN incidents: Clinical management and health protection.* London: Health Protection Agency, 2005. Revised version4, September 2008. Last accessed April 2, 2009. Available from: www.hpa.org.uk/web/HPAwebFile/HPAweb_C/1194947377166.
20. European Network of Infectious Diseases (EUNID). Compendium of national guidelines on highly infectious diseases. Last accessed April 5, 2009. Available from: www.eunid.com/privato/registered/guidelines2.asp.
21. Henderson DA, Inglesby TV, Bartlett JG et al. Smallpox as a biological weapon; medical and public health management. Working Group on Civilian Biodefense. *Journal of the American Medical Association.* 1999; **281**: 2127-37.
22. Centers for Disease Control and Prevention. Vaccinia (smallpox) vaccine: Recommendations of the Advisory Committee on Immunization Practices (ACIP), 2001. *Morbidity and Mortality Weekly Reports.* 2001; **50**: 1-25.
23. Centers for Disease Control and Prevention. Smallpox vaccination and adverse reactions: guidance for clinicians. *Morbidity and Mortality Weekly Reports.* 2003; **52**: 1-28.
24. Centers for Disease Control and Prevention. Recommendations for using smallpox vaccine in a pre-event smallpox vaccination program. Supplemental recommendations of ACIP and HICPAC. *Morbidity and Mortality Weekly Reports.* 2003; **52**: 1-16.
25. Strikas RA, Neff LJ, Rotz L et al. US Civilian Smallpox Preparedness and Response Program, 2003. *Clinical Infectious Diseases.* 2008; **46**: S157-67.
26. Center for Infectious Disease Research and Policy (CIDRAP) News. US military switching to new smallpox vaccine. February 8, 2008. Last accessed April 2, 2009. Available from: www.cidrap.umn.edu/cidrap/content/bt/smallpox/news/feb0808smallpox.html.
27. Morgan H, Roper MH, Sperling L et al. Myocarditis, pericarditis, and dilated cardiomyopathy after smallpox vaccination among civilians in the United States, January-October 2003. *Clinical Infectious Diseases.* 2008; **46**: S242-50.
28. Neff J, Modlin J, Birkhead GS et al. Monitoring the safety of a smallpox vaccination program in the United States: Report of the Joint Smallpox Vaccine Safety Working Group of the Advisory Committee on Immunization Practices and the Armed Forces Epidemiological Board. *Clinical Infectious Diseases.* 2008; **46**: S258-70.
29. Centers for Disease Control and Prevention. Notice to readers: Supplemental recommendations on adverse events following smallpox vaccine in the pre-event vaccination program: Recommendations of the Advisory Committee on Immunization Practices. *Morbidity and Mortality Weekly Reports.* 2003; **52**: 282-4.
30. Manchee RJ, Broster MG, Stagg AJ et al. Out of Gruinard Island. *Salisbury Medical Bulletin.* 1990; **68** (Special suppl.): 17-18.
31. Inglesby TV, O'Toole T, Henderson DA et al. for the Working Group on Civilian Biodefense. Anthrax as a biological weapon, 2002: Updated recommendations for management. *Journal of the American Medical Association.* 2002; **287**: 2236-52.
32. Bush LM, Abrams BH, Beall A, Johnson CC. Index case of fatal inhalational anthrax due to bioterrorism in the United States. *New England Journal of Medicine.* 2001; **50**: 973-6.
33. Borio L, Frank D, Mani V et al. Death due to bioterrorism-related anthrax; report of 2 patients. *Journal of the American Medical Association.* 2001; **286**: 2554-9.
34. Mayer TA, Bersoff-Matcha S, Murphy C et al. Clinical presentation of inhalational anthrax following bioterrorism

exposure: Report of 2 surviving patients. *Journal of the American Medical Association.* 2001; **286**: 2549–53.
35. Mina B, Dym JP, Kuepper *et al.* Fatal inhalational anthrax with unknown source of exposure in a 61-year old woman in New York City. *Journal of the American Medical Association.* 2002; **287**: 858–62.
36. Freedman A, Afonja O, Chang MW *et al.* Cutaneous anthrax associated with microangiopathic hemolytic anemia and coagulopathy in a 7-month old infant. *Journal of the American Medical Association.* 2002; **287**: 869–74.
37. Barakat LA, Quentzel HL, Jernigan JA *et al.* Fatal inhalational anthrax in a 94-year old Connecticut woman. *Journal of the American Medical Association.* 2002; **287**: 863–8.
38. Jernigan DB, Raghunathan PL, Bell BP *et al.* Investigation of bioterrorism-related anthrax, United States, 2001: Epidemiologic findings. *Emerging Infectious Diseases.* 2002; **8**: 1019–28.
39. Centers for Disease Control and Prevention. Update: Investigation of bioterrorism-related anthrax and interim guidelines for exposure management and antimicrobial therapy, October 2001. *Morbidity and Mortality Weekly Reports.* 2001; **50**: 909–19.
40. Shepard CW, Soriano-Gabarro M, Zell ER *et al.* Antimicrobial postexposure prophylaxis for anthrax: Adverse events and adherence. *Emerging Infectious Diseases.* 2002; **8**: 1124–32.
41. Centers for Disease Control and Prevention. Official Health Advisory. Interim recommendations for protecting workers from exposure to *Bacillus anthracis* in work sites where mail is handled or processed (updated from CDC Health Advisory 45 issued 10/24/01). October 31, 2001. Last accessed April 5, 2009. Available from: www2a.cdc.gov/HAN/ArchiveSys/ViewMsgV.asp?AlertNum=00051.
42. US Postal Inspection Service. Publication 166: Guide to Mail Center security. USPIS, March 2008. Last accessed April 5, 2009. Available from: www.usps.com/cpim/ftp/pubs/pub166/welcome.htm.
43. Centers for Disease Control and Prevention. Use of anthrax vaccine in the United States: Recommendations of the Advisory Committee on Immunization Practices. *Morbidity and Mortality Weekly Reports.* 2000; **40**: 1–20.
44. Srinivasan A, Kraus CN, DeShazer D *et al.* Glanders in a military research microbiologist. *New England Journal of Medicine.* 2001; **345**: 256–8.
45. Rusnak JM, Kortepeter MG, Aldis J, Boudreau E. Experience in the medical management of potential laboratory exposures to agents of bioterrorism on the basis of risk assessment at the United States Army Medical Research Institute of Infectious Diseases (USAMRIID). *Journal of Occupational and Environmental Medicine.* 2004; **46**: 801–11.
46. Barry MA. Report of pneumonic tularemia in three Boston university researchers, November 2004–March 2005. Boston Public Health Commission, Boston, March 28, 2005. Last cited April 2, 2009. Available from: www.bphc.org/reports/pdfs/report_202.pdf.
47. Rusnak JM, Kortepeter M, Ulrich R *et al.* Laboratory exposures to staphylococcal enterotoxin B. *Emerging Infectious Diseases.* 2004; **10**: 1544–9.
48. ProMed-mail. Ebola, laboratory accident death – Russia (Siberia) (04), August 23, 2004. Archive number 20040823.2350. Last accessed April 2, 2009. Available from: www.promedmail.org.
49. Kortepeter MG, Martin JW, Rusnak JM *et al.* Managing potential laboratory exposure to ebola virus by using a patient biocontainment care unit. *Emerging Infectious Diseases.* 2008; **14**: 881–7.
50. Pro-Med Mail. Ebola virus, needlestick injury – Germany (03) (Hamburg). Archive number 20090331.1243, March 31, 2009. Last accessed April 3, 2009. Available from: www.promedmail.org.
51. Centers for Disease Control and Prevention. Update: Cutaneous anthrax in a laboratory worker – Texas, 2002. *Morbidity and Mortality Weekly Reports.* 2002; **51**: 482.
52. Centers for Disease Control and Prevention. Update: Potential exposures to attenuated vaccine strain Brucella abortus RB51 during a laboratory proficiency test – United States and Canada, 2007. *Morbidity and Mortality Weekly Reports.* 2008; **57**: 36–9.
53. World Health Organization. *Laboratory biosafety manual*, 3rd edn. Geneva: World Health Organization, 2004. Last accessed April 29, 2009. Available from: www.who.int/csr/resources/publications/biosafety/Biosafety7.pdf.
54. Rusnak JM, Kortepeter MG, Hawley RJ *et al.* Management guidelines for laboratory exposures to agents of bioterrorism. *Journal of Occupational and Environmental Medicine.* 2004; **46**: 791–800.
55. Centers for Disease Control and Prevention, Richmond JY, Nesby-O'Dell SL. Laboratory security and emergency response guidance for laboratories working with select agents. *Morbidity and Mortality Weekly Reports.* 2002; **51**: 1–8.

Genetic modification and biotechnology

DAVID ROOMES

Introduction	782	Biotechnology processes and their health hazards	787
Development of biotechnology	783	Risk management of genetic modification work	791
Nanotechnology	784	Health surveillance	793
Genetic modification	784	Conclusion	796
Organisms used in biotechnology	785	Acknowledgements	796
Products and applications of biotechnology	786	References	797

INTRODUCTION

Biotechnology brings together the fields of biology and technology in order to harness the power of living organisms. Fermentation, one of the fundamental biotechnological processes has been known to man for millennia, although it was Carl Wehmer in 1893 who first patented the manufacture of citric acid using microorganisms, thus ushering in the modern era of commercialization of biological processes. The term 'biotechnology' has had many different meanings since its first use in 1919,[1] ranging from a branch of technology concerned with the development and exploitation of machines in relation to the various needs of human beings[2] to today's meaning, which is principally based on genetic modification. The definition is broad, but may be described as the use of biological processes for the production of goods and services, and for environmental management.[3,4] The United Nations Convention on Biological Diversity has defined it as 'any technological application that uses biological systems, living organisms or derivatives thereof to make or modify products or processes for specific use'.[5] As the uses and applications of biotechnologies have grown, it is becoming more common for the term to be used in the context of a specific industry, for example food biotechnology, pharmaceutical biotechnology and marine biotechnology. It is essentially a technology which integrates biology, microbiology, chemistry and biochemistry, as well as chemical and process engineering. A legally accepted definition of genetic modification is 'the alteration of genetic material in a way that does not occur naturally by mating or natural recombination or both'.[6]

This includes recombinant DNA techniques using viral or bacterial vectors, the direct introduction of DNA into any organism, e.g. by microinjection, and cell fusion or hybridization.

Biotechnology is widely employed in industry. It is estimated by the Department for Trade and Industry that over 23 000 people in the United Kingdom are directly employed in the industry in roles ranging from molecular biologists and biophysicists to technical and non-technical staff. In the United States, there were 1415 biotechnology companies at the end of 2005 with a market capitalization of US$410 billion, a ten-fold growth since 1994.[7] It is still growing rapidly and as it expands so does the range of biological, chemical and physical hazards to which employees may potentially be exposed. The rate of change and development within the industry is also rapid, necessitating frequent revision of health, safety and environmental management of the potential risks surrounding rapidly changing processes.[8]

In general, the view that 'biotechnology poses no risks that are fundamentally different from those faced by workers in other processing industries'[9] is still valid today, although the rapid development of new technologies, such as nanotechnology, may pose as yet undefined risks.[10] Product hazards are deemed 'not likely to differ qualitatively from those encountered in other sectors of the pharmaceutical and chemical industries; the fact that the molecules ... are the products of organisms rather than of synthetic catalysts will not alter their reactivity or toxicity'.[11] Risks from handling recombinant organisms may be considered to be no greater than those arising from handling unmodified pathogens.[12] Reports of illness or health effects attributable specifically to work with genetically modified microorganisms and recombinant DNA (rDNA) cells are rare.[13] Although exposure to these genetically modified microorganisms, biologically active products and processing chemicals constitutes a potentially serious risk to the health of employees, it is concluded that biotechnology processes are safe if practised with appropriate risk control measures in place.

DEVELOPMENT OF BIOTECHNOLOGY

Traditionally, biotechnology has been based on the purification and enhancement of the products of naturally occurring organisms through selection and mutation, in processes such as brewing and baking. Alcohol remains one of the main products of the biotechnology industry, not only ethanol, but also alcohol for industrial use.

In the last four decades, the introduction of genetic modification has improved the yield and purity of products, and allowed the development of new ones. In the 1950s, antibiotics and vaccines were produced using biotechnology methods, and in the 1960s, single cell protein as a source of food for animals and humans was developed. The early 1970s saw the development of recombinant DNA techniques. This had a major effect on biomedical research and diagnostics, on agriculture, and on food, chemicals and pharmaceutical manufacture.[14]

The first pharmaceutical products made were human insulin, somatostatin and growth hormone. Development since then has been in the area of pharmacologically active mammalian peptides, such as hormones, enzymes and antibodies. Biological response modifiers, such as the interferons, and growth factors, such as epidermal growth factor, fibroblast growth factor and platelet-derived growth factor, have also been manufactured using biotechnology techniques. Tissue plasminogen activator was a successful product of the late 1980s which has been used extensively as thrombolytic therapy for coronary artery disease. Erythropoietin was developed for use in the treatment of anaemia secondary to renal disease and various clotting factors have also been produced. Since the turn of the century, there has been a rapid growth in approvals for new pharmaceutical products made possible by new biotechnological techniques, most notably in the fields of vaccines and cancer treatments. A multitude of healthcare applications is currently in development utilizing techniques such as monoclonal antibody technology, stem cell technology, cell culture, cloning, nanobiotechnology, microarrays and protein engineering. Table 62.1 shows a list of peptides, their host systems and clinical indications.

There are many other industrial applications of biotechnology, including bacterial enzymes used in the manufacture of detergents, the treatment of leather, and the brewing and baking industries; fungal enzymes used in the preparation of fruit juices; and yeast enzymes in ice-cream manufacture. The water treatment industry also makes extensive use of biotechnology. Agriculture has seen a massive increase in

Table 62.1 Therapeutic or prophylactic products of biotechnology.

Protein	Date	Host system	Indication
Blood grouping reagents	1990	Hybridoma	Blood transfusion
Human insulin	1982	E. coli	Diabetes
Growth hormone	1985		
Interferon-a	1986	E. coli	Hypopituitarism/leukaemia
Hepatitis B surface antigen	1986	E. coli	Prevention of hepatitis B
Tissue plasminogen activator	1987	S. cerevisiae	Myocardial infarction
Erthropoietin	1989	CHO	Anaemia of renal failure
Factor IX	1992	CHO, hybridoma	Haemophilia B
Factor VIII	1992	CHO	Haemophilia A
Interferon-b	1993	E. coli	Multiple sclerosis

the use of biotechnology, including genetic modification of crops to increase yields and disease resistance. 2005 saw the planting of the billionth acre of biotech seed, an increase from only 5 million acres in 1997. Public interest (and concern) in biotechnology has been significantly heightened in the past ten years following a series of high profile advances, including the first cloned animal from an adult cell, a sheep named Dolly in Scotland in 1996[15] and the completion of the Human Genome Project in 2002.

The increasing use of genetically modified organisms in laboratory research and large-scale industrial processes resulted in concern about the potential health and environmental hazards of the organisms and their products. These concerns led to the introduction of legislative measures to ensure adequate control of any risks.

The traditional applications of biotechnology have usually been within the scope of general health and safety law. However, the European Union has legislation to cover work in this area; specifically European Directives 98/81/EC for Contained Use and 1990/220/EEC and 2001/18/EC for Deliberate Release of GM organisms. In the UK, these directives on GMOs and also the requirements of the Environmental Protection Act 1990, have been implemented by specific regulations made under the Health and Safety at Work Act 1974, namely the Genetically Modified Organisms (Contained Use) Regulations 2000 and the Genetically Modified Organisms (Contained Use) (Amendment) Regulations 2005 (for work involving contained use of GMOs) and also the Genetically Modified Organisms (Deliberate Release) Regulations 2002 (for work involving deliberate release of GMOs).

The EU also has a directive (EU86/609/EEC) (currently under active revision) covering the protection of laboratory animals, together with the European Convention for Protection of Vertebrate Animals (ETS No. 123), as amended in 1993 (ETS No. 170). These are implemented in the UK under the Animals (Scientific Procedures) Act 1986 and the Animals (Scientific Procedures) (Amendment) Order 1993, and are applicable to any work with laboratory animals, including any transgenic animals.

The UK regulations specify the following requirements:

1. To assess the risk to human health and the environment, and to keep records.
2. To establish a local genetic modification safety committee to advise on risk assessments.
3. To classify organisms and operations.
4. To notify the Health and Safety Executive (HSE) of the intention to use premises for genetic modification work for the first time and of subsequent individual activities above the lowest risk class and, in some cases of higher risk, to seek consent from the HSE.
5. To adopt controls, including suitable containment measures.
6. To inform the HSE of accidents involving genetically modified organisms.

Guidelines have been produced by the HSE and the Department for Environment, Food and Rural Affairs (DEFRA), which give further information on procedures for risk assessment and control. Independent expert committees have been established to advise government in this complex area (the Scientific Advisory Committee for Genetic Modification (SACGM) and the Advisory Committee for Releases to the Environment (ACRE), for contained use and deliberate release, respectively). In the UK, some techniques are exempt from the regulations, including mutagenesis, the construction and use of somatic hybridoma cells (for the production of monoclonal antibodies), plant cell fusion where the resultant organisms can be produced by traditional breeding methods and self-cloning.

In the United States, the Federal Government has developed a coordinated, risk-based system to ensure new biotechnology products are safe for the environment and human and animal health. Established as a formal policy in 1986, the Coordinated Framework for Regulation of Biotechnology[16] describes the federal system for evaluating products developed using modern biotechnology. The Coordinated Framework is based upon health and safety laws developed to address specific product classes and a number of different agencies are involved including the Food and Drug Administration (FDA), the Environmental Protection Agency (EPA) and the Department of Agriculture. The US Government has written new regulations, policies and guidance to implement these laws for biotechnology as products have developed. Additional guidance includes guidelines for research involving recombinant DNA molecules[17] and guidelines for biosafety in microbiological and biomedical laboratories.[18] The former constitutes regulatory guidelines for laboratory research which must be followed by organizations receiving federal funding, and the latter assigns biosafety levels to organisms and specifies the equipment and procedures to be used within each biosafety containment level.

NANOTECHNOLOGY

Nanotechnology (which includes the field of nanobiotechnology) is a rapidly developing area of science with a worldwide market for commercial application estimated to reach US$1 trillion by 2015.[19] Man-made nanoparticles have existed for many years, mainly in the form of inhaled air pollutants as a byproduct of the burning of fossil fuels or occupations such as welding and tyre manufacture. The health effects following inhalation of such particles have been widely studied and the detrimental effects thereof on the cardiorespiratory system are well understood.[20-23] The term 'nanotechnology' was first used in 1974 to refer to the ability to engineer materials precisely at the nanometer level,[24] although a more complete definition is 'the purposeful engineering of matter at scales of less than 100 nm to achieve size-dependent properties and functions'. It is believed that some of the health effects of inhaled nanoparticles may be predicted from the epidemiological study of available occupational and environmental aerosol exposure information and that an initial assessment of risk can be made using these data.[25] What is less well understood is the ability of manufactured nanoparticles to penetrate the system via the intestinal tract and skin and once taken up, the pharmacokinetics and end organ effects that may occur.[26] As the science advances, it is expected that nanobiotechnology will be a major area of development in biology and medicine with applications in current development including biological labelling, drug and gene delivery, tissue engineering and the biodetection of pathogens.[27] For the occupational health professional, it will be necessary to work closely with toxicologists and other experts in allied fields to understand the possible health effects and to implement appropriate controls and risk management strategies.[28]

GENETIC MODIFICATION

Genetic modification has proved an immensely powerful tool for the biotechnology industry enabling discovery of novel drugs, as well as directly being the driving force for production of biopharmaceuticals, such as human growth hormone and interferon. The development of organisms for use in biotechnology commonly involves the improvement of desirable properties, such as the level of production of a metabolite, as well as eliminating properties that are less useful. Such modification, either incidentally or deliberately as a control measure, may also reduce the ability of the organism to survive outside the bioreactor. Traditional methods for altering such characteristics included mutation by either chemical or physical means followed by selection of organisms with the desired properties.[29] Because mutagenesis is a random process, laborious and careful screening is necessary to isolate organisms with the required properties and thus it is rarely used today within the biotechnology industry. An alternative method for improving the process characteristics of organisms is hybridization; for example, by conjugation between closely related species or strains of bacteria, or by recombination between different mating types of yeast. Protoplast fusion offers an additional method of strain improvement, particularly between organisms of different species.

A specific example of hybridization is the formation of 'hybridomas' for the production of monoclonal antibodies. In this technique, antibody-producing cells from the spleen of an immunized animal (normally a rat or mouse) are fused with homologous myeloma cells and the resulting mixture of cell types grown in selective media. The fusion products are then screened to obtain clones of 'hybridoma' cells that produce useful amounts of antibody against the antigen used for the immunization. These clones are genetically identical and the resulting antibody will be a pure species, or 'monoclonal antibody'.

A more recent development for obtaining essentially similar antibodies has been 'phage display', where genes for an antibody with extensive variation of the 'variable regions' have been fused to a surface protein on a bacteriophage, to create a library of recombinant bacteriophages displaying the antibodies on their surfaces.[30,31] This library can be panned by trapping the phage on to the desired target, immobilized on a suitable support, and washing away the unbound bacteriophage before releasing the bound ones. These can then be grown up further, to produce a population enriched for those binding to the target protein, since the gene for the antibody is now linked to its presence on the surface of the bacteriophage, and the panning repeated until a population with high and specific affinity is obtained. Individual bacteriophage can then be cloned from this population, to give clones containing the wanted gene sequences, which can then be recloned into appropriate expression vectors for the production of the antibody.

Much of the current interest in biotechnology is over the use of techniques to develop microorganisms that produce products coded for by genes from a wide variety of sources. Potential donor organisms include viruses and eukaryotic microorganisms (i.e. microorganisms in which DNA is contained in a distinct nucleus), such as bacteria, plant and animal cells. The choice of organism is dependent on a number of factors including the ability to express functional products, the cost of manufacture and ultimate use of the product. Hormones and antibodies tend to be produced from animal cells, whereas biotechnology enzyme manufacturers, making components for polymerase chain reaction kits, might use a thermophilic microorganism, e.g. *Thermophilus aquaticus*, to produce the Taq enzyme. Virus donors include hepatitis B virus, whose DNA is used to make vaccines by expression in a heterologous organism.

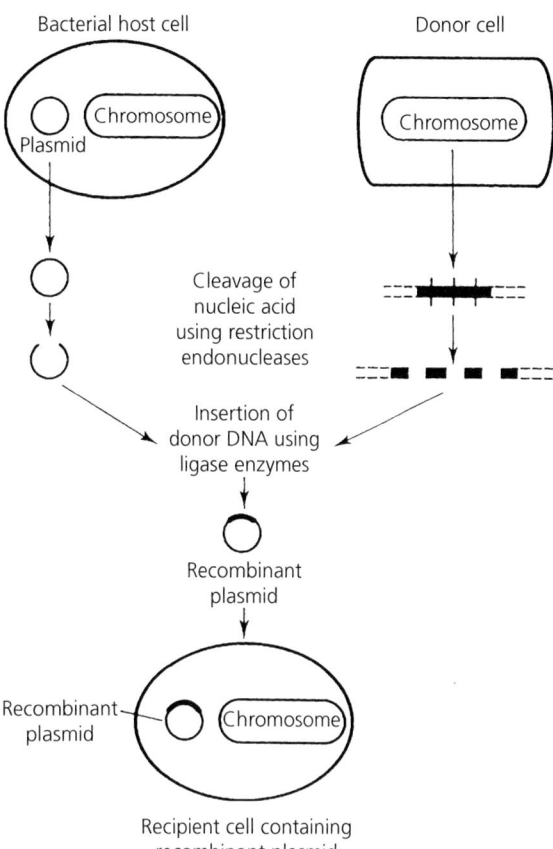

Figure 62.1 Principles of genetic modification.

The underlying technology for modern biotechnology is the ability to manipulate DNA. A typical manipulation is outlined in Figure 62.1. Initially, the target gene of interest is identified and isolated[32] and the selected gene is cleaved using restriction endonuclease enzymes and inserted into a vector capable of being inserted or incorporated into the recipient cell (either a circular piece of DNA termed a plasmid, or a virus). The 'new' gene is joined to the vector's nucleic acid using ligase enzymes. The vector can then be used to introduce the gene into the recipient or host cell, to which it is able to pass on the characteristics coded in the gene from the donor organism. Host species have included *Saccharomyces cerevisiae*, *Bacillus* spp. and *Streptomyces* spp., but the most frequently used is *Escherichia coli* through which nearly all genetic manipulations are made before using the vector DNA and introducing into the final destination host.

ORGANISMS USED IN BIOTECHNOLOGY

These come from a wide range of taxonomic groups, including bacteria, fungi and viruses, as well as animal and plant cells. The most common organisms used for biotechnology medicines are animal cells and bacteria; however, fungi are still widely used in other industrial (i.e. non-pharmaceutical) processes. Viruses can carry and donate DNA and are most commonly used during vaccine production. Viruses are also used extensively as vectors in molecular biological research and in therapeutic delivery systems. Routinely used organisms such as *Escherichia coli*, have been genetically modified, selected and improved to enable a number of factors. Examples include the inability to undergo homologous recombination, modification of biochemical pathways to enable growth on only certain types of media, removal of genes that might enable the bacteria to transfer genetic material to other cells by conjugation and removal of resistance genes from the chromosome. The resultant organism is optimized for genetic manipulation, but severely impeded in its ability to grow outside the laboratory environment, such that the safety profile for the worker and the environment is enhanced. The modification of host microorganisms in this way plays a major role in assessment of biosafety hazards.

PRODUCTS AND APPLICATIONS OF BIOTECHNOLOGY

The various applications of biotechnology can be divided into five main categories: biomass production, metabolite production, recombinant DNA pharmaceutical production, transformation processes and enzyme production.

Biomass production

Biomass production involves the use of the organism itself as the product, usually for animal feed, but in some cases as a human food product. Apart from the use of yeast cells in the baking industry, biomass production is often referred to in the UK as single-cell protein production. Examples include the use of *Fusarium graminearum* to produce Quorn® for human consumption and *Methylophilus methylotrophus* for the production of Pruteen® for animal feed.

Metabolite production

Metabolite production exploits the biosynthetic capabilities of organisms and has resulted in the establishment of many industrial processes. A metabolite is something that is produced during growth, stationary or even death phases of culture. Growth of an organism results in a range of metabolites being produced. Whether the desired metabolite will predominate depends upon the organism, its growth rate and the culture conditions used. The compounds produced may be either primary or secondary metabolites or, in the case of a genetically modified organism, they could be 'foreign' or 'novel' metabolites introduced from another organism. Primary metabolites are compounds produced in the logarithmic growth phase when cells are growing at constant, maximal rate.

Compounds produced during this phase are either essential to the growth of the organism, such as amino acids, lipids and carbohydrates, or are byproducts of catabolism, such as ethanol. Once the logarithmic growth phase has ceased, because either nutrients have been exhausted or toxic metabolites have built up, growth eventually stops and the culture enters the stationary phase. During the stationary phase, products termed 'secondary metabolites' are produced which play no obvious role in cell growth and are usually specific to particular groups of organisms. Secondary metabolites include the antibiotics, alkaloids and some other molecules. Genetic modification has extended the range of metabolites that may be produced by microorganisms. For example, microbial cells may be developed with the ability to synthesize compounds normally associated with plant or animal cells, including hormones, growth factors and proteins, such as serum albumin.

Recombinant pharmaceutical products

Following the discovery of recombinant DNA in the early 1970s, within four years, genetically modified bacteria were being used to make human insulin, somatostatin and growth hormone. Since then, the major thrust of recombinant DNA technology has been the production of rare mammalian peptides, which are pharmaceutically active hormones, enzymes, antibodies and biological response modifiers. Previously, these peptides were harvested from animal tissue. Large numbers of animals and a significant amount of processing activity were required to produce tiny amounts of the desired substance. Now they can be made on demand, in bacterial or yeast culture and quality is easier to control. The problems associated with contamination of the product with infectious agents present in the host animal can be eliminated (e.g. the risk of transmission of the Creutzfeldt–Jakob disease agent from growth hormone derived from human pituitary glands). The proteins yielded are purer and the process is more economical.

Examples of recombinant pharmaceutical products are human insulin, growth hormone, tissue plasminogen activator, erythropoietin, interferons and interleukins. Commonly used organisms are *E. coli*, *Bacillus subtilis*, *Saccharomyces cerevisiae* and *Aspergillus niger*. Occasionally, the rDNA product differs slightly from the natural product, but retains therapeutic activity, as with gamma interferon produced from *E. coli*.[33] In other cases, molecules or transformation steps can be added by the recombinant cell. Mammalian cells are frequently used and genes coding for reproductive hormones, such as human chorionic gonadotrophin and luteinizing hormone have been cloned and expressed in such cells. Recent advances in generating active proteins through refolding of bacterial inclusion body proteins has seen great improvements in the yield and purity of products, such as human TPA (tissue plasminogen activator) using bacterial cells.[34] The qualities and specific activities of some peptides can be modified by adding various ingredients to the culture broth.[35] The peptides themselves can be changed by recombinant technology, e.g. by recombination of hybrid genes to produce proteins (analogues) with different but more desirable properties.

The pharmaceutical industry is also using this technology to research the amino acid sequence of naturally occurring bioregulatory proteins. This will allow the development of analogues which act as inhibitors or promoters of activity. Many vaccines are now produced using biotechnology. Genes can be cloned and expressed, which code for specific antigens of viruses, bacteria and parasites. An early example of this is the hepatitis B vaccine which utilizes yeast to produce hepatitis B surface antigen. Also, DNA from genetically modified vaccinia virus has been used to produce protective antigens for hepatitis B, rabies and malaria vaccines.[36] With increasing concern regarding the possibility of a global influenza pandemic, the development of DNA vaccines whereby an individual is not given the protein antigen, but DNA encoding the antigen, is seen as a greatly improved method of delivering vaccination on a large scale.[37]

Monoclonal antibodies (produced from a combination of myeloma cells and antibody-producing cells from the spleen of an immunized mouse) are used in diagnostic kits, in protein purification and as therapeutic agents in cancer and organ transplant rejection. At present, monoclonal antibodies account for the largest product category of all biotechnology-derived drugs.[38]

Recombinant DNA technology has also been applied to the production of antibiotics, and in the development of direct-acting gene therapies, e.g. for cystic fibrosis and rheumatoid arthritis. The 'normal' gene is administered to patients with the aim of incorporating this 'good' genetic material into cells to influence the course of the disease. While there has been some success in obtaining expression of the new transgene, major problems have occurred due to the integration of the vector and further work is needed, to develop safer vectors, before this technique can be applied more generally.

Transformation processes

Transformation processes involve the enzymic conversion of one compound into another. This may involve, for example, isomerization, oxidation, hydroxylation or dehydrogenation. Examples of transformation processes include the oxidation of ethanol into acetic acid and the production of steroids, such as hydrocortisone or cortisone, from plant steroids.

Enzyme production

Enzyme production involves the isolation of useful enzymes from organisms either to use in transformation processes or for other purposes. Examples include proteases from *Bacillus subtilis* which are used in the manufacture of biological detergents and pectinases from *Aspergillus* spp., used in drink manufacture. These applications of biotechnology can be divided into four different types of process:

1. non-aseptic processes using indigenous organisms, such as in traditional wine production;
2. non-aseptic processes using specified inocula which include brewing and milk fermentation;
3. aseptic processes using specified inocula, as in antibiotic and single-cell protein production;
4. aseptic and contained processes using potentially hazardous organisms, such as vaccine production.

BIOTECHNOLOGY PROCESSES AND THEIR HEALTH HAZARDS

A typical industrial, biotechnology process involves a number of stages: inoculum preparation (for processes using specific inocula); large-scale growth of the organism in a bioreactor; separation of the organism from its growth medium; and product recovery and purification. These stages are summarized in Figure 62.2. The process may be aerobic or anaerobic, depending upon the organism used, and may be carried out in bioreactors ranging from open pan vessels to highly enclosed systems that may require mechanical agitation or aeration. Downstream processing depends on whether the product is intracellular or extracellular. Intracellular product requires extraction, whereas extracellular product is purified from spent medium (Figure 62.3) and the health hazard and effluent issues may be quite different. Extraction of intracellular product generally requires that the cells are disrupted, usually by chemical lysis or by physical disruption, such as homogenization. The potential for release of aerosols is greatest during disruption stages. The final processing stages are purification and concentration of the product, through some of the operations listed in Table 62.2.

Biotechnology processes may result in risk of exposure to biological, chemical, ergonomic, physical and other hazards.

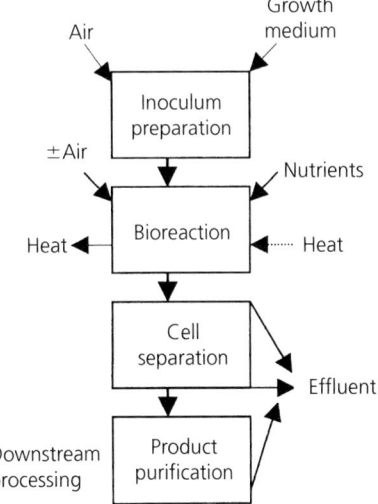

Figure 62.2 A generalized schematic representation of a typical biotechnology production process.

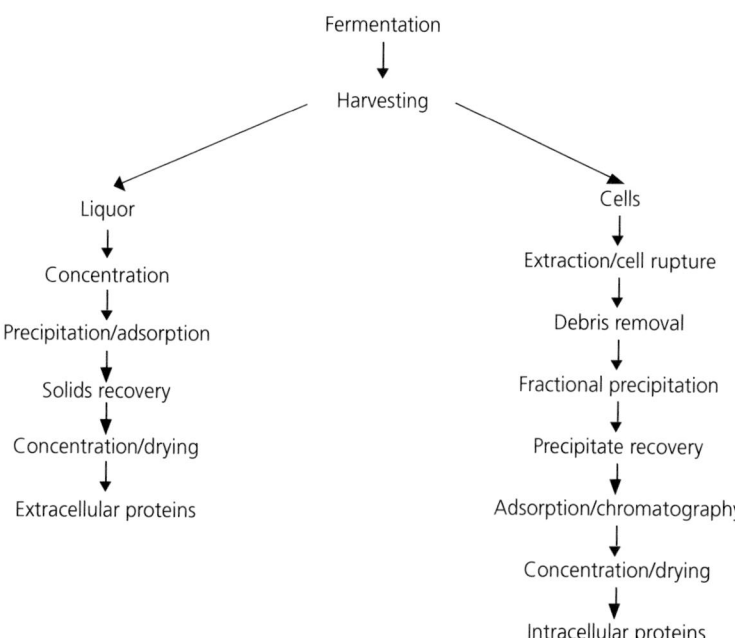

Figure 62.3 Purification of fermentation products.

Table 62.2 Typical unit operations in downstream processing.

Downstream processing stage	Typical process alternatives
Harvesting	Centrifugation
	Filtration
	Flocculation
	Membrane separation
Product separation	Homogenization
	Solvent extraction
	Ultrafiltration
	Distillation
	Affinity chromatography
	Lysis
Product purification	Ion exchange
	Chromatographic separation
	Gel filtration
	Electrophoresis
	Fractional crystallization
	Precipitation
Product concentration	Precipitation
	Crystallization
	Evaporation
	Ultrafiltration

Biological hazards

The organisms used in biotechnology processes present a number of potential hazards for consideration. These include infection, toxic effects, allergenic or other biological effects of the organisms or cells, its components or its naturally occurring metabolic products and other products expressed by the organism.[39–42] Occupational exposure may occur via inhalation, ingestion, inoculation or transmission through broken skin and mucous membranes.

The effect on health of exposure to an organism depends on the route of entry of the organism, its viability, transmissibility, dose received and immune status of the exposed individual. Most organisms used in industrial processes are unlikely to cause human disease or to cause significant harm to the environment. More risk may accompany the use of non-modified organisms than genetically modified microorganisms, which are often unable to survive outside the bioreactor. However, cases of ill health among individuals involved in genetic modification work may not always be attributed to occupational exposure, leading to under-reporting. Occupational infections are not always recognized as such, especially if the resulting disease or symptoms occur commonly in the community. Reports of ill health associated with biotechnology processes are summarized in Table 62.3.

The biotechnology industry has experienced a good health and safety record. The current consensus is that the potential risks of rDNA research, development and manufacturing activities were overstated initially.[11] The hazards associated with this work are similar to those associated with the organisms, vectors, DNA, chemicals and physical apparatus being used. This is supported by the fact that studies designed to test the capacity of a host organism to acquire novel hazardous properties from DNA donor cells failed to demonstrate the existence of this potential hazard, and no illness attributed to infection with a genetically modified microorganism has been reported.

Possible human health risks related to genetic modification work include:

1. Exposure to a genetically modified microorganism resulting in infection or delivery of expressed

Table 62.3 Incidents of ill health in biotechnology processes.

Organism	Process	Symptoms
Aspergillus penicillium	Fermentation: citric acid production, Czechoslovakia	Bronchitis
Pseudomonas aeruginosa	Downstream processing (centrifugation): enzyme isolation, UK	Flu-like symptoms, kidney/stomach pains
Methylophilus methylotrophus	Fermentation/downstream processing: single-cell protein production, UK	Flu-like symptoms, conjunctivitis
Methylophilus methonolica	Downstream processing (spray drying): single-cell protein production, Sweden	Flu-like symptoms, conjunctivitis
Aspergillus niger	Fermentation/downstream processing: citric acid production, UK; fermentation: citric acid production, USSR	Asthma, respiratory symptoms
Yeasts	Fermentation/downstream	Asthma, bronchitis
Streptomyces spp.	Downstream processing: single-cell protein production, USSR; antibiotic production, UK	Asthma, bronchitis, respiratory symptoms, conjunctivitis

biologically active molecules, such as enzymes, hormones or toxins to target tissues.
2. Risk of transmissible spongiform encephalopathy from exposure to modified prion genes.
3. Exposure to cloned human genes that could lead to an immune response and subsequent autoimmune disorders.
4. Exposure to a gene product, leading to induction of an immune response that could cause therapeutic complications if treatment with that product were required.
5. Respiratory sensitization related to exposure to foreign proteins, with the possibility that inclusion bodies and fusion proteins may increase the risk of sensitization.
6. Exposure to cloned oncogenic sequences or genetically modified retroviruses that could pose a carcinogenic risk.

Special consideration should be given to work with DNA-containing genes coding for potent toxins or for oncogenes. Theoretically, there is the possibility that the introduction of oncogenic sequences into a human, as a result of an occupational accident or cumulative exposure, could cause cell transformation and lead to tumour growth.[43] No cases of this have been reported. Particular concern has been raised about possible oncogene exposure through inhalation, since the newer potential therapies use airborne viruses, such as adenovirus.

Much recombinant DNA work has used *E. coli* K12 as the recipient organism. Its modification demonstrates how many rDNA organisms are disabled so that they can no longer survive in the human host. Because *E. coli* K12 lacks certain surface antigens, the fimbriae which enable it to adhere to gut epithelial walls, resistance to lysis by serum complement, resistance to phagocytosis and part of an important liposaccharide, it is thus unable to colonize the human gut and is non-pathogenic as a result of these modifications.

Another potential source of biological hazard is contaminating organisms present in the culture. This may be of particular concern in animal cell cultures, where viruses (retro, simian, polyoma, herpes or hepatitis), mycoplasma and prions may exist as contaminants. Tasks involving potential aerosol generation or manipulation of sharps could expose the employee to a risk of potentially serious infection.

Toxic effects

Toxic effects may result from inhalation of Gram-negative bacterial endotoxin.[44,45] The reaction may follow exposure to the dust of single-cell protein after it has been cultured in fermenters and subsequently dried in a spray drier. Workers exposed to the end-product as a result of inadequate protective measures can develop flu-like febrile reactions 4–12 hours later, with shivering, fever, tightness of the chest, aching limbs and cough. Blood tests reveal neutropenia followed by leukocytosis[46] and a decline in forced expiratory volume in one second (FEV_1)[47] has been described. These symptoms may start during the evening or the night after a day's work, but subside by the morning or over the next day. Acute symptoms of conjunctivitis, rhinitis or cough may start immediately after exposure. Sore red eyes with a persistent discharge have also been reported. Exposed workers can be found to have precipitating antibodies to the organism, but the responses have been regarded as more likely to be due to endotoxin rather than an immunological reaction to the organism. Endotoxin intolerance can develop on subsequent challenge.[48,49]

Inadequate protection against exposure to single-cell proteins (protein products developed for animal and human food (e.g. mycoprotein) or enzymes, may result in allergic effects such as asthma[50–53] or contact dermatitis. Extrinsic allergic alveolitis can follow exposure to fungal spores. Type 1 immediate or anaphylactic response is a theoretical possibility after exposure to enzymes or antibiotics.[54]

Table 62.4 Tissue culture additives.

Additives	
Antibiotics	**Antineoplastics and cytotoxins**
Chloramphenicol	Actinomycin
Gentamicin	Adriamycin
Rifampicin	Aminopterin
Streptomycin	Bleomycin
Tobramycin	Chlorambucil
Hormones	Cyclophosphamide
Dexamethasone	Daunorubicin
Growth hormones	Sodium azide
Prednisone	Vincristine

Table 62.5 Chemical solvents and extractants.

Chemical solvents and extractants
Ammonium compounds
2-Aminoethanol benzene
Chloroform
Carbon tetrachloride
Chloral hydrate
Chromic acid
Chromium trichloride
Cyanogen bromide
Cyanogen chloride
Cyclohexane
Chlorodifluoromethane
Diisopropylethylamine
Dimethoxybenzidine dihydrochloride
5-Bromo-4-chloro-3-indolyl phosphate p-toluidine
Cobalt chloride hexahydrate
EDTA
Ethanol
Ethers
Ethylene glycol
Hydrazine
Hydrochloric acid
Formic acid
Lithium compounds
2-Mercaptoethanol
Methanol
Naphthalene
Paraformaldehyde phenylhydrazine
Toluene

EDTA, ethylene diamine tetra-acetate.

The production of biologically active products, such as hormones, interleukins and interferon, is also potentially hazardous to workers either through direct effects on health or interference with existing disease treatment.

Chemicals

Although biological hazards are the primary focus of this chapter, it should be recognized that there are significant chemical hazards in the biotechnology industry. Potential chemical exposures may occur at many stages in the process.[55] There are differences in the type and volume of chemicals encountered in a research and development environment and a production environment, and the levels of risk of exposure in each also vary due to differences in the way the chemicals are handled.

Growth media used in tissue cultures and fermenters consist mostly of water, inorganic salts, carbohydrates, amino acids, vitamins and other nutrients. Selective cell growth is supported by the addition of steroids, antibiotics and anti-neoplastics, e.g. methotrexate (Table 62.4), all of which pose a significant health concern, even at low levels of exposure. Chronic low level exposure to antibiotics could lead to colonization with antibiotic-resistant organisms. It may also induce or activate drug allergy, which then becomes a problem when the employee is treated with that antibiotic at a later date. Process workers are at greater risk of exposure to chemical hazards than those involved in research scale work. Tasks involved in cell culture preparation, including weighing out of chemicals, creating and agitating solutions and cleaning up spills, all present a risk of exposure.

Extraction of nucleic acids from whole tissue or tissue culture is an important preliminary phase in virtually all biotechnology processes. Table 62.5 shows a list of solvents and precipitating agents used for these purposes. Trichloroacetic acid and perchloric acid are used commonly, the latter also being an explosion hazard. Dimethyl sulphate is widely used. Certain additives can be acutely hazardous, e.g. sodium azide used to suppress unwanted bacterial growth. Cyanide salts, such as cyanogen bromide, are used with the potential release of cyanide gas, and its attendant dangers.

High-pressure liquid chromatography is used for the identification of nucleic acid components and requires the use of toxic reagents.

Sequencing establishes the order of DNA pairs in a gene and can involve the use of toxic chemicals, such as dimethyl sulphate and hydrofluoric acid. Gel electrophoresis involves the use of acrylamide, but the risk of exposure can be reduced by using commercially prepared polyacrylamide gel or finished gel electrophoresis plates. Ethidium bromide, which is a mutagenic substance, is also added to electrophoresis gels, although other safer alternatives are now being used.

Sterilizing agents, such as formaldehyde, are frequently used. Potent solvent detergents, driven through by pressurized steam, are used to sanitize lines in manufacturing facilities. If this is not used in an enclosed system, inhalation exposure may cause respiratory irritation.

Ergonomic hazards

Working environments where genetic modification work is conducted range from laboratory to manufacturing plant housing large bioreactors. Employees may also work in traditional office environments and processes are increasingly computer controlled. In addition, the role of scientists has changed to the extent that much of a bioanalyst's job may be carried out using a computer outside the traditional biological laboratory environment.

These working arrangements mean that employees are exposed to a variety of ergonomic hazards. The importance of a good ergonomic fit for staff using display screen equipment is well known. Less well appreciated is the ergonomic challenge presented by a laboratory environment. The design of safety cabinets may make it difficult to sit comfortably with a suitable work posture. Pipettes vary in weight and efficiency and do not suit all operators equally. Tasks in biotechnology laboratories are often repetitive, requiring accuracy and speed and are carried out while maintaining the upper limbs in non-neutral postures. It is thus important to carry out an ergonomic assessment of these tasks, to minimize risks to health. The increasing trend to automate sample processing will help reduce ergonomic risks.

Media preparation involves a significant amount of material handling as sacks of powdered constituents are moved around, weighed, dispensed and added to solutions. The resulting liquids often have to be moved again to storage or to other parts of the plant. Manual handling risk assessment must be carried out, training delivered to handlers and recommendations adhered to. Despite the sophistication of the biotechnology industry and the emphasis on biological and genetic modification risks, manual handling accidents and musculoskeletal ill health are leading causes of work-related ill health in the industry.

Physical hazards

Another potential health hazard in biotechnology plants is noise, resulting in a risk of noise-induced hearing loss to exposed workers. The physical hazards of steam, heat, pressure and radiation, both ionizing and non-ionizing, must also be considered. It is still not uncommon for scalds to occur, as steam is used for sterilization of fermentation vessels and lines. Other physical hazards are combustion and explosion.

Mental stressors

Finally, this comprehensive list of hazards would not be complete without the inclusion of workplace stressors. Biotechnology employees are as susceptible as any other to mental health effects from exposure to excessive pressures at work, perhaps more than some, due to the rapid pace of change in their industry. There are the added fears and anxieties related to working with genetically modified organisms and substances which have the potential to cause lasting or heritable ill-health effects. The provision of information to staff is crucial to help allay these fears. The psychological aspects of lone working or shift working should also be considered.

Environmental considerations

To render process microorganisms non-viable and to inactivate other components, the waste stream may require treatment by physical, chemical or biological methods, or a combination of these. Effluent from biotechnology processes may include growth medium components, viable and non-viable organisms, suspended solids and waste water. It will also include such chemicals as inducers, solvents, detergents, cleaning agents, buffers and alkali and acids used for pH adjustment.

RISK MANAGEMENT OF GENETIC MODIFICATION WORK

The current European approach to risk assessment for genetic modification work is based upon a classification scheme which equates the hazards to those from pathogens, assigning a genetically modified microorganism to a class which is equivalent to an equally hazardous pathogen, in terms of risk to both humans and the environment, and then assigning the same level of containment. For non-microorganisms (e.g. transgenic animals or plants) the assessment is based upon whether there is any increased risk to humans, due to the transgene, together with minimization, or avoidance in higher risk cases, of any release to the environment. In the UK, this risk assessment is mandated by the Genetically Modified Organisms (Contained Use) Regulations 2000 (as amended in 2005) and the Genetically Modified Organisms (Deliberate Release) Regulations 2002. The required process for the risk assessment for contained use is set out in the Compendium of Guidance of the Scientific Advisory Committee for Genetic Modification, which includes much helpful advice about detailed systems and considerations.[56] The Compendium also includes limited advice on the assessment of risks for the products of 'synthetic biology' work.

A requirement of the Contained Use Regulations is the establishment of a Genetic Modification Safety Committee (GMSC), which should involve representatives from a range of relevant disciplines, representing both management and employees (e.g. union representatives), as well as appropriate safety personnel, while still not being too large and unwieldy. While the GMSC is specifically charged with considering and advising on all GM risk assessments, it may well also fulfil other functions, as a more general biological safety committee. The safety personnel will usually include the biological safety officer (BSO), who sometimes doubles up as the 'competent person' required, under the

Management of Health and Safety at Work Regulations (MHSWR), to advise the employer on safety of any GM work undertaken. However, for larger premises, where the total workload may be high, or when more specialist knowledge is required, it may be desirable to appoint a biological safety adviser to assist the BSO, as well as advising the employer.

In general, health surveillance will not be required for most GM activities and it is not a requirement under the Contained Use Regulations, although it might be under COSHH and MHSWR, depending upon the risks and benefits under particular circumstances. If a supervisory medical officer is appointed, then they would usually be a member of the GMSC, even if mainly receiving papers rather than attending meetings.

Previous regulations made a distinction between different scales of work at the risk assessment stage. This distinction has now been abandoned for the risk assessment, although it is clearly still relevant when deciding the details of the physical containment to be applied, in particular when large-scale production occurs outside usual laboratory style containment (e.g. during manufacture of GM influenza vaccine in embryonated eggs) or during clinical studies involving GM agents administered to humans in a hospital. Under the current regulations, the initial assessment is concerned to determine the relative risks to human health and the environment, considering the potential severity, likelihood of occurrence and any uncertainty. Based upon this initial assessment, the main assessment will then be aimed at reducing these factors and assigning sufficient containment measures to bring the likelihood to an acceptable probability. The GM class of the work is then determined from the containment measures required. Subsequently, consideration is given to whether these containment measures will also give sufficient protection to the lesser hazard, between human health and environment, and any necessary additional measures added. The final overall class is then reassessed, to allow for any such additional containment. The overall class determines whether it is necessary to notify the Health and Safety Executive of the particular project (initial notification of all GM centres is necessary) or even, for the higher risk classes, to seek consent before the work can be commenced.

In considering the potential hazards to human health from a genetically modified microorganism, the following should be considered:

1. Any hazard associated with the recipient strain of microorganism, particularly whether it has the potential to enter human cells or establish an infection in human hosts. Usually disabled host strains are employed, but this is not always the case and sometimes the wild-type host might be sufficiently pathogenic that even a disabled strain would still present a significant hazard. In general, the starting containment considered will be that required for the host alone.
2. Any hazard presented by the vector. While this will frequently be minimal (e.g. when the vector is a non-mobilizable plasmid which requires to be transfected into a bacterium), at other times the vector may be a virus with the potential to enter human cells and even insert into the genomic DNA, posing potential hazards not only from the genes which it contains, but also from the possibility of insertional mutation in the human genome. Examples of potentially hazardous vectors include any lentiviral, or even viral, vectors containing the enhancer of gene expression derived from woodchuck hepatitis virus.[57]
3. Hazards associated with the genomic insert. Often the inserted gene will code only for a harmless protein, which is to be produced in bulk for subsequent purification, but on occasion the inserted DNA itself, or its product, might be harmful. Hazardous DNA will include potentially oncogenic sequences, since these have been shown to be capable of causing increased tumours (e.g. when rubbed on to the skin of mice).[58]
4. Hazardous products from the inserted gene. These could include potentially hazardous RNA, such as siRNA targeted against tumour suppressor proteins (which would be potentially oncogenic if expressed in a human cell), and hazardous proteins, either because they are toxic or else have a physiological function (e.g. allergens, cytokines, growth factors or oncogenes).
5. Possible modification of the pathogenicity of the host microorganism. Obvious examples include pathogenicity-determining genes from a related microorganism (e.g. adhesion factors or transport factors) and any gene whose product might lower the susceptibility of the host to the immune system.

Assessment of potential hazards to the environment is less systematized, as clearly factors of the local environment are relevant, e.g. if the potential target for harm from the genetically modified microorganism is not in the immediate locality the likelihood of hazard may be substantially reduced. Risk assessment is carried out by assessing both the consequence of the hazard and also its likelihood separately, and then combining these to obtain an overall risk assessment. Among the factors which need to be considered are:

1. Any hazard associated with the recipient strain of microorganism, considering whether it might either infect or compete with any organism naturally present in the environment. Usually disabled host strains are employed, but this is not always the case and sometimes the wild-type host might be sufficiently pathogenic or dominant that even a disabled strain would still present a significant hazard. In general, the starting containment considered will be that required for the host alone.
2. Any hazard presented by the vector. While this will frequently be minimal (e.g. when the vector is a non-mobilizable plasmid which requires to be transfected into a bacterium), at other times the vector may be a

Table 62.6 Risk determination matrix for environmental hazards.

Consequence of hazard	Likelihood of hazard			
	High	Medium	Low	Negligible
Severe	High	High	Medium	Effectively zero
Modest	High	Medium	Medium/low	Effectively zero
Minor	Medium/low	Low	Low	Effectively zero
Negligible	Effectively zero	Effectively zero	Effectively zero	Effectively zero

Reproduced with permission from SACGM Compendium of Guidance, Health and Safety Executive, © Crown Copyright.[56]

virus with the potential to infect a host present in the environment.
3. Hazards associated with the genomic insert. Often the inserted gene will code only for a harmless protein, which is to be produced in bulk for subsequent purification, but on occasion the inserted DNA itself, or its product, might be harmful.
4. Hazards associated with products from the transgene. These will usually involve consideration of whether any protein product might be harmful to any species present in the environment.

The consequence and likelihood of hazard are combined, to produce an overall assessment of risk, as shown in Table 62.6, and additional containment measures are considered until the risk to the environment is 'low' or 'effectively zero'.

Once the appropriate containment measures have been determined for the more important of the human health or environmental risk, any additional measures necessary for the other risk are added, and then the appropriate GM class is determined from the containment measures.

The containment measures necessary for genetically modified microorganisms depend upon the scale of the work. Those for small scale (i.e. laboratory scale) activities are the same as those for different hazard group pathogens and a number of the main ones are summarized in Table 62.7. In the case of GM plants, the risk to the environment will almost always outweigh that to human health and the main assessment will be that necessary to protect the environment, paying particular attention to the possibilities of dispersal, whether of pollen or seed. In consequence, the health risks are usually negligible, unless some product of the plant poses such a risk, including potential allergenicity giving rise to hay fever symptoms.

For the majority of activities involving GM animals, the primary consideration is the potential of harm to the environment, should it be able to escape and become established in the environment (e.g. by breeding and passing on its transgene(s)), and the risk to human health is similar to that posed by the wild-type animal. The issues of containment are very different, with a range in sizes from farm animals to small invertebrates requiring very different consideration. In the case of laboratory animals, the methods employed for their maintenance in a barrier unit, to ensure their pathogen-free status, will be fully sufficient to ensure that the likelihood of escape is negligible, and the risk to the environment effectively zero.

The containment measures required by the risk assessment should be adequate to protect a worker of average susceptibility. However, additional consideration should be given to anyone who might be more vulnerable, particularly those on immunosuppressive therapy (e.g. under treatment for rheumatoid arthritis or following a transplant) or who are otherwise immunosuppressed. A wider category for whom special consideration should be given is women who are, or might be, pregnant or breastfeeding. Most low class GM work will not present any specific risks to such women, or their child, but consideration should be taken if work is planned with any host known to have adverse effects, or any transgene which codes for any agent which is suspected of affecting the fetus or newborn child.

An important aspect of risk assessment is the communication of any hazards which are found to the relevant members of the workforce, so that they have a good appreciation of why the containment measures are necessary, together with appropriate training so that they can use these measures for their own, and their colleagues', protection.

HEALTH SURVEILLANCE

Health surveillance was a prominent risk control measure in the past when the health risks arising from genetic modification were considered to be uncertain. National guidance in several countries promoted highly prescriptive health surveillance procedures, with a hierarchy of measures linked to categories of containment levels. However, with growing experience of occupational health outcomes showing little evidence of health problems related to genetic modification work,[10,59] it is clear that these traditional measures have been out of proportion to the risks to health.

The role of health surveillance has been revised in recently updated guidance, such as that produced by the Scientific Advisory Committee on Genetic Modification in the UK in 2007.[56] The emphasis has been placed on determining appropriate health surveillance procedures based on a risk assessment of the likelihood of health effects resulting from

Table 62.7 Examples of containment measures for small scale work with genetically modified microorganisms.

	Containment measure	Containment level 1	Containment level 2	Containment level 3	Containment level 4
Building/ physical measures	Laboratory suite isolation	Not required	Not required	Required	Required
	Laboratory sealable for fumigation	Not required	Not required	Required	Required
	Negative pressure relative to surroundings	Not required	Required where risk assessment shows	Required	Required
	Extract and input air HEPA filtered	Not required	Not required	HEPA filters required for extract	HEPA filters required for both input and extract
	Microbiological safety cabinet or enclosure	Not required	Required where and to extent risk assessment shows	Required, and all procedures with infective materials required to be contained within cabinet/enclosure	Class III cabinet required
	Laboratory to contain its own equipment	Not required	Not required	Required, so far as is reasonably practicable	Required
	Safe storage of GMMs	Required where and to extent risk assessment shows	Required	Required	Secure storage required
Staff	Access restricted to authorized personnel only	Not required	Required	Required	Required via air lock key procedure
	Written records of staff training	Not required	Required where and to extent risk assessment shows	Required	Required
Waste inactivation	Inactivation of GMMs in effluent from handwashing sinks, showers and similar effluent	Not required	Not required	Required where and to extent risk assessment shows	Required
	Inactivation of GMMs in contaminated material	Required by validated means	Required by validated means	Required by validated means, with waste inactivated in the laboratory suite	Required by validated means, with waste inactivated within the laboratory

Adapted with permission from SACGM Compendium of Guidance, HSE © Crown Copyright.[56]

exposure to all the potential hazards involved in genetic modification work. Health surveillance is likely to be appropriate when all of the following criteria are fulfilled:

1. An identifiable health effect may be related to exposure.
2. There is a reasonable likelihood that the disease or effect may occur under the conditions of the work.
3. There are valid techniques for detecting indications of the disease or health effect.

The purpose of any health surveillance programme could be to collect baseline information to assist in the identification of subsequent ill health, identify health factors which are likely to increase vulnerability or susceptibility to exposure-related health effects or permit early detection of such effects. Additional aims could be to evaluate the efficacy of control measures or provide data for subsequent epidemiological study. There is also an opportunity to communicate health risks and to counsel employees about any health concerns.

Decision-making on the indications for, and content of, health surveillance programmes should be made by an occupational physician who is experienced in this field and who is involved with the organization's biological safety committee that has responsibility for reviewing risk assessments of genetic modification work. If health assessment procedures are indicated, an occupational health nurse can perform these and obtain advice from the occupational physician overseeing the programme.

Low risk genetic modification work

For work with genetically modified microorganisms that present no identifiable risk to human health, it is unlikely that there will be any indication for health surveillance. However, health surveillance may still be appropriate if there are identifiable health effects related to an allergenic response to the genetically modified microorganism or to toxic effects from expressed products.

It may still be appropriate to conduct an initial health assessment to identify individuals who may be at greater risk because of pre-existing illness or an underlying medical condition. The aim of such an assessment would be to consider the need for additional control measures or to identify adjustments to allow the individual to carry out the work with tolerable control of health risks. The following factors may require special consideration:

- relevant medical history, such as a history of asthma or recurrent infections;
- health problems which reduce the efficacy of barriers to infection, such as disorders of the skin, respiratory tract and alimentary canal;
- reduced immune competence, including treatment with immunosuppressive therapies;
- treatment with antibiotics, in particular those used in the work, or systemic steroid therapy and other treatments that could increase susceptibility to infection.

Higher risk genetic modification work

Health surveillance may be indicated if there is likelihood that any of the following potential health hazards may result in exposure-related health effects:

- infection, particularly with modified viruses which exhibit altered tissue tropism, reduced susceptibility to therapeutic agents or where conventional immunization would result in reduced protection;
- oncogenic or tumorigenic sequences that could give rise to a risk of carcinogenesis if incorporated into human cells;
- modified prion protein genes that could cause transmissible spongiform encephalopathy;
- biologically active substances expressed by genetically modified microorganisms, such as enzymes, hormones or toxins;
- cloned human genes that may lead to an immune response and subsequent autoimmune disease;
- substances that are asthmagens.

There is a range of health surveillance procedures that could be applied. Periodic enquiry about respiratory symptoms and lung function assessment would be an appropriate method of surveillance if occupational asthma were assessed to be a foreseeable health effect. For lower risk situations, providing information about relevant symptoms and encouraging self-reporting may be all that is indicated.

Biological effect monitoring could be used to detect antibody to the genetically modified microorganism in use, either to establish immune status prior to exposure or to detect seroconversion after a period of potential exposure. Immunization may be indicated for work with certain organisms. In the past, immunization with smallpox vaccine was recommended for work with modified strains of vaccinia virus, but there would be few circumstances now when this would be indicated as a result of a risk assessment of work with this virus. Maintaining records of exposure may be an appropriate method of health surveillance for work with oncogenic sequences where there is likely to be a long latency period between exposure and possible carcinogenic effects.

Storage of serum samples

Long-term storage of serum samples taken prior to exposure as a baseline reference has been widely practised in the past. The idea was that if antibody responses relevant to the genetically modified microorganisms being handled were subsequently detected, the baseline sample could be tested for comparison. However, there are few circumstances when the health benefits to the individual justify conducting such an invasive procedure and the implementation of the Human Tissue Act 2004 in the United Kingdom reinforces the view that this practice should be restricted to situations where consideration of the risk assessment for the work indicates a justifiable health or social benefit to the individual.

Previously, it was believed that the immunological response to exposure to a genetically modified microorganism or an expressed product could cause confusion during diagnostic tests for infection with the same or a related microorganism. Examples include expressed HIV proteins, where antibodies to these proteins form the basis of serological tests for HIV infection; however, previously held concerns regarding the impact that having submitted for HIV testing could have on an individual's life insurance are no longer valid. In 2005 in the UK the Association of British Insurers implemented new practice[60] that ensures that applicants will not be penalized for having taken an HIV test and are not required to declare negative tests nor will occupation be used to assess HIV risk. In general, there is only likely to be an indication for baseline serum storage when the current diagnostic tests would have difficulty distinguishing true infection from immunological response to a related protein, or acute from chronic infection states, and where such confusion could have substantial health or social consequences. The usefulness of the baseline sample is of limited medicolegal value, however, when one considers the implication of the window period that an employee could be in at the time of submitting a sample.

If serum storage is practised, then it is important that the purpose of the procedure is explained to the employee and informed consent obtained. It should be emphasized that the individual is only consenting to the sample being stored and that subsequent testing would only be conducted with the individual's express consent, even after the individual has left the organization where the sample is stored. A sample of approximately 5 mL of serum should be labelled to allow later identification of the donor and stored in a secure freezer at −20°C or below, with arrangements made for dealing with sample salvage in the event of freezer malfunction. The period of long-term storage before discarding the sample should be agreed with the donor. It is unlikely that there would be advantages in storing such samples for longer than 40 years. As can be seen, a multitude of practical and legal considerations regarding ensuring cold custody, informed consent, maintenance of accurate registers, notification to the occupational health department of staff leavers and disposal of samples need to be weighed in the balance prior to embarking on any programme of serum storage.

Medical contact cards

In the past, issuing medical contact cards to employees involved in genetic modification work with higher hazard genetically modified microorganisms was common practice. The rationale for doing so was to alert other medical personnel to the possibility of occupationally acquired infection and provide details on how to contact someone at the employing organization who would be able to give the clinician information about relevant biohazards. In practice, however, there is the likelihood that employees may lose or not carry their cards and as any occupationally acquired infection is unlikely to present with unconsciousness or an acute confusional state, this practice would seem to be of limited benefit. Any unusual symptoms not readily diagnosed by standard means would lead to a thorough assessment that would include a complete occupational history, thus yielding the required information.

Health records

Health records should be maintained of all health assessments conducted as part of any health surveillance related to genetic modification work. Records that contain clinical information must be held in confidence by healthcare professionals.

Records of exposure may also be indicated for work which involves higher hazard microorganisms, prion proteins or oncogenic sequences where there is known to be a long latent period of many years between exposure and the onset of ill health related to infection or carcinogenesis. These records should include personal identifying information, details of the nature of the hazards, the dates when the work started and finished and information that links the record to the relevant risk assessment and any exposure monitoring data. Such non-clinical records can be maintained by the employer. The records could also be used to provide retrospective information on health and related exposures for epidemiological investigation.

CONCLUSION

The clinician may be puzzled at the contrast between the complexities of biotechnology with its surrounding myriad of regulations and control measures and the dearth of data on ill health in the scientists and production workers involved. The industry is perceived to have a good health record, but, to be able to demonstrate the absence of a problem or to provide early warning of an unforeseen health hazard in this novel and rapidly expanding technology, it will be important to ensure that health surveillance measures based on sound theoretical considerations, including epidemiological studies where appropriate, are maintained. The challenge for the future will be to ensure that any potential hazards to human health or the environment are controlled to the satisfaction of employees, health and safety professionals, regulatory authorities and, ultimately, the general public.

Key points

- The field of biotechnology has an excellent health and safety record, but consideration must be taken of associated traditional risks such as chemical, physical and ergonomic.
- Work with genetically modified microorganisms is highly regulated and occupational health practitioners should familiarize themselves with relevant legislation and guidance.
- Health surveillance activities should be risk-based and outdated practices such as routine serum save discontinued.
- The field of biotechnology is developing rapidly and the risks posed by emerging technologies such as nantechnology are as yet not fully characterized.

ACKNOWLEDGEMENTS

This chapter is updated from *Hunter's Diseases of Occupations*, ninth edition, Chapter 25 Genetic modification and biotechnology by AM Finn *et al*.

REFERENCES

1. Bud R. History of 'biotechnology'. *Nature.* 1989; **337**: 10.
2. Simpson JA, Weiner ESC (eds). *Oxford English Dictionary.* Oxford: Clarendon Press, 1989.
3. Kennedy MJ. The evolution of the word 'biotechnology.' *Trends in Biotechnology.* 1991; **9**: 218–20.
4. Advisory Council on Science and Technology. *Developments in biotechnology.* London: HMSO, 1990.
5. The Convention on Biological Diversity (Article 2. Use of Terms). United Nations. 1992.
6. Statutory Instrument 2000, No. 2831. The genetically modified organisms (contained use) regulations 2000. London: TSO.
7. Biotechnology Industry Organisation. Annual biotechnology industry reports. London: Ernst & Young LLP, 1995–2006.
8. Liberman OF, Ducatman AM, Fink R. Biotechnology: Is there a role for medical surveillance? In: Hyer WC (ed.). *Bioprocessing safety: Worker and community safety and health considerations.* Philadelphia: ASTM, 1990: 101–10.
9. Miller H. Report on the World Health Organization Working Group on Health Implications of Biotechnology. *Recombinant DNA Technical Bulletin.* 1983; **6**: 65–6.
10. Borm PJA. Hazards and risks of nanomaterials: A look forward. Proceedings of the First International Symposium on Occupational Health Implications of Nanomaterials, October 12–14, 2004, Buxton: Health and Safety Executive and the National Institute for Occupational Safety and Health, 2005.
11. Landrigan PJ, Cohen MI, Dowdle W *et al.* Medical surveillance of biotechnology workers: Report of the CD/NIOSH Ad Hoc Working Group on Medical Surveillance for Industrial Applications of Biotechnology. *Recombinant DNA Technical Bulletin.* 1982; **5**: 133–8.
12. Frommer W, Kraeme P. Safety aspects in biotechnology: Classifications and safety precautions for handling of biological agents, e.g. genetically engineered microorganism containment. *Drugs Made in Germany.* 1990; **33**: 128–32.
13. Cohen R, Hoerner CL. Occupational health perspective: Recombinant DNA technology – human gene therapy safety. *Biopharm Manufact.* 1994; **7**: 28–38.
14. Demain AL. An overview of biotechnology. *Occupational Medicine - State of the Art Review.* 1991; 157–68.
15. Campbell KHS, McWhir J, Ritchie WA, Wilmut A. Sheep cloned by nuclear transfer from a cultured cell line. *Nature.* 1996; **380**: 64–6.
16. Coordinated Framework for Regulation of Biotechnology. US Office for Science and Technology. June 1986. Available from: http://usbiotechreg.nbii.gov/CoordinatedFrameworkForRegulationOfBiotechnology1986.pdf.
17. National Institutes for Health. Guidelines for research involving recombinant DNA molecules. Washington, DC: Federal Register, 2002.
18. Centers for Disease Control. Biosafety in microbiological and biomedical laboratories, 4th edn. Washington, DC: US Government Printing Office, 1999.
19. Rocco MC. Environmentally responsible development of nanotechnology. *Environmental Science and Technology.* 2005; **39**: 106A–12A.
20. Antonini JM. Health effects of welding. *Critical Reviews in Toxicology.* 2003; **33**: 61–103.
21. Sferlazza SJ, Beckett WS. The respiratory health of welders. *American Review of Respiratory Disease.* 1991; **143**: 1134–48.
22. Seaton A, MacNee W, Donaldson K *et al.* Particulate air pollution and acute health effects. *Lancet.* 1995; **345**: 176–8.
23. Schwarz J. Morris R. Air pollution and hospital admissions for cardiovascular disease in Detroit, Michigan. *American Journal of Epidemiology.* 1995; **142**: 23–25.
24. Taniguchi N. On the basic concept of 'nanotechnology'. Proceedings of the International Conference on Production Engineering, Part II. Tokyo: Japan Society of Precision Engineering, 1974.
25. Maynard AD, Kuempel ED. Airborne nanostructured particles and occupational health. *Journal of Nanoparticle Research.* 2005; **7**: 587–614.
26. Hoet PHM, Brueske-Hohlfeld I, Salata OV. Nanoparticles – known and unknown health risks. *Journal of Nanobiotechnology.* 2004; **2**: 12.
27. Salata OV. Applications of nanoparticles in biology and medicine. *Journal of Nanobiotechnology.* 2004; **2**: 3.
28. Seaton A. Nanotechnology and the occupational physician. *Occupational Medicine.* 2006; **56**: 312–16.
29. Glover OM. *Gene cloning: The mechanics of DNA manipulation.* London: Chapman and Hall, 1984.
30. Clackson T, Hoogenboom HR, Griffiths AD, Winter G. Making antibody fragments using phage display libraries. *Nature.* 1991; **352**: 624–8.
31. Reichman L, Winter G. Novel folded proteins by combinatorial shuffling of peptide segments. *Proceedings of the National Academy of Sciences of the United States of America.* 2000; **97**: 10068–73.
32. Duffus JH, Brown CM. Health aspects of biotechnology. *Annals of Occupational Hygiene.* 1985; **29**: 1–12.
33. Rinderknecht E, O'Connor BH, Rodriguez H. Natural human interferon. Complete amino acid sequencing and determination of site of glycosylation. *Journal of Biological Chemistry.* 1984; **259**: 6790–7.
34. Vallejo LF, Rinas U. Strategies for the recovery of active proteins through refolding of bacterial inclusion body proteins. *Microbial Cell Factories.* 2004; **3**: 11.
35. Knight P. The carbohydrate frontier. *BioTechnology.* 1989; **7**: 35–40.
36. Brown F, Shild GC, Ada GL. Recombinant vaccinia viruses as vaccines. *Nature.* 1986; **319**: 549–50.
37. Forde GM. Rapid-response vaccines – does DNA offer a solution? *Nature Biotechnology.* 2005; **23**: 1059–62.
38. Pharmaceutical Research and Manufacturers of America. 2006 Report: medicines in development – biotechnology. Washington, DC: Pharmaceutical Research and Manufacturers of America, August 2006.
39. Dutkiewia J, Jabionski I, Olenchock SA. Occupational biohazards: A review. *American Journal of Industrial Medicine.* 1988; **14**: 605–23.

40. Lacey J, Crook B. Fungal and actinomycete spores as pollutants of the workplace and occupational allergen. *Annals of Occupational Hygiene.* 1988; **32**: 515-33.
41. Demain AL, Solomon NA. Industrial microbiology. *Scientific American.* 1981; **245**: 43-51.
42. World Health Organization. Health impact of biotechnology – report on a Working Group. *Swiss Biotech.* 1984; **2**: 7-32.
43. Burns PA, Jack A, Neilson F et al. Transformation of mouse skin endothelial cells *in vivo* by direct application of plasmid DNA encoding the human T24 H-ras oncogene. *Oncogene.* 1991; **6**: 1973-8.
44. Burrell R, Ye S-H. Toxic risks from inhalation of bacterial endotoxin. *Occupational and Environmental Medicine.* 1990; **47**: 688-91.
45. Palchak RB, Cohen R, Ainslie M, Hoerner CL. Airborne endotoxin associated with industrial scale production of protein products in Gram-negative bacteria. *American Industrial Hygiene Association Journal.* 1988; **49**: 420-42.
46. Birch K. *The role of endotoxin tolerance in byssinosis.* Morgan Town, WV: West Virginia University, 1983.
47. Pernis B, Vigliani EC, Cavagna C, Finulli M. The role of bacterial endotoxins in occupational disease caused by inhaling dusts. *British Journal of Industrial Medicine.* 1961; **18**: 120-9.
48. DeMaria TF, Burrell R. Effect of inhaled endotoxin-containing bacteria. *Environmental Research.* 1980; **23**: 87-97.
49. Lantz RC, Birch K, Hinton DE, Burrell R. Morphometric changes in the lung induced by inhaled bacterial endotoxin. *Experimental and Molecular Pathology.* 1985; **43**: 305-20.
50. Flindt MLH. Pulmonary disease due to inhalation of derivatives of *Bacillus subtilis* containing proteolytic enzyme. *Lancet.* 1969; **i**: 1177-81.
51. Pepys J, Hargreaves RE, Longbottom JL, Faux J. Allergic reactions of the lungs to enzymes of *Bacillus subtilis. Lancet.* 1969; **i**: 1181-4.
52. Newhouse ML, Tagg B, Pocock ST, McEwan AC. An epidemiological study of workers producing enzyme washing powders. *Lancet.* 1970; **i**: 689-93.
53. Milne J, Brand S. Occupational asthma after inhalation of dust of the proteolytic enzyme, papain. *British Journal of Industrial Medicine.* 1975; **32**: 302-7.
54. Nava C. Allergy. In: Parmeggiani L (ed.). *Encyclopaedia of occupational health and safety.* Geneva: International Labour Office, 1983: 124-6.
55. Ducatman AM, Columbis JJ. Chemical hazards in the biotechnology industry. *Occupational Medicine – State of the Art Review.* 1991; 193-225.
56. Scientific Advisory Committee on Genetic Modification. The SACGM compendium of guidance. Last accessed June 19, 2009. Available from: www.hse.gov.uk/biosafety/gmo/acgm/acgmcomp/index.htm.
57. Kingsman SM, Mitrophanous K, Olsen JC. Potential oncogene activity of the woodchuck hepatitis post-transcriptional regulatory element (WPRE). *Gene Therapy.* 2005; **12**: 3-4.
58. Burns PA, Jack A, Neilson F et al. Transformation of mouse skin endothelial cells *in vivo* by direct application of plasmid DNA encoding the human T24 H-ras oncogene. *Oncogene.* 1991; **6**: 1973-8.
59. Cohen R, Hoerner CL. Recombinant DNA technology: A 20-year occupational health retrospective. *Reviews on Environmental Health.* 1996; **11**: 149-65.
60. Association of British Insurers. Statement of best practice on HIV and insurance. London: ABI, October 2004.

PART SIX

WORK AND MENTAL HEALTH

Section One: Work and stress   801
Section Two: Work and psychiatric disorder   831
Section Three: Substance abuse   857

SECTION ONE

Work and stress

63	Introduction to work and stress *Peter J Baxter, Tar-Ching Aw and Anne Cockcroft*	803
64	Work, stress and sickness absence: a psychosocial perspective *Maurice Lipsedge and Michael Calnan*	804
65	Mental health at work: psychological interventions *Adrian Neal*	823

63

Introduction to work and stress

According to Hayward,[1] stress derives from the Latin word *stringo* (*stringere*), meaning to bind or draw tight. It entered the English language in the fourteenth century, when it referred to physical hardship and later, a form of injury. It was not until the seventeenth century that the word began to refer to an inner state.[1] Its modern usage to describe a combination of harmful environmental pressures and pathological physiological responses was popularized in the research work of the biochemist Hans Selye (1907–82). The notion that the body's response to the environment might have adverse health consequences, especially on the heart, was proposed by the famous clinician Sir William Osler (1849–1919).[1,2] Experimental evidence on the effects of stress emerged in the laboratory work of the physiologist Walter B Cannon in the 1930s, when he showed a range of physiological responses, such as adrenaline release and cardiac arrythmias, in response to external 'strains'.[1] These concepts, part developed by pioneers in an era that preceded modern scientific medicine, took firm root with the public and the medical profession.

Readers turning to *Hunter's Diseases of Occupations* for authoritative guidance on stress disorders arising out of work will find the following three chapters covering the topic from separate, but overlapping, angles: a review of the evidence base, the reflections of a psychiatrist on the psychosocial aspects and a clinical psychologist's perspective on intervention. Stress at work manifests in many different ways, but occupational physicians should have little difficulty in recognizing the 'work-stress victim' described by Lipsedge and Calnan. William Blake's 'dark, satanic mills' may have finally receded into history in high-income nations, where in this age of globalization the entrepreneur employer is seen less as a villain than as the wealth creator we desperately need. However, employees in almost all employment sectors complain increasingly of such problems as overwork, or fear of making mistakes, or of being marginalized, bullied and harassed, to the point of intolerable distress. These three chapters agree on at least two things: first, that the evidence on the management of individuals presenting with stress at work is still controversial, and second, most employees who have work-related distress do not need to be medicalized. In the chapters by Glozier and colleagues, and Lipsedge and Calnan, the mental effects of exposure to life-threatening trauma and involvement in warfare as part of work are also described, along with the medicolegal minefield of post-traumatic stress disorder.

Peter J Baxter
Tar-Ching Aw
Anne Cockcroft

REFERENCES

1. Hayward R. Historical keywords: Stress. *Lancet.* 2005; **365**: 2001.
2. Brotman DJ, Golden SH, Wittstein IS. The cardiovascular toll of stress. *Lancet.* 2007; **370**: 1089–100.

Work, stress and sickness absence: a psychosocial perspective

MAURICE LIPSEDGE AND MICHAEL CALNAN

Introduction	804
The discourse of work stress	804
Sickness absence as a form of resistance	806
Susto and the sick role: a way out?	807
Work stress as a culture-bound syndrome	808
Benign surveillance	809
Defining entitlement	810
Incapacity benefit claims and sick notes	810
Fitness to attend disciplinary hearings	811
Adverse workplace events and trauma	811
Workplace phobia	812
Depression, adjustment disorder and sickness absence	812
Post-traumatic stress disorder	814
Resilience	815
Work overload, distress and sickness absence	815
Counselling is not a substitute for mediation	816
Incivility in the workplace	816
Resentment and sickness absence	816
The positive role of mediation	817
Government policy on incapacity benefit and getting back to work	817
Summary and conclusion	818
Acknowledgements	819
References	819

INTRODUCTION

The main aim of this chapter is to identify the cultural and psychosocial influences on the illness behaviour of employees with problems that manifest under the title of 'work-related stress'. Much of the previous work on the relationship between work and stress has tended either to focus on the social epidemiological factors,[1] which put workers at risk of stress-related ill health, or has adopted a psychological approach and focused on the personal characteristics of the worker and their influence on the perception of threat and the ability to cope (see Ref. 2). What appears to have been neglected is the link between the two and how aspects of the structure of the working environment to do with social relations that affect health need to be incorporated into the psychiatric assessment of the individual. This psychosocial perspective combines occupational psychiatry and medical sociology and anthropology and is illustrated with case examples.

THE DISCOURSE OF WORK STRESS

The theoretical perspective adopted here provides a general framework for understanding the arguments and explanations which are presented for the relationship between work-stress and sickness absence. It draws, at least in part, on cultural sociology[3] as it focuses on the cultural construction of the 'epidemic' of work stress and the creation of the social identity of the 'work stress victim'. The argument runs as follows: The 'popular' discourse of work stress suggests that the labour process is being intensified and making greater demands on the worker, which may lead to poor mental and physical health. The apparent increases in strain and tension across workplaces are claimed to be due to changes in work characteristics, such as technological innovation, introduction of new managerial techniques, greater job insecurity or increases in working hours. These changes in the organization and character of work are increasingly conceptualized in terms of the 'medical' category of stress which emphasizes their consequences for the physical and mental health of the individual worker. There are essentially two strategies for addressing the work stress 'epidemic'.[3] The first emphasizes strengthening the individual through stress management techniques and therapeutic interventions, such as counselling or medication. The second focuses on job redesign as a means of reducing job strain, although even here the emphasis is still on health and safety at work.[3]

The reaction to problems at work depends mainly on how employees interpret their experiences, and how they decide to respond. However, employees do not make sense of their experiences in a vacuum, rather they make sense of their personal experiences by relating them to a broader pattern of assumptions and expectations. This broader pattern, according to Wainwright and Calnan,[3] might be referred to as the 'discourse of work stress', and it acts almost as a guide to action, or at least as a pre-existing framework within which experiences can be made sense of and decisions about future action can be taken. The discourse of work stress is an informal body of social knowledge built on a mixture of lay experience, professional and academic opinion and media representations. It tends to reflect current social and structural arrangements and is, therefore, historically specific.[3] This argument, however, has a further dimension in that it suggests that work stress is not entirely mediated at the level of consciousness or cognition.[3] Over the life course, social experiences become embodied or as Wainwright and Calnan propose 'become written on the body' in the form of learned emotional and physiological responses which can later be triggered independently of conscious assessment. Unaware that these reactions have been 'learned' since childhood, it is taken for granted that they represent a 'natural' limit on the body's capacity for endurance and resilience, further reinforcing the belief that work stress is basically a biomedical reaction to the excessive demands and strains of working in the current cultural context.

The work-stress discourse can be interpreted as an example of the medicalization of a social problem,[4,5] i.e. that adverse experiences at work which were previously seen as political or industrial relations issues are increasingly falling into the domain of medical jurisdiction. Medicalization operates at a number of different levels[4–7] with varying degrees of medical professional involvement. The work-stress discourse provides a conceptual framework for defining and understanding the problem in medical terms. Yet this medicalization process may also be evident at the institutional level where doctors can control access to and legitimate sickness absence and benefits and at the interactional level where they treat and diagnose those who consult them for work-related problems.

There is a range of different approaches to medicalization, but the more recent ones[5,8] have emphasized the way medical discourse might influence self-identity in a positive rather than a repressive way. Thus, the new self-identity of the work-stress victim might offer an accessible framework for making sense of and responding to, not just adverse experiences at work, but what appear to be their emotional and physiological manifestations. It not only provides a seemingly 'scientific' explanation of lived embodied experiences, it also offers a range of strategies for action: therapies and sick leave for some, exit from the workplace through early retirement on medical grounds for others, and for a few the opportunity to seek financial redress through the courts.

The adoption of the identity of a work-stress victim is a choice and thus the question is how far the discourse of work stress which appears to dominate public debate about changes in work at the macro level has been taken on by workers at the micro level. Evidence from studies[3] which explored the processes by which employees come to recognize adverse experiences at work as health problems and the extent to which they turn to medicalized solutions for dealing with these problems, suggest that the stress discourse is salient to workers (both men and women) when they are discussing adverse experiences at work, and that it is used to make sense of a wide range of experiences, from low morale and low job satisfaction, through to embodied manifestations, including physiological signs and symptoms. Moreover, the assumption that workers passively accept medical solutions, such as medication and counselling, was shown to be inaccurate and consultation was a way of getting sickness absence rather than treatment (for example, Ref. 3):

> ... he (the doctor) said, 'there are two ways of handling this, we can either give you some time off work, or, I can give you some medication, something to take.' And I said, 'I didn't want to take anything,' so he signed me off work for a week. And he said; 'come and see me in a week and we'll see how it goes (p. 185).

And

> the doctor was just a means to an end to get a sick note because I wasn't fit enough to work. I didn't feel that the doctor herself actually talked to me and helped me. At the time I couldn't continue to work (p. 181).

While some workers adhered to medical labels and followed an illness pathway which led to exit from the labour market through early retirement on medical grounds, others contested the medicalization process and resisted seeking professional medical help. The value attached to personal resilience coupled with the reluctance to adopt the self-identity of a work stress 'victim' appears to be an important factor in determining resistance to the medicalization process (for example, Ref. 3):

> *Interviewer*: How did you feel about going to the doctor with that kind of problem?
>
> Pathetic basically, you should be able to cope with life, shouldn't you, be stronger willed and get on with everything (p. 183).

> ... you feel you're letting yourself down because you haven't been able to cope. You feel that you have an image that you have to maintain. I've told a few close friends and the rest you tend not to talk to about it (p. 183).

A range of alternative strategies for addressing problems at work was identified, including informal mechanisms of support, 'emotion work' and informal relaxation techniques. In a related study of arm pain,[9] contrary to expectations, informants rarely invoked work and its effect on them as a cause of their problems and as a consequence did not always feel it was appropriate or possible to alert their work colleagues and employers to their condition. Some of this reticence stemmed from a fear of being seen as a trouble maker and others, who felt unable to discuss their condition at work, were more likely to feel this way because of the 'age factor':

> I'm just very conscious of my age and I work with a lot of young people, and I just don't take time off of work ... I've got a TENS machine for my back and I sit and work with my TENS machine on (A1217).

Why was there opposition or resistance to medicalization? Wainwright and Calnan[3] suggest that the answer seems to lie in the extent to which becoming a work-stress victim entails relinquishing control over one's mental life. Agency, or the ability to actively engage with the world as a conscious actor, depends fundamentally upon mental competence. To be unable to cope with the demands of a stressful job and to seek medical advice, is to give up one's identity as an independent social actor where being able to work is a fundamental part of social identity. The ability to cope with stressful life events without using medical therapy has traditionally been viewed as a positive personal trait, but the negative side of valuing the capacity to withstand pressure is that those who fail to cope are stigmatized as weak or inadequate. Hence, the reluctance among the informants to change from being a person who is suffering work stress but coping with the pressure, to someone who cannot cope without clinical support. Thus, it is argued[3] that for many experiencing work stress, the choice of consulting a doctor or coping alone is still available and consultation remains something to be struggled against or lapsed into. It also reflects the tension between the social benefits and disadvantages of the different statuses of 'health' and 'illness'.

SICKNESS ABSENCE AS A FORM OF RESISTANCE

This perspective on the construction of work stress and the response to it will be used to frame the approach taken here, although the emphasis is rather different as it focuses on those whose problems appear so incapacitating that they are physically or mentally unable to carry on working and thus have little choice but to seek sickness absence. However, the thesis of this chapter is that much work stress-related sickness absence is a form of resistance, when the employee, feeling weak and powerless in the face of perceived oppressive managerial practices, begins to interpret their subjective emotional reaction in terms of psychophysiological dysfunction and disorder. As Fineman[10] concludes (p. 126), resistance to organizational change arises from both the disruption of the moral/political order that binds the employee to the organization and from the apprehension and uncertainty caused to their sense of identity, security and self-worth. Sickness absence on the grounds of work-related stress is interpreted here as an oblique form of resistance, a covert acting out of indignation and anger. This, as the previous theoretical discussion suggested, is no easy or lightly taken option given the moral imperative to be resilient, to be able to cope and continue to work.

We would argue that paradoxically the new identity reinforced with a medical label (disorder or 'syndrome') can become a strategic tool to redress the balance for those employees who feel undervalued, exploited or discarded. The quest for a diagnostic label and the performance of a culturally standardized sequence of events and actions has the characteristics of a 'culture-bound syndrome'.[11] The necessary conditions for a culture-bound syndrome are a specific configuration of social expectations and a template of how to behave when oppressed. Culture-bound syndromes are local patterns of time-limited behaviour, specific to a particular culture, which while regarded as undesirable, have a problem-solving function for the dislocated individual who is not held to be aware or responsible in the everyday sense (p. 290).[12]

In the workplace, the employee who feels humiliated, whose dignity has been affronted or who feels that his work is over-controlled, is denied what Scott calls 'the ordinary luxury of negative reciprocity: trading a slap for a slap, an insult for an insult' (p. 23).[13] Being treated with respect and dignity might be more important at work than financial reward (p. xii).[13] When an individual is wronged by a person of inferior status they feel contempt, when the offender is of the same rank the victim becomes angry, but when a person is treated badly by a superior they feel bitterness and resentment,[14] which can become the state of chronic embitterment recently described by Tom Sensky.[15]

In his monograph, *Happiness and Unhappiness in the Workplace*, Warr[14] has defined the key characteristics of any job which lead to greater well-being and self-validation. These include opportunities for personal control, skills use, variety, clarity of role, social interaction, status, support, security and equity, as well as amount of pay.[16]

These ingredients are perceived to be lacking in the modern workplace, as in Franz Kafka's description of a large open-plan office:

People were criss-crossing the middle of the floor, in all directions, at great speed. No-one offered a greeting, greetings had been abolished, each one fell into the tracks of the man ahead of him and kept his eyes on the floor, across which he walked to make as rapid progress as possible (p. 34).

Kafka[17]

Employees' complaints about stress often reflect feeling undervalued and powerless within an organization.[18] Subjective well-being is undermined by a perception of organizational injustice and where there is thought to be a breach of the psychological contract. (This is defined as a set of expectations specifying what the individual and the employer expect to give and receive from each other in terms of rights, privileges, duties and obligations) (p. 149).[19]

Pinder[20] found that 'systemic injustice', i.e. the perception of unfairness within the organizational context, tends to induce fear, resentment, hopelessness and sadness (p. 122). Anger and hatred towards superiors were common in employees who felt they had been treated unfairly, especially if there had been an element of public humiliation (p. 123). 'Employees who feel locked into their jobs have limited constructive means for dealing with their frustration and, as a result, are more likely to resort to either aggression or displaced aggression in their jobs' (p. 125).

Pinder[20] (p. 277) describes what job dissatisfaction feels like: 'It often carries feelings of gloom and despair, sometimes anger and resentment, sometimes futility'. He adds that 'withdrawal in response to job dissatisfaction can take the form of tardiness, absenteeism and turnover, as well as passive compliance and minimal effort' (p. 278) and that the 'perception of unfair or unjust treatment by employers is a major cause of theft, sabotage, violence at work, absenteeism and lateness' (p. 313).

When the subordinate takes sick leave because of a breach of the psychological contract, they might be adopting a political strategy to redress the imbalance in the power relationship between employer and employee, by embodying a 'hidden transcript of the weak' (p. xii),[13] which covertly expresses their resentment and frustration'. 'Oh my Lord', he thought, 'If only I didn't have to follow such an exhausting profession! On the road, day in, day out. The work is so much more strenuous than it would be in head office, and then there's the additional ordeal of travelling, worries about train connections, the irregular meals, bad food, new people all the time, no continuity, no affection. Devil take it!' (p. 88).[21]

Historically, subordinates have disguised their resentful opposition by resorting to tactics such as foot-dragging and dissimulation which Scott describes as the 'infrapolitics of the powerless' (p.xiii),[13] 'a substitute for an act of assertion directly in the face of power' (p. 155).[13]

In his novella about Bartleby, the indolent scrivener, Herman Melville describes the predicament of the benign employer in the face of his employee's repeated refrain: 'I would prefer not to'. 'Nothing so aggravates an earnest person as a passive resistance ... mortified as I was at his behaviour, and resolved as I had been to dismiss him when he entered my office, nevertheless I felt some superstitious knocking at my heart, forbidding me to carry out my purpose and denouncing me for a villain if I dared to breathe one bitter word against this forlornest of mankind' (pp. 17–26).[22]

SUSTO AND THE SICK ROLE: A WAY OUT?

From a sociological perspective, the resort to sickness absence by employees with seemingly minor symptoms and distress is an example of both strategic manoeuvring and of illness behaviour. Taking sick leave is one of those conditions identified by Robert Edgerton which are 'culturally recognized and named as brief periods during which the temporarily ill, intoxicated, bereaved or possessed person is expected to behave in ways that would ordinarily be prohibited' (p. 49).[23] In advanced industrial societies, being on sick leave starts off as a temporary status which exempts people from their ordinary obligation of economic productivity (p. 6).[23] When the powerless individual is enmeshed in a situation that he cannot control, the passive appeal of helplessness affords room for manoeuvre and negotiation with management.[24]

As Brown[25] has asserted (p. 39), 'some people with the same symptoms and conditions as others choose widely disparate ways of dealing with their symptoms or conditions'. *Susto* is an example of the well-known 'sick role' as defined by Parsons and Fox[26] which provides a socially sanctioned exemption from the challenge of everyday responsibility and which is fashioned in accordance with the 'dominant social elements of medical knowledge' (p. 37).[25] As with stress in the West, *susto* is a culturally shaped idiom of distress.[27] Medical anthropology recognizes that bodily and psychological complaints are used as metaphors of personal, social or occupational stress, 'which give the sufferer a little more leverage in negotiating for a less difficult work situation ...' (p. 27).[27] Sometimes these temporary conditions can become long term, and evolve into eligibility for incapacity benefits and eventually early retirement on the grounds of ill health.

Among the Zapotec of the Oaxaca Valley of Mexico, *susto* ('fright sickness')[28] exempts the afflicted person from onerous duties for a limited period of time, before resumption of normal responsibilities. The 'clinical presentation' of *susto* includes unrefreshing sleep, low mood, lack of drive, energy and motivation, poor appetite and neglecting one's appearance, together with feeling overwhelmed by routine tasks and non-specific aches and pains. This amalgam of complaints is found throughout rural Latin America and is attributed to 'soul loss' in which the person's spiritual element departs from their body.[29] The victim has generally felt powerless and trapped in a stressful situation where they cannot meet social or personal obligations. *Susto* provides a socially respectable escape hatch from intolerable circumstances, by affording respite from normal social responsibilities.

Becoming an *asustado* appears to be a more or less conscious choice. Its potency in mobilizing privileges derives from the folk belief that *susto*, like hypertension and even stress in the West, is potentially fatal.[30] The status of *asustado* is arrived at through group negotiation, with cues provided by neighbours. Entitlement is sometimes challenged because not all temporary conditions that have the potential to provide exemption actually have clear criteria for entitlement and the claim for exemption has to be negotiated (p. 49).[23] As Edgerton points out (p. 74), exempting conditions such as grief, illness, intoxication and spirit possession 'can be readily exaggerated, prolonged or faked altogether'. He asks, 'Was someone really possessed, truly drunk, honestly grief-stricken?' In our society, a sceptical benefits gate-keeper might ask, 'Is this person genuinely sick and disabled?' or is this a case of 'strategic opportunism?' (p. 53).[23]

WORK STRESS AS A CULTURE-BOUND SYNDROME

The culture-bound nature of workplace stress reactions is illustrated by the epidemic of possession states described in Malaysian factories in the 1970s.

In one ethnographic account,[31] foreign-owned electronics factories enlisted single Muslim women from village communities. They lived in hostels at some distance from their rural homes. These young women were closely supervised on the factory floor by male managers from a different ethnic background. Their electronic assembly work was repetitive and monotonous and caused eye strain. The employees were motivated to work in these factories by the prospect of earning enough money to send to their families and to pay for their own further education. This was an attractive alternative career to traditional arduous physical labour in the rice fields. However, despite the attraction of regular wages and a degree of independence from the constraints of traditional village life, there were sporadic outbreaks of possession. These dramatic, but generally short-lived, episodes were characterized by sudden screaming and falling to the ground with violent convulsive movements.

A common theme was having a vision, while in the lavatory and especially when menstruating, of a Tamil male supervisor peering at the employee (both the toilet zone and menstruation are liminal and associated with pollution).[32] Several fellow workers would typically then see the same vision, collapse and make violent movements with their limbs. Work on the assembly line would be halted and production targets sabotaged.

At first, management called in *bomohs*, traditional healers, to exorcise the possessing spirit. The local interpretation of these bouts was that the factories had been built on virgin forest land which had offended and displaced tree spirits. These vengeful spirits were now possessing and punishing the factory workers.

Some possession cases proved to be refractory to priestly intervention and so company medical officers were invited to examine the afflicted workers. They made a diagnosis of mass hysteria and prescribed psychiatric drugs, mainly benzodiazepine tranquillizers. These biomedical interventions were only partially effective and some of the possessed women, after further episodes, were dismissed on medical grounds and returned to their villages.

In a foreign-owned factory in Malacca manufacturing trainers, there were 40 outbreaks of 'mass hysteria' in 1977–78 among poorly educated, badly paid female workers.[33] The hysterical behaviour included convulsions, aggression and apparent loss of consciousness. This behaviour was attributed by the employees to spirit possession due to violation of moral codes. Management labelled this as 'hysteria due to superstition'. Again they encouraged local traditional healers to carry out exorcisms at the factory water tanks. Private interviews with an anthropologist revealed a number of grievances: resentment about low wages, lack of subsidies for bus fares, strict and closely supervised work regimes, restricted leave and alleged harassment by male supervisors. The women expressed feelings of powerlessness, exploitation and job insecurity. Their wish to join a union had been thwarted.

In both cases, the Malay cultural disapproval of open display of anger prevented these workers from verbalizing their grievances and their resistance to management took an oblique form.[34]

Chew[35] who was director of the industrial health department in the Ministry of Labour in Singapore discusses the management of outbreaks of hysteria among factory workers in Malaysia. 'These mass hysteria episodes were treated like an epidemic disease of bacteriological origin. (p. 50)' Control of contagion was attempted by isolating the identifiable cases from the general factory population and injecting them with chlorpromazine. Isolation was required since they were considered to be 'infectious'. It was recognized that psychological factors were important and it was also concluded that as a long-term preventative measure 'a key factor seems to be education and raising the level of immunity in the susceptible community by "inculcating" the right notions and giving basic facts to eliminate superstitious beliefs' (p. 53).[35] There is no reference to conflict in the workplace. In this public health approach which was based on the principles of containing a microbial epidemic, tranquillizers were administered to control the activity of the disease in the victims.

In Ackerman and Lee's study[33] of a spirit possession event at a shoe factory in Malaysia, the authors emphasize the factory's policy of strong anti-unionism. The managing director had instructed management to listen for rumblings of discontent and indications of collective organization among the workers, whose leaders were to be identified and dismissed immediately to deter any would-be organizers. They describe episodes of violent convulsions, loss of consciousness, incoherent mumblings and aggressive behaviour among groups of Malay female workers which were interpreted as spirit possession. Fellow workers attempted to hold them down, applying cooling agents to their foreheads and accompanying them home after they had calmed down. Other workers were afraid to approach them in case the behaviour was contagious. The afflicted workers were all female. The managers had few complaints about the female production workers' job performance and discipline, but the male workers presented continual problems of insubordination and theft. Management were perplexed by the outbreaks of possession and did not hold these women workers responsible for their disruptive behaviour which on occasion led to the closure of the factory. The authors elicited antagonism towards management and both male and female workers' dissatisfaction with the incentive system and work conditions, but this antagonism was not perceived by either the workers or the management as a significant causal factor in the occurrence of possession. Thus, the assumed supernatural influences in the factory were not explicitly linked with the workers' grievances, i.e. the outbreaks of mass spirit possession and the resentment of the workers were perceived as two unrelated domains.[33]

From the perspective of medical anthropology, these outbreaks of possession in factories in the industrializing world can be interpreted as follows:

- As with other culture-bound syndromes,[36] the stylized behaviour has a shared meaning which articulates a personal predicament and represents a conflict, in this case the opposition between employer and employee.
- The culturally shaped resistance to pressure from managers has both a personal expressive meaning for the individual and an instrumental function.
- The resistance draws on locally available beliefs in possession which mainly afflicts non-dominant people, i.e. women of low status. As in other situations of frustration, 'the principal is able to adjust his or her situation by recourse to mystical pressure'.[37] 'Such spiritual afflictions … are to be found in circumstances where other secular means of ventilating grievances or pursuing vital interests are blocked, or very restricted' (p. 89).[38] This sideways recourse to transcendental action mobilizes the 'power of the weak',[39] invoking supernatural (or biomedical) pressure which permits personal adjustment of the situation and reduces frustration.
- Possession tends to occur during a visit to the factory lavatory. This is a liminal place invested with potency because of the contrast between purity and dirt. A woman's vulnerability in the toilet is enhanced if she is menstruating which is also associated with notions of pollution and danger.
- Furthermore, the recurrent theme of being spied on by hallucinated foreign male apparitions reflects the subordinate position of the female workers who are under close surveillance by male supervisors of a different ethnicity.

- Malaise due to the demands of working in an electronic assembly plant and a shoe factory provoking a sequence of 'symptoms' followed by traditional folk labelling and exorcism has parallels in the West, where the therapeutic quest for relief from work-induced medically unexplained symptoms often shifts from the biomedical to New Age methods: acupuncture, reiki, bioenergy, amygdala retraining, 'healing', Chinese herbal medication, multivitamins, reflexology, natural food remedies, Light Bath, vibration therapy, geodetic force analysis, massage and cranial osteopathy.

BENIGN SURVEILLANCE

The tension between productivity and employees' subjective well-being has been a core issue of industrial psychology and psychiatry since the early twentieth century.[40] 'Alex', the *Daily Telegraph* business pages strip cartoon for July 28, 2008, provides a good example of the stress discourse. A senior executive at Megabank asks the bank's stress counsellor if anybody from his department has consulted him recently. The stress counsellor replies that although his services are paid for by the bank, the names of the employees who consult him and the matters discussed have to remain strictly confidential. The executive replies, 'But I have decisions to make about the running of my department and I need to be forewarned if any of my team is cracking up or losing the plot …'. He adds, 'I mean I wouldn't want to fire a guy and waste a payoff on him if he was already planning to quit …'. The stress counsellor refuses to breach professional confidentiality and a day or two later he himself is made redundant.

Close surveillance in the workplace is familiar in the West[40] and even extends to toilet breaks. Thus, Gillian Howard in the Law Society Manual on drafting employment contracts writes, 'When you take lavatory breaks during the course of your working day, you are required to report to central office at the time of starting and finishing the break. This is required for safety reasons so that management knows where you can be located in the case of any emergency or safety issue' (p. 127).[41] According to an American Postal Workers' Union official, supervisors have the right to order emergency psychiatric examinations for employees who have 'increased bathroom use' or become 'argumentative'.[42] In these cases, the surveillance aspect is mitigated by the expressed concern for health and safety.

Psychological interpretations of sickness absence have inspired a number of management solutions over the past 100 years or so.[40] These approaches have attempted to work on the subjective experience of the private self, i.e. to socially organize and manage thoughts. Under the French insurance company AXA's 'My Budget Day' initiative, employees are given an hour off during a working day to check their financial planning and use the company's website to contact brokers, consultants and advisers to develop personal budget plans. The scheme was introduced by

AXA to improve relations with staff and to raise morale. The programme, interestingly, also helps managers to check whether money worries are affecting staff (the group human resources director describes the scheme as an employer's financial web-based 'health check tool'). This initiative is included in the employee's benefit programme (Daily Telegraph Business, Appointments section October 30, 2008, https://mybudgetday.axa.co.uk).

The programme has helped morale and reduced absenteeism and staff turnover and managers have reported an improvement in performance when employees were less worried about their personal finances. After the 'My Budget Day' in 2007, employee turnover rates fell from 12.8 to 11 per cent, while absenteeism which AXA uses as a 'stress indicator', fell by 10 per cent to just over 3 per cent.

DEFINING ENTITLEMENT

The sick role concept has long been criticized for having limited explanatory power for accounting for the social position of chronically sick people as it applies mainly to acute, physical short-term illness. Of more relevance is the way it might be used to control deviance by providing a set of rules, responsibilities and obligations which circumscribe eligibility and access.

The Employment Appeals Tribunal in the case of Morgan v Staffordshire University furnished practical guidance on the type of evidence needed to 'prove' that an individual is suffering from a mental impairment. For organizational and legal purposes, 'stress' is often too nebulous a concept and there is a requirement to produce a more focused diagnosis using WHO ICD-10 categories (Morgan v Staffordshire University[43] cited in D'Auria et al;[44] see also Jamdar and Byford[45]).

A diagnosis involves reified definitions of disease into which professionals fit their observations. This implies legal endorsement for medically 'organizing' a mishmash of disparate feelings, emotions and complaints to create a coherent entity[46] by a process of mapping reported symptoms onto available cultural models of illness and healing.[47,48] As Brown observes '… physicians are confronted with what is often an "unorganized illness" and a conglomeration of complaints and symptoms which may be unclear, unconnected and mysterious. Their job is to understand and interpret that material in order to arrive at an "organized" illness' (p. 39).[25]

However, although employment tribunals require specific medical diagnoses, categorical diagnostic classifications such as depressive disorder or anxiety states obscure the cultural shaping of symptoms. As Horwitz[49] points out, the basic assumption of the diagnostic framework is that the presence of sufficient particular symptoms, regardless of their cause, indicates an underlying disease. In reality, distress takes the form of generalized and non-specific symptoms which reflect expected reactions to challenging situations, unhappiness, frustration, demoralization and dissatisfaction (pp. 14–15).[49] Psychological and psychosomatic 'symptoms' develop as a reaction to a taxing social environment, such as problems in the workplace, but these symptoms are often appropriate flight or fight responses of the autonomic nervous system to challenge or threat, rather than evidence of specific disease entities or of an underlying mental disorder (p. 14).[47] Psychological symptoms of distress overlap across many diagnoses and lie on a spectrum of abnormality. As Kirmayer[50] writes (p. 331), 'Some milder forms of distress are coterminous with everyday emotions …'. Anxiety is on a continuum with worry and apprehension, and depression merges with grief and a sense of loss. It can be difficult to distinguish demoralization from depression. Demoralization often stems from lack of a sense of personal control in jobs where there is close supervision, reduced autonomy and little participation in decision-making (pp. 184–5).[51]

Entitlement can be falsely claimed. 'Someone skilled at strategic manipulation of the rules may successfully exaggerate the extent to which he is ill, emotionally distressed or intoxicated in order to claim the exemptions from responsibility that these conditions provide' (p. 53).[23] Psychiatric labels are a readily available source of mitigation and exculpation.[52] Clinical decisions about the presence of psychiatric disorder are somewhat subjective and are prone to influence by the social context, despite the 'technical rationality of the standard diagnostic systems' (p. 220).[53]

Case 1

A commercial property surveyor threatened a colleague in their office whom he suspected of making suggestive remarks to his girlfriend. He stormed out of the office, called at his doctor's surgery on his way home and was given a certificate for 'work-related stress'. Subsequently, a private psychiatrist submitted a report that he was suffering from mixed anxiety and depressive disorder (ICD-10, F41.2)[54] and was not fit to attend a disciplinary hearing. It was this specialist's opinion that his patient was 'unlikely to recover from his anxiety with depression unless the disciplinary charges are withdrawn'.

INCAPACITY BENEFIT CLAIMS AND SICK NOTES

Doctors are more minded to provide certificates to patients with a psychological problem.[55] The Health and Safety Executive has reported that work-related stress is now the most common cause of working days lost as a result of occupational injury and ill health.[56] The American anthropologist, Allan Young, has commented that, 'When faced with a diagnosis for which he has equally convincing reasons to believe that either his client is sick or he is not sick, the physician finds that the professional and legal risks are less if he accepts the hypothesis of sickness' (p. 15).[57]

Doctors have acted as gate-keepers to the benefit system since the 1911 National Insurance Act. They control access to the Department for Work and Pensions.[58,59] Sick leave is discussed with between one and six patients per doctor session,[60] but only a proportion may be regarded as genuinely unfit for work on medical grounds.[61] Family practitioners find consultations about sick notes problematic because of the threat to the doctor–patient relationship from a perceived conflict of roles and a suspicion that patients will 'doctor-shop' to obtain a sick note. Doctors might feel coerced into writing sick notes.[62] Many doctors issue certificates on demand, either on the grounds of speed or of acting as the patient's advocate,[63] believing that their responsibilities to the Department for Work and Pensions are outweighed by their commitment to their patient.

In a qualitative study of 19 primary care patients' perspective in South Wales, there was an expressed need to prove that they were genuinely disabled. This validation of their sick role was required for work, for family and for their community.[64] Only a quarter of the 19 participants wanted a passive role in the decision-making process, i.e. 'the doctor knows best', while an equal number said they would not work regardless of the doctor's opinion. The remainder were less committed to the sick role.

A study of sickness certification by 67 doctors in Scotland[63] found that the system was largely patient-led and most of them wanted a 'sick certificate on demand system' (p. 91).[63] The doctors themselves showed resistance to participation in a perceived flawed bureaucratic system. 'There seemed to be a code or language of sick lines developed by general practitioners' which fulfilled three purposes: to preserve patient confidentiality, to communicate with other agencies, and to deliberately misuse or sabotage the system by the use of vague diagnoses. Participants described writing "malaise", "debility", and TALOIA ("there's a lot of it about"), producing meaningless statistics' (p. 89).[63] The authors comment that the gate-keeping role is effectively sabotaged by the strategy of acquiescence to every patient. Doctors do not wish to jeopardize the doctor–patient relationship by confronting patients over sick note requests (p. 89).[63]

The chief medical officer to the Department for Work and Pensions has challenged the view that doctors 'should simply accede to the patient's wishes without any negotiation' (p. 461).[65]

FITNESS TO ATTEND DISCIPLINARY HEARINGS

Medical support for a claim of unfitness on mental health grounds to attend a disciplinary hearing is not uncommon. 'Withdrawal from everyday social responsibilities is made socially acceptable through some means of exculpation usually through mechanisms of biophysical determinism' (p. 298).[12] 'The mystical power of biomedicine as "external" justification for individual action, and the negotiated "space" it affords seem relevant to those other situations in which the patient enacts a *pas de deux* with the doctor' (p. 316),[12] such as requests for sick notes on the grounds of work-related stress.

Employers might suspend the disciplinary hearing because of fear of litigation and failure in their duty of care. In the case of Deadman v Bristol City Council,[66] the Court of Appeal decided that an employer is liable for stress caused to the employee during a grievance or disciplinary investigation if it is reasonably foreseeable that the investigation might cause personal injury (Howard, personal communication, 2008).

Nevertheless, in most cases, employees should be able to participate in disciplinary hearings, unless they are effectively unfit to plead. Fitness to attend disciplinary hearing requires answers to the following questions which are based on standard fitness to plead criteria:

- Does the employee have the ability to understand the allegations made against him or her?
- Does the employee have the ability to distinguish right from wrong?
- Is the employee able to instruct a friend or a lawyer to represent their interests?
- Does the employee have the ability to understand and follow the proceedings, if necessary with extra time and written explanation?

It is recognized that a protracted delay in attending a disciplinary hearing is likely to increase the probability of a normal reaction to stressful events (anxiety, low mood, insomnia and diminished concentration) becoming more severe (Staley, personal communication, 2009).

If necessary the hearing can be held at a neutral location or the employee can provide written submissions to be considered in their absence or send their representative to speak for them or ask their representative to read out their statements. Alternatively, they could attend a telephone or video conference from their home with the hearing taking place in the office (Howard, personal communication, 2008).

ADVERSE WORKPLACE EVENTS AND TRAUMA

Fraudulent or exaggerated claims to be suffering from an exemption condition are only likely to be successful when there are widespread examples of genuine disability to act as a template.[67] Post-traumatic stress disorder (PTSD) is a well-known model which provides the litigant with a specific incident as the cause of emotional distress (see Ref. 68, for incontrovertible work-related examples). Alexander lists the circumstances which foster the inclusion of 'imaginary and/or deceitful' complaints in the illness category.[69] These include 'monetary gain from disability insurance, workmen's compensation, private medical insurance and litigation; interpersonal gain – sympathy, attention, assurance of personal importance, excuse for inept or unsuccessful personal performance; [and] freedom – sanctioned release from onerous responsibility, from work and employment …'. Thus, there may be ambiguities over the attribution of personal agency with dispute over whether illness behaviour is 'pragmatic' or the result of trauma, whether it is volitional or the expression of disease (p. 26).[67]

A sophisticated typology of adverse events and their context has been developed by Brown et al.[70] and applied in a very large survey by Kendler et al.[71] Specific aversive experiences in the workplace are familiar precipitants of adverse psychological reactions. These events include public humiliation which in the workplace is often a 'put-down' which is defined as rejection or direct verbal attack by a person in authority. Events in which the subject themselves brought about the put-down are associated with a marked sense of shame and personal failure.[71] Another familiar workplace situation is entrapment when the individual feels that unpleasant circumstances will persist or even get worse with little or no possibility that a resolution can be achieved. Of particular relevance to the Walker v Northumberland County Council[72] case is a failed positive event which is defined as an 'event which suggests that a fresh start went disastrously wrong within one to two weeks, leaving the person stuck in a situation as bad as or worse than before, with seemingly no way forward'.[71]

WORKPLACE PHOBIA

Amorphous feelings of humiliation, helplessness, shame, insecurity and distress are shaped and organized by culturally available tools into culture-specific nosological entities, especially depression, anxiety, adjustment disorder and 'phobia of the workplace'. Just as shyness has been transformed into the psychiatric category of social phobia[73] and unhappiness into depression,[74] so an aversion for the workplace is now medicalized as a phobia.

Case 2

Frustration, humiliation and entrapment might make the prospect of returning to work intolerable.

A sales manager who had not achieved his targets because of a failure in the supply of his company's products was unjustly criticized and humiliated by his boss. He went off sick with 'anxiety and depression'. After months of cognitive-behavioural therapy (CBT), he felt much calmer and was less miserable but any mention or thought of his workplace triggered off intense worry and discomfort. The occupational health department recommended mediation with the employer to facilitate a graded return to work, but the patient's private psychiatrist submitted a report invoking ICD-10, F40.2. He stated that his patient's intractable 'specific phobia of the workplace' constituted a permanent barrier to any contact with his employers and that early retirement on medical grounds was the only solution.

Case 3

A 53-year-old chartered accountant in Stirling had been on sick leave for the previous four years. He went off sick when he felt severely stressed in his office after a heated confrontation with a colleague. He had recently reluctantly taken on additional managerial duties, but felt unable to cope. His 'breakdown' at work followed several days of irritability, poor concentration, unrefreshing sleep and worry about his future. He obtained a significant score on a depression self-rating scale, the PHQ 9-Health Questionnaire (the threshold for 'caseness' on this scale is very low) and the doctor made a diagnosis of mixed anxiety and depressive disorder (ICD-10, F40.2).

ICD-10 sounds a helpful note of caution in its annotation about anxiety with depression. This category is one of the most common diagnoses provided by GPs on Med 3 certificates for work-related stress. The description emphasizes that the category refers to a mixture of comparatively mild symptoms which are commonly seen in general practice settings. ICD-10 adds that 'many more cases exist among the population at large which never come to medical or psychiatric attention' (ICD-10, F41.2).[75]

A cognitive-behavioural therapist elicited the patient's lifelong aversion for his own profession. He had only become an accountant because of his parents' insistence. Despite his lack of passion about his career, he had succeeded in becoming a partner in his firm, but the requirement to take on managerial duties had been the last straw. The cognitive-behavioural therapist constructively recommended mediation with his partners to allow him to start a carefully graded return to his fee-earning work, while being spared any managerial duties. However, his general practitioner intervened, predicting that the very thought of even visiting his office would be bound to precipitate a relapse. She concluded that he would never be able to attempt any rehabilitation to work because this would only cause his health to deteriorate alarmingly. In the doctor's opinion he had to give up his profession altogether on the grounds of his refractory psychiatric illness which had failed to respond to CBT and to all the latest antidepressants. As the occupational psychologist, Bob Grove, has written,[76] CBT is not a magic bullet. CBT will not work if the workplace situation and relationships remain toxic or if the employee is in the wrong job.

DEPRESSION, ADJUSTMENT DISORDER AND SICKNESS ABSENCE

As Derek Summerfield points out,[7] 'the term "depression" tends to be used without qualification as if it was settled that we were always referring to a freestanding biologically based disorder' (p. 161). Apart from a small number of very severe cases (suffering from what used to be called 'melancholia'), 'there is no reliable demarcation of depression from ordinary unhappiness or misery …'.

It is a mistake to conceptualize normality and mental illness as dichotomous, i.e. as states of mind which are not distributed along a continuum. 'Depression' is a pervasive term which is applied to a variety of states of unhappiness and misery, including grief at a loss, demoralization, frustration, low self-esteem, disillusionment and finally a depressive illness which is assumed to have a biological basis.

In terms of DSM-IV, a distressed individual achieves 'caseness' if they experience more than the minimum number of symptoms in specific categories. The arbitrary nature of this diagnostic system is most apparent in the distinction between a severe reaction to bereavement and depressive illness. As Arthur Kleinman shows in *Rethinking psychiatry: From cultural category to personal experience*,[77] 'An anthropological sensibility regarding the cultural assumptions and social uses of the diagnostic process can be an effective check on its potential misuses and abuses' (p. 17).

The widespread belief that depression is under-recognized at the primary care level (prompted by the Royal Colleges of Psychiatrists and General Practitioners Defeat Depression Campaign)[78] has led doctors to prescribe more readily. However, there is now evidence that there is almost no difference between the effects of drug treatment and placebo at moderate levels of depression.[79]

As a study of psychiatric drug advertisements has shown, advertisements tend to individualize negative reactions to the workplace by ignoring the situation which provoked the distress.[80] Messages in these advertisements reinforce the view of distress that there must be pathology within the individual. The advertisements imply that the work context is either irrelevant or is an unchangeable situation to which the afflicted person must accommodate.

Psychotropic medication is presented as the panacea for the problems of adjustment to a stressful work environment.[80] Moving emotional distress out of the context of work and into the employee's neurochemistry diverts attention from factors in the workplace that might require challenge and alteration. With the current emphasis on cognitive-behavioural therapy as an alternative cure-all, the identification of 'faulty cognitions' and 'dysfunctional attitudes' can amplify the 'decontextualization' described by Kleinman and Cohen[80] so that a person's problems are defined as internal rather than external, individual rather than environmental, 'psycho' rather than 'social', with the option of adding antidepressants as a 'bio' solution if both belt and braces are required.[81]

Adjustment disorder is a disputed diagnosis because of the blurred distinction between the varied manifestations of adjustment disorder and normal adaptive reactions.[82] Casey et al. point out that 'transient depressive responses to stressful events are increasingly regarded as illness requiring specific intervention'. Furthermore, 'a low threshold for making a diagnosis of depression propels an individual towards a specific therapeutic approach. Distress and disorder remain conflated in clinical practice, and among the research communities we continue to medicalize the emotional vagaries of the human condition' (p. 480).

For the anthropologist and psychiatrist Arthur Kleinman, the increasing articulation of life problems as mental health conditions leads to a 'misguided search for magic bullets for complex social problems' (p. 38).[27] Kleinman also refers to the ideological influence of the modern medical scientific and technological programme which tends to convert suffering into a technical problem: 'Suffering is "euphemized" and distress is "medicalized" as a psychiatric condition, thereby transforming an inherently moral category into a technical one' (p. 35). He adds that psychiatric diagnostic systems provide far-reaching administrative and legal definitions of 'what is a problem and how it should be treated' (p. 39).[27]

In their critique of DSM-III and its successors, Kirk and Kutchins[53] write, 'The precise nature of a client's trouble is frequently ambiguous, its causes obscured by a lifetime of personal experiences, environmental stresses and psychological confusion' (p. 226).[53] However, psychiatrists may feel compelled to construe suffering in terms of a distinct nosological category rather than an existential response.

The symptoms of depression, of anxiety and of post-traumatic stress disorder are mostly subjective and they can be recited in a checklist fashion in the context of sickness absence, disciplinary hearings, applications for early retirement and litigation for compensation. These conditions are now amazingly common, with one in six of the adult population of the United Kingdom currently suffering from 'crippling depression' and chronic anxiety, according to the Depression Report published by the London School of Economics, Centre for Economic Performance.[83] One million people are in receipt of incapacity benefit because of mental illness, which accounts for 40 per cent of all disability, both physical and mental.[83] According to this report, poverty is a less significant cause of unhappiness than mental health problems. To address this problem, the proposed expanded psychological therapy service requires an extra 10 000 therapists to treat 800 000 people a year.

There is an increasing tendency for the normal and expectable consequences of stressful circumstances, which include low mood and worry, and which are a universal response to unpleasant situations, to be defined as mental illness. A low threshold for diagnosing clinical depression leads to the labelling of normal emotional states as illness. As Parker points out, 'The gravitas of the term "major depression" gave it a cachet with clinicians ... and helped patients get medical insurance cover' (p. 328).[84]

Regier et al.[85] warn that patients might receive a label of depression when in fact they are having 'appropriate homeostatic responses which are neither pathological nor in need of treatment'. For Crossley,[86] 'Mental distress is predefined in western culture by the discourses of psychiatry whose reach has extended beyond the realms of professional cliques into the domains of everyday discourse. Psychiatric schemas and practices enjoy widely taken-for-granted status. As such, they shape perceptions/conceptions of the lay public, some of whom will experience psychological difficulties first hand in relation to either self or significant others and may thus categorize self and others from the psychiatric point of view (p. 162).'

In theory, to qualify for 'caseness', these psychological difficulties have to be disproportionate to the trigger in terms of intensity and duration after the causative stressors have disappeared, but as Horwitz points out (p. 31):[49] 'disproportion can only be defined according to social judgements of the normal range of responses to various stressors in particular contexts'. In practice, the widespread use of psychiatric nomenclature to describe common reactions to personal problems in specific social contexts has contributed to the escalating number of people claiming incapacity benefits on the grounds of stress-related illness. The ready availability of these scientific-sounding diagnostic categories (which necessarily lack confirmatory laboratory and imaging evidence) contributes to 'the technological process of transforming a person with an ambiguous complaint into a client with a defined mental disorder' (p. 222).[51]

Furedi[87] describes the pervasive influence of the therapeutic culture, and the ever-expanding medicalization of adverse emotional experience, while Dalrymple laments the replacement of the concept of unhappiness in modern life by the word 'depression'. 'Of the thousands of patients I have seen, only two or three have ever claimed to be unhappy, all the rest have said they were depressed. This shift is deeply significant, for it implies that dissatisfaction with life is itself pathological, a medical condition, which it is the responsibility of the doctor to alleviate by medical means ... A marvellous *pas de deux* between doctor and patient ensues: the patient pretends to be ill and the doctor pretends to cure him (p. 9).'[88]

In the encounter between client and traditional healer in francophone creole society, the patient resorts to an explanatory system which absolves him of personal responsibility by identifying an external cause for his bad behaviour. The anthropologist Massé questions whether the afflicted person is 'lying' when he proposes to the healer that he is the victim of a hostile spirit, while the highly paid *quimboiseur* actively colludes with this mitigating interpretation.[89] As Kirmayer[50] writes (p. 335), 'The microdynamics of the negotiated encounter of patient and practitioner are embedded in larger political and economic systems that sanction some forms of distress while others are punished, suppressed or even made unthinkable'.

POST-TRAUMATIC STRESS DISORDER

The choice of the diagnosis of post-traumatic stress disorder (PTSD) as a cause of emotional distress has strategic advantages over the diagnosis of depression. With depression there may be a series of causes for the individual's distress, whereas the diagnosis of PTSD implies that all the litigant's psychological problems arise from one specific incident 'and not from a myriad other sources encountered in life' (p. 85).[90] Dr Henry Field has written that it is virtually impossible nowadays to study a medicolegal report prepared by a psychiatrist or psychologist instructed on behalf of the plaintiff in personal injury litigation where it is not concluded that he or she is suffering from PTSD.[91]

The fact that litigation might be based on a trivial incident is an affront to the survivors of truly horrific experiences, such as rape, torture or terrorist attacks. DSM-IV rightly requires the victim to have experienced intense horror, fear or helplessness in a life-threatening incident and any allegedly traumatic event that does not meet this criterion must be discounted. In the occupational health setting, one meets employees who claim to be suffering from intrusive imagery, avoidance behaviour and symptoms of autonomic arousal in the absence of a single acute overwhelming life-threatening trauma.[48]

The possibility of benefits or of compensation can have a pathoplastic effect after relatively minor injuries or disabilities. Allan Young in *Harmony of illusions* (p. 17)[92] cites Herbert Page, consulting physician to the London and Western Railway Company whose monograph on railway accidents identified a proportion of victims with minimal or invisible injuries whose recovery is retarded: 'The knowledge of compensation ... seems almost from the first moment of illness to colour the course and aspect of the case, with each successive day to become part and parcel of the injury in the patient's mind, and unwittingly to affect his feelings towards and his impressions of the sufferings he must undergo ...' (pp. 255–6, 261).[93,94]

Case 4

A bus driver who had been rebuked by his line manager threatened to deliberately crash his vehicle. He claimed that he was suffering from PTSD after seeing a friend being decapitated by a roadside bombing in Iraq. It transpired that he had never actually served in a war zone.

The diagnostic entity of PTSD was invented in 1980 by advocates for veterans of the war in Vietnam working with anti-war psychiatrists. Ben Shephard, the military historian, rebukes psychiatrists for medicalizing the human response to stressful situations and for creating a culture of trauma which is undermining resilience (p. 57).[95] Shephard decries the unitary concept of trauma which groups together under a common label a very wide range of stressors. 'Any unit of classification that simultaneously encompasses the experience of surviving Auschwitz and that of being told rude jokes at work must, by any reasonable lay standard, be a nonsense, a patent absurdity' (p. 57).[95]

In a comprehensive review of the unreliability of the PTSD diagnosis, Rosen and Davison warn about the trivialization of PTSD by 'criterion creep', the fallibility of self-reporting in the context of litigation, the routine use of checklists and of coaching by legal advisers, and 'parroting' or 'echo attribution' in which 'a false sense of validity is gained by attribution to a prestige source [a psychiatrist or psychologist] what is nothing more than an echo from the original communicator' (p. 94).[96]

RESILIENCE

There has been a tendency to neglect resilience in response to catastrophic events, such as the destruction of the World Trade Centre[97] and the July 2005 London bombings.[98] Between 11 and 13 days after the London bombings, 31 per cent of Londoners reported one or more symptoms of 'substantial stress' relating to the attacks,[99] but follow up seven to eight months later showed that the figure had fallen to 11 per cent.

As the psychologist, Bonanno[100] has shown, many people exposed to violent or life-threatening events show a significant degree of resilience that should not be interfered with by clinical intervention. His review of the published research shows that most individuals exposed to loss or violent or life-threatening incidents do not exhibit chronic symptom profiles and that very many, if not most, show significant resilience. He cites Ozer et al.[101] who found that while 50–60 per cent of the population of the United States was exposed to traumatic stress, only 5–10 per cent develop PTSD. Many individuals exposed to violent or life-threatening events might show evidence of short-lived PTSD or subclinical stress reactions, but these tend to abate over the course of several months.

The redoubtable Mr John Eke showed great fortitude in 1898 when the express train whose Westinghouse brakes he was adjusting left Kings Cross Station unexpectedly while he was under a carriage. He clung to the base of the carriage until the first stop which was at Grantham, where he climbed out on to the platform. After a restorative cup of tea with the station master, Mr Eke returned to London to go back on duty.[102]

Case 5

A 40-year-old man working in a safety-critical occupation went off sick with 'stress'. He was complaining of dizziness, backache, irritable bowel, poor sleep and nightmares. The doctor made a diagnosis of PTSD. He was found to have specific work-related issues which included representing his union during stressful strike negotiations, victimization by his manager because of the strike and investigation of an incident which caused friction with some of his colleagues.

His employer proposed a graded and supervised non-safety-critical return-to-work package which would have been viable and included the suggestion that he should be spared trade union duties which had led to his stress at work problems in the first place. On receipt of this proposal, the employee's psychosomatic symptoms became more severe.

Case 6

Sometimes, there is a combination of personal factors and an uncongenial work setting which acts as a deterrent to returning to work. A security guard in a risky area who had been subjected to intimidation on several occasions took sick leave on the grounds of work-related stress and PTSD. His wife from whom he was separated and who worked for the same employer and on the same site, was suing for divorce. In addition to his aversion to meeting her at work, the employee's solicitor warned him to remain on incapacity benefit because otherwise his wife would be entitled to a more generous settlement in the ongoing financial dispute resolution.

As Horwitz[49] observes, 'When symptoms are classified without regard to their causes or to whether they indicate a mental illness, there is no limit on the sort of conditions that could enter the new diagnostic manual. Chronic dissatisfaction with life could be renamed "dysthymia"; distress arising from problems with spouses or lovers could be called "major depression" … a symptom-based approach has the dual advantage of providing a seemingly objective and factual basis for diagnosis and of including any entity that mental health professionals currently treated' (p. 73).[49]

WORK OVERLOAD, DISTRESS AND SICKNESS ABSENCE

Overwork outside the control of the individual is a common complaint and is widely reported as a cause of work stress.

Case 7

A health service manager had three admissions to a private psychiatric clinic. Each admission lasted four weeks which reflects the maximum length permitted by private medical insurance. (The fact of a psychiatric hospital admission does not necessarily reflect the severity of the condition because the threshold for admission to the private sector is much lower than in the NHS. This patient's personal crisis would not have warranted voluntary inpatient treatment within the NHS.)

He was found to have a tendency to overwork and he was having to cover for a colleague who was on long-term sick leave. During one of his hospital admissions, he was invited by his employer's occupational health department to attend for review. However, his doctor provided him with a letter stating that such an assessment would be detrimental to his recovery.

After many weeks of sick leave, the doctor reported that he could not return to work because of residual problems which included poor concentration, feeling in a state of limbo about his job and 'not feeling up to a return to work as yet'. The non-medical obstacles to his return to work had not yet been addressed and he continued to experience understandable feelings of apprehension, worry and uncertainty about his future with some loss of self-confidence, pessimism and distractibility because of the challenging prospect of finding a new job in the present economic climate.

COUNSELLING IS NOT A SUBSTITUTE FOR MEDIATION

It is important not to medicalize these common emotions and attitudes which are entirely understandable in the circumstances of work overload but which do not in themselves constitute a disease. Furthermore, it is essential to address the causative problems in the workplace and the provision of personal counselling is not a legally sanctioned substitute for this.

Case 8

Mrs Daw was a pay roll integration analyst with 13 years of outstanding service, employed by Intel. She developed a depressive illness which was attributed to her excessive workload. Her reporting lines were confused and it was difficult to prioritize the demands of her different managers. She eventually won an award for personal injury caused by stress at work, but her employer appealed on the grounds that she had failed to use their external confidential counselling facility. The Court of Appeal[103] concluded that the counselling would not have attenuated the risk of her breakdown since it would not have reduced her workload, which was the only way the employer could provide a safe working environment. The Court of Appeal held that the provision of counselling was no substitute for putting in place measures to reduce Mrs Daw's workload (Howard, personal communication, 2008).

INCIVILITY IN THE WORKPLACE

The targets of incivility often feel alienated and become less committed to the employing organization.[104]

Case 9

A plumber went off sick from work with 'stress-related depression' after finding that his managers were giving him more work than he could cope with and imposing unrealistic deadlines. He had been rebuked by his line manager who had sworn at him in front of colleagues. He presented to his doctor with feelings of humiliation, anger and ideas of taking revenge. The doctor made a diagnosis of depression and he was prescribed various antidepressants and saw three different psychiatrists. He was reluctant to return to his job. A professional mediator attempted to work out a reconciliation, but it emerged that there was a financial disincentive to return to work and the company was not prepared to take him back until his doctor reported that he was completely symptom-free. By that time, he was taking out a compensation claim against his employer for causing his work stress-related illness. The principal precipitating and maintaining factors were his grievance against his employers. He felt overwhelmed by anger and resentment, but his doctor described him as suffering from anxiety with depression. He was referred for cognitive-behavioural therapy, but the therapist felt that because of the unresolved conflict with his employer he would not be able to return to work for the foreseeable future. (Organizational injustice increases the effects of psychosocial health risks on sickness absence.[105]) He became entrenched in the sick role and both he and his medical advisers interpreted his frustration and anger in medical terms. He consulted his solicitor who felt that following the case of Barlow v Borough of Broxbourne,[106] he would find it difficult to establish that the employer had been in breach of its duty to take reasonable care to ensure that he did not suffer psychiatric injury as a result of work-related stress, because it had not been foreseeable that he would suffer such an injury. He had previously coped perfectly well with his workload, the instances of swearing were not numerous and he had never reported 'symptoms of stress' and had not used the employer's counselling service.

RESENTMENT AND SICKNESS ABSENCE

The interpretations that employees make of their working conditions have a crucial role in determining psychological well-being.[107,108]

Case 10

A middle-aged executive had a very public falling out with her chief executive officer. She went off sick with a diagnosis of stress-induced depression. She was noted to have loss of self-esteem combined with anger and resentment at the way she had been treated. Her doctor elicited mild depressive symptoms, but over the following months she developed fatigue and lack of physical and mental energy. She had a long course of acupuncture with a Chinese medicine practitioner, who had identified a weak pulse and prescribed adrenal gland extract. She had also had reiki healing, reflexology and cranial osteopathy. This individual had excellent qualifications and an outstanding professional track record, but so far no attempt had been made to encourage her to resume her career with another employer. There was no objective evidence that she had been treated unfairly and her perception that she had been victimized would be insufficient for successful litigation on the grounds of work-related stress, since the judgement in Ian Richard Paterson v Surrey Police Authority.[109] In that case of a demoralized estate manager, the court concluded that the cause of his anxiety and depression was how he considered that he had been treated by his employer, rather than any breach of duty by the employing authority. During the trial, he evinced a strong sense of grievance about a perceived challenge to his personal worth to the organization, for which he had worked conscientiously for 26 years.

THE POSITIVE ROLE OF MEDIATION

The powerless individual enmeshed in an uncontrollable situation at work is afforded room for manoeuvre by the dominant biomedical symbolism of 'work stress' with its passive but potent appeal of helplessness.[12] The mystical power of biomedicine affords negotiating space to the disaffected employee.

However, long-term sick leave is demoralizing and stigmatizing and it induces its own morbidity.[59] A large power company, EDF, has developed a constructive way of redressing the imbalance which might otherwise push employees into the psychodrama of protracted sickness absence. They provide a negotiating forum, the facilitated round-table meeting, which employees with stress are invited to attend within a couple of weeks of going off sick. The participants include the employee and their representative, their line manager, together with representatives from human resources and occupational health.

The agenda is to ascertain the obstacles to a return to work and to negotiate practical solutions to the familiar precipitating problems of work overload, conflicting demands, lack of control over work, poor social support, ambiguity in management and work role, conflict with colleagues and tension between work and the demands of the family.[110]

The round-table meetings take place in a supportive environment which helps the employee and the manager to understand each other's interpretation of the particular work issue and to agree a way forward. There is constructive discussion about rehabilitation and agreement to reasonable adjustments that are acceptable to all parties.

The round-table system is one ingredient of a comprehensive intervention which is primarily educational and avoids medicalization and which has significantly reduced both sickness absence and early retirement on medical grounds. The programme is proactive and the aim is to create a risk-free way in which an employee can seek help when they feel under pressure or develop the psychophysiological feelings of distress. The company has circulated all the employees with information leaflets on the early identification of these 'symptoms'.

When employees return to work they are given a carefully graded re-entry and are provided with support and regular two-way appraisals focusing on the employee's adjustment and their work priorities. The incidence of work-related psychological ill health was reduced by 63 per cent over the three years following the introduction of this programme. This innovative round-table approach is in line with the Institute for Employment Studies' conclusion that 'improved communication, co-operation and common agreed goals between employers, employees, occupational health providers, and primary care professionals can result in faster recovery, less re-occurrence of ill health and less time out of work overall'.[111]

The success of this company's programme also shows the importance of the employer, the doctor and the occupational health professional asking, 'What are the barriers to recovery and return to work that this person is experiencing?' (p. 291).[76]

Unfortunately, there has been no published systematic assessment of the mediation/round-table model – see for example, *Workplace interventions for people with common mental health problems*[112] and *What works at work?*[111]

GOVERNMENT POLICY ON INCAPACITY BENEFIT AND GETTING BACK TO WORK

In recent years, there have been a number of UK Government policy initiatives,[113–117] aimed at getting people back to work. These policies are linked to a concern with the high level of uptake of Incapacity Benefit (IB) which appears to relate to the period between 1979 and 1995 when the number of recipients of Invalidity Benefit (IB) rose dramatically. However, the number has begun to fall of late at the latter period of economic growth since the 1990s recession.[59] Men are more likely to be claiming incapacity benefit than women and these male claimants have been characterized[116] as almost all having some kind of health limitations; only a quarter say they cannot do any work; half would like a job, but fewer than one-in-ten are looking; health was the main reason for job loss in only half of all cases, although age, skills and qualifications would anyway expose them to unemployment. However, there is also evidence of a rising number of women claimants and the explanation for this increase is similar to that of men, i.e. hidden unemployment, those who could be expected to have been in employment in a fully employed economy.[117] Other reasons for the marked increase in the uptake of IB might include the political need, at least at that time, to keep the number of registered unemployed at a low level. The concern for policymakers is not just that IB rates are high and therefore costly, but that the benefit might be being used by those whose intention is to malinger and avoid work, rather than by those who are genuinely incapacitated by health problems.[58] There is thus a moral element (a kind of 'moral hazard') to this policy of trying to ensure that IB is only available to those who are deserving of it.

The Pathways to Work programme, which was implemented throughout the country in 2008, is central to the government's IB reforms, which distinguish between those with severe health problems who are incapable of work and those with less severe problems who, with appropriate help, have the propenity to return to work.[113–115] This programme requires all new IB claimants to attend a work-focused interview (WFI) with an IB personal adviser. Those with severe medical conditions or deemed likely to return to work without support are exempt from further WFIs, others must attend up to five more WFIs. The other elements of the Pathways programme are optional and according to recent reports not well used.[115] They comprise the Choices package – a range of interventions aiming to improve labour market readiness and opportunities, including the New Deal for Disabled People and the Condition Management Programme; the Return to Work Credit; In-Work Support, and the Advisers' Discretionary Fund.

The Pathways programme has been introduced to promote employment, and to address psychosocial obstacles to return to work by therapeutic means. Those who refuse to participate in WFIs face benefit sanctions, while those who return to work receive the Return to Work Credit. Interventions, such as mentoring and job coaching, appear to aim to try to address the harm of being on long-term benefits to personal and social identity.

These proposals are the outcome of policy deliberations about the inappropriate uptake of IB which has led the government to set a target of one million IB recipients returned to work by 2015,[114] although this target figure appears to have increased in more recent policy documents.[115] These IB reform policies aim not only to reduce the number of new people applying for benefit, but also tries to encourage long-term recipients to go off benefits and back into paid employment.

Recent analysis suggests that these target figures may be untenable as there are marked geographical variations in the distribution of incapacity claimants and thus attainment of these targets depends on an accelerated revival in the economies of the North, Scotland and Wales.[118]

Is the programme effective? The limited evidence currently available suggest it might have some advantages for new IB claimants,[119] although the impact of the Pathways programme on existing IB recipients appears to be small.[120] However, further evidence is needed before the effectiveness of the Pathways initiative of returning long-term IB recipients to work can be fully assessed.

More recent policy has been less influenced by concerns with rising levels of unemployment and more with reducing those on IB, although this may change in the current economic climate. Thus, following on from the Pathways programme a new, more stringent assessment, the Work Capability Assessment (WCA), was introduced in 2008 for new IB claimants, to assess their eligibility for the Employment and Support Allowance (ESA) which will replace IB. Again, this aims to distinguish between applicants according to their capacity for work, with the less impaired assigned to the work-related activity group who will be expected to prepare for return to work, while the more severely disabled will receive a higher rate of benefit, but will still be able to volunteer for back-to-work support. These new initiatives, like the previous ones, combine 'stick and carrot' measures with pragmatic policies which intend to address some of the psychosocial barriers which hinder people returning to work.

A more recent White Paper, building on this policy, has been published[115] on the reform of the benefit system where the expectation is that most people on out-of-work benefits, such as ESA, will look for work and the proposal is for all existing IB claimants will be reassessed using the WCA. Early evidence[117] suggests that the vast majority (two thirds) of new applicants for benefits such as the ESA are being rejected at the WCA stage, although it is not clear what the consequences of this have been and if this has led to higher levels of those returning to or retaining employment.

SUMMARY AND CONCLUSION

This chapter has attempted to show how emotional distress is often translated into an idiom of suffering which is used to empower the employee who feels helpless.

The cultural and social construction of grievance in the workplace organizes negative feelings into psychiatric diagnoses. However, diagnosis is an imperfect means of representing psychological distress, disaffection and demoralization. The sociologists Mirowsky and Ross challenge this medicalization of distress. 'Psychological problems are real but are not entities. They are not discrete. They are not something that is entirely present or entirely absent without shades in between. They are not alien things that enter a person and wreak havoc. Nevertheless, psychiatrists often speak of depression and other psychological problems as if they are discrete entities entering the bodies or souls of hapless victims. An imagery of detection follows from such language of discrete entities. The psychiatrist detects the presence of an entity, determines its species and selects an appropriate weapon against it. This categorical language is the legacy of nineteenth century epidemiology and microbiology. A person is diseased or not. The disease is malaria or not, cholera or not, schistosomiasis or not. A language of categories fits some realities better than others; it fits the reality of psychological problems poorly (p. 11).'[51]

It is increasingly clear that psychiatric assessment in these cases should be taking into account the problem of the medicalization of grievance and of a sense of injustice. A typical sequence is:

> A loyal, hardworking employee is not given an informally promised promotion/bonus.
> ↓
> Confrontation with manager.
> ↓
> Employee feels very upset.
> ↓
> Employee goes off sick and sees doctor and mental health professionals, who reconceptualize anger, resentment, demoralization and a sense of injustice and of grievance.
> ↓
> These thoughts and feelings are translated into ICD-10/DSM-IV terms as anxiety/depression, adjustment disorder and even PTSD.
> Grievance and disciplinary proceedings and litigation help to crystallize the medicalization in terms of the impact of harassment/constructive dismissal.
> ↓
> The individual is rarely vindicated or might win a pyrrhic victory.
> ↓
> Mental health professionals become the employee's advocates with a mission to protect the patient from a return to the perceived noxious environment of the workplace.
> ↓
> Long-term incapacity with a 'phobia' of returning to paid employment. 'The thought of going back to work brings back all my symptoms.'
> ↓
> Referral for cognitive-behavioural therapy which often fails to assist a return to work because of the therapist's advocacy role.
> ↓
> Long-term sickness absence with certificated 'work-related stress'.

This chapter has identified the cultural and psychosocial influences on the illness behaviour of sufferers with work-related problems and the case studies have illustrated the complex and diverse circumstances that lead people to seek sickness absence from work. It is therefore questionable whether the package of measures and standardized assessments proposed in recent government policies will be sufficiently personalized and tailored to individual needs to effectively rebuild people's confidence and identity for them to be attracted back to work.

> **Key points**
>
> - The epidemic of work stress-related sickness absence is interpreted in terms of medical sociology and anthropology.
> - The distress of aggrieved, disgruntled and demoralized employees who feel powerless and exploited at work is commonly labelled as a morbid condition.
> - Understandable human reactions (frustration, humiliation, disappointment) are often located within the psychiatric diagnostic systems (ICD-10 and DSM-IV).
> - Entry into the sick role can be a form of passive resistance by employees which affords temporary relief and exemption, but which is self-defeating in the long term (e.g. so-called 'phobia of the workplace').
> - As a constructive alternative to the medicalization of everyday distress, we propose mediation and the resolution of grievances between employee and employer in the form of round-table dialogue and conflict resolution.

ACKNOWLEDGEMENTS

We wish to thank Gillian Howard LLB FFOM(Hon) for suggestions about cases and Charles Stewart and Roland Littlewood of the Department of Anthropology, University College London for discussions about epidemic possession states. We also wish to thank Samantha Durrell for her skilled and patient preparation of the manuscript. Thanks to Dr David Wainwright from Bath University for his contribution to the development of the ideas on the epidemic of work stress and policies on sickness absence. Finally, thanks to Dr Margaret Samuel and Dr William Mitchell of EDF.

REFERENCES

1. Calnan M, Wadsworth E, May M et al. Job strain, effort–reward imbalance and stress at work: Competing or complementary models. *Scandinavian Journal of Public Health*. 2004; **14**: 297–311.
2. Payne R. Stress at work. A conceptual framework. In: Firth-Cozens J, Payne R (eds). *Stress in health professionals: Psychological and organisational causes and interventions*. Chichester: John Wiley, 1999: 3–16.
3. Wainwright D, Calnan M. *Work stress: The making of a modern epidemic*. Buckingham: Open University Press, 2002.
4. Conrad P. Medicalization and social control. *Annual Review of Sociology*. 1992; **18**: 209–32.
5. Conrad P. *The medicalization of society: On the transformation of human conditions into treatable disorders*. Baltimore, MD: Johns Hopkins University Press, 2007.

6. Summerfield D. The invention of post-traumatic stress disorder and the social usefulness of a psychiatric category. *British Medical Journal.* 2001; **322**: 95-8.
7. Summerfield D. Depression: Epidemic or pseudo epidemic. *Journal of Royal Society of Medicine.* 2006; **99**: 161-2.
8. Lupton D. Foucault and the medicalisation critique. In: Peterson A, Bunton R (eds). *Health and medicine.* London: Routledge, 1997.
9. Calnan M, Wainwright D, O'Neil O et al. Making sense of aches and pains. *Family Practice.* 2005; **23**: 91-105.
10. Fineman S. *Understanding emotion at work.* London: Sage, 2003.
11. Simons RC, Hughes CC. *The culture-bound syndromes: Folk illnesses of psychiatric and anthropological interest.* Dordrecht: D Reidel, 1985.
12. Littlewood R, Lipsedge M. The butterfly and the serpent: Culture, psychopathology and biomedicine. *Culture, Medicine and Psychiatry.* 1987; **11**: 289-336.
13. Scott JC. *Domination and the arts of resistance: Hidden transcripts.* New Haven: Yale University Press, 1990.
14. Solomon R. *The passions.* New York: Anchor Press/Doubleday, 1976.
15. Sensky T. Chronic embitterment and organisational justice. *Psychotherapy and Psychosomatics.* 2010; **79**: 65-72.
16. Warr P. *Work, happiness and unhappiness.* London: Laurence Erlbaum, 2007.
17. Kafka F. *Amerika: The man who disappeared*, 1927. Hofmann M (trans). London: Penguin, 2007.
18. Barley SR, Knight DB. Toward a cultural theory of stress complaints. *Research in Organisational Behaviour.* 1992; **14**: 148.
19. Furnham A. *Psychology of behaviour at work: The individual in the organisation.* Hove: Psychology Press, 2005.
20. Pinder C. *Work motivation in organisational behaviour,* 2nd edn. Hove: Psychology Press, 2008.
21. Kafka F. *Metamorphosis and other stories,* 1913. Hofmann M (trans). London: Penguin, 2007.
22. Melville H. *Bartelby in Billy Budd, sailor, and other stories, 1853.* London: Penguin, 1986.
23. Edgerton RB. *Rules, exceptions and social order.* London: University of California Press, 1985.
24. Symonds A. Phobias after marriage: Women's declaration of independence. *American Journal of Psychoanalysis.* 1971; **31**: 144-52.
25. Brown P. Naming and framing: The social construction of diagnosis and illness. *Journal of Health and Social Behaviour.* 1995; (Extra issue): 34-52.
26. Parsons T, Fox R. Illness, therapy and the modern urban American. *Journal of Social Issues.* 1952; **13**: 31-44.
27. Kleinman A. *The illness narratives: Suffering, healing and the human condition.* London: Basic Books, 1988.
28. Uzzell D. *Susto* revisited: Illness as strategic role. *American Ethnologist.* 1974; **1**: 369-78.
29. Rubel RJ. The epidemiology of a folk illness: *Susto* in Hispanic America. *Ethnology.* 1964; **3**: 268-83.
30. Bosma H, Marmot M, Hemingway H et al. Low job control and risk of coronary heart disease in the Whitehall II (prospective cohort) study. *British Medical Journal.* 1997; **314**: 588-95.
31. Ong A. The production of possession: Spirits and the multinational corporation in Malaysia. *American Ethnologist.* 1988; **15**: 28-42.
32. Douglas M. *Purity and danger. An analysis of the concept of pollution and taboo.* Harmondsworth: Penguin, 1970.
33. Ackerman ASE, Lee RLM. Communication and cognitive pluralism in a spirit possession event in Malaysia. *American Ethnologist.* 1981; **8**: 789-99.
34. Lee R. Hysteria among factory workers. In: Hong E (ed.). *Malaysian women: Problems and issues.* Malaysia: Consumers Association of Penang, 1983: 76-8.
35. Chew PK. How to handle hysterical factory workers. *Occupational Health and Safety.* 1978; **47**: 50-3.
36. Littlewood R, Lipsedge M. Culture-bound syndromes. In: Granville-Grossman K (ed.). *Recent advances in clinical psychiatry, 5.* Edinburgh: Churchill Livingstone, 1985.
37. Lewis IM. *Ecstatic religion: An anthropological study of spirit possession and shamanism.* Harmondsworth: Penguin, 1971.
38. Lewis IM. *Social anthropology in perspective: The relevance of social anthropology.* Harmondsworth: Penguin, 1976.
39. Turner VW. *The ritual process: Structure and anti-structure.* London: Routledge & Kegan Paul, 1969.
40. Rose N. *Governing the soul: The shaping of the private self.* London: Routledge, 1990.
41. Howard G. *Drafting employment contracts.* London: The Law Society, 2004.
42. Downs P. Giving workers the treatment: If you raise a stink you go to a shrink. *The Progressive.* 2001; **65**: 24-7.
43. *Morgan v Staffordshire University* [2002] IRLR 190 EAT.
44. D'Auria D, Howard G, Verow P. Legal aspects of mental health in the workplace. In: Miller D, Lipsedge M, Litchfield P (eds). *Work and mental health: An employer's guide.* London: Gaskell and Faculty of Occupational Medicine, 2002.
45. Jamdar S, Byford J. *Workplace stress: Law and practice.* London: Law Society, 2003.
46. Balint M. *The doctor, his patient and the illness.* New York: International Universities Press, 1957.
47. Ware NC. Suffering and the social construction of illness: The deligitimation of illness experience and chronic fatigue syndrome. *Medical Anthropology Quarterly.* 1992; **6**: 347-61.
48. Lipsedge M. Compensation for psychiatric disorder, but not for ordinary suffering. Can this be justified? *Clinical Risk.* 1999; **5**: 155-9.
49. Horwitz AV. *Creating mental illness.* Chicago: University of Chicago Press, 2002.
50. Kirmayer LJ. Cultural variations and response to psychiatric disorders and emotional distress. *Social Science and Medicine.* 1989; **29**: 327-39.
51. Mirowsky J, Ross CE. *Social causes of psychological distress,* 2nd edn. New York: Aldine de Gruyter, 2003.
52. Lipsedge M. Jonathan Martin: Prophet and incendiary. *Mental Health, Religion and Culture.* 2003; **6**: 59-77.

53. Kirk SA, Kutchins H. *The selling of medicine: The rhetoric of science in psychiatry*. New York: Gruyters, 1992.
54. World Health Organization. ICD version 2007. F41.2 Mixed anxiety and depressive disorder. Available from: http://apps.who.int/classifications/apps/icd/icd10online/index.htm?gf30.htm.
55. Campbell A, Ogden J. Why do doctors issue sick notes? An experimental questionnaire study in primary care. *Family Practice*. 2006; **23**: 125–30.
56. Health and Safety Executive. Self-reported work-related illness and workplace injuries in 2007/08: Results from the Labour Force Survey. London: HSE, 2008.
57. Young A. Some implications of medical beliefs and practices for social anthropology. *American Anthropology*. 1976; **78**: 5–24.
58. Bambra Cl. Incapacity benefit reform and the politics of ill health. *British Medical Journal*. 2008; **337**: 452.
59. Waddell G, Aylward M. *The scientific and conceptual basis of incapacity benefits*. London: TSO, 2005.
60. Mowlam A, Lewis J. *Exploring how general practitioners work with patients on sick leave*. Department for Work and Pensions, Research Report No. 257. London: The Stationery Office, 2005.
61. McEwan IM. Absenteeism and sickness absence. *Postgraduate Medical Journal*. 1991; **67**: 1067–71.
62. Reiso H, Nygard JF, Brage S et al. Work ability assessed by patients and their GPs in new episodes of sickness certification. *Family Practitioner*. 2000; **17**: 139–44.
63. Hussey S, Hoddinot P, Wilson P et al. Sickness certification system in the United Kingdom: Qualitative study of the views of general practitioners in Scotland. *British Medical Journal*. 2004; **328**: 88–91.
64. O'Brien K, Canterbury N, Rollnick S, Wood F. Certification in the general practice consultation: The patients' perspective, a qualitative study. *Family Practice*. 2008; **25**: 20–6.
65. Aylward M. Sickness certification system in the United Kindom: Department for Work and Pensions is trying to address challenges. *British Medical Journal*. 2004; **328**: 461–2.
66. *Deadman v Bristol City Council* [2007] Court of Appeal.
67. Lipsedge M, Littlewood R. Psychopathology and its public sources: From a provisional typology to a dramaturgy of domestic sieges. *Anthropology and Medicine*. 1997; **4**: 25–43.
68. Lipsedge M. Bullying, post-traumatic stress disorder and violence in the workplace. In: Adams P, Baxter P, Aw TC et al. (eds). *Hunter's Diseases of occupations*, 9th edn. London: Arnold, 2000.
69. Alexander L. Illness maintenance and the new American sick role. In: Chrisman NJ, Maretzki TW, Reidel D (eds). *Clinically applied anthropology*. London: Springer, 1982.
70. Brown PW, Harris JO, Hepworth C. Loss, humiliation and entrapment among women developing depression: A patient and non-patient comparison. *Psychological Medicine*. 1995; **25**: 7–21.
71. Kendler KS, Hettema JM, Butera F et al. Life event dimensions of loss, humiliation, entrapment and danger in the prediction of onsets of major depression and generalised anxiety. *Archives of General Psychiatry*. 2003; **60**: 789–96.
72. *Walker v Northumberland County Council* [1995] AIR ER 737 HC.
73. Lane C. *Shyness: How normal behaviour became a sickness*. Newhaven, CT: Yale University Press, 2007.
74. Horwitz AV, Wakefield JC. *The loss of sadness: How psychiatry transformed normal sorrow into depressive disorder*. Oxford: Oxford University Press, 2007.
75. World Health Organization. International classification of diseases. Geneva: WHO, 1994.
76. Grove B. Common mental health problems in the workplace: How can occupational physicians help? *Occupational Medicine*. 2006; **56**: 291–2.
77. Kleinman A. *Rethinking psychiatry: From cultural category to personal experience*. New York: The Free Press, 1988.
78. Rix S, Paykel ES, Lelliott P et al. Impact of a national campaign on GP education: An evaluation of the Defeat Depression Campaign. *British Journal of General Practice*. 1999; **49**: 99–102.
79. Kirsch I, Deacon BJ, Huedo-Medina TB et al. Initial severity and antidepressant benefits: A meta-analysis of data submitted to the Food and Drug Administration. *PLoS Medicine*. 2008; **5**: e45.
80. Kleinman DL, Cohen LJ. The detextualisation of mental illness: The portrayal of work in psychiatric drug advertisements. *Social Science and Medicine*. 1991; **32**: 867–74.
81. Engel G. The clinical application of the biopsychological model. *American Journal of Psychiatry*. 1980; **137**: 535–44.
82. Casey P, Dowrick C, Wilkinson G. Adjustment disorders: Fault line in the psychiatry glossary. *British Journal of Psychiatry*. 2001; **179**: 479–81.
83. Layard R. *The depression report: A new deal for depression and anxiety disorders*. London: London School of Economics, 2006.
84. Parker G. Is depression over-diagnosed? *British Medical Journal*. 2007; **335**: 328.
85. Regier DA, Kaelber CE, Rey DS et al. Limitations of diagnostic criteria and assessment instruments for mental disorders. Implications for research and policy. *Archives of General Psychiatry*. 1998; **55**: 105–15.
86. Crossley N. Not being mentally ill: Social movements, system survivors and the oppositional habitus. *Anthropology and Medicine*. 2004; **11**: 161–80.
87. Furedi F. *Therapy culture: Cultivating vulnerability in an uncertain age*. London: Routledge, 2004.
88. Dalrymple T. *Our culture, what's left of it: The mandarins and the masses*. Chicago: Ivan R Dee, 2005.
89. Massé ER, 2002. Gadé deceptions and lies told by the ill: The Caribbean socio-cultural construction of truth in patient–healer encounters. *Anthropology and Medicine*. 2002; **9**: 175–88.

90. Slovenko R. Legal aspects of post-traumatic stress disorder. *Psychiatric Clinics of North America.* 1994; **17**: 439–46.
91. Field LH. Post-traumatic stress disorder: A reappraisal. *Journal of Royal Society of Medicine.* 1999; **92**: 35–7.
92. Young A. *The harmony of illusions: Inventing PTSD.* Princeton, NJ: Princeton University Press, 1995.
93. Page HW, 1883. Cited in Young A. *The harmony of illusions: Inventing post-traumatic stress disorder.* Chichester: Princeton University Press, 1995.
94. Page HW. *Injuries of the spine and spinal cord without apparent mechanical lesion, and nervous shock in their surgical and medico-legal aspects.* London: J and A Churchill, 1883.
95. Shephard B. Risk factors and PTSD. In: Rosen GM (ed.). *Historical perspective in PTSD: Issues and controversies.* Chichester: John Wiley & Sons, 2004.
96. Rosen GM. Malingering and the PTSD database. In: Rosen GM (ed.). *Post-traumatic stress disorder: Issues and controversies.* Chichester: John Wiley & Sons, 2004: 85–99.
97. Bonanno GA, Galea S, Bucciarelli A, Vlahov D. Psychological resilience after disaster: New York City and the aftermath of September 11th terrorist attack. *Psychological Science.* 2006; **17**: 971–85.
98. Rubin GJ, Brewin CR, Greenberg N et al. Enduring consequences of terrorism: 7-month follow up survey to reactions to bombings in London 7th July 2005. *British Journal of Psychiatry.* 2007; **190**: 350–6.
99. Rubin GJ, Brewin CR, Greenberg N et al. Psychological and behavioural reaction to the bombings in London on 7th July 2005: Cross-sectional survey of a representative sample of Londoners. *British Medical Journal.* 2005; **331**: 606–11.
100. Bonanno GA. Loss, trauma and human resilience. *American Psychologist.* 2004; **59**: 20–8.
101. Ozer EJ, Best SR, Lipsey TL, Weiss DS. Predictors of post-traumatic stress disorder and symptoms in adults: A meta-analysis. *Psychological Bulletin.* 2003; **129**: 52–71.
102. Safont P. *The Wide World Magazine: True adventures for men.* London: Macmillan, 2004.
103. *Intel Corporation (UK) Ltd v Daw* [2007] IRLR 355. Court of Appeal.
104. Pearson CM, Andersson LM, Wegner JW. When workers flout convention: Study of workplace incivility. *Human Relations.* 2001; **54**: 1387–419.
105. Elovanio M, van den Bos K, Linna A et al. Combined effects of uncertainty and organisational justice on employee health: Testing the uncertainty, management of model of fairness, judgments among Finnish public sector employees. *Social Science and Medicine.* 2005; **61**: 2501–12.
106. *Barlow v Borough of Broxbourne* [2003] High Court, Queen's Bench Division.
107. Briner R. Relationships between work environments, psychological environments and psychological well-being. *Occupational Medicine.* 2000; **50**: 299–303.
108. Daniels K, Harris C, Briner RB. Linking work conditions to unpleasant affect: Cognition, categorisation and goals. *Journal of Occupational and Organisational Psychology.* 2004; **77**: 343–63.
109. *Ian Richard Paterson v Surrey Police Authority* [2008] EWHC 2693 (QE).
110. Michie S, Williams S. Reducing work-related psychological ill health and sickness absence: A systematic literature review. *Occupational and Environmental Medicine.* 2003; **60**: 329.
111. Hill D, Lucy D, Tyers C, James L. *What works at work? Review of evidence assessing the effectiveness of workplace interventions to prevent and manage common health problems.* London: Institute for Employment Studies, HMSO, 2007.
112. Seymour L, Grove B. *Workplace interventions for people with common mental health problems: Evidence review and recommendations.* London: British Occupational Health Research Foundation, 2005.
113. Department of Works and Pension. A new deal for welfare: Empowering people to work, Cm 6730. London: The Stationery Office, 2006.
114. Department of Works and Pension. No one written off: Reforming welfare to reward responsibility, Cm 7363. London: The Stationery Office, 2008.
115. Department for Work and Pensions. Raising expectations and increasing support: Reforming welfare for the future. London: The Stationery Office, 2008.
116. Fothergill S. New forms of unemployment: The rise and rise of sickness and disability in the UK. Centre for Regional Economic and Social Research, Sheffield Hallam University PPT slides, 2010.
117. Sissons P. Welfare reform and recession: Past labour market responses to job losses and the potential impact of Employment Support Allowance. *People, Place and Policy* (online). 2009; **3**: 7–182.
118. Fothergill S, Wilson I. A million of Incapacity Benefit: How achievable is Labour's target? *Cambridge Journal of Economics.* 2007; **31**: 1007–23.
119. Bewley H, Dorsett R, Haile G. *The impact of Pathways to Work.* Department for Work and Pensions Research Report No. 435. London: HMSO, 2007.
120. Adam S, Bozio A, Emmerson C et al. *A cost-benefit analysis of Pathways to Work for new and repeat incapacity benefits claimants.* Department for Work and Pensions Research Report No. 498. London: HMSO, 2008.

65

Mental health at work: psychological interventions

ADRIAN NEAL

Introduction	823	Conclusions	829
Mental health problems and psychological interventions	823	Acknowledgements	829
Case formulation: making sense of people's distress	824	References	830
Formulation-based pragmatism: direct and indirect psychological interventions	825		

INTRODUCTION

The term 'work-related stress' can be misleading and seems to have become a generic label describing a range of mental health problems in the workplace. Commonly experienced mental health problems in the general adult population fit into a continuum of distress ranging from formal diagnoses (including disorders of mood and behaviour, such as depression, panic disorder, phobias and eating disorders) to varying levels of non-diagnostic emotional distress. Thus, many individuals who do not have a condition that fits into a formal psychiatric diagnosis can nevertheless experience marked emotional distress which may also reduce their ability to function, including at work. Indeed, it may be argued that emotional distress, even at subdiagnostic levels, may impact with the most significance in many occupational settings where high levels of physical and/or intellectual performance are required.

In addition, there is continuing confusion on what constitutes work-related mental ill health, and also inherent problems in understanding its mixed aetiology, including how or if the work environment has had an impact in a given individual. This level of uncertainty makes responding to and planning effective interventions difficult, even if the individual has clearly diagnosable mental health needs.

In light of all this, it can be useful to adopt a psychological approach that considers:

- the benefits of developing a biopsychosocial case formulation of an individual's mental health needs, which includes both diagnostic and psychological perspectives;
- the merits of using this process as the basis of an intervention plan;
- the use of direct or indirect psychological interventions as part of this plan.

This chapter will argue that psychological management can be helpful in reducing employee emotional distress and thus improve mental health in the workplace. It advocates that a case formulation approach is needed, which may then lead to either indirect and/or direct psychological interventions. Five case examples are used to support this argument and the chapter concludes by drawing attention to important issues, such as the limitations to psychological interventions, the value of prevention and the importance of the relationships between health providers, employee and employer.

MENTAL HEALTH PROBLEMS AND PSYCHOLOGICAL INTERVENTIONS

The evidence base for the effectiveness of psychological therapies for adults with mental health problems has gained momentum over the past decade. In the United Kingdom, the National Institute for Health and Clinical Excellence (NICE) guidelines have recommended that psychological therapy in the form of cognitive behavioural therapy (CBT) be provided as possible first-line treatment for mild to moderate depression and post-traumatic stress disorder.[1,2] NICE also made recommendations in support of specific psychological treatments for a range of mental health problems, such as panic disorder, adjustment disorder, complex grief, agoraphobia, generalized anxiety disorder, health anxiety, social phobia, obsessive compulsive disorder, eating disorders and phobias. The treatments currently practised, depending upon the condition, are interpersonal therapy, cognitive analytic therapy, dialectical behaviour therapy, eye movement desensitization and reprocessing, and brief psychodynamic therapy. Evidence is also emerging to indicate that mindfulness-based cognitive therapy can be helpful for people who experience reoccurring moderate clinical depression.[3] Psychological therapies can also contribute in the management of patients with complex mental health problems, including borderline personality disorder, psychosis and non-chronic bipolar disorder.

It is reasonable to suppose, in the light of these recommendations in the general population, that some of these methods may be applicable to the mental health problems that arise in the workplace. However, before it is possible to recommend psychological therapy in this context, caution is needed to ensure a tailored approach, including an acknowledgement of the potential role of the work environment and employer. Interestingly, it is this ability to tailor psychological interventions to the individual that makes them so potentially useful in a range of settings.

CASE FORMULATION: MAKING SENSE OF PEOPLE'S DISTRESS

Formulation is a tool used by clinical psychologists and many psychotherapists to conceptualize the difficulties of the individual, and as a rationale from which to frame the psychological intervention. The majority of contemporary case formulation literature comes from the cognitive behavioural tradition which has its roots in 1950s' behavioural models of aberrant behaviour and in particular functional analysis. Case formulation was seen as an alternative to psychiatric diagnosis aiming to identify and describe problems,[4] thus allowing an intervention to be designed which would directly address the maintaining mechanisms of the problem.

Beck[5] modified traditional behavioural models by putting increased emphasis on the role of internal events, such as thoughts and emotions, and developed CBT along with Albert Ellis. Case formulations from a cognitive behavioural perspective soon incorporated different levels of thoughts, and detailed how they interacted with emotions and behaviours to both trigger and maintain emotional distress. CBT approaches and case formulation have widened lately to include a biopsychosocial matrix that incorporates a range of biological, psychological and environmental or social factors. Biopsychosocial-based case formulation has thus evolved into a broad and inclusive clinical tool. Case formulation is viewed as the cornerstone of clinical psychology in the United Kingdom,[6] and although not all clinical psychologists are exclusively cognitive behavioural in their theoretical orientation, with many having an integrated approach, there is wide acknowledgement that the process of case formulation is central to understanding an individual's problems and thus developing effective interventions.

A formulation framework

Formulation begins as soon as the clinician receives information about their potential client(s). From this point, it may be helpful to use a simple framework to guide and organize information. The five P model[7] is a widely used generic cognitive behavioural formulation framework useful in all clinical areas. The framework requires information to be organized around five key areas, namely: presenting issues, precipitating issues, predisposing problems, perpetuating factors and protective factors, which are described in more detail below. The five P framework facilitates the identification of a wide range of information, allowing the clinician and client to develop a current and working conceptualization of the key problems, and thus begin to see hypothetically how they may be best addressed.

PRESENTING ISSUES

Identifying the individual's key current problem(s) is a primary task in the assessment, often these are linked to distressing and current emotions or behaviours. The ideal situation is to generate a list of clearly identified problems, even if they are not going to be addressed directly. It is useful to try and quantify these problems and anchor them in behaviour (e.g. I feel low in mood, I struggle to motivate myself and I avoid work). Providing clear examples of the problems helps to target future intervention, is useful as a measure of outcome and also illustrates the individual nature of the problems and how they may be connected.

PRECIPITATING FACTORS

Precipitating factors can be difficult to identify as not everyone is aware of what might have triggered their current problem(s). In addition, some precipitating factors may not be only recent events, but can be seen as related to past experiences, as is often the case in post-traumatic stress disorder. Hypothetical precipitating factors may also need to be identified, and these can be internal (thoughts, memories, feelings or physical sensations) and/or external (environmental).

PREDISPOSING FACTORS

Establishing a coherent model of a person's problems is enhanced by the identification, even hypothetically, of predisposing factors, which often consist of highly individual interactions between life experiences, personality traits and biologically based factors, including, one could argue, temperament, cognitive structures (beliefs), emotions and relationships. For many people, it is often helpful to explore their past to find related factors and events which can help give some meaning to their current distress.

PERPETUATING FACTORS

A useful way of understanding these is to consider the relationship between the factors which maintain and perpetuate the cycle of distress, and which can be internal or external to the individual, or a combination of both. Of all the perpetuating factors, the 'experiential avoidance' of distress[8] seems to be the most commonly identified across most mental health problems. Put simply, if an individual tries to avoid distress, or any experience that for them triggers distress, they are likely to experience a negative reinforcement of the problem.

For example, a woman felt highly fearful following an experience of breathing difficulty and believed she was at increased risk of choking, thus possibly dying, if she had any future breathing difficulties. If she were to experience being short of breath, she may well perceive this as the beginning of another choking episode, become fearful and then try to avoid any situation that triggers similar physical feelings. Over time, she successfully avoids 'risky' situations, but her fear actually increases.

In this example, avoidance-based coping plays the primary perpetuating factor in the person's catastrophic beliefs and predictions. Likewise, problems can also be in part maintained by external factors, such as financial difficulties, issues with family, friends, workplace and other environmental factors over which they may have minimal control.

Within the cognitive behavioural literature, there are disorder-specific maintenance patterns, particularly in anxiety problems.[9] For example, with panic disorder and health anxiety, there is a characteristic over-vigilance for bodily changes,[10] and for post-traumatic stress disorder, there is an active avoidance of stimuli that trigger distress.[11]

PROTECTIVE FACTORS

Often overlooked when trying to identify and plan how to approach emotional problems, protective factors can be very useful to client and clinician, both in the formulation process and also during the intervention. Protective factors are best framed as a person's strengths. These can be seen as factors that have protected them in the past, helped them to cope, or have acted to prevent them from experiencing even more distress than they are currently. As such, these are often highly individual and should be considered carefully as internal resources, such as humour, which could also be used as a means to avoid, as well as cope, and thus actually be a perpetuating factor in one instance and yet a protective factor in another.

The recent review of the resilience literature by Atkinson et al.[12] provides a useful overview of the psychological construct and its role as a protective factor. In their review, the authors identify a number of characteristics considered to be protective. These include having purpose, pragmatism, being able to goal plan, optimism, hope, good self-esteem, perceived control, flexibility and distress tolerance. The authors urge caution and add that this list is not exhaustive and other factors, such as biological, and chance are probably also important in making a person resilient.

Overview of the formulation process

The process of formulation, particularly if guided by the five P model, can offer an invaluable resource for both client and clinician. In addition to being useful in creating a framework to understand a problem and plan for intervention, there is an emerging literature looking at the impact of the formulation process itself on outcome. Although early, there is a growing recognition that formulation is an important process as it helps form a collaborative therapeutic alliance.[13] Indeed, for some individuals the formulation process is all the intervention they require.

Another aspect to consider and include in a formulation process are the accepted attributions that form part of the social and workplace milieu. These will differ from one work environment to the next and may differ between the type of work undertaken, e.g. information technology, medical, research, manufacturing, construction, etc. Attribution style based on attribution theory[14] is significant as it forms the basis of the individual's expectations of his employer and colleagues, and points to why the employee might have different values and expectations to their employer. An attribution style will help determine personal responsibility, role, and what an individual thinks they deserve. Formal industrial action, ongoing antagonistic relationships, sabotage, conflicts and bullying between employer and employee will be linked to the attributions of those involved.

FORMULATION–BASED PRAGMATISM: DIRECT AND INDIRECT PSYCHOLOGICAL INTERVENTIONS

There are many models of brief psychological therapy which focus on direct work with adult populations. The most documented and commonly used within clinical psychology in the United Kingdom currently include: CBT, interpersonal therapy, cognitive analytic therapy, Gestalt, humanistic and psychodynamic. These models typically centre around two individuals, a client and a clinician, identifying problems, agreeing goals and developing a therapeutic relationship. Although sharing common themes, the content, organization and nature of the stages of therapy will differ between models. Interestingly, these differences appear to be slowly becoming smaller as the trend towards briefer time-limited models develops.

Although traditional psychotherapeutic models tend to focus on working directly with one adult, there are a number that allow for working with the individual indirectly. Systemic models often encourage teamwork and working with more than one individual (e.g. a family) and are commonly seen in child and adolescent mental health services. More recently, traditional one-to-one models have been broadened to integrate systemic ideas, allowing the psychologist to work towards helping an individual through others within the system. In occupational settings, this may involve working with human resources, occupational health services, general practitioners, managers and even colleagues where necessary. As with traditional direct methods, indirect methods need to be based on a clear understanding of the problems, and have a formulation anchored in psychological theory.

Before embarking on a psychological intervention, it is important to consider, in the formulation process, what the aims are to be, how achievable they are and whether they are compatible with the needs of the referrer. This is a particular issue for occupational health services as returning an individual back to health in order that they return to work may not, in some instances, be ethical or indeed realistic, particularly if the work environment has in some way played an active part in the development or maintenance of their problem. Psychological interventions are more likely to be of help if these issues can be acknowledged early on.

The following case studies illustrate effective direct and indirect psychological interventions within different occupational health settings.

Case 1

Alan, a 48-year-old medical doctor, was referred by the occupational health service of the hospital where he practised. Alan reported feeling highly anxious, self-conscious, lacking in confidence and low in mood, although he was not apparently clinically depressed. All of these symptoms impacted on him negatively at work and he worried about them leading to a reduction in performance. His symptoms seemed to have developed over a period of a few months following an incident at work where he had made an error during a surgical procedure. The error was identified and corrected; however, Alan was temporarily suspended from surgical duties until an internal investigation had been carried out. Alan reported experiencing regular and distressing flashbacks to the events surrounding this incident and seemed to be stuck in a pattern of rumination.

The referral had asked for an assessment with treatment recommendations; however, it soon became evident that formal treatment was not necessary and that an extended assessment with an active formulation would be sufficient.

The generic cognitive behavioural formulation identified that most of Alan's distressing emotions were, at least to begin with, normal reactions to a difficult event (e.g. anxiety, fear, guilt, concern, shame). What appeared to have developed, however, was a number of distress maintaining patterns that seemed to have evolved as a consequence of how he had tried to cope with his distressing emotions. Alan had experienced marked anticipatory anxiety at the thought of running into colleagues who might know about the incident, so he had tried to cope by avoiding situations he considered to be 'risky'. As a result he changed his route to work, worried about the journey beforehand and arrived at work anxious. This anxious state triggered further anxiety as he worried that he might make a mistake, or that his anxiety would be seen by a colleague who might comment critically. The worries he had about being viewed negatively by others steadily increased, as did his efforts to cope until he felt he needed help.

Based on the formulation, a self-directed behavioural exposure programme was devised, and anxiety-based psychoeducation recommended. He later reported that the formulation process had allowed him to see his main problems more objectively, and to then feel able to address the self-maintaining mechanism of his anxiety, which he learnt were both understandable and changeable.

Case 2

Heather was a 43-year-old woman with 25 years' experience of working for her employers. She had recently taken a new role as team leader, a role she was well experienced in and qualified for, but she was struggling. Heather was referred by the occupational health department who explained in a referral letter that 'she was low in mood, felt on edge and unable to cope'.

During assessment, Heather explained that she was experiencing a 'crisis of confidence' and marked low mood, as well as other symptoms of moderate clinical depression. She explained that she had felt this way in the past, but had recovered quickly. She had been feeling this way for 'too long' and it was impacting on her ability to perform. Heather stressed how important it was that she should do her job well and explained that as a woman in a predominantly male work environment she could not afford to 'slack'. In addition to her low mood, she reported feeling marginalized and unfairly treated which is why she, in her eyes, had had angry outbursts.

Heather's low mood seems to have been initially triggered following an undermining comment from a colleague. This comment had suggested that Heather's team were underperforming. It was Heather's perception that this colleague wanted her role and that she was vulnerable. Normally, she would have been able to cope, but Heather explained that she was feeling increasingly vulnerable as the project the team were tasked with was simply too complex to do well. She felt a sense of failure in spite of the impossibility of the task.

Heather admitted that she was a perfectionist and that things had to be just right or she felt uncomfortable.

She had a reputation at work of being a hard worker, and always seemed to succeed. Faced with a task that was impossible, she began to feel low and vulnerable. The formulation identified, along with her protective factors (determination, creativity, drive and confidence) that she was also dependent upon success to support her self-worth. Thus, failing to maintain her standards posed grave risks to her self-worth. We also recognized that her perfectionism seemed to have its origins early in life. She experienced many physical problems as a child, but she was able to excel academically. She had also learnt that to be favourably viewed by those around her, she had to succeed. Thus, not to succeed was both unfamiliar and, from her perspective, highly frightening.

The intervention was highly pragmatic and aimed primarily at helping her cope with her day-to-day, work-related distress, and slowly she started to recover from her depression. Based on direct cognitive behavioural-based work, the focus was on identifying and adapting beliefs that underpinned her drive to be perfect (e.g. 'If I can't succeed I am a failure, no one likes a failure'), activity scheduling, increasing her distress tolerance, and being more able to directly communicate her emotions to others, rather than waiting until she felt uncontrollably angry. She was also helped to link present emotions, beliefs and behaviours to relevant past experiences. The collaborative relationship was vital as she felt a deep sense of shame for appearing to fail.

Later, it transpired that she had been right and her colleague had been trying to take her role, which was curiously reassuring to her as she no longer felt threatened, but consoled herself that at least she could still judge human nature.

Case 3

Julia was a 34-year-old woman who worked as an administrator in a university records department. She reported experiencing high levels of anxiety at work which impaired her ability to function. She also reported feeling low in mood. Julia was referred from the occupational health service, and during the initial assessment presented as highly distressed, she struggled to make eye contact and reported that she felt unable to cope and she believed that colleagues wanted to get rid of her. It seemed that Julia's anxiety had been getting worse over the past few months and that she had, in her opinion 'always been sensitive to criticism'. Following a critical annual appraisal, Julia had found her anxiety increasing, her capacity to cope reduced, and had eventually gone off work sick.

The formulation process suggested that she had a predisposition to feeling negatively evaluated, and although never having felt this scared before, she had often felt uncomfortable with others. Compounding matters further, she had also experienced severe stress-related alopecia that had further increased her self-consciousness.

The formulation further indicated that she was experiencing heightened social/performance anxiety underpinned by the belief that others would be critical and that she could not cope alone. Julia also explained that as a child her stepfather had been highly critical of her. It seems that these old experiences had had a direct effect on her developing self-worth and had also played a role in the formation of her beliefs about the criticalness of others. Following the annual appraisal, and to cope with feeling vulnerable due to a fear of further negative evaluation, Julia isolated herself, slowly disconnected from her social network, and reduced her assertiveness at work. Over time, her sleep deteriorated and she began to feel ashamed and highly self-conscious, and avoided more aggressively. In addition, she began to feel hopelessness having realized that she would probably struggle to find another job.

Although Julia struggled with the assessment, she was offered a cognitive behavioural-based intervention for her social anxiety. Her aims were to feel 'stronger' and return to work, and also to be able to make an active choice about staying in her current job. The intervention also involved close liaison with occupational health professionals and her line manager in planning her return to work. The intervention focused on helping her to feel more confident in identifying and challenging her primary negative predictions around negative social evaluation.

We used the formulation process, then behavioral experiments, to do this over a number of weeks. At the same time, we developed a graded exposure hierarchy combined with activity scheduling to increase her out of work positive experience. Julia kept records of her work and successes as evidence of progress and as a basis for supporting more compassionate self-beliefs. Julia also became aware that she was responding defensively to perceived and not necessarily actual threats. However, it was vital she accepted that at one time in her life she had needed to protect herself from actual threats. This was an important message to convey as it helped her feel less ashamed of her lifelong avoidant behaviour, which was once highly adaptive and protective, even if it acted to maintain her anxiety.

After 14 sessions, Julia successfully improved her understanding and management of her anxiety, increased her social network and confidence. She returned to work and finally resigned some months later with the confidence that she could find another job.

Case 4

Mary was a 35-year-old computer programmer referred from the occupational health department for help in dealing with anger at work, depressed mood and generally struggling to cope. She also had a history of self-harm and had recently been to Accident and Emergency having deeply cut one of her wrists with a broken wine glass.

During the assessment, Mary struggled to recognize any thoughts or feelings that might shed light on her problems from a cognitive behavioural perspective. She also reported long-standing problems with obsessional behaviour, restrictive eating and drinking alcohol. It quickly became clear that alcohol consumption preceded her risk behaviour, particularly at weekends. Mary identified her anger as a key problem and also explained she felt powerful feelings of guilt. These problems seem to permeate all parts of her life and negatively impacted on work, as there was a risk of her being disciplined and possibly made redundant.

In order to understand Mary's problems, the formulation needed to expand to include the cognitive analytic therapy (CAT) model.[15] The CAT model is a time-limited, integrative model incorporating cognitive, behavioural and psychodynamic components. CAT has been found to be a useful model for problems which have a chronic dysfunctional relationship component and where strong emotions are regularly activated. The evolving reformulation (CAT uses the idea of a reformulation, as opposed to formulation) suggested that Mary's overwhelming negative emotions (anger and guilt) were connected to her relationship with her parents, particularly her father. Interestingly, she also relied on her father to give her a lift into work each morning and described 'starting the day on edge'. The reformulation also suggested that she drank to avoid feeling strong emotions, but that it was also an indirect way of punishing her parents. This strategy, however, simply promoted conflict and critical behaviour in the family. Mary also explained that she hated going to her parents for a meal on Sunday, but felt compelled to. It was at these dinners that she would often drink too much, return home and self-harm.

The reformulation guided the 16-week long direct intervention in a number of ways. First, it allowed Mary to observe her unhelpful patterns and see how they were maintaining her very serious problems and distress. Second, it seems to have given her permission to make some simple behavioural changes, such as getting the bus to work, and becoming more assertive with her parents, so she began to politely decline her parents' offer of a Sunday meal, thus avoiding becoming angry and feeling guilty. Mary also began to accept that she could not change her parents, but that she had a choice to change how she reacted. At work, her mood improved. The anger outbursts decreased and she was generally happier – as were her managers.

Case 5

Tim was a 56-year-old laboratory technician who had worked for a university engineering department for 26 years. Tim was referred from the occupational health department having been off work for six months with 'stress'.

At assessment, Tim reported high levels of anxiety, mostly around feeling overwhelmed and physically weak, and not being able to cope with the demands of the job or indeed those of his day-to-day life. He reported that these symptoms had been getting worse since going off work sick.

Before going off work, Tim had had been ill with a cardiac problem and was undergoing tests. Psychological assessment revealed that Tim had been feeling increasingly stressed at work for at least four or five years. He reported changes in the work environment, management structure and job description that had left him feeling unsupported and at times unclear as to what his role involved. He added that his job used to be very important to him, as it provided structure and predictability, as well as enjoyment and a sense of achievement. He also explained that his wife was now ill and that he was very worried about her.

Much to his doctor's surprise, Tim's problems seemed to have worsened while off work. Rather than having time to recover and regain his confidence, his anxiety had deepened and he had become clinically depressed. It also became clear that he had stopped all forms of exercise for fear of setting off a 'heart attack'. He had subsequently invested a great deal of energy in trying to 'think himself better' in the form of ruminations, checking (scanning his body regularly for signs of danger, e.g. increased pulse rate) and he avoided anything that reminded him of his work or which triggered increased anxiety/low mood.

In addition, before going off work, Tim had been assessed for an autistic spectrum disorder, and been given a diagnosis of high functioning autism. While this diagnosis made sense to him and his doctor, it seemed to add to his sense of feeling overwhelmed, particularly as his work colleagues upon hearing the news had started to treat him differently.

Following the assessment and early formulation, Tim was offered a cognitive behavioural-based intervention and realistic goals were planned. These included: developing new ways of understanding and managing his anxieties, feeling more pleasure and less overwhelmed, and finally returning to work. The formulation suggested that he had gradually grown to feel increasingly overwhelmed at work as he had struggled to manage organizational changes. This was perhaps linked to his autism and the fact that he had done the same job for so long. Feeling overwhelmed meant he struggled to cope with the daily worries which soon became too much. His heart problems were just the final stressor and triggered an acute stress reaction. The time spent off work seems to have led to an avoidance (and hypervigilance) based maintaining cycle, which had led to a worsening of his distress.

The intervention focused on both direct and indirect work. Working directly with Tim using a cognitive behavioural framework, he was able to understand that his anxiety and depression was based on catastrophic predictions about his health and ability to cope in general. He also found that his avoidant coping style, i.e. rumination, active avoidance and hypervigilance were making him worse. This led to a graded exercise exposure programme under advice from his doctor, who was liaising with the cardiology department. Working with occupational health, a carefully graded return to work was planned and a clearer job description was negotiated. Occupational health also established an effective line of communication between Tim and his line manager which allowed Tim to feel listened to and more in control. He eventually returned to work successfully and negotiated a new role in his old department after being off for nearly nine months.

Case studies: A summary

These five case studies draw attention to the importance of systematically formulating an individual's psychological needs before embarking on a treatment plan. They also highlight the individual nature of mental illness. Most importantly, these cases illustrate the potential helpfulness of both formulation and psychological interventions, particularly when carried out in transparent coordination with other professional carers, and those working on behalf of the employer.

CONCLUSIONS

As mentioned previously in this chapter, there is not always a clear or even helpful relationship between employer, occupational health provider, psychologist and employee. It is important, therefore, to include these factors into any formulation process as they may have direct impact on the aims and outcome of any intervention and may also impact on client confidentiality.

Formulations are hypothesis based and remain 'work in progress' with no absolute declarations or truths. At best, they are helpful hypotheses which help individuals make sense of their problems, at worst they are a rigid, reductionist and patronizing list of a person's problems and do not contribute to recovery. However limited a poor formulation might be, it at least does not have the same stigmatizing potential as some psychiatric diagnoses, e.g. schizophrenia or borderline personality disorder. The potential normalizing effect of the distress-focused biopsychosocial formulation can help engage those individuals who feel stigmatized by the thought that they may have a mental illness and therefore avoid seeking help.

It is not hard to imagine a situation where an employer sends an anxious or depressed employee to occupational health, who then discovers that aspects of the work environment are directly linked to the individual's distress. This was similar to Heather's (case 2) experience. The formulation may reveal that there is little that can be done to change the individual and what is recommended is to change the environment. This can be very frustrating for all involved, especially if the employer disagrees or is actively attributing blame to the employee. This is a particularly difficult situation if the core problem is linked to ongoing bullying, harassment, disputes or relationship problems in the workplace. In these instances, there needs to be clear communication between professional carers involving the client, and an agreement about what is in the best interest of the employee, both ethically and clinically.

Where a work environment is psychologically toxic and thus part of the identified problem, the health professional should raise the issue under the duty of care of the employer. Occupational health practitioners have an important role here, but as advisers they may have limited ability to change the work set-up if the employer resists. In these cases, there is an ethical responsibility to raise the issue with the client and help them make the best informed choice they can: in Julia's situation (case 3) one of the aims was to help her regain her confidence so she could leave the job. It is important to be as open and pragmatic with clients as possible in order to facilitate their recovery and alleviate their distress.

Finally, it is important to raise the limitations of psychological therapies. Therapies should be chosen for a specific purpose by individuals who are competent in their ability and knowledge base. Psychological therapies and techniques have the potential to cause harm if used inappropriately. Referrers to psychologists should be aware that choosing a specific type of therapy, planning its individualized structure and ensuring quality is complex and often only possible after specialized training and ongoing supervision. Likewise, even CBT, in its many forms, can cause harm in the hands of an incompetent practitioner. It is important for practitioners and referrers to be aware of the contraindications to therapy, ongoing risk factors and the realistic limitations of psychological treatment so as not to give false hope to those in distress.

> **Key points**
>
> - Mental ill health, including 'work stress', can be conceptualized as being on a continuum of emotional distress ranging from mild to severe and enduring.
> - A biopsychosocial model of emotional distress is highly relevant in the workplace, given the range of diverse factors that may have an influence in any one case.
> - A problem-focused formulation can inform psychological, systemic and medical interventions in order to reduce emotional distress in the workplace.
> - Psychological interventions need to be pragmatic, realistic and supported by collaborative relationships between invested parties.

ACKNOWLEDGEMENTS

The author would like to thank Dr Julie Highfield for her support, ideas and for proof-reading.

REFERENCES

1. National Institute for Clinical Excellence. The management of PTSD in children and adults in primary and secondary care. Trowbridge: Cromwell Press, 2005.
2. National Institute for Clinical Excellence. Depression (amended): Management of depression in primary and secondary care. London: NICE, 2007.
3. Ma SH, Teasdale JD. Mindfulness-based cognitive therapy for depression: Replication and exploration of differential relapse prevention effects. *Journal of Consulting and Clinical Psychology.* 2004; **72**: 31–40.
4. Johnstone L, Dallos R. Introduction to formulation. In: Johnstone L, Dallos R (eds). *Formulation in psychology and psychotherapy.* London: Routledge, 2006.
5. Beck AT. *Cognitive therapy for emotional disorders.* New York: Meridian, 1976.
6. British Psychological Society, Division of Clinical Psychology. The core purpose and philosophy of the profession. Leicester: British Psychological Society, 2001.
7. Dudley R, Kuyken W. Formulation in cognitive behavioural therapy. In: Johnstone L, Dallos R (eds). *Formulation in psychology and psychotherapy.* London: Routledge, 2006.
8. Cullen C. Acceptance and commitment therapy (ACT): A third wave behaviour therapy. *Behavioural and Cognitive Psychotherapy. Special Issue: Developments in the Theory and Practice of Cognitive and Behavioural Therapies.* 2008; **36**: 667–73.
9. Wells A. Cognitive therapy of anxiety disorders: A practice manual and conceptual guide. Chichester: Wiley, 1996.
10. Clark DM. A cognitive approach to panic. *Behaviour Research and Therapy.* 1986; **24**: 461–70.
11. Elhers A, Clark DM. A cognitive model of post traumatic stress disorder. *Behaviour Research and Therapy.* 2000; **38**: 319–45.
12. Atkinson PA, Martin CR, Rankin J. Resilience revisited. *Journal of Psychiatric Mental Health Nursing.* 2009; **16**: 137–45.
13. Kuyken W, Padesky CA, Dudley R. *Collaborative case conceptualization.* New York: Guilford Press, 2009.
14. Heider F. *The psychology of interpersonal relations.* New York: John Wiley & Sons, 1958.
15. Ryle A, Kerr IB. *Introducing cognitive analytic therapy. Principles and practice.* Chichester: John Wiley & Sons, 2002.

SECTION TWO

Work and psychiatric disorder

66 Work and psychiatric disorder: an evidence-based approach 833
  Nick Glozier, Max Henderson, Neil Greenberg and Simon Øverland

66

Work and psychiatric disorder: an evidence-based approach

NICK GLOZIER, MAX HENDERSON, NEIL GREENBERG AND SIMON ØVERLAND

Introduction	833
Effect of work upon the development of psychiatric symptoms and disorder	833
Psychosocial work environment	836
Psychiatric disorder and work disability	842
Occupational impairment of psychiatric disorder	842
Organizational effects of psychiatric disorder	843
What influences the interface of occupational risks and psychiatric disorder?	845
What can be done in the workplace?	847
Conclusions	848
Acknowledgements	849
References	849

INTRODUCTION

This chapter will concentrate on the relative effect of work and its context upon psychiatric disorders, particularly those most commonly encountered in the working population (including depression and anxiety). It will then outline the impact of psychiatric disorder on functioning in the workplace, before evaluating the current knowledge on the value of health promotion interventions. Given the effect of different health, social and employment systems between countries, this review will concentrate on the United Kingdom and other northern European literature.

The UK government Foresight Project on Mental Capital and Wellbeing identified the importance of nurturing the 'mental capital' of a nation to maintain economic and social prosperity. Meanwhile, reports from the UK and other OECD (Organization for Economic Cooperation and Development) countries have also highlighted the problem of tackling the association between psychiatric disorder and the workplace.[1–4] One of the most important ways in which psychiatric disorders affect the lives of sufferers and their families is on their functioning in the workplace[5] and on their losing employment and receiving disability benefit.[6] At the same time, the public view work and 'work stress' as a primary, and increasing, cause of their ill health.[7] The body of literature on work stress is now substantial, with numerous definitions extending from well-being and resilience to stress and depression. Finding a way through this forest of data is a major challenge.

One issue that recurs repeatedly in evaluating the literature is that there is no standard definition of 'employment' or 'work'. It is often unclear whether a given rate refers to competitive, sheltered, voluntary, part-time or full-time employment, what time-frame has been used for measurement and how far definitions require sustained attendance at work for people to be categorized as employed. Also, there is often only scant mention of what sort of work people were engaged in outside specific occupational settings and whether this was for an open market rate of pay. The majority of reports do not explain how they have dealt with women who are working in the home, who may be classified as employed, as well as voluntary workers and students. These deficiencies make interpreting and comparing results from different studies difficult or impossible.

EFFECT OF WORK UPON THE DEVELOPMENT OF PSYCHIATRIC SYMPTOMS AND DISORDER

The potential experiences at work that might be related to poor mental health are legion. These have been postulated to range from discrete events, such as personal injury and witnessing disturbing events, through intermittent but repetitive events, e.g. bullying, encounters with aggressive or threatening clients in public services, through to more consistent job characteristics, e.g. physical discomfort, both overly onerous and overly undemanding roles, social support, perceptions of organizational injustice and imbalances between the efforts expended and the reward received. Some of these may be related to particular occupations, organizations or types of work, others to actual or perceived experience and all are impacted by a range of factors operating outside work.

Objectively assessed occupational risks

OCCUPATION

Surveys of occupations which would seem to carry a high chance of exposure to stressful events and violence, unsociable hours, shift work and many other features considered to constitute a 'toxic' working environment, consistently report levels of about one-quarter to one-third of respondents meeting criteria for psychiatric disorder. These levels have been determined, most usually, through studies in which respondents have reached a cut-off point on a screening tool. Examples of such studies include front-line ambulance staff and paramedics,[8–10] police,[11,12] doctors,[13] other hospital staff,[14] and veterinary practitioners.[15] In such studies, the prevalence of 'stress' in members of the occupational group are compared to the prevalence of psychiatric disorder, ascertained through interview in a rigorously sampled population-based study, such as the National Psychiatric Morbidity Survey in the United Kingdom or the National Comorbidity Survey in the United States. These studies get good publicity and are popular with the respective professional groups and unions, yet frequently suffer from poor response rates, different methods of determining disorder (self-report measures often derive higher prevalence rates than interview-based studies) and little information on the context that may lead to response bias. For instance, it is quite possible that the answers to a 'stress' survey may differ from identical questions asked in a 'well-being' survey. It is important to remember that prevalence estimates obtained in different groups using different study designs cannot be directly compared. Therefore, such studies are unlikely to provide a valid answer to the question of whether one group has a higher prevalence of psychiatric disorder compared to other occupational groups.

Attempts have been made to use broader based surveys to identify occupations in which employees are more or less likely to develop common psychiatric disorders. Using a large self-reported database, ambulance workers, teachers, social services, customer services (call centres), prison officers and police reported poorer than average scores on psychological well-being and job satisfaction measures.[16] More robust data come from population-based data in the UK where higher rates of psychiatric disorders are found among teachers, sales staff and managers in government organizations, and lower rates in plant operatives and health-associated professions, and few changes over the seven years between national surveys (Table 66.1).[17]

Other sources of routinely collected data have shown similar results – staff in certain public service occupations having higher levels of psychiatric disorders. Similar studies from Norway have also identified farmers at particular risk for anxiety and depression.[18] In Canada, a study using one simple question of self-reported mental health[19] suggested that risky occupations were concentrated in four of the ten major occupational groupings: (1) health; (2) sales and service; (3) trades, transportation and equipment operators and related occupations; (4) occupations unique to processing, manufacturing and utilities. Nevertheless, as the authors point out, 'the extent of the specific contribution of occupations in explaining variations in worker reporting of poorer mental health is rather low ...'. This would also appear to have informed Lady Justice Hale's determination that no occupation is inherently psychologically toxic when she said, 'The notion that some occupations are in themselves dangerous to mental health is not borne out by the literature to which we have already referred: it is not the job, but the interaction between the individual and the job which causes the harm'.[20] A more important observation in the literature, and in the above landmark judgement, appears to be the effect of being lower within the organizational hierarchy within each occupational grouping. The effect of occupational grouping virtually disappears when individual factors, such as personality and family strains, were included.[21] As shown below, it is aspects of the job rather than occupation *per se* which is important for mental health.

Studies evaluating the role of occupation in suicide in high income countries have shown two consistent patterns. First, not having a job is worse than having any type of job,[22–24] although less so in a period of high unemployment.[25] This was confirmed recently in a pan-European study.[26] Second, suicide registers consistently suggest that healthcare workers[27] are the only occupational groups consistently associated with raised suicide rates after adjusting for other known risk factors. For instance, among those who have previously been admitted with psychiatric disorders, minimal associations between occupation and suicide are observed except for doctors, who are at almost four-fold greater risk. This presumably reflects access to the means of suicide (drugs) and knowledge of how to use them. Some have suggested knowledge of the consequences of chronic illness or the effect of having people so dependent upon them as explanations.[27] In others, the risk may be due to economic factors, such as the transient nature of some occupations predisposing to periods of being unemployed and being in receipt of low income. Within such groups, however, the same risk factors operate for being vulnerable to suicide as in the rest of the population – psychiatric or personality disorder and previous deliberate self-harm being the most prominent.[28]

Table 66.1 The prevalence of psychological disorder by standard occupational classification group (reproduced with permission from Stansfeld et al.[17]).

	All (95% CI)	Males (95% CI)	Females (95% CI)
Overall prevalence	13 (12–15)	11 (9–12)	17 (15–19)
High prevalence group			
Buyers, brokers and sales representatives			30 (13–48)
Clerical occupations	16 (13–19)		20 (16–24)
Managers and administrators	15 (12–17)	14 (10–17)	
Other associate professional occupations	18 (14–22)	13 (7–19)	24 (16–31)
Other sales occupations	18 (14–22)	16 (7–25)	19 (14–24)
Personal service occupations	16 (13–20)	13 (6–20)	
Secretarial occupations	15 (10–20)		
Skilled construction trades		13 (6–19)	
Teaching professionals	15 (11–20)	13 (6–19)	
Low prevalence groups			
Buyers, brokers and sales representatives		6 (0–12)	
Clerical occupations		9 (5–14)	
Drivers and mobile machine operators	9 (4–14)	7 (2–11)	
Health associate professionals	11 (6–16)		11 (6–16)
Industrial plant and machine operators, assemblers	9 (6–12)	9 (5–12)	9 (3–15)
Managers and proprietors in agricultural services			12 (6–17)
Other elementary occupations		8 (4–13)	15 (10–20)
Other professional occupations	10 (5–15)	8 (2–14)	
Other skilled trades	10 (7–14)		
Protective service occupations	11 (4–18)		
Science and engineering associate professionals	11 (6–16)	6 (1–11)	
Science and engineering professionals	8 (3–13)		
Secretarial occupations			14 (9–19)
Skilled engineering trades	10 (5–15)		

The oft-quoted association of suicide with another large group with access to lethal means, farmers and farm workers, is less consistent with both positive and null associations, although veterinarians have high levels, presumably for similar reasons to other health professionals.[29] Groups such as the police and other front-line public sector workers have similar rates to the rest of the population. Much of the apparently high suicide rates in certain occupations are due to lower death rates from other causes.[29] Beyond this, it is difficult to make out a common job pattern, although Sanne et al.[18] suggest a strong effect of low skill use occupations being associated with depression in men suggesting job selection. Certain people are drawn to certain jobs, for example, there is a stronger relationship between a simple global measure of intelligence with future occupational level than the multitude of specific aptitudes often tested in the psychological selection processes used by many organizations.[30] Late adolescent personality characteristics also play a strong role in determining future occupation and attainment, with 'alienated and hostile adolescent's … personality dispositions leading them to work experiences that undermine their ability to make a successful and rewarding transition into the adult world'.[31]

POSITION IN THE ORGANIZATION

Within many workplaces or jobs, there is a hierarchy between higher and lower grades. A consistent finding is that those in lower status jobs have higher levels of psychological distress. In the Whitehall II study, this association was not explained by poorer mental health leading to employment grade changes (social causation), but rather supporting a selection into certain grades by factors that are also risks for psychiatric disorder.[31] The association with workplace position in fact appears stronger than broader objective measures of socioeconomic position in society as a whole.[32] Subjective measures of socioeconomic status also have a strong effect,[33] bolstering the idea that workplaces perceived to have flatter hierarchies may be less likely to engender negative health effects.

HOURS WORKED

Long hours and overtime have also been linked to psychiatric disorder in some studies (e.g. Ref. 34), which can receive media attention. However, the most comprehensive literature review in the area[35] showed that fewer than half of all longitudinal studies demonstrated any negative impact of long hours, indicating a need for more understanding and better determination of what long hours mean rather than a simplistic 'more work = bad' approach.

PSYCHOSOCIAL WORK ENVIRONMENT

Job strain and effort–reward imbalance

> Men are disturbed not by things, but by the view which they take of them
> Epictetus (AD55–135)

Two major models have emerged to describe the psychosocial work environment – both are determined by an individual's perception of their environment. In the 'job strain' model the 'demands' of work are contrasted with the level of control ('decision latitude') an individual has over how they work.[36] 'Job strain' is said to occur when high demands are associated with low decision latitude. Later, a third dimension was added to the model, namely, perceived social support at work, and was combined with the other two dimensions. Hence, a high-strain job in the context of low social support should produce the worst effects on health. This situation created the 'demand–control–support' or 'iso-strain' model. The second model is the 'effort–reward imbalance', in which stress responses are believed to occur when effort expended at work is not matched by rewards in terms of pay, self-esteem and sense of achievement.[37] Both job strain and effort–reward imbalance were shown to be associated with psychiatric disorder in numerous cross-sectional studies, e.g. Ref. 38. When objective, rather than self-reported, assessments of work demands are included, the association between the psychosocial work environment and psychological morbidity is attenuated.[39] Adversely perceived changes in these stressors, particularly control, are associated with future increased and longer spells of absenteeism.[40,41]

A meta-analysis of prospective studies from both Europe and North America[42] showed that there was consistent evidence for similar effects of job strain (summary OR 1.8 (95 per cent CI 1.1–3.1)) and effort–reward imbalance (summary OR 1.8 (95 per cent CI 1.4–2.3)), in predicting later psychological symptoms, termed 'common mental disorder', that was not explained by response bias (the tendency for certain individuals to report things more negatively). The individual components of these models, i.e. demands, decision authority and support, showed smaller but still significant effects of increasing the likelihood of later psychological distress by about 1.3 times. The effects were less strong generally among women than men.

When the outcome of a clinically defined diagnosis of depression is used, the evidence is less convincing. Bonde[43] identified seven studies where the risk of later depression was determined using a validated interview. The two studies assessing demands provided conflicting results of no or a strong association. There was no association of decision latitude on its own. The combined measure of high job strain (high demand and low control) did produce an effect, particularly in men, with a relative risk in the 1.5–2.5 range. A second systematic review in the same year[44] with the same objectives identified a slightly different, but generally overlapping, set of studies. This review concluded that there were consistent effects of job demands upon the development of depression with relative risks around 2.0, but conflicting results with respect to decision latitude. Social support at work was associated with a decrease in risk for future depression, as all four studies identified showed that high social support reduced the risk of future depression. Both of these latter reviews suggested less of a gender difference. One important point was the observation of a 'very strong' publication bias with only one negative study published which was attributed to a positive secondary outcome.

Another recent study across 11 large companies has bolstered the observation of the deleterious effects of people reporting either high strain or so-called 'passive' (low demand, low control) work stress patterns leading to later onset of prolonged sick leave for depression, particularly for men, a negative effect of low control for both genders,[45] but failed to show any protective effect of social support. A young birth cohort showed that higher levels of psychological, but not physical, job demands, poor support and low decision latitude (high strain) were associated with a recent onset of well-defined major depressive disorder and generalized anxiety disorder in 32 year olds.[46] Previous studies have highlighted the importance of adjusting for prior disorder given the social causation effect. Finally, recent Canadian work has shown that those exposed to chronic high job strain developed depression at twice the rate (8 per cent) as those with consistently low strain (4 per cent) and those who reported a change from high to low job strain had a risk of major depression similar to those exposed to persistently low job strain.[47] This would reinforce the idea that reducing an individual's perception of strain may have a positive impact on the risk of depression.

While the study of the perceived psychosocial work environment has deepened our understanding of the nature of the relationship between the individual and his work, the models have limitations. The reliance upon self-reported data is either a hindrance or the 'core of the issue' depending upon the viewpoint as it incorporates beliefs, perceptions and attitudes to work. More work is needed on validating methods of assessing work demands and the way in which the perceptions of demands and decision latitude are filtered or modified by individual factors, such as personality, temperament and previous experience. The literature has concentrated upon depression and depressive symptoms with little emphasis upon anxiety. Bonde's review demonstrated that not one of the 16 papers accounted for all common potential confounders of demography, life events/family demands, personality, previous disorder, chronic disease and family history. The similar findings of associations across widely varying measurements of both stressor and psychiatric disorder, with no apparent trend towards greater effect of early versus late onset (unlike other life event work), and the huge variation in outcome prevalence, led him to suggest that much of the association may represent bias and confounding.

Other specific elements of the psychosocial work environment have attracted research attention and seem important clinically.

Bullying (mobbing)

Despite two decades of intense work on workplace bullying and studies demonstrating significant personal,[48] organizational and societal sequelae, the field is somewhat hampered by lack of an agreed definition. The prevalence varies enormously depending upon the definition, but tight definitions of bullying consistently produce a figure of around 5 per cent.[49–51] Broader definitions of unwanted acts can lead to much higher rates, e.g. 40 per cent[52] or even 50 per cent.[53] The most comprehensive review in the area[54] used a definition of 'prolonged and repeated hostile behaviours conducted by at least one person toward one or more individuals when they are unable to resolve their workplace conflicts in non-hostile manners and can cause health problems for victims and affect their performance'. As can be seen, the definition of risk factor includes the outcome and so anyone experiencing such behaviour who does not endure a health or performance effect is not bullied by definition. Thus, the bullying occurs as a transaction between external behaviour and individual perception, much as with other psychosocial risk factors. Whether or not intentionality is a defining characteristic of bullying has been the subject of some debate. Keashly and Jagatic[55] argue that intent constitutes a key element of bullying and emotional abuse. On the contrary, Zapf et al.[56] point out that it would be difficult to include intentionality as a feature of bullying, given that intent may prove difficult to verify. There does, however, appear to be one consistent criterion which is the rule of thumb that the unpleasant behaviour must happen at least once a week for at least six months[57] to be classed as bullying. Despite a great deal of interest, conceptual articles and the presence of numerous websites on bullying and whistle blowing, the systematic review by Moayed et al.[54] found only 37 analytical papers, of which only seven met a moderate threshold of quality. Six of these were case control as probably befits such an outcome. A consistent finding was that those with certain personality and stress characteristics (lower levels of assertiveness and extraversion, higher levels of depressive symptoms) were more likely to report being victims of bullying at a later date. There were no consistent effects of gender, although men tended to be bullied by men, and women more likely to be bullied by women, potentially reflecting the gender-segregated composition of many work environments. In the only cohort study, less than half of those reporting bullying did so over the two-year time period, but this group had much poorer outcomes, being four times more likely to develop depressive symptoms.[48] Bullying has also been associated with insomnia[57] and a range of other health indices, although once again hampered by tautologous definitions and cross-sectional study designs with their inherent biases. One interesting observation is that people who report observation of the bullying of others have poorer mental health themselves, which may suggest either the presence of wide organizational issues or support the view that those with low mood perceive actions and workplaces in a less favourable light.[58]

Trauma and violence in the workplace

There is no *a priori* reason to presume that an experience of trauma or violence, that might be psychologically disabling in other areas of one's life, should not be so if experienced at work. While most people who experience such an event will experience short-lived symptoms, such as distress, insomnia, anxiety or unhappiness, only a minority will develop a mental health disorder. Responses to traumatic events have been suggested to comprise one of five groups with the first being by far the most common:

1. The normal stress response characterized by intense intrusive recollections, numbing, denial, feelings of unreality and arousal. If more severe and prolonged, this forms the adjustment disorder of the ICD.
2. Acute stress disorder/reaction which is characterized by feelings of panic, cognitive disorganization, disorientation, dissociation and severe insomnia, and infrequently paranoid or truly psychotic reactions, and difficulty in work and interpersonal functioning.
3. Uncomplicated post-traumatic stress disorder (PTSD). Where PTSD does occur, it usually has an onset within a month of the event. While PTSD may persist for months or even years, a substantial number of PTSD cases resolve without the need for formal intervention.
4. PTSD, comorbid with other disorders, is more common than uncomplicated PTSD and is usually associated with disorders such as depression, alcohol/substance abuse, panic disorder and anxiety disorders.
5. Personality change as a result of catastrophic experience which is suggested to be the result of exposure to prolonged, or in some cases highly intense, traumatic situations.

Some have suggested that other disorders, such as depression, are more common sequelae of traumatic events. For example, Fullerton et al.[59] studied the development of depression among rescue workers who were exposed to dead bodies and physical danger and who gave assistance to survivors in disaster situations. The study observed the rescue workers for one year and found a threefold increase in the risk of developing depression of 3.5.

A significant critique of the field in ascribing PTSD to an occupational cause, has been that the occurrence of 'a stressful event or situation of an exceptionally threatening nature, which is likely to cause pervasive distress in almost anyone' (the criterion A event necessary for a diagnosis) is common. The proportion of adults who report having experienced at least one such traumatic event includes the majority of people in the United States (61 per cent of men, 51 per cent of women),[60] such that many have suggested it does not provide a specific aetiology for a disorder.[61] The association between exposure to trauma and the development of symptoms of post-traumatic stress is not fully understood. It involves a complex interplay between factors related to the trauma, neurobiology and psychosocial influences. All of these determine an individual's vulnerability or resilience to developing PTSD as a result of exposure to a traumatic event. Certain sociodemographic factors, such as sex, age, ethnicity and income, have also been shown to be associated with vulnerability to developing PTSD.[62]

The majority of studies addressing work-related traumatic events has focused on specific occupational groups that obviously carry a much higher risk of experiencing such events, i.e. military, ambulance, fire and police staff. Surveys of emergency service personnel find a sizeable minority of fully operational employees who screen positive or meet criteria for PTSD. For example, in UK ambulance personnel between 5 and 20 per cent of paramedics still working screen positive for PTSD.[8,63,64] There is an extensive literature which suggests that many employees experience horrendous events but do not develop PTSD. Our survey of London ambulance staff in the aftermath of the July 2005 London bombings[63] suggested that the prevalence of PTSD as found on a screening tool was similar to that in the general population (2–3 per cent), with a higher prevalence of 6 per cent in those involved in the bombings directly. The failure to find substantially raised levels in emergency services[59] suggests either that affected staff rapidly leave the service or that people joining such organizations self-select for resilience.[65]

In the field of military operations, there are extensive texts best referred to, such as the PTSD Compensation and Military Service report.[66] Cohort studies of military personnel deployed in Iraq and Afghanistan suggest a threefold elevated incidence of PTSD among those reporting combat exposures of around 8 per cent.[67] As above, there are vulnerability factors – those with poor physical and mental health prior to deployment being the most likely to develop PTSD for any given level of combat exposure.[68] In United Kingdom, Gulf War veterans of low rank and leaving the service were the strongest determinants of poor mental health, with little effect of either pre-deployment training or post-deployment leave.[69] Studies which have looked at more recent operations found that among UK troops, about 4 per cent of the force, whether deployed or not, reported symptoms of probable PTSD, although troops engaged on combat duties reported higher rates (6 per cent),[70] suggesting that increased 'toxic' exposure may well have a significant, albeit small, effect upon PTSD rates.

A primary source of traumatic events outside the emergency services is violence at work which is more common in those working in the public sector: health and social work professionals. According to the British crime survey, 0.9 per cent of employees had been physically assaulted while they were working, a similar number threatened and 0.5 per cent of workers said that worrying about workplace violence had a 'great deal' of impact on their health, and 2 per cent said that it affected their health 'quite a bit'. Despite increasing attention, the reported rates in this frequently repeated survey have actually been falling since 1995.

A major issue besets the field of post-traumatic distress disorder and violence in medicolegal settings. If two people experience the same DSM-IV or ICD-10 criterion A event, yet only one goes on to develop a disorder, only this person is compensated for this experience with sickness absence, pension or some other form of social recompense. There has long been a suggestion that the presence of compensation claims can prolong the course of the disorder as seems to be the general pattern following a range of injuries.[71] The United States veterans' review suggested that compensation was not a barrier to help seeking, but did not address the issue of whether it was a disincentive to recovery. However, as shown by the rates of PTSD specific to trauma experienced at work in occupational groups, the presence of such a disorder does not preclude employment even in front-line operational posts. Work into the factors preventing the onset of PTSD[72] and enabling well-trained people to continue being gainfully employed, e.g. by tackling the stigma associated with help seeking,[73] are major foci of attention in the area.

Given the apparent lack of specificity of a traumatic event as a cause, the numerous vulnerability and resilience factors and the role that compensation and other benefits play in the development and persistence of symptoms of PTSD (and other disorders), the disorder can be a medicolegal minefield. Future research may help to clarify matters, although with more and more experiences being considered as potentially traumatic (www.hcp.med.harvard.edu/wmhcidi/instruments_papi.php) the threshold for traumatic events is likely to be lowered, making this group far more heterogenous.

Downsizing and job insecurity

In the Stansfeld meta-analysis,[42] job insecurity appeared to have a moderate effect on increasing the risk of future psychiatric disorder, primarily in men (OR 1.3) in the two studies that assessed this, both by simply asking a yes/no question.[74,75] As with many of these psychosocial risks, the effect seems stronger in cross-sectional surveys. The effect of current job insecurity seems stronger in men[51,76] and uncommonly observed in women[21] in population-based studies. The Finnish study also followed up those who left the workplace showing that for those who found employment elsewhere, their mental health improved and was in fact better on average than those who stayed, particularly after major restructuring.

Job insecurity is noted in two main areas: first when organizations are downsizing, retrenching or rightsizing ('making people redundant' as it used to be called). Although there are some studies from the mid-1990s suggesting positive health benefits during downsizing (e.g. Parker et al.[77]) in general, the remaining workforce appears to be consistently and negatively affected. One interesting observation is that the perception of job insecurity mediates the relationship between actual likelihood of being laid off, e.g. being given warning notices or having members of one's team laid off, and psychological problems.[78] This has also been suggested to be mediated through longer hours and work intensification across a range of countries and industries and occurs despite the observation that those still employed tend to be a healthier group than those who lose their jobs.[79] Chronic job insecurity seems to have a particularly strong effect.[80] In a large Scandinavian study group, the 4783 employees who worked in organizations undergoing change, but kept their jobs after downsizing, were at a higher risk of being prescribed psychotropic drugs (rate ratio 1.49, 95 per cent CI 1.10 to 2.02 in men and 1.12, 95 per cent CI 1.00 to 1.27 in women) than the 17 600 not exposed to downsizing.[81] The association of downsizing was strongest with hypnotics among the men and with anxiolytics among the women. Older workers, those more committed to their employer and potentially male gender were identified as riskier groups for the psychological effects of downsizing. Others have identified racial factors potentially indicating forms of discrimination or stigma.[82]

The other major area of job insecurity occurs in what is called 'contingent' or 'precarious' employment.[83] This term reflects the growth of flexible workers, such as fixed-term employees and workers without an employment contract in many OECD countries. These employees are more likely to have health problems on recruitment, particularly poorer mental health, and also to develop health problems later.[84] This effect is not explained by part-time, as opposed to full-time work, but rather contract type. In many OECD countries, contract workers constitute a sizeable minority of the workforce. As this practice spreads, there will be more work on this area of insecure employment and the broader impacts on health both within organizations and society.[6] Although some have suggested that increased focus on performance has reduced the tolerance of staff with health problems, the job market over the early part of this millennium was such that many with mental health problems re-entered employment. The effect of the recent economic downturn is likely to be felt most acutely in this group.

Stigma and discrimination

People with psychiatric disorders are among the stigmatized and the workplace is an important source of discrimination.[85] The 'concealability', attribution of blame and perceived unpredictability are key components of this work-placed risk.[86] Individuals with psychiatric disorders are less likely to enter the job market and, if they do, they are more likely to be underemployed, employed in low status or poorly remunerated jobs, or employed in roles which are not commensurate with their skills or level of education.[87] Many more have entered employment over the past few years of economic growth, but often in contingent and flexible roles.[88] They then become harder to identify and study, and are overlooked in reports where only data from the primary labour market are analysed. The flexible and short-term nature of these positions may be attractive to those returning to the workforce following a prolonged absence, but this comes at a price. Positions in the secondary labour market are often unstable, poorly remunerated or open to exploitation. Short-term employees have weaker legal protection, and poorer opportunities for training and career development.[89] They frequently report being denied opportunities for training, promotion or transfer. Others have been dismissed or forced to resign. Baldwin and Marcus identified over 5 per cent of workers with a psychiatric disorder who had been laid off, fired or told to resign because this fact became known.[90] Furthermore, those returning to work following a psychiatric disorder come under far greater scrutiny, such as vigilance for, or overinterpretation of, symptoms,[91] or more requests for further information from doctors than those returning after an apparently physical disorder.[92] There is, however, a spectrum of views – depression is better tolerated than psychosis, and individuals are viewed more charitably if they are taking medication, better still if they are not currently ill.[93]

When it comes to disclosure of a mental illness to an employer, most high-income countries have anti-discrimination policies and laws obliging employers to accommodate people despite health problems. The presence of such laws has made people aware of these processes, but covert discrimination is hard to detect and tackle.[94] As such, a challenge for those with psychiatric illness is if, how and when to disclose this to an employer.[95] Many patients are reluctant to disclose their psychiatric history[96] fearing being treated differently or having their job offer withdrawn, often with good reason. The Shaw Trust, a UK disability charity, recently conducted telephone interviews with CEOs, directors and human resources officers in 500 businesses of different sizes. A huge majority (89 per cent) believed that they did not have anyone with a diagnosis of mental illness working in their organization at present.

Furthermore, 80 per cent believed that 'potential employees should disclose mental health problems prior to recruitment', but when asked if they would employ someone with mental health problems, only one-third reported that they would (compared with 62 per cent for physical health disability).[97] In terms of what drives these discriminating views, work with human resources managers suggested these were based less on an expectation that those with a history of psychiatric disorder would take more time off, rather that they would be worse at their jobs.[92] Disclosure is therefore often delayed until a 'good impression' has been made.[98] In trying to keep problems secret, employees may be less likely to seek appropriate support from occupational health,[87] be reluctant to be seen taking medication or to seek time off for hospital or therapy sessions.

Emerging concepts

There has been a slew of very recent studies examining other psychosocial risks. Initial results suggest that employees with low workplace social capital, both vertical (lack of respectful and trusting relationships across power differentials at work) and horizontal components (lack of trust and reciprocity between employees at the same hierarchical level) increase the odds for newly diagnosed depression and antidepressant treatment by 30–50 per cent compared to their counterparts with high social capital at work.[99] Poor team climate and other group level indictors can also impact upon the mental health of employees,[100] as can perceptions of organizational injustice[101] and unfairness.

Psychosocial risk factors at work and physical disorders

The contribution of many of these psychosocial occupational risks to more physical disorders has been addressed. There are a number of reviews in pain conditions which generally show a tendency for higher job strain to be associated with development of back pain and neck/upper limb pain.[102] Working longer hours is associated with a range of adverse physical health outcomes.[103] Recent evidence suggests that long hours also make cognitive function decline faster in middle age.[104] Organizational injustice and unfairness at work has been linked to cardiovascular disease[105] and heavy drinking.[106]

Work stressors are entrenched in the public's perception as a cause of heart attacks, although the evidence is not consistent, e.g. Kivimaki et al.[107] and Eaker et al.[108] This has led to observations that it is the accumulated impact of chronic work-related stressors that are important.[109] Certainly, chronic job strain was shown to increase the risk of recurrent myocardial infarction[110] in a predominantly male cohort, independent of any demographic or medical risk factors. This was to the extent that the positive effect of returning to work on mortality seen over the first few years was reversed by year four. Any effect of job stressors on the health of women with cardiovascular disease has yet to be shown convincingly, although it has been examined.[111]

The potential pathways by which occupational stressors lead to physical disease are legion. Some have suggested that any effect of work stressors on cardiovascular health may be mediated by psychiatric disorder. Depression, for instance, has an independent effect upon the development of cardiovascular disease in otherwise healthy people[112] and for poorer outcome, in particular recurrent depressive episodes, after a cardiac event.[113] The psychiatric disorder may mediate this through health behaviours and poor adherence, social exclusion or reduced support. Cognitive models of harm avoidance, coping and self-efficacy appear useful in understanding work-related illness in pain conditions.[114] The Whitehall II study suggested that a combination of adverse health behaviours and the development of metabolic syndrome explained a significant part of the link between work stressors and cardiovascular disease.[115] Alternatively, linked (pro-) inflammatory and immune responses and hypothalamic–pituitary–adrenal axis dysfunction are being explored as either common determinants of psychiatric and physical disorders or as the mediating paths between psychosocial risks and disease.[116] There are whole textbooks in this emerging field of psychoneuroimmunology, but a useful introduction can be found in Ref. 117.

One emerging avenue is the impact of many of these occupational stressors, such as the effort–reward imbalance in men,[118] long hours[119] and organizational injustice,[120] on sleep disturbance and insomnia. Given that similar inflammatory and oxidative stress markers are apparent in people with sleep disturbance as in mood disorders and cardiovascular disease,[121] sleep disturbance may be one of the mediating paths by which health is affected.[122]

Toxic exposures and medically unexplained syndromes

Another important consequence of working in high threat locations is the potential for personnel who do so to develop a 'syndrome' of physical symptoms which lack a consistent pathophysiological base. Such syndromes are categorized in ICD-10 as somatoform disorders and also known as functional somatic syndromes or medically unexplained symptoms.[123] Probably the best known of these conditions afflicted, and continues to afflict, military personnel who served in the 1991 Gulf War.[124] Although it is not clear who first coined the term, initial media reports described so-called 'Gulf War Syndrome' (GWS) as being clusters of either unusual illnesses in veterans or their families, such as cancers in previously fit veterans, or birth defects in veterans' children. Soon, however, the term covered virtually any physical or psychological symptom, alone or in combination, occurring in anyone who had served in the region. Troops from almost all coalition nations, including the United States, United Kingdom, Canada, Australia and Denmark, reported suffering from the condition.[125] Numerous studies investigating GWS have repeatedly failed to find any definitive evidence of a syndrome that is specific to Gulf War service. Instead, studies repeatedly showed that personnel, who had served in the 1991 Gulf War, report two to three times more symptoms than those who did not, but the pattern of symptom reporting is the same irrespective of deployment to the Gulf in 1991.

Although there is no consistent evidence for a causative agent for GWS, medically unexplained symptoms were experienced by some 17 per cent of UK service personnel who served in the Gulf War.[126] Furthermore, those who suffer from the condition remain adamant that their work was the direct cause of their symptoms and disability. The suggested candidates for causative agents are legion and include pesticides, oil fires and vaccinations. One particular substance, depleted uranium (DU), has been frequently linked to the development of GWS. However, studies of military personnel who have been injured with DU fragments, and thus indisputably exposed, have not shown them to have suffered higher levels of adverse health consequences to date.[127] Evidence from the 2003 Iraq War has also failed to link exposure to DU with health problems in coalition forces.[128] Another putative cause was pyridostigmine bromide (PB), which was used, in tablet form, as a prophylactic against the possible effects of some chemical weapons. However, Canada sent three ships to the Gulf, the personnel of only two of which used PB prophylaxis, yet the rate of illness was the same in all three ships.[129]

In summary then, although multiple unexplained symptoms have been found to afflict substantial numbers of veterans of the 1991 Gulf War, those symptoms did not cluster in any particular pattern, nor has it been possible to demonstrate any definitive links with possible toxic, causative agents. The GWS legacy continues though, with a four-year follow up of UK veterans showing that the majority of those who had originally reported GWS symptoms remained unwell.[130] Although GWS is perhaps the most well known of the military somatization disorders, it is noteworthy that similar patterns of symptoms have been found in military personnel after many other conflicts.[131,132]

Moreover, the military is not the only occupation to be associated with an increased risk of controversial somatization disorders. Although these disorders go by many names, such as chronic fatigue syndrome, multiple chemical sensitivity or fibromyalgia, the constellation of symptoms, including fatigue, joint pain or dizziness, reported by those who suffer from them are similar, as are the frequent disagreements about what causes them.[133] These conditions tend to affect people of working age (between 20 and 50 years) and are more commonly seen in women. Multiple chemical sensitivity, for instance, is said to be associated with low level exposure to a variety of industrial substances, such as smoke, pesticides, plastics, synthetic fabrics, scented products, petroleum products and paints. However, blinded trials show that in fact those who are said to suffer with this condition do not react to chemicals.[134] A detailed review of 37 provocation studies concluded that 'persons with MCS do react to chemical challenges; however, these responses occur when they can discern differences between active and sham substances, suggesting that the mechanism of action is not specific to the chemical itself and might be related to expectations and prior beliefs'.[135]

Another important occupational consideration in these conditions is that they have a relatively poor prognosis. For instance, the UK's Health and Safety Executive suggests that while 40 per cent of those who suffer from chronic fatigue syndrome may improve with treatment, only few recover fully.[136] Once these syndromes are established, occupational outcomes tend to be even poorer.[137] Psychiatric medication, usually antidepressants, is generally not effective at treating these conditions, although comorbid depression and anxiety, which may be present in up to 50 per cent of cases, should respond to pharmacological approaches. However, there is evidence that cognitive behavioural therapy (CBT) is effective in some cases.[138] A 2007 meta-analysis of five CBT randomized controlled trials of chronic fatigue and chronic fatigue syndrome (CFS) reported 33–73 per cent of the patients improved to the point of no longer being clinically fatigued.[139] However, in keeping with the controversial nature of these disorders, the use of CBT has often been criticized by patients. For instance, a survey ($n = 285$) of CFS sufferers conducted by 'Action for ME' found that only 7 per cent of respondents reported CBT to be helpful, while 26 per cent reported that it made their condition worse.[140]

In summary, such medically unexplained symptoms and the associated syndromes are generally difficult to manage in the occupational environment because of controversy about their causation, their impairing effects on function and the poor response to treatment, particularly when the cause is perceived to be the workplace.

Future for psychosocial risk evaluation

Whereas the models of job strain and effort–reward imbalance have merits, the other psychosocial working conditions identified above have uncommonly been investigated in epidemiologic studies, with the exception of responses to traumatic events. In future research, more precise measures of risk and exposure are needed including duration or the intensity of a given exposure. Such evaluation cannot be obtained by means of postal or Internet-based questionnaires alone. In addition, standardized in-depth interviews can be applied in order to gather more information on the quality and quantity of occupational risks. These observations will need to be replicated in different countries and organizations and the relative effects of these versus other risks determined in well-conducted cohort studies that take the full range of mediators and confounders into account.

PSYCHIATRIC DISORDER AND WORK DISABILITY

Depression and phobic anxiety disorders are the most commonly identified psychiatric disorders in the workplace.[141] These can impact upon an individual's work through various ways: employment status, disability measured through extra effort, reduced performance, work cutback days, poor role functioning, sickness absence and being pensioned out of the workforce on a long-term or permanent basis. Assessment of each of these outcomes is conducted in different fashions. Much of the literature revolves around cross-sectional surveys with self-reporting of both disorder and work disability. Increasingly, the literature uses observable outcomes, routine data or validates the self-reported outcomes, although similar patterns are observed and self-reporting of outcomes, such as sickness absence, appears fairly reliable.

Two apparently conflicting, but consistent, findings make determining the association of any one individual's psychiatric disorder and work ability complex:

1. There is no direct relationship between the presence of psychiatric disorder and working, either as employment status or work performance. In the UK, for example, the employment rates of women with psychiatric disorder range from 42 per cent (phobias) to 59 per cent (panic disorder), compared to employment rates of 62 per cent overall. The comparable employment figures for men are 35 per cent and 70 per cent compared to 75 per cent overall.[142] The lack of association is well described by Wikman et al.[143] In this study, effectively a cross-sectional survey of people of working age in Sweden, respondents were asked to identify whether they had one or more of a range of common symptoms of illness, had a physician-made diagnosis and were identified as having been absent from work from the National Social Security Board. Each person could fit into none or any permutation of these groups. Only a minority of the population (25 per cent) had no illness symptoms. More (33 per cent) had symptoms, but had no diagnosis nor took sickness absence. Some 14 per cent had had a recent sickness absence of over two weeks, although 2 per cent of the whole population had been off sick without apparently experiencing symptoms or receiving a diagnosis (Figure 66.1).
2. In the general population, the more severe the disorder the more likely there is to be a limitation of working.[144] Employment rates for those with severe psychiatric illness (who comprised some 6.5 per cent of a US population-based study[145] and similar levels in other

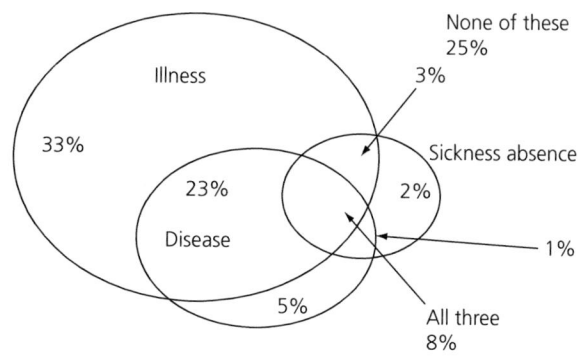

Figure 66.1 Relationship between illness, disease and sickness absence. Percentage of employed, aged 16–64 years, in Sweden 1998–2001 ($n = 13\,887$).

OECD countries) is between 5 and 20 per cent. This can lead to dramatically reduced earning capacity in those with more serious conditions. This was estimated to lead to approximately $27 000 per year less income for men and $9000 for women (at 2005 US dollar rates). Those with less serious conditions – who can presumably access sickness benefits, remain in work underachieving or take limited time off – were not as affected.

OCCUPATIONAL IMPAIRMENT OF PSYCHIATRIC DISORDER

What is it about a psychiatric disorder that impairs occupational functioning? As Mechanic eloquently pointed out, psychiatric disorder impairs exactly those functions most required in modern workplaces – concentration, cognitive function, energy, motivation and social interaction.[146] One aspect often raised in clinical situations, but rarely covered in research, is that of the extra effort that those with psychiatric disorder have to put in, in order to do their work, e.g. to overcome poor motivation or anxious cognitions.[147] Fatigue may also be one of the occupationally toxic elements of depression[148] and improvements of energy levels are associated with improved work productivity.[149] Most studies, though, have concentrated on cognitive function.[150] Depression is often associated with impaired cognitive function, aspects of which appear differentially affected. A meta-analysis of studies from a range of patient populations showed a strong and consistent effect for an association of depression severity with executive functioning (short-term working memory, cognitive flexibility, planning and problem solving), and weaker but consistent associations with learning, immediate and delayed recall and processing speed.[151] Scheid[152] cites these as potential barriers to both high status jobs and those where there are high levels of contact with the public. There was no consistently observed association with semantic memory or visuospatial functioning. Analysis of individual items on self-report questionnaires has shown that people with depression identified more disabilities in occupations requiring proficiency in decision-making and communication or frequent customer contact.[153] In the European ESMED study of 21 000 people in six countries,[154] attention and concentration and embarrassment in social situations were the mediators of the association between depression and occupational functioning. This finding has particular implications for making adjustments in allowing people to return to work following illness in that those with ongoing symptoms will experience poorer functioning and will require some degree of task modification.

Several studies have demonstrated temporal associations of work-related disability with relapse and remission in depression and anxiety.[155,156] These are not just limited to clinically diagnosable disorders, but appear to exist on a continuum, with people with subclinical disorders still having a significant occupational disability.[144,157] However, there is still a substantial amount of occupational disability that is not accounted for by either psychological or physical symptoms.[158] This may be because there appears to be a time lag effect, such that occupational functioning becomes impaired some time after the onset of symptoms and resolves later than the remission of symptoms.[159] The most important predictors of incomplete functional recovery are clinical and social, whereas personality and demographic characteristics are less important.[160] One important observation is that those who do make a recovery generally return to their premorbid level of functioning and only those with a severe and recurrent illness experience a decline in function – an important issue in determining eligibility for disability benefit.[155] Other relatively unexplored, but clinically relevant, issues include the impact of the disability associated with psychiatric disorder upon co-workers, for example through performance or absenteeism.

Severe mental illness such as schizophrenia, very disabling mood disorders and severe personality disorders, are dealt with predominantly by psychiatric services in most developed countries. The literature in this area over the past decade has almost exclusively focused upon rates of employment, vocational interventions with 'competitive employment' as an outcome and barriers to this, although much practice is still in the sheltered employment type of vocational rehabilitation facilities. In part, this reflects the consistent finding that in most OECD countries the proportion of people in paid employment with severe mental disorders, usually schizophrenia, but in some studies encompassing other psychoses, e.g. bipolar affective disorder, is very low (10–20 per cent) and has decreased over time compared to the rate of employment in the general population.[161] Again, cognitive and 'negative symptoms' of lack of motivation and anergia appear to drive this work disability, rather than the more obvious psychotic experiences. Many such people are able to be employed and the spreading practice of individual placement and support (IPS) has the strongest evidence base for maintaining stable employment.[162,163]

ORGANIZATIONAL EFFECTS OF PSYCHIATRIC DISORDER

Presenteeism

Most employees come to work with a range of symptoms which are best not medicalized.[143] Sickness presence, or 'presenteeism', describes a situation where an employee has a disorder, but nevertheless goes to work and may underperform.[164] A number of work (e.g. time pressure and working in a small company) and personal characteristics (e.g. level of commitment to work) affect the likelihood of such presenteeism behaviour,[165] but studies often combine types of disorder. A moment in time study showed that the decrements on task focus and productivity over a month in those with a diagnosis of depression was equivalent to two days per month absence.[166] An alternative approach is to measure 'work cut-back days'. Kessler and colleagues have consistently demonstrated the negative effect of both depression and anxiety,[167,168] whereby people with these common psychiatric disorders experience more cut-back days than many with other chronic conditions. The more chronic, but less severe diagnoses, such as dysthymia and mixed anxiety and depression, tend to have an even greater societal and organizational impact through lost productivity and presenteeism because of their greater prevalence.[144,157] Other studies confirm that the reduced productivity attributable to psychiatric illnesses is significant[166,169] and that depression, of all common conditions, has the greatest negative impact on time management and productivity and is equivalent to rheumatoid arthritis in its impact on physical tasks.[170]

Sickness absence

Short-term absences are by far the most common type of absence episode. The 'causes' of short-term absence appear to be different from longer-term sick leave. The Whitehall II study compared causes of different forms of sickness absence,[38] and although respiratory and gastrointestinal disorders were the most common causes of short-term absences by some margin, it is likely though that the role played by psychiatric disorders is underestimated. Job satisfaction and motivation, both linked to mental ill health have been shown to predict increased short-term absenteeism for colds.[171]

There is no agreed demarcation between short- and long-term sickness absence and this complicates comparisons between studies and countries.[172] Although long-term absence makes up only a small proportion of the incident number of absences, it accounts for up to a third of days off and 75 per cent of absence costs.[173] Although psychiatric disorder accounts for a small proportion of long-term absence, when it does it can be very long term and absence for this reason has a higher median cost. Once the employee has gone off sick with depression, there do not appear to be any work characteristics which predict the length of sick leave, although lower education and, surprisingly, being the main breadwinner, do seem to be associated with longer leave.[174]

Returning to work

A successful return to work is the desired outcome for most episodes of sick leave due to psychiatric disorder; however, there has been little research on how best to ensure that personnel do indeed return to work. The longer someone is off sick the less likely they are to return to work. This is partly due to factors related to the initial difficulties surrounding the decision to take time off, but also relates to obstacles implementing a return to work. Fear-avoidant and catastrophizing coping strategies[175] impact on the decision to leave work and are also likely to play a role in decisions on returning to work, particularly in workers who believe that their work has either caused their health problem or made it worse.[176] A commonly used technique to overcome some of these problems is a phased return to work. The employee starts back to work initially part-time and gradually builds up the hours and/or days over several weeks. While being apparently sensible, there is little evidence to suggest whether such an approach is the best one to use and, if so, in which circumstances.

Decisions about when to return to work are made more difficult by issues of timing – when is someone who has been off work with a psychiatric disorder ready to go back to work? Although obtaining reports from treating physicians is common practice, the only study of liaison between the employer and the employee's treating physicians found that doing so actually increased the time to return to work in those with psychiatric disorder, although communication between employer and employee only, had a positive effect.[177] There is also no standard way in which an individual moves through the 'stages' or 'phases'. Should the employee increase his hours in a preordained fashion decided at the start or should the increase depend on how well he is performing, or his level of symptoms? In many physical disorders, where the natural history of this aspect of recovery is relatively well understood, these dilemmas may be less important, but recovery from psychiatric disorders is less predictable, and might not fit into a rigid protocol. The attitudes of the individual's co-workers and resentment over covering their work or perceived underperformance might also play a role in making the return to work a success.[178] These effects appear even greater in those from minorities, compounding the discrimination.[179]

Ill health retirement and disability pensioning

In both the United Kingdom and many OECD countries, psychiatric disorders have now overtaken musculoskeletal disorders as the most common cause of ill health retirement and disability pensioning.[2,180] This rise has not occurred due to a fall in the prevalence of musculoskeletal disorders – they have just increased more quickly. Furthermore, this rise in benefit claims for symptom-related disorders does not reflect a similar rise in the incidence of such disorders in the population which have remained fairly static over the same period, suggesting a lowering of the severity at which retirement is awarded. More research is needed to discover what lies behind this discrepancy, but it seems probable that it has been brought about by a greater acceptance of psychiatric disorders on the part of claimants and their doctors. Even then, the true impact of psychiatric symptoms may be underestimated. A large prospective study found that anxiety and depression were strong predictors of ill health retirement awarded for physical disorders.[181] The same was found for insomnia, which only in rare cases is denoted as a cause for disability pensions.[182]

The evidence about the health impact of ill health retirement is mixed – some studies show an improvement over time.[183] However, this apparent improvement might instead be a return to normal after a temporarily increased level of symptoms around the time of being awarded the disability pension.[184] Given the potential harmful social and individual effects, it is surprising that many who are awarded ill health retirement for psychiatric illness report not having received treatment for it.[185] Nonetheless, several studies, most notably of health service employees in the UK, identify that a large minority of people supposedly retired for a (semi-) permanent incapacity are back in work a year later.[186]

Burnout

Burnout is defined as a 'prolonged response to chronic emotional and interpersonal stressors on the job' and is a widely used term in occupational psychology and even a qualifying 'diagnosis' for accessing social welfare benefits in some countries, such as Sweden.[187] The concept is almost universally measured by one or other version of the originator's assessment: the Maslach Burnout Inventory (MBI), the primary version of which has 22 items. The three key dimensions, as postulated by Maslach, are of 'overwhelming exhaustion', 'feelings of cynicism and detachment from the job' and 'reduced effectiveness/accomplishment'. There is an extensive literature associating burnout as an outcome of a range of negatively perceived work experiences. However, Wieclaw has identified conceptual and measurement difficulties with this concept, including the challenging issue, from an occupational health and preventive perspective, of providing convincing evidence of the relationship between burnout and specific occupational exposures.[188] There are strong correlations of burnout with psychiatric disorders, such as depression and anxiety, and personality traits like neuroticism and job satisfaction (from -0.40 to -0.75). The questions in the measure itself ask the respondent to attribute their response to their job which, it is argued, establishes that 'burnout is a problem that is specific to the work context, in contrast to depression which tends to pervade every domain of a persons life',[187] regardless of conflicting evidence showing the substantial contribution of non-work factors if assessed, e.g. life events.[189] This study of medical students also highlights problems with the term being used as an end point. Nearly 50 per cent of the medical students were already classified as 'burnt out' yet the vast majority will go on to long and productive careers in the same area. Recent work has shown that once labelled burnt out, someone has a greater risk of permanent disability in Finland even accounting for baseline diagnosable disorders.[190] While burnout is not a psychiatric disorder, and unlikely to become so in DSM-V or ICD-11, establishing the concept's utility and validity as potentially a mediator of work-related stressors and disorder is warranted.

Comorbidity of physical and psychiatric disorders

Psychiatric disorders are often comorbid with physical illness. Attributing sickness absence to a single physical 'cause' ignores the multiple factors that contribute to the process. The propensity for those with psychiatric disorders to have periods of absence '... not necessarily the type diagnosed as nervous', has been recognized for at least 80 years.[191] Many cross-sectional studies have shown higher unemployment or poorer occupational functioning in people who have comorbid depression and anxiety. For instance, the presence of a comorbid depression[192] and anxiety[193] is associated with greater degrees of work disability across all pain-related conditions.

For those who are employed and experience an episode of physical illness, even accounting for the physical impairment arising from that condition, the presence of mental ill health, usually defined by some cut-off point on a scale, has a deleterious impact upon returning to the workplace. Glozier et al.[194] showed that for the 20–25 per cent of people who have a stroke while of working age, over half return to work by six months. However, those with mental ill health were less than half as likely to return, even after adjusting for levels of physical disability and other factors. Similar findings have been shown after myocardial infarction.[195,196]

WHAT INFLUENCES THE INTERFACE OF OCCUPATIONAL RISKS AND PSYCHIATRIC DISORDER?

Most research into the effect of work characteristics upon the development or exacerbation of psychiatric disorder has focused either on the nature of the work or the nature of the disorder. As shown in Chapter 64, Work, stress and sickness absence: a psychosocial prespective (p. 804), a host of contextual factors plays a role in shaping these influences. More recent work has demonstrated the proximal effects of an individual's cognitive processes as the mediator between external factors and occupational dysfunction. Karasek and Theorell,[36] Marmot[197] and Stansfeld et al.[39] have all alluded to the role of such individual perceptions, which have been extensively studied in the field of musculoskeletal disorders, but less so in psychiatric disorders. What might influence such perceptions is difficult to study, but a range of related personal factors are important determinants of psychiatric disorder and are candidates for mediating the effects of work upon mental health.

Job satisfaction is strongly associated with mental health in meta-analyses,[198] as are many aspects of perception and personality.[199] These derive from a combination of temperament, mainly genetic, and a range of early experiences. Using lifecourse data, Henderson et al.[200] have shown that teachers' ratings of temperament in childhood and even whether the child's father was off sick were also strongly predictive of work disability in adult life, over and above accepted predictors such as IQ and education. This suggests there are early life influences upon health behaviours which affect the likelihood of an individual to take sick leave.

Individual perceptions on work functioning are influenced by a number of other contextual factors, the most notable being balancing demands between work and other aspects of life. Appreciation of this by researchers (lagging behind clinicians) has shown that such factors as perceiving an imbalance between work and family/personal lives was strongly associated with current mood problems in both genders and in anxiety in women, even making allowances for standard work stress measures,[201] a gender effect seen elsewhere.[202] In some cases, a specific home life pressure actually makes some people more likely to come to work.[165]

The interaction between work factors, the individual and their psychiatric disorder can best be understood using a dynamic model whereby individuals are seen as active agents making decisions about their status along a 'sickness journey' as shown below. This accords with what is called the 'voluntaristic' aspect of sickness behaviour in an occupational setting.[203] It provides a framework for thinking about how to manage an individual with psychiatric symptoms in a specific context as there will be a host of influences on the cognitive factors underlying each decision. Certainly tackling the cognitions that determine these decisions has been shown to improve such occupational disability as return to work after myocardial infarction.[204]

This dynamic model (Figure 66.2) suggests that an employee's perception of their symptoms and health occurs in a specific context leading to the person actively making a decision about their work status. The journey starts with perceiving sensations or feelings as symptoms of illness that may or may not have an effect upon function. Any reduced function can be expressed as either taking

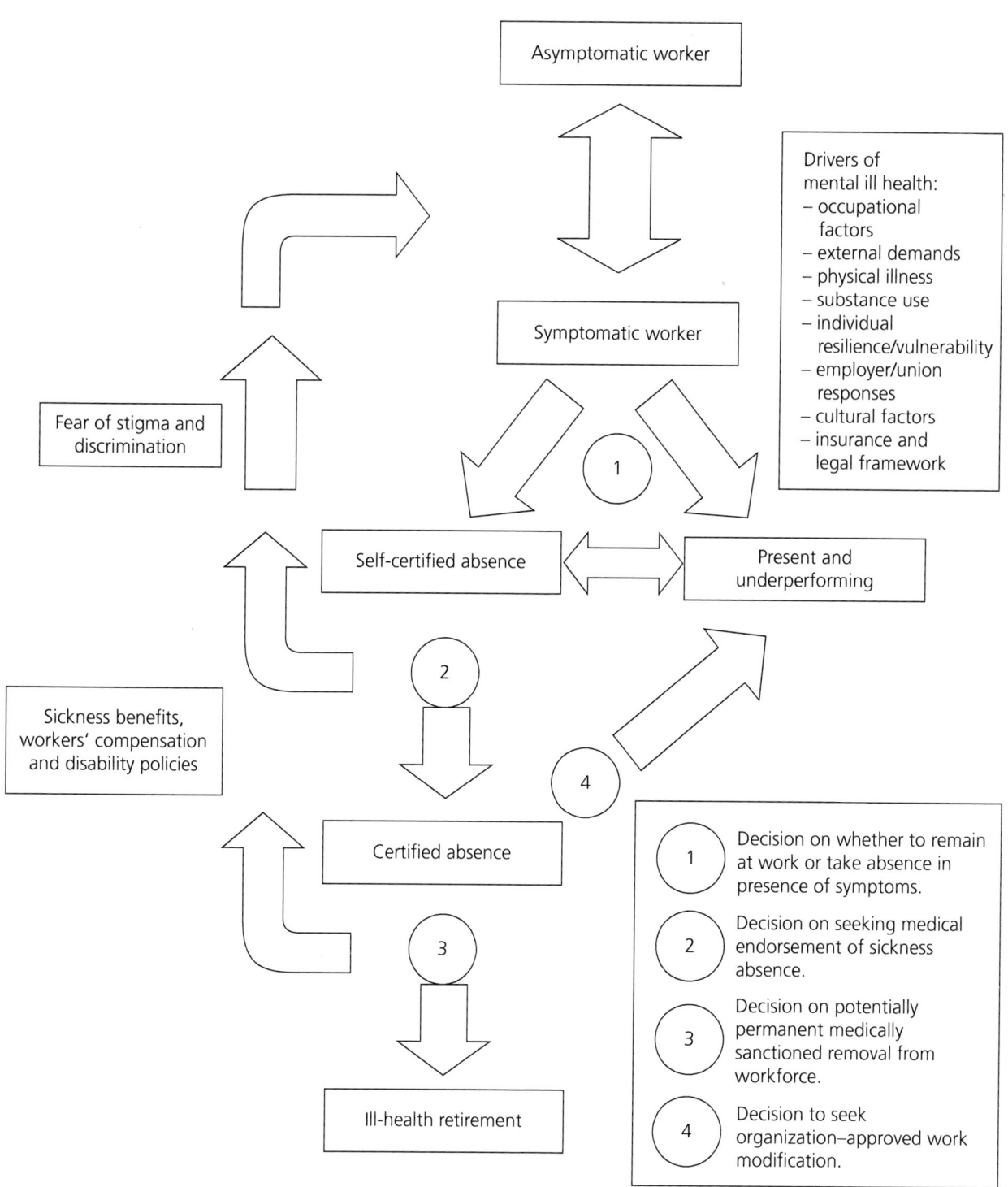

Figure 66.2 Decisions made by employees during their sickness pathway and potential influences.

leave from work or presenteeism. The decision (point 1) on which of these two options to take will, as shown above, be affected by a range of factors, e.g. personality (conscientiousness, for instance), background culture of working, organizational (team structure or flexibility) and social characteristics (level of unemployment), as well as perceived severity. Most countries allow some period of self-certified absence after which a doctor's confirmation is required. The decision to seek (point 2): this is also multifactorial and includes such factors as ease of access, benefit systems and perception of how likely the doctor is to concur with the patient. After a period of time on some form of sickness benefit, a decision has to be made upon returning to work – of either the original role in some form – full or modified (point 4) or of moving to another role, or seeking the more permanent support of a disability pension (point 3). These time periods, ease of access, level of support, etc., vary dramatically across countries, as do even the diagnoses allowable for compensation. It is the understanding of this sickness pathway that underpins much of what professionals in the field do (Figure 66.2).

WHAT CAN BE DONE IN THE WORKPLACE?

While it is clear that workplace factors have a moderate role in the development and perpetuation of psychiatric disorders, and that the public health impact of psychiatric symptoms on occupational outcomes is enormous, it is unclear how governments, insurers, employers and health services should respond. The most striking feature of the research to date is the paucity of high quality studies addressing these questions.[205] There are also differing views from reviews of the same literature, potentially dependent upon the views of the authors and the rigor of the review criteria which make any recommendations difficult.

Primary and indicated prevention through organizational interventions

A common conclusion from the epidemiological studies of psychosocial risk factors is that one or more of the identified factors should be tackled to prevent later psychiatric disorder. While there have been some examples of simple changes in the workplace, such as in the pattern of shift work, leading to lower levels of distress,[206] a recent systematic review concluded that there was currently insufficient evidence to judge the effectiveness of any specific organizational changes.[207] Graveling et al.[207] identified a range of participatory approaches to changing organizational practices in 11 studies, fewer than half of which showed a positive benefit upon 'mental well-being'. A systematic review of organizational interventions to improve employee control could not identify a single randomized controlled trial (RCT) in this field of study.[208] A small majority of the studies showed some benefit and two studies which ran concurrently with redundancies reported worsening health. An interesting observation from a second review by this team[209] suggested that task-restructuring interventions increasing team working had minimal or no effect and that working in autonomous groups in fact caused deterioration in the psychosocial work environment, with resulting health effects. Interventions that did manage to improve employee control appear to have a positive effect, but the processes by which this is achieved have not been identified, making any replication of the study very difficult.[210]

Educating and training individual managers about psychiatric illness and the potential importance of job strain through web-based or more traditional formats, although attractive, does not seem to reduce either job strain or psychiatric illness when evaluated.[211,212] One intensive 40-hour programme did appear to have a beneficial effect,[207] suggesting a major commitment was needed to make an impact.

Primary and indicated prevention through individually focused interventions

Alternative approaches have focused on the individual worker, rather than the work environment, with interventions aimed at increasing an individual's ability to cope with stressful work situations. Two separate systematic reviews have concluded that the heterogeneity of individually focused prevention programmes and the limited methodological quality prevent any definite recommendations being made.[207,213] Nevertheless, both reviews reported that the majority of stress management programmes have a modest or short-term impact on a range of variables associated with individual distress. Other reviews have concluded that interventions which reduce psychological distress among workers will also reduce levels of sickness absence.[214] A meta-analysis of 48 experimental studies agreed that individually focused interventions designed to reduce or prevent psychological consequences of occupational stress tended to be more effective than organizational interventions,[215] and that cognitive behavioural therapy had the best evidence for effectiveness.[213,215] New linked interventions, such as acceptance and commitment therapy (ACT) may have a role in reducing psychiatric disorders in employees via increasing their acceptance of undesirable thoughts and feelings.[216] A similar review in healthcare workers suggested a positive effect of individual interventions, generally cognitive and behaviourally based, on 'stress and burnout'.[217]

A number of employers have instigated general 'healthy lifestyle' programmes to improve employee health and, presumably, occupational performance. Undertaking regular exercise and maintaining a healthy weight may help prevent psychiatric disorders,[218] but no reliable studies have been able to demonstrate that exercise programmes in the workplace reduce levels of psychiatric illness.[213] There is, however, some evidence from observational studies that workers in sedentary jobs who engage in regular strenuous leisure-time physical activity outside the work environment, have a lower risk of sickness absence due to psychological complaints.[219]

Screening and treatment of established cases of psychiatric disorder

Health screening is an established part of risk management in many larger organizations. A large trial[220] demonstrated that screening for depression in the workplace, followed by a systematic programme of telephone outreach and care management (encouraging employees to enter appropriate treatment and monitoring treatment quality) resulted in decreased symptoms, higher job retention and more hours worked. There is also some theoretical evidence that screening programmes may be cost-effective for purchasers.[221]

Established guidelines on the treatment of depression and anxiety[222,223] are based on the broad research evidence from primary and secondary care trials. However, few of these trials have measured occupational outcomes. It is therefore difficult to assess the occupational benefits of interventions recommended in such guidelines, particularly as symptom improvement does not necessarily correlate with return to work.

The Cochrane collaboration has published a systematic review of all randomized controlled trials of work or worker-directed interventions for depression.[224] The authors identified 11 studies, involving 2556 individuals, which evaluated the effectiveness of a range of pharmacological and psychological interventions. They concluded there was no evidence that medication, enhanced primary care or psychological interventions have any impact on the amount of sickness absence taken by depressed individuals, although the interventions might have been effective in reducing symptoms. For instance, employers changing an employee's tasks seems to have a positive effect upon depressive symptoms, while reducing hours or tasks, changing department and sending people on courses had no such effect.[174] A recent meta-analysis showed that while a range of different treatments can cause significant reductions in symptom severity, the associated gain in labour output was only a third as large as the reductions in symptoms,[225] an observation that does not bode well for any future economic analyses. The apparent lack of an effect of standard treatments on occupational outcomes suggests that additional specific interventions addressing return to work issues may be needed. When occupational health practitioners are available, training them in cognitive behavioural approaches such as graded activity, can result in employees returning to work more rapidly.[226]

Employee assistance programmes (EAPs) or counselling services are commonly provided by many organizations and these usually use relatively unstructured psychological support offered on a voluntary basis, delivered by individuals from a range of professional backgrounds. An English Appeal Court ruling in 2002 suggested the provision of a counselling service was likely to satisfy an employer's duty of care, which may have led many employers to implement a counselling scheme as a form of 'insurance' against stress at work claims.[227] In a 2001 systematic review, the British Association of Counselling and Psychotherapy claimed such counselling could reduce sickness absence,[228] although the poor quality of studies included, including no RCTs, has been highlighted.[229] Workplace counselling may be helpful for some, but better quality evidence is needed to guide further use of this intervention.

Population-based interventions

Interventions at a societal level, such as improving mental health literacy,[230] have been credited with increasing help seeking and treatment for psychiatric disorders. Such campaigns may have a role in tackling the occupational consequences of disease and health promotion advocated as a method of reducing the impact of work stressors on psychiatric disorder.[231] In 1997, a public health campaign was undertaken in Victoria, Australia, which aimed to educate the population on the importance of staying active and remaining at work when they suffered back pain.[232] Interestingly, a later evaluation of those physicians who claimed to have a special interest in the management of back pain showed that these physicians were most likely to advocate bed rest and avoidance for acute low back pain contrary to recommendations.[233] Such potential pitfalls to this approach are also highlighted by Coggon,[234] who suggested that the back pain epidemic of the 1970s and 1980s was partly a result of the very interventions aimed to make workers aware of the risk of harm to their backs.

CONCLUSIONS

Over the past two decades, there has been an accumulation of evidence that both objective and subjective characteristics of workplaces are associated with increased risks of psychiatric disorder and mental ill health. None of these have been demonstrated to be sufficient in their own right to cause these disorders, not even catastrophic life-threatening trauma. As with many epidemiologically identified 'risk factors' for disease, demonstrating that interventions designed to reduce these risks actually improve health has proven a far more difficult task. Reviews of a range of approaches have yet to demonstrate any repeatable significant impacts of organizational interventions despite their widespread adoption. Individually focused interventions show more promise in improving mental ill health, although how these are to be delivered has yet to be adequately defined. However, the notion that attempts to improve health in an occupational setting actually brings tangible benefits to an organization seems to have been widely accepted with little evidential support.

The lack of a one-to-one correlation between occupational risk factors and psychiatric disorder means that other factors are required for the development of a disorder. These include genetic predisposition, personality, early life events and brain development, substance misuse, and stressors such as illness and other demands, e.g. family, caring and financial. Conversely, there is also no one-to-one relationship of the presence of psychiatric disorder with an inability to work: most people with the common illnesses work and many of those with more serious illness would like to, although the number who do is woeful. We suggest that the increasing levels of work-related disability (a social construct) across OECD countries, without a demonstrable rise in the population prevalence of these conditions, indicate that there are a range of social factors that are having a major impact. It may be that, at one level, a reduction of stigma and increased health literacy may lead to workers being more accepting of psychological conditions, while the actions of media, professions, employers, unions and government in perpetuating occupationally related mental ill health as a disorder is potentially understated. Much of the public perception of the complex interplay of work and mental health is based upon a relatively poor, or at times non-existent, evidence base upon which to base occupational and medicolegal practice and policy, yet the societal costs of dealing with these conditions are staggering. Understanding the complexity of this topic may be helped by viewing the individual employee as an active agent who makes decisions about their ability to work in the context of their symptoms and perceived stressors, which in themselves are influenced by the medicolegal and sociocultural context in which they reside.

Key points

- Psychiatric disorder has been increasingly attributed to work-related causes and designated as a reason for work disability over the past two decades without any observable change in overall prevalence of these disorders.
- There is little consistent evidence for any independent effect of occupation or profession upon psychiatric disorders when compared to other measures of inequality, such as grade and income.
- There is moderate evidence that a range of perceived psychosocial stressors, including job strain, effort–reward imbalance, perceived bullying, job insecurity and organizational injustice, are associated with psychiatric disorder and mental ill health.
- A range of personal factors, such as early experience of sickness behaviour, personality and education, and contextual factors, such as medical, legal and social security practices, have at least as strong an effect on the expression and development of work-related psychiatric disorder as work and occupational characteristics.
- Successful interventions need to identify how best to balance individual and organizational needs and should view an individual as an active decision-making agent in determining their work and health-related behaviours.
- Persuasive evidence for the effectiveness, and especially cost-effectiveness, of workplace interventions is generally lacking.

ACKNOWLEDGEMENTS

We would like to acknowledge the invaluable assistance of Dr Arnstein Mykletun, Dr Sam Harvey, and Professors Matthew Hotopf, Simon Wessely, Philip Bohle and Michael Quinlan.

REFERENCES

1. Black C. *Working for a healthier tomorrow*. London: The Stationery Office, 2008.
2. Henderson M, Glozier N, Holland Elliott K. Long term sickness absence. *British Medical Journal*. 2005; **330**: 802–3.
3. Organisation for Economic Co-operation and Development. Sickness, disability and work: Breaking the barriers. Norway, Poland and Switzerland. Paris: Organisation for Economic Corporation and Development, 2006.
4. Royal College of Psychiatrists. Mental health and work. London: The Stationery Office, 2008.
5. Harvey SB, Henderson M, Lelliott P, Hotopf M. Mental health and employment: Much work still to be done. *British Journal of Psychiatry*. 2009; **194**: 201–3.
6. Organisation for Economic Co-operation and Development. Employment outlook: Tackling the jobs crisis. Paris: OECD, 2009.
7. Paoli P, Merllié D. Third European survey on working conditions. Dublin: European Foundation for the Improvement of Living and Working Conditions, 2003.
8. Clohessy S, Ehlers A. PTSD symptoms, responses to intrusive memories and coping in ambulance service workers. *British Journal of Clinical Psychology*. 1999; **38**: 251–65.
9. Alexander DA, Klein S. Ambulance personnel and critical incidents. Impact of accident and emergency work on mental health and emotional well-being. *British Journal of Psychiatry*. 2001; **178**: 78–81.
10. Bennett P, Williams Y, Page N *et al*. Levels of mental health problems among UK emergency ambulance workers. *Emergency Medicine Journal*. 2004; **21**: 235–6.
11. Brown JM, Campbell EA. Sources of occupational stress in the police. *Work Stress*. 1990; **4**: 305–18.
12. Alexander D, Walker L, Innes G, Irving B. Police stress at work. The Police Foundation Series 1993; 15–38, 74–77.
13. Firth-Cozens J. The psychological problems of doctors. In: Firth-Cozens J, Payne R (eds). *Stress in health professionals: Psychological and organizational causes and interventions*. London: Wiley, 1999.
14. Wall TD, Bolden RI, Borrill CS *et al*. Minor psychiatric disorders in NHS trust staff: Occupational and gender differences. *British Journal of Psychiatry*. 1997; **171**: 519–23.
15. Gardner DH, Hini D. Work-related stress in the veterinary profession in New Zealand. *New Zealand Veterinary Journal*. 2006; **54**: 119–24.

16. Johnson S, Cooper C, Cartwright S *et al*. The experience of work related stress across occupations. *Journal of Managerial Psychology*. 2005; **20**: 178-87.
17. Stansfeld SA, Head J, Rashul S *et al*. Occupation and mental health: Secondary analysis of the ONS Psychiatric Morbidity Survey of Great Britain. London: HSE Books, 2003.
18. Sanne B, Mykletun A, Dahl AA *et al*. Occupational differences in levels of anxiety and depression: The Hordaland Health Study. *Journal of Occupational and Environmental Medicine*. 2003; **45**: 628-38.
19. Marchand A. Mental health in Canada: Are there any risky occupations and industries? *International Journal of Law and Psychiatry*. 2007; **30**: 272-83.
20. *Sutherland v Hattoner* [2002] EWCA Civ 76.
21. Marchand A, Demers A, Durand P. Do occupational and work conditions really matter? A longitudinal analysis of psychological distress experiences among Canadian workers. *Sociology of Health and Illness*. 2005; **27**: 602-27.
22. Platt S, Hawton K. Suicidal behaviour and the labour market. In: Hawton K, van Heeringen K (eds). *The international handbook of suicide and attempted suicide*. New York: Wiley, 2000: 310-84.
23. Blakely TA, Collings SCD, Atkinson J. Unemployment and suicide: Evidence for a causal association? *Journal of Epidemiology and Community Health*. 2003; **57**: 594-600.
24. Agerbo E. Effect of psychiatric illness and labour market status on suicide: A healthy worker effect? *Journal of Epidemiology and Community Health*. 2005; **59**: 598-602.
25. Martikainen PT, Valkonen T. Excess mortality of unemployed men and women during a period of rapidly increasing unemployment. *Lancet*. 1996; **348**: 909-12.
26. Stuckler D, Basu S, Suhrcke M *et al*. The public health effect of economic crises and alternative policy responses in Europe: An empirical analysis. *Lancet*. 2009; **374**: 315-23.
27. Agerbo E, Gunnell D, Bonde J *et al*. Suicide and occupation: The impact of socio-economic, demographic and psychiatric differences. *Psychological Medicine*. 2007; **37**: 1131-40.
28. Hawton K, Simkin S, Rue J *et al*. Suicide in female nurses in England and Wales. *Psychological Medicine*. 2002; **32**: 239-50.
29. Meltzer H, Griffiths C, Brock A *et al*. Patterns of suicide by occupation in England and Wales: 2001-2005. *British Journal of Psychiatry*. 2008; **193**: 73-6.
30. Schmidt FL, Hunter J. General mental ability in the world of work: Occupational attainment and job performance. *Journal of Personality and Social Differences*. 2004; **86**: 162-73.
31. Roberts B, Caspi A, Moffitt T. Work experiences and personality development in young adulthood. *Journal of Personality and Social Psychology*. 2003; **84**: 582-93.
32. Skapinakis P, Weich S, Lewis G *et al*. Socio-economic position and common mental disorders: Longitudinal study in the general population in the UK. *British Journal of Psychiatry*. 2006; **189**: 109-17.
33. Demakakos P, Nazroo J, Breeze E, Marmot M. Socieconomic status and health: The role of subjective social status. *Social Science and Medicine*. 2008; **67**: 330-40.
34. Kleppa E, Sanne B, Tell G. Working overtime is associated with anxiety and depression: The Hordaland Health Study. *Journal of Occupational and Environmental Medicine*. 2008; **50**: 658-66.
35. Fujino Y, Horie S, Hoshuyama T *et al*. A systematic review of working hours and mental health burden. *Sangyo Eiseigaku Zasshi*. 2006; **48**: 87.
36. Karasek R, Theorell T. *Healthy work: Stress, productivity and the reconstruction of working life*. New York: Basic Books, 1990.
37. Siegrist J. Adverse health effects of high-effort/low-reward conditions. *Journal of Occupational Health Psychology*. 1996; **1**: 27-41.
38. Stansfeld SA, Fuhrer R, Shipley MJ, Marmot MG. Work characteristics predict psychiatric disorder: prospective results from the Whitehall II Study. *Occupational and Environmental Medicine*. 1999; **56**: 302-7.
39. Stansfeld S, Feeney A, Head J *et al*. Sickness absence for psychiatric illness: The Whitehall II Study. *Social Science and Medicine*. 1995; **40**: 189-97.
40. Head J, Kivimaki M, Martikainen P *et al*. Influence of change in psychosocial work characteristics on sickness absence: the Whitehall II study. *Journal of Epidemiology and Community Health*. 2006; **60**: 55-61.
41. Roelen C, Koopmans P, de Graaf J *et al*. Job demands, health perception and sickness absence. *Occupational Medicine*. 2007; **57**: 499-504.
42. Stansfeld S, Candy B. Psychosocial work environment and mental health. A meta analytic review. *Scandinavian Journal of Work, Environment and Health*. 2006; **32**: 443-62.
43. Bonde JPE. Psychosocial factors at work and risk of depression: A systematic review of the epidemiological evidence. *Occupational and Environmental Medicine*. 2008; **65**: 438-45.
44. Netterstrøm B, Conrad N, Bech P *et al*. The relation between work-related psychosocial factors and the development of depression. *Epidemiologic Reviews*. 2008; **30**: 118-32.
45. Clumeck N, Kempenaers C, Godin I *et al*. Working conditions predict incidence of long-term spells of sick leave due to depression: Results from the Belstress I Prospective Study. *Journal of Epidemiology and Community Health*. 2009; **63**: 286-92.
46. Melchior M, Caspi A, Milne B *et al*. Work stress precipitates depression and anxiety in young working women and men. *Psychological Medicine*. 2007; **37**: 1119-29.
47. Wang J, Schmitz N, Dewa C, Stansfeld S. Changes in perceived job strain and the risk of major depression: Results from a population-based longitudinal study. *American Journal of Epidemiology*. 2009; **169**: 1085-91.
48. Kivimaki M, Virtanen M, Vartia M *et al*. Workplace bullying and the risk of cardiovascular disease and depression. *Occupational Environment Medicine*. 2003; **60**: 779-83.

49. Kivimaki M, Elovainio M, Vahtera J. Workplace bullying and sickness absence in hospital staff. *Occupational Environment Medicine*. 2000; **57**: 656-60.
50. Mikkelsen EG, Einarsen S. Relationships between exposure to bullying at work and psychological and psychosomatic health complaints. *Scandinavian Journal of Psychology*. 2002; **43**: 397-405.
51. Kivimaki M, Vahtera J, Elovainio M et al. Human costs of organizational downsizing: Comparing health trends between leavers and stayers. *American Journal of Community Psychology*. 2003; **32**: 57-67.
52. Quine L. Workplace bullying in NHS community trust: Staff questionnaire survey. *British Medical Journal*. 1999; **318**: 218-32.
53. Rayner C. The incidence of workplace bullying. *Journal of Community and Applied Social Psychology*. 1997; **7**: 199-208.
54. Moayed FA, Daraisheh N, Shell R, Salem S. Workplace bullying: A systematic review of risk factors and outcomes. *Theoretical Issues in Ergonomic Science*. 2006; **7**: 311-22.
55. Keashly L, Jagatic K. By any other name: American perspectives on workplace bullying. In: Einarsen S, Hoel H, Zapf D, Cooper CL (eds). *Bullying and emotional abuse in the workplace*. International Perspectives in Research and Practice. London: Taylor & Francis, 2003: 31-61.
56. Zapf D, Einarsen S, Hoel H, Vartia M. Empirical findings on bullying in the workplace. In: Einarsen S, Hoel H, Zapf D, Cooper CL (eds). *Bullying and emotional abuse in the workplace*. International Perspectives in Research and Practice. London: Taylor & Francis, 2003: 102-26.
57. Niedhammer I, David S, Degioanni S et al. Workplace bullying and sleep disturbances: Findings from a large scale cross-sectional survey in the French working population. *Sleep*. 2009; **32**: 1211-19.
58. Mogen S, Agervold A, Mikkelsen E. Relationships between bullying, psychosocial work environment and individual stress reactions. *Work and Stress*. 2004; **18**: 336-51.
59. Fullerton CS, Ursano RJ, Wang L. Acute stress disorder, posttraumatic stress disorder, and depression in disaster or rescue workers. *American Journal of Psychiatry*. 2004; **161**: 1370-6.
60. Stein MB, Walker JR, Hazen AL, Forde DR. Full and partial posttraumatic stress disorder: Findings from a community based survey. *American Journal of Psychiatry*. 1997; **154**: 1114-19.
61. Breslau N, Davis GC. Posttraumatic stress disorder: The stressor criterion. *Journal of Nervous and Mental Disease*. 1987; **175**: 255-64.
62. Bonanno GA, Galea S, Bucciarelli A, Vlahov D. What predicts psychological resilience after disaster? The role of demographics, resources and life stress. *Journal of Consulting and Clinical Psychology*. 2007; **75**: 671-81.
63. Misra M, Greenberg N, Hutchinson C et al. Psychological impact upon London Ambulance Service of the 2005 bombings. *Occupational Medicine*. 2009; **59**: 428-33.
64. Smith A. *Post traumatic stress disorder, stress and emergency ambulance personnel: A semi-systematic review of the literature*. Cardiff: The Wales Office of Research and Development for Health and Social Care, 2009.
65. Whally M, Brewin C. Mental health following terrorist attacks. *British Journal of Psychiatry*. 2007; **190**: 94-96.
66. Committee on Veterans Compensation for Post-traumatic Stress Disorder, Institute of Medicine and National Research Council. PTSD compensation and military service. Washington DC: The National Academies Press, 2007.
67. Smith TC, Ryan MAK, Wingard DL et al. New onset and persistent symptoms of post-traumatic stress disorder self reported after deployment and combat exposures: Prospective population based US military cohort study. *British Medical Journal*. 2008; **336**: 366-71.
68. Leard Mann CA, Smith TC, Smith B et al. for the Millennium Cohort Study Team. Baseline self-reported functional health and vulnerability to post-traumatic stress disorder after combat deployment: Prospective US military cohort study. *British Medical Journal*. 2009; **338**: b1273.
69. Ismail K, Blatchley N, Hotopf M et al. Occupational risk factors for ill health in Gulf veterans of the United Kingdom. *Journal of Epidemiology and Community Health*. 2000; **54**: 834-8.
70. Hotopf M, Hull L, Fear N et al. The health of UK military personnel who deployed to the 2003 Iraq War. *Lancet*. 2006; **367**: 1731-41.
71. Cameron P, Gabbe B. The effect of compensation claims on outcomes after injury. *Injury*. 2009; **40**: 905-6.
72. Feldner MT, Monson CM, Friedman MJ. A critical analysis of approaches to targeted PTSD prevention: Current status and theoretically derived future directions. *Behavioral Modification*. 2007; **31**: 80-116.
73. Jones N, Roberts P, Greenberg N. Peer-group risk assessment: A post-traumatic management strategy for hierarchical organizations. *Occupational Medicine*. 2003; **53**: 469-75.
74. Bultmann U, Kant IJ, van den Brandt PA et al. Psychosocial work characteristics as risk factors for the onset of fatigue and psychological distress: Prospective results from the Maastricht Cohort Study. *Psychological Medicine*. 2002; **32**: 333-45.
75. Wang JL. Work stress as a risk factor for major depressive episode(s). *Psychological Medicine*. 2005; **35**: 865-71.
76. Plaisier I, de Bruijn JG, De Graaf R et al. The contribution of working conditions and social support to the onset of depressive and anxiety disorders among male and female employees. *Social Science and Medicine*. 2007; **64**: 401-10.
77. Parker S, Chmiel N, Wall T. Work characteristics and employee well-being within the context of strategic downsizing. *Journal of Occupational and Health Psychology*. 1997; **2**: 289-303.
78. Grunberg L, Moore S, Greenberg E. Differences in psychological and physical health amongst layoff survivors: The effect of layoff contact. *Journal of Occupational and Health Psychology*. 2001; **6**: 15-25.

79. Quinlan M, Bohle P. Overstretched and unreciprocated commitment: Reviewing research on the occupational health and safety effects of downsizing and job insecurity. *International Journal of Health Services.* 2009; **39**: 1-44.
80. Ferrie JE, Shipley MJ, Stansfeld SA, Marmot MG. Effects of chronic job insecurity and change in job security on self reported health, minor psychiatric morbidity, physiological measures, and health related behaviours in British civil servants: The Whitehall II study. *Journal of Epidemiology and Community Health.* 2002; **56**: 450-4.
81. Kivimaki M, Honkonen T, Wahlbeck K et al. Organisational downsizing and increased use of psychotropic drugs among employees who remain in employment. *Journal of Epidemiology and Community Health.* 2007; **61**: 154-8.
82. Zimmerman FJ, Christakis DA, Vander Stoep A. Tinker, tailor, soldier, patient: Work attributes and depression disparities among young adults. *Social Science and Medicine.* 2004; **58**: 1889-901.
83. Benach J, Muntaner C. Precarious employment and health: Developing a research agenda. *Journal of Epidemiology and Community Health.* 2007; **61**: 276-7.
84. Benach J, Amable M, Muntander C, Benavides FG. The consequences of flexible work for health: Are we looking at the right place? *Journal of Epidemiology and Community Health.* 2002; **56**: 405-6.
85. Thornicroft G. *Shunned: Discrimination against people with mental illness.* Oxford: Oxford University Press, 2006.
86. Beatty JE, Kirby SL. Beyond the legal environment: How stigma influences invisible identity groups in the workplace. *Employee Responsibilities and Rights Journal.* 2006; **18**: 29-44.
87. Stuart S. Mental illness and employment discrimination. *Current Opinion in Psychiatry.* 2006; **19**: 522-26.
88. Catalano R, Drake RE, Becker DR, Clark RE. Labor market conditions and employment of the mentally ill. *Journal of Mental Health Policy and Economics.* 1999; **2**: 51-4.
89. Hudson K. The disposable worker. *Monthly Review.* 2001; **52**: 43-55.
90. Baldwin ML, Marcus SC. Perceived and measured stigma among workers with serious mental illness. *Psychiatric Services.* 2006; **57**: 388-92.
91. Michalak EE, Yatham LN, Maxwell V et al. The impact of bipolar disorder upon work functioning: A qualitative analysis. *Bipolar Disorders.* 2007; **9**: 126-43.
92. Glozier N. Workplace effects of the stigmatization of depression. *Journal of Occupational and Environmental Medicine.* 1998; **40**: 793-800.
93. Manning C, White P. Attitudes of employers to the mentally ill. *Psychiatric Bulletin.* 1995; **19**: 541-3.
94. Sainsbury Centre for Mental Health. Mental health and employment. Briefing No. 33. London: SCMH, 2007.
95. MacDonald-Wilson K. Managing disclosure of psychiatric disabilities to employers. *Journal of Applied Rehabilitation Counselling.* 2005; **36**: 11-21.
96. Mental Health Foundation. Out at work. A survey of the experiences of people with mental health problems within the workplace. London: Mental Health Foundation, 2002.
97. The Shaw Trust. *Mental health: The last workplace taboo.* Chippenham: The Shaw Trust, 2006.
98. Goldberg S, Killeen M, O'Day B. The disclosure conundrum: How people with psychiatric difficulties navigate employment. *Psychology, Public Policy and Law.* 2005; **11**: 463-500.
99. Oksanen T, Kouvonen A, Vahtera J et al. Prospective study of workplace social capital and depression: Are vertical and horizontal components equally important? *Journal of Epidemiology and Community Health.* 2010, May 12. [Epub ahead of print] Available from: www.ncbi.nlm.nih.gov/pubmed/19692720.
100. Sinokki M, Hinkka K, Ahola K et al. The association between team climate at work and mental health in the Finnish Health 2000 Study. *Occupational and Environmental Medicine.* 2009; **66**: 523-8.
101. Kivimaki M, Vahtera J, Elovainio M et al. Effort-reward imbalance, procedural injustice and relational injustice as psychosocial predictors of health: Complementary or redundant models? *Occupational and Environmental Medicine.* 2007; **64**: 659-65.
102. Macfarlane GJ, Pallewatte N, Paudyal P et al. Evaluation of work-related psychosocial factors and regional musculoskeletal pain: Results from a EULAR Task Force. *Annals of the Rheumatic Diseases.* 2009; **68**: 885-91.
103. Shields M. Long working hours and health. *Health Reports.* 1999; **11**: 33-48.
104. Virtanen M, Singh-Manoux A, Ferrie JE et al. Long working hours and cognitive function: The Whitehall II study. *American Journal of Epidemiology.* 2009; **169**: 596-605.
105. de Vogli R, Ferrie J, Chandola T et al. Unfairness and health: Evidence from the Whitehall II study. *Journal of Epidemiology and Community Health.* 2007; **61**: 513-18.
106. Kouvonen A, Kivimaki M, Elovainio M et al. Low organisational justice and heavy drinking: A prospective cohort study. *Occupational and Environmental Medicine.* 2008; **65**: 44-50.
107. Kivimaki M, Leino-Arjas P, Luukkonen R et al. Work stress and risk of cardiovascular mortality: Prospective cohort study of industrial employees. *British Medical Journal.* 2002; **325**: 857.
108. Eaker ED, Sullivan LM, Kelly-Hayes M et al. Does job strain increase the risk for coronary heart disease or death in men and women?: The Framingham Offspring Study. *American Journal of Epidemiology.* 2004; **159**: 950-8.
109. Kivimaki M, Head J, Ferrie JE et al. Why is evidence on job strain and coronary heart disease mixed? An illustration of measurement challenges in the Whitehall II Study. *Psychosomatic Medicine.* 2006; **68**: 398-401.
110. Aboa-Eboule C, Brisson C, Maunsell E et al. Job strain and risk of acute recurrent coronary heart disease events. *Journal of the American Medical Association.* 2007; **298**: 1652-60.
111. Orth-Gomer K. Job strain and risk of recurrent coronary events. *Journal of the American Medical Association.* 2007; **298**: 1693-4.

112. Nicholson A, Kuper H, Hemingway H. Depression as an aetiologic and prognostic factor in coronary heart disease: A meta-analysis of 6362 events among 146 538 participants in 54 observational studies. *European Heart Journal*. 2006; **27**: 2763–74.
113. Frasure-Smith N, Lesperance F. Depression and anxiety as predictors of 2-year cardiac events in patients with stable coronary artery disease. *Archives of General Psychiatry*. 2008; **65**: 62–71.
114. Iles RA, Davidson M, Taylor NF. Psychosocial predictors of failure to return to work in non-chronic non-specific low back pain: A systematic review. *Occupational and Environmental Medicine*. 2008; **65**: 507–17.
115. Chandola T, Britton A, Brunner E et al. Work stress and coronary heart disease: What are the mechanisms? *European Heart Journal*. 2008; **29**: 640–8.
116. Cohen S, Janicki-Deverts D, Miller GE. Psychological stress and disease. *Journal of the American Medical Association*. 2007; **298**: 1685–7.
117. Steptoe A (ed.). *Depression and physical illness*. New York: Cambridge University Press, 2007.
118. Rugulies R, Norborg M, Sørensen TS et al. Effort–reward imbalance at work and risk of sleep disturbances. Cross-sectional and prospective results from the Danish Work Environment Cohort Study. *Journal of Psychosomatic Research*. 2009; **66**: 75–83.
119. Virtanen M, Ferrie JE, Gimeno D et al. Long working hours and sleep disturbances: The Whitehall II prospective cohort study. *Sleep*. 2009; **32**: 737–45.
120. Elovainio M, Ferrie JE, Gimeno D et al. Organizational justice and sleeping problems: The Whitehall II Study. *Psychosomatic Medicine*. 2009; **71**: 334–40.
121. Patel SR, Zhu X, Strofer-Isser A et al. Sleep duration and biomarkers of inflammation. *Sleep*. 2009; **32**: 200–4.
122. Glozier N, Grunstein R. Losing sleep over work? Does it matter? *Sleep*. 2009; **32**: 11–15.
123. Wessely S, Nimnuan C, Sharpe M. Functional somatic syndromes: One or many? *Lancet* 1999; **354**: 936–9.
124. Greenberg N, Wessely S. Gulf War Syndrome: An emerging threat or a piece of history? *Emerging Health Threats Journal*. 2008; **1**: e10.
125. Tarn M, Greenberg N, Wessely S. Gulf War syndrome – has it gone away? *Advances in Psychiatric Treatment*. 2008; **14**: 414–22.
126. Unwin C, Blatchley N, Coker W et al. The health of United Kingdom servicemen who served in the Persian Gulf War. *Lancet*. 1999; **353**: 169–78.
127. McDiarmid MA, Squibb K, Engelhardt SM. Health effects of depleted uranium on exposed Gulf War veterans: A 10-year follow up. *Journal of Toxicology and Environmental Health. Part A*. 2004; **67**: 277–96.
128. Bland D, Coggon D, Anderson J et al. Urinary isotopic analysis in the UK Armed Forces: No evidence of depleted uranium absorption in combat and other exposed personnel in Iraq. *Occupational and Environmental Medicine*. 2007; **64**: 834–8.
129. Goss Gilroy Inc. Health study of Canadian forces personnel involved in the 1991 conflict in the Persian Gulf, vol. I. Ottawa: Goss Gilroy Inc., 1998.
130. Hotopf M, David AS, Hull L et al. Gulf war illness – better, worse, or just the same? A cohort study. *British Medical Journal*. 2003; **327**: 1370–2.
131. Hyams KC, Wignall FS, Roswell R. War syndromes and their evaluation: From the US Civil War to the Persian Gulf War. *Annals of Internal Medicine*. 1996; **125**: 398–405.
132. Scott WJ. PTSD and Agent Orange: Implications for a sociology of veterans issues. *Armed Forces and Society*. 1992; **18**: 592–612.
133. Miller CS, Prihoda TJ. A controlled comparison of symptoms and chemical intolerances reported by Gulf War veterans, implant recipients and persons with multiple chemical sensitivity. *Toxicology and Industrial Health*. 1999; **15**: 386–97.
134. Bornschein S, Hausteiner C, Römmelt H et al. Double-blind placebo-controlled provocation study in patients with subjective multiple chemical sensitivity (MCS) and matched control subjects. *Clinical Toxicology*. 2008; **46**: 443–9.
135. Das-Munshi J, Rubin GJ, Wessely S. Multiple chemical sensitivities: A systematic review of provocation studies. *Journal of Allergy and Clinical Immunology*. 2006; **118**: 1257–64.
136. Health and Safety Executive: Occupational aspects of the management of chronic fatigue syndrome – employer's leaflet. Last accessed December 14, 2009. Available from: www.hse.gov.uk/chronicfatigue/index.htm.
137. Glozier N. Chronic Fatigue Syndrome: It's tiring not knowing much – an in depth review for occupational health professionals. *Occupational Medicine*. 2005; **35**: 10–12.
138. Jackson JL, O'Malley PG, Kroenke K. Antidepressants and cognitive-behavioral therapy for symptom syndromes. *CNS Spectrums*. 2006; **11**: 212–22.
139. Malouff JM, Thorsteinsson EB, Rooke SE et al. Efficacy of cognitive behavioral therapy for chronic fatigue syndrome: A meta-analysis. *Clinical Psychology Review*. 2008; **28**: 736–45.
140. Department of Health. Report of the Working Party on CFS/ME to the Chief Medical Officer for England and Wales. January 2002. Last accessed December 14, 2009. Available from: www.doh.gov.uk/cmo/cfsmereport/cfsmereport.pdf.
141. Sanderson K, Andrews G. Common mental disorders in the workforce: Recent findings from descriptive and social epidemiology. *Canadian Journal of Psychiatry*. 2006; **51**: 63–75.
142. Office for National Statistics. National psychiatric morbidity survey. London: ONS, 2002.
143. Wikman A, Marklund S, Alexanderson K. Illness, disease, and sickness absence: An empirical test of differences between concepts of ill health. *Journal of Epidemiology and Community Health*. 2005; **59**: 450–4.
144. Das-Munshi J, Goldberg D, Bebbington PE et al. Public health significance of mixed anxiety and depression: Beyond current classification. *British Journal of Psychiatry*. 2008; **192**: 171–7.

145. Kessler RC, Heeringa S, Lakoma MD et al. Individual and societal effects of mental disorders on earnings in the United States: Results from the National Comorbidity Survey Replication. *American Journal of Psychiatry*. 2008; **165**: 703–11.
146. Mechanic D. Cultural and organisational aspects of the ADA to persons with psychiatric disabilities. *Millbank Quarterly*. 1998; **76**: 5–23.
147. Dewa CS, Lin E. Chronic physical illness, psychiatric disorder and disability in the workplace. *Social Science and Medicine*. 2000; **51**: 41–50.
148. Janssen N, Kant IJ, Swaen GM et al. Fatigue as a predictor of sickness absence: Results from the Maastricht cohort study on fatigue at work. *Occupational and Environmental Medicine*. 2003; **60** (Suppl. 1): 71–6.
149. Swindle R, Kroenke K, Braun L. Energy and improved workplace productivity in depression. In: Farquhar I, Summers K, Sorkin A (eds). *Research in human capital and development investing in health: The social and economic benefits of health care innovation*. Stamford, CT: JAI Press, 2001; **14**: 323–41.
150. Mancoso L. Reasonable accomodation for workers with psychiatric disabilities. *Psychosocial Rehabilitation Journal*. 1990; **14**: 3–19.
151. McDermott LM, Ebmeier KP. A meta-analysis of depression severity and cognitive function. *Journal of Affective Disorders*. 2009; **119**: 1–8.
152. Scheid TL. Stigma as a barrier to employment: Mental disability and the Americans with Disabilities Act. *International Journal of Law and Psychiatry*. 2005; **28**: 670–90.
153. Lerner D, Adler DA, Chang H et al. The clinical and occupational correlates of work productivity loss among employed patients with depression. *Journal of Occupational and Environmental Medicine*. 2004; **46**: S46–55.
154. Buist-Bouwman MA, Ormel J, de Graaf R et al. Mediators of the association between depression and role functioning. *Acta Psychiatrica Scandinavica*. 2008; **118**: 451–8.
155. Ormel J, Von Korff M, Van den Brink W et al. Depression, anxiety, and social disability show synchrony of change in primary care patients. *American Journal of Public Health*. 1993; **83**: 385–90.
156. Judd L, Akiskal HS, Zeller PM et al. Psychosocial disability during the long term course of unipolar major depressive disorder. *Archives of General Psychiatry*. 2000; **57**: 375–80.
157. Broadhead WE, Blazer DG, George LK, Tse CK. Depression, disability days, and days lost from work in a prospective epidemiologic survey. *Journal of the American Medical Association*. 1990; **264**: 2524–8.
158. Øverland S, Glozier N, Mæland J et al. Employment status and perceived health in the Hordaland Health Study (HUSK). *BMC Public Health*. 2006; **6**: 219.
159. Mintz J, Mintz LI, Arruda MJ, Hwang SS. Treatments of depression and the functional capacity to work. *Archives of General Psychiatry*. 1992; **49**: 761–8.
160. Buist-Bouwman MA, Ormel J, de Graaf R, Vollebergh WA. Functioning after a major depressive episode: Complete or incomplete recovery? *Journal of Affective Disorders*. 2004; **82**: 363–71.
161. Marwaha S, Johnson S. Schizophrenia and employment. A review. *Social Psychiatry and Psychiatric Epidemiology*. 2004; **39**: 337–49.
162. Bond GR, Drake RE, Becker DR. An update on randomized controlled trials of evidence-based supported employment. *Psychiatric Rehabilitation Journal*. 2008; **31**: 280.
163. Catty J, Lissouba P, White S et al. EQOLISE Group. Predictors of employment for people with severe mental illness: Results of an international six-centre randomised controlled trial. *British Journal of Psychiatry*. 2008; **192**: 224–31.
164. Vingard E, Alexanderson K, Norlund A. Chapter 10. Sickness presence. *Scandinavian Journal of Public Health*. 2004; **32**: 216–21.
165. Hansen C, Andersen J. Going to work ill – what persoanl circumstances, attitudes and work-related factors are associated with sickness presenteeism. *Social Science and Medicine*. 2008; **67**: 956–64.
166. Wang PS, Beck AL, Berglund P et al. Effects of major depression on moment-in-time work performance. *American Journal of Psychiatry*. 2004; **161**: 1885–91.
167. Kessler RC, Greenberg PE, Mickelson KD et al. The effects of chronic medical conditions on work loss and work cutback. *Journal of Occupational and Environmental Medicine*. 2001; **43**: 218–25.
168. Kessler RC, Ormel J, Demler O, Stang PE. Comorbid mental disorders account for the role impairment of commonly occurring chronic physical disorders: Results from the National Comorbidity Survey. *Journal of Occupational and Environmental Medicine*. 2003; **45**: 1257–66.
169. Stewart WF, Ricci JA, Chee E et al. Cost of lost productive work time among US workers with depression. *Journal of the American Medical Association*. 2003; **289**: 3135–44.
170. Burton WN, Pransky G, Conti DJ et al. The association of medical conditions and presenteeism. *Journal of Occupational and Environmental Medicine*. 2004; **46**: S38–45.
171. Mohren DCL, Swaen GMH, Kant IJ et al. Fatigue and job stress as predictors for sickness absence during common infections. *International Journal of Behavioral Medicine*. 2005; **12**: 11–20.
172. Hensing GR. Methodological aspects in sickness-absence research. *Scandinavian Journal of Public Health*. 2004; **32**: 44–8.
173. Spurgeon P, Mazelan P, Barwell F, Flanagan H. *New directions in managing employee absence: An evidence based approach*. London: Chartered Institute of Personnel and Development, 2007.
174. Brenninkmeijer V, Houtman I, Blonk R. Depressed and absent from work: Predicting prolonged depressive symptomatology among employees. *Occupational Medicine*. 2008; **58**: 295–301.
175. Severeijns R, Vlaeyen JW, van den Hout MA, Picavet HS. Pain catastrophizing is associated with health indices in

musculoskeletal pain: A cross-sectional study in the Dutch community. *Health Psychology*. 2004; **23**: 49–57.
176. Jones J, Huxtable C, Hodgson J. Self-reported work-related illness in 2004/2005: Results from the Labour Force Survey. London: Health and Safety Executive, 2005.
177. Nieuwenhuijsen K, Verbeek JHAM, de Boer AGEM et al. Supervisory behaviour as a predictor of return to work in employees absent from work due to mental health problems. *Occupational and Environmental Medicine*. 2004; **61**: 817–23.
178. Glozier N, Hough C, Henderson M, Holland-Elliott K. Attitudes of nursing staff towards co-workers returning from psychiatric and physical illnesses. *International Journal of Social Psychiatry*. 2006; **52**: 525–34.
179. Alexandre PK, Patrick R, Beauliere A, Martins SS. Race differentials in employment effects of psychological distress: A study of non-Hispanic Whites and African-Americans in the United States. *The Social Science Journal*. 2009; **46**: 201–10.
180. Salminen JK, Saarijarvi S, Raitasalo R. Depression and disability pension in Finland. *Acta Psychiatrica Scandinavica*. 1997; **95**: 242–3.
181. Mykletun A, Overland S, Dahl AA et al. A population-based cohort study of the effect of common mental disorders on disability pension awards. *American Journal of Psychiatry*. 2006; **163**: 1412–18.
182. Sivertsen B, Overland S, Neckelmann D et al. The long-term effect of insomnia on work disability. The HUNT-2 historical cohort study. *American Journal of Epidemiology*. 2006; **163**: 1018–24.
183. Ejlertsson G, Eden L, Leden I. Predictors of positive health in disability pensioners: A population-based questionnaire study using positive odds ratio. *BMC Public Health*. 2002; **2**: 20.
184. Øverland S, Glozier N, Henderson M et al. Health status before, during and after disability pension award. The Hordaland Health Study (HUSK). *Occupational and Environmental Medicine*. 2008; **65**: 769–73.
185. Øverland S, Glozier N, Krokstad S, Mykletun A. Undertreatment before the award of a disability pension for mental illness: The HUNT study. *Psychiatric Services*. 2007; **58**: 1479–82.
186. Pattani S, Constantinovici N, Williams S. Predictors of re-employment and quality of life in NHS staff one year after early retirement because of ill health. A national prospective study. *Occupational and Environmental Medicine*. 2004; **61**: 572–6.
187. Maslach C, Schaufeli WB, Leiter MP. Job burnout. *Annual Review of Psychology*. 2001; **52**: 397–422.
188. Wieclaw JW. Can burnout measure be useful in screening for disability pensions? *Occupational and Environmental Medicine*. 2009; **66**: 282–3.
189. Dyrbye LN, Thomas MR, Huntington JL et al. Personal life events and medical student burnout: A multicenter study. *Academic Medicine*. 2006; **81**: 374–84.
190. Ahola K, Gould R, Virtanen M et al. Occupational burnout as a predictor of disability pension: A population-based cohort study. *Occupational and Environmental Medicine*. 2009; **66**: 284–90.
191. Culpin M, Smith M. *The nervous temperament – A report for the Industrial Health Research Board*. London: His Majesty's Stationery Office, 1930.
192. Demyttenaere K, Bonnewyn A, Bruffaerts R et al. Comorbid painful physical symptoms and depression: Prevalence, work loss, and help seeking. *Journal of Affective Disorders*. 2006; **92**: 185–93.
193. Demyttenaere K, Bonnewyn A, Bruffaerts R et al. Comorbid painful physical symptoms and anxiety: Prevalence, work loss and help-seeking. *Journal of Affective Disorders*. 2008; **109**: 264–72.
194. Glozier N, Hackett M, Parag V, Anderson S for the Auckland Regional Community Stroke (ARCOS) Study Group. The influence of psychiatric morbidity on return to paid work after stroke in younger adults. *Stroke*. 2008; **39**: 1526–32.
195. Bhattacharyya MR, Perkins-Porras L, Whitehead DL, Steptoe A. Psychological and clinical predictors of return to work after acute coronary syndrome. *European Heart Journal*. 2006; **28**: 160–5.
196. Maeland JG, Havik OE. Psychological predictors for return to work after a myocardial infarction. *Journal of Psychosomatic Research*. 1987; **31**: 471–81.
197. Marmot MG. *Status syndrome*. London: Times Books, 2004.
198. Faragher EB, Cass M, Cooper CL. The relationship between job satisfaction and health: A meta-analysis. *Occupational and Environmental Medicine*. 2005; **62**: 105–12.
199. Judge T, Heller D, Mount M. The Five Factor Model of personality and job satisfaction: A meta-analysis. *Journal of Applied Psychology*. 2002; **87**: 530–41.
200. Henderson M, Hotopf M, Leon D. Childhood temperament and long term sickness absence – data from the Aberdeen Children of the1950s cohort study. *British Journal of Psychiatry*. 2009; **194**: 220–3.
201. Wang J. Perceived work stress, imbalance between work and family/personal life and mental disorders. *Social Psychiatry and Psychiatric Epidemiology*. 2006; **41**: 541–8.
202. Väänänen A, Kumpulainen R, Kevin MV et al. Work-family characteristics as determinants of sickness absence: A large-scale cohort study of three occupational grades. *Journal of Occupational Health Psychology*. 2008; **13**: 181–96.
203. Kristinsen T. Sickness absence and work strain amongst Danish slaughterhouse workers: An analysis of absence from work regarded as coping behaviour. *Social Science and Medicine*. 1991; **32**: 15–27.
204. Petrie KJ, Cameron LD, Ellis CJ et al. Changing illness perceptions after myocardial infarction: An early intervention randomized controlled trial. *Psychosomatic Medicine*. 2002; **64**: 580–6.
205. Alexanderson K, Norlund A. Swedish Council on Technology Assessment in Health Care (SBU). Chapter 12. Future need for research. *Scandinavian Journal of Public Health*. 2004; **63** (Suppl.): 256–8.
206. Totterdell P, Smith L. Ten-hour days and eight-hour nights: Can the Ottawa Shift System reduce the problems of shiftwork? *Work and Stress*. 1992; **6**: 139–52.

207. Graveling RA, Crawford JO, Cowie H et al. *A review of workplace interventions that promote mental wellbeing in the workplace*. Edinburgh: Institute of Occupational Medicine, 2008.
208. Egan M, Bambra C, Thomas S et al. The psychosocial and health effects of workplace reorganisation. 1. A systematic review of organisational-level interventions that aim to increase employee control. *Journal of Epidemiology and Community Health*. 2007; **61**: 945–54.
209. Bambra C, Egan M, Thomas S et al. The psychosocial and health effects of workplace reorganisation. 2. A systematic review of task restructuring interventions. *Journal of Epidemiology and Community Health*. 2007; **61**: 1028–37.
210. Murta SG, Sanderson K, Oldenburg B. Process evaluation in occupational stress management programs: A systematic review. *American Journal of Health Promotion*. 2007; **21**: 248–54.
211. Kawakami N, Takao S, Kobayashi Y, Tsutsumi A. Effects of web-based supervisor training on job stressors and psychological distress among workers: A workplace-based randomized controlled trial. *Journal of Occupational Health*. 2006; **48**: 28–34.
212. Takao S, Tsutsumi A, Nishiuchi K et al. Effects of the job stress education for supervisors on psychological distress and job performance among their immediate subordinates: A supervisor-based randomized controlled trial. *Journal of Occupational Health*. 2006; **48**: 494–503.
213. British Occupational Health Research Foundation. *Workplace interventions for people with common mental health problems: Evidence review and recommendations*. BOHRF: London, 2005.
214. Michie S, Williams S. Reducing work related psychological ill health and sickness absence: A systematic literature review. *Occupational and Environmental Medicine*. 2003; **60**: 3–9.
215. van der Klink JJ, Blonk RW, Schene AH, van Dijk FJ. The benefits of interventions for work-related stress. *American Journal of Public Health*. 2001; **91**: 270–6.
216. Bond FW, Bunce D. Mediators of change in emotion-focused and problem-focused worksite stress management interventions. *Journal of Occupational Health Psychology*. 2000; **5**: 156–63.
217. Marine A, Ruotsalainen JH, Serra C, Verbeek JH. Preventing occupational stress in healthcare workers. *Cochrane Database of Systematic Reviews*. 2006; (**4**): CD002892.
218. Wiles NJ, Haase AM, Gallacher J et al. Physical activity and common mental disorder: results from the Caerphilly study. *American Journal of Epidemiology*. 2007; **165**: 946–54.
219. Bernaards CM, Jans MP, van den Heuvel SG et al. Can strenuous leisure time physical activity prevent psychological complaints in a working population? *Occupational and Environmental Medicine*. 2006; **63**: 10–16.
220. Wang PS, Simon GE, Avorn J et al. Telephone screening, outreach, and care management for depressed workers and impact on clinical and work productivity outcomes: A randomized controlled trial. *Journal of the American Medical Association*. 2007; **298**: 1401–11.
221. Wang PS, Patrick A, Avorn J et al. The costs and benefits of enhanced depression care to employers. *Archives of General Psychiatry*. 2006; **63**: 1345–53.
222. National Institute for Health and Clinical Excellence. *Anxiety: Management of anxiety (panic disorder, with or without agoraphobia, and generalised anxiety disorder) in adults in primary, secondary and community care)*. London: NICE, 2004.
223. National Institute for Health and Clinical Excellence. *Depression: Management of depression in primary and secondary care*. London: NICE, 2004.
224. Nieuwenhuijsen K, Bultmann U, Neumeyer-Gromen A et al. Interventions to improve occupational health in depressed people. *Cochrane Database of Systematic Reviews*. 2008; (**2**): CD006237.
225. Timbie JW, Horvitz-Lennon M, Frank RG, Normand SL. A meta-analysis of labor supply effects of interventions for major depressive disorder. *Psychiatric Services*. 2006; **57**: 212–18.
226. van der Klink JJ, Blonk RW, Schene AH, van Dijk FJ. Reducing long term sickness absence by an activating intervention in adjustment disorders: A cluster randomised controlled design. *Occupational and Environmental Medicine*. 2003; **60**: 429–37.
227. Royal Courts of Justice. *Supreme Court of Judicature Court of Appeal (Civil Division) on appeal from Liverpool County Court*. London: Royal Courts of Justice, 2002.
228. McLeod J. *Counselling in the workplace: The facts. A systematic study of the research evidence*. Lutterworth: British Association for Counselling and Psychotherapy, 2001.
229. Henderson M, Hotopf M, Wessely S. Workplace counselling. An appeal for evidence. *Occupational and Environmental Medicine*. 2003; **60**: 899–900.
230. Kelly CM, Jorm AF, Wright A. Improving mental health literacy as a strategy to facilitate early intervention for mental disorders. *Medical Journal of Australia*. 2007; **187**: S26–S30.
231. Martin A, Sanderson K, Scott J, Brough P. Promoting mental health in small-medium enterprises: An evaluation of the 'Business in Mind' program. *BMC Public Health*. 2009; **9**: 239.
232. Buchbinder R, Jolley D, Wyatt M. Population based intervention to change back pain beliefs and disability: Three part evaluation. *British Medical Journal*. 2001; **322**: 1516–20.
233. Buchbinder R, Staples M, Jolley D. Doctors with a special interest in back pain have poorer knowledge about how to treat back pain. *Spine*. 2009; **34**: 1218–26.
234. Coggon D. Occupational medicine at a turning point. *Occupational and Environmental Medicine*. 2005; **62**: 281–3.

SECTION THREE

Substance abuse

67 Substance abuse and the workplace
Jonathan D Chick

859

67

Substance abuse and the workplace

JONATHAN D CHICK

Introduction	859	Ingredients of successful treatment	866
Definitions	859	Substance misuse and the medical profession	867
Workplace problems related to alcohol	860	Prevention	868
Work factors contributing to alcohol-related problems	861	References	868
Identification of the problem drinker/drug addict	861	Further reading	870
Management of substance abuse in the workplace	865		

INTRODUCTION

This chapter explores for clinicians the relation between substance abuse and health and performance at work. It also considers clinical management of substance abuse, company policies that may be available to help abusers and implications for the occupational physician. Numerous substances are abused, including cannabis, cocaine, opiates and benzodiazepines, but the most common in the working population is alcohol, which is the main focus of this chapter.

DEFINITIONS

Employees with a substance misuse problem can be defined as those whose regular or intermittent use of a substance or mix of substances repeatedly interferes with their work, or the work of others, their job performance or their ability to work, their relationships with colleagues or clients, or their health.

As in the general population, alcohol-related problems in the workplace can be considered as: heavy drinking, acute problems, chronic effects and dependence on alcohol. These overlap in different people in different ways (Figure 67.1). Dependence is a state in which an individual experiences difficulty controlling the intake of the substance, and experiences withdrawal symptoms on reduction or cessation of intake. An affected person may move in and out of periods of dependence. The syndrome tends to be reinstated if, after a period of abstinence, the individual begins to use the drug again.

The terms 'drug addict', 'alcoholic' and 'alcoholism' are still widely used, and usually connote chronic excessive use of the substance, either regular or periodic; an admitted or an inferred difficulty in controlling when and how much is consumed; and usually the experience of social or medical problems (Figure 67.2).

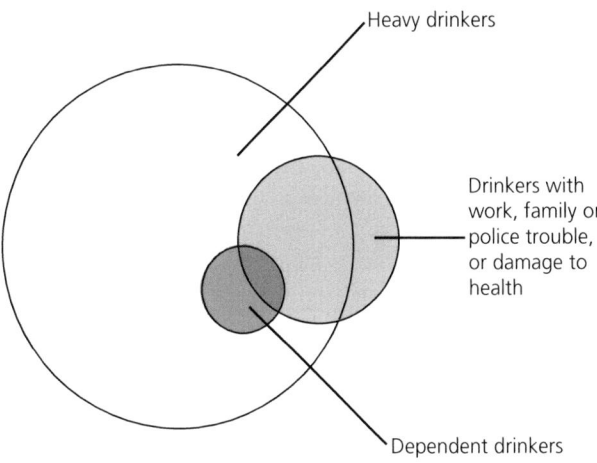

Figure 67.1 The interrelation of heavy drinking, alcohol-related problems and dependence on alcohol.

- Loss of control
- Compulsion or desire and craving
- Tolerance, requiring increasing doses
- Withdrawal state and use to avoid this state
- Neglect alternative pleasures or interests
- Persistence despite harm to relationships, work, crime, health and finance

Figure 67.2 Features of the substance dependence syndrome.

WORKPLACE PROBLEMS RELATED TO ALCOHOL

Work competence and safety

The acute effects of alcohol are chiefly those of a central nervous system depressant, leading to impairment of reasoning, perception, reaction time, balance and co-ordination. In some drinkers, in the appropriate social setting, a transient disinhibition gives the feeling of enhanced interpersonal communication and well-being. This is partly due to culturally defined expectations. However, in this state, decision-making, operating machinery, driving and other skilled activities are compromised.

Even before the burgeoning of UK alcohol consumption in the late 1900s, surveys found that 24 per cent of company executives in a variety of organizations and 14 per cent of manual workers in alcohol production industries admitted to occasional impaired work efficiency due to drinking in the preceding six months.[1] The dose-related effects of alcohol on motor/perceptual skills and judgement have been shown in American drivers.[2] A blood alcohol level of 60 mg/dL (produced by approximately two consecutive pints of 3.5 per cent alcohol by volume beer, i.e. 4 UK units, where 1 unit contains 8 g ethanol) doubled the risk of involvement in an accident compared with drivers with no alcohol in the blood; levels of 100 mg/dL (consumption of 7 units) and of 150 mg/dL (consumption of 10 units) were associated with increased risk of six and 25 times, respectively. Laboratory experiments show that risk-taking increases and perceptual decision-making skills begin to decline at blood alcohol levels as low as 25–50 mg/dL. After a major train accident in California, a survey of drinking among railroad workers revealed that more than 33 per cent of employees reported seeing a co-worker drinking on duty in the preceding year and 20 per cent reported seeing a colleague too drunk to work.[3]

Workers seeking medical attention after an accident often refuse a blood alcohol test. Thus, estimates of the role of alcohol in industrial accidents are very approximate. In an autopsy study of cases where the death certificate recorded 'injury at work', 9.2 per cent were found to have a blood alcohol level of over 100 mg/dL; workers in the transport industry were the most commonly affected. Diazepam was detected in 15.6 per cent of cases, although the extent of its use in the local population of working age was not available for comparison.[4] An autopsy study of fatal occupational injuries in Maryland found that 11 per cent of cases had a blood alcohol concentration of at least 80 mg/dL.[5] Since alcohol continues to be metabolized after death, these rates might underestimate the true prevalence.

Laboratory studies of 'hangover' have examined cognitive function the next day after a 'normal' evening's drinking by university students, when the blood alcohol level has returned to zero. They find that performance is impaired on tests of vigilance and reaction time, and possibly memory.[6,7]

Although heavy drinkers are most at risk of accidents at work, it is moderate drinkers who, because they are more numerous, account for most of the cases; hence 'the preventive paradox'.[1] Harm at work will be reduced if all employees reduce their alcohol consumption, not only the heaviest drinkers. When a port authority reduced availability of alcohol at lunchtime, it removed a peak of accidents in dock employees in the afternoon and reduced the overall rate of accidents.

Chronic use of alcohol and performance

Light drinking of up to 4 units/day in middle age and above is associated with better cognitive functioning than abstinence, even after adjusting for basic educational attainment, social and health confounders.[8–10] It is suspected that there are inefficiencies of cognition in those drinking between 8 and 16 units/day, while above 16 units/day impairments of the degree seen in alcohol treatment clinics will sometimes occur, the early signs being impaired problem-solving, rigidity of thought, impaired recent memory and difficulty with spatial tasks.[11]

Epilepsy

'Rum fits' were well known in the British Navy, usually occurring two to three days after the ship left port. An analogous situation occurs now in oil rig workers. Oil rigs are alcohol-free zones to which workers return after two weeks on shore. In drinkers who develop chemical dependence, an epileptic seizure can occur when alcohol consumption is reduced or ceases. Although this may be an immediate indication for a change of job if machinery is involved, clinical experience shows that affected individuals do not have recurrence of fits if they maintain long-term abstinence from alcohol (or if, after some months of abstinence, they eventually resume drinking but keep consumption below, say, 10 units per week).

This may be the first presentation of alcohol dependence. Investigations might be necessary to exclude other causes of late onset of fits. The electroencephalogram in alcohol dependence does not show epileptic foci.

Absenteeism

General practitioners are sometimes asked by drug or alcohol users for medical certificates to cover absence from work actually spent seeking drugs or drinking, or recovering from the effects thereof. Clinicians should be aware of the typical pattern. Where weekend drinking is the culture, Monday morning is the most common day for alcohol-related absenteeism, usually because of hangover or gastrointestinal upset. If pay day is on Thursday rather than Friday for the weekly paid staff, some drinkers will not appear for work on Friday. Such absenteeism is common even among those whose alcohol-related problems are not severe.

The study of Scottish company executives/alcohol production workers, mentioned above,[1] found that 4 per cent of the executives and 23 per cent of the workers admitted to being off work because of alcohol in the two-year period before the survey interview. A higher than average medical consultation rate was noted in the ten years that preceded a diagnosis of alcoholism in a sample of US Navy personnel.[12] Drinkers whose problems are sufficient to lead to attendance at an alcohol problem clinic have twice the sickness absenteeism rate of the general population.[13,14] Sickness absence certificates covering alcohol-related absenteeism span a wide range of diagnoses, including gastritis, anxiety state, nervous disability and injuries.[13] In the New South Wales police force, heavy drinkers were found to have more sickness absenteeism.[14]

Mortality

The famous J-shaped curve of alcohol consumption versus mortality is only seen above age 35.[15] This is presumably because deaths from accidents begin to occur in young people whose average consumption is low, and when they drink heavily they lack tolerance, as well as being inexperienced drivers. The contribution of alcohol has been discussed above. Among new conscripts to the Swedish army (aged 18), those who admitted to drinking over 250 g of alcohol per week (30 units) had a mortality rate over the subsequent 15 years five times greater than the remainder.[16]

The risks of several cancers are increased in drinkers: cancer of the mouth, pharynx, larynx and oesophagus, colorectum and breast cancer in women.[17] Rates of death among heavy drinkers are increased for haemorrhagic stroke, liver disease, suicide and violence. This increased mortality commences with consumption as low as 4 units per day. However, after middle age, abstainers have a higher mortality than light drinkers. Thus, the mortality risk curve for alcohol consumption is J-shaped. Care has to be taken in interpreting these data because the group of 'abstainers' may include ex-drinkers (and often ex-smokers) who have commenced abstaining because of diagnosed illnesses such as heart disease, rather than being life-long abstainers. Moderate drinkers (1–3 units/day) may be people with better social adjustment and a healthier lifestyle than either abstainers or heavy drinkers, but even taking this into account the evidence is increasingly persuasive that moderate ethanol consumption in those over four years of age protects against coronary artery disease and possibly ischaemic stroke.[18]

WORK FACTORS CONTRIBUTING TO ALCOHOL-RELATED PROBLEMS

Mortality rates from hepatic cirrhosis vary with occupational group and are highest in the alcohol manufacturing and retailing industries. Brewery workers were found to have a higher average intake of alcohol at recruitment than biscuit factory workers, but the brewery workers also increased their consumption to a greater extent during the next two years.[19] Thus, both selective recruitment and exposure contribute to the alcohol-related risks in the brewing industry. Both may also be important in seamen (officers and crew) and fishermen, who have mortality rates for hepatic cirrhosis three or four times the average. Absence from home and family, and lack of a normal social and sexual life, are clear risk factors; they may also contribute to the higher rates of cirrhosis in the armed services and the construction industry. In the latter occupation in England, recruitment of labourers from Ireland and Scotland is also relevant, because among them there is a higher proportion of heavy drinkers than among indigenous labourers.

Professions with higher risks include insurance, finance, law and journalism. In the most recent decennial report, UK doctors were for the first time in 40 years no longer showing an increased mortality from alcohol-related causes.[20] Freedom from supervision at work, high incomes and the emotionally demanding nature of their work have been proposed as reasons why these professions have increased rates of alcoholism. The culture at work presumably explains some of the journalists' problems, just as the business lunch routine and the after-business wine bar have contributed to alcoholism among executives.

Other contributing factors

Clinicians assessing individual patients with alcohol and drug problems must consider the following factors outside the occupational sphere: other psychiatric disorder to which substance misuse is secondary, such as anxiety, phobic or panic disorder, and depressive illness; family history of alcohol or drug misuse (alcohol problems are highly heritable); living alone; or death of a spouse. Divorce or legal separation from a spouse can, of course, be a cause or consequence of substance misuse.

IDENTIFICATION OF THE PROBLEM DRINKER/DRUG ADDICT

The workplace is often where an alcohol or drug problem is first identified. Accidents, illnesses or a drink/drive conviction may make the diagnosis clear. Unreliable timekeeping, coming to work smelling of alcohol and (or) arguments with colleagues are earlier signs, but are often missed. 'Denial' of the contribution of alcohol or drugs to such difficulties is common and such overt signs as shaky hands in the morning might wrongly be attributed to 'stress of the morning business meeting'. The individual may evade any discussion that could implicate alcohol as the cause of his difficulties. The drinker or drug user is likely to perceive any discussion of his habit as one of

Questions	Scoring system					Your score
	0	1	2	3	4	
How often do you have 8 (men)/ 6 (women) or more drinks on on occasion?	Never	Less than monthly	Monthly	Weekly	Daily or almost daily	
Only answer the following questions if your answer above is monthly or less						
How often in the last year have you not been able to remember what happened when drinking the night before?	Never	Less than monthly	Monthly	Weekly	Daily or almost daily	
How often in the last year have you falled to do what was expected of you because of drinking?	Never	Less than monthly	Monthly	Weekly	Daily or almost daily	
Has a relative/friend/doctor/health worker been concerned about your drinking or advised you to cut down?	No		Yes, but not in the last year		Yes, during the last year	

Figure 67.3 The FAST Alcohol Use Disorders Screening Test. Score of 3 or more suggests a hazardous or harmful drinker.[21]

moral disapproval: any comment about his behaviour is seen as an insult. He/she may be practised at evasion and colleagues at work may be misled or afraid of upsetting the cantankerous employee, and minimize the problem or cover up. Yet it is the manager at work who is well placed to intervene when an alcohol- or drug-related problem occurs.

Because alcohol has a legitimate and accepted role in Western society, the manager who confronts an employee about smelling of alcohol at work may be made to feel a 'killjoy' or 'wet blanket'. Managers may become more motivated to involve the personnel staff or occupational physician as soon as work performance is affected if they can be persuaded that early intervention for substance misuse can prevent later, more difficult and perhaps costly problems which might arise when the employee is involved in an incident – or long-suffering workmates finally lose their tolerance.

The manager must, however, take a delicate and confidential approach. The manager's role is not the diagnosis of alcohol or drug problems, but the assessment of work performance. He or she should firmly encourage the individual to consult the occupational physician or general practitioner, who should then deal with the patient with the usual care about confidentiality.

Any clinician assessing a patient with a drink or drug problem should ask about comments or complaints from colleagues and managers at work as well as from those at home, and if disciplinary action has commenced, know what stage has been reached.

When a health screening opportunity arises, a useful questionnaire for alcohol screening is FAST (Figure 67.3).[21] The test identifies problems with alcohol at an early stage, as well as later cases of alcohol dependence.

Assessment

Within the confidential interview (Figure 67.4), the clinician discusses with the employee information from management about performance and attendance. A full history, including a non-judgemental, objective enquiry into drinking patterns and drug use, should eventually be elicited:

- What is your current main concern?
- Help me understand how this came about.
- What are the various factors in your view?
- Where does your use of alcohol fit in? Have you used alcohol to help with stress/insomnia?
- What would your partner say if he/she were here?

The clinician might specifically enquire into the past seven days, work and leisure time, to determine what and where drinking (or drug use) took place. Ask about injuries at home, at work, on the road or at leisure, and enquire about any relation to alcohol. Specifically, ask about police involvement or convictions. Ideally also, information from the family is obtained, because in this situation it is common for individuals to minimize their alcohol or drug intake and the problems caused.

Clinical features

Intoxication with alcohol or sedatives may manifest as slurred speech or disinhibited behaviour. Inappropriate giggling or elation might indicate cannabis intoxication (Figure 67.5). At physical examination, the heavy drinker may show excessive capillarization of the conjunctivae and skin of the cheeks and nose. Close examination of the tongue may reveal the smell of alcohol on the breath. In the dependent drinker, tremor of the tongue and mouth can be seen before it is visible in the outstretched fingers. Intoxication with sedatives may cause nystagmus. Opiates cause constriction of the pupils; there may be venepuncture marks. The drinker may have an enlarged liver, signs of parenchymal liver disease, cerebellar ataxia particularly affecting the gait, weakness of the proximal shoulder and pelvic girdle muscles, or evidence of peripheral neuropathy.

Identification of the problem drinker/drug addict 863

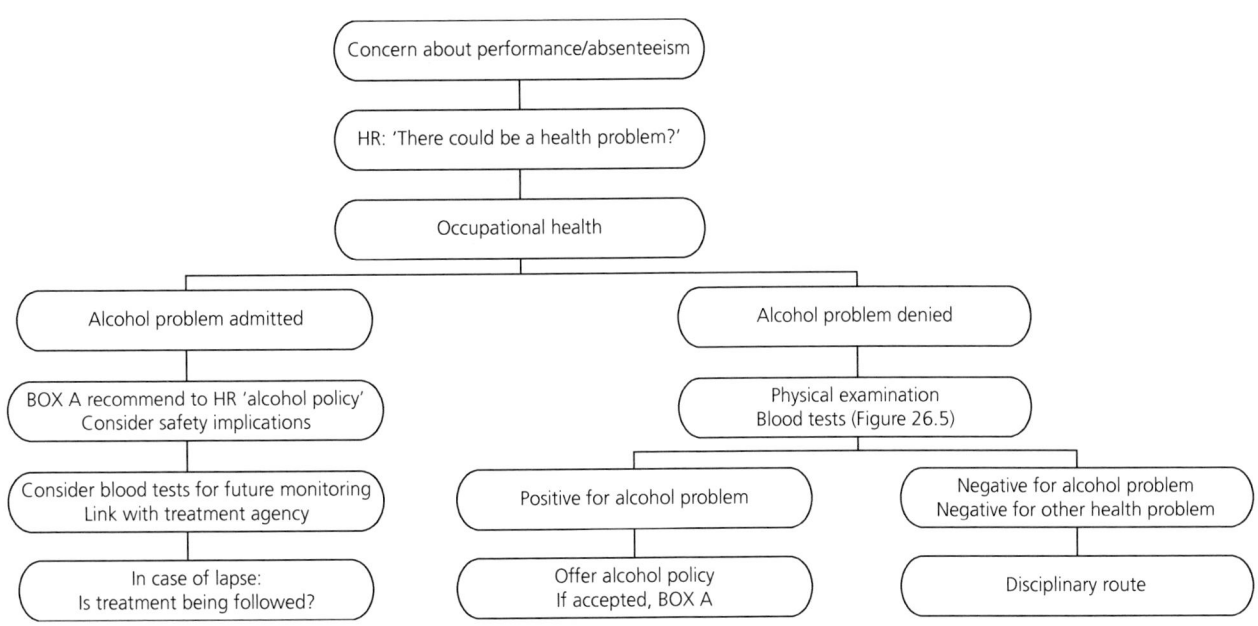

Figure 67.4 Managing the employee with a suspected alcohol problem. HR, Human resources/personnel manager.

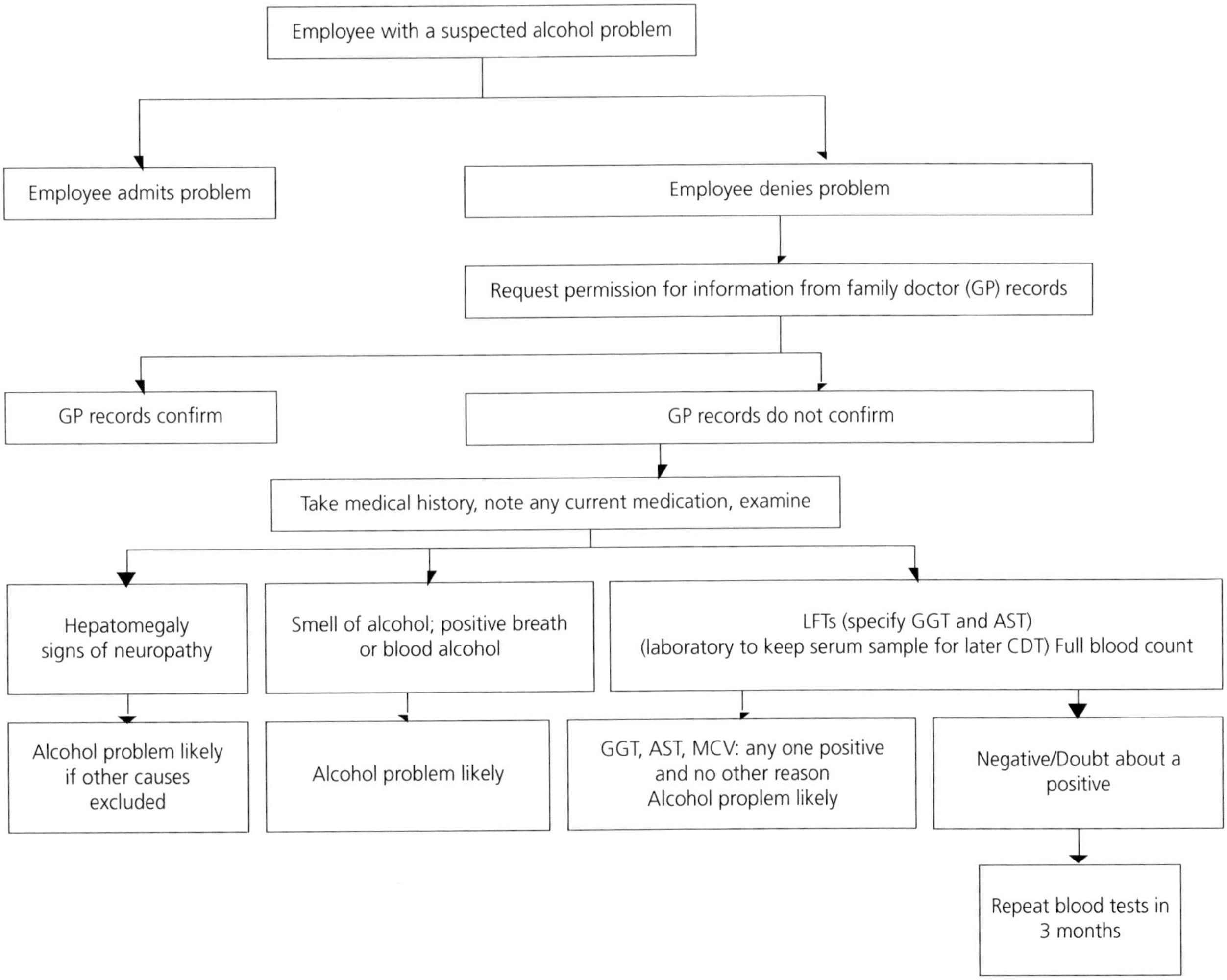

Figure 67.5 Investigation of an employee with a suspected alcohol problem.

Objective markers

DRUGS

Workplace urine screening

The UK Transport and Works Act 1992 has led to most operators of passenger transport systems in the United Kingdom introducing urine drug screening for operational staff. Police are empowered to test for alcohol and drugs in railway staff associated with a train accident. Similar legislation was passed in the United States in the 1980s and later federal employees became subject to screening.

That safety is thereby improved has, however, proved difficult to demonstrate. For example, to assess the potential preventive impact of recruitment drug screening, the US Postal Service in Boston monitored industrial accidents, occupational injuries, disciplinary actions and turnover in 2537 new employees. Positive testing for cocaine in the urine at recruitment predicted a raised incident rate in the first and the second year of employment, but testing positive for cannabis was no longer predictive of incidents after the first year.[22] Perhaps cannabis users gradually change their lifestyle as they develop job responsibility. Interpretation of a positive result requires experience and sometimes further analysis.

Reliability of testing

Cannabis metabolites can be detected in urine several weeks after the last dose, but only in very heavy regular users. Traces can be found for three or four hours after passive smoking. Eating biscuits containing poppy seeds can cause a trace of morphine to be found in urine. The concordance between urine analysis and self-reports of drug use in workplace samples tends to be low, suggesting that these detection methods should be regarded as complementary and not alternatives.

Hair grows about 1 cm per month. Drugs and their metabolites are absorbed into hair and can be extracted and measured, for example, by radioimmunoassay.[23] There is doubt about how accurately, if at all, hair analysis can distinguish between frequent and occasional use, and about whether the timing of use can be specified since drug metabolites might 'move along' the hair shaft. Evasion or manipulation of the results is easy with urine tests, but not possible with saliva or hair analysis. Both are available through several commercial laboratories.

Legal and ethical pitfalls

An employee's job could be threatened if a test is positive. Occupational physicians and physicians functioning as 'medical review officers' should be familiar with the recommendations given by the Faculty of Occupational Medicine (UK) in its Guidelines for Testing for Drugs of Abuse in the Workplace[24] or those of an experienced forensic toxicologist[25] which are:

1. If, at a recruitment examination or an examination at the request of the employer, blood or urine is to be tested for alcohol or drugs, informed consent must be obtained to collect and analyse the specimen, and to report the results to the employer.
2. Employees should list all medications currently taken.
3. The specimen is collected under supervision, to avoid adulteration or substitution, placed in a tamper-evident container and the steps to testing and recording of the result are audited (the 'chain of custody' must be observed).
4. It is good practice to divide the sample into two parts, for analysis at the employee's laboratory of choice if desired (the specimen cannot be deemed owned by the employer).
5. The employee will have the right to see the result.
6. The medical reviewer or occupational physician, in the view of Forrest,[25] 'cannot be exempt from the requirement to act in good faith in the best interests of the patients, even though paid by the employer ...'.

Establishing a drug-testing programme

Before a drug-testing programme of any kind is announced in a company, the employer should be clear about its objectives. These may be public safety, employee safety, financial or information security, or improved performance and quality. The Faculty of Occupational Medicine[24] recommends that companies take legal advice before embarking on a programme. Testing may be in various circumstances, which also need specifying in advance, for example, pre-employment, in-house promotion or transfer, 'for cause' (i.e. if there has been unsatisfactory behaviour or performance, post-incident, 'periodic', during or after rehabilitation, or as part of a clinical assessment by the company physician).

Monitoring drug abuse treatment

Drug testing should not be an end in itself. It has a use in clinical decision-making, for feedback to patients on progress, and for programme evaluation. However, for patients who are 'doing well' (e.g. complying with therapy, employed) a strong or punitive response by the clinician who had detected merely a brief 'slip' could be harmful overall.

Alcohol

The mean erythrocyte cell volume (MCV) is greater than 98 fL in 30 per cent of men drinking over 50 units per week; serum gamma-glutamyl transferase (GGT) is raised above 45 IU/L in 70 per cent, and in these drinkers rises and falls with changes in consumption.[26] If serum aspartate aminotransferase (AST) is also raised, the clinician can attach greater confidence to the diagnosis of alcohol abuse. Clearly there are other medical conditions, and medication effects which can cause false positives, obesity is associated with slight elevations of GGT. Two abnormal findings are a stronger indication of heavy drinking than any single abnormality.

Serum carbohydrate-deficient transferrin (CDT) is a marker used by some specialists. A standard 5 mL venous blood sample is required. Only selected clinical chemistry laboratories run the test routinely. The percentage of transferrin which is deficient in its carbohydrate moiety is calculated. This is raised in some 60 per cent of those recently drinking above 60 g per day. It may be elevated in primary biliary cirrhosis, but is only rarely raised in other non-alcoholic liver disease and is not affected by common medications.[22] Although sensitivity for detecting excessive drinking is only slightly greater for CDT than for GGT, specificity is greater (i.e. fewer false positives). It is useful when the cause of a raised GGT is being explored.

An indirect method of screening for people in whom it might be clinically relevant to ask about drinking, is to ask about fractures or dislocations, head injuries, assaults or road traffic accidents since the age of 18. When sports injuries are excluded, it is found that people who answer 'yes' to two or more of the above, and then answer positively to the question 'Have you been injured after drinking alcoholic beverages', are likely to have an alcohol problem.[27]

MANAGEMENT OF SUBSTANCE ABUSE IN THE WORKPLACE

Intervention should occur early, before harm accumulates and dismissal or medical retirement needs to be contemplated. Substance misuse policies and treatment referral procedures have evolved in most organizations. This is partly humanitarian, partly for legal reasons and partly because employers realize it may be cheaper for the company to encourage the employee to have treatment than to put up with his behaviour or to dismiss him.

Workplace policies

The main statements in such policies are:

1. An alcohol or drug problem can be regarded as a health matter, with the corollary that the employee is expected to pursue and comply with treatment.
2. If disciplinary action was indicated, it can be postponed if the employee seeks treatment.
3. If sick leave is required for treatment, the firm will grant it.
4. Information about compliance and success of treatment may be communicated from treatment agency to employer. Evidence of relapse visible at work should be passed to the treatment agency if the employee is still being dealt with under the policy. Supervision, independent of the treating agency, with objective testing, is recommended. (This is important for the success of such policies, but not always enshrined in the policy.)
5. If there is poor cooperation with treatment, or if treatment fails, the employer may return to the disciplinary route if this were justified (i.e. the ultimate sanctions of disciplinary action or termination of employment on health grounds remain when all efforts at help have failed).

Some large companies in North America employ staff to run the alcohol and drug policy, and to make assessments of drug and alcohol problems. Elsewhere, the responsibility for the policy is with the human resources department, the health and safety team or the occupational health team, and assessments are made by outside agencies including, in the United Kingdom, by the National Health Service. Guidance in the United Kingdom has been provided by the Health and Safety Executive.[28] It is important that clinicians clarify at the first interview whether such workplace policies exist, and especially whether point 4 (above) applies.

Coercion? – ethics

If there are clear grounds to dismiss an employee, but management postpones this to allow assessment and treatment of an alcohol- or drug-related problem, this may be regarded as 'constructive coercion'. It is not regarded as ethical for the employer to nudge an employee into medical assessment or treatment with the threat of dismissal if there are as yet no clear grounds for dismissal.

Coercion? – efficacy

'Motivation to change' is one predictor of outcome of treatment for substance abuse. An ultimatum from the spouse or the threat of a serious physical illness will often influence motivation, as will an unequivocal statement from an employer.[29] It is important that such statements are clear – that the obligations and intentions of the firm are delineated and that what is expected of the employee is spelt out. It is possible to do this in a way that is not felt by the employee as punitive.

Several North American studies have shown that the outcome of patients mandated into treatment from the courts or the workplace is no worse than the outcome of 'voluntary' patients. In the United States, physicians on probation because of drug or alcohol abuse have, in general, a better outcome than most populations of substance abusers. In part, this may be due to their greater social resources, but may also be because a licensing board has had a role in their coming for treatment (see under Helping a fellow physician, p. 867).

When treating an employed substance misuser, if his or her problem is already known to the employer, it can sometimes improve the outcome of therapy to recommend such supervision by the employer or his nominee.

When substance abuse has led to doubt about fitness to work in very critical posts, for example in the airline industry (pilots, traffic controllers) and medicine, continued supervision of compliance with abstinence, including random monitoring of breath, sputum, urine or blood tests, contributes to good outcome.

INGREDIENTS OF SUCCESSFUL TREATMENT

Perhaps the most important element of treatment is for the individual to enter a non-judgemental, objective relationship in which he can weigh up the advantages and disadvantages of continuing the alcohol or drug habit. Only then is it possible for him to make a firm decision to alter his habit and obtain support to stick to that decision.

It was common practice in North America, to offer the employee residential treatment with an emphasis on group therapy lasting between four and six weeks. Controlled studies demonstrating the advantage of such relatively expensive treatment over outpatient care are lacking. However, specific psychological treatments such as marital counselling, anxiety management and social skills training have been shown to be effective.

Alcoholics Anonymous has helped thousands of alcoholics, in many countries, and a stable fellow employee who is an AA member may be a great help in introducing a colleague. Narcotics Anonymous (NA), for drug abusers, can be found in some cities.

Psychotropic medication to reduce relapse may occasionally have a place if other psychiatric disorders are found to persist after the drug use has ceased.

Two compounds (naltrexone and acamprosate) are now licensed in many countries to help prevent relapse in newly abstaining alcoholics. Their neuropharmacological actions, while different from each other, are consistent with current knowledge of the neurotransmitter basis of dependence and relapse. The characteristics of patients most likely to respond are still to be specified. However, when patients are willing to take disulfiram, in a supervised arrangement to improve compliance (see under Deterrent medication), and are randomly allocated to either that treatment or to supervised acamprosate or naltrexone, disulfiram has been shown to be more effective than either naltrexone or acamprosate.[30]

Medically assisted withdrawal

Withdrawal from alcohol can often be successfully and safely achieved at a specialist outpatient clinic, or at home guided by the general practitioner or nurse. Ideally, the patient is seen daily to monitor the dosage of the medication (usually benzodiazepine) and to ensure that drinking is not continuing. Admission to hospital is appropriate if this fails, or if the individual is liable to severe withdrawal symptoms and lives alone. (A patient drinking 25 or more units per day may require 50 mg of diazepam or equivalent in the first 24 hours, reducing to zero over 5 days.)

Subjects can also withdraw from benzodiazepines, opiates and stimulant drugs as outpatients. The socially unstable young abuser often takes a very wide variety of substances, including alcohol, and discussion during a drug-withdrawal regimen should include strategies of developing a different lifestyle.

Medical aid for the opiate abuser who requests detoxification is necessary only if chemical dependence exists – often such abusers are only intermittent users and hope to obtain more drugs (sometimes to sell) by requesting detoxification. Treatment will consist of either substituting a reducing dose of oral liquid methadone or sublingual buprenorphine, with controls to check other continuing drug use, or attempting to reduce withdrawal symptoms with clonidine or lofexidine, perhaps with a benzodiazepine to aid sleep. A specialist clinic should advise about appropriate doses. Ultra-rapid withdrawal by giving an opiate antagonist while the patient is unconscious under anaesthetic is possible, but is rarely practised because of the risk of respiratory or circulatory failure. It requires full intensive care facilities, an experienced addiction specialist and an experienced anaesthetist. In such hands, the patient's discharge and return home after being prescribed naltrexone can be achieved in a few days.

Deterrent medication

When an employee has been given his final warning, the treatment agency may suggest that he takes disulfiram supervised at work or at a clinic. The occupational physician or employer's representative can request assurance that the employee is complying in swallowing the medication as required, which might be daily, or in double doses if administered three days per week. The deterrent effect of this drug is its highly unpleasant alcohol interaction and depends on taking it regularly in sufficient dosage. Counselling on changing lifestyle during the disulfiram-induced abstinence is important if relapse is not to occur when the disciplinary period ends. Naltrexone can be used in the same way with an opiate abuser. Naltrexone blocks the rewarding mental effects of opiates, rather than causing an aversive reaction, and, if taken regularly (perhaps three times per week), greatly reduces the risk of relapse.

Abstinence?

Early, not severely dependent, problem drinkers can sometimes resume problem-free drinking. Those with social supports (family and job) and without impulsive personalities and many social problems are those who might succeed to control their drinking. Abstinence is the appropriate goal for most other alcohol and drug abusers. Services for opiate addicts, because of the imperative of reducing the spread by needles of AIDS, have emphasized 'harm reduction' and offered substitution therapy to many injecting opiate users. Although many opiate users state to research interviewers that they would like to become abstinent, the relapse rate among those who are helped to withdraw is high. Therefore, oral methadone or buprenorphine is offered, to satiate the opioid neuroreceptors and thus to reduce injecting, and stabilize the user's pattern of life. Patients taking regular doses of substitute opiates may be able to perform satisfactorily at work, unless they are also using additional *ad hoc* street drugs, which treatment clinics try to prevent but cannot rule out. Maintenance prescribing of benzodiazepine to benzodiazepine addicts is common, and some users continue functioning effectively at work, but should not drive vocationally or operate machinery because reaction time and cognitive function may be impaired.

Prognosis

In individuals who have reached criteria for dependence and/or have come for treatment, a period of abstinence from drugs or alcohol of less than a year has no prognostic value.[31] Abstinence for one year begins to indicate a good outcome. Individuals do best when they still have a job and a close relationship. In the emerging life story of males who at some stage in their life abused alcohol, it can be seen that an abstinent period of five years is only very rarely followed by a relapse, but nevertheless can still occur.[32] It is clearly very difficult to decide when it will be safe for a recovering alcohol or drug misuser to resume work, especially if when the job is responsible for public safety, for example as a driver, pilot, ship's captain or a doctor. Monitoring is essential and might reasonably continue for up to five years, although some US medical boards recommend 15 years.

Vocational driving licences

In the European Union and in many other countries, employees with an alcohol or drug problem are not permitted to drive large goods- or passenger-carrying vehicles. A minimum of several years (three years in the United Kingdom) since cessation of treatment, and evidence of recovery, is required before renewal of the licence.

The driver who develops a drug or alcohol problem should declare this to the licensing authorities. Opiate addicts maintained on oral methadone and patients receiving regular benzodiazepines may not hold vocational licences in the UK and the European Community. It is a debated point whether such individuals may hold ordinary driving licences, although studies of psychomotor performance in patients on a stable dose of methadone have not shown impairment.

Ordinary licence – The high risk offender scheme

On reapplication for an ordinary UK driving licence following disqualification for drink/driving, a driver must satisfy the Secretary of State for Transport's medical advisers that he or she is not, or never was, alcohol dependent, if (1) the blood alcohol at the time of the offence was 200 mg/L or more, or (2) he or she refused the tests, or (3) he or she has been disqualified more than once in ten years.

SUBSTANCE MISUSE AND THE MEDICAL PROFESSION

The annual reports of the UK regulatory authority, the General Medical Council (GMC), show that alcohol and drug misuse, with or without other psychiatric disorders, is a common cause of unfitness to practise.

'Stress' in the medical profession was widely researched and discussed in the 1990s[33,34] and it appears that personality features may contribute both to an attraction to a medical career and to a vulnerability to stress.[35] Stress can be a factor in substance misuse in doctors, but should not be too readily assumed to be the central issue. For some, addiction has simply begun as a great liking for a drug's euphoric effects. Medical student life in Western countries can involve heavy drinking. Later on, doctors not only have sufficient income to subsidize heavy drinking, but they also have relatively easy access to other addictive substances. Anaesthetists are at particular risk of opiate misuse (oral or injected) or misuse of anaesthetics (sniffing), and may experiment to the point of dependence. Pharmacists and veterinarians share the high risk of drug dependence due to the availability of addictive drugs.

Helping a fellow physician

Work colleagues may have maintained a blanket of secrecy, so that the addiction is well advanced when help is eventually sought. Your support and understanding may be needed, but you may also need to take a firm stance (easier if disciplinary action is pending) to shift the misusing doctor to the point of acceptance that there is a problem to be addressed.[36,37] This requires courage and compassion, not covering up. If he or she is a work colleague, leave the treatment to a specialist. If the doctor makes no attempt to seek advice, then others who can bring some coercion to bear may need to be involved, for example, the hospital managers, the appropriate section of the local health authority or, when none of these are relevant and fitness to practise is in question, the GMC or appropriate licensing board.

In helping a substance-misusing doctor, the dialogue should be as with an intelligent layman, without assuming he or she has special knowledge. Commence with his or her main concerns, using a non-judgemental style. Avoid secrecy. Be ready to set limits and prevent too early discontinuation of treatment. Beware too ready an acceptance of the view that 'stress' or 'depression' are the main issues: the main issue may be the substance dependence itself, but this is not yet identified/accepted by the individual. It is easy to collude in a way that only postpones dealing with the dependence on the drug, that is, to making a commitment to abstinence and following methods to achieve that. Monitor progress using objective markers such as breath, blood and urine tests. If matters have reached a point where the professional licensing board is involved, evidence will be required that treatment is being followed and abstinence achieved before limitations on practice are rescinded. The UK General Medical Council appoints supervisors, separate from the treating specialist.

Doctors who resume work tend to have a better outcome than other substance misusers; supervision, with testing, may be a helpful ingredient.[38,39] Professional mutual support networks should be accessed.[37] In the United Kingdom, there is the Doctors' and Dentists' Group, c/o Medical Council on Alcoholism, Tel: 0207 487 4445. In addition, in the United Kingdom, there is the National Counselling Service for Sick Doctors, Tel: 0207 935 5982.

PREVENTION

Limiting the availability of alcohol in the workplace is important and can reduce accidents; similarly, regulations about the taking of psychotropic drugs or alcohol at work or before coming to work can be helpful. One strategy is to provide free hot lunches inside the plant to discourage lunch hour and 'parking lot' drinking by blue-collar workers.

Hazardous drinkers, detected opportunistically at family practices, have been shown to respond favourably to fairly minimal medical intervention (such as feedback about their level of drinking or their serum GGT).[40] In one four-year follow-up study, a reduction of sickness absenteeism was demonstrated.[41] Transferring this model to the workplace has been disappointing. In the New South Wales police force, 251 hazardous drinkers attended a brief appointment with a health worker, but this appeared to have no impact on their drinking when compared with a sample of heavy drinkers from police districts where no intervention was being offered.[14] A similar negative result was obtained among Australian male postal workers, although some female staff appeared to have reduced their consumption slightly, related to the intervention.[42] Employee assistance programmes may aim to recruit problem drinkers early, but except in the United States where seeking help for personal problems is perhaps more accepted, self-referrals to these programmes are rare and managers still tend to refer only when impaired work performance is severe or chronic.

Employee committees, when consulted about health promotion they would see as relevant, tend not to mention drugs or alcohol. They perceive organizational stressors as the most important: deadlines, unrealistic expectations, excessive supervision, inadequate supervision, poor feedback and harassment.[43] Health promotion in the workplace should be broad and look at links between personal health practices (eating, smoking, exercise, weight control, stress management) and factors at the workplace. Programmes should help participants to develop or regain a sense of control, efficacy and competence in their health practices, and to use support from family, friends and fellow workers if trying to change these. Such projects are most likely to be successful when the workforce is involved in their development. Health promotion programmes applied in group sessions to workers have not had a striking impact.[43] Didactic teaching that comes down from personnel departments or management is unlikely to succeed in individualistic Western society. It is not known whether more success would be obtained by education projects initiated by the workforce.[44]

Key points

- Alcohol misuse and drug misuse are a cause of absenteeism, inefficiency and work accidents.
- Early identification can be helped by blood tests.
- Abstinence must usually be the goal.
- Workplace policies agreed by employer and employee representatives are helpful.
- Success of an intervention can be helped by sanctions and monitoring which may involve the employer or professional regulator.
- Workplace health education around substances seems to have little effect.

REFERENCES

1. Kreitman N. Alcohol consumption and the preventive paradox. *British Journal of Addiction*. 1986; **81**: 353–63.
2. National Highway Traffic Safety Administration, National Center for Statistics and Analysis. Drunk driving facts. Washington DC: NHTSA, 1988.
3. Seaman FJ. Problem drinking among American railroad workers. In: Hore B, Plant M (eds). *Alcohol problems in employment*. London: Croom Helm, 1981: 118–28.
4. Lewis RJ, Cooper SP. Alcohol, other drugs and fatal work-related injuries. *Journal of Occupational Medicine*. 1989; **31**: 23–8.

5. Baker S, Sankoff IS, Fisher RS et al. Fatal occupational injuries. *Journal of the American Medical Association.* 1982; **248**: 692–7.
6. Finnigan F, Schulze D, Smallwood J, Helander A. The effects of self-administered alcohol-induced 'hangover' in a naturalistic setting on psychomotor and cognitive performance and subjective state. *Addiction.* 2005; **100**: 1680–9.
7. McKinney A, Coyle K. Next day effects of a normal night's drinking on memory and psychomotor performance. *Alcohol and Alcoholism.* 2004; **39**: 509–13.
8. Lang IF, Wallace RB, Huppert FAF, Melzer D. Moderate alcohol consumption in older adults is associated with better cognition and well-being than abstinence. *Age and Ageing.* 2007; **36**: 256–61.
9. Richards M, Hardy R, Wadsworth MEJ. Alcohol consumption and midlife cognitive change in the British 1946 Birth Cohort Study. *Alcohol and Alcoholism.* 2005; **40**: 112–17.
10. Stampfer MJ, Kang JH, Chen J et al. Effects of moderate alcohol consumption on cognitive function in women. *New England Journal of Medicine.* 2005; **352**: 245–53.
11. Parsons OA, Nixon SJ. Cognitive functioning in sober social drinkers: A review of the research since 1986. *Journal of Studies on Alcohol.* 1998; **59**: 180–90.
12. Kolb D, Gunderson EKE. Medical histories of problem drinkers during their first twelve years of naval service. *Journal of Studies on Alcohol.* 1983; **44**: 84–94.
13. Saad E, Madden J. Certificated incapacity and unemployment in alcoholics. *British Journal of Psychiatry.* 1976; **128**: 340–5.
14. Richmond RL, Kehoe L, Hailstone S et al. Quantitative and qualitative evaluations of brief interventions to change excessive drinking, smoking and stress in the police force. *Addiction.* 1999; **94**: 1509–21.
15. White IR, Altmann DR, Nanchahal K. Alcohol consumption and mortality: Modelling risks of men and women of different ages. *British Medical Journal.* 2002; **325**: 191–4.
16. Andreasson S, Alleback P, Romelsjo A. Alcohol consumption and mortality among young men: Longitudinal study of Swedish conscripts. *British Medical Journal.* 1988; **296**: 1021–5.
17. World Cancer Research Fund. Food, nutrition, physical activity and the prevention of cancer: A global perspective. London: WCRF, 2007.
18. Connor J. The life and times of the J-shaped curve. *Alcohol and Alcoholism.* 2007; **41**: 583–4.
19. Plant M. Alcoholism and occupation: Cause or effect? A controlled study of recruits to the drink trade. *International Journal of Addiction.* 1978; **13**: 605–26.
20. Baker A. Alcohol-related deaths by occupation: What do data for England and Wales in 2001–2005 tell us about doctors' mortality? *Alcohol and Alcoholism.* 2008; **43**: 121–2.
21. Hodgson R, Alwyn T, John B et al. The FAST alcohol screening test. *Alcohol and Alcoholism.* 2002; **37**: 61–6.
22. Ryan J, Zwerling C, Jones M. The effectiveness of preemployment drug screening in the prediction of employment outcome. *Journal of Occupational Medicine.* 1992; **34**: 1057–63.
23. Magura S, Freeman RC, Siddiqui Q, Lipton DS. The validity of hair analysis for detecting cocaine and heroin use among addicts. *International Journal of Addiction.* 1992; **27**: 51–69.
24. Faculty of Occupational Medicine. Guidelines for testing for drugs of abuse in the workplace. London: Royal College of Physicians, 1994.
25. Forrest ARW. Ethical aspects of workplace urine screening for drug abuse. *Journal of Medical Ethics.* 1977; **23**: 12–17.
26. Chick J, Kemppainen E. Estimating alcohol consumption. *Pancreatology.* 2007; **7**: 157–61.
27. Israel Y, Hollander O, Sanchez-Craig M et al. Screening for problem drinking and counseling by the primary care physician-nurse team. *Alcoholism, Clinical and Experimental Research.* 1996; **20**: 1443–50.
28. Health and Safety Executive. Alcohol and drugs at work. Last accessed December 28, 2007. Available from: www.hse.gov.uk/alcoholdrugs/.
29. Chick J. Treatment of alcoholic violent offenders: Ethics and efficacy. *Alcohol and Alcoholism.* 1998; **33**: 20–5.
30. Laaksonen E, Koski-Jannes A, Salaspuro M et al. A randomized multicentre open label comparative trial of disulfiram, naltrexone and acamprosate in the treatment of alcohol dependence. *Alcohol and Alcoholism.* 2008; **43**: 53–61.
31. Yates WR, Reed DA, Booth BM et al. Prognostic validity of short-term abstinence. *Alcoholism, Clinical and Experimental Research.* 1994; **18**: 280–3.
32. Vaillant GE. A long-term follow-up of male alcohol abuse. *Archives of General Psychiatry.* 1996; **53**: 243–9.
33. Ramirez AJ, Graham J, Richards MA et al. Mental health of hospital consultants: The effects of stress and satisfaction at work. *Lancet.* 1996; **347**: 724–8.
34. Caplan RP. Stress, anxiety, and depression in hospital consultants, general practitioners and senior health service managers. *British Medical Journal.* 1994; **309**: 1261–3.
35. Brooke D. Why do some doctors become addicted? *Addiction.* 1996; **91**: 317–19.
36. Chick J. Doctors with emotional problems: How can they be helped? In: Hawton K, Cowen P (eds). *Practical problems in clinical psychiatry.* Oxford: Oxford University Press, 1992: 242–52.
37. Lloyd G. Supporting the addicted doctor. *Practitioner.* 1990; **234**: 989–91.
38. Morse RM, Martin MA, Swenson WM, Niven RG. Prognosis of physicians treated for alcoholism and drug dependence. *Journal of the American Medical Association.* 1984; **251**: 743–6.
39. Shore JH. The Oregon experience with impaired physicians on probation: An 8 year follow-up. *Journal of the American Medical Association.* 1987; **257**: 2931–4.
40. Bertholet N, Daeppen JB, Wietlisbach V. Reduction of alcohol consumption by brief alcohol intervention in primary care: Systematic review and meta-analysis. *Archives of Internal Medicine.* 2005; **165**: 986–95.
41. Kristenson H, Ohlin H, Huttin-Nosslin MB et al. Identification and intervention of heavy drinking in middle-aged men: Result and follow-up of 24–60 months of long term study

with randomised controls. *Alcoholism, Clinical and Experimental Research*. 1983; **7**: 203–9.
42. Richmond R, Kehoe L, Heather N, Wodak A. Evaluation of a workplace brief intervention for excessive alcohol consumption: The workscreen project. *Preventive Medicine.* 2000; **30**: 51–63.
43. Bennett JB, Patterson CR, Reynolds GS *et al.* Team awareness, problem drinking, and drinking climate: Workplace social health promotion in a policy context. *American Journal of Health Promotion.* 2004; **19**: 103–13.
44. Shain M. Worksite community processes and the prevention of alcohol abuse: Theory to action. In: Giesbrecht N, Conley P, Denniston RW *et al.* (eds). *Research, action and the community: Experiences in the prevention of alcohol and other drug problems*. US Dept of Health and Human Services OSAP Prevention monograph. Washington DC: US Government Printing Office, 1990: 106–12.

FURTHER READING

Edwards G, Marshall J, Cook C. *The treatment of drinking problems*, 3rd edn. Oxford: Oxford University Press, revised, 1997.

Department of Health. Drug misuse and dependence: Guidelines on clinical management. London: Department of Health. Last accessed December 17, 2005. Available from: www.dh.gov.uk/en/Publicationsandstatistics/Publications/PublicationsPolicyAndGuidance/DH_4009665.

PART SEVEN

RESPIRATORY DISORDERS

Section One: General issues   873
Section Two: Organic dust diseases   939
Section Three: Inorganic dust diseases   983

//
SECTION ONE

General issues

68	Imaging in occupational lung disease *Paul M Taylor*	875
69	Work and chronic air flow limitation *David J Hendrick*	889
70	Health effects of ultrafine/nanoparticles *Ken Donaldson, Robert J Aitken, Jon G Ayres, Brian G Miller and C Lang Tran*	903
71	Health effects related to non-industrial workplace indoor environments *Jouni JK Jaakkola and Maritta S Jaakkola*	921

68

Imaging in occupational lung disease

PAUL M TAYLOR

Introduction	875	Magnetic resonance	878
Chest radiography	875	Radionuclide studies	879
Computed tomography	876	Coalworker's pneumoconiosis	879
High-resolution computed tomography	877	International Labour Organization classification	885
Ultrasound	878	References	886

INTRODUCTION

The developments in imaging technology that have occurred over the last two decades have provided valuable insights into the body's structure and function. Despite this, the chest radiograph remains the primary and, in many cases, the only radiological investigation performed. The use of more complex imaging techniques often carries a financial and radiation penalty and these must be balanced against the expected benefits.

CHEST RADIOGRAPHY

Conventional radiography

Within a year of Roentgen's discovery of x-rays chest radiography had been used as a diagnostic tool. The initial images of the chest were crude, but progress was rapid and by the early part of the twentieth century the chest radiograph was a recognized part of clinical investigation. Its validity in occupational lung disease was established as a result of correlative radiological and pathological studies.

The principles of chest radiography are well known. The patient is positioned with the anterior chest placed against a cassette containing the film and the x-ray tube approximately 2 metres from the film, behind the patient. The film is exposed during maximum inspiration. Exposure factors can radically alter the appearance of the resultant radiograph. The radiographer can alter the kilo voltage (kV) of the x-rays produced by the tube. Higher kV x-rays possess more energy and pass more easily through all tissues, producing a 'flatter' image with less intrinsic contrast. A high kV exposure may be preferred since it produces clearer images of the mediastinum and the overlying lung. However, this is at the expense of clarity of the ribs and intrathoracic calcifications. The converse occurs with a lower kV exposure.

Radiographic film varies in quality. In order to reduce radiation dose to the patient, manufacturers have developed more sensitive films which produce a similar level of radiographic density at a lower exposure to x-rays. This development, although desirable, is not without its drawbacks and these films may produce a coarser image. This is of particular relevance in occupational disease where subtle alterations in the parenchymal pattern may be significant. The practical impact of these considerations is that in longitudinal studies of workers, no effort should be spared in ensuring that exposure factors and film quality vary as little as possible.

Of equal importance to technical factors are patient variables involved in the radiograph and before any attempt is made at interpretation, the observer should consider the following:

- Is the patient rotated? Rotation produces asymmetry in the size and density of the lungs. Rotation is assessed by noting the position of the medial ends of the clavicles with respect to the spinous processes of the upper thoracic spine.
- Has the patient achieved a satisfactory inspiration? A poor inspiration causes crowding of the basal lung

markings, an increase in density of the lower zone of the lungs and enlargement of the cardiac silhouette. These changes are often misinterpreted as basal fibrosis. In a normal full inspiration, the dome of the right hemidiaphragm should lie between the anterior ends of the 6th and 7th ribs.
- Is the film adequately exposed? An overexposed film causes the lungs to appear dark with loss of normal vascular markings, which is often misinterpreted as 'emphysematous lungs'. Underexposure causes the lungs to appear pale, often misinterpreted as due to pulmonary infiltration. Exposure is difficult to assess objectively and depends upon body habitus. It may be necessary to take two films at different exposures to demonstrate the lungs and mediastinum.

Digital imaging

Conventional radiography using radiographic film remains the most frequent method of imaging. However, in the developed world, radiography, including chest radiography, is now increasingly undertaken using digital methods of image acquisition. These include computed radiography (CR) and direct radiography (DR).

In CR, an imaging plate replaces the radiographic film. After exposure, the image produced on the plate is scanned and read by a computer system. The image is then wiped from the plate which is subsequently reused. Direct radiography systems are analogous to digital cameras in that the image is captured directly by the imaging system and transmitted to a computer system without the need for an intermediate plate reading process. The advantages of digital imaging are well described and include a potential reduction in radiation dose, greater reproducibility of the image and the ability to manipulate, process and store the image using one of a variety of storage media. Digital systems may stand alone, with the digital image being printed on to a film to be handled in a similar way to a conventional radiograph, or they may form part of a picture archiving and communication system (PACS)[1] where digital images from several sources, e.g. CR, DR, ultrasound and angiography, are stored, manipulated and distributed within the radiology department and beyond. Digital techniques and PACS are still evolving, but it is likely that within the next decade most radiology departments in the developed world will have some form of PACS system. Detailed descriptions of digital imaging systems are available in several comprehensive reviews.[2–4]

Whatever system is used, the appearance of the resulting digital image will differ from a conventional radiograph. In its most obvious form this is because the image is displayed on a monitor rather than on a transilluminated film. Even when the image is printed on to film, differences persist and the explanation for this is seen in Figure 68.1.

Figure 68.1 shows that the relationship between the x-ray exposure and the film density on a conventional radiograph

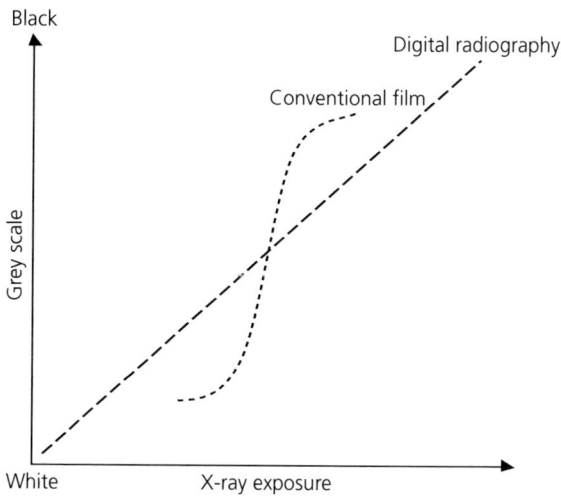

Figure 68.1 A graph showing the relationship between the x-ray exposure and the degree of blackening of the image using a conventional x-ray film and a computed radiography system. The conventional film has a non-linear response to exposure, which means that at high or low exposure rates the effect on the film is reduced. It also has a narrower range in which it functions (exposure latitude). For these reasons, computed radiography systems offer more consistent and reliable images.

is non-linear. In a digital system, there is a linear relationship which ensures a more consistent density to the image, a greater reproducibility between exposures and a wider exposure latitude. It is also possible to manipulate the image using system software. Image manipulation is often referred to as post-processing. Post-processing allows the image to be optimized by changing parameters, such as the image contrast, or adding features, such as edge enhancement, which increases the conspicuity of small structures. In the context of occupational lung disease where early detection of subtle abnormalities is important, the software in the system should be optimized to permit this.

COMPUTED TOMOGRAPHY

The introduction of computed tomography (CT) into clinical practice was a milestone in radiological development.[5] First, it introduced computing into radiology, thus laying the foundations for the development of digital imaging. Second, it established the utility of cross-sectional imaging as a method of displaying anatomy.

The initial CT scanners were suitable only for brain imaging with the system aperture large enough to accommodate only the head. Moreover, the long image acquisition times made them suitable only for immobile structures. By the late 1970s, general purpose CT systems were available and the first reports of their use in the chest were published.[6,7]

CT has assumed an increasing role in thoracic imaging; however, the principles remain unchanged despite continuing technological development.

During the acquisition of a CT image, the patient lies on the examination table and the area of the body to be examined is positioned within the CT gantry. The CT gantry contains the x-ray tube and an array of x-ray detectors. These are mounted on opposite sides of a ring which surrounds the patient. During the exposure, the x-ray tube rotates around the patient emitting a tightly collimated beam of x-rays. The x-rays emerging from the patient strike the detectors and the data from these are fed to a computer. The computer calculates the attenuation of the beam by the patient's body to produce a matrix (typically 512×512) in which the attenuation value of each cell in the matrix is determined. Attenuation values are measured in Hounsfield units (HU). Air has a value of -1000 HU and water 0 HU. Soft tissues in the body range in value between 40 and 80 HU, their attenuation varies depending on factors such as the subject's haemoglobin level, the amount of fat in the tissue and the presence of any calcification. The matrix is displayed as an image by correlating the calculated attenuation values with a grey scale, in which the higher the attenuation value the brighter the shade of grey. Thus, the image consists of many thousands of picture elements (pixels) each one of which represents the attenuation value of a small volume of tissue (voxel). Because of the wide range of calculated attenuation values and the limited number of shades of grey detectable by the human eye, it is not practicable to display each attenuation value as a separate level of grey and the range of attenuation values to be displayed must be selected. The range selected can be altered by changing the window width and level. The window width describes the range of attenuation values that are allocated to the available levels of grey. A narrow window width ensures that tissues of slightly different attenuation are displayed as different levels of grey; this is suitable for demonstrating the mediastinal structures. A wider window is selected to demonstrate the lungs to accommodate the large range of attenuation present. Attenuation values above and below the chosen range appear white and black, respectively. The window level is defined as the attenuation value at the midpoint of the window width. A low level is selected for predominantly low attenuation regions, such as the lung, and a high level for higher attenuation tissues, such as bone.

In common with other digital imaging systems, CT images can be post-processed. Post-processing procedures include changing algorithms to smooth or filter the image, reformatting the data in different planes and statistical analysis of the attenuation data.

HIGH-RESOLUTION COMPUTED TOMOGRAPHY

Introduced in the mid-1980s, high-resolution computed tomography (HRCT) of the lungs is now the preferred CT technique in the investigation of diffuse lung disease.[8–10]

HRCT differs from conventional CT in two key respects:[11,12]

1. Section thickness. In conventional CT, the sections are approximately 10 mm in thickness. In HRCT, the sections are typically no more than 1 mm thick. The beneficial effect of this is that partial volume averaging is reduced. Partial volume averaging occurs when a structure only partially fills a voxel. When the attenuation value for the voxel is calculated an average value is obtained lying between the true attenuation value of the structure and its background. As a result, small structures, such as peripheral pulmonary vessels or small nodules, can be 'lost' because they occupy only a small fraction of a voxel. By reducing slice thickness, the voxels are made smaller and the percentage occupied by these small structures increases, thus decreasing partial volume averaging. The disadvantages of thinner sections are two-fold. First, if the section thickness is reduced from 10 to 1 mm, ten times as many sections would be required to image the same volume of the body. In practice, this is not a problem since the images although 1 mm thick are usually acquired at 10-mm increments rather than contiguously. In effect only 10 per cent of the lung is imaged and this therefore is a second sampling technique problem, inherent in all CT systems, that reducing the section thickness decreases the signal to noise ratio. This makes the images appear rather 'noisy' with variations in pixel density even in homogenous body tissue. The problem can be overcome to some extent by increasing the output of the x-ray tube, although this results in a higher radiation dose to the patient.

2. Reconstruction algorithm. In calculating the attenuation values of the voxels the computer has to deal with biological heterogeneity of body tissue, variation in x-ray output and other factors which produce variations in the calculated attenuation of ostensibly homogenous structures. To overcome this software used in conventional CT smoothes these variations, reducing the differences between adjacent voxels. However, in heterogeneous tissues, such as the lung, smoothing results in loss of clarity of the margins of small structures making them appear blurred. In HRCT, however, a high spatial frequency processing algorithm is used which has a much reduced smoothing function.

The majority of HRCT images are obtained with the patient supine during maximum inspiration. However, in some circumstances, it may be preferable to perform prone or expiratory images.

Due to the greater hydrostatic pressure in the supine position, the vessels in the posterior lung become distended and there is an increase in the extravascular fluid. This produces an increase in the attenuation of the posterior lung which can obscure underlying structural change

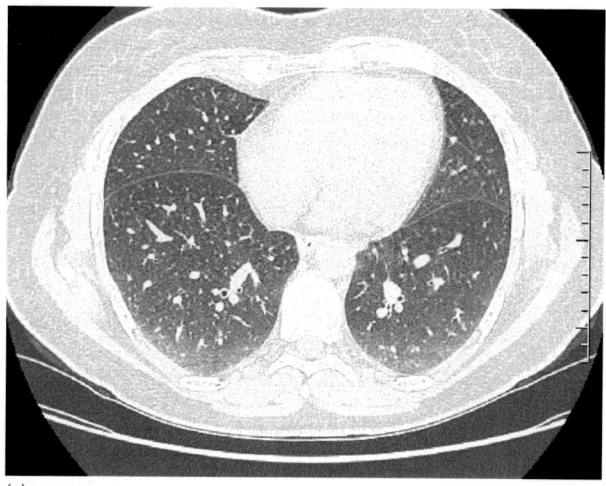

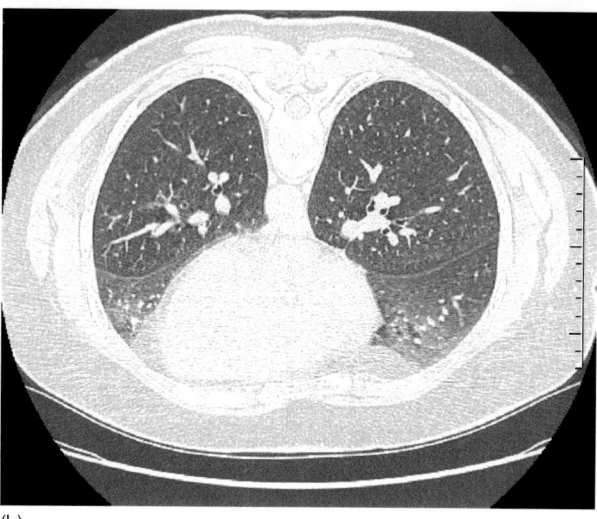

Figure 68.2 (a) A CT section through the lung bases in a patient with normal lungs demonstrating hypostatic change. Note the gradation in density through the lung with the posterior dependent lung appearing denser and the pulmonary vessels larger. (b) The same patient as has been turned to the prone position, with the dependent changes now present in the anterior lung.

(Figure 68.2a,b). This is of particular importance in asbestosis since the posterior lung bases are the most frequently involved portions of the lung.

By turning the patient prone and repeating the sections, the hypostatic changes are repositioned anteriorly. A period of 5–10 minutes is required for full reversal of these changes. Failure to undertake this manoeuvre can result in fibrosis being obscured by the hydrostatic changes or normal lung being misinterpreted as abnormal.

Air trapping in the gas exchange spaces of the lungs occurs in several conditions including extrinsic allergic alveolitis.[13] It is difficult to detect air trapping on inspiratory scans, but expiratory sections are helpful. On expiration, the normal lung decreases in cross-section and increases in attenuation. In regions of air trapping, these changes fail to occur and they become highlighted against the normal lung.

In recent years, multislice CT has become established in clinical practice. Multislice CT systems subdivide each acquired axial section into multiple (typically 32 or 64) subsections. This produces images of similar resolution in the sagittal and coronal planes, as in the axial planes.[14] The potential benefits of this technique in respect of pulmonary anatomy are under evaluation.[15,16]

Enhancement of the mediastinal structures by intravenous contrast plays a key role in differentiating normal from abnormal structures, particularly lymphadenopathy. This is not usually required in patients with occupational lung disease, but is invaluable in staging patients with occupationally induced bronchial carcinoma.

ULTRASOUND

Outside the cardiovascular system, the applications of ultrasound in the thorax are limited by its inability to pass through the gas-filled lung. However, ultrasound is helpful in imaging the pleura.[17] It is often difficult to differentiate pleural fluid from solid pleural masses on chest radiography; moreover, the two can coexist. Real-time ultrasound allows detection and quantification of pleural fluid and is a highly sensitive method of detecting small effusions. It can identify pleural masses and permits accurate percutaneous biopsy of lesions including mesothelioma.[18] Pleural plaques can be identified by ultrasound, but CT is the preferred technique.

MAGNETIC RESONANCE

The ability of magnetic resonance (MR) to image in multiple planes with high intrinsic soft tissue contrast without using ionizing radiation has made it an essential imaging tool in many areas of the body, in particular the brain, spine and skeleton.[19] Within the thorax, it has established a role in cardiovascular and mediastinal imaging.[20,21] Its use in the lung is restricted for several reasons.[22]

1. Magnetic resonance primarily images protons. Within the lung, the large amount of air produces a very low proton density.
2. The combination of air-containing spaces and interlacing vessels produces heterogeneity in the magnetic field which significantly degrades the image.
3. There are physiological movements, in particular cardiac and respiratory motion, which produce artefacts.

Despite these problems, several studies have demonstrated the ability of MR to image patients with diffuse lung disease. It is likely that further developments in MR will be directed at improving our knowledge of pathophysiological events rather than replicating CT and providing structural data. In this context, the high intrinsic soft tissue contrast of MR may enable the differentiation of active pulmonary infiltrates from more indolent fibrotic processes.

RADIONUCLIDE STUDIES

The most frequently performed radionuclide studies of the lung are ventilation/perfusion lung scans in patients with suspected pulmonary embolic disease. In occupational lung disease, two other less frequently used techniques should be considered.

1. Gallium-67 (^{67}Ga) is produced by cyclotron. When injected intravenously, it is accumulated, by a variety of mechanisms, into inflammatory tissue including pulmonary inflammation. The process is slow and scans are obtained one to three days after the injection. Several inflammatory processes, including drug-induced lung disease, sarcoidosis, fibrosing alveolitis and asbestosis, have been shown to take up ^{67}Ga. The resulting scans are sensitive, but not specific.[23–25]
2. Technetium-99m diethylenetriamine penta acetic acid (Tc^{99}m DTPA) aerosols can be used to assess alveolar integrity. The patient inhales the aerosol and the lungs are imaged by the gamma camera. From the resultant images, the rate of clearance of the radionuclide from the lungs is calculated. This is normally less than 4 per cent per minute. Increased rates are seen in patients with a variety of conditions, including extrinsic allergic alveolitis.[26] Higher rates of clearance are also seen in smokers and in patients with respiratory infections.[27]

Although these techniques provide elegant demonstrations of pathophysiology, their role in clinical investigation is limited. Structural changes are more clearly demonstrated by HRCT and conventional pulmonary function tests provide a more practical alternative to assess functional impairment.

COALWORKER'S PNEUMOCONIOSIS

Simple coalworker's pneumoconiosis

In addition to coal dust, miners frequently inhale quantities of silica dust from adjacent rock strata. The composition of the coal dust and the proportion of silica affect the radiological appearances of coalworker's pneumoconiosis (CWP).

The prime radiological feature of simple CWP is the development of well-defined, relatively discrete pulmonary nodules. The nodules tend to spare the extreme lung bases and do not calcify (Figure 68.3).[28] Unlike in pure silicosis, mediastinal and hilar lymph node enlargement does not

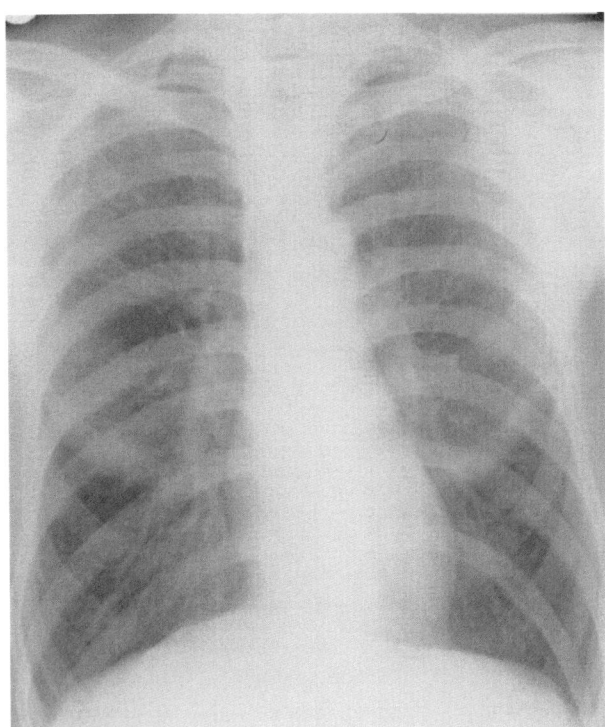

Figure 68.3 A chest radiograph in a former miner with coalworker's pneumoconiosis. There is fine nodularity in the upper and mid zones with the lung bases appearing relatively unaffected.

occur as part of simple CWP. The size and clarity of the nodules is related to the composition of the dust. Nodules tend to be larger in those miners exposed to dust with a high silica content. It is now recognized that irregular small opacities can also occur in simple CWP and are associated with dust exposure, the presence of emphysema and impairment of lung function.[29,30] The profusion of nodules is related to the degree of exposure. HRCT is more sensitive than chest radiography in the detection of the nodules.[31] The extent of CWP demonstrated by HRCT is also related to the severity of pulmonary functional impairment.[32,33] At least one study has demonstrated an increased incidence of bronchiectasis in workers with CWP, the severity of which is related to the degree of exposure.[34]

Caplan's syndrome

Caplan's syndrome is a rare condition occurring in dust-exposed workers with rheumatoid diathesis (with or without clinical arthritis). Although first described in coalworkers, it has also been observed in workers exposed to silica and silicates. It is characterized by the development of single or multiple well-defined nodules within the lungs, which may be calcified. These are typically 0.5–2 cm in diameter and occur in crops or clusters (Figure 68.4). The nodules may cavitate, enlarge and coalesce, although they often remain static over several years.

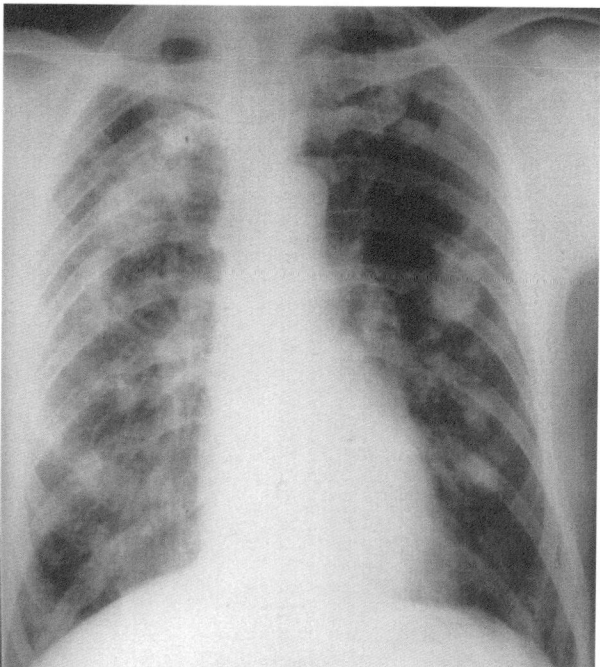

Figure 68.4 A chest radiograph in a patient with Caplan's syndrome demonstrating multiple nodules in both lungs.

Complicated coalworker's pneumoconiosis

The defining process in the development of complicated CWP is the formation of areas of progressive massive fibrosis (PMF). Characteristically, the lesions occur in the mid and upper zones of the lung and are frequently bilateral. They are ovoid or 'sausage'-shaped and enlarge over many years to reach several centimetres in diameter. In advanced cases of PMF, there is often distortion and marked emphysema in the surrounding lung. PMF usually occurs on a background of nodules of simple CWP of at least category 2 profusion (see Table 68.1), but the background nodules may become less apparent as the emphysema becomes more advanced. The lesions of PMF rarely cavitate and there may be hilar lymph node enlargement. In clinical practice, the prime differential diagnosis is bronchial carcinoma which has an occurrence, even in miners, many times that of PMF.

Silicosis

The appearances of silicosis are not dissimilar to CWP.[35] However, the degree of fibrosis present in the lung is greater and as a result the nodules are larger, more discrete, and tend to become confluent. Hilar and mediastinal node enlargement occurs and the periphery of the nodes calcifies producing an 'eggshell' appearance. Silicosis is now an uncommon condition in developed countries and sarcoidosis is a more common cause of these appearances. However, silicosis remains a problem in less developed countries. PMF occurs infrequently in silicosis (Figure 68.5).[36]

Table 68.1 International Labour Organization classification.

Feature	Code	Definition
Small opacities		
Rounded		
Size	p	Up to 1.5 mm diameter
	q	1.5–3 mm diameter
	r	3–10 mm diameter
Profusion	1[a]	Few in number
	2[a]	Numerous, lung markings visible
	3[a]	Very numerous, lung markings obscured
Irregular		
Type	s	Fine irregular or linear
	t	Medium irregular
	u	Coarse irregular
Profusion	1[a]	Few, lung markings visible
	2[a]	Numerous, lung markings partially obscured
	3[a]	Very numerous, lung markings totally obscured
Large opacities		
Size	A	1–5 cm
	B	Larger than 5 cm, but smaller than area of the right upper lobe
	C	Larger than the area of the right upper lobe
Pleural thickening		Site, calcification, extent and width
Pleural calcification		Site, calcification, extent and width

[a]Each point on the scale is subdivided, e.g. 1/2.

People with silicosis are at increased risk of tuberculosis; this may lead to new upper lobe shadowing on serial radiographs and cavitation of confluent silicotic nodules.

HRCT demonstrates changes not appreciable on chest radiography. These include emphysema, bronchial dilatation and, on expiratory sections, air trapping.[37]

Asbestos exposure

With the decline in coal mining in the United Kingdom, asbestosis is now the most frequently encountered pneumoconiosis. The radiological features can be considered under three headings: pleural disease, pulmonary diseases and extrathoracic manifestations.

PLEURAL DISEASE

Pleural plaques are the most frequent radiological feature of asbestos exposure. They form well-defined, rather angular densities. These are most easily seen on the chest radiograph when they lie along the lateral chest wall or over the diaphragm, since in these positions they lie tangential to the x-ray beam rather than *en face*. The plaques may calcify

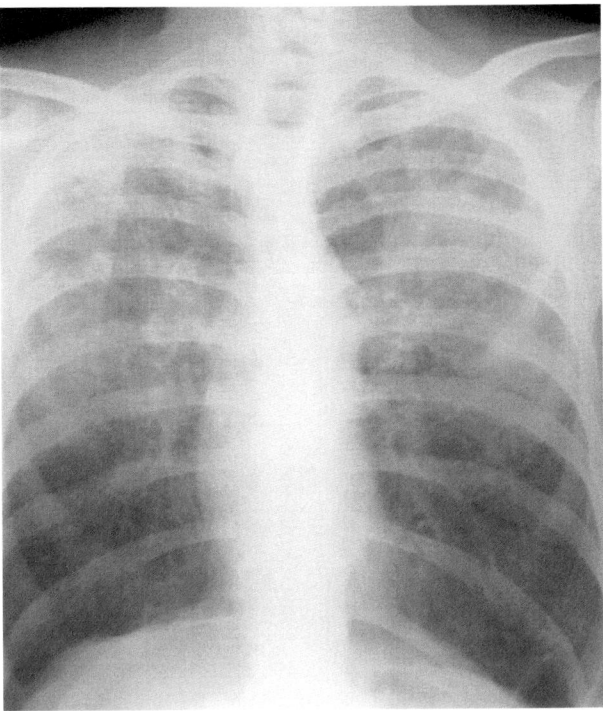

Figure 68.5 Chronic silicosis in a patient who had worked in the china clay industry. Confluent nodules are present in the upper lobes of both lungs with fibrosis producing loss of volume in the upper lobes and upward displacement of the pulmonary hila.

producing a 'holly leaf' appearance (Figure 68.6). The full extent of plaque deposition is most reliably assessed by CT (Figure 68.7).[38] On chest radiographs, the appearance of plaques can be mimicked by subpleural fat deposits and prominent intercostal muscles; however, CT can differentiate these appearances.[39] Pleural plaques are almost specific to asbestos exposure, although they are occasionally seen in workers exposed to other silicates.[40]

Diffuse pleural thickening is less common than pleural plaques, but unlike pleural plaques it may lead to a restrictive functional abnormality if it encases the lung. The thickening varies in thickness and has tapered, ill-defined margins. Asbestos-induced pleural thickening uncommonly calcifies and this helps to differentiate it from thickening secondary to empyemas and haemothoraces (Figure 68.8). As with pleural plaques, the extent of pleural thickening is best assessed by CT.[41]

Pleural effusions, as a manifestation of asbestos exposure, are indistinguishable radiologically from other pleural effusions. Although they are the most frequent radiographic manifestation of asbestos exposure in the first decade after the onset of exposure, they are not common, occurring in only 3 per cent of workers in one series.[42] However, in some areas, asbestos exposure is an important cause of pleural effusions with no other obvious cause. Not uncommonly an effusion in an asbestos worker is secondary to an underlying bronchial carcinoma or mesothelioma.

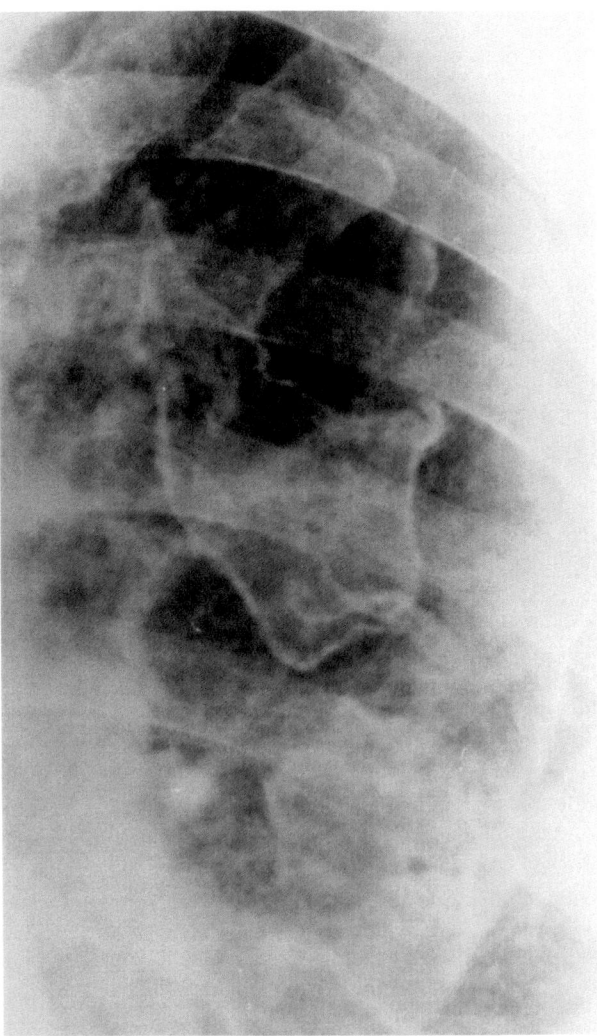

Figure 68.6 Part of a chest radiograph in an asbestos worker, demonstrating a calcified pleural plaque. The plaque has a typical 'holly leaf' appearance.

Malignant mesothelioma is accompanied by a pleural effusion in approximately two-thirds of cases and this is often the main radiographic feature, obscuring the underlying tumour. The tumour itself forms a well-defined lobular mass with tongues of tissue extending over the pleural surface producing encasement of the lung in the affected hemithorax. The ribs appear crowded due to the shrinkage of the underlying lung, but rib destruction is an uncommon feature (Figure 68.9). The tumour can spread through the diaphragm. The features are most easily appreciated on CT (Figure 68.10).[43,44] Although biopsy can be obtained by CT or ultrasound guidance, this is one of the few tumours which can seed along the biopsy track and prophylactic radiotherapy should be administered to the biopsy site.[45] The main radiological differential diagnosis is of metastatic pleural tumour, particularly adenocarcinomas. Pleural thickening and thymic tumours, which have a predilection to extend into the pleura, can produce similar appearances.

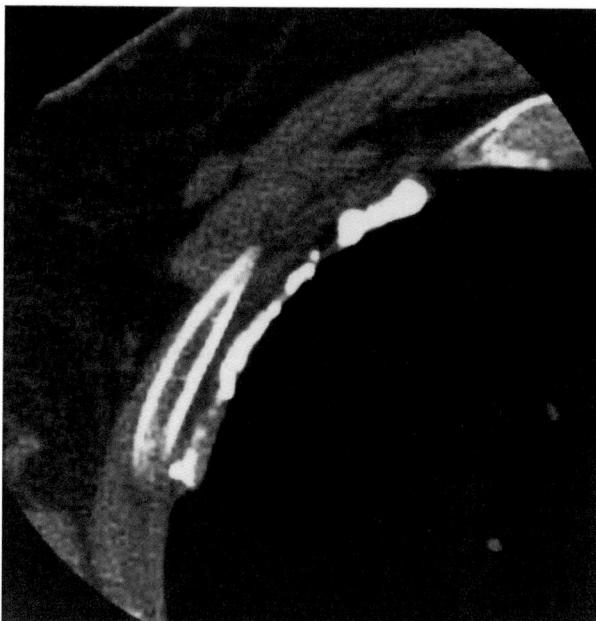

Figure 68.7 Magnified section from a CT scan demonstrating a pleural plaque. The lesion shows the typical well-defined margin and is of uniform thickness.

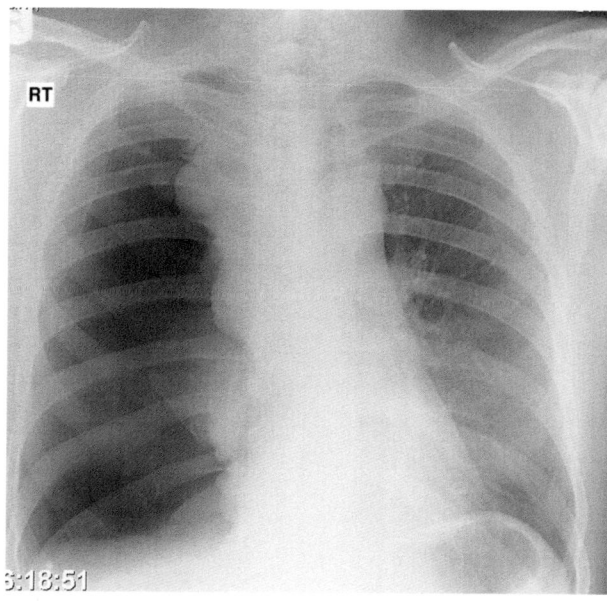

Figure 68.9 A chest radiograph in a patient with a malignant mesothelioma in the right thorax who has developed a large pneumothorax following pleural aspiration. The tumour is clearly outlined by the adjacent air and is seen to produce an extensive lobulated mass extending over the pleural surface.

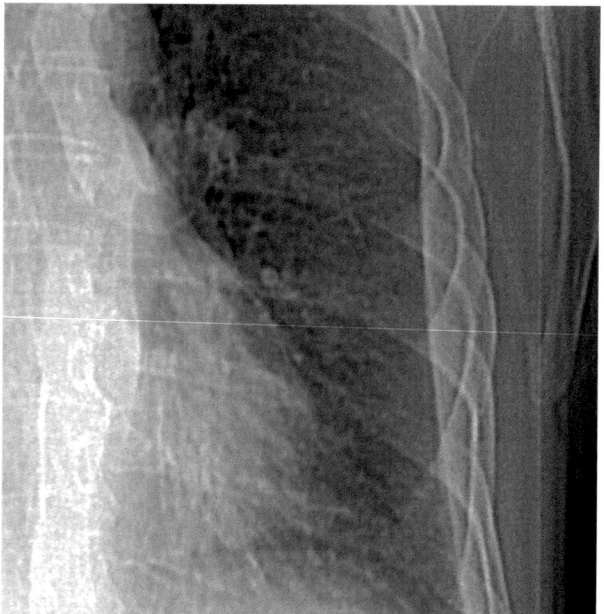

Figure 68.8 Part of a chest radiograph showing an extensive pleural thickening in an asbestos worker. Unlike pleural plaques, pleural thickening usually has a tapered margin, is variable in thickness and often extends over a much greater area.

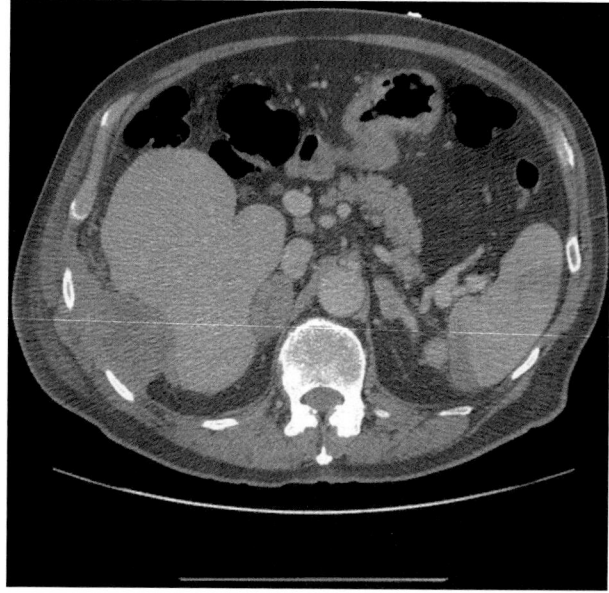

Figure 68.10 A CT section through the upper abdomen in a patient with a right pleural malignant mesothelioma. The tumour has extended through the diaphragm and is seen to lie between the liver and the posterolateral abdominal wall.

PULMONARY DISEASE

Asbestosis is characterized, on the chest radiograph, by the presence of fine reticular basal shadowing producing loss of clarity of the cardiac silhouette. Increased public awareness in North America and Europe has meant that patients are often investigated when the extent of pulmonary fibrosis is mild, frequently before the radiographic features are visible on a standard chest radiograph and the radiological changes are detectable only on HRCT.

The main HRCT features are ill-defined areas of subpleural high attenuation, linear parenchymal band opacities due to fibrotic strands, peripheral reticulation and curvilinear subpleural densities.[46,47] These features are most commonly encountered at the posterior lung base and for this reason prone HRCT sections should be performed to prevent them being obscured by hypostatic change (Figure 68.11a,b). Although typical of asbestosis, the features described are not specific and are seen in other fibrotic lung conditions, particularly usual interstitial pneumonia (UIP) and differentiation can be problematic.[48]

Pulmonary pseudotumour, also referred to as round atelectasis or folded lung, is caused by a severe local inflammatory reaction occurring in the lung periphery adjacent to an area of pleural thickening. It produces a well-defined rounded opacity, usually in the lower lobes and more commonly on the right.[49] HRCT shows the adjacent pulmonary vessels dragged into the mass producing a whorled appearance described as the 'comet tail' or 'vacuum cleaner' sign (Figure 68.12).[50]

Bronchial carcinoma, occurring in patients with asbestosis, has no distinguishing radiological features from bronchial carcinoma occurring in other patients, although there is an increased incidence of synchronous and metachronous tumours.

EXTRATHORACIC MANIFESTATIONS

Peritoneal mesothelioma occurs almost exclusively after asbestos exposure. The tumour forms a dense cicatrizing mass that encases loops of small bowel and mesenteric vessels. Barium studies show areas of strictured bowel with fixity and loss of peristaltic activity. The tumour mass and any associated ascites are well seen on CT.[51,52]

Siderosis and stannosis

Iron and tin are both inert dusts and do not excite an inflammatory reaction when they are inhaled. However, they produce striking radiological features. Due to their relatively high atomic number (iron = 26, tin = 50) compared to the majority of elements in the soft tissues (carbon = 6, nitrogen = 7 and oxygen = 8), they are radiographically dense and produce a myriad of small, high-density nodules. The nodules of stannosis tend to be smaller but denser than those of siderosis (Figure 68.13). The appearances can appear similar to other causes of miliary mottling, such as miliary tuberculosis or miliary metastatic deposits. However, the density of the nodules should allow differentiation.

Berylliosis

The main adverse effects of beryllium are observed in the lung. Acute exposure to high concentrations of beryllium can cause an acute pneumonitis. The chest radiograph

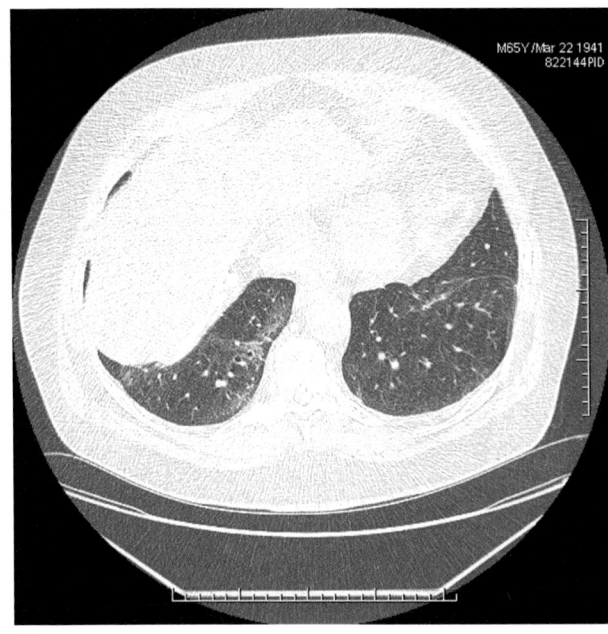

(a)

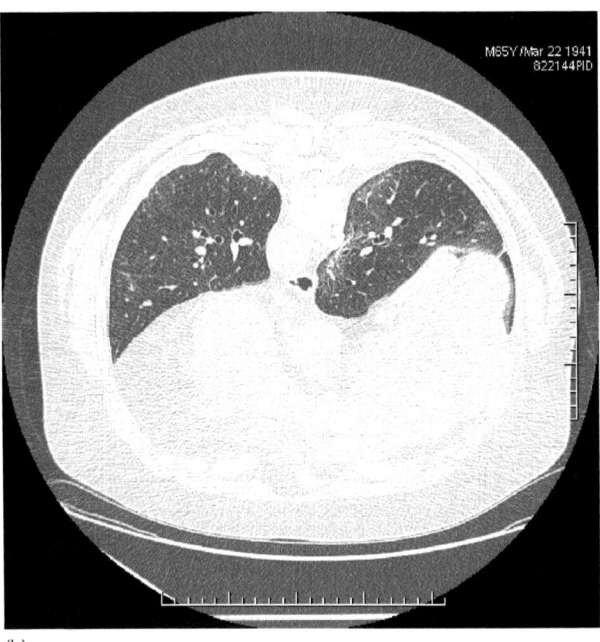

(b)

Figure 68.11 (a) A CT section through the lung bases in a patient with asbestosis demonstrating fine reticular changes at the right base. Note the dilatation of the adjacent bronchi due to traction. Less severe changes are also present at the left base. (b) A prone CT section in the same patient confirms that the abnormalities observed at the right base are constant and are not due to hypostatic changes.

shows patchy airspace opacities which resolve rapidly on removal from exposure. More frequently occurring is chronic beryllium lung disease. Prolonged low-dose exposure produces, in a minority of individuals, a chronic granulomatous reaction affecting the lungs and thoracic

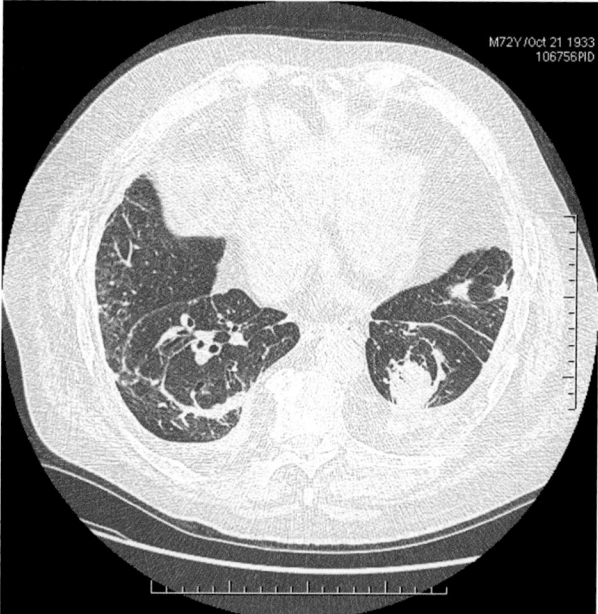

Figure 68.12 A CT section in a patient with severe asbestosis and an area of round atalectasis at the left base. The atalectatic mass typically lies adjacent to an area of pleural thickening and shows indrawing of the local pulmonary vessels to produce a 'comet tail' appearance.

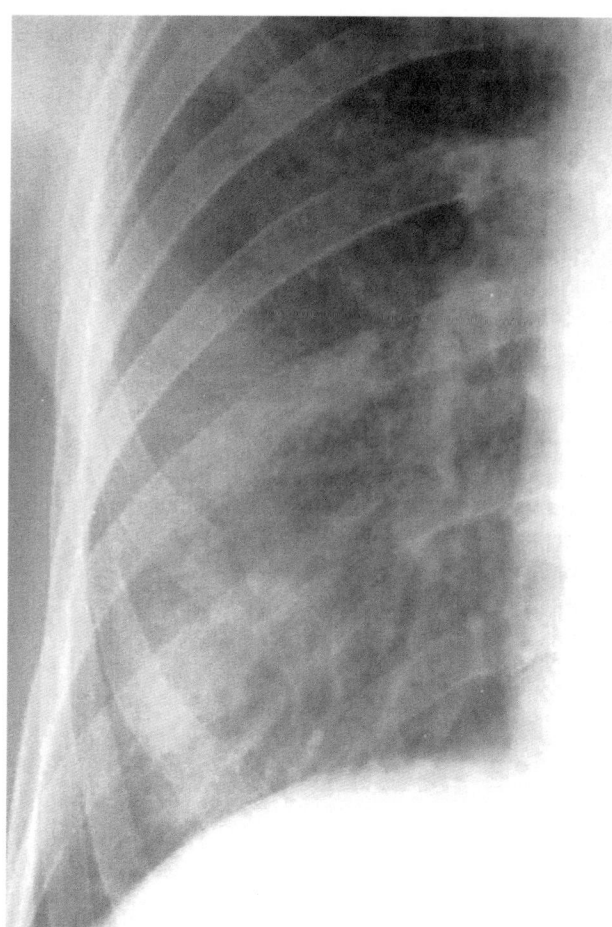

Figure 68.14 A section of a chest radiograph in a woman with extrinsic allergic alveolitis. There is fine hazy 'ground-glass' opacification at the right base. She had a budgerigar at home and the area of abnormality resolved rapidly on admission to hospital. Her avian precipitins were strongly positive.

lymph nodes. The radiological features are similar to those seen in sarcoidosis with bilateral nodular pulmonary infiltrates predominantly affecting the mid and upper zones of the lungs often with associated hilar and mediastinal lymphadenopathy.[53]

Extrinsic allergic alveolitis

In its acute form, extrinsic allergic alveolitis (EAA) produces widespread, ill-defined, small opacities. These are almost invariably bilateral, although the extreme lung bases and apices are often spared.[54] The opacities are not particularly dense and produce a hazy veiled appearance to the lungs, described as 'ground-glass' opacification (Figure 68.14). The opacities are fleeting and in a substantial proportion of patients, the chest radiograph is normal at the time of presentation. HRCT shows abnormalies more frequently than the chest radiograph and is particularly effective in demonstrating the 'ground-glass' appearances (Figure 68.15).[55]

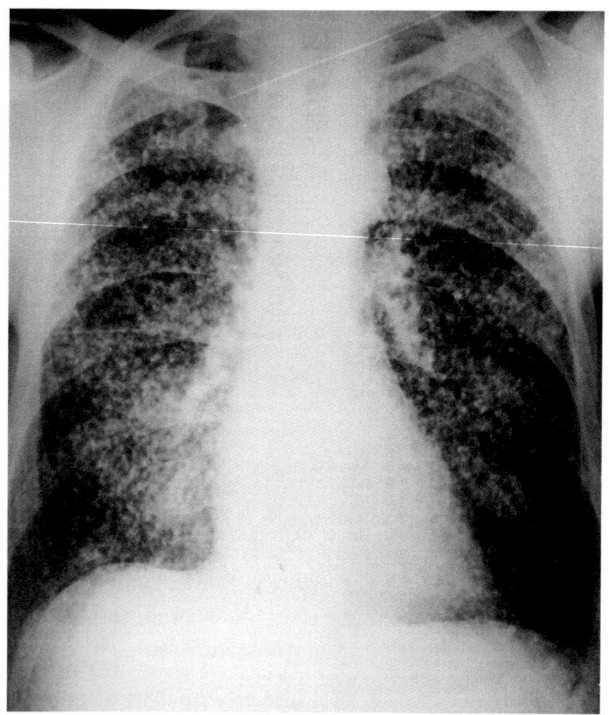

Figure 68.13 A chest radiograph in a patient with extensive stannosis. There are multiple small, well-defined high density nodules present within the lungs. Despite these appearances, the patient was asymptomatic.

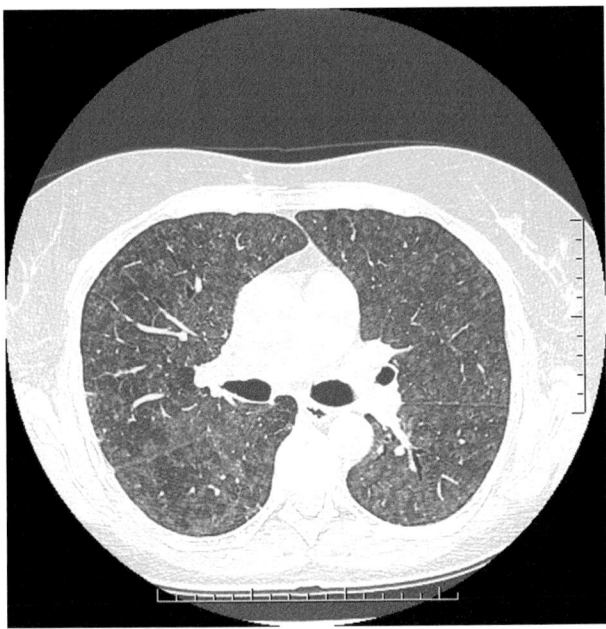

Figure 68.15 A CT section in a patient with extrinsic allergic alveolitis. There is extensive 'ground-glass' opacification with small foci of lower density within them, due to areas of air trapping. These features are often more conspicuous on sections obtained during expiration.

Pleural effusions and nodal enlargement are uncommon and this helps differentiate the condition from infective pneumonias.

In the chronic form of EAA, fibrosis occurs, typically in the upper lobes. The radiological differentiation from other causes of upper zone fibrosis, including sarcoidosis and tuberculosis, may be difficult, but pleural thickening, pulmonary and nodal calcification do not occur in EAA.

Pulmonary infections

A wide variety of animal workers are at potential risk of contracting animal-borne infections.[56] The most common are brucellosis, psittacosis and Q fever.

Brucella infection produces an acute pneumonic illness with areas of consolidation visible on the chest radiograph. Hilar and mediastinal lymph node enlargement occurs. In chronic brucellosis, multiple bilateral nodular opacities are present and the appearances can resemble sarcoidosis.

Psittacosis and Q fever both produce pneumonic changes. The radiographic features are indistinguishable from other forms of pneumonia, although Q fever can pursue a chronic course.

Some workers are at increased risk of infection from human sources. Examples include an increased incidence of tuberculous infection in mortuary attendants and influenza in healthcare workers. The radiographic appearances in these workers are identical to those observed in non-occupational cases of infection.

INTERNATIONAL LABOUR ORGANIZATION CLASSIFICATION

In 1930 the International Labour Organization (ILO) published a system for the classification of radiographs of the pneumoconioses. This has been revised on several occasions, most recently in 2002.[57] The system combines qualitative descriptions with qualitative assessments. In order to standardize the classification, the ILO publishes a series of reference radiographs. In addition, the ILO recommends the technical parameters which must be met to allow the radiograph to be classified. These parameters include the type of film used and the exposure of the film. In the United States, radiologists and physicians wishing to apply the classification must attend a training programme to become accredited readers. The widespread use of digital imaging will have an impact on the use of the ILO classification as the conspicuity and appearances of lesions are modified by these techniques. At the time of writing, the National Institute of Occupational Safety and Health in the United States recommends the continued use of conventional radiographs, although it is likely that in the near future a revised ILO classification based on digital radiographs will be introduced.

The aim of the classification is to standardize radiographic classification of the pneumoconioses. It is intended for use in research, epidemiological or statutory investigations; it is not a tool for routine clinical practice.

There are several components which are considered and coded in the classification:

1. Film quality. The quality of the radiograph, which is recorded on a three-point scale. Grade 1 is optimal and abnormalities in exposure, position or processing artefacts, which affect the film quality, are recorded.
2. Small opacities. These are divided into regular and irregular opacities. The regular opacities are graded by size, the irregular opacities by width. The profusion of these opacities is then assessed. Using the short form of the classification, a four-point profusion scale is used, a 12-point scale is used in the extended form.
3. Large opacities. These are graded by size. They are usually few in number and profusion is not considered.
4. Pleural plaques. These are assessed for site, calcification, extent and width.
5. Pleural thickening. In the short form, this is assessed as present or absent. In the extended form, the position, thickness and extent of thickening are recorded for each hemithorax.
6. Additional features. There is a list of additional features which are also recorded. These include the presence of cancer, bullae, effusions and cavities.

Table 68.2 Additional features.

	Feature		Feature
aa	Atherosclerotic aorta	em	Marked emphysema
at	Apical pleural thickening	es	Eggshell calcification of hilar or mediastinal lymph nodes
ax	Coalescence of small rounded opacities	hi	Enlargement of hilar or mediastinal lymph nodes
bu	Bullae	ho	Honeycomb lung
ca	Cancer of lung or pleura	kl	Septal (Kerley) lines
cn	Calcification in small pneumoconiotic opacities	me	Mesothelioma
co	Abnormality of cardiac size or shape	pa	Plate atelectasis
cp	Cor pulmonale	od	Other significant disease. This includes disease not related to dust exposure
cg	Calcified granuloma	px	Pneumothorax
cv	Cavity	ra	Round atelectasis
di	Marked distension of intrathoracic organs	tb	Tuberculosis
ef	Effusion		

The ILO classification (Table 68.2) was designed to be applied to chest radiographs. However, it has been applied to HRCT images.[58] The results, although correlated, are not transposable since HRCT demonstrates higher sensitivity for most of the components.[59]

Key points

- Chest radiography in occupational lung disease requires meticulous attention to detail to ensure standardization and reproducibility of the images.
- Digital radiography has largely replaced conventional radiography in developed countries.
- High resolution computed tomography is more sensitive than chest radiography in the assessment of the majority of patients with occupational lung disease.
- The radiographic appearances of many occupational lung diseases are similar to other, more common, non-occupational diseases.
- The International Labour Organization classification is a tool for epidemiological, research and statutory compliance, rather than clinical evaluation.

REFERENCES

1. Reynolds RA. Digital radiology and PACS. In: Grainger RG, Allison DJ (eds). *Diagnostic radiology: A textbook of medical imaging.* London: Churchill Livingstone, 1997: 5–19.
2. Glazer HS, Muka MA, Sagel SS, Jost RG. New techniques in chest radiography. *Radiological Clinics of North America.* 1994; **32**: 711–29.
3. Cowen AG, Davies AG, Kengyelics SM. Advances in computed radiography systems and their physical imaging characteristics. *Clinical Radiology.* 2007; **62**: 1132–41.
4. Aberle DR, Hansell D, Huang HK. Current status of digital projection radiography of the chest. *Journal of Thoracic Imaging.* 1990; **5**: 10–18.
5. Ambrose J. Computerised transverse axial scanning (tomography). Part 2: Clinical applications. *British Journal of Radiology.* 1973; **46**: 1023–47.
6. Katz D, Kreel L. Computed tomography in asbestosis. *Clinical Radiology.* 1979; **30**: 207–13.
7. McLoud TC, Wittenberg J, Ferucci JT. Computed tomography of the thorax and standard radiographic evaluation of the chest – a comparative study. *Journal of Computer Assisted Tomography.* 1979; **3**: 170–80.
8. Nakata H, Kimoto T, Nakayama T et al. Diffuse peripheral lung disease: Evaluation by high resolution computed tomography. *Radiology.* 1985; **157**: 181–5.
9. Muller NL. Clinical value of high resolution CT in chronic diffuse lung disease. *American Journal of Roentgenology.* 1991; **157**: 1163–70.
10. Padley SPG, Adler B, Muller NL. High resolution computed tomography of the chest: Current indications. *Journal of Thoracic Imaging.* 1993; **8**: 189–99.
11. Mayo JR, Webb WR, Gould R, Stein MG, Bass I, Gamsu G et al. High resolution CT of the lungs: An optimal approach. *Radiology.* 1987; **163**: 507–10.
12. Mayo JR. High resolution computed tomography: Technical aspects. *Radiologic Clinics of North America.* 1991; **26**: 1043–9.
13. Desai SR, Hansell DM. Small airways disease: Expiratory computed tomography comes of age. *Clinical Radiology.* 1997; **52**: 332–7.
14. Chooi WK, Morcos SK. High resolution volume imaging of airways and lung parenchyma with multislice CT. *British Journal of Radiology.* 2004; **77** (Spec No 1): S98–105.
15. Nishino M, Kuroki M, Boiselle PM et al. Sagittal reformations of volumetric inspiratory and expiratory high-resolution CT of the lung. *Academic Radiology.* 2004; **11**: 1282–90.
16. Rydberg J, Sandrasegaran K, Tarver RD et al. Routine isotropic computed tomography scanning of chest: Value of coronal and sagittal reformations. *Investigational Radiology.* 2007; **42**: 23–8.
17. Lipscombe DJ, Flower CDR, Hadfield JW. Ultrasound of the pleura: An assessment of its clinical value. *Clinical Radiology.* 1981; **32**: 289–90.

18. Chang DB, Yang PC, Luh KT et al. Ultrasound guided pleural biopsy with Tru-Cut needle. *Chest.* 1991; **100**: 1328–33.
19. Bradley WG, Bydder GM, Worthington BS. Magnetic resonance imaging: Basic principles. In: Grainger RG, Allison DJ (eds). *Diagnostic radiology: A textbook of medical imaging.* London: Churchill Livingstone, 1997: 63–81.
20. Webb WR, Sostman HD. MR imaging of thoracic disease: Clinical uses. *Radiology.* 1992; **182**: 621–30.
21. Mohiaddin RH, Longmore DB. Functional aspects of cardiovascular nuclear magnetic resonance imaging: Techniques and application. *Circulation.* 1993; **88**: 264–81.
22. Mayo JR. Magnetic resonance imaging of the chest. *Radiologic Clinics of North America.* 1994; **32**: 795–809.
23. Moiuddin M, Rockett J. Gallium scintigraphy in the detection of amiodarone lung toxicity. *American Journal of Roentgenology.* 1986; **147**: 607.
24. Kramer EL, Sanger JH, Garay SM et al. Diagnostic implications of Ga^{67} chest scan patterns in HIV seropositive patients. *Radiology.* 1989; **170**: 671–6.
25. Hayes AA, Mullan B, Lovegrove FT et al. Gallium lung scanning and broncho alveolar lavage in crocidolite exposed workers. *Chest.* 1989; **96**: 22–6.
26. Bourke SJ, Banham SW, McKillop JH, Boyd G. Clearance of ^{99m}Tc DTPA in pigeon fanciers hypersensitivity pneumonitis. *American Review of Respiratory Disease.* 1990; **142**: 1168–71.
27. Minty BD, Jordan C, Jones JG. Rapid improvement in abnormal pulmonary permeability after stopping cigarettes. *British Medical Journal.* 1981; **282**: 1183–6.
28. Stark P, Jacobson F, Schaffer K. Standard imaging in silicosis and coal workers pneumoconiosis. *Radiologic Clinics of North America.* 1992; **30**: 1147–54.
29. Cockcroft A, Berry G, Cotes JE, Lyons JP. Shape of small opacities and lung function in coalworkers. *Thorax* 1982; **37**: 765–9.
30. Collins HPR, Dick JA, Bennett JG et al. Irregularly shaped small shadows on chest radiographs, dust exposure, and lung function in coalworkers' pneumoconiosis. *British Journal of Industrial Medicine.* 1988; **45**: 43–55.
31. Savranlar A, Altin R, Mahmutyazicioğlu K et al. Comparison of chest radiography and high-resolution computed tomography findings in early and low-grade coal worker's pneumoconiosis. *European Journal of Radiology.* 2004; **51**: 175–8.
32. Wang X, Yu IT, Wong TW, Yano E. Respiratory symptoms and pulmonary function in coal miners: Looking into the effects of simple pneumoconiosis. *American Journal of Industrial Medicine.* 1999; **35**: 124–31.
33. Akkoca Yildiz O, Eris Gulbay B, Saryal S, Karabiyikoglu G. Evaluation of the relationship between radiological abnormalities and both pulmonary function and pulmonary hypertension in coal workers' pneumoconiosis. *Respirology.* 2007; **12**: 420–6.
34. Altin R, Savranlar A, Kart L et al. Presence and HRCT quantification of bronchiectasis in coal workers. *European Journal of Radiology.* 2004; **52**: 157–63.
35. Prendergrass EP. Silicosis and a few of the other pneumoconioses: Observations on certain aspects of the problem with emphasis on the role of the radiologist. *American Journal of Roentgenology.* 1958; **80**: 1–41.
36. Marchiori E, Ferreira A, Saez F et al. Conglomerated masses of silicosis in sandblasters: high-resolution CT findings. *European Journal of Radiology.* 2006; **59**: 56–9.
37. Arakawa H, Gevenois PA, Saito Y et al. Silicosis: Expiratory thin-section CT assessment of airway obstruction. *Radiology.* 2005; **236**: 1059–66.
38. Friedman AC, Fiel SB, Fisher MS et al. Asbestos related pleural disease: A comparison of CT and chest radiography. *American Journal of Roentgenology.* 1988; **150**: 269–75.
39. Sargent EN, Boswell WD, Ralls PW. Subpleural fat pads in patients exposed to asbestos: Distinction from non calcified pleural plaques. *Radiology.* 1984; **152**: 273–7.
40. Aberle DR, Gamsu G, Ray CS. Asbestos related pleural and parenchymal fibrosis: Detection with high resolution computed tomography. *Radiology.* 1986; **166**: 729–34.
41. Aberle DR, Balmes JR. Computed tomography of asbestos related pulmonary parenchymal and pleural disease. *Clinics in Chest Medicine.* 1991; **12**: 115–31.
42. Epler GR, McLoud TC, Gaensler EA. Prevalence and incidence of benign asbestos pleural effusion in a working population. *Journal of the American Medical Association.* 1982; **247**: 617–22.
43. Kawashima A, Libshitz H. Malignant pleural mesothelioma: CT manifestations in 50 cases. *American Journal of Roentgenology.* 1990; **155**: 965–9.
44. Ng CS, Munden RF, Libshitz HI. Malignant pleural mesothelioma: the spectrum of manifestations on CT in 70 cases. *Clinical Radiology.* 1999; **54**: 15–21.
45. Boutin C. Prevention of malignant seeding after invasive diagnostic procedures in patients with pleural mesothelioma. A randomised trial of local radiotherapy. *Chest.* 1995; **108**: 754–8.
46. Jones RN. The diagnosis of asbestosis. *American Review of Respiratory Disease.* 1991; **144**: 477–8.
47. Akira M, Yokoyama K, Yamamoto S et al. Early asbestosis: Evaluation with high resolution CT. *Radiology.* 1991; **178**: 409–16.
48. Akira M, Yamamoto S, Inoue Y, Sakatani M. High-resolution CT of asbestosis and idiopathic pulmonary fibrosis. *American Journal of Roentgenology.* 2003; **181**: 163–9.
49. Tylen U, Nilsson U. Computed tomography in asbestos pseudotumours and their relation to asbestos exposure. *Journal of Computer Assisted Tomography.* 1982; **6**: 229–37.
50. McHugh K, Blaquiere RM. CT features of rounded atelectasis. *American Journal of Roentgenology.* 1989; **153**: 257–60.
51. Whitley NO, Bohlman ME, Baker LP. CT patterns of mesenteric disease. *Journal of Computer Assisted Tomography.* 1982; **6**: 490–6.
52. Puvaneswary M, Chen S, Proietto T. Peritoneal mesothelioma: CT and MRI findings. *Australasian Radiology.* 2002; **46**: 91–6.

53. Meyer KC. Beryllium and lung disease. *Chest.* 1994; **106**: 942–6.
54. Cook PG, Wells IP, McGavin CR. The distribution of pulmonary shadowing in farmer's lung. *Clinical Radiology.* 1988; **39**: 21–27.
55. Hansell DM, Moskovic E. High resolution computed tomography in extrinsic allergic alveolitis. *Clinical Radiology.* 1991; **43**: 8–12.
56. Esposito AL. Pulmonary infection aquired in the workplace. *Clinics in Chest Medicine.* 1992; **13**: 355–65.
57. International Labour Office (ILO). Guidelines for the Use of the ILO International Classification of Radiographs of Pneumoconioses, rev edn 2000 (Occupational Safety and Health Series, No. 22). Geneva: International Labour Office: Geneva, 2002.
58. Kraus T, Raithell HG, Hering KG. Evaluation and classification of high resolution computed tomographic findings in patients with pneumoconiosis. *International Archives of Environmental and Occupational Health.* 1996; **68**: 249–54.
59. Remy-Jardin M, Degreef JM, Beuscart R *et al.* Coal workers pneumoconiosis: CT assessment in exposed workers and correlation with radiographic findings. *Radiology.* 1990; **177**: 363–7.

69

Work and chronic air flow limitation

DAVID J HENDRICK

Introduction	889	Chronic obstructive pulmonary disease and agents known to induce asthma	895
Definitions and epidemiology	889	Chronic obstructive pulmonary disease and agents not known to induce asthma	896
Historical background	890		
Uncertainties and controversies	890	Chronic obstructive pulmonary disease of subacute onset	898
Cigarette smoking – confounding and interactions	891		
Pathophysiology	892	Perspective in the population at large	899
Recognition of excessive decline in ventilatory function	892	Conclusions	900
		References	900

INTRODUCTION

Chronic air flow limitation results from a persistent diffuse reduction in airway calibre relative to the degree of lung inflation (i.e. airway obstruction), which cannot be reversed by treatment. The fixed nature of this obstruction is the cardinal feature, but this is shared by several pathogenically distinct disorders. They are recognized collectively to produce chronic obstructive pulmonary disease (COPD). The importance of COPD lies with its tendency to progress and to cause a disabling, even life-threatening, loss of lung function. It seems likely that 10–20 per cent of current cases can be attributed to occupational causes, but the evidence to confirm this has proved to be illusive. The investigatory difficulties that have arisen will consequently be reviewed in some detail, as will persisting uncertainties and controversies.

It has been conventional to apply the term COPD to fixed airway obstruction which develops insidiously over many years – long before any symptoms are recognized. Recent experience demands an adjustment to accommodate a few novel subacute causes which produce fixed airway obstruction over a matter of weeks or months at bronchiolar level (bronchiolitis obliterans). Bronchiolitis obliterans may also arise acutely as a rare complication of toxic lung injury (e.g. from gassing accidents or warfare), but this has been recognized for many decades and is beyond the scope of this chapter.

DEFINITIONS AND EPIDEMIOLOGY

Airway obstruction which responds partially, but not fully, to treatment implies there may be an asthmatic or acute bronchitic component to the disorder, of which the fixed component alone should be identified as COPD. The fixed component may itself be a consequence of long-standing asthma, but more commonly it is a consequence of emphysema or obstructive bronchiolitis. Bronchiectasis too often leads to COPD, but is an uncommon cause of COPD overall. Whether chronic bronchitis should be considered a cause depends on whether it is defined solely by a persistent, otherwise unexplained, productive cough – as it usually is. Many subjects with mucus hypersecretion (and hence chronic productive cough) have no airway obstruction, implying that when both chronic bronchitis and COPD do occur together, they are usually independent effects of the same inducing cause – for example, cigarette smoking.

It is estimated that about 10 per cent of adults are affected by COPD globally, depending on the diagnostic criteria used.[1] The prevalence is higher (about 14 per cent) in industrially developed countries,[2,3] with 1–2 per cent affected severely. Although most are smokers, as many as 3 per cent of never-smokers have COPD to some degree. COPD is currently the sixth leading cause of death globally and is projected to become fourth by 2020.[4] It is already ranked fourth in individuals aged over 45 years in Europe and the United States, and is responsible for 200–300 deaths per 100 000 per year in industrially developed countries.

Data from the third National Health and Nutrition Examination Survey (NHANES 3) suggest that 19 per cent of COPD in the United States overall can be attributed to work, while among never-smokers the percentage climbs to 31 per cent.[5] The American Thoracic Society estimates independently that about 15 per cent of COPD in the United States is occupationally induced.[6]

The recent Global Initiative on Obstructive Lung Disease (GOLD) adopted the commonly used value of 70 per cent for the ratio of forced expired volume in 1 second (FEV_1) to forced vital capacity (FVC) as the defining point for airway obstruction – that is, the lower limit of normality.[7] It is recognized that the ratio tends to fall as a normal consequence of ageing and so this definition may lead to the prevalence of COPD being underestimated in young adults, but overestimated in the elderly.

HISTORICAL BACKGROUND

That COPD might arise as a consequence of the occupational environment is a matter of evolving interest and importance, and not a little controversy. The possibility of COPD of occupational origin, unassociated with complicated pneumoconiosis, first gained widespread acceptance as recently as the 1960s as a result of a series of investigations in cotton workers by Schilling and Bouhuys and colleagues.[8,9] They suggested that cotton dust-induced airway disease (byssinosis) could be usefully classified into three distinct clinical grades. Workers who developed chest tightness and breathing difficulty only on the first working day of each week were said to have byssinosis grade 1; those who had similar symptoms on additional working days of the week, but who recovered fully away from the workplace, were said to have byssinosis grade 2; and those who had symptoms of persisting respiratory disability were said to have byssinosis grade 3. Physiological studies indicated that byssinosis grades 1 and 2 were associated with reversible airways obstruction, while byssinosis grade 3 was associated with fixed airways obstruction. It was assumed that affected workers followed an orderly progression through these escalating grades. Cotton dust was consequently a potential cause of COPD, and byssinosis grade 3 was the first documented example of occupational COPD.

The specific effects of cotton dust are discussed in detail in Chapter 73, Byssinosis and other cotton-related diseases, and so cotton dust and byssinosis will be mentioned here only to provide a convenient historical focus for reviewing the claims and controversies which have arisen subsequently from many occupational environments concerning COPD.

Many (perhaps most) authorities would now regard byssinosis grades 1 and 2 as occupational asthma attributable to cotton dust. The physiological correlates (acute, but reversible episodes of airway obstruction) are diagnostic of asthma, and the curious work-related periodicity of the symptoms (which had been considered particularly characteristic of byssinosis) has since been observed with other types of occupational asthma. As with active asthma of any aetiology, airway hyper-responsiveness can be demonstrated to a variety of bronchoconstrictor agents at times when byssinosis grade 1 or grade 2 is active. If, then, byssinosis grades 1 and 2 are examples of occupational asthma, is occupational COPD (i.e. byssinosis grade 3) simply a consequence of occupational asthma? This is certainly plausible, since long-standing asthma of non-occupational origin often results in fixed airway obstruction.

The relation of byssinosis grade 3 to byssinosis grades 1 and 2 may, however, be looked at from a different viewpoint to that adopted by Schilling and Bouhuys. The investigations which led to their grading classification were cross-sectional not longitudinal in structure. Grade 1 byssinosis was not, in fact, observed to progress to grade 3 byssinosis, and so it is conceivable that byssinosis grade 3 is a fundamentally different disorder from byssinosis grades 1 and 2, albeit one which is also induced by occupational exposure to cotton dust. If this is so, byssinosis grade 3 could be regarded as the prototype for occupational COPD, and the question arises whether it is likely that cotton dust alone among occupational agents would have this effect on the airways?

Most of the cotton workers of the 1960s had been heavy cigarette smokers for many years, and doubts were expressed subsequently whether the confounding effect of this on the development of COPD (which was barely recognized in the 1960s) was adequately taken into account.[10] Although recent investigations have confirmed that COPD does arise as a consequence of occupational exposure to cotton dust independently of smoking,[11,12] this relationship remained uncertain for many years, and the confounding role of cigarette smoking came to lie at the centre of current controversies.

UNCERTAINTIES AND CONTROVERSIES

The experience with the cotton industry provides invaluable lessons for the assessment of occupational COPD, and for evaluating today's inevitable controversies. In essence, they centre on whether an excess prevalence of COPD in a given working population has arisen from some other cause (such as smoking or asthma), rather than the working environment, and whether, if the workplace is responsible, COPD arises independently of occupational asthma or as a direct consequence of it – or both (Figure 69.1).[13]

There is a further source of confusion – regular exposure to respirable dusts and irritant gases/vapours commonly leads to mucus hypersecretion and to chronic productive cough (i.e. chronic bronchitis). In an occupational setting, this is often termed 'industrial bronchitis'. When chronic bronchitis develops coincidentally alongside asthma (whether occupational or not), the emergence of obstructive

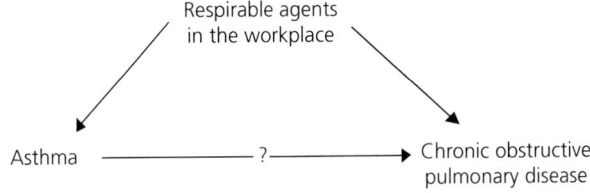

Figure 69.1 Pathways to chronic obstructive pulmonary disease. From: *Thorax*, 1995, **50** (Suppl. 1), S16–S21, reproduced with permission from the BMJ Publishing Group.

symptoms (wheeze, chest tightness, undue shortness of breath) is often attributed, not unreasonably, to COPD and to the cause of the productive cough.

The possible presence of coincidental asthma (now a common disease at all ages in the population at large) may consequently simulate occupational COPD. This is particularly likely if industrial bronchitis or smoker's bronchitis coexists. Asthma of non-occupational origin may also simulate occupational asthma because it is likely to worsen transitorily in the workplace if there are respirable irritants, and in some occupational settings (e.g. cotton mills) the development of occupational asthma is as plausible as the development of occupational COPD. If it is true that there are substantial differences in the prevalence of asthma from region to region, from population to population and from birth cohort to birth cohort, as is now suggested, formidable difficulties must be expected in allowing for this if a given working population appears to show an excess of COPD.

The difficulty in distinguishing between asthma and COPD is compounded by the common occurrence of both disorders in the same individual. When this does occur, however, the clinical features tend to resemble those of COPD alone much more closely than asthma alone – as pointed out in the recent American Thoracic Society statement, 'Occupational contribution to the burden of airway disease'.[6]

CIGARETTE SMOKING – CONFOUNDING AND INTERACTIONS

The relative effects of smoking and occupation on COPD can only be assessed from epidemiological investigations where study populations include smokers and non-smokers, and workers with different levels of the relevant occupational exposure (some, ideally, with none). There may be difficulty in finding such a balanced population, and there may be difficulty in avoiding bias in the exposure histories which are obtained. The investigation of possible occupationally induced disease often leads to anxiety, anger and claims for compensation in at least some of the study population. Once these arise, memory for the noxious nature of former workplace environments may prove to be better preserved than that of former tobacco consumption.

Table 69.1 Current or former smoking habits of apprentices compared with workers.

	No.	Smokers (per cent)
Workers		
Low exposure	179	30
Medium exposure	219	39
High exposure	284	58
School leavers		
Low exposure	53	9
Medium exposure	126	21
High exposure	75	36

Data taken from Ref. 14.

An important additional tendency is for those who are best able to tolerate the heaviest levels of tobacco consumption to take on jobs with the most noxious occupational exposures (and vice versa), or for cultural or family influences to link smoking with recruitment to particular types of work. This inevitably confounds any potential effect of the work environment with that of smoking, and is illustrated in Table 69.1.[14] Here, the smoking habits of 15- to 16-year-old school leavers applying for a range of apprenticeships associated with three levels of exposure to noxious working environments (low, medium, high concentrations of welding fume) are compared with established workers aged 19–26 years in the same trade groups. The clear differences in current smoking prevalence seen between the occupational exposure groups of the workers can also be observed in the school leavers before any occupational exposure occurred, though age exerted an additional effect and increased the prevalences in the older workers in all work-exposure categories.

Smoking is thus likely to be associated with the very occupational environments which are themselves suspected of causing COPD. This may lead not only to confounding, but to an exaggerated survival bias. The most susceptible workers are likely to leave the particular working environment prematurely if they develop COPD (whether from smoking, occupational exposure or both), thereby producing a surviving population which is less severely affected. Investigation of the surviving workers will underestimate the occupational hazard involved. Furthermore, those workers who are initially less able (or less willing) to tolerate noxious exposures will avoid the relevant working environments and this will exert an additional bias (healthy-worker effect) on the selection of populations who work with the risk of developing occupational lung disease. Investigators, regulating bodies, employers and employees may be hard-pressed to recognize when longitudinal loss of ventilatory function in a working population is truly excessive once the idiosyncratic effect of cigarette smoking is taken into account. Full smoking histories are consequently essential in research, and should include a quantitative measure of cumulative consumption.

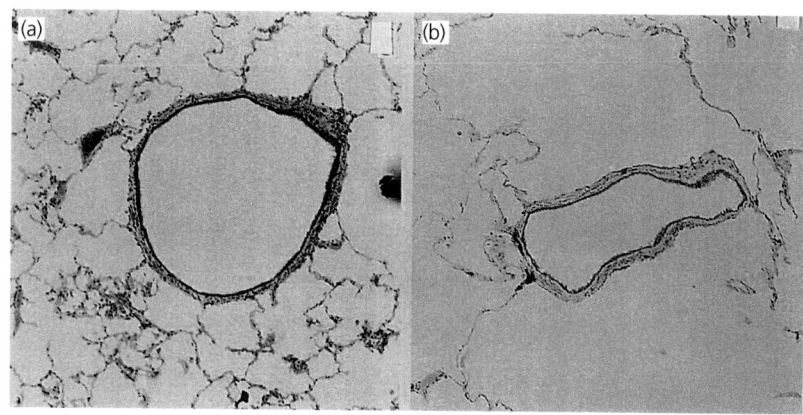

Figure 69.2 Histology of a bronchiole and the surrounding lung tissue in (a) normal lung and (b) emphysema.

The issue is unduly complicated because only a minority of smokers (15–20 per cent) appear to develop COPD (hence the idiosyncrasy) and because doubts over the accuracy of past smoking histories may invalidate, or at least weaken, the statistical analyses involved. There may be strong justification for such doubts. In a UK study of the population at large, it was concluded that up to 7 per cent of smokers and former smokers had described themselves incorrectly as never-smokers,[15] while in an American study of coal miners seeking compensation, as many as 15 per cent claimed to be never-smokers despite recording in earlier assessments that they were regular smokers.[16]

PATHOPHYSIOLOGY

Fixed airway obstruction, when not due to chronic asthma, may be a consequence of either destructive disease of the lung parenchyma and interstitium (emphysema), or of intrinsic inflammatory/fibrotic disease of the small intrathoracic airways (obstructive bronchiolitis). It is questionable whether mucus hypersecretion alone (chronic bronchitis) has this effect. With emphysema, airway obstruction and air trapping are associated additionally with impairment of gas transfer and loss of elastic recoil. It is this loss of elastic support to the smaller airways, whose walls are not supported by cartilage, which leads to airway collapse and obstruction (Figure 69.2), particularly during expiration. Most surveys attributing COPD to occupation have not included measurements of parenchymal function (gas transfer) and so it is unclear whether emphysema was the chief underlying mechanism.

Extensive work with COPD attributable to smoking has shown that emphysema is not always present. Even in the absence of emphysema, the smaller unsupported airways provide the most probable primary site for the obstruction to airflow, there being a mixed pathological picture of inflammation and fibrosis chiefly in and around the bronchioles. The disorder is more accurately described as obstructive bronchiolitis or bronchiolitis obliterans, than as chronic obstructive bronchitis (Figure 69.3). However, bronchial inflammation is often seen, especially when there is chronic productive cough. This is best regarded as an independent phenomenon and is often unassociated with airflow limitation. COPD is also associated with bronchiectasis, but the underlying mechanism is at present uncertain.

The potential importance of obstructive bronchiolitis has taken a new twist over the last few years with the recognition of subacute causes among workers inhaling certain food-flavouring materials, synthetic fibre flock and garment printing dyes. Disablement occurs within a matter of weeks or months of exposure onset, rather than years.

RECOGNITION OF EXCESSIVE DECLINE IN VENTILATORY FUNCTION

An epidemiological approach to estimating the rate of decline in ventilatory function offers the only practical means of identifying insidious occupational causes of COPD in living populations, though the evidence obtained has been tested experimentally in a number of animal models.[6] If the occupational contribution to COPD in a given workforce is relatively small and if COPD itself is uncommon (often the case in populations subjected to healthy worker and survivor biases), the investigation of large numbers of subjects will be necessary if an occupational effect is to be shown convincingly. Such investigations are necessarily time-consuming and expensive. They must also be complex if multiple regression techniques are to take adequate account of all the various factors which may independently influence the measured end point (i.e. the level of ventilatory function) or interact with environmental exposures of relevance. Otherwise, there is the risk that these factors (e.g. age, height, race, gender, social grouping, changing body mass, smoking, passive smoking, air pollution, viral infections, atopy, airway responsiveness) might be distributed unevenly between subgroups of the study population which differ also in the levels of exposure to the agent suspected of inducing COPD. If such unevenness occurs it

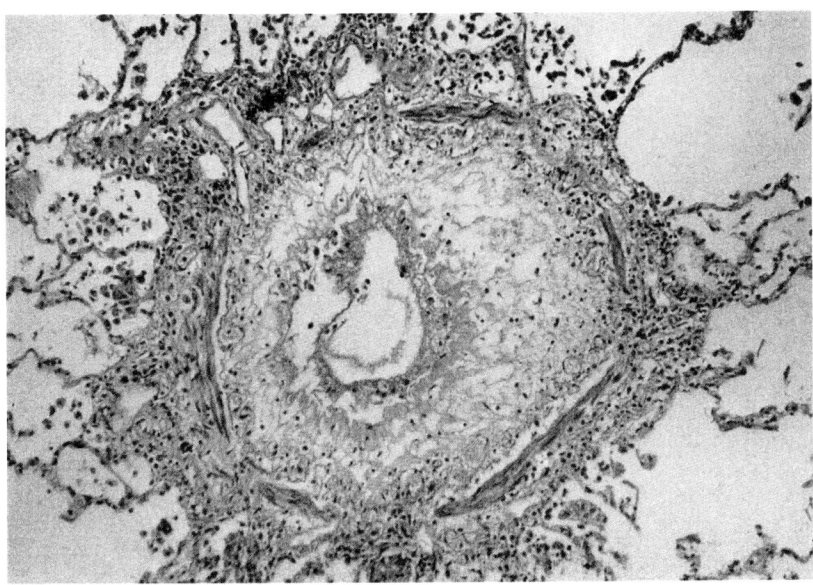

Figure 69.3 Histology of a bronchiole and the surrounding lung tissue in obstructive bronchiolitis.

might explain or exaggerate significant differences which appear otherwise to be a consequence of the occupational agent. Conversely, it might mask a true occupational effect in investigations which appear to give negative results.

Chronic obstructive pulmonary disease and cigarette smoking

From a series of pioneering epidemiological investigations of COPD attributable to cigarette smoking, Fletcher and colleagues[17] showed during the 1960s that the majority of smokers appeared to experience no adverse effect on ventilatory function. In the minority who were seen to be adversely affected, an excess annual decline in FEV_1 could be deduced from cross-sectional data (i.e. FEV_1 appeared to be excessively diminished in older subjects who had smoked). The magnitude of the apparent decline in FEV_1 with age (FEV_1 slope) was related to the level of smoking consumption. The mean annual decline among symptomatic smokers appeared to be approximately twice that of the non-smokers. The excess rate of decline could be detected after as little as five years of regular smoking and its cumulative dose-related effect was readily quantified by the degree of fixed airway obstruction evident already at the time of the initial measurement of ventilatory function.

A cohort of the men investigated cross-sectionally by Fletcher and colleagues (male transport and postal workers in London) was followed longitudinally, so that the actual annual changes in FEV_1 could be measured. The mean decline in FEV_1 (when standardized for height) was about 30 mL/year. The actual rates of decline were related to height, smoking and symptoms, and they appeared to increase a little with increasing age. The excess rate of decline in smokers ceased when they gave up the habit, but the damage already sustained was permanent (Figure 69.4). A similar natural history is to be expected from any cause of

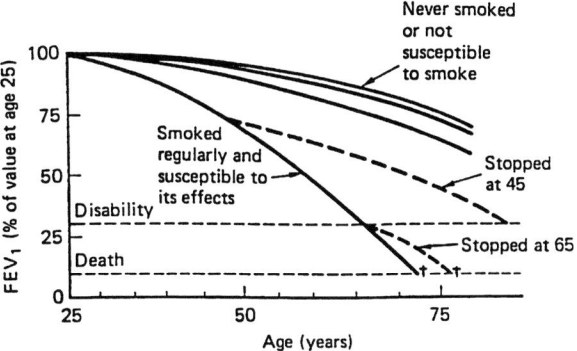

Figure 69.4 Decline in FEV_1 with age: Smokers versus non-smokers (reproduced from Ref. 80, where it was adapted from Ref. 17).

COPD, though there will be much variability from individual to individual, and in some of those affected many exposure years will pass before the disease becomes evident.

Discrepancy between cross-sectional and longitudinal data

When data from the London workers were analysed from the initial cross-sectional study, regression of FEV_1 on age suggested a rather greater mean annual decline of 46 mL/year. That is to say, the differences in FEV_1 between the youngest and oldest participants in the initial study suggested that the mean annual decline in FEV_1, after allowing for differences in height, was about 1.5 times the rate actually measured during the subsequent longitudinal phase of the investigation. The discrepancy was not readily explained at the time. It is a discrepancy which has since

Table 69.2 Age-related changes in ventilatory function: Cross-sectional versus longitudinal data.

Cross-sectional regressions of mean FEV_1 against age	Mean of longitudinal regressions of FEV_1 against time
1974 −42.6 mL/year	1974–79 (5 years) −12.4 mL/year
1975 −47.2 mL/year	1975–79 (4 years) −17.4 mL/year
1976 −44.9 mL/year	
1977 −50.5 mL/year	
1979 −44.6 mL/year	

Reproduced with permission from Ref. 18.
The investigation involved a 'normal' population of 52 adult caucasian males, aged 30–58 years, of whom nine were current smokers, 16 former smokers and 27 never-smokers. There were no relevant occupational exposures. Three subjects reported chronic cough and seven undue breathlessness. The initial 1974 measurements were slightly less than those of 1975, possibly reflecting inexperience with spirometric manoeuvres and so the period 1975–79 may provide a more accurate estimate of longitudinal change than 1974–79.

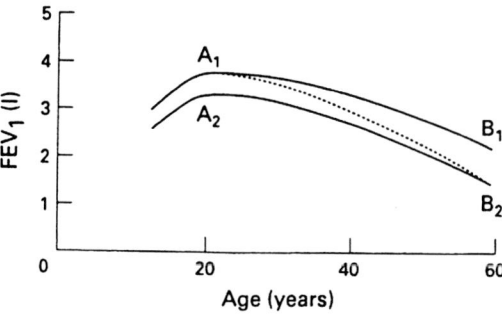

Figure 69.5 Discrepant mean decline in FEV_1 from cross-sectional and longitudinal data.
A1→B1 represents true (future) longitudinal decline in subjects currently aged 20 years.
A2→B2 represents true (completed) longitudinal decline in subjects currently aged 60 years.
A1→B2 represents apparent (current) decline using cross-sectional data from subjects currently aged 20–60 years.
From: *Thorax* 1996, **51**, 947–55 reproduced with permission from the BMJ Publishing Group.

been recognized by a number of investigators. Those from Tulane University demonstrated a more striking discrepancy when estimating the annual decline in FEV_1 from a longitudinal study over five years of a normal population of males aged 30–58 years.[18] The cross-sectional data from each survey year indicated a mean decline of 40–50 mL/year with increasing age, once the effect of height was taken into account, while the mean of the actual longitudinal declines measured in each participant was only 12.4 mL/year (Table 69.2).

Thus cross-sectional data cannot be extrapolated to predict longitudinal change with any precision and should not be compared directly with longitudinal data from other investigations. Much of the discrepancy arises because subjects at the younger end of an age spectrum of, say, 20–60 years from a current cross-sectional investigation do not necessarily have the same mean FEV_1 as did those at the older end of the spectrum some 40 years earlier when they were of a similar young age. In fact, the currently young subjects are likely to have greater values of FEV_1 at a standardized young age, partly because they have larger lungs and partly because they are less likely to have sustained respiratory diseases (e.g. tuberculosis, bronchiectasis) which impair ventilatory function. The difference in FEV_1 between younger and older subjects at the time of a cross-sectional study therefore exaggerates the true declines which were experienced by the older subjects during the preceding years. Furthermore, the currently young subjects are likely to encounter less lung damaging insults as they age to 60 years, compared with subjects who had already attained 60 years. Thus, mean longitudinal decline in lung function in populations is not wholly a consequence of increasing age and of cumulative exposure to cigarette smoke or occupational agents.

It depends also on the cumulative burden of all damaging pulmonary insults throughout the ageing period (Figure 69.5).

By using study subjects as their own controls and avoiding the problems which arise from mismatching in cross-sectional studies (i.e. by eliminating between-worker variability), longitudinal studies are inherently more satisfactory. They are less 'sensitive', however, because they detect change over the period of longitudinal surveillance only. By contrast, cross-sectional studies quantify the changes which have occurred throughout the lifetimes of the participants. Longitudinal studies may also be more vulnerable to diminishing participation rates, and this may introduce new risks of bias. They are also lengthy and very expensive.

Other non-occupational factors of possible relevance

The study of London transport and postal workers usefully suggested that although intercurrent episodes of respiratory tract viral infection (i.e. episodes of acute bronchitis, exacerbations of COPD) caused significant reductions in ventilatory function, the effect was only temporary. Full recoveries to former levels of ventilatory function were noted within a few weeks, after which the rate of longitudinal decline returned to its usual level. Repeated viral infections do not therefore influence the assessment of occupational COPD from either cross-sectional or longitudinal studies, provided there are no acute infections at the time of study. Whether intercurrent episodes of acute bronchitis following brief exposure to toxic chemicals at work (e.g. gassing accidents) will prove to be equally benign is currently a matter of much speculation, concern and ongoing investigation. Major accidents which produce life-threatening pulmonary toxicity are recognized to cause bronchiolitis obliterans in a small proportion of survivors, although the majority of survivors appear to recover fully. A few develop asthma, which may persist indefinitely and so pose a further pathway for the emergence of COPD.

This asthmatic complication of acute pulmonary toxicity (it may also follow a series of less toxic exposures, one alone having insufficient potency) has been termed the reactive airways dysfunction syndrome (RADS).[19,20] The term is unhelpful in one sense because it suggests, incorrectly, that RADS is a disorder distinct from asthma. However, it is helpful in another sense because it neatly categorises a major subgroup of occupational asthma cases (some 5–10 per cent overall) for which the mechanism is reasonably clear. For the remaining cases, the mechanism(s) is generally assumed to involve hypersensitivity pathways, but confirmatory evidence has been illusive for many causal agents (particularly low molecular weight chemicals) and with certain organic dusts (e.g. from cotton, grain, animal confinement buildings) endotoxin from contaminating Gram-negative microorganisms may play a critical role in inducing asthmatic responsiveness.[6]

Age, height, race, gender, smoking and increasing body mass all exert important influences on the measurement of ventilatory function, and it may be that passive smoking and air pollution during the course of longitudinal investigation will also exert potentially important (adverse) effects. The wide range of apparent individual susceptibility to COPD suggests a dependence on genetic factors and there is supportive evidence for this especially from twin studies.[21,22] Genetically determined atopy has not generally been found to influence COPD, but this depends on how COPD is defined and how vigorously an asthmatic contribution is excluded.

Analysis of data from the American Multicentre Lung Health Study suggests that airway responsiveness (to methacholine) may prove to be almost as important as cigarette smoking in exerting an adverse influence on the rate of decline in ventilatory function.[23] If it is confirmed that a measure of asthmatic activity is relevant to predicting the development of COPD (a relationship enshrined in what became known as the Dutch hypothesis of the 1970s and 1980s, but disputed thereafter), then factors of aetiological relevance to asthma may also need to be taken into account when studying COPD.[24,25] It may be useful, therefore, to consider the occupational agents (or environments) that have been associated with COPD in two categories – those which are also believed to cause asthma through 'non-RADS' pathways and those which are not. It may also be useful to classify them according to whether current evidence identifies them as 'definite or probable' causes of occupational COPD (Table 69.3) or merely 'possible' causes (Table 69.4).

Table 69.3 Definite and probable causes of occupational chronic obstructive pulmonary disease.

Agents thought to induce occupational asthma by hypersensitivity pathways

Cotton dust	Di-isocyanates
Grain dust	
Farm dusts	
Flour	

Other agents

Acramin dye – Ardystil syndrome	Flock (nylon, rayon, polypropylene)
Cadmium	Food (popcorn) flavouring – diacetyl
Coal mine dust	
Cotton dust	Silica

Table 69.4 Possible causes of occupational chronic obstructive pulmonary disease.

Agents thought to induce occupational asthma by hypersensitivity pathways

Wood dust

Other agents

Ammonia	Printing
Carbon black	Rubber and plastics manufacture
Concrete dust	Smoke (fire fighting)
Endotoxin	Sulphur dioxide/paper pulp dust and fume
Iron and steel foundry fume/dust	Vanadium
Leather work	Welding fume
Metal ore processing and smelting	Wollastonite
Nitrogen oxides	Wood/biomass smoke

CHRONIC OBSTRUCTIVE PULMONARY DISEASE AND AGENTS KNOWN TO INDUCE ASTHMA

Naturally occurring inducers of occupational asthma

Respiratory disease in grain workers has been widely recorded since the eighteenth century and the time of Ramazzini. Grain dust has become a particularly well-recognized cause of occupational asthma, although the precise causative agent (or agents) remains unclear. Storage mites, microbial contaminants, pesticides and fungicides, and even rodent urinary proteins have all been incriminated together with allergenic material derived from the grain itself. A number of investigators have produced impressive evidence that occupational exposure to grain dust may also lead to COPD, though none has suggested that this is a direct consequence of occupational asthma and most have found some inconsistencies among their data.[26,27] The uncertainty as to the precise causal agent extends to many other settings associated with occupational COPD (and asthma), and thus Tables 69.3 and 69.4 refer either to a particular agent or to a particular setting.

The experience of Chan-Yeung and colleagues[28] in the port of Vancouver provides a useful illustrative example. They followed port grain workers and control subjects working in civic centre posts between 1978 and 1990. After six years, the annual rates for the decline in FEV_1 were significantly greater among the grain workers (−31 mL/year) than the controls (+4 mL/year), but when the smokers alone were studied little difference was noted between grain workers and controls (−36 mL/year versus −31 mL/year). In this particular investigation, therefore, the grain–COPD effect was seen largely in the non-smokers (in whom asthma was not satisfactorily excluded though atopy proved to be irrelevant) and it appeared to be of similar magnitude to the smoking–COPD effect in the control workers. Furthermore, its demonstration depended on there being an unusually small annual decline in FEV_1 among the controls (in fact, there was a trivial increase). After 12 years, significant differences between grain workers and controls were no longer evident, but this may have been a consequence of survivor bias or of the greatly diminishing levels of grain dust exposure during the course of the investigation. Not all investigators have found this COPD effect. When it was observed, it was generally clearer among the smokers than non-smokers, contrary to the Vancouver experience.

Grain dust is also encountered by farm workers, who additionally encounter other types of occupational dust from harvesting and storing crops, hay and straw, and from handling and feeding livestock. Several asthmagenic agents may contribute to their risk of COPD, which has been demonstrated from a number of studies.[29] The refined product of grain, flour, is encountered by many workers beyond the farming community, and has proved to be a potent cause of allergic asthma and rhinitis. It too appears to cause COPD, not necessarily in association with asthma.

With wood dust, a further common cause of occupational asthma, evidence for a COPD effect is less strong. Again there is evidence that smokers may be unduly susceptible to it. This is noteworthy in view of the curious 'protective' effect of smoking observed with occupational asthma attributable to western red cedar.[30] A similar protective effect in smokers, for which there are plausible immunological explanations, has been observed with extrinsic allergic alveolitis and sarcoidosis, and so should not be dismissed too hastily.[31,32]

Chemical inducers of occupational asthma

In the United Kingdom in recent years, di-isocyanates have been a common cause of occupational asthma and di-isocyanate asthma continues to provide a typical example of asthma attributable to occupational chemicals. Not unnaturally, di-isocyanate workers have provided a focus for investigations, of which there have been many, of possible occupational COPD. The results have been conflicting. A major multicentre surveillance programme in the United Kingdom revealed no hint of a COPD effect, while study of a single di-isocyanate-producing plant in the United States suggested a crippling occupationally induced mean decline in FEV_1 exceeding 100 mL/year.[33,34] Both investigations may have been flawed: the one because there was an implausibly low prevalence of occupational asthma (and possibly a major survivor bias), the other because the levels of ventilatory function observed initially were too well preserved for an excessive decline of such a degree to have been occurring before the investigation commenced.

The five-year investigation of Diem and colleagues of workers in a new toluene di-isocyanate-manufacturing plant included an extensive series of exposure measurements, from which the workforce was usefully separated into categories of low–average cumulative exposure (<68.2 ppb-months) and high cumulative exposure (>68.2 ppb-months).[35] The high exposure group showed a significantly greater annual decline in FEV_1 (−37 mL/year) than the non-smokers of the low exposure group (+1 mL/year), but it was not influenced by smoking. Smoking did, however, lead to a similar excessive decline in those with low levels of di-isocyanate exposure. Thus, similar excessive declines in FEV_1 of modest degree appeared to result from either di-isocyanate exposure or smoking, without there being any additive or multiplicative effects (Figure 69.6). These conclusions differ from the general consensus, which does favour an interaction between smoking and the occupational environment, but they mirror those derived from the grain workers in the port of Vancouver. Interestingly, Diem and colleagues attempted to identify asthmatics from their study population, and showed no weakening of the COPD effect when these workers were excluded from the analysis.

CHRONIC OBSTRUCTIVE PULMONARY DISEASE AND AGENTS NOT KNOWN TO INDUCE ASTHMA

Cadmium

Cadmium-induced emphysema was first described in 1952.[36] For some years, doubts persisted as to whether the apparently excess prevalences of COPD noted among some, but not all, cadmium-exposed working populations might instead be a consequence of smoking.[37] More recent investigations involving long-term surveillance have provided more convincing evidence that cadmium does indeed cause emphysema. Thus, in a case–control study, Davison and colleagues[38] found radiographic and spirometric evidence of emphysema in twice as many men manufacturing copper–cadmium alloy for at least one year than in

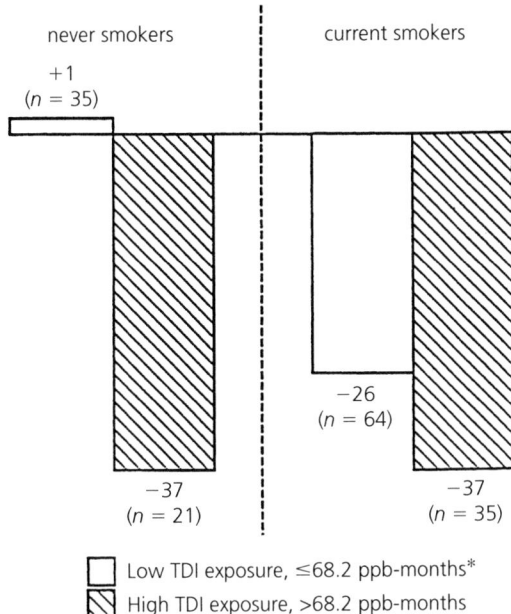

Figure 69.6 Longitudinal loss of FEV_1 versus toluene di-isocyanate (TDI) exposure. Compiled from data in Ref. 35. *ppb-months is the net result of multiplying the mean exposure in parts per billion (ppb) by the number of months over which the exposure was sustained.

unexposed controls with similar smoking habits, and they identified a significant dose–response relationship linking cumulative measures of exposure to decline in gas transfer.

Although cadmium is a trace component of cigarette smoke, cumulative exposures from smoking alone are not likely to approach those sustained occupationally. It seems improbable that smoking-induced emphysema could be attributed to cadmium.[39]

Mineral dusts

Although airway obstruction was quickly recognized to be a feature of complicated pneumoconiosis and of its accompanying emphysema, COPD in the absence of complicated pneumoconiosis was until recently attributed to other, coincidental, disorders. High mortality rates from respiratory disease in some groups of miners led to early and intensive investigations of large numbers in many countries.[40–43] Although complicated pneumoconiosis and occupational tuberculosis were associated with excess respiratory mortality and morbidity, the pattern of respiratory disease in miners seemed otherwise similar to that in their families and in suitably matched control populations.[44–47] It appeared to be related more to social circumstances (and particularly to smoking) than to the working environment.

The largest investigations involved coal miners, principally because of the enormous populations employed over the years in the coal mining industry and partly because of political influence. Particularly detailed cross-sectional studies from British and American coal mines both showed excess declines in FEV_1 related to estimated cumulative levels of exposure to coal mine dust, after appropriate adjustments for the effects of smoking and other potential confounders.[48–51] Similar associations between lung function impairment and exposure were subsequently reported from other countries. In the most heavily exposed miners, the severity of the dust effect approached that of smoking. The conclusion that coal mine dust causes COPD was partly but not fully supported by subsequent longitudinal studies – FEV_1 decline during the surveillance period being related to the cumulative (lifetime) levels of exposure, but not exposure sustained during the actual periods of surveillance.[52,53] The cumulative level of exposure from employment onset was calculated from measured levels during the studies together with estimates of earlier levels using extrapolations and so could include inaccuracies. The relation might also have been confounded by factors exerting an accumulated effect over the years of exposure (for example, air pollution, passive smoking and weight gain), for which adjustments were not made. For some, uncertainty persists. It may prove to be irresolvable because exposure levels (hence risk) and the numbers of active coal miners (hence epidemiological power) have diminished too profoundly. The optimal opportunity to demonstrate a COPD effect from coal dust may already have passed.

The evidence does, nevertheless, point to a COPD effect from coal dust.[54] This led to it becoming a prescribed industrial disease in the United Kingdom in 1992 (Prescribed Disease D12: 'Chronic bronchitis or emphysema' in underground coal miners, see www.opsi.gov.uk/ si/si1993/ Uksi_19931985_en_1.htm, for more information), providing the claimant has worked underground for at least 20 years and severity is sufficient to reduce the FEV_1 by 1 litre from its predicted value. An amendment of 1996 catered for miners of short stature and benefit became payable as soon as the FEV_1 fell to or below 1 litre. The UK's prescribed diseases legislation requires that the relevant occupational exposure doubles, at least, the risk which already exists within the population at large (thereby making it more likely than not in an affected individual that the disease in question would not otherwise have arisen). At present, only occupational exposure to coal mine dust is considered to meet these requirements, although COPD from occupational exposure to cotton dust or cadmium is already covered by separate state legislation. A possible need for wider 'prescription' was considered by the UK's Industrial Injuries Advisory Council in 2007. It recommended that surface work with coal dust should also qualify for state compensation, provided the worker has exposure for a minimum of 40 years. This implies that two years of surface work has roughly the same adverse effect as one year underground, and so surface and underground work can now be aggregated to satisfy the minimum requirement for cumulative exposure.

Similar events were experienced in South Africa in relation to exposure to respirable silica in gold mines. Although state compensation became available there from 1952, later investigations did not provide uniformly supportive evidence of a silica-related loss of ventilatory function.[55,56] More recently, cross-sectional and longitudinal studies have shown an excess of COPD in silica-exposed workers which could not be attributed to smoking, but there was no clear relationship with intensity of exposure.[57–59] In one investigation, silica and smoking appeared to exert effects of similar magnitude, while in another, the influence of smoking on FEV_1 decline was approximately twice that of silica exposure. In the severe cases which led to death, an interaction between the two environmental factors seemed likely.

Both siliceous and non-siliceous ore is encountered in the refining and smelting of metals generally, and exposure to a number of airborne mineral dusts is inevitable during the processing of iron and steel. The dusts involved are considered 'mixed', and in some circumstances have posed excess risks for pneumoconiosis, lung cancer and COPD.

Investigation of some groups of asbestos-exposed populations has suggested asbestos-induced impairment of ventilatory function at the small airway level, thought not of sufficient degree for asbestos to be considered a cause of COPD.

So far there is not convincing evidence to suggest that man-made (ceramic) mineral fibre poses a risk for COPD. The issue could change, however, as fibres of increasingly smaller diameter are produced. Some exposed populations have shown an excess prevalence of pleural plaques, but this was possibly a consequence of earlier, coincidental, exposure to asbestos.

Welding fume

Welding fume is conveniently considered separately from other minerals, partly because the circumstances of exposure are rather different, partly because a possible COPD effect in welders is a matter of considerable topical interest and partly because evidence of an additional asthmagenic effect is now emerging. The latter is convincing for stainless steel welding fume (where hypersensitivity to chromium is presumed), but most welders work with mild steel or other metals, not stainless steel, and the evidence for asthma here is less convincing.

Consistent with the investigation of numerous workforces exposed regularly to respirable irritant or noxious dusts, vapours or fumes, many investigations of welders have demonstrated a clear excess prevalence of chronic productive cough (industrial bronchitis). Until recently, none has found convincing evidence of an excess of airway obstruction implying, perhaps, that if there is a COPD effect it must be of relatively small degree.[60–62]

A small but significant COPD effect was the conclusion of a cross-sectional study of 607 shipyard workers carried out by Cotes and colleagues.[63] The workforce spanned an age range of 17–69 years. After allowing for age and height, the trades associated with welding fume exposure showed a mean and significant overall loss in FEV_1 of 250 mL compared with the unexposed trades. This effect was noted only among the smokers.[63] From the original study population, 487 were re-examined seven years later.[64] Multiple regression analyses suggested that FEV_1 was declining at an annual rate of 16.2 mL for a 50-year-old non-smoking worker without occupational exposure to welding fume. The additional losses attributable to smoking and welding fume exposure were 17.7 and 16.4 mL/year, respectively. Interactions were noted between welding fume and smoking, and between welding fume and atopy. There was no effect from welding fume on gas transfer. The longitudinal study consequently suggested that a mild COPD effect attributable to welding fume might also occur in non-smokers, but it confirmed that this effect was greater in smokers. The further enhancement of the effect in atopic subjects provides a hint of an asthmatic component, and the lack of any effect on gas transfer suggests that COPD was not occurring as a consequence of emphysema. In the absence of smoking and atopy, the risk of COPD was not clearly doubled by welding fume.

Non-tobacco smoke

Although welding fume usually contains smoke (particulate products of combustion) from surface coatings or contaminants, its probable adverse respiratory effects are chiefly consequences of metal fume itself. Smoke (and oxides of nitrogen and sulphur) from sources other than welding and tobacco may nevertheless contribute to COPD, whether encountered in industrial settings, during firefighting,[65] in polluted air generally[66] or in poorly ventilated domestic environments where biomass (e.g. wood, crop residue, charcoal, dung) is used as a cooking fuel. Biomass smoke, in particular, was thought to explain the higher prevalence of COPD in a rural compared with an urban area of China, both in the study populations as a whole (12.0 versus 7.4 per cent) and in the non-smoking women who did most of the cooking (7.2 versus 2.5 per cent).[67] A further Chinese study demonstrated a significantly diminished relative risk of COPD in both men (0.58) and women (0.75) when efficient chimneys were installed for cooking stoves that were previously unvented.[68]

CHRONIC OBSTRUCTIVE PULMONARY DISEASE OF SUBACUTE ONSET

The unusual experience of observing COPD develop over a matter of weeks or months only, has made it much easier to identify a number of interesting and recently emerged causes of subacute bronchiolitis obliterans. Because of moderate or severe (even life-threatening) disablement, the identities of the causal agents were quickly established. Evidence that bronchiolitis obliterans could result from inhaled popcorn-flavouring ingredients was first published in 2002.[69] Its recognition in eight former workers from a single American factory packaging popcorn for microwave use led to the term 'popcorn worker's lung'. It was sufficiently severe in four that lung transplantation was considered. Investigations by the National Institute for Occupational Safety and Health (NIOSH) showed that the prevalence of fixed airway obstruction among continuing employees was 3.3-fold that expected, that bronchiolitis obliterans could be detected in workers from four of five subsequently studied microwave popcorn plants and that a prominent ingredient providing a butter taste (the oily organic chemical 2,3-butanedione [diacetyl]) could cause airway necrosis when inhaled by laboratory animals. Subsequent publications have shown that occupational exposure to diacetyl, as a food-flavouring ingredient, has caused obstructive bronchiolitis in settings other than popcorn manufacture and in countries other than the United States.[70,71] The Industrial Injuries Advisory Council in the United Kingdom has recommended prescription of bronchiolitis obliterans in association with exposure to diacetyl.[72]

No evidence at present suggests that diacetyl is hazardous when ingested, but the possibility is not lightly dismissed. Inhaled diacetyl causes a relatively pure form of obliterative (or constrictive) bronchiolitis as does the ingestion, as an appetite suppressant, of leaf extracts from the Asian shrub, *Sauropus androgynus*, in the population at large.[73] Occupational exposures to the sprayed garment print dye, acramin (Ardystil syndrome) and dust-containing fragmented synthetic polymer fibres (flock worker's lung), carry the potential for more widespread parenchymal lung disease. Some affected subjects show a lymphocytic pneumonitis or bronchiolitis obliterans organizing pneumonia (BOOP), while in others the subacute inflammatory response is largely confined to the bronchioles.[74,75] Acramin is no longer used as a transport chemical for the dyes used for garment printing, and flock worker's lung appears to occur only when rotary cutters (rather than guillotine cutters) are used to produce flock. In consequence, both diseases should be readily controllable. It remains to be seen whether a suitable substitute will be found for diacetyl within the food-flavouring industry (perhaps butter itself) and whether the sporadic cases of obstructive bronchiolitis identified so far may prove in an epidemiological sense to be tips of icebergs. In any event, physicians need to be aware that COPD is not always an insidious disease which progresses slowly over many years. Some cases, and perhaps many, are subacute in nature and they may arise in unexpected settings.

PERSPECTIVE IN THE POPULATION AT LARGE

The relative risk posed to the general population by common allergens, outdoor air pollution, air pollution within the home and respirable agents at work is a matter of increasing public concern, particularly with regard to the aetiology and progression of COPD and asthma. Both disorders are clearly dependent on changing patterns of life within industrially developed countries and so environmental factors must be of great relevance. It may be that many different respirable agents are capable of exerting an influence and that in different individuals the measured COPD effects are due to different combinations of these agents (the 'multiple hit' hypothesis) together with inherent susceptibility.

Recent investigations in the former east and west regions of Germany provide interesting comparisons within the developed world between, respectively, an area of high smoking prevalence and relatively high outdoor air pollution from industrial emissions, and one of high domestic affluence.[76,77] It appears that COPD dominated in the former and asthma in the latter, although in the more affluent societies there is greater not lesser outdoor pollution from vehicle exhausts. This is thought to be of relevance to asthma in Los Angeles where such pollution is persistently high and intermittently dramatically so, but a recent comparative study using measurements of airway responsiveness between an urban area with more modest exposure to vehicle exhaust (Newcastle upon Tyne, UK) and a rural area with low exposure (Cumbria and the English Lake District) showed no difference.[78] Vehicle exhausts are changing qualitatively as well as quantitatively, however, and it remains to be seen whether the products of catalytic converters will pose new hazards despite eliminating those associated with lead.

Further perspectives regarding the possible role of occupational exposures in the aetiology of COPD in the population at large can be seen from the results of an epidemiological investigation of urban (Bergen) and rural (Hordaland) communities in western Norway.[79] A postal survey first sampled 5000 individuals from a total population of 250 000, and from the respondents an age-stratified sample of 1500 was invited to undertake a more detailed investigation that included respiratory symptoms, smoking history, work history and spirometry. In all, 1275 individuals participated. When COPD was defined from strict spirometric parameters alone ($FEV_1/FVC < 70$ per cent and $FEV_1 < 80$ per cent of predicted), smoking proved to be the only explanatory variable of clear relevance from multiple regression analyses.

When COPD was defined less stringently but more clinically from objective spirometry ($FEV_1/FVC < 70$ per cent) or subjective symptoms (chronic productive cough together with undue breathlessness or wheeze), the odds ratios for participants reporting specific occupational exposure to aluminium, welding/metal fume, quartz or asbestos all increased to significant levels; so too did the odds ratio for heavy exposure to any source of occupational dust. An increased prevalence of COPD was also noted in the urban compared with rural communities, but this was attributable to the greater number of elderly individuals (who were affected disproportionately) living in the city of Bergen.

The study population was consequently sufficiently large for subjective evidence of occupational productive cough to be demonstrated. However, the excess prevalences of strictly defined airway obstruction, which were noted among certain groups of workers, did not reach conventional levels of statistical significance.

In its 2007 review, the UK's Industrial Injuries Advisory Council did not identify any further occupational causes, other than coal mine dust, cotton dust and cadmium fume, which it considered should qualify for state compensation. This should not be interpreted to mean that the council does recognize additional causes of occupational COPD. Its tasks are to recognize causes of COPD which are likely to cause significant disability (i.e. a loss of FEV_1 of at least 1 litre or a loss in short subjects so that the FEV_1 is no more than 1 litre) and to identify which circumstances of cumulative exposure increase this risk of COPD at least two-fold. This implies, in the individual satisfying these criteria, that it is more likely than not that he/she has become significantly disabled by COPD because of occupational exposure. As the council acknowledged, there is evidence that many other occupational exposures may well cause COPD, and it may be that evidence will emerge in due course to show that some do indeed pose a risk of such a magnitude as to justify state compensation within the United Kingdom.

CONCLUSIONS

Evidence relating occupational environments to COPD is extensive but often conflicting, and this inevitably stimulates controversy. Any summary is necessarily influenced by personal, biased and possibly preconceived views[81] and so it should be emphasized that the following key points reflect a changing scene and a personal interpretation of it.

Some occupational environments are likely to exert a COPD effect and it may be that 10–20 per cent of all cases of COPD in industrially developed countries are occupational in origin.

Key points

- Differences in individual susceptibility play an important role.
- The impact of occupational exposures on COPD is likely to be less than that of smoking (perhaps much less), but will vary from industry to industry depending on potency and exposure level of the agent involved.
- Complex adverse interactions probably exist with smoking and (presumably) with other environmental agents.
- It is plausible that both asthmatic and non-asthmatic pathways play a role.
- Occupational COPD will be found uncommonly in the absence of both smoking and asthma.
- Some cases of fixed airway obstruction are subacute rather than chronic in their development, and have surprising and unexpected causes.

REFERENCES

1. Halbert RJ, Natoli JL, Gano A et al. Gobal burden of COPD: Systemic review and meta-analysis. *European Respiratory Journal.* 2006; **28**: 523–32.
2. Mannino DM, Gagnon RC, Petty TL, Lydick E. Chronic obstructive pulmonary disease surveillance – United States, 1971–2000. *Morbidity and Mortality Weekly Report, Surveillance Summaries.* 2002; **51**: 1–16.
3. Celli BR, MacNee W, Force AET. Standards for the diagnosis and treatment of patients with COPD: A summary of the ATS/ERS position paper. *European Respiratory Journal.* 2004; **23**: 932–46.
4. Murray CJL, Lopez AD, Mathers CD, Stein C. The global burden of disease 2000 project: Aims, methods, and data sources, vol. 36. In: *Global programme on evidence for health policy discussion paper.* Geneva: World Health Organization, 2001: 1–57.
5. Hnizdo E, Sullivan PA, Bang KM, Wagner G. Association between chronic obstructive pulmonary disease and employment by industry and occupation in the US population: A study of data from the Third National Health and Nutrition Examination Survey. *American Journal of Epidemiology.* 2002; **156**: 738–46.
6. Balmes J, Becklake M, Blanc P et al. American Thoracic Society Statement: Occupational contribution to the burden of airway disease. *American Journal of Respiratory and Critical Care Medicine.* 2003; **167**: 787–97.
7. Pauwels RA, Buist AS, Ma P et al. Global strategy for the diagnosis, management, and prevention of chronic obstructive pulmonary disease: National Heart, Lung, and Blood Institute and World Health Organization Global Initiative for Chronic Obstructive Lung Disease (GOLD): Executive summary. *Respiratory Care.* 2001; **46**: 798–825.
8. Schilling RSF, Vigliani EC, Lammers B et al. Report on a conference on byssinosis. In: 14th International Conference on Occupational Health. Madrid: Excerpta Medica, 1963.
9. Bouhuys A, Heaphy LJ, Schilling RSF, Welborn JW. Byssinosis in the United States. *New England Journal of Medicine.* 1967; **227**: 170–5.
10. Parkes WR. Occupational asthma (including byssinosis). In: Parkes WR (ed.). *Occupational lung disorders.* London: Butterworths, 1983: 415–53.
11. Glindmeyer HW, Lefante JJ, Jones RN et al. Exposure-related declines in the lung function of cotton textile workers. Relationship to current workplace standards. *American Review of Respiratory Disease.* 1991; **144**: 675–83.
12. Glindmeyer HW, Lefante JJ, Jones RN et al. Cotton dust and across-shift change in FEV_1 as predictors of annual change

in FEV$_1$. *American Journal of Respiratory and Critical Care Medicine.* 1994; **149**: 584–90.
13. Becklake MR. Relationship of acute obstructive airway change to chronic (fixed) obstruction. *Thorax.* 1995; **50** (Suppl. 1): S16–21.
14. Hendrick DJ, Beach JR, Avery AJ et al. *An epidemiological investigation of asthma in apprentice (shipyard) welders.* London: Medical Research Council, 1994.
15. Wald NJ, Nanchahal K, Thompson SG, Cuckle HS. Does breathing other people's tobacco smoke cause lung cancer? *British Medical Journal.* 1986; **293**: 1217–22.
16. Lapp NL, Morgan WKC, Zaldivar G. Airways obstruction, coal mining, and disability. *Occupational and Environmental Medicine.* 1994; **51**: 234–8.
17. Fletcher CM, Peto R, Tinker C, Speizer F. *The natural history of chronic bronchitis and emphysema.* Oxford: Oxford University Press, 1976.
18. Glindmeyer HW, Diem JE, Jones N, Weill H. Noncomparability of longitudinally and cross-sectionally determined annual change in spirometry. *American Review of Respiratory Disease.* 1982; **125**: 544–8.
19. Brooks SM, Weiss MA, Bernstein IL. Reactive airways dysfunction syndrome. Case reports of persistent airways hyperreactivity following high-level irritant exposures. *Journal of Occupational Medicine.* 1985; **27**: 473–6.
20. Brooks SM, Weiss MA, Bernstein IL. Reactive airways dysfunction syndrome (RADS). Persistent asthma syndrome after high level irritant exposures. *Chest.* 1985; **88**: 376–84.
21. Cohen BH, Diamond EL, Graves CG et al. A common familial component in lung cancer and chronic obstructive pulmonary disease. *Lancet.* 1977; **2**: 523–6.
22. Redline S, Tishler PV, Lewitter FI et al. Assessment of genetic and nongenetic influences on pulmonary function. A twin study. *American Review of Respiratory Disease.* 1987; **135**: 217–22.
23. Tashkin DP, Altose MD, Connett JE et al. Methacholine reactivity predicts changes in lung function over time in smokers with early chronic obstructive pulmonary disease. The Lung Health Study Research Group. *American Journal of Respiratory and Critical Care Medicine.* 1996; **153**: 1802–11.
24. Van der Lende R, Rijcken B, Scaf-Klomp W, Schouten JP. Epidemiology of chronic obstructive pulmonary disease (COPD). *European Journal of Respiratory Diseases.* 1986; **146** (Suppl.): 49–60.
25. Postma DS, de Vries K, Koeter GH, Sluiter J. Independent influence of reversibility of air-flow obstruction and nonspecific hyperreactivity on the long-term course of lung function in chronic air-flow obstruction. *American Review of Respiratory Disease.* 1986; **134**: 276–80.
26. doPico GA, Reddan W, Flaherty D et al. Respiratory abnormalities among grain workers: A clinical, physiologic and immunologic study. *American Review of Respiratory Diseases.* 1977; **115**: 915–27.
27. Becklake MR. Grain dust and health. In: Dosman JA, Cotton DJ (eds). *Occupational pulmonary disease in grain workers: Focus on grain dust and health.* New York: Academic Press, 1980: 189–200.
28. Chan-Yeung M, Enarson DA, Kennedy SM. The impact of grain dust on respiratory health. *American Review of Respiratory Disease.* 1992; **145**: 476–87.
29. Christiani DC. Organic dust exposure and chronic airway disease. *American Journal of Respiratory and Critical Care Medicine.* 1996; **154**: 833–4.
30. Chan-Yeung M, Lam S, Koerner S. Clinical features and natural history of occupational asthma due to Western Red Cedar (*Thuja plicata*). *American Journal of Medicine.* 1982; **72**: 411–15.
31. Warren CPW. Extrinsic allergic alveolitis: A disease commoner in non-smokers. *Thorax.* 1977; **32**: 567–9.
32. Valeyre D, Soler P, Clerici C et al. Smoking and pulmonary sarcoidosis: Effect of cigarette smoking on prevalence, clinical manifestations, alveolitis, and evolution of the disease. *Thorax.* 1988; **43**: 516–24.
33. Adams WGF. Long-term effects on the health of men engaged in the manufacture of tolylene di-isocyanate. 1975; **32**: 72–8.
34. Peters JM, Murphy RLH, Pagnotto LD, Whittenberger JL. Respiratory impairment in workers exposed to 'safe' levels of toluene diisocyanate (TDI). *Archives of Environmental Health.* 1970; **20**: 364–7.
35. Diem JE, Jones RN, Hendrick DJ et al. Five-year longitudinal study of workers employed in a new toluene diisocyanate manufacturing plant. *American Review of Respiratory Disease.* 1982; **126**: 420–8.
36. Baader EW. Chronic cadmium poisoning. *Industrial Medicine and Surgery.* 1952; **21**: 427–30.
37. Anonymous. Leading article: Cadmium and the lung. *Lancet.* 1973; **ii**: 1134–5.
38. Davison AG, Fayers PM, Taylor AJ et al. Cadmium fume inhalation and emphysema. *Lancet.* 1988; **i**: 663–7.
39. Hendrick DJ. Smoking, cadmium, and emphysema. *Thorax.* 2004; **59**: 184–5.
40. Registrar-General. *Decennial Supplement, England and Wales, 1951.* London: HMSO, 1958.
41. Enterline P. Mortality rates among coal miners. *American Journal of Public Health.* 1964; **54**: 758–68.
42. Atuhaire LK, Campbell MJ, Cochrane AL et al. Mortality of men in the Rhondda Fach 1950–80. *British Journal of Industrial Medicine.* 1985; **42**: 741–5.
43. Finkelstein M, Kusiak R, Suranyi G. Mortality among miners receiving workmen's compensation for silicosis in Ontario: 1940–1975. *Journal of Occupational Medicine.* 1982; **24**: 663–7.
44. Anonymous. Chronic bronchitis and occupation. *British Medical Journal.* 1966; **1**: 101–2.
45. Miller GJ. Dust exposure, pneumoconiosis, and mortality of coal miners. *British Journal of Industrial Medicine.* 1985; **42**: 723–33.
46. Foxman B, Higgins ITT, Oh MS. The effects of occupation and smoking on respiratory disease mortality. *American Review of Respiratory Disease.* 1986; **134**: 649–52.
47. Ortmeyer CE, Costello J, Morgan WKC et al. The mortality of Appalachian coal miners, 1963 to 1971. *Archives of Environmental Health.* 1974; **29**: 67–72.
48. Rogan JM, Attfield MD, Jacobsen M et al. Role of dust in the working environment in development of chronic bronchitis in British coal miners. *British Journal of Industrial Medicine.* 1973; **30**: 217–26.

49. Attfield MD, Hodous TK. Pulmonary function of US coal miners related to dust exposure estimates. *American Review of Respiratory Disease*. 1992; **145**: 605–9.
50. Marine WM, Gurr D, Jacobsen M. Clinically important respiratory effects of dust exposure and smoking in British coal miners. *American Review of Respiratory Disease*. 1988; **137**: 106–12.
51. Soutar C, Campbell S, Gurr D et al. Important deficits of lung function in three modern colliery populations: Relations with dust exposure. *American Review of Respiratory Disease*. 1993; **147**: 797–803.
52. Love RG, Miller BG. Longitudinal study of lung function in coal-miners. *Thorax*. 1982; **37**: 193–7.
53. Seixas NS, Robbins TG, Attfield MD, Moulton LH. Longitudinal and cross sectional analyses of exposure to coal mine dust and pulmonary function in new miners. *British Journal of Industrial Medicine*. 1993; **50**: 929–37.
54. Coggon D, Newman Taylor A. Coal mining and chronic obstructive pulmonary disease: A review of the evidence. *Thorax*. 1998; **53**: 398–407.
55. Sluis-Cremer GK, Walters LG, Sichel HS. Ventilatory function in relation to mining experience and smoking in a random sample of miners and non-miners in a Witwatersrand Town. *British Journal of Industrial Medicine*. 1967; **24**: 13–25.
56. Manfreda J, Sidwall G, Maini K et al. Respiratory abnormalities in employees of the hard rock mining industry. *American Review of Respiratory Disease*. 1982; **126**: 629–34.
57. Hnizdo E. Combined effect of silica dust and tobacco smoking on mortality from chronic obstructive lung disease in gold miners. *British Journal of Industrial Medicine*. 1990; **47**: 656–64.
58. Hnizdo E. Loss of lung function associated with exposure to silica dust and with smoking and its relation to disability and mortality in South African gold miners. *British Journal of Industrial Medicine*. 1992; **49**: 472–9.
59. Cowie RL, Mabena SK. Silicosis, chronic airflow limitation, and chronic bronchitis in South African gold miners. *American Review of Respiratory Disease*. 1991; **143**: 80–4.
60. Barhad B, Teculescu D, Crciun O. Respiratory symptoms, chronic bronchitis, and ventilatory function in shipyard welders. *International Archives of Occupational and Environmental Health*. 1975; **36**: 137–50.
61. McMillan GH, Pethybridge RJ. A clinical, radiological and pulmonary function case–control study of 135 Dockyard welders aged 45 years and over. *Journal of the Society of Occupational Medicine*. 1984; **34**: 3–23.
62. Simonato L, Fletcher AC, Andersen A et al. A historical perspective study of European stainless steel, mild steel, and shipyard workers. *British Journal of Industrial Medicine*. 1991; **48**: 145–54.
63. Cotes JE, Feinmann EL, Male J et al. Respiratory symptoms and impairment in shipyard welders and caulker/burners. *British Journal of Industrial Medicine*. 1989; **46**: 292–301.
64. Chinn DJ, Stevenson IC, Cotes JE. Longitudinal respiratory survey of shipyard workers: Effects of trade and atopic status. *British Journal of Industrial Medicine*. 1990; **47**: 83–90.
65. Sparrow D, Bosse R, Rosner B, Weiss ST. The effect of occupational exposure on pulmonary function: A longitudinal evaluation of fire fighters and nonfire fighters. *American Review of Respiratory Disease*. 1982; **125**: 319–22.
66. Kauffmann F, Drouet D, Lellouch J, Brille D. Occupational exposure and 12-year spirometric changes among Paris area workers. *British Journal of Industrial Medicine*. 1982; **39**: 221–32.
67. Liu S, Zhou Y, Wang X et al. Biomass fuels are the probable risk factor for chronic obstructive pulmonary disease in rural South China. *Thorax*. 2007; **62**: 889–97.
68. Chapman RS, He XZ, Blair AE, Lan Q. Improvement in household stoves and risk of chronic obstructive pulmonary disease in Xuanwei, China: Retrospective cohort study. *British Medical Journal*. 2005; **331**: 1050.
69. Kreiss K. Flavoring-related bronchiolitis obliterans. *Current Opinion in Allergy and Clinical Immunology*. 2007; **7**: 162–7.
70. van Rooy FG, Rooyackers JM, Prokop M et al. Bronchiolitis obliterans syndrome in chemical workers producing diacetyl for food flavourings. *American Journal of Respiratory and Critical Care Medicine*. 2007; **176**: 498–504.
71. Hendrick DJ. 'Popcorn worker's lung' in Britain in a man making potato crisp flavouring. *Thorax*. 2008; **63**: 267–8.
72. Industrial Injuries Advisory Council, Department for Work and Pensions. *Bronchiolitis obliterans and food flavouring agents*. Cm 7439. London: HMSO, 2008.
73. Chang H, Wang JS, Tseng HH et al. Histopathological study of *Sauropus androgynus* associated constrictive bronchiolitis obliterans: A new cause of constrictive bronchiolitis obliterans. *American Journal of Surgical Pathology*. 1997; **21**: 35–42.
74. Moya C, Antó JM, Taylor AJ. Outbreak of organising pneumonia in textile printing sprayers. *Lancet*. 1994; **343**: 498–502.
75. Kern DG, Crausman RS, Durand KT et al. Flock worker's lung: Chronic interstitial lung disease in the nylon flocking industry. *Annals of Internal Medicine*. 1998; **129**: 261–72.
76. Von Mutius E, Fritsch C, Weiland SK et al. Prevalence of asthma and allergic disorders among children in united Germany: A descriptive comparison. *British Medical Journal*. 1992; **305**: 1395–9.
77. Krämer U, Behrendt H, Dolgner R et al. Airway diseases and allergies in East and West German children during the first 5 years after reunification: Time trends and the impact of sulphur dioxide and total suspended particles. *International Journal of Epidemiology*. 1999; **28**: 865–73.
78. Devereux G. An investigation of geographic, gender and other factors on asthma prevalence in the Northern Health Region. Work carried out at Newcastle University, DM thesis, Cambridge University, 1996.
79. Bakke PS, Batse V, Hanoa R, Gulsvik A. Prevalence of obstructive lung disease in a general population: Relation to occupational title and exposure to some airborne agents. *Thorax*. 1991; **46**: 863–70.
80. Parkes WR. Chronic bronchitis, airflow obstruction, and emphysema. In: Parkes WR (ed.). *Occupational lung disorders*. London: Butterworth-Heinemann, 1994: 223.
81. Hendrick DJ. Occupation and chronic obstructive pulmonary disease (COPD). *Thorax*. 1996; **51**: 947–55.

70

Health effects of ultrafine/nanoparticles

KEN DONALDSON, ROBERT J AITKEN, JON G AYRES, BRIAN G MILLER AND C LANG TRAN

Introduction	903	Risk assessment and the challenge of measuring exposures to nanoparticles in the workplace	913
Toxicology	904	Conclusion	916
Chamber studies with nanoparticles in humans	909	References	917
Epidemiological studies	910		

INTRODUCTION

Nanoparticles (NP) and ultrafine particles are interchangeable terms used to describe particles less than 100 nm in size. It has been suggested that the term 'ultrafine' be constrained to accidental or naturally occurring particles of this size and that the term 'nanoparticles' be used for manufactured particles of this size, but there is no general agreement on this, and the terms are used interchangeably in this chapter.

Occupational lung disease has long been associated with exposures to low aspect ratio (roughly spherical or globular) particles such as silica, coalmine dust, or high aspect ratio particles (fibres) like asbestos. Chronic diseases such as pneumoconiosis, chronic obstructive pulmonary disease (COPD) and cancer are the typical end points. Such 'conventional' (in the sense of long-recognized) particles tend to be in the size range 0.1–10 μm. Since the last edition of *Hunter's Diseases of Occupations*, particle toxicology has undergone a shift in thinking to focus on the finer fractions where the most inflammatory potential seems to lie, according to the recent findings of epidemiological studies into the health effects of urban air pollution and experimental studies in laboratory animals. Thus, recent experience with combustion-derived nanoparticles (CDNP), such as diesel soot, suggests that additional acute end points, such as acute coronary syndrome and exacerbations of airways disease, may need to be considered in addition to the long-term end points of lung disease, such as pneumoconiosis. Such different end points imply that nanoparticles act by different mechanisms from conventional particles. Additionally, research into the potential hazard of nuisance dust (dust of low toxicity and low solubility) has demonstrated that surface area, rather than mass, is a better dose metric for explaining the inflammatory reaction in the lung. This finding is directly relevant to nanoparticles which have a very large surface area to volume ratio. Recent concerns regarding risks from nanoparticles stem from the rise of nanotechnologies and the potential for new types of nanoparticles to be developed. However, experiences with ambient particles (particles found in the general environment) and nuisance dust have also contributed to the present state of concern over nanoparticles. Nanoparticles are a challenge for occupational medicine because of the rise of nanotechnologies and the increasing use of nanoparticles in manufacturing and research, as well as the realization that exposure to nanoparticles has been a feature of some conventional occupations, such as welding and driving. Trying to define the risk in occupations with exposure to nanoparticles is difficult at present, and not only because the technology is relatively new. This chapter includes a section on exposure measurement to explain how uncertain current measurement techniques are, and hence the limitations of trying to apply occupational exposure limits to protect workers. As well as being difficult to measure and markedly heterogeneous, nanoparticles have a propensity to translocate in the body and could therefore have effects distal to their portal of entry through the lungs, nose, gut or skin.

The main occupational exposures to nanoparticles occur in the situations shown in Table 70.1.

There is a small but increasing toxicology database on the new types of manufactured (or engineered) nanoparticles, but the predominance of human studies, chamber exposure and epidemiology, have focused on other types of 'traditional' nanoparticles, such as bulk-manufactured nanoparticles like carbon black or TiO_2 and diesel particles and welding fumes. The measurement of nanoparticles in

Table 70.1 Different nanoparticle types, potentially exposed populations and their potential effects.

Nanoparticle type	Example of exposed population	Recorded adverse effects
Diesel exhaust particles	Drivers	Exacerbation of asthma and COPD, lung cancer
Bulk manufactured nanoparticles, e.g. carbon black, silica, alumina	Workers in the carbon black, titanium dioxide industries	Increased prevalence of productive cough
Welding fume	Welders	Metal fume fever Bronchitis Airway irritation Chemical pneumonitis Lung cancer
Nanotechnology applications, e.g. carbon nanotubes, fullerenes, quantum dots	Workers in manufacture of carbon nanotubes	Unknown

COPD, chronic obstructive pulmonary disease.

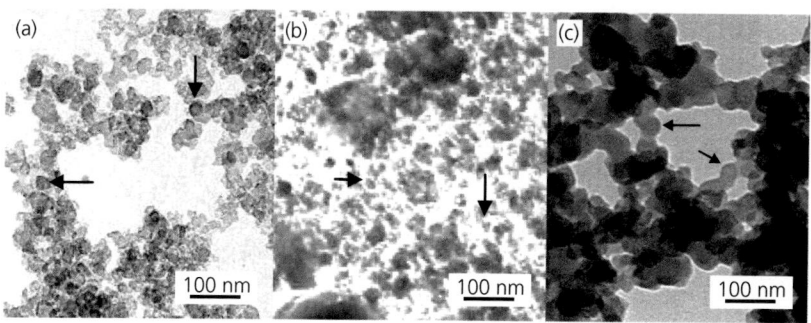

Figure 70.1 Transmission electron microscope images of nanoparticles of (a) carbon black; (b) welding fume; (c) diesel soot. Arrows indicate individual nanoparticles, but note the occurrence of the nanoparticles commonly in the form of aggregates and chains, especially evident in the carbon black and diesel soot. The welding fume particles are more heterogeneous in size and shape than the two carbon-based nanoparticle samples.

the air poses a difficult problem that is being addressed in ongoing research (Figure 70.1).

TOXICOLOGY

Origins of concern over ultrafine/nanoparticle exposure in the workplace

PARTICULATE MATTER

Concern regarding the potential adverse effects of nanoparticles came to the fore in the 1990s when the environmental air pollution literature highlighted the importance of particulate matter (PM) (PM_{10}, particles in ambient air collected using a sampling convention that has 50 per cent efficiency for particles with an aerodynamic diameter of 10 μm) as the most potent component of the air pollution cocktail. Adverse effects of PM_{10} were seen in some susceptible populations with increases of as little as 10 μg/m³, suggesting that this was a potently toxic exposure. This sparked off substantial research into which component(s) of PM_{10} might be most important. This research highlighted the ultrafine fraction as a likely major arbiter of adverse effects,[1] although not the only potentially harmful component of particulate matter in air pollution.[2] The ultrafine component of PM in urban air is dominated by combustion-derived nanoparticles (CDNP) like diesel soot. CDNP have a number of components and properties that enable them to be potent producers of free radicals and oxidative stress in the environment of the lungs, leading to inflammation (Figure 70.2) (reviewed in Ref. 3). Although adverse effects are seen in asthmatics and patients with COPD, the lead adverse effects of PM_{10} are seen in patients with cardiovascular disease, where increases in PM_{10} and $PM_{2.5}$ ($PM_{2.5}$, particles in ambient air collected using a sampling convention that has 50 per cent efficiency for particles with an aerodynamic diameter of 5 μm) were found to exacerbate atherothrombosis leading to deaths and hospitalizations.

A potential mechanistic link was made between ultrafine particles and cardiovascular effects[4] that has developed into more generic hypotheses regarding the impact of nanoparticles on atherothrombosis and heart rate variability (see under Effects of nanoparticles on extrapulmonary sites, p. 908).

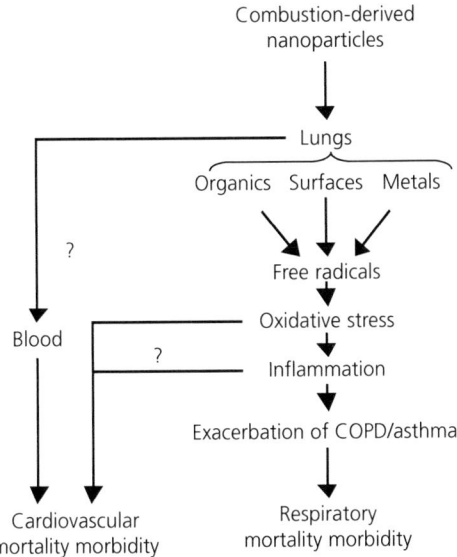

Figure 70.2 Mechanism of the effects of combustion-derived nanoparticles in causing inflammation and how this leads to adverse respiratory and cardiovascular disease. Dotted lines represent alternative pathways for the effects of inhaled combustion-derived nanoparticles (CDNP) on the cardiovascular system, i.e. effects emanating from the pulmonary response via inflammatory mediators and oxidative stress versus direct transfer of particles to the blood.

NUISANCE DUSTS

In the 1980s, concern arose regarding 'nuisance dusts'. These low toxicity low solubility materials, such as carbon black, titanium dioxide and zinc oxide are regulated in workplaces at a few *milligrams*/m^3, in recognition of their low intrinsic harmfulness. However, rat studies showed that after lifetime exposure to clouds of particles at these concentrations, rats developed pulmonary fibrosis and lung cancer. A considerable research effort was put into the relation this had to human risk and the conclusions were as follows:

- Rats suffer from an unusually florid inflammatory response to nuisance particles – so-called rat lung overload.[5]
- Surface area is the metric driving the onset of the inflammatory response, indicating rat lung overload, not mass or volume or particle number.[6]

This latter finding immediately raises concern regarding nanoparticles, because of their high surface area per unit volume. Indeed, nanoparticles caused a more rapid onset of rat lung overload, at lower mass burden, than seen with larger particles of the same material.[7] Although 'overload' has not been demonstrated in humans, the general principle of particle surface being a driver of inflammation is generalizable.

THE RISE OF NANOTECHNOLOGIES

There has been a great deal of specialist and public interest in the 'nanotechnology revolution'. Nanotechnology can be defined as the manipulation, precision placement, measurement, modelling or manufacture of sub-100 nm scale matter. Manipulation of matter at the nanoscale will greatly influence most areas of our life, such as manufacturing, engineering, health, pharmaceuticals and information technology.[8] While much of the nanotechnology endeavour is applied to surfaces and matrices, it has also led to development and accelerated production of a wide range of nanoparticles of different types and different properties. These include a range of metal oxides, metals such as silver, carbon-based nanoparticles, such as carbon black and fullerenes, and complex nanoparticles, such as quantum dots. One of the principal reasons why nanoparticles are such a focus for research and development is the propensity for particle properties to change as particle size decreases. As metal particles become progressively smaller, for example, a higher percentage of the atoms in the particle are found on the surface of the particle instead of being locked away inside the metal where they cannot interact with other chemicals. Fine palladium has less than 4 per cent of the palladium atoms on the surface of the particle, but pure palladium nanoparticles have 24 per cent of the metal atoms available on the surface. Thus, below 100 nm and particularly below about 10 nm, properties such as the dynamics of dispersion, rate of dissolution and/or aggregation, particle number, surface area and potential to adsorb and react with other substances can all change and these different properties can all be exploited industrially.

For this reason, discovery and development of new nanoparticles for various applications is likely to increase. However, the changing properties alluded to above may also have toxicological implications if the particles enter the body. A rapid expansion in new and different types of nanoparticles that are being developed and the potential for their large-scale production brings with it potential risk to human health and to the environment.[9] In the initial phase, this will occur predominantly in the workplace as these nanoparticles are handled during integration into products. Eventually, however, the particles can be released during wear and destruction throughout the product life where there will be more widespread environmental exposure. Diverse use and numerous potential exposure scenarios mean that manufactured nanoparticles (MNP) are likely to make contact with the body via the lungs, gut and skin. In the UK, the Royal Society/Royal Academy of Engineering report on nanotechnology and its risks[8] was the starting point for concern regarding the potential harmful effects of nanoparticles and the term 'nanotoxicology' was quickly coined to embrace this aspect of particle toxicology which might represent a unique class of particulate toxins that differed from conventional pathogenic particles.[10] More recently, 'grand challenges' for safe nanotechnologies have been published.[11]

Nanotubes and high aspect ratio nanoparticles

Asbestos and fibre toxicology, in general, has considerable resonance in the public and scientific mind. There is thus added concern regarding the toxicology of fibre-shaped or high aspect ratio nanoparticles (HARN).[8] Carbon nanotubes (CNT) are HARN whose production is increasing dramatically, because of their potentially useful properties and the fact that they can be made as very long fibrils (Figure 70.3).[12]

Research to date has shown CNT to be highly fibrogenic after instillation into rodent lungs,[13–16] but these were not individual 'fibre-shaped' nanotube particles, but rather bundled, particulate aggregates. The question regarding whether nanotubes can be present in the air as long thin particles has not been addressed at the time of writing. However, one study[17] has addressed the likely impact of such long nanotube fibres in relation to the 'fibre pathogenicity paradigm' which includes asbestos. The current paradigm for fibre pathogenicity is that fibres are pathogenic if they are thin, biopersistent and longer than around 20 µm.[18] As regards thinness and biopersistence, there is good evidence that nanotubes satisfy these components of the paradigm as a result of their intrinsic structure (thinness) and being composed of highly durable graphene (biopersistence). The study[17] examined the third component of the paradigm, i.e. the length-dependence of pathogenicity. A direct mesothelial model was chosen that measured the inflammation and granulomatous response to long and short nanotubes and relevant controls. Essentially, the results showed that carbon nanotubes conformed to the length-dependent paradigm in that long (greater than 15–20 µm) nanotubes were highly pathogenic but that short (<5 µm) had no pathogenicity. The end points were inflammation and granuloma formation following direct exposure of the peritoneal mesothelium in mice. Long and short asbestos showed exactly the same length-dependent behaviour with 'frustrated' or incomplete phagocytosis of the long fibres of either asbestos or nanotubes being an important underlying stimulus to inflammation (Figure 70.4).

There are a number of caveats in interpreting this work to mean that exposure to long nanotubes in workplaces might lead to mesothelioma: it is not known whether nanotubes are present in the air in workplaces in appreciable numbers; it is not known whether nanotubes that deposit in the air spaces of the lung can find their way to the pleural mesothelium in the way that asbestos does, nor whether, even if they did, they would cause mesothelioma.[17] However, these data do sound a warning bell that HARN may behave like asbestos in some ways.

Other types of high aspect ratio nanoparticles need to be considered for their conformity with the fibre paradigm.

Deliberate exposure to nanoparticles: nanomedicine, cosmetics and food technology

There are a number of scenarios where there is use of nanoparticles with a high or certain likelihood of penetration into the body. They are mentioned here for completeness. The use of nanoparticles in medicine is developing and holds out promise for therapeutics, imaging and tissue engineering. The types of particles used in nanomedicine generally differ from the types of 'hard' nanoparticles discussed so far. They include liposomes, dendrimers and polymers, but carbon-based nanoparticles such as C60 and carbon nanotubes have been advanced as potentially useful medical nanoparticles. Nanoparticles are also present in some cosmetics, such as sunscreen (TiO_2 and ZnO) and anti-ageing face cream (C60). There is a possibility that such particles could cross the skin and enter the body, or be toxic to the skin, but this has not been convincingly

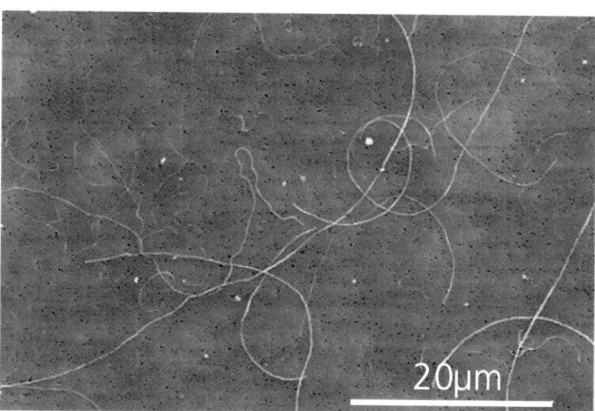

Figure 70.3 Scanning electron microscope view of multi-walled carbon nanotubes showing the extreme thinness of the fibres and their length compared to the scale bar; the similarity with asbestos is obvious. Image courtesy of Craig Poland, The Queen's Medical Research Institute, Edinburgh, UK.

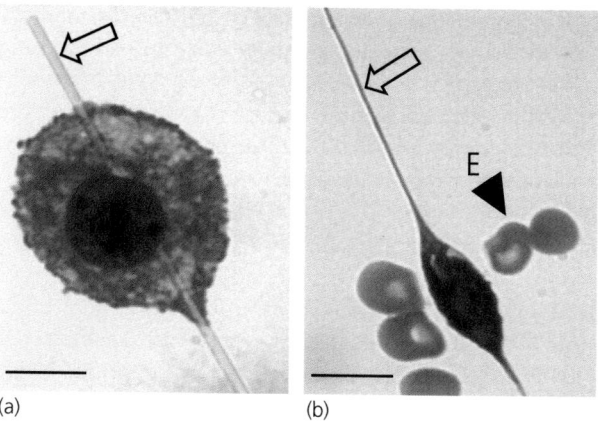

(a)   (b)

Figure 70.4 Macrophages that are undergoing frustrated or incomplete phagocytosis of long amosite asbestos (a) or long multi-walled carbon nanotubes (b). E, erythrocytes.

demonstrated so far. Nanoparticles are also present in food but risks, if any, associated with this are not well characterized. The direct introduction of such nanoparticles into or on to the human body means that their toxicokinetics, toxicity and fate are potentially quite different from those of nanoparticles encountered accidentally in the workplace or the general environment.

TOXICOLOGY OF NANOPARTICLES

The toxicology of MNP is at a very early stage and relies at present on (1) analogy with CDNP and (2) experience gained with a limited number of nanoparticle types that have been bulk-produced for decades, e.g. carbon black, titanium dioxide, and (3) limited *in vitro* and *in vivo* studies with new MNP. It remains to be seen whether general rules will emerge that will allow us to generalize on the extent or mechanism of toxicity for any untested nanoparticle sample. Currently, the hazard of nanoparticles is defined on a case-by-case basis, but the concept of a structure/activity relationship for nanoparticles that would allow prediction of toxicity from physicochemical analysis is attractive. This goal, however, lies some time in the future.

ANIMAL AND CELLULAR STUDIES

Exposure, dose and response together with ADME (absorption, distribution, metabolism and excretion) produce toxicokinetic data that allow us to describe the detailed history of a toxin in the body of a rodent species and extrapolate to humans. Mass balance toxicokinetic analysis is not available for any pathogenic particle, including nanoparticles. Most pathogenic particles have not been considered to be metabolized and excreted in any conventional way. However, because of their small size, nanoparticles may undergo transformation and excretion by such routes.[19,20] Mechanistic toxicologists are especially focused on 'dose' as a key to understanding molecular and cellular toxicity, as well as contributing to understanding the best metric. For nanoparticles, the optimal dose-metric is not yet elucidated, but mass is probably not the best metric and surface area is often assumed to be a better index. However, surface reactivity is also important and is likely to vary with different particle types since they can be composed of a range of materials and can be different sizes and shapes. Our understanding of the responses to nanoparticles in humans is based entirely on CDNP as the most-studied exposed population. The PM$_{10}$/CDNP literature suggests that atherothrombosis and airways diseases and cancer are the most likely responses. The proclivity of MNP to translocate to different sites in the cell and within the body could mean that exposure to nanotechnology-derived NP might produce extra risks to other target organs (brain, liver, etc.). For example, if nuclear translocation is seen with some NP,[21] then neoplastic outcomes might be anticipated, and if HARN behave like asbestos fibres then the pleura could be a target, with mesothelioma production.

EXPOSURE AT PORTAL OF ENTRY

In the past, particle toxicology concerned exclusively the lungs, but with the advent of nanoparticle toxicology there has been a seismic shift in perception of what qualifies as 'target tissue' and, following inhalation of nanoparticles, the blood and brain are seen as secondary targets for particle effects.[19] Aerodynamic diameter is the key particle parameter that predicts whether any particle gains access to the lungs and it also determines the site of particle deposition in the lungs. Nanoparticles deposit with moderate efficiency throughout the lower respiratory tract and with high efficiency in the nose and upper respiratory tract.[22,23] Nanoparticles may be formed as inseparable aggregates and group together in agglomerates with time and so their aerodynamic diameter may change. The fate of agglomerates in terms of de-agglomeration or further agglomeration in the lining fluid of the lungs following deposition is unknown, but is likely to depend on particle type.

TRANSLOCATION FROM THE PORTAL OF ENTRY

Animal studies show small but definite translocation of radioactive nanoparticles from the lungs to the blood following instillation exposure,[24–27] and to the brain following inhalation exposure.[28] There is no evidence for this type of translocation following inhalation of any nanoparticle type in man at the time of writing and a previous report that this does occur[29] has been disputed.[30] A flow diagram of the hypothetical fate and effects of nanoparticles is shown in Figure 70.5, based on limited animal studies with a few selected nanoparticle types.

Nanoparticles in the lungs

INFLAMMATION AND OXIDATIVE STRESS

The dominant hypothesis for the mechanism of lung injury caused by CDNP is that oxidative stress produced at the particle surface leads to intracellular oxidative stress, cell injury and lung inflammation. The oxidative stress is produced as a consequence of the properties of the combustion-derived NP, principally the large surface-area metals and organic molecules (reviewed in Ref. 31). Oxidative stress–responsive transcription factors, such as NF-κB and AP-1, then translate this oxidative stress into pro-inflammatory proteins, a sequence of events described for a number of pathogenic particle types.[31,32] Inflammation can then set in train a number of pathological processes, such as airways disease, cardiovascular disease, fibrosis or cancer.[33] This is also the dominant paradigm for MNP and we recently reviewed the data on MNP in terms of this paradigm.[34] The literature on carbon nanotubes, metal oxides, fullerenes, quantum dots and other NP types was reviewed and despite the very different particle samples used and different models, such as cell-free, cellular and animal, there was evidence of oxidative stress, cell injury and

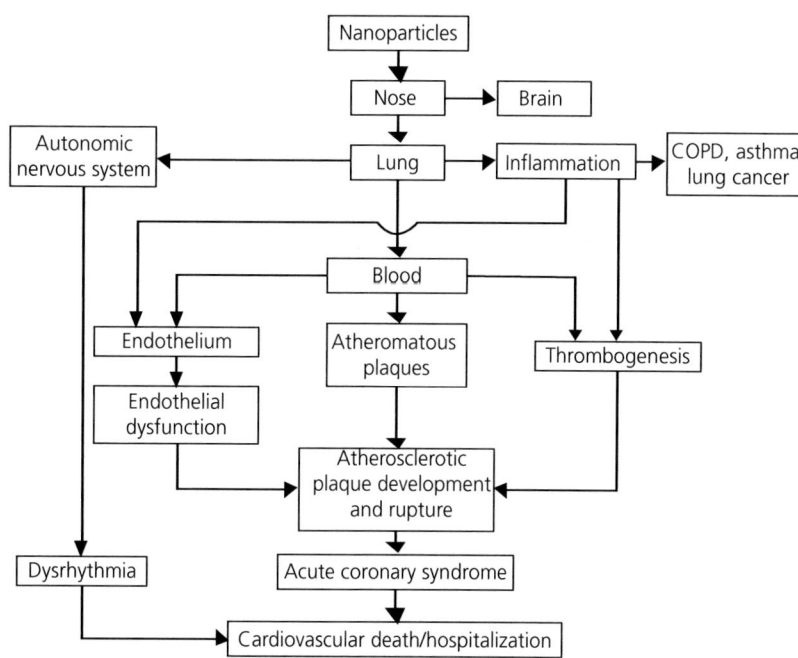

Figure 70.5 Diagram of the potential toxicokinetics and subsequent pathological responses that might arise; based on PM_{10} literature, and toxicology studies in animals and humans using a limited range of nanoparticles.

inflammation with all the different nanoparticle types.[34] Additionally, NP have been seen to inhibit phagocytosis,[35] which could allow enhanced interaction of NP with epithelial cells with pro-inflammatory consequences.

FIBROGENICITY

Carbon nanotubes have been found to be especially efficient at causing pulmonary fibrosis after instillation.[14,16,36] These fibrogenic effects have been seen after instillation into rat lungs and could be a consequence of high doses and dose rates. Inhalation studies would be very illuminating, but none has been published at the time of writing.

GENOTOXICITY AND CARCINOGENICITY

Earlier carcinogenesis studies with ultrafine carbon black and TiO_2 in rats did show lung cancer with high exposures, but these were complicated by rat lung overload, a non-specific response of the rat lung to high levels of even low toxicity particles that probably does not operate in humans.[5,37,38] However, the findings that some types of nanoparticle can cross the nuclear membrane and gain close proximity to the genetic material, pose the question as to whether such nanoparticles might have an increased genotoxicity hazard.[21]

Effects of nanoparticles on extrapulmonary sites

CARDIOVASCULAR SYSTEM

Inflammation in the lungs may also affect cardiovascular risk and so explain the increased risk of cardiovascular death and hospitalization with increased PM_{10} (reviewed in Refs 39–42). Atherosclerosis is widely recognized to be an inflammatory process.[43] There are two possible patterns of association: a link between chronic low-grade inflammation and the slow process of atherogenesis, and an association between an acute systemic inflammatory response and a transiently increased risk of an acute atheromatous plaque rupture. Toxicology studies have shown that ambient particles that are concentrated to cause high exposure (concentrated ambient particles, CAPs) can influence atherogenesis in the AopE mouse model.[44,45] The mechanism is unknown, but could include lung inflammation or systemic inflammation and oxidative stress, translocation of NP to the blood and direct interaction with endothelium or the processes within plaques could also play a role. A recent study showed that three intratracheal injections of nanotubes into mouse lungs could cause oxidative stress in the aorta.[46] Further research on this is warranted. Microvascular/endothelial dysfunction in rodents exposed to ultrafine/nanoparticles has been demonstrated.[47,48] Nemmar and colleagues have demonstrated that nanoparticles delivered into both the blood and the lungs enhanced the size of an experimentally produced thrombus.[24] Radomski et al.[49] showed that MNP of various sorts could increase platelet aggregation *in vitro* and so could enhance thrombosis. Some of these effects could be mediated by inflammation in the lungs since systemic inflammation is a risk factor for ischaemic heart disease, and predicts long-term cardiovascular risk in both patients and healthy populations.[50–53]

In addition to frank inflammatory effects in the lungs and particle translocation, there is another mechanism whereby pulmonary deposition of nanoparticles might affect the cardiovascular response. Deposited nanoparticles may cause activation of pulmonary neural reflexes via interaction with receptors present in the lungs, and may initiate changes in the autonomic function and cause a change in heart rate variability (HRV). These changes in parasympathetic input may contribute to increases in arrhythmias and subsequently to cardiovascular morbidity and mortality associated with particle exposure. Many studies have demonstrated an association between environmental particle exposure and changes in heart rate variability[54–56] and this is a potential mechanism for adverse effects of MNP in workplaces.

BRAIN

Limited studies indicate that nanoparticles can gain access to the brain following deposition in the nose, via the nerves that run from the olfactory epithelium into the olfactory lobes of the brain.[28,57] Nothing is known of the dosimetry in relation to exposure nor whether this is a generic property of nanoparticles. However, if this is a general property of NP, then given the ubiquitousness of combustion-derived nanoparticles in our environment, it is likely that most urban dwellers have a burden of nanoparticles in their brains. Indirect evidence that this is indeed true and that there might be adverse effects on the brain comes from studies in Mexico City, an area with very high particle pollution, describing unusual brain pathology in the young.[58] It is not known if nanoparticles can generally cross the blood–brain barrier, but medical nanoparticles have been designed to translocate efficiently to the brain from the blood.[59]

OTHER EFFECTS

Very small particles and structures could have a range of other effects that are not seen with conventional particles. For instance, they may not be detected by the normal phagocytic defences allowing them to gain access to the blood or the nervous system. Very small particles are smaller than some molecules and could act like haptens to modify protein structures: either altering their function or rendering them antigenic, raising the potential for autoimmune effects.[60]

Nanoparticles at the cellular level

The various compartments of the cell, evolved to isolate various functions and structures in order to control and effect efficient cell function, normally operate also to contain particles in a few compartments and exclude them from others. Depending on the particle size phagosomes, phagolysosomes, pinocytotic vesicles and clathrin-coated vesicles all may contain particles, while particles are normally excluded from the nuclei and mitochondria. However, recent work has suggested that NP may penetrate membranes that act as a barrier to bigger particles and can relocate within cells, finding potential new targets for toxicity. Li and colleagues have demonstrated that the ultrafine fraction of air pollution can enter mitochondria and cause respiration and oxidative stress effects.[61] Geiser and colleagues have shown that, unlike larger particles, nanoparticles can enter macrophages by non-microfilament-mediated processes[62] and that they can freely diffuse within the lungs, as if there were no membrane barriers.[63] They have also demonstrated that nanoparticles can enter erythrocytes, which have no normal particle uptake mechanisms.[64] Li et al.[61] showed that nanoparticles of silica, but not larger particles of the same material, were able to enter the nucleus and form aggregates with nucleoproteins.

Once inside cells, MNP can have a range of effects that depend on the surface dose and surface reactivity. The ability of the particles to produce oxidative stress and pro-inflammatory gene expression are typical responses.[34,65] However, cell-specific functional impairment is to be expected, e.g. inhibition of the ability of phagocytes to phagocytose.[66]

Oxidative stress from other particles can stimulate proliferation[67] and cause genotoxicity.[68] As well as having unusual toxicokinetics at the whole body level, NP may therefore show unusual 'microtoxicokinetics' and so may affect cellular structures not targeted by larger particles; particle-derived oxidative stress may thus result in toxicity, inflammation, proliferation and genotoxicity.

CHAMBER STUDIES WITH NANOPARTICLES IN HUMANS

Toxicity of ultrafine particles/nanoparticles can be studied using controlled exposures in the laboratory. These are complex and expensive studies which raise some ethical concerns, so the literature is small.

Diesel exhaust challenge

Laboratory exposures to diesel exhaust replicates real-life exposure, but it is difficult to separate out the effect of the particle from the gaseous components so attribution of specific outcomes to specific components needs to be undertaken with caution. There have been two broad types of study – those involving nasal challenge and those involving inhalational challenge. There are two main caveats when considering this approach to toxicity:

1. While diesel exhaust contains a substantial fraction of ultrafine particles, absolute attribution of toxicity to the ultrafine fraction using this approach cannot be made with complete confidence.
2. Studies are usually limited to healthy volunteers rather than putative at-risk groups of subjects (such as the elderly, or those with existing cardiovascular disease).

NASAL STUDIES

Studies of diesel exhaust particle instillation into the nose have shown induction of mucosal inflammatory changes and nasal hyper-reactivity and allergen potentiation by induction of specific IgE formation[69,70] and by steering cytokine production towards a T_H2 profile. These responses are likely to be mediated by the production of reactive oxidant species as the phase II enzymes, GSTM1 and GSTP1, modify these effects.[71] It is difficult to be sure about the relevance of the local lining fluid concentrations of these particles produced in these studies compared with those achieved in real life, but this mechanism does cohere with animal work and findings from studies involving larger particles in ambient air pollution.

INHALATIONAL CHALLENGE

Exposures of healthy volunteers to doses ranging between 100 and 300 $\mu g/m^3$ of PM_{10} from diesel exhaust for an hour, usually without exercise, is associated with airway neutrophilia.[72–76] In some studies, there has also been an increase in lymphocyte numbers in bronchoalveolar lavage[72,76] in mast cells[72,75] and, in one study, evidence of increased migration of macrophages into the airways and potentiation of their phagocytic capacity.[73] There is also some evidence to suggest that these neutrophils are activated with elevations of myeloperoxidase.[74,75,77]

Ozone may enhance this response. In one study in healthy volunteers, one hour of 300 $\mu g/m^3$ diesel exhaust particles followed five hours later by two hours of ozone at 200 ppb showed,[77] apart from an increase in neutrophils and myeloperoxidase (MPO) in induced sputum, a clear association between neutrophil counts and levels of MPO and matrix metalloproteinase 9 (MMP9) suggesting neutrophil activation. Increased levels of interleukin 8 with enhancements of IL-8 gene expression was also seen in one study at low-dose exposure,[75] IL-8 also being elevated in an ozone enhancement study.[75] Intriguingly, in asthmatic subjects, no such changes are seen. In one study, the only change in asthmatics after exposure to 100 $\mu g/m^3$ of diesel exhaust for two hours was an increase in IL-10 levels in bronchial mucosa.[75] However, in a study of higher-dose diesel exhaust exposure (300 $\mu g/m^3$ for an hour), 14 atopic asthmatics showed enhanced bronchial responsiveness and increased levels of sputum IL-6 at 24 hours.[78] Use of a ceramic filter had no abrogating effect on the inflammatory response to diesel exhaust in ten healthy volunteers,[73] which might suggest a role for the ultrafine component of the mix.

Thus, diesel exhaust appears to cause an inflammatory response at relatively low levels of exposure for short periods of time. However, this is seen only in normal individuals not in asthmatics, perhaps reflecting either a different time course for asthmatics or a different mechanism of inflammation, bearing in mind that the epidemiological evidence suggests that exacerbations of asthma can be caused by exposure to diesel exhaust particles.

Studies of the effects on the cardiovascular system have been variable. There are inconsistent reports of changes in heart rate variability, but perhaps a more consistent effect on endothelial responsiveness as judged by modulation of tests of forearm vasodilatation. In 30 healthy volunteers exposed to 300 $\mu g/m^3$ of diesel exhaust with intermittent exercise for an hour, endothelial responsiveness was attenuated after diesel exhaust exposure with a suggestion of an initial and delayed increase in plasminogen activator activity. At 24 hours, there appeared to be an increase in the circulating levels of TNFα and IL-6 and a reduction in acetycholine-induced vasodilatation.[79,80] This suggests that there is a dynamic component to the effects of diesel exposure, although it should be noted that not all studies are consistent, with one other study showing no effects of 100 or 200 $\mu g/m^3$ diesel on 13 healthy volunteers on a wide range of clotting factors.[81]

Chamber studies are helpful in understanding the response to diesel exhaust, but do not necessarily point to the active component being in the ultrafine fraction. Extraction of the ultrafine component from a diesel engine for subsequent challenge has not been undertaken and this would be the logical next study, although this is difficult to achieve.

ULTRAFINE CARBON CHALLENGE

Studies have also been undertaken of ultrafine carbon exposure in healthy volunteers or subjects with mild asthma, at higher doses than ambient when considered in mass terms. These have shown inconsistent influences on heart rate variability, with evidence of increased adhesion molecule expression in peripheral blood monocytes, but no acute phase response which would be compatible with retention of white cells within the lung following exposure.[82,83] A study of 20 patients with severe coronary artery disease (i.e. those who are likely to be more at risk) exposed to carbon particles with a median diameter of 60 nm and a range of up to 300 nm for an hour at concentrations equivalent to those achieved on a day when ambient PM_{10} levels would be 100 $\mu g/m^3$ showed no change in any cardiac parameter with carbon alone in diseased patients, but in healthy controls showed an increase in the high frequency power component of heart rate variability. This suggests that the diseased patients on treatment may show a loss of the protective effect of a vagal response to a stimulus.[84]

EPIDEMIOLOGICAL STUDIES

Epidemiological studies of ultrafine particle/nanoparticle exposure are limited to welding fume and diesel exhaust exposures.

Welding fume

Welding fume constitutes an aerosol which includes combustion products from the base metals, electrode coatings, shielding gases, fluxes and paint or surface coatings. Heat produces metal oxides, but these will be of differing valency and information on the relative proportion of these different valencies is not available. Very small particle (tens of nanometres in size) are produced in the primary process and these tend to aggregate into chains of primary particles.

EXPOSURE ASSESSMENT

A number of different approaches to quantification of exposure to welding fume have been employed. Personal exposures to mass of particles have been used, but as ultrafine particles are of very low mass this may not be the best approach. Personal inhaled exposures to metals (particularly nickel and aluminium) may be more relevant than urinary levels of metals, but both are logistically troublesome. Finally, magnetopneumography, the amount of metal in lungs is assessed using magnetic resonance and is assumed to be an indicator of overall exposure, has been used. However, how this truly relates to relevant exposures is not known.

In general terms, welding in confined spaces (such as by shipyard workers and tunnel workers) is associated with higher exposures, and lack of local exhaust ventilation system is associated with much higher exposures.

METAL FUME FEVER

This condition is one of the most common reactions reported by welders and may be of relevance to the specific exposure to ultrafine particles, potentially by generation of acute phase reactants.[85]

RESPIRATORY SYMPTOMS

There is consistent evidence that exposure to welding fume is associated with an increased prevalence of cough, productive of sputum. In countries where control of occupational exposures is poor, the prevalence is higher, often even into the 90 per cent range, but in general the prevalence of productive cough ranges between 20 and 40 per cent, being usually around three times higher than controls. The risk of chronic productive bronchitis is also reported to be higher in welders than non-welders, usually by a factor of about two.

LUNG FUNCTION

Reductions in lung function are more variably reported. Some studies show a reduction in FEV_1 and the presence of an obstructive defect (using the criteria of a reduced FEV_1 and a reduced forced expiratory ratio), but in most studies there are no measurable changes in basic spirometric variables. However, reductions in maximum mid-expiratory flows, usually to the order of 10–15 per cent below controls, are fairly consistently reported. In absolute terms, around two-thirds of this decrement is due to smoking with one-third due to welding fumes.

OCCUPATIONAL ASTHMA

Welding fumes are recognized as a cause of occupational asthma, but the evidence to support this is mixed. The evidence is strongest in stainless steel welders where workers are likely to be exposed to known respiratory sensitizers, notably chrome, nickel and vanadium. It is reasonable to suggest that where welders are exposed to metal fumes containing these elements, there is a significantly increased risk of occupational asthma. There is some evidence that exposure to welding fume increases bronchial responsiveness in one study from Newcastle (in the UK) showing a dose–response relationship.[86] Following specific bronchial challenge in stainless steel welders, late responses typical of occupational asthma have been seen.[87]

In some welders, particularly stainless steel welders, cross-shift falls in lung function have been recorded. This has been well characterized by Fishwick and colleagues[88] who specified that a fall in FEV_1 of >5 per cent after 15 minutes welding was significant and found this detriment more frequently in exposed welders than among welders non-exposed over a similar time period. Some welders show persistent cross-shift falls in lung function even after 20 years or more of welding, although others show attenuation of this effect with time.

While it is assumed that the causal agent for welding-induced occupational asthma will be in the base metal, it is also possible that other factors associated with the welding process might be risk factors for the development of asthma. These could include exposures to other agents other than welding fume, such as cleaning agents involved in the welding process, or possibly fume arising from the electrode coatings, the content of which is often unclear. However, asthma is a disease which characteristically affects the medium-sized airways where deposition of ultrafine particles is limited, which might point to factors other than the ultrafine particles being important in its genesis among welders.

INTERSTITIAL LUNG DISEASE

There have been a number of cases reported of restrictive ventilatory defects in welders. This effect, allowing for technical issues, seems to be real, although unusual. Again, this seems to be more frequent in those countries where control of exposure to welding fume is less effective. A study from the 1970s in the United Kingdom showed that 7 per cent of welders had pneumoconiosis on the basis of radiography and lung function.[89] Siderosis from welding fume, although well recognized, has no clinical implications. As deposition of ultrafine particles in the alveoli is high, an alveolar disease is a logical potential outcome of exposures to such particles.

Diesel exhaust

EXPOSURE

The internal combustion engine is an important source of nanoparticles in the general and working environments. The diesel engine produces exhaust containing 20–100 times more particles than that from petrol (gasoline) engines and a proportion of these are sized in the nanoparticle range. The exhaust is a mixture of soot, gases including oxides of sulphur and of nitrogen, vapours and liquid aerosols, and the particles are either soot or condensates of the other phases. The mixture varies with the type, age, condition and operating temperature of the diesel engine, and with the composition of the fuel itself. Precise characterization of the size distribution is made difficult by the propensity of the particles to form, dissolve, agglomerate and attract other molecules, e.g. polycyclic aromatic hydrocarbons (PAHs) to their surfaces, in a dynamic process. Therefore, the totality of any health risk from diesel exhaust does not necessarily derive from the nano fraction alone, as measured in air.

Occupations with exposure to diesel exhaust include trucking and transportation, and underground mining, where both transport systems and other mechanical equipment may be diesel powered. Of course, traffic exhaust pollution is a major contributor to the ambient particulate concentrations to which whole populations are exposed.

Because the primary route of exposure to diesel exhaust is respiratory and because some of its components are known carcinogens, interest in the past has focused mainly on possible lung cancer risks. Toxicological evidence from exposed rats has convincingly demonstrated carcinogenic activity, but not consistently in mice nor in hamsters. In addition, results from exposing rats to carbon black, as a surrogate for diesel soot without organic compounds, showed similar tumour incidence, suggesting that carcinogenicity was not due to the organics. Evidence with other particles suggests that the carcinogenicity at experimental doses may be a function simply of physically overloading the rat lung with ultrafine particles and not relevant to human risks.

Evidence from human epidemiology suggests that long-term exposure to diesel exhaust in a variety of occupational circumstances is weakly associated with lung cancer (relative risk, 1.2–1.5 compared with unexposed workers) and that the association persists where adjustment for smoking is possible. However, poor exposure assessment in most of these studies severely limits the possibility of using these results for quantitative risk assessment.[90] The largest and most informative studies of railroad workers and teamsters (truck drivers) in the United States, reviewed by the Health Effects Institute (HEI)'s Diesel Epidemiology Expert Panel,[90] showed differences in lung cancer risk between job categories in the railroad workers, but no increase in risk with duration of employment. The teamster studies showed an exposure–response association. The gravimetric exposures used differed between the studies, but in both cases would have been dominated by particles larger than the nano range.

Studies of cancer end points are facilitated by the death and cancer incidence registration systems which collect outcome data routinely in many countries. No such systems exist for other respiratory conditions, such as asthma and COPD, so occupational studies of these conditions are difficult and risks are assessed largely by analogy from non-occupational investigations. However, one study of COPD mortality in diesel-exposed railroad workers[91] reported increased odds of mortality from this cause with increasing length of employment, with an odds ratio of 1.6 for workers with >16 years' work.

Concern is often voiced over the possible role of particles in the causation or exacerbation of asthma. The incidence of childhood asthma has increased steadily as traffic volumes have increased, but the increase has been seen even in communities with very low pollution, so the evidence for particulate pollution as a primary cause is weak. However, there are numerous studies showing that episodes of exacerbation of asthma are more frequent on high-pollution days and in subjects living in proximity to higher than average exposure sources, e.g. near main roads. In addition, animal experiments and human volunteer studies in healthy adults have shown clear inflammatory effects on the lungs and other tissues following exposure to diesel fumes.

These inflammatory responses link to current knowledge regarding the effects of particulate air pollution in the general population. The data come from two types of study, i.e. 'time-series' and 'cohort'. In the former, the association between daily totals of events, such as deaths or hospital admissions, is related to current and recent pollution levels measured locally. These studies typically can detect effects over days or possibly a few weeks, and they may have no information on the characteristics of those affected, except possibly age and sex. Cohort studies, on the other hand, usually have good baseline information on each subject, and they typically compare event incidence between subgroups; particularly relevant are studies which compare between locations with different average concentrations of particulate pollution.

Both types of study have demonstrated effects of particles, but the magnitude of effects in the cohort studies is much greater than in time-series studies, presumably reflecting the long-term build up of damage from chronic exposures. Both types of study have identified that the largest and most consistent effects are in mortality from cardiovascular and respiratory causes, with some additional evidence from the cohort studies for increased lung cancer risks in locations with higher average pollution.

Initially, the finding of a cardiovascular mortality effect from inhaled pollution was puzzling, because no mechanism had been identified. The body of recent research reviewed above has now suggested possible mechanisms. However, we know of no studies of these effects in occupational settings.

To summarize, diesel exhaust fumes include a proportion of nanoparticles. Diesel exhaust is an irritant and is classified by a number of authorities in different countries as a probable human carcinogen of the lung. It has inflammatory effects and these increase the risks of asthmatic exacerbations, and may also increase cardiovascular risks, including cardiovascular mortality. In the main, these health effects are not specific to diesel exhaust, which will have the effect of modifying the risks from other causes contributing to these disease processes. It seems likely that the cardiovascular effects are associated primarily with the nanoparticle fraction, but this may not be true of the carcinogenicity, which has been ascribed to the adsorbed PAHs and is less likely to be mediated by particle size.

Given the evidence, action and regulation to minimize human exposure to diesel exhaust is justified, both in the environment and in the workplace. Although there have been many improvements to diesel engines over recent decades, some of these have increased the number of smaller particles produced, and it is not known whether these changes have decreased or increased the risks described above.

RISK ASSESSMENT AND THE CHALLENGE OF MEASURING EXPOSURES TO NANOPARTICLES IN THE WORKPLACE

Nanoparticle types

As indicated under Introduction (p. 903), it is overly simplistic to regard nanoparticles as a single class of material. In practice, nanoparticles include a diverse range of chemical composition, size and structural form. In addition to established ultrafine particles which have been manufactured for several decades, such as TiO_2, many new variants of existing materials and entirely new materials are being developed. These include metals, metal oxides, ceramics, semiconductors and organic particles. They can include composites, having for example a metal core with an oxide coating or alloys in which mixtures of metals are present.[92] Carbon-based particles include fullerenes, the best known of which is C60 (buckminsterfullerene), which has a cage-like structure.[93] Carbon nanotubes,[94] mentioned under Nanotubes and high aspect ratio nanoparticles (p. 906), exist in a variety of forms, but primarily comprise rolled-up sheets of graphene which form high aspect ratio particles. These particles may also be functionalized by addition of molecular groups.

Potentially, exposure may occur to the particles themselves, or to agglomerations of these particles or to particles in the presence of a formulation material, such as a liquid carrier. These nanostructured particles may be much larger than the size limits which are currently used to define nanoparticles. Maynard and Aitken[95] suggested a classification scheme for these nano objects which potentially may be helpful in the development of risk management strategies (Figure 70.6). Production methods include gas phase processes, such as flame pyrolysis and chemical vapour deposition, and liquid phase emulsion reactions. They vary from laboratory scale to full industrial production. Uses and applications of nanomaterials are growing rapidly.[96]

Occupational hygiene practice

As with other particles and chemicals, risks to health may be reduced by understanding and controlling exposures in at-risk populations. In an occupational context, this will include those involved in the development, production and use of these materials. Currently, there is a substantial gap in knowledge about the likely exposure scenarios and the relevant exposure levels, duration or population size. Published guidance to support good occupational hygiene practice is only just beginning to emerge. The British Standards Institute's Nanotechnologies Guide to Safe Handling document[97] provides a coherent framework by which potential risks may be addressed. It is based on a conventional risk assessment framework and incorporates a hierarchical approach to exposure control (eliminate, substitute, enclosure, engineering control, procedural control and personal protective equipment). Overall, the approach is intended to be conservative, as well as giving

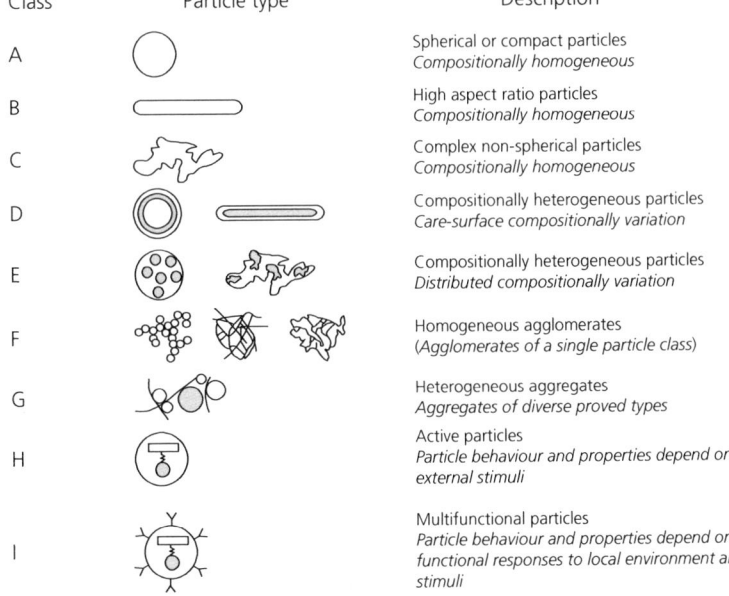

Figure 70.6 A proposed working classification scheme for nanostructured particles.

Measurement of nanoparticles in the workplace

In most early epidemiology studies, dust (particle) samples were collected on to a filter or other media and subsequently analysed off-line to define estimates of exposure, expressed as a concentration in air. In some of the early studies in the coal industry, the samples were analysed by counting particles on the filter under a light microscope.[98] This resulted in an estimate of exposure in terms of particle number concentration. Epidemiology studies in the coal industry later showed a good correlation between pneumoconiosis and mass concentration. Subsequently, the use of mass concentration measurements to demonstrate compliance with established occupational exposure limits has become the norm in most occupational scenarios.

A range of sampling instruments are available which may be used to collect samples for analysis. Usually these are small devices, comprising a selection stage, a filter (the combination often referred to as the sampling head) and a sampling pump mounted on the torso of a wearer. The sampling head is typically positioned in the 'breathing zone', normally on the upper chest, of the wearer and the samples collected referred to as 'personal samples'. The use of personal sampling is widespread, since aerosol concentrations in workplaces can have wide spatial variability and a personal sample represents the closest approximation to actual exposures. This approach has typically been used to assess exposure to ultrafine particles, such as welding fume or carbon black in the workplace. For welding fume, however, the breathing zone is modified by the presence of a welding helmet and the sample is therefore collected inside the helmet.[99]

A further refinement of this approach is collection of a 'biologically relevant aerosol fraction'. In this context, biological relevance is characterized by where in the respiratory tract a particle can potentially deposit, and determined as a function of particle size, measured in terms of aerodynamic diameter. For this reason, international standards[100–102] have been developed which define the size of particles capable of penetrating to the various regions of the respiratory tract. The three most commonly used standards relating to occupational exposure are the inhalable fraction (representing that fraction of aerosol which can enter the respiratory tract), the thoracic fraction (particles capable of penetrating to the airways below the larynx typically defined according to a selection curve with a 50 per cent cut off at 10 μm (10 000 nm) and the respirable fraction (particles defined according to a selection curve with a 50 per cent cut off at 4 μm (4000 nm), which can penetrate beyond the ciliated airways to the gas exchange region of the lung.

Sampling aerosols with instruments that match one of the three size fractions is generally accepted as good practice, and occupational exposure limits typically apply to mass concentrations of a specific fraction, in almost all cases either the inhalable or thoracic fraction.

One exception is the class of fibrous particles, such as asbestos or glass fibre. Although some of the toxic mechanisms associated with asbestos exposure remain unclear, it is known that ill health following exposure is associated with physicochemical properties, such as fibre length and surface chemistry, and the persistence of the fibres in the lungs. As a result, exposure is not characterized in terms of averaged mass and composition, but rather by the number (concentration) of fibres in the air with a specific shape and composition.[103]

Currently, measurement of nanoparticles in workplaces is problematic and there are no established guidelines or protocols and very little published experience. A critical issue is the choice of measurement metric (i.e. mass, number or surface area concentration). As in the earlier coal industry example, it is necessary to choose a metric which is correlated with the health effect of concern. However, emerging toxicological evidence suggests that, for at least some nanoparticles, potential health effects are more likely to be correlated with surface area concentration, rather than mass concentration. For some high aspect ratio nanomaterials, it is probable that, like larger fibres, number concentration will prove to be the most appropriate metric. Although instruments are available to measure each of these metrics, there are in each case a number of limitations to the utility of these.

MEASUREMENT OF PARTICLE NUMBER CONCENTRATION

Optical particle counters in which light scattered from a particle is counted as a pulse, are used routinely for counting larger particles (Figure 70.7). However, these devices do not operate well in the nanoparticle size range, since the

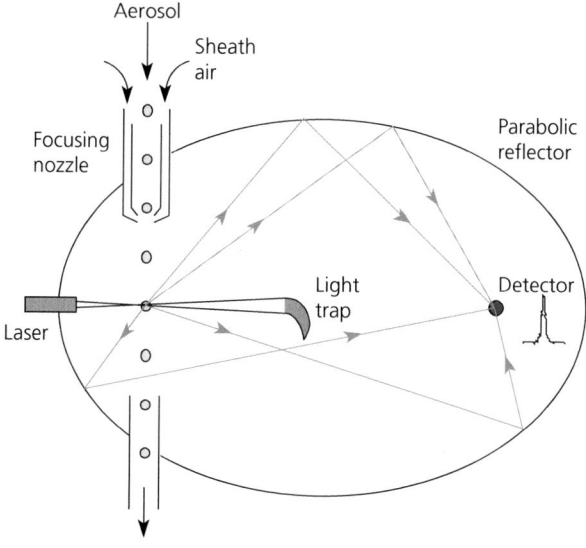

Figure 70.7 Diagrammatic representation of the mechanism of operation of optical particle counters.

wavelength of the light used in them is greater that the particle size, and so the light is not scattered. Condensation particle counters (CPCs) overcome this limitation by passing sampled particles through a chamber containing a saturated atmosphere (usually of alcohol or water) which condenses on to the particles, forming larger droplets which can be detected by the optical system and counted.[95] This largest particle size detected by the device is set using a size-selecting inlet, and the lower size limit depends on the specific instrument, but is typically in the range of 10 nm. These devices are typically fairly robust, hand-held instruments which can therefore be used to provide real-time information on particle number concentration, but no information on particle size. Although they are hand held, CPCs are not yet at a size which can be incorporated into a personal sampler.

CPCs may also be used as a counter in series with instruments which can select differing size fractions as a function of time. One such device is the differential mobility particle sizer (DMPS).[95] This instrument sequentially selects particles according to their electrical mobility by stepping the voltage across a pair of electrodes. By sequentially counting these particles using a CPC, a particle size distribution can be produced.

Measuring particle number concentration in isolation can, however, be misleading. In all particle number concentration measurements, the integration limits over which a particular instrument operates are critical in interpreting the reported results. CPC instruments become increasingly insensitive to particles smaller than 10–20 nm. Concentrations measured with instruments with different sensitivities might therefore differ substantially, particularly if the particle count median diameter is close to or in this range, which is often the case.

A further complication relates to the ambient aerosol. Unless the workplace is operating under clean room conditions other nanoscale aerosols, for example from combustion sources, may be present in the workplace and result in overestimation of the levels of nanoparticles emitted from the process under investigation. In the same way, CPCs do not provide any information about particle shape and so cannot discriminate between HARN and compact nanoparticle forms.

Off-line assessment of nanoparticle number concentrations is feasible by collecting particles on to suitable media and analysis by electron microscopy, although this approach has to date not been validated. Despite the difficulties, this is currently the only practicable approach for assessing HARN number concentration.

MEASUREMENT OF PARTICLE MASS CONCENTRATION

In principle, assessment of the mass of nanoparticles can be achieved using a personal sampler with an appropriate size-selecting cut-off point to collect a sample on to appropriate media for subsequent off-line gravimetric or chemical analysis. Currently, however, there are no commercial devices of this type available. One issue to be resolved in a device of this type is the size at which the cut point would be set. Although nanoparticles are currently defined[104] as particles having one dimension less than 100 nm, agglomerates of such nanoparticles are still likely to be biologically relevant but would be excluded by such a device. A second issue relates to the actual masses which would be collected by a device with a 100-nm cut. It is probable that these masses would be substantially below those typically collected in current occupational hygiene practice presenting great challenges in relation to limits of detection.

MEASUREMENT OF SURFACE AREA CONCENTRATIONS

In recent years, emerging methods such as diffusion charging provide a more viable approach to measuring aerosol surface area *in situ* (Figure 70.8). The instrument works principally by the mechanism of unipolar diffusion charging. Ions are produced in the carrier gas by a corona discharge. The ions attach to the surface of the particles in proportion to the total surface area and are collected in an electrically insulated particle filter. The electric charge is converted to a DC voltage signal in an electrometer amplifier. Good agreement has been shown[105] between diffusion chargers from Matter Engineering (LQ1-DC; Matter Engineering, Wohlen, Switzerland) and EcoChem (DC2000CE; EcoChem, Delia, CA, USA), TEM-derived surface area and size distribution-derived surface area for sub-100 nm particles.

Active surface area does not scale directly with geometric surface area above 100 nm. Diffusion chargers are

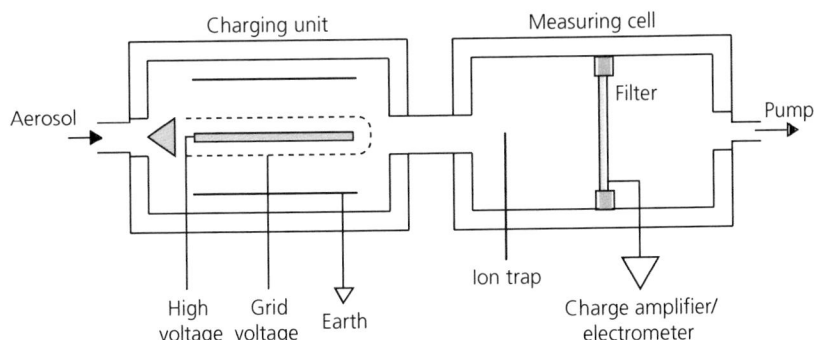

Figure 70.8 Diagrammatic representation of the mechanism of operation of a diffusion charging aerosol surface area counter.

specific to nanoparticles only if used with an appropriate inlet preseparator.

A recent variant of this approach is the TSI Nanoparticle Surface Area Monitor (NSAM) Model 3550 (TSI Inc, Shoreview, MN, USA). In this device, the instrument response has been tuned by changing the voltage on the ion trap, such that the signal has been shown to relate to the human lung deposited surface area (expressed in cm^2/m^3) of the tracheobronchial or alveolar regions of the lung. Although this is a promising device, its utility has yet to be fully investigated.

Recommended sampling strategy for risk assessment

While all of these devices are capable of providing useful information on mass, number or size concentrations, none provides the utility of taking personal samples and all require careful interpretation of the data obtained to provide useful and comparable information. Maynard and Aitken[95] have suggested the concept of an idealized sampler. Such a device would be capable of measuring all the attributes of interest relating to the physical, chemical properties of engineered nanomaterials-related particles: (1) it would be portable to allow it to be worn by potentially exposed subjects; (2) it would be capable of providing time-differentiated information; and (3) it would be inexpensive, to allow large numbers of such instruments to be purchased for any given study. No such instrument is currently available, nor is it likely that in the short term such an instrument will become available. Until such time then, any attempt to characterize workplace exposure to nanoparticles should preferably involve a multifaceted approach incorporating many of the sampling techniques mentioned above. Brouwer et al.[106] recommend that all relevant characteristics of nanoparticle exposure be measured and a sampling strategy similar to theirs would provide a reasonable approach to characterizing workplace exposure.

The first step would involve identifying the source of nanoparticle emissions using a CPC. It is critical to determine ambient or background particle counts before measuring particle counts during the manufacture or processing of the nanoparticles involved. If a specific nanoparticle is of interest, then area sampling with a filter suitable for analysis by electron microscopy should also be employed. Electron microscopy can be used to identify specific particles and can estimate the size distribution of the particles.

Once the source of emissions is identified, aerosol surface area measurements should be conducted with a portable diffusion charger and aerosol size distributions should be determined with a DMPS or ELPI using static (area) monitoring. The location of these instruments would need to be be considered carefully, ideally as close to the work areas of the workers as possible.

Finally, personal sampling using filters or grids suitable for analysis by electron microscopy or chemical identification should be employed, particularly if measuring exposures to specific nanoparticles is of interest. Electron microscopy can be used to identify the particles and can provide an estimate of the size distribution of the particle of interest.

By using a combination of these techniques, an assessment of worker exposure to nanoparticles can be conducted. This approach will allow a determination of the presence and identification of nanoparticles and the characterization of the important aerosol metrics.

CONCLUSION

Ultrafine particles/nanoparticles form a diverse group of materials that share a similar small size, but have varied compositional characteristics and so different adverse health outcomes might be expected. They pose a threat to the lungs because of their potential to become airborne where they can be easily inhaled, in view of their small size. There are long-standing exposures to some types of nanoparticles, such as diesel soot and welding fume and epidemiology studies document a range of adverse pulmonary effects in such exposed workers. Exposure in chamber studies confirms a range of inflammatory effects. Less well understood hazards and risks are attached to new and emerging nanoparticles, products of the nanotechnologies industries. These nanotechnological particles, aimed at specific industrial usages, can be complex and can have diverse sizes, composition and coating to support their industrial applications. The impact of such modifications on toxicity is poorly understood in general. In addition, some 'engineered nanoparticles', such as carbon nanotubes, have a high aspect ratio and the potential parallels with asbestos are clear. One area of research focus is the cardiovascular system as a target for inhaled nanoparticles, a concern extrapolated from the PM_{10}/combustion-derived nanoparticles experience, where cardiovascular effects are the main health impact. The potential for nanoparticles to translocate from their portal of entry in the lungs poses new targets and mechanisms for the effects of nanoparticles, such as the blood and the brain, that are ill understood. These new types of hazard from inhaled nanoparticles are currently the focus of considerable research.

Effective exposure assessment is absolutely necessary for the determination of risk. While welding fume and diesel soot are measured in the air by mass, the best metric for relating nanoparticle exposure to health effects remains under debate. Measurement of low mass concentrations of manufactured and engineered nanoparticles in the air, against a changing background of ambient nanoparticles from sources such as fuel combustion, presents a challenge that is currently being addressed at national and international level.

Ultrafine/nanoparticles represent an interesting and ubiquitous category of potentially pathogenic particles whose adverse effects could be substantial. Additions to the list of candidate particles requiring testing are to be anticipated, in view of the burgeoning nanotechnologies. Viewing ultrafine/nanoparticles as a class of particles with both common and diverse pathogenic mechanisms, reflecting their origin and structure, should provide impetus and direction to research. There is an urgent need for greater understanding of these ubiquitous industrial materials and their hazard, so that there is improved understanding of the risks for those who work with them.

Key points

- Nanoparticles are a subclass of particles defined on the basis of having one dimension less than 100 nm (0.1 microns). Nanoparticles have received increased attention over the last few years, especially because of the rise of nanotechnologies, which produce novel types of nanoparticle for industrial use and subsequent potential for inhalation exposure.
- Exposures to nanoparticles of diesel soot and other combustion-derived nanoparticles also occur in the general environment. In the occupational environment, nanoparticle exposures also include welding fume, carbon black, amorphous silica, and other bulk-manufactured nanoparticle types.
- The toxicological effects of nanoparticles appear to be related to their large surface area per unit mass, which leads to an ability to cause oxidative stress and inflammation in lung tissue. Some nanoparticle types have a fibrous shape and so there is concern over whether they might pose an asbestos-type hazard. The small dimensions of nanoparticles give them potential for translocation from their site of deposition to the blood and brain and other potential target tissues.
- Human epidemiological studies and chamber studies have predominantly addressed the effects of diesel soot and welding fume. Exposures to both of these nanoparticles is associated with lung cancer in epidemiology studies, while exposure to welding fume is associated with a number of other end points, including systemic effects and lung fibrosis. Chamber studies show pro-inflammatory effects and also systemic effects of both exposures.
- There is a pressing need for portable samplers that allow real-time quantification of nanoparticle mass, number, or surface area in the workplace. A number of different types of instrumentation are undergoing research and development for this purpose.

REFERENCES

1. Utell MJ, Frampton MW. Acute health effects of ambient air pollution: the ultrafine particle hypothesis. *Journal of Aerosol Medicine*. 2000; **13**: 355–9.
2. Brunekreef B, Forsberg B. Epidemiological evidence of effects of coarse airborne particles on health. *European Respiratory Journal*. 2005; **26**: 309–18.
3. Donaldson K, Tran L, Jimenez L et al. Combustion-derived nanoparticles: A review of their toxicology following inhalation exposure. *Particle and Fibre Toxicology*. 2005; **2**: 10.
4. Seaton A, MacNee W, Donaldson K, Godden D. Particulate air-pollution and acute health-effects. *Lancet*. 1995; **345**: 176–8.
5. Mauderly JL, Cheng YS, Snipes MB. Particle overload in toxicological studies – friend or foe. *Journal of Aerosol Medicine*. 1990; **3** (Suppl. 1): S169–S187.
6. Tran CL, Buchanan D, Cullen RT et al. Inhalation of poorly soluble particles. II. Influence of particle surface area on inflammation and clearance. *Inhalational Toxicology*. 2000; **12**: 1113–26.
7. Oberdorster G. Significance of particle parameters in the evaluation of exposure–dose-response relationships of inhaled particles. *Inhalational Toxicology*. 1996; **8** (Suppl.): 73–89.
8. Royal Society and Royal Academy of Engineering. *Nanoscience and nanotechnologies: Opportunities and uncertainties*. London: The Royal Society, 2004.
9. Maynard AD, Kuempel E. Airborne nanostructured particles and occupational health. *Journal of Nanoparticle Research*. 2005; **7**: 587–614.
10. Donaldson K, Stone V, Tran CL et al. Nanotoxicology. *Occupational and Environmental Medicine*. 2004; **61**: 727–8.
11. Maynard AD, Aitken RJ, Butz T et al. Safe handling of nanotechnology. *Nature*. 2006; **444**: 267–9.
12. Donaldson K, Aitken R, Tran L et al. Carbon nanotubes: A review of their properties in relation to pulmonary toxicology and workplace safety. *Toxicological Sciences*. 2006; **92**: 5–22.
13. Shvedova AA, Kisin ER, Mercer R et al. Unusual inflammatory and fibrogenic pulmonary responses to single-walled carbon nanotubes in mice. *American Journal of Physiology. Lung Cellular and Molecular Physiology*. 2005; **289**: L698–L708.
14. Muller J, Huaux F, Moreau N et al. Respiratory toxicity of multi-wall carbon nanotubes. *Toxicology and Applied Pharmacology*. 2005; **207**: 221–31.
15. Warheit DB, Laurence BR, Reed KL et al. Comparative pulmonary toxicity assessment of single-wall carbon nanotubes in rats. *Toxicological Sciences*. 2004; **77**: 117–25.
16. Lam CW, James JT, McCluskey R, Hunter RL. Pulmonary toxicity of single-wall carbon nanotubes in mice 7 and 90 days after intratracheal instillation. *Toxicological Sciences*. 2004; **77**: 126–34.
17. Poland C, Duffin R, Kinloch I et al. High aspect ratio carbon nanotubes display asbestos-like pathogenic behaviour. *Nature Nanotechnology*. 2008; **3**: 423–8.

18. Donaldson K, Tran CL. An introduction to the short-term toxicology of respirable industrial fibres. *Mutation Research*. 2004; **553**: 5–9.
19. Oberdorster G, Oberdorster E, Oberdorster J. Nanotoxicology: An emerging discipline evolving from studies of ultrafine particles. *Environmental Health Perspectives*. 2005; **113**: 823–39.
20. Singh R, Pantarotto D, Lacerda L et al. Tissue biodistribution and blood clearance rates of intravenously administered carbon nanotube radiotracers. *Proceedings of the National Academy of Sciences of the United States of America*. 2006; **103**: 3357–62.
21. Chen M, von Mikecz A. Formation of nucleoplasmic protein aggregates impairs nuclear function in response to SiO_2 nanoparticles. *Experimental Cell Research*. 2005; **305**: 51–62.
22. Kreyling WG, Moller W, Semmler-Behnke M, Oberdorster G. Particle dosimetry: Deposition and clearance from the respiratory tract and translocaton to extra-pulmonary sites. Chapter 3. In: Donaldson K, Borm P (eds). *Particle toxicology*. Boca Raton, FL: CRC Press, 2007: 47–74.
23. Gehr P, Brand P, Heyder J. Particle deposition in the repiratory tract. In: Gehr P, Heyder J (eds). *Particle lung cell interactions*, vol. 143 in Lung biology in health and disease. (Executive editor, C Lenfant). New York: Marcel Dekker, 2000: 229–322.
24. Nemmar A, Hoylaerts MF, Hoet PH, Nemery B. Possible mechanisms of the cardiovascular effects of inhaled particles: Systemic translocation and prothrombotic effects. *Toxicology Letters*. 2004; **149**: 243–53.
25. Semmler M, Seitz J, Erbe F et al. Long-term clearance kinetics of inhaled ultrafine insoluble iridium particles from the rat lung, including transient translocation into secondary organs. *Inhalational Toxicology*. 2004; **16**: 453–9.
26. Kreyling W, Semmler M, Erbe F et al. Minute translocation of inhaled ultrafine insoluble iridium particles from lung epithelium to extrapulmonary tissues. *Annals of Occupational Hygiene*. 2002; **46** (Suppl. 1): 223–6.
27. Nemmar A, Vanbilloen H, Hoylaerts MF et al. Passage of intratracheally instilled ultrafine particles from the lung into the systemic circulation in hamster. *American Journal of Respiratory and Critical Care Medicine*. 2001; **164**: 1665–8.
28. Oberdorster G, Sharp Z, Elder AP et al. Translocation of inhaled ultrafine particles to the brain. *Inhalational Toxicology*. 2004; **16**: 437–45.
29. Nemmar A, Hoet PH, Vanquickenborne B et al. Passage of inhaled particles into the blood circulation in humans. *Circulation*. 2002; **105**: 411–14.
30. Mills N, Amin N, Robinson S et al. Inhaled ^{99m}Technetium-labeled carbon nanoparticles do not translocate into the circulation in man. *American Journal of Respiratory and Critical Care Medicine*. 2006; **173**: 426–31.
31. Donaldson K, Jimenez LA, Rahman I et al. Respiratory health effects of ambient air pollution particles: Role of reactive species. In: Vallyathan V, Shi X, Castranova V (eds). *Oxygen/nitrogen radicals: Lung injury and disease*, vol. 187 in Lung biology in health and disease. (Executive editor, C Lenfant). New York: Marcel Dekker, 2004.
32. Schins RP, McAlinden A, MacNee W et al. Persistent depletion of I kappa B alpha and interleukin-8 expression in human pulmonary epithelial cells exposed to quartz particles. *Toxicology and Applied Pharmacology*. 2000; **167**: 107–17.
33. Mauderly JL, Snipes MB, Barr EB et al. Pulmonary toxicity of inhaled diesel exhaust and carbon black in chronically exposed rats. Part I: Neoplastic and nonneoplastic lung lesions. Research report (Health Effects Institute). 1994; **68** (Pt 1): 1–75.
34. Donaldson K, Stone V. Toxicological properties of nanoparticles and nanotubes. *Issues in Environmental Science and Technology, Nanotechnology*. 2007; **24**: 81–96.
35. Renwick LC, Brown D, Clouter A, Donaldson K. Increased inflammation and altered macrophage chemotactic responses caused by two ultrafine particle types. *Occupational and Environmental Medicine*. 2004; **61**: 442–7.
36. Warheit DB. What is currently known about the health risks related to carbon nanotube exposures? *Carbon*. 2006; **44**: 1064–9.
37. Lee KP, Henry NW III, Trochimowicz HJ, Reinhardt CF. Pulmonary response to impaired lung clearance in rats following excessive TiO_2 dust deposition. *Environmental Research*. 1986; **41**: 144–67.
38. Lee KP. Lung response to particulates with emphasis on asbestos and other fibrous dusts. *Critical Reviews in Toxicology*. 1985; **14**: 33–86.
39. Brook RD, Brook JR, Rajagopalan S. Air pollution: The 'heart' of the problem. *Current Hypertension Reports*. 2003; **5**: 32–9.
40. Brook RD, Franklin B, Cascio W et al. Air pollution and cardiovascular disease: A statement for healthcare professionals from the Expert Panel on Population and Prevention Science of the American Heart Association. *Circulation*. 2004; **109**: 2655–71.
41. Glantz SA. Air pollution as a cause of heart disease. Time for action. *Journal of the American College of Cardiology*. 2002; **39**: 943–5.
42. Routledge HC, Ayres JG, Townend JN. Why cardiologists should be interested in air pollution. *Heart*. 2003; **89**: 1383–8.
43. Ross R. Atherosclerosis is an inflammatory disease. *American Heart Journal*. 1999; **138**: S419–S420.
44. Chen LC, Nadziejko C. Effects of subchronic exposures to concentrated ambient particles (CAPs) in mice. V. CAPs exacerbate aortic plaque development in hyperlipidemic mice. *Inhalational Toxicology*. 2005; **17**: 217–24.
45. Sun Q, Wang A, Jin X et al. Long-term air pollution exposure and acceleration of atherosclerosis and vascular inflammation in an animal model. *JAMA*. 2005; **294**: 3003–10.
46. Li Z, Hulderman T, Salmen R et al. Cardiovascular effects of pulmonary exposure to single-wall carbon nanotubes. *Environmental Health Perspectives*. 2007; **115**: 377–82.

47. Nurkiewicz TR, Porter DW, Barger M et al. Particulate matter exposure impairs systemic microvascular endothelium-dependent dilation. *Environmental Health Perspectives*. 2004; **112**: 1299–306.
48. Nurkiewicz TR, Porter DW, Barger M et al. Systemic microvascular dysfunction and inflammation after pulmonary particulate matter exposure. *Environmental Health Perspectives*. 2006; **114**: 412–19.
49. Radomski A, Jurasz P, Alonso-Escolano D et al. Nanoparticle-induced platelet aggregation and vascular thrombosis. *British Journal of Pharmacology*. 2005; **146**: 882–93.
50. Das I. Raised C-reactive protein levels in serum from smokers. *Clinica Chimica Acta*. 1985; **153**: 9–13.
51. Bermudez E, Rifai N, Buring JE et al. Relation between markers of systemic vascular inflammation and smoking in women. *American Journal of Cardiology*. 2002; **89**: 1117–19.
52. Gotsman I, Lotan C, Soskolne WA et al. Periodontal destruction is associated with coronary artery disease and periodontal infection with acute coronary syndrome. *Journal of Periodontology*. 2007; **78**: 849–58.
53. Modica A, Karlsson F, Mooe T. Platelet aggregation and aspirin non-responsiveness increase when an acute coronary syndrome is complicated by an infection. *Journal of Thrombosis and Haemostasis*. 2007; **5**: 507–11.
54. Rhoden CR, Wellenius GA, Ghelfi E et al. PM-induced cardiac oxidative stress and dysfunction are mediated by autonomic stimulation. *Biochimica et Biophysica Acta*. 2005; **1725**: 305–13.
55. Gong H Jr, Linn WS, Terrell SL et al. Altered heart-rate variability in asthmatic and healthy volunteers exposed to concentrated ambient coarse particles. *Inhalational Toxicology*. 2004; **16**: 335–43.
56. Devlin RB, Ghio AJ, Kehrl H et al. Elderly humans exposed to concentrated air pollution particles have decreased heart rate variability. *European Respiratory Journal*. 2003; **40** (Suppl.): 76s–80s.
57. Elder A, Gelein R, Silva V et al. Translocation of inhaled ultrafine manganese oxide particles to the central nervous system. *Environmental Health Perspectives*. 2006; **114**: 1172–8.
58. Calderon-Garciduenas L, Reed W, Maronpot RR et al. Brain inflammation and Alzheimer's-like pathology in individuals exposed to severe air pollution. *Toxicologic Pathology*. 2004; **32**: 650–8.
59. Kreuter J, Shamenkov D, Petrov V et al. Apolipoprotein-mediated transport of nanoparticle-bound drugs across the blood–brain barrier. *Journal of Drug Targeting*. 2002; **10**: 317–25.
60. Borm PJ, Kreyling W. Toxicological hazards of inhaled nanoparticles – potential implications for drug delivery. *Journal of Nanoscience and Nanotechnology*. 2004; **4**: 521–31.
61. Li N, Sioutas C, Cho A et al. Ultrafine particulate pollutants induce oxidative stress and mitochondrial damage. *Environmental Health Perspectives*. 2003; **111**: 455–60.
62. Geiser M, Rothen-Rutlshauser B, Kapp N et al. Ultrafine particles cross cellular membranes by non-phagocytic mechanisms in lungs and in cultured cells. *Environmental Health Perspectives*. 2006; **114**: A211–12.
63. Gehr P, Blank F, Rothen-Rutishauser BM. Fate of inhaled particles after interaction with the lung surface. *Paediatric Respiratory Reviews*. 2006; **7** (Suppl. 1): S73–S75.
64. Rothen-Rutishauser BM, Schurch S, Haenni B et al. Interaction of fine particles and nanoparticles with red blood cells visualized with advanced microscopic techniques. *Environmental Science and Technology*. 2006; **40**: 4353–9.
65. Nel A, Xia T, Madler L, Li N. Toxic potential of materials at the nanolevel. *Science*. 2006; **311**: 622–7.
66. Renwick LC, Donaldson K, Clouter A. Impairment of alveolar macrophage phagocytosis by ultrafine particles. *Toxicology and Applied Pharmacology*. 2001; **172**: 119–27.
67. Shukla A, Ramos-Nino M, Mossman B. Cell signaling and transcription factor activation by asbestos in lung injury and disease. *International Journal of Biochemistry and Cell Biology*. 2003; **35**: 1198–209.
68. Schins RP. Mechanisms of genotoxicity of particles and fibers. *Inhalational Toxicology*. 2002; **14**: 57–78.
69. Nikasinovic L, Momas I, Just J. A review of experimental studies on diesel exhaust particles and nasal epithelium alterations. *Journal of Toxicology and Environmental Health. Part B, Critical Reviews*. 2004; **7**: 81–104.
70. Diaz-Sanchez D, Garcia MP, Wang M et al. Nasal challenge with diesel exhaust particles can induce sensitization to a neoallergen in the human mucosa. *Journal of Allergy and Clinical Immunology*. 1999; **104**: 1183–8.
71. Wan J, Diaz-Sanchez D. Phase II enzymes induction blocks the enhanced IgE production in B cells by diesel exhaust particles. *Journal of Immunology*. 2006; **177**: 3477–83.
72. Salvi S, Blomberg A, Rudell B et al. Acute inflammatory responses in the airways and peripheral blood after short-term exposure to diesel exhaust in healthy human volunteers. *American Journal of Respiratory and Critical Care Medicine*. 1999; **159**: 702–9.
73. Rudell B, Blomberg A, Helleday R et al. Bronchoalveolar inflammation after exposure to diesel exhaust: Comparison between unfiltered and particle trap filtered exhaust. *Occupational and Environmental Medicine*. 1999; **56**: 527–34.
74. Nightingale JA, Maggs R, Cullinan P et al. Airway inflammation after controlled exposure to diesel exhaust particulates. *American Journal of Respiratory and Critical Care Medicine*. 2000; **162**: 161–6.
75. Behndig AF, Mudway IS, Brown JL et al. Airway antioxidant and inflammatory responses to diesel exhaust exposure in healthy humans. *European Respiratory Journal*. 2006; **27**: 359–65.
76. Stenfors N, Nordenhall C, Salvi SS et al. Different airway inflammatory responses in asthmatic and healthy humans exposed to diesel. *European Respiratory Journal*. 2004; **23**: 82–6.

77. Bosson J, Pourazar J, Forsberg B et al. Ozone enhances the airway inflammation initiated by diesel exhaust. *Respiratory Medicine*. 2007; **101**: 1140–6.
78. Nordenhall C, Pourazar J, Ledin MC et al. Diesel exhaust enhances airway responsiveness in asthmatic subjects. *European Respiratory Journal*. 2001; **17**: 909–15.
79. Tornquist S, Nicklasson M, Soderkvist P et al. Bioavailability of benzo(a)pyrene deposited in the lung. Correlation with dissolution from urban air particulates and covalently bound DNA adducts. *Drug Metabolism and Disposition*. 1988; **16**: 842–7.
80. Mills NL, Tornqvist H, Robinson SD et al. Diesel exhaust inhalation causes vascular dysfunction and impaired endogenous fibrinolysis. *Circulation*. 2005; **112**: 3930–6.
81. Carlsten C, Kaufman JD, Peretz A et al. Coagulation markers in healthy human subjects exposed to diesel exhaust. *Thrombosis Research*. 2007; **120**: 849–55.
82. Frampton MW, Stewart JC, Oberdorster G et al. Inhalation of ultrafine particles alters blood leukocyte expression of adhesion molecules in humans. *Environmental Health Perspectives*. 2006; **114**: 51–8.
83. Pietropaoli AP, Frampton MW, Hyde RW et al. Pulmonary function, diffusing capacity, and inflammation in healthy and asthmatic subjects exposed to ultrafine particles. *Inhalational Toxicology*. 2004; **16** (Suppl. 1): 59–72.
84. Routledge HC, Manney S, Harrison RM et al. Effect of inhaled sulphur dioxide and carbon particles on heart rate variability and markers of inflammation and coagulation in human subjects. *Heart*. 2006; **92**: 220–7.
85. Kim JY, Chen JC, Boyce PD, Christiani DC. Exposure to welding fumes is associated with acute systemic inflammatory responses. *Occupational and Environmental Medicine*. 2005; **62**: 157–63.
86. Beach JR, Dennis JH, Avery AJ et al. An epidemiologic investigation of asthma in welders. *American Journal of Respiratory and Critical Care Medicine*. 1996; **154**: 1394–400.
87. Hannu T, Piipari R, Kasurinen H et al. Occupational asthma due to manual metal-arc welding of special stainless steels. *European Respiratory Journal*. 2005; **26**: 736–9.
88. Fishwick D, Bradshaw LM, Slater T, Pearce N. Respiratory symptoms, across-shift lung function changes and lifetime exposures of welders in New Zealand. *Scandinavian Journal of Work and Environmental Health*. 1997; **23**: 351–8.
89. Attfield MD, Ross DS. Radiological abnormalities in electric-arc welders. *British Journal of Industrial Medicine*. 1978; **35**: 117–22.
90. Health Effects Institute. Diesel exhaust: A critical analysis of emissions, exposure and health effects. A special report of the Institute's diesel working group. HEI research report. Boston, MA: Health Effects Institute, 1995.
91. Hart JE, Laden F, Schenker MB, Garshick E. Chronic obstructive pulmonary disease mortality in diesel-exposed railroad workers. *Environmental Health Perspectives*. 2006; **114**: 1013–17.
92. Aitken RJ, Creely KS, Tran CL. *Nanoparticles: An occupational hygiene review*. HSE Book Reseach Report 274. London: HSE Books, 2004.
93. Kroto H. Fullerene science – a most international endeavour. *Journal of Molecular Graphics and Modelling*. 2001; **19**: 187–8.
94. Iijima S. Helical microtubules of graphite carbon. *Nature*. 1991; **354**: 56.
95. Maynard AD, Aitken R. Assessing exposure to airborne nanomaterials: Current abilities and future requirements. *Nanotoxicology*. 2007; **1**: 26–41.
96. Aitken RJ, Chaudhry MQ, Boxall AB, Hull M. Manufacture and use of nanomaterials: Current status in the UK and global trends. *Occupational Medicine*. 2006; **56**: 300–6.
97. British Standards Institute. Nanotechnologies – Part 2: Guide to the safe handling and disposal of engineered nanomaterials. British Standards Institute published document, PD 6699-2, 2007.
98. Walton WH, Vincent JH. Aerosol instrumentation in occupational hygiene: An historical perspective, aerosol science and technology. *Aerosol Science and Technology*. 1998; **28**: 417–38.
99. British Standards Institute. Health and safety in welding and allied processes – Sampling of airborne particles and gases in the operator's breathing zone. Part 1: Sampling of airborne particles. BS EN ISO 10882-1. London: BSI, 2001.
100. CEN. Workplace atmospheres: Size fraction definitions for measurement of airborne particles in the workplace. CEN standard EN481. Brussels: CEN, 1993.
101. ISO. Air quality: Particle size fraction definitions for health-related sampling. CD7708. Geneva: International Standards Organization, 1993.
102. ACGIH. Threshold limit values of chemical substances and physical agents. Cincinatti, OH: American Conference of Governmental Occupational Hygienists, 1993.
103. WHO. Determination of airborne fibre number concentrations: A recommended method by phase constrast optical microscopy. Geneva: World Health Organization, 1997.
104. British Standards Institute. Publicly available specification PAS 136:2007. Terminology for nanomaterials. London: BSI, 2007.
105. Ku BK, Maynard AD. Comparing aerosol surface area measurements of monodisperse ultrafine silver agglomerates by mobility analysis, transmission electron microscopy and diffusion charging. *Journal of Aerosol Science*. 2008; **36**: 1108–24.
106. Brouwer DH, Gijsbers JH, Lurvink MW. Personal exposure to ultrafine particles in the workplace: Exploring sampling techniques and strategies. *Annals of Occupational Hygiene*. 2004; **48**: 439–53.

71

Health effects related to non-industrial workplace indoor environments

JOUNI JK JAAKKOLA AND MARITTA S JAAKKOLA

Introduction	921	Specific diseases or syndromes related to non-industrial indoor environments	925
Sources of occupational hazards in non-industrial environments	921	Public health impact and economic consequences	933
Occupational exposures in non-industrial workplace environments and health	923	Management and prevention	933
		References	934

INTRODUCTION

An increasing proportion of the workforce is working in non-industrial indoor environments, among which the modern office environment is becoming the most common workplace. Other similar environments include schools and other educational institutions, day-care centres and hospitals, as well as care homes. These environments have traditionally been considered as safe, because occupants are usually not exposed to high levels of physical, chemical or biological compounds potentially hazardous to health. This view has been based on simple causal models where an identifiable single agent causes a well-defined occupational disease. In multifactorial causal webs, several component causes create complex environmental conditions, which may increase the risk of developing well-defined diseases or the occurrence of a set of symptoms and signs, which form disease-like entities. The idea of a safe office environment was already being strongly challenged in the early 1980s by reports of a high prevalence of symptoms in employees working in modern office buildings. These health problems were often related to indoor air quality and ventilation. A World Health Organization working group on indoor air and health characterized these in their report on 'sick' building syndrome.[1] These observations have stimulated long-term research programmes, which have provided more insight into the type of specific diseases, symptoms, signs and syndromes, which can be caused by modern non-industrial environments. This chapter provides a presentation of these problems. First, the determinants of indoor air quality are presented. Second, the most common occupational exposures in non-industrial environments and their health effects are presented systematically. Third, specific diseases related to non-industrial workplaces are presented. A discussion of their impact on public health and their economic consequences concludes the chapter.

SOURCES OF OCCUPATIONAL HAZARDS IN NON-INDUSTRIAL ENVIRONMENTS

Components of the indoor environment

The determinants of indoor air quality in the non-industrial workplace can be divided into the following: (1) outdoor sources, (2) type of building, (3) occupants and their activities, (4) physical indoor sources and (5) heating, ventilation and air conditioning. In addition, psychological and social factors are important determinants of health.

The main route of exposure to the physical environment is inhalation, but skin exposure may also be relevant. Social environment causes both psychological and physical effects via psychological processes.[2]

OUTDOOR SOURCES

The air, water and soil surrounding the building have the potential to have an impact on the indoor air quality.

Industry, traffic, heating and natural sources contribute to outdoor air pollution and indirectly to indoor air quality, but outdoor–indoor penetration has not been sufficiently studied. The geographic location of the building is therefore an important determinant of many indoor factors. The proximity of busy traffic routes or industrial plants may contribute substantially to total exposure to various environmental pollutants in the non-industrial work environment, but the type of building and ventilation system plays an important role in managing these exposures.

THE TYPE OF BUILDING

The type of building, the structure, openings and the type of ventilation system influence the penetration of outdoor pollutants into buildings, as well as the elimination of air pollutants from indoor sources. In a sealed building, penetration and elimination depend mainly on the function of the ventilation system. The location of an air inlet in a building can be important, because it may influence the penetration of outdoor pollutants from local sources back into the building. For example, an air inlet facing a bus stop may result in high concentrations of diesel exhaust gases and particles indoors.

OCCUPANTS AND THEIR ACTIVITIES

Occupants are an important source of indoor air pollution in non-industrial workplaces. Human metabolism results in carbon dioxide, carbon monoxide, ammonia, acetone, alcohol and various other odorous organic gases, which are released into the indoor air through breathing and perspiration. In addition, occupants release bacteria and viruses, which may cause infections. Clothing textiles may release various types of particles and clothes may carry animal dander from one environment to another. Munir and colleagues[3] measured substantial concentrations of cat and dog allergens in Swedish day-care centres. The levels were related to the number of children and staff with cats or dogs at home. Cleaning method or cleaning frequency had little effect on allergen levels which were higher than in homes without pets, but lower than in homes with pets. Office activities, such as paper handling, including carbonless copy paper, photocopying and printing may generate important exposures to gases and particles. Studies in paper industries with high paper dust levels have suggested that paper dust can be highly irritative.[4–7] Carbonless copy papers contain solvents and colour-forming chemicals and these have been suggested to be potential sensitizers.[8–12] In many countries, tobacco smoking is still an important source of indoor air pollution, although national smoke-free workplace legislation is shown to be a valuable tool to protect people against the adverse health effects of environmental tobacco smoke exposure.[13] When non-smokers occupy the same indoor space as smokers, they inhale tobacco combustion products that are released into the air, i.e. they undergo passive smoking.[14] The smoke inhaled by these non-smokers is called environmental tobacco smoke (ETS), tobacco-smoke pollution or second-hand smoke, and it is formed mainly of sidestream smoke (SS) and, to a small extent, exhaled mainstream smoke (MS). SS is smoke released into the air from the smouldering end of a cigarette between puffs, whereas MS is smoke inhaled by a smoker during a puff. Both types of smoke contain thousands of chemicals, including approximately 50 carcinogenic and tens of irritative and toxic substances.[15] The concentrations of many harmful substances are higher in undiluted SS than in MS,[16] but the final concentrations of hazardous compounds inhaled by non-smokers are determined by factors such as the number of smokers, the number of cigarettes smoked and the volume of the space.

PHYSICAL INDOOR SOURCES

There is increasing evidence that interior surface materials used in floors, walls and ceilings, as well as furnishing are potential sources of indoor air pollution.

In the 1970s, exposure to formaldehyde from building materials emerged as a large-scale health problem.[17] Formaldehyde (HCHO) is present in several building materials (particleboard, fibreboard and plywood), paintings and wall paints, glued wallpapers, coatings, fabrics, draperies, carpets and insulation materials, and is emitted significantly from pressed wood products (particleboard, hardwood plywood panelling, medium density fibreboard) which are made using adhesives that contain urea-formaldehyde and wood products containing phenol-formaldehyde resins, conversion varnishes and latex paints. With available measurement techniques and being a singular chemical compound, regulatory processes have lead to reduction of formaldehyde use in building material and hence to dramatic reduction of indoor air formaldehyde concentrations in non-industrial workplaces and homes.

However, interior surface materials are potential sources of a large number of other volatile organic compounds (VOCs). VOC emissions are categorized into primary and secondary sources. Primary emissions refer to non-bonded or free VOCs within building and surface materials and normally found as additives, or solvents, or monomers of low molecular weight. Secondary emissions are physically or chemically bounded VOCs which are emitted or formed through mechanisms, such as reactions between ozone and aliphatic hydrocarbons (in photocopiers and laser printers), or reactions between ozone and fitted carpets or limonene, or microbiological emissions on damped surfaces (MVOCs), or hydrolysis of wet PVC flooring materials or degradation of building and interior surface materials. The most reported VOCs include ethanol, limonene, carbonyls (aldehydes and ketones), aliphatic, cylic and aromatic hydrocarbons, methylene chloride, terpenes, glycols, acids and esters and their individual concentrations vary from 5 to 50 $\mu g/m^3$.

Polyvinyl chloride (PVC) is a polymer and a major building material in which phthalates are used extensively as plasticizers to enhance the flexibility, viscosity, stability and other desirable physical properties of PVC.[18] Plasticized PVC is used extensively indoors as wall and flooring covering in kitchens, bathrooms and children's playrooms and bedrooms, because it is inexpensive and is easy to clean. Other uses of plasticized PVC indoors are as roofing materials, shower curtains, electric cables, adhesives and synthetic leather. Because phthalate esters are not covalently bonded to the polymer with which they are mixed, they can migrate from PVC material and adhere to the surfaces of indoor particulate matter (PM), as well as house dust. Phthalate may also migrate to PM surfaces, following wear and tear of PVC materials or use of other PVC products, such as nail polish.

Dampness and moisture from building structures and interior surfaces is an important source of indoor pollution, not only in the home, but also in non-industrial workplaces, including office buildings, schools and day-care centres. Damp or moisture accumulates in building structures and/or interior finishes via leaks in roofs, windows or pipes; or moisture from the ground penetrating into the building structure by capillary movement; or moisture from humans and indoor activities such as cooking, bathing, human expiration and humidifiers; or moisture already present in the building material from the time the building was erected. The usual signs are colour changes in and loosening of the surface materials, wet spots on the surfaces, visible moulds and mould odour. Air humidity influences the materials where the climate is moist and warm throughout the year, but has little influence in a cold climate where outdoor air humidity is relatively low throughout the year.

Indoor environments constitute a complex mixture of viable and non-viable microorganisms, which produce fragments, toxins, allergens, microbial volatile compounds (MVOCs) and other chemicals. Dampness is likely to enhance indoor concentration of some of these organisms, in particular dust mites and fungi. Fungi also produce a number of toxins and irritants with suspected respiratory health effects. Dampness may also enhance chemical emissions from buildings and interior surface materials, sometimes compromising the integrity of the material. Emissions of irritants and odorous substances from microbiological and chemical processes on building structures and interior finishes following dampness have also been noted.

HEATING, VENTILATION AND AIR CONDITIONING

Heating, ventilation and air conditioning influence indoor air quality in different ways. Changing the air dilutes the concentration of pollutants from indoor sources when the outdoor concentrations are lower than indoor concentrations. Ventilation systems may also serve as sources of indoor air pollution. Air humidification equipment, used to alleviate the effects of dry air, may serve as source of microbial pollutants some of which may have adverse health effects.

OCCUPATIONAL EXPOSURES IN NON-INDUSTRIAL WORKPLACE ENVIRONMENTS AND HEALTH

Changing the air

The main purpose of a ventilation system is to maintain good indoor air quality in buildings by changing the air by removal and dilution of pollutants and supply of fresh air. In naturally ventilated buildings, air moves into and out of the building through intentionally provided openings, such as windows or doors, or through non-powered ventilators, or by infiltration.

Air change influences the concentrations of indoor air pollutants according to the following formula:

$$C = G/Q_v \varepsilon_v$$

where C is the concentration of the contaminant, G is the generation of contaminant (volume flow), Q_v is the clean air flow to the room and ε_v is the efficiency of pollutant removal.

Insufficient air change or ventilation may lead to accumulation of contaminants and moisture problems, which may lead to adverse health effects. There is also evidence that excessive ventilation may increase emission rates from some materials,[19,20] as well as increase the resuspension of sedimented particulate matter into indoor air.[21] Insufficient air change is a common problem in office buildings,[22–24] schools[25] and day-care centres.[26] Air change rates measured as air flow in volume units per hour have been measured as relatively low, but air flows in particular calculated per person were very low in schools and day-care centres.[26] Carbon dioxide concentrations reflect excessive human burden. Studies in day-care centres in Denmark, Finland, Norway and Canada have reported low air flows per person and high carbon dioxide concentrations.[26] Ventilation rates below 5 litres/s per person are likely to cause indoor air pollution problems in non-industrial facilities with high emission rates. Based on several epidemiologic studies, the minimum ventilation rate for office buildings is recommended to be 10–15 litres/s per person.[22,24,27]

Thermal environment

The thermal environment, including temperature, relative humidity and air velocity, may influence human health, well-being and performance both directly and indirectly. Thermal environment may act indirectly by either influencing sources, emissions and indoor concentrations of indoor pollutants or by possibly modifying the adverse effects of exposures. Temperature is probably the most important indoor air quality parameter in non-industrial workplaces. Temperature can be considered suitable if the occupants feel comfortable and do not wish to be warmer or cooler. Satisfaction with temperature depends on several factors, including indoor air temperature, radiation temperature from the sun and from cold and warm surfaces and equipment, and surface temperature.[28] Thermal comfort is a function of the total body heat exchange with the environment. Individuals vary substantially in satisfaction with temperature, which means that in a given space it is virtually impossible to achieve conditions where 100 per cent of the occupants are satisfied. In an environment of 22°C with negligible radiant temperature and lower than moderate air movement, approximately 80 per cent of the occupants in sedentary work with light clothing feel comfortable. The remaining 20 per cent would prefer a lower or higher temperature, thus a 100 per cent occupant satisfaction rate can only be achieved by personal control of temperature. The optimal temperature in office work is 22 ± 2°C.[29,30]

Perceptions of dry air may be caused by low relative humidity, but such sensations may also be related to other indoor air parameters, such as high temperature, particles and organic gases. Humans do not have a special sense to perceive humidity, and perception of dry air is related to irritation of conjunctivae, mucosae and skin.[31] Perceived temperature is strongly related to relative humidity: the sensation of warmth decreases in lower relative humidity. A controlled crossover trial showed that perceived air dryness is alleviated by steam humidification for relative humidity of 29–39 per cent during winter when the relative humidity in non-humidified periods varied between 12 and 28 per cent.[32]

The thermal environment directly affects the neural sensors of mucous membranes and skin, and may provoke neuron–sensoral responses indirectly by changes in blood circulation.[33] There is evidence that symptoms affecting the eyes, airways, skin and central nervous system are related to temperature and relative humidity. The concept 'sick building syndrome' (SBS) has been used to describe a set of symptoms common among office workers in buildings with indoor air problems.[1] The occurrence of SBS symptoms is related to temperature[29,30] and relative humidity,[34] and the relation between the occurrence of SBS symptoms and temperature is U-shaped, with lowest prevalence in temperature between 21 and 23°C.[29]

Dampness and mould problems

Based on a 2004 literature review including studies from several European countries, the United States and Canada, it was estimated that at least 20 per cent of buildings had one or more signs of dampness problems.[35] Many non-industrial workplaces including office buildings, schools and day-care centres have dampness problems and the prevalence of dampness problems is likely to vary from 10 to 50 per cent, depending on building type, location and the criteria used.

A large number of epidemiological studies have assessed the relation between dampness and moulds at home and the risk of health effects. In the most recent systematic review and meta-analysis by Fisk et al.,[36] dampness and moulds increased the risk of upper respiratory tract symptoms (summary odds ratio (OR) of 13 studies: 1.70, 95 per cent CI, 1.44–2.00), cough (summary OR of six studies in adults: 1.52, 95 per cent CI, 1.18–1.96), wheeze (summary OR of five studies in adults: 1.39, 95 per cent CI, 1.04–1.85), current asthma (summary OR of ten studies: 1.56, 95 per cent CI, 1.30–1.86) and development of asthma (summary OR of four studies: 1.34, 95 per cent CI, 0.86–2.10). Few studies have assessed the effects of workplace dampness and mould problems.[37–41] Moisture and debris in ventilation systems, possibly by supporting microbiologic growth, may increase adverse respiratory effects, particularly among asthmatics. The risk of lower respiratory symptoms, throat irritation and rash/itchy skin have been shown to be related to the fungal and endotoxin levels in floor dust.[40] Non-specific symptoms were positively associated with unidentified chair fungi.[41] Upper respiratory symptoms were positively associated with total fungal concentrations recovered from chair dust. There is also evidence that dampness and mould problems in schools increase the risk of respiratory symptoms[42] and general symptoms, such as headache and concentration problems.[43] The effects of dampness and moulds on asthma and asthma-related symptoms are discussed under Asthma, p. 925. In summary, dampness and mould problems are common in non-industrial workplaces and have similar health effects as these problems in the home.

Allergens

Traditionally, relevant exposures to allergens have been thought to take place in the home where the most important sources include dander from cats, dogs and other hairy and feathered pets, house dust mites and excretions, insects, pollen and dust from clothes and other textiles. Studies in day-care centres have shown that occupants can also be exposed to common domestic allergens probably via transportation on children's clothes.[3] Outdoor pollen via openings and ventilation systems is also a likely allergen in non-industrial workplaces. Exposures to indoor allergens usually cause IgE-mediated type I immunological reactions in the airways of individuals who have propensity to specific sensitization. Thus, allergens in the workplace may contribute to an increase in the risk of asthma and allergic rhinitis. The authors did not find any empirical studies focusing on this occupational health problem in non-industrial work environments.

Volatile organic compounds

The potential effects of exposure to VOCs in the levels appearing in non-industrial indoor environments range from sensory irritation at low and medium levels of exposure to airway inflammation, to neurotoxic, organotoxic and carcinogenic effects at high exposure levels. Some of the VOCs, including benzene and vinyl chloride, have been identified as human carcinogens in much higher levels than occurring in non-industrial environments and others, such as chloroform, have been found to be carcinogenic in animals.[44]

VOCs may affect the airways and induce inflammation and airway obstruction. Molhave[45] suggested three mechanisms for the effects of exposure to low-level VOCs: sensory perceptions of the environment, weak inflammatory reactions and environmental stress reactions. Humans use several senses to identify VOCs: the sense of smell in the nasal cavity, the sense of taste on the tongue and/or the stimulation of sensory nerves in the skin surface. The perception of air quality is an integration of these sensations. Sensory nerves in the skin mediate irritation, smarting or stinging (i.e. symptoms). Eyes may form tears as a protective reflexion (i.e. signs). Chemical mediators usually cause acute reversible inflammatory reactions leading to dilatation of vessels and changes in colour and temperature of the tissue. Environmental stress from complex perceptions may lead to increases in stress hormone levels and blood pressure and consequently to fatigue, irritability, reduced tolerance, as well as psychological processes and symptoms.

VOC from water-based paint was shown to increase the prevalence of asthma by two-fold in a study of healthy Swedish adults.[46] Work-related symptoms of eye irritation, cough with sputum and itchy hands are also common among workers using water-based paints.

Office equipment

An increasing amount of equipment and supplies are used in modern offices. Carbonless copy paper can be a source of various particles and volatile organic compounds, such as solvents and colour-forming chemicals.[47] Exposure can be direct through contaminated air to the eyes, nasal mucosa and or indirect through fingers used for handling the paper. Photocopying is also a potential source of chemicals, including VOCs, ozone, particles and resin.[48]

Epidemiological studies conducted in northern Europe and the United States have consistently shown an increased risk of SBS symptoms related to handling of carbonless copy paper.[48–50] Exposure to carbonless copy paper, paper dust and fumes from photocopiers and printers (FPP) may increase the occurrence of SBS-related symptoms, chronic respiratory symptoms, chronic bronchitis, general symptoms (headache and fatigue) and respiratory infections.[50,51] There is also evidence that exposure to paper dust and to FPP increases the risk of upper respiratory and skin symptoms, breathlessness, tonsillitis and middle ear infections.[51] Effects on asthma are discussed under Asthma, p. 925.

Environmental tobacco smoke or secondhand tobacco smoke

Sidestream smoke contains the same carcinogenic, irritative and toxic compounds as mainstream smoke and on a biologic basis, it is likely that ETS has similar respiratory effects to active smoking. Exposure to ETS ten years ago was still common in most European and North American countries, as shown in Table 71.1, but is now radically decreasing due to progressive smoke-free workplace legislation.[13] However, ETS remains a major global occupational health problem in both non-industrial and industrial workplaces. Table 71.2 summarizes the evidence of the health effects of occupational exposure to ETS. There is abundant evidence that workplace ETS exposure is causally linked to lung cancer and coronary heart disease, and there is strong evidence that such exposure is related to increased risk of asthma in adults. Strong evidence also links reduced birthweight in newborns to ETS exposure of their mothers during pregnancy. In addition, relatively strong evidence links ETS exposure to chronic obstructive pulmonary disease (COPD) and stroke and one study suggests its association with severe pneumonia.

SPECIFIC DISEASES OR SYNDROMES RELATED TO NON-INDUSTRIAL INDOOR ENVIRONMENTS

Asthma

Many studies have suggested that the prevalence of asthma has increased at least in western countries in the late twentieth century.[52] There are several possible explanations for this, including changes in environmental exposures, changes in lifestyle habits, changes in diagnostic and management practices of asthma, as well as methodological issues.[53] There is a trend towards an increasing proportion of the workforce working in an office-type environment, where they may be exposed to indoor pollutants. Energy-saving measures have sometimes led to reduced ventilation of the indoor spaces, which can increase the levels of indoor pollutants. Both development of adult-onset asthma and exacerbations of underlying asthma have been linked to many exposures in non-industrial indoor environments.

Occupational asthma is asthma where the probable principal cause is a chemical, physical or biological exposure at work. It can be induced by a sensitizer or long-term or intermittent exposure to low levels of irritants. The diagnostic criteria of occupational asthma are presented in Chapter 72, Occupational asthma, p. 941. The diagnostic procedures include a thorough occupational history and inventory of exposures in the workplace, which in some cases may include environmental measurements of exposures at work, serial peak expiratory flow recordings on work days and days off work, spirometry, histamine or methacholine challenge, and for some exposures immunological tests (specific IgE and/or skin prick tests).[54,55] When hypersensitivity is suspected as the underlying mechanism, specific bronchial challenge tests can be carried out in expert centres. Comparison of lung function during exposure and away from it can also be tested in a workplace challenge. As many of the non-industrial indoor

Table 71.1 Occurrence of environmental tobacco smoke exposure at work.

Region/country	Type of study	Occurrence of workplace ETS exposure	Reference
Europe			
15 European Union countries	CAREX database used to assess exposure to known or probable carcinogens	7.5 million workers exposed to ETS at least 75% of their working time	105
Spain	ECRHS cross-sectional survey (20–44 years)	32–54%	111
Italy	ECRHS	30–42%	111
Netherlands	ECRHS	29–38%	111
Belgium	ECRHS	28–30%	111
Germany	ECRHS	25–29%	111
Ireland	ECRHS	29%	111
France	ECRHS	18–28%	111
UK	ECRHS	11–24%	111
Switzerland	ECRHS	20%	111
Norway	ECRHS	19%	111
Iceland	ECRHS	18%	111
Estonia	ECRHS	13%	111
Sweden	ECRHS	3–10%	111
Finland	Longitudinal follow up of a random population sample (15–64 years)	In 2000, 8% of employed men and 4% of employed women	112
United States of America			
	Estimated impact of a national smoke-free workplace legislation in the USA	Currently, 31% of 24.6 million non-smoking indoor workers are not covered by smoke-free legislation and are exposed to ETS at work	106
	Cross-sectional study of 7301 non-smokers from California	31%	113
	Cross-sectional study of 20 801 US employees from 114 worksites	52%	114
Australia			
	ECRHS	8%	111
New Zealand			
	ECRHS	5–10%	111

ECRHS, European Community Respiratory Health Survey; ETS, environmental tobacco smoke.

Table 71.2 Summary of health effect estimates for workplace exposure to environmental tobacco smoke.

Disease	OR (95% CI)	No. studies	Reference
Lung cancer	1.17 (1.04–1.32)	16 (meta-analysis)	115
Coronary heart disease	1.21 (1.04–1.41)	5 (meta-analysis)	116
Asthma	2.16 (1.26–3.72)	9	59
COPD	1.36 (1.002–1.84)	9	117
Low birth-weight	1.43 (0.50–4.12)	17	97
Stroke	1.82 (1.34–2.49)	6	118
Severe pneumonia	2.5 (1.2–5.1)	1	119

environmental exposures are likely to induce irritant, rather than hypersensitivity-induced asthma, specific bronchial challenges may not be the way to proceed in the diagnostics and the role of a good-quality serial peak expiratory flow (PEF) recording is emphasized. The recently studied known or potential causes of occupational asthma in non-industrial indoor environments are reviewed briefly in this section.

Occupational asthma is a medicolegal concept and remediating environmental measures should be taken when appropriate from the disease management point of view even if the legal definition of occupational asthma may not be met. Many countries have compensation systems covering occupational asthma, but the systems vary between different countries, so information to be given to the patient depends on the local system.

Work-aggravated asthma is a concept more recently introduced to the literature. It means that work exposures aggravate the symptoms of pre-existing asthma and lead to less well-controlled asthma, even if they are not the principal cause of the asthma. This is likely to affect the employee's work ability. The control of asthma can be improved by reducing the workplace exposures and ensuring that the asthma medication is adequate.

SECONDHAND TOBACCO SMOKE EXPOSURE

Among children, the causal role of secondhand smoke (SHS) exposure at home for both onset of asthma and exacerbation of asthma has been established.[56,57] In recent years, an increasing number of studies have also addressed the relationship between SHS and adult asthma.[13,57,58] SHS exposure at work and at home was related to adult-onset asthma in a large Finnish population-based case–control study, the OR estimates being 2.16 (95 per cent CI, 1.26–3.72) in relation to workplace exposure and 4.77 (95 per cent CI, 1.29–17.7) in relation to home SHS exposure in the previous 12 months.[59] Cumulative SHS exposure over lifetime at work and at home was linked to increased risk of asthma showing an exposure–response relation. The risk estimates, usually OR, from other studies varied between 1.15 and 4.7.[13] Several studies found a stronger effect related to workplace SHS exposure than home exposure.

The mechanisms by which SHS induces asthma are not well known. SHS contains many irritant substances that can induce mucus hypersecretion and inflammation in the airways. Long-term exposure could lead to irritant-induced asthma.[59] Tobacco smoke also seems to cause epithelial damage and to increase epithelial permeability to environmental allergens and has been shown to enhance allergic reactions to some inhalable allergens. There is also some evidence that SHS exposure may cause bronchoconstriction and increased microvascular leakage, which are typical for asthma.[60]

Subjects with asthma have chronic inflammation in their airways and consequently, may be particularly susceptible to the adverse effects of SHS exposure, so SHS may be a cause of work-aggravated asthma. The review by Jaakkola and Jaakkola[61] and another by the Californian Environmental Protection Agency[57] identified a total of nine studies on the role of SHS exposure for exacerbation of a pre-existing asthma. The studies showed that in adult subjects with asthma, SHS exposure at home and/or at work is related to increased occurrence of respiratory symptoms, increased use of bronchodilator and steroid medications, reduced general health, increased health-care use including emergency department visits and hospitalizations, increased bronchial hyper-responsiveness and reduced spirometric lung function. The Third National Health and Nutrition Examination Survey (NHANES III) found that adult asthmatics with the highest serum creatinine levels had significantly lower lung function levels, especially in women, compared to those with low SHS exposure levels.[62]

INDOOR DAMPNESS AND MOULD PROBLEMS

In 2007, Fisk and colleagues[36] reported a meta-analysis of 33 studies on dampness and mould problems in homes and asthma and respiratory symptoms. In analyses combining studies of children and adults, the estimated OR of lifetime asthma was 1.37 (95 per cent CI, 1.23–1.53) and that of current asthma 1.56 (1.30–1.86). Thus, the results suggested a 30–50 per cent increased risk of asthma in relation to indoor dampness and mould problems. The risks of cough and wheeze were also statistically significantly increased, the effects being usually slightly larger among children.

In 2004, Jaakkola and Jaakkola[63] reviewed the literature on indoor moulds and asthma in adults. They concluded that there is strong evidence that indoor moulds at home increase the risk of asthma, as epidemiological studies have consistently found a relation between exposure to dampness and moulds at home and the risk of asthma in adults. The OR of asthma has ranged between 1.3 and 2.2 and there is some evidence of a dose–response relationship with more severe mould problems being related to a higher OR. They also concluded that there is increasing evidence that indoor moulds at work increase the risk of wheezing, with an OR between 1.3 and 2.8. A recent Finnish incident case–control study showed evidence that indoor moulds at work significantly increase the risk of asthma, with an OR of 1.54 (95 per cent CI, 1.01–2.31).[64] That study indicated that women, young adults and smokers are particularly susceptible to the adverse effects of workplace indoor moulds.

The mechanisms by which indoor dampness and mould problems could lead to asthma are not yet fully understood, but several potential mechanisms have been suggested. These include IgE-mediated hypersensitivity reactions to fungal allergens or to mite allergens,[65] toxic effects of mycotoxins produced by fungi and non-specific inflammatory reactions caused by fungal cell wall components, such as 1,3-β-D-glucan and ergosterol.[66,67] It is not known whether these mechanisms are specific for different species of moulds.

In Finland, indoor moulds have been a rather common cause of occupational asthma according to the Finnish Register of Occupational Diseases. However, this is a difficult diagnosis to make, as hypersensitivity reactions seem to be the underlying mechanism only in a minority of mould-induced cases. Thus, specific bronchial challenge tests may not be very useful. Currently, the diagnosis of occupational asthma due to mould problems is based mainly on serial PEF recording, while at work and off work, in conjunction with a history that asthma started in a workplace where there is clear evidence of mould problems.

In addition to the role of indoor moulds for inducing asthma, there is some evidence that indoor moulds also increase the severity of a pre-existing asthma, suggesting that it may cause work-aggravated asthma.

Overall, it can be concluded that there is increasing evidence suggesting that prevention and prompt repair of indoor dampness and mould problems in both the home and work environments prevents asthma. There is some evidence that correction of indoor and dampness problems leads to alleviation of asthma symptoms in damaged workplaces. The long-term prognosis of occupational asthma from indoor moulds is not well understood, but minimizing mould exposure by repair of the damage or relocation of the affected individual is recommended as management.

OTHER OFFICE ENVIRONMENT EXPOSURES

The recent Finnish Environment and Asthma study on adult-onset asthma also investigated the relationship between some office work exposures and asthma. Regular occupational exposure to self-copying paper that contains inks and solvents was linked to significantly increased risk of asthma, with an OR of 1.66 (1.03–2.66).[68] No exposure–response relationship was detected with increasing number of hours working with self-copying paper per week. A significant increase in asthma risk was observed among those with an exposure of between 1 and <15 hours. It was speculated that this could suggest a hypersensitivity reaction, so that even small amounts of exposure might induce the reaction. Exposure to paper dust, in general, was significantly related to the risk of adult-onset asthma, with an OR of 1.97 (95 per cent CI, 1.25–3.10).[68] An increasing risk of asthma was observed with increasing hours of exposure to paper dust at work. More studies are needed to investigate the mechanisms behind this observation. A case–control study from Sweden has also reported increased risk of asthma in relation to paper dust exposure.[69] In contrast, exposure to fumes from copying machines and printers was not significantly associated with asthma in the Finnish study.

Some individual cases of occupational asthma in relation to acrylate glues used in flooring have been detected. Indoor plants in offices have also been reported as identified causes of occupational asthma, a commonly involved plant being the weeping fig (*Ficus benjamina*).[70]

The Finnish Environment and Asthma Study also evaluated potential links between interior surface materials and adult-onset asthma.[71] It found a significantly increased risk of asthma in office workers who reported that at least half of the wall surface area in their office was plastic (OR 2.43, 95 per cent CI, 1.03–5.75). It was speculated that phthalates contained in PVC materials could be the mechanism explaining this finding. Plasticizers of PVC have been shown to induce inflammation in the airways of humans and in animal models.[72] The risk of asthma was also somewhat increased in relation to large areas of textile wall material and wall-to-wall carpet.

CLEANING CHEMICALS

Recent studies have detected increased risk of asthma among cleaners.[73–75] Jaakkola and Jaakkola[75] reviewed the studies on cleaners in 2006 and concluded that there is accumulating, consistent evidence that the risk of asthma is significantly increased among domestic and industrial cleaners. The OR from the studies ranged between 1.42 and 8.1. The agents that have been identified as important exposures include cleaning chemicals containing ammonium, bleach (containing chlorine) and some disinfecting substances. In addition, long-term exposure to a mixture of irritating chemicals may induce asthma via an irritant-induced mechanism. There are also reports in the literature of occupational asthma of personnel other than the cleaners themselves, where the exposure was attributed to residues of cleaning chemicals after the cleaning had taken place.[76]

Extrinsic allergic alveolitis

Extrinsic allergic alveolitis, also known as hypersensitivity pneumonitis, is type III and IV hypersensitivity reaction of the alveolar and bronchiolar tissue and interstitium of the lungs, in response to inhaled antigens. Farmer's lung caused by mouldy forage is the best investigated form of extrinsic allergic alveolitis, but it can be related to a range of environmental allergens in the workplace and at home, including fungi, bacteria, some animal species (e.g. pigeons, rodents), plant proteins and less commonly reactive chemicals.[77–79] Microbiological contamination of air conditioners or humidifiers in indoor environments has been reported as causes of extrinsic allergic alveolitis in office environments and printing works. Contaminated water, for example in washers, has also been reported as a source of outbreaks of extrinsinc allergic alveolitis in some factories, such as car manufacturing.[80] Spraying or vaporization of recycled or stored water has often been involved. The causative microbes identified include fungi, such as *Micropolyspora faeni*, *Aspergillus* and *Penicillium* species, and bacteria, such as *Thermoactinomyces vulgaris* or *Klebsiella* species. In addition, bacterial endotoxins and in some cases amoebae have been detected as significant contaminants. Extrinsinc allergic alevolitis caused by contaminated humidifiers is often called 'Humidifier lung'.

Extrinsinc allergic alveolitis presents as an acute, subacute and chronic form. The acute form is easiest to recognize, as the patient typically experiences cough, chest tightness, febrile chills, malaise and flu-like symptoms three to eight hours after exposure. The symptoms wane spontaneously over a few hours, but recur on subsequent exposure. This is the form most commonly described in outbreaks of humidifier lung. The subacute form develops without obvious episodes of flu-like illness and presents as progressive shortness of breath, dry cough and weight loss. The chronic form is the least well described, presenting as slow development of interstitial fibrosis. The subacute and chronic forms of this disease may well go undetected.

The diagnosis of extrinsic allergic alveolitis from indoor contaminants includes the same diagnostic tests as other forms of extrinsic allergic alveolitis. The diagnostic criteria are presented in Chapter 74, Extrinsic allergic alveolitis, p. 970. The key point is to find the source of exposure and, to investigate this, it is important to take a thorough exposure history and if needed, to conduct a worksite visit, including environmental measurements. Immunoglobulin G (IgG) antibodies (i.e. precipitins) can often be measured to the causal antigen, for example to many moulds and birds. However, IgG antibodies have also been measured in asymptomatic exposed workers, so they may simply be indicators of exposure and not necessarily of disease.

In physical examination, a typical finding is crackles in the lower fields of the lungs. Standard chest x-ray is abnormal in about 80 per cent of cases of extrinsic allergic alveolitis, so a normal finding does not rule out the disease. In acute and subacute forms, the typical findings are fine interstitial infiltrates, while in the chronic form of the disease the radiological appearance is irregular scarring, related to diffuse pulmonary fibrosis or even diffuse emphysema.[81] High-resolution chest computed tomography (CT) shows patchy ground glass opacities, decreased attenuation due to air trapping and a mosaic pattern. In lung function tests, a typical finding is restrictive ventilatory function impairment (with both forced vital capacity (FVC) and forced expiratory volume in 1 second (FEV_1) reduced with normal FEV_1/FVC, as well as reduced total lung capacity), although sometimes a combined restrictive and obstructive pattern may be observed. As extrinsic allergic alveolitis is a diffuse parenchymal disease, the diffusion capacity of the lungs is typically reduced (both DL_{co} and K_{co}). With a mild form of the disease, arterial blood gases show hypoxia only in relation to exercise, while in more advanced disease the patient may be hypoxic even at rest. Carbon dioxide tension may be lowered due to hyperventilation stimulated by low oxygen tension. The lung function findings reflect the interstitial nature of the disease and are not specific for extrinsic allergic alveolitis. It should be borne in mind that all the physiological findings may have subsided if the patient has not been exposed for some time before the investigations.

It is usually recommended that bronchoscopy with bronchoalveolar lavage (BAL) and sometimes transbronchial biopsy be carried out when investigating a patient with suspected extrinsic allergic alveolitis. Surgical lung biopsy is rarely needed for the diagnosis of this disease. BAL typically shows increased total cell count, with an increased proportion of lymphocytes (>40 per cent). T-helper to T-suppressor ratio is usually reduced to less than 1. After acute exposure, neutrophils are transiently increased in BAL. The characteristic histopathologic findings of EAA include diffuse interstitial infiltrate, scattered non-caseating granulomas and cellular inflammation of the bronchioles. A specific inhalation provocation test with the relevant specific antigen can be performed to confirm the diagnosis, but this is rarely needed to establish the diagnosis. Such challenge tests should only be conducted in centres with considerable experience with them. A more common approach to this is to carry out a worksite challenge test with lung function testing before and after workplace exposure.

The most important in the management of extrinsic allergic alveolitis is to remove the source of exposure from the work environment or, if this is not possible, to remove the patient to another, uncontaminated work environment. If the source of exposure is a contaminated humidifier or air conditioning system, cleaning of this is essential. It is important to remember that those performing this cleaning should wear respiratory protection equipment. Oral corticosteroids may be given at the acute episodes, as they have been shown to shorten the recovery time and reduce the probability and severity of recurrence, but currently there is no evidence that they would affect the long-term outcome of extrinsic allergic alveolitis. In the case of farmer's lung, reduction of exposure by using motorized respirators is an option for treatment, but this is not a solution for extrinsic allergic alveolitis related to indoor sources. Prevention of extrinsic allergic alveolitis focuses on prevention of exposure. In the case of indoor microbiological contaminants, preventive actions include adequate building techniques and maintenance of the buildings, and ventilation and humidification systems. Any dampness or mould problems detected should be repaired promptly.

Humidifier fever

Humidifier fever is a disease with similar symptoms to those experienced in extrinsic allergic alveolitis. The patient typically experiences fever, nausea, sweating and myalgia, sometimes with breathlessness, four to eight hours after exposure. However, the subject typically develops tolerance on continued exposure, so the symptoms diminish towards the end of the working week. After a break from work, for example over the weekend, the attack is usually worse again (i.e. Monday morning fever). Outbreaks have been reported in relation to bioaerosol exposure from contaminated humidifier water in offices and printing houses, but this disease differs from extrinsic allergic alveolitis (i.e. humidifier lung) in that the disease mechanism seems to be a toxic alveolitis, usually due to bacterial endotoxins.[82] The patients may have specific IgG antibodies to the microorganisms growing in water reservoirs as a sign of exposure.[83] The patient may present with fine crackles from the lungs in physical inspection and show reduced diffusing capacity of the lungs and/or mild restriction. The chest x-ray is often normal. The patient should monitor their body temperature twice a day (in the morning and after work) and work days should be compared to days off work.

Cessation of exposure leads to improvement of symptoms spontaneously.[84] For example, when the humidifier equipment is turned off, airborne levels of bacteria and endotoxin fall. It is important to detect the source of exposure and to clean the contaminated humidifier or air conditioning system (with the cleaners wearing adequate respiratory protection equipment). According to current thinking, humidifier fever does not lead to any long-term health problems. Regular maintenance of humidifiers and air conditioners is the best approach to prevent humidifier fever.

Legionnaires' disease

Legionella pneumophila is a bacterial microorganism that is found widely in nature in wet surroundings and it is capable of colonizing cooling towers and hot water systems. Infection presents in two forms: pneumonia called 'Legionnaires' disease' and acute self-limiting influenza-like illness called 'Pontiac fever'.

An outbreak of pneumonia occurred at the American Legion Convention in Philadelphia in 1976.[85] *Legionella pneumophila* was identified as the causative organism and its spread was linked to the hotel's air conditioning system. Of 221 persons affected in this outbreak, as many as 19.5 per cent died. Other outbreaks have subsequently been described related to cooling towers and hot water systems, for example in hospitals and office buildings. Recently, an outbreak of Legionnaires' disease was related to poorly maintained air conditioning equipment in Cumbria, UK. The outbreak caused several fatalities and resulted in prosecution of the individual who was responsible for deciding how frequently the air conditioning system was serviced. Infections linked to Legionella were also detected among individuals who had passed through the alley where the system vented.

The incubation period for Legionnaires' disease is between two and ten days. The clinical development of the disease varies from mild cough and fever to widespread pulmonary infiltrates and multiorgan failure.[86,87] The early symptoms include malaise, myalgia, fever and mild cough, sometimes with blood in the sputum. Neurological symptoms range from headache to severe encephalopathy. Watery diarrhoea occurs in 25–50 per cent of cases. In chest x-ray, a typical initial finding is unilateral lobe infiltrate, although it may present in a wide variety of manifestations. *Legionella* is typically associated with rapidly progressive infiltrations. Complete recovery of the infiltrates may take between one and four months. In chest CT, *Legionella* presents as ground glass appearance in the affected lobes, the patient typically having hyponatraemia and being bradycardic and hypotensive. C-reactive protein increases in the early phases of disease. The definitive diagnosis is based on isolation of the organism by culturing respiratory secretion on buffered charcoal yeast extract agar with four days of incubation. Urinary antigen detection is a good rapid test, but it is less sensitive than culture. Serological detection of antibodies is less useful.

Legionnaires' disease requires treatment in hospital. Erythromycin used to be the drug of choice, but the second-generation macrolides, such as azithromycin and clarithromycin, quinolones, and telithromycin have replaced its use. In severe cases and in immunocompromised patients, a combination of a second-generation macrolide and quinolone may be used.

Outbreaks of Pontiac fever have also been reported in hospitals and offices. The incubation period is 24–48 hours and the attack rate of the exposed seems to be as high as 90 per cent. The symptoms include malaise, myalgias, fever, chills and headache, non-productive cough and nausea. There is no pneumonia in this milder form of *Legionella pneumophila* infection. The therapy is symptomatic and recovery usually takes place within one week.

Superheating of hot water to >50°C and flushing are the most important methods to disinfect the water distribution systems and prevent *Legionella* infections. In hospitals where organ and bone marrow transplants are performed, it is recommended that routine environmental culturing of *Legionella* be carried out.

Sick building syndrome

The concept of sick building syndrome (SBS) was first applied in the 1980s as a health problem related to indoor air quality.[1] A UK epidemiological study characterized empirically the main components of SBS: nasal, eye and mucous membrane symptoms, dry skin, lethargy and headache.[88] The WHO working group suggested that there was an association between the symptoms and forced (mechanical) ventilation systems, and the British study reported an excess of symptoms related to air handling, especially air conditioning. The concept of SBS has also been used to characterize work-related health problems in non-industrial workplaces, such as day-care centres, schools and hospitals. Research has revealed a complex set of modern occupational health problems underlying the SBS. It has been postulated that there is no single disease entity which could be diagnosed within individuals.[2,89] The symptoms of SBS are symptoms and signs of a number of different health outcomes with different manifestations and aetiological factors. One, or a set of environmental determinants of different ontological nature, i.e. physical or social, can cause the symptoms and signs. Therefore, the phenomenon SBS consists of several types of relations between environmental determinants and health outcomes, and a singular exposure can cause different health outcomes and a given symptom can be caused by one, several or a combination of different exposures and exposure patterns.

Figure 71.1 presents the worker (inner circle) and the office environment (outer circle–inner circle) and illustrates phenomena in the office environment or non-industrial work environment in general.[2,89] First, the work environment is divided into physical and social environments, which both include determinants of human health and well-being. Second, man can be viewed to constitute two different domains, the one belonging to the physical phenomena and the other to the psychological phenomena, and the health outcomes related to the environmental determinants are thus either physical or psychological, or both. The purpose of this simplified model is to elaborate the different types of phenomenon. The relationship between these phenomena theoretically describes how the environmental determinants can affect human health and well-being and can cause both physical (objective) and mental (subjective) outcomes. A disease or health state can have physiological and/or psychological underlying mechanisms and manifestations.

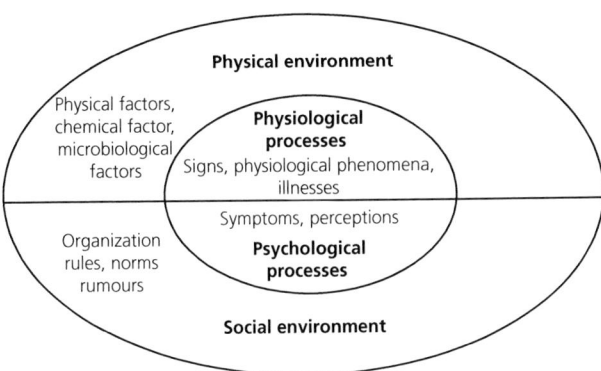

Figure 71.1 The office environment model: the worker (inner circle), the office environment (outer circle – inner circle), and phenomena of different ontological nature involved in the sick building syndrome. Adapted with permission from Jaakkola JJK. The office environment model: A conceptual analysis of sick building syndrome. *Indoor Air*, Wiley-Blackwell.

Table 71.3 Dimensions of the outcomes related to the sick building syndrome.

Dimension	Symptoms and signs
Anatomic site	Eyes
	Respiratory tracts, including nose, airways and parenchyma
	Skin
	Central nervous system
Possible underlying mechanism	Mechanical irritation and inflammation
	Allergic reactions (type I and III)
	Toxicity
	Infectious
	Environmental psychological stress

The first step to identify relevant relations between possible health problems and their environmental or constitutional determinants is to consider the components of the SBS (Table 71.3). The symptoms and signs of interest can be categorized into two dimensions: anatomical site and hypothesized underlying mechanism. The main anatomic sites are the eyes, the respiratory tract (nose, airways, lung parenchyma), the skin and the central nervous system. Possible underlying mechanisms include mechanical irritation and inflammation, immunological/allergic reactions, toxicity, infection and environmental psychological stress.

The symptoms arising at the different anatomic sites are non-specific as to their causes. Inference about their causes and underlying mechanisms can be made by characterizing the type and intensity of the symptoms and the time and place of their occurrence. Therefore, a number of environmental factors, e.g. artificial mineral fibres, formaldehyde and pollen, can cause similar eye symptoms via mechanical irritation and/or chemical toxicity and/or allergic reactions. Biochemical or immunological investigation of tear fluid or conjunctiva, and/or measurements of indoor air quality may help to identify the underlying mechanisms and environmental causes of the symptoms. Exposure to a given environmental factor may cause different symptoms and signs in different individuals or environmental conditions. For example, the effect of a complex mixture of office air could cause different types of symptoms and different health outcomes in different individuals depending on personal susceptibility and, in addition, one or several mechanisms could be involved.

Table 71.4 summarizes different physical exposures and social factors, which may cause one or several symptoms and signs of SBS. The role of thermal environment and air change is discussed under Thermal environment, p. 923. Dampness and mould problems have also been linked to increases in the risk of several of the typical symptoms related to SBS, including irritation of eyes, nose and throat. There is increasing epidemiological evidence that the risk of asthma, asthma-like symptoms and allergic rhinitis is related to the presence of PVC materials which are sources of di-ethyl-hexyl-phthalate and its metabolic products.[72]

According to the occupational stress model, stress arises when there is perceived imbalance between external demand and response capabilities, especially under conditions where failure to meet demands has important consequences.[90] The job strain or 'demand–control model' developed by Karasek in 1979[91] suggests that the joint effect of high demand and low control will lead to negative health outcomes. Baker et al.[90] developed the demand–control model by emphasizing the role of social support in moderating the adverse effects of occupational stress. Jaakkola[2,85] suggested that the demand–control model characterizes both conceptually and empirically the effects of social environment on the SBS-related symptoms. This is supported by results from epidemiological studies conducted among Finnish[27,92] and British office workers.[93] A Swedish cross-sectional study of 532 office workers showed that the three-dimensional model of demand–control–support can predict symptoms compatible with SBS.[94]

Adverse pregnancy outcomes

An increasing number of women are working outside the home during pregnancy. This increasing trend of women working in pregnancy underlines the need to understand the potential adverse effects of prenatal exposures taking place in workplaces. Workers in non-industrial workplaces are exposed to several factors which are potential causes of reduced fetal growth, preterm delivery, spontaneous abortion and congenital malformations. The concentrations of individual compounds of exposures are typically lower in non-industrial compared to industrial workplaces, but exposures may comprise complex mixtures in which the compounds act synergistically. In this section, known or potential, recently investigated occupational causes of adverse pregnancy outcomes are discussed in brief.

Table 71.4 A summary of environmental exposures and social factors which may cause symptoms and signs related to sick building syndrome.

Sources	Potential exposures/factor
Physical environment	
	High indoor temperature (>23°C)
	Low relative humidity
	Low air change
Water damage or leakage	Dampness and mould
Occupants' clothing	Allergens
PVC flooring	Phthalates
Carpets	Particles, vinyl acetate, styrene, dodecanol, acetaldehyde
Plastic wall materials	Phthalates
Textile wall material	Particles, VOCs
Furniture: Plywood, plastic	Formaldehyde, 2-pentyl furan, banzaldehyde, hexanal, pentanal
Photocopying	Xylenes, benzene, 2-ethyl-1-hexanol
Cleaning agents: Detergents	Fatty acid salts (soap), organic sulphonates
Cleaning agents: Complexing agents (water softeners)	EDTA, tripolyphosphates
Cleaning agents: Alkaline agents	Silicates, carbonates, sodium hydroxide, ammonia
Cleaning agents: Acids	Phosphoric, acetic, citric, sulphamic, hydrochloric acid
Disinfectants	Hypochlorite, aldehydes, quaternary ammonium compounds
Carbonless copy paper	Trimellitic anhydride, phenol-formaldehyde resins, azo dyes, diisopropyl naphtalenes, formaldehyde, isocyanates, hydrocarbon-based solvents, polycyclic aromatic hydrocarbons, polyoxypropylene diamine, epoxy resins, aliphatic isocyanates, Bisphenol A, diethylene triamine
Paints (fresh)	Toluene, propylene, glycol, ethylene glycol, butyl propionate, methyl propanol
Smoking	ETS includes 4000 chemicals, many irritants
Work at video display terminals	Ergonomic factors
Social environment	
	Reported work stress
	Reported work atmosphere
	High job demand
	Low support

EDTA, ethylenediaminetetraacetic acid; ETS, environmental tobacco smoke; VOC, volatile organic compounds.

SECONDHAND TOBACCO SMOKE

There is substantial evidence that exposure to secondhand tobacco smoke of the mother during pregnancy increases the risk of low birth weight and preterm delivery. Although individual studies were often inconclusive, a meta-analysis by Windham and colleagues[95] suggested that exposure to SHS during pregnancy has a small, but significant adverse effect on birthweight and increases the risk of low birthweight. The evidence of effect on preterm delivery was weaker,[96] but supported by a Californian[95] and a Finnish study.[97] In the latter, work exposure was a stronger determinant of adverse pregnancy outcomes than home exposure.

ORGANIC SOLVENTS AND VOLATILE ORGANIC COMPOUNDS

There is evidence that work exposure to organic solvents may reduce intrauterine growth and increase the risk of small-for-gestational age infants. Previous epidemiologic studies conducted in laboratory workers,[98] drycleaners,[99] pharmacy assistants[100] and workers in the petrochemical industry[101] have suggested an association between exposure to organic solvents and fetal growth. These observations are based on studies in industrial work and laboratories, where the exposure levels for singular compounds exceeds those of non-industrial workplace levels. However, workers in non-industrial environments may be exposed to rather high concentrations of a complex mixture of VOC, i.e. total VOC concentrations, but the effects of such exposures on the risk of adverse pregnancy outcomes have not been studied.

STRESS

Based on a recent systematic review, the overall evidence is indicative of an independent association between prenatal maternal stress and adverse pregnancy outcomes.[102] Evidence consistently suggests that exposure to stressful stimuli increases the risk of preterm delivery. The effect on low birthweight and fetal growth was mediated by the absence of psychosocial resources, such as positive personality characteristics and social support.

Cancer

The International Agency for Research in Cancer (IARC) summarized the available evidence on the effects of exposure to secondhand smoke on cancer in 2004.[103] They found sufficient evidence to conclude that involuntary smoking is a cause of lung cancer in never-smokers. The excess risk was estimated to be of the order of 20 per cent for women and 30 per cent for men. The evidence on the effects on cancers of the nasopharynx, nasal cavity, paranasal sinuses, cervix and gastrointestinal tract was found to be sparse and conflicting.

Several volatile organic compounds, including benzene and vinyl chloride, are shown to be potential human carcinogens at levels taking place in industrial workplaces. There is no evidence that levels of such exposures in non-industrial workplaces increase the risk of cancer.

PUBLIC HEALTH IMPACT AND ECONOMIC CONSEQUENCES

There are no reports of an overall estimate of the impact of non-industrial occupational hazards. The public health impact and economic consequences from the two most common hazards, dampness and mould problems and secondhand tobacco smoke exposure have been assessed recently.

Mudarri and Fisk[104] assessed the public health risk and economic impact of dampness and mould exposures in the United States on current asthma using effect estimates for current asthma from exposure to dampness and mould in homes from Fisk et al.[36] They assessed the proportion of current asthma cases in the United States that are attributable to dampness and mould exposure to be 21 per cent (95 per cent CI, 12–29). Based on the literature covering dampness and mould problems in schools, offices and institutional buildings, the risks from exposure in these buildings are similar to risks from exposures in homes. Of the 21.8 million people reported to have asthma in the United States, approximately 4.6 (2.7–6.3) million cases are estimated to be attributable to dampness and mould exposure in the home. The national annual cost of asthma that is attributable to dampness and mould exposure in the home is estimated to be $3.5 billion ($2.1–4.8 billion).

According to recent estimates from Europe and the United States, significant numbers of workers are exposed to secondhand tobacco smoke in their workplaces: approximately 7.5 million workers in 15 EU countries[105] and 24.6 million workers in the United States.[106] Experience from different parts of the world with national, state-wide or local smoke-free workplace legislations has shown that such legislation is feasible to implement and leads to significant decline in SHS exposure of employees in the short and long term, compared to situations where there are no, or only a few, voluntary smoking restrictions.[13] These reductions in SHS exposure have been accompanied by health benefits, including reduced respiratory symptoms and acute myocardial infarctions, and increased lung function levels.[13,106–108] Experience from Finland[109] shows that following implementation of national smoke-free workplace legislation, smokers' attitudes become more favourable towards smoking restrictions in the workplace. A body of evidence also shows that such legislation leads to reduced active smoking, by increasing the number of smokers who cease and by reducing the tobacco consumption of continuing smokers.[109,110] The weight of evidence suggests that smoke-free workplace legislation will result in a considerable reduction in the burden from several chronic diseases and substantially reduce health care costs.

MANAGEMENT AND PREVENTION

The location of the building is an important determinant of indoor exposures. Therefore, health issues should be taken into account when deciding on the location of the building and when designing it. The building and its ventilation system can be used to protect its occupants from high levels of ambient air pollution. Use of building materials with low chemical emission is an important aspect of source control to reduce indoor air pollution in non-industrial workplaces. Several macroscale activities are likely to reduce population exposure from material emissions and producers of building materials should develop and produce materials with lower emissions. Testing of new materials entering the market is a critical factor, but can be difficult, because the number of surface materials used can vary in different micro-environments and emission rates depend on air change, temperature, humidity and building structures. Special emphasis should be placed on materials covering large surfaces, such as walls and floors. Consumers should be informed about the emission rates of different materials and they should be educated to demand the least damaging materials, as this is the most efficient way to influence the market. Classification of materials, paints and chemicals would help the consumer to choose products and provide guidance to the builders and producers.

Many typical dampness and mould problems can be prevented in the planning, construction and maintenance of buildings. These problems can lead to serious health effects and therefore should be mitigated at an early phase.

Sufficient air change, at least 10 litres/s per person in sedentary work, is the most important characteristic of a good non-industrial indoor environment. Both emissions from occupants, their activities and other sources, e.g. surface materials, should be taken into account when defining the minimum ventilation rate.

In many developed countries in colder climates, overheating of non-industrial workplaces is common, whereas in warm climates, the cooling during the summer is often excessive. The optimal indoor temperature for sedentary work is 21–23°C. Thus, less winter heating and less summer cooling may reduce acute symptoms and improve thermal comfort, while providing substantial energy conservation benefits.

Finally, maintenance of buildings and heating, ventilation and air conditioning systems is an important aspect of primary prevention of the harmful effects of indoor environmental problems.

As is the case in industrial workplaces, the same is true for those in non-industrial work environments, if an individual worker or a group of workers become ill from an occupational cause, it is important to assess the potential risk from the exposure to the health of other workers, in order to prevent further cases of occupational disease.

Key points

- An increasing proportion of the workforce is working in non-industrial indoor environments which have traditionally been considered as safe, because occupants are not exposed to high levels of physical, chemical or biological compounds traditionally thought to be hazardous to health.
- In non-industrial environments, such as offices, day-care facilities, schools, hospitals and nursing homes, several physical, chemical, microbiological and/or social factors create complex environmental conditions which may increase the risk of developing well-defined diseases or occurrence of a set of symptoms and signs often through multifactorial causal webs.
- Occupational exposures in non-industrial workplaces can cause several diseases including asthma, extrinsic allergic alveolitis, humidifier fever, Legionnaires' disease, as well as reduced fetal growth, and non-specific symptoms and signs of the eyes, airways, skin and central nervous system denoted as 'sick building syndrome'.
- The most common occupational health problems are related to the physical environment, including the thermal environment, insufficient air change, dampness and mould problems, environmental tobacco smoke and emissions from office equipment and paper handling and from interior surface materials, especially in new buildings or after recent refurbishment, and factors of the social environment including occupational stress and organizational factors.
- Action points for the prevention of indoor-related health problems include maintenance of sufficient air change (>10 litres/s per person) and optimal temperature (21–23°C), use of low emitting surface materials, isolation of unnecessary pollution sources from work space (e.g. photocopying, excessive paper handling, storage of solvents and cleaning agents), prompt mitigation of dampness and mould problems and good management of the workforce.

REFERENCES

1. WHO. Indoor air pollutants: Exposure and health effects. EURO Report and Studies No 78: Report on a WHO meeting, Copenhagen. Geneva: World Health Organization Regional Office for Europe, 1983.
2. Jaakkola JJK. The office environment model: A conceptual analysis of sick building syndrome. *Indoor Air.* 1998; **9**: 7–16.
3. Munir AKM, Einarson R, Dreborg SKG. Mite (*Der p I*, *Der f I*), cat (*Fel d I*) and dog (*Can f I*) allergens in dust from Swedish day-care centers. *Clinical and Experimental Allergy.* 1995; **25**: 119–26.
4. Hellgren J, Eriksson C, Karlsson G et al. Nasal symptoms among workers exposed to soft paper dust. *International Archives of Occupational and Environmental Health.* 2001; **74**: 129–32.
5. Järvholm B, Torén K, Brolin I et al. Lung function in workers exposed to soft paper dust. *American Journal of Industrial Medicine.* 1988; **14**: 457–64.
6. Kraus T, Pfahlberg A, Gefeller O, Raithel HJ. Respiratory symptoms and diseases among workers in the soft tissue producing industry. *Occupational and Environmental Medicine.* 2002; **59**: 830–5.
7. Torén K, Järvholm B, Sällsten G, Thiringer G. Respiratory symptoms and asthma among workers exposed to paper dust: A cohort study. *American Journal of Industrial Medicine.* 1994; **26**: 489–96.
8. Jäppinen P, Kanerva L. Pulp and paper workers, and paper dermatitis. In: Kanerva L, Elsner P, Wahlberg JE (eds). *Handbook of occupational dermatology.* New York: Springer Verlag, 2000: 1036–7.
9. LaMarte FP, Merchant JA, Casale TB. Acute systemic reactions to carbonless copy paper associated with histamine release. *JAMA.* 1988; **260**: 242–4.
10. Marks JG, Trautlein JJ, Zwillich CW, Demers LM. Contact urticaria and airway obstruction from carbonless copy paper. *JAMA.* 1984; **252**: 1038–41.
11. Norbäck D, Wieslander G, Göthe C-J. A search for discomfort-inducing factors in carbonless copying paper. *American Industrial Hygiene Association Journal.* 1988; **49**: 117–20.
12. Shehade SA, Beck MH, Chalmers RJG. Allergic contact dermatitis to crystal violet in carbonless copy paper. *Contact Dermatitis.* 1987; **17**: 310–26.
13. Jaakkola MS, Jaakkola JJK. Impact of smoke free workplace legislation on exposures and health: Possibilities for prevention. *European Respiratory Journal.* 2006; **28**: 397–408.
14. Jaakkola MS, Jaakkola JJK. Assessment of exposure to environmental tobacco smoke. *European Respiratory Journal.* 1997; **10**: 2384–97.
15. Jaakkola MS, Samet JM. Occupational exposure to environmental tobacco smoke and health risk assessment. *Environmental Health Perspectives.* 1999; **107** (Suppl. 6): 829–35.
16. US Environmental Protection Agency. Respiratory health effects of passive smoking: Lung cancer and other disorders. EPA/600/6-90/006F. Washington DC: US Environmental

Protection Agency, Office of Health and Environmental Assessment, Office of Research and Development, 1992.
17. Marbury MC, Krieger RA. Formaldehyde. In: Samet JM, Spengler JD (eds). *Indoor air pollution. A health perspective.* Baltimore, MD: The Johns Hopkins University Press, 1991: 223-51.
18. Jaakkola JJ, Oie L, Nafstad P et al. Interior surface materials in the home and the development of bronchial obstruction in young children in Oslo, Norway. *American Journal of Public Health.* 1999; **89**: 188-92.
19. Tichenor BA, Guo Z. The effect of ventilation on emission rates of wood finishing materials. *Environment International.* 1991; **17**: 317-23.
20. Wolkoff P, Clausen PA, Nielsen JB et al. The influence of specific ventilation rate on the emissions from construction products. In: Saarela K, Kalliokoski P, Seppänen O (eds). *Indoor Air '93*, vol. 2, Chemicals in indoor air, material emissions. Juväskylä, 1993: 9-14.
21. Thatcher TL, Layton DW. Deposits, resuspension, and penetration of particles within a residence. *Atmospheric Environment.* 1995; **29**: 1487-97.
22. Jaakkola JJK, Miettinen P. Ventilation rate in office buildings and sick building syndrome. *Occupational and Environmental Medicine.* 1995; **52**: 709-14.
23. Bluyssen P, DeOliveiro Fernandes E, Groes L et al. European indoor air quality audit project in 56 office buildings. *Indoor Air.* 1996; **6**: 221-38.
24. Fisk WJ, Mirer AG, Mendell MJ. Quantitative relationship of sick building syndrome symptoms with ventilation rates. *Indoor Air.* 2009; **19**: 159-65.
25. Jaakkola JJK. Temperature and humidity. In: Frumkin H, Geller RJ, Rubin IL (eds). *Safer and healthy school environment.* Oxford: Oxford University Press, 2006: 46-57.
26. Jaakkola JJK. Day-care environment and health. In: Spengler JD, Samet JM (eds). *Indoor air quality handbook.* Chapter 69. New York: McGraw-Hill, 2001.
27. Jaakkola JJK, Heinonen OP, Seppänen O. Mechanical ventilation in office buildings and the sick building syndrome. An experimental and epidemiological study. *Indoor Air.* 1991; **1**: 111-22.
28. Fanger PO. Calculations of thermal comfort, introduction of a basic comfort equation. *ASHRAE Transactions.* 1967; **73** (Suppl. II): 4.1-4.20.
29. Jaakkola JJK, Heinonen OP, Seppänen O. Sick building syndrome, sensation of dryness and thermal comfort in relation to room temperature in an office building: Need for individual control of temperature. *Environment International.* 1989; **15**: 163-8.
30. Menzies R, Tamblyn R, Farant JP et al. The effect of varying levels of outdoor-air supply on the symptoms of the sick building syndrome. *New England Journal of Medicine.* 1993; **328**: 821-7.
31. Andersen I, Lundqvist GR, Proctor DF. Human perception of humidity under four controlled conditions. *Archives of Environmental Health.* 1973; **26**: 22-7.
32. Reinikainen LM, Jaakkola JJK, Seppänen O. The effect of air humidification on symptoms and the perception of air quality in office workers. A six period cross-over trial. *Archives of Environmental Health.* 1992; **47**: 8-15.
33. Berglund B, Gustafsson L, Lindvall T. Thermal climate. *Environment International.* 1991; **17**: 185-204.
34. Reinikainen LM, Aunela-Tapola L, Jaakkola JJK. Humidification and perceived indoor air quality in the office environment. *Occupational and Environmental Medicine.* 1997; **54**: 322-7.
35. Institute of Medicine (IOM). *Damp indoor spaces and health.* Washington, DC: The National Academies Press, 2004.
36. Fisk WJ, Lei-Gomez Q, Mendell MJ. Meta-analyses of associations of respiratory health effects with dampness and molds in homes. *Indoor Air.* 2007; **17**: 284-96.
37. Ruotsalainen R, Jaakkola N, Jaakkola JJK. Dampness and molds in day-care centers as an occupational health problem. *International Archives of Occupational and Environmental Medicine.* 1995; **66**: 369-74.
38. Li CS, Hsu CW, Lu CH. Dampness and respiratory symptoms among workers in daycare centers in a subtropical climate. *Archives of Environmental Health.* 1997; **52**: 68-71.
39. Mendell MJ, Naco GM, Wilcox TG, Sieber WK. Environmental risk factors and work-related lower respiratory symptoms in 80 office buildings: An exploratory analysis of NIOSH data. *American Journal of Industrial Medicine.* 2003; **43**: 630-41.
40. Park JH, Cox-Ganser J, Rao C, Kreiss K. Fungal and endotoxin measurements in dust associated with respiratory symptoms in water-damaged office buildings. *Indoor Air.* 2006; **16**: 192-203.
41. Chao HJ, Schwartz J, Milton DK, Burge HA. The work environment and workers health in four large office buildings. *Environmental Health Perspectives.* 2003; **111**: 1242-8.
42. Dangman KH, Bracker AL, Storey E. Work-related asthma in teachers in Connecticut: Association with chronic water damage and fungal growth in schools. *Connecticut Medicine.* 2005; **69**: 9-17.
43. Ebbehøj NE, Meyer HW, Würtz H et al. Members of a Working Group under the Danish Mold in Buildings program (DAMIB). Molds in floor dust, building-related symptoms, and lung function among male and female schoolteachers. *Indoor Air.* 2005; **15** (Suppl. 10): 7-16.
44. Golden RJ, Holm SE, Robinson DE et al. Chloroform mode of action: Implications for cancer risk assessment. *Regulatory Toxicology and Pharmacology.* 1997; **26**: 142-55.
45. Molhave L. Volatile organic compounds, indoor air quality, and health. In: Proceeding of the 5th International Conference on Indoor Air Quality and Climate. Vol. 5, *Indoor Air '90*, Toronto, 1990: 15-34.
46. Wieslander G, Norbäck D, Björnsson E et al. Asthma and the indoor environment: The significance of emission of formaldehyde and volatile organic compounds from newly painted indoor surfaces. *International Archives of Occupational and Environmental Health.* 1997; **69**: 115-24.

47. Buring JE, Hennekens CH. Carbonless copy paper: A review of published epidemiologic studies. *Journal of Occupational Medicine.* 1991; **33**: 486-95.
48. Stenberg B. *Office illness. The worker, the work and the workplace.* Umeå University Medical Dissertations, New Series No. 399. Umeå, Sweden: Umeå Universty Press, 1994.
49. Skov P, Valbjørn O, Pedersen BV. Influence of personal characteristics, job-related factors and psychosocial factors on the sick building syndrome. Danish Indoor Climate Study Group. *Scandinavian Journal of Work and Environmental Health.* 1989; **15**: 286-95.
50. Jaakkola MS, Jaakkola JJK. Office equipment and supplies – a modern occupational health concern? *American Journal of Epidemiology.* 1999; **150**: 1223-8.
51. Jaakkola MS, Yang L, Ieromnimon A, Jaakkola JJ. Office work, SBS and respiratory and sick building syndrome symptoms. *Occupational and Environmental Medicine.* 2007; **64**: 178-84.
52. Eder W, Ege MJ, von Mutius E. The asthma epidemic. *New England Journal of Medicine.* 2006; **355**: 2226-35.
53. Magnus P, Jaakkola JJK. Secular trend in the occurrence of asthma among children and young adults – critical appraisal of repeated cross sectional surveys. *British Medical Journal.* 1997; **314**: 1795-9.
54. Fishwick D, Barber CM, Bradshaw LM *et al.* Standards of care for occupational asthma. *Thorax.* 2008; **63**: 240-50.
55. Tarlo SM, Balmes J, Balkissoon R *et al.* Diagnosis and management of work-related asthma. American College of Chest Physicians Consensus Statement. *Chest.* 2008; **134**: 1S-41S.
56. Jaakkola JJK, Jaakkola MS. Effects of environmental tobacco smoke on respiratory health in children. *Scandinavian Journal of Work and Environmental Health.* 2002; **28** (Suppl. 2): 71-83.
57. California Environmental Protection Agency. Proposed identification of environmental tobacco smoke as a toxic air contaminant. Art B: Health effects assessment for environmental tobacco smoke. California EPA, Office of Environmental Health Hazard Assessment, Air Toxicology and Epidemiology Branch, 2005.
58. Gilmour MI, Jaakkola MS, London SJ *et al.* How exposure to environmental tobacco smoke, outdoor air pollutants, and increased pollen burdens influences the incidence of asthma. *Environmental Health Perspectives.* 2006; **114**: 627-33.
59. Jaakkola MS, Piipari R, Jaakkola N, Jaakkola JJK. Environmental tobacco smoke and adult-onset asthma: A population-based incident case-control study. *American Journal of Public Health.* 2003; **93**: 2055-60.
60. US Department of Health and Human Services. The health consequences of involuntary exposure to tobacco smoke. A report of the Surgeon General. Atlanta, GA: US Department of Health and Human Services, Centers for Disease Control and Prevention, Coordinating Center for Health Promotion, National Center for Chronic Disease Prevention and Health Promotion, Office on Smoking and Health, 2006.
61. Jaakkola MS, Jaakkola JJK. Effects of environmental tobacco smoke on respiratory health in adults. *Scandinavian Journal of Work and Environmental Health.* 2002; **28** (Suppl. 2): 52-70.
62. Eisner MD. Environmental tobacco smoke exposure and pulmonary function among adults in NHANES III: Impact on the general population and adults with current asthma. *Environmental Health Perspectives.* 2002; **110**: 765-70.
63. Jaakkola MS, Jaakkola JJK. Indoor molds and asthma in adults. *Advances in Applied Microbiology.* 2004; **55**: 309-38.
64. Jaakkola MS, Laitinen S, Piipari R *et al.* IgG antibodies against dampness-related microbes and adult-onset asthma: A population-based incident case-control study. *Clinical and Experimental Immunology.* 2002; **129**: 107-12.
65. Jaakkola MS, Ieromnimon A, Jaakkola JJK. Are atopy and specific IgE to mites and molds important for adult asthma? *Journal of Allergy and Clinical Immunology.* 2006; **117**: 642-8.
66. Husman T. Health effects of indoor air micro-organisms. *Scandinavian Journal of Work, Environment and Health.* 1996; **22**: 5-13.
67. Jaakkola MS, Nordman H, Piipari R *et al.* Dampness and molds in the workplace and development of adult-onset asthma: A population-based incident case-control study. *Environmental Health Perspectives.* 2002; **110**: 543-7.
68. Jaakkola MS, Jaakkola JJK. Office work exposures and adult-onset asthma. *Environmental Health Perspectives.* 2007; **115**: 1007-11.
69. Toren K, Balder B, Brisman J *et al.* The risk of asthma in relation to occupational exposures: A case-control study from a Swedish city. *European Respiratory Journal.* 1999; **13**: 496-501.
70. Axelsson IG. Allergy to *Ficus benjamina* (weeping fig) in nonatopic subjects. *Allergy.* 1995; **50**: 284-5.
71. Jaakkola JJK, Ieromnimon A, Jaakkola MS. Interior surface materials and asthma in adults: A population-based incident case-control study. *American Journal of Epidemiology.* 2006; **164**: 742-9.
72. Jaakkola JJK, Knight TL. The role of exposure to phthalates from polyvinyl chloride products in the development of asthma and allergies: A systematic review and meta-analysis. *Environmental Health Perspectives.* 2008; **116**: 845-53.
73. Jaakkola JJK, Piipari R, Jaakkola MS. Occupation and asthma: A population-based incident case-control study. *American Journal of Epidemiology.* 2003; **158**: 981-7.
74. Zock JP. World at work: Cleaners. *Occupational and Environmental Medicine.* 2005; **62**: 581-4.
75. Jaakkola JJK, Jaakkola MS. Professional cleaning and asthma. *Current Opinion in Allergy and Clinical Immunology.* 2006; **6**: 85-90.
76. Burge PS, Richardson MN. Occupational asthma due to indirect exposure to lauryl dimethyl benzyl ammonium chloride used in a floor cleaner. *Thorax.* 1994; **49**: 842-3.

77. Patel AM, Ryu JH, Reed CE. Hypersensitivity pneumonitis: Current concepts and future questions. *Journal of Allergy and Clinical Immunology.* 2001; **108**: 661–70.
78. Cormier Y. Hypersensitivity pneumonitis. In: Hendrick D, Beckett WS, Burge PS, Churg A (eds). *Occupational disorders of the lung.* London: Saunders/Harcourt Publishers, 2002: 229–39.
79. Simon-Nobbe B, Denk U, Pöll V *et al.* The spectrum of fungal allergy. *International Archives of Allergy and Immunology.* 2008; **145**: 58–86.
80. Robertson W, Robertson AS, Burge CB *et al.* Clinical investigation of an outbreak of alveolitis and asthma in a car engine manufacturing plant. *Thorax.* 2007; **62**: 981–90.
81. Erkinjuntti-Pekkanen R, Rytkönen H, Kokkarinen JI *et al.* Long-term outcome of farmer's lung evaluated by high resolution computed tomography: A case-control study. *American Journal of Respiratory and Critical Care Medicine.* 1998; **158**: 662–5.
82. Rylander R, Haglind P. Airborne endotoxins and humidifier disease. *Clinical Allergy.* 1984; **14**: 109–12.
83. Baur X, Dewair M, Ehret W *et al.* Humidifier lung and humidifier fever. *Lung.* 1988; **166**: 113–24.
84. Pal TM, de Moncgy JG, Groothoff JW, Post D. Exposure and acute exposure-effects before and after modification of a contaminated humidification system in a synthetic-fibre plant. *International Archives of Occupational and Environmental Health.* 2000; **73**: 369–75.
85. Fraser DW, Tsai TR, Orenstein W *et al.* Legionnaires' disease: Description of an epidemic of pneumonia. *New England Journal of Medicine.* 1977; **297**: 1189–97.
86. Ong V. Non-tuberculous infections. In: Hendrick D, Beckett WS, Burge PS, Churg A (eds). *Occupational disorders of the lung.* London: Saunders/Harcourt Publishers, 2002.
87. Cunha BA. Atypical pneumonias: Current clinical concepts focusing on Legionnaires' disease. *Current Opinion in Pulmonary Medicine.* 2008; **14**: 183–94.
88. Finnegan MJ, Pickering CAC, Purge PS. The sick building syndrome: Prevalence studies. *British Medical Journal.* 1984; **289**: 1573–5.
89. Jaakkola JJK. Sick building syndrome: The phenomenon and its air-handling etiology. PhD thesis. Department of Epidemiology and Biostatistics, McGill University, Montreal, 1995. Helsinki University of Technology, Laboratory of Heating, Ventilating and Air-Conditioning, Report A2, Espoo, 1995: 121.
90. Baker E, Israel B, Schurman S. Role of control and support in occupational stress: An integrated model. *Social Science and Medicine.* 1996; **7**: 1145–59.
91. Karasek RA. Job demands, job decision latitude, and mental strain: Implications for job redesign. *Administrative Science Quarterly.* 1979; **4**: 285.
92. Jaakkola JJK, Tuomaala P, Seppänen O. Textile wall materials and the sick building syndrome. *Archives of Environmental Health.* 1994; **49**: 175–81.
93. Marmot AF, Eley J, Stafford M *et al.* Building health: An epidemiological study of 'sick building syndrome' in the Whitehall II study. *Occupational and Environmental Medicine.* 2006; **63**: 283–9.
94. Runeson R, Wahlstedt K, Wieslander G, Norbäck D. Personal and psychosocial factors and symptoms compatible with sick building syndrome in the Swedish workforce. *Indoor Air.* 2006; **16**: 445–53.
95. Windham GC, Eaton A, Hopkins B. Evidence for an association between environmental tobacco smoke exposure and birth weight: A meta-analysis and new data. *Pediatric and Perinatal Epidemiology.* 1999; **13**: 35–57.
96. Windham GC, Hopkins B, Fenster L, Swan SH. Prenatal active or passive tobacco smoke exposure and the risk of preterm delivery or low birth weight. *Epidemiology.* 2000; **11**: 427–33.
97. Jaakkola JJK, Jaakkola N, Zahlsen K. Fetal growth and length of gestation in relation to exposure to environmental tobacco smoke measured by hair nicotine concentration. *Environmental Health Perspectives.* 2001; **109**: 557–61.
98. Taskinen H, Kyyrönen K, Hemminki K *et al.* Laboratory work and pregnancy outcomes. *Journal of Occupational Medicine.* 1994; **36**: 311–19.
99. Olsen J, Hemminki K, Ahlborg G *et al.* Low birth weight, congenital malformations, and spontaneous abortions among dry cleaning workers in Scandinavia. *Scandinavian Journal of Work and Environmental Health.* 1990; **16**: 163–8.
100. Schaumburg I, Olsen J. Birth weight and gestational age among children of Danish pharmacy assistants. *Journal of Epidemiology and Community Health.* 1990; **45**: 49–51.
101. Ha E, Cho SI, Chen D *et al.* Parental exposure to organic solvents and reduced birth weight. *Archives of Environmental Health.* 2002; **57**: 207–14.
102. Beydoun H, Saftlas AF. Physical and mental health outcomes of prenatal maternal stress in human and animal studies: A review of recent evidence. *Paediatric and Perinatal Epidemiology.* 2008; **22**: 438–66.
103. IARC 2004. IARC monographs, vol. 83. Tobacco smoke and involuntary smoking. Lyon: IARC, 2004: 1409–13.
104. Mudarri D, Fisk WJ. Public health and economic impact of dampness and mold. *Indoor Air.* 2007; **17**: 226–35.
105. Kauppinen T, Toikkanen J, Pedersen D *et al.* Occupational exposure to carcinogens in the European Union. *Occupational and Environmental Medicine.* 2000; **57**: 10–18.
106. Ong MK, Glantz SA. Cardiovascular health and economic effects of smoke-free workplaces. *American Journal of Medicine.* 2004; **117**: 32–8.
107. Allwright S, Paul G, Greiner B *et al.* Legislation for smoke-free workplaces and health of bar workers in Ireland: Before and after study. *British Medical Journal.* 2005; **331**: 1117–20.
108. Sargent RP, Shepard RM, Glantz SA. Reduced incidence of admissions for myocardial infarction associated with public smoking ban: Before and after study. *British Medical Journal.* 2004; **328**: 997–80.

109. Heloma A, Jaakkola MS. Four-year follow-up of smoke exposure, attitudes and smoking behaviour following enactment of Finland's national smoke-free workplace law. *Addiction*. 2003; **98**: 1111–17.
110. Fichtenberg CM, Glantz SA. Effect of smoke-free workplaces on smoking behaviour: Systematic review. *BMJ*. 2002; **325**: 188–94.
111. Janson C, Chinn S, Jarvis D *et al.* for the European Community Respiratory Health Survey. Effect of passive smoking on respiratory symptoms, bronchial responsiveness, lung function, and total serum IgE in the European Community Respiratory Health Survey: A cross-sectional study. *Lancet*. 2001; **358**: 2103–9.
112. Jousilahti P, Helakorpi S. Prevalence of exposure to environmental tobacco smoke at work and at home: 15-year trends in Finland. *Scandinavian Journal of Work and Environmental Health*. 2002; **28** (Suppl. 2): 16–20.
113. Borland R, Pierce JP, Burns DM *et al.* Protection from environmental tobacco smoke in California. A case for smoke-free workplace. *JAMA*. 1992; **268**: 749–52.
114. Thompson B, Emmons K, Abrams D *et al.* ETS exposure in the workplace. Perceptions and reactions by employees in 114 work sites. Working Well Research Group (corrected). *Journal of Occupational and Environmental Medicine*. 1995; **37**: 1086–92.
115. Boffetta P. Involuntary smoking and lung cancer. *Scandinavian Journal of Work and Environmental Health*. 2002; **28** (Suppl. 2): 30–40.
116. Steenland K. Risk assessment for heart disease and workplace ETS exposure among nonsmokers. *Environmental Health Perspectives*. 1999; **107** (Suppl. 6): 859–63.
117. Eisner MD, Balmes J, Katz PP *et al.* Lifetime environmental tobacco smoke exposure and the risk of chronic obstructive pulmonary disease. *Environmental Health*. 2005; **4**: 7–14.
118. Bonita R, Duncan J, Truelsen T *et al.* Passive as well as active smoking increases the risk of acute stroke. *Tobacco Control*. 1999; **8**: 156–60.
119. Nuorti JP, Butler JC, Farley MM *et al.* and the Active Bacterial Core Surveillance Team. Cigarette smoking and invasive pneumococcal disease. *New England Journal of Medicine*. 2000; **342**: 681–9.

SECTION TWO

Organic dust diseases

72	Occupational asthma *Paul Cullinan and Anthony Newman Taylor*	941
73	Byssinosis and other cotton-related diseases *CAC Pickering and Robert Niven*	958
74	Extrinsic allergic alveolitis *Paul Cullinan and Anthony Newman Taylor*	970

# 72

Occupational asthma

PAUL CULLINAN AND ANTHONY NEWMAN TAYLOR

Introduction	941	Prevention of occupational asthma	946
Causes of occupational asthma	942	Identification and diagnosis of occupational asthma	947
Mechanisms of occupational asthma	943	Management of occupational asthma	951
Frequency of occupational asthma	944	Outcome of occupational asthma	951
Determinants of occupational asthma	945	References	952

INTRODUCTION

It is estimated that exposures in the workplace account for around one in ten cases of new or recurrent asthma in adulthood. Many general respiratory physicians may be surprised by the magnitude of this proportion which is derived from meta-analysis of epidemiological studies that have examined, in the main, the distribution of asthma in different occupations.[1] Their scepticism probably reflects not only differences in the way that clinicians and epidemiologists understand 'attribution' and the geographical variation in all occupational lung diseases, but also the frequency with which an occupational aetiology for asthma is overlooked.[2] On the other hand, physicians with an interest in occupational disease and especially those concerned directly with the health of employees in high-risk workforces will not be taken aback. Indeed most will agree that work-related asthma is among the most common of occupational respiratory diseases, particularly in the industrialized world.

There are two broad categories of work-related asthma. First, the disease may be induced anew by exposure to an airborne sensitizing or irritant agent encountered at work. This, the focus of this chapter, is generally termed 'occupational asthma'. Such asthma may develop in an employee who has or does not have a previous history of asthma from another cause. Alternatively, pre-existing asthma may be provoked by workplace exposure(s) to 'exacerbating' agents which commonly include irritant fumes or dusts, cold air and physical exercise. This, termed 'work-exacerbated asthma', is probably very common and is generally manageable with careful attention to workplace exposures, protective equipment and appropriate pharmacological treatment of the underlying disease.

Occupational asthma almost always develops as an immune response to an airborne sensitizing agent in the workplace. The nature of this 'hypersensitive' response is such that there is a latent ('sensitizing') period of several months between initial exposure and the development of symptoms and subsequently the provocation of symptoms by very low exposures to the inducing agent. Presumably a reflection of variations in innate susceptibility, not all exposed employees will become sensitized although, depending on the levels of exposure in a workplace, very high proportions may do so.[3,4] In most cases of occupational asthma caused by airborne proteins, the immunological response is characterized by the production of specific IgE antibodies. In cases arising from exposure to chemical agents, the type of immunological response is far less well understood.

Occupational asthma may also arise – albeit uncommonly – from very high exposures to respiratory irritants. The mechanism of this response, originally termed 'reactive airways dysfunction syndrome',[5] but now more commonly referred to as 'irritant-induced' asthma, is primarily non-immunological. Most well-characterized cases follow single 'toxic' exposures to agents such as chlorine or oxides of nitrogen. It remains unclear whether more frequent, but less intense exposures to irritants in the workplace can give rise to asthma, although domestic exposures – to cleaning sprays, etc. – have been associated with incident 'asthmatic' symptoms.[6]

Respiratory sensitization to an occupational agent is one of very few well-established causes of adult asthma. It is thus potentially preventable and furthermore offers a rare opportunity to cure an asthmatic patient of their disease. Moreover, it seems to be a costly disease. In the UK, the total lifetime costs of cases of occupational asthma reported to a national surveillance scheme each year (a fraction only of the true number of cases) are estimated to be up to £100 million.[7] Only a small proportion of these costs are borne by employers, the rest accruing to the state and the individual. For these reasons, the disease has a high profile in industrial legislation in most of the developed world.

CAUSES OF OCCUPATIONAL ASTHMA

The published literature includes between 300 and 400 workplace agents reported to have caused occupational asthma. In some instances, the number of cases of asthma is very small. Those agents, and the occupational circumstances under which exposure to them occurs, which are widely recognized to cause a substantial burden of disease are listed in Table 72.1. Occupational asthmagens are generally categorized as being of either high or low molecular mass. The former are usually proteins that act as complete allergens; the latter are 'chemical' agents, which probably become antigenic only after conjugation with a body protein such as human serum albumen.

Currently, the respiratory allergenicity of all recognized chemical allergens is identified, for example on a safety data sheet, by the risk label 'R42' ('may cause sensitization by inhalation'). This signifies either that there is published evidence in humans that the substance can induce specific respiratory sensitization, or that there have been positive results from appropriate animal tests or that the agent is an isocyanate (unless there is evidence that it does *not* cause hypersensitivity). In the future, the familiar R42 label is likely to be replaced, under the Globally Harmonized

Table 72.1 Selected high and low molecular mass causes of occupational asthma by occupational group.

Occupational group	Agent(s)
(a) High molecular mass	
Laboratory technicians, research scientists, animal handlers	Small animal proteins (urine, dander, serum): rats, mice, guinea pigs, ferrets, etc. Insect proteins: cockroach, locust, housefly, fruit fly, gypsy moth, mealworm, etc. Other animal proteins: latex
Bakers and millers	Flour (wheat, barley, rye, oat, soya), fungal α-amylase, egg proteins, milk proteins, storage mites
Food processors	Linseed, green coffee bean, castor bean, tea dust, tobacco leaf, rosehip, shellfish proteins, fish proteins, milk proteins, egg proteins, cocoa proteins, proteolytic enzymes
Detergent powder manufacturers	Detergent enzymes: protease, amylase, lipase, cellulase
Nurses, dental workers, other healthcare workers	Latex
Farmers, farm workers and agriculturists	Storage mites, meal worms, spider mite, poultry mite, cow dander, cow β-lactoglobulin, pig urine, mink urine, insect larvae, poultry feathers, silkworm larvae, fruit, vegetable and flower pollens, fungi, grain dust
Florists, botanists	Pollens, weeping fig, baby's breath, spider mite, vine weevil
(b) Low molecular mass	
Spray painters	Hexamethylene diisocyanate, various amines
Plastics workers	Diphenylmethane diisocyanate, toluene diisocyanate, monomer acrylates, various amines, azodicarbonamide
Hairdressers	Persulphate salts, henna
Chemical processors	Phthalic anhydride, trimellitic anhydride, maleic anhydride, azodicarbonamide
Welders, solderers, electronic workers	Colophony fume, stainless steel welding fume, aminoethylethanolamine, cyanoacrylates, toluene diisocyanate, persulphate salts
Woodworkers	Hard wood dusts: western red cedar, iroko, African maple, mahogany, manosonia, obeche, etc.
Pharmaceutical workers, pharmacists	Psyllium, ispaghula, methyl-dopa, penicillins, cephalosporins, tetracycline, sulphathiazole, spiramycin, isoniazid, piperazine, cimetidine, dichloramine, ipecacuanha, bromelain, morphine
Nurses, dental workers, other healthcare workers	Glutaraldehyde, formaldehyde, monomer acrylates, antibiotics, psyllium, hexachlorophane, pancreatic extracts, N-acetyl cysteine
Metal refiners, electroplaters	Complex platinum salts, hexavalant chromium, nickel
Food processors	Chloramine-t, metabisulphite
Textile/fabric workers	Reactive dyes, gum acacia

System of Classification and Labelling of Chemicals, by 'H334' ('may cause allergy or asthma symptoms or breathing difficulties if inhaled'). Under the new regulations, a respiratory sensitizer is defined as a substance that will induce hypersensitivity of the airways following inhalation on the basis of evidence in humans or positive results from an appropriate animal test.

The list of agents which can cause occupational asthma is, necessarily, ever expanding. Fairly comprehensive information is available in specialist textbooks and websites.[8-11] It is in any case prudent to assume that any airborne protein (of either animal or vegetable origin) and any highly reactive chemical is capable of inducing respiratory sensitization.

MECHANISMS OF OCCUPATIONAL ASTHMA

Disease that is induced by exposure to a sensitizing agent encountered at work is the most common form of occupational asthma. It has the characteristic features of an acquired, immunological ('hypersensitive') reaction. Thus, specific sensitization and asthma develop only in a proportion (usually a minority) of exposed subjects and only after an asymptomatic (latent) period of exposure lasting several weeks or months, but occasionally years. Once asthma has developed, symptoms are provoked by concentrations of the sensitizing agent which are too low to provoke symptoms in non-sensitized workers and which the affected individual would previously have tolerated.

Most, if not all, protein respiratory sensitizing agents have the capacity of stimulating a T_H2 lymphocyte, IgE-associated immune response. IgE sensitization is ascertained by skin prick testing with water-soluble extracts of the responsible allergen or a search for specific antibodies in serum. Assuming equivalence of the antigens used in the different methods and with appropriate interpretation of test findings, skin prick and serum IgE tests produce broadly comparable results. On the grounds that occupational asthma from high molecular mass (protein) allergens is an immediate-type hypersensitivity, it should in all cases be accompanied by specific sensitization to the causative allergen. Thus, tests for IgE sensitization, if carried out properly, have a high diagnostic sensitivity and a very low false negative rate.

The same cannot be claimed for low molecular mass chemicals which are 'incomplete' allergens. Identifiable immune responses to such agents are usually not to the chemical itself, but to hapten–protein conjugates. For example, serum IgE antibodies to antigen–human serum albumen (HSA) conjugates may be detected in most cases of occupational asthma caused by acid anhydrides and in some cases of asthma attributable to diisocyanates and reactive dyes. An exception is platinum salt hypersensitivity which is almost always accompanied by positive responses to skin prick testing – but not by demonstrable specific IgE production – with dilute solutions of complex platinum–halide salts.

Such examples, however, are rare among the many chemical causes of occupational asthma suggesting that the relevant allergen–protein conjugate has yet to be identified or that alternative mechanisms are responsible. Specific IgE to diisocyanate–protein conjugates is detectable in only around 25 per cent of cases of asthma caused by this important group of chemicals,[12] and a study of patients with a confirmed asthmatic reaction to controlled exposures, but absent IgE responses did not detect upregulation of IgE receptors.[13] Other important causes of occupational asthma in which specific IgE responses are apparently absent include colophony fumes[14] and plicatic acid.[15] In some cases where 'specific' IgE antibodies are detected, it is unclear that they have any pathological or diagnostic specificity.[16]

Consequently, alternative immunological mechanisms for occupational chemical sensitization have been postulated. For example, most T-cell clones collected by bronchial biopsy of patients with diisocyanate-induced asthma are of CD8 phenotype producing gamma interferon and IL-5, rather than IL-4.[17] Such T cells may represent a $CD3^+/CD4^-/CD8^+$ population expressing a γ/δ T-cell receptor specific for the diisocyanate.[18]

Alternatively, non-immunological pathways may (also) be important in some causes of occupational asthma.[19] For example, plicatic acid in western red cedar can directly activate complement[20] and toluene diisocyanate may have direct actions on bronchial smooth muscle acting as a bronchoconstrictor or as a beta-2 adrenergic blocking agent.[21,22] Neurogenic mechanisms may also be relevant in some instances. Toluene diisocyanate, in addition to its postulated pharmacological effects (above in this section) stimulates, in animal models, neuropeptide release and inhibits neutral endopeptidase.[23,24]

Such non-immunological mechanisms do not readily explain the typical pattern of hypersensitivity-induced asthma, arising after a period of latency and associated with increasing sensitivity to low exposures, but they may have important secondary roles in explaining the clinical picture. Alternatively, some chemical agents may be capable of inducing more than one asthma phenotype, one immunological (through IgE-associated mechanisms) and one non-immunological. The distinction of these will require more careful clinical and epidemiological study than is currently available.

Irritant-induced asthma

Asthma developing shortly after exposure to high concentrations of inhaled respiratory irritants probably reflects non-immunological mechanisms. A small number of bronchial biopsies have been carried out in patients with irritant-induced asthma and indicate bronchial inflammation with lymphocytes and plasma cells, but not eosinophils,[25-27] suggesting that the clinical response is a manifestation of direct epithelial cell injury. Importantly, there have been no reports which include histological data prior to the initiating event in these cases.

FREQUENCY OF OCCUPATIONAL ASTHMA

Estimates of the prevalence – and less frequently incidence – of occupational asthma are available for both occupational and community populations.

Occupational populations

WORKPLACE STUDIES

Most workplace-based studies use standard cross-sectional epidemiological methods; occasionally longitudinal (cohort) designs, most of them prospective, are used. Data may be derived from a purposeful study or by analysis of the records of routine health surveillance. If the methods of surveillance are insensitive, then the latter approach will underestimate the true frequency of disease. In any case, a 'healthy worker effect', reflecting selection into and survival within a workforce, is likely and cross-sectional approaches to estimation of the prevalence of occupational asthma in a workplace – or to examination of its determinants – will generally underestimate both disease frequency and the effects of risk factors, such as exposure. This can be overcome, to some extent, by focusing attention on relatively new employees. Despite these important reservations – and the further uncertainty of how far findings from one setting can be generalized to others – workplace-based estimates of disease frequency have provided much of our knowledge of the detailed epidemiology of occupational asthma.

SURVEILLANCE SCHEMES

Several countries – notably Finland, the UK and France (Table 72.2), but also Ireland, South Africa and parts of Spain, the United States, Canada and Australia – have established surveillance schemes for occupational asthma. These measure disease that is newly recognized and reported by specialized physicians, usually in occupational or respiratory medical practice. In some instances, the schemes are closely linked to compensation claims. Where workforce denominators are available, occupation-specific incidence rates may be estimated, although these are often crude and probably underestimate the true incidence.[28] Reports from the longer running surveillance schemes are sometimes used to examine temporal trends or geographical variations in disease incidence within certain industries or in relation to specific agents. The findings of such analyses need to be interpreted with great care. The numerators for specific incidence rates are usually very small and there is good evidence of international variations in diagnostic practice. Nonetheless, surveillance schemes provide valuable information on the approximate size and distribution of the problem at a national level and a good estimate of the relative frequencies of important causes. In any case they have proved to be a powerful incentive for regulators.

Table 72.2 Numbers of cases of occupational asthma and estimated annual incidence rates per million workers in the UK, France and Finland from reports to national surveillance schemes, by occupational groups (may be defined differently in different countries).

Occupational group	UK 1989–90[110]		France 1996–99[111]		Finland 1989–95[112,a]	
	No. of cases	Annual incidence	No. of cases	Annual incidence	No. of cases	Annual incidence
Coach and spray painters	65	658	111	326	45	223
Chemical processors	54	364	NA		12	146
Plastics workers	47	337	NA		18	68
Bakers	50	334	410	683	101	444
Metal treatment workers	43	267	NA		NA	
Laboratory workers	50	188	NA		52	116
Welders and electronic assemblers	78	175	NA		68	76
Food processors (excluding bakers)	35	108	NA		7	99
Hairdressers	16	81	138	308	1	33
Painters (excluding spray painters)	28	66	NA		NA	
Wood workers	51	54	89	218	NA	
Farmers	23	28	NA		591	120
Healthcare workers	22	16	213	41	10	5
Veterinary surgeons	NA		NA		5	171
Cleaners	15	10	74	55	1	4
Teachers	NA		NA		6	5
All groups	1985	20	2178	24	2602	17

[a]Men only.
NA, not available.

General population studies

A number of epidemiological studies have set out to measure, in general (non-occupational) populations, the proportion of asthma in adulthood that is 'attributable' to workplace exposures. Studies of this sort estimate the prevalence of asthma, usually by self-report, in a representative sample of the community. By comparison with a referent group, usually office workers, any excess risks of asthma in specific occupational groups can be estimated and then summed to generate a measure of the proportion of communal asthma that is attributable to occupational exposures. Meta-analyses of such studies[1,29] indicate attributable proportions of between 10 and 15 per cent for all incident or relapsing cases of adult asthma. Studies of incident asthma are fewer, but provide essentially similar estimates.[30]

Epidemiological approaches of this kind employ a probabilistic, rather than individual, approach to the issue of causation. They cannot easily distinguish asthma that is induced from asthma that is provoked by an occupational exposure, nor examine whether there is selection by or of people with asthma into certain occupations. However, they are valuable in quantifying the communal risk of work-related asthma and in identifying increased risks of disease among occupational groups not traditionally recognized in clinical practice.[31,32]

DETERMINANTS OF OCCUPATIONAL ASTHMA

An understanding of the determinants of occupational asthma beyond its distributions is essential in the development of strategies to reduce its incidence. Broadly, the potential determinants that have been studied in detail include those relating to the environment (the level of workplace exposure to the sensitizing agent) and those that reflect host susceptibility (atopic status and genotype). The limited information on any interaction between host and environment suggests that susceptible individuals have a heightened – and perhaps accelerated – response to allergen exposure. One important consequence of this is that under conditions of relatively low exposure those factors that determine individual susceptibility are more prominent.[33] This is likely to have important implications in settings where exposure control is improving, while the population prevalence of susceptibility (for example, atopy) is either stable or rising.

Exposure

Direct relationships between the intensity of workplace allergen exposure and symptoms indicative of occupational asthma have been described for a variety of sensitizing agents. These, and studies confined to the risks of allergic sensitization alone, are summarized in Table 72.3.

Table 72.3 Studies demonstrating positive relationships between antigen exposure and either occupational asthma or specific sensitization, by antigen group.

Antigen group	References
Flour and enzymes (bakery and mill employees)	113–121
Enzymes (detergent manufacturers)	3, 56, 57, 121, 122
Laboratory animals (research workers)	123–126
Shellfish proteins (seafood processors)	127, 128
Castor bean (processors)	129
Diisocyanates (spray painters, plastics manufacturers)	130–133
Acid anhydrides (manufacturers, various)	62, 134, 135
Colophony fume (electronic assemblers)	136
Pharmaceuticals (manufacture)	137, 138
Complex platinum salts (precious metal refiners)	139
Western red cedar (lumber workers)	140

Most are of high molecular mass agents; there are fewer data relating to the exposure-related risks of work with low molecular mass agents.

While the existence of a relationship between exposure and occupational asthma is well established, there is little information on its detailed nature and almost none on meaningful threshold values. This probably reflects the difficulties in measuring relevant exposure intensities and their timing. On biological grounds alone, a 'sigmoid' relationship would be expected whereby the risk rises relatively steeply at the lower end of the exposure range and less steeply (or not at all) at the higher end. While this is likely to be true for most agents, there is evidence for laboratory animal exposures that the risk may be attenuated at very high exposures[34] – possibly reflecting a form of immunotolerance.

Most studies examining exposure–response relationships are of prevalent disease in cross-sectional, occupational populations. Few have studied incident disease in working cohorts. The findings of cross-sectional surveys need to be interpreted cautiously since they are prone to an unquantifiable bias from survivor effects. Survival biases, notably the movement of employees who have become sensitized away from situations of continuing exposure, are likely to lead to an underestimate of the effects of exposure. Furthermore, few studies of any design have succeeded in measuring directly the levels of sensitizing agents in exposed workforces and fewer still have characterized the nature, in terms of particle size and deposition of these exposures.

There is very little information on the relationship between exposure and response in irritant-induced asthma. Following a spill of glacial acetic acid in a US hospital, the frequency of subsequent asthma was higher (21 per cent) in those who had incurred the greatest exposure than that in those with medium or low exposures

(3 and 0 per cent, respectively), suggesting both that the relationship was causal and that it was dependent on the intensity of exposure.[35]

Several studies suggest that in some settings cigarette smoking increases the risk of sensitization or of asthmatic symptoms. They include studies of workforces exposed to ispaghula,[36] snow-crab proteins,[37] tetrachlorophthalic anhydride,[38] laboratory animals[39] and complex platinum salts.[40] It is not always clear, however, that the effects attributed to smoking are independent of other determinants, such as allergen exposure.

Individual susceptibility

Even at exposures well above any threshold, not all employees develop respiratory hypersensitivity – although in some instances the proportion of workers who are affected can be very high.[3,4] Thus, some employees appear to have an innately high risk.

Atopic workers are at increased risk of occupational asthma from a number of workplace allergens. The most consistent evidence is for allergens that induce an identifiable specific IgE response. Thus, atopy increases the risk of asthma or sensitization in workers exposed to flour, laboratory and other animals, detergent and other enzymes, sea foods, castor and green coffee bean, acid anhydrides and some reactive dyes. A useful summary of the evidence is provided by Nicholson et al.[41] In contrast there is little consistent evidence that atopy increases the risk for those who work with western red cedar, glutaraldehyde, complex platinum salts or diisocyanates. As with studies of exposure, the findings from cross-sectional surveys should be interpreted cautiously since reported associations, negative or positive, may reflect selection and survival pressures which are perhaps stronger among atopic employees.

The rapid advances in genotyping have been applied, in a limited fashion, to the study of occupational asthma. Two classes of gene have received most attention: those that determine specific antigen responsiveness (genes of the HLA class II complex) and those that relate to antioxidant respiratory responses. In each case, the presence or absence of candidate genes have been compared in case–control studies of employees with or without occupational asthma. Studies of this type require very large populations and most have probably been underpowered. All the same, associations – sometimes strong – between HLA genes and specific sensitization have been reported in workers exposed to trimellitic anhydride,[42] laboratory animal proteins,[43,44] western red cedar,[45] complex platinum salts[33] and diisocyanates.[46–48] The findings from the last of these are not entirely consistent.[49]

Similarly, genetic polymorphisms of the glutathione-S-transferase and N-acetyltransferase groups, important in determining the antioxidant status of the respiratory tract, have been associated with occupational asthma from a number of diisocyanates.[50–52]

PREVENTION OF OCCUPATIONAL ASTHMA

Primary prevention

Primary prevention eradicates or reduces incident disease. In the context of occupational asthma, it is achieved by elimination of the sensitizing agent from the workplace or where this is not possible by the reduction of exposures to levels at which sensitization does not occur. The former may be impossible, as in the example of flour in a bakery, but notable success has been achieved in some settings including occupational asthma from latex in hospitals – either by the substitution of latex gloves with synthetic alternatives or by the use of powder-free gloves which essentially prevent the release of latex particles into the air.[53,54] Because there are important variations in individual susceptibility, reductions in exposure rarely eliminate incident disease altogether, but they may be highly effective in maintaining disease rates at a very low level.

The details of the exposure–response relationships for most workplace allergens are poorly understood. In all cases it is unclear whether relationships are linear or whether a 'threshold' of zero incidence at low exposures exists. In practice, effective prevention of occupational asthma requires the maintenance of exposures, including occasional 'peak' values, at as low an intensity as is feasible and lower than that which incites symptoms in sensitized subjects. Much current legislation is based on this premise and very little of it includes specified 'safe' thresholds – a reflection not only of the paucity of evidence in this area, but also of the essentially immunological nature of the disease.

There is very little evidence that the use of protective respiratory equipment alone is effective in the primary prevention of occupational asthma.[55]

Published examples of the primary prevention of occupational asthma are few and most describe programmes that include not only improvements in exposure control but also procedures such as targeted pre-employment screening, enhanced surveillance and the increased use of personal protective equipment. It is seldom possible to disentangle the separate effects of different components. Nonetheless, success has been reported in the detergent industry[56,57] and with workforces exposed to laboratory animals,[58,59] diisocyanates,[38,60] acid anhydrides[61,62] and latex.[53,54] In most instances, a reduction in the number of newly identified cases following intervention(s) is reported without reference to the denominator, at-risk population and it is not always clear that this reflects a true reduction in disease incidence.

An alternative approach to primary prevention focuses on restricting the exposure or even employment of perceived 'high-risk' persons. Such restrictions are usually based on evidence of prior asthma or other allergy, usually but not always obtained by self-report. The discriminant performance of these methods – their ability to predict who will and who will not develop an occupational respiratory sensitization – is poor. Increasing understanding of the genetic determinants of occupational asthma may result in the extension of such techniques.

Secondary and tertiary prevention

Respiratory surveillance of employees working with respiratory sensitizing agents is widely practised and in many countries is mandated by legislation. The process, which aims to identify workers with occupational asthma at an early stage of their disease and thus allows appropriate action to prevent deterioration ('tertiary prevention'), is based on the premise that early recognition and avoidance of further exposure improve the prognosis of the disease. The most widely used surveillance methods are the questionnaire and regular spirometry. Almost certainly, self-completed questionnaires are an insensitive measure of work-related respiratory symptoms.[63] Similarly, routine measurement of spirometry is insensitive since many employees with occupational asthma will have a normal FEV_1, particularly if it is measured when they are not directly exposed to the causative allergen. There is evidence that routine spirometry detects very few cases of disease that would not otherwise or also have been recognized on the basis of reported symptoms.[64,65]

In some settings, surveillance includes the use of immunological methods to measure specific sensitization: either skin prick testing or specific IgE assay directed to the workplace allergen(s). The purpose of such immunological surveillance varies. In some parts of the platinum refining industry, for example, regular skin prick testing with complex platinum salts forms part of a health surveillance programme. A positive prick test result, highly specific for platinum salt asthma, is used to identify employees who require rapid relocation away from exposure. Similarly respiratory surveillance in much of the detergent manufacturing sector includes a measure of immunological sensitization. There, however, where sensitization is a highly sensitive but not wholly specific adjunct of detergent enzyme asthma, the practice is designed to identify areas of the workplace where further attention to exposure control is necessary. A further example, in the baking sector as described by Brant et al.[63] is the assay of serum-specific IgE antibodies to flour and α-amylase for employees who report work-related respiratory symptoms. This improves the specificity of the surveillance programme and aids the selection of those employees who require further investigation.

Any use of immunology in routine surveillance requires access to validated test methods and an intimate knowledge of their diagnostic properties, and an explicit understanding of the purpose of testing. In carefully selected instances, immunological approaches can be a useful adjunct to other methods and are likely to be increasingly used in the future.

IDENTIFICATION AND DIAGNOSIS OF OCCUPATIONAL ASTHMA

Accuracy in the diagnosis of occupational asthma is critically important. A positive diagnosis frequently leads to a change in job and too frequently to the loss of current employment or a major change in occupation. A false positive diagnosis can lead to unnecessary financial and social hardship and a lack of clinical improvement once exposure has ceased. In legal terms the burden of proof is generally set at a level of 'more likely than not'. Most occupational health practitioners and their patients will prefer a more certain standard than this.

On the other hand, the early and accurate identification of an occupational cause of asthma has several advantages. First, it will explain the onset of new or recurrent asthma in adult life and make a search for alternative causes unnecessary. Second, it allows a rational approach to both pharmacological and non-pharmacological management, and third, it identifies, for other employees, potential risks that may be prevented.

Guidelines to the diagnosis of occupational asthma, derived from systematic review of the published literature, are available both electronically[66] and in print.[41] Other, consensus-developed, guidance is also available.[67–70] An outline of available methods in the diagnostic pathway is shown in Figure 72.1. In essence the process is iterative and should include each of the following: an assessment of relevant exposures, the identification of an asthmatic airway response in relation to exposure(s) and, where appropriate, the identification of specific immunological sensitization. None of these is sufficient alone.

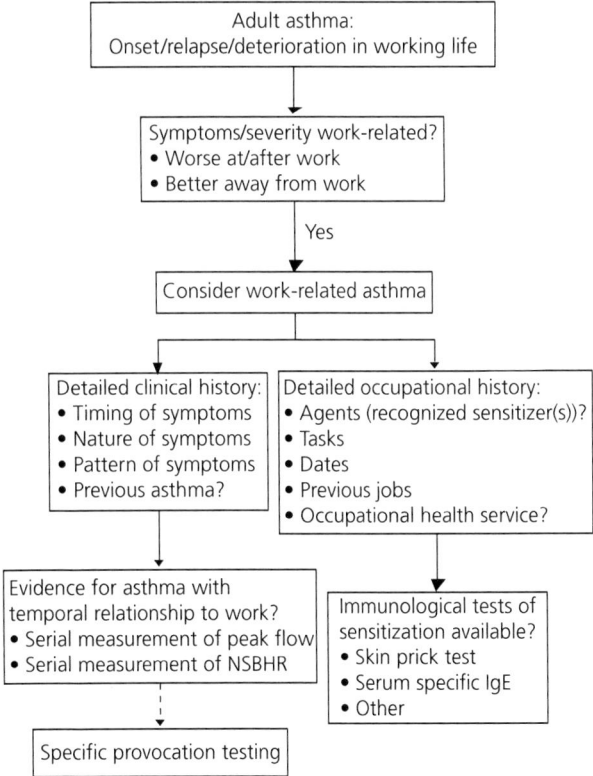

Figure 72.1 Summary of diagnostic approaches to occupational asthma. NSBHR, non-specific bronchial hyperreactivity.

History

The prior likelihood of occupational asthma is higher in employees with exposure to a recognized sensitizing agent and familiarity with these agents and the occupations in which they are encountered is important. At the same time, patients may develop sensitivity to a rare or previously unrecognized agent and in all cases a low threshold of suspicion is sensible. Patients with occupational respiratory sensitization characteristically develop symptoms after a relatively short latent period following first exposure to the sensitizing agent. 'First' exposure often reflects a new job, but may reflect a qualitative or quantitative change in exposure in a long-held job. The latent, asymptomatic period, during which sensitization is presumed to be developing, is usually between three and 24 months. Symptoms that develop sooner after a new exposure are more likely to have an irritant mechanism. Thus careful attention to the timing of the onset of symptoms and any changes in exposure that may have preceded them, is diagnostically helpful.

The symptoms themselves are characteristic of asthma, but are frequently accompanied by upper respiratory symptoms of nasal obstruction, sneezing and discharge and itching or running of eyes – as well as, if the causative agent is a protein, by itching of the skin or even urticaria. Occupational rhinitis is probably more common than occupational asthma, but the two conditions frequently occur together.[71] The frequency and intensity of nasal symptoms may be greater in cases caused by sensitization to high molecular mass agents.[72]

A history of previous or coexistent respiratory disease does not preclude a diagnosis of occupational asthma, but raises the possibility of aggravation of pre-existing asthma or other airways disease by one of the many workplace respiratory irritants.

In cases of occupational asthma, symptoms are typically present during or immediately after periods of exposure at work and improve when away from work. This pattern may be complicated by varying shift patterns, by isolated 'late-phase' symptoms that are present only after a period at work and in cases where, with repeated exposures, recovery is only achieved, if at all, by an absence from work of several days or more. Further confusion can arise when the non-specific bronchial hyperreactivity that is typical of asthma gives rise to symptoms provoked by a variety of irritants encountered at and away from the workplace. In these cases, employees (and their clinicians) frequently attribute the cause of the disease to the obviously irritant exposure rather than the sensitizing agent.

In cases of irritant-induced asthma (reactive airways dysfunction syndrome (RADS)), the history is very different, partly because of constraints imposed by the current disease definition. Here symptoms develop within minutes or hours after a defined, high-intensity and sometimes dramatic exposure to a respiratory irritant, frequently in an individual without known previous respiratory disease. Unlike those with occupational sensitization, patients with irritant-induced asthma can usually identify precisely the time of onset of their disease which may or may not be many years after the onset of employment and of exposure, at lower levels, to the responsible agent.

Investigations

Relevant investigations are, broadly, either immunological or functional. The former aim to identify a specific immunological response to the putative agent, the latter to establish a relationship between variable airflow obstruction ('asthma') and one or more specific occupational exposures.

IMMUNOLOGICAL TESTS

As described above under Mechanisms of occupational asthma (p. 943), sensitization to almost all high molecular mass occupational agents and to some of low molecular mass is accompanied by the presence of specific IgE antibody production. This can be identified through skin prick tests with extracts of soluble antigens or in serum using standardized immunoassays. In cases of occupational asthma caused by exposure to a high molecular mass agent, the test is highly sensitive. In other words, it is almost always positive and a negative result makes the diagnosis improbable. On the other hand, a positive result can occur in the absence of clinical disease, presumably reflecting an asymptomatic state of specific sensitization. In all cases, it is important to include well-validated tests for all relevant allergens and liaison with an experienced (specialized) laboratory is valuable.

The general absence of an identifiable IgE response in diisocyanate asthma has prompted the search for alternative immunological tests for this common type of occupational asthma. They include the measurement of monocyte chemotactic protein-1 (MCP-1) produced by peripheral blood mononuclear cells after stimulation with a relevant isocyanate conjugate. The results of a pilot study suggest that this method has a sensitivity of about 80 per cent and a specificity of 91 per cent, respectively far higher than and similar to methods based on specific IgE production.[73] This technique requires replication in other populations before it can be widely applied.

FUNCTIONAL TESTS OF VARIABLE, WORK-RELATED AIRFLOW OBSTRUCTION

The most sensitive and specific method of examining the existence and pattern of airflow limitation is through the use of serial, self-recorded measurements of peak flow or FEV_1.[74–79] Workers under investigation are supplied with a portable meter and invited to make repeated measurements over a period of time including both periods at and away from work. A protocol that demands, during waking hours, two-hourly measurements for four weeks has higher sensitivity than less frequent measurements[78,80] and is generally acceptable to patients. Where possible, especially in cases

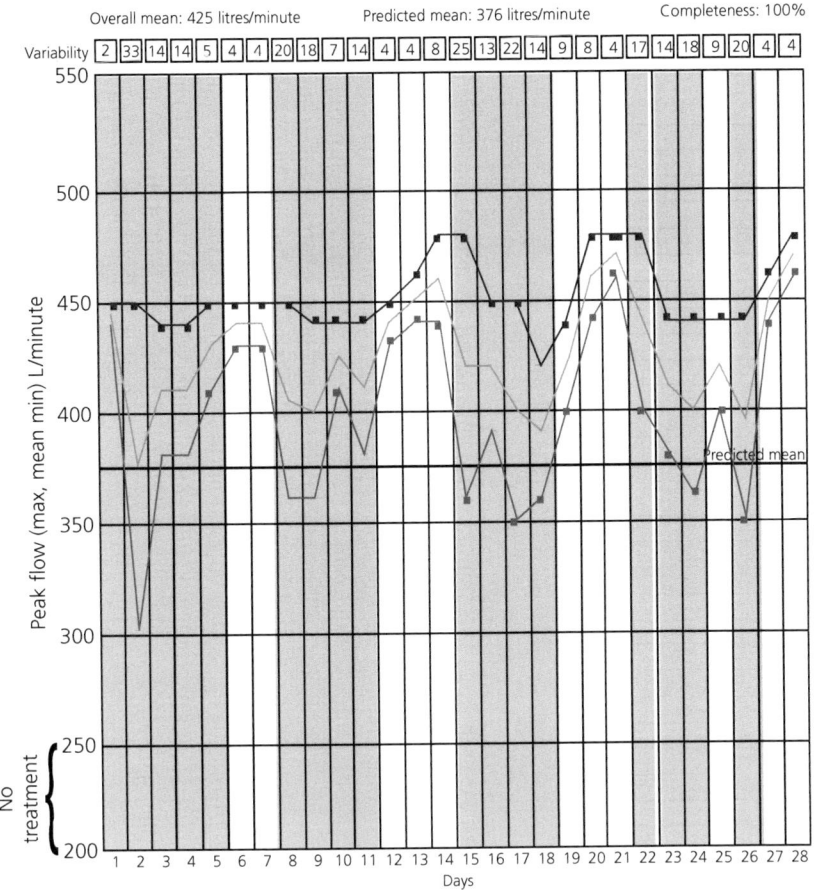

Figure 72.2 Serial peak flow record of an employee with laboratory-animal asthma. The shaded columns represent days at work. On each day the mean, maximum and minimum peak flow measurements only are plotted. The figures in boxes are measurements of peak flow variability.

where symptoms have been present for many months or years, it is helpful to include within the period of measurement a prolonged absence from work, such as a holiday of several days or more. Potential confounding by concurrent asthma treatment is avoided by asking patients to maintain the same treatment throughout the measurement period.

On completion, the readings are best plotted on a daily basis as the maximum, minimum and mean values from each day. An example of such a plot, using peak flow, is shown in Figure 72.2. The pattern of lung function in relation to work is then examined – usually visually, but sometimes by computed statistical analysis.[81] Agreement of visual analyses by experienced clinicians is high, but there are important variations among less-experienced observers. Statistical analyses, intended to provide a more objective analysis, have proved to be little more valid or reliable than visual inspection.[76,79,82]

Confusion and even misdiagnosis may arise if, particularly through early morning shift patterns, readings are made at different times on work and rest days.[83] Serial measurements of lung function may also fail to distinguish immunologically mediated occupational asthma from asthma that is provoked by workplace-irritant exposures. Thus, the method should only be interpreted in the light of other diagnostic evidence.

Other techniques for assessing the pattern of airflow obstruction include the 'cross-shift' measurement of lung function (FEV_1 or peak flow) or non-specific bronchial responsiveness immediately before and after one or more periods at work. These methods may be less time consuming than a lengthy series of functional measurements, but have lower diagnostic specificity and sensitivity and produce a higher proportion of false positive and false negative results.[75,79,84–86] As with FEV_1, bronchial responsiveness may be normal in patients with confirmed occupational asthma if measurements are made outside periods of exposure to the causative allergen.

SPECIFIC PROVOCATION (INHALATIONAL) TESTING

The gold standard of diagnostic tests for occupational asthma is often claimed to be the specific provocation test, whereby patients are observed and their lung function measured during and after carefully controlled exposures, under laboratory conditions, to the suspected sensitizing agent. The first use of such tests, for the diagnosis of occupational asthma, was in 1972.[87]

Indications for specific provocation testing vary between centres. In some jurisdictions it is conducted as a necessary step in the process of establishing a diagnosis and thereby allocating compensation. In others, such as the United Kingdom and many other European countries, it is used as an occasional adjunct to the diagnostic process, particularly when other, simpler techniques have failed or cannot be used to establish a diagnosis with sufficient accuracy. If, for example, a patient is not currently exposed to

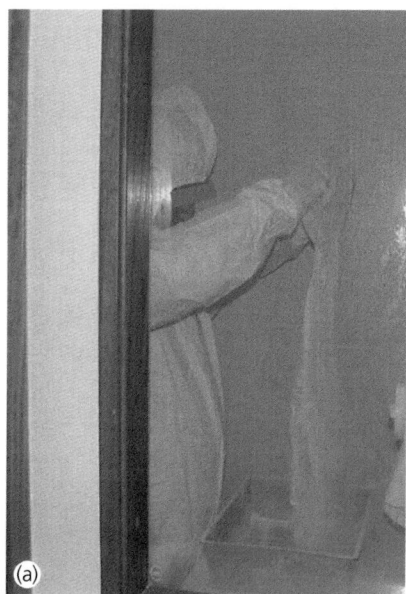
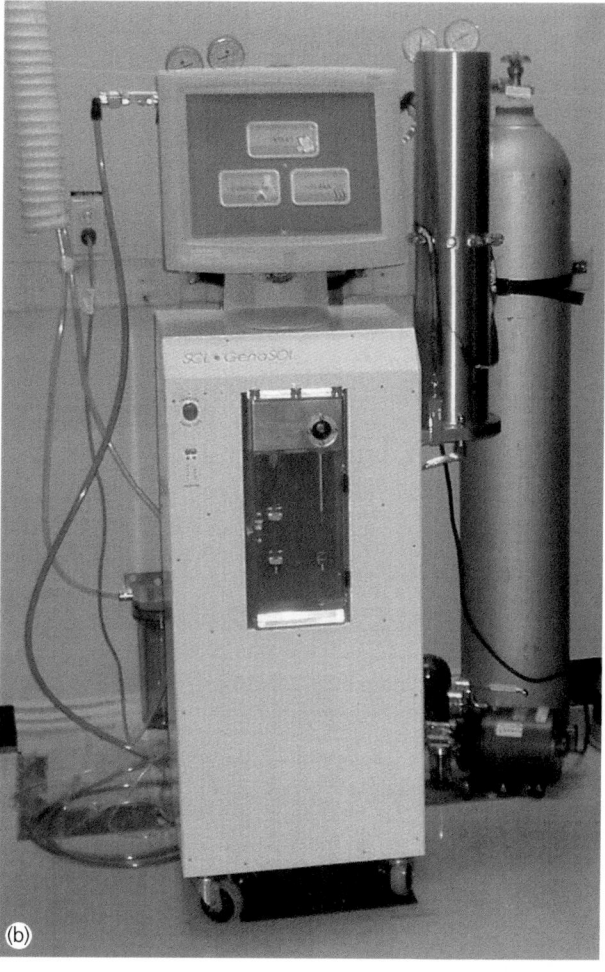

Figure 72.3 Specific provocation testing using (a) traditional ('Pepys') method in which the patient is asked to recreate, in a sealed chamber, exposures at their workplace (in this case a baker is tipping a mixture of flour and lactose to create a dust cloud) and (b) machine for generating controlled exposures to vapours. Figure 72.3(b) courtesy of J-L Malo, Hôpital du Sacré-Coeur de Montréal, Montreal, Canada.

the suspected agent, but an accurate diagnosis is still required to assist in decisions about continuing employment, serial measurement of lung function as described above will be uninformative. Alternatively, a patient may be exposed to more than one sensitizing agent at work and it may be considered important to identify which (if any) is responsible for their disease. In rare cases, the symptoms provoked by exposure at work are too severe (or unpleasant) to justify serial measurement of lung function. In such cases, the judicious use of specific provocation testing can be an appropriate and even essential diagnostic method. Finally, a further indication may be the investigation of response to an agent that is not recognized to be a respiratory sensitizer. Provocation testing solely in support of a legal claim for personal injury is difficult to justify.

Specific provocation tests are hazardous and should be undertaken only by experienced staff in specialist centres where the risks are very low. Most tests use a single-blind[88] methodology which aims to recreate as closely as possible exposures encountered by the patient in the workplace (Figure 72.3). More recently, some centres have developed sophisticated delivery techniques of mechanized dust or fume generation.[89] The advantage of these over the simpler techniques is yet to be established. Whichever method is used, great care must be taken over the dosing and frequency of exposures which should be of lower intensity than those in the workplace and several orders lower than occupational safety limits.

Responses to inert and active exposures are generally assessed and compared by the subsequent measurement of FEV_1 at frequent intervals. This is more reliable than peak flow measurement. The measurement of changes in non-specific bronchial responsiveness following exposure (using histamine or metacholine) is a very useful additional test, helping to distinguish irritant from immunologically mediated responses. The specificity of provocation testing is increased if reproducibility of the responses to repeated active and control exposures is confirmed (Figure 72.4).

Several patterns of response are taken to be indicative of specific sensitization, but their interpretation requires an experienced clinician. An immediate or early response is one in which a fall in baseline lung function occurs and recovers within one or two hours of provocation. If isolated and unaccompanied by evidence of a concurrent

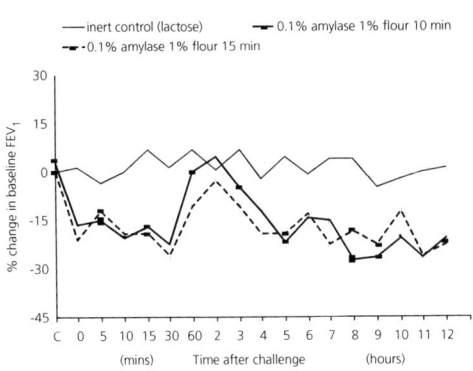
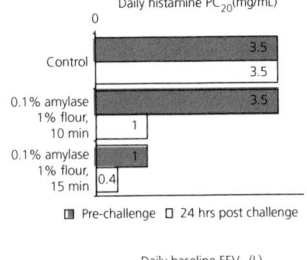
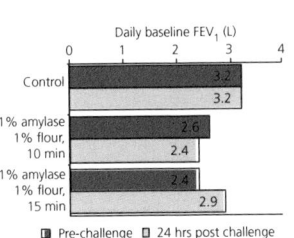

Figure 72.4 Specific inhalation challenge to bakers' flour and α-amylase: positive result with dual asthmatic response and increase in non-specific bronchial reactivity. Note the reproducible findings and the lack of any consistent change in baseline FEV_1.

increase in bronchial responsiveness, an immediate response may be an indication of either respiratory sensitization or reflex irritation. Late reactions are those that develop only one or more hours after exposure. They may persist for 24 hours or longer and are frequently accompanied by an increase in bronchial reactivity measurable three[90] or 24 hours after provocation. Dual (combined early and late) responses are common, especially in cases of sensitization to high molecular mass agents.

Specific provocation testing is very difficult in patients with unstable baseline asthma when it can be difficult to distinguish an irritant from a hypersensitivity response. False negative results may occur when patients have been away from workplace exposures for prolonged periods,[37,91] if an inappropriate form of the test material is used or if patients continue to use anti-inflammatory asthma treatments during the period of testing.

MANAGEMENT OF OCCUPATIONAL ASTHMA

Optimal management of occupational asthma will in most cases abolish or control symptoms and prevent the development of persistent disease. In general, these are achieved only by complete avoidance of exposure to the causative allergen, ideally through a change in work practice or relocation within the same workplace or industry to a non-exposed area – but in practice often requiring a major change in occupation.

Some patients, particularly those who are self-employed or those who have significant investment in a current occupation – such as research scientists working with animal models – are especially reluctant to make changes sufficient to prevent further exposure.[92] At present, further allergen exposure even at very low intensity cannot be advised, but support to those determined to continue can be provided by the prevention, as far as is possible, of exposure at levels high enough to incite symptoms or changes in lung function. Repeated, serial measurements of peak flow during periods at and away from work are often helpful in these situations, as is good pharmacological control of symptoms. (Enhanced)

respiratory protective equipment is often considered, but is only effective if it is worn appropriately and if it is removed, stored and maintained correctly. There is some evidence that helmet-type respirators can improve symptoms in some but not all employees who continue to work in conditions where there may be further allergen exposure.[93–98]

Pharmacological treatment is as for non-occupational asthma, but is generally ineffective in the face of continuing allergen exposure. Conversely, little or no treatment may be needed once allergen exposure has ceased. There is only limited evidence that treatment with inhaled steroids improves the prognosis in occupational asthma, whether allergen exposure continues or otherwise.[99]

OUTCOME OF OCCUPATIONAL ASTHMA

Following avoidance of further exposure to the causative allergen, the symptoms of most patients with occupational asthma improve, and many recover completely. However, this is not always the case. Most studies of the outcome of occupational asthma are of patients attending specialist centres. These are likely to have more severe and more refractory disease and their experience may not be representative. A systematic review of 39 publications with a median length of follow up of 31 months following diagnosis suggests that only one-third of patients recovered completely from their asthma after the cessation of exposure. Individual estimates ranged however from 0 to 100 per cent.[100] The same review examined a number of potential determinants of recovery. Complete symptomatic recovery was significantly lower with increasing age at diagnosis, in studies of patients seen in specialist clinics and in patients with the longest durations of employment, or of symptomatic exposure (Figure 72.1). No studies examined the independent effects of age and exposure duration. There were no clear differences in recovery between patients with disease caused by agents of different molecular mass or between those who were or were not smokers.

Any recovery in lung function and bronchial hyperresponsiveness seems to take place in the first two years after avoidance of exposure.[101] Persistence of longer duration is associated with continuing eosinophil and lymphocyte infiltration of the airways and may be related to fixed airway remodelling.[102-104] However, it remains unclear why disease should persist after exposure avoidance. Retention of allergen or hapten within the lung – or extrapulmonary tissue – may promote persistent IgE production after the cessation of workplace exposure to acid anhydrides.[105]

Other outcomes are common in occupational asthma and may be equally or even more important to the patient. Surveys suggest that about a third of patients are unemployed soon after diagnosis – a figure which is probably higher than that among other adults with asthma[92,106,107] – but that the rate of unemployment falls with passing time.[108] Nonetheless the necessary change in job or occupation is commonly associated with a loss of income and many patients will struggle to find suitable alternative employment.[92,107,109]

Most industrialized countries operate a compensation scheme for those who have developed occupational asthma. In some countries, such as Germany, this is funded by employers' contributions to a central insurance association. In others, such as the UK, the scheme is financed and administered by the state. The features, criteria of eligibility and benefits of schemes vary widely between jurisdictions: some, for example, provide only a financial pension while others include provision for retraining or even primary preventive programmes in the workplace.

Key points

- Workplace exposures account for around 10 per cent of cases of new or recurrent asthma in adulthood. These cases include those where symptoms of pre-existing asthma are provoked by irritant exposures at work ('work-exacerbated asthma') and cases of new asthma arising directly from a – generally sensitizing – workplace agent ('occupational asthma').
- Several hundred agents in the workplace have been identified as capable of inducing occupational asthma; most are airborne proteins or highly reactive chemicals.
- Occupational asthma usually has a short latency and tends to afflict relatively young employees who will need expert advice on career options. An accurate diagnosis is essential.
- In most cases, a sufficiently accurate diagnosis can be achieved through a combination of a careful history, appropriate immunology and the comparison of serial measurements of lung function made at work and at home.
- Occupational asthma is (potentially) preventable. Preventive action should be focused on exposure control.

REFERENCES

1. Blanc PD, Toren K. How much adult asthma can be attributed to occupational factors? *American Journal of Medicine.* 1999; **107**: 580-7.
2. de Bono J, Hudsmith L. Occupational asthma: A community-based study. *Occupational Medicine.* 1999; **49**: 217-19.
3. Cullinan P, Harris JM, Newman Taylor AJ et al. An outbreak of asthma in a modern detergent factory. *Lancet.* 2000; **356**: 1899-900.
4. Dille JR, Gibbons HL, Spikes GA. Allergic problems in screw worm fly eradication program personnel. *Aerospace Medicine.* 1968; **39**: 1116-19.
5. Brooks SM, Weiss MA, Bernstein IL. Reactive airways dysfunction syndrome (RADS). Persistent asthma syndrome after high level irritant exposures. *Chest.* 1985; **88**: 376-84.
6. Zock JP, Plana E, Jarvis D et al. The use of household cleaning sprays and adult asthma: An international longitudinal study. *American Journal of Respiratory and Critical Care Medicine.* 2007; **176**: 735-41.
7. Health and Safety Executive. The true cost of occupation asthma in Great Britain, 2006. Available from: www.hse.gov.uk/RESEARCH/rrpdf/rr474.pdf.
8. Palmarès des Hopitaux. Occupational asthma. Cited 2006. Available from: www.asmanet.com.
9. Asthme professionnel. Cited 2008. Available from: www.asthme.csst.qc.ca.
10. European Academy of Allergy and Clinical Immunology. Cited 2008. Available from: www.eaaci.net.
11. Malo J-L, Chan-Yeung M. Agents causing occupational asthma with key references. In: Bernstein IL, Chan-Yeung M, Malo J-L, Bernstein D (eds). *Asthma in the workplace*, 3rd edn. London: Taylor & Francis, 2006: 852-66.
12. Tee RD, Cullinan P, Welch J et al. Specific IgE to isocyanates: A useful diagnostic role in occupational asthma. *Journal of Allergy and Clinical Immunology.* 1998; **101**: 709-15.
13. Jones MG, Floyd A, Nouri-Aria KT et al. Is occupational asthma to diisocyanates a non-IgE-mediated disease? *Journal of Allergy and Clinical Immunology.* 2006; **117**: 663-9.
14. Malo JL, Bernstein IL. Other chemical substances causing occupational asthma. In: Bernstein IL, Chan-Yeung M, Malo JL, Bernstein D (eds). *Asthma in the workplace.* New York: Marcel Dekker, 1992: 481-582.
15. Tse KS, Chan H, Chan-Yeung M. Specific IgE antibodies in workers with occupational asthma due to western red cedar. *Clinical Allergy.* 1982; **12**: 249-58.
16. Vyas A, Pickering CA, Oldham LA et al. Survey of symptoms, respiratory function, and immunology and their relation to glutaraldehyde and other occupational exposures among endoscopy nursing staff. *Occupational and Environmental Medicine.* 2000; **57**: 752-9.
17. Maestrelli P, Del Prete GF, De Carli M et al. CD8 T-cell clones producing interleukin-5 and interferon-gamma in

bronchial mucosa of patients with asthma induced by toluene diisocyanate. *Scandinavian Journal of Work, Environment and Health.* 1994; **20**: 376–81.
18. Wisnewski AV, Herrick CA, Liu Q et al. Human gamma/delta T-cell proliferation and IFN-gamma production induced by hexamethylene diisocyanate. *Journal of Allergy and Clinical Immunology.* 2003; **112**: 538–46.
19. Raulf-Heimsoth M, Baur X. Pathomechanisms and pathophysiology of isocyanate-induced diseases – summary of present knowledge. *American Journal of Industrial Medicine.* 1998; **34**: 137–43.
20. Chan-Yeung M, Lam S, Koener S. Clinical features and natural history of occupational asthma due to western red cedar (*Thuja plicata*). *American Journal of Medicine.* 1982; **72**: 411–15.
21. Davies RJ, Butcher BT, O'Neil CE, Salvaggio JE. The *in vitro* effect of toluene diisocyanate on lymphocyte cyclic adenosine monophosphate production by isoproterenol, prostaglandin, and histamine: A possible mode of action. *Journal of Allergy and Clinical Immunology.* 1977; **60**: 223–9.
22. McKay RT, Brooks SM, Johnson C. Isocyanate-induced abnormality of beta-adrenergic receptor function. *Chest.* 1981; **80** (Suppl. 1): 61–3.
23. Mapp CE, Chitano P, Fabbri LM et al. Evidence that toluene diisocyanate activates the efferent function of capsaicin-sensitive primary afferents. *European Journal of Pharmacology.* 1990; **180**: 113–18.
24. Sheppard D, Thompson JE, Scypinski L et al. Toluene diisocyanate increases airway responsiveness to substance P and decreases airway neutral endopeptidase. *Journal of Clinical Investigation.* 1988; **81**: 1111–15.
25. Bardana EJ Jr. Reactive airways dysfunction syndrome (RADS): Guidelines for diagnosis and treatment and insight into likely prognosis. *Annals of Allergy, Asthma and Immunology.* 1999; **83**: 583–6.
26. Lemiere C, Malo JL, Boulet LP, Boutet M. Reactive airways dysfunction syndrome induced by exposure to a mixture containing isocyanate: functional and histopathologic behaviour. *Allergy.* 1996; **51**: 262–5.
27. Lemiere C, Malo JL, Boutet M. Reactive airways dysfunction syndrome due to chlorine: Sequential bronchial biopsies and functional assessment. *European Respiratory Journal.* 1997; **10**: 241–4.
28. Draper A, Newman TA, Cullinan P. Estimating the incidence of occupational asthma and rhinitis from laboratory animal allergens in the UK, 1999-2000. *Occupational and Environmental Medicine.* 2003; **60**: 604–5.
29. Balmes J, Becklake M, Blanc P et al. American Thoracic Society Statement: Occupational contribution to the burden of airway disease. *American Journal of Respiratory and Critical Care Medicine.* 2003; **167**: 787–97.
30. Kogevinas M, Zock JP, Jarvis D et al. Exposure to substances in the workplace and new-onset asthma: An international prospective population-based study (ECRHS-II). *Lancet.* 2007; **370**: 336–41.
31. Jaakkola JJ, Piipari R, Jaakkola MS. Occupation and asthma: A population-based incident case-control study. *American Journal of Epidemiology.* 2003; **158**: 981–7.
32. Kogevinas M, Anto JM, Sunyer J et al. Occupational asthma in Europe and other industrialised areas: A population-based study. European Community Respiratory Health Survey Study Group. *Lancet.* 1999; **353**: 1750–4.
33. Newman Taylor AJ, Cullinan P, Lympany PA et al. Interaction of HLA phenotype and exposure intensity in sensitization to complex platinum salts. *American Journal of Respiratory and Critical Care Medicine.* 1999; **160**: 435–8.
34. Jeal H, Draper A, Harris J et al. Modified Th2 responses at high-dose exposures to allergen: Using an occupational model. *American Journal of Respiratory and Critical Care Medicine.* 2006; **174**: 21–5.
35. Kern DG. Outbreak of the reactive airways dysfunction syndrome after a spill of glacial acetic acid. *American Review of Respiratory Disease.* 1991; **144**: 1058–64.
36. Zetterstrom O, Osterman K, Machado L, Johansson SG. Another smoking hazard: Raised serum IgE concentration and increased risk of occupational allergy. *British Medical Journal.* 1981; **283**: 1215–17.
37. Cartier A, Malo JL, Forest F et al. Occupational asthma in snow crab-processing workers. *Journal of Allergy and Clinical Immunology.* 1984; **74**: 261–9.
38. Venables KM, Dally MB, Burge PS et al. Occupational asthma in a steel coating plant. *British Journal of Industrial Medicine.* 1985; **42**: 517–24.
39. Venables KM, Upton JL, Hawkins ER et al. Smoking, atopy, and laboratory animal allergy. *British Journal of Industrial Medicine.* 1988; **45**: 667–71.
40. Venables KM, Dally MB, Nunn AJ et al. Smoking and occupational allergy in workers in a platinum refinery. *British Medical Journal.* 1989; **299**: 939–42.
41. Nicholson PJ, Cullinan P, Taylor AJ et al. Evidence based guidelines for the prevention, identification, and management of occupational asthma. *Occupational and Environmental Medicine.* 2005; **62**: 290–9.
42. Young RP, Barker RD, Pile KD et al. The association of HLA-DR3 with specific IgE to inhaled acid anhydrides. *American Journal of Respiratory and Critical Care Medicine.* 1995; **151**: 219–21.
43. Jeal H, Draper A, Jones M et al. HLA associations with occupational sensitization to rat lipocalin allergens: A model for other animal allergies? *Journal of Allergy and Clinical Immunology.* 2003; **111**: 795–9.
44. Sjostedt L, Willers S, Orbaek P. Human leukocyte antigens in occupational allergy: A possible protective effect of HLA-B16 in laboratory animal allergy. *American Journal of Industrial Medicine.* 1996; **30**: 415–20.
45. Horne C, Quintana PJ, Keown PA et al. Distribution of DRB1 and DQB1 HLA class II alleles in occupational asthma due to western red cedar. *European Respiratory Journal.* 2000; **15**: 911–14.
46. Balboni A, Baricordi OR, Fabbri LM et al. Association between toluene diisocyanate-induced asthma and DQB1

markers: A possible role for aspartic acid at position 57. *European Respiratory Journal.* 1996; **9**: 207–10.
47. Bignon JS, Aron Y, Ju LY et al. HLA class II alleles in isocyanate-induced asthma. *American Journal of Respiratory and Critical Care Medicine.* 1994; **149**: 71–5.
48. Mapp CE, Beghe B, Balboni A et al. Association between HLA genes and susceptibility to toluene diisocyanate-induced asthma. *Clinical and Experimental Allergy.* 2000; **30**: 651–6.
49. Rihs HP, Barbalho-Krolls T, Huber H, Baur X. No evidence for the influence of HLA class II in alleles in isocyanate-induced asthma. *American Journal of Industrial Medicine.* 1997; **32**: 522–7.
50. Mapp CE, Fryer AA, De Marzo N et al. Glutathione S-transferase GSTP1 is a susceptibility gene for occupational asthma induced by isocyanates. *Journal of Allergy and Clinical Immunology.* 2002; **109**: 867–72.
51. Piirila P, Wikman H, Luukkonen R et al. Glutathione S-transferase genotypes and allergic responses to diisocyanate exposure. *Pharmacogenetics.* 2001; **11**: 437–45.
52. Wikman H, Piirila P, Rosenberg C et al. N-Acetyltransferase genotypes as modifiers of diisocyanate exposure-associated asthma risk. *Pharmacogenetics.* 2002; **12**: 227–33.
53. Allmers H, Schmengler J, Skudlik C. Primary prevention of natural rubber latex allergy in the German health care system through education and intervention. *Journal of Allergy and Clinical Immunology.* 2002; **110**: 318–23.
54. Tarlo SM, Easty A, Eubanks K et al. Outcomes of a natural rubber latex control program in an Ontario teaching hospital. *Journal of Allergy and Clinical Immunology.* 2001; **108**: 628–33.
55. Grammer LC, Harris KE, Yarnold PR. Effect of respiratory protective devices on development of antibody and occupational asthma to an acid anhydride. *Chest.* 2002; **121**: 1317–22.
56. Cathcart M, Nicholson P, Roberts D et al. Enzyme exposure, smoking and lung function in employees in the detergent industry over 20 years. Medical Subcommittee of the UK Soap and Detergent Industry Association. *Occupational Medicine.* 1997; **47**: 473–8.
57. Juniper CP, How MJ, Goodwin BF, Kinshott AK. Bacillus subtilis enzymes: A 7-year clinical, epidemiological and immunological study of an industrial allergen. *Journal of the Society of Occupational Medicine.* 1977; **27**: 3–12.
58. Botham PA, Davies GE, Teasdale EL. Allergy to laboratory animals: a prospective study of its incidence and of the influence of atopy on its development. *British Journal of Industrial Medicine.* 1987; **44**: 627–32.
59. Fisher R, Saunders WB, Murray SJ, Stave GM. Prevention of laboratory animal allergy. *Journal of Occupational and Environmental Medicine.* 1998; **40**: 609–13.
60. Tarlo SM, Liss GM, Yeung KS. Changes in rates and severity of compensation claims for asthma due to diisocyanates: A possible effect of medical surveillance measures. *Occupational and Environmental Medicine.* 2002; **59**: 58–62.
61. Drexler H, Schaller KH, Nielsen J et al. Efficacy of measures of hygiene in workers sensitised to acid anhydrides and the influence of selection bias on the results. *Occupational and Environmental Medicine.* 1999; **56**: 202–5.
62. Liss GM, Bernstein D, Genesove L et al. Assessment of risk factors for IgE-mediated sensitization to tetrachlorophthalic anhydride. *Journal of Allergy and Clinical Immunology.* 1993; **92**: 237–47.
63. Brant A, Nightingale S, Berriman J et al. Supermarket baker's asthma: How accurate is routine health surveillance? *Occupational and Environmental Medicine.* 2005; **62**: 395–9.
64. Bernstein DI, Korbee L, Stauder T et al. The low prevalence of occupational asthma and antibody-dependent sensitization to diphenylmethane diisocyanate in a plant engineered for minimal exposure to diisocyanates. *Journal of Allergy and Clinical Immunology.* 1993; **92**: 387–96.
65. Kraw M, Tarlo SM. Isocyanate medical surveillance: Respiratory referrals from a foam manufacturing plant over a five-year period. *American Journal of Industrial Medicine.* 1999; **35**: 87–91.
66. British Occupational Health Research Foundation. Cited 2008. Available from: www.bohrf.org.uk/downloads/asthevre.pdf.
67. Guidelines for the diagnosis and evaluation of occupational lung disease. *Journal of Allergy and Clinical Immunology.* 1989; **84**: 791–844.
68. Ad Hoc Committee on Occupational Asthma of the Standards Committee, Canadian Thoracic Society. Occupational asthma: Recommendations for diagnosis, management and assessment of impairment. *Canadian Medical Association Journal.* 1989; **140**: 1029–32.
69. Burge PS. Diagnosis of occupational asthma. *Clinical and Experimental Allergy.* 1989; **19**: 649–52.
70. Chan-Yeung M. Occupational asthma update. *Chest.* 1988; **93**: 407–11.
71. Siracusa A, Desrosiers M, Marabini A. Epidemiology of occupational rhinitis: Prevalence, aetiology and determinants. *Clinical and Experimental Allergy.* 2000; **30**: 1519–34.
72. Malo JL, Lemiere C, Desjardins A, Cartier A. Prevalence and intensity of rhinoconjunctivitis in subjects with occupational asthma. *European Respiratory Journal.* 1997; **10**: 1513–15.
73. Bernstein DI, Cartier A, Cote J et al. Diisocyanate antigen-stimulated monocyte chemoattractant protein-1 synthesis has greater test efficiency than specific antibodies for identification of diisocyanate asthma. *American Journal of Respiratory and Critical Care Medicine.* 2002; **166**: 445–50.
74. Bright P, Newton DT, Gannon PF et al. OASYS-3: Improved analysis of serial peak expiratory flow in suspected occupational asthma. *Monaldi Archives for Chest Disease.* 2001; **56**: 281–8.
75. Cote J, Kennedy S, Chan-Yeung M. Sensitivity and specificity of PC20 and peak expiratory flow rate in cedar asthma. *Journal of Allergy and Clinical Immunology.* 1990; **85**: 592–8.

76. Leroyer C, Perfetti L, Trudeau C et al. Comparison of serial monitoring of peak expiratory flow and FEV$_1$ in the diagnosis of occupational asthma. *American Journal of Respiratory and Critical Care Medicine.* 1998; **158**: 827–32.
77. Liss GM, Tarlo SM. Peak expiratory flow rates in possible occupational asthma. *Chest.* 1991; **100**: 63–9.
78. Malo JL, Cote J, Cartier A et al. How many times per day should peak expiratory flow rates be assessed when investigating occupational asthma? *Thorax.* 1993; **48**: 1211–17.
79. Perrin B, Lagier F, L'Archeveque J et al. Occupational asthma: Validity of monitoring of peak expiratory flow rates and non-allergic bronchial responsiveness as compared to specific inhalation challenge. *European Respiratory Journal.* 1992; **5**: 40–8.
80. Blainey AD, Ollier S, Cundell D et al. Occupational asthma in a hairdressing salon. *Thorax.* 1986; **41**: 42–50.
81. Gannon PF, Newton DT, Belcher J et al. Development of OASYS-2: A system for the analysis of serial measurement of peak expiratory flow in workers with suspected occupational asthma. *Thorax.* 1996; **51**: 484–9.
82. Cote J, Kennedy S, Chan-Yeung M. Quantitative versus qualitative analysis of peak expiratory flow in occupational asthma. *Thorax.* 1993; **48**: 48–51.
83. Venables KM, Davison AG, Browne K, Newman Taylor AJ. Pseudo-occupational asthma. *Thorax.* 1989; **44**: 760–1.
84. Bardy JD, Malo JL, Seguin P et al. Occupational asthma and IgE sensitization in a pharmaceutical company processing psyllium. *American Review of Respiratory Disease.* 1987; **135**: 1033–8.
85. Burge PS. Occupational asthma in electronics workers caused by colophony fumes: Follow-up of affected workers. *Thorax.* 1982; **37**: 348–53.
86. Tarlo SM, Broder I. Outcome of assessments for occupational asthma. *Chest.* 1991; **100**: 329–35.
87. Pickering CA. Inhalation tests with chemical allergens: Complex salts of platinum. *Proceedings of the Royal Society of Medicine.* 1972; **65**: 272–4.
88. Stenton SC, Beach JR, Dennis JH et al. Glutaraldehyde, asthma and work – a cautionary tale. *Occupational Medicine.* 1994; **44**: 95–8.
89. Cloutier Y, Lagier F, Lemieux R et al. New methodology for specific inhalation challenges with occupational agents in powder form. *European Respiratory Journal.* 1989; **2**: 769–77.
90. Durham SR, Graneek BJ, Hawkins R, Taylor AJ. The temporal relationship between increases in airway responsiveness to histamine and late asthmatic responses induced by occupational agents. *Journal of Allergy and Clinical Immunology.* 1987; **79**: 398–406.
91. Carroll KB, Secombe CJ, Pepys J. Asthma due to non-occupational exposure to toluene (tolylene) di-isocyanate. *Clinical Allergy.* 1976; **6**: 99–104.
92. Cannon J, Cullinan P, Newman Taylor A. Consequences of occupational asthma. *British Medical Journal.* 1995; **311**: 602–3.
93. Laoprasert N, Swanson MC, Jones RT et al. Inhalation challenge testing of latex-sensitive health care workers and the effectiveness of laminar flow HEPA-filtered helmets in reducing rhinoconjunctival and asthmatic reactions. *Journal of Allergy and Clinical Immunology.* 1998; **102**: 998–1004.
94. Muller-Wening D, Neuhauss M. Protective effect of respiratory devices in farmers with occupational asthma. *European Respiratory Journal.* 1998; **12**: 569–72.
95. Obase Y, Shimoda T, Mitsuta K et al. Two patients with occupational asthma who returned to work with dust respirators. *Occupational and Environmental Medicine.* 2000; **57**: 62–4.
96. Pisati G, Baruffini A, Zedda S. Toluene diisocyanate induced asthma: Outcome according to persistence or cessation of exposure. *British Journal of Industrial Medicine.* 1993; **50**: 60–4.
97. Slovak AJ, Orr RG, Teasdale EL. Efficacy of the helmet respirator in occupational asthma due to laboratory animal allergy (LAA). *American Industrial Hygiene Association Journal.* 1985; **46**: 411–15.
98. Taivainen AI, Tukiainen HO, Terho EO, Husman KR. Powered dust respirator helmets in the prevention of occupational asthma among farmers. *Scandinavian Journal of Work, Environment and Health.* 1998; **24**: 503–7.
99. Malo JL, Cartier A, Cote J et al. Influence of inhaled steroids on recovery from occupational asthma after cessation of exposure: An 18-month double-blind crossover study. *American Journal of Respiratory and Critical Care Medicine.* 1996; **153**: 953–60.
100. Rachiotis G, Savani R, Brant A et al. Outcome of occupational asthma after cessation of exposure: A systematic review. *Thorax.* 2007; **62**: 147–52.
101. Malo JL, Cartier A, Ghezzo H et al. Patterns of improvement in spirometry, bronchial hyperresponsiveness, and specific IgE antibody levels after cessation of exposure in occupational asthma caused by snow-crab processing. *American Review of Respiratory Disease.* 1988; **138**: 807–12.
102. Paggiaro P, Bacci E, Paoletti P et al. Bronchoalveolar lavage and morphology of the airways after cessation of exposure in asthmatic subjects sensitized to toluene diisocyanate. *Chest.* 1990; **98**: 536–42.
103. Saetta M, Maestrelli P, Di Stefano A et al. Effect of cessation of exposure to toluene diisocyanate (TDI) on bronchial mucosa of subjects with TDI-induced asthma. *American Review of Respiratory Disease.* 1992; **145**: 169–74.
104. Saetta M, Maestrelli P, Turato G et al. Airway wall remodeling after cessation of exposure to isocyanates in sensitized asthmatic subjects. *American Journal of Respiratory and Critical Care Medicine.* 1995; **151**: 489–94.
105. Venables KM, Topping MD, Nunn AJ et al. Immunologic and functional consequences of chemical (tetrachlorophthalic anhydride)-induced asthma after four years of avoidance of exposure. *Journal of Allergy and Clinical Immunology.* 1987; **80**: 212–18.
106. Axon EJ, Beach JR, Burge PS. A comparison of some of the characteristics of patients with occupational and non-occupational asthma. *Occupational Medicine.* 1995; **45**: 109–11.

107. Larbanois A, Jamart J, Delwiche JP, Vandenplas O. Socioeconomic outcome of subjects experiencing asthma symptoms at work. *European Respiratory Journal.* 2002; **19**: 1107-13.
108. Ross DJ, McDonald JC. Health and employment after a diagnosis of occupational asthma: A descriptive study. *Occupational Medicine.* 1998; **48**: 219-25.
109. Venables KM, Davison AG, Newman Taylor AJ. Consequences of occupational asthma. *Respiratory Medicine.* 1989; **83**: 437-40.
110. Meredith S. Reported incidence of occupational asthma in the United Kingdom, 1989-90. *Journal of Epidemiology and Community Health.* 1993; **47**: 459-63.
111. Ameille J, Pauli G, Calastreng-Crinquand A et al. Reported incidence of occupational asthma in France, 1996-99: The ONAP programme. *Occupational and Environmental Medicine.* 2003; **60**: 136-41.
112. Karjalainen A, Martikainen R et al. Risk of asthma among Finnish patients with occupational rhinitis. *Chest.* 2003; **123**: 283-8.
113. Brisman J, Jarvholm B, Lillienberg L. Exposure-response relations for self reported asthma and rhinitis in bakers. *Occupational and Environmental Medicine.* 2000; **57**: 335-40.
114. Cullinan P, Lowson D, Nieuwenhuijsen MJ et al. Work related symptoms, sensitisation, and estimated exposure in workers not previously exposed to flour. *Occupational and Environmental Medicine.* 1994; **51**: 579-83.
115. Cullinan P, Cook A, Nieuwenhuijsen MJ et al. Allergen and dust exposure as determinants of work-related symptoms and sensitization in a cohort of flour-exposed workers; a case-control analysis. *Annals of Occupational Hygiene.* 2001; **45**: 97-103.
116. Heederik D, Houba R. An exploratory quantitative risk assessment for high molecular weight sensitizers: Wheat flour. *Annals of Occupational Hygiene.* 2001; **45**: 175-85.
117. Houba R, Heederik DJ, Doekes G, van Run PE. Exposure-sensitization relationship for alpha-amylase allergens in the baking industry. *American Journal of Respiratory and Critical Care Medicine.* 1996; **154**: 130-6.
118. Houba R, Heederik D, Doekes G. Wheat sensitization and work-related symptoms in the baking industry are preventable. An epidemiologic study. *American Journal of Respiratory and Critical Care Medicine.* 1998; **158**: 1499-503.
119. Musk AW, Venables KM, Crook B et al. Respiratory symptoms, lung function, and sensitisation to flour in a British bakery. *British Journal of Industrial Medicine.* 1989; **46**: 636-42.
120. Nieuwenhuijsen MJ, Heederik D, Doekes G et al. Exposure-response relations of alpha-amylase sensitisation in British bakeries and flour mills. *Occupational and Environmental Medicine.* 1999; **56**: 197-201.
121. Vanhanen M, Tuomi T, Nordman H et al. Sensitization to industrial enzymes in enzyme research and production. *Scandinavian Journal of Work, Environment and Health.* 1997; **23**: 385-91.
122. Weill H, Waddell LC, Ziskind M. A study of workers exposed to detergent enzymes. *Journal of the American Medical Association.* 1971; **217**: 425-33.
123. Cullinan P, Cook A, Gordon S et al. Allergen exposure, atopy and smoking as determinants of allergy to rats in a cohort of laboratory employees. *European Respiratory Journal.* 1999; **13**: 1139-43.
124. Heederik D, Venables KM, Malmberg P et al. Exposure-response relationships for work-related sensitization in workers exposed to rat urinary allergens: Results from a pooled study. *Journal of Allergy and Clinical Immunology.* 1999; **103**: 678-84.
125. Kruize H, Post W, Heederik D et al. Respiratory allergy in laboratory animal workers: A retrospective cohort study using pre-employment screening data. *Occupational and Environmental Medicine.* 1997; **54**: 830-5.
126. Platts-Mills TA, Longbottom J, Edwards J et al. Occupational asthma and rhinitis related to laboratory rats: serum IgG and IgE antibodies to the rat urinary allergen. *Journal of Allergy and Clinical Immunology.* 1987; **79**: 505-15.
127. McSharry C, Anderson K, McKay IC et al. The IgE and IgG antibody responses to aerosols of *Nephrops norvegicus* (prawn) antigens: The association with clinical hypersensitivity and with cigarette smoking. *Clinical and Experimental Immunology.* 1994; **97**: 499-504.
128. Ortega HG, Daroowalla F, Petsonk EL et al. Respiratory symptoms among crab processing workers in Alaska: Epidemiological and environmental assessment. *American Journal of Industrial Medicine.* 2001; **39**: 598-607.
129. Osterman K, Zetterstrom O, Johansson SG. Coffee worker's allergy. *Allergy.* 1982; **37**: 313-22.
130. Meredith SK, Bugler J, Clark RL. Isocyanate exposure and occupational asthma: A case-referent study. *Occupational and Environmental Medicine.* 2000; **57**: 830-6.
131. Petsonk EL, Wang ML, Lewis DM et al. Asthma-like symptoms in wood product plant workers exposed to methylene diphenyl diisocyanate. *Chest.* 2000; **118**: 1183-93.
132. Pronk A, Preller L, Raulf-Heimsoth M et al. Respiratory symptoms, sensitization, and exposure response relationships in spray painters exposed to isocyanates. *American Journal of Respiratory and Critical Care Medicine.* 2007; **176**: 1090-7.
133. Tarlo SM, Liss GM, Dias C, Banks DE. Assessment of the relationship between isocyanate exposure levels and occupational asthma. *American Journal of Industrial Medicine.* 1997; **32**: 517-21.
134. Barker RD, van Tongeren MJ, Harris JM et al. Risk factors for sensitisation and respiratory symptoms among workers exposed to acid anhydrides: A cohort study. *Occupational and Environmental Medicine.* 1998; **55**: 684-91.
135. Grammer LC, Shaughnessy MA, Lowenthal M, Yarnold PR. Risk factors for immunologically mediated respiratory disease from hexahydrophthalic anhydride. *Journal of Occupational Medicine.* 1994; **36**: 642-6.

136. Burge PS, Edge G, Hawkins R *et al.* Occupational asthma in a factory making flux-cored solder containing colophony. *Thorax.* 1981; **36**: 828-34.
137. Coutts IL, Lozewicz S, Dally MB *et al.* Respiratory symptoms related to work in a factory manufacturing cimetidine tablets. *British Medical Journal.* 1984; **288**: 1418.
138. Hagmar L, Bellander T, Ranstam J, Skerfving S. Piperazine-induced airway symptoms: Exposure–response relationships and selection in an occupational setting. *American Journal of Industrial Medicine.* 1984; **6**: 347–57.
139. Calverley AE, Rees D, Dowdeswell RJ *et al.* Platinum salt sensitivity in refinery workers: Incidence and effects of smoking and exposure. *Occupational and Environmental Medicine.* 1995; **52**: 661–6.
140. Brooks SM, Edwards JJ Jr, Apol A, Edwards FH. An epidemiologic study of workers exposed to western red cedar and other wood dusts. *Chest.* 1981; **80** (Suppl. 1): 30–2.

73

Byssinosis and other cotton-related diseases

CAC PICKERING AND ROBERT NIVEN

Historical background	958	Management	964
Acute byssinosis	958	Chronic bronchitis and chronic obstructive pulmonary	
Chronic byssinosis	959	disease in cotton workers	964
Atopic status and bronchial hyper-reactivity	961	Mortality and morbidity in cotton and textile workers	965
Genetic factors	962	Measurement of dust exposure	965
Clinical features	962	Prevention	965
Physical signs	963	References	966
Pathology	963		

HISTORICAL BACKGROUND

Respiratory disease associated with exposure to textile dusts was first recognized by Ramazzini amongst flax and hemp workers. The term 'byssinosis', which is derived from the Greek (flax), was first used by the Parisian physician A Proust in 1877.[1] Earlier in 1831 Kay, a Manchester physician, described cotton spinners phthisis.[2] This condition was characterized by a work-related cough, which initially resolved on leaving the mill, later becoming more severe and persistent and associated with a sensation of uneasiness beneath the sternum. The first description of the symptom pattern now associated with byssinosis, that is respiratory symptoms most severe at the start of the working week, was given in 1845 by Mareska and Heyman.[3]

> All the workers have told us that the dust bothered them much less on the last days of the week than on the Monday and Tuesday. The masters find the cause of this increased sensitivity to be in the excesses of the Sunday, but the workers never fail to attribute it to the interruption of work which, they say, makes them lose, in part, their habituation to the dust.

In 1860, in response to concern about the high death rates from respiratory disease in some Lancashire towns, Greenhow[4] investigated the causes of this excess of pulmonary disease and described an asthma-like condition in cotton workers worse at the beginning of the working week and most severe on returning to work after a longer period away from work than a weekend. This syndrome is now generally referred to as byssinosis. Subsequently, byssinosis has been reported from most countries with a textile industry.[5–8]

ACUTE BYSSINOSIS

Acute byssinosis is an acute response to cotton dust. It can be replicated in artificial cardrooms in subjects exposed to cotton dust or extracts of cotton dust for the first time. The relationship of this acute, fully reversible response to the chronic changes which develop in cotton workers exposed to cotton dust for many years remains uncertain. It was long postulated that this acute response contributed to the high labour turnover which was seen in the first year of employment[9] in cotton spinning mills with heavy dust exposures. A recent study in a new cotton spinning factory with low levels of exposure to cotton dust and endotoxin, found that 40 per cent of new workers, naive to cotton dust, reported work-related symptoms, with cross-shift and cross-week falls in lung function. A tolerance effect was noted with continued exposure.[10]

Textile workers may also experience other acute symptoms (mill fever) on exposure to cotton, flax or hemp dust. Mill fever characteristically occurs following a worker's first exposure to cotton, flax or hemp dust. It consists of a fever with a non-productive cough, malaise and sneezing, which usually lasts for a few hours, resolving despite continued exposure to dust.[11] It is thought that mill fever is caused by the endotoxins from Gram-negative bacteria contaminating the cotton. This idea is supported by endotoxin exposure studies in healthy volunteers, where at high levels a febrile response is seen, similar to the symptoms described as mill fever.[12]

CHRONIC BYSSINOSIS

Prevalence

The prevalence of byssinosis amongst cotton workers depends on the quality and airborne concentration of cotton dust to which workers are exposed and to the duration of their exposure. The majority of prevalence studies have been cross-sectional in design and have thus been looking at 'survivor' populations and, therefore, likely to underestimate the true prevalence of this disease. The reduction in dust levels over the past 30 years has led to a fall in the prevalence of byssinosis. In the late 1950s in the United Kingdom, the prevalence amongst male cardroom workers (coarse cotton) was 43 per cent and in blowroom workers 66 per cent.[13] By the 1970s the prevalence (combined) had fallen to 24 per cent.[14] The prevalence of byssinosis, at the time the cotton spinning industry in Lancashire cotton mills essentially ceased was 4 per cent.[15]

In Australia, the prevalence of byssinosis has been reported to be low: 1.1 per cent (two of 176 employees) exposed to mean dust levels of between $0.14\,mg/m^3$ to $0.25\,mg/m^3$.[16] An earlier study[17] revealed similarly low prevalence. In most developing countries, the prevalence of byssinosis remains high: Indonesia, 21–30 per cent;[18] Ethiopia, 24–43 per cent;[19] Sudan, 37 per cent;[20] India, 30–38 per cent;[21] Nigeria, 2–6.4 per cent;[22] and Pakistan, 19 per cent.[23]

The prevalence of byssinosis is influenced by the occupational group, being most frequent amongst opening room operatives and cardroom workers (strippers and grinders), followed by drawframe tenters, and least common amongst ring spinners.[24] These occupational relationships appear to follow the early processes where contaminants are common, rather than being related to total levels of personal dust exposure.[25]

In flax workers, the prevalence of byssinosis is also related to occupational group, the dustiest jobs being associated with the highest prevalences: pre-preparers, 54 per cent; other preparers, 27 per cent; wet finishers, 0.4 per cent.[26] A similar relationship between dust level and prevalence has been noted in Egyptian flax workers.[27]

Smoking may increase the risk of developing byssinosis and exacerbate the reduction in ventilatory capacity.[24,28,29] Byssinosis is reported to be up to four times more common in smoking workers than in non- and ex-smoking workers.[24] However, other studies have found no association between smoking and the prevalence of byssinosis.[17,30] Where the prevalence of byssinosis is low, there may be insufficient power to demonstrate weak co-factor effects, such as from smoking.

Pathogenesis

Although byssinosis has been recognized for over a century, and a considerable research effort has examined possible mechanisms by which textile dusts can cause airways narrowing, the pathogenesis of byssinosis is still not fully understood. The ability of textile fibres to produce byssinosis is determined by fibre type, cotton being the most potent, followed by flax, hemp and finally possibly sisal. Harvested cotton consists of a mixture of plant materials including: leaves, bracts and stems, fibre, bacteria, fungi, and other contaminants. The particles of bract have attracted particular attention since exposure to aerosols of extracts of bracts, but not other plant components, can cause acute symptoms similar to those of byssinosis and can lead to release of significant amounts of histamine from human lung tissue. The cotton bract is a specialized leaf at the base of the cotton flower. As these leaves mature they become hard and brittle and tend to shatter into small particles during harvesting, becoming adherent to the cotton fibre, later forming a major constituent of cotton dust in the mill. Many different compounds have been examined as potential causes of byssinosis. It seems definite that the compounds which cause byssinosis are water soluble. The biological activity of cotton can be greatly reduced by either steaming[31] or washing[32] the cotton before processing.

A number of different mechanisms have been proposed to explain the pathogenesis of byssinosis: bacterial endotoxin activity, immunological and para-immunological responses, the non-immunological release of histamine and fungus enzymes.

Bacterial endotoxins

The presence of large quantities of Gram-negative bacteria in cotton mills was first reported by a Home Office Commission in 1932.[33] Ten years later, the relationship between the grade of the cotton and the degree of contamination by Gram-negative bacteria was first described.[34] This group also identified an endotoxin-like substance in extracts from contaminated cotton and from the organism cultured from the cotton. Subsequently, a role for endotoxin in the aetiology of byssinosis was proposed.[35] The predominant species of Gram-negative bacteria found in cotton dust is of the *Enterobacter* genus. Endotoxin is derived from the lipopolysaccharide (LPS) component of the outer membrane of Gram-negative bacteria, and its release has been described, both *in vivo* and *in vitro*, from various genera of Gram-negative bacteria. A number of airway responses, on challenge testing with endotoxin, have been described, indicating the presence of airway inflammation and immune responses. These include neutrophilic bronchitis and alveolitis, alveolar-macrophage activation, complement activation and mast cell release of histamine.

The relationship between the prevalence of byssinotic symptoms, dust concentrations and airborne Gram-negative bacteria[36,37] has been studied. In a UK study, the prevalence of byssinosis was shown to correlate better with airborne bacterial levels than with dust concentrations, although the correlation with endotoxin was strong.[38]

In a study of mill workers with and without a history of byssinosis, the authors challenged the workers with varying levels of endotoxin and cotton dust in an experimental cardroom. They reported a dose–response relationship between endotoxin levels, symptoms of byssinosis and mean group changes in FEV_1.[39] A prospective study of Chinese cotton workers over 15 years measured cumulative exposures to endotoxin, and demonstrated an exposure–response trend between endotoxin exposure and byssinosis. The exposure–response trend for cotton dust was less clear.[28]

Challenge studies using healthy volunteers have cast doubt on the role of endotoxin in the acute airway constrictor response on first exposure to cotton dust.[40,41] In a group of healthy volunteers challenged with aqueous extracts of cotton bracts containing 0.086–50 µg/mL of endotoxin, no correlation was found between the severity of the airway constrictor response and the concentration of endotoxin. After almost complete elimination of endotoxin from the extracts, airway responses greater than 60 per cent of the responses seen with crude bract extract, continued to occur.[40] In a group of normal subjects, challenge tests were carried out using flax dust containing a known concentration of endotoxin and using pure endotoxin at an equivalent concentration. While an airway constrictor response was demonstrated to flax dust, there was no significant airways constriction following pure endotoxin challenge.[41]

More recently, challenge tests in healthy volunteers using cotton dust extract (CDE) (endotoxin level 31.88 EU/mg) and cotton bract extract (CBE) (endotoxin level 5.71 EU/mg) measured the response to methacholine challenge, and demonstrated similar physiological responses to CDE and CBE.[42]

These types of exposure studies, however, do not reproduce the cumulative effects in mill workers of inhaling, over many years, dusts capable of inducing airway inflammation.

Immunological mechanisms

The hypothesis that a specific immunological response is involved in the causation of byssinosis has been extensively investigated. However, the majority of studies have failed to show convincing evidence of an immunological mechanism. Skin tests using cotton dust extracts failed to differentiate between normal, atopic and byssinotic subjects.[43] The authors used an intracutaneous skin test technique, which produced both immediate and late skin responses. There was no difference in the frequency of positive responses between any of the groups tested. Some 90 per cent of normal subjects gave a late skin response, suggesting a non-immunological mechanism. A study of groups of workers with byssinosis, asthma and chronic bronchitis, demonstrated immediate skin responses and frequent late responses.[44] The positive skin responses were not specific to those individuals with byssinosis. The authors also performed inhalation tests with textile allergens, and only four of 39 subjects with byssinosis gave a positive reaction. Intradermal skin tests in naive subjects with cotton bract extract induced both immediate and late skin reactions.[45] Skin biopsies taken during both responses revealed an initial oedematous phase followed by a perivascular infiltration with polymorphonuclear and mononuclear cells. Eosinophils were not a feature and mast cells were seen to degranulate during both phases.

Other authors[46] have compared serum concentrations of total IgE in textile mill workers both with and without byssinosis. They found no difference in total IgE concentrations between the groups, and no relationship between the clinical grade of byssinosis and the level of IgE.

It has been suggested that fungal antigens may play a role in the aetiology of byssinosis. A study of the antigenic composition of aqueous cotton extracts demonstrated a significant portion of the immune response directed against known fungal contaminants of cotton dust: *Alternaria tenuis*, *Aspergillus niger* and *Fusarium solani*.[47] A preliminary study using a crossed radio-immunoelectrophoretic technique suggested that some of these fungi were antigenic in man. However, skin tests using fungal extracts in textile workers have demonstrated no correlation between positive skin responses and symptoms of byssinosis.

There is at present no good evidence that atopy plays a direct role in the aetiology of byssinosis. The association between atopic status and the presence of increased airway reactivity may have a role, in rendering an individual susceptible to the chronic inhalation of a pro-inflammatory/irritant dust and the subsequent development of increasing airway reactivity associated with airway dysfunction.

The finding of late skin responses raises the possibility of IgG-mediated pulmonary responses. Precipitating IgG antibody to cotton antigen has been found in both cotton and non-cotton workers. The titre is highest in grade 2 byssinotics, lower in non-byssinotic workers and lowest in unexposed subjects.[48,49] These elevated IgG antibody titres seem to be markers of exposure to cotton dust rather than indicators of disease.

A condensed polyphenol (leucocyanidin) has been isolated from the bracts of cotton plants and used in inhalation studies in byssinotic and non-byssinotic subjects.[50] The inhalation challenge produced symptoms similar to those that they experienced in the mill, without changes in lung function, in five of six byssinotic subjects, and in none of 11 non-byssinotic workers. A study in a group of 29 byssinotic workers and 31 normal controls used the same polyphenol.[50] The authors did not find any differences in symptoms or pulmonary function changes between the byssinotic workers and the normal controls.

Extracts of cotton mill dust have been shown to activate complement by the classical and alternative pathways.[51,52] The activation of both complement pathways will generate biologically active fragments capable of releasing histamine and recruitment of polymorphonuclear leukocytes (PMN). Other *in vitro* experiments have demonstrated the release of prostaglandin F2 alpha from rat fundal smooth muscle and rabbit cultured alveolar macrophages, on challenge with cotton dust extract.[53,54] Prostaglandin F2 alpha is a potent broncho-constrictor of human respiratory smooth muscle.

It is clear from these experimental studies that cotton dust is highly biologically active and capable of mediating an inflammatory response via a variety of different pathways. However, it remains unclear which of these pathways or combination of pathways is involved in the pathogenesis of byssinosis.

Non-immunological histamine release

The release of pharmacological mediators, such as histamine, has been postulated as an explanation for the acute symptoms of byssinosis occurring on the first day back at work. Histamine is found in the respirable fraction of cotton dust itself. However, the amounts present in a work situation are considered too small to produce airways narrowing. The levels of blood histamine have been shown to be elevated in both flax and cotton workers. This elevation occurred within two hours of starting work and was seen in all workers.[55] Histamine levels had fallen to prechallenge levels by the second morning in all workers except those with grade 2 byssinotic symptoms. A comparison between exposures to equivalent levels of cotton and flax dusts showed cotton exposure produced significantly higher levels of blood histamine compared to flax. The histamine metabolite, L-methyl-imidazole-4-acetic acid was also found to be elevated in the 24-hour urinary specimens of control subjects challenged with cotton dust.

The release of histamine alone clearly does not explain the development of byssinosis, since histamine release can be demonstrated in all those exposed and immediate pulmonary responses occur on bronchial challenge with histamine, whereas byssinosis takes years to develop and immediate-type responses during a working shift are usually not demonstrable.

Fungal enzymes

Cotton dust has been demonstrated to have proteolytic enzyme activity. This activity probably originates from contaminating microorganisms. It has been suggested that airborne enzyme concentrations in cotton dust correlate better than cotton dust with airway responses in cotton workers. However, there is a low incidence of byssinosis in cotton willowing and woollen mills where there are high enzyme levels.[56,57]

ATOPIC STATUS AND BRONCHIAL HYPER-REACTIVITY

One might expect that atopic individuals would be more likely to develop an allergic respiratory disease after exposure to cotton dust. There is some evidence this may be the case. Cross-sectional studies of cotton workers have revealed a low prevalence of atopy (defined by positive skin tests to common environmental allergens) compared with the prevalence in the general population. A survey of 30 workers in four cotton seed-crushing mills found a prevalence of atopy (positive skin tests to two or more of 10 common inhalant antigens) of 15 per cent.[58] A study of 324 byssinotic subjects found a prevalence of atopy of 14.5 per cent, compared with 23.5 per cent in an age- and sex-matched control population.[59] The prevalence of atopy in the general population depends on the age of the groups studied; at the time these studies were performed it varied from 20 to 40 per cent. The reduced prevalence of atopy among cotton-exposed populations implies they are survivor populations from which atopic subjects have been selected out.

Jones *et al.*[58] evaluated the effect of atopy on the ventilatory decline across a working shift in three groups of cotton workers. In one group (those exposed to linter dust), there was a positive association between atopic status and mean declines in FEV_1 and FEF_{25-75} across the working shift.

Atopic subjects frequently possess a high degree of bronchial hyper-reactivity and this may be an important determinant of the bronchoconstrictor response to cotton dust. Cotton workers who develop asthma and known asthmatic subjects who enter a cotton mill tend to develop rapidly increasing airways obstruction and have to leave the work (personal observation). A recent study of newly hired workers failed to demonstrate an effect of atopy on early leaving from the mill, but only included small numbers of atopic workers.[10]

Relatively little research has examined the effect of airway reactivity on the pulmonary responses of cotton workers, although it may be important in determining the development of early respiratory disease, and perhaps the degree of disability associated with byssinosis. One study considered the acute airways constrictor response to cotton bract extract in normal subjects and its relationship to airways reactivity.[60] The subjects who responded to cotton bract extract were significantly more reactive on methacholine challenge than the non-responder group. The baseline measurements of pulmonary function were, however, significantly lower in the responder group, and this could explain the difference between the two groups. An earlier study by the same authors, using histamine to measure airways reactivity, failed to show any significant difference in airways reactivity between responders and non-responders to cotton bract extract challenge in a group of healthy subjects.

Studies of airways reactivity in byssinotic subjects have produced inconclusive results. One study reported on histamine challenge tests in 26 byssinotic card-room workers.[61] The workers with 'bronchitic byssinosis' (byssinosis with cough and sputum) showed an important increase in airways reactivity; this was not seen in the workers with pure byssinosis. However, the bronchitic byssinotics also had higher grades of byssinosis, longer exposure to cotton dust and impaired lung function. Another study of the bronchoconstrictive effect of inhaled histamine demonstrated a response in two of 11 byssinotic subjects, in ten of 13 asthmatic subjects, and in none of ten control subjects.[52] Haglind et al.[62] used methacholine challenge to examine cross-shift changes in airway reactivity in cotton workers with and without byssinosis. Baseline airway reactivity was increased in the byssinotics, and 11 of the 16 showed an increase in airway reactivity across the shift. Fishwick et al.[63] reported an increase in airway reactivity in 18 of 23 cotton workers with symptoms of byssinosis, 21 of 56 symptomatic non-byssinotic workers and 14 of 84 asymptomatic workers. The responders among the byssinotic group were more likely to have bronchitic symptoms. The proportion with atopy did not differ between the three groups.

GENETIC FACTORS

Endotoxin exposure is known to generate reactive oxygen species in the airways, which may induce oxidative lung injury and lung function decline. Reactive oxygen species are detoxified by the enzyme microsomal epoxide hydrolase (mEH). A recently reported 20-year prospective study of cotton workers examined the associations between mEH polymorphisms, endotoxin exposure and lung function decline.[64] Endotoxin exposure was associated with more rapid lung function decline in individuals with the mEH His/His genotypes of both Tyr11is and His139Arg polymorphisms, both associated with lower enzyme activities. This association was noted in both smokers and non-smokers.

CLINICAL FEATURES

Symptoms

Cross-sectional studies of textile spinning operatives have documented a variety of work-related ocular and upper and lower respiratory tract symptoms on exposure to cotton and synthetic fibres.[65,66] These include ocular and nasal irritation, byssinosis, chronic bronchitis, persistent cough, work-related chest tightness and work-related wheeze. Work-related ocular symptoms (17.5 per cent) and work-related nasal irritation (11 per cent) seem to be the most common symptoms among both cotton and synthetic textile workers, occurring more often in cotton workers than in synthetic fibre workers.

The development of symptoms of byssinosis is rare in the first ten years of exposure to cotton, hemp or flax dusts and usually requires a period of dust exposure of between 20 and 25 years. The classical symptoms of byssinosis consist of chest tightness and breathlessness, characteristically

Table 73.1 Roach and Schilling[67] clinical grading of byssinosis.

Grade	Features
0	No symptoms
½	Occasional chest tightness on Mondays[a] or mild symptoms, such as irritation of the respiratory tract, on Mondays
1	Chest tightness and/or breathlessness on Mondays only
2	Chest tightness and/or breathlessness on Mondays and other days
3	Grade 2 symptoms with evidence of permanent respiratory impairment from reduce ventilatory capacity

[a]'Monday' means the first day back at work after the weekly break. The original version of the classification did not include grade 3.

developing on the first day of the working week over the second half of the working shift, and experienced most severely with the exertion of returning home in the evening. Others have described a rapid onset of symptoms within 30 minutes of starting work, which may be most severe over the first half of the shift. Roach and Schilling[67] devised a scheme for grading the clinical stages of byssinosis (Table 73.1). The original description did not include grade 3 and this was added later.[68] The Roach–Schilling clinical grading has been widely accepted and used for many epidemiological studies. However, it does not take into account the irritant effects of dust exposure or the lung function changes which may occur even in asymptomatic workers. A later classification grades byssinosis, respiratory tract irritation and acute and chronic lung function changes separately (Table 73.2).[69]

A characteristic feature of byssinosis is that it is most severe on the first day of the working week. Surveys of cotton workers have revealed a group of workers experiencing chest tightness on each working day with no variation in severity across the working week.[66] The relationship between these symptoms and the classic symptoms of byssinosis is not clear.

It used to be thought that individuals progressed through the clinical grades of byssinosis, starting at grade ½ and, depending on their individual susceptibility and dust exposure, perhaps finishing at grade 3. However, the pattern and progression of symptoms in cotton workers has changed over the past 60 years, with the progressive reduction in cotton dust exposure. A 15-year prospective study in a Chinese cotton spinning mill, including enquiry about respiratory symptoms on four occasions, documented the intermittent nature of respiratory symptoms.[28] There was a cumulative incidence of byssinosis of 24 per cent and of chest tightness of 23 per cent. Symptoms of byssinosis were reported once by 23 per cent of workers, twice by 10 per cent, and three times or more by only 1 per cent of workers. There was a similar picture for symptoms of chronic bronchitis, chronic cough and breathlessness.

Table 73.2 Revised clinical classification of adverse effects from cotton dust exposure.

Grade/effect	Features
0	No symptoms or adverse effects
Byssinosis	
B1	Chest tightness and/or breathlessness on most of first days back at work
B2	Chest tightness and/or breathlessness on the first and other days of the working week
Respiratory tract irritation	
RTI1	Cough associated with dust exposure
RTI2	Persistent phlegm (on most days during three months of the year) initiated or exacerbated by dust exposure
RTI3	Persistent phlegm initiated or exacerbated by dust exposure with either exacerbations of chest illness or persisting for two years or more
Lung function	
1. Acute changes	
No effect	Decline in FEV_1 of less than 5% or an increase in FEV_1 across the working shift
Mild effect	Consistent decline in FEV_1 of 5–10% across the working shift
Moderate effect	Consistent decline in FEV_1 of 10–20% across the working shift
Severe effect	Consistent decline in FEV_1 of more than 20% across the working shift
2. Chronic changes	
No effect	FEV_1 is 80% or more of the predicted value
Mild to moderate effect	FEV_1 is 60–79% of the predicted value
Severe effect	FEV_1 is less than 60% of the predicted value

Consistent decline means a decline in at least three consecutive tests made after an absence from dust exposure of two days or more.
Predicted values should be based on data from local populations, or groups of similar ethnicity and social class.
The FEV_1 to assess chronic changes should be measured in a preshift test after an absence from dust exposure of two days or more.

Remission of symptoms of byssinosis, despite continued exposure to cotton dust, has been described in other studies.[24] Workers may complain of chest tightness in the absence of changes in FEV_1, and others may have significant decrements in FEV_1 with no associated chest tightness.[24] However, one study reported that among cotton workers without byssinosis, those with the greatest decrements in FEV_1 were the most likely to go on to develop symptomatic byssinosis.[70]

PHYSICAL SIGNS

On physical examination, there are no specific abnormalities associated with byssinosis. When physical signs are present they simply indicate the presence of airflow limitation. For example, there may be signs of chest hyperinflation, prolonged expiration and expiratory wheeze.

Radiology

There are no specific abnormalities on the chest radiograph in byssinosis.

Lung function

The changes in lung function associated with the symptoms of byssinosis were first documented in 1958.[71] There is a decline in FEV_1 across the working shift in grades 1 and 2 byssinosis. The maximum decline in lung function across a working shift occurs on the first day of the working week, but this does not necessarily imply that the overall level of airways obstruction improves over the remainder of the week. In a study of 25 carders, including asymptomatic workers and grades ½ and 2 byssinotics, the greatest across-shift decline in FEV_1 occurred on the first day of the working week, but the mean FEV_1 was lowest towards the end of the week.[72] Serial peak expiratory flow rate (PEFR) measurements in grade 3 byssinotic card-room workers may show a variety of patterns (Figure 73.1a,b) associated with wide diurnal variations in PEFR consistent with a diagnosis of asthma. Reduced mid-expiratory flow rates seem to be a sensitive indicator of airways obstruction in cotton workers.[73,74] Gas transfer measurements[74] were within normal limits when measured preshift in a small group of hemp, flax and cotton workers. Impairment of gas transfer, when present, appears to be related to smoking habits rather than exposure to cotton dust.[75]

PATHOLOGY

No specific pathological abnormalities have been described associated with byssinosis. Macroscopically, the lungs show heavy black pigmentation. In a study of 43 byssinotic subjects, mucous gland hyperplasia and hypertrophy of smooth muscle were found in upper and lower lobe bronchi, but not to a significant degree in segmental bronchi. Emphysema was present in less than half the cases. Some 23 per cent showed evidence of centrilobular emphysema and 14 per cent had panacinar emphysema.[76] The finding of smooth muscle hypertrophy and mucus gland hyperplasia is of interest, since it is a pathological finding associated with bronchial asthma rather than chronic bronchitis.[77] An autopsy study in 1980 again did not find emphysema associated with cotton dust exposure.[78] These pathological findings are supported by physiological studies in smoking and non-smoking byssinotics, which reported the presence and severity of lung function changes consistent with emphysema be related to smoking habits and unrelated to cotton dust exposure.[75]

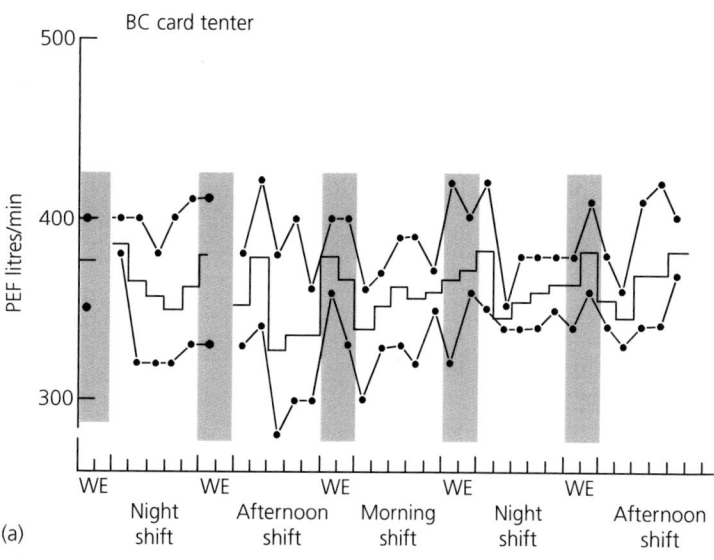

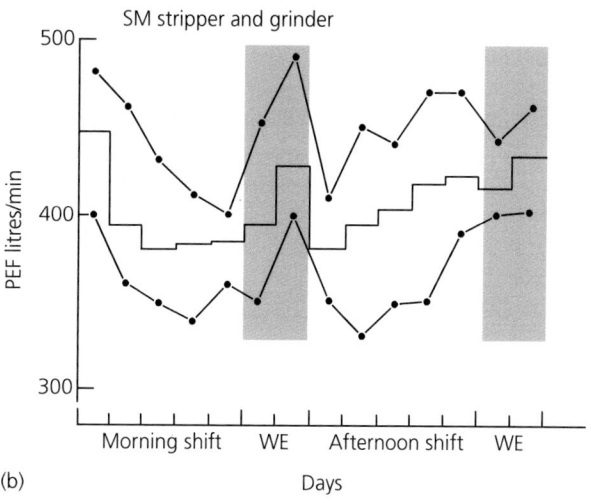

Figure 73.1 (a,b) Daily maximum, mean and minimum peak expiratory flow (PEF) rates in two cardroom workers with grade 3 byssinosis. WE, weekend.

MANAGEMENT

Antihistamine and a bronchodilator may reduce or prevent falls in FEV_1 across the working shift. In a comparison of the effects of disodium cromoglycate, beclomethasone dipropionate and salbutamol on the ventilatory response to cotton dust in mill workers, salbutamol was found to be the most effective and disodium cromoglycate the least effective in preventing symptoms and changes in ventilatory capacity.[79]

The finding in the study of Chinese cotton workers[28] that repeated cross-shift declines in lung function were associated with large declines in FEV_1, compared with a control population of silk workers, suggests that regular monitoring of lung function may identify this susceptible group of workers before they develop disabling loss of lung function. Ideally, their exposure to cotton dust should then cease, either by transfer to a mill handling pure man-made fibre or by finding a new job. Cessation of exposure has been found to have a protective effect on respiratory health that is independent of age, duration of exposure and smoking status.[28] In practice, new employment is often difficult to find and many affected workers continue their exposure to cotton dust. This exposure should be kept to a minimum by using respiratory protection and by moving the worker to the least dusty work area.

CHRONIC BRONCHITIS AND CHRONIC OBSTRUCTIVE PULMONARY DISEASE IN COTTON WORKERS

Molyneux and Tombleson[80] observed that bronchitis (mucous hypersecretion) occurred more frequently amongst cotton workers than man-made fibre workers. A later study of 14 cotton mills and two man-made fibre mills reported a prevalence of bronchitis of between 18 and 45 per cent in cotton workers and between 23 and 26 per cent in man-made fibre workers.[81] There was an association between the length of exposure and bronchitis in women, but not in men. A study of 2991 textile workers found an increased prevalence of chronic bronchitis in cotton workers aged more than 45 years, and an association with cumulative cotton dust exposure.[82] The presence of chronic bronchitis was associated with a small decrement in lung function. The authors estimated that the effect of cotton dust exposure in a non-smoking cotton worker was the equivalent of moderate smoking in a man-made fibre worker.

A study in Lancashire mills reported the prevalence of bronchitis was higher in byssinotics than non-byssinotics, after allowing for age and smoking habits.[80]

There is evidence that even at low levels of exposure to textile dusts, a small excess loss of lung function is demonstrable, which may be greater in man-made fibre than in cotton workers. In a longitudinal study of a large population of cotton and man-made fibre workers, with low cotton dust exposures (only 1 per cent of the population had symptoms of byssinosis), a dose–response accelerated decline in FEV_1 and FVC was observed in smoking cotton yarn workers (the highest exposure group), but not in non-smokers in the same work area, nor in workers in other cotton work areas.[83] The declines demonstrated in current smokers were 41.2 mL per year at average dust exposures of $150\,\mu g/m^3$, 49.3 mL per year at $200\,\mu g/m^3$, and 57.4 mL per year at $250\,\mu g/m^3$. Exposure measurements in this US study are not equivalent to personal dust exposures measured in UK studies. Accelerated declines in FEV_1 among cotton workers appear to be produced by a synergistic effect between cotton dust exposure and current smoking. Accelerated lung function decline is also related to higher across-shift decreases in FEV_1.[83,84]

MORTALITY AND MORBIDITY IN COTTON AND TEXTILE WORKERS

The long-term effects of exposure to cotton and flax dusts on lung function in textile workers, with and without byssinosis, have been a matter of some controversy. Early epidemiological studies in the United Kingdom, when exposure levels to cotton dust were high, revealed evidence of excess morbidity amongst cotton workers. In 1908, Collis[85] reported a study of strippers and grinders from 31 mills, with a prevalence of an asthma-like condition of 74–91 per cent. He noted that it was unusual for these men to remain in the cardroom after the age of 45 years. In 1930, Hill[86] reported high death rates from respiratory disease amongst strippers and grinders, compared with ring room workers and warehousemen. A survey of cardroom workers in 1955 reported a high prevalence (14 per cent) of severe respiratory disease.[87] More recently, Elwood et al.[88] reported that prevalence and incidence of disability pensions for respiratory and other diseases were increased among cotton mill workers with a minimum exposure to cotton dust of five years.

Early mortality figures are difficult to interpret, as the occupation of the deceased was recorded as their last occupation, and many individuals with respiratory disability left the cotton industry to take up lighter jobs. Over the last 30 years there have been improvements in working conditions in textile mills, with marked reductions in dust levels. More recent mortality studies have failed to demonstrate an increased mortality amongst textile workers[89,90] or workers with byssinosis.[91] Given this failure to demonstrate an excess mortality amongst textile workers and the evidence from studies of normal populations that respiratory symptoms and lung function are strongly associated with mortality,[90] one possible conclusion is that under prevailing industrial conditions exposure to cotton dust is not associated with significant permanent respiratory impairment. A Finnish study of disability pensions found no excess in mortality for respiratory disease in a cohort of cotton workers.[92] A study of a group of cotton workers initially identified between 1968 and 1970 reported that both the total mortality and the mortality due to respiratory disease were less than expected.[93] However, respiratory disease mortality was raised in those who had reported symptoms of byssinosis.

The available evidence suggests there is a small subgroup of textile workers (those with byssinosis) who develop respiratory disability with an associated excess mortality due to respiratory disease.

MEASUREMENT OF DUST EXPOSURE

Measurement of cotton dust exposure has not been internationally standardized. The United States standards for dust exposure monitoring have involved the use of work area dust sampling, but using a vertical elutriator to allow measurement of the respirable fraction of dust. This has the advantage of targeting the proportion of dust which is most likely to penetrate the lower airways. The disadvantage is that the equipment is large and cumbersome and can only be used to measure area samples. The samplers may be positioned some distance from the individual worker and therefore may give poor estimates of actual exposure in the personal breathing zone. The UK used a similar work area sampling technique until the 1990s and it is the basis for all the early literature about byssinosis and cotton dust exposure.

A comparison of area and personal sampling techniques in cotton workers found a nearly eight-fold difference in measured dust levels between the two techniques in the opening processes, with personal sampling exposures being much higher than area sampling exposure estimates.[94] The difference between area and personal sampling was less in other processes: five-fold in carding, four-fold in other cardroom processes, 1.4 times in ring spinning and 2.5-fold in winding. Since respiratory disease in cotton workers is much more frequent in the early stages of processing, this difference between area and personal sampling is important in terms of setting exposure standards. There is now a personal exposure dust standard for cotton in the UK.

PREVENTION

The most important preventive measure is a reduction in dust levels. It was originally calculated that approximately

10 per cent of workers exposed to cotton dust for 40 years at a concentration of 0.5 mg/m^3 (as measured using work area dust sampling with a 2-mm pitch gauze prefilter) would develop byssinosis.[95] Efficient exhaust ventilation with filtering of recirculated air is an important preventive measure. Over the past ten years, there have been progressive reductions in cotton dust exposure levels in the USA, such that now byssinosis is a rare disease. Attention is focused on preventing dust-related chronic decline in lung function. The results of the Tulane longitudinal study suggest that to achieve this, smokers should be excluded from the high dust exposure areas (yarn manufacture) and that dust exposure should be reduced to approximately 100 µg/m^3.[96] This exposure level is based on area sampling measurements using a vertical elutriator.

The pre-processing of cotton to prevent byssinosis has also been investigated. Cotton steaming reduced the biological activity of cotton dust and also the dust levels in the early stages of processing.[97] However, fine dust particles may be released later in the manufacturing process, leading to an increased incidence of byssinosis in these work areas. More recently, the bactericidal treatment of raw cotton in the field before harvesting has been evaluated and shown to be highly efficient at reducing the growth of bacteria during transportation and storage, thus potentially reducing endotoxin exposure during the cotton spinning process.[98]

Key points

- Byssinosis is a disease of occupational aetiology which is asthma-like, with bronchial reactivity and airways obstruction, developing after many years of occupational exposure to cotton dust.
- The aetiological agent involved in causing byssinosis is unknown; however, the agent is water-soluble and is likely to be a contaminant of cotton rather than the fibre itself. Bacterial endotoxin is the most likely agent.
- Chronic cotton dust exposure is associated with symptoms other than those known as classical byssinosis. COPD and chronic bronchitis are more common in cotton workers irrespective of smoking habit.

REFERENCES

1. Proust A. *Traite d'hygiene publique et privée*. Paris: Masson, 1877: 171–7.
2. Kay JP. Observations and experiments concerning molecular irritation of the lungs as one source of tubercular consumption; and on spinner's phthisis. *North of England Medical and Surgical Journal*. 1831; **1**: 348–63.
3. Mareska J, Heyman J. Enquête sur le travail et la condition physique et morale des ouvriers employés dans les manufacturers de coton, à Gand. *Annals of the Society of Medicine of Gand*. 1845; **16**: 11: 5, 199.
4. Greenhow H. *Third Report of the Medical Officer of the Privy Council. Sir John Simon*. 1861: 152.
5. Bouhuys A, Heaphy LJ Jr, Schilling RSF, Welborn JW. Byssinosis in the United States. *New England Journal of Medicine*. 1967; **277**: 170–5.
6. Gandevia B, Milne J. Ventilatory capacity changes on exposure to cotton dust and their relevance to byssinosis in Australia. *British Journal of Industrial Medicine*. 1965; **22**: 295–304.
7. Tsai SY. Study of byssinosis in cotton textile workers in Taiwan. *Journal of the Formosan Medical Association*. 1964; **63**: 10–15.
8. Morgan PGM, Ong SC. First report of byssinosis in Hong Kong. *British Journal of Industrial Medicine*. 1981; **38**: 290–2.
9. Koskela R-S, Klockars M, Jarvinen E. Mortality and disability among cotton mill workers. *British Journal of Industrial Medicine*. 1990; **47**: 384–91.
10. Bakirci N, Kalaca S, Francis H et al. Natural history and risk factors of early respiratory responses to cotton dust in newly exposed workers. *Journal of Occupational and Environmental Medicine*. 2007; **49**: 853–61.
11. Gill CIC. Byssinosis in the cotton trade. *British Journal of Industrial Medicine*. 1947; **4**: 48–55.
12. Loh LC, Vyas B, Kanabar V et al. Inhaled endotoxin in healthy human subjects: Dose-related study on systemic and peripheral CD4 and CD8$^+$ T cells. *Respiratory Medicine*. 2006; **100**: 519–28.
13. Schilling RSF, Hughes JPW, Dingwall-Fordyce I, Gilson JC. An epidemiological survey of byssinosis amongst cotton workers. *British Journal of Industrial Medicine*. 1955; **12**: 217–27.
14. Fox AJ, Tombleson JBL, Watt A, Wilkie AG. A survey of respiratory disease in cotton operatives. *British Journal of Industrial Medicine*. 1973; **30**: 42–53.
15. Cinkotai FF, Rigby A, Pickering CAC et al. Recent trends in the prevalence of byssinotic symptoms in the Lancashire textile industry. *British Journal of Industrial Medicine*. 1988; **45**: 782–9.
16. Gun RT, Janckewiez G, Esterman A et al. Byssinosis: A cross-sectional study in an Australian textile factory. *Journal of the Society of Occupational Medicine*. 1983; **33**: 119–25.
17. Field GB, Owen P. Respiratory function in an Australian cotton mill. *Bulletin Européen de Physiopathologie Respiratoire*. 1979; **15**: 455–68.
18. Baratawidjaja K. Byssinosis study among 250 textile mill workers in Jakarta. *American Journal of Industrial Medicine*. 1990; **17**: 71–2.
19. Abebe Y, Seboxa T. Byssinosis and other respiratory disorders among textile mill workers in Bahr Dar northwest Ethiopia. *Ethiopian Medical Journal*. 1995; **33**: 37–49.
20. elKarim A. Prevalence of byssinosis and respiratory symptoms in Sudanese cotton mills. *American Journal of Industrial Medicine*. 1987; **12**: 281–9.

21. Murldhar V, Murlidhar VJ, Kanhere V. Byssinosis in a Bombay textile mill. *National Medical Journal of India*. 1995; **8**: 204–7.
22. Osibogun A, Oseji MI, Isah EC, Iyawe V. Prevalence of byssinosis and other respiratory problems among textile mill workers in Asaba, Nigeria. *Nigerian Postgraduate Medical Journal*. 2006; **13**: 333–8.
23. Farooque MI, Khan B, Aziz E et al. Byssinosis: As seen in cotton spinning mill workers of Karachi. *Journal of the Pakistan Medical Association*. 2008; **58**: 95–8.
24. Berry C, Molyneux MKB, Tombleson JBL. Relationships between dust levels and byssinosis and bronchitis in Lancashire cotton mills. *British Journal of Industrial Medicine*. 1974; **31**: 18–27.
25. Niven RMcL, Fishwick D, Pickering CAC et al. A study of the performance and comparability of the sampling response to cotton dust of the work area and personal sampling techniques. *Annals of Occupational Hygiene*. 1992; **36**: 349–62.
26. Elwood PC, Pemberton J, Merrett JD et al. Byssinosis and other respiratory symptoms in flax workers in Northern Ireland. *British Journal of Industrial Medicine*. 1965; **22**: 27–37.
27. Noweir MH, El-Sadik YM, El-Dakhakhny AA, Osman HA. Dust exposure in manual flax processing in Egypt. *British Journal of Industrial Medicine*. 1975; **32**: 147–54.
28. Wang X-R, Eisen EA, Zhang H-X et al. Respiratory symptoms and cotton dust exposure; results of a 15 year follow up observation. *Occupational and Environmental Medicine*. 2003; **60**: 935–41.
29. Merchant JA, Lumsden JC, Kilburn KH et al. An industrial study of the biological effects of cotton dust and cigarette smoke exposure. *Occupational Medicine*. 1973; **15**: 212–21.
30. Noweir MH, Noweir KH, Osman HA, Moselhi M. An environmental and medical study of byssinosis and other respiratory conditions in the cotton textile industry in Egypt. *American Journal of Industrial Medicine*. 1984; **6**: 173–83.
31. Imbus HR, Suh MW. Steaming of cotton to prevent byssinosis – a plant study. *British Journal of Industrial Medicine*. 1974; **31**: 209–19.
32. Merchant JA, Lumsden JC, Kilburn KH et al. Preprocessing cotton to prevent byssinosis. *British Journal of Industrial Medicine*. 1973; **30**: 237–47.
33. Home Office. *Report of the Departmental Committee on dust in card-rooms in the cotton industry*. London: Home Office, 1932.
34. Schneiter R, Neal PA, Caminita BH. Etiology of acute illness among workers using low grade stained cotton. *American Journal of Public Health*. 1942; **32**: 1345–52.
35. Cavagna C, Foa V, Vigliani EC. Effects in man and rabbits of inhalation of cotton dust or extracts and purified endotoxins. *British Journal of Industrial Medicine*. 1969; **26**: 314–21.
36. Cinkotai FF, Whitaker CJ. Airborne bacteria and the prevalence of byssinotic symptoms in 21 cotton spinning mills in Lancashire. *Annals of Occupational Hygiene*. 1978; **21**: 239–50.
37. Rylander R, Haglind P, Lundholm M. Endotoxin in cotton dust and respiratory function decrement among cotton workers in an experimental card room. *American Review of Respiratory Disease*. 1985; **131**: 209–13.
38. Niven RMcL, Fletcher AM, Pickering CAC et al. Endotoxin exposure and respiratory symptoms in Lancashire cotton spinning mills. Proceedings of the 16th Beltwide Research Conference, National Cotton Council, Memphis, TN, 1992: 222–4.
39. Rylander R, Haglind P, Lundholm M. Endotoxin in cotton dust and respiratory function decrement among cotton workers in an experimental cardroom. *American Review of Respiratory Disease*. 1985; **131**: 209–13.
40. Buck MG, Wall JH, Schachter EN. Airway constrictor response to cotton bract extracts in the absence of endotoxin. *British Journal of Industrial Medicine*. 1986; **43**: 220–6.
41. Jamison JP, Lowry RC. Bronchial challenge of normal subjects with the endotoxin of *Enterobacter agglomerans* isolated from cotton dust. *British Journal of Industrial Medicine*. 1986; **43**: 327–31.
42. Schachter EN, Zuskin E, Buck M et al. Airway responses to the inhalation of cotton dust and cotton bract extracts. *Respiration*. 2006; **73**: 41–7.
43. Cayton HR, Furness G, Maitland HB. Studies in cotton dust in relation to byssinosis. Part 11. Skin tests for allergy with extracts of cotton dusts. *British Journal of Industrial Medicine*. 1952; **9**: 186–96.
44. Popa V, Gavrilescu N, Preda N et al. An investigation of allergy in byssinosis: Sensitisation to cotton, hemp, flax and jute antigens. *British Journal of Industrial Medicine*. 1969; **26**: 101–8.
45. Schachter EN, Buck MG, Merrill WW et al. Skin testing with an aqueous extract of cotton bract. *Journal of Allergy and Clinical Immunology*. 1985; **76**: 481–7.
46. Petronio L, Bovenzi M. Byssinosis and serum IgE concentrations in textile workers in an Italian cotton mill. *British Journal of Industrial Medicine*. 1983; **40**: 39–44.
47. O'Neil CE, Reed MA, Aukrust L, Butcher BT. Studies on the antigenic composition of aqueous cotton dust extracts. *International Archives of Allergy and Applied Immunology*. 1983; **72**: 294–8.
48. Taylor C, Massoud A, Lucas F. Studies on the aetiology of byssinosis. *British Journal of Industrial Medicine*. 1971; **28**: 145–51.
49. Norweir MH. Studies on the etiology of byssinosis. *Chest*. 1981; **79**: 62S–67S.
50. Edwards JH, Alzubaidy TS, Altikriti R, Bunni H. Byssinosis. Inhalation challenge with polyphenol. *Chest*. 1984; **85**: 215–17.
51. Massoud AE, Altounyan REC, Howell JBL, Lane RE. Effects of histamine aerosol in byssinotic subjects. *British Journal of Industrial Medicine*. 1967; **24**: 38–40.
52. Bouhuys A. Response to inhaled histamine in bronchial asthma and in byssinosis. *American Review of Respiratory Disease*. 1967; **95**: 89–93.
53. Mundie TG, Cordova-Salinas M, Bray VJ, Ainsworth SK. Bioassays of smooth muscle contracting agents in cotton mill dust and bract extracts: Arachidonicacid metabolites as possible mediators of the acute byssinotic reaction. *Environmental Research*. 1983; **32**: 62–71.

54. Fowler SR, Ziprin RI, Elissalde MH, Greenblatt GA. The etiology of byssinosis – possible role of prostaglandin F_2 alpha synthesis by alveolar macrophages. *American Industrial Hygiene Association Journal*. 1981; **42**: 445–8.
55. Noweir MH, Abdel-Kader HM, Omran F. Role of histamine in the aetiology of byssinosis. Blood histamine concentrations in workers exposed to cotton and flax dusts. *British Journal of Industrial Medicine*. 1984; **41**: 203–8.
56. Chinn DJ, Cinkotai FF, Lockwood MC. Airborne dust: Its protease content and byssinosis in willowing mills. *Annals of Occupational Hygiene*. 1976; **19**: 101–8.
57. Cinkotai FF. The size-distribution and protease content of airborne particles in textile mill cardrooms. *American Industrial Hygiene Association Journal*. 1976; **37**: 234–8.
58. Jones RN, Butcher BT, Hammond YY et al. Interaction of atopy and exposure to cotton dust in the bronchoconstrictor response. *British Journal of Industrial Medicine*. 1980; **37**: 141–6.
59. Honeybourne D, Finnegan MJ, Pickering CAC. Does atopy matter in byssinosis? In: *New light on byssinosis*. Cardiff: MRC Epidemiology Unit, 1985: 57–60.
60. Schachter EN, Zuskin E, Buck MG et al. Airway reactivity and cotton bract-induced bronchial obstruction. *Chest*. 1985; **87**: 51–5.
61. Massoud AE, Altounyan REC, Howell JBL, Lane RE. Effects of histamine aerosol in byssinotic subjects. *British Journal of Industrial Medicine*. 1967; **24**: 38–40.
62. Haglind P, Bake B, Belin L. Is mild byssinosis associated with small airways disease? *European Journal of Respiratory Diseases*. 1983; **64**: 449–59.
63. Fishwick D, Fletcher AM, Pickering CAC et al. Lung function, bronchial reactivity, atopic status and dust exposure in Lancashire mill operatives. *American Review of Respiratory Disease*. 1992; **145**: 1103–8.
64. Zhou W, Wang X, Zhang H et al. Microsomal epoxide hydrolase, endotoxin, and lung function decline in cotton textile workers. *American Journal of Respiratory and Critical Care Medicine*. 2005; **171**: 165–70.
65. Fishwick D, Fletcher AM, Pickering CAC et al. Ocular and nasal irritation in operatives in Lancashire cotton and synthetic fibre mills. *Occupational and Environmental Medicine*. 1994; **51**: 744–8.
66. Fishwick D, Fletcher AM, Pickering CAC et al. Respiratory symptoms and dust exposure in Lancashire cotton and man-made fiber mill operatives. *American Journal of Respiratory and Critical Care Medicine*. 1994; **150**: 441–7.
67. Roach SA, Schilling RSF. A clinical and environmental study of byssinosis in the Lancashire cotton industry. *British Journal of Industrial Medicine*. 1960; **17**: 1–9.
68. Schilling RSF, Vigliani EC, Lammers B et al. A report on a conference on byssinosis. (14th International Conference on Occupational Health. Madrid, 1963). International Congress Series, No. 62. Amsterdam: Exerpta Medica, 1963: 137–44.
69. World Health Organization. Report of a World Health Organization study group. *Recommended health-based occupational exposure limits for selected vegetable dusts*. WHO Technical Report Series 684. Geneva: World Health Organization, 1983.
70. Berry C, McKerrow CB, Molyneux MKB et al. A study of the acute and chronic changes in ventilatory capacity of workers in Lancashire cotton mills. *British Journal of Industrial Medicine*. 1973; **30**: 25–36.
71. McKerrow CB, McDermott M, Gilson JC, Schilling RSF. Respiratory function during the day in cotton workers: A study in byssinosis. *British Journal of Industrial Medicine*. 1958; **15**: 75–83.
72. Merchant JA, Halprin GM, Hudson AR et al. Evaluation before and after exposure – the pattern of physiological response to cotton dust. *Annals of the New York Academy of Sciences*. 1974; **221**: 38–43.
73. Merchant JA, Halprin GM, Hudson AR et al. Responses to cotton dust. *Archives of Environmental Health*. 1975; **30**: 222–9.
74. Zuskin E, Valic F, Butkovic D, Bouhuys A. Lung function in textile workers. *British Journal of Industrial Medicine*. 1975; **32**: 283–8.
75. Honeybourne D, Pickering CAC. Physiological evidence that emphysema is not a feature of byssinosis but is due to concomitant cigarette smoking. *Thorax*. 1986; **41**: 6–11.
76. Edwards C, Macartney J, Rooke C, Ward F. The pathology of the lung in byssinotics. *Thorax*. 1975; **30**: 612–23.
77. Takizawa T, Thurlbeck WM. Muscle and mucous gland size in the major bronchi of patients with chronic bronchitis, asthma and asthmatic bronchitis. *American Review of Respiratory Disease*. 1971; **104**: 331–6.
78. Pratt PC, Volmer RT, Miller JA. Epidemiology of pulmonary lesions in nontextile and cotton textile workers: A retrospective autopsy analysis. *Archives of Environmental Medicine*. 1980; **35**: 133–7.
79. Fawcett IW, Merchant IA, Simmonds SP, Pepys J. The effect of sodium cromoglycate, beclomethasone dipropionate and salbutamol on the ventilatory response to cotton dust in mill workers. *British Journal of Diseases of the Chest*. 1978; **72**: 29–37.
80. Molyneux MKB, Tombleson JBL. An epidemiological study of respiratory symptoms in Lancashire mills 1963–1966. *British Journal of Industrial Medicine*. 1970; **27**: 225–34.
81. Berry G, Molyneux MKB, Tombleson JBL. Relationship between dust level and byssinosis and bronchitis in Lancashire cotton mills. *British Journal of Industrial Medicine*. 1974; **31**: 18–27.
82. Niven RMcL, Fletcher AM, Pickering CAC et al. Chronic bronchitis in textile workers. *Thorax*. 1997; **52**: 22–7.
83. Glindmeyer HW, Lefante JJ, Jones RN et al. Exposure-related declines in the lung function of cotton textile workers. *American Review of Respiratory Disease*. 1991; **144**: 675–83.
84. Wang X, Zhang H-Z, Sun B-X et al. Cross-shift airway responses and long-term decline in FEV_1 in cotton workers. *American Journal of Respiratory and Critical Care Medicine*. 2008; **177**: 316–20.
85. Collis EL. *Annual Report of Chief Inspector of Factories for 1908*. London: HMSO, 1909.
86. Hill AB. Sickness among operatives in Lancashire cotton mills (with special reference to the cardroom). Report of the

Industrial Health Research Board Report, No 59. London: HMSO.

87. Schilling RSF, Hughes JPW, Dingwall-Fordyce I, Gilson JC. An epidemiological survey of byssinosis amongst cotton workers. *British Journal of Industrial Medicine.* 1955; **12**: 217–27.

88. Elwood PC, Sweetnam PM, Bevan C, Saunders MJ. Respiratory disability in ex-cotton workers. *British Journal of Industrial Medicine.* 1986; **43**: 580–6.

89. Berry G, Molyneux MKB. A mortality study of workers in Lancashire cotton mills. *Chest.* 1981; **79** (Suppl.): 11S–15S.

90. Elwood PC, Thomas HF, Sweetnam PM, Elwood JH. The mortality of flax workers. *British Journal of Industrial Medicine.* 1982; **39**: 18–22.

91. Peto R, Speizer FE, Fletcher E. The relevance in adults of airflow obstruction but not of mucous hypersecretion to mortality from chronic lung disease: 20 year results from prospective surveys. *American Review of Respiratory Disease.* 1983; **128**: 491–500.

92. Koskela R-S, Klockars M, Jarvinen E. Mortality and disability among cotton mill workers. *British Journal of Industrial Medicine* 1990; **47**: 384–91.

93. Hodgson JT, Jones RD. Mortality of workers in the British cotton industry in 1964–1984. *Scandinavian Journal of Work and Environmental Health.* 1990; **16**: 113–20.

94. Niven RMcL, Fishwick D, Pickering CAC *et al.* A study of the performance and comparability of the sampling response to cotton dust of the work area and personal sampling techniques. *Annals of Occupational Hygiene.* 1992; **36**: 349–62.

95. Fox AJ, Tombleson JBL, Watt A, Wilkie AG. A survey of respiratory disease in cotton operatives. Part 11 Symptoms, dust estimations and the effect of smoking habit. *British Journal of Industrial Medicine.* 1973; **30**: 48–53.

96. Glindmeyer HW, Lefante JL, Jones RN *et al.* Exposure-related declines in the lung function of cotton textile workers. Relationship to current workplace standards. *American Review of Respiratory Disease.* 1991; **144**: 675–83.

97. Merchant JA, Lumsden JC, Kilburn KH. Intervention studies of cotton steaming to reduce biological effects of cotton dust. *British Journal of Industrial Medicine.* 1984; **31**: 261–74.

98. Hend IM, Milnera M, Milnera SM. Bactericidal treatment of raw cotton as the method of byssinosis prevention. *American Industrial Hygiene Association Journal.* 2003; **64**: 88–94.

Extrinsic allergic alveolitis

PAUL CULLINAN AND ANTHONY NEWMAN TAYLOR

Introduction	970
Disease frequency	970
Causes of extrinsic allergic alveolitis	971
Pathology	971
Immunopathology	973
Clinical, radiological and physiological features	973
Diagnosis of extrinsic allergic alveolitis	975
Outcome of extrinsic allergic alveolitis	977
Management of extrinsic allergic alveolitis	977
Statutory compensation	978
Particular types of extrinsic allergic alveolitis	978
References	980

INTRODUCTION

Extrinsic allergic alveolitis (EAA) is an immunological disease of the gas-exchanging parts of the lung and the connecting small airways in response to an external antigen. The disease is also known as hypersensitivity pneumonitis (HP), the two labels being synonymous. In most cases, the antigen is airborne and exposure is through inhalation; most such antigens are biological in nature, but the disease may also occur after exposure to an airborne, low molecular mass chemical. Occasionally EAA is attributed to an ingested medicine.

DISEASE FREQUENCY

A firm diagnosis of EAA requires an appropriate history of exposure. This may sometimes be difficult to elicit, especially in chronic cases. It also requires access to fairly sophisticated immunological, radiological and pathological technology. As a result of these diagnostic challenges, information on the frequency and distribution of the disease is patchy and particularly so in general populations. Perhaps the best source of community-based data is a general practice register in the UK covering several million.[1] Analysis of 271 new cases between 1991 and 2003 suggested an overall annual incidence of 1 per 100 000 total population. This rate varied from 0.4 per 100 000 in those aged less than 45 years to 2.4 per 100 000 in those aged 65–74 years. There was very little difference in overall incidence between males and females and little evidence of temporal variation across the 12 years of study. The data did not allow any identification of causative agents. Population-based information derived from mortality data is available from the United States for a period covering 22 years. Age-adjusted death rates increased from 0.9 per 100 000 in 1980 to 2.9 per 100 000 in 2002; the highest rates were in Wisconsin (10 per 100 000). It is unclear whether this rise reflects a true increase in disease incidence or a change in the methods of disease ascertainment or labelling. In 26 states with information on occupation, proportional mortality rates were significantly higher among agricultural production workers, especially those working with livestock in whom the proportional mortality rate was increased almost 20-fold.[2]

Other information on disease frequency is largely from groups with specific exposures, most of them occupational. In general, estimates of disease prevalence are derived from cross-sectional surveys, often with incomplete information on the size of the base population – and thus response rates. 'Healthy worker' survival pressures may also operate,[3] but are difficult to quantify. There are fewer longitudinal studies from which measures of incidence can be derived. In all cases measures of the frequency of EAA depend on the methods by which it was ascertained. Although the number of reported causes of EAA is large, most are uncommon. Furthermore, the risk of many of the classical microbial causes of extrinsic allergic alveolitis has been considerably reduced by changes and improvements in work practices.

EAA can be common among farmers with exposure to hay, but the frequency of disease depends closely on farming practices, climate and probably other factors. In Ireland the annual incidence of hospital-diagnosed EAA among farmers was estimated at about 1.5 per 100 000 between 1982 and 1996. Rates fell to about one-quarter of this level between 1997 and 2002, a decline attributed to changes in the production methods of cattle feeds.[4] In Finland, between 1980 and 1982, 512 new cases of farmer's lung were registered – two-thirds of them in women. Estimates of annual incidence were far higher than in Ireland (ranging from 8 to 60 per 100 000), but varied both geographically and temporally, being closely related to daily rainfall and season – the highest incidence rates were in the spring (April).[5] Similar patterns have been identified in Japan.[6]

EAA is often persistent but rarely fatal; hence its prevalence is generally higher than its incidence. Estimates of the prevalence of disease among farmers tend to vary in the manner above. In Scotland, the prevalence of EAA in farmers – identified by questionnaire alone – varied between 23 per 1000 farm workers in East Lothian and 86 per 1000 in the wetter Ayrshire and Orkneys. About half of the cases in the latter two regions had serum-specific precipitating antibodies to an appropriate antigen.[7] Similar prevalence rates have been measured among English,[8] French[9,10] and US dairy farmers.[11]

There are fewer data on apparently less common forms of occupational EAA. In 1978, budgerigar fancier's lung was described as the most important cause of EAA in Britain, with an estimated prevalence among current budgerigar owners of between 0.5 and 7.5 per cent.[12]

CAUSES OF EXTRINSIC ALLERGIC ALVEOLITIS

The list of recognized causes of EAA is long; several of the more common are shown in Table 74.1. Most occupational causative agents are organic, but the list also includes a small number of low molecular mass chemicals, the most important of which are diisocyanates. The colourful names given to EAA caused by many different organic dusts reflect the varied work settings in which exposure occurs. However, by definition, the tissue response in the lungs and the clinical manifestations of the disease are essentially the same, whatever the cause.

The attribution of cause to a particular agent is rarely simple. In general, it is dependent on the identification of the agent in the workplace environment – most convincingly in air – and on the recognition of a specific serum immune response in those with clinical manifestations of the disease. Serum immunological responses are not, however, specific for the disease, being found in variable proportions of exposed workers without evidence of disease. Moreover, different agents may be responsible for EAA in the same occupational setting, apparently dependent on local conditions and working practices. Thus, in addition to its most commonly recognized causes (*Saccharopolyspora rectivirgula* and *Thermoactinomyces vulgaris*) farmer's lung may be attributable to a wide variety of bacterial and fungal species.[13] To complicate matters further, the nomenclature of some important causative agents changes frequently. Thus, *S. rectivirgula* was formerly known as *Faeni rectivirgula*, and before that as *Micropolyspora faeni*.

Some important varieties of EAA are of unknown cause; indeed the diagnosis is not infrequently made on clinical, radiological or pathological grounds without an identified causative agent. For example, several outbreaks of EAA among metal workers in the United States and the United Kingdom have been described. Although it seems that in each outbreak the source of the antigen was a water-based, metalworking fluid, it remains unclear which component – or more probably microbiological contaminant – was responsible. Finally, EAA is not necessarily an occupational disease. The most common type of disease in Japan is known as 'summer-type EAA (or HP)' and is attributed to domestic exposures to *Trichosporon cutaneum* and possibly *Cryptococus albidus*.[14] This form of disease appears to be confined to southern Japan and has a strong seasonal pattern, being clinically evident only in summer months. It has been linked to residence in older, wooden homes. Domestic exposures to *Aspergillus* and other species have also been reported to cause EAA,[15–17] as have *Cladosporium* and other species in 'hot tub' lung.[18]

These issues aside, there are some conditions that appear to be necessary for the induction of EAA:

- Antigen size: The aerodynamic diameters of the causative agent must be sufficiently small to allow penetration into and retention within the alveoli; for example, the spores of *S. rectivirgula*, the major cause of farmer's lung, are about 2 μm in diameter and those of *Aspergillus clavatus*, the cause of malt worker's lung, are about 3.5 μm in diameter. These dimensions are considerably smaller than those of the moulds, such as *Alternaria alternata* and *Cladosporium herbarum*, that give rise to asthma.
- Antigen persistence: The organic dusts (spores and animal proteins) which cause EAA are poorly degradable and able to persist in the lungs for long periods.
- Exposure conditions: EAA usually occurs in circumstances where the inhaled dose of organic dusts is very high. For example, measurements in barns when bales of mouldy hay are opened suggest that up to 750 000 spores of respirable size may be deposited in the lungs during each minute of exposure.[19]

Nonetheless, only a proportion of exposed persons develops EAA. This may be a reflection of innate susceptibility (or resistance), perhaps related to genetic factors located in the major histocompatibility complex region.[20,21]

PATHOLOGY

Relatively little is known about the pathology of acute EAA since histological specimens are rarely collected in that

Table 74.1 Selected causes of extrinsic allergic alveolitis.

Eponym	Source (probable) of antigen	Antigen(s)
Organic dusts of occupational origin		
Farmer's lung	Mouldy hay, straw or grain	Thermophilic actinomycetes (*Saccharaplyspora recitvirgula*) and other fungi
Malt worker's lung	Mouldy maltings (barley)	*Aspergillus clavatus, Aspergillus fumigatus*
Mushroom grower's lung	Mushroom spores	Thermophilic actinomycetes
Maple bark stripper's lung	Bark from stored maple	*Cryptostroma corticale*
Bagassosis	Mouldy bagasse	Thermophilic actinomycetes (*Saccharaplyspora recitvirgula*)
Suberosis	Mouldy cork	*Penicillium frequentens*
Cheese washer's lung	Mouldy cheese	*Penicillium casei*
Wood pulp worker's lung	Mouldy wood pulp	*Altenaria*
Sequoiosis	Mouldy redwood sawdust	*Aureobasidium pullulans*
Paprika splitter's lung	Mouldy paprika	*Mucor stolonifer*
Roof thatcher's lung	Mouldy thatch	*Sacchoromonospora viridis*
Stipatosis	Esparto dust	*Aspergillus fumigatus*, thermophilic actinomycetes
Ventilation pneumonitis/humidifier lung/hot tub lung	Contaminated, water-cooled air conditioning	Thermophilic actinomycetes, *Cladosporium*
Metal worker's lung	Metal-working fluids (?contaminated)	Unclear
(Nacre) button maker's lung	Mollusc (sea snail) shell	Unclear
Fish meal worker's lung	Fish meal	Unclear
Organic dusts of non-occupational origin		
Summer-type EAA	Domestic (Japan)	*Trichosporon cutaneum, Cryptococcus albidus*
Bird fancier's lung	Avian bloom and excreta	Avian serum proteins
Pituitary snuff taker's lung	Therapeutic 'snuff'	Porcine/bovine proteins
Inorganic		
Occupational	Hexamethylene diisocyanate	
	Diphenyl methane diisocyanate	
	Toluene diisocyanate	
	Copper sulphate fungicide (Bordeaux mixture)	
	Phthalic anhydride	
	Trimellitic anhydride	
	Sodium diazobenzenesulphate (pauli's reagent)	
Pharmacological	Methotrexate	
	Propanolol	
	Amiodarone	

setting. The pathological changes in chronic disease are better described. The characteristic pathological finding in EAA is a granulomatous inflammatory response centred on the peripheral bronchioles and extending peripherally – and often patchily – into adjacent alveoli (Figure 74.1). The inflammatory exudate consists primarily of plasma cells, lymphocytes, macrophages and monocytes; characteristically, foamy macrophages are more abundant in alveoli and lymphocytes in the interstitium. Macrophages and cells derived from them (epithelioid and giant cells) accumulate in foci ('granulomata') within the bronchiolar and interstitial inflammation. Although the appearances of the non-necrotizing granulomata are similar to those found in sarcoidosis, they tend to be smaller and more poorly differentiated than in that disease. Moreover, the bronchocentric nature of EAA and the formation of granulomata within areas of interstitial inflammation distinguish the granulomatous response from that of sarcoidosis.

With avoidance of exposure, the granulomata resolve in some three to four months. If avoidance of exposure occurs at a sufficiently early stage in the disease process the remaining inflammatory response in the lungs can resolve.

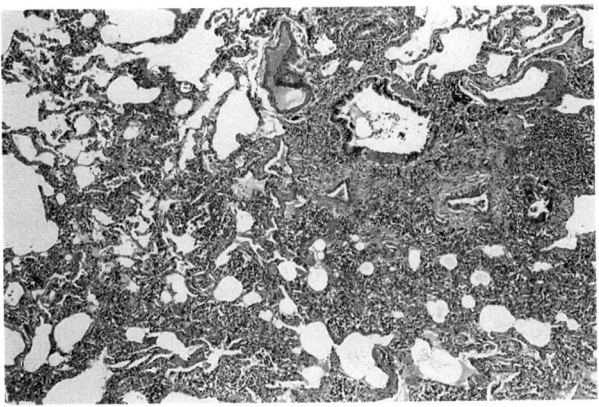

Figure 74.1 Bronchocentric inflammatory response in extrinsic allergic alveolitis.

In other cases, the inflammatory exudate may organize by interstitial fibrosis, causing irreversible damage to the lungs. For reasons which are unknown, fibrosis in allergic alveolitis, as in other granulomatous lung diseases, such as tuberculosis and sarcoidosis, predominantly involves the upper lobes causing lobar shrinkage and cyst formation. The determinants of progression to fibrosis are not clear, but it may particularly occur after repeated symptomatic exposures to the specific cause.[22]

IMMUNOPATHOLOGY

Understanding of the immunological basis of EAA has advanced considerably in recent years but remains incomplete. The original hypothesis that the disease was the outcome of local complement-fixing immune complexes formed between inhaled antigen and circulating antibody deposited in the lungs, was based on several observations:

- the presence of specific, precipitating IgG antibodies (precipitins) in the sera of patients with EAA;
- the provocation by inhaled antigens of a late alveolar response with a time of onset and duration which paralleled the time course of the late 'oedematous' skin reaction;
- the finding of immunoglobulin and complement by immunofluorescence in lung tissue of patients with farmer's lung 36 hours after inhalation of the causative agent.[23]

However, the explanation of EAA solely as an immune complex-mediated response was unsatisfactory for two major reasons. First, granuloma formation, a characteristic component of the pathological response in EAA, was more typical of a T-lymphocyte than immune complex-dependent inflammatory reaction. Second, depending on the sensitivity of the serum assay, IgG antibody could be detected in up to 50 per cent of individuals exposed to causes of EAA but without disease.

The nature of the immunological response in EAA and, in particular, the role of the T-lymphocyte has been clarified by the study of fluid recovered from the lungs during bronchoalveolar lavage (BAL). The proportion of lymphocytes recovered at BAL from patients with EAA is, as in sarcoidosis, greatly increased above normal. Whereas in normal individuals some 85–90 per cent of the cells recovered are macrophages, in sarcoidosis the proportion of lymphocytes may be increased to 50 per cent and in allergic alveolitis to 60–70 per cent or more. In sarcoidosis, the ratio of CD4:CD8 T lymphocytes is increased from the normal value of about 2:1 to 5:1. In EAA, the CD4:CD8 ratio can be normal or low and CD8 T-lymphocytes can comprise 40 per cent and CD4 T lymphocytes 30 per cent of the total lymphocytes recovered to give a CD4:CD8 ratio of less than one.[24] Incubation with pigeon serum of T-lymphocytes recovered by lavage from the lungs of a patient with pigeon fancier's lung stimulated their transformation,[25] and in animal models, the disease can be reproduced by transfer of sensitized T-lymphocytes.[26]

The increase in the proportion of lymphocytes recovered at BAL and the reversed CD4:CD8 T-lymphocyte ratio has, however, also been observed in healthy asymptomatic farmers and pigeon breeders. In one study of 28 farmers with increased BAL lymphocytes, none of 27 studied two to three years later – all of whom had remained on their farms – had developed farmer's lung.[27] Thus the T-lymphocyte response in the lungs by itself is no more able to explain the disease than the presence of IgG antibody in serum.

The explanation for the apparently contradictory evidence above is probably complex and possibly differential.[28] Thus, humoral mechanisms may be relatively more important in the early stages of acute disease, whereas T-cell mediated responses may predominate in more chronic forms. It is likely that in the latter the regulation of responses – and the genetic variants that determine this – is important.[29] For example, pigeon fanciers with EAA differ from asymptomatic exposed individuals with similar increases in BAL lymphocytes in that they show a defect in antigen-specific T-lymphocyte suppressor function.[30] This defect may allow inhaled allergen to provoke a T-lymphocyte dependent inflammatory response; in the asymptomatic person with BAL lymphocytosis, translation of the immunological response into granulomatous inflammation may be inhibited by antigen-specific suppressor T-lymphocytes.

The risk of developing both specific IgG antibody and allergic alveolitis in those exposed to its causes has been consistently reported to be lower in cigarette smokers than in non-smokers.[8,31] This apparent protection may be a reflection of impaired alveolar macrophage function.

CLINICAL, RADIOLOGICAL AND PHYSIOLOGICAL FEATURES

The clinical features of EAA, however caused, depend on the pattern of exposure to the cause and on variation in the severity and nature of the individual response. Although several clinical classifications of the disease have been proposed, they are used inconsistently and in practice the distinction of just two presentations is useful: *acute* (or subacute) EAA that is potentially reversible and *chronic* disease that is irreversible. Even these labels should be used with care since it is not necessarily the case that 'chronic' disease follows 'acute' disease.

Acute (reversible) extrinsic allergic alveolitis

Acute allergic alveolitis typically follows exposure to antigen in high concentration. In a typical case, as in the farmer who feeds mouldy hay to cattle in a cowshed, symptoms do not occur during the period of exposure, but several hours later when breathlessness and 'flu-like symptoms – fever, constitutional upset, muscle pains and headache – develop and predominate. With recurrent attacks, considerable weight loss may also occur. In the absence of further exposure to their cause, symptoms usually start to improve within 48 hours, but may persist for a week or more before resolving completely. Where exposure continues, the (subacute) symptoms do not resolve, but become increasingly severe. On examination during the acute episode, scattered inspiratory crackles and on occasions inspiratory squeaks may be heard over the lungs, but in some cases no abnormal sounds are audible.

A variety of patterns of changes, including no visible changes, on the chest radiograph may develop during the acute disease.[32] A patchy, bilateral ground glass pattern can occur, which is often difficult to detect unless a previous (or subsequent) radiograph is available for comparison. The generalized haze is associated with a loss of sharpness of outline of the vascular shadows, particularly in the lower lung zones; the apices may be spared. Micronodular (less than 3 mm) or nodular shadows, either widespread or more prominent in the lower zones may also occur (Figure 74.2). On occasions, nodules can merge into larger areas of patchy consolidation. In the absence of further antigen exposure, these acute shadows can take four to six weeks or longer to resolve.

High resolution computed tomography (HRCT) scanning of the chest is more sensitive than standard chest radiography and is abnormal in almost all cases.[33] The changes reflect those seen on chest x-ray and presumably the underlying pathological processes. In acute EAA, the typical findings are of a ground glass patchy infiltration predominantly in the lower lobes. A 'mosaic' pattern, most evident on expiratory scans, may be apparent (Figure 74.3). With avoidance of further exposure to the causative agent, the changes of consolidation are the first to resolve; micronodules tend to clear less rapidly.[34]

The important abnormalities of lung function in acute allergic alveolitis are a reduction in lung volumes ('small, stiff lungs') and impairment of gas transfer. Total lung

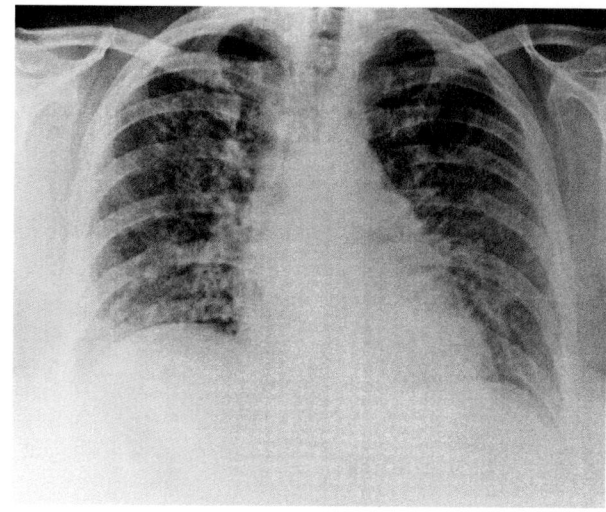

Figure 74.2 Chest radiograph in acute extrinsic allergic alveolitis (farmer's lung).

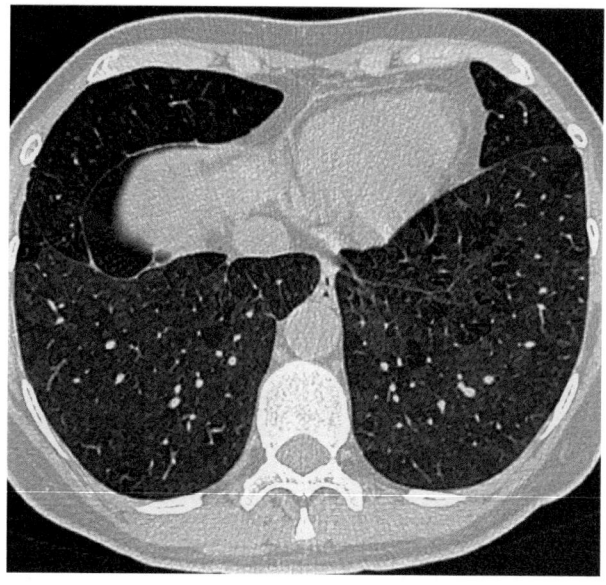

Figure 74.3 High resolution computed tomography scan of chest in acute extrinsic allergic alveolitis with mosaic pattern.

capacity (TLC) and residual volume (RV) are reduced as are vital capacity (VC) and forced expiratory volume in 1 second (FEV_1). The FEV_1/FVC ratio is maintained or increased. Both transfer factor for carbon monoxide (TLCO) and gas transfer coefficient (KCO) are reduced. Of these abnormalities, the reduction in TLCO is the most sensitive indicator of disease severity. In addition, the alveolar–arterial Po_2 gradient is increased at rest and widens with exercise. In severe cases, Po_2 at rest may be sufficiently reduced for patients to be cyanosed; Pco_2 is normal or reduced. Lung function in patients with acute alveolitis generally improves during four to six weeks of avoidance of exposure, but can continue to improve for up to six months. During the acute illness the blood neutrophil count, erythrocyte sedimentation rate (ESR) and C-reactive protein are usually increased, but rarely by very much.

Recurrent episodes of alveolitis follow intermittent exposures to antigenic dust in high concentration and may give rise to a 'subacute' presentation. While it is widely believed that progressive disease occurs in those continuously exposed to high concentrations of antigen, the evidence for this – from longitudinal study of individual patients or populations – is very limited.[22]

Chronic (irreversible) extrinsic allergic alveolitis

Chronic allergic alveolitis is distinguished from acute disease by the development of irreversible pulmonary fibrosis. It may result from recurrent episodes of acute alveolitis or repeated exposures, over a long period, to antigen in concentrations insufficient to provoke acute symptoms, but sufficient to cause progressive pulmonary damage. The commonly cited example of this latter pattern of presentation is the budgerigar fancier exposed to low concentrations of bird dust in her home, who only comes to medical attention when pulmonary fibrosis has caused sufficient loss of respiratory reserve to cause symptoms.

The dominant symptom of chronic allergic alveolitis is breathlessness on exertion. Other than weight loss which can be considerable, systemic symptoms are usually absent. Finger clubbing is unusual. Scattered inspiratory crackles and squeaks may be audible over the lungs.

Chronic irreversible changes develop on the chest radiograph. Linear shadows, honeycombing and lung shrinkage occur, particularly in the upper lobes, with compensatory dilatation in the lower lobes (Figure 74.4). These findings are mirrored with greater sensitivity on HRCT (Figure 74.5).

The abnormalities of lung function are similar to those in acute alveolitis, but may improve little with avoidance of exposure to their cause, and can progress in its absence. Lung volumes (TLC, RV and VC) are reduced, FEV_1/FVC is maintained or increased and TLCO and KCO are reduced. The magnitude of the reduction in TLC and TLCO correlate with the profusion of abnormalities on the chest radiograph.[35] Arterial Po_2 is reduced and in severe cases patients are cyanosed. The alveolar–arterial gradient is increased and widens on exercise. Pulmonary hypertension can develop in patients with widespread pulmonary fibrosis and patients may present at this stage of the disease.

DIAGNOSIS OF EXTRINSIC ALLERGIC ALVEOLITIS

The diagnosis of extrinsic allergic alveolitis is based on a combination of the following:

1. Identification of a potential source of antigen in the patient's working (or domestic) environment.

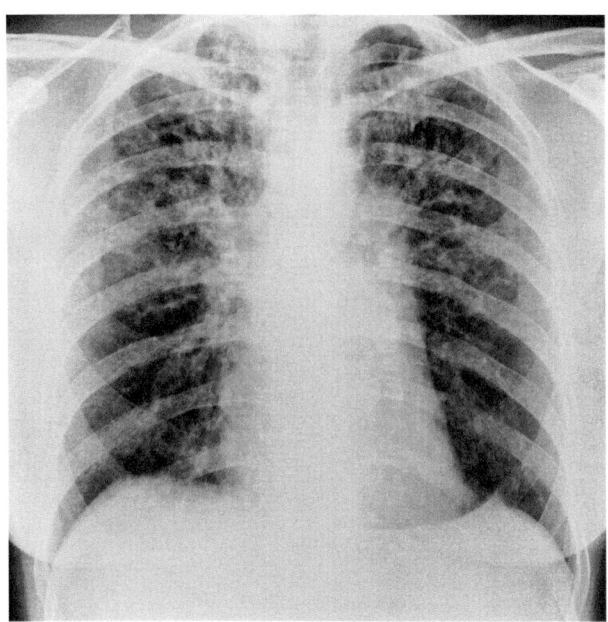

Figure 74.4 Chest radiograph in chronic extrinsic allergic alveolitis (parakeet breeder).

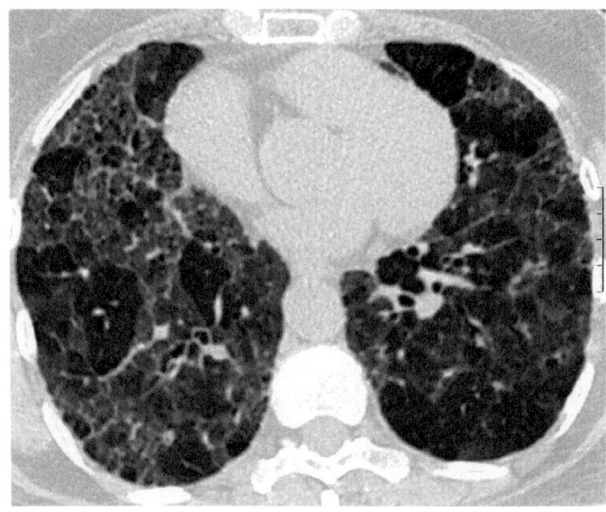

Figure 74.5 High resolution computed tomography scan of chest in chronic, fibrotic extrinsic allergic alveolitis.

2. A pattern of clinical symptoms linked to exposure to the above with, importantly, a pattern of improvement after avoidance of exposure to the causative antigen. Such improvement may be confounded by hospitalization and treatment.
3. Characteristic clinical, radiographic and functional changes of the disease.
4. Characteristic cytology of BAL (lymphocyte count >30–40 per cent), where available.
5. Characteristic histopathological changes, where the appropriate material is available.
6. Demonstration of specific IgG antibodies, including precipitins, to the causal antigen in the patient's serum.

Table 74.2 Diagnostic algorithm for distinguishing acute extrinsic allergic alveolitis from other interstitial lung disease; the figures are disease probabilities given a set of clinical and laboratory characteristics.

Exposure to known antigen	Recurrent episodes	Symptoms 4–8 hours after exposure	Weight loss	Inspiratory crackles (%)			
				Yes Serum precipitins		No Serum precipitins	
				Yes	No	Yes	No
Yes	Yes	Yes	Yes	98	92	93	72
Yes	Yes	Yes	No	97	85	87	56
Yes	Yes	No	Yes	90	62	66	27
Yes	Yes	No	No	81	45	49	15
Yes	No	Yes	Yes	95	78	81	44
Yes	No	Yes	No	90	64	68	28
Yes	No	No	Yes	73	33	37	10
Yes	No	No	No	57	20	22	5
No	Yes	Yes	Yes	62	23	26	6
No	Yes	Yes	No	45	13	15	3
No	Yes	No	Yes	18	4	5	1
No	Yes	No	No	10	2	2	0
No	No	Yes	Yes	33	8	10	2
No	No	Yes	No	20	4	5	1
No	No	No	Yes	6	1	1	0
No	No	No	No	3	1	1	0

Adapted from Ref. 37.

7. A positive response to specific inhalation challenge under experimental conditions.

Few of the above are diagnostically specific for EAA and in any case it is rare that all are available. Specific inhalation challenge testing, for example, is very rarely undertaken and the response to antigen avoidance is often confounded by concurrent steroid treatment. Thus, in many cases, a diagnosis is made on incomplete evidence and there is almost certainly wide variation in diagnostic practice.[36]

Nonetheless, the diagnostic value of the combination of various clinical, laboratory and other tests in distinguishing acute EAA from other interstitial lung disease has been studied in considerable detail.[37] In the absence of an independent, gold standard diagnostic test, there is a certain circularity of argument in any such study, but its findings are instructive. Just six measures, most of them derived from a clinical history, were significantly associated with a diagnosis of acute EAA, the most powerful of them being an appropriate exposure history. Estimates of the probability of disease using these simple measures are summarized in Table 74.2.

Traditionally, reflecting early studies of the immunopathology of EAA, specific laboratory tests have focused on the identification of precipitating IgG antibodies ('precipitins') using methods based on the Ouchterlony technique. This method is essentially qualitative and is time consuming. More recently, indirect enzyme immunoassay methods for the detection of any specific IgG antibodies have become available, some of them commercially so. These are far more easily automated and provide a quantitative measure. Broadly speaking, the two approaches are in agreement, although the latter may be diagnostically more sensitive, and less specific.[38,39]

Specific IgG antibodies, whether precipitating or otherwise, are in general a more sensitive than specific index of EAA. In cases of EAA, their detection is further dependent on the interval since last exposure to the causative antigen. In farmer's lung, precipitins to causative antigens are found in the serum of between 75 and 100 per cent of cases during an acute episode, but in only about 50 per cent after two years from the last acute episode and in only one-third of cases after five years.[22] In pigeon fancier's lung, IgG titres fall rapidly after allergen avoidance.[38] Thus, in acute disease with recent exposure, the test has a high sensitivity with a low false negative rate. In chronic disease, the sensitivity is far lower. For example, precipitating antibodies may be found in just 20 per cent of farmers with EAA whose last acute attack was more than 36 months previously.[40]

Conversely, the measurement of specific IgG antibodies has a low specificity (a high false positive rate); the majority of farmers, for example, who have serum precipitins do not have farmer's lung. In a random sample of Quebec dairy farmers, 8 per cent had serum precipitins, but only four of the 56 with precipitins had farmer's lung.[41] Similarly, one-third of US dairy farmers without overt evidence of disease had specific precipitins.[42] While the great majority of pigeon breeders with acute allergic alveolitis have been reported to have serum precipitins, so have some 15 per cent of healthy breeders without disease.[43] A Bayesian analysis of the value of avian precipitins in the diagnosis of bird breeder's lung suggested that the test was most useful in clinical situations of low or medium prior probability.[44]

Differential diagnosis

The most important differential diagnoses in acute EAA are febrile microbial respiratory illnesses which cause widespread shadows on chest radiograph. These include pneumonias caused by influenza virus, by *Mycoplasma* and by *Legionnella*, psittacosis and Q fever. In the immunocompromised patient infection with *Pneumonocystis carinii* should be excluded before starting treatment with corticosteroids. Important differential diagnoses in chronic EAA include other forms of interstitial lung disease, such as non-specific interstitial pneumonitis (NSIP), usual interstitial pneumonitis (UIP) and sarcoidosis.

OUTCOME OF EXTRINSIC ALLERGIC ALVEOLITIS

The important long-term consequence of EAA is pulmonary fibrosis which can be disabling and shorten life. Because of its relative frequency and important economic consequences, the risk of developing disabling pulmonary fibrosis and the factors determining its occurrence have been particularly investigated in farmer's lung. One large study followed up 144 patients for an average period of 15 years during which time some 10 per cent died of causes associated with their disease. Of those alive at the end of follow up, 40 per cent had radiographic evidence of chronic alveolitis, less than one-quarter had exertional dyspnoea, and about one-third reduced TLCO, the most sensitive index of impaired lung function in EAA. The development of disabling fibrosis particularly occurred in those with a history of recurrent (more than five) episodes of acute alveolitis. Continuing to farm and disease of long duration were not associated with worse lung function. Provided adequate precautions were taken to minimize exposure to mouldy hay and other sources of thermophilic actinomycetes, the majority of farmers were able to remain on their farms without developing disabling pulmonary fibrosis.[22] The results of several other studies support this finding. One compared the outcome five years after an attack of acute EAA in 24 farmers who had left their farms with 37 who had remained. Mean TLCO improved in those who had left their farms, but not in those who remained. However, there was wide variation between subjects in both groups and the majority of farmers were able to continue to farm without developing disabling disease.[45] A similar follow-up study of 86 cases of farmer's lung in Finland found that lung function improves during the six months after an acute episode, but that after five years there was no difference in lung function between the two-thirds who had continued to farm as compared to those who had left. Corticosteroid treatment accelerated the rate of improvement following an acute attack, but did not produce any long-term improvement in lung function.[46]

In 1981–82, 43 asymptomatic Quebec dairy farmers were identified; 23 had serum-specific precipitins and 19 had an increased lymphocyte count on BAL – none had abnormal radiology or lung function. Twenty-seven were re-examined 20 years later; none had stopped farming for reasons of respiratory ill health.[47] There was no evidence of clinically important disease or of reductions in lung function in any suggesting that the presence of precipitins or BAL lymphocytosis alone have no adverse consequences.

The prognosis of acute pigeon fancier's lung seems to be good. A decade of observation of 21 patients with the disease (18 of whom continued to keep pigeons) suggested a favourable clinical course in most. Continuing high levels of specific IgG antibodies suggested that avoidance of exposure could not easily explain this pattern.[48] In contrast, in a cohort of 78 patients with chronic pigeon fancier's lung, almost 30 per cent died of their disease within five years of diagnosis.[49] These observations suggest that those with insidious disease, without acute symptoms, may develop more severe pulmonary fibrosis.

MANAGEMENT OF EXTRINSIC ALLERGIC ALVEOLITIS

The aims in management of cases of EAA are to ensure maximum restoration of lung function and to prevent the development or progression of pulmonary fibrosis. Patients with acute EAA should avoid all exposure to the cause of their disease until maximum restoration of lung function has occurred. Corticosteroids accelerate the rate of recovery in acute disease, but do not seem to provide additional long-term benefit.[50] Treatment should be discontinued within six months of an acute episode. An initial dose of prednisolone of 1 mg/kg body weight should be reduced within four to eight weeks to 20 mg on alternate days which can be continued for three to six months. The starting high dose should be maintained until maximum resolution of the chest radiograph and sustained improvement in lung function are obtained.

Occasionally, patients develop a progressively fibrosing disease which should be treated with longer-term, regular oral steroids supplemented when appropriate by an immunosuppressant drug, such as azathioprine or cyclophosphamide.

Long-term management is primarily based on avoidance of exposures which are believed to increase the risk of progressive pulmonary fibrosis. It is clear from studies of farmers that only a minority with EAA develops disabling pulmonary fibrosis and the majority is able to continue to farm without this occurring. If a farmer wishes to continue in employment it is reasonable to support this provided: (1) he or she takes appropriate measures to minimize exposure to mouldy hay (including the use of effective respiratory protection, such as laminar flow equipment when handling stored hay, straw and grain); (2) lung function is monitored regularly, at the minimum before and after each winter season. Should lung function show progressive deterioration during the winter and incomplete resolution in the summer, he or she should be strongly advised against continuing farm work.

A similar approach may be taken with other occupational causes of extrinsic allergic alveolitis, where complete avoidance of exposure is only obtained at the expense of an individual's job.

The situation is less straightforward in situations, such as bird fancier's lung, where an exposure is unrelated to occupation, and thus continuation, or otherwise, of exposure is not contingent on employment. In these situations, it seems more reasonable to advise avoidance of all further contact with the source of exposure. However, particularly in the case of pigeon fanciers, the birds may be the focus of a social life with which the individual is unwilling to part. In this situation, it may be appropriate to apply the same rules as for occupational alveolitis: minimal exposure with the use of respiratory protection when exposed and serial measurement of lung function (in particular of gas transfer) to monitor the effectiveness of this strategy.

STATUTORY COMPENSATION

In the UK, extrinsic allergic alveolitis is prescribed for 'employed earners' in certain occupations. These are defined as those that involve:

- exposure to moulds or fungal spores, or heterologous proteins by reason of employment in agriculture, horticulture, forestry, cultivation of edible fungi or maltworking, or
- loading or unloading, or handling in storage of mouldy vegetable matter or edible fungi, or
- caring for or handling birds, or
- handling bagasse or
- exposure to metal-working fluids.

Employed earners (i.e not the self-employed) who develop EAA as a consequence of employment in which they have been exposed to one of these groups of agents are entitled to disablement benefit.

PARTICULAR TYPES OF EXTRINSIC ALLERGIC ALVEOLITIS

Farmer's lung

Farmer's lung is the most frequently recognized occupational form of EAA. It is usually, but not always, the outcome of an allergic response to thermophilic actinomycetes which cause vegetable matter to mould during storage. Actinomycetes are Gram-positive, filamentous bacteria that resemble fungi in their morphology and are the only known bacteria to produce antigenic spores. Species that are thermophilic, with growth favoured by high humidity and temperatures of between 30 and 65°C, include *S. rectivirgula* (formerly *Micropolyspora faeni*), *Thermoactinomycetes vulgaris*, *Saccharomonospora viridis* and *Thermoactinomycetes sacchari*, among others. Inhalation of spores and mycelial fragments typically occurs when mouldy hay, straw or grain is handled in enclosed and poorly ventilated buildings. Crops become mouldy when they are harvested damp and stored with a high water content. Moulding generates heat, the maximum temperature achieved being dependent upon the water content of the hay. Stored with a water content of between 35 and 50 per cent, the temperature of hay can reach 65°C, sufficiently high to permit the growth of thermophilic actinomycetes. This general relationship between water content, heating and microbial growth applies also to other crops and vegetable matter, such as straw, grain, bagasse and mushroom compost, which can support the growth of microorganisms whose spores cause EAA.

The prevalence of farmer's lung is related to local rainfall and to farming methods. In general, the disease is most prevalent in areas of high rainfall and where economic circumstances (as on small and undercapitalized farms) do not allow drying of crops before storage or the prevention of wetting during storage. Opening bales of hay and straw during animal feeding and bedding, especially in under-ventilated buildings, is the most common circumstance incurring high exposure. The estimated prevalence of the disease will also vary with the criteria used to identify cases. It appears to be uncommon in contemporary UK farming.

Farmer's lung can be prevented by drying crops adequately before storage, by preventing their becoming damp and ensuring good ventilation during storage. To prevent significant moulding, hay must be stored with a water content of less than 20 per cent. The disease can also be prevented by the substitution of silage for hay. Respiratory protection should be worn by farm workers when working with mouldy crops in conditions likely to generate spores into the air in high concentration and in particular by those who have experienced an attack of farmer's lung in the past.

Bird fancier's lung

Bird fancier's (or breeder's) lung is caused by inhaled avian serum proteins (IgA may be most important) present in the birds' excreta and secreta, and in pigeons particularly, the bloom from their feathers. It primarily occurs amongst individuals who breed and keep pigeons for racing and those who share their homes with caged birds, especially, although not exclusively, budgerigars. EAA has also been reported in those exposed to chickens, turkeys, ducks, geese, pheasants, parrots and turtle doves.

Typically, protein containing dust is disseminated into the air during the cleaning of pigeon lofts and budgerigar cages. Antigenic dust is also generated continuously by birds when active and inhaled by owners and others observing the birds in their cages. Budgerigar fancier's lung may be the most important cause of EAA in Britain, with an estimated prevalence among current budgerigar owners (in 1978) of between 0.5 and 7.5 per cent.[12] This is similar to the prevalence of farmer's lung among farm workers; the greater number of budgerigar owners in the community, however, suggests that alveolitis caused by birds is the more common disease.[51]

Metal-working fluids and extrinsic allergic alveolitis

Metal-working fluids (MWF) are used for lubrication, cooling and waste removal during high-speed metal machining processes. Their use is very widespread in manufacturing occupations. In the United States, for example, there are estimated to be more than a million workers with potential exposure.[52] Traditional MWF were 'straight' insoluble petroleum oils, but these have been replaced by emulsions of water with soluble, synthetic or semi-synthetic oils. During machining and similar processes, the MWF is readily aerosolized and both respiratory and dermal exposure can occur. Modern fluids are designed to reduce such 'misting'. A significant problem with MWF, and perhaps particularly with synthetic varieties, is contamination by bacterial, mycobacterial and fungal organisms.[53] Effective management of MWF systems requires processes designed to reduce or eliminate microbial contamination, including regular biocidal treatment.

In addition to a limited number of case reports, there is literature describing several outbreaks of extrinsic allergic alveolitis among metal machinists. Most of these have been in US factory populations,[54–57] but there are also reports from the UK,[58] including one of a relatively large outbreak in a car engine plant.[59,60] Investigations using simple epidemiological approaches suggest a causative role for a component of metal-working fluids, but immunological studies have failed consistently to identify any particular agent.

Mushroom worker's lung

Mushroom worker's lung is caused by the inhalation of microbial spores generated during commercial mushroom cultivation. Mushrooms are cultivated commercially on compost, a mixture of wheat straw and fresh animal manure. After decomposition outdoors, the compost is heated indoors by steam to 60°C at 100 per cent humidity, conditions ideal for the growth of thermophilic organisms. After around five days of these conditions, mushroom spawn is added to the compost and mechanically mixed, generating large numbers of spores. The mushrooms are grown in sheds at a temperature of about 20°C and 90 per cent humidity. After the mushroom crop is picked, the spent compost is removed and dumped outdoors. Exposure to microbial spores primarily occurs during spawning, particularly when done by hand and during disposal of spent compost. The specific microorganisms responsible for the disease have not been identified with any certainty, but may be microbes growing in the compost, from the mushrooms or both.

Activities that lead to high mould exposure include mixing compost, spawning and compost disposal. The risk of developing mushroom worker's lung has decreased since the introduction of mechanical, as opposed to manual, spawning. Chronic mushroom worker's lung appears to be very uncommon.

Malt worker's lung

Malt worker's lung is caused by *Aspergillus clavatus*, a contaminant of barley to which maltmen in whisky distilleries or breweries may be exposed during malting. In a distillery, barley is dried in hot air kilns, stored in silos for at least eight weeks and dehydrated in steeping tanks with a mild fungicide. In the traditional 'open floor' malting process, the barley is then spread out on open floors and allowed to germinate. Heat is generated by respiration of the germinating barley and the temperature maintained by regular turning and raking of the barley. Germination is stopped by putting the barley into a hot air kiln, in which the malt is dried and turned.

Exposure to the spores of *A. clavatus* occurs primarily among those turning barley on the malt floor and in the malt kilns. In modern maltings, these processes have been partly or wholly mechanized and both exposure to *Aspergillus* and the risk of malt worker's lung have been greatly reduced. Chronic malt worker's lung seems to be very uncommon.

Bagassosis

Bagasse is the fibrous cellulose residue of sugar cane which remains after the sugar has been extracted. It is used in the manufacture of several different materials which include paper and particle boarding. After sugar extraction, bagasse is stored for about a year, often outdoors, in bales. Storage with a water content above 27 per cent permits moulding, heat generation and the growth of thermophilic microorganisms including *T. sacchari*.

Exposure to *T. sacchari* primarily occurs in those involved in the removal, opening and milling of stored bagasse. Moulding of bagasse can be prevented by pretreating the fresh material with 1 per cent propionic acid. Bagassosis is now uncommon, although sporadic outbreaks continue to be reported.

'Ventilation pneumonitis'

Extrinsic allergic alveolitis can occur in the inhabitants of air-conditioned homes and among those working in air-conditioned office blocks.[61] The majority of cases reported to date have occurred in the United States where the disease is caused by thermophilic *Actinomycetes* growing in reservoirs of humidification systems where water recirculates at temperatures which are sufficiently high to permit their growth. The conditioned air acts as the vehicle of antigen dissemination. 'Ventilation pneumonitis', like other forms of extrinsic allergic alveolitis, can cause progressive pulmonary fibrosis. It should be distinguished from 'humidifier fever' which causes similar acute symptoms and changes in lung function, but is associated with humidification systems whose reservoir of water is cold.[62] The symptoms of humidifier fever have a characteristic periodicity: they occur on the first day back at work after a weekend or holiday absence and improve, despite continuing exposure during the working week. Abnormalities on the chest radiograph and progressive pulmonary fibrosis do not develop in humidifier fever.[63]

Key points

- In the general population extrinsic allergic alveolitis – synonymous with hypersensitivity pneumonitis – has an annual incidence of about 1 per 100 000.
- Rates are higher among those working in the many occupations where a risk of disease has been identified; but are very dependent on local behavioural, climatic, microbiological and other factors.
- The disease has 'reversible' (acute) and 'irreversible' (chronic) presentations; the relationship between these types is uncertain.
- While immunological measurements of specific IgG antibodies are undoubtedly helpful in identifying a causative antigen, they must be interpreted in the light of a careful clinical history with particular attention to environmental exposures.
- Most causes of EAA are microbial; both occupational and respiratory specialists should be alert to new sources of exposure – recently identified examples include with metal-working fluids and residence in a mouldy home.

REFERENCES

1. Solaymani-Dodaran M, West J, Smith C, Hubbard R. Extrinsic allergic alveolitis: Incidence and mortality in the general population. *Quarterly Journal of Medicine*. 2007; **100**: 233–7.
2. Bang KM, Weissman DN, Pinheiro GA *et al*. Twenty-three years of hypersensitivity pneumonitis mortality surveillance in the United States. *American Journal of Industrial Medicine*. 2006; **49**: 997–1004.
3. Sanderson W, Kullman G, Sastre J *et al*. Outbreak of hypersensitivity pneumonitis among mushroom farm workers. *American Journal of Industrial Medicine*. 1992; **22**: 859–72.
4. Arya A, Roychoudhury K, Bredin CP. Farmer's lung is now in decline. *Irish Medical Journal*. 2006; **99**: 203–5.
5. Terho EO, Heinonen OP, Lammi S, Laukkanen V. Incidence of clinically confirmed farmer's lung in Finland and its relation to meteorological factors. *European Journal of Respiratory Diseases*. 1987; **152** (Suppl.): 47–56.
6. Takahashi T, Ohtsuka Y, Munakata M *et al*. Occurrence of farmer's lung disease is relevant to meteorological conditions: A 20-year follow-up field survey analysis. *American Journal of Industrial Medicine*. 2002; **41**: 506–13.
7. Grant IW, Blyth W, Wardrop VE *et al*. Prevalence of farmer's lung in Scotland: A pilot survey. *British Medical Journal*. 1972; **1**: 530–4.
8. Morgan DC, Smyth JT, Lister RW *et al*. Chest symptoms in farming communities with special reference to farmer's lung. *British Journal of Industrial Medicine*. 1975; **32**: 228–34.
9. Dalphin JC, Debieuvre D, Pernet D *et al*. Prevalence and risk factors for chronic bronchitis and farmer's lung in French dairy farmers. *British Journal of Industrial Medicine*. 1993; **50**: 941–4.
10. Depierre A, Dalphin JC, Pernet D *et al*. Epidemiological study of farmer's lung in five districts of the French Doubs province. *Thorax*. 1988; **43**: 429–35.
11. Marx JJ, Guernsey J, Emanuel DA *et al*. Cohort studies of immunologic lung disease among Wisconsin dairy farmers. *American Journal of Industrial Medicine*. 1990; **18**: 263–8.
12. Hendrick DJ, Faux JA, Marshall R. Budgerigar-fancier's lung: The commonest variety of allergic alveolitis in Britain. *British Medical Journal*. 1978; **2**: 81–4.
13. Reboux G, Piarroux R, Mauny F *et al*. Role of molds in farmer's lung disease in Eastern France. *American Journal of Respiratory and Critical Care Medicine*. 2001; **163**: 1534–9.
14. Ando M, Suga M, Nishiura Y, Miyajima M. Summer-type hypersensitivity pneumonitis. *Internal Medicine*. 1995; **34**: 707–12.
15. Bryant DH, Rogers P. Allergic alveolitis due to wood-rot fungi. *Allergy Proceedings*. 1991; **12**: 89–94.
16. Enriquez-Matas A, Quirce S, Hernandez E *et al*. Hypersensitivity pneumonitis caused by domestic exposure to molds. *Journal of Investigational Allergology and Clinical Immunology*. 2007; **17**: 126–7.

17. Jacobs RL, Andrews CP, Coalson JJ. Hypersensitivity pneumonitis: Beyond classic occupational disease-changing concepts of diagnosis and management. *Annals of Allergy, Asthma and Immunology.* 2005; **95**: 115–28.
18. Jacobs RL, Thorner RE, Holcomb JR et al. Hypersensitivity pneumonitis caused by *Cladosporium* in an enclosed hot-tub area. *Annals of Internal Medicine.* 1986; **105**: 204–6.
19. Lacey J, Lacey ME. Spore concentrations in the air of farm buildings. *Transactions of the British Mycological Society.* 1964; **47**: 547–52.
20. Ando M, Hirayama K, Soda K et al. HLA-DQw3 in Japanese summer-type hypersensitivity pneumonitis induced by *Trichosporon cutaneum*. *American Review of Respiratory Disease.* 1989; **140**: 948–50.
21. Camarena A, Juarez A, Mejia M et al. Major histocompatibility complex and tumor necrosis factor-alpha polymorphisms in pigeon breeder's disease. *American Journal of Respiratory and Critical Care Medicine.* 2001; **163**: 1528–33.
22. Braun SR, doPico GA, Tsiatis A et al. Farmer's lung disease: Long-term clinical and physiologic outcome. *American Review of Respiratory Disease.* 1979; **119**: 185–91.
23. Ghose T, Landrigan P, Killeen R, Dill J. Immunopathological studies in patients with farmer's lung. *Clinical Allergy.* 1974; **4**: 119–29.
24. Salvaggio JE, Robert A. Cooke memorial lecture. Hypersensitivity pneumonitis. *Journal of Allergy and Clinical Immunology.* 1987; **79**: 558–71.
25. Schuyler MR, Thigpen TP, Salvaggio JE. Local pulmonary immunity in pigeon breeder's disease. A case study. *Annals of Internal Medicine.* 1978; **88**: 355–8.
26. Bice DE, Salvaggio J, Hoffman E. Passive transfer of experimental hypersensitivity pneumonitis with lymphoid cells in the rabbit. *Journal of Allergy and Clinical Immunology.* 1976; **58**: 250–62.
27. Cormier Y, Belanger J, Laviolette M. Prognostic significance of bronchoalveolar lymphocytosis in farmer's lung. *American Review of Respiratory Disease.* 1987; **135**: 692–5.
28. Selman M. Hypersensitivity pneumonitis. In: Schwarz MI, King TE (eds). *Interstitial lung disease*, 4th edn. London: BC Decker; 2003: 452–84.
29. Facco M, Trentin L, Nicolardi L et al. T cells in the lung of patients with hypersensitivity pneumonitis accumulate in a clonal manner. *Journal of Leukocyte Biology.* 2004; **75**: 798–804.
30. Keller RH, Swartz S, Schlueter DP et al. Immunoregulation in hypersensitivity pneumonitis: Phenotypic and functional studies of bronchoalveolar lavage lymphocytes. *American Review of Respiratory Disease.* 1984; **130**: 766–71.
31. Warren CP. Extrinsic allergic alveolitis: A disease commoner in non-smokers. *Thorax.* 1977; **32**: 567–9.
32. Hodgson MJ, Parkinson DK, Karpf M. Chest X-rays in hypersensitivity pneumonitis: A metaanalysis of secular trend. *American Journal of Industrial Medicine.* 1989; **16**: 45–53.
33. Lynch DA, Rose CS, Way D, King TE Jr. Hypersensitivity pneumonitis: Sensitivity of high-resolution CT in a population-based study. *American Journal of Roentgenology.* 1992; **159**: 469–72.
34. Akira M, Kita N, Higashihara T et al. Summer-type hypersensitivity pneumonitis: Comparison of high-resolution CT and plain radiographic findings. *American Journal of Roentgenology.* 1992; **158**: 1223–8.
35. Cormier Y, Belanger J, Tardif A et al. Relationships between radiographic change, pulmonary function, and bronchoalveolar lavage fluid lymphocytes in farmer's lung disease. *Thorax.* 1986; **41**: 28–33.
36. Farebrother MJ, Kelson MC, Heller RF. Death certification of farmer's lung and chronic airway diseases in different countries of the EEC. *British Journal of Diseases of the Chest.* 1985; **79**: 352–60.
37. Lacasse Y, Selman M, Costabel U et al. Clinical diagnosis of hypersensitivity pneumonitis. *American Journal of Respiratory and Critical Care Medicine.* 2003; **168**: 952–8.
38. McSharry C, Dye GM, Ismail T et al. Quantifying serum antibody in bird fanciers' hypersensitivity pneumonitis. *BMC Pulmonary Medicine.* 2006; **6**: 16.
39. Van Hoeyveld E, Dupont L, Bossuyt X. Quantification of IgG antibodies to *Aspergillus fumigatus* and pigeon antigens by ImmunoCAP technology: An alternative to the precipitation technique? *Clinical Chemistry.* 2006; **52**: 1785–93.
40. Hapke EJ, Seal RM, Thomas GO et al. A clinical, radiographic, functional, and serological correlation of acute and chronic stages. *Thorax.* 1968; **23**: 451–68.
41. Cormier Y, Belanger J, Durand P. Factors influencing the development of serum precipitins to farmer's lung antigen in Quebec dairy farmers. *Thorax.* 1985; **40**: 138–42.
42. Roberts RC, Wenzel FJ, Emanuel DA. Precipitating antibodies in a midwest dairy farming population toward the antigens associated with farmer's lung disease. *Journal of Allergy and Clinical Immunology.* 1976; **57**: 518–24.
43. Barboriak JJ, Sosman AJ, Reed CE. Serological studies in pigeon breeder's disease. *Journal of Laboratory and Clinical Medicine.* 1965; **65**: 600–4.
44. Reynaud C, Slosman DO, Polla BS. Precipitins in bird breeder's disease: How useful are they? *European Respiratory Journal.* 1990; **3**: 1155–61.
45. Cormier Y, Belanger J. Long-term physiologic outcome after acute farmer's lung. *Chest.* 1985; **87**: 796–800.
46. Monkare S, Haahtela T. Farmer's lung – a 5-year follow-up of eighty-six patients. *Clinical Allergy* 1987; **17**: 143–51.
47. Cormier Y, Letourneau L, Racine G. Significance of precipitins and asymptomatic lymphocytic alveolitis: A 20-yr follow-up. *European Respiratory Journal.* 2004; **23**: 523–5.
48. Bourke SJ, Banham SW, Carter R et al. Longitudinal course of extrinsic allergic alveolitis in pigeon breeders. *Thorax.* 1989; **44**: 415–18.
49. Perez-Padilla R, Salas J, Chapela R et al. Mortality in Mexican patients with chronic pigeon breeder's lung compared with those with usual interstitial pneumonia. *American Review of Respiratory Disease.* 1993; **148**: 49–53.

50. Kokkarinen JI, Tukiainen HO, Terho EO. Effect of corticosteroid treatment on the recovery of pulmonary function in farmer's lung. *American Review of Respiratory Disease.* 1992; **145**: 3-5.
51. Ismail T, McSharry C, Boyd G. Extrinsic allergic alveolitis. *Respirology.* 2006; **11**: 262-8.
52. National Institute for Occupational Safety and Health. National occupational hazard survey. Washington, DC: United States Department of Health, Education, and Welfare, 1977.
53. Passman FJ, Rossmore HW. Reassessing the health risks associated with employee exposure to metalworking fluid microbes. *Lubrication Engineering.* 2002; **58**: 30-8.
54. Bernstein DI, Lummus ZL, Santilli G et al. Machine operator's lung. A hypersensitivity pneumonitis disorder associated with exposure to metalworking fluid aerosols. *Chest.* 1995; **108**: 636-41.
55. Fox J, Anderson H, Moen T et al. Metal working fluid-associated hypersensitivity pneumonitis: An outbreak investigation and case-control study. *American Journal of Industrial Medicine.* 1999; **35**: 58-67.
56. Gupta A, Rosenman KD. Hypersensitivity pneumonitis due to metal working fluids: Sporadic or under reported? *American Journal of Industrial Medicine.* 2006; **49**: 423-33.
57. Hodgson MJ, Bracker A, Yang C et al. Hypersensitivity pneumonitis in a metal-working environment. *American Journal of Industrial Medicine.* 2001; **39**: 616-28.
58. Friend JA, Gaddie J, Palmer KN et al. Extrinsic allergic alveolitis and contaminated cooling-water in a factory machine. *Lancet.* 1977; **1**: 297-300.
59. Dawkins P, Robertson A, Robertson W et al. An outbreak of extrinsic alveolitis at a car engine plant. *Occupational Medicine.* 2006; **56**: 559-65.
60. Robertson W, Robertson AS, Burge CB et al. Clinical investigation of an outbreak of alveolitis and asthma in a car engine manufacturing plant. *Thorax.* 2007; **62**: 981-90.
61. Banaszak EF, Thiede WH, Fink JN. Hypersensitivity pneumonitis due to contamination of an air conditioner. *New England Journal of Medicine.* 1970; **283**: 271-6.
62. Robertson AS, Burge PS, Wieland GA, Carmalt MH. Extrinsic allergic alveolitis caused by a cold water humidifier. *Thorax.* 1987; **42**: 32-7.
63. Newman Taylor A, Pickering CA, Turner-Warwick M, Pepys J. Respiratory allergy to a factory humidifier contaminant presenting as pyrexia of undetermined origin. *British Medical Journal.* 1978; **2**: 94-5.

SECTION THREE

Inorganic dust diseases

75	Inorganic dusts: general aspects *Anne Cockcroft*	985
76	Asbestos and asbestos-related diseases *David Weill and Anne Cockcroft*	990
77	Epidemiology of asbestos-related diseases *Robin M Rudd*	1000
78	Other fibrous mineral dusts *Anne Cockcroft*	1011
79	Silica and silica-related diseases *Anne Cockcroft*	1014
80	Epidemiology of silica-related disease *Kyle Steenland*	1021
81	Other non-fibrous mineral dusts *Anne Cockcroft*	1029
82	Metal dusts and fumes *Benoit Nemery*	1040
83	Berylliosis *Holly M Christensen and Lee S Newman*	1050

75

Inorganic dusts: general aspects

ANNE COCKCROFT

Pathogenesis of inorganic dust diseases	985	Acknowledgements	989
Investigation and diagnosis	986	References	989

PATHOGENESIS OF INORGANIC DUST DISEASES

The effects of inorganic dusts on the lung airways are relatively minor compared with those produced by the organic dusts (see Chapter 42, Organic chemicals) and by cigarette smoking. The main effects of inorganic dusts are in the lung parenchyma. The term 'pneumoconiosis' is used for all dust damage to the alveolar part of the lung, including the airways that have no mucociliary lining. By convention, the term does not include bronchitis, asthma or cancers. Exposure to inorganic dusts can also lead to effects outside the lung, such as cancers associated with asbestos, and cardiovascular effects of exposure to very small particles (see Chapter 70, Health effects of ultrafine particles). The features of lung disease due to occupational exposure to inorganic dusts depend not only on the dust itself, but also on features of the exposed individual, such as cigarette smoking, infection with tuberculosis, and genetic susceptibility. Relevant features of the dust, apart from its chemical composition, include the particle size; very small particles (less than 0.1 microns), such as encountered in general air pollution, are toxic at much lower levels of exposure than the conventional particles (0.1–10 microns) more usually encountered in the occupational setting (Chapter 70, Health effects of ultrafine particles). The shape of the dust particles is also important; fibrous dusts have different effects related to the length and width of the fibres. According to the World Health Organization (WHO) definition, a fibre is any particle longer than 5 μm, thinner than 3 μm, and with an aspect ratio greater than 3:1.

There are several common features in the process of lung damage due to retained inorganic dusts. The timing and relative importance of these depends on the dust load and the toxicity of the particular dust.

- The lung is damaged when alveolar macrophages die and the system fails to clear the dust landing beyond the mucociliary system.
- Where macrophages die, substances are released from the dying cells that provoke an inflammatory reaction – reactive oxygen species, cytokines and growth factors – all of which contribute to the damaging of the surrounding epithelial cells and stimulating abnormal growth of fibroblasts, for example. While often initially reversible, if this process occurs repeatedly in the same site, permanent damage is done to the structure of the lung. The site of the damage is determined by how far the macrophages get before they die. In a few cases, the macrophages die in the alveoli and the damage occurs there. However, it is more usual for them to die in aggregations around the centrilobular bronchioles or along the lymphatics leading to the hilar lymph nodes either via the interlobular septa and the pleura or along the bronchovascular bundles.
- The severity and form of the damage depends on the toxicity of the dust and the amount of exposure. Although cumulative exposure (exposure × time) is important, prolonged low level exposure is not necessarily as damaging as a short-term high exposure, especially if the dust is inherently very toxic.
- If the dust is of low toxicity, the pathological process may halt after exposure. However, for most dusts there is a progression (even if slow) of the pathology after exposure ceases, due to continuing reaction to the retained dust.
- The accumulation of dust in the phagocytic cells of the lung leads to release of inflammatory mediators from neutrophils and other cells.[1] The resulting migration and activation of leukocytes leads to proteolysis of fibronectin and subsequent laying down of fibrin,

reticulin and even collagen. The toxicity of mineral dusts at cellular level involves reactive oxygen species, cytokines, growth factors and proteases.[2,3] Some of the mediators involved have been proposed as suitable biomarkers of effect of dust inhalation.[4] The balance between tissue destruction and fibrosis differs depending on the nature of the dust. With coal dust and other relatively low toxicity dusts, there is typically some fibrosis in the form of a nodule, or macule, around the terminal bronchiole with some mild surrounding centrilobular emphysema. This causes little problem unless it progresses to more marked fibrotic changes or to more severe emphysema, as happens in some cases with heavy coal dust exposure. Silica, a more toxic dust, causes a more severe fibrotic reaction, but still mainly in discrete nodules. Adjacent foci of scarring may link up to form masses, and blood vessel walls may become involved leading to thrombosis and patchy necrosis. Asbestos more typically leads to a more diffuse fibrotic reaction, giving a form of interstitial fibrosis. In some cases, immune mechanisms may be involved in the tissue reaction to retained dust and this is discussed below in relation to specific dusts.

INVESTIGATION AND DIAGNOSIS

The diagnosis of occupational lung disease may be delayed or missed altogether because it is not considered. Without a history of exposure, the clinical features and radiographic appearances may be non-specific or suggestive of non-occupational disease.

Occupational history

Unlike diseases due to inhalation of organic dusts, most forms of pneumoconiosis do not cause immediate symptoms and most require prolonged exposure and have a long latency after first exposure. Therefore, the cause must be sought in past occupations (see Chapter 3, The occupational history). A general job classification, such as 'joiner' or 'fitter', is of no help without hearing what the worker actually did, what the industry was and what the dust conditions and the nature of the materials were.

The symptoms of bronchitis (persistent productive cough) may develop early, but it is usually many years before the worker notices either symptoms or disablement from the underlying disease. Radiographic changes may not develop until 10–20 years after exposure starts and may appear and progress long after exposure ceases. By the time the breathlessness of the pneumoconiosis is noticed, the radiographic changes are usually well advanced. In mild cases, symptoms may be attributed by the worker to 'old age' and may indeed be due to falling respiratory reserve (ageing of the normal lung) rather than progression of the dust disease. In the case of the asbestos-related cancers, the latent interval may average 40 years or more. Recent occupations are often unimportant, but past and present smoking habits are always important.

Symptoms

Breathlessness on exertion is often the only symptom. Cough and sputum can occur due to the dust exposure itself, but are frequently due to concomitant smoking. Complicated pneumoconiosis with cavitation of necrotic masses leads to the expectoration of large volumes of dirty material (once euphemistically called 'melanoptysis' in coalworkers) and sometimes to serious haemoptysis. The cavities left behind may become secondarily infected, causing a cough productive of copious foul sputum, similar to bronchiectasis.

Pneumoconiosis almost never causes pain. However, the chest tightness of a restrictive pathology (as in asbestosis or severe silicosis) can be mistaken for the 'tightness' of angina pain.

Signs

There are no physical signs in simple pneumoconiosis. They begin to appear as the disease becomes 'complicated'. Chest movement will be restricted a little if there is interstitial fibrosis or extensive pleural scarring which may also cause some dullness. Even the large masses of complicated pneumoconiosis before and after cavitation are usually not detectable on physical examination because they are relatively central and are surrounded by emphysematous lung.

Confluent fibrosis, such as occurs in asbestosis, is indistinguishable from other interstitial fibrotic lung disease and is associated with limited chest expansion, basal end-inspiratory 'dry' crepitations, cyanosis, polycythaemia and sometimes clubbing of the fingers.

Investigations

Ordinary haematological and biochemical tests are of no value in pneumoconiosis as they become abnormal only in extreme situations. The erythrocyte sedimentation rate and the plasma angiotensin converting enzyme level may indicate the activity of the destructive lesion in the lung, but have no diagnostic specificity. Tuberculin and Kveim tests, if positive, may indicate that the chest disease is tuberculosis or sarcoidosis, respectively, but there is no reliable way of distinguishing between beryllium pneumoconiosis and sarcoidosis in a worker with exposure to beryllium, except by performing a beryllium lymphocyte transformation test.

Examination of the sputum and bronchial lavage may yield confirmation of the occupational history in that the dust cells (dust-loaded macrophages) can be examined under the electron microscope and the nature of the dust identified. Asbestos bodies can be detected with the light microscope. They usually indicate amphibole exposure (which may be confirmed with the analytic electron microscope) and their profusion is a useful indication of the lung asbestos burden, but is not necessarily indicative of active disease. The cell count in the lavage fluid is increased in various forms of pneumoconiosis, but this is non-specific.

The role of biopsy is discussed below for individual diseases. On the whole, because of the focal nature of dust diseases, percutaneous and transbronchial biopsy have proved disappointing for diagnosis because the biopsy may miss the foci of disease. To determine the precise nature of the dust and its relationship to the pathology may require sophisticated electron microscopy of material taken at thoracotomy. However, it is rarely justifiable to undertake a thoracotomy to obtain a biopsy for diagnostic purposes. Biopsies obtained by thoracoscopy are less invasive and may represent an acceptable alternative in selected patients. On the other hand, in modern pneumology, 'crystals' or 'fibres' are often found in lung biopsies obtained for diagnosing interstitial lung disease, and it is not always easy in such cases to assign a causal role to these materials, which may or may not be incidental.

Chest radiography

Fortunately, most patients with a chest complaint have a chest radiograph and it is at this stage that either the radiologist or the clinician may realize that the disease is occupational. Even then, because many occupational lung diseases have non-specific radiographic features, cases are missed (see Chapter 33B1, Asbestos and asbestos-related diseases). The radiograph is useful in the diagnosis of the individual case, although the degree of radiographic abnormality is poorly related to the pathological severity of disease or the loss of lung function for many dusts. Some dusts produce dramatic radiographic shadows with little or no loss of lung function. In simple coalworkers' pneumoconiosis, the radiographic appearance of small, rounded opacities relates well to dust exposure, but almost not at all to lung function. In asbestosis, the radiographic abnormality is a poor guide to the pathological severity of disease. However, the chest radiograph is of particular value for epidemiological purposes. Radiographic surveys combined with exposure, lung function and pathology information have helped to determine whether certain patterns of change are associated with particular occupations. This sort of research has also helped to establish the relationships between radiology, lung function and pathology in groups of workers.

The ILO classification of radiographs of the pneumoconioses

Since 1930, the International Labour Office (ILO) in Geneva has sponsored a classification of the radiographic changes in pneumoconiosis which is used to describe the pattern and severity of the change in groups of workers. In principle, it is not intended as a method of diagnosis or of estimating the severity of an individual case. Despite many modifications, most recently in 2002,[5] there remains a subjective element in how an individual reader classifies a particular film. The reading is also dependent on the quality of the film (in particular how dark or light it is). Films should be read in batches mixed with controls and 'trigger' films. The readings are then analysed statistically to examine the relationship, if any, between radiographic changes and dust exposure measurements (or estimates of level of dust exposure). It is also possible to relate the radiographic changes to measurements of lung function in the population. Each batch of radiographs should be read independently by three trained observers and all the readings should be taken into account in the analysis. The readers should not be aware of any other information about the individuals whose films they read, to avoid bias. The method of reading is to compare each film with a set of standard films supplied by the ILO in Geneva. A brief description of the classification is given in Chapter 68, Imaging in occupational lung disease.

Lung function tests

Lung function tests are used in two ways in inorganic dust diseases: (1) to study exposed populations of workers and to follow individuals over time (in which case spirometry is the suitable measure) and (2) to diagnose individual cases of lung disease, in which case a battery of tests and comparison with predicted values is useful.

FOR SURVEYS AND MONITORING

In spite of their lack of specificity, the simple spirometric tests (forced vital capacity (FVC) and forced expiratory volume in 1 second (FEV_1)) are useful measures for either population surveys or long-term monitoring. Comparison with 'predicted' values for age, sex and height is not especially helpful. Measurements in groups of exposed workers can be compared with those in non-exposed workers and individuals can be compared with themselves over time. These tests are not particularly good indicators of parenchymal lung disease and they can be markedly affected by other conditions, such as asthma and chronic obstructive pulmonary disease due to smoking. They have proved useful and robust measures for several reasons:

- The equipment is cheap, easy to keep standardized and widely available.
- The tests are easy to learn and not frightening for the subject so that reliable, repeatable readings can usually be achieved after a few minutes' practice. Repeat tests at six-monthly or yearly intervals take less than five minutes.

- It is easy to train technicians to do the test properly, maintain the apparatus and calculate the results. Modern spirometers usually do the calculation automatically.

Electronic spirometers, now widely available, also give information about the whole of the flow-volume curve, allowing more sophisticated analysis of the curve to study dysfunction of the smaller airways. Unfortunately, the predicted results for the indices of small airways function from the flow-volume curve are much less reliable than the simple FEV_1 and FVC.

FOR DIAGNOSIS IN INDIVIDUAL CASES

In the diagnosis or assessment of the lung function deficit and disability in an individual case, a wide range of tests can be useful. Simple pneumoconiosis with dust macules forming around the centrilobular airways may or may not produce abnormalities in tests for small airways narrowing or compliance, depending on the severity. Early alveolar lesions or interstitial fibrosis may produce a reduction in gas transfer capacity. In practice, damage at either level produces abnormalities in both types of test, and either can be used as a measure of loss of lung function. Both types of test have proved useful in the detection of early disease in relatively young workers. Increasing age increases the scatter of findings in the 'normal' population. Much of this is due to cigarette smoking (and in the past to urban atmospheric pollution). The high proportion of smokers among workers in dusty occupations means that these tests may be of little diagnostic value in older individuals.

When lung function tests are used in individual diagnosis it is useful to compare with the values predicted for age, height and sex, derived from large studies for normal individuals. The normal populations used usually do not include smokers. Predicted values derived from one population may not be applicable to another ethnic group and it is important to use the most appropriate predicted values for an individual.

Post-mortem examination

Histological examination of autopsy material and the study of the dust extracted from the lung after death have been major sources of information about the nature and causes of occupational lung disease in the last 100 years. Although chest physicians with special experience may have little difficulty with the diagnosis of a pneumoconiosis during life, in the light of the occupational history, the chest radiograph and the pattern of lung function loss, the diagnosis is still often made by the pathologist on the basis of the post-mortem appearances and histology.

Until the 1990s, because of the arrangements in the United Kingdom for the granting of widows' pensions, most compensated cases of occupational lung disease came to autopsy, providing a source of important information to further understanding of these conditions. Similar material has been available in South Africa, but in many other countries it is difficult to obtain autopsy material and this has limited the study of the pathology of the pneumoconioses. With the discontinuation of the pension for widows of men dying with a pneumoconiosis, many fewer cases of suspected or confirmed occupational lung disease now come to autopsy in the UK. Studies comparing post-mortem lung pathology with radiographic appearances and lung function during life would now be very hard to mount.

A special technique helps the study of post-mortem lung pathology in suspected cases of occupational lung disease. The lungs are removed *en bloc* with the trachea and with the parietal pleura still attached if it is adherent. Any tears in the visceral pleura are oversewn and the lungs are fixed in inflation via the trachea either with formol-saline or with formalin vapour. After fixation (which takes several days) the lungs are cut into 1.0-cm thick slices and examined in detail before taking representative histological blocks. The slices may be recolourized with alcohol and photographed under water to provided a permanent record of the texture of the lung. Alternatively, they can be impregnated with gelatine and used to prepare 'Gough' paper-mounted whole lung sections (Figure 75.1).

Key points

- Disease related to inhalation of dusts occurs when the lung defences are overwhelmed; cellular mechanisms result in a mixture of tissue destruction and fibrosis, depending on the characteristics of the dust.
- Diagnosis requires a careful occupational history; the relevant exposure may have occurred many years ago and may not be apparent without a good knowledge of likely exposures in different occupations.
- Symptoms and signs are usually non-specific, but radiographic changes can be helpful, although they are often not a good indicator of disease severity.
- Lung biopsy is generally not appropriate for diagnostic purposes and may be unhelpful because it may miss the affected areas; lung histology with mineral analysis can be diagnostic.

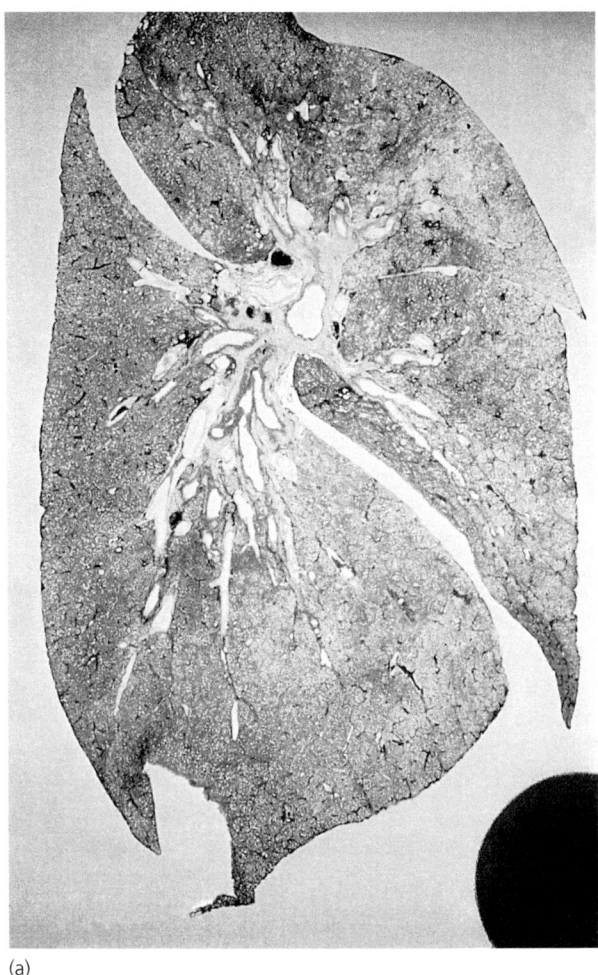 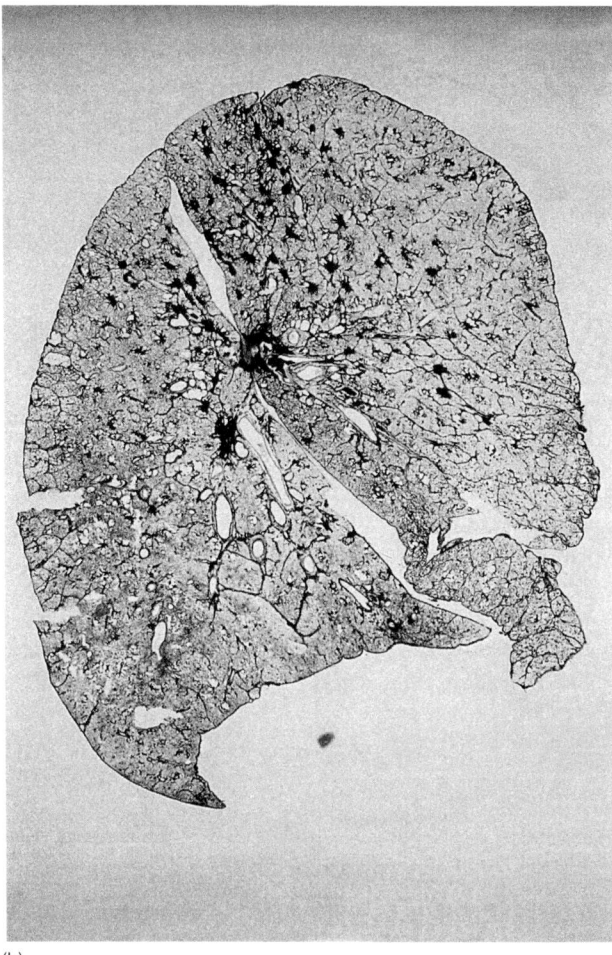

Figure 75.1 (a) Gough paper-mounted whole lung section of a normal lung. (b) Gough paper-mounted whole lung section of a lung with dust macules of simple coalworkers' pneumoconiosis.

ACKNOWLEDGEMENTS

Anne Cockcroft would like to acknowledge the contribution of the late Peter Elmes who authored the chapter on inorganic dusts in the seventh and eighth editions of *Hunter's Diseases of Occupations*.

REFERENCES

1. Rom WN. Relationship of inflammatory cell cytokines to disease severity in individuals with occupational inorganic dust exposure. *American Journal of Industrial Medicine.* 1991; **19**: 15–27.
2. Schins RPF, Borm PJA. Mechanisms and mediators in coal dust induced toxicity: A review. *Annals of Occupational Hygiene.* 1999; **43**: 7–33.
3. Castranova V, Vallyathan V. Silicosis and coal workers' pneumoconiosis. *Environmental Health Perspectives.* 2000; **108** (Suppl. 4): 675–84.
4. Gulumian M, Borm PJA, Vallyathan V et al. Mechanistically identified suitable biomarkers of exposure, effect, and susceptibility for silicosis and coal-worker's pneumoconiosis: A comprehensive review. *Journal of Toxicology and Environmental Health, Part B.* 2006; **9**: 357–95.
5. International Labour Office (ILO). Guidelines for the use of the ILO International Classification of Radiographs of Pneumoconioses, rev edn. Occupational Safety and Health Series, No. 22. Geneva: International Labour Office, 2002.

Asbestos and asbestos-related diseases

DAVID WEILL AND ANNE COCKCROFT

Introduction	990	Parietal pleural plaques	995
Asbestos minerals	990	Diffuse pleural thickening	995
Asbestosis	991	Benign asbestos pleural effusion	996
Mesothelioma	993	Chronic airways obstruction	996
Lung cancer	994	Health surveillance for asbestos workers	996
Benign asbestos-associated pleural disease	994	References	997

INTRODUCTION

Long ($>8\,\mu m$), thin ($<0.25\,\mu m$) particles (fibres) inhaled into the lung, especially if more than ten times as long as they are thick, are potentially capable of causing fibrosis and cancer, depending upon their chemical composition, toxicity and biopersistence. By far the most important are the asbestos family. Their industrial use started in the 1870s and there has been increasing awareness of the frequency and severity of their health hazards since 1930. Asbestos-related diseases have a long latency and remain common, and in many countries are continuing to increase in frequency.

Asbestos has been used in a wide variety of end products, including insulation materials, cement, brake linings, paint, textiles, gas masks and gaskets, until it was banned in the United States and European Union in the 1990s. Since then, in these countries, the most important exposures to asbestos have been to the material used in the past in the construction industry when it becomes disturbed by maintenance workers or during the demolition of old buildings. However, in much of the developing world, asbestos remains widely used and chrysotile asbestos continues to be mined in and exported from Russia and Canada.

ASBESTOS MINERALS

'Asbestos' is the general industrial term encompassing six different fibrous silicates and includes the serpentine mineral chrysotile which is structurally different from the rest, which are the amphiboles. They all result from the leaching by water of siliceous minerals and recrystallization in the interstices of the parent rock. Therefore, their metal content shows some variability within the limits set by the crystal lattices; the nomenclature is not very precise. Four varieties of asbestos have been used commercially: chrysotile (white), crocidolite (blue), amosite (brown) and anthophyllite. However, a number of other amphiboles, tremolite and actinolite, occur in a variety of commercially exploited minerals. They are all relatively inert to chemical attack, are poor conductors of heat and withstand temperatures up to 300–400°C, a property which has made them widely used to increase the fire resistance of buildings, ships and protective clothing.

Chrysotile (white asbestos)

Chrysotile is relatively abundant and easy to mine, producing bundles of soft flexible fibres up to several centimetres long. The longer fibres have been, and in some countries still are, used to make textiles and the shorter fibres for reinforcing cement and plastics and for insulation, friction materials and filters. The fibres split up easily to smaller bundles and eventually to individual fibrils. Each fibril consists of double sheets of brucite ($Mg(OH)_2$) and silica (SiO_2) rolled up like a scroll around a small core of amorphous magnesium silicate and forming a curved tube between 25 and 50 nm in diameter. The brucite forms the outer surface; in acid conditions, magnesium leaches out and the fibre disintegrates.

Chrysotile has always provided at least 90 per cent of the asbestos in commercial use and is mined in large deposits in central Russia and Quebec in Canada. Smaller deposits are mined in western Canada and the United States, in the Mediterranean basin, in southern Africa and in Australia. Some deposits, particularly those in the Mediterranean basin and a large one in western China, are associated with fibrous tremolite. This is less obvious in the Quebec deposits and it is not clear to what extent this has contaminated the chrysotile. Tremolite is a calcium magnesium silicate which crystallizes either as a platey talc (see Chapter 81) or as an amphibole fibre.

Crocidolite (blue asbestos)

Blue asbestos is mined in the Republic of South Africa, mainly in the Northern Cape and Western Cape provinces. Other deposits, notably one at Wittenoom in Western Australia, have been mined on a smaller scale. Crocidolite is found in banded ironstone which also yields commercial iron ore which crocidolite may contaminate. It is the fibrous form of the sodium iron silicate riebeckite. The bundles of fibres are much shorter and stiffer than chrysotile and readily split to straight fibrils with a minimum diameter of about 100 nm. It is much more resistant to acid and has slightly higher heat tolerance, but is not easily used for textiles unless supported by chrysotile. It was used where acid resistance was important and is still used in some countries in the manufacture of large-diameter asbestos cement pipes.

Amosite (brown asbestos)

Amosite is the commercial name for the fibrous grunerite (iron magnesium silicate), an amphibole mined in the Republic of South Africa; there are deposits elsewhere, but few are commercially viable. As mined, the fibres are coarse, but split down to 100 nm in use. It is used in insulation and as a reinforcement for plastic tiles, etc. It is too harsh for some forms of machine processing and is seldom used in cement or textiles for that reason.

Anthophyllite

This amphibole is the fibrous form of another iron magnesium silicate. It has been used mixed with clay for making pottery in Finland from prehistoric times and the same deposit was still worked until the end of the twentieth century. Its properties are similar to amosite and it has ceased to have any commercial value. Its occurrence is widespread and occasionally causes environmental problems where it contaminates the soil and becomes airborne.

ASBESTOSIS

Famously, the first report was by a woman factory inspector in 1898. William Cooke published a report of asbestos being associated with disease in 1924.[1] He described a patient who had worked in the Rochdale asbestos factory and developed a fibrotic lung disease. Thomas Oliver subsequently termed the lung condition 'asbestosis'.

Diagnosis of asbestosis

Asbestosis is a non-malignant, fibrotic parenchymal lung disease which can be static or slowly progressive. Progressive asbestosis can lead to profound respiratory disability and death from respiratory failure. Because histopathology is often not available in suspected cases of asbestosis, the diagnosis is usually based on clinical features and a history of significant occupational exposure. When pathologic material is available, the diagnosis is confirmed by the presence of both asbestos bodies and parenchymal fibrosis.[2] Asbestos bodies can also be found in the lung tissue of urban dwellers, but are not associated with surrounding lung parenchymal fibrosis.

The features that lead to a diagnosis of asbestosis include a history of asbestos exposure with a latent interval between exposure and disease (usually 15 years or longer); chest radiograph evidence of small irregular opacities; a restrictive pattern demonstrated by pulmonary function testing; and a diffusion capacity below normal.[2,3] Not all the features need be present to establish a diagnosis.

Physical signs and symptoms

FINGER CLUBBING

Finger clubbing can be associated with asbestosis, but it may also be a feature of other lung diseases, including idiopathic pulmonary fibrosis, cystic fibrosis and bronchogenic carcinoma. Less common causes of finger clubbing include bronchiectasis, cirrhosis, tuberculosis and lung abscess. In fact, finger clubbing is rare in asbestosis. However, when present, it is associated with a poor prognosis.[4]

BREATHLESSNESS

Breathlessness of insidious onset is a common early symptom of asbestosis. Chest pain occurs occasionally in advanced cases, with a significant restrictive defect or extensive pleural thickening. The presence of persistent chest pain should prompt an investigation to exclude an asbestos-related pleural effusion, lung cancer metastatic to the chest wall, or a mesothelioma.

NON-PRODUCTIVE COUGH

Non-productive cough is common, particularly as the disease advances, but a productive cough can be present in cigarette smokers who also have chronic bronchitis. Haemoptysis is not a feature of asbestosis. If haemoptysis occurs, it is important to exclude a concomitant bronchogenic carcinoma or other lung diseases commonly associated with haemoptysis (e.g. tuberculosis, pneumonia or pulmonary embolus).

WEIGHT LOSS

As with many lung diseases, advanced asbestosis usually results in weight loss, due to the significant caloric expenditure associated with tachypnea.

INSPIRATORY CRACKLES

The most consistent physical finding in patients with asbestosis is inspiratory crackles. Crackles (or rales) heard on chest auscultation are usually present in asbestosis, but can also be heard in patients with any interstitial lung disease, heart failure, bronchiectasis or pneumonia. Determining at what part of the respiratory cycle crackles are present has been suggested to be helpful in distinguishing among the lung diseases associated with this physical finding, but in fact there is considerable overlap. Crackles associated with asbestosis are typically fine and occur with each inspiratory effort, but this does not distinguish them from crackles due to any diffuse pulmonary fibrotic lung disease. In early disease, the crackles are mainly heard over the lower lung zones, but as the disease progresses they can be heard over all lung zones.

OTHER PHYSICAL SIGNS

Wheezes are not a feature of asbestosis and, if present, suggest the presence of chronic obstructive pulmonary disease or asthma. Both these conditions can coexist with asbestosis. A pleural rub can be heard in patients with diffuse pleural thickening. Cyanosis can be present in severe disease, as in any cardiopulmonary disorder that causes hypoxia. In advanced asbestosis, signs of right-sided heart failure (with raised jugular venous pressure, ascites and lower extremity oedema) develop.

Radiographic appearance

Chest radiographs are essential in the diagnosis of asbestosis. Asbestosis is generally characterized by lower lobe involvement with the presence of small irregular opacities (s, t, or u lesions). In advanced disease, these parenchymal abnormalities can be seen in all lung zones, but the first abnormalities are typically seen in the lower zones. As the disease progresses, the linear opacities become thicker and may ultimately obliterate the vascular markings; honeycombing can be seen, especially in the subpleural areas of the lower lobes. Large opacities are not seen in asbestosis, unless silica or coal dust exposure also occurred; the presence of large opacities raises the possibility of a lung malignancy.

The radiographic changes of asbestosis are similar to those of other diseases causing diffuse pulmonary fibrosis. The clinical course can give some hint about the aetiology of the diffuse lung infiltrates. For instance, rapid clinical progression would favour a diagnosis of idiopathic pulmonary fibrosis, rather than asbestosis.

Pleural abnormalities (either thickening or plaques) are commonly present together with the parenchymal changes of asbestosis. Diffuse pleural thickening is usually seen in the lower and middle third of the chest and is often asymmetric. It often leads to costophrenic angle obliteration and is, in fact, distinguished from pleural plaques by the presence of costophrenic angle abnormalities. Pleural plaques, either calcified or non-calcified, are discrete and do not extend into the costophrenic angle. Oblique radiographs can help to distinguish pleural thickening from overlying fat.

Rounded atelectasis is a radiographic finding highly characteristic of asbestosis. It represents a folded area of pleura which traps the adjacent lung tissue. Rounded atelectasis may be mistaken for a lung mass and lead to unnecessary further investigation. Because of its characteristic appearance on computed tomography (CT) ('comma sign'), rounded atelectasis can usually be confidently diagnosed by experienced chest radiologists based on CT findings (see Chapter 68, Imaging in occupational lung disease, Figure 68.12). If uncertainty remains, serial CT scanning can help exclude a malignancy.

Computed tomography scanning has increased the diagnostic sensitivity for asbestosis (see Chapter 68, Imaging in occupational lung disease, Figure 68.11a,b).[5] High-resolution computed tomography (HRCT) scanning reveals parenchymal and pleural abnormalities not detected by plain radiography. CT scanning can help to distinguish *en face* pleural plaques from parenchymal lesions and to identify parenchymal abnormalities when pleural changes obscure the lung parenchyma on plain chest radiographs. Unfortunately, CT scanning does little to help distinguish asbestosis from other fibrotic lung diseases, such as idiopathic pulmonary fibrosis, collagen vascular-associated interstitial lung disease, and drug-induced lung diseases. Studies that support the higher sensitivity of HRCT in diagnosing asbestosis[6–8] are limited by low specificity. When using HRCT, the challenge to the clinician is whether or not to assign clinical significance to marginally abnormal CT scans.

Pathophysiology

The physiological abnormalities associated with asbestosis are due to the parenchymal fibrosis that characterizes the disease. Typically with advanced asbestosis, there is reduced lung compliance with a restrictive ventilatory defect. There is usually a reduction in the residual volume (RV) and the total lung capacity (TLC). However, because some patients with asbestosis also have emphysema (characterized by increased RV and TLC), a normal or even increased RV and TLC can be present, depending on the relative contribution of each disease. This situation results in a mixed obstructive–restrictive defect. Because of replacement by scarring of the gas exchange surface at the alveolar level, a reduction of the diffusing capacity is often present, and some authors have identified a reduced diffusing capacity as an early indicator of disease. Furthermore, because of the presence of low lung compliance, minute ventilation is increased, with an increased respiratory rate and reduced tidal volume. The ventilation changes are particularly marked at the lung bases, the area of the lung most involved in asbestosis. All the abnormalities of respiratory mechanics are exacerbated by exercise and exercise testing is one way to unmask occult disease. The pathophysiological findings associated with asbestosis are non-specific and can be found in any of the restrictive lung diseases.

The role of the small airways in the pathophysiology associated with asbestosis remains unclear, largely because much of the information comes from cohorts with a high prevalence of cigarette smoking. While structural abnormalities have been demonstrated in the small airways of exposed workers,[9] the findings are often confounded by the effects of cigarette smoking in the populations studied. Furthermore, studies which purportedly demonstrated a small airways effect from asbestos exposure relied on the FEF_{25-75}, which is an effort-dependent test that has large variability. In a study by Begin et al. analysing a non-smoking asbestos-exposed cohort, the workers did have an increase in airflow resistance, but this predominantly occurred in patients who also had restriction. In the non-smoking workers who did not have restriction, physiological abnormalities in the small airways were small.[10]

Pathological findings

When other causes of diffuse interstitial lung disease are a serious possibility, a lung biopsy (preferably by obtaining adequate tissue through a surgical approach) should be considered. A diagnosis of asbestosis is confirmed by the finding of asbestos bodies together with parenchymal fibrosis. However, asbestos bodies are mainly formed on amphibole fibres over 20 μm long and their number underestimates the lung burden of thinner fibres. They are a poor indicator of the presence of chrysotile. Lavage of the airways in asbestosis yields increased numbers of polymorphs, as well as asbestos bodies and fibres.

Prognosis

While asbestosis itself may progress to respiratory failure and death, the major cause of death in individuals with asbestosis is asbestos-related malignancy: lung cancer or mesothelioma. Between 1952 and 1976, an analysis of men certified as having asbestosis in the United Kingdom reported that for all causes the observed number of deaths was 2.6 times expectation and for lung cancer 9.1 times expectation; 39 per cent of the deaths were from lung cancer, 9 per cent mesothelioma and 20 per cent asbestosis.[11]

MESOTHELIOMA

Mesothelioma can be either benign or malignant. Nearly all malignant mesotheliomas are due to asbestos exposure. Such exposure can be brief and low level, such as living near an asbestos factory or a wife washing the clothes of an asbestos worker (Chapter 77, Epidemiology of asbestos-related diseases). Diffuse malignant mesothelioma is a progressive disease, which can affect the pleura, peritoneum, pericardium or tunica vaginalis.

Radiographic appearance

Pleural mesotheliomas generally present radiographically as a unilateral pleural effusion. In some cases, the pleural effusion is accompanied by the appearance of a pleural-based mass, or masses, which may look nodular (see Chapter 68, Imaging in occupational lung disease, Figures 68.9 and 68.10). Mediastinal structures may be shifted away from the side of the tumour or toward the tumour side when the predominant tissue reaction to the mesothelioma is pleural fibrosis. Pleural mesotheliomas may or may not be associated with concomitant pleural plaques or asbestosis. As the tumour advances, compression of adjacent organs, such as the heart, can occur, as can distortion of the central airways and destruction of adjacent ribs.

Pathology

Pleural biopsy, ideally by video-assisted thoracoscopic surgery (VATS), is the diagnostic gold standard for mesothelioma. Using VATS, tumour studding of the pleural surface can be appreciated, and the surgeon is able to perform biopsies under direct vision. Another benefit of this procedure is the ability to mobilize the lung and to perform cytoreductive pleurectomy.[12] The diagnosis can be difficult in individual cases. There are several types of malignant mesothelioma: an epithelial type, which can be mistaken for adenocarcinoma; a sarcomatous type, which can mimic other sarcomatous cancers; and a mixed type.[13] Immunochemical staining techniques can help to confirm the diagnosis in individual cases.

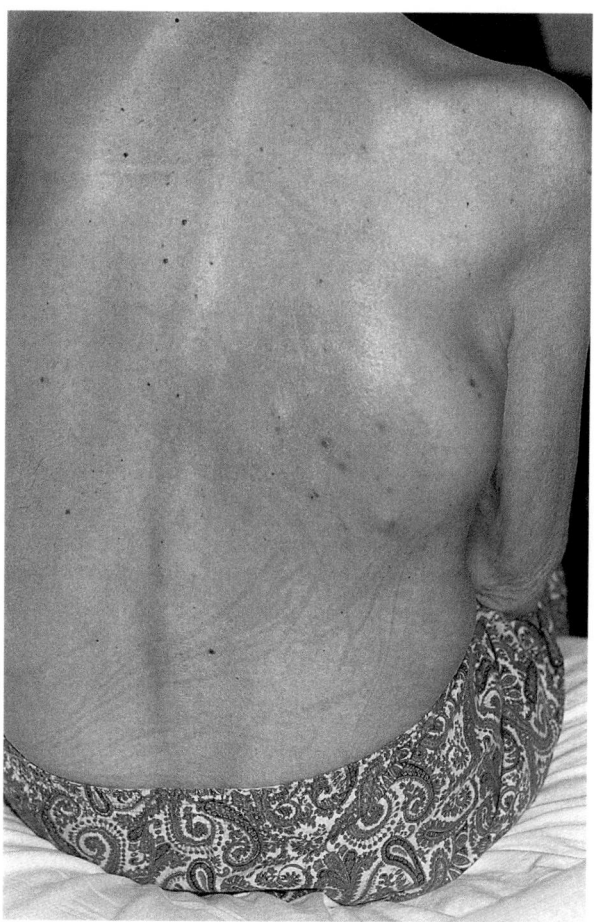

Figure 76.1 Mesothelioma that has grown through the chest wall along the track of needles used to aspirate the pleural fluid.

Prognosis

The prognosis for patients with diffuse malignant mesothelioma is very poor. The tumour grows inexorably, compressing the lungs and mediastinal structures. Distal metastasis is rare, but the tumour may spread into the chest wall, sometimes along the track of needles used to aspirate pleural fluid (Figure 76.1). Most patients die within two years, usually of respiratory failure or bronchopneumonia. Extrapleural pneumonectomy has been the traditional operative approach, but the results have been discouraging. Response rates to chemotherapy have traditionally not exceeded 30 per cent, but newer agents, for example antimetabolites such as pemetrexed, appear more promising. Response rates of up to 45 per cent have been achieved when these agents are used in combination with platinum compounds.

LUNG CANCER

From a clinical perspective, lung cancer in an asbestos-exposed individual is similar to that found in non-exposed people. For example, it might present with haemoptysis, or a mass detected on the chest radiograph, or with the effects of secondary spread elsewhere.

Pathogenesis

The role of asbestos in lung cancer development probably involves common biochemical pathways that lead to both fibrosis and carcinogenesis. While initially thought to be 'scar carcinomas' (i.e. tumours that arise in a scarred area of lung due to transformation of the fibrotic tissue into cancerous tissue), lung cancers that occur in association with asbestos exposure probably do so as a result of molecular pathways that cause damage to DNA, leading either to fibrosis or to cancer development. Whether an individual patient develops fibrosis or cancer or both probably depends on the nature and the extent of the cellular damage. In a study of lung cancer in patients with cryptogenic (idiopathic) fibrosing alveolitis, Turner-Warwick et al.[14] found a relative risk of lung cancer of 14 in male smokers with lung fibrosis, compared with smokers without lung fibrosis. This suggests that lung fibrosis, from whatever cause, may be a marker for those with excess cancer risk. Similar studies have shown an excess cancer risk in patients with another fibrosing lung disease (scleroderma), allowing for age and smoking.[15,16]

In support of the idea that lung fibrosis and lung cancer may be due to a common mechanism, rather than the cancer arising from the fibrotic process, it is notable that, while the fibrosis of asbestosis affects predominantly the lower lung zones, lung cancers associated with asbestosis do not seem to have a predilection for any particular lung zone.[17,18] Furthermore, while most 'scar carcinomas' are adenocarcinomas, the lung cancers associated with asbestosis can be of any cell type[19] and are pathologically indistinguishable from cancers attributable to cigarette smoking.[18,20]

BENIGN ASBESTOS-ASSOCIATED PLEURAL DISEASE

Benign asbestos-associated pleural disease includes parietal pleural plaques, diffuse pleural fibrosis and benign asbestos pleural effusions. In any individual patient, a combination of the pleural diseases may be present. While most cases of pleural disease are seen after asbestos exposure in the occupational setting, there can be pleural changes in individuals with lower levels of exposure occurring in the non-occupational environment. The precise mechanism by which asbestos exposure leads to pleural disease occurring is poorly understood but probably involves the translocation of inhaled fibres to the pleura, where they cause an inflammatory reaction on the parietal pleural surface. The inflammatory reaction can lead to fibrosis or development of a pleural effusion.

PARIETAL PLEURAL PLAQUES

The association of pleural plaques with asbestos exposure was first described by Sparks in 1931.[21] Pleural plaques are localized, discrete areas of dense fibrosis located on the parietal pleural surface, generally on the diaphragmatic pleural surface or along the lateral chest wall or, more rarely, on the pericardium. They may calcify.[22] Plaques on the lateral chest wall are usually sharply demarcated from the adjacent lung parenchyma and are termed 'in profile' plaques. Plaques on the anterior or posterior chest wall are known as 'en face' plaques. There is a long latency and it is uncommon for pleural plaques to occur within 20 years of first exposure to asbestos.

Radiographic appearance

Pleural plaques appear on the chest radiograph as areas of discrete pleural thickening with or without calcification (Chapter 68, Imaging in occupational lung disease, Figure 68.12). They are more easily detected when calcium is present, creating a dense, 'white' appearance on the chest radiograph. The revised 2000 International Labor Office (ILO) classification describes plaques as, by definition, not involving the costophrenic angle. Pleural plaques are most easily seen when in profile. The width of in profile plaques can vary from about 0.5 to 1.0 cm. En face plaques on the anterior and posterior thoracic wall appear as hazy, ill-defined opacities overlying the lung parenchyma. Pleural plaques can be confused radiographically with shadows due to the serratus anterior muscle or due to excess subpleural fat in obese individuals.[23] Pleural fat pads typically start at the lung apex and extend down the lateral chest wall. Other diseases which cause pleural calcification and which can be confused with pleural plaques due to asbestos exposure include tuberculosis, chronic empyema and trauma to the chest wall; in all of these cases, the pleural changes are typically unilateral. If there is uncertainty about the presence of pleural plaques, oblique chest radiographs can be helpful. CT scans are more sensitive in detecting pleural abnormalities (Chapter 68, Imaging in occupational lung disease, Figure 68.7).[24-26] However, due to cost, the use of routine CT scanning is impractical.

Functional significance

Most individuals with pleural plaques are asymptomatic and have no measurable physiologic impairment.[27,28] Many of the studies purporting to demonstrate functional impairment due to pleural plaques did not make a distinction between individuals with localized pleural plaques alone and those who also had diffuse pleural thickening, or were unable to exclude the presence of concomitant parenchymal lung disease not detected by routine chest radiography.[29] Several authors have reported no additional functional impairment associated with pleural plaques, over and above those associated with underlying parenchymal abnormalities.[30,31] A study of railroad workers exposed to asbestos reported a decrease in FVC associated with the presence and the extent of the plaques.[32] However, there were more smokers and older workers in the group with plaques. The presence of parenchymal fibrosis in individuals with pleural plaques seems to be the important factor leading to lung function deficits.[33]

Prognosis

Some studies have shown a higher risk of mesothelioma among people with pleural plaques.[34] However, it remains unclear whether this is simply because both pleural plaques and mesothelioma are associated with asbestos exposure, or whether the presence of pleural plaques actually indicates sufficient exposure to increase the risk of mesothelioma development.

The association between pleural plaques and lung cancer has also been debated in the medical literature. A study of asbestos cement workers found the presence of pleural plaques was not associated with an increased lung cancer risk.[35] A meta-analysis of 13 studies concluded that people with asbestos-related pleural plaques did not have an increased risk of lung cancer in the absence of parenchymal asbestosis.[36] A more recent study of Finnish construction workers also concluded the risk of lung cancer was not increased by the presence of pleural plaques. However, a study from Sweden, which controlled for the presence of asbestosis, concluded that pleural plaques not only implied significant exposure to asbestos, but also were associated with an increased risk for mesothelioma and a small increased risk of lung cancer.[37]

DIFFUSE PLEURAL THICKENING

Radiographic appearance

Diffuse pleural thickening can be seen on plain chest radiographs (Chapter 68, Imaging in occupational lung disease, Figure 68.8), but is more easily seen on CT scans.[26] According to the 2000 ILO classification system, diffuse pleural thickening by definition includes involvement of the costophrenic angle. Thickening of the visceral pleura can be either unilateral or bilateral. If unilateral, the differential diagnosis includes pleural fibrosis from previous pneumonia with pleural reaction, empyema, trauma and mesothelioma. Bilateral pleural thickening can also be seen in collagen vascular diseases, such as rheumatoid arthritis, scleroderma or systemic lupus erythematosus. Up to one-third of patients with diffuse pleural thickening may have had a previous benign asbestos-related pleural effusion or pleurisy.[38]

Functional significance

Several authors have reported an association between diffuse pleural thickening and restrictive lung function abnormalities[38] or a reduction in diffusing capacity.[39] One study reported obstructive lung function loss in men with pleural disease.[40] Overall, most patients with diffuse pleural thickening are asymptomatic. Some may have breathlessness, cough with sputum production and chest pain.[41–43]

BENIGN ASBESTOS PLEURAL EFFUSION

An asbestos-related pleural effusion was first reported in the medical literature in 1964.[44] The pathophysiology of these effusions is not entirely clear, but probably involves pleural inflammation from direct toxicity to mesothelial cells by asbestos fibres. Inhaled asbestos fibres can also indirectly cause pleural injury by the release of growth factors and inflammatory cytokines from the lung.

Patients who present with a pleural effusion, particularly those with a history of asbestos exposure, should undergo diagnostic thoracentesis with cytological analysis. If a clear aetiology of the effusion is not forthcoming, pleural biopsy should be considered, particularly to exclude the presence of mesothelioma.

Several authors have studied pleural effusions among asbestos-exposed populations, sometimes in comparison with non-exposed populations.[45–48] The latent period for the development of these effusions is relatively short, often less than 20 years, and they are the most common asbestos-related abnormality within 20 years of first exposure. The incidence increases with increasing degrees of asbestos exposure, up to around nine per 1000 person-years for heavy exposure. The effusions may be recurrent. Many are asymptomatic and transient (lasting a matter of months), so their true incidence is probably higher than that estimated in prevalence studies. Those with symptoms most commonly complain of chest pain, fever, cough and breathlessness. The effusions are usually blood-stained. Follow-up studies of cases of asbestos pleural effusion over two to three decades have reported a low incidence of subsequent mesothelioma, not necessarily on the same side as the effusion. Asbestos effusions do seem to be a risk factor for the development of diffuse pleural thickening.

CHRONIC AIRWAYS OBSTRUCTION

Although asbestos has traditionally been considered to cause a restrictive lung function impairment, some authors have reported airways obstruction in asbestos-exposed workers who have normal radiographs with no clinical evidence of asbestosis.[49,50] The mechanism by which asbestos may cause airway obstruction is unclear, but may involve the deposition of asbestos in the small airways, leading to an inflammatory response that causes airway fibrosis.[51–53] Whatever the mechanism, the confounding effects of cigarette smoking have been a limitation of many of the studies investigating this issue. One such study by Weill et al.[54] reported a dose–response relationship between asbestos exposure and small airways dysfunction, but did not find evidence of clinically significant obstructive disease. In a study of asbestos insulators, the authors concluded that reduced FVC and reduced FEV_1/FVC were both more frequent in insulators who smoked (compared with non-smoking insulators or smokers in the general population), suggesting an interaction between asbestos and smoking in producing both these physiologic abnormalities. However, airways obstruction in the absence of radiographic abnormalities and/or cigarette smoking was uncommon.[50] Other studies have been unable to find differences in the prevalence of obstruction in smoking and non-smoking groups.[55,56] Some authors have concluded that there is evidence of airways obstruction related to asbestos exposure,[57,58] but others have challenged this conclusion.[59]

If there is a direct asbestos effect on the airways, it probably only involves the small airways, and is small and clinically insignificant, particularly when compared to the effect of cigarette smoke on airway function.[60,61] Airway fibrosis following asbestos inhalation has been demonstrated in animal models, but the significance of this for humans is unclear. Significant respiratory disability in asbestos-exposed workers is due to a restrictive, rather than an obstructive, process.

HEALTH SURVEILLANCE FOR ASBESTOS WORKERS

Although the importation and use of asbestos is now banned in industrialized countries, exposure to old asbestos, especially in the construction industry, remains a potential hazard. As well as strict controls to prevent exposure and protect workers, health surveillance of those working with asbestos-containing materials is a requirement in most industrialized countries. In the United Kingdom, work with asbestos (e.g. stripping old asbestos-containing materials from buildings) requires a licence from the Health and Safety Executive, and the licence requires employers to provide health surveillance and maintain the records for 40 years.[62] The pre-employment and periodic examination of workers includes enquiry about respiratory symptoms, examination of the chest, chest radiography when indicated and lung function testing.[63]

People who are not asbestos workers, but discover they have been inadvertently exposed to asbestos (for example, from frayed insulation material), or have had some other unforeseen but minimal exposure to asbestos at work, are understandably anxious and concerned about possible effects on their health. Although the type of asbestos may be known, there is often little, if any, reliable information concerning the amount of asbestos which may have been inhaled. They can be reassured that the risk to their health is very low; it is advisable that their general practitioner documents the incident in their medical record.[63] Chest radiography and lung function testing are not appropriate after an inadvertent exposure, given the very low risk and the long latency of asbestos-related lung effects.

Key points

- Four varieties of asbestos have been used commercially: chrysotile (white), crocidolite (blue), amosite (brown) and anthophyllite.
- Asbestosis is a type of interstitial fibrosis; it can lead to death from respiratory failure, but the major cause of death in people with asbestosis is lung cancer or mesothelioma.
- Mesothelioma is a tumour of the pleura (or rarely peritoneum) that usually leads to death within two years; diagnosis is confirmed by histology, but sometimes it is difficult to differentiate mesothelioma from other cancers.
- Lung cancer related to asbestos exposure is clinically similar to lung cancer from other causes.
- Pleural plaques, which may calcify, are a marker of asbestos exposure, but do not themselves cause any loss of function.
- Diffuse pleural thickening, by definition, includes involvement of the costophrenic angle on the chest radiograph; extensive pleural thickening may lead to some restrictive lung function deficit.
- Asbestos exposure has little, if any, effect on the airways.

REFERENCES

1. Cooke W. Fibrosis of the lungs due to inhalation of asbestos dust. *British Medical Journal*. 1924; **2**: 147.
2. American Thoracic Society. Medical Section of the American Lung Association. The diagnosis of nonmalignant diseases related to asbestos. *American Review of Respiratory Disease*. 1986; **134**: 363-8.
3. Ohar J, Sterling DA, Bleecker E *et al*. Changing patterns in asbestos-induced lung disease. *Chest*. 2004; **125**: 744-53.
4. Coutts II, Gilson JC, Kerr IH *et al*. Significance of finger clubbing in asbestosis. *Thorax*. 1987; **42**: 117-19.
5. Lozewicz S, Reznek RH, Herdman M *et al*. Role of computed tomography in evaluating asbestos related lung disease. *British Journal of Industrial Medicine*. 1989; **46**: 777-81.
6. Neri S, Antonelli A, Falaschi F *et al*. Findings from high resolution computed tomography of the lung and pleura of symptom free workers exposed to amosite who had normal chest radiographs and pulmonary function tests. *Occupational and Environmental Medicine*. 1994; **51**: 239-43.
7. Neri S, Boraschi P, Antonelli A *et al*. Pulmonary function, smoking habits, and high resolution computed tomography (HRCT) early abnormalities of lung and pleural fibrosis in shipyard workers exposed to asbestos. *American Journal of Industrial Medicine*. 1996; **30**: 588-95.
8. Staples CA, Gamsu G, Ray CS, Webb WR. High resolution computed tomography and lung function in asbestos-exposed workers with normal chest radiographs. *American Review of Respiratory Disease*. 1989; **139**: 1502-8.
9. Churg A, Wright JL, Wiggs B *et al*. Small airways disease and mineral dust exposure. Prevalence, structure, and function. *American Review of Respiratory Disease*. 1985; **131**: 139-43.
10. Begin R, Cantin A, Berthiaume Y *et al*. Airway function in lifetime-nonsmoking older asbestos workers. *American Journal of Medicine*. 1983; **75**: 631-8.
11. Berry G. Mortality of workers certified by pneumoconiosis medical panels as having asbestosis. *British Journal of Industrial Medicine*. 1981; **38**: 130-7.
12. Grossebner MW, Arifi AA, Goddard M, Ritchie AJ. Mesothelioma: VATS biopsy and lung mobilization improves diagnosis and palliation. *European Journal of Cardiothoracic Surgery*. 1999; **16**: 619-23.
13. Corson JM. Pathology of mesothelioma. *Thoracic Surgery Clinics*. 2004; **14**: 447-60.
14. Turner-Warwick M, Lebowitz M, Burrows B *et al*. Cryptogenic fibrosing alveolitis and lung cancer. *Thorax*. 1980; **35**: 496-9.
15. Roumm AD, Medsger TA Jr. Cancer and systemic sclerosis. An epidemiologic study. *Arthritis and Rheumatology*. 1985; **28**: 1336-40.
16. Peters-Golden M, Wise RA, Hochberg M *et al*. Incidence of lung cancer in systemic sclerosis. *Journal of Rheumatology*. 1985; **12**: 1136-9.
17. Weiss W. Asbestosis and lobar site of lung cancer. *Occupational and Environmental Medicine*. 2000; **57**: 358-60.
18. Brodkin CA, McCullough J, Stover B *et al*. Lobe of origin and histologic type of lung cancer associated with asbestos exposure in the Carotene and Retinol Efficacy Trial (CARET). *American Journal of Industrial Medicine*. 1997; **32**: 582-91.
19. Churg A. Lung cancer cell type and asbestos exposure. *Journal of the American Medical Association*. 1985; **253**: 2984-5.
20. Auerbach O, Garfinkel L, Parks VR *et al*. Histologic type of lung cancer and asbestos exposure. *Cancer*. 1984; **54**: 3017-21.
21. Gloyne S. Pathology. In: Lanza A (ed.). *Silicosis and asbestosis*. New York: Oxford University Press, 1938: 120-35.
22. Rubino GF, Scansetti G, Pira E *et al*. Pleural plaques and lung asbestos bodies in the general population: An autoptical and clinical-radiological survey. *IARC Scientific Publications*. 1980; **30**: 545-51.

23. Sargent EN, Boswell Jr WD, Ralls PW, Markovitz A. Subpleural fat pads in patients exposed to asbestos: Distinction from non-calcified pleural plaques. *Radiology.* 1984; **152**: 273–7.
24. Aberle DR, Gamsu G, Ray CS. High-resolution CT of benign asbestos-related diseases: Clinical and radiographic correlation. *American Journal of Roentgenology.* 1988; **151**: 883–91.
25. Friedman AC, Fiel SB, Fisher MS *et al.* Asbestos-related pleural disease and asbestosis: A comparison of CT and chest radiography. *American Journal of Roentgenology.* 1988; **150**: 269–75.
26. al Jarad N, Poulakis N, Pearson MC *et al.* Assessment of asbestos-induced pleural disease by computed tomography: Correlation with chest radiograph and lung function. *Respiratory Medicine.* 1991; **85**: 203–8.
27. Copley SJ, Wells AU, Rubens MB *et al.* Functional consequences of pleural disease evaluated with chest radiography and CT. *Radiology.* 2001; **220**: 237–43.
28. Van Cleemput J, De Raeve H, Verschakelen JA *et al.* Surface of localized pleural plaques quantitated by computed tomography scanning: No relation with cumulative asbestos exposure and no effect on lung function. *American Journal of Respiratory and Critical Care Medicine.* 2001; **163**: 705–10.
29. Schwartz DA, Fuortes LJ, Galvin JR *et al.* Asbestos-induced pleural fibrosis and impaired lung function. *American Review of Respiratory Disease.* 1990; **141**: 321–6.
30. Sette A, Neder JA, Nery LE *et al.* Thin-section CT abnormalities and pulmonary gas exchange impairment in workers exposed to asbestos. *Radiology.* 2004; **232**: 66–74.
31. Gaensler EA, Jederlinic PJ, McLoud TC. Lung function with asbestos-related pleural plaques, Part I. Proceedings of the VIIth International Pneumoconiosis Conference, 1990: 696–702.
32. Oliver LC, Eisen EA, Greene R, Sprince NL. Asbestos-related pleural plaques and lung function. *American Journal of Industrial Medicine.* 1988; **14**: 649–56.
33. Fridriksson HV, Hedenstrom H, Hillerdal G, Malmberg P. Increased lung stiffness of persons with pleural plaques. *European Journal of Respiratory Diseases.* 1981; **62**: 412–24.
34. Hillerdal G. Pleural plaques and risk for bronchial carcinoma and mesothelioma. A prospective study. *Chest.* 1994; **105**: 144–50.
35. Hughes JM, Weill H. Asbestosis as a precursor of asbestos related lung cancer: Results of a prospective mortality study. *British Journal of Industrial Medicine.* 1989; **46**: 537–40.
36. Weiss W. Asbestos-related pleural plaques and lung cancer. *Chest.* 1993; **103**: 1854–9.
37. Koskinen K, Pukkala E, Martikainen R *et al.* Different measures of asbestos exposure in estimating risk of lung cancer and mesothelioma among construction workers. *Journal of Occupational and Environmental Medicine.* 2002; **44**: 1190–6.
38. Yates DH, Browne K, Stidolph PN, Neville E. Asbestos-related bilateral diffuse pleural thickening: Natural history of radiographic and lung function abnormalities. *American Journal of Respiratory and Critical Care Medicine.* 1996; **153**: 301–6.
39. Kee ST, Gamsu G, Blanc P. Causes of pulmonary impairment in asbestos-exposed individuals with diffuse pleural thickening. *American Journal of Respiratory and Critical Care Medicine.* 1996; **154**: 789–93.
40. Kilburn KH, Warshaw RH. Abnormal lung function associated with asbestos disease of the pleura, the lung, and both: A comparative analysis. *Thorax.* 1991; **46**: 33–8.
41. Ameille J, Matrat M, Paris C *et al.* Asbestos-related pleural diseases: Dimensional criteria are not appropriate to differentiate diffuse pleural thickening from pleural plaques. *American Journal of Industrial Medicine.* 2004; **45**: 289–96.
42. Kouris SP, Parker DL, Bender AP, Williams AN. Effects of asbestos-related pleural disease on pulmonary function. *Scandinavian Journal of Work, Environment and Health.* 1991; **17**: 179–83.
43. McGavin CR, Sheers G. Diffuse pleural thickening in asbestos workers: Disability and lung function abnormalities. *Thorax.* 1984; **39**: 604–7.
44. Eisenstadt HB. Asbestos pleurisy. *Diseases of the Chest.* 1964; **46**: 78–81.
45. Robinson BW, Musk AW. Benign asbestos pleural effusion: Diagnosis and course. *Thorax.* 1981; **36**: 896–900.
46. Epler GR, McLoud TC, Gaensler EA. Prevalence and incidence of benign asbestos pleural effusion in a working population. *Journal of the American Medical Association.* 1982; **247**: 617–22.
47. Hillerdal G, Ozesmi M. Benign asbestos pleural effusion: 73 exudates in 60 patients. *European Journal of Respiratory Diseases.* 1987; **71**: 113–21.
48. Cookson WO, De Klerk NH, Musk AW *et al.* Benign and malignant pleural effusions in former Wittenoom crocidolite millers and miners. *Australian and New Zealand Journal of Medicine.* 1985; **15**: 731–7.
49. Zejda JE. Occupational exposure to dusts containing asbestos and chronic airways disease. *International Journal of Occupational Medicine and Environmental Health.* 1996; **9**: 117–25.
50. Miller A, Lilis R, Godbold J *et al.* Spirometric impairments in long-term insulators. Relationships to duration of exposure, smoking, and radiographic abnormalities. *Chest.* 1994; **105**: 175–82.
51. Dai J, Gilks B, Price K *et al.* Mineral dusts directly induce epithelial and interstitial fibrogenic mediators and matrix components in the airway wall. *American Journal of Respiratory and Critical Care Medicine.* 1998; **158**: 1907–13.
52. Filipenko D, Wright JL, Churg A. Pathologic changes in the small airways of the guinea pig after amosite asbestos exposure. *American Journal of Pathology.* 1985; **119**: 273–8.
53. Wright JL, Churg A. Morphology of small-airway lesions in patients with asbestos exposure. *Human Pathology.* 1984; **15**: 68–74.
54. Weill H, Morton M, Waggenspack C, Rossiter CE. Lung function consequences of dust exposure in asbestos cement manufacturing plants. *Archives of Environmental Health.* 1975; **30**: 88–97.

55. Griffith DE, Garcia JG, Dodson RF *et al.* Airflow obstruction in nonsmoking, asbestos- and mixed dust-exposed workers. *Lung.* 1993; **171**: 213–24.
56. Dossing M, Groth S, Vestbo J *et al.* Small-airways dysfunction in never smoking asbestos exposed Danish plumbers. *International Archives of Occupational and Environmental Health.* 1990; **62**: 209–12.
57. Kilburn KH, Warshaw RH, Einstein K *et al.* Airway disease in non-smoking asbestos workers. *Archives of Environmental Health.* 1985; **40**: 293–5.
58. Kilburn KH, Warshaw RH. Airways obstruction from asbestos exposure. Effects of asbestosis and smoking. *Chest.* 1994; **106**: 1061–70.
59. Jones RN, Glindmeyer 3rd HW, Weill H. Review of the Kilburn and Warshaw chest article: Airways obstruction from asbestos exposure. *Chest.* 1995; **107**: 1727–9.
60. Wang XR, Yano Y, Wang M *et al.* Pulmonary function in long-term asbestos workers in China. *Journal of Occupational and Environmental Medicine.* 2001; **43**: 623–9.
61. Wang X, Araki S, Yano E *et al.* Effects of smoking on respiratory function and exercise performance in asbestos workers. *Industrial Health.* 1995; **33**: 173–80.
62. Health and Safety Executive. Work with material containing asbestos. Control of asbestos regulations 2006. Approved code of practice and guidance. London: Health and Safety Executive, 2006.
63. Health and Safety Executive. Asbestos: Medical guidance note MS13, 4th edn. London: Health and Safety Executive, 2005.

Epidemiology of asbestos-related diseases

ROBIN M RUDD

Introduction	1000	Malignant mesothelioma	1002
Asbestosis	1000	Non-industrial mesothelioma	1005
Asbestos-induced airway disease	1001	Lung cancer	1005
Benign pleural disease	1002	Other malignant diseases	1006
Acute asbestos pleurisy and pleural effusion	1002	References	1007
Diffuse pleural thickening	1002		

INTRODUCTION

During the first half of the twentieth century, there was a rapid increase in the use of asbestos for a variety of purposes, exploiting its properties of fire resistance and poor conduction of heat, electricity and sound. The hazards to health were first recognized in factories manufacturing asbestos products. In the United Kingdom, the Asbestos Industry Regulations (1931) was the first legislation to control asbestos exposure at work in such factories. However, perhaps strangely in retrospect, it was not until much later that it was widely recognized that end users and bystanders to use of asbestos materials were also at risk. Use of asbestos continued to increase until the late 1960s to early 1970s in industrialized countries. In the UK, stricter controls were imposed by the Asbestos Industry Regulations (1969), but it was not until the mid-1970s that use of more effective precautions became widespread. Peak asbestos imports into the UK occurred in 1973. In 1979, the Advisory Committee on Asbestos recommended the gradual substitution of asbestos by other materials, a ban on the use of sprayed asbestos and control of the asbestos removal industry.[1] In the UK, the Asbestos (Prohibition) Regulations (1985) banned the importation, supply and use of amosite and crocidolite and, in 1999, an amendment to the regulations extended them to chrysotile with certain exceptions in safety specific areas until January 1, 2005, by which date the marketing and use of all asbestos became illegal throughout the European Union. The use of asbestos has also virtually ceased in North America, but its use is still widespread throughout the developing world to which the epidemic of asbestos-related disease will spread.

By the time precautions began to be introduced in the late 1960s, a 'second wave' of asbestos disease was becoming rampant among workers in ship building and repair, and the construction industry who had worked with, or in proximity to, those using asbestos materials. Later, a 'third wave' affected those less directly exposed, such as building maintenance personnel who incidentally encountered and disturbed asbestos in place, the hazards of which were widely recognized later with measures to enforce mandatory documentation of asbestos in buildings and a requirement for removal or effective encapsulation. A 'fourth wave' of disease now may be affecting those who merely worked in buildings where asbestos materials were poorly maintained, with cases of mesothelioma appearing among staff at hospitals and schools.

ASBESTOSIS

In subjects heavily exposed to asbestos, such as insulators, a very high prevalence of radiographic evidence of asbestosis has been recorded. A study of 2907 US insulators between 1981 and 1983 found that 11.6 per cent had pulmonary opacities without pleural abnormalities and 48.7 per cent had pulmonary and pleural abnormalities.[2] Because of the reduction in exposures from the 1970s onwards, the nature of asbestosis diagnosed is changing. There are fewer cases of severe disease and more cases of mild disease. This changing picture is reflected in UK statistics where the annual number of new awards of Industrial Injuries Disablement benefit for asbestosis increased from 335 in 1996 to 575 in 2006, a 72 per cent increase, while the annual number of deaths attributed on death certificates to asbestosis rose from 68 in 1996 to 104 in 2006, a 53 per cent increase.[3] In a recent French study of 5545 subjects exposed to asbestos in various occupations, asbestosis was identified on high resolution computed tomography (HRCT) in 6.8 per cent.[4] The prevalence of asbestosis increased with cumulative exposure estimated from the occupational history.

Latency

The latency between commencement of exposure and appearance of asbestosis is inversely related to the dose of asbestos received. Dose is usually expressed as the product of mean airborne fibre concentration encountered and duration of exposure in working years, commonly taken to be 2000 hours per year. The interval between the onset of exposure to asbestos and the development of symptoms of asbestosis is commonly 20 years or longer, although in earlier years when continuous heavy exposure occurred, fibrosis occasionally became evident as early as five years after the first exposure. New lung and pleural lesions continue to appear more than 40 years after first exposure.[2] Asbestos fibres remain in the lungs for long periods, many permanently, and disease may appear and progress long after exposure has ceased.

Dose and response

The long latent period contributes to the difficulty in determining the attack rate among exposed people and its relation to the dose of asbestos inhaled. There are relatively few studies in which reliable estimates of exposure are provided. An additional complicating factor is the variable means of ascertainment of the disease. In early years, it was diagnosed on variable combinations of detection of basal crackles on auscultation of the lungs, chest x-ray abnormalities and lung function abnormalities. The minimum criteria for the diagnosis varied between studies. In recent years, asbestosis has often been diagnosed on the basis of minor abnormalities on a computed tomography (CT) scan without clinical or plain radiographic signs.

In 1985, Doll and Peto[5] adjudged the best evidence concerning the relation between incidence of asbestosis and dose to be a study of Rochdale asbestos textile factory workers.[6] The frequency and severity of asbestosis increased with increasing dose of asbestos where dose comprises the product of intensity of exposure in fibres per millilitre and duration of exposure in working years. Among these workers who were exposed predominantly to chrysotile, there was a 1 per cent prevalence of certified asbestosis, possible asbestosis and lung crackles after doses of 72, 55 and 43 fibres/mL per year, respectively. This study was relied upon by the UK Advisory Committee on Asbestos (1979)[1] which concluded that the annual incidence of certified (i.e. clinically evident) asbestosis after a cumulative dose of less than 100 fibres/mL per year, i.e. a working life of exposure to less than 2 fibres/mL, was 0.5 per cent and that cases of 'possible asbestosis' occurred after less than 50 fibres/mL per year. The Royal Commission on Matters of Health and Safety Arising from the Use of Asbestos in Ontario (1984)[7] concluded that the minimum threshold dose for the development of clinical asbestosis is around 25 fibres/mL per year, and Doll and Peto agreed.[5] These conclusions were based largely on studies of workers exposed to chrysotile.

However, there is evidence that asbestosis may occur after lower levels of exposure exclusively to amphiboles. In a study of 807 South African amphibole miners among 64 men who had sustained cumulative exposures between 2 and 5 fibres/mL per year, five cases were found.[8] These may be questioned on grounds of possible erroneous diagnosis, but diagnoses of asbestosis in 16 and 28 per cent of men with cumulative exposures in the ranges 5–10 and 10–20 fibres/mL per year, respectively, are harder to ignore. In Western Australian crocidolite miners, mortality from asbestosis began to increase with exposures of less than 4 fibres/mL per year.[9]

A study of 678 household contacts of American amosite asbestos workers found that compared with controls there was a significantly increased prevalence of small opacities on the chest x-ray (17 versus 3 per cent), as well as of benign pleural changes (26 versus 2 per cent).[10] Among those with small opacities, crackles were heard over the lungs in 10 per cent. The frequency of radiographic abnormalities was higher in wives than in other relatives, reflecting their heavier exposure from laundering work clothes. These observations imply that household exposure could be quite heavy rather than minor as sometimes suggested.

There is variation in individual susceptibility to asbestosis. Smoking increases the risk of development of radiographic signs suggesting asbestosis[11] and of progression of asbestosis.[12] Lung structure is probably also important in determining individual susceptibility. A case–control study in Quebec showed that cases were shorter than controls, possibly because shorter men have shorter tracheas which are less effective in trapping inhaled fibres, so that more fibres reach alveolar areas.[13] Differences between subjects in retention of asbestos fibres probably contributes to differences in susceptibility to disease.[14] Increasing knowledge of the genetic basis for disease suggests that genetic polymorphisms which determine the response to oxidative stress, an important mechanism in asbestos-induced disease, affect susceptibility to asbestosis.

ASBESTOS-INDUCED AIRWAY DISEASE

Evidence of small airways dysfunction has been found in asbestos workers who have never smoked, in studies including unexposed non-smoking control subjects.[15,16]

Patients with asbestos-related pleural disease commonly have airflow limitation, even when non-smokers, reflecting asbestos airway disease.[17] This is generally of insufficient degree to cause breathlessness, however.

BENIGN PLEURAL DISEASE

Pleural plaques

Pleural plaques occur much more frequently in subjects with known exposure than in the general population without identified exposure to asbestos. Plaques may occur after occupational exposure at a lower level than is required to cause asbestosis, and are found in household contacts of asbestos workers and in people exposed to environmental contamination with asbestos. The frequency of plaques reported varies according to method of ascertainment. Autopsy studies show a higher prevalence of plaques than plain radiographic surveys, because direct observation is diagnostically more sensitive than chest x-ray, and partly because a population studied at autopsy is generally older and more likely to have sustained occupational exposure than one undergoing chest radiography. For example, in a Swedish study, plaques were found in 6.8 per cent of autopsies, of which only 12.5 per cent were detected by radiography.[18] In a UK study of a general urban population, plaques were reported from 4.2 per cent of routine autopsies, but this figure rose to 11.2 per cent when a specific search for plaques was made in a subsequent series.[19] Computed tomography is more sensitive than plain radiography. In a study of 5545 subjects exposed to asbestos in various occupations, plaques were identified on HR CT in 15.9 per cent.[4] The prevalence of plaques increased with time since first exposure and with cumulative exposure, in accordance with findings from an earlier study using chest x-rays.[20]

In certain areas, such as parts of Finland, Turkey and Greece, plaques occur with much increased frequency. This has been attributed to the presence of asbestos in the soil and outcropping rocks.[21] Plaques are more common in urban than in rural dwellers.[22] Among an urban population, the frequency and extent of plaques at autopsy increases in relation to lung asbestos fibre content.[23]

The latent period between first exposure and appearance of plaques is similar to that for asbestosis. In a group of 624 asbestos workers from various industries, plaques were seen in none within ten years, in 10 per cent by 19 years, in 29 per cent by 29 years, in 32 per cent by 39 years and in 58 per cent by 49 years.[24] In a study of 1117 insulation workers, pleural calcification was found in none of 346 men less than ten years after first exposure, in only 1.1 per cent of 379 men less than 20 years, in 10.4 per cent up to 30 years, in 34.5 per cent up to 40 years and in 57.9 per cent more than 40 years after first exposure.[25] The prevalence of plaques has been reported to be higher in smokers,[26] but among insulation workers this relationship was not apparent.[27]

ACUTE ASBESTOS PLEURISY AND PLEURAL EFFUSION

In an early study, a history of pleural effusion thought to be due to asbestos was found in 21 per cent of subjects recorded to have had asbestos exposure.[28] A history of asbestos exposure was significantly more common in subjects with otherwise labelled 'idiopathic' pleural effusion than in control subjects, supporting a causal link.[29] Benign pleural effusion may occur less than ten years after first exposure to asbestos, but the mean latency from first exposure was 26 years in a series of 20 cases.[30] The risk of benign effusion increases with the dose of asbestos received.[24]

DIFFUSE PLEURAL THICKENING

Diffuse pleural thickening is a less common manifestation than pleural plaque formation. A survey of 5545 asbestos-exposed subjects by HRCT which found pleural plaques in 15.9 per cent identified diffuse pleural thickening in only 0.7 per cent.[4] It is less clearly dose related than asbestosis or the malignant diseases[31–33] and its occurrence may be determined largely by host susceptibility factors. A wide range of fibre counts is observed in association with the condition, but mean counts appear to be somewhat lower than in groups of patients with asbestosis.[34] Amphibole counts were higher than usually seen in non-occupationally exposed individuals in six of seven cases in this series. In another series, in which fibre counts were comparable to those seen in mild asbestosis, amphiboles were the main fibre type in the lungs, although chrysotile was the main fibre type in the pleura.[35]

MALIGNANT MESOTHELIOMA

In 1960, Wagner and colleagues described 33 cases of diffuse pleural mesothelioma and all but one had experienced probable exposure to crocidolite.[36] In 1964, a case–control study of patients who had died of mesothelioma at the London Hospital found evidence of asbestos exposure in a majority of cases.[37] Interestingly, some of the patients had not worked with asbestos but had been exposed via dust brought home on the clothes of asbestos workers or from residence in the vicinity of a local asbestos factory.

Much evidence has since accumulated indicating that asbestos exposure is responsible for the great majority of mesotheliomas. The risk of mesothelioma is not affected by smoking.[38] Among subjects with no history of asbestos exposure, the annual incidence has been estimated at around one per million population[39,40] and a few childhood cases, apparently unrelated to asbestos have been described.[41] A review suggested that the estimated background risk may be inflated by cases due to unsuspected environmental exposure.[42]

A recent study in the United Kingdom obtained occupational and residential histories from 622 mesothelioma patients and 1420 population controls.[43] This reported a lifetime risk among apparently unexposed people of one in 1000, much higher than has been reported previously. Approximately half the male cases were construction workers with the highest lifetime risk of one in 17 for carpenters. The risk was doubled in relatives of exposed workers. Surprisingly, the study found that 14 per cent of male and 62 per cent of female cases were not attributable to identified asbestos exposure. The authors pointed out that their findings show a female mesothelioma death rate by age 70 more than three times higher than in the United States. If, as seems likely, this difference reflects greater asbestos exposure sustained by UK women, this implies that more than two-thirds of mesotheliomas in UK women are due to asbestos, far more than were identified by the occupational and residential histories obtained. The authors suggested that the other asbestos-induced cases may be a result of environmental asbestos exposure or unidentified occupational exposures. The latter is very probably at least a contributory factor because the main analysis was based upon job titles rather than self-reported exposure in order to minimize the effect of recall bias. This is likely to have missed less obvious exposures, for example those sustained as a result of working in what would appear to be low risk occupations, but in buildings containing poorly maintained asbestos. The male death rate for men aged 45–49 is also three times higher in the United Kingdom than in the United States and this is thought likely to be a result of much greater use of amosite in the UK.[43] Australia's death rates for mesothelioma are similar to the UK and so were their use of amosite and crocidolite.[44]

In the recent UK study, residence within one mile of a source of environmental exposure was not associated with a significantly increased risk of mesothelioma.[43] However, sites such as asbestos product factories, disposal sites, power plants and shipyards were lumped together, and the effect of high exposure sources, such as asbestos product factories, is likely to have been diluted by inclusion of the other sites. A case–control study suggested that exposure derived only from residence in the vicinity of asbestos plants in Yorkshire (United Kingdom) accounted for 3 per cent of mesothelioma cases in the area.[45] A population case–control study in three European countries found an odds ratio for mesothelioma of 11.5 for living within 2000 m of an asbestos source.[46] A population-based case–control study in Italy found that residents around an asbestos cement plant had a relative risk of 10.5 for mesothelioma.[47]

In people with heavy exposure, the risk of mesothelioma is high. Mortality from mesothelioma among employees at an asbestos textile factory before 1964 was estimated at 7.3–10.8 per cent for men and 9.1–12.0 per cent for women.[48] In insulation workers whose exposure began before age 20, the death rate from mesothelioma may be as high as 15 per cent.[49] Situations which might be assumed to be associated with low level exposure, such as domestic contact with contaminated clothing and working in an office with a deteriorating sprayed asbestos ceiling, have been shown to be capable of giving rise to fibre levels in the lung comparable to those found in people with occupational exposure.[45,50,51]

The incidence of mesothelioma in the UK and other industrial countries is still rising and it is likely to continue to do so (Figure 77.1). In Great Britain in 2006, there were 1740 male and 316 female deaths.[3] The expected number of mesothelioma cases among males is projected to increase to a peak of 2038 in the year 2016, decreasing thereafter (Figure 77.2).[3] Projections for females are more uncertain. This increase reflects the increasing use of asbestos, largely without protection, until the early 1970s. A similar picture applies to Western Europe, where asbestos use remained high until 1980 and where it has been predicted that mesothelioma deaths will almost double from 5000 in 1998 to 9000 by 2018.[52]

Dose and response

Several studies have shown an increase in risk of mesothelioma with increasing cumulative exposure. However,

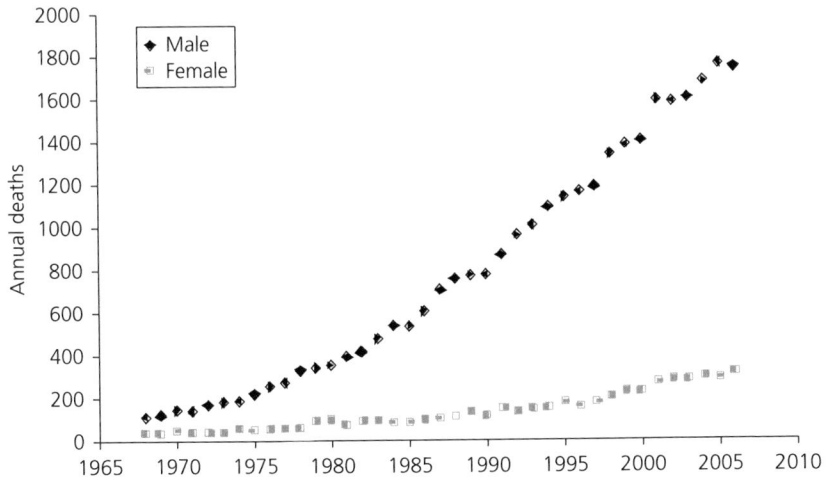

Figure 77.1 Male and female mesothelioma annual deaths in Great Britain 1968–2006. Data from the Health and Safety Executive.[3]

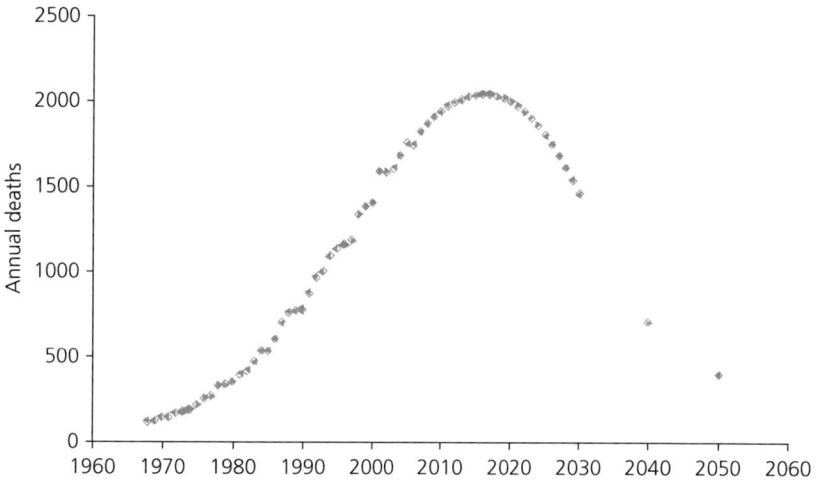

Figure 77.2 Actual to 2006 and future projected male mesothelioma deaths in Great Britain 2007–50. Data from the Health and Safety Executive.[3]

there is no clear evidence for a threshold dose of asbestos below which there is no risk of mesothelioma.[5,7,53] Among workers at an asbestos factory in east London, where approximately 8 per cent of deaths were due to mesothelioma, the risk increased with both the duration of exposure and the estimated intensity of exposure.[54] Similar findings were reported in and among gas mask assemblers[55] and in crocidolite miners in Western Australia.[56] A case–control study found a significant excess of mesothelioma at levels of exposure far below limits adopted in most industrial countries during the 1980s and an increasing risk with estimated cumulative exposure.[57] A review of cohort studies found evidence for a non-linear relation between dose and risk of mesothelioma.[58] The peritoneal mesothelioma risk was proportional to the square of cumulative exposure and the pleural mesothelioma risk was sublinear.

Pleural mesothelioma is much more common than the peritoneal form, although the ratio between the sites is variable from entirely pleural to only about 2:1 in favour of pleural in different series.[59] Factors favouring the peritoneal site are longer and heavier exposure, and exposure to amphiboles. Clinical evidence of asbestosis of the lungs is found in association with peritoneal mesothelioma more commonly than with pleural mesothelioma[59,60] supporting the observation that, on average, exposure has been heavier in peritoneal cases.

Latency

Using data from a study of North American insulation workers, a model was formulated for predicting mesothelioma incidence in a cohort.[49] The incidence of mesothelioma increased with time since first exposure to asbestos in proportion to a power function of the time elapsed. This could be explained on the assumption that each brief period of exposure causes an addition to subsequent incidence which increases approximately as the cube of time since the exposure occurred. The formula derived from the study was consistent with evidence from other studies, although any power of time between 2.5 and 4 fitted as well. This means that a dose of asbestos received early in life produces a much larger lifetime risk of mesothelioma than the same dose received later in life. The formula also implies that inhaling a given dose over a shorter period gives rise to a larger risk than the same dose over a longer period. There is some evidence to suggest that the risk does not increase indefinitely and there may be some decline after 35–50 years.[58]

In two UK series in which 85 per cent[61] and 87 per cent[62] of cases had a history of definite or probable asbestos exposure, mean latent intervals between first exposure and death were 38 (range, 3.5–53) years[61] and 41 (15–67) years.[62] The case with the shortest latency of 3.5 years was not well documented[61] and there must be doubt as to its validity. The latency between first exposure and appearance of disease is unrelated to the heaviness of exposure.[63]

Fibre type

A review of cohort studies concluded that relative potencies for crocidolite:amosite:chrysotile are 500:100:1.[58] It has been suggested that the mesotheliomas occurring in workers exposed only to chrysotile may have been caused by small quantities, usually less than 1 per cent, of tremolite contaminating the chrysotile. This forms part of the so-called 'amphibole hypothesis' to the effect that most, if not all, asbestos-induced mesotheliomas are caused by amphiboles.[64] The main evidence for this hypothesis has come from Canadian studies.[65] In Quebec, the risk of mesothelioma was higher among workers in central mines where tremolite contamination was higher than among workers in peripheral mines where it was lower.[66] Analysis of lung tissue from chrysotile workers showed that tremolite was the predominant fibre type retained compared with controls.[67] The amphibole hypothesis has been questioned[64] and it has been argued that even though chrysotile is a less potent cause of mesothelioma than amphiboles, because it accounts for a large majority of asbestos used commercially, it may nevertheless be an important cause of pleural mesothelioma.[68]

There is evidence of some risk from chrysotile. A case–control study from Australia demonstrated an increase in risk of mesothelioma with increasing counts of crocidolite, amosite and chrysotile, including cases in which only chrysotile was present.[69] Human cases in which chrysotile was the only type of asbestos in the lungs have been reported from Japan.[70] A World Health Organization review of the evidence concluded that chrysotile poses a risk for mesothelioma in a dose-dependent manner with no evidence of a threshold below which there is no risk.[52] Another recent review concluded that the evidence that chrysotile causes mesothelioma fulfils the criteria for causation according to the Bradford Hill causation model.[71]

NON-INDUSTRIAL MESOTHELIOMA

In the Cappadocian region of central Anatolia in Turkey there are two villages, Karain and Tuzkoy, where mesothelioma causes approximately 50 per cent of all deaths.[72] Many of the deaths occur in middle-aged subjects, although the youngest cases occurred in a 12-year-old boy and in a 15-year-old girl.[73] Exposure to a carcinogenic agent from birth was suspected. The materials responsible were found to be a fibrous zeolite called erionite and possibly tremolite present in the volcanic tuff which is quarried and used for building. The observation that mesothelioma occurred in certain families prompted detailed kinship studies which implicated a genetic factor determining susceptibility, probably in an autosomal dominant way.[70] This observation may help to explain variation in susceptibility to asbestos-induced mesothelioma. Naturally occurring asbestos minerals, including tremolite and perhaps chrysotile, have also been reported to cause mesothelioma in other countries, including in Greece and Cyprus.[74,75]

LUNG CANCER

Since the 1930s, there have been anecdotal reports of an increased incidence of lung cancer in asbestos workers. In 1955, Doll and colleagues reported a high risk of lung cancer in workers in an asbestos textile factory.[76] In this study, subsequently extended,[77] men exposed to asbestos for ten years or more before 1933 had a ten-fold increased risk of lung cancer. Many other studies have subsequently confirmed an increased risk in asbestos workers.

There is an important synergistic interaction between asbestos and smoking in the causation of lung cancer. A study of mortality among insulation workers in the United States demonstrated that the mortality from lung cancer was five times greater in men exposed to asbestos and there was a multiplicative interaction with a ten-fold increase from smoking, so that mortality was increased greater than 50-fold in asbestos-exposed smokers.[78] Saracci[79] reviewed several studies and concluded that the data support the view that the effects of asbestos exposure and smoking on the risk of lung cancer are multiplicative. Since this review, several other studies have been published and the conclusions remain broadly similar.[80–83] The excess risk of lung cancer from asbestos is higher in non-smokers and very light smokers than in heavier smokers.[84]

Dose–response relation

Most epidemiological studies, which have considered the relation between dose of asbestos and the risk of lung cancer, have produced results consistent with an approximately linear relation between dose and mortality with no threshold dose below which there is no increased risk of lung cancer.[5,7,79] However, a review of cohort studies found the lung cancer risk increased in proportion to somewhere between the dose of asbestos and its square.[58] Age at the time of exposure does not affect the relative risk produced by asbestos exposure.[5]

Fibre type

Amphiboles are substantially more potent than chrysotile in causing lung cancer in humans. A review of cohort studies estimated that the risk of lung cancer increases by about 5 per cent for each fibre/mL per year of exposure to commercial amphiboles, i.e. amosite or crocidolite. The relative risk associated with chrysotile varies between industries. South Carolina chrysotile textile workers were at a much higher risk of lung cancer than miners and millers of the same variety of asbestos.[85] It has been hypothesized that the physical characteristics of fibres, depending on the processes to which they have been subjected, may affect the lung cancer risk. However, an electron microscopic study of lung tissue from these two populations indicated that differences in fibre dimensions could not explain the higher risk of lung cancer in asbestos textile workers.[86] A co-carcinogenic effect of mineral oils used in textile plants to control dust has been suggested as another possible explanation and an increase in risk of cancer after mineral oil spraying was introduced in the Rochdale textile plant in the UK lends some support to this hypothesis.[58] However, the size of the risk observed could not fully explain the very high risk in the Carolina cohort of chrysotile textile workers. For chrysotile cohorts, there is wide variation in risk estimates. Doll and Peto estimated a 1 per cent increase in cancer risk per fibre/mL per year for chrysotile textile workers, based on the Rochdale and Carolina data.[5] In a review of cohort studies, an estimate of 0.5 per cent per fibre/mL per year has been suggested as the upper limit to the risk from chrysotile with a best estimate of 0.1 per cent per fibre/mL per year, for other than the Carolina cohort.[58]

Latent period between exposure and onset of lung cancer

The latent period is variable. Some cases may occur as soon as five to nine years after first exposure. Doll and Peto suggested the risk rises until at least 30 years after first exposure.[5] However, Hodgson and Darnton[58] suggested there is probably little change in lung cancer risk between ten and 40 years from first exposure with a possible decline thereafter.[58] A study of American amosite factory workers suggested that the latent period may be shorter when first exposure occurs at older ages.[87] A study of Quebec chrysotile miners and millers found no evidence for a relation between latency and dose.[88]

Lung cancer and asbestosis

The risk of asbestosis and the risk of lung cancer are both related to the dose of asbestos inhaled, so the conditions frequently occur in the same individual. The risk of asbestos-induced lung cancer was first identified in people with asbestosis and in the context of ideas about 'scar cancers' which were then current, but now anachronistic, the view became prevalent that the lung fibrosis of asbestosis led to the development of cancer. Twenty-five years ago, Doll and Peto suggested that in the light of modern knowledge of carcinogenesis the idea no longer seemed plausible,[5] and with increasing knowledge of the molecular basis of carcinogenesis, the idea that causation of cancer is wholly dependent upon the presence of fibrosis has become increasingly implausible.[89] A detailed discussion of the biological evidence is beyond the scope of this article.

A review of older epidemiological studies noted that two supported the view that asbestosis was necessary for the attribution of lung cancer to asbestos and seven supported the view that it was not.[90] All the studies had methodological weaknesses and none was considered definitive. Additional information comes from case–control studies which suggest a doubling of risk at levels of exposure lower than suggested by the cohort studies reviewed by Hodgson and Darnton.[58] A German population-matched, case–control study found a relative risk of 1.94 (95 per cent CI 1.1–3.43) for men with cumulative exposure exceeding 10 fibres/mL per year after adjusting for smoking.[91] A Swedish population-matched, case–control study found significantly elevated cancer risk at levels of exposure far below those necessary to cause asbestosis.[92] For exposure of 4 fibres/mL per year, the relative risk of cancer was 1.90 (95 per cent CI 1.32–2.74). The demonstration of a significantly elevated risk of cancer at levels of exposure below those necessary to cause asbestosis clearly invalidates the proposition that asbestosis is a necessary precursor of asbestos-induced lung cancer.

However, recent evidence has substantiated the suggestion from the reanalysis of the South African data that the presence of asbestosis further increases the risk of lung cancer above that arising from asbestos exposure.[93,94] In a study of former workers and residents exposed to crocidolite at Wittenoom in Western Australia, there was a significant increase in risk of lung cancer with dose of asbestos in those without radiographic evidence of asbestosis, but the presence of asbestosis was associated with a further increment in risk.[95]

Criteria for attribution of lung cancer to asbestos

The Helsinki criteria[96] were formulated by an international panel of experts. The presence of asbestosis diagnosed on radiological or pathological evidence is a sufficient, but not necessary, criterion for attribution of lung cancer to asbestos. In the absence of asbestosis, an alternative criterion is sufficient cumulative exposure to asbestos to more than double the risk of lung cancer, assessed on the basis of the occupational history, or by measurement of the asbestos content of lung tissue. The most precise occupational history criterion was an estimated cumulative exposure of 25 fibres/mL per year or more. This criterion was later criticized on the grounds that account was not taken of fibre type and the level chosen represented the upper end of the estimated range of risk of lung cancer in relation to dose. Several of the senior authors reviewed the position in the light of more recent evidence and reaffirmed the criterion where exposure has been predominantly to amphiboles, but acknowledged that the threshold is higher for other mixtures of fibre types.[89] From the risk estimates estimated from the review of cohort studies by Hodgson and Darnton,[58] exposure to around 40 fibres/mL per year for an equal mixture of amphiboles and chrysotile is sufficient to more than double the risk of lung cancer. Cumulative exposure is the basis for the award of state benefit for asbestos-induced lung cancer in Germany, France, Belgium, Norway, Sweden, Finland, Denmark, Quebec and Australia (AWARD criteria)[97] and Japan. In the United Kingdom, it is accepted by the Industrial Injuries Advisory Council that asbestosis is not necessary to attribute lung cancer to asbestos and exposure for designated periods in prescribed occupations is sufficient for the award of state benefit.[98]

OTHER MALIGNANT DISEASES

There is controversy as to whether asbestos increases the risks of other cancers. The 1987 International Agency for Research on Cancer (IARC) review of the strength of evidence for a causal relationship between asbestos exposure and various cancers found 'sufficient' evidence to infer a causal relation between asbestos exposure and both laryngeal cancer and gastrointestinal cancer.[99] The 2006 US Institute of Medicine (US IoM) Committee on Asbestos found the evidence was 'sufficient' for laryngeal cancer and 'suggestive but not sufficient' for gastrointestinal cancer.[100] In the UK, the Industrial Injuries Advisory Council reviewed the evidence in 2008 and noted that, although some studies had shown an increased risk of laryngeal cancer, few had shown a risk factor of greater than two-fold and the council concluded that there was insufficient evidence to make laryngeal cancer a prescribed disease, eligible for state compensation.[101]

In the Great Britain Asbestos Survey, which from 1971 onwards monitored mortality among workers covered by regulations to control asbestos exposure, standard mortality rates (SMR), but not proportional mortality rates (PMR) were elevated for cancers of the larynx, oesophagus and colorectum.[102] These disparities suggest that the elevated SMRs were likely to have been due to confounding factors, such as smoking. However, both the SMR (166) and PMR (114) were significantly elevated for stomach cancer raising the possibility of a weak causal link.

Key points

- All types of asbestos cause all the asbestos-related diseases.
- Amphibole asbestos, e.g. crocidolite (blue) and amosite (brown), are far more potent than chrysotile (white) in causation of mesothelioma and lung cancer.
- There is no evidence of a threshold dose of asbestos below which there is no increase in risk of mesothelioma.
- A much larger dose of asbestos is needed to cause asbestosis than is capable of causing benign pleural disease and mesothelioma.
- A dose of asbestos sufficient to cause asbestosis is sufficient to approximately double the risk of lung cancer.
- The risk of lung cancer from asbestos exposure increases with cumulative dose and is not confined to people who have developed asbestosis of the lungs, although the presence of asbestosis further increases the risk.

REFERENCES

1. Health and Safety Commission. Asbestos: Final Report of the Advisory Committee, vol. 1. London: HMSO, 1979.
2. Lilis R, Miller A, Godbold J et al. Radiographic abnormalities in asbestos insulators: Effects of duration from onset of exposure and smoking. Relationships of dyspnea with parenchymal and pleural fibrosis. *American Journal of Industrial Medicine*. 1991; **20**: 1–15.
3. Health and Safety Executive. Mesotheolioma deaths in Great Britain. Last accessed October 11, 2009. Available from: www.hse.gov.uk/statistics.
4. Paris C, Thierry S, Brochard P et al. Pleural plaques and asbestosis: dose– and time–response relationships based on HRCT data. *European Respiratory Journal*. 2009; **34**: 72–9.
5. Doll R, Peto J. *Asbestos: Effects on health of exposure to asbestos*. London: HMSO, 1985.
6. Berry G, Gilson JC, Holmes S et al. Asbestosis: A study of dose–response relationships in an asbestos textile factory. *British Journal of Industrial Medicine*. 1979; **36**: 98–112.
7. Report of the Royal Commission on Matters of Health and Safety Arising from the Use of Asbestos in Ontario. Ontario: Ministry of the Attorney General, 1984.
8. Sluis-Cremer GK. Asbestos disease at low exposures after long residence times. *Annals of the New York Academy of Sciences*. 1991; **643**: 182–93.
9. de Klerk NH, Musk AW, Cookson WOCM et al. Radiographic abnormalities and mortality in subjects with exposure to crocidolite. *British Journal of Industrial Medicine*. 1993; **50**: 902–6.
10. Anderson HA, Lilis R, Daum SM, Selikoff IJ. Asbestosis among household contacts of asbestos factory workers. *Annals of the New York Academy of Sciences*. 1979; **330**: 387–99.
11. McMillan GHG, Pethybridge RJ, Sheers G. Effect of smoking on attack rates of pulmonary and pleural lesions related to exposure to asbestos dust. *British Journal of Industrial Medicine*. 1980; **37**: 268–72.
12. Samet JM, Epler GR, Gaensler EA, Rosner B. Absence of synergism between exposure to asbestos and cigarette smoking in asbestosis. *American Review of Respiratory Disease*. 1979; **120**: 75–82.
13. Becklake MR, Toyota B, Stewart M et al. Lung structure as a risk factor in adverse pulmonary responses to asbestos exposure. *American Review of Respiratory Disease*. 1983; **128**: 385–8.
14. Begin R, Sebastien P. Excessive accumulation of asbestos fibre in the bronchoalveolar space may be a marker of individual susceptibility to developing asbestosis: Experimental evidence. *British Journal of Industrial Medicine*. 1989; **46**: 853–5.
15. Hjortsberg U, Orbaek P, Arborelius M Jr et al. Railroad workers with pleural plaques: II. Small airway dysfunction among asbestos-exposed workers. *American Journal of Industrial Medicine*. 1988; **14**: 643–7.
16. Dossing M, Groth S, Vestbo J, Lyngenbo O. Small airway dysfunction in never smoking asbestos exposed Danish plumbers. *International Archives of Occupational and Environmental Health*. 1990; **62**: 209–12.
17. Kilburn KH, Warshaw R. Pulmonary functional impairment associated with pleural asbestos disease: Circumscribed and diffuse thickening. *Chest*. 1990; **98**: 965–72.
18. Hillerdal G, Lindgren A. Pleural plaques: Correlation of autopsy findings to radiographic findings and occupational history. *European Journal of Respiratory Diseases*. 1980; **61**: 315–19.
19. Hourihane DO'B, Lessof L, Richardson PC. Hyaline and calcified pleural plaques as an index of exposure to asbestos. A study of radiological and pathological features of 100 cases with a consideration of epidemiology. *British Medical Journal*. 1966; **1**: 1069–74.

20. Harries PG, Mackenzie FA, Sheers G et al. Radiological survey of men exposed to asbestos in naval dockyards. *British Journal of Industrial Medicine.* 1972; **29**: 274–9.
21. Craighead JE, Abraham JL, Churg A et al. The pathology of asbestos-associated diseases of the lungs and pleural cavities: Diagnostic criteria and proposed grading schema. Report of the Pneumoconiosis Committee of the College of American Pathologists and the National Institute for Occupational Safety and Health. *Archives of Pathology and Laboratory Medicine.* 1982; **106**: 544–96.
22. Zitting AJ, Karjalainen A, Impivaara O et al. Radiographic small lung opacities and pleural abnormalities in relation to smoking, urbanization status, and occupational asbestos exposure in Finland. *Journal of Occupational and Environmental Medicine.* 1996; **38**: 602–9.
23. Karjalainen A, Karhunen PJ, Lalu K et al. Pleural plaques and exposure to mineral fibres in a male urban necropsy population. *Occupational and Environmental Medicine.* 1994; **51**: 456–60.
24. Epler GR, McLoud TC, Gaensler EA. Prevalence and incidence of benign asbestos pleural effusion in a working population. *Journal of the American Medical Association.* 1982; **247**: 617–22.
25. Selikoff IJ. The occurrence of pleural calcification among asbestos insulation workers. *Annals of the New York Academy of Sciences.* 1965; **132**: 351–67.
26. Weiss W, Levin R, Goodman L. Pleural plaques and cigarette smoking in asbestos workers. *Journal of Occupational Medicine.* 1981; **23**: 427–30.
27. Lilis R, Selikoff IJ, Lerman Y et al. Asbestosis. Interstitial pulmonary fibrosis and pleural fibrosis in a cohort of asbestos insulation workers: Influence of cigarette smoking. *American Journal of Industrial Medicine.* 1986; **10**: 459–70.
28. Gaensler EA, Kaplan AI. Asbestos pleural effusion. *Annals of Internal Medicine.* 1971; **74**: 178–91.
29. Martensson G, Hagberg S, Pettersson K, Thiringer G. Asbestos pleural effusion: A clinical entity. *Thorax.* 1987; **42**: 646–51.
30. Lilis, R Lerman Y, Selikoff IJ. Symptomatic benign pleural effusions among asbestos insulation workers: Residual radiographic abnormalities. *British Journal of Industrial Medicine.* 1988; **45**: 443–9.
31. Becklake MR, Case BW. Fiber burden and asbestos-related lung disease: Determinants of dose-response relationships. *American Journal of Respiratory and Critical Care Medicine.* 1994; **150**: 1488–92.
32. Finkelstein MM. A study of dose–response relationships for asbestos associated disease. *British Journal of Industrial Medicine.* 1985; **42**: 319–25.
33. Smith KA, Sykes LJ, McGavin CR. Diffuse pleural fibrosis – an unreliable indicator of heavy asbestos exposure? *Scandinavian Journal of Work, Environment and Health.* 2003; **29**: 311–16.
34. Stephens M, Gibbs AR, Pooley FD, Wagner JC. Asbestos induced diffuse pleural fibrosis: Pathology and mineralogy. *Thorax.* 1987; **42**: 583–8.
35. Gibbs AR, Stephens M, Griffiths DM et al. Fibre distribution in the lungs and pleura of subjects with asbestos related diffuse pleural fibrosis. *British Journal of Industrial Medicine.* 1991; **48**: 762–70.
36. Wagner JC, Sleggs CA, Marchand P. Diffuse pleural mesothelioma and asbestos exposure in the North Western Cape Province. *British Journal of Industrial Medicine.* 1960; **17**: 260–71.
37. Newhouse ML, Thompson H. Mesothelioma of the pleura and peritoneum following exposure to asbestos in the London area. *British Journal of Industrial Medicine.* 1965; **22**: 261–9.
38. Muscat JE, Wynder EL. Cigarette smoking, asbestos exposure, and malignant mesothelioma. *Cancer Research.* 1991; **51**: 2263–7.
39. Hillerdal G. Mesothelioma: Cases associated with non-occupational and low dose exposures. *Occupational and Environmental Medicine.* 1999; **56**: 505–13.
40. Tan E, Warren N. Projection of mesothelioma mortality in Great Britain. Health and Safety Laboratory. Health and Safety Executive Research Report. Last accessed October 11, 2009. London: HSE, 2009: RR728. Available from: www.hse.gov.uk/research/rrpdf/rr728.pdf.
41. Brenner J, Sordillo PP, Magius GB. Malignant mesothelioma in children: Report of seven cases and review of the literature. *Medical and Pediatric Oncology.* 1981; **9**: 367–73.
42. Hillerdal G. Mesothelioma: Cases associated with non-occupational and low dose exposures. *Occupational and Environmental Medicine.* 1999; **56**: 505–13.
43. Rake C, Gilham C, Hatch J et al. Occupational, domestic and environmental mesothelioma risks in the British population: A case–control study. *British Journal of Cancer.* 2009; **100**: 1175–83.
44. Leigh J, Driscoll T. Malignant mesothelioma in Australia, 1945–2002. *International Journal of Occupational and Environmental Health.* 2003; **9**: 206–17.
45. Howel D, Arblaster L, Swinburne L et al. Routes of asbestos exposure and the development of mesothelioma in an English region. *Occupational and Environmental Medicine.* 1997; **54**: 403–9.
46. Magnani C, Agudo A, Gonzalez CA et al. Multicentric study on malignant pleural mesothelioma and non-occupational exposure to asbestos. *British Journal of Cancer.* 2000; **83**: 104–11.
47. Maule MM, Magnani C, Dalmasso P et al. Modeling mesothelioma risk associated with environmental asbestos exposure. *Environmental Health Perspectives.* 2007; **115**: 1066–71.
48. Newhouse ML, Berry G. Predictions of mortality from mesothelial tumours in asbestos factory workers. *British Journal of Industrial Medicine.* 1976; **33**: 147–51.
49. Peto J, Seidman H, Selikoff IJ. Mesothelioma mortality in asbestos workers: Implications for models of carcinogenesis and risk assessment. *British Journal of Cancer.* 1982; **45**: 124–35.
50. Stein RC, Kitajewska JB, Kirkham N et al. Pleural mesothelioma resulting from exposure to amosite asbestos in a building. *Respiratory Medicine.* 1989; **83**: 237–9.

51. Gibbs AR, Griffiths DM, Pooley FD, Jones JSP. Comparison of fibre types and size distributions in lung tissues of paraoccupational and occupational cases of malignant mesothelioma. *British Journal of Industrial Medicine*. 1990; **47**: 621–6.
52. Peto J, Decarli A, La Vecchia C et al. The European mesothelioma epidemic. *British Journal of Cancer*. 1999; **79**: 666–72.
53. World Health Organization. Chrysotile asbestos. Environmental Health Criteria 203. Geneva: World Health Organization, 1998.
54. Newhouse ML, Berry G, Wagner JC. Mortality of factor workers in East London 1933–1980. *British Journal of Industrial Medicine*. 1985; **42**: 4–11.
55. Jones JSP, Smith PG, Pooley FD et al. The consequences of exposure to asbestos dust in a wartime gas-mask factory. In: Wagner JC, Davis W (eds). *Biological effects of mineral fibres*, No. 30. Lyon: IARC Scientific Publications, 1980: 637–53.
56. Hobbs MST, Woodward SD, Murphy B et al. The incidence of pneumoconiosis, mesothelioma and other respiratory cancer in men engaged in mining and milling crocidolite in Western Australia. In: Wagner JC, Davis W (eds). *Biological effects of mineral fibres*, No. 30. Lyon: IARC Scientific Publications, 1980: 615–24.
57. Iwatsubo Y, Pairon JC, Boutin C et al. Pleural mesothelioma: Dose–response relation at low levels of asbestos exposure in a French population-based case–control study. *American Journal of Epidemiology*. 1998; **148**: 133–42.
58. Hodgson JT, Darnton A. The quantitative risks of mesothelioma and lung cancer in relation to asbestos exposure. *Annals of Occupational Hygiene*. 2000; **44**: 565–601.
59. Browne K, Smither WJ. Asbestos-related mesothelioma: Factors discriminating between pleural and peritoneal sites. *British Journal of Industrial Medicine*. 1983; **40**: 145–52.
60. Elmes PC, Simpson MJC. The clinical aspects of mesothelioma. *Quarterly Journal of Medicine*. 1976; **179**: 427–49.
61. Greenberg M, Davies TAL. Mesothelioma register 1967–68. *British Journal of Industrial Medicine*. 1974; **31**: 91–104.
62. Yates DH, Corrin B, Stidolph PN, Browne K. Malignant mesothelioma in south east England: Clinicopathological experience of 272 cases. *Thorax*. 1997; **52**: 507–12 (published erratum appears in *Thorax* 1997; **52**: 1018).
63. Mowe G, Gylseth B, Hartveit F, Skaug V. Occupational asbestos exposure, lung-fiber concentration and latency time in malignant mesothelioma. *Scandinavian Journal of Work, Environment and Health*. 1984; **10**: 293–8.
64. Stayner LT, Dankovic DA, Lemen RA. Occupational exposure to chrysotile asbestos and cancer risk: A review of the amphibole hypothesis. *American Journal of Public Health*. 1996; **86**: 179–86.
65. McDonald JC, McDonald AD. The epidemiology of mesothelioma in historical context. *European Respiratory Journal*. 1996; **9**: 1932–42.
66. McDonald JC, McDonald AD. Chrysotile, tremolite and carcinogenicity. *Annals of Occupational Hygiene*. 1997; **41**: 699–705.
67. Churg A, Wiggs B, Depaoli L et al. Lung asbestos content in chrysotile workers with mesothelioma. *American Review of Respiratory Disease*. 1984; **130**: 1042–5.
68. Smith AH, Wright CC. Chrysotile asbestos is the main cause of pleural mesothelioma. *American Journal of Industrial Medicine*. 1996; **30**: 252–66.
69. Rogers AJ, Leigh J, Berry G et al. Relationship between lung asbestos fiber type and concentration and relative risk of mesothelioma; a case control study. *Cancer*. 1991; **67**: 1912–20.
70. Morinaga K, Kohyama N, Yokoyama K et al. Asbestos fibre content of lungs with mesotheliomas in Osaka, Japan: A preliminary report. In: Bignon J, Peto J, Saracci R (eds). *Non-occupational exposure to mineral fibres*, No. 90. Lyon: IARC Scientific Publications, 1989: 438–43.
71. Lemen RA. Chrysotile asbestos as a cause of mesothelioma. Application of the Hill causation model. *International Journal of Occupational and Environmental Health*. 2004; **10**: 233–9.
72. Roushdy-Hammady I, Siegel J, Emri S et al. Genetic-susceptibility factor and malignant mesothelioma in the Cappadocian region of Turkey. *Lancet*. 2001; **357**: 444–5.
73. Baris YI. The clinical and radiological aspects of 185 cases of malignant pleural mesothelioma. In: Wagner JC, Davis W (eds). *Biological effects of mineral fibres*, No. 30. Lyon: IARC Scientific Publications, 1980: 937–47.
74. Sakellariou K, Malamou-Mitsi V, Haritou A et al. Malignant pleural mesothelioma from nonoccupational asbestos exposure in Metsovo (north-west Greece): Slow end of an epidemic? *European Respiratory Journal*. 1996; **9**: 1206–10.
75. McConncohie K, Simonato L, Mavrides P et al. Mesothelioma in Cyprus: The role of tremolite. *Thorax*. 1987; **42**: 342–7.
76. Doll R. Mortality from lung cancer in asbestos workers. *British Journal of Industrial Medicine*. 1955; **12**: 81–6.
77. Knox JF, Holmes S, Doll R, Hill ID. Mortality from lung cancer and other causes among workers in an asbestos textile factory. *British Journal of Industrial Medicine*. 1968; **25**: 293–303.
78. Hammond EC, Selikoff IJ, Seidman H. Asbestos exposure, cigarette smoking and death rates. *Annals of the New York Academy of Sciences*. 1979; **330**: 473–90.
79. Saracci R. Asbestos and lung cancer: An analysis of the epidemiological evidence on the asbestos–smoking interaction. *International Journal of Cancer*. 1977; **20**: 323–31.
80. Berry G, Newhouse ML, Antonis P. Combined effect of asbestos and smoking on mortality from lung cancer and mesothelioma in factory workers. *British Journal of Industrial Medicine*. 1985; **42**: 12–18.
81. Lee PN. Relation between exposure to asbestos and smoking jointly and the risk of lung cancer. *Occupational and Environmental Medicine*. 2001; **59**: 494–5.
82. Vainio H, Bofetta P. Mechanisms of the combined effect of asbestos and smoking in the etiology of lung cancer. *Scandinavian Journal of Work, Environment and Health*. 1994; **20**: 235–42.
83. Henderson DW, de Klerk NH, Hammar SP et al. Asbestos and lung cancer: Is it attributable to asbestosis or to asbestos

fiber burden? In: Corrin B (ed.). *Pathology of lung tumours.* London: WB Saunders, 1997: 83–118.
84. Berry G, Liddell FD. The interaction of asbestos and smoking in lung cancer: A modified measure of effect. *Annals of Occupational Hygiene.* 2004; **48**: 459–62.
85. McDonald AD, Fry JS, Woolley AJ, McDonald J. Dust exposure and mortality in an American chrysotile textile plant. *British Journal of Industrial Medicine.* 1983; **40**: 361–7.
86. Sebastien P, McDonald JC, McDonald AD et al. Respiratory cancer in chrysotile textile and mining industries: Exposure inferences from lung analysis. *British Journal of Industrial Medicine.* 1989; **46**: 180–7.
87. Seidman H, Selikoff IJ, Hammond EC. Short-term asbestos work exposure and long-term observation. *Annals of the New York Academy of Sciences.* 1979; **330**: 61–89.
88. Liddell FDK. Latent periods in lung cancer mortality in relation to asbestos dose and smoking. In: Wagner JC, Davis W (eds). *Biological effects of mineral fibres*, No. 30. Lyon: IARC Scientific Publications, 1980: 661–5.
89. Henderson DW, Rodelsperger K, Worrowitz H-J, Leigh J. After Helsinki: A multidisciplinary review of the relationship between asbestos exposure and lung cancer, with emphasis on studies published during 1997–2004. *Pathology.* 2004; **36**: 517–50.
90. Hessel PA, Gamble JF, McDonald JC. Asbestos, asbestosis, and lung cancer: A critical assessment of the epidemiological evidence. *Thorax.* 2005; **60**: 433–6.
91. Pohlabeln H, Wild P, Schill W et al. Asbestos fibre years and lung cancer: A two phase case–control study with expert exposure assessment. *Occupational and Environmental Medicine.* 2002; **59**: 410–14.
92. Gustavsson P, Nyberg F, Pershagen G et al. Low-dose exposure to asbestos and lung cancer: Dose-reponse relations and interaction with smoking in a population-based case-referent study in Stockholm, Sweden. *American Journal of Epidemiology.* 2002; **155**: 1016–22.
93. Sluis-Cremer GK, Bezuidenhout BN. Relation between asbestosis and bronchial cancer in amphibole asbestos miners. *British Journal of Industrial Medicine.* 1989; **46**: 537–40.
94. Rudd RM. Relation between asbestosis and bronchial cancer in amphibole asbestos miners. *British Journal of Industrial Medicine.* 1990; **47**: 215–16.
95. Reid A, de Klerk N, Ambrosini GK et al. The effect of asbestosis on lung cancer risk beyond the dose related effect of asbestos alone. *Occupational and Environmental Medicine.* 2005; **62**: 885–9.
96. Consensus Report: Asbestos, asbestosis and cancer: The Helsinki criteria for diagnosis and attribution. *Scandinavian Journal of Work, Environment and Health.* 1997; **23**: 311–16.
97. Henderson DW, Jones ML, De Klerk N et al. The diagnosis and attribution of asbestos-related diseases in an Australian context: Report of the Adelaide Workshop on Asbestos-Related Diseases. October 6–7, 2000. *International Journal of Occupational and Environmental Health.* 2004; **10**: 40–6.
98. Department for Work and Pensions. Social Security Administration Act 1992. Asbestos-related diseases. London: Department for Work and Pensions, 2005: Cm 6553.
99. International Agency for Research on Cancer. Overall evaluations of carcinogenicity. Lyon: IARC, 1987.
100. Committee on Asbestos: Selected health effects. Asbestos: Selected cancers. New York: National Academies Press, 2006.
101. Industrial Injuries Advisory Council Position Paper 22. Laryngeal cancer and asbestos exposure. 2008. Available from: http://www.iiac.org.uk/pdf/pos_papers/pp22.pdf.
102. Harding A-H, Darnton A, Wegerdt J, McElvenny D. Mortality among British asbestos workers undergoing regular medical examinations (1971–2005). *Occupational and Environmental Medicine.* 2009; **66**: 487–95.

78

Other fibrous mineral dusts

ANNE COCKCROFT

Zeolites	1011	Synthetic mineral fibres	1012
Fibrous clays	1011	References	1012

ZEOLITES

This group of commercially valuable minerals is formed by recrystallization from water which has percolated through sedimentary deposits of volcanic ash (tuffs), or basic lavas originally formed in fresh water and marine environments. They are hydrated aluminium silicates with other metal ions within their open crystal lattice and act as catalysts, absorbents, etc., in the petrochemical industry, filters for sewage and water, water softeners, soil improvers and nitrogen adsorbers for oxygen concentrators. For most of these purposes, non-fibrous zeolites with an amorphous or cuboidal crystal structure are used. They are even synthesized in this form with the precise characteristics needed for the particular use. The mineral deposits contain a mixture of volcanic glass and a variety of crystalline forms of zeolite, and may be associated with small amounts of quartz and silicates. There are many different fibrous crystal forms, but they are seldom present in sufficient quantity for commercial exploitation, some only occurring in geodes. However, one, erionite, has been found in large workable deposits in several places between the mountain ranges of the western United States and in the North Island of New Zealand.

The risk due to erionite was recognized from the studies of Baris et al.[1] on the incidence of mesothelioma in scattered villages in Cappadocia in Turkey. The whole area consists of narrow valleys cut into the thick layer of volcanic tuff with flat uplands in between. The incidence of mesothelioma varied from nil to over 50 per cent of the adult population in villages within a few miles of each other. Only the villages where fine fibrous erionite was present were affected and the average age at death from mesothelioma was 45 years. A 23-year prospective study found mesothlioma accounted for 45 per cent of deaths in two exposed villages.[2]

Experimental studies have confirmed that erionite fibres are very active in producing mesotheliomas and that this activity is very strongly size-dependent.[3] Environmental exposure to erionite should be prevented, and commercial exploitation should be prevented completely.

FIBROUS CLAYS

There is a group of clays and soft rocks which are used in the manufacture of quality tiles and ceramics. They are of special value because they consist of very fine fibre crystals, mostly less than 0.1 mm in diameter and 5 mm long. However, many of the deposits contain a proportion of fibres long enough to cause mesothelioma, and this has been confirmed by intrapleural studies in animals. It is not known how long these fibres survive in the lung.

The clays are often extracted damp and then dried, milled and marketed as a fine powder with or without calcining. Other uses are as adsorbents for insecticides, for mopping up oil spills and as cat litter. There is a wide range of potential exposure which is continuous only for small groups of workers and occasional for the rest. Little information about fibre exposure is available and what epidemiological information exists indicates pneumoconiosis with some high exposures, but as yet no evidence of lung cancer or mesothelioma.

The main group are the aluminium silicates sepiolite, attapulgite, palygorskite and meerschaum, names which do not seem to correspond to different clearly defined minerals. The fibres break up easily and may not survive the normal milling procedure.

Wollastonite is a harder material mined mainly in the United States for use in the ceramics industry and as a filler to prevent cracking in cements, plasters and paints. It is a calcium silicate which formed into a mixture of platey and fibre-like crystals. Again the commercial product is milled and contains few if any 'fibres' sufficiently long to cause concern. Problems may arise if the method of processing or use is changed to preserve the elongated crystals or if other deposits are exploited.

SYNTHETIC MINERAL FIBRES

The health risks associated with the industrial use and consequent environmental contamination by asbestos led to an increased production and use of man-made fibres to replace asbestos for uses such as insulation, filtration, fire protection and friction materials. The most common man-made (or manufactured or synthetic or artificial) fibres are man-made vitreous fibres (MMVF), but there are also a number of other synthetic fibres, such as carbon/graphite fibres and silicon carbide fibres and whiskers, as well as synthetic polymers, such as Kevlar para-aramid fibres.

Also called (inappropriately) man-made mineral fibres (MMMF), MMVFs comprise glass fibres (glass wool, continuous glass filament and special purpose glass fibre), mineral wool (i.e. rock wool and slag wool) and refractory ceramic fibres. More than 80 per cent of the total production of MMVFs is made up by the insulation wools (glass, rock and slag wool). They are obtained by melting glass (with stabilizers and modifiers or fluxes), rock (basalt, granite, slate, limestone), slag (from metallic ore refining) or kaolin clay (or combinations of alumina/silica often with zirconium), and producing fibres by rotary or other processes. Various materials are used as additives and the fibres are often held together with binders (e.g. phenol-formaldehyde resin). The size characteristics of MMVFs are such that their mean diameters exceed the sizes considered to be respirable (3 µm), except for refractory ceramic fibres and glass microfibres. In addition, airborne concentrations have been reported to be generally lower than 1 fibre/mL air during manufacture, although higher levels are possible during applications. Another reassuring feature of MMVFs compared with asbestos is that their biopersistence (durability) in the lung is much lower, again with the exception of refractory ceramic fibres.

A number of structural similarities between some of these fibres and asbestos, as well as experimental data *in vitro* and in laboratory animals, led to concern that these asbestos substitutes may in fact be as hazardous as asbestos. Fortunately, this does not appear to be the case, although working with man-made fibre is not free from health risks.[4,5]

Occupational (and residential) exposure to MMVFs is well known to lead to acute skin and eye irritation, as well as upper respiratory tract irritation. However, neither interstitial fibrosis nor chronic obstructive pulmonary disease has been demonstrated to result from exposure to them. Pleural changes have not been shown to occur either, except in the case of the more persistent refractory ceramic fibres, for which a study of a cohort of production workers found a progressive relationship between plaques and cumulative exposure to refractory ceramic fibres, taking into account the possible exposure to asbestos.[6] With regard to malignant lung disease, an IARC monograph published in 2002[7] concluded that there is inadequate evidence in humans for carcinogenicity of various forms of MMMF, although there is evidence of carcinogenicity in animals for some types of MMMF; the committee classified special-purpose glass fibres such as E-glass and '475' glass fibres and refractory ceramic fibres as possibly carcinogenic to humans, while insulation glass wool, continuous glass filament, rock (stone) wool and slag wool were not classifiable as to their carcinogenicity to humans.

The human health effects of synthetic fibres other than MMVFs, are much less well studied. With the exception of silicon carbide fibres, which may lead to pneumoconiosis, no human disease has been reported following exposure to these fibres. However, an outbreak of interstitial lung disease (mainly non-specific interstitial pneumonia) has been described in workers exposed to microfibres made of nylon.[8] Nylon is not generally included among the man-made fibres, but like Kevlar, it is a synthetic fibre.

> **Key points**
>
> - Environmental exposure to erionite has led to an epidemic of mesothelioma, for example in Cappadocia in Turkey.
> - While human evidence of carcinogenicity is lacking, the IARC has classified certain types of man-made fibres as possibly carcinogenic to humans.

REFERENCES

1. Baris YI, Sahin AA, Ozesmi M. An outbreak of pleural mesothelioma and chronic fibrosing pleurisy in the village of Karain/Urgup in Anatolia. *Thorax.* 1978; **33**: 181–92.
2. Baris YI, Grandjean P. Prospective study of mesothelioma mortality in Turkish villages with exposure to fibrous zeolite. *Journal of the National Cancer Institute.* 2006; **98**: 414–17.
3. Wagner JC, Pooley FD. Mineral fibres and mesothelioma. *Thorax.* 1986; **41**: 161–6.
4. De Vuyst P, Dumortier P, Swaen GMH *et al.* Respiratory health effects of man-made vitreous (mineral) fibres. *European Respiratory Journal.* 1995; **8**: 2149–73.
5. Lockey JE. Man-made fibers and non-asbestos fibrous silicates. In: Harber P, Schenker MB, Balmes JR (eds). *Occupational and environmental respiratory disease.* St Louis: Mosby, 1996: 330–44.

6. Lockey J, Lemasters G, Rice C et al. Refractory ceramic fiber exposure and pleural plaques. *American Journal of Respiratory and Critical Care Medicine*. 1996; **154**: 1405–10.
7. World Health Organization, International Agency for Research on Cancer. IARC monographs on the evaluation of carcinogenic risks to humans, vol. 81. Man-made vitreous fibres. Lyon: IARC Press, 2002.
8. Kern DG, Crausman RS, Durand KTH et al. Flock worker's lung: Chronic interstitial lung disease in the nylon flocking industry. *Annals of Internal Medicine*. 1998; **129**: 261–72.

79

Silica and silica-related diseases

ANNE COCKCROFT

Quartz and related dust	1014	Risks and prevention of silicosis in different occupations	1017
Acute silicosis	1015	Health surveillance of workers exposed to silica dust	1019
Chronic (active) silicosis	1015	References	1019
Chronic (inactive) silicosis	1016		

QUARTZ AND RELATED DUST

Quartz dust is among the most toxic of the non-fibrous mineral dusts and can cause fatal disease (acute silicosis) after exposure for only a few months to very high concentrations which may not even be perceptible to the naked eye. Heavy exposure to fine dusts containing quartz in the drilling of rock in mining and quarrying can therefore be highly dangerous and workplace exposure to quartz containing dusts has been subject to regulation for many decades in industrialized countries. Longer-term exposure to lower concentrations of quartz can lead to fibrogenic disease and silicosis used to be commonplace in many dusty industries; it remains common in less developed countries. Many mixed dusts produce disease due to their quartz content.

Silicon dioxide (SiO_2) is ubiquitous in the earth's crust. Silicosis results from the inhalation of one of the three crystalline forms of silicon dioxide. Quartz is by far the most common, the other two being cristobalite and tridymite. Amorphous (non-crystalline) forms of silica dusts dissolve fairly rapidly in the tissue and do not cause the progressive pulmonary disease produced by crystalline forms, although the dissolved silica may damage other tissues, such as the kidney.

Quartz is found free as (silica) sand which is the residue left by the erosion of igneous rocks, like granite, in which the quartz crystals formed when larva cooled. Pure quartz is colourless, but traces of metal in the melt have produced various gemstones, such as citrine and cairngorm. Quartz is very hard and is virtually insoluble in tissue fluids and in most acids and alkalis.

Toxicity of quartz

The mechanisms by which apparently inert insoluble particles of quartz damage cells include direct cytotoxicity, with release of lipases and proteases, activation of oxidant production by pulmonary macrophages, activation of mediator release from alveolar macrophages leading to production of cytokines and reactive species, and secretion of growth factors from alveolar macrophages.[1–3] Freshly ground respirable particles will kill phagocytic cells in culture, and kill the cells lining the alveoli of experimental animals and of humans at high levels of exposure. At lower levels, especially when the quartz is diluted with an inert dust, the macrophages will take up a few active particles with the inert ones and survive long enough to move into the alveolar wall or to the centrilobular interstitium before dying. At greater dilution, some of the quartz mixed in with the other dust will be cleared by the macrophages to the bronchial mucus escalator.

Resuspended quartz dust, such as that which blows off the Sahara desert, is relatively inert and much of it is cleared from the lung without causing damage, although pneumoconiosis in Bedouin has been described.[4] Similarly, quartz mixed with metal oxides, as encountered in iron ore mining, does not show the expected toxicity. Experimentally, this has been shown to be due to the adsorption of a layer of the metal oxide on to the crystal. Experimental studies have since shown that these coatings, applied before inhalation, will delay the onset of fibrosis and reduce its severity, but that the coating is eventually lost and the particles become actively fibrogenic.[5]

In the hope that metals, such as aluminium, and some polymers might make quartz dust less toxic, such compounds have even been administered to workers who have already inhaled quartz dust in the hope that silicosis may be prevented or even cured. Long-term use of aluminium powder as a prophylactic inhalation in Canadian uranium miners was abandoned after 30 years because of lack of evidence of its efficacy. (Metallic aluminium powder has been shown to be fibrogenic in animals in the same size range as quartz (0.5–5 mm) and cases of pulmonary fibrosis have been reported from industry.) Aluminium citrate given parenterally has been shown both in laboratory animals and on clinical trial in humans to reduce the severity of silicosis. However, the known toxicity of aluminium to the central nervous system precludes its long-term parenteral use (see Chapter 13, Aluminium).

ACUTE SILICOSIS

This is also known as 'silicotic alveolar proteinosis' or even 'silicotic alveolar lipoproteinosis'. High level exposure to active dust causes immediate damage in the alveolus with death of the type I and II alveolar lining cells, as well as the macrophages. Protein fluid, followed by inflammatory cells, leaks from the capillaries into the alveoli, mingling with the surfactant. Resolution does not occur and the alveoli become obliterated with fibrous tissue. This acute alveolitis may present within weeks of the start of exposure. The first symptoms are breathlessness and dry cough which get gradually worse despite all treatment. The radiograph shows patchy pulmonary oedema, but with the shadows gradually hardening and the affected areas shrinking. Lung function tests indicate a restrictive lesion with falling gas transfer leading to hypoxia and cyanosis. The disease is often fatal, sometimes within a few months, the prognosis being dependent on the amount of active dust already retained before the exposure stopped.

As there is no safe or effective treatment for this (or any other) form of silicosis, acute silicosis should never be allowed to occur in any country. There are documented incidents of large numbers of men dying of acute silicosis in the face of high, uncontrolled silica exposure in tunnelling, the most notorious being at Hawk's Nest in the United States.[6] Acute silicosis is still reported, for instance, where a small enterprise is set up to sand blast metal parts or to make silica flour without dust control.

The lesions of acute silicosis can also be seen in parts of the lung in cases of chronic active silicosis when the exposure has been high and recent. This intermediate disease is known as 'accelerated silicosis' and outbreaks of this condition have occurred even recently in the United Kingdom.[7]

CHRONIC (ACTIVE) SILICOSIS

This disease was once widespread in industrial countries. It is now uncommon in developed countries mainly due to the use of safer alternative materials. Where this is not possible (hard rock mining, tunnelling, etc.), the adoption of modern methods of dust control and the enforcement of international standards have minimized the risk. In developing countries, many sources of risk still exist and the disease is still a major problem.

In the late 1980s, the pathology of silicosis and silicate dust pneumoconiosis was reviewed in some detail by an international panel of pathologists and much of this is still relevant.[8]

Symptoms are a late manifestation of the disease. By the time breathlessness is noticed or is sufficient to interfere with labouring work, the radiograph shows widespread change. The first shadows to appear are the medium to large size of small, rounded opacities ('q' or 'r' on the International Labour Organization (ILO) scale) and are either evenly distributed or more frequent in the upper zones. Hilar node enlargement is common. The histology of the lesions in the lung is diagnostic; they are discrete nodules made of concentric layers of dense collagen tissue with a core containing birefringent quartz particles. They seldom grow to more than 1 cm in diameter. Larger masses consist of a conglomeration of these nodules as do the enlarged hilar lymph nodes. The nodules first form in the centrilobular area and then along the lymphatics both to the pleura and the hilar nodes with lines of less organized fibrous tissue linking them together. In the absence of further exposure, the nodules may become inactive and calcify from the periphery inwards. However, it may take 20–30 years for nodules to form, become quiescent and calcify; few workers with active silicosis live this long. A similar phenomenon in the hilar nodes gives rise to the appearance of 'eggshell calcification' ('ec' in the ILO symbols). A short period of relatively high exposure can give rise to hilar gland enlargement and nodules in the pleura with adhesions and pleural thickening, before there is a build up of nodules in the lung parenchyma. Figure 79.1 is a chest radiograph showing the appearances of silicosis.

The onset of breathlessness is usually due to the beginning of coalescence of individual nodules through the contraction of the linking fibrous bands. In the absence of complicating tuberculosis, there may be a dry cough and no pain. Lung function testing shows a restrictive pattern with loss of gas transfer capacity. Eventually, hypoxia and cyanosis occur, first on exercise and then at rest. Death is usually due to cor pulmonale. There are usually no physical signs in the chest and clubbing is not a feature. Depending possibly on the presence of amorphous silica in the dust, severe silicosis may be associated with liver and renal damage.[9]

The accelerated form of silicosis can produce symptoms within a year of the start of exposure, when the lungs may show some of the features of acute silicosis, and when some deaths may occur within five years. In the last 50 years, it has been uncommon in the United Kingdom to see radiographic changes starting before 10–20 years from first exposure and leading (in the absence of tuberculosis) to life-threatening lung impairment before the retiring age. The longer the interval between first exposure and the onset

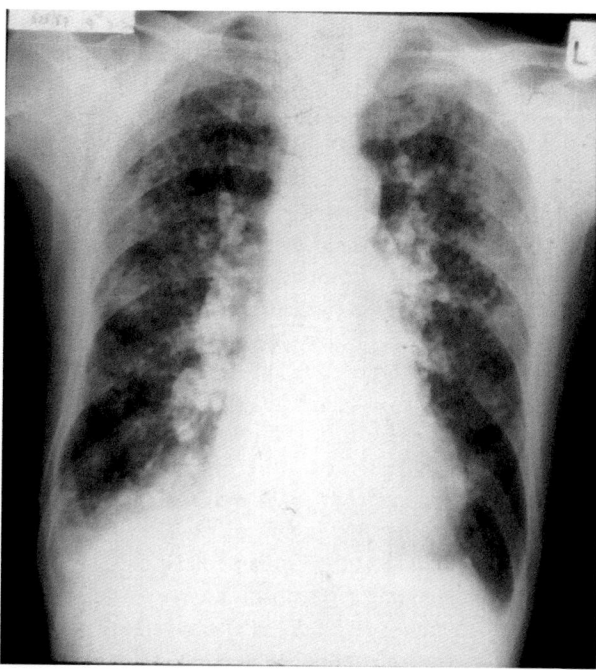

Figure 79.1 Chest radiograph of silicosis, with small rounded opacities in the lung fields and enlargement and 'egg shell' calcification of the hilar lymph nodes.

of symptoms, the slower they tend to progress and the greater the likelihood of the subject living to the retiring age and beyond. If the dust is relatively pure quartz, then little will be seen on the radiograph until the first nodules ('r' shadows) appear 5–15 years after first exposure. When there is heavy admixture of inert dust then a simple small opacity pneumoconiosis ('p' or 'q') may appear first. It is possible for workers exposed to quartz to leave their occupation after five or more years, free of symptoms, with a normal chest radiograph and lung function tests at that time, and then to develop classical silicosis and die of respiratory failure or complicating tuberculosis many years later.

CHRONIC (INACTIVE) SILICOSIS

Just as there is no clear distinction between acute and chronic (active) disease so there is none between chronic (active) and chronic (inactive). It is a matter of the level and duration of exposure. The presence of other dusts, cigarette smoking and environmental pollution outside the workplace can also modify the effect of the quartz.

When workers are exposed for many years to a dust which is occasionally contaminated with quartz or which contains, most of the time, a very small proportion of quartz (or quartz activity is being suppressed by the presence of other minerals such as aluminium, iron oxide, etc.), their pneumoconiosis shows mixed features. On the radiograph, a simple pneumoconiosis with mainly 'p'- and 'q'-sized rounded opacities may be present after 20–30 years. A few workers may show 'r' shadows in the upper zone and hilar gland enlargement. These 'r' shadows may become more profuse, tend to coalesce to form irregular masses or they may remain static and calcify. The hilar nodes may show eggshell calcification without obvious 'r'-sized parenchymal shadows ever appearing. In workers with a long exposure history and who show these mixed features, it is unwise to give a good prognosis without following the case for at least ten years after exposure has ceased. Histology of such lungs often shows silicotic nodules in various stages of development, some dating from early exposure and others arising more recently with scope for further development. Calcification is probably the only sure indication that a silicotic lesion is no longer active.

Silicotuberculosis

When active tuberculosis is common in the community, many patients with silicosis develop a combined disease with an extremely poor prognosis called 'silicotuberculosis'. This is now rare in developed countries, but remains common in many developing countries,[10] and is even increasing in developing countries with a serious HIV epidemic.[11] Conventional chemotherapy for tuberculosis may delay progression, but patients can die with their infection still active in spite of chemotherapy that would eradicate the disease in patients without silicosis. Among South African gold miners, the presence of silicosis has been shown to increase the risk of tuberculosis and to exacerbate its clinical course.[12,13] Some years ago Westerholm[14] calculated that the risk of developing tuberculosis after the diagnosis of silicosis in Sweden was up to 15 times the risk for the general population. A study of mortality among silicosis claimants in California (cases from 1945 to 1975 followed from 1946 to 1991) found a grossly elevated mortality from tuberculosis among these patients with silicosis.[15] The risk in the individual is related to the severity of the silicosis. It remains high for at least 15 years after the diagnosis of silicosis and probably for a lifetime. The mechanism is unknown, but *in vitro* studies indicate that macrophages are less able to engulf and kill tubercle bacilli when quartz dust is present. Silicosis causes damage to the lymphatic drainage of the lung which is important for the control of tuberculous infections; there may be an additional constitutional factor.

The detection of active tuberculosis in patients with early asymptomatic silicosis is not difficult because the onset of cough, sputum, night sweats, malaise and weight loss may be enough to bring the patient to the clinic. On the chest radiograph, new soft upper zone shadowing should show up clearly against the pre-existing 'r'-sized rounded opacities. A raised sedimentation rate and the presence of tubercle bacilli in the sputum confirm the diagnosis. The diagnosis is difficult in advanced silicosis, especially patients who smoke, as they probably already have a cough, sputum and loss of weight. Confluent silicotic nodules in the upper zone with associated emphysema may mimic the appearance of cavities and make new infiltrates difficult to see on conventional radiographs. Confluent silicotic nodules (unlike the masses of progressive massive fibrosis in coal miners and those of Caplan's syndrome) rarely cavitate in the absence of tuberculosis. Haemoptysis and cavitation of the lung masses (confirmed by computed tomography (CT) scan, if possible) are strong indications of active tuberculosis. The organisms may be hard to identify on sputum smear or culture from the sputum and it is often necessary to treat such cases on suspicion, without microbiological confirmation of the diagnosis. Treatment is as for pulmonary tuberculosis (for example, following the British Thoracic Society guidelines in the United Kingdom). There is evidence that treatment should be more prolonged than for tuberculosis in the absence of silicosis.[16] It can be difficult to gauge effectiveness of treatment in the absence of organisms in the sputum, as the radiographic shadows may not regress.

Prevention of silicotuberculosis

Prevention of silicotuberculosis is difficult. The main risk of silicosis now is in developing countries where the general risk of tuberculosis is high and most of the population are exposed to the tubercle bacillus in childhood. Occupational exposure to quartz dust then carries the risk of reactivation of latent infection or new infection. The overcrowded and insanitary conditions prevailing for migrant workers in mine compounds contribute to the spread of the disease. In a developing country where most children are already tuberculin skin test positive before they start breathing in quartz dust, there is obviously no point in giving BCG when work starts. The use of BCG among tuberculin skin test negative mine workers exposed to silica in Eastern Europe apparently had an adverse effect,[17] although a benefit was reported for copper miners in Africa.[18] Some authors have reported benefit from prophylactic chemotherapy, for example with isoniazid for people with silicosis, and recommended its use;[19] but this may be impractical in developing countries where the majority of the cases now occur. Careful monitoring of patients with silicosis is important, with treatment on suspicion of infection, even without microbiological confirmation.

RISKS AND PREVENTION OF SILICOSIS IN DIFFERENT OCCUPATIONS

Grinders

When the cause of lung disease in grinders (Figure 79.2) was recognized as being due to their exposure to silica dust (for example, knife grinders in Sheffield), the first move was to change from dry to wet working; later, sandstone or millstone grit grinding wheels were replaced by synthetic silicon carbide. Although harder than quartz, this produces a dust which is very much less fibrogenic and its use has virtually eradicated silicosis from this occupational group. As even silicon carbide dust can cause lung fibrosis, most grinding work should still be done wet and exposure must be kept well below the limits for 'nuisance dusts'.

Masons and polishers

Wet working can be effective in controlling silicosis among monumental masons and men who polish granite and other quartz-containing rock for architectural and decorative use, but failure to control dust exposure can lead to accelerated disease.

In some traditional workplaces, materials like precious stones, jade and metals are polished with dangerous powders. Silicosis has been reported from a workshop where jade was polished (dry), using a mixture containing silica flour.[20] The silicosis risk can be avoided by using a non-fibrogenic polishing powder.

Miners

Hard rock mining for metals, such as tin, gold and copper, was another occupation recognized early as causing silicosis, and similarly the cutting of shafts and 'drivages' (passages or roadways) through hard rock to gain access to coal seams and other ores. Civil engineering tunnelling first for canals and then railways and now for motorways and underground railways, hydroelectric schemes, etc., are situations where the risk may vary from week to week depending on the rock strata encountered. The most important step was the introduction of hollow drills which could not be used without water flowing down the centre (Figure 79.3). However, in hard rock situations, it is not possible to inject water into the rock face to prevent dust formation when charges are fired. This can be dealt with by positive ventilation and waiting periods after shot firing to allow the dust and toxic fumes to be cleared by the ventilation before the workers go back in.

Pottery and refractory making

Silicosis was common in the UK area in Staffordshire known as the 'Potteries' where the making of crockery and ceramics was concentrated. It resulted partly from the grinding of quartz-containing minerals, like 'china stone', for mixing with the clay for making porcelain. The main problem was the use of silica sand and silica flour as a parting medium to prevent the pots from sticking together or to the stands while they were being fired. Not only did the dust from applying the silica sand and flour cause silicosis, but by the time firing was complete the quartz was converted to cristobalite and the workers handling the items after firing were at even greater risk. Refractory bricks for

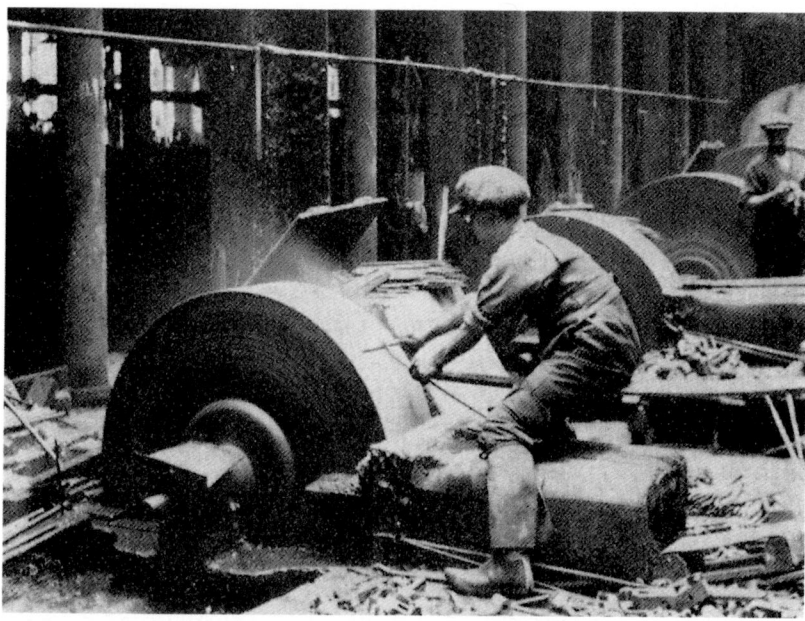

Figure 79.2 Grinding with a sandstone wheel; wet working was not by itself sufficient to prevent silicosis. Courtesy Platt Bros & Co. Ltd

cristobalite, as well as quartz, and fibres of mullite are also formed which may contribute to the lung damage. All these risks could be avoided by dust suppression, but this is technically very difficult especially when cleaning the lining out of an old furnace. Alternatives for prevention include automation and changing to ingredients and parting media that are not fibrogenic.

Moulders and fettlers

Traditionally, iron and brass were cast by pouring the metal into moulds formed of damp sand. When cool, the mould was broken open, leaving some of the sand embedded in the surface of the metal. This was first knocked off with a hammer and chisel (fettled) and the surface finished by grinding. Both these processes released sufficient quartz dust to cause chronic active silicosis in a proportion of the workers. It was a slow, labour-intensive process and was replaced by sand blasting, which caused acute silicosis. The sand was replaced by steel shot, but there was still the sand on the casting and silicosis still occurred. Even the replacement of silica sand as a main casting medium by less fibrogenic material such as 'green sand' has not completely solved this problem. If castings are to be cleaned in this manner, the work has to be completely enclosed in a specially ventilated cabinet. High-precision casting, such as is demanded of the light alloy components for the motor industry, has moved towards the use of binders in the moulding medium and various separating agents to produce a clean smooth casting.

There are a number of other jobs with likely exposure to quartz, including work in geology laboratories, or in mineralogy, road work and construction work. There is a wide variation in risk of exposure and in the type of controls required to control the exposure effectively.

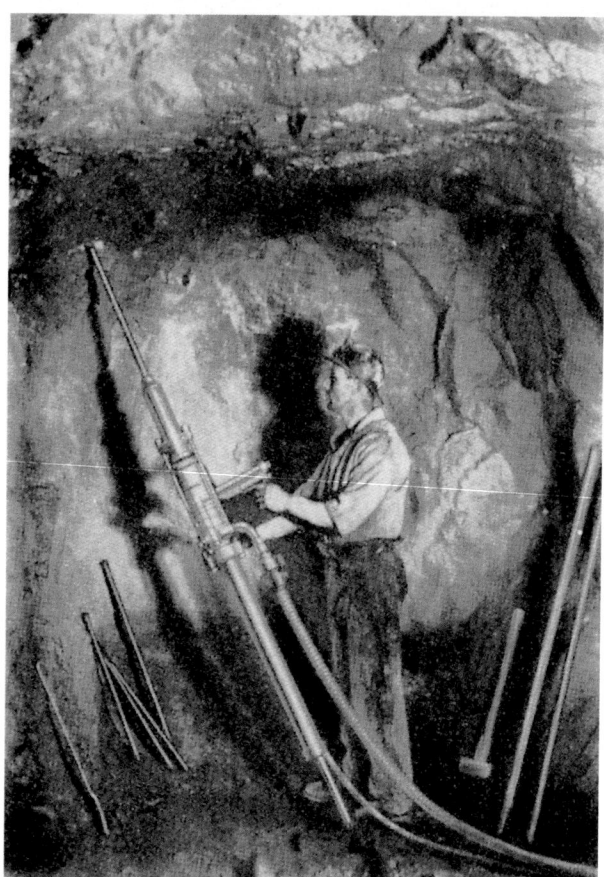

Figure 79.3 Wet drilling of hard rock using a drill which will only rotate when the water running down the middle is turned on. Courtesy Mr T Holman.

lining furnaces were made of silica sand and caused silicosis during manufacture and use when the lining of furnaces had to be renewed at regular intervals by digging out the old bricks (a very dusty job). The spent bricks contained

HEALTH SURVEILLANCE OF WORKERS EXPOSED TO SILICA DUST

As described in Chapter 80, Epidemiology of silica-related disease, current exposure limits, although already stringent in developed countries, may still be not be stringent enough to prevent development of silica-related diseases in some industries. Therefore, health surveillance of exposed workers is still important and is a legal requirement in most industrialized countries for workers with more than minimal exposure to respirable crystalline silica. In the United Kingdom, in certain occupational settings where the risk of exposure to quartz is known to be insignificant and with good controls in place, such as in mineralogy laboratories, health surveillance is not required under the Control of Substances Hazardous to Health (COSHH) regulations.

The details of recommended health surveillance for silica-exposed workers vary between countries. Recommended pre-employment screening includes enquiry about previous exposure to silica and other dusts and about respiratory symptoms, examination of the chest, a chest radiograph and ventilatory lung function testing.[21] Because of the increased risk of tuberculosis, in many countries a tuberculin skin test is recommended;[21,22] this is not recommended in situations where the community rate of tuberculosis is high or where there is a programme of BCG vaccination, where a positive skin reaction is not helpful as an indicator of active tuberculosis. In the United Kingdom, tuberculin skin testing is not recommended as part of health surveillance for silica-exposed workers.[23] A positive history or radiological evidence of past or present pulmonary tuberculosis are good reasons for advising against employment involving significant exposure to quartz, for example in mining. At follow-up examinations, the cumulative dust exposure for each individual, details of respiratory illnesses and changes in smoking habits should be added to the results of the clinical examination, radiograph and ventilatory lung function tests.

The recommended frequency of health surveillance varies between countries.[21] Follow-up examinations with a chest radiograph, spirometry and a clinical examination of the chest are recommended every one to four years, with the recommended frequency increasing after longer exposure, when silicosis is more likely to develop. Guidelines in many industrialized countries recommend that workers with a significant cumulative exposure to respirable crystalline silica should be offered continued follow up after they leave or retire, even if they have a normal chest radiograph and lung function at the time, as progression of silicosis can continue after exposure ceases, and they are at risk of developing silicotuberculosis or lung cancer (see Chapter 80, Epidemiology of silica-related diseases).

The development of radiographic changes suggestive of silicosis, especially if accompanied by an unexpected drop in ventilatory capacity, should lead to the worker being removed from dusty work and to a re-examination of the working conditions. The worker should be advised against further exposure to quartz in any employment, and acquainted with the procedure for claiming appropriate statutory benefit where such a scheme exists (see Chapter 8, Compensation schemes). Chemoprophylaxis against tuberculosis should also be considered.

> **Key points**
>
> - Acute silicosis due to high exposure to quartz is a rapidly developing acute alveolitis which is often fatal. This disease is now rare.
> - Chronic silicosis is now rare in developed countries, but remains a serious problem in developing countries with poor dust control mechanisms.
> - The chest radiograph in silicosis shows small rounded opacities with hilar lymph node enlargement and sometimes 'egg shell' calcification; coalescence to mass lesions may occur later.
> - Silicosis greatly increases the risk of tuberculosis; silicotuberculosis is a serious complication and can be difficult to treat. Tuberculosis chemoprophylaxis should be considered for people with silicosis, where this is feasible.

REFERENCES

1. Vanhee D, Gosset P, Boitelle A *et al*. Cytokines and cytokine network in silicosis and coal workers' pneumoconiosis. *European Respiratory Journal*. 1995; **8**: 834–42.
2. Vallyathan V. Generation of oxygen radicals by minerals and its correlation to cytotoxicity. *Environmental Health Perspectives*. 1994; **102** (Suppl. 10): 111–15.
3. Castranova V, Vallyathan V. Silicosis and coal workers' pneumoconiosis. *Environmental Health Perspectives*. 2000; **108** (Suppl. 4): 675–84.
4. Hirsch M, Bar-Ziv J, Lehmann E, Goldberg GM. Simple siliceous pneumoconiosis of Bedouin females in the Negev desert. *Clinical Radiology*. 1974; **25**: 507–10.
5. Le Bouffant L, Daniel H, Martin JC, Bruyere S. Effect of impurities and associated minerals on quartz toxicity. *Annals of Occupational Hygiene*. 1982; **26**: 625–32.
6. Cherniack M. *The Hawk's Nest incident: America's worst industrial disaster*. New Haven: Yale University Press, 1986.
7. Seaton A, Legges IS, Henderson J, Kerr KM. Accelerated silicosis in Scottish stone masons. *Lancet*. 1991; **337**: 341–4.
8. Craighead JE, Kleinerman J. Silicosis and silicate committee, NIOSH. Diseases associated with exposure to silica and non-fibrous silicate minerals. *Archives of Pathology and Laboratory Medicine*. 1988; **112**: 673–720.

9. Sluis-Cremer GK, Hessel PA, Nizdo EH et al. Silica, silicosis and progressive systemic sclerosis. *British Journal of Industrial Medicine.* 1985; **42**: 838-43.
10. Tiwari RR, Sharma YK. Respiratory health of female stone grinders with free silica dust exposure in Gujarat, India. *International Journal of Occupational and Environmental Health.* 2008; **14**: 280-2.
11. Mulenga EM, Miller HB, Sinkala T et al. Silicosis and tuberculosis in Zambian miners. *International Journal of Occupational and Environmental Health.* 2005; **11**: 259-62.
12. Hnizdo E, Murray J. Risk of pulmonary tuberculosis relative to silicosis and exposure to silica dust in South African gold miners. *Occupational and Environmental Medicine.* 1998; **55**: 496-502.
13. teWaterNaude JM, Ehrlich RI, Churchyard GJ et al. Tuberculosis and silica exposure in South African gold miners. *Occupational and Environmental Medicine.* 2006; **63**: 187-92.
14. Westerholm P. Silicosis, observations on a case register. *Scandinavian Journal of Work and Environmental Health.* 1980; **6** (Suppl. 2): 1-86.
15. Goldsmith DF, Beaumont JJ, Morrin LA, Schenker MB. Respiratory cancer and other chronic disease mortality among silicotics in California. *American Journal of Industrial Medicine.* 1995; **28**: 459-67.
16. Lam CW. Comparison of 6- and 8-month chemotherapy in the treatment of silicotuberculosis. Singapore: Proceedings of the International Union against Tuberculosis, 1986.
17. Pramatarov I. Investigation of the incidence of silicosis and silicotuberculosis among BCG vaccinated underground workers in the Rodopsk mine basin. *Gigiena Truda i Professional'nye Zabolevaniia.* 1965; **9**: 41-9.
18. Paul R. Silicosis in Northern Rhodesia copper mines. *Archives of Industrial Health.* 1961; **2**: 96.
19. Barboza CE, Winter DH, Seiscento M et al. Tuberculosis and silicosis: Epidemiology, diagnosis and chemoprophylaxis. *Jornal Brasileiro de Pneumologia.* 2008; **34**: 959-66.
20. Ng TP, Allan WGL, Tsin TW, O'Kelly FJ. Silicosis in jade workers. *British Journal of Industrial Medicine.* 1985; **42**: 761-4.
21. Wagner GR. *Screening and surveillance of workers exposed to mineral dust.* Geneva: World Health Organization, 1996.
22. Raymond LW, Wintermeyer S. Medical surveillance of workers exposed to crystalline silica: ACOEM evidence-based statement. *Journal of Occupational and Environmental Medicine.* 2006; **48**: 95-101.
23. Health and Safety Executive. Health surveillance for those with exposure to respirable crystalline silica (RCS): G404. London: Health and Safety Executive, 2006.

80

Epidemiology of silica-related disease

KYLE STEENLAND

Introduction	1021	Autoimmune disease	1024
Silicosis	1021	Comparative risks	1025
Lung cancer	1022	References	1026
Kidney disease	1024		

INTRODUCTION

Crystalline respirable silica is one of the best known and well-characterized occupational toxins, because of its long history of causing silicosis. In the last 20 years, epidemiologic data are reasonably conclusive that silica also causes lung cancer and quite suggestive that silica leads to renal disease. Furthermore, some data also link silica to autoimmune diseases, such as rheumatoid arthritis (RA), systemic lupus erythematosis and scleroderma.

Exposure to silica is still common. For example, in the United States about 2 million workers (2 per cent of the workforce) are estimated to be exposed, principally in foundries, ceramic and brick, granite, mining and sandblasting. It is estimated that 100 000 of these workers have exposure above the National Institute for Occupational Safety and Health (NIOSH) recommended exposure limit of 0.05 mg/m^3.[1,2] While high-silica exposure has been traditionally associated with dusty trades, such as mining and brickmaking, significant exposure also occurs in construction, a common occupation.[3]

SILICOSIS

Silicosis is perhaps the best-known of all occupational diseases. Although it was once thought to have been largely eliminated in developed countries by the 1950s, we now know that appreciable numbers of cases continue to occur there, and much larger numbers occur in less-developed countries. A recent review[4] estimates 8800 silicosis deaths a year worldwide. The number of worldwide incident cases are not known, but there are probably several hundred thousand cases annually.

Silicosis usually refers to chronic (or 'simple') silicosis, defined by the presence of small rounded opacities of ILO category 1/1 or greater on x-rays.[5] This disease may be asymptomatic, but can often progress to symptomatic disease. Acute silicosis is symptomatic disease resulting from a short-term, very high exposure and is rare nowadays. Progressive massive fibrosis characterized by large opacities on x-ray may also occur as a complication of chronic silicosis. Another sequel can be tuberculosis; rates of tuberculosis are higher among silicotics ('tuberculo-silicosis').

That silica causes silicosis is not in doubt. However, despite a large body of epidemiologic literature documenting silicosis in different populations, not until the last 10–15 years have we had quantitative exposure–response data allowing us to evaluate whether current exposure standards are adequately protective.

Table 80.1 provides estimates of the risk of silicosis morbidity (defined as an x-ray with ILO category 1/1 or greater) from studies with quantitative exposure–response data. These risks are those estimated to occur after an exposure of 45 years at the current standard for 100 per cent pure quartz in the United States (0.1 mg/m^3 respirable crystalline silica). Studies without follow up after employment (when many cases occur), or without sufficient time since first exposure, may substantially underestimate the risk. Acute silicosis can occur rapidly after short-term high exposures, but chronic silicosis has a variable latency period (time since first exposure), so that some cases occur much later than others even given equivalent cumulative exposure. Cross-sectional studies tend to underestimate risk, because workers with disease may not survive or may not be present in the workplace if the survey is workplace based.

Lifetime risks in Table 80.1 vary widely, but all are above the risk level that many regulatory agencies accept. For

Table 80.1 Silicosis morbidity. Lifetime risk, ILO category 1/1 or higher (small rounded opacities on radiograph).

Follow up after employment	Study design	Estimated lifetime risk at 0.1 mg/m³ for 45 years (%)	Reference
No, current workers	Longitudinal	2	61
Some retirees	Cross-sectional	3	62
Some retirees	Cross-sectional	15–20	63
Yes	Longitudinal	47	64
Yes	Longitudinal	77	65
Yes	Cross-sectional	92	66
Yes	Longitudinal	55	67
No	Cross-sectional	95	10
Yes	Longitudinal	15–20	9

example, the US Occupational Safety and Health Administration (OSHA) generally accepts an excess risk of up to one in 1000 (0.1 per cent) (of exposed individuals developing disease).[6] Given that there is no background risk for silicosis among the non-exposed, absolute and excess risk are the same. The wide variation of risk between studies in Table 80.1 probably mainly reflects differences in study design and length of follow up, but may also reflect the different capacity of different types of silica to produce silicosis. In a number of settings, appreciable clay coatings of the silica may occur, which may decrease the risk of silicosis and other diseases caused by silica. There is support from animal data for this phenomenon,[7] and International Agency for Research on Cancer (IARC)[8] cited it in noting the variation in lung cancer risk across silica studies. Chen et al.[9] for example, provide data on not only respirable silica but also cumulative surface-available respirable silica, for which the estimated lifetime risk of silicosis increases from 15–20 to 25–30 per cent.

Churchyard et al.[10] studied South African gold miners with an average silica exposure level of 0.05 mg/m³, half the current standard in many countries. They typically had a long duration of exposure (median 21 years). Even though the study was cross-sectional and did not include follow up after employment, these miners had a 19 per cent prevalence of silicosis. These data again strongly indicate that the current exposure standard in many countries is too high to prevent silicosis, and suggest that in fact the standard needs to be below 0.05 mg/m³ (the current NIOSH recommended level). Greaves[5] has recommended a standard of 0.01 mg/m³ under the assumption that such a level would reduce lifetime risk of silicosis to approximately two in 100, still too high but a compromise with what is technologically feasible and practically possible.

There are additional data from three studies regarding exposure–response analyses for silicosis mortality. The largest of these is by t'Mannetje et al.,[11] which analyses silicosis mortality from an IARC study of 18 000 workers in six cohorts (170 deaths, underlying cause). The estimated risk of death by age 75 years due to silicosis was 1.9 per cent after a lifetime of work (age 20–65 years) at the current standard (0.1 mg/m³). This result, this time for death rather than x-ray abnormality, is again well above the one in 1000 risk accepted by US OSHA. A second study by Hedlund et al.[12] studied 7729 miners, with 58 deaths from silicosis. The crude death rate from silicosis as an underlying cause was 20/100 000, similar to that in the IARC study by t'Mannetje (29/100 000). A third study by Tse et al.[13] analyses non-malignant respiratory disease mortality, a category broader than silicosis mortality, and does not provide detailed results for exposure–response by cumulative silica exposure.

LUNG CANCER

Since the 1980s, there have been many cohort studies focusing on lung cancer and silica exposure. A meta-analysis of 17 studies of silica and lung cancer by Steenland et al.[14] found a modest combined relative risk for the exposed versus non-exposed of 1.3, after excluding studies with known confounders (e.g. studies of foundry workers, who are exposed to many other known carcinogens). A similar meta-analysis of 19 studies of silicotics (with presumably high levels of silica exposure) found a relative risk of lung cancer of 2.3, compared with non-exposed populations.[14]

In 1997, IARC classified silica as a definite lung carcinogen (group 1), but noted that not all studies were consistent, and the carcinogenic potential of silica might be affected by the physical properties of the silica particles.[8] The US NIOSH and the US National Toxicology Program (NTP) later also decided that silica was a human carcinogen.[1,15]

Another recent meta-analysis covers 45 studies published after the 1997 IARC classification and after the previous meta-analysis by Steenland et al. Pelucchi et al.[16] found a pooled relative risk for lung cancer among the silica-exposed compared with non-exposed of 1.34 and 1.41 for cohort and case–control studies, respectively. For silicotics compared with non-exposed populations, these relative risks increased to 1.69 and 3.27, respectively. Thus, these results are broadly similar to the earlier literature and tend to confirm the decisions by IARC, NTP and NIOSH to classify silica as a known human carcinogen. Another meta-analysis restricted to silicotics was published by Lacasse et al.,[17] and found a combined standardized mortality ratio (SMR) of 2.45 (1.63–3.66) across 27 studies comparing silicotics with non-exposed populations. This was reduced to 1.52 (1.02–2.26) for never-smokers (ten studies had never-smokers).

Since the Pelucchi et al. meta-analysis,[16] there have been a few more publications regarding silica and lung cancer, the most important of which is a recent large case–control study in Eastern Europe.[18] This study included 2800 lung cancer cases, about 15 per cent had been occupationally exposed to silica during their lifetime (based on self-reported work history, followed by expert review and creation of a job–exposure matrix), compared with 10 per cent among controls. The odds ratio for occupational exposure to silica was 1.37 (95 per cent confidence interval (CI) 1.14–1.65).

Despite the many epidemiologic studies showing an increased lung cancer risk, the overall conclusion about silica's carcinogenicity has remained somewhat controversial (for example, see Hessel et al.[19]) due to some inconsistency in the literature, where not all studies show a positive association with lung cancer. Nonetheless, controversy has been receding as the evidence has mounted.[20] One element which has diminished the controversy has been several studies showing positive exposure–response relationships. Positive exposure–response trends are important supporting evidence for a causal relationship.

Steenland et al.[21] published a large exposure–response analysis of silica exposure and lung cancer based on ten occupational cohorts with good exposure data assembled by NIOSH. This was a pooled analysis (using original data) of 65 000 workers and over 1000 lung cancer deaths. Lung cancer rates increased with increased cumulative exposure in internal categorical analyses. Odds ratios by quintiles of cumulative exposure were 1.0, 1.0 (0.9–1.3), 1.3 (1.1–1.7), 1.5 (1.2–1.9), 1.6 (1.3–2.1), using cutpoints if <0.4, 0.4–2.0, 2.0–5.4, 5.4–12.8, >12.8 mg/m^3 years. A number of these studies controlled indirectly for smoking, which had little impact on results. These exposure–response data, based on almost all cohort studies with quantified exposure data, showing a significant positive trend between silica exposure and lung cancer, strengthen the case that silica is a human lung carcinogen.

Four other exposure–response analyses have been published based on data not included in the IARC pooled analysis. Two of these showed significant positive exposure–response trends.[18,22] Yu et al.[23] studied a cohort of silicotic workers in Hong Kong and did not see a positive exposure–response trend, but since all silicotics have generally had high exposure, it may be difficult to detect exposure–response trends within this cohort with relatively small exposure variation. Brown and Rushton[24] published an analysis of silica sand workers in England and

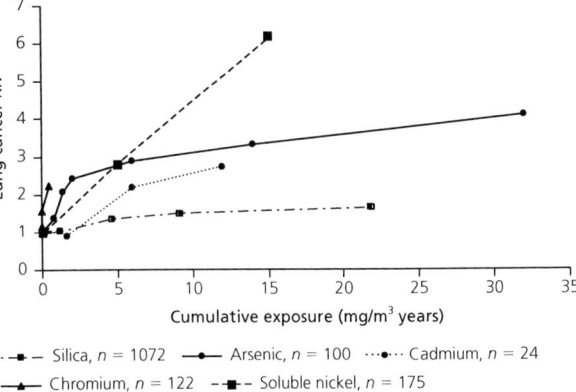

Figure 80.1 Lung cancer relative risk by mg/mm^3, five agents; n = lung cancers. RR, relative risk.

failed to find a positive exposure response, but the exposure levels in this study were very low, and hence this study might not be expected to result in positive exposure–response trends.[25]

Overall, the data suggest that silica is a relatively weak carcinogen compared with other classic lung carcinogens. Figure 80.1 shows the exposure response for silica compared with several metals. This low relative potency is one of the reasons why the lung carcinogenicity of silica has been somewhat controversial and difficult to establish.

It has been speculated that the risk of lung cancer among the silica-exposed is restricted to those who develop silicosis, or that silicosis is a risk factor for lung cancer independent of exposure.[26] Silicosis is a marker of high exposure, and it is therefore logical (under the assumption that silica per se increases lung cancer risk) that silicotics would have higher risk than non-silicotics, even without any independent role for silicosis. However, existing epidemiologic data are not, and probably never will be, sufficient to disentangle this issue.[26] One would need very good longitudinal data on exposure and silicosis throughout the follow-up period in a large cohort, i.e. very good exposure assessment of silica levels and repeated chest x-rays. Existing data to date have not been sufficient to answer this question. In the UK scheme for Industrial Injuries Disability Benefit, lung cancer with silica exposure is only recognized for benefits in individuals who have silicosis.[27]

A common method of expressing risk of lung cancer in a silica-exposed population consists of calculating an excess risk of death from lung cancer by the age of 75, above the already existing background risk for the non-exposed. Based on the spline model from Steenland et al.'s exposure–response analysis,[21] the excess lifetime risk of lung cancer (to age 75) after a 45-year exposure at current standard (0.1 mg/m^3) is 1.7 per cent (0.2–3.6 per cent), above a background risk of lung cancer death of 7.5 per cent (in a non-exposed population, including smokers and non-smokers).

By way of comparison, to get some feeling for the magnitude of these excess risks, consider never smokers and current smokers. Never smokers have a background risk of dying of lung cancer by age 75 of about 1 per cent, while current smokers (assuming a rate ratio of 15 for current smokers versus never smokers) have an excess risk of about 9 per cent (or an absolute risk of about 10 per cent), of dying of lung cancer by age 75, after taking into account competing causes of death.

KIDNEY DISEASE

In the last 10–15 years, several studies have linked crystalline silica with renal disease (particularly glomerulonephritis). Five occupational cohort studies (three mortality studies, two incidence studies) and one proportional mortality ratio (PMR) study have shown two- to three-fold excesses of renal disease among those with silica exposure, based on relatively small numbers.[28–33] Two population-based case–control studies of incident renal disease[34,35] have shown odds ratio of two or more for silica exposure. One study of silicotics found an increased risk of high creatinine compared with controls without silica exposure.[36] Another report from England found a higher incidence of renal disease, particularly glomerulonephritis, among those living in mining areas.[37] Overall, the evidence is too sparse to be conclusive, but it seems likely that silica causes kidney disease.

Again, exposure–response studies can provide additional evidence in support of causality. Cohort studies of rare diseases often suffer from small numbers of cases, but on the other hand, exposure is usually better defined and measured than in case–control studies, where past exposure is self-reported and difficult to quantify. For renal disease and silica, there are three cohort studies with sufficient numbers to evaluate exposure response, two of which have been positive and one negative. In a cohort incidence study of 4620 industrial sand workers with good historical exposure information and relatively high silica exposure, Steenland et al.[29] found significantly elevated risk of mortality for chronic renal disease (SMR 2.22 for underlying cause, 10 deaths; SMR 1.61 for any mention on the death certificate, 36 deaths). These authors then matched their cohort to a US national end-stage renal disease (ESRD) registry, which covered a more limited time period than the mortality follow up. They found 23 ESRD incident cases versus 11.7 expected (standardized incidence ratio (SIR) 1.97 (1.25–2.96). Exposure–response analyses revealed a strong positive exposure–response trend; rate ratios were 1.00, 3.09, 5.33 and 7.79 for categories of cumulative exposure (0–0.10, 0.10–0.51, 0.51–1.28 and 1.28+ mg/m^3 years). In a pooled study of three silica-exposed cohorts which examined mortality ($n = 13\,000$), Steenland et al.[38] found 51 deaths from kidney disease as an underlying cause, and 151 deaths considering any mention on the death certificate (multiple cause). The overall comparison of the exposed workers to the US population yielded an SMR of 1.41 (1.05–1.85) for underlying cause, and 1.28 (1.10–1.47) for multiple cause. These authors found significant positive trends in exposure–response analyses for both underlying and multiple causes. On the other hand, McDonald et al.[28] studied 2670 industrial sand workers and, while finding a significantly elevated SMR of 2.39 based on 19 cases, found a negative trend in mortality risk with increased cumulative exposure.

Under the assumption that using incident cases is preferable to using mortality data and relying on the exposure–response found for ESRD in Steenland et al.,[29] the estimated excess risk of ESRD incidence after a 45-year working lifetime under the current OSHA silica standard (0.1 mg/m^3), as of age 75 for males, is a high 5.1 per cent (3.3–7.3 per cent), above a background risk of 2 per cent. However, the data are too sparse and contradictory at this point to consider this figure as anything more than suggestive.

Silica damage to the kidney can result from direct toxicity of silica particles reaching the kidney, deposition in the kidney of immune complexes (IgA) following inflammation, or an autoimmune mechanism.[39] Silica-exposed patients often have high levels of antibodies (IgA, IgG) and immune complexes have been seen in the glomerulus. Others have anti-nuclear antibodies (ANA) and anti-neutrophil cytoplasmic antibodies (ANCA), suggesting an autoimmune mechanism.[35]

AUTOIMMUNE DISEASE

There is increasing evidence that silica can cause autoimmune disease, particularly rheumatoid arthritis, systemic lupus erythematosis (SLE) and scleroderma (see reviews in Parks et al.,[40] Cooper et al.,[41] Cooper and Parks,[42] Pernis[43] and Parks and Cooper[44]). It is possible that the strong immune response to silica in the lung, which has immune effects outside the lung, can trigger an autoimmune reaction.[41] There are mice models showing increased autoantibodies and other indices of an autoimmune process after silica exposure.[45–47]

The majority of epidemiology in this regard, and perhaps the strongest evidence, has been for rheumatoid arthritis. Khuder et al.[48] reviewed 15 studies published from 1986 to 2001 in a meta-analysis, and found a combined relative risk for rheumatoid arthritis (RA) with silica exposure of 3.43 (2.25–5.22). Cooper et al.[41] also provide an overview of the literature, citing five occupational cohort studies with a relative risk of three or more. Several of these studies were based on disability claims among members of exposed cohorts, while others were based on mortality, and one was based on a medical record review of patients with silicosis. However, not all studies have reported positive associations with RA. Turner and Cherry[49] found no relation between cumulative silica exposure and RA (58 cases) among 8300 workers under medical surveillance in the pottery industry in England. Limitations of this study included its restriction to currently employed workers, relatively low levels of silica insufficient to result in silicosis and matching of cases to controls on age of employment tending to decrease variation in cumulative exposure. Since the two 2002 reviews mentioned above, there have been three new reports. In one of the largest and most thorough studies to date, Stolt et al.[50] conducted a population-based case–control study of RA in males in Sweden from 1996 to 2001 (276 cases, 276 controls). Men working in jobs with presumed exposure to silica (rock drilling, stone crushing, exposure to stone dust) had an odds ratio of 2.2 (1.2–3.9). Calvert et al.[51] analysed US death certificate data and found a significant association between RA and work in jobs assumed to have silica exposure. Finally, Cooper et al.[52] measured anti-nuclear antibodies in the general population and found a significant two-fold increased risk of high titer antibodies for those with a past history of occupational silica exposure.

Increasingly strong evidence also links SLE to silica exposure. This evidence has been summarized recently by Parks and Cooper,[44] who cite six studies of various designs and quality, all of which show some evidence linking silica exposure to SLE. Perhaps the strongest evidence comes from a population-based large case–control study by Cooper et al.[53] These authors compared 265 incident SLE cases from rheumatology practices in southeastern United States with 355 controls. Nineteen per cent of SLE cases reported occupational silica exposure compared with 8 per cent of controls, and the odds ratio for SLE for medium versus no silica exposure was 2.1 (1.1–4.3) and for high versus no silica exposure the odds ratio was 4.6 (1.4–15.4). A newer report by Finckh et al.[54] described a case–control study of 115 SLE cases, which showed a significant four-fold increased risk with occupational silica exposure, as ascertained via a job–exposure matrix (4 per cent exposure prevalence among controls).

Evidence linking scleroderma and systemic sclerosis to silica was reviewed by Cooper et al.[41] Four occupational cohort studies showed a three-fold increased risk, while five population-based case–control studies had mixed results. Since this 2002 review, there are three new studies.

Magnant et al.[55] reported that in a case series of 39 silica-exposed and 66 non-exposed patients with systemic sclerosis, severe disease was significantly more common among the silica-exposed. Bovenzi et al.[56] and Diot et al.[57] both conducted relatively small case–control studies of systemic sclerosis, the former finding a statistically non-significant excess risk with silica exposure, and the latter finding a significant positive association with silica exposure.

A fourth autoimmune disease associated with silica is ANCA-associated vasculitis. Vasculitis, an inflammation of the blood vessels, may occur by itself, but is also often a feature of RA or SLE. Vasculitis can arise from infection or from immune complexes which form after infection. A third type is associated with an autoimmune process, characterized by the presence in the blood of ANCA. ANCA-associated vasculitis has been associated with silica exposure in several studies (for example, see Hogan et al.,[58] Beaudreuil et al.[59] and Lane et al.[60]

COMPARATIVE RISKS

Silica has now joined a handful of other toxic exposures which cause multiple serious diseases, such as tobacco smoke, dioxin and asbestos. Table 80.2 presents a summary of the excess (or absolute) risk due to a 45-year lifetime of exposure to silica at the current standard (0.1 mg/m^3) as of age 75, for silicosis, lung cancer and kidney disease. The risk estimates for lung cancer, silicosis mortality and end-stage renal disease incidence, and kidney disease mortality are based, respectively, on exposure–response data from Steenland et al.,[21] t'Mannetje et al.,[11] Steenland et al.[29] and Steenland et al.,[38] while the risk estimates for silicosis morbidity are based on the broad assumption that lifetime cumulative risk at the current standard is somewhere between 0.47 and 0.77 (Table 80.1). These risk estimates should be considered tentative, especially for silicosis morbidity where studies have given heterogeneous results, and for end-stage renal disease where there is only one incidence study with large enough

Table 80.2 Comparative lifetime risks (age 75 years) after 45 years exposure.[a]

Disease	Absolute or excess risk, 0.1 mg/m^3 exposure (%)	Absolute or excess risk, 0.01 mg/m^3 exposure (%)	Background risk of non-exposed US males (%)
Silicosis (1/1 or more)	47–77	0.8 (0.1–1.6)	None
Silicosis death	1.9 (0.8–2.9)	0.3 (0.0–0.6)	None
Lung cancer death	1.7 (0.2–3.6)	0.3 (0.1–0.6)	7.5
End-stage renal disease incidence	5.1 (3.3–7.3)	0.5 (0.3–0.8)	2
Kidney disease mortality (underlying)	1.8 (0.8–9.7)	0.8 (0.1–3.4)	0.3

[a]Usual Occupational Safety and Health Administration (OSHA) permissible excess (or absolute) risk, 0.1%.

numbers. Furthermore, no risk estimates for rheumatoid arthritis, lupus or scleroderma/systemic sclerosis are presented, as detailed exposure–response data are generally not available for these diseases.

Also presented in Table 80.2 are the corresponding risks at levels a tenth of the current standard (0.01 mg/m^3), as well as the corresponding background risks for the non-exposed population. These absolute risks and excess risks are calculated solely for men, because there were negligible numbers of women in the cohorts which were studied.

Keeping in mind that the usual acceptable excess risk of serious disease or death for workers for US OSHA is 0.1 per cent,[6] it is clear from Table 80.2 that the current standard is far from sufficiently protective of worker's health. Lowering the standard to a tenth of the current one still results in risks that are above the usual US OSHA permitted excess (or absolute) risk. Nonetheless, it seems unlikely that it is currently feasible to lower the standard to this level, both because it would be quite difficult to lower actual exposure levels in many work sites to this level, and because of increased measurement difficulties.[5] However, the perfect is the enemy of the good: any significant lowering of the standard would be an important step forward in light of the evidence.

Key points

- Crystalline silica has long been known to cause silicosis. A large number of epidemiologic studies are now available to estimate exposure–response relationships. These studies suggest that the common standard in many countries of 0.1 mg/m^3 needs to be lowered by at least half and probably more to protect exposed workers from a lifetime risk in excess of 1 per 1000.
- The epidemiologic data linking silica to lung cancer have increased over recent years and there are increasing numbers of studies with exposure–response data. The studies are rather consistent in showing that silica is a human lung carcinogen. However, it appears to be a weaker one per unit dose than many classic lung carcinogens, which has led to controversy and a slower acceptance of silica's carcinogenicity than other lung carcinogens.
- The epidemiologic data linking silica to non-malignant kidney disease have also increased in recent years. Although not as conclusive as the data for silicosis and lung cancer, the data are reasonably consistent and point in the direction of causality.
- There are also epidemiologic data linking silica with a variety of autoimmune diseases, such as lupus, sclerodema and rheumatoid arthritis. Again, these data have not reached the point where causality can be reasonably assumed, but they point in that direction.
- Silica is linked to many diseases. Exposure–response data sufficient for risk assessment are available for silicosis, lung cancer and non-malignant kidney disease. Of these, the lifetime risk of silicosis and non-malignant renal disease is greater than the lifetime risk of lung cancer at the existing occupational standard of 0.1 mg/m^3, but all three outcomes point towards the need for a substantial reduction of that standard.

REFERENCES

1. National Institute for Occupational Safety and Health (NIOSH). Health effects of occupational exposure to respirable crystalline silica. NIOSH publication No 2002-129. Atlanta, GA: NIOSH.
2. Linch KD, Miller WE, Althouse RB. Surveillance of respirable crystalline silica dust using OSHA compliance data (1979–1995). *American Journal of Industrial Medicine*. 1998; **34**: 547.
3. Rappaport S, Goldberg M, Susi P, Herrick RF. Excessive exposure to silica in the US construction industry. *Annals of Occupational Hygiene*. 2003; **47**: 111–22.
4. Driscoll T, Nelson D, Steenland K et al. The global burden of non-malignant respiratory disease due to occupational airborne exposures. *American Journal of Industrial Medicine*. 2005; **48**: 432–45.
5. Greaves IJ. Not-so-simple silicosis: A case for public health action. *American Journal of Industrial Medicine*. 2000; **37**: 245–51.
6. Rodricks J, Brett S, Wrenn G. Significant risk decisions in federal regulatory agencies. *Regulatory Toxicology and Pharmacology*. 1987; **7**: 307–20.
7. Bolsaitis F, Wallace W. The structure of silica surfaces in relation to cytotoxicity. In: Castranova V, Vallyathan V, Wallace W (eds). *Silica and silica-inducted lung diseases*. Boca Raton: CRC Press, 1996: 79–89.
8. International Agency for Research on Cancer (IARC). *Monographs on the evaluation of carcinogenic risks to humans*, vol. 68. Silica, some silicates, coal dust and para-aramid fibrils. Lyon: International Agency for Research on Cancer, 1997.
9. Chen W, Hnizdo E, Chen J et al. Risk of silicosis in cohorts of Chinese tin and tungsten miners, and pottery workers (I): An epidemiological study. *American Journal of Industrial Medicine*. 2005; **48**: 1–9.
10. Churchyard G, Ehrlich R, teWaterNaude J et al. Silicosis prevalence and exposure–response relations in South African goldminers. *Occupational and Environmental Medicine*. 2004; **61**: 811–16.

11. t'Mannetje A, Steenland K, Attfield M et al. Exposure-response analysis and risk assessment for silica and silicosis mortality in a pooled analysis of six cohorts. *Occupational and Environmental Medicine*. 2002; **59**: 723–8.
12. Hedlund U, Jonsson H, Eriksson K, Jarvholm B. Exposure–response of silicosis mortality in iron ore miners. *Annals of Occupational Hygiene*. 2008; **52**: 3–7.
13. Tse L, Yu I, Leung C et al. Mortality from non-malignant respiratory diseases among people with silicosis in Hong Kong: Exposure-response analyses for exposure to silica dust. *Occupational and Environmental Medicine*. 2007; **64**: 87–92.
14. Steenland K, Stayner L, Dankovic D. Silica, asbestos, man-made mineral fibers and cancer. *Cancer Causes and Control*. 1997; **8**: 494–506.
15. National Toxicology Program (NTP). Report on carcinogens, 11th edn. USDHHS, Public Health Service, January 31, 2005.
16. Pelucchi C, Pira E, Piolatto G et al. Occupational silica exposure and lung cancer risk: A review of epidemiological studies 1996–2005. *Annals of Oncology*. 2006; **17**: 1039–50.
17. Lacasse Y, Martin S, Simard S, Desmeules M. Meta-analysis of silicosis and lung cancer. *Scandinavian Journal of Work and Environmental Health*. 2005; **31**: 450–8.
18. Cassidy A, 't Mannetje A, van Tongeren M et al. Occupational exposure to crystalline silica and risk of lung cancer: A multicenter case-control study in Europe. *Epidemiology*. 2007; **18**: 36–43.
19. Hessel P, Gamble J, Gee J et al. Silica, silicosis, and lung cancer: a response to a recent working group report. *Journal of Occupational and Environmental Medicine*. 2000; **42**: 704–20.
20. Stayner L. Silica and lung cancer: When is enough evidence enough? *Epidemiology*. 2007; **18**: 23–4.
21. Steenland K, Mannetje A, Boffetta P et al. Pooled exposure-response and risk assessment for lung cancer in 10 cohorts of silica-exposed workers: An IARC multi-centric study. *Cancer Causes and Control*. 2001; **12**: 773–84.
22. Cherry N, Burgess G, Turner S, McDonald J. Crystalline silica and risk of lung cancer in the potteries. *Occupational and Environmental Medicine*. 1998; **55**: 779–85.
23. Yu IT, Tse LA, Leung CC et al. Lung cancer mortality among silicotic workers in Hong Kong – no evidence for a link. *Annals of Oncology*. 2007; **18**: 1056–63.
24. Brown TP, Rushton L. Mortality in the UK industrial silica sand industry: 2. A retrospective cohort study. *Occupational and Environmental Medicine*. 2005; **62**: 446–52.
25. Steenland K, Silica: Déjà vu all over again? *Occupational and Environmental Medicine*. 2005; **62**: 430–2.
26. Checkoway H, Franzblau A. Is silicosis required for silica-associated lung cancer? *American Journal of Industrial Medicine*. 2000; **37**: 252–9.
27. Industrial Injuries Advisory Council. Lung cancer in relation to occupational exposure to silica. Cm 2043. London: The Stationery Office, 1992.
28. McDonald JC, McDonald AD, Hughes JM et al. Mortality from lung and kidney disease in a cohort of North American industrial sand workers: An update. *Annals of Occupational Hygiene*. 2005; **49**: 367–73.
29. Steenland K, Sanderson W, Calvert G. Kidney disease and arthritis among workers exposed to silica. *Epidemiology*. 2001; **12**: 405–12.
30. Steenland K, Brown D. Mortality study of gold miners exposed to silica and non-asbestiform amphibole mineral: An update with 14 more years of follow-up. *American Journal of Industrial Medicine*. 1995; **27**: 217–29.
31. Calvert G, Steenland K, Palu S. End-stage renal disease among silica-exposed gold miners. *Journal of the American Medical Association*. 1997; **277**: 1219–23.
32. Rapiti E, Sperati A, Miceli M et al. End stage renal disease among ceramic workers exposed to silica. *Occupational and Environmental Medicine*. 1999; **56**: 559–61.
33. Steenland K, Nowlin S, Ryan B, Adams S. Use of multiple-cause mortality data in epidemiologic analyses. *American Journal of Epidemiology*. 1992; **136**: 855–62.
34. Steenland K, Thun M, Ferguson B, Port F. Occupational and other exposures associated with end-stage renal disease: A case-control study. *American Journal of Public Health*. 1990; **80**: 153–7.
35. Gregorini G, Feriola A, Donato F et al. Association between silica exposure and necrotizing crescentic glomerulonephritis with p-ANCA and anti-MPO antibodies: A hospital-based case-control study. *Advances in Experimental Medicine and Biology*. 1993; **336**: 435–40.
36. Rosenman KD, Moore-Fuller M, Reilly MJ. Kidney disease and silicosis. *Nephron*. 2000; **85**: 14–19.
37. Fenwick S, Main J. Increased prevalence of renal disease in silica-exposed workers. *Lancet*. 2000; **356**: 913–14.
38. Steenland K, Mannetje A, Attfield M. Pooled analysis of kidney disease mortality and silica exposure in three cohorts. *Annals of Occupational Hygiene*. 2002; **46** (Suppl.): 14–19.
39. Calvert GM, Steenland K, Paul S. End-stage renal disease among silica-exposed gold miners. A new method for assessing incidence among epidemiologic cohorts. *Journal of the American Medical Association*. 1997; **278**: 546–7.
40. Parks C, Conrad K, Cooper G. Occupational exposure to crystalline silica and autoimmune disease. *Environmental Health Perspectives*. 1999; **107** (Suppl. 5): 793–802.
41. Cooper GS, Miller FW, Germolec DR. Occupational exposures and autoimmune diseases. *International Immunopharmacology*. 2002; **2**: 303–13.
42. Cooper GS, Parks CG. Occupational and environmental exposures as risk factors for systemic lupus erythematosus. *Current Rheumatology Reports*. 2004; **6**: 367–74.
43. Pernis B. Silica and the immune system. *Acta Biomedica*. 2005; **76** (Suppl. 2): 38–44.
44. Parks CG, Cooper GS. Occupational exposures and risk of systemic lupus erythematosus: A review of the evidence and exposure assessment methods in population- and clinic-based studies. *Lupus*. 2006; **15**: 728–36.
45. Brown JM, Archer AJ, Pfau JC, Holian A. Silica accelerated systemic autoimmune disease in lupus-prone New Zealand mixed mice. *Clinical and Experimental Immunology*. 2003; **131**: 415–21.

46. Brown JM, Pfau JC, Holian A. Immunoglobulin and lymphocyte responses following silica exposure in New Zealand mixed mice. *Inhalation Toxicology*. 2004; **16**: 133–9.
47. Brown JM, Schwanke CM, Pershouse MA *et al*. Effects of rottlerin on silica-exacerbated systemic autoimmune disease in New Zealand mixed mice. *American Journal of Physiology. Lung Cellular and Molecular Physiology*. 2005; **289**: L990–8.
48. Khuder SA, Peshimam AZ, Agraharam S. Environmental risk factors for rheumatoid arthritis. *Reviews on Environmental Health*. 2002; **17**: 307–15.
49. Turner S, Cherry N. Rheumatoid arthritis in workers exposed to silica in the pottery industry. *Occupational and Environmental Medicine*. 2000; **57**: 443–7.
50. Stolt P, Källberg H, Lundberg I *et al*. and EIRA study group. Silica exposure is associated with increased risk of developing rheumatoid arthritis: Results from the Swedish EIRA study. *Annals of the Rheumatic Diseases*. 2005; **64**: 582–6.
51. Calvert GM, Rice FL, Boiano JM *et al*. Occupational silica exposure and risk of various diseases: An analysis using death certificates from 27 states of the United States. *Occupational and Environmental Medicine*. 2003; **60**: 122–9.
52. Cooper GS, Parks CG, Schur PS, Fraser PA. Occupational and environmental associations with antinuclear antibodies in a general population sample. *Journal of Toxicology and Environmental Health. Part A*. 2006; **69**: 2063–9.
53. Cooper GS, Parks CG, Treadwell EL *et al*. Occupational risk factors for the development of systemic lupus erythematosus. *Journal of Rheumatology*. 2004; **31**: 1928–33.
54. Finckh A, Cooper GS, Chibnik LB *et al*. Occupational silica and solvent exposures and risk of systemic lupus erythematosus in urban women. *Arthritis and Rheumatism*. 2006; **54**: 3648–54.
55. Magnant J, de Monte M, Guilmot JL *et al*. Relationship between occupational risk factors and severity markers of systemic sclerosis. *Journal of Rheumatology*. 2005; **32**: 1713–18.
56. Bovenzi M, Barbone F, Pisa FE *et al*. A case–control study of occupational exposures and systemic sclerosis. *International Archives of Occupational and Environmental Health*. 2004; **77**: 10–16.
57. Diot E, Lesire V, Guilmot JL *et al*. Systemic sclerosis and occupational risk factors: A case–control study. *Occupational and Environmental Medicine*. 2002; **59**: 545–9.
58. Hogan SL, Cooper GS, Savitz DA *et al*. Association of silica exposure with anti-neutrophil cytoplasmic autoantibody small-vessel vasculitis: A population-based, case–control study. *Clinical Journal of the American Society of Nephrology*. 2007; **2**: 290–9.
59. Beaudreuil S, Lasfargues G, Lauériere L *et al*. Occupational exposure in ANCA-positive patients: A case–control study. *Kidney International*. 2005; **67**: 1961–6.
60. Lane SE, Watts RA, Bentham G *et al*. Are environmental factors important in primary systemic vasculitis? A case–control study. *Arthritis and Rheumatism*. 2003; **48**: 814–23.
61. Muir D, Shannon J, Julian J *et al*. Silica exposure and silicosis among Ontario hardrock miners III: Analysis and risk estimates. *American Journal of Industrial Medicine*. 1989; **16**: 29–43.
62. Rosenman K, Reillly M, Rice C *et al*. Silicosis among foundry workers. *American Journal of Epidemiology*. 1996; **144**: 890–9.
63. Ng T, Chan S. Quantitative relations between silica exposure and development of radiological small opacities in granite workers. *Annals of Occupational Hygiene*. 1994; **38** (Suppl.): 857–63.
64. Steenland K, Brown D. Silicosis among gold-miners: An exposure–response analysis. *American Journal of Public Health*. 1995; **85**: 1372–7.
65. Hnizdo E, Sluis-Cremer G. Risk of silicosis in a cohort of white South African gold miners. *American Journal of Industrial Medicine*. 1993; **24**: 447–57.
66. Kreiss K, Zhen B. Risk of silicosis in a Colorado mining community. *American Journal of Industrial Medicine*. 1996; **30**: 529.
67. Chen W, Zhuang Z, Attfield M *et al*. Exposure to silica and silicosis among tin miners in China: Exposure–response analyses and risk assessment. *Occupational and Environmental Medicine*. 2001; **58**: 31–7.

81

Other non-fibrous mineral dusts

ANNE COCKCROFT

Introduction	1029	The micas and vermiculite	1035
Coalworkers' pneumoconiosis	1029	Other non-fibrous clays	1036
Slate workers' pneumoconiosis	1033	Carbon black	1037
Kaolin pneumoconiosis	1034	References	1037
Talc	1035		

INTRODUCTION

Most of the other non-fibrous mineral dusts leading to occupational lung diseases are mixed dusts containing quartz. Much of their toxicity is related to their quartz content, but modified according to the other components of the dust and the form of the quartz.

COALWORKERS' PNEUMOCONIOSIS

Coal mining and dust exposure

Coal mining as an occupation is historically important; coal was the fuel that supported the Industrial Revolution. The British coal mines at one time employed nearly a million men. While there is now little coal mining in the United Kingdom, there are still many men with lung disease resulting from their exposure as coalworkers. Coal mining remains an important industry worldwide, and many countries continue to rely on coal as a main energy source. The top five producers of hard coal are China, the United States, India, Australia and South Africa. Some 60 pert cent of world coal production comes from underground mining; some countries, such as Australia, have most of their production from surface (opencast) mining.

Workers in the coal mining industry, particularly those who work in underground coal mines, are exposed to a variety of mineral dusts besides coal. To open up or extend and maintain a coal mine, shafts and roadways must be driven though other strata which may contain hard rock with 75 per cent or more of quartz. This quartz exposure can lead to silicosis (see Chapter 79, Silica and silica-related diseases). This work may be done by specialized teams or by men who also work on the coalface itself. When the coal seams are two metres or more thick, the rock above and below the seam is left undisturbed. One of the reasons that most mines in the UK became uneconomic is because the coal seams are thin and frequently faulted, so the rock must be cut above and below to allow the men and machines access to the coal (hard heading). All underground workers are exposed to some extent to this rock dust, which may contain high proportions of quartz.

Coal was formed when forests were crushed under the weight of sedimentary rock. It therefore includes stones from the forest floor and from above. This is a source of rock dust exposure to surface and transport workers, as well as those down the mine.

The proportions of quartz and other mineral dusts vary from mine to mine and from job to job within a coalfield and even more between different coalfields. The greatest differences in dust exposure, however, are between countries where the work practices and the regulations controlling exposure are different. This can have profound effects on the prevalence and characteristics of the occupational lung disease among coalworkers in different places.

The exposure to dust in opencast mining is much lower than in underground mining. However, there is evidence that some workers in opencast coal mines develop radiological changes of pneumoconiosis, perhaps contributed to by the quartz content of the dust.[1]

Simple coalworkers' pneumoconiosis

This condition develops after relatively high cumulative exposures to underground coal mine dust, usually over a period of more than 20 years (see below). It has been a source of continuing controversy in the UK and internationally, with some people arguing that it is not associated with any respiratory disability unless the relatively rare complicated form of the disease is present. Others have presented convincing evidence of a loss of lung function related to cumulative dust exposure in coalworkers and ex-coalworkers without complicated pneumoconiosis,[2,3] which can be severely disabling in some men[4] as a result of the associated chronic airflow limitation (mainly emphysema). During the last three decades, much evidence has accumulated in favour of the proposition that coal dust exposure can produce serious respiratory disability in the absence of complicated coalworkers' pneumoconiosis, and this is now generally accepted.[5]

The features of simple coalworkers' pneumoconiosis result from accumulation of dust in the lung parenchyma and the tissue reaction to that dust. Typically, the chest radiograph shows small, rounded opacities scattered through the lung fields (see Chapter 68, Imaging in occupational lung disease, Figure 68.3). In the early stages, there is little or no impairment of lung function. Pathologically, there are simple coal macules: collections of dust-laden macrophages around the terminal bronchioles in the centre of the acinus, with a little surrounding centrilobular emphysema ('focal' emphysema).

If men are removed from dust exposure at this stage, very few will progress to complicated pneumoconiosis and most will not suffer respiratory impairment. However, even without further dust exposure, some men have a progression of disease. The opacities on the chest radiograph tend to become more irregular in shape,[6] an obstructive pattern of lung function loss occurs and the lungs pathologically show increasing emphysema and fibrosis around the centrilobular collections of dust-laden cells. The picture is often complicated by the effects of cigarette smoking, but severe pathological emphysema can occur even in non-smoking coalworkers (or, more usually, retired coalworkers) with heavy dust exposure.[7] There is good evidence of an excess of pathological emphysema, including severe degrees, in coalworkers compared with non-coalworkers, taking smoking into account.[8] Studies from the Institute of Occupational Medicine in Edinburgh demonstrated a dose–response relationship between pathological emphysema and dust exposure in coalworkers[9] and showed there could be important loss of lung function associated with coal dust exposure in non-smoking coalworkers.[10]

Research on the relationship between radiographic appearances, pathology and lung function in coalworkers has shown that small irregular opacities are better associated with emphysema and loss of lung function than small rounded opacities.[11] Research in South Wales demonstrated an association between years of coalwork and small irregular opacities[6] and evidence from the Pneumoconiosis Field Research scheme set up by British Coal confirmed a relationship between small irregular opacities, as well as small rounded opacities, and cumulative dust exposure.[12]

The main cause of lung function loss and disability in men with simple coalworkers' pneumoconiosis is emphysema, sometimes with associated fibrosis. Cases of interstitial fibrosis, with or without changes of simple coalworkers' pneumoconiosis, have been reported in coalworkers,[13] but there is no evidence that interstitial fibrosis is more common among coalworkers than non-coalworkers. Until relatively recently, the prevalent belief, in the UK at least, was that emphysema in men with simple coalworkers' pneumoconiosis was due to other factors, mainly cigarette smoking, and not related to the pneumoconiosis process. However, in 1993, emphysema and chronic bronchitis became prescribed diseases in coalworkers under the UK Industrial Injuries Disablement Benefit (IIDB) scheme (see under Disability benefit for coalworkers' pneumoconiosis and Chapter 8, Compensation schemes). Coggon et al.[14] found that the mortality from coalworkers' pneumoconiosis varied greatly between coalfields in the UK, whereas the mortality from chronic bronchitis and emphysema varied less and did not correlate with the pneumoconiosis mortality, and suggested that this indicated the two conditions were related to different features of the coal dust. Another approach is to consider both conditions as part of the overall picture of the lung reaction to accumulated dust, with variation according to features of the dust itself and to individual susceptibility factors.

Complicated coalworkers' pneumoconiosis

This describes cases in which simple pneumoconiosis is complicated by additional (related) pathology. As a group, coalworkers do not have an increased risk of tuberculosis or lung cancer. However, coalworkers with high exposure to hard rock dust and with features of silicosis are at increased risk of tuberculosis, and possibly also lung cancer (see Chapter 80, Epidemiology of silica-related disease). The pneumoconiosis 'complication' usually takes the form of large masses of solid tissue within the parenchyma, and is disabling. There are three main causes: coal mine dust itself, quartz encountered in coal mines, and dust plus rheumatoid disease.

PROGRESSIVE MASSIVE FIBROSIS

The most frequent type of mass occurring in the lungs of coalworkers with heavy dust exposure is circumscribed, smooth in outline and a uniform black or dark grey. It is usually in the upper or middle zone, oval in shape, with the long axis parallel to the pleura and the outer surface initially 2 or 3 cm from the pleura. It is convex, the inner surface can be flattened or slightly concave and is clearly separate from the hilum (Figure 81.1). Size ranges from around 3 cm to over 10 cm long. The masses may appear singly or one in each lung and others may appear some years later. They may be missed (except in retrospect) for several years because each first shows as a faint but clearly defined area of increased density which becomes denser and slightly smaller as the years go by. Due to emphysematous change in the lung between the mass and the pleura, they appear to move towards the hilum over time. They are not detectable on physical examination, but are associated with a definite loss of lung function. The lung function loss is mainly obstructive, partly because the lesions distort and produce scar emphysema in the surrounding lung and partly because they usually occur on a background of heavy simple pneumoconiosis with associated emphysema.[15] Some loss of lung volume can occur due to the space occupied by large progressive massive fibrosis (PMF) masses.

After many years, these masses may cavitate and yield, once or repeatedly, large quantities of material like black ink (so-called 'melanoptysis'), which is necrotic tissue and dust. Death may occur from aspiration of the black material or from associated haemoptysis, but this is uncommon. The cavity may shrink and cause no further trouble or become infected with fungi (to form a mycetoma) or with opportunistic mycobacteria. Both can be life shortening in spite of treatment and are indications for surgery if lung function permits. Infection with *Mycobacterium tuberculosis* is not a feature of straightforward PMF and the lesions are not prone to malignant change.

Pathologically, before they cavitate, the lesions are firm and rubbery with no definite capsule. On microscopic examination, there is a great deal of amorphous ground substance mixed with the dust and the ghosts of macrophages, but no collagen. At the periphery, there are living macrophages and other mononuclear cells set in a reticulin network. The blood vessels within the mass show a low-grade inflammatory change leading to obliteration. The siting and shape of the mass suggests that the vascular occlusions are secondary. Immunoreactive cells and immune complexes are present in the lesions, especially around the periphery. PMF may result at least in part from an immune reaction to dust in the hilar lymph nodes, with passage of activated material back into the lung parenchyma by invasion of bronchi or branches of the pulmonary artery.[16]

The attack rate of PMF among coalworkers is strongly influenced by the cumulative dust exposure and the radiographic category of simple pneumoconiosis.[17–21] Development of PMF is unlikely in men with less than category 2/2 simple pneumoconiosis. However, it can occasionally occur at low profusions of simple pneumoconiosis. A few men may develop it long after they have stopped being exposed to dust.[22] Reported rates of PMF

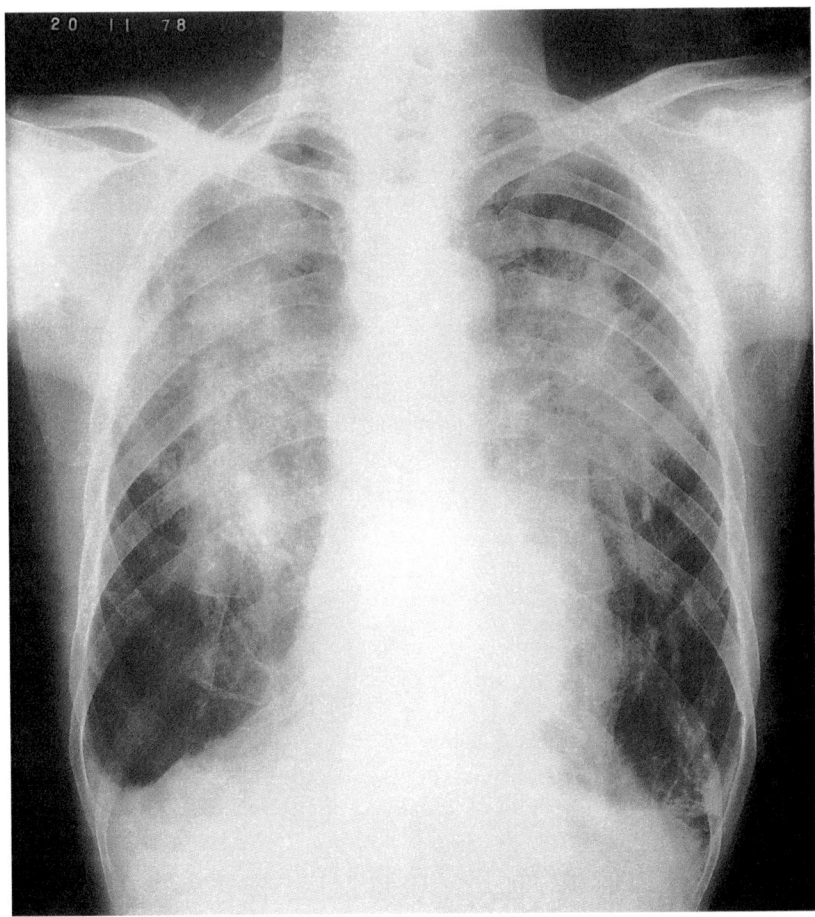

Figure 81.1 Bilateral progressive massive fibrosis on the chest radiograph of a coalworker. There is emphysema in the lower lobes.

have varied considerably over time and between coalfields. PMF was especially common in South Wales from the 1930s to the 1960s: in the 1950s, 30 per cent or more of coalworkers with category 3 simple pneumoconiosis developed PMF over an eight-year follow up.[17] In individual men, the risk of PMF is also related to the amount of quartz in the dust,[23] and to tuberculosis.[20] Studies of genetic markers involved in inflammatory and fibrotic processes have so far failed to identify specific genetic variations related to the risk of developing PMF.[24]

SILICOSIS IN COALWORKERS

The lesions of subacute or chronic silicosis may be seen in coalworkers. They can usually be traced to exposure to quartz in work on shafts and drivages, or to coalface dust with an exceptionally high quartz content (more than 10–15 per cent) due to hard heading or to working rock-contaminated coal. Coalworkers with these exposures may show larger, rounded ('r') opacities in the lung fields, subsequently leading to confluent irregular massive shadows in the upper zones with pleural thickening, hilar enlargement, calcification of the parenchymal shadows and eggshell calcification of the hilar nodes (see Chapter 79, Silica and silica-related diseases). More commonly, coalworkers with relatively high quartz exposure have the features of coalworkers' pneumoconiosis, with or without typical PMF lesions, mixed with some features of silicosis, or they may have a few typical silicotic nodules found in the lung or hilar nodes at autopsy.

RHEUMATOID PNEUMOCONIOSIS

At the peak of the surge in PMF cases in the mid-twentieth century, Caplan,[25] working in South Wales, noticed atypical shadows on the radiograph of coalworkers who also had rheumatoid arthritis. The shadows could appear at any level of dust exposure, being relatively common in young miners with little or no simple coalworkers' pneumoconiosis and with short exposure.

The lesions were round, 1–4 cm in diameter, and usually about 2 cm in from the pleura (Chapter 68, Imaging in occupational lung disease, Figure 68.4). There was no definite change in the surrounding lung so that they looked like secondary cancer deposits. They often remained the same size for months or years and then enlarged by perhaps 0.5 cm, sometimes at the same time as new lesions appeared. Clinical arthritis often developed later than the lung lesions and was relatively mild, but the men were seropositive for rheumatoid factor. After perhaps five or ten years, the lesions sometimes cavitated (with a brief flu-like illness followed by the coughing up of inky sputum often with haemoptysis, which could be severe). The cavities that formed often closed and the lesions recavitated at intervals. As they enlarged, lesions lying close together often used to form large lumpy masses which were difficult to distinguish from PMF or confluent silicosis. The distinction could only be made histologically. It is not known whether the treatments given for rheumatoid arthritis affected the course of the lung lesions. The prognosis in the absence of further dust exposure depended on when the rheumatoid disease became inactive, but the risk of cavitation remained.

The histology of the early lung lesions showed the same regular arrangement of subacute inflammatory cells as rheumatoid nodules in other tissues. Older lesions showed central necrosis with new concentric layers of inflammatory reaction surrounding it. This layered pattern is so characteristic that rheumatoid lesions causing massive shadows or adding to the lesions produced by coal dust or quartz could be identified easily. Rheumatoid pneumoconiosis was not necessarily associated with the other lung lesions of rheumatoid arthritis.

Between 100 and 200 cases of this syndrome were identified in South Wales. In the rest of the United Kingdom, and indeed the rest of the world, only isolated cases have been reported. It seems to have been a characteristic of South Wales at that time and few new cases from the area have been reported since. Rheumatoid pneumoconiosis has also been reported rarely in men with silicosis or asbestosis.

Disability benefit for coalworkers' pneumoconiosis

Coalworkers' pneumoconiosis is covered by occupational disability benefit schemes in countries that have such schemes. In the UK, it is a prescribed disease and attracts benefit under the Industrial Injuries Disability Benefit scheme. Prior to 1993, Industrial Disability Benefit was payable to coalworkers with simple pneumoconiosis if their chest radiograph showed at least category 2/2 profusion of small rounded opacities. The level of benefit was low since it was argued that the simple pneumoconiosis itself did not lead to disability. Sometimes, a small amount of additional benefit was granted for concomitant emphysema and chronic bronchitis, but only if the radiograph showed the qualifying changes (category 2/2 rounded opacities). Severely disabled men were generally considered to be suffering the effects of cigarette smoking and men who claimed to smoke little or not at all were usually not believed.

In 1992, the UK Industrial Injuries Advisory Council (IIAC) recommended prescription of chronic bronchitis and emphysema in coalworkers with 20 years' underground exposure, a loss of lung function (FEV_1) of at least 1 litre below the predicted value, and evidence of dust retention (category 1/1 changes on the chest radiograph).[26] In 1996, IIAC recommended removing the requirement for evidence of dust retention on the chest radiograph.[27] The new system was criticized on the grounds that the radiograph is a better index of actual exposure and dust retention in the lungs than the length of time underground.[28]

SLATE WORKERS' PNEUMOCONIOSIS

Exposure to slate dust

The slate quarries and mines in North Wales supplied most of the slate for the roofing of factories and houses in the United Kingdom during the nineteenth century, and produced slate for export in large quantity. Because explosives and machines tended to shatter the slate and make it unsuitable for roofing or cladding, most of the work had to be done by hand. At its peak at the end of the nineteenth century, the industry employed about 100 000 people in many small businesses. The industry subsequently dwindled because it could not compete with synthetic roofing and cladding material made close to the point of use.

Slate is formed by the sedimentation of a mixture of finely divided mineral particles in layers on to a flat surface. The mixture varies from layer to layer and site to site. The North Wales slate contains mica, feldspar and anything from 15 to 35 per cent crystalline quartz (other deposits may contain over 60 per cent crystalline quartz).

When splitting slate by hand, a little puff of respirable dust is released every time the rock is split along the plane of cleavage (Figure 81.2). The pneumoconiosis among slate workers was recognized over 100 years ago when 'silicosis' was diagnosed and attributed to the use of mechanical saws to cut slabs dry and the dry engraving of tombstones. That work was often done in sheds and was very dusty. The introduction of wet working (Figure 81.3) some 100 years ago was thought to have solved the problem of lung disease in slate workers.

The disease

Up to the 1950s, the high rate of chest disease in the slate-working areas of North Wales was attributed to tuberculosis. However, a subsequent study,[29] which included men who had left the slate industry, found evidence of radiographic change and loss of lung function related to time spent in slate work. The jobs with most exposure were 'getting' of slate underground (as opposed to open quarrying) and 'dressing' of roof slates indoors.

The radiographic changes in slate pneumoconiosis are somewhat different from silicosis seen in other industries. The findings in North Wales were as follows: Against a clear background or a low profusion of smaller rounded opacities ('q' or 'p'), 'r' shadows appeared in the upper zones in the older men. These sometimes remained static and calcified and sometimes coalesced to form irregular massive shadows. The massive shadows were difficult to distinguish during life from cavitating tuberculosis because the associated emphysema looked like cavitation. There was sometimes patchy pleural thickening overlying the irregular coalescent masses in the upper zone or evidence of more extensive pleurisy. However, the most unusual feature was the amount of bilateral hilar gland enlargement with eggshell calcification which was found even in some men with no radiological evidence of parenchymal disease. The lung dust burden at autopsy is high, perhaps 100 g per lung, and the proportion of quartz higher than in the inspired dust. The radiographic changes and pathology were those of a mixed dust pneumoconiosis with only part of the abnormality in the lung and the hilar nodes in the form of silicotic nodules.

The risk of tuberculosis in men with radiological slate pneumoconiosis in North Wales seems to have been at least as high as that reported by Westerholm[30] in patients with silicosis in Sweden. Many of the cases were treated with conventional courses of chemotherapy.

Despite the reduced exposure to dust in the North Wales slate industry, a 24-year cohort mortality study (1975–98) found an excess of deaths among slate workers compared with controls, mainly due to respiratory disease and pneumoconiosis.[31] Dust measurements in the slate industry in Norway found up to 41 per cent quartz in the respirable dust and levels of quartz exposure often above the Norwegian limit value, leading to concern about development of silicosis among the exposed workers.[32] Silicosis has been reported in small-scale slate pencil manufacture in India,[33] where the workers, often teenagers,

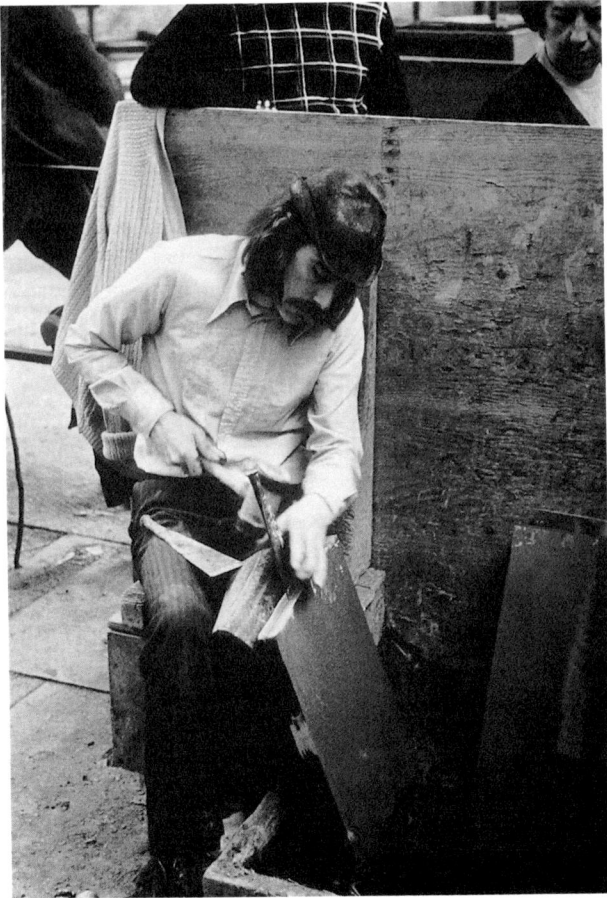

Figure 81.2 Splitting slate by hand. A puff of dust is released as the sheets separate, creating a risk when performed in a poorly ventilated shed, but not at the open quarry face.

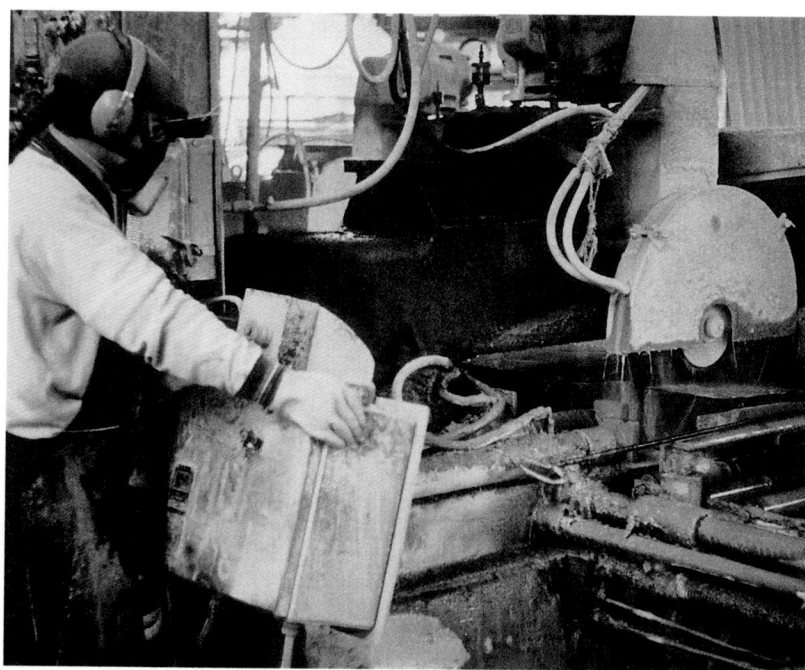

Figure 81.3 Sawing slabs of slate for tombstones. When this process was converted to wet working about 100 years ago, the problem of silicosis in slate workers was thought to have been solved.

sawed pencils from blocks of slate containing up to 60 per cent quartz. Gross disease and early deaths resulted.

KAOLIN PNEUMOCONIOSIS

Kaolin (china clay) is formed by the action of water on granite. In Cornwall, in the United Kingdom, the deposits of clay are still in the cone-shaped holes in the granite where they formed. They are associated with silica sand, mica, fluorspar and undegraded granite (china stone). In other parts of the world, such as in the southern United States, the clay was washed out of the granite and sedimented into layers of pure clay millions of years ago. Such pure deposits are sufficiently free of parent minerals that clay can be dug out, dried and sold without purification. However, in the main Cornish industry, the clay is extracted with high pressure hoses and the contaminating mica and silica sand removed by sedimentation before drying and marketing as a fine powder. The level of contamination of the product by quartz and mica depends both upon the nature of the original deposit and the method of extraction. The exposure in one country may be quite different from that in others. Whereas, by the time it is handled dry, Cornish kaolin seldom contains as much as 1 per cent of quartz (with up to 7 per cent fluorspar and 6 per cent mica), some of the 'ball clays' which are dried directly may contain up to 20 per cent quartz.

The kaolin itself (kaolinite) is a multilayered particle made up of alternating plates of aluminium hydroxide and silicon oxide and is a powerful adsorbent. Nowadays, more is used as a filler for paper than for making crockery. It is also used as a thickener for paints, as an ingredient of special plasters and as a medication for treating diarrhoea. In Cornwall, a byproduct of the industry was 'china stone'. Lumps of quartz-containing stone in the kaolin deposit were either shipped unground to the potteries for milling or were milled locally and added to the kaolin before it was sent to the potteries.

In the pottery industry, any hazard from kaolin was swamped by the effect of silica. In Cornwall, most of the workers lived well beyond retiring age so that the occasional case of serious chest disease was attributed to tuberculosis, to silicosis from working in the tin mines or from milling 'china stone'. Early animal studies compared the effect of inhaled kaolin with inhaled quartz. The kaolin effect was described as minor with a reticulin reaction, but no true fibrosis. As a result, kaolin was classified as a nuisance dust (nuisance dusts are low toxicity dusts regulated in the UK to 4 mg/m^3 respirable).

The disease

An early survey by Sheers[34] described changes on the radiograph in men working with kaolin who had not had any obvious exposure to quartz. Kaolin workers develop an exposure-related simple pneumoconiosis similar to that seen in British coal miners. Even though the dust appears to have contained considerably less than 1 per cent quartz, the simple rounded opacity change appeared earlier than for coalworkers. Men who had worked a lifetime in the dustiest jobs could reach category 2/2 change by retiring age. Although some coalescence is seen, calcification and hilar gland changes are rare. Progressive massive fibrosis is not now seen in working and recently retired men, but has been found in men seeking compensation after leaving the industry in the past. The massive shadows tend to be smooth outlined, resembling those seen in coalworkers' pneumoconiosis rather than those seen in silicosis.

Further detailed surveys of ventilatory capacity, respiratory symptoms, radiographic changes and exposure to kaolin, confirmed radiographic changes and a small loss of lung function related to exposure.[35,36] They confirmed that the effects seen were mainly due to earlier, higher dust exposures and that men employed after 1971 in the Cornish china clay industry were unlikely to develop radiographic changes or lung function loss after a full working life in the industry.

In a post-mortem study of china clay workers, some of whom had ground china stone, three types of pathological change were noted: (1) nodular fibrosis similar to that seen in silicosis, related to high amounts of quartz in the lung dust; (2) diffuse or interstitial fibrosis similar to that resulting from mica exposure; and (3) massive lesions similar to those seen in coalworkers and not showing the histological characteristics of either silicosis or rheumatoid pneumoconiosis.[37]

Adherence to the exposure limit for nuisance dust (4 mg/m^3 respirable dust) greatly reduced the risk of kaolin pneumoconiosis in the china clay industry. More recently, in view of the evidence for an exposure–response effect, a somewhat lower, specific occupational exposure standard was set for kaolin (2 mg/m^3 respirable). Concerns have been raised about the possibility of an excess lung cancer risk among kaolin workers because of the quartz content of the dust, but there is no evidence of such an excess of lung cancer, which would be expected to be small if any.

TALC

Talc is a form of magnesium silicate that has crystallized into thin plates which readily split and slide over each other. Powdered talc is used as a lubricant and parting medium in industrial processes varying from the moulding of tyres to the making of chocolate-coated toffee bars. It is also used as a filler in heat-resistant ceramics, refractories and insulators. It is perhaps best known as the fine white powder (talcum powder) used for powdering babies (and others) after bathing.

The disease

The quarrying and mining of talc and its subsequent milling to a powder have been known to be risky occupations for over a hundred years. Early reports described a disabling disease affecting a high proportion of the workers with heavy dust exposure. Talc deposits are often contaminated with other minerals and at first it was assumed that the disease was really silicosis due to quartz in the ore, but radiographs showed a fine nodular pneumoconiosis with either rounded ('p' and 'q') or irregular opacities ('s' and 't'), unlike those usually seen in silicosis. The histology also showed a more diffuse granulomatous lesion with more interstitial fibrosis and few if any of the typical silicotic nodules.

Talc was the traditional coating for surgeons' gloves to prevent them sticking together during autoclaving. Unless carefully washed off at the beginning of an operation, some was left in the wound. Granulomas filled with talc were recognized as the cause of intra-abdominal adhesions and similar late complications of operation. In the 1950s, talc was replaced by starch powder for surgical gloves. More recently still, latex surgical gloves without any powder are recommended to reduce the risk of occupational asthma (see Chapter 72, Occupational asthma).

In 1949, McLaughlin et al.[38] described fibrous particles and coated fibres resembling asbestos bodies in a case of talc pneumoconiosis arising in the motor tyre industry. In the early 1960s, when the full extent of the risks of asbestos was being explored, the situation with regard to talc was reviewed because some ore deposits contain fibrous forms of calcium and magnesium silicates (tremolite, actinolite and anthophyllite), which are really forms of asbestos. Regulations were introduced in the United Kingdom to restrict the importation of talc for cosmetic use to material completely free of fibres. No such controls, however, were applied to talc for industrial purposes.

Epidemiological work in the United States clarified the situation. Talc from Montana, Texas and North Carolina is almost free from fibres and contains very little quartz. Heavily exposed workers showed a simple rounded opacity pneumoconiosis without significant loss of lung function, although some develop disabling pleural changes. There was no increase in cancer.[39] Talc is also produced in New England where the deposits vary in their tremolite content. In exposed workers, there was a variable incidence of disabling interstitial fibrosis leading to right heart failure in some workers and a simple non-disabling pneumoconiosis in others.[40] The evidence suggests that the severe disease is associated with fibre (tremolite, actinolite or anthophyllite) contamination; exposed workers also have an increased risk of lung cancer and mesothelioma (see Chapter 77, Epidemiology of asbestos-related diseases).

Tremolite falls into the group of asbestos minerals with no safe limits of exposure. Therefore, talc deposits containing respirable tremolite fibres should not be worked and the use of talc from such deposits in industry is banned in developed countries. On the other hand, there appear to be adequate deposits of fibre-free talc and there is no reason why talc from these sources should not continue to be used for industrial and cosmetic purposes.

THE MICAS AND VERMICULITE

This family of silicates shares the same crystal structure (monoclinic with basal cleavage) which forms flat sheets like talc but often on a much larger scale. They are aluminium and potassium silicates with varying amounts of magnesium, iron, lithium and sodium, and have a number of geological names such as muscovite, biotite and phlogopite.

The large transparent sheet material (mostly mined in India) was used as window glass in stoves and furnaces because of its heat resistance. Other sheet material was used as an insulator in the electrical industry and the waste material was ground and used instead of talc. Synthetic materials have replaced mica for most purposes, except perhaps as a filler in iridescent paints and in those countries where mica is produced, such as India and South America.

A benign simple pneumoconiosis has been reported in men mining and milling mica,[41] as well as the occasional more serious case.[42] Animal experiments have not given a clear answer about whether pure mica is fibrogenic; it is likely that the pneumoconiosis in humans exposed to mica dust is usually due to contaminating minerals, including quartz.[43]

Vermiculite

Vermiculite is a poorly compacted form of mica which exfoliates to occupy more than ten times its original volume when heated. It is then used as an insulator for roof spaces, domestic stoves, etc., and in lightweight materials which combine fire resistance with insulation. Like the other micas, pure vermiculite does not appear to be a significant risk.

Amandus and colleagues[44] described a cluster of mesotheliomas around a commercial deposit of vermiculite in Montana. Although the recent product does not contain easily detectable quantities of tremolite, apparently sufficient tremolite fibre was released in the past to have caused primary lung cancers and mesotheliomas. Not all vermiculite deposits are contaminated with fibrous tremolite.

Diatomite (Kieselgahr)

Diatomite, or diatomaceous earth, is a soft rock or clay resulting from the dust deposition of dead plankton (diatoms) on the floors of lakes and shallow seas. It is of geologically recent origin, so that the skeletons of the diatoms are still easily seen under the microscope. The main constituent is amorphous silica with some calcium, magnesium and aluminium silicates. Depending on how dry the deposit is, the extraction may or may not be dusty. Heat processing is carried out in two stages: (1) drying and burning off the residual organic content; then (2) treatment at about 1200°C (calcining) which converts the amorphous silica to cristobalite (see below).

Diatomite is milled and marketed as a fine powder after either stage 1 or 2. The stage 1 material is used in face powder, as an improver for heavy soils, as a filter aid and to clarify soft drinks. The stage 2 material can be used (dry) for polishing or in special plasters and cements and ceramics.

Serious progressive pneumoconiosis leading to respiratory failure and with a high risk of tuberculosis has occurred with exposure to diatomite.[45] Histology showed silicotic nodules in some cases, but a more diffuse cellular reaction (similar to that found with talc) in others.

Epidemiological investigations indicate that the serious risk comes from the calcined product, which contains cristobalite. There may be a risk after stage 1 if this process is carried out at too high a temperature (above 600°C). In a follow-up study of diatomite mine and mill workers in California, radiographic abnormalities were rare and definite pneumoconiosis was not found in workers with less than 25 years of service, despite the fact that the processing included flux-calcination with opportunity for exposure to cristobalite.[46] More recent studies in workers in the diatomaceous earth industry have demonstrated radiographic evidence of silicosis related to the exposure of respirable crystalline silica (in the form of cristobalite)[47] and a dose–response relationship between exposure to cristobalite and risk of lung cancer, even in the absence of silicosis.[48]

OTHER NON-FIBROUS CLAYS

Bentonites, montmorillonite and Fuller's earth

This ill-defined group comprises mixtures of poorly crystallized and amorphous silicates of sodium, potassium, aluminium and magnesium. Bentonites are versatile clays consisting predominantly of montmorillonite, a clay mineral of the smectite group, and are almost always contaminated in their raw state with crystalline silica. Extensive deposits are linked to large volcanic eruptions. Bentonite rocks form mainly from the devitrification of volcanic glass in pyroclastic and/or volcaniclastic rocks subject to hydrothermal activity or other aqueous environments, such as alkaline lakes, marine sediments or by percolating groundwater.

Today, bentonite is a key raw material in the production of energy and metal castings, and other applications of great importance to the world economy. These clays are used in many building materials and as drilling muds, for example in oil exploration and mining. They also have adsorbent qualities and were traditionally used since Roman times in cleaning raw wool (fulling). They are used in treating patients who have swallowed poisons or have diarrhoea, as a vehicle for pesticides, to prevent workers slipping on oil spills and as cat litter. They are nearly always processed and marketed according to the uses they are designed for. High-end products containing contaminant-free bentonite include paint, ink, cosmetics and pharmaceuticals.

Epidemiological data are scarce. Some operations seem to cause a simple pneumoconiosis,[49] but more aggressive disease has been reported.[50] It is not clear whether the disease reported is due to the clay itself, to the contaminating crystalline materials or to the products of calcining. Overall, the limited data available suggest that the toxicity of bentonite particles in the lung is low.[51]

Gypsum, plaster of Paris

Gypsum is a hydrated calcium sulphate in microcrystalline form that is used in the building industry, especially in plaster board. Careful heating will drive off part of the water to produce 'plaster of Paris' which sets when mixed with sufficient water to return it to the fully hydrated state. Gypsum is found in many places and varies from rock (alabaster and selenite) to soft clay. Some deposits are contaminated with quartz and others contain elongated crystals (needles) that might resemble fibres. Long crystals also form when gypsum is processed to make plaster board. Gypsum is mined, dried and sometimes 'calcined' before being milled and marketed in powder form. The mines may be opencast or deep; the level of dust exposure and the quartz contamination vary considerably.

Gypsum is classified as a nuisance dust because workers survive many years of exposure without serious respiratory difficulty and animal studies using pure gypsum have failed to produce lung fibrosis. However, study of two English deposits reported that pneumoconiosis can occur.[52] A simple pneumoconiosis with radiological changes up to category 2/1 was seen with only minor loss of lung function; disability occurred in the most heavily exposed. Disease was more frequent in the area where the quartz content of the dust was higher.

Gypsum needles are unlikely to be pathogenic in the lungs because of their short half-life (estimated at minutes) as a result of their high solubility.[53,54] Epidemiological studies of workers exposed to pure-phase gypsum dust have not found evidence of lung fibrosis or pneumoconiosis (see, for example, Refs 55 and 56). In tests on rat and guinea pig lungs, aerosols of calcium sulphate fibres were quickly cleared via dissolution and mechanisms of particle clearance.[57] In a chronic inhalation study, Schepers et al.[58] found that calcined gypsum dust produced minor effects in the lungs of guinea pigs.

CARBON BLACK

Carbon black is produced by the incomplete combustion of heavy petroleum products, and a small amount from vegetable oil. It is a form of amorphous carbon with a high surface area to volume ratio, although its surface area to volume ratio is low compared with activated carbon. It differs from soot because of its much higher surface area to volume ratio and significantly less (negligible and non-bioavailable) polynuclear aromatic hydrocarbons (PAH) content. Carbon black is used as a pigment and as reinforcement in rubber and plastic products. Its main use is in tyres.

Studies of lung cancer among carbon black manufacturing workers have been inconclusive. The International Agency for Research on Cancer classifies carbon black as possibly carcinogenic to humans.[59] Studies of workers in European carbon black production plants have found symptoms of chronic bronchitis, small lung function reductions and small opacities on the chest radiograph associated with measures of current and cumulative dust exposure.[60] There is evidence that the radiographic abnormalities may be reversible after reduction or cessation of exposure.[61]

Key points

- Coal dust exposure, usually over ten years or more, leads to both simple coalworkers' pneumoconiosis and to chronic bronchitis and emphysema; serious disability can result, mostly due to the emphysema.
- Radiographically, the small rounded opacities of simple coalworkers' pneumoconiosis relate to the dust exposure but not to lung function loss, while small irregular opacities relate to exposure, lung function loss and degree of emphysema.
- The development of progressive massive fibrosis is mainly related to cumulative dust exposure; immune mechanisms are also involved, and high quartz content of the dust and tuberculosis increase the risk.
- In rheumatoid pneumoconiosis (Caplan's syndrome), rheumatoid nodules, which may cavitate, develop in the lungs of coalworkers with rheumatoid diathesis. The syndrome may also occur rarely in silicosis and asbestosis.
- Slate workers' pneumoconiosis is related to the quartz content of the dust; serious disease can occur with heavy exposure to slate dust.
- Kaolin pneumoconiosis is similar to simple coalworkers' pneumoconiosis; the quartz exposure is generally low and there is no evidence of an increased risk of lung cancer in china clay workers.
- Talc pneumoconiosis is a mild condition, but some talc deposits are contaminated with asbestos and this exposure can lead to interstitial fibrosis and lung cancer.
- Exposure to carbon black may lead to a mild pneumoconiosis; studies of lung cancer have been inconclusive, but carbon black is classified by IARC as possibly carcinogenic to humans.

REFERENCES

1. Love RG, Miller BG, Groat SK et al. Respiratory health effects of opencast coalmining: A cross-sectional study of current workers. *Occupational and Environmental Medicine*. 1997; **54**: 416–23.
2. Soutar CA, Hurley JF. Relation between dust exposure and lung function in miners and ex-miners. *British Journal of Industrial Medicine*. 1986; **43**: 307–20.

3. Seixas NS, Robins TG, Attfield MD et al. Exposure–response relationships for coal mine dust and obstructive lung disease following enactment of the federal Coal Mine Health and Safety Act of 1969. *American Journal of Industrial Medicine.* 1992; **21**: 715-34.
4. Hurley JF, Soutar CA. Can exposure to coal mine dust cause severe impairment of lung function? *British Journal of Industrial Medicine.* 1986; **3**: 150-7.
5. Coggon D, Newman Taylor A. Coal mining and chronic obstructive pulmonary disease: A review of the evidence. *Thorax.* 1998; **53**: 398-407.
6. Cockcroft A, Lyons JP, Andersson N, Saunders MJ. Prevalence and relation to underground exposure of radiological irregular opacities in South Wales coalworkers with pneumoconiosis. *British Journal of Industrial Medicine.* 1983; **40**: 169-72.
7. Lyons JP, Ryder RC, Seal RME, Wagner JC. Emphysema in smoking and non-smoking coalworkers with pneumoconiosis. *Bulletin Européen de Physiopathologie Respiratoire.* 1981; **17**: 75-85.
8. Cockcroft A, Seal RME, Wagner JC et al. Post-mortem study of emphysema in coalworkers and non-coalworkers. *Lancet.* 1982; **ii**: 600-3.
9. Ruckley VA, Gauld JS, Chapman JMC et al. Emphysema and dust exposure in a group of coalworkers. *American Review of Respiratory Disease.* 1984; **4**: 528-32.
10. Marine WM, Gurr D, Jacobsen M. Clinically important effects of dust exposure and smoking in British coal miners. *American Review of Respiratory Disease.* 1988; **137**: 106-12.
11. Cockcroft A, Berry G, Cotes JE, Lyons JP. Shape of small opacities and lung function in coalworkers. *Thorax.* 1982; **37**: 765-9.
12. Collins HPR, Dick JA, Bennett JG et al. Irregularly shaped small shadows on chest radiographs, dust exposure, and lung function in coalworkers' pneumoconiosis. *British Journal of Industrial Medicine.* 1988; **45**: 43-55.
13. McConnochie K, Green FHY, Vallyathan V et al. Interstitial fibrosis in coal workers: Experience in Wales and West Virginia. *Annals of Occupational Hygiene.* 1988; **32** (Suppl. 1): 553-60.
14. Coggon D, Inskip H, Winter P, Pannett B. Contrasting geographical distribution of mortality from pneumoconiosis and chronic bronchitis and emphysema in British coal miners. *Occupational and Environmental Medicine.* 1995; **52**: 554-5.
15. Lyons JP, Campbell H. Relation between progressive massive fibrosis, emphysema and pulmonary dysfunction in coalworkers' pneumoconiosis. *British Journal of Industrial Medicine.* 1981; **38**: 125-9.
16. Seal RME, Cockcroft A, Kung I, Wagner JC. Central lymph node involvement and progressive massive fibrosis in coalworkers. *Thorax.* 1986; **41**: 531-7.
17. Cochrane AL. The attack rate of progressive massive fibrosis. *British Journal of Industrial Medicine.* 1962; **19**: 52-64.
18. Maclaren WM, Hurley JF, Collins HP, Cowie AJ. Factors associated with the development of progressive massic fibrosis in British coalminers: A case-control study. *British Journal of Industrial Medicine.* 1989; **46**: 597-607.
19. Gautrin D, Auburtin G, Alluin F et al. Recognition and progression of coalworkers' pneumoconiosis in the collieries of northern France. *Experimental Lung Research.* 1994; **20**: 395-410.
20. Yi Q, Zhang Z. The survival analyses of 2738 patients with simple pneumoconiosis. *Occupational and Environmental Medicine.* 1996; **53**: 129-35.
21. Soutar CA, Hurley JF, Miller BG et al. Dust concentrations and respiratory risks in coalminers: Key risk estimates from the British Pneumoconiosis Field Research. *Occupational and Environmental Medicine.* 2004; **61**: 477-81.
22. Maclaren WM, Soutar CA. Progressive massive fibrosis and simple pneumoconiosis in ex-miners. *British Journal of Industrial Medicine.* 1985; **42**: 734-40.
23. Jacobsen M, Maclaren WM. Unusual pulmonary observations and exposure to coal mine dust: A case-control study: Inhaled particles, V. *Annals of Occupational Hygiene.* 1982; **26**: 753-65.
24. Yucesoy B, Johnson VJ, Kissling GE et al. Genetic susceptibility to progressive massive fibrosis in coal miners. *European Respiratory Journal.* 2008; **31**: 1177-82.
25. Caplan A. Certain unusual radiological appearances in the chest of coal-miners suffering from rheumatoid arthritis. *Thorax.* 1953; **8**: 29-37.
26. Industrial Injuries Advisory Council. Chronic bronchitis and emphysema, Cm 2091. London: The Stationery Office, 1992.
27. Industrial Injuries Advisory Council. Chronic bronchitis and emphysema, Cm 3240. London: The Stationery Office, 1996.
28. Seaton A. The new prescription: Industrial injuries benefits for smokers? *Thorax.* 1998; **53**: 335-6.
29. Clover JR, Bevan C, Cotes JE et al. Effects of exposure to slate dust in North Wales. *British Journal of Industrial Medicine.* 1980; **37**: 152-62.
30. Westerholm P. Silicosis, observations on a case register. *Scandinavian Journal of Work, Environment and Health.* 1980; **6** (Suppl. 2): 1-86.
31. Campbell M, Thomas H, Hodges N et al. A 24 year cohort study of mortality in slate workers in North Wales. *Occupational Medicine.* 2005; **55**: 448-53.
32. Bang BE, Suhr H. Quartz exposure in the slate industry in northern Norway. *Annals of Occupational Hygiene.* 1998; **42**: 557-63.
33. Saiyed HN, Parikh DJ, Ghodasara NB et al. Development and progression of silicosis in an Indian slate pencil manufacturing industry: A longitudinal study. Proceedings of the VIth International Pneumoconiosis Conference 1983, Bochum, Germany. Geneva: ILO, 1984: 1959-75.
34. Sheers G. Prevalence of pneumoconiosis in Cornish kaolin workers. *British Journal of Industrial Medicine.* 1964; **21**: 21-5.
35. Ogle CJ, Rundle EM, Sugar ET. China clay workers in the south west of England: Analysis of chest radiograph readings, ventilatory capacity, and respiratory symptoms in relation to type and duration of occupation. *British Journal of Industrial Medicine.* 1989; **46**: 261-70.

36. Rundle EM, Sugar ET, Ogle CJ. Analyses of the 1990 chest health survey of china clay workers. *British Journal of Industrial Medicine*. 1993; **50**: 913–19.
37. Wagner JC, Pooley FD, Gibbs A *et al.* Inhalation of china stone and china clay dust: Relationship between the mineralogy of dust retained in the lungs and pathological changes. *Thorax*. 1986; **41**: 190–6.
38. McLaughlin AIG, Rogers E, Dunham KC. Talc pneumoconiosis. *British Journal of Industrial Medicine*. 1949; **6**: 184–94.
39. Gamble J, Griefe A, Hancock J. An epidemiological industrial hygiene study of talc workers. *Annals of Occupational Hygiene*. 1982; **26**: 841–59.
40. Dement JM, Zumwalde RD, Gamble IF *et al*. *Occupational exposure to talc containing asbestos*. DHEW (NIOSH) publication No. 80–115. Washington DC: US Government Printing Office, 1980.
41. Venter E, Nyantumbu B, Solomon A, Rees D. Radiologic abnormalities in South African mica millers: A survey of a mica milling plant in the Limpopo province. *International Journal of Occupational and Environmental Health*. 2004; **10**: 278–83.
42. Zinman C, Richards GA, Murray J *et al*. Mica dust as a cause of severe pneumoconiosis. *American Journal of Industrial Medicine*. 2002; **41**: 139–44.
43. Skulberg KR, Gylseth B, Skaug V, Hanoa R. Mica pneumoconiosis – a literature review. *Scandinavian Journal of Work and Environmental Health*. 1985; **11**: 65–74.
44. Amandus HE, Wheeler R, Armstrong B *et al*. Mortality of vermiculite workers exposed to tremolite. VI International Symposium on Inhaled Particles, British Occupational Hygiene Society, Cambridge 1985. *Annals of Occupational Hygiene*. 1988; **32** (Suppl. 1): 459–67.
45. Clark WC, Cralley LJ. *Pneumoconiosis in diatomite mining and processing*. US Department of Health/Education and Welfare Public Health Service, Publication No. 601. Washington DC: US Department of Health, 1958.
46. Cooper WC, Sargent EN. A 26-year radiographic follow-up of workers in a diatomite mine and mill. *Journal of Occupational Medicine*. 1984; **26**: 456–60.
47. Hughes JM, Weill H, Checkoway H *et al*. Radiographic evidence of silicosis risk in the diatomaceous earth industry. *American Journal of Respiratory and Critical Care Medicine*. 1998; **158**: 807–14.
48. Checkoway H, Hughes JM, Weill H *et al*. Crystalline silica exposure, radiological silicosis, and lung cancer mortality in diatomaceous earth industry workers. *Thorax*. 1999; **54**: 56–9.
49. Gibbs AR, Pooley FD. Fuller's earth (montmorillonite) pneumoconiosis. *Occupational and Environmental Medicine*. 1994; **51**: 644–6.
50. McNally WD, Trostler IS. Severe pneumoconiosis caused by the inhalation of fullers earth. *Journal of Industrial Hygiene and Toxicology*. 1941; **23**: 118–26.
51. IPCS EHC 231. *Bentonite, kaolin, and selected clay minerals*. Geneva: World Health Organization, 2005.
52. Oakes D, Douglas R, Knight K *et al*. Respiratory effects of prolonged exposure to gypsum dust. *Annals of Occupational Hygiene*. 1982; **26**: 833–40.
53. Hoskins JA. Mineral fibres and health. *Indoor and Built Environment*. 2001; **10**: 244–51.
54. US Department of Heath and Human Service. EPA/IRIS United States Environmental Protection Agency/Integrated Risk Information System database, 2006. Last accessed March 25, 2009. Available from: http://cfpub.epa.gov/ncea/iris/index.cfm.
55. Burilkov T, Michailova-Dotschewa L. Dangers of exposure to dust extraction and production of natural gypsum. *Wissenschaft und Umwelt*. 1990; **2**: 89–91 (Abstract from EMBASE 91094689).
56. Einbrodt HJ. The health risks by dusts of calcium sulfate (Ger.). Burilkov T, Michailova-Dotschewa L. Dangers of exposure to dust extraction and production of natural gypsum. *Wissenschaft und Umwelt*. 1988; **4**: 179–81 (Abstract from EMBASE 89261036).
57. Clouter A, Houghton CE, Bowskill CA *et al*. An *in vitro/in vivo* study into the short-term effects of exposure to mineral fibres. *Experimental and Toxicologic Pathology*. 1996; **48**: 484–6.
58. Schepers GW, Durkan TM, Delahant AB. The biological effects of calcined gypsum dust: An experimental study on animal lungs. *AMA Archives of Industrial Health*. 1955; **12**: 329–47.
59. Baan R, Straif K, Grosse Y *et al*. on behalf of the WHO International Agency for Research on Cancer Monograph Working Group. Carcinogenicity of carbon black, titanium dioxide, and talc. *Lancet Oncology*. 2006; **7**: 295–6.
60. Gardiner K, Trethowan NW, Harrington JM *et al*. Respiratory health effects of carbon black: A survey of European carbon black workers. *British Journal of Industrial Medicine*. 1993; **50**: 1082–96.
61. van Tongeren MJ, Gardiner K, Rossiter CE *et al*. Longitudinal analyses of chest radiographs from the European Carbon Black Respiratory Morbidity Study. *European Respiratory Journal*. 2002; **20**: 417–25.

Metal dusts and fumes

BENOIT NEMERY

Introduction	1040
Acute toxic effects	1040
Pneumoconioses and specific interstitial lung disorders caused by metals	1044
References	1046

INTRODUCTION

The subject of metal-induced lung diseases is complex, not only because there are so many different agents to be considered, but also because the conditions caused are quite diverse. Pulmonary diseases caused by occupational exposures to metals involve more than 'pneumoconioses'; they encompass almost the entire spectrum of respiratory conditions, ranging from acute inhalation injury to lung cancer, from airway disease to parenchymal disorders. The clinical experience and epidemiological understanding of metal-induced pulmonary disease is much less extensive than for silicosis, coal pneumoconiosis or asbestos-related disease. This section is an update of the same section in the previous edition, which was itself an updated summary of an older review article containing specific references to the older literature.[1]

The toxicity of a metallic compound is heavily dependent on its physicochemical form, also called 'metal speciation'. Inhalation of metallic compounds does not necessarily lead to significant pulmonary damage. Lung disorders in workers occupationally exposed to metals (or metal-containing ores) are not always due to these metals, but may be due to cigarette smoking, concomitant exposure to silica (particularly in mining), asbestos, irritant gases (as in welding), organic chemicals (such as degreasing solvents, or isocyanates) or microorganisms (such as fungi or mycobacteria in metal working fluids).[2] Exposure to metals is not confined to metal mining or metallurgy, but may take place in almost every sector of industry, for example as paint pigments, as catalysts in chemical processes, as well as in the general or domestic environment.

It is customary to divide metals and their alloys into ferrous metals (iron and various types of steels) and non-ferrous metals. The first category is the most widely encountered and does not pose much specific respiratory hazard, whereas non-ferrous metals can cause a number of specific respiratory conditions.

ACUTE TOXIC EFFECTS

Metal fume fever

Metal fume fever (see Chapter 44, Welding) is a non-allergic, influenza-like reaction following a single exposure to high concentrations of metal fumes. The syndrome consists of fever, chills, muscle pains and malaise, generally with relatively mild respiratory symptoms, and classically little or no radiographic or functional abnormalities, although this is not always the case. The symptoms usually begin a few hours after a heavy exposure to metal oxides and they subside spontaneously after 24 hours or a night's sleep. Peripheral leukocytosis is present during the acute illness, and studies using bronchoalveolar lavage have showed marked neutrophil infiltration and cytokine release in the lungs.[3]

Although metal fume fever is said to occur after exposure to the fumes of many different sorts of metals, it has been documented mainly following exposure to fumes of zinc (i.e. zinc oxide, ZnO) and to a lesser extent copper. Zinc fume fever commonly occurs, for example, after the smelting or thermal spraying of zinc without adequate exhaust, or after welding or flame cutting galvanized steel in a confined space. Workers at risk of metal fume fever are usually quite familiar with the condition; however, few cases come to the attention of physicians. No specific treatment is required, except preventive hygiene measures.

Metal fume fever is said not to lead to sequelae, but this has not been adequately investigated.

Acute inhalation injury

As indicated in Table 82.1, the inhalation of various metallic compounds can cause severe inhalation injury, involving the upper and/or lower respiratory tract. Depending on the agent and the intensity of exposure, the injury may manifest itself as rhinitis, laryngitis, tracheobronchitis or chemical pneumonitis and non-cardiogenic pulmonary oedema.[4] Symptoms will, therefore, possibly include lacrimation, nose irritation with sneezing and bleeding, sore throat, hoarseness, cough, wheezing, chest pain or tightness, and dyspnoea. In severe cases, the clinical picture may be that of the adult respiratory distress syndrome. When the deep lung is involved, respiratory distress is often delayed for several hours (without any alarming symptoms) until severe non-cardiogenic pulmonary oedema develops.

METAL OXIDES

Exposure to metal oxides (see Chapter 12, Metals) may result from the smelting, welding, flame-cutting or thermal spraying of pure metals or alloys, but sometimes also through direct exposure to dust particles (e.g. V_2O_5, MnO) or vapours (e.g. Os_3O_4). Inhalation injury may occur with new technologies, such as those involving the thermal spraying of metals, as shown by a fatal case caused by spraying nickel.[5]

CADMIUM

The best documented metallic agent causing toxic pneumonitis is cadmium. Cadmium is a byproduct of the zinc and lead industry; it is used in metal plating and in special alloys; it is also used in the production of batteries, pigments and plastic stabilizers. Cadmium oxides may be liberated, often unknown to the worker, from the welding or burning of cadmium-containing alloys and cadmium-plated metal, from the use of hard solders, or from the smelting of zinc or lead (or scrap metal), which often contain significant levels of contaminating cadmium. It is important to distinguish acute toxic pneumonitis from simple metal fume fever.

MERCURY

Acute pneumonitis after the inhalation of high quantities of mercury vapours has been described as a consequence of the refining of gold or silver (using amalgams) in confined spaces, which is often the case in the cottage industry, and after accidents involving (large quantities of) mercury lamps. However, there is no risk of acute lung injury after exposure to the small quantities of mercury (about 4 mg) – compared with 500 mg in a mercury thermometer – that may be released when a single energy-efficient compact fluorescent lamp (CFL) is broken.[6]

VANADIUM

Vanadium pentoxide (V_2O_5) may be present in significant quantities in slags from the steel industry (ferrovanadium) and, because some fuel oils contain high quantities of vanadium, in furnace residues from oil refineries or in soot from oil-fired boilers. Dust containing V_2O_5 may cause upper and lower airway irritation: rhinitis with sneezing and nose bleeds, pharyngitis, acute tracheobronchitis, with cough, wheeze and (possibly) airway hyper-reactivity ('boilermaker's bronchitis'),[7] as well as possibly bronchopneumonia.

ZINC

Cases of adult respiratory distress syndrome, some with a protracted course, have been reported in military or civilian personnel accidentally exposed to smoke bombs which liberate zinc chloride ($ZnCl_2$).[8]

OTHER METALLIC AGENTS

Accidental exposure, for example as a result of explosions, burst pipes or leaks in chemical plants, to antimony trichloride ($SbCl_3$) and pentachloride ($SbCl_5$), zirconium tetrachloride ($ZrCl_4$), titanium tetrachloride ($TiCl_4$) and uranium hexafluoride (UF_6) may also lead to inhalation injury. Nickel carbonyl [$Ni(CO)_4$] is a volatile liquid of very high toxicity for the lungs and brain. Acute inhalation may cause haemorrhagic pulmonary oedema.[9]

Lithium hydride (LiH), phosphine (hydrogen phosphide, PH_3, used as a doping agent for the manufacture of silicon crystals, or released from aluminium phosphide grain fumigants or zinc phosphide rodenticides), hydrogen selenide (SeH_3) and diborane (B_2H_5, used as high energy fuel) have also been reported to cause acute inhalation injury with, possibly, pulmonary oedema.[10]

Table 82.1 Non-exhaustive list of metallic agents described as possible causes of acute lung injury.

Oxides of cadmium (Cd), manganese (Mn), nickel (Ni), osmium (Os), vanadium (V), cobalt (Co), beryllium (Be)
Mercury (Hg) vapours
Zinc chloride ($ZnCl_2$) and other metal chlorides ($TiCl_4$, $SbCl_3$, $SbCl_5$, $ZrCl_4$, UF_6)
Nickel carbonyl [$Ni(CO)_4$]
Hydrides (B_2H_6 or diborane, LiH, PH_3, AsH_3, SbH_3, ...)

See also specific metals under Part two, Diseases associated with chemical agents, Section two, Metals.

Inhalation of the hydrogenated forms of arsenic (arsine, AsH_3) or antimony (stibine, SbH_3) can also be lethal as a result of fulminant haemolysis, which may sometimes manifest itself initially as dyspnoea, abdominal and lumbar pain, and haemoglobinuria.

Chronic obstructive lung disease

Occupational exposures may have a significant impact on the incidence of chronic obstructive pulmonary disease (COPD), independently of or in synergy with cigarette smoking. In general, epidemiological studies have concerned workers exposed to mine dust or to poorly specified mineral dusts. The overall conclusions of these studies are that the population attributable risk of COPD caused by occupational exposures is around 15 per cent (at least in industrially developed countries).[11–13]

There is good evidence that exposure to high concentrations of cadmium may cause pulmonary emphysema. This was demonstrated in a study of a group of 101 workers and ex-workers from a cadmium alloy factory in England, in which a clear excess of functional and radiological signs of emphysema were found compared with appropriate controls.[14] The study found evidence of a dose–response relationship, with dose being estimated both by past hygiene measurements and by the internal (liver) cadmium burden. Other studies have found an increased mortality from non-malignant respiratory disease in cadmium-exposed workers.[15]

There have been many surveys of the prevalence of chronic obstructive lung disease in workers from the iron and steel industry, as well as among metal welders (see Chapter 44, Welding and Chapter 74, Extrinsic allergic alveolitis). Although exposure in the iron and steel industry is mainly to iron dust, many other metallic and non-metallic particulates (including silica and asbestos), as well as gases, may be inhaled. During welding, even of steel, the plume is not so much composed of the metals being welded together, but of the materials which make up the electrode, the filler wire and the fluxes used. Despite the generally consistent finding of an increase in the prevalence of chronic bronchitis, as defined by questionnaire, among welders and steelworkers, the results regarding ventilatory function have been largely negative, inconclusive or showing only small effects.[16,17] However, because of the healthy-worker effect and various methodological issues, one should not conclude from these studies that there are no specific work processes within these broad categories which entail a risk of significant obstructive respiratory impairment in susceptible subjects. Population studies indicate that there is an excess mortality[18] and morbidity[19,20] from non-malignant respiratory disease among steelworkers and welders. A longitudinal study of shipyard workers has shown a faster annual decline in FEV_1 in welders and caulker/burners than in controls.[21] Recent studies from Norway demonstrate increased declines in pulmonary function in workers exposed to dusts from the metal smelting industry.[22] In any case, the absence of certainty regarding the magnitude of the risk of chronic obstructive lung disease in welders and steelworkers should not lead to complacency about the need for adequate surveillance and prevention of dust exposure in these jobs, also because chronic obstructive lung disease is not the only risk incurred.

Cross-sectional studies have indicated an excess of chronic bronchitis and a loss of ventilatory function, sometimes mainly of FVC, associated with chronic exposure to beryllium, aluminium, cobalt (or hard metal), manganese and titanium dioxide (TiO). This seems to be independent of the other respiratory diseases associated with some of these metals (see Bronchial asthma). However, other surveys of workers exposed to these compounds have not reached the same conclusions, possibly because of differences in total dust, in concomitant exposures, or in population characteristics and study designs. The absence of demonstrable effects does not exclude the existence of a preventable health risk.

Bronchial asthma

Several metals are known to be capable of causing bronchial asthma.[23] Metal-induced asthma is a particular case of an occupational asthma caused by agents of low molecular weight, a topic which is covered elsewhere in this book (see Chapter 72, Occupational asthma). In essence, the clinical characteristics of metal-induced asthma are similar to those of occupational asthma caused by other agents. With some metals (as in fact with some organic molecules), alveolitis and asthma may coexist, as has been described with cobalt. Other forms of metal-related occupational asthma are more likely to belong to the category of non-immunologic asthma, i.e. 'irritant-induced asthma' or 'occupational asthma without latency'.

The best known cause of metal-induced occupational asthma is that caused by complex platinum salts, which has mainly been described in workers from precious metal refineries. However, significant exposure to platinum may also occur in the manufacture of catalysts,[24] in photographic applications and in electroplating. Platinum salts are extremely potent sensitizers and are generally considered to do so via IgE-mediated pathway. Palladium[25] and rhodium salts[26] are other precious metal salts that may occasionally cause occupational asthma (see Chapter 12, Metals).

Nickel, chromium and cobalt are also potential causes of occupational asthma, although the number of reported cases is not high, certainly compared with the high prevalence of allergic sensitization of the skin caused by these metals. This may be partly due to differences in mechanisms of immunological sensitization, but there is probably also some degree of underdiagnosis. Patients with asthma caused by nickel or chromium often also have urticaria or allergic contact dermatitis.[27] Significant exposure to hexavalent chromium occurs mainly in chromate production industries, in chrome plating, during stainless steel welding, but also in the building industry because cement often contains small amounts of chromates, which is not only a frequent source of allergic contact dermatitis, but occasionally also an unsuspected cause of occupational asthma.[28]

Most cases of cobalt asthma have been described in relation to the manufacture or grinding of sintered hard metal, in which cobalt is used as a binder for tungsten carbide.[29,30] Coolants used in wet grinding of hard metal tools may contain a high concentration of dissolved (i.e. ionized) cobalt, thus leading to the paradox that wet grinding may be more 'harmful' than dry grinding.[31] Cobalt asthma has also been found in relation to the production of cobalt,[32] the manufacture or use of cobalt pigments or additives, and in diamond polishers. It is possible that cobalt asthma is but an 'airway variant' of hard metal disease (see Hard metal lung disease – 'cobalt lung', p. 1045) and there are occasional subjects who exhibit both asthmatic reactions and parenchymal involvement.

Pot room asthma is a particular form of occupational asthma described in aluminium smelters (see Chapter 13, Aluminium), who are exposed to the fumes evolving from the 'pots' in which aluminium ore is molten after the addition of fluoride salts. Several clinical and epidemiological studies carried out mainly in the Norwegian aluminium industry,[33] but also elsewhere,[34] have described 'pot room asthma'. The exact causal agent of this form of asthma is not known and it probably does not involve allergic mechanisms. It seems more likely that pot room asthma is a form of irritant-induced asthma, with the irritants being most probably the fluorides present in the fumes. Occupational asthma has also been reported as a result of exposure to aluminium fluoride salts.

There are rare reports[35] of asthma in subjects welding galvanized metal, with sensitization to zinc being postulated on the grounds of a positive bronchial challenge. Similarly, occupational asthma due to soldering fluxes containing zinc chloride has been described.[36] However, no immunological support for sensitization to zinc has been provided. It is conceivable that (some) individuals with non-specific bronchial hyperreactivity exhibit asthmatic reactions when they have a bout of metal fume fever. The possible presence of metals other than zinc should also be considered in such instances.

Exposure to vanadium, usually as vanadium pentoxide (V_2O_5), has been reported as a possible cause of occupational asthma. This exposure has been described in workers who maintain, clean or dismantle oil-fired boilers, because the fly ash produced by some types of fuel oil may be very rich in vanadium (see Chapter 37, Vanadium). From the available evidence it appears that this form of asthma essentially results from the strong irritation produced by V_2O_5 which may cause nasal ulceration and acute bronchitis, with more or less lasting non-specific bronchial hyper-reactivity as a result.

In addition to the specific causes of occupational asthma described above, steel welding is often mentioned as a cause of occupational asthma or as a risk factor of asthma.[37–41] It is not clear whether these are cases of asthma from metal sensitization, 'irritant-induced' asthmas due to irritant gases, or work-related asthmas (see Chapter 44, Welding). A study from Finland described a series of 34 workers (welders, fitters, plumbers and others) with a history of occupational asthma occurring after many years (22 years on average) of being exposed to stainless steel welding fumes, and whose occupational asthma was confirmed by challenge tests with fumes from stainless steel welding; none of these subjects had positive skin prick tests to metal salts.[42]

Lung cancer

Several metallic compounds are proven lung carcinogens in humans and include radioactive metals (and their decay products) and non-radioactive metals (see Chapter 85, Occupational cancer: Epidemiology, biological mechanisms and biomarkers). The increased incidence of lung cancer observed in uranium miners has been causally linked with the inhalation of radon daughters.[43] However, the underground mining of other compounds may also be associated with significant exposure to radioactivity, if there is insufficient ventilation of the radon which leaks from igneous rocks.[44] This factor has been implicated in the higher incidence of lung cancer seen in various groups of mine workers, such as Swedish iron ore miners,[45] although it does not seem to play a role in the similarly increased lung cancer incidence of French iron ore miners.[46] Domestic radon gas exposure is also implicated in the causation of bronchial cancer.

The epidemiologic evidence of the relation between exposure to specific metallic agents and lung cancer has been reviewed in detail by Wild et al.[47] Epidemiological and experimental studies have clearly established the carcinogenic risk of exposure to arsenic, chromates and nickel, at least to some of their chemical forms. Thus, the relationship of arsenic to increased lung cancer risk in copper smelting workers is unequivocal. This is also the case for other occupational exposures to arsenic, such as the manufacture or spraying of arsenical pesticides. A greatly increased risk of lung cancer has also been demonstrated for workers in the primary chromate production and in the chromate pigment industry. Epidemiological studies of the carcinogenic risk of exposure to chromium during metal plating or during stainless steel welding have been inconclusive. Occupational exposure to nickel compounds in nickel smelters and refineries is clearly associated with an increase in cancer of the lung and the nasal sinuses. Cadmium and beryllium are also considered as human lung carcinogens. A re-evaluation of the carcinogenicity of cobalt compounds by the IARC concluded that occupational exposure to cobalt with tungsten carbide is possibly carcinogenic for humans (group 2A),[48] mainly based on epidemiological studies showing increased lung cancer risks in workers from the hard metal industry.[49,50]

Moreover, in many epidemiological studies, occupations involving exposure to (less well specified) metallic agents appear to be associated with increased risks of lung cancer.[51–54] Studies of iron and steel foundry workers have consistently found an increased risk of lung cancer, but this may be due to other agents, such as silica or asbestos, or to polycyclic aromatic hydrocarbons emitted as pyrolysis products of organic materials used.

PNEUMOCONIOSES AND SPECIFIC INTERSTITIAL LUNG DISORDERS CAUSED BY METALS

Some epidemiological surveys have revealed that subjects with 'idiopathic' lung fibrosis are more likely than controls to have been occupationally exposed to metals (and also to wood).[55,56] This means either that many patients receive a diagnosis of idiopathic lung disease because no good occupational and environmental history has been taken, or that some metals may play a hitherto unrecognized role in the causation of interstitial lung disease. Both explanations are probably valid to some extent.

Documentation of exposure to metals may be obtained from the analysis of metal concentrations in blood or urine (or even hair or nails) taken for biological monitoring. In addition, elemental analysis may be carried out on bronchoalveolar lavage fluid, on biopsy tissue or on autopsy material. Both macroanalytical (or bulk) and microanalytical techniques may be applied. The former are destructive techniques which allow the detection, quantitation and/or characterization of the crystalline structure of inorganic elements. The latter techniques allow *in situ* analysis of individual cells and particles. Several sophisticated microanalytical techniques, coupled with scanning or transmission electron microscopy, exist: energy dispersive x-ray analysis (EDXA), particle-induced x-ray emission (PIXE), electron energy loss spectrometry (EELS) and laser microprobe mass analysis (LAMMA). These techniques have been successfully applied in both bronchoalveolar lavage (BAL) fluid and lung biopsies, and databases of 'normal' values of inorganic particles are available.[57,58] Of course, the presence of a particular element, even in abnormally high quantities, does not in itself constitute proof that it is causally involved in the disease, but it may reveal unsuspected past exposures or confirm such exposures.

Siderosis

Of the metallic pneumoconioses, the most frequent and best (although still poorly) studied is siderosis, which is caused by the inhalation of iron compounds. More than 90 per cent of the total world production of metallic materials is in the form of steels and cast irons, and occupational exposure to iron is, therefore, extremely widespread. It occurs during iron (hematite) mining and related operations, during iron refining and at various stages in steel-making, during welding, cutting and abrading of iron-containing materials, as well as during the manufacture or use of iron-containing abrasives (such as emery). Despite the large number of workers who are exposed to iron-containing dust, little research has been carried out in recent years regarding the pulmonary effects of occupational exposure to iron dust. Yet, in the past decade there has been considerable interest in the possible role of iron in pulmonary diseases, because ferrous/ferric ions catalyze the Fenton reaction, whereby the very toxic hydroxyl radical (OH°) is produced. It is noteworthy that workers exposed to iron have a higher risk of (lobar) pneumonia.[18,19]

There is a widespread belief that siderosis is only a 'radiological disorder' which manifests itself by the presence of small, very radiodense opacities with uniform distribution throughout the lungs, without coalescence. With cessation of exposure, the radiographic opacities may gradually disappear. Pure siderosis is not associated with respiratory symptoms or functional impairment, and does not predispose to tuberculosis. However, exposure to silica or asbestos is not uncommon in many jobs that involve exposure to iron, thus giving rise to mixed dust fibrosis ('siderosilicosis') or to asbestosis, with their associated morbidity. The view that the symptomatic interstitial fibrosis which is sometimes found in welders ('welder's pneumoconiosis'), is simply siderosis with coexisting silicosis has been challenged on the grounds that the pulmonary silicon content of such cases did not differ from that of control lungs.[59] There are case reports of siderosis with significant fibrosis in welders.[16]

Aluminium lung

The existence of 'aluminium lung' has been the subject of some controversy. Indeed in view of the extensive industrial use of aluminium, parenchymal lung disease caused by exposure to this metal appears to be very uncommon, both at the stage of its production and during its use. On the basis of animal experimental data showing that aluminium counteracts the toxic effects of silica, inhalation of aluminium was proposed and even implemented (without real success, but also without apparent pulmonary adverse effects) for the prevention of silicosis and even for its therapy. Dinman[60] concluded that fibrosis only occurred in workers who were heavily exposed to submicron-sized aluminium plates during the production of fireworks and explosives and in workers involved in the smelting of bauxite for the production of Al_2O_3 (corundum) abrasive (Shaver's disease). The second group was perhaps also exposed to crystalline silica. An extensive review also concluded that pulmonary fibrosis was not a significant problem in aluminium smelter workers.[34] The conclusion is that exposure to aluminium dust does not pose an important risk of interstitial lung disease.

Nevertheless, there is still a risk. Severe interstitial fibrosis was described in three workers (out of a workforce of about 1000 workers) who had been heavily exposed for 19–33 years mainly, but not exclusively, to Al_2O_3 in the production of abrasives.[61] There are reports of isolated cases of granulomatous lung disease, fibrosis and alveolar proteinosis in aluminium welders or polishers. The physical characteristics of the aluminium particles, notably their surface area, or even their possibly fibrous nature, have been suggested as important determinants of their bioreactivity and hence fibrogenicity.

Other metal pneumoconioses

Other rare 'benign' pneumoconioses include those caused by tin (stannosis), barium (baritosis) and antimony (antimoniosis). These pneumoconioses were described many years ago and few recent clinical and epidemiological data are available.

'Dental technician's pneumoconiosis' is an interstitial fibrosis of many potential origins,[62–70] including silica and beryllium, but possibly also vitallium, an alloy consisting of chromium, cobalt and molybdenum. The synthetic abrasive silicon carbide (SiC) or carborundum is not actually a metallic compound – in contrast to some other abrasives such as corundum (Al_2O_3) or emery (corundum with iron oxides). Respiratory disease, including pneumoconiosis with fibrosis, has been associated with exposure to silicon carbide, during its manufacture or use.[71,72]

Recently, cases of interstitial pulmonary disease have been described in workers exposed to 'indium tin oxide' (ITO), a sintered material consisting mainly of indium oxide (In_2O_3, 90 per cent) doped with tin oxide (SnO_2, 10 per cent) which is used for making flat panel and liquid crystal displays. Cases of serious interstitial lung disease, with features of pulmonary alveolar proteinosis, have been reported from Japan[73,74] and the United States.[75] Experimental studies[76] and epidemiologic surveys[77,78] confirm the pneumotoxic potential of this new material.

Although no instances of pneumoconioses or interstitial lung disease caused by engineered nanomaterials have been reported as yet, the development, manufacture and use of various types of (insoluble) metal oxides as nanoparticles represent a potential threat of occupational lung disease for researchers, production and maintenance workers, if exposure to such novel materials becomes significant (see Chapter 70, Health effects of ultrafine/nanoparticles).

Interstitial lung disease with granuloma formation

Granulomatous lung disease has been attributed, mainly in case reports, to exposure to zirconium (Zr), during the manufacture of ceramic tiles,[79] the welding of nuclear fuel rods,[80] or lens grinding.[81] Exposure to titanium[82] and aluminium[83] are also said to have led to sarcoid-like lung granulomatosis. Beryllium lung is discussed separately in Chapter 83, Berylliosis.

Exposure to rare earth metals (or lanthanides), of which cerium (Ce) is the most abundant element, has also been associated with interstitial fibrosis in a small number of subjects.[84,85] Rare earths are essential components of carbon arc lamps used for photoengraving, and the majority of cases of this pneumoconiosis have been described in photoengravers. Deposits of rare earths have also been found, without radiologic abnormalities, in the lung of a movie projectionist.[86] Rare earths are also used in the fabrication and polishing of glass, where they have been associated with pneumoconiosis.[85,87] The presence of granulomatous interstitial alterations is mentioned occasionally, but this is not the case in most available pathologic descriptions of cerium pneumoconiosis.

Hard metal lung disease – 'cobalt lung'

Hard metal (lung) disease (sometimes also called hard metal pneumoconiosis) is a specific form of interstitial lung disease, which may occur in workers as a result of exposure to cobalt-containing dusts during the manufacture or use of hard metal or diamond tools.[88,89] Hard metal-induced bronchial asthma, which may coexist with interstitial disease in the same patient, is sometimes included in the clinical entity of hard metal lung disease, but usually the term 'hard metal lung disease' is restricted to the parenchymal form of the disease.

Hard metal is a composite material composed mainly of tungsten carbide and varying amounts (5–25 per cent) of cobalt, which functions as a binder. Besides tungsten carbide, other carbides (e.g. with tantalum, titanium, niobium) may also be used and small amounts of other metals (e.g. nickel, chromium) may also be present. Hard metals are also designated as sintered carbides or cemented carbides. Sintering refers to a process by which a powder compact is converted into a solid polycrystalline material by pressing under specific conditions of temperature and pressure. Hard metals are mainly utilized in tools used for drilling, sawing, cutting, grinding or polishing various materials, such as stones, concrete, metals, wood, etc. In recent years, diamonds have also been increasingly used to make grinding tools or saw blades and here too, the binder used for the microdiamond powder is cobalt, which makes up to 90 per cent of the grinding surface. Although these diamond tools are not composed of 'hard metal', they pose a similar hazard (see Chapter 19, Cobalt).[90]

The highest exposures to cobalt dust take place during the various stages of the manufacture of hard metal or diamond tools. However, hazardous exposure to cobalt may also occur during the filing and resharpening of hard metal tools, particularly during wet grinding,[31] as well as during the polishing of diamonds with diamond-cobalt disks. Coating with hard metal by the detonation gun process and related operations may also give rise to significant exposure.[91] All these activities often take place in small- or medium-sized factories with poor hygiene conditions, and even in large plants, tool-sharpening is often not recognized as a significant health risk.

Hard metal lung disease shares many clinical features with hypersensitivity pneumonitis: the presentation may be that of a subacute alveolitis with fever, cough, dyspnoea and a clear exposure-related clinical course, while in other instances a more insidious course with progressive diffuse fibrosis may be found. Overt disease only occurs in a minority of exposed workers and those affected may be young subjects with only a short exposure. These features clearly point to a condition caused mainly by a specific, perhaps immunological, susceptibility, as opposed to a simple process of chronic accumulation of dust in the lungs, as in the classical mineral pneumoconioses. On the other hand, hard metal lung disease also exhibits characteristics which make it distinct from hypersensitivity pneumonitis caused by organic antigens. Thus, no precipitating antibodies are found in the serum and the lung pathology and cellular findings in the bronchoalveolar lavage fluid generally differ from those of hypersensitivity pneumonitis.

The most characteristic finding in the lungs, as well as in bronchoalveolar lavage, is the presence of numerous so-called 'bizarre' giant multinucleated cells with 'cell in cell' or 'cannibalistic' features. The latter feature, i.e. giant cell interstitial pneumonitis, is pathognomonic for hard-metal disease.[92,93] However, these giant cells may be absent and histology may exhibit desquamation of numerous cells in the alveoli (desquamative interstitial pneumonitis), lymphoplasmocyte infiltration, and varying degrees of interstitial, mainly centrilobular fibrosis.[94] Except for the possible presence of giant cells, bronchoalveolar lavage fluid findings are non-specific, with all cell types – macrophages, lymphocytes, neutrophils or eosinophils, and even mast cells – being possibly increased. The finding of the constituents of hard metal (usually only tungsten) in the bronchoalveolar lavage fluid or lung tissue is a useful indicator of (past) exposure, but there is no quantitative relation with disease.[93]

The evolution of hard metal lung disease is variable, but cessation of exposure usually results in clinical improvement and good recovery, but some patients progress to end-stage fibrosis. Although corticosteroids have been given, their benefit has not been established.

While the role of cobalt in the causation of interstitial lung disease in hard metal workers and diamond polishers is undisputed, exposure to cobalt alone does not appear to be sufficient to lead to parenchymal disease and fibrosis.[95–98] Thus, occupational exposure to even high levels of 'pure' cobalt dust is apparently not associated with interstitial lung disease (although pure cobalt and cobalt salts may cause asthma).

The mechanisms for the pulmonary toxicity of cobalt have not yet been entirely elucidated.[99] The relative rarity of the condition and the fact that it may arise after short and apparently low exposures plead for an important role of individual susceptibility. The known dermal and respiratory sensitizing properties of cobalt and some of the clinical features of the disease, including the recurrence of giant cell interstitial pneumonitis in a transplanted lung despite cessation of exposure,[100] favour immunological sensitization as a possible mechanism. However, unlike the situation with beryllium, no hard evidence for immunological sensitization to cobalt as a cause for 'cobalt lung' is available. Experimental data and the observation that oxygen administration may be detrimental in 'cobalt lung'[101] suggest that poor defence against oxidants may also be involved.

Key points

- Although exposure to zinc fumes leads to a generally mild condition ('metal fume fever'), exposure to some metallic fumes, most notably cadmium fumes, can lead to severe, potentially fatal lung injury (chemical pneumonitis).
- Occupational asthma may be caused by sensitization to complex platinum salts, as well as by cobalt, nickel and chromium.
- Working in the iron and steel industry is a risk factor for pneumonia, chronic airways disease, lung cancer and, rarely, pneumoconiosis (siderosis).
- Some metals, most notably beryllium, may cause granulomatous lung disease that is clinically similar to sarcoidosis.
- Exposure to dust from hard metal (sintered tungsten carbide with cobalt) or diamond-cobalt tools may lead to interstitial lung disease, characterized by cannibalistic multinucleated giant cells in the alveoli ('giant cell interstitial pneumonitis').

REFERENCES

1. Nemery B. Metal toxicity in the respiratory tract. *European Respiratory Journal.* 1990; **3**: 202–19.
2. Robertson W, Robertson AS, Burge CB et al. Clinical investigation of an outbreak of alveolitis and asthma in a car engine manufacturing plant. *Thorax.* 2007; **62**: 981–90.
3. Blanc PD, Boushey HA, Wong H et al. Cytokines in metal fume fever. *American Review of Respiratory Disease.* 1993; **147**: 134–8.
4. Nemery B. Occupational diseases: Inhalation injury, Chemical. In: Laurent GJ, Shapiro SD (eds). *Encyclopedia of respiratory medicine.* London: Elsevier, 2006: 208–16.
5. Rendall REG, Phillips JI, Renton KA. Death following exposure to fine particulate nickel from a metal arc process. *Annals of Occupational Hygiene.* 1994; **38**: 921–30.

6. Johnson NC, Manchester S, Sarin L et al. Mercury vapor release from broken compact fluorescent lamps and in situ capture by new nanomaterial sorbents. *Environmental Science and Technology.* 2008; **42**: 5772–8.
7. Levy BS, Hoffman L, Gottsegen S. Boilermakers bronchitis. Respiratory tract irritation associated with vanadium pentoxide exposure during oil-to-coal conversion of a power plant. *Journal of Occupational Medicine.* 1984; **26**: 567–70.
8. Allen MB, Crisp A, Snook N, Page RL. 'Smoke-bomb' pneumonitis. *Respiratory Medicine.* 1992; **86**: 165–6.
9. Zhicheng S. Acute nickel carbonyl poisoning: A report of 179 cases. *British Journal of Industrial Medicine.* 1986; **43**: 422–4.
10. Cordasco EM, Stone FD. Pulmonary edema of environmental origin. *Chest.* 1973; **6497**: 182–5.
11. Balmes J, Becklake M, Blanc P et al. American Thoracic Society Statement: Occupational contribution to the burden of airway disease. *American Journal of Respiratory and Critical Care Medicine.* 2003; **167**: 787–97.
12. Blanc PD, Toren K. Occupation in chronic obstructive pulmonary disease and chronic bronchitis: an update. *International Journal of Tuberculosis and Lung Disease.* 2007; **11**: 251–7.
13. Blanc PD, Iribarren C, Trupin L et al. Occupational exposures and the risk of COPD: dusty trades revisited. *Thorax.* 2009; **64**: 6–12.
14. Davison AG, Newman Taylor AJ, Darbyshire J et al. Cadmium fume inhalation and emphysema. *Lancet.* 1988; **i**: 663–7.
15. Kazantzis G, Lam TH, Sullivan KR. Mortality of cadmium-exposed workers. *Scandinavian Journal of Work, Environment and Health.* 1988; **14**: 220–3.
16. Billings CG, Howard P. Occupational siderosis and welders' lung: A review. *Monaldi Archives for Chest Disease.* 1993; **48**: 304–14.
17. Sferlazza SJ, Beckett WS. The respiratory health of welders. *American Review of Respiratory Disease.* 1991; **143**: 1134–48.
18. Coggon D, Inskip H, Winter P, Pannett B. Lobar pneumonia: An occupational disease in welders. *Lancet.* 1994; **344**: 41–3.
19. Palmer KT, Poole J, Ayres JG et al. Exposure to metal fume and infectious pneumonia. *American Journal of Epidemiology.* 2003; **157**: 227–33.
20. Valentin H, Smidt U. *Research project: Chronic bronchitis and occupational dust exposure.* Boppard: Harald Boldt Verlag, 1978.
21. Chinn DJ, Stevenson IC, Cotes JE. Longitudinal respiratory survey of shipyard workers: Effect of trade and atopic status. *British Journal of Industrial Medicine.* 1990; **47**: 83–90.
22. Soyseth V, Johnsen HL, Benth JS et al. Production of silicon metal and alloys is associated with accelerated decline in lung function: A 5-year prospective study among 3924 employees in Norwegian smelters. *Journal of Occupational and Environmental Medicine.* 2007; **49**: 1020–6.
23. Bernstein DL, Brooks SM, Nemery B. Metals. In: Bernstein DL, Chan-Yeung M, Malo JL, Bernstein IL (eds). *Asthma in the workplace*, 2nd edn. New York: Dekker, 1999.
24. Merget R, Kulzer R, Dierkes-Globisch A et al. Exposure-effect relationship of platinum salt allergy in a catalyst production plant: Conclusions from a 5-year prospective cohort study. *Journal of Allergy and Clinical Immunology.* 2000; **105**: 364–70.
25. Daenen M, Rogiers P, Van de Walle C et al. Occupational asthma caused by palladium. *European Respiratory Journal.* 1999; **13**: 213–16.
26. Merget R, Sander I, van Kampen V et al. Occupational immediate-type asthma and rhinitis due to rhodium salts. *American Journal of Industrial Medicine.* 2010; **53**: 42–6.
27. Fernandez-Nieto M, Quirce S, Carnes J, Sastre J. Occupational asthma due to chromium and nickel salts. *International Archives of Occupational and Environmental Health.* 2006; **79**: 483–6.
28. De Raeve H, Vandecasteele C, Demedts M, Nemery B. Dermal and respiratory sensitization to chromate in cement floorer. *American Journal of Industrial Medicine.* 1998; **34**: 169–76.
29. Davison AG, Haslam PL, Corrin B et al. Interstitial lung disease and asthma in hard-metal workers: Bronchoalveolar lavage, ultrastructural, and analytical findings and results of bronchial provocation tests. *Thorax.* 1983; **38**: 119–28.
30. Kusaka Y, Yokoyama K, Sera Y et al. Respiratory diseases in hard metal workers: An occupational hygiene study in a factory. *British Journal of Industrial Medicine.* 1986; **43**: 474–85.
31. Sjögren I, Hillerdal G, Andersson A, Zetterström O. Hard metal lung disease: Importance of cobalt in coolants. *Thorax.* 1980; **35**: 653–9.
32. Linna A, Oksa P, Palmroos P et al. Respiratory health of cobalt production workers. *American Journal of Industrial Medicine.* 2003; **44**: 124–32.
33. Kongerud J, Boe J, Soyseth V et al. Aluminium potroom asthma: The Norwegian experience. *European Respiratory Journal.* 1994; **7**: 165–72.
34. Abramson MJ, Wlodarczyk JH, Saunders NA, Hensley MJ. Does aluminum smelting cause lung disease? *American Review of Respiratory Disease.* 1989; **139**: 1042–57.
35. Malo JL, Cartier A. Occupational asthma due to fumes of galvanized metal. *Chest.* 1987; **92**: 375–7.
36. Weir DC, Robertson AS, Jones S, Burge PS. Occupational asthma due to soft corrosive soldering fluxes containing zinc chloride and ammonium chloride. *Thorax.* 1989; **44**: 220–3.
37. Beach JR, Dennis JH, Avery AJ et al. An epidemiologic investigation of asthma in welders. *American Journal of Respiratory and Critical Care Medicine.* 1996; **154**: 1394–400.
38. Vandenplas O, Dargent F, Auverdin JJ et al. Occupational asthma due to gas metal arc welding on mild steel. *Thorax.* 1995; **50**: 587–8.
39. Wang ZP, Larsson K, Malmberg P et al. Asthma, lung function and bronchial responsiveness in welders. *American Journal of Industrial Medicine.* 1994; **26**: 741–54.

40. Hannu T, Piipari R, Kasurinen H et al. Occupational asthma due to manual metal-arc welding of special stainless steels. *European Respiratory Journal.* 2005; **26**: 736-9.
41. Hannu T, Piipari R, Tuppurainen M, Tuomi T. Occupational asthma due to welding fumes from stellite. *Journal of Occupational and Environmental Medicine.* 2007; **49**: 473-4.
42. Hannu T, Piipari R, Tuppurainen M et al. Occupational asthma caused by stainless steel welding fumes: A clinical study. *European Respiratory Journal.* 2007; **29**: 85-90.
43. Samet JM, Kutvirt DM, Waxweiler RJ, Key CR. Uranium mining and lung cancer in Navajo men. *New England Journal of Medicine.* 1984; **310**: 1481-4.
44. Archer VE. Lung cancer risks of underground miners. Cohort and case-control studies. *Yale Journal of Biology and Medicine.* 1988; **61**: 183-94.
45. Radford EP, Renard SKG. Lung cancer in Swedish iron miners exposed to low doses of radon daughters. *New England Journal of Medicine.* 1984; **310**: 1485-94.
46. Mur JM, Meyer-Bisch C, Pham QT et al. Risk of lung cancer among iron ore miners; a proportional mortality study of 1,075 deceased miners in Lorraine, France. *Journal of Occupational Medicine.* 1987; **29**: 762-8.
47. Wild P, Bourgkard E, Paris C. Lung cancer and exposure to metals: The epidemiological evidence. *Methods in Molecular Biology.* 2009; **472**: 139-67.
48. IARC Working Group on the Evaluation of Carcinogenic Risks to Humans, International Agency for Research on Cancer. Cobalt in hard metals and cobalt sulfate, gallium arsenide, indium phosphide and vanadium pentoxide. Lyon: International Agency for Research on Cancer, 2006.
49. Moulin JJ, Wild P, Romazini S et al. Lung cancer risk in hard-metal workers. *American Journal of Epidemiology.* 1998; **148**: 241-8.
50. Wild P, Perdrix A, Romazini S et al. Lung cancer mortality in a site producing hard metals. *Occupational and Environmental Medicine.* 2000; **57**: 568-73.
51. Bardin-Mikolajczak A, Lissowska J, Zaridze D et al. Occupation and risk of lung cancer in Central and Eastern Europe: The IARC multi-center case-control study. *Cancer Causes and Control.* 2007; **18**: 645-54.
52. MacArthur AC, Le ND, Fang R, Band PR. Identification of occupational cancer risk in British Columbia: A population-based case-control study of 2,998 lung cancers by histopathological subtype. *American Journal of Industrial Medicine.* 2009; **52**: 221-32.
53. Siew SS, Kauppinen T, Kyyronen P et al. Exposure to iron and welding fumes and the risk of lung cancer. *Scandinavian Journal of Work, Environment and Health.* 2008; **34**: 444-50.
54. Veglia F, Vineis P, Overvad K et al. Occupational exposures, environmental tobacco smoke, and lung cancer. *Epidemiology.* 2007; **18**: 769-75.
55. Taskar VS, Coultas DB. Is idiopathic pulmonary fibrosis an environmental disease? *Proceedings of the American Thoracic Society.* 2006; **3**: 293-8.
56. Hubbard R, Lewis S, Richards K et al. Occupational exposure to metal or wood dust and aetiology of cryptogenic fibrosing alveolitis. *Lancet.* 1996; **347**: 284-9.
57. Abraham JL, Burnett BR, Hunt A. Development and use of a pneumoconiosis database of human pulmonary inorganic particulate burden in over 400 lungs. *Scanning Microscopy.* 1991; **5**: 95-108.
58. Dumortier P, De Vuyst P, Yernault JC. Non-fibrous inorganic particles in human bronchoalveolar lavage fluids. *Scanning Microscopy.* 1989; **3**: 1207-18.
59. Funahashi A, Schlueter DP, Pintar K et al. Welders' pneumoconiosis: Tissue elemental microanalysis by energy dispersive X-ray analysis. *British Journal of Industrial Medicine.* 1988; **45**: 14-18.
60. Dinman BD. Alumina-related pulmonary disease. *Journal of Occupational Medicine.* 1988; **30**: 328-35.
61. Jederlinic PJ, Abraham JL, Churg A et al. Pulmonary fibrosis in aluminum oxide workers. Investigation of nine workers, with pathologic examination and microanalysis in three of them. *American Review of Respiratory Disease.* 1990; **142**: 1179-84.
62. Choudat D. Occupational lung diseases among dental technicians. *Tubercle and Lung Disease.* 1994; **75**: 99-104.
63. De Vuyst P, Van de Weyer R, Decoster A et al. Dental technician's pneumoconiosis. A report of two cases. *American Review of Respiratory Disease.* 1986; **133**: 316-20.
64. Fireman E, Kramer MR, Priel I, Lerman Y. Chronic beryllium disease among dental technicians in Israel. *Sarcoidosis, Vasculitis, and Diffuse Lung Diseases.* 2006; **23**: 215-21.
65. Kotloff RM, Richman PS, Greenacre JK, Rossman MD. Chronic beryllium disease in a dental laboratory technician. *American Review of Respiratory Disease.* 1993; **147**: 205-7.
66. Nayebzadeh A, Dufresne A, Harvie S, Bégin R. Mineralogy of lung tissue in dental laboratory technicians' pneumoconiosis. *American Industrial Hygiene Association Journal.* 1999; **60**: 349-53.
67. Rom WN, Lockey JE, Jeffrey LS et al. Pneumoconiosis and exposure of dental laboratory technicians. *American Journal of Public Health.* 1984; **74**: 1252-7.
68. Selden A, Sahle W, Johansson L et al. Three cases of dental technician's pneumoconiosis related to cobalt-chromium-molybdenum dust exposure. *Chest.* 1996; **109**: 837-42.
69. Selden AI, Persson B, Bornberger-Dankvardt SI et al. Exposure to cobalt chromium dust and lung disorders in dental technicians. *Thorax.* 1995; **50**: 769-72.
70. Sherson D, Maltbaek N, Heydorn K. A dental technician with pulmonary fibrosis: A case of chromium-cobalt alloy pneumoconiosis? *European Respiratory Journal.* 1990; **3**: 1227-9.
71. Funahashi A, Schlueter DP, Pintar K et al. Pneumoconiosis in workers exposed to silicon carbide. *American Review of Respiratory Disease.* 1984; **129**: 635-40.
72. Peters JM, Smith TJ, Bernstein L et al. Pulmonary effects of exposures in silicon carbide manufacturing. *British Journal of Industrial Medicine.* 1984; **41**: 109-14.

73. Homma S, Miyamoto A, Sakamoto S et al. Pulmonary fibrosis in an individual occupationally exposed to inhaled indium-tin oxide. *European Respiratory Journal*. 2005; **25**: 200–4.
74. Homma T, Ueno T, Sekizawa K et al. Interstitial pneumonia developed in a worker dealing with particles containing indium-tin oxide. *Journal of Occupational Health*. 2003; **45**: 137–9.
75. Cummings KJ, Donat WE, Ettensohn DB et al. Pulmonary alveolar proteinosis in workers at an indium processing facility. *American Journal of Respiratory and Critical Care Medicine*. 2010; **181**: 458–64.
76. Lison D, Laloy J, Corazzari I et al. Sintered indium-tin-oxide (ITO). particles: A new pneumotoxic entity. *Toxicological Sciences*. 2009; **108**: 472–81.
77. Chonan T, Taguchi O, Omae K. Interstitial pulmonary disorders in indium-processing workers. *European Respiratory Journal*. 2007; **29**: 317–24.
78. Hamaguchi T, Omae K, Takebayashi T et al. Exposure to hardly soluble indium compounds in ITO production and recycling plants is a new risk for interstitial lung damage. *Occupational and Environmental Medicine*. 2008; **65**: 51–5.
79. Liippo KK, Anttila SL, Taikina-Aho O et al. Hypersensitivity pneumonitis and exposure to zirconium silicate in a young ceramic tile worker. *American Review of Respiratory Disease*. 1993; **148**: 1089–92.
80. Schneider J, Freitag F, Rödelsperger K. Durch Zirkonium-Einwirkung am Arbeitsplatz verursachte exogen-allergische Alveolitis (Nr. 4201 BeKV). *Arbeitsmedizin, Sozialmed und Umweltmedizin*. 1994; **29**: 382–5.
81. Bartter T, Irwin RS, Abraham JL et al. Zirconium compound-induced pulmonary fibrosis. *Archives of Internal Medicine*. 1991; **151**: 1197–201.
82. Redline S, Barna BP, Tomashefski JF Jr, Abraham JL. Granulomatous disease associated with pulmonary deposition of titanium. *British Journal of Industrial Medicine*. 1986; **43**: 652–6.
83. De Vuyst P, Dumortier P, Schandené L et al. Sarcoidlike lung granulomatosis induced by aluminium dust. *American Review of Respiratory Disease*. 1987; **135**: 493–7.
84. Haley PJ. Pulmonary toxicity of stable and radioactive lanthanides. *Health Physics*. 1991; **61**: 809–20.
85. Pairon JC, Roos F, Sébastien P et al. Biopersistence of cerium in the human respiratory tract and ultrastructural findings. *American Journal of Industrial Medicine*. 1995; **27**: 349–58.
86. Waring PM, Watling RJ. Rare earth deposits in a deceased movie projectionist. A new case of rare earth pneumoconiosis? *Medical Journal of Australia*. 1990; **153**: 726–30.
87. McDonald JW, Ghio AJ, Sheehan CE et al. Rare earth (cerium oxide). Pneumoconiosis: Analytical scanning electron microscopy and literature review. *Modern Pathology*. 1995; **8**: 859–65.
88. Cugell DW, Morgan WKC, Perkins DG, Rubin A. The respiratory effects of cobalt. *Archives of Internal Medicine*. 1990; **150**: 177–83.
89. Nemery B, Verbeken EK, Demedts M. Giant cell interstitial pneumonia (hard metal lung disease, cobalt lung). *Seminars in Respiratory and Critical Care Medicine*. 2001; **22**: 435–47.
90. Demedts M, Gheysens B, Nagels J et al. Cobalt lung in diamond polishers. *American Review of Respiratory Disease*. 1984; **130**: 130–5.
91. Figueroa S, Gerstenhaber B, Welch L et al. Hard metal interstitial pulmonary disease associated with a form of welding in a metal parts coating plant. *American Journal of Industrial Medicine*. 1992; **21**: 363–73.
92. Ohori NP, Sciurba FC, Owens GR et al. Giant-cell interstitial pneumonia and hard-metal pneumoconiosis. A clinicopathologic study of four cases and review of the literature. *American Journal of Surgical Pathology*. 1989; **13**: 581–7.
93. Naqvi AH, Hunt A, Burnett BR, Abraham JL. Pathologic spectrum and lung dust burden in giant cell interstitial pneumonia (hard metal disease/cobalt pneumonitis): Review of 100 cases. *Archives of Environmental and Occupational Health*. 2008; **63**: 51–70.
94. Moriyama H, Kobayashi M, Takada T et al. Two-dimensional analysis of elements and mononuclear cells in hard metal lung disease. *American Journal of Respiratory and Critical Care Medicine*. 2007; **176**; 70–7.
95. Lison D. Human toxicity of cobalt-containing dust and experimental studies on the mechanism of interstitial lung disease (hard metal disease). *Critical Reviews in Toxicology*. 1996; **26**: 585–616.
96. Lison D, Lauwerys R, Demedts M, Nemery B. Experimental research into the pathogenesis of cobalt/hard metal lung disease. *European Respiratory Journal*. 1996; **9**: 1024–8.
97. Swennen B, Buchet JP, Stanescu D et al. Epidemiological survey of workers exposed to cobalt oxides, cobalt salts, and cobalt metal. *British Journal of Industrial Medicine*. 1993; **50**: 835–42.
98. Verougstraete V, Mallants A, Buchet JP et al. Lung function changes in workers exposed to cobalt compounds: A 13-year follow-up. *American Journal of Respiratory and Critical Care Medicine*. 2004; **170**: 162–6.
99. Nemery B, Abraham JL. Hard metal lung disease: Still hard to understand. *American Journal of Respiratory and Critical Care Medicine*. 2007; **176**: 2–3.
100. Frost AE, Keller CA, Brown RW et al. Giant cell interstitial pneumonitis. Disease recurrence in the transplanted lung. *American Review of Respiratory Disease*. 1993; **148**: 1401–4.
101. Nemery B, Nagels J, Verbeken E et al. Rapidly fatal progression of cobalt-lung in a diamond polisher. *American Review of Respiratory Disease*. 1990; **141**: 1373–8.

83

Berylliosis

HOLLY M CHRISTENSEN AND LEE S NEWMAN

Introduction	1050	Prevention	1052
Epidemiology	1050	Future research	1052
Mechanisms of disease	1050	References	1052
Clinical disease	1051		

INTRODUCTION

Beryllium has chemical and physical properties that make it an excellent material for highly technological applications. Unfortunately, it continues to cause a significant burden of illness among those who work with the metal and its alloys. Exposure occurs during the extraction and the processing of beryllium into metal alloys and ceramic raw materials, as well as during the production of beryllium-containing products that may involve heating and machining operations, and the recycling of beryllium-containing products. The spreading use of beryllium in modern industries has created a serious public health problem worldwide.[1]

EPIDEMIOLOGY

Berylliosis takes two principal forms: acute and chronic. The major, persisting problem in modern industry is with chronic beryllium disease (CBD) which was first described in the United States in the 1940s, when fluorescent lamp workers presented with pulmonary granulomatous disease.[2] A large, but imprecisely known number of workers internationally have been exposed to beryllium, with estimates exceeding 800 000.[1] A recent review placed a low end estimate for current US workers at 134 000.[3,4] The prevalence of CBD, from epidemiologic studies, has been variously estimated at 1 per cent to greater than 15 per cent of exposed workers, depending on the group of workers studied. On average, CBD develops six to ten years after exposure, but has been reported to occur with a latency up to 40 years and as early as three months after initial exposure. Beryllium sensitization precedes CBD and affects approximately 1–5 per cent of exposed workers.[5–24] The rate of progression from sensitization to CBD is estimated at 6–8 per cent per year.[25]

While the precise exposure–response relationship for CBD is not linear, certain beryllium industrial processes and job tasks with high beryllium exposures carry a higher risk.[6–10,12,14,16,22,24] CBD has been detected in workers with evidence of only very low levels and short duration of exposure, with sensitization being seen at levels as low as $0.02\,\mu g/m^3$ lifetime-weighted exposure.[1,7,8,15–17,22,24,26–28]

MECHANISMS OF DISEASE

Beryllium induces immunologic reactions in exposed and sensitized individuals, by triggering an adaptive immune response to beryllium antigen in T lymphocytes.[29–31] In the presence of beryllium salts *in vitro*, both blood and bronchoalveolar lavage lymphocytes proliferate, forming the basis of the beryllium lymphocyte proliferation test (BeLPT), the preferred diagnostic and screening test. This response is specific for beryllium and is not induced by other metals.[30,32]

Lung mononuclear cell inflammation and granuloma formation is maintained by the accumulation in the lung of $CD4^+$ memory T cells specific for beryllium, presented to those cells by human leukocyte antigen (HLA) molecules found on antigen-presenting cells.[33]

The progression from exposure to sensitization to CBD hinges partly on genetic susceptibility. Research has demonstrated that HLA-DPB1 with a glutamic acid residue at position 69 (E69) is associated with beryllium sensitization and CBD.[34–42] Regardless of an individual's genetics, CBD does not occur unless a worker has been exposed to beryllium.

CLINICAL DISEASE

Acute disease

Although acute disease is rare, exposure to elevated concentrations of beryllium can result in nasopharyngitis, tracheobronchitis and a lymphocyte-predominant acute pneumonitis.[43–46] Signs and symptoms are non-specific and include cough, occasionally productive of blood-tinged sputum, dyspnoea and chest discomfort. Examination may reveal airway hyperaemia, as well as rales or rhonchi. The chest radiograph may show increased bronchovascular markings, diffuse bilateral alveolar infiltrates or severe bilateral pulmonary oedema. Management is mainly supportive for acute upper airway disease and should include removal from exposure. Corticosteroids, oxygen, rest and even ventilatory support may be part of the treatment regimen, although no controlled clinical trials have been published of their efficacy.

Skin disease

Beryllium can induce a number of dermatologic conditions, depending on the form of beryllium and severity of exposure. Contact dermatitis can occur on exposed areas of skin. It generally resolves with cessation of exposure and recrudesces with re-exposure. If the contact dermatitis involves the face, conjunctivitis, periorbital oedema and upper respiratory tract involvement may occur concomitantly.[44,46] Ulceration or granulomatous nodular skin lesions may occur after accidental beryllium inoculation. These persist until the beryllium material is excised and the lesion debrided.

Lung cancer

A number of large epidemiologic studies have shown an increased risk of lung cancer among beryllium-exposed workers and among workers with acute beryllium disease.[47–51] The International Agency for Research on Cancer (IARC) classifies beryllium as a class I human carcinogen.[52,53]

Chronic beryllium disease

Chronic beryllium disease may be asymptomatic and detected through medical surveillance, including testing for immune response in the BeLPT. Such cases typically have normal chest radiographs and resting pulmonary function, but often have abnormal gas exchange with exercise.

CBD shares many clinical and histopathological features with pulmonary sarcoidosis. It is estimated that up to 6 per cent of patients diagnosed with sarcoidosis may actually have CBD.[54,55] CBD typically has a gradual course and insidious onset of non-specific respiratory and systemic symptoms, with most patients presenting with some combination of fatigue, non-productive cough, and gradually progressive shortness of breath, especially upon exertion.[44–46] Anorexia, weight loss, fevers, night sweats, chest pains and arthralgias are fairly common. Dry bibasilar rales, cyanosis, clubbing, lymphadenopathy and skin changes may be present on examination, with other findings depending on the severity. With advancing disease, symptoms associated with pulmonary hypertension, cor pulmonale or respiratory failure develop.

PULMONARY PHYSIOLOGY

The pulmonary function abnormalities seen in CBD are typical of many interstitial lung diseases. A restrictive pattern with decreased lung volumes occurs in advanced disease; however, normal volumes with a mild obstructive pattern is common early in CBD.[56,57] The diffusing capacity for carbon monoxide (D_LCO) is reduced in more advanced disease. Common abnormalities noted on exercise testing include reduced exercise tolerance, decreased oxygen consumption (VO_2), an abnormal fall in oxygen saturation, and widening alveolar–arterial gradient. Reduced oxygenation at rest and during exercise is a sensitive indicator of physiologic impairment.

IMAGING FINDINGS

The chest radiograph may be normal or show hilar adenopathy with reticulonodular opacification especially in mid- and upper lung zones. Thin-section computed tomography (CT) is more sensitive than chest radiography in identifying parenchymal nodules, septal lines, ground glass opacities and hilar or mediastinal adenopathy.[58] Pleural thickening can be observed adjacent to areas of dense subpleural parenchymal nodules.

BRONCHOALVEOLAR LAVAGE AND TRANSBRONCHIAL BIOPSY

In CBD, bronchoalveolar lavage (BAL) shows increased total white cells with $CD4^+$ T lymphocyte predominance.[30,59–61] The extent of BAL cellularity, lymphocytosis, and BAL BeLPT response correlates with disease severity, suggesting that the magnitude of the inflammatory and antigenic response in the lung may help predict disease progression.[62]

PATHOLOGY

The non-caseating granuloma is a hallmark of CBD, but is histologically indistinguishable from the granulomas found in sarcoidosis. Other pathologic abnormalities commonly found include a mononuclear cell interstitial infiltrate and varying degrees of fibrosis.[44,45,63,64] The absence of granulomas on either transbronchial biopsy or thoracoscopic lung biopsy does not exclude CBD. The presence of multinucleated giant cells and mononuclear cell interstitial infiltrates is also consistent with CBD.

DIAGNOSTIC EVALUATION

The diagnosis of CBD is confirmed by demonstrating a beryllium-specific immune response, through the BeLPT on blood or, preferably, on BAL fluid, together with finding pathologic changes consistent with CBD on transbronchial biopsy.[61,65,66] Bronchoscopy is not essential for diagnosis; the presence of a beryllium-specific immune response in the blood, together with a chest radiograph or CT scan showing changes consistent with CBD provide sufficient evidence. Patients who demonstrate a beryllium-specific immune response with normal lungs are considered to have beryllium sensitization without CBD.

TREATMENT AND FOLLOW UP

There is no known cure for CBD. The goals of treatment are to inhibit inflammation and slow disease progression. Removal from exposure is important. Corticosteroids are the first-line therapy for CBD, reducing symptoms and improving lung function.[67–81] Indications for treatment include (1) severe symptoms, such as debilitating cough or dyspnoea; (2) abnormal gas exchange, diminished exercise tolerance or abnormal pulmonary physiology; (3) progressive decline in these tests of impairment; or (4) evidence of pulmonary hypertension or cor pulmonale. Initial therapy includes oral prednisone at a dose of approximately 20–40 mg either daily or on alternate days. After three to six months, the response to therapy should be reassessed and the prednisone dose tapered gradually to the minimum dose required to sustain symptomatic improvement. Therapy is usually required lifelong, because relapses occur after steroid withdrawal.[44–46] More severe cases may require additional supportive measures, such as supplemental oxygen, to improve hypoxaemia and treat pulmonary hypertension and cor pulmonale, or diuretics for right heart failure. Obstructive ventilatory defects and cough may respond to inhaled bronchodilators and steroids. In patients who fail to respond to corticosteroids or who experience severe side effects, other immunosuppressive agents such as methotrexate (up to 20 mg orally per week) may prove effective.

Less severe cases not requiring steroid therapy should be examined and tested annually to monitor for disease progression. Patients who are beryllium sensitized without granulomatous disease should be checked for evidence of CBD, perhaps every two years, because of the risk of progression to clinical disease.

PREVENTION

The current US Occupational Safety and Health Administration (OSHA) exposure limit for beryllium is not protective.[3,6,9–13,82–84] As a result, many beryllium-using industries have minimized exposure by using safer metals, improving ventilation systems, implementing administrative controls, requiring personal protection equipment, educating workers concerning the hazards and offering medical monitoring using the BeLPT.[23,85] As dermal exposure might also contribute to risk, measures should also be taken to protect the skin.[86,87]

FUTURE RESEARCH

Current and future research efforts are focused on identifying additional non-invasive tests to confirm a diagnosis of CBD,[88–91] as well as seeking new treatments. Tumour necrosis factor-alpha blockers appear to be promising therapeutic agents, but no clinical trials of this approach have been completed to date.

> **Key points**
>
> - Broader use of beryllium in modern industry has created an increasing public health problem globally, affecting 1–15 per cent of exposed workers.
> - Chronic and acute forms of berylliosis continue to occur as a result of immunologic recognition of beryllium antigen.
> - Beryllium sensitization and chronic beryllium disease can be detected in workplace surveillance programmes and can be distinguished from other granulomatous disorders using the beryllium lymphocyte proliferation test.
> - Chronic beryllium disease is a latent disorder preferentially affecting the lungs and immune system, as well as other organs.
> - Exposure to beryllium at levels below current permissible exposure limits results in disease, necessitating strict attention to ventilation, use of personal protective equipment, administrative controls, exposure monitoring and substitution of beryllium with safer materials whenever possible.

REFERENCES

1. Infante PF, Newman LS. Beryllium exposure and chronic beryllium disease. *Lancet.* 2004; **363**: 415–16.
2. Hardy HL, Tabershaw IR. Delayed chemical pneumonitis in workers exposed to beryllium compounds. *Journal of Industrial Hygiene and Toxicity.* 1946; **28**: 197–211.
3. Cullen MR, Kominsky JR, Rossman MD *et al.* Chronic beryllium disease in a precious metal refinery. Clinical epidemiologic and immunologic evidence for continuing risk

from exposure to low level beryllium fume. *American Review of Respiratory Disease*. 1987; **135**: 201–8.
4. Henneberger PK, Goe SK, Miller WE *et al*. Industries in the United States with airborne beryllium exposure and estimates of the number of current workers potentially exposed. *Journal of Occupational and Environmental Hygiene*. 2004; **1**: 648–59.
5. Kreiss K, Newman LS, Mroz MM, Campbell PA. Screening blood test identifies subclinical beryllium disease. *Journal of Occupational Medicine*. 1989; **31**: 603–8.
6. Henneberger PK, Cumro D, Deubner DD *et al*. Beryllium sensitization and disease among long-term and short-term workers in a beryllium ceramics plant. *International Archives of Occupational and Environmental Health*. 2001; **74**: 167–76.
7. Kreiss K, Mroz MM, Zhen B *et al*. Epidemiology of beryllium sensitization and disease in nuclear workers. *American Review of Respiratory Disease*. 1993; **148**: 985–91.
8. Kreiss K, Wasserman S, Mroz MM, Newman LS. Beryllium disease screening in the ceramics industry. Blood lymphocyte test performance and exposure–disease relations. *Journal of Occupational Medicine*. 1993; **35**: 267–74.
9. Kreiss K, Mroz MM, Newman LS *et al*. Machining risk of beryllium disease and sensitization with median exposures below 2 micrograms/m^3. *American Journal of Industrial Medicine*. 1996; **30**: 16–25.
10. Kreiss K, Mroz MM, Zhen B *et al*. Risks of beryllium disease related to work processes at a metal, alloy, and oxide production plant. *Occupational and Environmental Medicine*. 1997; **54**: 605–12.
11. Kelleher PC, Martyny JW, Mroz MM *et al*. Beryllium particulate exposure and disease relations in a beryllium machining plant. *Journal of Occupational and Environmental Medicine*. 2001; **43**: 238–49.
12. Schuler CR, Kent MS, Deubner DC *et al*. Process-related risk of beryllium sensitization and disease in a copper-beryllium alloy facility. *American Journal of Industrial Medicine*. 2005; **47**: 195–205.
13. Rosenman K, Hertzberg V, Rice C *et al*. Chronic beryllium disease and sensitization at a beryllium processing facility. *Environmental Health Perspectives*. 2005; **113**: 1366–72.
14. Stange AW, Hilmas DE, Furman FJ, Gatliffe TR. Beryllium sensitization and chronic beryllium disease at a former nuclear weapons facility. *Applied Occupational and Environmental Hygiene*. 2001; **16**: 405–17.
15. Sackett HM, Maier LA, Silveira LJ *et al*. Beryllium medical surveillance at a former nuclear weapons facility during cleanup operations. *Journal of Occupational and Environmental Medicine*. 2004; **46**: 953–61.
16. Welch L, Ringen K, Bingham E *et al*. Screening for beryllium disease among construction trade workers at Department of Energy nuclear sites. *American Journal of Industrial Medicine*. 2004; **46**: 207–18.
17. Eisenbud M, Lisson J. Epidemiologic aspects of beryllium-induced non-malignant lung disease. *Journal of Occupational Medicine*. 1983; **25**: 196–202.
18. Kriebel D, Sprince NL, Eisen EA. Beryllium exposure and pulmonary functions: A cross-sectional study of beryllium workers. *British Journal of Industrial Medicine*. 1988; **45**: 167–73.
19. Deubner D, Kelsh M, Shum M *et al*. Beryllium sensitization, chronic beryllium disease, and exposures at a beryllium mining and extraction facility. *Applied Occupational and Environmental Hygiene*. 2001; **16**: 579–92.
20. Stanton ML, Henneberger PK, Kent MS *et al*. Sensitization and chronic beryllium disease among workers in copper-beryllium distribution centers. *Journal of Occupational and Environmental Medicine*. 2006; **48**: 204–11.
21. Stange AW, Furman FJ, Hilmas DE. Rocky Flats Beryllium Health Surveillance. *Environmental Health Perspectives*. 1996; **104** (Suppl. 5): 981–6.
22. Newman LS, Mroz MM, Maier LA *et al*. Efficacy of serial medical surveillance for chronic beryllium disease in a beryllium machining plant. *Journal of Occupational and Environmental Medicine*. 2001; **43**: 231–7.
23. Cummings KJ, Deubner DC, Day GA *et al*. Enhanced preventive programme at a beryllium oxide ceramics facility reduces beryllium sensitisation among new workers. *Occupational and Environmental Medicine*. 2007; **64**: 134–40.
24. Rodrigues EG, McClean MD, Weinberg J, Pepper LD. Beryllium sensitization and lung function among former workers at the Nevada Test Site. *American Journal of Industrial Medicine*. 2008; **51**: 512–23.
25. Newman LS, Mroz MM, Balkissoon R, Maier LA. Beryllium sensitization progresses to chronic beryllium disease: A longitudinal study of disease risk. *American Journal of Respiratory and Critical Care Medicine*. 2005; **171**: 54–60.
26. Newman LS, Lloyd J, Daniloff E. The natural history of beryllium sensitization and chronic beryllium disease. *Environmental Health Perspectives*. 1996; **104** (Suppl. 5): 937–43.
27. Newman LS. Immunology, genetics, and epidemiology of beryllium disease. *Chest*. 1996; **109** (Suppl. 3): 40S–43S.
28. Newman LS. Significance of the blood beryllium lymphocyte proliferation test. *Environmental Health Perspectives*. 1996; **104** (Suppl. 5): 953–6.
29. Curtis GH. Cutaneous hypersensitivity due to beryllium; a study of thirteen cases. *Archives of Dermatology and Syphilology*. 1951; **64**: 470–82.
30. Saltini C, Winestock K, Kirby M *et al*. Maintenance of alveolitis in patients with chronic beryllium disease by beryllium-specific helper T cells. *New England Journal of Medicine*. 1989; **320**: 1103–9.
31. Fontenot AP, Maier LA. Genetic susceptibility and immune-mediated destruction in beryllium-induced disease. *Trends in Immunology*. 2005; **26**: 543–9.
32. Hanifin JM, Epstein WL, Cline MJ. In vitro studies on granulomatous hypersensitivity to beryllium. *Journal of Investigative Dermatology*. 1970; **55**: 284–8.
33. Fontenot AP, Canavera SJ, Gharavi L *et al*. Target organ localization of memory CD4(+) T cells in patients with chronic beryllium disease. *Journal of Clinical Investigation*. 2002; **110**: 1473–82.

34. McCanlies EC, Kreiss K, Andrew M, Weston A. HLA-DPB1 and chronic beryllium disease: A HuGE review. *American Journal of Epidemiology.* 2003; **157**: 388-98.
35. Richeldi L, Sorrentino R, Saltini C. HLA-DPB1 glutamate 69: A genetic marker of beryllium disease. *Science.* 1993; **262**: 242-4.
36. Newman LS. To Be2+ or not to Be2+: Immunogenetics and occupational exposure. *Science.* 1993; **262**: 197-8.
37. Maier LA, McGrath DS, Sato H et al. Influence of MHC class II in susceptibility to beryllium sensitization and chronic beryllium disease. *Journal of Immunology.* 2003; **171**: 6910-18.
38. Rossman MD, Stubbs J, Lee CW et al. Human leukocyte antigen class II amino acid epitopes: Susceptibility and progression markers for beryllium hypersensitivity. *American Journal of Respiratory and Critical Care Medicine.* 2002; **165**: 788-94.
39. Wang Z, White PS, Petrovic M et al. Differential susceptibilities to chronic beryllium disease contributed by different Glu69 HLA-DPB1 and -DPA1 alleles. *Journal of Immunology.* 1999; **163**: 1647-53.
40. Weston A, Snyder J, McCanlies EC et al. Immunogenetic factors in beryllium sensitization and chronic beryllium disease. *Mutation Research.* 2005; **592**: 68-78.
41. Amicosante M, Berretta F, Rossman M et al. Identification of HLA-DRPhebeta47 as the susceptibility marker of hypersensitivity to beryllium in individuals lacking the berylliosis-associated supratypic marker HLA-DPGlubeta69. *Respiratory Research.* 2005; **6**: 94.
42. McCanlies EC, Ensey JS, Schuler CR et al. The association between HLA-DPB1Glu69 and chronic beryllium disease and beryllium sensitization. *American Journal of Industrial Medicine.* 2004; **46**: 95-103.
43. Kim Y. Acute beryllium disease in metal workers. *European Respiratory Journal.* 2004; **24**: 149S.
44. Tepper LB, Hardy HL, Chamberlin RI. Toxicity of beryllium compounds. In: Browning E (ed.). *Elsevier Monographs on toxic agents.* Amsterdam: Elsevier Science, 1961: 1-190.
45. Hardy HL. Beryllium poisoning – lessons in control of man-made disease. *New England Journal of Medicine.* 1965; **273**: 1188-99.
46. Finkel AJ, Hamilton A, Hardy HL. *Hamilton and Hardy's industrial toxicology,* 4th edn. Boston: John Wright, 1983.
47. Mancuso TF, el-Attar AA. Epidemiological study of the beryllium industry. Cohort methodology and mortality studies. *Journal of Occupational Medicine.* 1969; **11**: 422-34.
48. Mancuso TF. Mortality study of beryllium industry workers' occupational lung cancer. *Environmental Research.* 1980; **21**: 48-55.
49. Mancuso TF. Occupational lung cancer among beryllium workers. In: Lemen R, Dement J (eds). *Dust and diseases.* Forest Park: Pathatox Publishers, 1979: 463-72.
50. Infante PF, Wagoner JK, Sprince NL. Mortality patterns from lung cancer and nonneoplastic respiratory disease among white males in the beryllium case registry. *Environmental Research.* 1980; **21**: 35-43.
51. Wagoner JK, Infante PF, Bayliss DL. Beryllium: An etiologic agent in the induction of lung cancer, nonneoplastic respiratory disease, and heart disease among industrially exposed workers. *Environmental Research.* 1980; **21**: 15-34.
52. Cancer IAfRo. *Monographs on the evaluation of the carcinogenic risk of chemicals to humans.* Lyon: IARC, 1980.
53. IARC. Meeting on the IARC Working Group on Beryllium, Cadmium, Mercury, and Exposures of the Glass Manufacturing Industry. *Scandinavian Journal of Work and Environmental Health.* 1993; **19**: 60-363.
54. Fireman E, Haimsky E, Noiderfer M et al. Misdiagnosis of sarcoidosis in patients with chronic beryllium disease. *Sarcoidosis, Vasculitis, and Diffuse Lung Diseases.* 2003; **20**: 144-8.
55. Rossman MD, Kreider ME. Is chronic beryllium disease sarcoidosis of known etiology? *Sarcoidosis, Vasculitis, and Diffuse Lung Diseases.* 2003; **20**: 104-9.
56. Andrews JL, Kazemi H, Hardy H. Patterns of lung dysfunction in chronic beryllium disease. *American Review of Respiratory Disease.* 1969; **100**: 791-800.
57. Pappas GP, Newman LS. Early pulmonary physiologic abnormalities in beryllium disease. *American Review of Respiratory Disease.* 1993; **148**: 661-6.
58. Naccache JM, Marchand-Adam S, Kambouchner M et al. Ground-glass computed tomography pattern in chronic beryllium disease: Pathologic substratum and evolution. *Journal of Computer Assisted Tomography.* 2003; **27**: 496-500.
59. Epstein PE, Dauber JH, Rossman MD, Daniele RP. Bronchoalveolar lavage in a patient with chronic berylliosis: Evidence for hypersensitivity pneumonitis. *Annals of Internal Medicine.* 1982; **97**: 213-16.
60. Rossman MD. Chronic beryllium disease. In: Daniele RP (ed.). *Immunology and immunologic diseases in the lung.* Boston: Blackwell Science, 1988: 351-9.
61. Newman LS, Kreiss K, King TE Jr et al. Pathologic and immunologic alterations in early stages of beryllium disease. Re-examination of disease definition and natural history. *American Review of Respiratory Disease.* 1989; **139**: 1479-86.
62. Newman LS, Bobka C, Schumacher B et al. Compartmentalized immune response reflects clinical severity of beryllium disease. *American Journal of Respiratory and Critical Care Medicine.* 1994; **150**: 135-42.
63. Freiman DG, Hardy HL. Beryllium disease: The relation of pulmonary pathology to clinical course and prognosis based on a study of 130 cases from the U.S. Beryllium Case Registry. *Human Pathology.* 1970; **1**: 25-44.
64. Dutra FR. The pneumonitis and granulomatosis peculiar to beryllium workers. *American Journal of Pathology.* 1948; **24**: 1137-65.
65. Bobka CA, Stewart LA, Engelken GJ et al. Comparison of *in vivo* and *in vitro* measures of beryllium sensitization. *Journal of Occupational and Environmental Medicine.* 1997; **39**: 540-7.

66. Kreiss K, Miller F, Newman LS et al. Chronic beryllium disease – from the workplace to cellular immunology, molecular immunogenetics, and back. *Clinical Immunology and Immunopathology.* 1994; **71**: 123–9.
67. Stoeckle JD, Hardy HL, Weber AL. Chronic beryllium disease: Long-term follow-up of sixty cases and selective review of the literature. *American Journal of Medicine.* 1969; **46**: 545–61.
68. Kennedy BJ, Pare JA, Pump KK, Stanford RL. The effect of adrenocorticotropic hormone on beryllium granulomatosis; a preliminary report. *Canadian Medical Association Journal.* 1950; **62**: 426–8.
69. Thorn GW, Forsham PH, Frawley TF et al. The clinical usefulness of ACTH and cortisone. *New England Journal of Medicine.* 1950; **242**: 865–72.
70. DeNardi JM. Chronic pulmonary interstitial granulomatosis: Preliminary report on two patients treated with ACTH. *Archives of Industrial Hygiene and Occupational Medicine.* 1951; **3**: 543–6.
71. Hardy HL. General discussion on the treatment of chronic beryllium poisoning with ACTH and cortisone. *Archives of Industrial Hygiene and Occupational Medicine.* 1951; **3**: 629–30.
72. Kennedy BJ, Pare JA, Pump KK et al. Effect of adrenocorticotropic hormone (ACTH) on beryllium granulomatosis and silicosis. *American Journal of Medicine.* 1951; **10**: 134–55.
73. Wright GW. Interpretation of results of ACTH and cortisone therapy in chronic beryllium poisoning; data obtained by pretherapy and post-therapy studies of pulmonary function. *Archives of Industrial Hygiene and Occupational Medicine.* 1951; **3**: 617–21.
74. Hardy HL. Epidemiology, clinical character, and treatment of beryllium poisoning; progress report. *Archives of Industrial Health.* 1955; **11**: 273–9.
75. Denardi JM. Long-term experience with beryllium disease. *Archives of Industrial Health.* 1959; **19**: 110–16.
76. Gaensler EA, Verstraeten JM, Weil WB et al. Respiratory pathophysiology in chronic beryllium disease; review of thirty cases with some observations after long-term steroid therapy. *Archives of Industrial Health.* 1959; **19**: 132–45.
77. Hall TC, Wood CH, Stoeckle JD, Tepper L. Case data from the beryllium registry. *Archives of Industrial Health.* 1959; **19**: 100–3.
78. Kline EM, Moir TW. Long-term experience with beryllium disease; a report of twenty patients. *Archives of Industrial Health.* 1959; **19**: 104–9.
79. Sood A, Beckett WS, Cullen MR. Variable response to long-term corticosteroid therapy in chronic beryllium disease. *Chest.* 2004; **126**: 2000–7.
80. Seeler AO. Treatment of chronic beryllium poisoning. *Archives of Industrial Health.* 1959; **19**: 164–8.
81. Dattoli JA, Lieben J, Bisbing J. Chronic beryllium disease. A follow-up study. *Journal of Occupational Medicine.* 1964; **6**: 189–94.
82. Izumi T, Kobara Y, Inui S et al. The first seven cases of chronic beryllium disease in ceramic factory workers in Japan. *Annals of the New York Academy of Sciences.* 1976; **278**: 636–53.
83. Shima S, Watanabe K, Tachikawa S. Experimental study on oral administration of beryllium compounds. *Rodo Kagaku.* 1983; **59**: 463–73.
84. Borak J. The beryllium occupational exposure limit: Historical origin and current inadequacy. *Journal of Occupational and Environmental Medicine.* 2006; **48**: 109–16.
85. Madl AK, Unice K, Brown JL et al. Exposure–response analysis for beryllium sensitization and chronic beryllium disease among workers in a beryllium metal machining plant. *Journal of Occupational and Environmental Hygiene.* 2007; **4**: 448–66.
86. Tinkle SS, Antonini JM, Rich BA et al. Skin as a route of exposure and sensitization in chronic beryllium disease. *Environmental Health Perspectives.* 2003; **111**: 1202–8.
87. Day GA, Stefaniak AB, Weston A, Tinkle SS. Beryllium exposure: Dermal and immunological considerations. *International Archives of Occupational and Environmental Health.* 2006; **79**: 161–4.
88. Maier LA, Kittle LA, Mroz MM, Newman LS. Beryllium-stimulated neopterin as a diagnostic adjunct in chronic beryllium disease. *American Journal of Industrial Medicine.* 2003; **43**: 592–601.
89. Pott GB, Palmer BE, Sullivan AK et al. Frequency of beryllium-specific, TH1-type cytokine-expressing CD4+ T cells in patients with beryllium-induced disease. *Journal of Allergy and Clinical Immunology.* 2005; **115**: 1036–42.
90. Farris GM, Newman LS, Frome EL et al. Detection of beryllium sensitivity using a flow cytometric lymphocyte proliferation test: The Immuno-Be-LPT. *Toxicology.* 2000; **143**: 125–40.
91. Milovanova TN, Popma SH, Cherian S et al. Flow cytometric test for beryllium sensitivity. *Cytometry. Part B, Clinical Cytometry.* 2004; **60**: 23–30.

PART EIGHT

OTHER EFFECTS OF WORKPLACE EXPOSURES

Section One: Occupational diseases of the skin	1059
Section Two: Occupational cancers	1079
Section Three: Other systemic effects	1123
Section Four: Shift work	1231

SECTION ONE

Occupational diseases of the skin

84 Occupational diseases of the skin 1061
John English and Jason Williams

84

Occupational diseases of the skin

JOHN ENGLISH AND JASON WILLIAMS

Introduction	1061		Contact urticaria	1069
Epidemiology	1061		Protein contact dermatitis	1069
Clinical range	1062		Oil folliculitis (oil acne)	1069
Contact dermatitis	1062		Chloracne	1069
Irritant contact dermatitis	1062		Leukoderma	1070
Allergic contact dermatitis	1063		Psoriasis	1070
Clinical diagnosis of occupational contact dermatitis	1064		Scleroderma-like diseases	1070
Patch testing	1065		Ulcerations	1071
Other investigations	1066		Skin carcinomas	1071
Treatment	1067		Cold urticaria	1071
Prevention	1067		Pseudo-epidemics	1071
Prognosis	1068		Major occupations causing dermatoses	1071
Non-eczematous occupational dermatoses	1069		References	1074

INTRODUCTION

The history of modern occupational dermatology begins in 1915 with the first edition of Prosser White's classic text,[1] followed in 1939 with publications by Poul Bonnevie[2] and Schwartz, Tulipan and Peck (and later Birmingham).[3] Since the Second World War, the major impetus came first from Europe[4] (and, in particular, from Sigfrid Fregert,[5] Foussereau[6] and Zschunke[7]). Adams[8] in the United States and Kanerva et al.[9] have since produced further major texts.

There is no universally accepted definition of an occupational skin disease (or dermatosis). A broad definition is a dermatosis due wholly or partially to the patient's occupation. Occupation must be a major factor in stricter definitions,[10] and essential to causation in still stricter definitions.[11]

EPIDEMIOLOGY

Dermatoses are perceived as following musculoskeletal and psychiatric conditions in the ranking of their frequency among occupational disorders.[12] A 1995 self-reported survey in the United Kingdom led to an estimate of over 50 000 work-related conditions involving the skin.[13] Reports to EPIDERM and OPRA (Occupational Physicians Reporting Activity) surveillance schemes in the UK between 1996 and 2001, suggested an annual rate of 720 new cases of occupational dermatoses per million at risk, according to reports to the scheme by dermatologists and occupational physicians.[14] Reports between 2002 and 2005 suggest overall rates of 406 per million workers.[12] These rates probably represent only the tip of the iceberg, with most cases going unreported. Data on the economic impact of occupational skin disease are limited, but the annual costs of occupational dermatoses in the United States have been estimated at up to 1000 million dollars.[15] A study of occupational dermatitis claims in Oregon has shown an average claim cost of $3552.[16] Financial costs will vary greatly from country to country depending on the social security systems in place, and also how the figures are estimated. The cost to the working community is a human as well as a financial one, with the disablement from an occupational dermatosis sometimes approaching that from loss of a limb.[17] Many high-risk occupations have been identified in which the prevalence of occupational dermatoses rises as high as 15 per cent.[18]

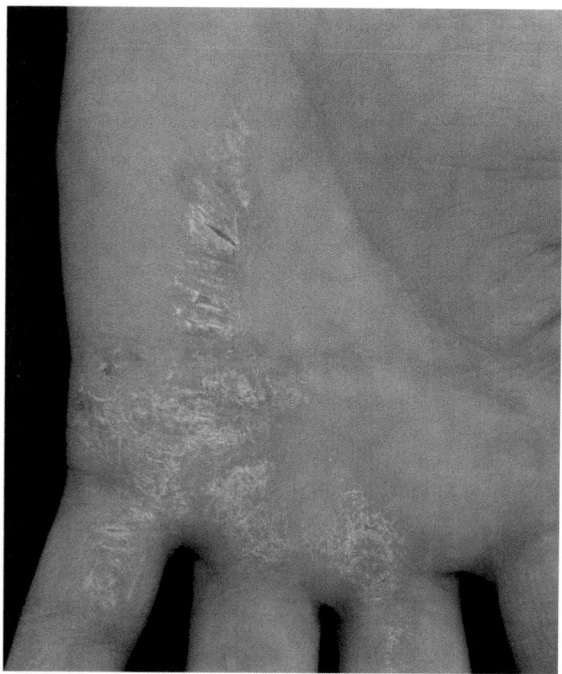

Figure 84.1 Frictional psoriasis from repetitive use of a spanner (for colour image, see www.hodderplus.com/hunters).

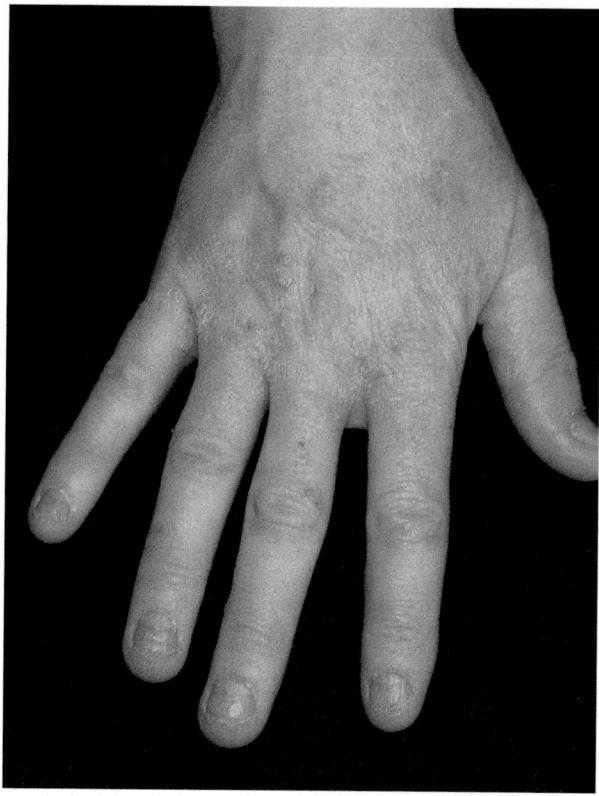

Figure 84.2 Scabies mimicking contact eczema (for colour image, see www.hodderplus.com/hunters).

CLINICAL RANGE

While 90–95 per cent[12] of occupational dermatoses are contact dermatitis, their clinical spectrum also includes contact urticaria, oil folliculitis, chloracne, leukoderma, scleroderma, ulcerations and neoplasia. Many substances that cause occupational dermatoses are also capable of causing respiratory and other disorders, for example rosin (colophony), chromium, formaldehyde, (meth)acrylates and isocyanates.[18] Psoriasis may be aggravated, or even initiated for the first time on the hands, by physical or chemical occupational irritants (Figure 84.1) and contact dermatitis may koebnerize into psoriasis. Scabies, though rarely occupational, may mimic contact dermatitis (Figure 84.2).

CONTACT DERMATITIS

Contact dermatitis is dermatitis caused by skin contact with external substances (Figure 84.3). It is distinguished from endogenous (constitutional) dermatitis not by morphology or histopathology, but only by aetiology. The term 'dermatitis', as used above, is synonymous with the term 'eczema', although the latter term might best be reserved for endogenous or constitutional dermatitis. Not only must dermatitis be divided into endogenous or contact (that is, exogenous), or a mixture of the two, but it must carefully be distinguished from clinically similar dermatoses, such as psoriasis and tinea. Practical experience is essential, but can usefully be supplemented by reference to well-illustrated textbooks[19] and other helpful publications.[20]

To cause contact dermatitis a substance must first be capable of penetrating the superficial layers of the epidermis, known as the barrier layer. This is the most superficial layer of the skin and is a paper-thin lipoprotein membrane, remarkably resistant to penetration, although vulnerable to substances of molecular weight below 1000. If a substance does penetrate to the living tissues beneath, it may then cause contact dermatitis by one of two mechanisms, contact irritation and contact sensitization (or contact allergy), which may go on to provoke irritant contact dermatitis and allergic contact dermatitis, respectively. Both forms of contact dermatitis may be morphologically indistinguishable from each other, as well as from endogenous dermatitis. Because of their predominance as the site of occupational contact, the hands are involved in as many as 90 per cent of cases of occupational contact dermatitis.[21]

IRRITANT CONTACT DERMATITIS

A contact irritant is a chemical (or physical) agent capable of causing cell damage (cytotoxicity) if applied to the skin for sufficient time and in sufficient concentration. The precise mechanisms of cytotoxicity are still not yet well

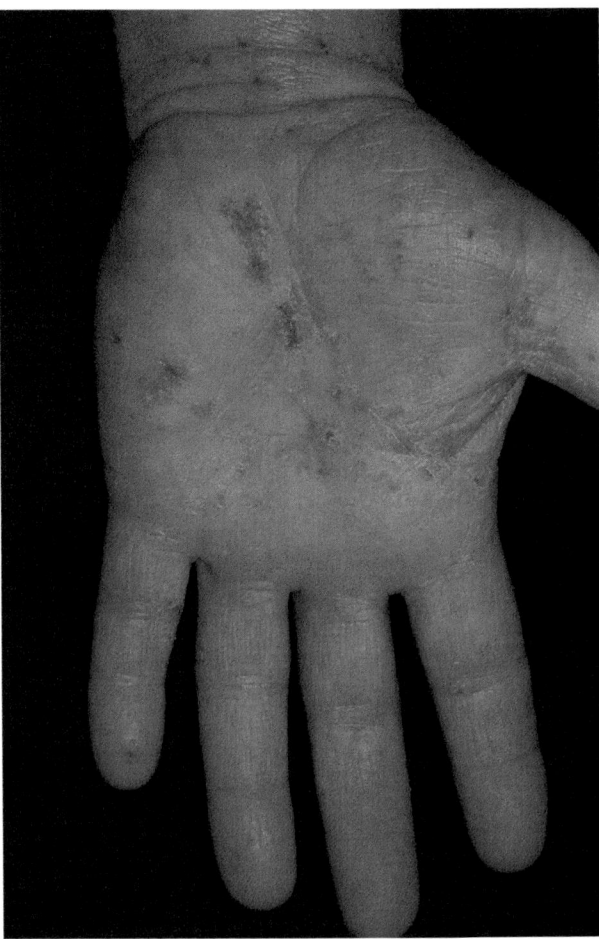

Figure 84.3 Allergic contact dermatitis from MCI/MI in cutting fluids in a machinist (for colour image, see www.hodderplus.com/hunters).

defined, although they are already known to differ from one irritant to another.[22]

Due to the increasing use of protective gloves, acute (or strong) irritants are becoming a less common cause of irritant contact dermatitis and chemical burns.[24] Occupational irritant contact dermatitis is caused most frequently by chronic (weak, mild or marginal) irritants, the damage from which is insidious and insensible, but cumulative with time.[23] Chronic irritant contact dermatitis is often the result of more than one occupational irritant (multifactorial), with common factors being wet work and the use of soaps and cleansers.[14]

Individual susceptibility to chronic irritant contact dermatitis varies very widely, though still largely unpredictably.[23] One high-risk group that has been identified are subjects with a previous history of severe childhood eczema, particularly if this involved the hands.[24,25] Susceptibility to one irritant, however, does not necessarily imply susceptibility to another.[23] Variation in susceptibility to weak irritants results in chronic irritant contact dermatitis involving only a certain proportion of an exposed workforce, which rarely rises in practice above a third.[18]

Age of onset varies from one occupation to another, sometimes showing a bimodal curve, with those at both ends of working life seeming to be at higher risk than those in mid-career,[20] and other times increasing with age (or sometimes even apparently decreasing). One example of this is the apprentice hairdresser or the student nurse who presents with occupational irritant contact dermatitis (ICD) of the hands due to more frequent wet work (washing hair, cleaning, etc.) involved in the personal care of patients. Individuals susceptible to ICD may often present early under these circumstances. Conversely, motor mechanics often present later in their occupational life, when 20–30 years of exposure to irritants (solvents and friction, etc.) lead to chronic hand eczema. Similarly, length of exposure prior to onset varies widely, depending both on the irritant and the degree of contact with it, but sometimes being years rather than, more commonly, months. Any apparent difference in susceptibility between the sexes arises from the different type of work that they do, rather than from any inherently increased susceptibility in either sex.[23]

The principal occupational irritants[18,23,26] may be grouped broadly into soaps and detergents, alkalis and acids, metalworking fluids (cutting oils), organic solvents, other petroleum products, oxidizing agents, reducing agents, animal and plant products, and physical factors, such as friction and low relative humidity, as well as desiccant powders. The more frequent wearing of occlusive gloves results in increased sweating of the hands, in itself a cause of irritation. German wet work regulations now legislate for those at increased risk of occupationl dermatitis due to wet work (described as over two hours' exposure of the hands to water, wearing of occlusive gloves for over two hours/day or frequent hand washing). Individuals at risk need to undergo annual surveillance for occupational dermatitis.[27] Common high-risk occupations for chronic irritant contact dermatitis[18,23,26] are catering, cleaning, construction, hairdressing, horticulture and floristry, metalworking, nursing, painting, printing, and vehicle maintenance and repair.

ALLERGIC CONTACT DERMATITIS

Although probably not as common as occupational irritant contact dermatitis, occupational allergic contact dermatitis is often less amenable to subsequent prevention, because of the much smaller quantities of allergen that may sustain a contact dermatitis in a sensitized individual, compared with the quantities required of irritants. It may therefore become much more difficult to manage than irritant contact dermatitis. Conversely, if the allergen can be identified and removed from the workplace, then prognosis may be excellent.

A contact allergen (or contact sensitizer), after penetrating the barrier layer of the skin, is chemically reactive enough to provoke delayed, cell-mediated or type IV allergy.[28,29] The first stage of this process is termed 'induction' and, once initiated, takes around seven days to be completed. After such time, further skin contact with that particular allergen results in the second stage of the process, called 'elicitation', that results in allergic contact dermatitis within a few hours to a day or two of the subsequent exposure, depending on both degree of contact and degree of sensitivity. Allergic contact dermatitis is usually morphologically indistinguishable from irritant contact dermatitis.

Sensitization may be induced after only one contact,[30] or after many contacts over a prolonged period. Occupationally, it is often induced after a few months of repeated contact, although sometimes it can occur after many years of well-tolerated contact, as with chromate sensitization in bricklayers.[18] There is a very wide individual variation in susceptibility to contact sensitization, and susceptibility to one allergen does not necessarily imply any general susceptibility to contact sensitization. Age and sex are not significant influences.

Knowledge of the mechanism of type IV hypersensitivity has accumulated in the last three decades to a fascinating degree.[28,29] Allergic contact dermatitis depends primarily on the activation of specifically sensitized T cells, an untoward side effect of a well-functioning immune system.

Induction of contact sensitization begins with the binding of allergen to major histocompatibility complex (MHC) class II molecules on the surface of allergen-presenting cells. These MHC class II molecules are present on Langerhans' cells within the epidermis, which migrate via the lymphatics to the paracortical areas of the regional lymph nodes. Here, T cells specifically recognize the allergen-class II molecule complexes and are activated to proliferate within the node, subsequently to be released into the circulation and enter the skin. The process of induction is then complete, having taken around seven days.

Elicitation of allergic contact dermatitis then depends on allergen-presenting cells and specific T cells subsequently meeting in the skin and leading there to cytokine production. Release of such mediators results in the arrival of more T cells, thus further amplifying local mediator release. This leads to a dermatitic reaction, peaking after one to two days.

Several thousand contact allergens are now recognized.[31] Rubber accelerators, epoxy resins and hardeners, (meth)acrylates, formaldehyde and formaldehyde-releasers, other biocides (preservatives), and plants and woods are common occupational examples.[18,29] High-risk occupations include chemical and pharmaceutical manufacture (Figure 84.4), construction, dyeing, electronics, hairdressing and tanning.[18] Chromium (in cement) used to be a common cause of occupational allergic contact dermatitis (ACD) in construction workers, but rates are now falling, as legislation in Europe and elsewhere has led to the addition of ferrous sulphate to cement powder to reduce the amount of free hexavalent chromate present.[32]

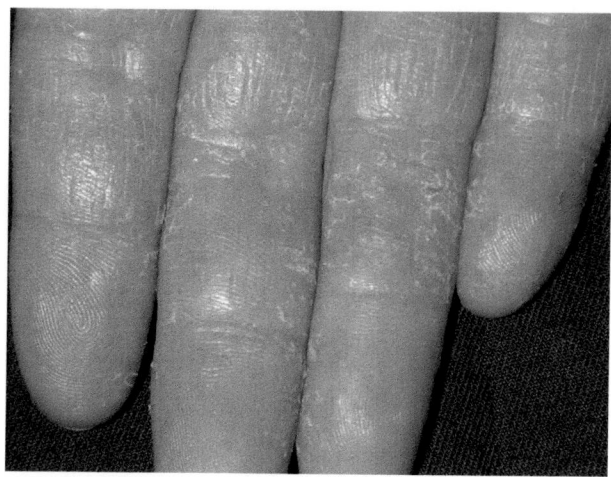

Figure 84.4 Allergic contact dermatitis from oxycodone in a pharmaceutical worker (for colour image, see www.hodderplus.com/hunters).

CLINICAL DIAGNOSIS OF OCCUPATIONAL CONTACT DERMATITIS

Establishing the occupational causation of contact dermatitis can be far from straightforward.[33–35] The foundation remains a thorough dermatological and occupational history, coupled with a close examination of the whole skin. There are certain essential facts that form the basis of every such history.

The time of onset of the earliest signs

The shorter the history, the more likely is the diagnosis of contact dermatitis. However, there is an important proviso to this general statement. Patients initially tend to underestimate the length of history, remembering the exacerbation that finally led them to seek medical advice rather than the original onset of the earliest signs. Many patients do not seek medical advice until they have had milder degrees of contact dermatitis for considerable periods (Figure 84.5). In Fregert's study,[5] 22 per cent of cases of occupational contact dermatitis had a history of less than one month, yet 29 per cent had a history of more than one year.

The primary site of onset

In occupational cases, this is usually the hands.[21] In a few cases, the wrists, forearms, lower legs or face are the primary site. The covered areas of the trunk or feet are rare primary sites.[21]

The route and timing of any secondary spread

Spread from one hand to the other and from the hands to the forearms is common, even in the absence of contact

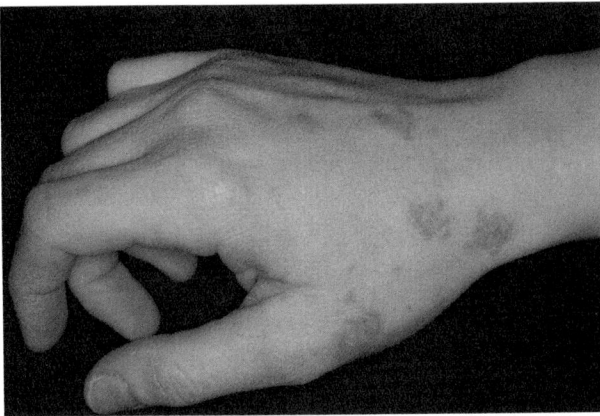

Figure 84.5 Irritant contact dermatitis in a healthcare worker (for colour image, see www.hodderplus.com/hunters).

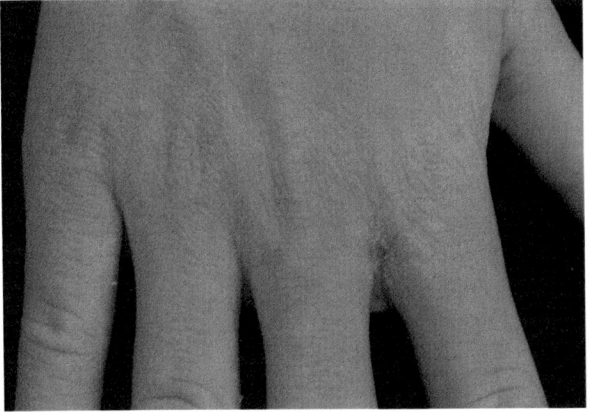

Figure 84.6 Irritant contact dermatitis in an atopic chef (for colour image, see www.hodderplus.com/hunters).

with the causal agent at such secondary sites.[36] Distant spread from the hands to the feet or to the face is more common in allergic contact dermatitis rather than irritant.[37] Photocontact dermatitis is rarely occupational, but primarily involves the face and backs of the hands.[38]

Atopy

Those with a history of severe childhood eczema, particularly if this involved the hands, are at higher risk as a group, of developing occupational irritant, though not allergic, contact dermatitis (Figure 84.6).[24,25]

Occupation

The essential questions that need to be asked of the patient are their occupational title, length of time in this job and precisely what work tasks are involved. As exact a picture as possible must be acquired of the degree of skin contact, as well as simply the substances involved. Personally visiting the workplace and actually looking at the work being done can increase the understanding of a dermatitis problem.[18,33]

Work-relatedness

The question as to whether the dermatitis improves away from work and worsens on return to work is clearly fundamental, but can usefully be refined a little further. Primarily endogenous eczema may also show such a pattern, but occupational contact dermatitis usually shows greater and more consistent work-relatedness. Occupational allergic contact dermatitis tends to relapse more rapidly on return to work than does irritant contact dermatitis, and allergic may sometimes be slower than irritant to improve away from work. As occupational contact dermatitis of either type becomes chronic, its initial work-relatedness tends to become increasingly less clear-cut.[39]

Preventive measures

Attempts to prevent or remove skin contamination and the use of personal protective equipment should be enquired about, as well as the amount of success achieved by such methods. Occupational contact dermatitis may sometimes be aggravated further by the irritancy of skin cleansers or allergy to protective gloves.[12]

Fellow workers

The involvement of a substantial proportion of working colleagues is more suggestive of irritant than allergic contact dermatitis. Patients' own assessments of the similarity of their workmates' dermatoses are, understandably, often unreliable, and a personal examination of any such additional cases is always to be recommended.[40]

Diagnosis

Mathias has previously described criteria for diagnosing occupational contact dermatitis (Box 84.1).[41]

PATCH TESTING

While there is no routine skin test to confirm the diagnosis of irritant contact dermatitis, patch testing is the only way of confirming the diagnosis of allergic contact dermatitis. The principle of patch testing is relatively straightforward, yet its reliability is highly dependent on the abilities of the person(s) carrying it out.

Patch testing is based on the dilution of potential contact allergens to below their threshold for either induction

> **Box 84.1 Diagnostic criteria for occupational contact dermatitis**[16]
>
> 1. Is the clinical appearance consistent with contact dermatitis?
> 2. Are there workplace exposures to potential cutaneous irritants or allergens?
> 3. Is the anatomical distribution consistent with cutaneous exposure in relation to the job task?
> 4. Is the temporal relationship between exposure and onset consistent with contact dermatitis?
> 5. Are non-occupational exposures excluded as probable causes?
> 6. Does dermatitis improve away from work exposure to the suspected irritant or allergen?
> 7. Do patch or provocation tests identify a probable causal agent?

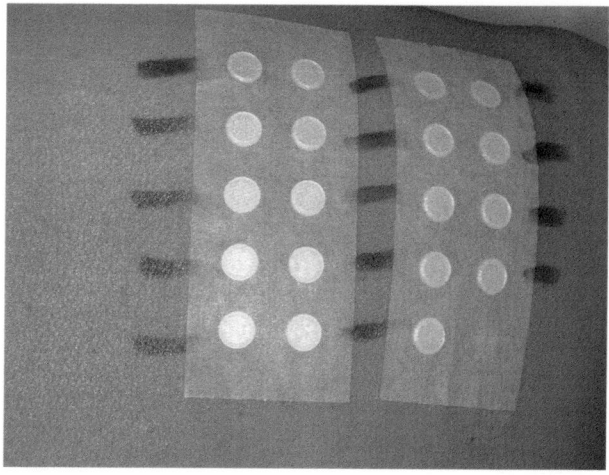

Figure 84.7 Patch tests are applied to the upper back (for colour image, see www.hodderplus.com/hunters).

of contact sensitivity or for contact irritancy under the conditions of the test, down to a level at which they nevertheless remain capable of an elicitation reaction in an already sensitized patient.[29]

The appropriate dilution for patch testing varies widely from substance to substance. Its selection is crucial to the reliability of the test. Underdilution may result in a positive reaction in the absence of contact allergy (false-positive reaction), whereas overdilution may result in a negative reaction in the presence of contact allergy (false-negative reaction).

A set of between 30 and 45 common allergens (standard series) and some additional series directed towards specific occupations are available commercially, but in occupational cases these will frequently need to be supplemented by patch tests to a patient's own contactants.[42] It is here that dilutional errors are easily made. Reference sources are a guide to correct patch test dilution,[31] but there is no substitute for training and experience; even commercial patch test preparations may occasionally give false-positive or false-negative reactions. The value of testing to patients' own samples has recently been shown.[43] It is essential, when taking the history, to identify as many of the chemicals as possible to which a worker is exposed. Ideally, small quantities of each substance are obtained, with the relevant material safety data sheeet, and these are used to decide how to dilute and test to the substance. Some substances are not tested because of their known irritancy.

Appropriate dilutions are occluded against the skin (Figure 84.7), usually in shallow aluminium chambers and usually on the back, for either one or (more usually) two days. Readings are made of any reactions that are present after removal of the tests and, preferably, again at between three and seven days after application. The interpretation of such reactions requires trained skills.[18,42] Positive reactions also require further informed assessment of their

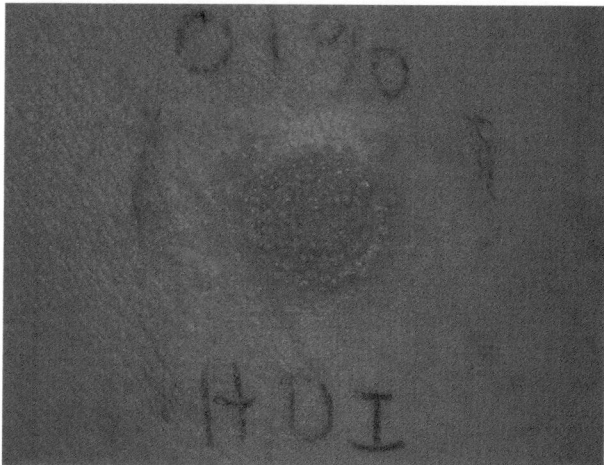

Figure 84.8 A positive patch test to HDI (for colour image, see www.hodderplus.com/hunters).

relevance to the current dermatitis, which may involve substantial investigation of potential occupational sources (Figure 84.8). A positive patch test only indicates allergy to the substance. It is then necessary to show its relevance to the workplace and the worker's contact dermatitis.

OTHER INVESTIGATIONS

As well as patch testing, other special investigations may be required in order to make an accurate diagnosis. Radioallergosorbent testing (RAST) or prick testing (Figure 84.9) may be indicated in contact urticaria and protein contact dermatitis (see under Contact urticaria, p. 1069 and Protein contact dermatitis, p. 1069). Skin biopsy may be needed in certain other non-eczematous dermatoses. Skin scrapes may be used to exclude tinea infection (fungal infection).

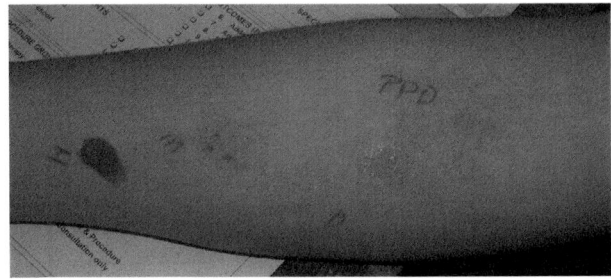

Figure 84.9 A positive prick test to PPD (for colour image, see www.hodderplus.com/hunters).

Simple chemical tests for the identification of specific allergens, more advanced chemical analytical techniques and methods for measuring the degree of skin contamination are reviewed.[18,33] Such chemical elucidation has considerably advanced our understanding of contact sensitization by such occupational allergens as chromate, epoxy resin, phenol-formaldehyde resin and colophony.

In recent years, non-invasive measurement techniques have come to play an increasing role in contact dermatitis research,[29] including transepidermal water loss, skin reflectance and conductance, and laser Doppler flowmetry. As yet, these have no routine applications in clinical dermatology.

In vitro tests for sensitization, such as the migration inhibition and lymphocyte transformation tests, are described,[29] but have not yet reached the level of reliability required to replace patch testing.

TREATMENT

The treatment of occupational contact dermatitis rests on the foundation of accurate diagnosis combined with partial or complete separation of the patient from the cause.

Acute contact dermatitis may sometimes require a period away from work, everything possible being done to minimize the length of any such period. Dermatological treatment is essentially the same as for any other acute eczema.[42,44] Hospital clinicians and general practitioners should be aware of the demoralization that can be produced by periods off work – even if only for a few weeks.

Chronic contact dermatitis, with certain exceptions indicated below, can usually be treated while the patient continues to work, even if this is in a temporary alternative location. Again, dermatological therapy is as for other chronic eczemas.[42,44]

Isolated uncomplicated allergic contact dermatitis may, however, respond so well to a permanent change of occupation that, if substitution of an allergen cannot be achieved,[45] this may become the best advice. Also, atopic individuals who find themselves with dermatitis from unavoidable irritants, such as in metalworking, hairdressing, catering and healthcare work may be best advised to look for a permanent alternative.

Irritant contact dermatitis may often respond better to the regular use of emollients (moisturizers) than to potent topical corticosteroids, the latter being more likely to be needed in **allergic contact dermatitis**. In either type of contact dermatitis, secondary bacterial infection may require additional treatment with topical or systemic antibiotics.

PREVENTION

The prevention of occupational contact dermatitis[18] is based on the same hierarchy of measures as for other occupational diseases, usefully considered under the headings of reduction of exposure, reduction of the effects of exposure and reduction of the effects of disease.

While substitution will always remain the ideal exposure control,[45] clinicians will more often find themselves involved in advising on personal protective equipment, and this largely in the form of gloves. Awareness is required here, both because in some jobs gloves are either unsafe or impracticable, as well as the fact that the choice of glove material can be crucial for certain substances.[18]

The effectiveness of 'barrier' creams remains controversial, but data are beginning to accumulate on their role in preventing at least some of the effects of skin contact, particularly from irritants.[46] The benefit of emollient (moisturizer) application following skin cleansing is also beginning to receive some experimental support, again particularly with respect to irritants.[47]

The preventive role of pre-employment assessment[24] remains limited by our lack of reliable indicators of susceptibility, although a partial exception to this is that subjects with a history of severe childhood eczema are, as a group, more susceptible to skin irritation.[24,25] Such susceptibility does not appear to extend, however, to those with a history of only mucosal atopy (hay fever and asthma).

The primary objective in reducing the long-term effects of occupational contact dermatitis is to enable the patient to remain at work.[11] Clinicians should therefore strive to reduce periods of work absence to a minimum, with any unavoidable breaks in work being regularly monitored. Delay in diagnosis is a prime contributor to dermatological disability.[48] One exception to this is when a period off work (taken as sick leave or annual leave) can be used to assess the work-relatedness of a skin condition. Occupational contact dermatitis would be expected to improve with a period of time away from work, at least in its early stages. Evidence-based skin care recommendations have been published (summarized in Box 84.2).[49] If improvements are made to the working conditions by intensified preventative measures, then this is likely to lead to a reduction in cases of occupational contact dermatitis.[50,51] It is also important to assess and give relevant advice on factors in the home, where there may be additional sources of ICD or exposure to relevant allergens.

> **Box 84.2 Basic workplace skin care principles**
>
> - Luke-warm water for washing
> - Use correct gloves before exposure for the shortest time
> - Remove rings
> - Cotton liners underneath protective gloves
> - Avoid disinfectant hand cleansers
> - Apply emollient hand creams
> - Protect hands at home
> - Workforce education

PROGNOSIS

In his pioneering questionnaire study, Fregert[5] found that only 25 per cent of his patients diagnosed as having occupational contact dermatitis had completely healed two to three years later: 50 per cent still had intermittent symptoms, while as many as 25 per cent still had continuous symptoms. Although 40 per cent had changed their occupation, the change had not improved their prognosis. These considerations applied to irritant as much as to allergic contact dermatitis.

Wall and Gebauer[52] refined this study by increasing the number of patients followed up, examining the majority of these, and establishing more precisely what their change of job had entailed. More than half their patients still had their dermatitis to some degree. Again, around 40 per cent had changed their jobs, but of these more than 25 per cent had chosen new jobs in which the work environment further aggravated their skin. Of the 57 per cent who were either in the same job or deemed to be still in the same type of occupation, as many as 68 per cent were still symptomatic, whereas of the 43 per cent who had changed to an entirely different work environment, from the dermatological point of view, only 37 per cent were still symptomatic. Overall, 11.5 per cent of the patients had an ongoing skin disease for which there was no identifiable present cause: this the authors termed 'persistent post-occupational dermatitis'.

Rosen and Freeman[53] took such studies still further by documenting improvement as well as complete healing, establishing improvement in 82 per cent of those who changed duties within the same industry, 76 per cent of those who changed industry altogether, and 61 per cent of those who remained with the same duties in the same industry.

The main findings of all three of these major studies can be summarized as follows. The prognosis of occupational contact dermatitis severe enough to be referred to a dermatologist (known to have a special interest in occupational dermatoses) is one of persistence in more than half, although with improvement in around half of these. This applies to irritant as much as to allergic contact dermatitis. Appropriate occupational changes improve the prognosis for most, but around 10 per cent of patients overall develop persistent

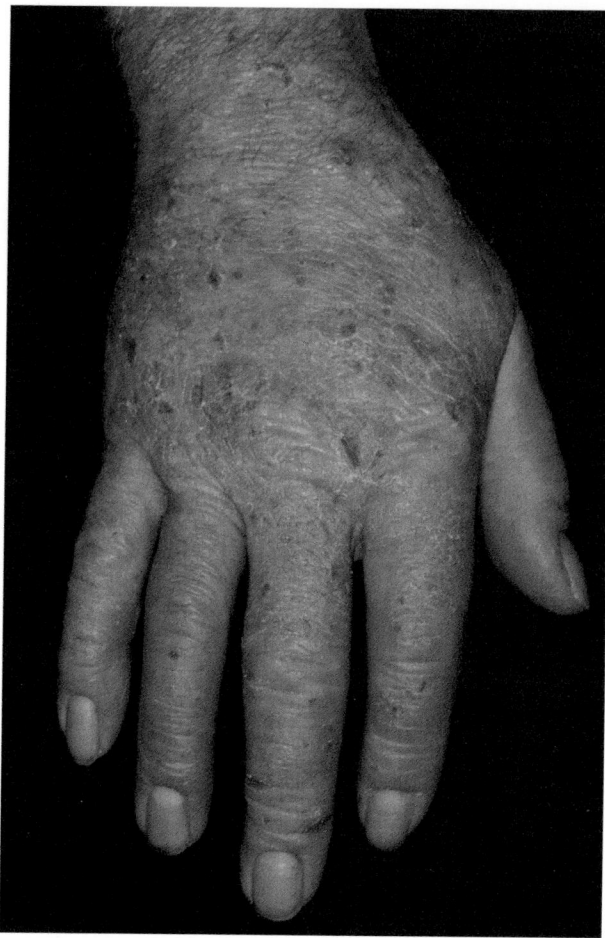

Figure 84.10 Persistent (allergic) contact dermatitis from chromium in cement (for colour image, see www.hodderplus.com/hunters).

post-occupational dermatitis. Chromate was the major allergen in all studies causing persistent post-occupational dermatitis (Figure 84.10), allergic contact dermatitis from plastics and resins having the best prognosis.[5]

Questionnaire studies of cutting fluid dermatitis (mainly irritant) have shown varying results. In a small study in Birmingham, UK, clearance was found in 45 per cent of patients followed for up to 2.5 years after diagnosis: only one of 40 patients had been obliged to change their job.[54] In a similar larger study in London, of those who continued to work with water-based metalworking fluids, 78 per cent had not healed after two years, and of those who had stopped working with soluble oils, 70 per cent had still not healed two years after discontinuing contact; a generally poor prognosis was found whether or not such patients continued in their work.[55]

The prognosis for catering workers studied by Cronin[56] was also poor. Of 32 such patients followed up for around two years, 12 had been obliged to give up their work because of their contact dermatitis. Of the 19 who remained in catering, only four healed completely; of the 13 who left, only four healed.

The reasons for this generally poor prognosis, which applies to irritant as much as to allergic contact dermatitis, remained debatable.[57] However, many less severe cases than those having to be referred to specialist dermatologists have a much better prognosis,[58] as occupational physicians will be well aware. Also, even in such severe cases, dermatitis may become significantly more manageable after adequate investigation and treatment.

NON-ECZEMATOUS OCCUPATIONAL DERMATOSES

There are a number of non-eczematous skin disorders that, even together, constitute only a minority of occupational dermatoses.[12] Nevertheless, some have serious implications that demand their accurate diagnosis.

CONTACT URTICARIA

This is a wheal-and-flare reaction usually within 20–30 minutes of contact between certain substances and the skin surface (Figure 84.9). It may be of immunological (allergic), non-immunological (irritant), or uncertain aetiology. The most frequent occupational cause currently is immunological (type I) contact urticaria from natural rubber latex, the main at-risk group being healthcare professionals who wear rubber gloves.[29,59] Clinical symptoms of type I allergy to natural rubber latex may extend from contact urticaria, conjunctivitis and rhinitis, to asthma and anaphylaxis. Two major latex allergens have been identified, the important one for healthcare professionals being a soluble protein, hevein.[60] Cross-reacting proteins are present in many fruits and vegetables, including avocado, banana, sweet pepper, potato, kiwi fruit and tomato. Atopics are at greater risk. Latex allergens are adsorbed on to cornstarch glove powder, thus increasing airborne exposure: powdered natural rubber latex gloves should therefore no longer be used. Guidance is increasingly available as to how to control this problem, particularly in the healthcare setting.[61] This has led to a tailing off of the latex allergy epidemic seen in the 1990s.[62,63]

The most common other causes of occupational contact urticaria are cow dander[64] and foodstuffs,[26] which are considered below under Protein contact dermatitis.

Confirmation of the diagnosis of immunological contact urticaria may be obtained by use tests, prick tests or RASTs, guided by clinical assessment of the extent and severity of symptoms.[26] Prick testing should never be conducted without appropriate resuscitation equipment to hand.

PROTEIN CONTACT DERMATITIS

Food handlers[29,64,65] and those working closely with animals may have hand dermatitis, either as well as or rather

Figure 84.11 Oil folliculitis on the thigh (for colour image, see www.hodderplus.com/hunters).

than contact urticaria, yet show positive prick tests or RASTs, rather than positive patch tests, to foodstuffs or animal products, a phenomenon first termed 'protein contact dermatitis' in 1976, where it was described in a cohort of sandwich makers.[66] The underlying allergic mechanism may depend on specific immunoglobulin-E being bound on the surface of epidermal Langerhans' cells.[67] Testing for type I as well as type IV allergy may therefore be required in chefs, animal laboratory technicians, farmers and veterinarians with hand dermatitis, as well as in the natural rubber latex glove wearers.

OIL FOLLICULITIS (OIL ACNE)

Petroleum oils exert a localized irritant effect on hair follicles, which causes a folliculitis of the hair-bearing skin of the backs of the hands, arms, thighs (Figure 84.11), abdomen, face and neck.[68] The primary lesions are open comedones ('blackheads'), causing mechanical blockage of the follicular openings. Second, inflammatory papules and pustules may develop. Metalworking machine operatives are the prime at-risk group, although adequate industrial and personal hygiene should nowadays make it rare. Those with previous cystic acne are more susceptible.

CHLORACNE

This is both clinically and aetiologically distinct from oil acne. It might better be termed 'halogenacne', in that, as well as polychlorinated aromatic hydrocarbons of a highly specific molecular structure, brominated, iodinated and fluorinated homologues are also causal.[69] These uncommon chemicals, of which the dibenzodioxins are an example (see Chapter 43, Pesticides and other agrochemicals), may be encountered in pesticide manufacture, chemical disposal plants and, sporadically, in other chemical and pharmaceutical work.[70,71] Chloracne may be differentiated

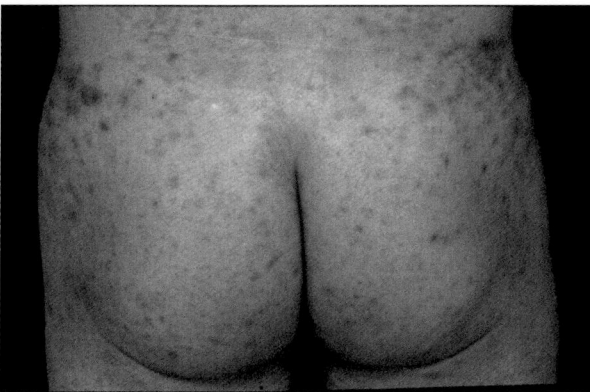

Figure 84.12 Extensive chloracne on the buttocks (for colour image, see www.hodderplus.com/hunters).

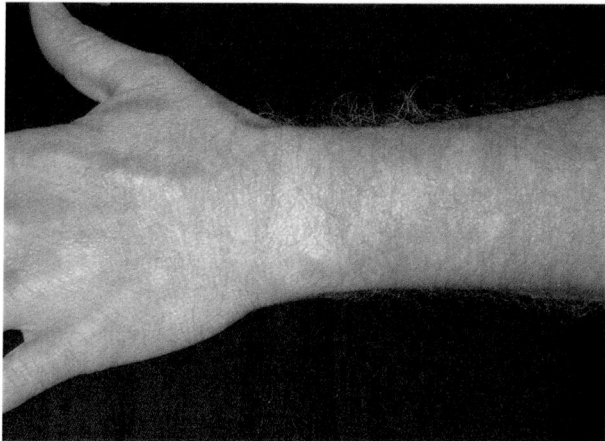

Figure 84.14 Chemical depigmentation from a phenol formaldehyde resin adhesive (for colour image, see www.hodderplus.com/hunters).

LEUKODERMA

Chemical depigmentation of the skin can arise occupationally from exposure either to various chemicals themselves or to their residues in products, such as adhesives (Figure 84.14).[74] The chemicals responsible include phenols, catechols and hydroquinones.[75,76] Because of systemic absorption, white patches may appear well beyond sites of direct skin contact, thus closely mimicking idiopathic vitiligo. There are several possible explanations for the effects of such chemicals on the pigmentary system, their structures being very similar to melanin precursors.[75] Death of melanocytes results in depigmentation usually being permanent. Associated changes in liver function tests of uncertain significance have been reported.[77] Occupational leukoderma is a prescribed disease in its own right (see Chapter 8, Compensation schemes).

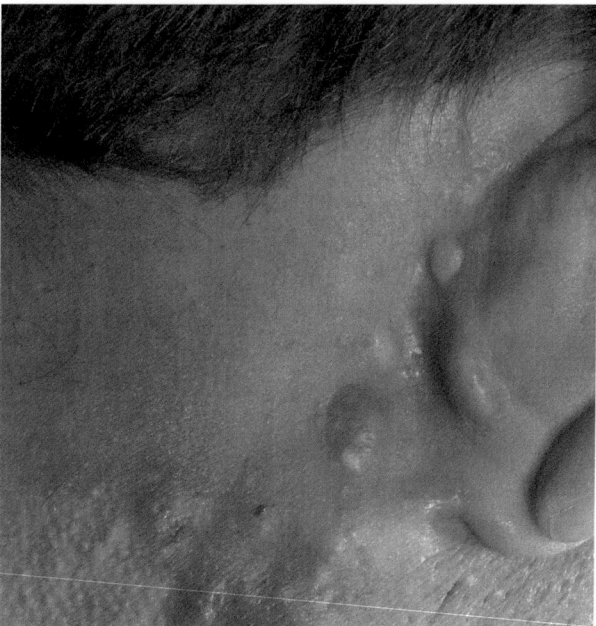

Figure 84.13 Comedones and pale yellow cysts are typical features of halogen acne (for colour image, see www.hodderplus.com/hunters).

PSORIASIS

Psoriasis can koebnerize in areas of skin inflammation – that is to say that any inflamed skin can develop into psoriasis in a predisposed individual. In patients with, for example, hand or fingertip psoriasis, it may be prudent to patch test to potential allergens in the workplace and home to exclude an ACD koebnerizing into psoriasis. In the same way, an ICD of the hands, including one with frictional features, could also koebnerize into psoriasis.

SCLERODERMA-LIKE DISEASES

Vinyl chloride monomer, silica dust, organic solvents and epoxy resins have all been reported as associated with scleroderma-like conditions.[78] Exposure to vinyl chloride monomer has also caused acro-osteolysis and angiosarcoma of the liver in polymerization vessel cleaners,[79] and

from other causes of chemical acne. Lesions are distributed typically over the temples, behind the ears and on the male genitals, and may spread to the trunk and limbs (Figure 84.12). The primary lesions are open comedones and pale-yellow cysts (Figure 84.13). In more severe cases, inflammatory lesions are also seen. The condition is notoriously chronic, even after complete removal of the cause, and may be extremely resistant to treatment.[71] Chloracne is always a symptom of systemic absorption[69] and may be associated with systemic morbidity.[72] Many substances causing chloracne may also cause hepatotoxicity. The most potent chloracnegenic agent known is 2,3,7,8-tetrachlorodibenzo-p-dioxin.[73] Exposure to relevant chemicals and the pattern of comedogenic acne is important in making the diagnosis.

miners exposed to silica dust may have associated silicosis.[80] A patient was reported with a sclerodermatous syndrome following occupational exposure to herbicides.[81] The mechanism remains obscure. In a recent study of 82 cases of scleroderma in France, up to 10 per cent were found to be potentially work related, with relevant occupational exposures present.[82] No clear diagnostic criteria were given.

ULCERATIONS

There are two main occupational causes of ulcerations, hexavalent chromium compounds and wet cement, in both cases the cause being toxic (irritant) rather than allergic. Chrome ulcers are mainly seen on the hands in those exposed to chromic acid in electroplating,[83] although regulation has generally made them rarer, and may occur from other sources, such as porcelain enamel paints.[84] Nasal septal ulceration, proceeding to perforation, may be associated.

Cement ulcers (or cement burns) are a rapid effect of wet cement trapped against the skin, for example by kneeling in it or by it entering footwear.[85] Symptoms may appear within an hour or two, the resulting ulceration then inexorably progressing and often requiring skin grafting. Precautions to avoid the occlusion of wet cement against the skin should be preventive, but inexperienced, amateur or heavily exposed professional cement users[86] may still be affected.

SKIN CARCINOMAS

Although now largely of historical interest,[87] except in outdoor workers from sun exposure,[12] cancerous and precancerous skin lesions can still present, for example in elderly machine operatives exposed to cutting oils in the 1950s and 1960s, as well as sporadically from previously unsuspected causes.[88] The characteristic skin lesions are keratoses ('oil warts') and squamous cell carcinomata. They affect particularly the scrotum in machine operatives, and also commonly the hands and forearms, but rarely the face and neck. The carcinogens in mineral oils have been identified as polycyclic aromatic hydrocarbons. Solvent refining is considered to have reduced these to an adequately safe level, which epidemiological analysis of new cases has since begun to reflect.[89] Those occupationally exposed to polycyclic aromatic hydrocarbons in coal tar pitch may be similarly affected.[90]

The risk of skin lesions that could turn cancerous due to occupational solar exposure is becoming increasingly recognized. In some parts of the world, sunscreen is routinely available to outdoor workers. Proving work-relatedness is often difficult, due to the long delay between solar exposure and the development of skin cancer (basal cell carcinoma (BCC), squamous cell carcinoma (SCC) and melanoma). A recent Bavarian study showed increased rates of BCC and SCC in outdoor workers than indoor workers, although there was no difference in rates for melanoma.[91]

COLD URTICARIA

Cold urticaria is an uncommon occupational skin disease.[92] In general, patients with cold urticaria are advised to avoid exposure to the cold in their work.

PSEUDO-EPIDEMICS

It is not uncommon for pseudo-epidemics of skin problems to present in a workplace or factory. The presentation of a few cases of actual work-related skin problems often leads to increased reporting of common skin problems unrelated to occupation among work colleagues. It is essential for a dermatologist to assess all workers with skin complaints to confirm the diagnoses. Where multiple patients are involved, it may be necessary to patch test the most severely affected to screen for ACD, and then widen the testing to include the others if positives are found.

MAJOR OCCUPATIONS CAUSING DERMATOSES[9,18,33]

Agriculture[93]

Irritant contact dermatitis can arise from disinfectants and cleansers for milking equipment, and from diesel oil powering machinery. Allergic contact dermatitis is seen mainly from rubber chemicals, including N-isopropyl-N'-phenyl-p-phenylenediamine (IPPD), in gloves, boots and milking equipment; plants, including Compositae (Asteraceae) such as the common weeds dandelion and thistle; pesticides; antibiotics in animal feeds and veterinary use; cobalt in fertilizers and animal feeds; other animal feed additives such as ethoxyquin and quinoxaline derivatives; and chromate in cement. Contact urticaria or protein contact dermatitis may be caused by animal hair and dander.[64] Zoonoses include cattle ringworm and orf in sheep.

Catering[65,94]

Detergents, as well as fish, meat, fruit and vegetable juices, and dough, can all cause irritant contact dermatitis. Allergic contact dermatitis is caused mainly by onion and garlic, spices, formaldehyde and other preservatives, and rubber chemicals in gloves. Contact urticaria or protein contact dermatitis[66] is common from fish, shellfish, meat, fruit, vegetables, flour and flour improvers, and natural rubber latex in gloves. Candidal paronychia and viral warts also occur.

Chemical and pharmaceutical[95,96]

Irritants and sensitizers are specific to each process. Sensitization is often more common during research and development than in later full-scale production. Halogenated chemical intermediates are potent allergens. Inadvertent synthesis of new chloracnegens may result in sporadic outbreaks of chloracne.[71]

Cleaning[97]

Detergents and cleansers containing organic solvents, acids or alkalis are irritant. Rubber chemicals in gloves, formaldehyde and other preservatives, and fragrance chemicals cause allergic contact dermatitis. Contact urticaria and protein contact dermatitis arise mainly from natural rubber latex in gloves.[60] Candidal paronychia is also a problem.

Construction[98]

Cement, fibreglass and wood preservatives can all cause irritant contact dermatitis, as well as mould oil in brickmaking. Cement burns are caused by wet cement trapped against the skin. Chromate (and cobalt) in cement, epoxy resin in special cements,[99] softwoods and hardwoods, and rubber chemicals in boots and sealing strips are the main allergens. Leptospirosis is an infectious hazard of open watercourses. A European Union directive (2003/53/EC) requires ferrous sulphate to be added to cement to reduce chromium (VI) to less soluble (therefore less allergenic) chromium (III).[100] The incidence of chromium allergy in construction workers should fall over the next few years as it has done so in Scandinavian countries, since ferrous sulphate has been added to cement in Scandinavian countries for many years.

Electronics[101]

Soldering fluxes are a cause of irritancy, sensitization and contact urticaria. Warm dry air causes itchy dry skin. Epoxy resin and anaerobic acrylic sealants are other important sensitizers.

Fishing[102]

Irritant contact dermatitis arises from wet work, especially in the cold, friction, oils and fuels, and fish juice itself. The major sensitizers, apart from rubber chemicals in boots, are marine organisms, such as those responsible for Dogger Bank itch, and plants. Dogger Bank itch is an allergic contact dermatitis to the (2-hydroxyethyl) dimethylsulphoxonium ion, a metabolite produced by the marine Bryozoan *alcyonidium diaphanum*. This marine organism is commonly found off the waters of the United Kingdom and despite the reduction in the size of the local fishing fleet, is likely to cause significant ongoing problems in fishermen and trawlermen.

Contact urticaria and protein contact dermatitis can also be caused by fish, marine organisms and plants.

Hairdressing[103]

Shampoos, permanent-wave solutions and bleaches are all irritant. The principal allergens are p-phenylenediamine (PPD) in hair dyes, glyceryl thioglycolate (GTG) in acid/pH-balanced permanent-wave solutions, and formaldehyde or isothiazolinones as preservatives in hair gels and mousses. Contact urticaria or protein contact dermatitis can arise from ammonium persulphate in bleaches, as well as natural rubber latex in gloves and even PPD.[104]

Apprentice hairdressers are at particular risk of developing hand eczema due to their relatively greater exposure to washing clients hair, etc. Studies have shown poor knowledge within the workforce of the potential skin hazards.[105]

Health care[106]

The main irritants are skin cleansers, disinfectants and prolonged wearing of occlusive gloves. Warm dry air in hospitals causes itchy skin dryness. Rubber gloves cause allergic contact dermatitis from their chemical content (rubber accelerators and natural rubber latex), contact urticaria or protein contact dermatitis from their natural rubber latex and potentially irritant contact dermatitis from prolonged wearing and subsequent sweating in occlusive gloves.[54] Hand cleansers are potential sources of allergens. There has been a recent increase in the use of alcohol-based hand rubs. While many workers complain of stinging and soreness when using these, one study has shown low rates of cutaneous adverse reactions to these products.[107] In general, occupational dermatologists feel that these products are less drying than frequent hand washing. The stinging and soreness tends only to occur when they are used on already broken skin. Dentistry sensitizes to local anaesthetics, resins and catalysts.[108] Orthopaedic surgeons run the risk of sensitization from acrylic cement. The cold sterilant glutaraldehyde has been a sensitization hazard in, for example, endoscopy units. Propacetamol (a prodrug of paracetamol given in i.v. formulation, often in post-operative patients) is the latest in a long line of drugs to sensitize their handlers.

The presence of dermatitis affecting the hands in healthcare workers provides potential sources of entry for pathogens and for increased colonization of the skin. Rapid assessment and treatment is therefore recommended in healthcare workers presenting with hand dermatitis.

It is important to bear in mind that in many patients the hand eczema may be mutifactorial, with ICD, ACD, possibly contact urticaria and constitutional eczema all playing a role. There has been a recent increase in the use of vinyl medical examination gloves – these do not provide adequate protection for blood-borne infections and their use should be reserved for low-risk exposures.

Horticulture and floristry[109]

Irritant contact dermatitis arises from wet work, friction from manipulating wire, handling bulbs and certain plants, such as *Dieffenbachia*, daffodils and spurges. Many other plants and flowers are sensitizers: *Primula obconica*, chrysanthemum, other Compositae (including common weeds), tulip and alstroemeria. Daffodils (and narcissi) may also sensitize. Dermatitis provoked by exposure to sunlight following contact with plants (phytophotodermatitis) occasionally occurs occupationally.[110] In the United Kingdom, the two main families of plants responsible are the Apiaceae (Umbelliferae), including celery, parsley, parsnip and carrot, as well as giant Russian hogweed; and the Rutaceae, including rue. In hotter climates, the Moraceae (figs) and Leguminosae (pea) may also be causal. The level of phototoxic furocoumarins (psoralens) is increased in response to fungal disease. Tending plants in aquaria may result in *Mycobacterium marinum* infection. Rubber gloves may cause the same problems as in other occupations. Contact urticaria and protein contact dermatitis may also be caused by plants such as *Schlumbergera* cacti.

Metalworkers[111]

So-called 'soluble oils' are the major irritants, as well as organic solvents and aggressive skin cleansers. The irritancy of soluble oils may be increased by the overaddition of alkaline biocides. Both soluble oils and neat cutting oils also contain potential sensitizers, such as biocides (including formaldehyde-releasers) and tall-oil-based emulsifiers (which cross-react with colophony in the patch test standard series) in the former and epoxides in the latter. The usually trace amounts of nickel, cobalt and chromate in cutting oils rarely sensitize.

Mining[112]

Mineral dusts, oils and hydraulic fluids, and cement can all cause irritant contact dermatitis. Rubber chemicals in boots and chromate (and cobalt) in cement sensitize. Tinea pedis tends to be endemic, because of shared washing facilities at the surface, and may spread to the hands, among other areas. Scleroderma-like disease has been documented in miners in Eastern Europe and South Africa.

Office workers[113]

Low relative humidity may dry out the skin in air-conditioned offices, leading to intense pruritus and asteatotic eczema. Allergic contact dermatitis may arise from nickel (paper clips and staplers), rubber chemicals (rubber bands, thimbles and sponges) and colophony (used in paper sizing, where modified rosins are added to paper to alter the wear and durability characteristics of the paper).

Painting[114]

Thinners (especially when used for skin cleansing), emulsion paints and wallpaper adhesives are irritant. Organotin compounds in anti-fouling paints for ships are highly irritant. Turpentine is now a sensitizer only in arts and crafts painters (e.g. porcelain). Other sensitizers include D-limonene (the 'citrus solvent'),[115] organocobalt paint driers, epoxy, acrylic and polyurethane resins, preservatives, such as chlorothalonil in water-based paints, and triglycidyl isocyanurate (TGIC) in polyester powder paints.

Photographic processing[116]

Photographic processing chemicals include many sensitizers, such as metol (*p*-aminophenol) in black-and-white processing, and substituted para-phenylenediamines in colour developing (sometimes causing lichenoid eruptions). Rubber gloves cause the same problems as in other occupations. However, with the advent of universal high quality video and digital photography sensitization to photographic chemicals is an increasingly rare occurrence.

Printing[117]

Irritant contact dermatitis arises from organic solvents and multifunctional acrylates in ultraviolet curing inks, lacquers and printing plates. Colophony is a sensitizer in paper size (see under Office workers, p. 1073), rubber chemicals in offset printing roller blankets, formaldehyde or isothiazolinones as preservatives in gum arabic and fountain solutions, and multifunctional acrylates in the ultraviolet-curing products already discussed. Rubber gloves are also a source of sensitization.

Tanning[118]

Acids, alkalis, reducing and oxidizing agents are all irritant, while chromate, formaldehyde, glutaraldehyde, vegetable tannins, dyes and resins are potential allergens. Formaldehyde may also be a source of contact urticaria, in addition to rubber gloves. Anthrax remains a risk from hides from endemic areas.

Veterinary care[119]

Disinfectants may irritate. Rubber gloves, antibiotics and antimycotics, glutaraldehyde and preservatives in rectal lubricants may all sensitize. Sources of contact urticaria and protein contact dermatitis include animal hair and dander, obstetric fluids and animal tissues, as well as rubber gloves. Zoonoses are clearly also a risk (see under Agriculture, p. 1071).

Woodworking[120,121]

Irritation may arise from certain hardwoods, wood preservatives and formaldehyde resins in fibreboard and chipboard. Other woods (both soft and hard) are sensitizers, as may also be formaldehyde resins, and frullania and lichens may in addition sensitize forestry workers.

Key points

- Irritant contact dermatitis is the commonest occupational skin health problem.
- The prognosis of allergic contact dermatitis is not always good.
- The morphology of allergic and irritant contact dermatitis is indistinguishable.
- Irritant contact dermatitis is treated with exposure reduction and allergic contact dermatitis with elimination.
- Atopy is a major risk factor for developing occupational contact dermatitis but there are other as yet not defined (genetic) factors.
- Non-eczematous dermatoses are important but very rare.

REFERENCES

1. White RP. *The dermatergoses or occupational affections of the skin*, 3rd edn. London: Lewis, 1928.
2. Bonnevie P. *Aetiologie und Pathogenese der Eczemkrankheiten*. Copenhagen: Busck, 1939.
3. Schwartz L, Tulipan L, Birmingham DJ. *Occupational diseases of the skin*, 3rd edn. London: Kimpton, 1957.
4. Calnan CD. Dermatology and industry (Prosser White oration). *Clinical and Experimental Dermatology*. 1977; **3**: 1–16.
5. Fregert S. Occupational dermatitis in a 10-year material. *Contact Dermatitis*. 1975; **1**: 96–107.
6. Foussereau J, Benezra C, Maibach HI. *Occupational contact dermatitis*. Copenhagen: Munksgaard, 1982.
7. Zschunke E. *Grundriss der Arbeitsdermatologie*. Berlin: VEB Verlag Volk und Gesundheit, 1985.
8. Adams RM. *Occupational skin disease*, 3rd edn. Philadelphia: WB Saunders, 1999.
9. Kanerva L, Elsner P, Wahlberg JE, Maibach HI. *Handbook of occupational dermatology*. Berlin: Springer, 2000.
10. Agrup G. Hand eczema and other dermatoses in South Sweden. *Acta Dermato-Venereologica*. 1969; **49** (Suppl.): 61.
11. Calnan CD, Rycroft RJG. Rehabilitation in occupational skin disease. *Transactions of the Medical College of South Africa*. 1981; **25** (Suppl.): 136–42.
12. Turner S, Carder M, van Tongeren M et al. The incidence of occupational skin disease as reported to The Health and Occupation Reporting (THOR) network between 2002 and 2005. *British Journal of Dermatology*. 2007; **157**: 713–22.
13. Health and Safety Commission. Health and safety statistics, 1996/97. London: HSE, 1997.
14. McDonald JC, Beck MH, Chen Y, Cherry NM. Incidence by occupation and industry of work-related skin diseases in the United Kingdom, 1996–2001. *Occupational Medicine*. 2006; **56**: 398–405.
15. Mathias CGT. The cost of occupational skin disease. *Archives of Dermatology*. 1985; **121**: 332–4.
16. McCall BP, Horwitz IB, Feldman SR, Balkrishnan R. Incidence rates, costs, severity, and work-related factors of occupational dermatitis: a workers compensation analysis of Oregon, 1990–1997. *Archives of Dermatology*. 2005; **141**: 713–18.
17. Burry JN, Kirk J. Environmental dermatitis: Chrome cripples. *Medical Journal of Australia*. 1975; **2**: 720–1.
18. Rycroft RJG. Occupational contact dermatitis. In: Rycroft RJG, Menné T, Frosch PJ, Lepoittevin JP (eds). *Textbook of contact dermatitis*, 3rd edn. Berlin: Springer, 2001: 555–80.
19. English JSC. *A colour handbook of occupational dermatology*. London: Manson Publishing, 1999.
20. Calnan CD. Eczema for me. *Transactions of the St. John's Hospital Dermatological Society*. 1968; **54**: 54–64.
21. Fregert S. *Manual of contact dermatitis*, 2nd edn. Copenhagen: Munksgaard, 1981.
22. Wilkinson SM, Beck MH. Contact dermatitis: Irritant. In: Burns DA, Breathnach SM, Cox NH, Griffiths CME (eds). *Textbook of dermatology*, 7th edn. Oxford: Blackwell Science, 2004: 19.1–19.30.
23. Lisby S, Baadsgaard O. Mechanisms of irritant contact dermatitis. In: Rycroft RJG, Menné T, Frosch PJ, Lepoittevin JP (eds). *Textbook of contact dermatitis*, 3rd edn. Berlin: Springer, 2001: 91–110.
24. Davies NF, Rycroft RJG. Dermatology. In: Cox RAF, Edwards FC, McCallum RI (eds). *Fitness for work. The medical aspects*, 2nd edn. Oxford: Oxford University Press, 1995: 102–12.
25. Coenraads P-J, Diepgen TL. Risk for hand eczema in employees with past or present atopic dermatitis. *International Archives of Occupational and Environmental Health*. 1998; **71**: 7–13.
26. Rycroft RJG. Principal irritants and sensitizers. In: Champion RH, Burton JL, Burns DA, Breachnach SM (eds). *Textbook of dermatology*, 6th edn. Oxford: Blackwell Science, 1998: 821–60.

27. Fartasch M. Skin protection. From TRGS 401 to guidelines on 'occupational skin protection products'. *Hautarzt*. 2009; **60**: 702–7.
28. Rustmeyer T, van Hoogstraten IMW, von Blomberg BME, Scheper RJ. Mechanisms in allergic contact dermatitis. In: Rycroft RJG, Menné T, Frosch PJ, Lepoittevin JP (eds). *Textbook of contact dermatitis*, 3rd edn. Berlin: Springer, 2001: 13–58.
29. Beck M, Wilkinson SM. Contact dermatitis: Allergic. In: Burns DA, Breathnach SM, Cox NH, Griffiths CME (eds). *Textbook of dermatology*, 7th edn. Oxford: Blackwell Science, 2004: 20.1–20.124.
30. Kanerva L, Tarvainen K, Pinola A et al. A single accidental exposure may result in a chemical burn, primary sensitization and allergic contact dermatitis. *Contact Dermatitis*. 1994; **31**: 229–35.
31. De Groot AC. *Patch testing: Test concentrations and vehicles for 3700 chemicals*, 2nd edn. Amsterdam: Elsevier, 1994.
32. Johansen J, Menne T, Christophersen J et al. Changes in the pattern of sensitization to common contact allergens in Denmark between 1985–86 and 1997–98, with a special view to the effect of preventive strategies. *British Journal of Dermatology*. 2000; **142**: 490–5.
33. English JSC. Occupational dermatoses. In: Burns DA, Breathnach SM, Cox NH, Griffiths CME (eds). *Textbook of dermatology*, 7th edn. Oxford: Blackwell Science, 2004: 21.1–21.25.
34. Wilkinson DS. Some causes of error in the diagnosis of occupational dermatoses. In: Griffiths WAD, Wilkinson DS (eds). *Essentials of industrial dermatology*. Oxford: Blackwell Science, 1985: 47–57.
35. Freeman S. Diagnosis and differential diagnosis. In: Adams RM (ed.). *Occupational skin disease*, 3rd edn. Philadelphia: Saunders, 1999: 189–207.
36. Meneghini CL, Angelini G. Primary and secondary sites of occupational contact dermatitis. *Dermatosen*. 1984; **32**: 205–7.
37. Dooms-Goossens A, Debusschere KM, Gevers DM et al. Contact dermatitis caused by airborne agents. A review and case reports. *Journal of the American Academy of Dermatologists*. 1986; **15**: 1–10.
38. Ferguson J. Occupational skin disorders associated with sun or artifical light exposure. In English JSC (ed.). *A colour handbook of occupational dermatology*. London: Manson Publishing, 1999: 53–62.
39. Williams J, Cahill J, Nixon R. Occupational autoeczematization or atopic eczema precipitated by occupational contact dermatitis? *Contact Dermatitis*. 2007; **56**: 21–6.
40. Rycroft RJG. Occupational dermatoses in perspective. *Lancet*. 1980; **ii**: 24–6.
41. Mathias CG. Contact dermatitis and workers' compensation: Criteria for establishing occupational causation and aggravation. *Journal of the American Academy of Dermatologists*. 1989; **20**: 842–8.
42. Bourke J, Coulson I, Engish J. British Association of Dermatologists, Therapy Guidelines and Audit Subcommittee. Guidelines for the management of contact dermatitis: An update. *British Journal of Dermatology*. 2009; **160**: 946–54.
43. Slodownik D, Williams J, Frowen K et al. The additive value of patch testing with patients on products at an occupational dermatology clinic. *Contact Dermatitis*. 2009; **61**: 231–5.
44. Wilkinson JD. The management of contact dermatitis. In: Rycroft RJG, Frosch PJ (eds). *Textbook of contact dermatitis*, 2nd edn. Berlin: Springer, 1995: 659–92.
45. Calnan CD. Studies in contact dermatitis. XXIII. Allergen replacement. *Transactions of the St. John's Hospital Dermatological Society*. 1970; **56**: 131–8.
46. Frosch PJ, Kurte A, Pilz B. Efficacy of skin barrier creams (III). The repetitive irritation test (RIT) in humans. *Contact Dermatitis*. 1993; **29**: 113–18.
47. Zhai H, Maibach HI. Moisturizers in preventing irritant contact dermatitis: An overview. *Contact Dermatitis*. 1998; **38**: 241–4.
48. Pryce DW, Irvine D, English JSC, Rycroft RJG. Soluble oil dermatitis: A follow-up study. *Contact Dermatitis*. 1989; **21**: 28–35.
49. Agner T, Held E. Skin protection programmes. *Contact Dermatitis*. 2002; **47**: 253–6.
50. Dickel H, Kuss O, Schmidt A, Diepgen TI. Impact of preventative strategies on trend of occupational skin disease in hairdressers: Population-based register study. *British Medical Journal*. 2002; **324**: 1422–3.
51. Brown TP, Rushton L, Williams HC et al. Intervention development in occupational research: An example from the printing industry. *Occupational and Environmental Medicine*. 2006; **63**: 261–6.
52. Wall LM, Gebauer KA. A follow-up study of occupational skin disease in Western Australia. *Contact Dermatitis*. 1991; **24**: 241–3.
53. Rosen RH, Freeman S. Prognosis of occupational contact dermatitis in New South Wales, Australia. *Contact Dermatitis*. 1993; **29**: 88–93.
54. Grattan CEH, Foulds IS. Outcome of investigation of cutting fluid dermatitis. *Contact Dermatitis*. 1989; **20**: 377–8.
55. Pryce DW, Irvine D, English JSC, Rycroft RJG. Soluble oil dermatitis: A follow-up study. *Contact Dermatitis*. 1989; **21**: 28–35.
56. Cronin E. Dermatitis of the hands in caterers. *Contact Dermatitis*. 1987; **17**: 265–9.
57. Sajjachareonpong P, Cahill J, Keegel T et al. Persistent post-occupational dermatitis. *Contact Dermatitis*. 2004; **51**: 278–83.
58. Cahill J, Keegel T, Nixon R. The prognosis of occupational contact dermatitis in 2004. *Contact Dermatitis*. 2004; **51**: 219–26.
59. Turjanmaa K, Alenins H, Mäkinen-Kiljunen S et al. Natural rubber latex allergy. *Allergy*. 1996; **51**: 593–602.
60. Posch A, Chen Z, Raulf-Heimsoth M, Baur X. Latex allergens. *Clinical and Experimental Allergy*. 1998; **28**: 134–40.

61. Medical Devices Agency (UK). Device Bulletin 9601. Latex sensitisation in the health care setting (use of latex gloves). London: MDA, 1996.
62. Allmers H, Schmengler J, John SM. Decreasing incidence of occupational contact urticaria caused by natural rubber latex allergy in German health care workers. *Journal of Allergy and Clinical Immunology.* 2004; **114**: 347–51.
63. Clayton TH, Wilkinson SM. Contact dermatoses in healthcare workers: Reduction in type I latex allergy in a UK center. *Clinical and Experimental Dermatology.* 2005; **30**: 221–5.
64. Kanerva L, Susitaival P. Cow dander: The most common cause of occupational contact urticaria in Finland. *Contact Dermatitis.* 1996; **35**: 309–10.
65. Cronin E. Dermatitis in food handlers. In: Callen JP, Dahl MV, Golitz LE *et al.* (eds). *Advances in Dermatology*, vol. 4. Chicago: Year Book, 1989: 113–24.
66. Hjorth N, Roed-Petersen J. Occupational protein contact dermatitis in food handlers. *Contact Dermatitis.* 1976; **2**: 28–42.
67. Lahti A, Basketter D. Immediate contact reactions. In: Rycroft RJG, Menné T, Frosch PJ, Lepoittevin JP (eds). *Textbook of contact dermatitis*, 3rd edn. Berlin: Springer, 2001: 111–32.
68. Rycroft RJG. Petroleum and petroleum derivatives. In: Adams RM (ed.). *Occupational skin disease*, 3rd edn. Philadelphia: WB Saunders, 1999: 553–66.
69. Tindall JP. Chloracne and chloracnegens. *Journal of American Academy of Dermatologists.* 1985; **13**: 539–58.
70. Poskitt LB, Duffill MB, Rademaker M. Chloracne, palmoplantar keratoderma and localized scleroderma in a weed sprayer. *Clinical and Experimental Dermatology.* 1994; **19**: 264–7.
71. Scerri L, Zaki I, Millard LG. Severe halogen acne due to a trifluoromethylpyrazole derivative and its resistance to isotretinoin. *British Journal of Dermatology.* 1995; **132**: 144–8.
72. Zober A, Ott MG, Messerer P. Morbidity follow up study of BASF employees exposed to 2,3,7,8-tetrachlorodibenzo-p-dioxin (TCDD) after a 1953 chemical reactor incident. *Occupational and Environmental Medicine.* 1994; **51**: 470–86.
73. Rozman K. A critical view of the mechanism(s) of toxicity of 2,3,7,8-tetrachlorodibenzo-p-dioxin. Implications for human safety assessment. *Dermatosen.* 1989; **37**: 81–92.
74. Stevenson CJ. Environmentally induced vitiligo (leucoderma) from depigmenting agents and chemicals. *Cutaneous and Ocular Toxicology.* 1984; **3**: 299–307.
75. Wattanakrai P, Miyamoto L, Taylor JS. Occupational pigmentary disorders. In: Kanerva L, Elsner P, Wahlberg JE, Maibach HI (eds). *Handbook of occupational dermatology.* Berlin: Springer, 2000: 280–94.
76. Gawkrodger DJ. Pigmentary changes due to occupation. In: English JSC (ed.). *A colour handbook of occupational dermatology.* London: Manson, 1999: 147–58.
77. James O, Mayes RW, Stevenson CJ. Occupational vitiligo induced by *p*-tert-butylphenol. A systemic disease? *Lancet.* 1997; **ii**: 1217–19.
78. Black CM, Welsh KI. Occupationally and environmentally induced scleroderma-like illness: Etiology, pathogenesis, diagnosis, and treatment. *Internal Medicine Specialist.* 1988; **9**: 135–54.
79. Walker AE. Clinical aspects of vinyl chloride disease: Skin. *Proceedings of the Royal Society of Medicine.* 1976; **69**: 286–9.
80. Ziegler V, Haustein UF. Die progressive Sklerodermie – eine quarzinduzierte Berufskrankheit? *Dermatologische Monatschrift.* 1992; **178**: 34–43.
81. Dunnill MGS, Black MM. Sclerodermatous syndrome after occupational exposure to herbicides – response to systemic steroids. *Clinical and Experimental Dermatology.* 1994; **19**: 518–20.
82. Granel B, Zemour F, Lehucher-Michel MP *et al.* Occupational exposure and systemic sclerosis. Literature review and result of a self-reported questionnaire. *Revue de Médecine Interne.* 2008; **29**: 891–900.
83. Williams N. Occupational skin ulceration in chrome platers. *Occupational Medicine.* 1997; **47**: 309–10.
84. Fleeger AK, Deng J-F. A case study of chromium VI-induced skin ulcerations during a porcelain enamel curing operation. *Applied Occupational and Environmental Hygiene.* 1990; **5**: 378–82.
85. Rycroft RJG. Acute ulcerative contact dermatitis from Portland cement. *British Journal of Dermatology.* 1980; **102**: 487–9.
86. Irvine C, Pugh CE, Hansen EJ, Rycroft RJG. Cement dermatitis in underground workers during construction of the Channel Tunnel. *Occupational Medicine.* 1994; **44**: 17–23.
87. Cruickshank CND, Squire JR. Skin cancer in the engineering industry from the use of mineral oil. *British Journal of Industrial Medicine.* 1950; **7**: 1–11.
88. Bowra GT, Duffield DP, Osborn AJ, Purchase IFH. Premalignant and neoplastic skin lesions association with occupational exposure to 'tarry' byproducts during manufacture of 4,4'-bipyridyl. *British Journal of Industrial Medicine.* 1982; **39**: 76–81.
89. Waldron HA, Waterhouse JAH, Tessema N. Scrotal cancer in the West Midlands, 1936–76. *British Journal of Industrial Medicine.* 1984; **41**: 437–44.
90. Voelter-Mahlknecht S, Scheriau R, Zwahr G *et al.* Skin tumors among employees of a tar refinery: The current data and their implications. *International Archives of Occupational and Environmental Health.* 2007; **80**: 485–95.
91. Radespiel-Troger M, Meyer M, Pfahlberg A *et al.* Outdoor work and skin cancer incidence: A registry based study in Bavaria. *International Archives of Occupational and Environmental Health.* 2009; **82**: 357–63.
92. Fitzgerald DA, Heagerty AH, English JS. Cold urticaria as an occupational dermatosis. *Contact Dermatitis.* 1995; **32**: 238.
93. Susitaival P. Farmer and farm workers. In: Kanerva L, Elsner P, Wahlberg JE, Maibach HI (eds). *Handbook of occupational dermatology.* Berlin: Springer, 2000: 924–31.
94. Veien NK. Bakers. In: Kanerva L, Elsner P, Wahlberg JE, Maibach HI (eds). *Handbook of occupational dermatology.* Berlin: Springer, 2000: 817–20.

95. Sherertz EF. Occupational skin disease in the pharmaceutical industry. *Dermatologic Clinics.* 1994; **12**: 533–6.
96. Bircher AJ. Pharmaceutical drug allergens. In: Kanerva L, Elsner P, Wahlberg JE, Maibach HI (eds). *Handbook of occupational dermatology.* Berlin: Springer, 2000: 479–89.
97. Nilsson E. Contact sensitivity and urticaria in 'wet' work. *Contact Dermatitis.* 1985; **13**: 321–8.
98. Bock M, Schmidt A, Bruckner T, Diepgen TL. Occupational skin disease in the construction industry. *British Journal of Dermatology.* 2003; **149**: 1165–71.
99. Van Putten PB, Coenraads PJ, Nater JP. Hand dermatoses and contact allergic reactions in construction workers exposed to epoxy resins. *Contact Dermatitis.* 1984; **10**: 146–50.
100. Athavale P, Shum KW, Chen Y *et al.* Occupational dermatitis related to chromium and cobalt: Experience of dermatologists (EPIDERM) and occupational physicians (OPRA) in the UK over an 11-year period (1993–2004). *British Journal of Dermatology.* 2007; **157**: 518–22.
101. Tucker SC, English JSC. The electronics industry. In: Kanerva L, Elsner P, Wahlberg JE, Maibach HI (eds). *Handbook of occupational dermatology.* Berlin: Springer, 2000: 650–61.
102. Ashworth J, Curry FM, White IR, Rycroft RJG. Occupational allergic contact dermatitis in east coast of England fishermen: Newly described hypersensitivities to marine organisms. *Contact Dermatitis.* 1990; **22**: 185–6.
103. Van der Walle HB, Brunsveld VM. Dermatitis in hairdressers (I). The experience of the past 4 years, II. Management and prevention. *Contact Dermatitis.* 1994; **30**: 217–21, 265–70.
104. Birnie AJ, English JS. Immediate hypersensitivity to paraphenylenediamine. *Contact Dermatitis.* 2007; **56**: 240.
105. Nixon R, Roberts H, Frowen K, Sim M. Knowledge of skin hazards and the use of gloves by Australian hairdressing students and practising hairdressers. *Contact Dermatitis.* 2006; **54**: 112–16.
106. Jungbauer FH, Lensen GJ, Groothoff JW, Coenraads PJ. Exposure of the hands to wet work in nurses. *Contact Dermatitis.* 2004; **50**: 225–9.
107. Wallenhammar LM, Ortengren U, Andreasson H *et al.* Contact allergy and hand eczema in Swedish dentists. *Contact Dermatitis.* 2000; **43**: 192–9.
108. Graham M, Nixon R, Burrell LJ *et al.* Low rates of cutaneous adverse reactions to alcohol-based hand hygiene solution during prolonged use in a large teaching hospital. *Antimicrobial Agents and Chemotherapy.* 2005; **49**: 4404–5.
109. Zug KA, Marks JG. Plants and woods. In: Adams RM (ed.). *Occupational skin disease,* 3rd edn. Philadelphia: WB Saunders, 1999: 567–96.
110. Lovell CR. *Plants and the skin.* Oxford: Blackwell Science, 1993: 86–95.
111. Pryce DW, White J, English JSC, Rycroft RJG. Soluble oil dermatitis: A review. *Journal of the Society of Occupational Medicine.* 1989; **39**: 93–8.
112. Puttick LM. Skin disorders in the mining industry. London: University of London, 1989 (dissertation).
113. Rycroft RJG. Occupational dermatoses among office personnel. *Occupational Medicine. State of the Art Review.* 1986; **1**: 323–8.
114. Högberg M, Wahlberg JE. Health screening for occupational dermatoses in house painters. *Contact Dermatitis.* 1980; **6**: 100–6.
115. Karlberg A-T, Dooms-Goossens A. Contact allergy to D-limonene among dermatitis patients. *Contact Dermatitis.* 1997; **36**: 201–6.
116. Rustemeyer T, Frosch PJ. Allergic contact dermatitis from colour developers. *Contact Dermatitis.* 1995; **32**: 59–60.
117. Livesley EJ, Rushton L, English JS, Williams HC. The prevalence of occupational dermatitis in the UK printing industry. *Occupational and Environmental Medicine.* 2002; **59**: 487–92.
118. Burrows D. Adverse chromate reactions on the skin. In: Burrows D (ed.). *Chromium: Metabolism and toxicity.* Boca Raton, FL: CRC Press, 1983: 137–63.
119. Falk ES, Hektoen H, Thune PO. Skin and respiratory tract symptoms in veterinary surgeons. *Contact Dermatitis.* 1985; **12**: 274–8.
120. Hausen BM. *Woods injurious to human health. A manual.* Berlin: Walter de Gruyter, 1981.
121. Estlander T, Jolanki R, Alanko K, Kanerva L. Occupational allergic contact dermatitis caused by wood dusts. *Contact Dermatitis.* 2001; **44**: 213–17.

SECTION TWO

Occupational cancers

85 Occupational cancer: epidemiology, biological mechanisms and biomarkers 1081
Manolis Kogevinas, J Malcolm Harrington and Roel Vermeulen

85

Occupational cancer: epidemiology, biological mechanisms and biomarkers

MANOLIS KOGEVINAS, J MALCOLM HARRINGTON AND ROEL VERMEULEN

Introduction	1081	Methodological issues in epidemiological research on occupational cancer	1104
Occupational carcinogens and exposure to occupational carcinogens	1082	Biomarkers and mechanisms	1111
Occupational cancers	1085	Acknowledgements	1115
Clinical assessment of occupational cancer and prevention	1100	References	1115

INTRODUCTION

Occupational carcinogens have an important role in the identification and prevention of cancer. They were the first human carcinogens to be identified and a large proportion of the carcinogens currently identified originate in the workplace. In England in 1771, Percival Pott, in his work *Chirurgical works*, described a higher frequency of cancer in the scrotum among chimney sweeps and associated the disease with exposure to soot. Bladder cancer, which is among the major cancers attributed to occupational exposures, occupies an important place in the history of occupational cancer epidemiology since the highest cumulative incidence of any cancer ever reported is for bladder cancer among workers in the dye industry. In addition, studies on occupational cancer have been among the first to develop methods for the conduct of historical cohort studies applying the concept of person-years[1] through the pioneering work of Bradford Hill in 1948 and Richard Doll in 1952. Occupational cancers should be considered as preventable and this makes their identification even more necessary. The benefits of prevention go beyond occupational settings since the general population is also exposed to several of these compounds, for example asbestos, benzene, diesel exhaust and formaldehyde.

On the basis of the evaluations made by the International Agency for Research on Cancer (IARC), about 400 agents can be considered as carcinogens and about 150 occur in the workplace. In addition, employment in 18 industries or occupations has been identified as conveying an increased risk for cancer.

In industrialized countries, about a quarter of all deaths are due to cancer. Nowadays, the tumour sites more frequently associated with occupational exposure are lung, urinary bladder, nasal cavity, liver (angiosarcoma), mesothelioma, leukaemia and non-melanocytic skin cancer.[2–6] Associations between industrial exposures and many other cancer sites, such as the pancreas, brain, pharynx, prostate, colon, breast, kidney, soft tissue sarcomas, lymphomas, multiple myeloma and others, have also been described, although the evidence is not always conclusive, or alternatively the proportion of cancers attributed to occupational exposures is low.

There is some controversy in relation to the percentage of all cancers attributable to occupational exposures. Most of the researchers and evaluating agencies consider that around 5 per cent of all cancer is attributable to exposures considered in the occupational setting, but there are also other (higher and lower) estimates. In most countries, occupational diseases are not regularly and completely identified. In industrialized countries it has been estimated that more than 80 per cent of occupational diseases, including cancer, are not recognized as such. This is despite the identification of numerous carcinogenic exposures in the workplace. The EU includes, for example, 15 agents related to cancer: asbestos, aromatic amines, arsenic and its derivates, benzene, beryllium, bis-(chloro-methyl) ether, cadmium, vinyl chloride, chromium IV and chromium VI compounds, polycyclic aromatic hydrocarbons (PAHs) and products of distillation of coal, nickel and nickel compounds, wood dust, silica, radon and ionizing radiation. Despite this list, the number of cancers notified as occupational is very low, in most countries being less than 1 per cent or even less than 0.1 per cent of all cancers.

Epidemiological research on occupational cancer has traditionally focused on men, although it has been decades since women entered the labour market on a massive scale.[7] In the past, there were relatively few extensive studies focused on occupational cancer in women. The dramatic changes in work conditions of the last decades have also resulted in a reshaping and widening of epidemiological research on occupational health and recent studies have also focused on the work environment of women. The effects of shift work on breast cancer incidence have been among the most important recent findings in relation to women's work.

In this chapter, we will review the evidence on occupational cancer and specifically refer to the major exposures and the main cancers caused by occupational exposures, present estimates of cancers attributable to occupational exposures, discuss the main issues related to epidemiological cancer research and, finally, extensively discuss mechanisms of disease and the use of biomarkers in studies on occupational cancer.

OCCUPATIONAL CARCINOGENS AND EXPOSURE TO OCCUPATIONAL CARCINOGENS

IARC classification of carcinogens

The IARC monograph series is the most well-known reference source for carcinogens, including carcinogens in the workplace. National health agencies extensively use this information as scientific support for their actions to prevent exposure to potential carcinogens. The monograph series of the IARC (available from www.iarc.fr) has been functioning since 1971 and has the objective of identifying environmental factors that can increase the risk of human cancer. Evaluations of the epidemiological and experimental evidence of the carcinogenicity are performed for chemicals, complex mixtures, occupational exposures, physical and biological agents, and lifestyle factors. Agents are selected by the IARC to be evaluated if there is evidence that exposure occurs in humans, and also if there is suspicion that the agent could cause cancer. The evidence used in the IARC monographs is based on exposure data, epidemiological studies, studies in experimental animals and also data on mechanisms of action (e.g. kinetics, mutagenicity). The IARC groups agents into five categories (Table 85.1). From 1972 to 2009, the IARC has published 100 volumes and has evaluated approximately 1000 agents, mixtures or exposure circumstances. Until January 2009, 108 have been classified into

Table 85.1 The International Agency for Research on Cancer (IARC) groups of carcinogenicity.

Group	
1	The agent, mixture, or exposure circumstance is carcinogenic to humans
2A	The agent, mixture, or exposure circumstance is probably carcinogenic to humans
2B	The agent, mixture, or exposure circumstance is possibly carcinogenic to humans
3	The agent, mixture, or exposure circumstance is not classifiable as to its carcinogenicity to humans
4	The agent, mixture, or exposure circumstance is probably not carcinogenic to humans

group 1 (carcinogenic to humans), 66 in group 2A (probably carcinogenic to humans), and 248 in group 2B (possibly carcinogenic to humans).[8]

The IARC does not categorize the carcinogens evaluated as for the source of exposure and therefore does not indicate which should be considered as occupational. To identify which carcinogens could be classified as occupational, it is necessary to review the text of the monographs and then apply *ad hoc* criteria. The identification and listing of exposures that could be defined as occupational can be complex. Many occupational exposures also occur in the general environment and, vice versa, many predominantly environmental exposures occur in the occupational environment. For example, asbestos exposure is considered predominantly occupational but undoubtedly also occurs in the environment and numerous cases of mesothelioma have been reported among residents close to asbestos mines and asbestos-cement plants. Exposure to medical drugs is another example of agents to which most people are not exposed as a consequence of their work environment, but those working in the health sector may be exposed. Another issue refers to the evaluation of exposures among workers in an occupation or industry with a known increased risk. On most occasions, a specific exposure can be identified, for example benzene provokes a higher risk of leukaemia in shoe workers. However, although an increased risk of cancer can be identified for an occupation, e.g. lung cancer in painters, the specific exposures associated with this increased risk cannot be confidently identified.

In recent reviews, Siemiatycki et al.[4] and Rousseau et al.[9] categorized the IARC carcinogens in relation to whether they could be identified as occupational. They used various criteria, but the most important was whether this exposure occurs in the work environment among more than 10 000 workers in the world or 1000 workers in any specific country. Due to difficulties in undertaking an accurate estimation, they excluded exposures to medical drugs and to biological agents such as HIV or the hepatitis B and C

Table 85.2 Substances and mixtures that have been evaluated by IARC as definite (group 1) human carcinogens and that are occupational exposures (data from Ref. 4).

	Substance or mixture	Site(s)
Physical agents	Ionizing radiation and sources thereof, including, notably, x-rays, γ-rays, neutrons and radon gas	Bone, leukaemia, lung, liver, thyroid, others
	Solar radiation	Melanoma, skin
Polycyclic aromatic hydrocarbons	Benzo[a]pyrene	Lung, bladder, skin
Respirable dusts and fibres	Asbestos (chrysotile, crocidolite, amosite, tremolite, actinolite and anthophyllite)	Lung, mesothelioma, larynx, ovary, colorectum, pharynx, stomach
	Erionite	Mesothelioma
	Leather dust	Nasal cavity and paranasal sinuses
	Silica dust, crystalline in the form of quartz or crystobalite	Lung
	Talc containing asbestiform fibres	Lung, mesothelioma
	Wood dust	Nasal cavity and paranasal sinuses, nasopharynx
Metal and metal compounds	Arsenic and inorganic arsenic compounds	Skin, lung, urinary bladder, liver, kidney, prostate
	Beryllium and beryllium compounds	Lung
	Cadmium and cadmium compounds	Lung, prostate, kidney
	Chromium compounds, hexavalent	Lung, nasal cavity and paranasal sinuses
	Nickel compounds	Lung, nasal cavity and paranasal sinuses
Wood and fossil fuels and their byproducts	Benzene	Leukaemia and lymphomas (AML, ALL, CLL, MM, NHL)
	Coal tars and pitches (paving, roofing)	Lung, bladder
	Mineral oils	Skin
	Shale oils	Skin
	Soot (chimney sweeping)	Skin, lung, bladder
Monomers	Vinyl chloride	Liver (angiosarcoma), liver (hepatocellular)
	1,3-Butadiene	Haematolymphatic organs
Intermediates in plastics and rubber manufacturing	Bis(chloromethyl) ether and chloromethyl methyl ether (technical grade)	Lung (oat cell)
Aromatic amine dyes	4-Aminobiphenyl	Bladder
	Benzidine	Bladder
	Dyes metabolized to benzidine	Bladder
	2-Naphthylamine	Bladder
	Ortho-toluidine	Bladder
Pesticides	Ethylene oxide	Lymphoid tumours (NHL, MM, CLL), breast
	2,3,7,8-Tetrachlorodibenzo-para-dioxin (TCDD)	All sites combined, lung, non-Hodgkin lymphoma, sarcoma
Others	Aflatoxin	Liver (HCC)
	Formaldehyde	Nasopharynx, leukaemia, sinonasal cancer
	Involuntary (passive) smoking	Lung
	Mustard gas	Lung, larynx
	Strong inorganic-acid	Larynx, lung

ALL, Acute lymphocytic leukaemia; AML, acute myeloid leukaemia; CLL, chronic lymphocytic leukaemia; HCC, hepatocellular carcinoma; MM, malignant melanoma; NHL, non-Hodgkin lymphoma.

viruses, although it is proven that healthcare workers may be exposed to these agents in their work environment. Using these criteria, they identified as occupational carcinogens (lists modified using more recent evidence):

- 34 definitive human carcinogens (group 1 of IARC; Table 85.2, modified from original publication);
- 21 probable carcinogens (group 2A of IARC; Table 85.3, modified from original publication);
- 114 possible carcinogens (group 2B of IARC);
- 16 occupations or industries where an increased cancer risk has been identified among workers but no specific agent could be identified (Table 85.4, modified from original publication).

Table 85.3 Substances and mixtures that have been evaluated by IARC as probable (group 2A) human carcinogens and that are occupational exposures (data from Ref. 4).

	Substance or mixture	Site(s)
Physical agents	Ultraviolet radiation (A, B and C) from artificial sources	Melanoma
Polycyclic aromatic hydrocarbons	Benz[a]anthracene	Lung, bladder, skin
	Dibenz[a,h]anthracene	Lung, bladder, skin
Wood and fossil fuels and their byproducts	Creosotes	Skin
	Diesel engine exhaust	Lung, bladder
Intermediates in plastics and rubber manufacturing	4,4′-methylene bis(2-chloroaniline)	Bladder
	styrene-7,8-oxide	
Chlorinated hydrocarbons	α-Chlorinated toluenes	Lung
	Polychlorinated biphenyls	Liver and biliary tract
	Tetrachloroethylene	Cervix, oesophagus, non-Hodgkin lymphoma
	Trichloroethylene	Liver and biliary tract, non-Hodgkin lymphoma, renal cell
Monomers	Acrylamide	Pancreas
	Epichlorohydrin	Lung, central nervous system
	Vinyl bromide	
	Vinyl fluoride	
Aromatic amine dyes	4-chloro-ortho-toluidine	Bladder
Intermediates in the production of dyes	Dimethylcarbamoyl chloride	
Pesticides	Captafol	
	Ethylene dibromide	
	Non-arsenical insecticides	Brain, leukaemia, lung, multiple myeloma, non-Hodgkin lymphoma
Others	Diethyl sulphate	
	Tris(2,3-dibromopropyl)	

Table 85.4 Occupations or industries that have been evaluated by IARC as definitely (group 1) or probably (group 2A) entailing excess risk of cancer among workers (data from Refs 4 and 10).

Occupation or industry	Site(s)
Aluminium production	Lung, bladder
Auramine manufacture	Bladder
Boot and shoe manufacture and repair	Leukaemia, nose and sinuses, bladder
Coal gasification	Lung
Coal tar distillation	Skin
Coke production	Lung
Furniture and cabinet making	Nose and sinonasal cavities
Hairdressers and barbers	Bladder, lung, non-Hodgkin lymphoma, ovary
Hematite mining underground with radon exposure	Lung
Iron and steel founding	Lung
Isopropyl alcohol manufacture using strong acids	Nasal cavity
Magenta manufacture	Bladder
Painters	Lung, urinary bladder, pleural mesothelioma, childhood leukaemia
Petroleum refining	Bladder, brain, leukaemia
Production of art glass, glass containers and pressed ware	Lung
Rubber manufacturing industry	Leukaemia, lymphoma, urinary bladder, lung, stomach, prostate, larynx, oesophagus

Prevalence of exposure to occupational carcinogens: CAREX estimates

Effective prevention of occupational cancer requires knowledge on the occurrence of exposure, but information on the numbers of workers exposed is seldom available. An information system called CAREX (carcinogen exposure) has been constructed for EU countries for the estimation of the numbers of workers exposed to established and suspected human carcinogens.[11] CAREX includes data on agents evaluated by the IARC (all agents in groups 1 and 2A and selected agents in group 2B) and on ionizing radiation, displayed across 55 industrial classes. CAREX provides selected exposure data and documented estimates of the number of workers exposed to carcinogens by country, carcinogen and industry. It was estimated that in the 1990s about 32 million workers (23 per cent of those employed) in the EU were exposed to agents covered by CAREX. At least 22 million workers were exposed to IARC group 1 carcinogens. The most common exposures (Figure 85.1) were solar radiation (9.1 million workers exposed at least 75 per cent of working time), environmental tobacco smoke (ETS, 7.5 million workers exposed at least 75 per cent of working time), crystalline silica (3.2 million exposed), diesel exhaust (3.0 million), radon (2.7 million) and wood dust (2.6 million). Exposure to ETS has been drastically reduced in recent years in many countries, since the CAREX estimates were done prior to the establishment of legislation limiting workplace exposure to ETS.

Since the original publication which included 15 EU countries, CAREX has been updated[12] and applied in other countries, including some developing countries. In Costa Rica,[13] CAREX was adapted for 27 carcinogens and seven groups of pesticides. Widespread workplace carcinogens in the 1.3 million workforce of Costa Rica are similar to those in industrialized countries, including solar radiation (333 000 workers) and diesel engine exhaust (278 000) as the most common exposures. Among pesticides, the most common exposures were to paraquat and diquat (175 000) and mancozeb, maneb and zineb (49 000). Among women, formaldehyde, radon and methylene chloride were the most common exposures.

OCCUPATIONAL CANCERS

Lung

Among men, lung cancer is the most important tumour to present to the clinician. In many industrialized countries, it has also become among the most common tumours in women. Its association with tobacco consumption requires no further emphasis. It is important to note, however, that certain workplace exposures that cause respiratory tumours may act additively or even synergistically with cigarette exposure (see under Issues in design and analysis, p. 1107). In particular, asbestos and cigarette consumption is, perhaps, the best known example of interaction in occupational health, as the two agents have a possible multiplicative effect on the risk of developing lung cancer. Mortality rates in workers exposed to smoking and asbestos are shown in Table 85.5. Those exposed to asbestos but who are non-smokers have around five times the risk of non-smokers/non-asbestos exposed. Smokers/non-asbestos exposed have around ten times higher risk, while smokers who are exposed have around 60 times higher risk.

Although the clinician might seem to be looking for a needle in a haystack when contemplating occupational factors for yet another lung cancer case, it is worth noting that estimates for occupational attributability vary between 0.6 and 40 per cent, depending on the place and the time. The most generally accepted estimates indicate that around 15 per cent of all lung cancers in men are due to occupational exposures, while a lower percentage has been

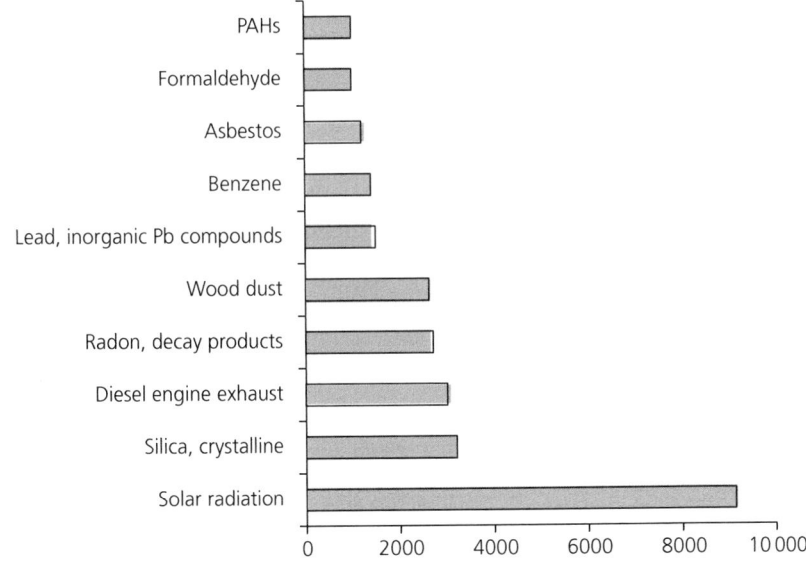

Figure 85.1 The ten most common occupational carcinogenic exposures (in thousands) among workers in the European Union (15 countries) in 1990–93.[11] Exposure to secondhand smoke with an estimated 7 500 000 exposed is not included in the graph.

Table 85.5 Mortality rates for lung cancer among asbestos-exposed workers in relation to their smoking habits (American Cancer Society cohort, United States and Canada). Mortality rates are adjusted for age (data from Ref. 14).

Asbestos	Tobacco smoking	Mortality rates (100 000 persons-years)
No	No	11.3
No	Yes	122.6
Yes	No	58.4
Yes	Yes	601.6

Rate ratios (exposed to asbestos versus non-exposed)
Smokers	4.91
Non-smokers	5.17

estimated in women.[5] In many countries, exposure to asbestos fibres has been the occupational exposure causing most lung cancers in the population.

For the clinician, the presenting features of lung cancer are all too well known and the confirmatory investigations usually demonstrate extensive and often inoperable spread at the time of diagnosis. The prognosis is frequently poor. Histopathologically, 90 per cent of all lung cancers are covered by four main categories: squamous, small cell, large cell and adenocarcinoma. Attempts to tease out a relationship between histopathology and putative lung carcinogens have not proved particularly successful. For example, adenocarcinoma or small cell carcinoma predominate in beryllium-exposed cases, while small cell types are in excess in uranium miners and in patients with exposure to bis(chloromethyl) ether, but this biological specificity is the exception rather than the rule.

There are many proven causes of lung cancer. Table 85.6 shows substances, mixtures, occupations and industries that have been classified by the IARC as group 1 or group 2A carcinogens. The list includes exposure circumstances (occupations or industries). For many of them, the specific exposures cannot be identified with certainty. For example, epidemiological studies of painters have consistently found increases in the risk of lung cancer, and studies evaluating mechanisms have frequently identified increased levels of genetic damage among painters. The specific exposures, however, causing these increases are not well identified since painters are exposed to numerous chemical solvents, pigments and additives and are also exposed to other hazards, such as asbestos and crystalline silica. The available information in the epidemiological studies is not detailed enough to identify specific agents as the cause of the excess lung cancer. A similar situation is observed in the rubber industry where studies, particularly those conducted in earlier periods, have identified excess lung cancer risk without being able to specify which agents cause this increase.

Such a list (Table 85.6) is less extensive than many, but even as it stands it begs some questions. Arsenic exposure these days can occur in smelting metalliferous ores or manufacturing certain pesticides. As for nickel, it is in nickel refining that the excess risk of lung (and nasal sinus) cancer has been observed. The precise compound has not been fully elucidated, but the available evidence points to the carcinogenicity of nickel sulphate and of the combination of nickel sulphides and oxides encountered in the

Table 85.6 Substances, mixtures, occupations and industries associated with lung cancer (IARC group 1 and 2A).

Category	
Physical agents	Ionizing radiation and sources thereof, including, notably, x-rays, γ-rays, neutrons and radon gas
Respirable dusts and fibres	Asbestos
	Silica, crystalline
	Talc containing asbestiform fibres
Metal and metal compounds	Arsenic and arsenic compounds
	Beryllium and beryllium compounds
	Cadmium and cadmium compounds
	Chromium compounds, hexavalent
	Nickel compounds
Wood and fossil fuels and their byproducts	Diesel engine exhaust
	Coal tars and pitches
	Soots
Polycyclic aromatic hydrocarbons	Benz[a]anthracene
	Benzo[a]pyrene
	Dibenz[a,h]anthracene
Monomers	Bis(chloromethyl) ether and chloromethyl methyl ether (technical grade)
	Epichlorohydrin
Pesticides and related compounds	2,3,7,8-Tetrachlorodibenzo-para-dioxin(TCDD)
	Non-arsenical insecticides
Others	Involuntary (passive) smoking
	Mustard gas
	Strong inorganic acids
Chlorinated hydrocarbons	α-Chlorinated toluenes
Occupation or industry	Aluminium production
	Coal gasification
	Coke production
	Hairdressers and barbers
	Hematite mining underground with radon exposure
	Iron and steel founding
	Painters
	Production of art glass, glass containers and pressed ware
	Rubber industry

Data from Siemiatycki et al.[4]

nickel refining industry. However, an exhaustive review of the processes, feedstock and procedures at the Clydach nickel refinery in South Wales over a 70-year period suggests that the main culprit in the lung and nasal cancer excess might be nickel arsenide. For chromium, it appears that the sparingly soluble hexavalent chromium compounds are the culprits and of these, the pigments, strontium, calcium and zinc chromate seem to be the most potent. Evidence of excess lung cancer in chrome platers suggests that chromic acid may be carcinogenic to humans as well. Ionizing radiation exposure also subsumes many studies of underground miners of metalliferous ores where relevant exposure is probably related to radon gas. These include uranium, haematite and exposures in tin mining.

The interest in the carcinogenicity of the chloromethyl ethers (which are of importance in the production of ion exchange resins) is out of proportion to their incidence. These chemicals seem to be particularly potent lung carcinogens, producing symptomatic neoplastic change in as short a latency period as 10–15 years, and with relative risks for heavily exposed workers as high as 20-fold. Their apparent association with small cell carcinoma has already been noted.

Polycyclic aromatic hydrocarbons are well-known lung (and skin) carcinogens and their presence in soot, tar, pitch and petroleum product exhaust fumes provides a potential opportunity for a wide variety of workplace exposures. The relevant worksites include gas retort and coke oven processes, the steel industry, the printing industry, aluminium refining sites, iron and steel foundries, as well as the motor vehicle transport industry and possibly the rubber industry. Chimney sweeping has re-emerged as an occupation at risk of cancer, as recent studies in Sweden and Denmark have shown a lung cancer excess in chimney sweeps. Welders are potentially exposed to a wide variety of gases and fumes, including nickel, chromium (VI) and nitrogen oxides.

The evidence for beryllium being a lung carcinogen rests, to some extent, on the excess risk associated with relatively short (one to five years) exposure and a latency period of two decades. Some authorities doubted the biological relevance of such short exposures, but it appears that these exposures were short because the affected individuals developed acute berylliosis. The exposures would therefore have been high and the inhaled dose, if not readily removed, could have lain there long enough to induce neoplastic change.

There is extensive epidemiological evidence associating exposure to silica with lung cancer. The IARC has evaluated crystalline silica as a group I human carcinogen,[15] based on lung cancer findings across a large number of existing occupational studies and positive animal studies. In many studies, the excess seems to be found in silicotics, but not in silica-exposed workers without silicosis. Whether this simply reflects an average higher exposure to silica among the silicotics, the role of fibrosis or itself as an intermediate stage in the causation of cancer remains unclear. Although evidence is not entirely consistent, it

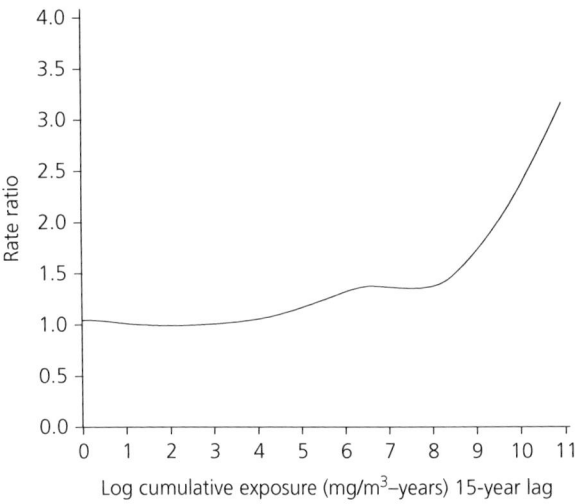

Figure 85.2 Lung cancer and silica exposure in the IARC international study. Spline curve showing log lung cancer rate ratio versus log cumulative exposure to silica in mg/m^3-years, applying a 15-year lag. With kind permission from Springer Science and Business Media: Cancer Causes and Control. Pooled exposure–response analyses and risk assessment for lung cancer in 10 cohorts of silica-exposed workers: An IARC multicentre study. 12: 2001; 773. Steenland K, Mannetje A, Boffetta P et al.

appears that lung cancer occurs only after considerable exposure to silica and this may not necessarily have to follow a diagnosis of silicosis. The most informative study evaluating dose–response is a pooled analysis of ten large silica-exposed cohorts with around 65 000 workers and 1000 lung cancer deaths.[16] This multicentric study found a significant positive exposure–response trend with cumulative silica exposure (Figure 85.2), but the lung cancer rate ratios did not increase in categorical analyses until after a cumulative exposure of 2 mg/m^3-years. Overall, there are still many inconsistencies in findings of different cohorts. For example, a recent study from the United Kingdom[17] did not identify an increased risk among workers in the industrial sand industry. These inconsistencies probably are due to several factors, including differences in the specific mineralogical properties of the silica that might result in varying levels of toxicity, and also may be due to differences in exposure levels. This is particularly so since exposure–response analysis showed that silica is not a strong lung carcinogen compared with the classic occupational carcinogens, such as nickel, arsenic and asbestos and that risk increases only after considerable exposure occurs.

The first modern description of pathology (fibrosis) associated with exposure to the naturally occurring crystalline fibres of asbestos, in its different varieties, goes back to the beginning of the twentieth century,[18] soon after the start of the mining and the exploitation of asbestos on an industrial scale. In 1931, this led to the Asbestos Industry Regulations to control exposure to asbestos dust. The first cases of pulmonary carcinomas superimposed on asbestosis were reported in the mid-1930s. The first clear epidemiological evidence of an increased risk of lung cancer from exposure to asbestos in a textile industry came, in the early 1950s, from a historical cohort study in a British factory, where 11 cases of lung cancer against an expectation of less than one were observed. This seminal paper by Sir Richard Doll,[19] confirmed by numerous other studies,[20] studied asbestos insulation workers in New Jersey and found a seven-fold excess of lung cancer. By the end of the 1960s, it had been shown that the lung cancer excess, in many circumstances of exposure to asbestos fibres, reflected an interactive effect of asbestos and tobacco smoking. Although asbestos use has been banned in many industrialized countries there remains a risk of exposure to unrecognized residual asbestos. An evaluation of exposure to carcinogens in Europe through the CAREX system[11] identified that those working in the construction industry were the primary occupations exposed in Europe. However, of even more concern is the exposure to asbestos in developing countries.[21] Precise estimates are not available of the number of workers in developing countries who are exposed to occupational carcinogens. Official statistics of the number of workers in specific industries are not fully reliable, since they may not cover major sections of the workforce, such as artisans, small-scale industrial production and illegal and migrant workers. At present, asbestos production is mainly done outside Western Europe, Australia and the United States,[22] with Russia, Brazil and Kazakhstan being among the largest producers (Table 85.7). Among industrialized countries, only Canada has been producing asbestos on a large scale and has mostly been exporting this production to developing countries.

Mention must be made of the controversy surrounding the carcinogenic potential of the asbestos substitute products, such as synthetic mineral fibres. For the clinician, it may well emerge that a worker with a history of using the newer insulation material was, in a previous job, using the older insulation products – namely, asbestos. This may even apply to those engaged in manufacture rather than use. Early cohort studies have found an elevated risk of lung cancer among rock and slag wool production workers.[23] However, retrospective analyses including nested case–control studies indicate that exposure to man-made mineral fibres is not associated with lung cancer risk.

A nested case–control study within the IARC multicentric study included 133 lung cancer cases and 513 matched controls in seven plants in Denmark, Norway, Sweden and Germany. After adjusting for smoking, there was no association with level of exposure to rock and slag wool fibres.[24]

Many of the above assertions on occupations are disputed and the arguments revolve around the quality of the human epidemiological studies. Nevertheless, the clinician has plenty of occupational aetiologies to consider even when contemplating the cause of a common tumour predominantly associated with cigarette smoking.

Urinary bladder

The occupational exposures classified by the IARC as being associated with a higher risk of bladder cancer are listed in Table 85.8. Aromatic amines, PAHs and diesel engine exhaust are the exposures most consistently found to

Table 85.7 Main countries currently producing asbestos (in tonnes). Data from World Mineral Production, 1999–2003.[22]

Country	2001	2002	2003
World	1900	2000	2000
Russia	735	775	878
Kazakhstan	271	291	353
Brazil	173	195	231
China	258	220	210
Canada	262	216	174
Zimbabwe	119	168	130

Table 85.8 Occupational carcinogens, occupations and industries that have been associated with bladder cancer, classified by the strength of the evidence. Included are definite (group 1) and probable (group 2A), as well as selected possible carcinogens (2B) as classified by IARC (data from Ref. 4).

Evidence strength	
Strong evidence	Aluminium production
	4-Aminobiphenyl
	Arsenic and inorganic arsenic compounds
	Auramine manufacture
	Benzidine
	Dyes metabolized to benzidine
	Magenta manufacture
	2-Naphthylamine
	Ortho-toluidine
	Painters
	Rubber industry
Suggestive evidence	Benz[a]anthracene
	Benzo[a]pyrene
	Boot and shoe manufacture and repair
	4-Chloro-ortho-toluidine
	Coal tars and pitches
	Coke production
	Dibenz[a,h]anthracene
	Diesel engine exhaust
	Dry cleaning (group 2B)
	Hairdressers and barbers
	4,4'-Methylene bis(2-chloroaniline)
	Petroleum refining
	Printing processes (group 2B)
	Soots (chimney sweeping)
	Tetrachloroethylene
	Textile manufacturing industry (group 2B)

increase the risk. Occupational exposures had been identified in the past as the second most important risk factor for bladder cancer after smoking.[25,26] Studies in the 1980s and 1990s suggest that certain high-risk occupations may be responsible for 4–10 per cent of bladder cancer cases in men[27] and a lower percentage in women.[28]

Aromatic amines are among the first identified occupational carcinogens. In 1954, a study among dyestuff-manufacturing workers in the United Kingdom was the first large occupational epidemiology study directly examining aromatic amines.[29] Exposure to b-naphthylamine entailed a 90-fold and to benzidine a 14-fold excess risk of bladder cancer. Numerous other studies of dyestuff-manufacturing workers confirmed these findings[30] and provided analyses of the exposure–response patterns for these chemicals. Among workers manufacturing aromatic amines, including b-naphthylamine, benzidine, 4-aminobiphenyl and 4-o-toluidine, relative risks ranging from 6 to 70 have been found. Findings for users of dyes are less consistent.[31] An excess risk of bladder cancer identified in the rubber industry in the early 1950s[32] was associated with the use of an antioxidant containing b-naphthylamine (Figure 85.3). The withdrawal of this compound in the rubber industry led to a reduction of bladder cancer risk among rubber workers, although an excess risk in the order of 50 per cent (Figure 85.4) appears to persist.[33] Aromatic amines are present in lower quantities in many other occupations, including aluminium production, hairdressing, painting, printing and shoemaking.

A moderately increased risk of bladder cancer has been associated with heavy exposure to PAHs, particularly from coal tars and pitches, and to diesel exhaust,[34] although the evidence is not entirely consistent. Exposure to PAH is high for workers in several industries, such as the pot rooms in aluminium production, coal gasification, roofing, road paving and the transport industry. Many case–control studies provided evidence of excess risk among transport workers exposed to engine exhausts, including diesel exhausts.[35] Cohort studies among workers exposed to diesel engine exhaust, such as taxi and truck drivers and operators of heavy equipment, however, have not confirmed a positive relationship between exposure to PAHs or diesel exhausts and bladder cancer risk.

Employment in several occupations has been identified as entailing an increased bladder cancer risk. Among the most consistent findings are those for painters, machinists, mechanics, workers in the metal industry such as sheet metal work and blacksmiths, workers in the textile industry, leather work and shoemaking, hairdressing, dry cleaning and transport work. These occupational relationships reflect, in part, past exposure to chemicals not currently used, such as benzidine or b-naphthylamine, but also more current exposures, possibly to aromatic amines, PAHs, cutting oils and solvents. Among the most consistent findings are those for painters.[10] A recent meta-analysis,[36] which included more than 2900 incident cases or deaths from bladder cancer among painters reported in 41 studies, identified a summary relative risk for bladder cancer in painters of 1.25 (95 per cent confidence interval (CI) 1.2–1.3; 41 studies) overall and 1.28 (95 per cent CI, 1.2–1.4; 27 studies) when including only estimates that were adjusted for smoking. Exposure–response analyses suggested that the risk increased with duration of employment. Metal workers are exposed to a heterogeneous group of potential carcinogens, including cuttings oils (a category including numerous agents), PAHs, metal fumes and dusts, as well as combustion gases and vapours. In European Union countries, metal workers appear to be the largest occupational group associated with increased bladder cancer risk.[27] An excess risk associated with metal working, although only moderately high, is among the most consistent epidemiologic findings. An elevated risk of bladder cancer has frequently been found among aluminium smelter workers, blacksmiths, foundry workers, furnace operators, machinists, welders and others.[37,38]

Various studies have also observed excess risks in white-collar occupations, such as sales workers, even after adjusting for potential confounding variables, an observation

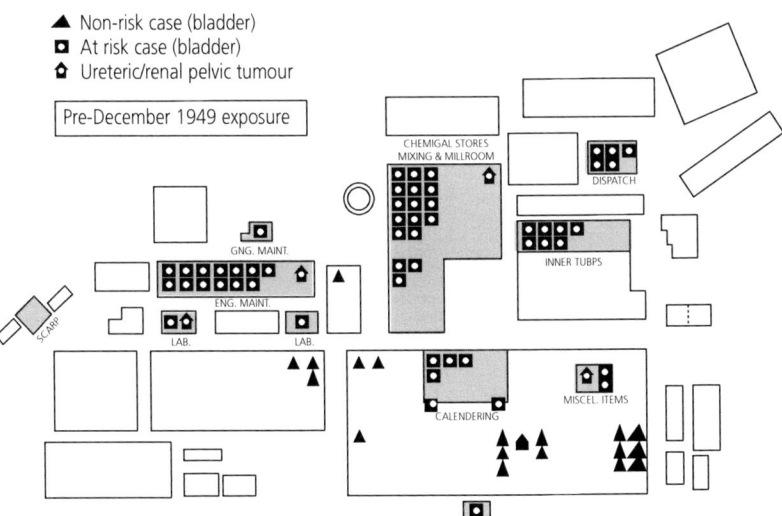

Figure 85.3 Map of rubber tyre production in England and deaths from bladder cancer (squares and triangles). Shaded areas indicate departments of the plant where 2-naphthylamine exposure occurred. From Veys CA, Bladder tumours in rubber workers: A factory study 1946–1995. *Occupational Medicine* 2004; **54**: 322 by permission of Oxford University Press.

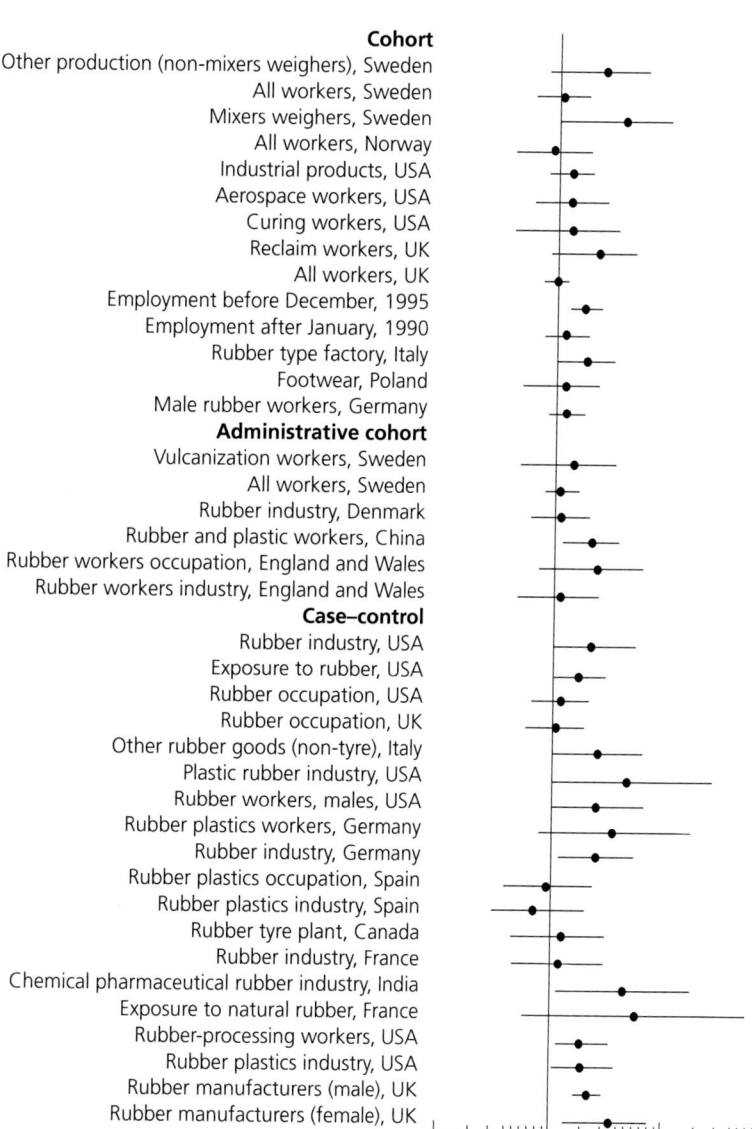

Figure 85.4 Bladder cancer risk in workers employed in the rubber industry. Odds ratios (95% CIs) for studies including greater than five exposed cases. For information on the studies cited in the artwork, see Ref. 33. Reproduced from *Occupational and Environmental Medicine*, Kogevinas M, Sala M, Boffetta P et al. 55, 1–12, 1998 with permission from BMJ Publishing Group Ltd.

compatible with the socioeconomic pattern of this disease.[39] These excess risks are difficult to attribute directly to exposures in the workplace and may be more likely related to general lifestyle factors. Less consistent are the findings for people in numerous other occupations, such as construction workers, electrical fitters, engine drivers, food processors and preservers, garage workers, plumbers and welders, railway workers, slaughterers and meat processors, cooks and waiters.

An open question is whether occupational exposures in industries identified in the past as high risk can still be linked to an excess risk of bladder cancer. In a pooled analysis,[27] attributable risks were higher for subjects first employed in a high-risk occupation before the 1950s than for those employed later. The attributable risk was also related to age, with higher estimates for people younger than 50 years.

Mesothelioma

Mesothelioma of the peritoneum and pleura has been shown to occur following both environmental and occupational (mining) exposure to crocidolite in South Africa and was subsequently shown to occur also after exposure to other varieties of asbestos. Although the risk of both lung cancer and mesothelioma have been documented for all main varieties of asbestos (chrysotile – the most widely used variety – amosite and crocidolite), several issues still remain open. For example, data are inadequate for quantitative comparisons on a fibre by fibre basis, and on a mass basis, between the potency of different fibres in respect of lung cancer and mesothelioma.

An estimation from an International Expert Meeting on Asbestos, Asbestosis and Cancer in 1997 indicated that around 10 000 cases of mesothelioma in Western Europe,

North America, Japan and Australia could be attributed to asbestos exposure.[40] Mesothelioma is strongly related to exposure to asbestos fibres and mortality from mesothelioma can be taken as an indicator of past exposure to mesothelioma. An international ecological analysis (Figure 85.5) of mesothelioma mortality in men in 32 countries showed a very close correlation with historical consumption of asbestos with an R^2 of 0.74 and p value <0.0001.[41]

Some salient features emerge from the long epidemiological history of asbestos in the working environment. First, there was a substantial lag between the first clinical case reports of cancers (in the mid-1930s) and the epidemiological evidence (mid-1950s), which led to an even longer delay in taking cancer into account when establishing hygiene standards. Second, the large volume of studies on a variety of exposed workers – such as miners and millers, textile workers, shipyard workers, including replicated cohort studies in several countries, which have contributed substantive evidence on the carcinogenic role of asbestos (and mineral fibres in general) – prompted methodological developments in occupational epidemiology and played a central role in demonstrating the need to prevent occupational cancers, as well as the effectiveness of exposure controls. Third, and notwithstanding this mass of data, there is a residual substantial uncertainty in the quantitative exposure–response relationships, which is in part likely to persist for ever, as in any case the information accruing from a longer follow up of worker cohorts is limited by the mediocre quality of past exposure measurements (while today exposure levels have been lowered and should, hopefully, produce no detectable effects). Finally, although asbestos has now been banned in most industrialized countries, there is still an observed increase in deaths from mesothelioma, due to the long latency period between exposure and occurrence of mesothelioma. An analysis of time trends in mesothelioma mortality in Britain in 1995[42] resulted in a prediction that the peak of deaths from mesothelioma would occur around 2020 (Figure 85.6).

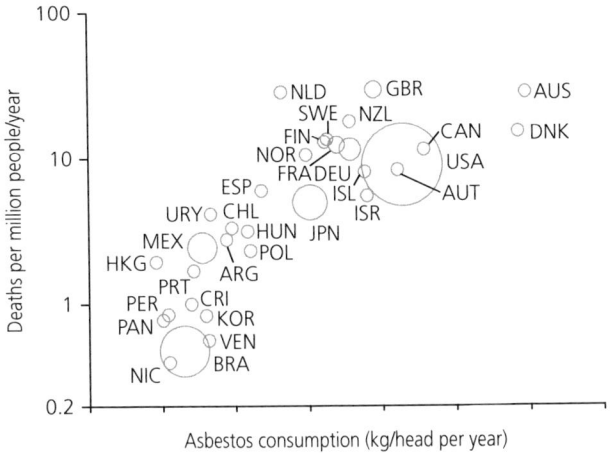

Figure 85.5 Ecological relations between current mortality rates from mesothelioma in men (deaths per million persons per year) and historical asbestos consumption weighted by the size of sex-specific national populations in 32 countries. Reprinted from *The Lancet* **369**, Lin RT, Takahashi K, Karjalainen A et al., Ecological association between asbestos-related diseases and historical asbestos consumption: An international analysis, 844–9, Copyright (2007), with permission from Elsevier.[41]

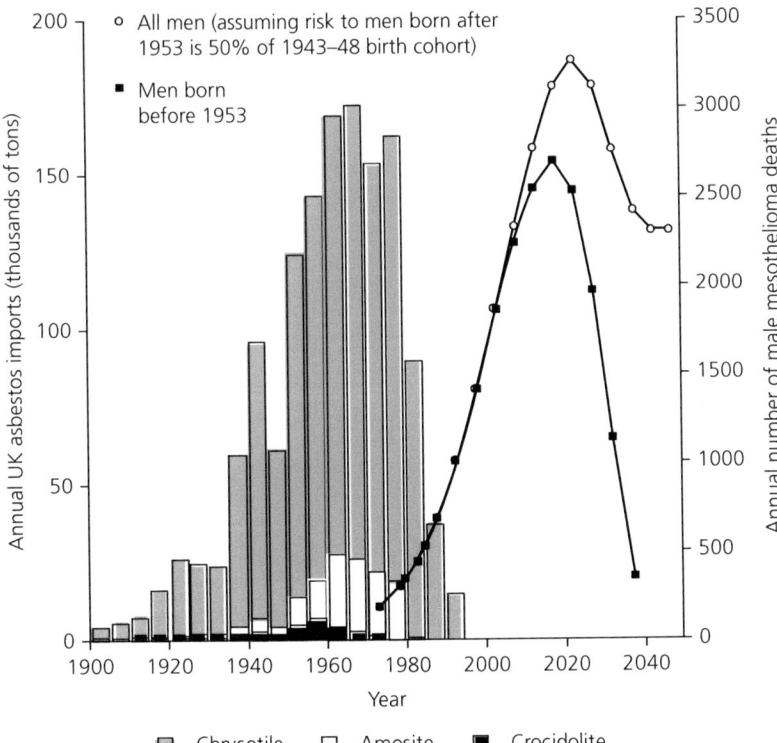

Figure 85.6 Predicted mesothelioma deaths in British men and UK asbestos imports. Reprinted from *The Lancet*, **345**, Peto J, Matthews FE, Hodgson JT, Jones JR, Continuing increase in mesothelioma mortality in Britain, 535–9, Copyright (1995), with permission from Elsevier.[42]

Haematopoietic system

Tumours of the blood-forming organs make up a complex group in which frequent changes in the nomenclature add to the complexity. Ionizing radiation is associated with non-lymphocytic leukaemia, multiple myeloma and non-Hodgkin's lymphoma. Non-Hodgkin's lymphoma has been associated with exposure phenoxy acid herbicides and dioxins,[10,43] benzene and some chlorinated organic compounds, such as trichloroethylene, tetrachloroethylene and polychlorinated biphenyls. The main occupational exposures with any degree of certainty of neoplastic effect are, however, associated with leukaemia.

LEUKAEMIAS

Leukaemias are a heterogeneous group of diseases. Epidemiological studies tended to group all leukaemias in one category. Recently, the use of new molecular techniques has resulted in new classifications and leukaemias are evaluated separately for the myeloid and lymphoid lineage. It is noteworthy that chronic lymphocytic leukaemia (CLL) is currently classified as a B-cell lymphoma.

Occupational ionizing radiation has been consistently associated with myeloid leukaemia through studies on radiologists and x-ray technicians working in the first half of the twentieth century.[44,45] A combined recent analysis of approximately half a million nuclear workers[46] indicated a small excess for myeloid leukaemia. Of special interest is the consistent finding of an increased risk of leukaemia associated with 'electrical' occupations. While electricians, telephone, radio and telegraphic staff are potentially exposed to a number of volatile solvents and resins, much interest has now centred on the possible role of electromagnetic field exposure in the leukaemogenic process. Improved exposure assessments and control of confounding factors has enhanced the quality of the latest studies. The best available studies indicate that there is no evidence that exposure to non-ionizing radiation and specifically extremely low frequency electromagnetic fields is associated with myeloid leukaemia (see Chapter 55, Extremely low frequency electric and magnetic fields).[47]

Benzene has been the first chemical agent identified to cause leukaemia and specifically acute myeloid leukaemia.[48] Numerous case reports and series have suggested a relationship between exposure to benzene and the occurrence of various types of leukaemia. Early studies in Finland[49] and more widely known studies in Turkey[50] identified increased leukaemia risks among shoe and other workers exposed to benzene. These studies were confirmed with both cohort and case–control studies, including the key pliofilm cohort which has been extensively used for benzene risk assessment.[51,52] Numerous studies in the last 20 years which have followed earlier or new cohorts with quantitative data on benzene exposure show fairly consistent dose–response relationship between exposure to benzene and risk of acute myeloid leukaemia.[10] Recent mechanistic studies have provided convincing evidence on the haematotoxicity of benzene at low exposure levels.[53]

Workplace exposures identified as being associated with a leukaemia risk – at least in the past – include much of the petrochemical industry. Apart from the chemical industry and exposure to benzene, there are several other occupations and industries with increased risks of leukaemia including painters, those working in the rubber industry and those working with formaldehyde.[54] A variety of other chemicals have been implicated as possible leukaemogens. Apart from the antineoplastic drugs, the most frequently cited chemicals are styrene, butadiene, epichlorhydrin and ethylene oxide. The source studies are often small, however, or the workplace exposures are confounded by benzene. An increased risk among farm workers has been identified in many countries, but the evidence is not consistent. The potential exposures among farmers include pesticides or exposure to biological agents.[55]

Chronic lymphocytic leukaemia is currently classified together with lymphomas (B-cell lymphoma). CLL is not associated with ionizing radiation.[56] There is little evidence that CLL is associated with chemical exposures. Recently, the IARC evaluated that there is limited evidence that benzene is associated with CLL. There is some evidence of an increased risk associated with exposure to styrene[57] and also limited evidence that CLL is associated with exposure to ethylene oxide from studies in nurses or other exposed workers.[10,58,59]

Acute lymphocytic leukaemia (ALL) is more common in young ages. There exists some evidence that ALL in children may be associated with parental exposure to pesticides and solvents. The IARC recently evaluated that there is limited evidence that exposure to benzene in the workplace is associated with ALL. However, this evidence is based on studies in adults with relatively small number of cases.[10]

The investigation of a possible occupational aetiology for the leukaemia patient can frequently be a difficult one. In our experience, while the disease is in no doubt, the exclusion of cytotoxic drug exposure, as well as benzene and ionizing radiation, provides little opportunity for further progress. Nevertheless, the patients are frequently younger than many with occupationally associated cancers and the failure to identify a causative agent is frustrating for the physician and harrowing for the patient.

Non-melanocytic skin cancer

There are three major forms of skin cancer, basal cell carcinoma (BCC), squamous cell carcinoma (SCC) and melanoma. Skin cancer has been historically one of the first cancers related to occupation, with the description by Percival Pott in the late eighteenth century of a higher incidence of cancer in the scrotum among chimney sweeps due to their exposure to soot. Sunlight exposure is the main risk factor for these cancers and many occupations currently at high risk for skin cancer are those with high

Table 85.9 Agents or mixtures classified by the IARC as carcinogens (group 1) or probable carcinogens (group 2A) associated with basal cell or squamous cell carcinoma of the skin (data from Ref. 4).

Agent/mixture	Occupation or industry where the exposure occurs	IARC classification
Solar radiation	Outdoor work	1
Arsenic and arsenic compounds	Non-ferrous metal smelting, production, packaging and use of arsenic-containing pesticides, sheep dip manufacture, wool fibre production, mining of ores containing arsenic	1
Coal tars and pitches	Production of refined chemicals and coal tar products (patent-fuel), coke production, coal gasification, aluminium production, foundries, road paving and construction (roofers and slaters)	1
Mineral oils, untreated or mildly treated	Production, used as lubricant by metal workers, machinists, engineers, printing industry (ink formulation), used in cosmetics, medicinal and pharmaceutical preparations	1
Shale oils or shale-derived lubricants	Mining and processing, used as fuels or chemical-plant lubricants, feedstocks, lubricant in cotton textile industry	1
Soots	Chimney sweeps, heating-unit service personnel, brick masons and helpers, building demolition workers, insulators, fire-fighters, metallurgical workers, work involving burning of organic materials	1
Benzo(a)anthracene, Benzo(a)pyrene, Dibenzo(a,h)anthracene	Work involving combustion of organic matter, foundries, steel mills, fire-fighters, vehicle mechanics	1, 2A
Creosote	Brick making, wood preserving	2A

exposure to ultraviolet radiation.[60] There are no reliable data worldwide on the incidence of keratinocyte cancers of the skin (BCC and SCC). In the United States, it has been estimated that about one million cancers occur annually. The highest incidence rates are observed among white-skinned populations. In this chapter, we will focus on BCC and SCC since the link of melanoma with occupational exposures is still uncertain.

Apart for solar radiation, BCC and SCC have been associated with several other occupational exposures, including mineral oils and coal-tar containing products, although risks nowadays tend to be relatively low in industrialized countries. The agents or mixtures classified by the IARC as carcinogens (group 1) or probable carcinogens (group 2A) and that have been associated with non-melanocytic skin cancer are shown in Table 85.9.

Squamous cell carcinoma has been most clearly associated with cumulative exposure to solar radiation, while the association with BCC is less clear and possibly associated with intermittent exposure to high doses. Epidemiological studies examining workplace exposure to solar radiation and non-melanocytic skin cancer are shown in Table 85.10. In most studies, workers most exposed to solar radiation are at higher risk of skin cancer, although these risks are frequently not very high and not statistically significant. Of the 13 studies published before 2008, six found an increased risk among outdoor workers compared to those working indoors. Five more studies identified a positive association, although this was not statistically significant. Finally, two studies evaluated the risk of BCC and SCC in relation to specific occupations.[61,62] The study by Suarez et al. was carried out in several EU countries and identified high risks for non-melanocytic skin cancer (NMSC) among miners and quarrymen, secondary education teachers and masons (Table 85.10). Railway engine drivers and firemen, specialized farmers and salesmen were associated with BCC only. Occupations with a high risk for SCC only were those involving direct contact with livestock, masons and others. In a study from the United States,[62] elevated risks of both BCC and SCC in men were found among groundskeepers and gardeners, except farm and for garage and service station-related occupations for BCC only. Women in health service occupations had elevated risks for both tumours, and administrative support occupations were related only to BCC risk. Only one study[71] provided measurements of ultraviolet (UV) radiation and estimated cumulative dose, while the remaining studies base the evaluation of exposure on questionnaires. A recent evaluation of occupational cancer in the United Kingdom[74] identified occupational exposure to solar radiation, mineral oils and coal tars/pitches as the main occupational causes of skin cancer.

Other cancers

CANCERS OF THE SINUSES AND NASAL CAVITY

Cancers of the sinuses and nasal cavity are rare neoplasms with an incidence of around one per 100 000 per year and are strongly associated with occupational exposures. Classical early studies in the 1950s identified a higher risk among nickel refiners who had worked at the Clydach plant in South Wales before certain process changes occurred in the late 1920s. An early study also identified a high risk of ethmoid

Table 85.10 Studies on non-melanocytic skin cancer and solar radiation exposure in the work environment.

Author, year	Place	Type study	Cancer	Results (odds ratios and 95% CI)
Lancaster and Nelson[63]	Australia	Case–control	NMSC	OR = 1.9 for 5–10 years occupational exposure OR = 4.2 for >10 years
Silverstone and Searle[64]	Queensland, Australia	Cross-sectional	NMSC	OR outdoor work = 1.29 ($p > 0.1$)
Aubry and MacGibbon[65]	Montreal, Canada	Case–control	SCC	OR = 1.08 moderate occupational exposure OR = 1.64 high occupational exposure
O'Loughlin et al.[66]	Ireland	Case–control	NMSC	OR = 1.5 (not significant) outdoor work
Green et al.[67]	Queensland, Australia	Cross-sectional	NMSC	OR = 1.01 (0.44–2.31) indoor and outdoor OR = 1.79 (0.77–4.05) outdoor work
Hogan et al.[68]	Canada	Case–control	BCC	OR = 1.29 (1.12–1.46) farmers OR = 1.13 (1.01–1.27) outdoor work >3 hours/day in winter
Marks et al.[69]	Australia	Cohort	NMSC	Outdoor work: CB: OR = 1.6 (significant) CE: OR = 1.7 (not significant)
Green and Battistutta[70]	Queensland, Australia	Cross-sectional	NMSC	OR = 1.5 (0.8–2.9) indoor and outdoor OR = 1.3 (0.6–2.8) outdoor work
Vitasa et al.[71]	United States	Cross-sectional, fishermen	NMSC	Dose above median: CE: OR = 2.05 (0.84–5.01) CB: OR = 0.69 (0.31–1.53)
Freedman et al.[72]	United States	Case–control	NMSC	OR = 0.95 (0.85–1.05) indoor and outdoor OR = 1.14 (0.96–1.36) outdoor work
Freedman et al.[73]	United States	Case–control (1985–1995)	NMSC	OR = 1.01 (0.93–1.09) indoor and outdoor OR = 1 OR = 1
Marehbian et al.[62]	United States	Case–control	NMSC	Trend by duration of employment: OR >1 gardeners (male) (p-trend <0.05) CB: OR > 1 mechanics (male) (p-trend <0.05) CE: OR > 1 farmers (male) (p-trend <0.05) CB: OR > 1 administrative women (p-trend <0.05)
Suarez et al.[61]	Europe, multicentric	Cancer registry based	BCC	OR = 1.76 (1.02–2.94) professors (secondary) OR = 3.02 (1.05–8.66) sales persons OR = 1.65 (1.05–2.59) farmers, specialized OR = 7.96 (2.72–23.23) miners and fire-fighters OR = 4.55 (0.96–21.57) train drivers
			SCC	OR = 2.11 (1.11–4.03) animal breeder OR = 3.64 (1.22–10.83) farmers (dairy) OR = 4.98 (1.23–20.18) miners OR = 2.41 (1.33–4.36) construction workers OR = 2.53 (1.03–6.23) construction OR = 4.75 (1.33–16.92) machine operators

BCC, basal-cell carcinoma; NMSC, non-melanocytic skin cancer; SCC, squamous cell carcinoma.

sinus cancer in furniture makers in Buckinghamshire. This study led to a major epidemiological exercise involving data linkage in the Oxford region. A further cluster of mixed cell type, mixed-site sinus cancers emerged in the Northampton area, thus leading to the assertion that leather goods manufacture – in particular, boots and shoes – carried a risk of neoplasia of the sinuses and nasal cavity.

Since the 1960s, a large excess risk for sinonasal cancer, particularly adenocarcinomas, has been repeatedly documented among workers in wood-related occupations.[8,75,76]

A high risk for sinonasal cancer has also been identified among workers in the leather industry, workers exposed to formaldehyde, workers in nickel refining and those exposed to hexavalent chromium compounds and also studies in the textile industry. Besides these exposures, elevated risks for sinonasal cancer were found in case–control studies for a variety of other occupations.[77] Most studies, however, lacked the power to demonstrate statistically significant associations of this rare disease with specific jobs. Few other risk factors have been identified for

Table 85.11 Relative risk for sinonasal cancer in men by wood dust exposure category and histology. Pooled analysis of 12 case–control studies (data from Ref. 78).

Wood dust category	All histologies		Adenocarcinoma		Squamous	
	Exposed case-controls	OR (95% CI)	Exposed cases	OR (95% CI)	Exposed cases	OR (95% CI)
Men (any exposure)	216/567	2.2 (1.8–2.7)	119	14.9 (10.0–22.2)	59	0.9 (0.6–1.2)
Low exposure	14/83	0.8 (0.4–1.5)	1	0.6 (0.1–4.7)	6	0.5 (0.2–1.2)
Moderate exposure	76/402	1.2 (0.9–1.6)	14	3.1 (1.6–6.1)	42	1.0 (0.7–1.4)
High exposure	126/82	5.8 (4.2–8.0)	104	45.5 (28.3–72.9)	11	0.8 (0.4–1.6)

sinonasal cancer, apart from occupational exposures and smoking.

Studies that provided results by histology, mostly distinguishing squamous cell carcinoma and adenocarcinoma, indicate that some of the identified risk factors for sinonasal cancer are related to specific histological types. In a number of individual studies and in a pooled analysis of case–control studies,[78] the higher risk for wood workers was specifically associated with sinonasal adenocarcinoma (Table 85.11). The increased risks for smoking have mostly been found for squamous cell carcinomas and, in some cases, with undifferentiated carcinomas. The findings of this study indicate that the two major risk factors for sinonasal cancer (SNC) are tobacco smoking causing about 20 per cent of all SNCs and occupation causing about 30 per cent. These results also indicate that in the case of SNC specific exposures can be linked to morphology. Wood dust and, to a lesser extent, leather dust and formaldehyde were predominantly associated with adenocarcinomas, a pattern which appears to be specific to this tumour.

NASOPHARYNGEAL CANCER

Cancer of the nasopharynx is a very rare neoplasm with an incidence of less than one per 100 000 in most populations, although it is more common in some geographical regions and ethnic groups in Southeast Asia. Formaldehyde has been shown to be associated with cancer of the nasal cavity in rodents.[10] A large study in the United States among 25 619 workers (865 708 person-years) employed in ten US formaldehyde-producing or -using facilities among workers exposed to formaldehyde with extensive quantitative exposure assessment has shown an increased risk of nasopharyngeal cancer.[79] Although findings are not entirely consistent among studies, it is generally accepted that formaldehyde causes this cancer and the IARC has evaluated formaldehyde as a human carcinogen on the basis of this evidence.[10]

LARYNGEAL CANCER

Several occupations have been associated with increased risks of laryngeal cancers including truck drivers, leather workers, metal workers and others, but few of these findings have been consistent. Among carcinogens identified by IARC, only exposure to strong inorganic mists, including sulphuric acid, is accepted as a group 1 carcinogen causing laryngeal cancer. Industries with exposure to these acids include manufacture of isopropanol (isopropyl alcohol), synthetic ethanol (ethyl alcohol), sulphuric acid, nitric acid, phosphate fertilizer, soap, detergent, lead batteries, copper smelting, pickling and other acid treatment of metals. The strongest evidence comes from studies of workers in pickling operations within the steel industry both in Europe and the United States. There has been a long controversy about whether exposure to asbestos is associated with laryngeal cancer. In 2009, the IARC classified as sufficient the evidence on asbestos and laryngeal cancer.[80] The most comprehensive meta-analysis on laryngeal cancer,[81] including 27 asbestos-exposed occupational cohorts, identified a meta-SMRs of 1.3 (95 per cent CI, 1.1–1.6), which rose to 1.6 when a latency analysis was applied. However, there was no evidence of a dose–response effect. Several other exposures or exposure circumstances have been associated with an increased risk for laryngeal cancer, including exposure to sulphur mustard and employment in the rubber industry.[10]

STOMACH CANCER

The main clinical epidemiological feature of stomach cancer is the falling incidence of the condition in developed countries, which has been linked to better nutrition. *Helicobacter pylori* infection has been identified as one of the main risks for gastric cancer. Nitrosamines, which are proven and potent animal carcinogens, have been linked to human exposure in that the secondary amines in fish and preserved meat and vegetables could be converted to nitrosamines by gastric hydrochloric acid. Most epidemiologic studies of stomach cancer have focused on diet and lifestyle factors. There are numerous studies which have identified increased risks in various occupations and industries, including quarrymen and stone cutters, coal and metal miners, rubber workers, construction workers, chemical and petrochemical workers, workers exposed to dioxins and farmers.[10,82] The specific exposures evaluated are asbestos, coal dust and nitrogen oxides, mineral and metal dusts, wood dusts, nitrosamines and others.[82] However, the evidence is not convincing for any of these exposures.

HEPATOCELLULAR CARCINOMA

The most important causes of liver cancer are infections with hepatitis B and C viruses and exposure to aflatoxins that have been consistently shown to be risk factors for hepatocellular carcinoma. Recent evidence[83] has also shown that exposure to vinyl chloride is associated with hepatocellular carcinoma. Among the occupational exposures that are suspected to cause hepatocellular carcinoma are polychlorinated biphenyls and trichloroethylene. The available evidence, however, does not allow firm conclusions.

ANGIOSARCOMA OF THE LIVER

Angiosarcoma of the liver is a tumour that is extremely rare in the general population, and that has been unequivocally associated with exposure to vinyl chloride monomer. A case report of three cases of angiosarcoma of the liver in men who had been employed in the manufacture of PVC resins provided the first evidence of an association between vinyl chloride and cancer in humans.[84] The case report was particularly informative because of the rarity of the tumour. Epidemiological evidence for the carcinogenicity of vinyl chloride in humans derives principally from two large, multicentric cohort studies, one of which was carried out in the United States[85] and the other in Europe.[83] Both studies found a substantial increase in the relative risk for angiosarcoma of the liver, and the European study, which had carried out extensive quantitative exposure assessment, also showed a clear trend of higher risk with increasing cumulative exposure (Table 85.12).

CANCER OF THE PANCREAS

Occupational exposures associated with cancer of the pancreas include studies of chemists and also radiologists. In the latter case, the excess risk appears to be for those exposed before 1929. This cohort effect may thus be a legacy of earlier, less well-controlled workplace exposures, although the absence of such a finding from other large-scale studies of workers exposed to ionizing radiation weakens the assertion that this physical agent alone was the responsible carcinogen. Among the chemical agents suspected to cause pancreatic cancer are some chlorinated organic solvents and chlorinated pesticides, including DDT (dichlorodiphenyltrichloroethane). The most complete meta-analysis of occupational exposures to chlorinated hydrocarbon (CHC) solvents and pancreatic cancer[86] included 24 studies and was based primarily on studies that addressed exposure directly. Suggestive weak excesses were found for trichloroethylene (meta-relative risk (MRR) = 1.24, 95 per cent CI, 0.79, 1.97), polychlorinated biphenyls (MRR = 1.37, 95 per cent CI, 0.56, 3.31), methylene chloride (MRR = 1.42, 95 per cent CI, 0.80, 2.53) and vinyl chloride (MRR = 1.17, 95 per cent CI, 0.71, 1.91), but not for carbon tetrachloride. Job title studies on metal degreasing and dry cleaning revealed significant MRRs (2.0 and 1.4, respectively).

COLORECTAL CANCERS

Occupational exposures have rarely been implicated in colorectal cancers. There has, however, been a recent flurry of interest in whether workers in the polypropylene production industry could be at increased risk. However, earlier cluster reports appear not to be confirmed on further review. Intriguingly, a recent report suggests a tentative association between colorectal cancer and the manufacture of the anti-knock agent, tetraethyl lead. One of the few established risk factors of colon cancer, however, is lack of physical activity: since occupation is one of the main determinants of physical exercise in adult populations, it can be indirectly implicated in the causation of this neoplasm.

BRAIN TUMOURS

Brain tumours show a bimodal frequency distribution with a small peak in childhood and a second, larger peak in the seventh decade. The majority of adult malignant tumours are astrocytoma or undifferentiated glioblastoma. Mortality rates are rising in industrialized countries, but this may be, at least in part, due to improved accuracy of certification. Occupational factors have been invoked in recent years and both professional and manual occupations had been reported to be at increased risk. These include laboratory workers, petrochemical plant workers and embalmers. Potential chemical exposures include certain organic solvents, as well as ionizing radiation. Recent additions to this list might include lead, but the greatest interest of late has centred on the possibility that electric fields or magnetic fields (or both) from residential or occupational exposure might be associated with an increased risk of brain tumours. Thorough reviews of residential exposure studies and meta-analysis of the brain cancer risks from occupational exposures have failed to resolve

Table 85.12 Risk of angiosarcoma in the European cohort study of workers exposed to vinyl chloride monomer (VCM). Data from Ref. 83.

Exposure to vinyl chloride	No. cases	Relative risk and 95% CI
Cumulative exposure (ppm years)		
0–734	4	1.00
735–2379	6	6.56 (1.85–23.3)
2380–5188	8	13.6 (4.05–45.5)
5189–7531	7	28.0 (8.00–98.2)
≥7532	12	88.2 (26.4–295)
		Trend test, $p < 0.001$
Autoclave workers		
Never	4	1.0
Ever	6	25.5 (8.86–73.2)

the issue. Ongoing large international studies with extensive exposure assessment will provide new information (see Chapter 55, Extremely low frequency electric and magnetic fields).

BREAST CANCER

Breast cancer risk has been reported in women employed in jobs that entail exposure to organic solvents.[87] These include dry cleaners, hairdressers, aircraft maintenance, textiles, electronics manufacturing and others. In addition, animal experimentation has shown that organic solvents have been associated with mammary gland tumours in rodents. However, the overall evidence for an association between occupational exposure to organic solvents is weak.[88]

Studies in recent years have identified that women engaged in shift work may have an increased risk of breast cancer. About 15–20 per cent of the working population in Europe and the United States is engaged in shift work that involves night work. Shift work is more prevalent in some occupations, such as the healthcare, industrial manufacturing, mining, transport, communication, leisure and hospitality sectors. Night work is disruptive for the circadian clock. There are several rodent models that have shown an association of tumour development with a disruption of the circadian system and with reduced nocturnal melatonin concentrations or removal of the pineal gland where melatonin is produced.[89] Epidemiological studies on nurses engaged in shift work at night and of female flight attendants have shown a modest increased risk (Figure 85.7). Most of these studies suffer from potential uncontrolled confounding by reproductive factors and cosmic radiation. If these risks are proven, given the high prevalence of shift work and the high background incidence of breast cancer, night shift may prove to be among the most important occupation-related risk factors for cancer. Further research on potential modification of effect in relation to light intensity may help evaluate aetiology of the disease and also potential preventive measures.

Estimates of risk of cancer attributed to occupational exposures

There exist several estimates of the proportion of cancers that can be attributed to occupational exposures (Table 85.13). These include the estimates for the US population by Doll and Peto[5] and by Harvard University,[92] by Dreyer et al.[93] for the Nordic countries, by Nurminen and Karjalainen[91] for Finland, a recent estimation for the UK[74] and also estimates by the WHO (WHO Comparative Risk Assessment).[94] Attributable risk estimates have also been provided in specific countries/areas for selected cancers for the EU,[95] the United States[6] and France,[96] among others.

Two approaches have mainly been followed to estimate the proportion of occupational cancers among all cancers. One is based on the estimation of attributable risk fractions for specific cancers (usually based on case–control studies) that are then applied directly to the number of deaths from cancer (see, for example Ref. 5). The second is based on an estimation of the number of workers exposed, an evaluation of the cancer risk associated with each exposure and a subsequent estimation of the number of cancer cases or deaths attributed to this exposure (e.g. Ref. 74).

The most well-known estimates are those by Doll and Peto[5] for the population of the United States that concludes that 4 per cent of all cancers could be attributed to occupational exposures. This estimate is an average and may differ in subgroups of the population and for different types of cancer. Doll and Peto defined three categories of cancers: those definitely produced by occupational exposures with an attributable risk (AR) of more than 1 per cent, those possibly produced with an AR of 0.5–1 per cent and those not associated with occupational exposures. The first category included neoplasms of the mesentery and peritoneum, liver and intrahepatic bile ducts, larynx, lung, pleura, nasal sinuses and remaining respiratory, bone, skin other than melanoma, prostate, bladder and leukaemia. The attributable risks for each of these cancers are shown

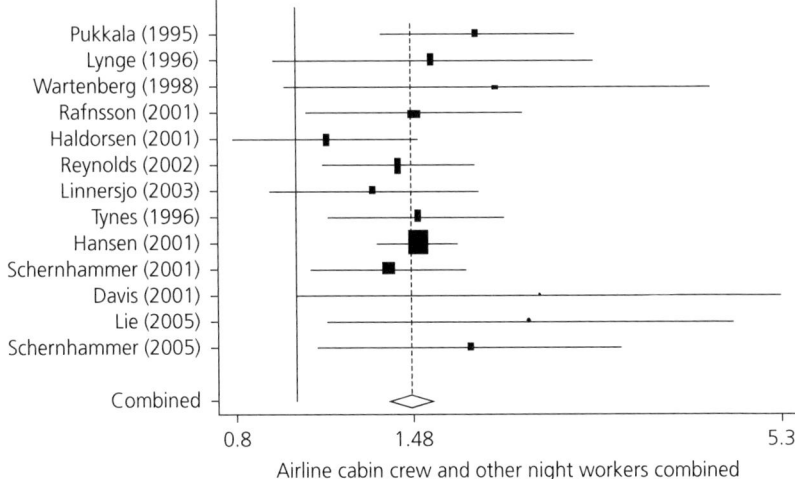

Figure 85.7 Meta-analysis of female night workers and breast cancer risk in 13 studies. Reprinted from *European Journal of Cancer*, 41, Megdal SP, Korenke CH, Laden F et al., Night work and breast cancer risk: A systematic review and meta-analysis, 2023–32, Copyright (2005), with permission from Elsevier.[90]

Table 85.13 Number of deaths per year from all cancers, lung cancer and bladder cancer in Europe and North America in 2002, attributable to occupational exposure according to different estimates. Estimates for number of deaths in each region were retrieved from GLOBOCAN (www-dep.iarc.fr/).

Cancer site (estimate)	Ref.	Percentage of deaths attributable to occupational exposures	Sex	Deaths (Europe)	Deaths (North America)
All cancers					
United States (35)	5	4	Both	68 059	25 279
Finland (122)	91	13.8	Male	132 238	45 709
		2.2	Female	16 351	6616
United Kingdom (144)	74	8	Male	76 660	26 498
		1.5	Female	11 148	4511
Lung cancer					
United States	5	15	Male	40 625	15 858
		5	Female	3538	3632
Finland	91	29	Male	78 541	30 658
		5.3	Female	3750	3849
United Kingdom	74	21.6	Male	58 499	22 835
		5.5	Female	3892	3995
Bladder cancer					
United States	5	10	Male	3827	952
		5	Female	625	217
Finland	91	14.2	Male	5435	1352
		0.7	Female	88	30
United Kingdom	74	11.6	Male	4440	1104
		2	Female	250	87

in Table 85.14. According to the Doll and Peto estimates, the proportion of cancer attributed to work is higher for men than for women, and also higher for manual workers compared to non-manual. It has been pointed out[97] that the 4 per cent estimated is much higher if this percentage is calculated for preventable cancers. The estimates of Doll and Peto were mainly based on studies evaluating exposure of the 1950s and 1960s and also reflected the knowledge on occupational carcinogens of that time. Since then, knowledge on occupational cancer has considerably expanded and has also included populations not previously studied, particularly women. This would tend to result in higher estimates of the attributable risk than those estimated by Doll and Peto. On the other hand, in industrialized countries exposure to 'classical' occupational carcinogens has been drastically reduced by controlling exposure in the work environment or by transporting dangerous occupations and industries to developing countries. This would tend to result in lower estimates of the attributable risk than those estimated by Doll and Peto.

Rushton et al.[74] provided for the population of the United Kingdom among the most complete and recent estimates of the proportion of cancer attributed to occupational exposures (Table 85.15). Attributable fractions and numbers were estimated for mortality and incidence in 2004 for bladder, lung, non-melanoma skin, sinonasal cancers, leukaemia and mesothelioma. The agents and occupations selected were those classified by the IARC as group 1 and 2A carcinogens. In 2004, 7317 deaths (4.9 per cent of the total) were estimated to be attributable to work-related carcinogens for the six cancers assessed. Of those, 6259 were in men (8 per cent) and 1058 in women (1.5 per cent). The estimates for cancer incidence were 13 338 cases (4.0 per cent) of the total cancer registrations. Of those, 11 284 were in men (6.7 per cent) and 2054 in women (1.2 per cent). The attributable risk percentages by cancer site are shown in Table 85.15. Asbestos contributed to over half the occupational attributable deaths, followed by silica, diesel engine exhaust, radon, work as a painter, mineral oils in metal workers and in the printing industry, environmental tobacco smoke (in non-smokers), work as a welder and dioxins. Occupational exposure to solar radiation, mineral oils and coal tars/pitches contributed significantly to skin cancer incidence. Industries and occupations that contributed a large number of deaths and/or registrations include construction, metal working, personal and household services, mining (not metals), land transport and services allied to transport, roofing, road repair/construction, printing, farming, the Armed Forces, some other service industry sectors and manufacture of transport equipment, fabricated metal products, machinery, non-ferrous metals and metal products, and chemicals.

Table 85.14 Attributable risks for cancers definitely associated with occupation according to the evaluation by Doll and Peto.[5]

Cancers definitely associated with workplace exposures	Sex	Percentage attributed to work (%)
Mesentery and peritoneum (including mesothelioma)	Male	15
	Female	5
Liver and intrahepatic bile ducts (including angiosarcoma)	Male	4
	Female	1
Larynx	Male	2
	Female	1
Lung	Male	15
	Female	5
Nasal sinuses	Male	25
	Female	5
Bone	Male	4
	Female	1
Skin (non-melanoma)	Male	10
	Female	2
Prostate	Male	1
Bladder	Male	10
	Female	5
Leukaemia	Male	10
	Female	5

Table 85.15 Estimated attributable fractions, deaths and registrations by cancer site in 2004 (2003 for registrations) in the UK for established and uncertain carcinogens (IARC group 1 and 2A carcinogens). Data from Ref. 74.

Cancer site	Attributable fraction (%)		Total
	Male	Female	
Bladder	11.6	2.0	8.3
Leukaemia	2.7	0.8	1.7
Lung	21.6	5.5	15.0
Mesothelioma	98	90	97
NMSC	11.8	3.0	8.4
Sinonasal	64.3		
Total based on deaths	8.0	1.5	4.9
Total based on registrations	6.7	1.2	4.0

Other estimates (Table 85.13) include those by Harvard University that used a very similar approach to that of Doll and Peto and concludes that 5 per cent of all cancer can be attributed to occupational carcinogens. The evaluation of Dreyer for the Nordic countries in 1997 estimates lower percentages of about 3 per cent for men and less than 1 per cent for women. The evaluation by Nurminen and Karjalainen[91] for Finland is among the most extensive and calculates that around 8 per cent of all cancers can be attributed to occupation. Kogevinas et al.[95] conducted pooled analyses of epidemiological studies in EU countries for four cancers (lung, bladder, larynx, sinonasal) including more than 13 000 subjects. They found similar estimates as those proposed by Doll and Peto.

The number of cancer deaths (all cancers, lung cancer, bladder cancer) attributed to occupational exposures using the estimates by Doll and Peto, Nurminen and Karjalainen and by Rushton are shown in Table 85.13 for Europe and for North America. Estimates for number of deaths in each region were retrieved from GLOBOCAN (www-dep.iarc.fr/). Cancer deaths due to occupational exposures vary from around 68 000 to 1 480 000 for Europe and from around 25 000 to 52 000 for North America. The estimated numbers for lung cancer range from 44 000 to 82 000 for Europe and 19 000 to 34 000 for North America, and those for bladder cancer from 4500 to 5500 for Europe and 1200 to 1400 for North America.

Existing estimates indicate that most occupational cancers occur among men due to the historically higher prevalence of exposure to occupational carcinogens among men. In most countries, the largest number of cancers attributed to occupational exposures is due to cancers of the lung and bladder. Numerous agents are associated with these two cancers including fibres and dusts, metals, radiation, combustion products and aromatic amines. Other specific cancers that contribute to the total number of occupational cancers are mesothelioma attributed nearly entirely to exposure to asbestos, sinonasal cancer attributed to wood dust, metals and formaldehyde, leukaemia and lymphomas attributed to solvents, pesticides, radiation and others. Mesothelioma contributes a significant number of occupational cancers in those countries where asbestos fibres have been extensively used such as the United States and the United Kingdom. In the United States, 85 per cent of all mesotheliomas can be attributed to asbestos exposure mostly in the occupational environment.[6,98]

According to Naud and Brugere,[99] in European Union countries, the number of occupational cancers officially notified in 1999–2000 was far below the estimated numbers of occupational cancers, similar to the pattern observed for other occupational diseases (Table 85.16). In those countries with the most extensive systems of notification of occupational cancers, around 10 per cent of all cancers that could be attributed to occupational exposures are notified as such. In most countries, this percentage is far lower and the under-reporting of cancers is extreme in some countries, such as Spain, where fewer than ten cancer deaths per year are notified as being of occupational origin.[100]

Although the estimates for occupational cancers vary considerably, all main estimates indicate that some tens of thousands of cancer deaths in Europe and in the United States can be attributed to exposures in the workplace. There are no valid estimates for developing or newly developed countries. It can be expected that the number of cancer cases due to occupational exposures in countries such as China,

India or Brazil, will significantly increase in the coming years.[101] Of those, only a minor fraction are recognized as of occupational origin. This under-reporting severely undermines any attempt to prevent further cases.

Contribution of occupational cancers to social inequalities

The occurrence of social class differences in cancer incidence and mortality is well documented.[102] Wide differences by socioeconomic status are observed in industrialized countries for all cancers combined and for many specific cancers, such as the lung, stomach and others. Occupational exposures are responsible for about 5 per cent of the total of human cancers in industrialized countries and these cancers are concentrated among manual workers and in the lower social classes. Occupational exposures are therefore one of the contributing factors for the occurrence of social class differentials in cancer.[103] Direct evidence on the extent of the contribution of occupational exposure to carcinogens to social class differences is lacking. Boffetta et al.[104] estimated the contribution of occupational exposures to the occurrence of social class differentials using 1971 cancer mortality data for England and Wales based on 25–64 years cumulative rates reported by Logan.[105] Proportions of cancers attributable to occupation were derived from Doll and Peto,[5] taking into account cancer sites that have been strongly related with occupational exposures. All occupational cancers were assumed to occur among manual workers. One-third of social class differences in all cancer mortality between non-manual social classes (categories I, II and III non-manual of the Registrar General's classification) and manual social classes (categories III manual, IV and V) could be attributed to occupational exposures (Table 85.17). For lung and for bladder cancer, about one-half of the differences could be attributed to occupation.

CLINICAL ASSESSMENT OF OCCUPATIONAL CANCER AND PREVENTION

Clinical assessment of occupational cancer

The recognition of work-related factors is vital in the effective diagnosis, treatment and prevention of ill health. Occupational diseases are most likely to be suspected by those closest to the patient or the workplace. This could be the workers themselves, although this is more likely to be the case for illness of short latency, such as asthma and dermatitis. Cancer, with its long latency – induction often extending to two or three decades – is less likely to be recognized as work related by the employee unless previous local instances have conditioned them to look for it and/or the agent responsible has a high carcinogenic potential.

Table 85.16 Estimated number and officially recognized occupational cancers in different EU countries (data from Ref. 99, with data for Spain from Kogevinas et al.[100]).

Country	Estimated number of occupational cancers	Recognized occupational cancers	No. recognized (%)
France	10 000	900	9
UK	9670	806	8.3
Germany	14 700	1889	12.9
Belgium	1850	149	8.1
Denmark	1180	79	6.7
Finland	890	110	12.4
Spain	6500–13 600	6	<0.1

Table 85.17 Ratios of cancer mortality in manual and non-manual social classes, with and without excluding cancers attributable to occupational exposures.

Cancer site	Mortality rate ratio for manual versus non-manual social classes	Rate ratio for the proportion of cancers non-attributable to occupation[a]	Excess risk (%) attributable to occupation
All cancers	1.40	1.27	32
Liver	1.16	1.09	42
Larynx	1.76	1.71	5
Lung	1.71	1.37	48
Nose	1.38	0.90	100
Skin (non-melanoma)	1.77	1.55	29
Prostate	1.19	1.17	9
Bladder	1.36	1.17	52

[a]Rate ratio, after excluding cancers attributable to occupation.
Proportions of cancers attributable to occupation were derived from Doll and Peto.[5] England and Wales, 1971 (data from Boffetta et al.[104]).

It is the clinician of first or second referral who has to take this responsibility. In view of the limited number of trained occupational physicians, the doctor consulted by the worker is likely to be a family doctor or a hospital consultant who has had little or no training in occupational medicine.

In other chapters of this book, considerable attention is given to the clinical presentation and management of occupational diseases. Such an approach is unlikely to be as helpful in the identification of occupation-related cancers. As a general rule, cancers that are of occupational origin are not distinguishable from non-occupational cancers whether in clinical features, natural history, pathological findings or other special investigations. A patient with lung or bladder cancer due to occupational factors will be diagnosed in the same way and using the same procedures as one without occupational factors. Where distinguishing features are relevant, they will be cited in the text.

One feature which has been noted with a number of occupationally related tumours is the possibility that the occupational cancer may present earlier than the non-occupational varieties. Thus, a patient aged 45 years with bladder cancer or one in his 30s with lung cancer – particularly if there is no history of tobacco consumption – should heighten the suspicion of the clinician that this might be an occupationally related tumour. For rarer tumours, such as angiosarcoma of the liver, pleural or peritoneal mesothelioma and nasal sinus cancer, for example, the occupational causes may outweigh the chances of finding such a tumour from other causes – known or unknown. The clinician thus needs to be aware of these varieties and their close links with occupation.

Given that occupation accounts for all or part of the tumour process in 5 per cent of cancers, physicians should contemplate occupation as a possible aetiological factor each time they see a new case of cancer. The rarity of the tumour may be the intellectual stimulus needed to consider workplace causes. It was occupational physicians at an American tyre manufacturer who were alerted to the carcinogenic potential of vinyl chloride monomer because of four cases of the extremely rare angiosarcoma of the liver in their workforce. However, it was an ear, nose and throat surgeon who first realized that woodworking was the common factor in her small series of rare adenocarcinoma of the ethmoid sinus.

A patient with a common tumour, such as lung or urinary bladder cancer, presents greater diagnostic difficulty. Nevertheless, many urothelial surgeons are now aware that occupation should be investigated when dealing with bladder cancer, where occupational exposures currently cause around 10 per cent of all tumours in Western Europe and North America. Similarly, it is our experience that haematologists commonly consider occupation when reviewing the possible causes of adult leukaemia, particularly the myeloid varieties.

The identification of work-related medical problems depends most importantly on the occupational history. Physical examination and special investigations may lead to a suspicion of a workplace agent as the cause of the disease but, ultimately, it is essential to obtain a thorough occupational history. A sentence or two in the family and social section of the medical history is not good enough.

The standard texts in occupational medicine have sections on the information that needs to be elicited in a good occupational history. This book on occupational diseases is no exception (see Chapter 3, The occupational history). From the point of view of occupational cancer, it is essential that this enquiry of 'work relatedness' goes back far enough in the patient's life to be sure of including relevant exposures. That means at least 20 years and sometimes as many as 40. Several databases and publications available on the internet may help in the identification of occupational causes of cancer. These include lists and frequency of occurrence of carcinogenic exposures by industry, such as CAREX,[11] or lists of carcinogens by cancer site as identified by the IARC.

Figure 85.3 shows a spot map of cases of bladder cancer occurring in a tyre factory in England where the association with exposure to 2-naphthylamine was clearly shown.[32] All cases of bladder cancer occurred in sectors of the plant where 2-naphthylamine had been used. A simple visual inspection gave strong clues for aetiology. In current times in industrialized countries, it is (fortunately) extremely rare to identify occupational causes of cancer in similar ways. First, exposures to carcinogens have diminished. Second, employment patterns have changed and it is less common to have the same job in the same department for decades. Work mobility together with changes in production practices seriously complicates the identification of carcinogens. In addition, both big and small industries tend to subcontract several jobs/tasks, such as cleaning or maintenance, that were previously done within the industry. This poses serious problems in the control of exposures and the identification of hazards since many of the subcontracted companies performing tasks such as cleaning do not tend to be stable and in addition may have a high turnover of personnel.

Three examples seen by us illustrate complications in the identification of occupational causes of cancer.

EXAMPLE 1. THE SUSPICION THAT OCCUPATION MIGHT BE OF AETIOLOGICAL RELEVANCE

A 70-year-old man was admitted to hospital for a cardiological assessment following symptoms likely to be due to coronary artery disease. At routine examination on the ward, the junior member of the medical team undertook the 'standard' clinical history and proceeded to the physical examination. She, quite properly, did not restrict the physical assessment to the cardiovascular system and, as a result, discovered an indolent ulcer on the patient's scrotum. Further enquiry revealed that the patient's family doctor had been treating this lesion with emollient creams for over two years, without success. The examining physician, working in an area of the country where scrotal cancer was no rarity, then turned again to the occupational history. The question: 'What is your job?' received the answer: 'I am retired'. She persisted (rightly) 'Yes, but what did you do before you retired?' The reply gave the answer: 'I was a multispindle lathe operator for 30 years.' The patient's mineral oil-induced scrotal cancer was excised the following day. Fortunately, in this case, the junior doctor was not put off by the 'retired' answer, and, equally fortunately, the patient had an uncomplicated work history which gave the occupational link straight away. Detailed questioning may be required, as the second case demonstrates.

EXAMPLE 2. THE NEED FOR A THOROUGH LIFETIME REVIEW OF OCCUPATIONAL HISTORY

A 65-year-old woman was admitted to hospital with breathlessness and chest pain. A pleural effusion was clinically detectable and a pleural tap revealed a blood-stained fluid which on microscopy was found to contain mesothelioma cells. In this case, the suspicion of an asbestos-related aetiology was readily apparent, but as a 'housewife' the exposure history appeared to be lacking. There began a painstaking review of the patient's life experiences. Finally, a crucial fact emerged. For a brief period of her early married life she was employed outside the home. She had worked during the Second World War for a short time and, for six months of that time, had filled gas masks with a 'blue fibrous material' 40 years before the onset of her symptoms of pleural mesothelioma.

EXAMPLE 3. INSPECTION OF WORKPLACE PRACTICES MAY BE IMPORTANT: OTHERS MAY BE POTENTIALLY AT RISK IN THE WORKPLACE

A third case, again of scrotal cancer, highlights a further area for the clinician. While working as a part-time occupational physician for a small engineering company, one of us saw an employee for a routine post-sickness absence medical. At that consultation, the employee stated that he was well, but asked for the form from 'the Social Security' to be completed so that he 'would get money'. The form – for Industrial Injuries Disability – stated that the man had undergone surgery for scrotal cancer. In this case, the diagnosis and treatment in the individual case was complete. What was now needed was a review of workplace practices for others at potential risk in the multispindle lathe section of the factory. On inspection, conditions were not good: there was poor hygiene for both skin and lung exposure to oils and oil mist, no formal policy for personal protection and no health surveillance for skin pathology.

These cases illustrate the importance of three aspects of a good clinical history:

- the suspicion that occupation might be of aetiological relevance;
- the need for a thorough lifetime review of those occupations;
- the need for somebody to consider others potentially at risk in the workplace.

Recognition of the importance of the first two aspects may not solve the problem even if occupation is the cause of the cancer. Thist is because patients may not know the relevant chemical (or physical) agents to which they were exposed or they may know them only by trade names or even nicknames. Second, the job titles used by patients may shed no light on the exposure issues and, finally, even if the employing company was known, it is possible that it has ceased to trade by the time of the enquiry. Use of certain chemicals is a problem, but employment in the chemical manufacturing industry compounds these difficulties. While the final product may be known and the exposures well documented, the range and complexity of possible exposure to intermediates can be staggering and may defy analysis even by the company's chemists. A fourth example might illustrate this point.

EXAMPLE 4. IDENTIFYING THE CAUSAL AGENT MAY BE COMPLEX: THERE MAY BE MORE THAN ONE EXPOSURE CAUSING THE SAME CANCER IN THE SAME WORKPLACE

A chemical company manufacturing a range of pesticides noted, in the course of its sophisticated and extensive health surveillance programme, that some workers had developed skin lesions reminiscent of solar keratoses. Cursory statistical analysis suggested that the risk for these workers of developing these premalignant skin lesions was in excess of what might be expected. A thorough review of the manufacturing process, the worker exposure profiles and the intermediates involved suggested that certain plant improvements would eliminate some suspect agents and greatly diminish worker exposure to others. Action was prompt and health surveillance stepped up. A decade later, further cases of keratosis were noted – some in plant operatives who had never worked with the old process. The disturbing message was that the previous plant review had either failed to reduce exposure to the putative carcinogen(s) or, more likely and more disturbing, those suspect agents were not the cause of the keratosis. The problem here is not ignorance nor incompetence, but the sheer complexity of the chemical process with hundreds of organic chemicals, alone or in combination, being potential sources of risk and exposure.

In such cases, the clinician has every reason to fail to find an aetiological agent, but, for every case like that, there are many more where a simple careful account of workplace experience can pay dividends.

Finally, two practical points about investigating a patient with suspected occupational cancer: (1) These investigations can be very time consuming. Not only is it necessary to obtain a detailed lifetime occupational history in order to clarify whether a workplace factor is responsible for the tumour – and, if so, which one(s) – but it is also necessary to ask about workmates who may have a similar disease. In our experience, a patient with an occupational disease is rarely, if ever, an isolated finding. Few patients are uniquely exposed at work and thus a case of occupational cancer should be assessed to be, in effect, the index case of what might turn out, on further enquiry, to be a cluster of cases. However, given the relative rarity of cancer, most cases will be individual cases particularly in smaller enterprises. (2) The clinician should, if possible, acquire information about the worksite either directly from the occupational health service or, if this is not possible or not sanctioned by the patient, make enquiries from the employer about the job and about any other relevant workplace exposures which might cast some light on the suspected association with occupation. While textbooks may help here, much useful assistance can be gained from talking to the local representatives of the national government agency responsible for health and safety at work. In the UK, this is the Employment Medical Advisory Service of the Health and Safety Executive. They might confirm the clinical suspicion or the enquiries may stimulate their investigations, locally and nationally, for further cases in similar workplaces. Where available, academic departments of occupational health serve a similar function and should be capable of providing the clinician with a second opinion on the case, as well as literature searches for published evidence of occupational risks for that cancer site, in addition to information on whether the suspect agent or process has been reported to be linked with tumours at that site.

In summary, the difficulties of identifying occupational factors in relation to cancer in the clinical setting are:

- ignorance of the risk by the worker – or management;
- failure of the clinician to consider an occupationally related aetiology – for that patient or for others at risk in the same workplace;
- diversity of chemical nomenclature;
- variable degrees of worker exposure to single or complex chemical mixtures;
- movement of workers between jobs, work areas or industries;
- failure to record previous occupations to the current (or last) one;
- long latency-induction times for cancer;
- job obsolescence;
- company closure;
- busy clinical workload.

Finally, it is important to note that for a clinician a new case might be yet another example of an occupational cancer already extensively reported in the specialist literature. It might, however, be the first case.

Prevention of occupational cancer

There are numerous examples of successful prevention of occupational cancer. Prevention may be primary or secondary. For primary prevention to be a practical proposition, it is necessary to know of the existence of proven aetiological agents and then to know that separation of humans from exposure to the agent is feasible. Primary prevention may also be efficient through the implementation of general measures for control of exposures as has happened in many industries in Europe and North America after the 1970s–1980s. Such measures were not necessarily focusing on one agent, but through improvements in work practices and changes in industrial processes may have resulted in efficient measures of primary prevention through a control of a wide range of occupational exposures. Secondary prevention usually means early detection of the disease process, and, most important, presumes that early detection will lead to an improved prognosis following treatment.

In this context, several regulatory actions exist both at the national and international level. The European Parliament regulates the protection of workers from the risks related to exposure to carcinogens or mutagens at work through Directive 2004/37/EC. The directive indicates that any activity likely to carry the risk of exposure to carcinogens or mutagens, the nature, degree and duration of workers' exposure must be determined on a regular basis in order to assess any risk to workers' health or safety and decide the steps to be taken. All routes of exposure must be taken into account, including absorption into and/or through the skin. Particular attention must be paid to workers who are especially at risk. The directive lays down exposure limit values, as well as preventive measures.

In addition to this more standard approach to the protection of workers and consumers, the European Union has implemented the REACH initiative. REACH is a new European Community Regulation on chemicals and their safe use (EC 1907/2006) that entered into force on June 1, 2007 and that deals with the registration, evaluation, authorization and restriction of chemical substances. REACH is based on the idea that industry itself is best placed to ensure that the chemicals it manufactures and puts on the market in the EU do not adversely affect human health or the environment. This requires that industry has certain knowledge of the properties of its substances. The benefits of the REACH system are not yet apparent and it is expected that they will come gradually, as more and more substances are phased into REACH. REACH also calls for the progressive substitution of the most dangerous chemicals when suitable alternatives have been identified.

In industrialized countries, there have been significant improvements in prevention and control of exposure to occupational carcinogens.[106] Improvement of work conditions and control of occupational carcinogens in newly industrialized countries or in developing countries is a major challenge.[107]

PRIMARY PREVENTION

In theory, all occupational cancers are preventable in that they result from workplace exposure. This is particularly so, since many occupational carcinogens have been successfully identified. All that is required to prevent the disease is elimination or drastic reduction in the level of exposure. Thus, the most efficient policy would be to ban the offending agent. In practice, this is less straightforward, for a number of reasons:

- The exposure may be defined only in terms of a very complex mixture, for example organic solvents or polycyclic aromatic hydrocarbons, or as a whole industrial process or even as a section of an industry or a large occupational category, for example painters. This may make it difficult to envisage, apart from general hygiene measurements (often effective in themselves), what more targeted control procedures one could adopt.
- The substance/process may be perceived to be of great societal importance. Benzene would be a good example here. It is the basic building block for so much of the aromatic organic chemical industry that its 'exclusion' from industry is difficult to conceive. It is also a natural ingredient of fossil fuels and thus would be difficult to eliminate even if the desire to do so were prevalent. In these situations, it is crucial to reduce the level of exposure to very low levels that are unlikely (with available knowledge) to cause disease.
- The substance has substitutes, but substitution is either expensive or the substitutes themselves are not without risk. Asbestos is undoubtedly a major cause of occupational cancer. Some of the more hazardous (amphibole) varieties have been largely excluded from commercial use, but it took a much longer period to exclude chrysotile asbestos from use. Chrysotile asbestos is believed to be less hazardous than other types of asbestos, at least in relation to mesothelioma, and has a combination of valuable properties not easily found in synthetic substitutes. Substitutes for chrysotile, such as man-made vitreous (mineral) fibres, may not be without risk, although it appears that this risk (if existent) is far lower than that of asbestos. All types of asbestos have been banned in many areas of the industrialized world.
- The agent itself is of limited economic importance, but its presence in an economically important industry is difficult to control. Radon exposure in metalliferous mining serves as an example here: effective control of radon exposure is extremely difficult, yet the need to mine for metals in these environments remains.

Nevertheless, the principle remains that reduction, substitution or, ideally, elimination of the known workplace carcinogens is of great public health importance. The lesson of vinyl chloride monomer shows that exposure to a vital chemical agent can be reduced sufficiently to eliminate a relevant tumour – even if one doubts in theory that a 'threshold' exposure exists. In other cases, such as 2-naphthylamine, purer ingredients or effective substitutes have been formed, thereby reducing workplace-related disease and death. However, even in the case of 2-naphthylamine and bladder cancer, analyses conducted many years after this ban identified an excess bladder risk in nearly all studies available (Figure 85.4). This could be due to a continuous increased risk among workers exposed in the past to 2-naphthylamine or probably to the presence of other carcinogenic substances in this industry. Where exposure, albeit at a reduced level, continues, every effort should be made to shorten the duration of exposure and to reduce exposure to very low levels. The earlier the action, the earlier the effect of reduction of exposure will be recorded.

SECONDARY PREVENTION

Primary prevention, although ideal, will never in the real world be the answer in every case. Therefore, secondary prevention in the form of early detection of human effect needs to be involved as well (not instead of). On the face of it, the earlier the neoplastic process is detected, the easier it should be to cure the patient. In practice, this is not so clear cut. This is not the place to discuss the general question of screening nor to describe in detail the attributes of a good screening test. For some cancer sites, screening is effective in leading to prevent cancer or to better cure/survival rates, as is the case of cervical cancer or breast cancer. However, there are no efficient secondary prevention strategies for occupational cancers, although there has been extensive research on the prevention of, for example, lung cancer and mesothelioma in asbestos-exposed workers through x-rays or cytological examination of sputum.

In summary, the whole purpose of detecting cancer is to cure or prevent other cases of cancer. Discovery of new workplace-related cancers by clinical acumen and the establishment of causative factors by epidemiological study provide the firm scientific basis for vigorous preventive action. Treating the cause of cancer has variable success. Eliminating a known cause ensures that, at least for the future, the need for treatment is obviated.

METHODOLOGICAL ISSUES IN EPIDEMIOLOGICAL RESEARCH ON OCCUPATIONAL CANCER

Epidemiological studies have significantly contributed to the recognition and control of occupational diseases and work exposure to carcinogens. In addition, studies on occupational cancer have been among the first to develop methods for the conduct of (historical) cohort studies applying the concept of person-years.[1] A report on lung cancer and mortality in an arsenical powder-producing factory published at the *British Journal of Industrial Medicine* in 1948 by A Bradford Hill and E Lewis Faning constitutes probably the first description of how to perform a historical cohort study. Note that the authors did not have the information to conduct such a study and instead performed a proportional mortality study. The first historical cohort study was published by Sir Richard Doll in 1952, evaluating the mortality among gas workers.

The main characteristics of studies on occupational cancer are similar to those in other areas of epidemiology.[108,109] There exists similarity on the basic principles such as that of the study base (the population from which the study population originates) or the fact that incidence is the main measure for disease. In this part of the chapter, we discuss specific items related to the design and analysis of epidemiological studies on occupational cancer. We do not discuss designs that are rarely applied on studies on occupational cancer, such as cross-sectional studies (although many biomarker-based studies are essentially cross-sectional). We also discuss some aspects related to exposure assessment that have considerably developed in recent years.

Formally, case series should not be considered as epidemiological studies. Frequently, what is reported is an accumulation (cluster) of cases in an industry or job, mostly concerning rare diseases. The report of a series of cases of liver angiosarcoma among workers in the polymerization of vinyl chloride is a classical example.[83] Case series can help identify new carcinogens as was the case for angiosarcoma of the liver and vinyl chloride monomer (VCM), benzene and leukaemia in shoe workers, or mesothelioma in asbestos-exposed workers, and may lead to a successful intervention. However, a case series can also represent an anecdotal occurrence and can be affected by reporting bias. Most of the time, case series do not refer to defined populations and frequently do not identify causal associations.

Types of study in occupational cancer

COHORT STUDIES

The cohort design is the one that has most frequently been applied in occupational cancer epidemiology. In these studies, populations of specific industrial sectors are examined or, occasionally, a sample of the general population is examined. Once a specific population has been identified, exposure information is collected and subjects are followed up to evaluate cancer incidence or mortality. In prospective cohort studies, information on exposure of each individual is selected and workers are followed in time. Retrospective cohort studies can only be conducted if complete registers of workers are available in an industry and also if mortality or cancer incidence data are available.

Identification of the cohort

The identification of the cohort is the first step in the design of the study. In most of the studies, the exposed group is usually identified through the payroll registry of the industry. Sometimes, labour union registries are also used. For example, in a study of wood workers in the United States, the exposed population was identified through its labour union (United Furniture Workers of America). Nevertheless, the usual lack of detailed and complete information about the occupational history of the workers in this type of registry makes it difficult to interpret the results. Finally, occupational disease registries have been used occasionally, for instance, when studying workers suffering silicosis or mercury poisoning in relation to the later occurrence of lung or other cancers.

The main concern in the design of an epidemiological study is the internal validity. For this reason, it might be necessary to apply restrictive criteria in the cohort identification. This will, in turn, depend on multiple factors, like the cost and the time of the feasibility of the study. For instance, sometimes it is not possible to identify and follow up the temporary or emigrant workers, mainly because the occupational registries for these groups of workers are neither complete nor precise. The restriction of a cohort to a subgroup of workers does not affect the validity of the study, but it implies an important loss of information. Once the inclusion criteria have been defined, each subject that fits in these criteria should be included in the study, and followed up until the end of the follow-up period. If the study population does not include all eligible subjects according to the criteria established initially, it is possible that individuals that were not identified have a difference with respect to the exposure characteristics and/or their vital status.

Determination of the vital status

In mortality studies, the research of the vital status (follow up) is performed by matching the personal identifiers of the cohort members (name, date of birth, registry number, national identity number, social security number, tax number, etc.) with the national mortality registries. One of the main concerns in cohort studies is the identification of the vital status of most of the individuals participating in the study. Although no strict criteria have been established to define the acceptable losses to follow up, the validity of results should be treated with caution if the loss to follow up is more than 20 per cent. There are different options to deal with losses to follow up and its contribution to the study in persons-year: (1) Delete from the study all individuals that have been lost during follow up, although this results in an unnecessary loss of information. (2) Assume that all subjects lost to follow up will be free from the disease at the end of the study, contributing to the persons-year at that particular moment; this will result in an underestimation of the disease risk of the cohort. (3) Count only the persons-years of the subjects lost to follow up only to the date of the last contact. This third option is the most justifiable, since all known information (persons-year) is included in the analysis.

Cause of death is usually obtained from death certificates and, in many industrialized countries, this information is relatively accurate. Most retrospective cohort studies on occupational cancer have not validated cause of death using other information, such as clinical records. However, validity of cause of death information may depend on type of tumour examined. In a study of dioxins and cancer, an excess risk for soft-tissue sarcoma was observed, with a standardized mortality ratio (SMR) of 338, including four deaths identified through death certificates.[110] The histological review of the tissue samples indicated that two of the four sarcomas were misclassified as such, and other sarcomas have not been diagnosed correctly. When comparing national mortality rates, the SMR should be calculated from the information in the death certificates registry, and not be based in a review of the cause of death by a group of experts. As a result, in the dioxins study, the risk of sarcoma was calculated correctly on the basis of the four deaths from sarcoma, but the validity of the results could have been questioned due to the large classification error.

Selection of a comparison group

In the occupational cohort studies, two comparison groups are used: (1) external comparison groups (usually country mortality rates) and (2) internal comparison groups, identified in the same cohort. Occasionally, both types of comparison groups might be used in the same study.

The use of an external comparison group has been extensive, particularly in the past in historical (retrospective) cohort studies on occupational cancer. The most common procedure is to choose the population of the country as a comparison group and then calculate the SMR. The indirect standardization (analysis of the SMR) is the technique most commonly used to adjust the rates in the occupational cohort studies. The SMR is the ratio of the total number of observed deaths to the number of expected deaths, provided that the study population has mortality rates similar to the comparison population group. There are some advantages to use the population of the country as a reference population. First, it is of interest to know how the cohort rates behave before the country rates. Second, the mortality rates per age group, sex and calendar year are usually available to both at national and international level (World Health Organization). Finally, the use of national mortality rates has the statistical advantage that they are stable, which is especially important when studying rare diseases. Nevertheless, the use of national mortality rates has some disadvantages. Where working populations are the object of study, the comparisons may be biased due to the healthy worker effect. Another disadvantage is the difficulty of controlling for potentially confounding factors that have not been measured, such as lifestyle-related factors in the study region. This problem can be partially solved when using other defined external populations as the reference population. In this case, comparisons can be made only with the working population rates, as in northern European countries, in regional or local populations, or with other external cohorts, for instance, other industrial populations. The use of regional rates is recommended when there is a prior knowledge that morbidity or mortality will vary considerably between different regions. The main advantage of using an external industrial cohort as a reference is the reduction in the bias due to the healthy worker effect, and that the two populations will probably be very similar in their lifestyle factors. In consequence, the importance of potentially confounding factors, such as tobacco, will probably be lessened. In summary, the selection of an external occupational cohort as a reference group has several advantages. However, the selection should be made carefully with the aim of making the two groups as comparable as possible in relation to factors such as age, gender, social class or average duration of the job, and that the reference group is not exposed to occupational risk factors related to the study disease. Moreover, unstable rates in the reference group (regional or local population, external industrial cohort) may limit the accuracy of the effect estimates, especially when examining rare diseases such as leukaemia or lymphoma.

Internal comparison group

When using an internal reference group, the comparisons are restricted to the experience of persons-time of the same cohort. In this situation, the reference category will be the disease rate associated with the persons-time of the non-exposed or low-exposed subjects. In this type of study, the quantity and quality of the data are similar in both comparison groups. Selection bias (including healthy worker effect) will also be similar between exposed and non-exposed individuals. However, unstable rates in the reference group might be a limiting factor in the accuracy of the risk estimates, specifically when rare diseases are under study. In addition, the variability of the exposure might be small in the same cohort, so it might not be possible to identify an internal reference group of non-exposed subjects. For instance, in an international cohort study of styrene workers, it was not possible to identify adequately an internal group of non-exposed workers. In this study, the comparisons were limited to exposed individuals classified into quintiles of the cumulative exposure, being the lowest quintile exposure group (less than 10 ppm-year) of the reference group.

CASE–CONTROL STUDIES

In case–control studies, exposures in the past of people with a disease (cases) are compared to those of subjects without the disease (controls). The main features of case–control studies on occupational cancer are similar to those of other risk factors. Two types of case–control studies on occupational cancer epidemiology can be distinguished: (1) community (population)-based studies and (2) nested case–control studies within an industrial cohort.

The only unique feature of community-based studies on occupational cancer is the measurement of occupational exposures. Questionnaires are the most frequently used methods to obtain information on occupational exposures, specifically information on occupation, industry, tasks at the job and dates of employment. While workers may fully recall the jobs they have performed, they may not recall or know the specific substances to which they were exposed. Studies based on cancer registries or death certificate data, are primarily used to generate new hypotheses on exposure disease relationships or are used for surveillance purposes. These studies are based on existing records, such as mortality or cancer incidence records. The main advantage of these studies is their low cost and the availability of already collected data. The main problem is the lack of detailed exposure information on occupational exposures even in studies that may do extensive record linkage between different registers as has been frequently performed in Scandinavian countries.

Nested case–control studies within a cohort is a study design that has been frequently used in occupational cancer epidemiology. Many occupational cohorts collect only limited occupational and disease information and may not have more detailed information both on the exposures in the workplace or of other exposures, such as smoking, alcohol, etc. This information could be obtained for a small subsample of the occupational cohort within the context of a nested case–control study in which cases occurring in the cohort are compared with a set of controls (rather than with the total cohort). For example, a nested case–control study on non-Hodgkin lymphomas and soft-tissue sarcomas was conducted within an international study of 25 000 workers exposed to phenoxy herbicides, chlorophenols and dioxins. Thirty-two cases of lymphoma and 111 of sarcoma were matched to 158 and 55 controls, respectively.[43] A panel of three industrial hygienists examined the detailed work records of these subjects regarding their exposure to 21 chemical agents. An increased risk both for lymphomas and sarcomas was found for exposure to the herbicides and to dioxins. This type of detailed evaluation would have been impossible if it were to be done among the 25 000 workers of the original cohort. In addition, an evaluation of the total cohort would have added very little in terms of statistical power.

The case–cohort design is another type of nested case–control study. The main feature of the case–cohort design is that the controls are selected randomly from the subjects present at baseline, i.e. when the cohort started. Case–cohort studies may include multiple cancers as their outcome, using the same set of controls. Among the advantages of case–cohort studies is that one control group can be used for many cancers making this design more efficient in terms of cost. Also, this design allows the calculation of absolute risks (in comparison to relative risks). A case–cohort study on several cancers was conducted in Shanghai, nested within a cohort of 267 000 women employed at the Shanghai Textile Industry Bureau (STIB) and that had originally been enrolled in an intervention study on breast cancer screening.[111] Complete occupational history was obtained for 102 incident cases of oesophageal cancer and 646 cases of stomach cancer, and for a reference group of 3188 women. A wide range of occupational exposures were evaluated by industrial hygienists and an increased risk of oesophageal cancer was associated with exposure to silica (HR = 15.8, 95 per cent CI, 3.5–70), while a protective effect was found for exposure to the endotoxins that are present in cotton dust.

Issues in design and analysis

HEALTHY WORKER EFFECT

The healthy worker effect (HWE) refers to the lower mortality observed in many worker studies compared to that of the general population. The lower rates observed among workers is, in part, due to the fact that people with serious diseases or those who are disabled are excluded from the labour market. Therefore, a comparison of workers' health with that of the general population may be inappropriate if this effect is not taken into account. This bias has been traditionally described as a selection bias, although it can also be described as a problem of confounding.[108]

The healthy worker effect can be determined by three components:

1. **Selection in employment.** The HWE occurs mainly due to the initial selection of healthy subjects in the labour force. Healthy individuals have more chance of searching to occur and for getting selected. In one of the first studies describing the HWE,[112] the overall SMR for the workers in a vinyl chloride polymerization plant was 0.75 and the SMRs were low for most specific diseases.
2. **Selection out of employment.** This aspect of the HWE (also called the healthy worker survivor effect) may occur when prolonged exposures are examined. Workers with longer duration of employment may have lower disease rates than those with shorter employment periods. This happens because sick workers tend to abandon employment. An increased disease risk in the first years after leaving employment has been observed in several studies.
3. **Duration of follow up.** The HWE is stronger during the first period after employment and diminishes as employment becomes longer. In the study by Fox and Collier,[112] mortality from all causes increased with duration of follow up: for 0–4 years the SMR was 0.37, for 5–9 it was 0.63, for 10–14 it was 0.75 and for more than 15, 0.94.

Different methods can be applied to control for the HWE. The most direct method is to take into account the initial employment status and compare the cancer risk of the study population with that of workers in other jobs/departments in the same or in another cohort. Given the inverse correlation of the HWE with length of follow up, this effect can be examined through stratification by follow-up time. When cancer mortality is examined, the HWE becomes very much attenuated after around 20 years of follow up.

Selection out of the labour force can be partially controlled by taking into account employment status. In the classical study by Fox and Collier,[112] they examined mortality depending on whether workers continued working in the industry or not. Mortality among those who left the industry was about 50 per cent higher than that of workers continuing working. More recently, Steenland and Stayner[113] examined the same problem by categorizing person-years into those active (years during employment) and those non-active (years after leaving employment) and found the same pattern as Fox and Collier only for ages before retirement.

CONFOUNDING IN OCCUPATIONAL CANCER STUDIES

In occupational cancer studies, general factors, such as tobacco smoking or obesity, can be considered as alternative explanations to increased cancer mortality in an occupational cohort. This is plausible since several lifestyle factors vary within a population by socioeconomic status. In many countries, tobacco smoking is more frequent, for example, in lower socioeconomic classes at least among males and those same classes have a higher prevalence of exposure to occupational carcinogens. It is noteworthy, however, that studies of occupation and lung cancer have found smoking to be a relatively infrequent confounder even though the association of smoking with lung cancer is as large as that of any potential confounder in the occupational setting.

Confounding in epidemiological studies can be controlled either at the design phase or, on most occasions, in the analysis provided information is available for the confounding factor. In most occupational cancer cohort studies, and particularly retrospective cohorts, such information is rarely available. In this event, several approaches can be applied to estimate the magnitude of a potential confounding effect.[114]

One of the simplest methods to indirectly and approximately evaluate confounding has been proposed by Axelson.[115] In this method, it is necessary to estimate the prevalence of exposure to the potential confounder in the study population and also in the reference population, e.g. the general population. It is also necessary to know the strength of the association of the potential confounder with the disease, e.g. smoking and lung cancer. This information allows estimation of the amount of the increased risk among exposed workers that could be explained by the confounder.

Internal analyses within the cohort of workers among those exposed and those non-exposed to a specific agent, in part, overcome the problem of confounding since a relatively safe assumption can be that lifestyle does not vary systematically among manual workers employed in different departments of the same industry.

LATENCY ANALYSIS

A cancer due to an occupational exposure will occur on most occasions, many years after first exposure. Analysis of epidemiological data should take into account the latency period of the disease and should evaluate the time periods during which exposures could have caused the disease.

One of the methods used to evaluate latency is to perform a lagged analysis.[108] In this approach, exposures occurring in periods that are not evaluated to be relevant for the occurrence of a cancer, are ignored, as for example exposures during the last period before diagnosis. It is assumed that the induction of the cancer had occurred at an earlier period and therefore any posterior exposure would be considered irrelevant. For example, in a worker exposed to asbestos fibres from 1960 to 1990 and diagnosed with lung cancer in the year 1990, a classical analysis would calculate his exposure to asbestos during the whole 30-year period. By contrast, a lagged analysis applying a five-year lag would assume that any disease occurring shortly after diagnosis (in this example five years) could not have been caused by the exposure. Therefore, the real period at risk would start at the fifth year of follow up, at which time the worker would be assigned his exposure of five years earlier.

The use of time-windows is an extension of the lagged analysis.[116] This approach intends to identify the most relevant exposure period for the occurrence of disease. With the time-windows approach, exposure occurring at both early and late periods may be ignored. Identification of the most relevant time-window is made empirically by examining risk in consecutive windows. Table 85.18 shows an example of the application of this methodology in a study on asbestos exposure and lung cancer. The highest risk is observed in the time-window from 20 to 24 years before disease occurrence, particularly when risk estimates for different periods are mutually adjusted. This indicates that the increased risk of cancer in this study could be attributed to exposures occurring mainly before 20 years from diagnosis.

INTERACTION

Diseases are caused by more than one factor and the risk of acquiring a disease depends not only on the separate effects of each factor, but also on the way different factors

Table 85.18 Rate ratios for lung cancer in subjects with exposure to asbestos at levels higher versus lower than 5.000 fibres/cm³, in relation to different time-windows (data from Ref. 116).

Exposure window (years)	Rate ratios[a]	Mutually adjusted rate ratios[b]
0–4	1.5	0.8
5–9	2.8	1.3
10–14	3.9	1.3
15–19	4.9	1.4
20–24	5.7	4.6
25–29	3.9	0.7
30+	3.4	1.2

[a]Adjusted for age and calendar period.
[b]As above but also adjusted for exposures in other time windows.

combine. How to define and measure the combined action of two or more factors has been long discussed in epidemiology and different terms have been used: interaction, effect modification, synergism (and antagonism), biological or statistical interaction. There is confusion in the use of the term 'interaction' mainly due to the different meaning of this term in statistical theory and in biology.

It serves no practical purpose to use the term 'interaction' in epidemiology without specifying what type of model (or scale) was used to evaluate the association of exposure and disease. The additive and the multiplicative models are those most used. There are arguments for using both models, although the multiplicative model has been used more frequently in aetiological cancer epidemiology both for empirical and theoretical reasons.

There are only a few examples of well-studied interactive effects in the causation of disease.[14,117] In occupational cancer, epidemiological interaction has mostly been investigated between tobacco consumption and exposure to asbestos and to ionizing radiation. In recent years, the interaction between occupational exposures and genetic polymorphisms has also been examined.

Table 85.5 shows incidence rates for lung cancer among workers exposed to asbestos in relation to smoking. The pattern observed indicates a possible multiplicative pattern of interaction with asbestos-related risk being equally elevated among non-smokers and smokers, i.e. around five times. However, note that because smokers not exposed to asbestos (122.6/100 000) have a much higher risk than non-smokers unexposed to asbestos (11.3/100 000), the multiplication of this risk by approximately 5 due to asbestos exposure results, in absolute terms, to a very great increase in risk among exposed smokers. There are a few, although not well-proven, examples of interactions of occupational exposures and smoking, including arsenic and nickel and lung cancer.

Evaluation of exposure in occupational cancer studies

Methods to evaluate occupational exposures have been considerably improved in recent years and incorporate modelling techniques and the application of biomarkers. New approaches have also been applied in the construction of questionnaires and methods to evaluate them.

Strategies applied to evaluate occupational exposures depend on the study design applied, the population studied and the resources and prior information available. Exposure could be directly measured at the workplace in a prospective study, could be estimated using questionnaires in a case–control study or based on job records in a retrospective cohort study. Several techniques can be further applied to estimate past exposures, for example use expert opinions, job exposure matrices (JEM) or applying exposure models. Modern exposure assessment methods may evaluate pathways of exposure including, for example, sources of exposure, personal exposure estimates, use of protective equipment and also incorporate uncertainty in the measurements (Figure 85.8). Many occupational cancer studies have been retrospective cohorts that have based exposure estimates on existing job records and, occasionally, additional exposure information from the workplace. In cancer case–control studies, questionnaires have been the main source of information used, frequently in combination with expert opinions and JEMs.

QUESTIONNAIRES

Questionnaires have been extensively used in case–control studies irrespective of whether these are community based or nested within a cohort and usually request detailed information on jobs, tasks, industries worked, specific exposures, use of protective equipment, etc. It has generally

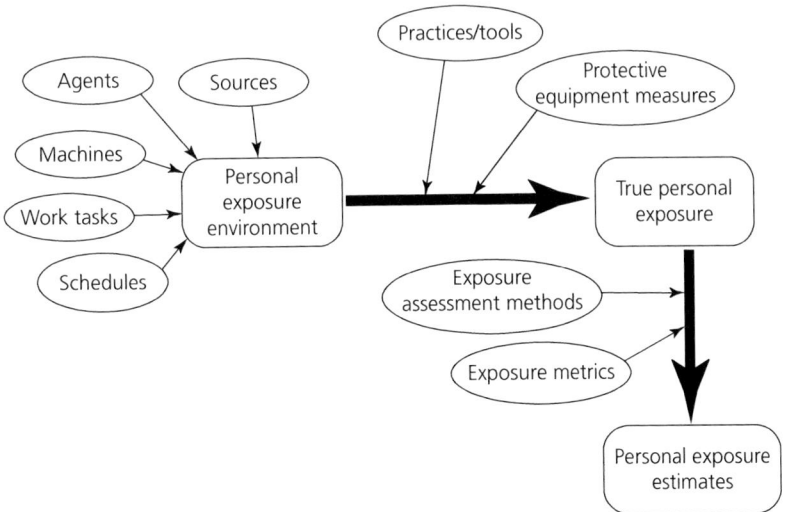

Figure 85.8 Exposure assessment pathway from sources to personal exposure estimates, showing determinants of exposure estimates. Reproduced with permission from Ref. 118.

been observed that questions on specific chemical exposures have a low sensitivity, i.e. many exposed subjects do not report that they have been exposed. In nested case–control studies, exposure assessment is easier mainly because the number of jobs, tasks and exposures is more limited than those observed in a general population study.

Supplementary questionnaires have been used in several occupational cancer case–control studies to retrieve more detailed information for specific carcinogens, e.g. asbestos, or to a whole list of carcinogens.[119] These supplementary questionnaires are used in subjects who report having worked in jobs or industries in which a specific carcinogenic exposure may occur. Specific questions relate to the materials used, tools, machinery, tasks performed, so as to evaluate with more certainty the probability and level of exposure. These detailed questionnaires are further analysed using a predetermined algorithm or through a case-by-case evaluation by experts.

For example, a study on occupational causes of bladder cancer in Spain[120] used 63 supplementary questionnaires for specific occupations, e.g. welders and machinists, or for specific industries, e.g. the textile industry.[121] These modules covered several exposures of interest, e.g. PAHs, diesel engine exhaust and solvents, that could occur in multiple workplaces. The use of such questionnaires, undoubtedly, provides important exposure information, but requires considerable expenditure in terms of time and money and also requires good knowledge of the workplace in order to prepare the questionnaires.

Industry questionnaires which collect information on industrial processes, exposures and accidents of specific industries have been used in studies on occupational cancer, for example the study in the pulp and paper industry of the IARC.[122] In this IARC study, information was collected in industries worldwide which participated in the study of industrial processes, volumes of production of specific compounds, use of primary materials, circumstances of industrial accidents, use of protective equipment, etc. This information was later coupled with information from the workers in the cohort to develop exposure estimates.

JOB EXPOSURE MATRICES

Job exposure matrices have been extensively used in occupational cancer epidemiology. JEMs are simply a matrix (or table) showing which occupations are exposed to specific chemicals and this information is based on prior knowledge of exposures of specific occupations. This method allows a nearly automatic assignment of exposures in the matrix to the subjects of the study, provided a complete occupational history is available for each subject. There exist several general and specific JEMs, using different methodologies, designed to cover different objectives and exposure areas.[123–127] Some have been constructed on the basis of expert opinion,[123,124] while others are based mostly on measurements in the workplace.[127] FINJEM, which was developed in Finland, is among the most widely used general JEMs (FINJEM)[128] and has been applied in several other countries. Some JEMs have been constructed for specific industries or exposures, such as a JEM on electromagnetic fields in the occupational environment.

The main advantages of JEMs is the low cost of using them once they have been created and the high repeatability of the estimates, since for a specific job one would attribute the same specific exposure estimate. The main disadvantage of JEMs is the potentially important exposure misclassification even though, in principle, this should be non-differential. This is a result of the fact that the same exposure is attributed to workers of the same job, even though it is known that exposure may vary considerably between workers or between workplaces among those doing the exactly the same job. This type of misclassification tends to reduce the risk estimates of a study towards null (i.e. to no association).

EVALUATION OF EXPOSURE BY EXPERTS

Evaluation by experts is considered among the most valid approaches when examining occupational exposure assessment.[129] In this approach, a group of experts (industrial hygienists, chemists) use their professional experience to evaluate if a worker has been exposed to a chemical or physical agent, on the basis of information they have on the occupational history of the worker and their own knowledge on exposures in the specific occupation/industry. The most quoted study was a multisite case–control study in Montreal which examined around 260 specific exposures.[130] The occupational history of the subjects in the study was examined by a group of experts who attributed to each subject the probability and extent of exposure to each chemical. In most case–control studies applying such an approach, the number of chemicals evaluated is much smaller. Frequently, the evaluation by experts is used in combination with other methods. For example, a JEM can first be applied and then experts evaluate only those subjects classified by the JEM as potentially exposed. This approach considerably reduces the experts' workload, which otherwise is one of the main disadvantages of this method. In addition, a problem of this method is potentially the lack of repeatability, particularly if the experts are not very experienced.

EXPOSURE MODELS

The most precise methods for evaluating occupational exposures are those using direct measurements in the workplace sometimes combined with the use of biomarkers. However, in most cases, this type of information is not available, or is available only for a subgroup of workers. In these cases, the use of exposure models can be considered to attribute exposure levels to the whole study population. Stochastic models are those that are based on existing measurements in a subgroup of workers that are then applied through regression or other modelling to the total

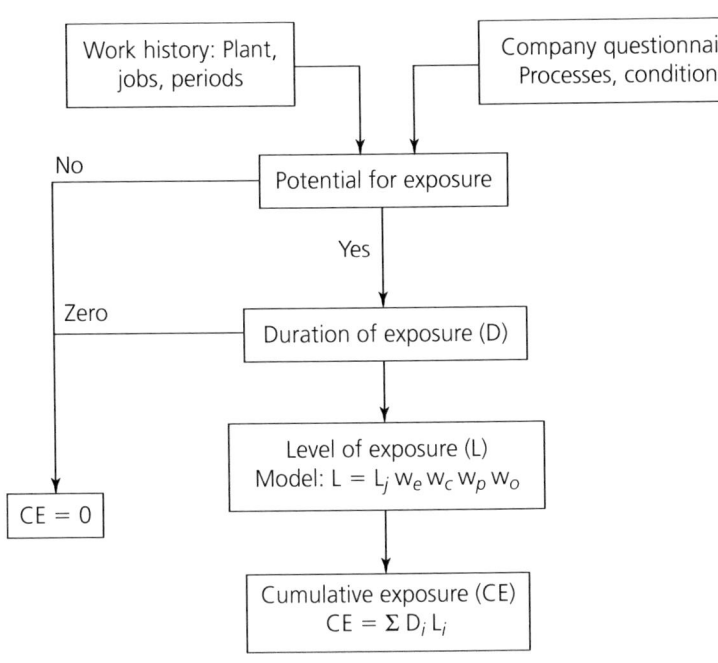

Figure 85.9 Model for the evaluation of exposures in the herbicide industry that were used in a nested case–control study. Reproduced with permission from Ref. 131. w_e, emission factors; w_c, contact factors; w_p, personal protection factors; w_o, other factors.

population. These models may incorporate an estimate of the error. By contrast, when measurements are not available for part of the population, but there is knowledge that may allow an evaluation of parameters affecting exposure (say closed production methods or use of ventilation), then a different type of model, sometime called deterministic, can be applied. These are based on fixed, 'arbitrary' criteria concerning factors affecting exposure in an industrial setting and are less precise than stochastic models.

A study on chlorophenoxy herbicides and dioxins applied such a deterministic model to evaluate several exposures within the herbicide industry and this was then applied to a nested case–control study.[131] The model applied (Figure 85.9) took into account the job history of each worker and then applied fixed weights to determine the relative exposure level of the workers. These factors involve, for example, the type of job (production worker, truck driver), knowledge on emissions in each factory and job, existence of personal protective equipment, accidents in the factory, etc. Exposure scores in these models are usually relative, so a production worker in this model had an initial exposure score of 10, while a worker in the shipping department had an exposure score of 1. These initial scores were then modified according to the other weights applied.

BIOMARKERS AND MECHANISMS

Carcinogenesis is a multistep process driven by carcinogen-induced genetic and epigenetic damage in susceptible cells that gain a selective growth advantage and undergo clonal expansion as a result of proto-oncogenes or the inactivation of tumour suppressor genes. The first stage of carcinogenesis, tumour initiation, involves the exposure of normal cells to a chemical, physical or viral carcinogen that causes a genetic change or changes resulting in 'initiated cells' (Figure 85.10). The next step, tumour promotion, is related to the acquisition of increased survival or proliferation of the 'initiated cells' as compared to normal cells. This process enhances the probability of additional genetic damage in the expanding population of these cells and might move the initiated cell, to pre-neoplastic lesions, to a malignant tumour and finally a clinical cancer.

Biomarkers can play an important role in the identification of key events in this multistep carcinogenesis process. More specifically within occupational cancer, biomarkers can be used to enhance exposure assessment, identify key events along the pathway from exposure to disease, determine sources of genetic susceptibility, and categorize tumours into more homogenous entities at the molecular level.[132–138] Furthermore, new discovery technologies, including whole genome analysis, mRNA expression arrays, proteomics and metabolomics/metabonomics (i.e. the study of cellular metabolites)[139–145] now enable investigators to broadly explore biologic responses to exogenous exposures, to evaluate potential modification of those responses by variants in essentially the entire genome, and to define tumours at the chromosomal, DNA, mRNA and protein levels. It is beyond the scope of this chapter to describe all biomarkers related to specific cancers and occupational exposures. Instead, we will describe the different types of biomarker that have been applied within occupational cancer research and provide some examples.

Tumour biomarkers

Both genetic changes (e.g. mutations and cytogenetic abnormalities) and epigenetic changes (e.g. altered transcription

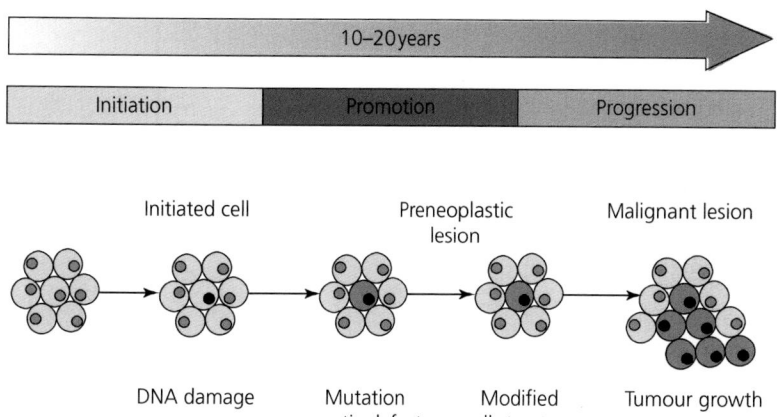

Figure 85.10 Schematic model of multistage carcinogenesis.

secondary to methylation and acetylation) in tumours that affect gene expression may provide important aetiologic clues. It has been postulated that certain chemical carcinogens can cause specific somatic mutations in oncogenes and tumour suppressor genes, leaving a DNA 'fingerprint' that can help identify tumours caused by this mechanism. Over the last decade, one of the most studied genes in epidemiology has been the *TP53* tumour suppressor gene because of its multiple important roles in carcinogenicity, and the high frequency and broad spectrum of mutations observed in most types of cancer. A database of all somatic p53 mutations reported to date maintained at the IARC has been particularly useful for detecting relationships between particular types of cancer, mutations and exposures (www.iarc.fr/p53).[146–148] Studies of *TP53* mutations as DNA fingerprints of exposures in several tumour types support the rationale of inferring environmental exposures from tumour gene mutations.[149] A well-established example is the G:C→T:A transversion mutation in codon 249 of *TP53* in hepatocellular carcinomas, which has been attributed to dietary aflatoxin B_1 exposure in high-risk populations.[150] Another commonly cited example is the high frequency of G:C→T:A transversion mutations of *TP53* found in lung tumours from smokers.[147,151] Hepatic angiosarcomas in people with occupational exposure to vinyl chloride carry *TP53* mutations almost exclusively at A:T base pairs,[152] while skin cancers associated with exposure to sunlight have *TP53* mutations at diprymidine sites that are usually G:C to A:T transitions. Comparing mutational spectra of a given tumour from a patient with a well-documented occupational exposure to the mutational spectra of the same genes from the same kind of tumours in patients with no history of occupational exposure could thus render some insight into the chemical carcinogens involved.

Endogenous or exogenous exposures might increase the risk of cancer by causing epigenetic changes, such as DNA hypermethylation of cytosine in CpG-rich promoter regions in tumour suppressor genes, leading to loss of function and tumorigenesis.[153–155] Several environmental exposures have been associated with altered levels of gene methylation. In one study, decreased repeated-element methylation in gene LINE-1 was observed after exposure to traffic particles.[156] Hypermethylation in p15 and hypomethylation in MAGE-1 were associated with increasing airborne benzene levels.[157] In another study,[158] inverse correlations were found between global methylation levels and persistent organic pollutant concentrations in the blood of Inuit populations.

Comparison of chromosomal alterations in tumour tissues from subjects with different exposures might provide insight into the molecular mechanisms by which exposures promote cancer. For instance, high levels of arsenic exposures have been found to be associated with an increased number of chromosomal gains and losses detected by comparative genomic hybridization (CGH) in bladder tumours.[159] This could reflect that arsenic-related tumours are less genetically stable than tumours unrelated to arsenic exposure. Conventional cytogenetic techniques, such as fluorescent *in situ* hybridization (FISH), have enabled the detection of chromosomal sites that might contain critical genes in haematological malignancies and other types of cancer, such as specific translocation breakpoints and subtypes of leukaemia, and lymphoma.[160] For instance, translocation t(14;18), the long-arm deletion of chromosome 6 [del(6q)], and trisomy 12 are frequently observed in lymphoma patients. Rearrangements of the *MLL* gene located on chromosome 11q23, such as t(4;11) and t(6;11), are common in therapy-related leukaemias resulting from treatment with topoisomerase II-inhibiting drugs. In addition, FISH virtual karyotyping with SNP arrays has become available recently facilitating high-throughput investigations of numerical alterations in specific chromosomal regions or whole chromosomes. These techniques can be applied in the future to investigate if there are chemical-specific chromosomal alterations in tumours.

Intermediate end points

Intermediate biomarkers directly or indirectly represent events on the continuum between exposure and disease.[132,138,161–163] One group of intermediate biomarkers, biomarkers of early biologic effect,[132] generally measure early biologic changes that reflect early, non-clonal and generally non-persistent effects. Examples of early biologic effect biomarkers include measures of cellular toxicity, chromosomal alterations, DNA, RNA and protein expression, and early non-neoplastic alterations in cell function (e.g. altered DNA repair, altered immune function). Generally, early biologic effect markers are measured in substances such as blood and blood components (red blood cells, white blood cells, DNA, RNA, plasma, sera, etc.) because they are easily accessible and because, in some instances, it is reasonable to assume that they can serve as surrogates for other organs. Early biological effect markers can also be measured in other accessible tissues such as skin, cervical and colon biopsies, epithelial cells from surface tissue scrapings or sputum samples, exfoliated urothelial cells in urine, colonic cells in faeces, and epithelial cells in breast nipple aspirates. Other early effect markers include measures of circulating biologically active compounds in plasma that may have epigenetic effects on cancer development (e.g. hormones, growth factors, cytokines).

Chromosomal aberrations in peripheral blood lymphocytes have been extensively used as the classic biomarker of early genotoxic effects in cross-sectional studies of populations exposed to occupational carcinogens.[164–166] Several cohort studies have reported that the prevalence of chromosomal aberrations in peripheral lymphocytes can predict subsequent risk of cancer.[167–171] The predictive performance of this biomarker was shown to be similar irrespective of whether the subjects had been smokers or occupationally exposed to carcinogenic agents.[172] Similar observations have been made for micronuclei (MN) frequency in peripheral blood lymphocytes of disease-free individuals. In some studies, MN frequency was found to be predictive for future cancer death.[173,174] In contrast, such associations were not observed for the sister chromatid exchange assay, another biomarker of genotoxicity also measured in peripheral lymphocytes.[167–169] These results do suggest that the identification of chromosomal aberrations and/or micronuclei due to occupational exposures should be seen as an indication of a possible increased risk for the development of cancer. Besides these aspecific markers of chromosomal damage, other studies have focused on the occurrence of specific chromosomal aberrations due to occupational exposures. An example of this is a study on translocations t(14;18), t(4;11) and t(6;11), which are associated with lymphoma and therapy-related leukaemias, among benzene-exposed subjects.[175] Interestingly, besides aneuploidy (both monosomy and trisomy) of all seven chromosomes studied (2, 4, 6, 11, 12, 14 and 18), benzene also induced translocations between chromosomes 14 and 18, t(14;18), known to be associated with follicular non-Hodgkin lymphoma among the highly exposed workers. Data obtained from this study add to the evidence that benzene might be related to the occurrence of lymphoma.

There are a wide range of other biological markers that have been applied as markers of possible carcinogenic mechanisms associated with occupational exposures. These include, among others, the measurements of DNA and protein adducts, oxidative stress markers, immunological and hormonal factors. Although these studies can provide important mechanistic insights into possible disease mechanisms, they have not been formally validated as intermediate markers. As such, the interpretation of these studies has to be performed with some reservation as the exact relevance to cancer remains often unknown.

Susceptibility markers

Traditionally, family history has been used in epidemiological studies as a crude marker for inherited susceptibility to cancer; however, identification of specific susceptibility factors requires the use of biomarkers. Susceptibility biomarkers can be measured at the genotypic level (variations in DNA base sequences) or at the functional/phenotypic level (e.g. metabolic phenotypes, DNA repair capacity). While phenotypic measures are closer to the disease process and can integrate the influences of multiple genetic and post-transcriptional influences on protein expression and function, genotypic measures are considerably easier to study in epidemiological studies since they are stable over time and less prone to measurement error.[176]

The most common types of genetic variation are single nucleotide polymorphisms (SNPs) and over a million already have been identified.[177] Most published occupational epidemiological studies on possible interactions between occupational exposures and genetic polymorphisms on cancer risk have evaluated one or a few promising candidate genes mostly related to the metabolic pathway. These studies have rendered largely inconsistent findings mostly due to the limited size of these studies. One of the few positive examples is the possible interaction between NAT2 acetylation status and benzidine exposure on the risk of developing bladder cancer. In a pooled analysis of two studies on the possible interaction between NAT2 acetylation status and bladder cancer risk among benzidine-exposed workers, a lower risk for developing bladder cancer was found among subjects with a slow NAT2 genotype (OR = 0.3, 95 per cent, CI 0.1–1.0).[178,179]

Currently, technological advances are enabling researchers to move beyond evaluating only a few genetic variants, to a more comprehensive evaluation of hundreds of variants in important aetiologic pathways (e.g. carcinogen activation and detoxification, DNA repair, inflammation, apoptosis), to the entire genome through genome-wide association studies (GWAS). An illustration of the progress of the use of genotyping methods in occupational research can be found in a study on haematological effects among a cohort of 250 workers exposed to benzene and 140 controls.[53] Initial gene–environment analyses in this study were based on candidate gene approaches focusing on genes involved in the metabolism of benzene (four genes, four SNPs),[53] DNA double-strand break repair (seven genes, 24 SNPs) and cytokine and cellular adhesion molecule pathways (20 genes, 40 SNPs).[180] A more recent analysis of the same study population,[181] used a chip-based assay (GoldenGate assay) for genotyping which allowed for a larger number of SNPs to be assessed (414 genes, 1433 SNPs). These SNPs were selected from the SNP500Cancer database, and were, therefore, hypothesized to be involved in the development of cancer. However, the influence of these SNP on benzene-induced haematotoxicity was largely unknown for most SNPs. This study should, therefore, primarily be seen as hypothesis-generating and indeed has provided information on several putative genes involved in benzene haematotoxity that went well beyond the more classical focus in occupational health research on metabolic genes. Studies on genome-wide interactions (GEWIS) are forthcoming. However, it is questionable if occupational studies will be amendable for these large-scale approaches given the inherent limited size of industry-based studies. Hospital- and population-based case–control studies might be more suitable given the much larger number of cases. However, the prevalence of specific occupational exposures are likely to be low in these studies resulting in low power to investigate gene–environment interactions. This could be solved by establishing large consortia of case–control studies; however, successful standardization of the exposure assessment across these studies will determine the eventual success of GEWIS in occupational research.

Exposure markers

Biomarkers of exposure generally aim at measuring the level of an external agent or its metabolites, in either the free state or bound to macromolecules. The range of biological samples that can be obtained and analysed includes blood, urine, exhaled breath, hair, nails, milk, faeces, sweat, saliva, semen and cerebrospinal fluid. The choice of biological sample depends on the substance of interest, its characteristics (e.g. solubility, metabolism, transformation and excretion), and how invasive the method to obtain it is. As such, several biomarkers can be available to represent the same exposure, including the parent compound itself, a metabolite, or a macromolecular DNA or protein adduct.

Whereas 'classical' methods of exposure assessment provide an estimate for exposure from one route of exposure only (e.g. inhalation through the respiratory system, ingestion through the gastrointestinal system, or absorption through the skin), biological monitoring has the theoretical advantage of integrating exposures from all exposure routes. In addition, it also covers unexpected or accidental exposures and reflects interindividual differences in uptake, metabolism, genetic susceptibility and excretion.[182,183] However, some exposure biomarkers can also be formed endogenously and levels may then reflect both endogenous formation and exogenous exposures.[184] Nonetheless, the use of exposure markers in occupational

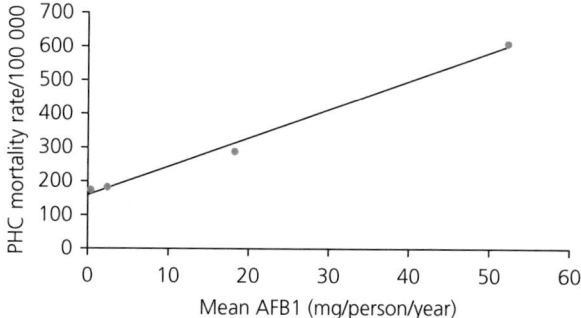

Figure 85.11 The relationship between hepatocellular carcinoma mortality rate and dietary aflatoxin B1 exposure in four communes in southern Guangxi, China (Adapted and reprinted by permission from the American Association for Cancer Research from Yeh FS et al. Hepatitis B virus, aflatoxins, and hepatocellular carcinoma in Southern Guangxi, China. *Cancer Research*. 1989; **49**: 2506–9).

epidemiology could potentially lead to more accurate and/or more biologically relevant exposure estimates than 'classical' methods. Examples of this are the studies on hepatocellular carcinoma (HCC) and aflatoxin exposures. In an early ecological study, mean aflatoxin B1 (AFB1), estimated through analysis of market samples of commonly eaten foods, showed an almost perfect linear relation when plotted against mortality rates of liver cancer (Figure 85.11).[185] However, when exposure was assessed on an individual basis via a structured questionnaire in a later study, no association was found between AFB1 exposure and HCC.[186] This finding stood in sharp contrast to the very strong association between the presence of urinary aflatoxin biomarkers, especially aflatoxin-N^7-guanine (AFB-N^7-gua) and risk of HCC in the same population. These data highlighted that in this particular case the assessment of AFB1, a food contaminant, by questionnaire is inadequate and that the use of urinary markers improved the exposure classification of the study subjects.

It is certainly not a given that the use of biomarkers of exposure will lead to a better assessment of exposure. The successful application of exposure markers depends both on assay performance and on intrinsic properties of the marker itself (half-life, intra- and interindividual variation). It is beyond the scope of this chapter to discuss these points in detail and we refer to textbooks that discuss these issues in more detail.[187,188] Before deciding to use a specific biological marker to assess exogenous exposures to investigate a specific hypothesis, there are a number of factors that should be assessed. One should verify that the marker is indeed detectable in human populations and that its kinetics are known. A repeated-measurements sampling strategy should be designed to be able to evaluate interindividual variation relative to intraindividual variation, and in addition duplicate samples should be included in the design to assess laboratory variation. Furthermore, the timing of sample collection in combination with the biological half-life of the biomarker should be optimized.

The effect of modifiers should be known and all major sources of variance should be quantified.

In summary increasing knowledge of the biological mechanisms involved in the development of occupational cancer, together with the technological advances in analytical platforms for genetic polymorphisms, gene transcripts, proteins and small molecular weight compounds, will allow a broad exploration of aetiologic factors in biologic samples from subjects in occupational studies.[189] Clearly, the statistical analysis and interpretation of study findings and their effective and ethically appropriate translation to the individual and general population will be challenging.[190,191] We are optimistic, however, that the application of biomarkers in occupational cancer research will lead to better identification of new risks, the identification of potential susceptible populations and might lead to the detection of cancer-exposure specific markers.

Key points

- Cancers of the lung, urinary bladder, mesothelioma, nasal cavity, liver (angiosarcoma), leukaemia and non-melanocytic skin are among those most consistently associated with occupational exposures.
- About 150 agents occurring in the workplace are considered as carcinogens.
- Around 5 per cent of all cancers are attributable to workplace exposures.
- Occupational cancers are preventable and this makes their identification even more necessary. However, the number of cancers notified as occupational is extremely small.
- In industrialized countries, the work environment is much more secure than it was in the past. An increasing number of workers in developing countries are exposed to occupational carcinogens.

ACKNOWLEDGEMENTS

Parts of this chapter have been adapted and updated from a book chapter entitled Application of biomarkers in cancer epidemiology, by Garcia-Closas *et al.* in *Cancer epidemiology and prevention* and from a book chapter entitled Urinary bladder cancer, by Kogevinas *et al.* in *A textbook of cancer epidemiology*, 2nd edn, edited by Adami *et al.*

REFERENCES

1. Lynge E. From cross-sectional survey to cohort study. *Occupational and Environmental Medicine*. 2009; **66**: 428–9.
2. Boffetta P, Saracci R Kogevinas M *et al.* Occupational carcinogens. In: Stellman JM (ed.). *Encyclopaedia on occupational health and safety*, 2nd edn. Geneva: International Labour Organization, 1998: 4–18.
3. International Agency for Research on Cancer. *Cancer: Causes, occurrence and control.* Tomatis L (ed.). Lyon: IARC Scientific Publications, 1990.
4. Siemiatycki J, Richardson L, Straif K *et al.* Listing occupational carcinogens. *Environmental Health Perspectives.* 2004; **112**: 1447–59.
5. Doll R, Peto R. The causes of cancer: Quantitative estimates of avoidable risks of cancer in the United States today. *Journal of the National Cancer Institute.* 1981; **66**: 1191–308.
6. Steenland K, Burnett C, Lalich N *et al.* Dying for work: The magnitude of US mortality from selected causes of death associated with occupation. *American Journal of Industrial Medicine.* 2003; **43**: 461–82.
7. Messing K, Punnett L, Bond M *et al.* Be the fairest of them all: Challenges and recommendations for the treatment of gender in occupational health research. *American Journal of Industrial Medicine.* 2003; **43**: 618–29.
8. International Agency for Research on Cancer. IARC Monographs on the Evaluation of the Carcinogenic Risk of Chemicals to Humans, vols 1–88. Lyon: IARC, 1972–2005. Available from: www.iarc.fr.
9. Rousseau MC, Straif K, Siemiatycki J. IARC carcinogen update. *Environmental Health Perspectives.* 2005; **113**: A580–1.
10. International Agency for Research on Cancer. Part F: Chemical agents and related occupations. IARC Monographs on the Evaluation of Carcinogenic Risks to Humans, vol. 100. Lyon: IARC Publications, 2009.
11. Kauppinen T, Toikkanen J, Pedersen D *et al.* Occupational exposure to carcinogens in the European Union. *Occupational and Environmental Medicine.* 2000; **57**: 10–18.
12. Mirabelli D, Kauppinen T. Occupational exposures to carcinogens in Italy: An update of CAREX database. *International Journal of Occupational and Environmental Health.* 2005; **11**: 53–63.
13. Partanen T, Chaves J, Wesseling C *et al.* Workplace carcinogen and pesticide exposure in Costa Rica. *International Journal of Occupational and Environmental Health.* 2003; **9**: 104–11.
14. Saracci R. The interactions of tobacco smoking and other agents in cancer etiology. *Epidemiologic Reviews.* 1987; **9**: 175–93.
15. International Agency for Research on Cancer. Silica: Some silicates, coal dust, and paraaramid fibrils. Monographs on the Evaluation of Carcinogenic Risks to Humans, vol. 68. Lyon: IARC, 1997.
16. Steenland K, Mannetje A, Boffetta P *et al.* Pooled exposure–response analyses and risk assessment for lung cancer in 10 cohorts of silica-exposed workers: An IARC multicentre study. *Cancer Causes and Control.* 2001; **12**: 773–84.

17. Brown T, Rushton T. Mortality in the US industrial silica sand industry: 2. A retrospective cohort study. *Occupational and Environmental Medicine.* 2005; **62**: 446–52.
18. Newman Taylor A. Asbestos, lung cancer and mesothelioma in the British Journal of Industrial Medicine. *Occupational and Environmental Medicine.* 2009; **66**: 426–7.
19. Doll R. Mortality from lung cancer in asbestos workers. *British Journal of Industrial Medicine.* 1955; **12**: 81–6.
20. Selikoff IJ, Churg J, Hammond EC. Asbestos exposure and neoplasia. *Journal of the American Association.* 1964; **188**: 22–6.
21. Kogevinas M, Boffetta P, Pearce N. Occupational exposure to occupational carcinogens in developing countries. In: Pearce N, Matos E, Vainio H et al. (eds). *Occupational cancer in developing countries.* IARC Scientific Publications No. 129. Lyon: IARC, 1994: 63–95.
22. Taylor LE, Hillier JA, Benham AJ. *World mineral production, 1999–2003.* Keyworth: Bristish Geological Survey, 2005.
23. Boffetta P, Saracci R, Andersen A et al. Lung cancer mortality among workers in the European production of man-made mineral fibres – A Poisson regression analysis. *Scandinavian Journal of Work and Environmental Health.* 1992; **18**: 279–86.
24. Kjaerheim K, Boffetta P, Hansen J et al. Lung cancer among rock and slag wool production workers. *Epidemiology.* 2002; **13**: 445–53.
25. Kogevinas M, Garcia-Closas M, Trichopoulos D. Urinary bladder cancer. In: Adami HO, Hunter D, Trichopoulos D (eds). *Textbook of cancer epidemiology,* 2nd edn. Oxford: Oxford University Press, 2007: 573–96.
26. Silverman DT, Devesa SS, Moore LE, Rothman N. Bladder cancer. In: Schottenfeld D, Fraumeni JF Jr (eds). *Cancer epidemiology and prevention.* New York: Oxford University Press, 2006: 1156–79.
27. Kogevinas M, 't Mannetje A, Cordier S et al. Occupation and bladder cancer among men in Western Europe. *Cancer Causes and Control.* 2003; **14**: 907–14.
28. Mannetje A, Kogevinas M, Chang-Claude J et al. Occupation and bladder cancer in European women. *Cancer Causes and Control.* 1999; **10**: 209–17.
29. Case RA, Hosker ME, McDonald DB, Pearson JT. Tumours of the urinary bladder in workmen engaged in the manufacture and use of certain dyestuff intermediates in the British chemical industry. Part I. The role of aniline, benzidine, alpha-naphthylamine, and beta-naphthylamine. *British Journal of Industrial Medicine.* 1993; **50**: 389–411.
30. Vineis P, Pirastu R. Aromatic amines and cancer. *Cancer Causes and Control.* 1997; **8**: 346–55.
31. International Agency for Research on Cancer. Occupational exposures of hairdressers and barbers and personal use of hair colourants; some hair dyes, cosmetic colourants, industrial dyestuffs and aromatic amines. IARC Monographs on the Evaluation of Carcinogenic Risks to Humans, vol. 57. Lyon: IARC, 1994.
32. Veys CA. Bladder tumours in rubber workers: A factory study 1946–1995. *Occupational Medicine.* 2004; **54**: 322–9.
33. Kogevinas M, Sala M, Boffetta P et al. Cancer risk in the rubber industry. A review of the recent epidemiological evidence. *Occupational and Environmental Medicine.* 1998; **55**: 1–12.
34. Boffetta P, Silverman DT. A meta-analysis of bladder cancer and diesel exhaust exposure. *Epidemiology.* 2001; **12**: 125–30.
35. Silverman DT, Hoover RN, Mason TJ, Swanson GM. Motor exhaust-related occupations and bladder cancer. *Cancer Research.* 1986; **46**: 2113–16.
36. Guha N, Steenland NK, Merletti F et al. Bladder cancer risk in painters: A meta-analysis. *Occupational and Environmental Medicine.* 2009 (in press).
37. Silverman DT, Levin L, Hoover RN. Occupational risks of bladder cancer among white women in the United States. *American Journal of Epidemiology.* 1990; **132**: 453–61.
38. Gaertner RR, Trpeski L, Johnson KC and the Canadian Cancer Registries Epidemiology Research Group. A case–control study of occupational risk factors for bladder cancer in Canada. *Cancer Causes and Control.* 2004; **15**: 1007–19.
39. Samanic C, Kogevinas M, Dosemeci M et al. Smoking and bladder cancer in Spain: Effects of tobacco type, timing, environmental tobacco smoke, and gender. *Cancer Epidemiology, Biomarkers and Prevention.* 2006; **15**: 1348–54.
40. Anonymous. Asbestos, asbestosis, and cancer: The Helsinki criteria for diagnosis and attribution. *Scandinavian Journal of Work and Environmental Health.* 1997; **23**: 311–16.
41. Lin RT, Takahashi K, Karjalainen A et al. Ecological association between asbestos-related diseases and historical asbestos consumption: An international analysis. *Lancet.* 2007; 369: 844–9.
42. Peto J, Hodgson JT, Matthews FE et al. Continuing increase in mesothelioma mortality in Britain. *Lancet.* 1995; **345**: 535–9.
43. Kogevinas M, Kauppinen T, Winkelmann R et al. Soft tissue sarcoma and non-Hodgkin's lymphoma in workers exposed to phenoxy herbicides, chlorophenols, and dioxins: Two nested case–control studies. *Epidemiology.* 1995; **6**: 396–402.
44. Smith PG, Doll R. Mortality from cancer and all causes among British radiologists. *British Journal of Radiology.* 1981; **54**: 187–94.
45. Matanoski GM, Sartwell P, Elliott E et al. Cancer risks in radiologists and radiation workers. In: Boice JD Jr, Fraumeni JF Jr (eds). *Radiation carcinogenesis: Epidemiology and biological significance.* New York: Raven Press, 1984: 83–96.
46. Cardis E, Vrijheid M, Blettner M et al. Risk of cancer after low doses of ionising radiation: Retrospective cohort study in 15 countries. *British Medical Journal.* 2005; **331**: 77.
47. Savitz DA, Loomis DP. Magnetic field exposure in relation to leukemia and brain cancer mortality among electric utility workers. *American Journal of Epidemiology.* 1995; **141**: 123–34.
48. Kelsey KT. Perspectives on research and practice in occupational and environmental health: The case of

benzene. *Occupational and Environmental Medicine.* 2010; **67**: 74–5.
49. Hernberg S, Savilahti K, Ahlman K, Asp S. Prognostic aspects of benzene poisoning. *British Journal of Industrial Medicine.* 1966; **23**: 204–9.
50. Aksoy M, Dincol K, Akgün T et al. Hematological effects of chronic benzene poisoning in 217 workers. *British Journal of Industrial Medicine.* 1971; **28**: 296–302.
51. Infante PF, Rinsky RA, Wagoner JK, Young RJ. Leukaemia in benzene workers. *Lancet* 1977; **2**: 76–8.
52. Rinsky RA, Smith AB, Hornung R et al. Benzene and leukemia. An epidemiologic risk assessment. *New England Journal of Medicine.* 1987; **316**: 1044–50.
53. Lan Q, Zhang L, Li G et al. Hematotoxicity in workers exposed to low levels of benzene. *Science.* 2004; **306**: 1774–6.
54. Beane Freeman L, Blair L, Lubin JH et al. Mortality from lymphohematopoietic malignancies among workers in formaldehyde industries: Update of the NCI cohort. *Journal of the National Cancer Institute.* 2009; **101**: 751–61.
55. Pearce N, Smith AH, Reif JS. Increased risks of soft tissue sarcoma, malignant lymphoma, and acute myeloid leukemia in abattoir workers. *American Journal of Industrial Medicine.* 1988; **14**: 63–72.
56. UNSCEAR (United Nations Scientific Committee on the Effects of Atomic Radiation). Sources and effects of ionizing radiation. United Nations Publication No. E. 00. IX. 3. Annex I. Epidemiological evaluation of radiation-induced cancer. New York: UNSCEAR, 2000: 297–431.
57. Kogevinas M, Ferro G, Andersen A et al. Cancer mortality in a historical cohort study of workers exposed to styrene. *Scandinavian Journal of Work and Environmental Health.* 1994; **20**: 249–59.
58. Hogstedt C, Malinqvist N, Wadman B. Leukemia in workers exposed to ethylene oxide. *Journal of the American Medical Association.* 1979; **241**: 1132–3.
59. Steenland K, Stayner L, Griefe A et al. Mortality among workers exposed to ethylene oxide. *New England Journal of Medicine.* 1991; **324**: 1402–7.
60. Gawkrodger DJ. Occupational skin cancers. *Occupational Medicine.* 2004; **54**: 458–63.
61. Suarez B, Lopez-Abente G, Martinez C et al. Occupation and skin cancer: The results of the HELIOS-I multicenter case–control study. *BMC Public Health.* 2007; **7**: 180.
62. Marehbian J, Colt JS, Baris D et al. Occupation and keratinocyte cancer risk: A population-based case–control study. *Cancer Causes and Control.* 2007; **18**: 895–908.
63. Lancaster HO, Nelson J. Sunlight as a cause of melanoma. A clinical survey. *Medical Journal of Australia.* 1957; **44**: 452–6.
64. Silverstone H, Searle JH. The epidemiology of skin cancer in Queensland: The influence of phenotype and environment. *British Journal of Cancer.* 1970; **24**: 235–52.
65. Aubry F, MacGibbon B. Risk factors of squamous cell carcinoma of the skin. A case–control study in the Montreal region. *Cancer.* 1985; **55**: 907–11.
66. O'Loughlin C, Moriarty MJ, Herity B, Daly L. A re-appraisal of risk factors for skin carcinoma in Ireland. A case–control study. *Irish Journal of Medical Science.* 1985; **154**: 61–5.
67. Green A, Beardmore G, Hart V et al. Skin cancer in a Queensland population. *Journal of the American Academy of Dermatologists.* 1988; **19**: 1045–52.
68. Hogan DJ, To T, Gran L et al. Risk factors for basal cell carcinoma. *International Journal of Dermatology.* 1989; **28**: 591–4.
69. Marks R, Jolley D, Dorevitch AP, Selwood TS. The incidence of non-melanocytic skin cancers in an Australian population: Results of a five-year prospective study. *Medical Journal of Australia.* 1989; **150**: 475–8.
70. Green A, Battistutta D. Incidence and determinants of skin cancer in a high-risk Australian population. *International Journal of Cancer.* 1990; **46**: 356–61.
71. Vitasa BC, Taylor HR, Strickland PT et al. Association of nonmelanoma skin cancer and actinic keratosis with cumulative solar ultraviolet exposure in Maryland watermen. *Cancer.* 1990; **65**: 2811–17.
72. Freedman DM, Zahm SH, Dosemeci M. Residential and occupational exposure to sunlight and mortality from non-Hodgkin's lymphoma: composite (threefold) case–control study. *British Medical Journal.* 1997; **314**: 1451–5.
73. Freedman DM, Dosemeci M, McGlynn K. Sunlight and mortality from breast, ovarian, colon, prostate, and non-melanoma skin cancer: A composite death certificate based case–control study. *Occupational and Environmental Medicine.* 2002; **59**: 257–62.
74. Rushton L, Hutchings S, Brown T. The burden of cancer at work: Estimation as the first step to prevention. *Occupational and Environmental Medicine.* 2008; **65**: 789–800.
75. Hayes RB, Raatgever JW, de Bruyn A, Gerin M. Cancer of the nasal cavity and paranasal sinuses, and formaldehyde exposure. *International Journal of Cancer.* 1986; **37**: 487–92.
76. Vaughan TL. Occupation and squamous cell cancers of the pharynx and sinonasal cavity. *American Journal of Industrial Medicine.* 1989; **16**: 493–510.
77. Leclerc A, Luce D, Demers PA et al. Sinonasal cancer and occupation. Results from the reanalysis of twelve case–control studies. *American Journal of Industrial Medicine.* 1997; **31**: 153–65.
78. Demers PA, Kogevinas M, Boffetta P et al. Wood dust and sino-nasal cancer: Pooled reanalysis of twelve case–control studies. *American Journal of Industrial Medicine.* 1995; **28**: 151–66.
79. Hauptmann M, Lubin JH, Stewart PA et al. Mortality from solid cancers among workers in formaldehyde industries. *American Journal of Epidemiology.* 2004; **159**: 1117–30.
80. Straif K, Benbrahim-Tallaa L, Baan R et al. On behalf of the WHO International Agency for Research on Cancer Monograph Working Group. A review of human carcinogens – Part C: Metals, arsenic, dusts, and fibres. *Lancet Oncology.* 2009; **10**: 453–4.
81. Goodman M, Morgan RW, Ray R et al. Cancer in asbestos-exposed occupational cohorts: A meta-analysis. *Cancer Causes and Control.* 1999; **10**: 453–65.

82. Cocco P, Ward MH, Buiatti E. Occupational risk factors for gastric cancer: An overview. *Epidemiologic Reviews.* 1996; **18**: 218–34.
83. Ward E, Boffetta P, Andersen A *et al.* Update of the follow-up of mortality and cancer incidence among European workers employed in the vinyl chloride industry. *Epidemiology.* 2001; **12**: 710–18.
84. Creech JL Jr, Johnson MN. Angiosarcoma of liver in the manufacture of polyvinyl chloride. *Journal of Occupational Medicine.* 1974; **16**: 150–1.
85. Mundt KA, Dell LD, Austin RP *et al.* Historical cohort study of 10 109 men in the North American vinyl chloride industry, 1942–72: Update of cancer mortality to 31 December 1995. *Occupational and Environmental Medicine.* 2000; **57**: 774–81.
86. Ojajärvi A, Partanen T, Ahlbom A *et al.* Risk of pancreatic cancer in workers exposed to chlorinated hydrocarbon solvents and related compounds: A meta-analysis. *American Journal of Epidemiology.* 2001; **153**: 841–50.
87. Goldberg MS, Labreche F. Occupational risk factors for female breast cancer: A review. *Occupational and Environmental Medicine.* 1996; **53**: 145–56.
88. Peplonska B, Stewart P, Szeszenia-Dąbrowska N *et al.* Occupational exposure to organic solvents and breast cancer in women. *Occupational and Environmental Medicine.* October 9, Epub ahead of print 2009.
89. Straif K, Baan R, Grosse Y *et al.* Carcinogenicity of shift-work, painting, and fire-fighting. *Lancet Oncology.* 2007; **8**: 1065–6.
90. Megdal SP, Kroenke CH, Laden F *et al.* Night work and breast cancer risk: A systematic review and meta-analysis. *European Journal of Cancer.* 2005; **41**: 2023–32.
91. Nurminen M, Karjalainen A. Epidemiological estimate of the proportion of fatalities related to occupational factors in Finland. *Scandinavian Journal of Work, Environment and Health.* 2001; **27**: 161–213.
92. Colditz G, Hunter D, Trichopoulos D, Willett W. Harvard report on cancer prevention. *Cancer Causes and Control.* 1996; **7**: S3–S58.
93. Dreyer L, Andersen A, Pukkala E. Occupation. Avoidable cancers in the Nordic countries. *Acta Pathologica, Microbiologica, et Immunologica Scandinavica.* 1997; **105**: 68–79.
94. Driscoll T, Takala J, Steenland K *et al.* Review of estimates of the global burden of injury and illness due to occupational exposures. *American Journal of Industrial Medicine.* 2005; **48**: 491–502.
95. Kogevinas M, Kauppinen T, Boffetta P, Saracci R. Estimation of the burden of occupational cancer in Europe. Final Report to the European Commission of a project funded by the programme 'Europe Against Cancer' (Contract SOC 96-200742-05F02). Barcelona: IMIM, 1998.
96. Imbernon E. *Estimation de certains cancers professionnels.* Paris: Institut de Veille Sanitaire, April, 2003.
97. Nicholson WJ. Quantitative estimates of cancer in the workplace. *American Journal of Industrial Medicine.* 1984; **5**: 341–2.
98. Spirtas R, Heineman EF, Bernstein L *et al.* Malignant mesothelioma: Attributable risk of asbestos exposure. *Occupational and Environmental Medicine.* 1994; **51**: 804–11.
99. Naud C, Brugere J. La reconnaissance des cancers professionnels en Europe. *British Toxicology Society Newsletter.* 2003.
100. Kogevinas M, Castaño-Vinyals G, Rodríguez Suárez MM *et al.* Estimación de la incidencia y mortalidad por cáncer laboral en España, 2002. *Archivos de Prevención de Riesgos Laborales.* 2008; **11**: 180–7.
101. Vineis P, Cantor K, Gonzales C *et al.* Occupational cancer in developed and developing countries. *International Journal of Cancer.* 1995; **62**: 655–60.
102. Faggiano F, Partanen T, Kogevinas M, Boffetta P. Socioeconomic differences in cancer incidence and mortality. In: Kogevinas M, Pearce N, Susser M, Boffetta P (eds). *Social inequalities in cancer.* IARC Scientific Publications No. 138. Lyon: International Agency for Research on Cancer, 1997: 65–176.
103. Marmot MG, Kogevinas M, Elston MA. Social/economic status and disease. *Annual Reviews of Public Health.* 1987; **8**: 111–35.
104. Boffetta P, Saracci R, Westerholm P, Kogevinas M. Exposure to occupational carcinogens and social class differences in cancer occurrence. In: Kogevinas M, Pearce N, Susser M, Boffetta P (eds). *Social inequalities in cancer.* IARC Scientific Publications No. 138. Lyon: International Agency on Research in Cancer, 1997: 331–41.
105. Logan WPD. Mortality from cancer in relation to occupation and social class. IARC Scientific Publication No. 36. Lyon: International Agency for Research on Cancer, 1982.
106. Symanski E, Kupper LL, Hertz-Picciotto I, Rappaport SM. Comprehensive evaluation of long-term trends in occupational exposure. Part 2: Predictive models for declining exposures. *Occupational and Environmental Medicine.* 1998; **55**: 310–6.
107. Pearce N, Matos E, Vainio H *et al.* (eds). *Occupational cancer in developing countries.* IARC Scientific Publications No. 129. Lyon: IARC, 1994: 1–191.
108. Checkoway H, Pearce N, Kriebel D. *Research methods in occupational epidemiology.* New York: Oxford University Press, 2004.
109. Breslow NE, Day NE. The design and analysis of cohort studies. In: Esteve J, Benhamou E, Raymond L (eds). *Statistical methods in cancer research*, vol. II. IARC Scientific Publication No. 82. Lyon: International Agency for Research on Cancer, 1987.
110. Fingerhut MA, Halperin WE, Marlow DA *et al.* Cancer mortality in workers exposed to 2,3,7,8-tetrachlorodibenzo-p-dioxin. *New England Journal of Medicine.* 1991; **324**: 212–18.
111. Wernli KJ, Fitzgibbons ED, Ray RM *et al.* Occupational risk factors for esophageal and stomach cancers among female textile workers in Shanghai, China. *American Journal of Epidemiology.* 2006; **163**: 717–25.

112. Fox AJ, Collier PF. Low mortality rates in industrial cohort studies due to selection for work and survival in the industry. *British Journal of Preventive and Social Medicine.* 1976; **30**: 225–30.

113. Steenland K, Stayner L. The importance of employment status in occupational cohort mortality studies. *Epidemiology.* 1991; **2**: 418–23.

114. Blair A, Stewart P, Lubin JH, Forastiere F. Methodological issues regarding confounding and exposure misclassification in epidemiological studies of occupational exposures. *American Journal of Industrial Medicine.* 2007; **50**: 199–207.

115. Axelson O. Aspects on confounding in occupational health epidemiology. *Scandinavian Journal of Work and Environmental Health.* 1978; **4**: 98–102.

116. Pearce N. Multistage modelling of lung cancer mortality in asbestos textile workers. *International Journal of Epidemiology.* 1988; **17**: 747–52.

117. Kaldor JM, L'Abbé KA. Interaction between human carcinogens. In: Vainio H, Sorsa M, McMichael AJ (eds). *Complex mixtures and cancer risk.* Lyon: IARC, 1990.

118. Kennedy SM, Koehoorn M. Exposure assessment in epidemiology: Does gender matter? *American Journal of Industrial Medicine.* 2003; **44**: 576–83.

119. Ahrens W, Jöckel KH, Brochard P *et al.* Retrospective assessment of asbestos exposure I. Case–control analysis in a study of lung cancer: Efficiency of job-specific questionnaires and job exposure matrices. *International Journal of Epidemiology.* 1993; **22**: S83–S95.

120. Stewart WF, Stewart PA. Occupational case–control studies: I. Collecting information on work histories and work-related exposures. *American Journal of Industrial Medicine.* 1994; **26**: 297–312.

121. Serra C, Kogevinas M, Silverman DT *et al.* Work in the textile industry in Spain and bladder cancer. *Occupational and Environmental Medicine.* 2008; **65**: 552–9.

122. Teschke K, Ahrens W, Andersen A *et al.* Occupational exposure to chemical and biological agents in the nonproduction departments of pulp, paper, and paper product mills: An international study. *American Industrial Hygiene Association Journal.* 1999; **60**: 73–83.

123. Pannett B, Coggon D, Acheson ED. A job-exposure matrix for use in population based studies in England and Wales. *British Journal of Industrial Medicine.* 1985; **42**: 777–83.

124. Hoar SK, Morrison AS, Cole P *et al.* An occupation and exposure linkage system for the study of occupational carcinogenesis. *Journal of Occupational Medicine.* 1980; **22**: 722–6.

125. Plato N, Steineck G, Norell SE. Construction of a job exposure matrix for epidemiological studies of urothelial cancer. In: *Progress in occupational epidemiology.* Amsterdam: Excerpta Medica, 1988.

126. Ferrario F, Continenza D, Pisani P *et al.* Description of a job exposure matrix for sixteen agents which are or may be related to respiratory cancer. In: *Progress in occupational epidemiology.* Amsterdam: Excerpta Medica, 1988.

127. Sieber WK, Sundin DS, Frazier TM *et al.* Development, use, and availability of a job exposure matrix based on national occupational hazard survey data. *American Journal of Industrial Medicine.* 1991; **20**: 163–74.

128. Kauppinen T, Toikkanen J, Pukkala E. From cross-tabulations to multipurpose exposure information systems: A new job–exposure matrix. *American Journal of Industrial Medicine.* 1998; **33**: 409–17.

129. Bouyer J, Hémon D. Retrospective evaluation of occupational exposures in population based case–control studies. General overview with special attention to job exposure matrices. *International Journal of Epidemiology.* 1993; **22**: S57–S67.

130. Siemiatycki J (ed.). *Risk factors for cancer in the workplace.* Boca Raton, FL: CRC Press, 1991.

131. Kauppinen T, Pannett B, Marlow D *et al.* Retrospective assessment of exposure by modelling in a collaborative study on cancer risks among workers exposed to phenoxy herbicides and chlorophenols. *Scandinavian Journal of Work and Environmental Health.* 1994; **20**: 260–9.

132. National Research Council. Biological markers in environmental health research. Committee on Biological Markers of the National Research Council. *Health Perspectives.* 1987; **74**: 3–9.

133. Rothman N, Wacholder S, Caporaso NE *et al.* The use of common genetic polymorphisms to enhance the epidemiologic study of environmental carcinogens. *Biochimica et Biophysica Acta – Reviews on Cancer.* 2001; **1471**: C1–C10.

134. Rothman N, Stewart WF, Schulte PA. Incorporating biomarkers into cancer epidemiology: A matrix of biomarker and study design categories. *Cancer Epidemiology Biomarkers and Prevention.* 1995; **4**: 301–11.

135. Schulte PA. Methodologic issues in the use of biologic markers in epidemiologic research. *American Journal of Epidemiology.* 1987; **126**: 1006–16.

136. Perera FP. Molecular cancer epidemiology: A new tool in cancer prevention. *Journal of the National Cancer Institute.* 1987; **78**: 887–98.

137. Perera FP. Molecular epidemiology: On the path to prevention? *Journal of the National Cancer Institute.* 2000; **92**: 602–12.

138. Toniolo P, Boffetta P, Shuker DEG *et al.* Application of biomarkers to cancer epidemiology. IARC Scientific Publications. Lyon: IARC, 1997: 142.

139. Aardema MJ, MacGregor JT. Toxicology and genetic toxicology in the new era of 'toxicogenomics': Impact of '-omics' technologies. *Mutation Research – Fundamental and Molecular Mechanisms of Mutagenesis.* 2002; **499**: 13–25.

140. Wang W, Zhou H, Lin H *et al.* Quantification of proteins and metabolites by mass spectrometry without isotopic labeling or spiked standards. *Analytical Chemistry.* 2003; **75**: 4818–26.

141. Hanash S. Disease proteomics. *Nature.* 2003; **422**: 226–32.

142. Baak JPA, Path FRC, Hermsen MAJA *et al.* Genomics and proteomics in cancer. *European Journal of Cancer.* 2003; **39**: 1199–215.

143. Sellers TA, Yates JR. Review of proteomics with applications to genetic epidemiology. *Genetic Epidemiology*. 2003; **24**: 83–98.
144. Strausberg RL, Simpson AJG, Wooster R. Sequence-based cancer genomics: Progress, lessons and opportunities. *Nature Reviews. Genetics.* 2003; **4**: 409–18.
145. Staudt LM. Molecular diagnosis of the hematologic cancers. *New England Journal of Medicine.* 2003; **348**: 1777–85.
146. Hollstein M, Hergenhahn M, Yang Q et al. New approaches to understanding p53 gene tumor mutation spectra. *Mutation Research – Fundamental and Molecular Mechanisms of Mutagenesis.* 1999; **431**: 199–209.
147. Hainaut P, Pfeifer GP. Patterns of p53 G->T transversions in lung cancers reflect the primary mutagenic signature of DNA-damage by tobacco smoke. *Carcinogenesis.* 2001; **22**: 367–74.
148. Olivier M, Eeles R, Hollstein M et al. The IARC TP53 database: New online mutation analysis and recommendations to users. *Human Mutation.* 2002; **19**: 607–14.
149. Greenblatt MS, Bennett WP, Hollstein M, Harris CC. Mutations in the p53 tumor suppressor gene: Clues to cancer etiology and molecular pathogenesis. *Cancer Research.* 1994; **54**: 4855–78.
150. Staib F, Hussain SP, Hofseth LJ et al. TP53 and liver carcinogenesis. *Human Mutation.* 2003; **21**: 201–16.
151. Pfeifer GP, Hainaut P. On the origin of G -> T transversions in lung cancer. *Mutation Research – Fundamental and Molecular Mechanisms of Mutagenesis.* 2003; **526**: 39–43.
152. Barbin A, Froment O, Boivin S et al. p53 Gene mutation pattern in rat liver tumors induced by vinyl chloride. *Cancer Research.* 1997; **57**: 1695–8.
153. Jones PA. Epigenetics in carcinogenesis and cancer prevention. *Annals of the New York Academy of Sciences.* 2003; **983**: 213–19.
154. Esteller M. Cancer epigenetics: DNA methylation and chromatin alterations in human cancer. *Advances in Experimental Medicine and Biology.* 2003; **532**: 39–49.
155. Moore LE, Huang WY, Chung J, Hayes RB. Epidemiologic considerations to assess altered DNA methylation from environmental exposures in cancer. *Annals of the New York Academy of Sciences.* 2003; **983**: 181–96.
156. Baccarelli A, Wright RO, Bollati V et al. Rapid DNA methylation changes after exposure to traffic particles. *American Journal of Respiratory and Critical Care Medicine.* 2009; **179**: 572–8.
157. Bollati V, Baccarelli A, Hou L et al. Changes in DNA methylation patterns in subjects exposed to low-dose benzene. *Cancer Research.* 2007; **67**: 876–80.
158. Rusiecki JA, Baccarelli A, Bollati V et al. Global DNA hypomethylation is associated with high serum-persistent organic pollutants in Greenlandic inuit. *Environmental Health Perspectives.* 2008; **116**: 1547–52.
159. Moore LE, Smith AH, Eng C et al. Arsenic-related chromosomal alterations in bladder cancer. *Journal of the National Cancer Institute.* 2002; **94**: 1688–96.
160. Rowley JD. The role of chromosome translocations in leukemogenesis. *Seminars in Hematology.* 1999; **36** (Suppl. 7): 59–72.
161. Schatzkin A, Freedman LS, Schiffman MH, Dawsey SM. Validation of intermediate end points in cancer research. *Journal of the National Cancer Institute.* 1990; **82**: 1746–52.
162. Schulte PA, Rothman N, Schottenfeld D. Design considerations in molecular epidemiology. In: Schulte PA, Perera PP (eds). *Molecular epidemiology – Principles and practices.* San Diego: Academic Press, 1993: 159–98.
163. Schatzkin A, Gail M. The promise and peril of surrogate end points in cancer research. *Nature Reviews. Cancer.* 2002; **2**: 19–27.
164. Zhang L, Rothman N, Wang Y et al. Benzene increases aneuploidy in the lymphocytes of exposed workers: A comparison of data obtained by fluorescence *in situ* hybridization in interphase and metaphase cells. *Environmental and Molecular Mutagenesis.* 1999; **34**: 260–8.
165. Zhang L, Eastmond DA, Smith MT. The nature of chromosomal aberrations detected in humans exposed to benzene. *Critical Reviews in Toxicology.* 2002; **32**: 1–42.
166. Tucker JD, Eastmond DA, Littlefield LG. Cytogenetic end-points as biological dosimeters and predictors of risk in epidemiological studies. IARC Scientific Publications, vol. 142. Lyon: IARC, 1997: 185–200.
167. Hagmar L, Brogger A, Hansteen IL et al. Cancer risk in humans predicted by increased levels of chromosomal aberrations in lymphocytes: Nordic study group on the health risk of chromosome damage. *Cancer Research.* 1994; **54**: 2919–22.
168. Bonassi S, Abbondandolo A, Camurri L et al. Are chromosome aberrations in circulating lymphocytes predictive of future cancer onset in humans? Preliminary results of an Italian cohort study. *Cancer Genetics and Cytogenetics.* 1995; **79**: 133–5.
169. Liou SH, Lung JC, Chen YH et al. Increased chromosome-type chromosome aberration frequencies as biomarkers of cancer risk in a blackfoot endemic area. *Cancer Research.* 1999; **59**: 1481–4.
170. Smerhovsky Z, Landa K, Rössner P et al. Risk of cancer in an occupationally exposed cohort with increased level of chromosomal aberrations. *Environmental Health Perspectives.* 2001; **109**: 41–5.
171. Bonassi S, Norppa H, Ceppi M et al. Chromosomal aberration frequency in lymphocytes predicts the risk of cancer: Results from a pooled cohort study of 22 358 subjects in 11 countries. *Carcinogenesis.* 2008; **29**: 1178–83.
172. Bonassi S, Hagmar L, Stromberg U et al. Chromosomal aberrations in lymphocytes predict human cancer independently of exposure to carcinogens. *Cancer Research.* 2000; **60**: 1619–25.
173. Bonassi S, Znaor A, Ceppi M et al. An increased micronucleus frequency in peripheral blood lymphocytes predicts the risk of cancer in humans. *Carcinogenesis.* 2007; **28**: 625–31.

174. Murgia E, Ballardin M, Bonassi S *et al.* Validation of micronuclei frequency in peripheral blood lymphocytes as early cancer risk biomarker in a nested case-control study. *Mutation Research - Fundamental and Molecular Mechanisms of Mutagenesis.* 2008; **639**: 27-34.
175. Zhang L, Rothman N, Li G *et al.* Aberrations in chromosomes associated with lymphoma and therapy-related leukemia in benzene-exposed workers. *Environmental and Molecular Mutagenesis.* 2007; **48**: 467-74.
176. Ahsan H, Rundle AG. Measures of genotype versus gene products: Promise and pitfalls in cancer prevention. *Carcinogenesis.* 2003; **24**: 1429-34.
177. Sachidanandam R, Weissman D, Schmidt SC *et al.* A map of human genome sequence variation containing 1.42 million single nucleotide polymorphisms. *Nature.* 2001; **409**: 928-33.
178. Carreon T, Ruder AM, Schulte PA *et al.* NAT2 slow acetylation and bladder cancer in workers exposed to benzidine. *International Journal of Cancer.* 2006; **118**: 161-8.
179. Hayes RB, Bi W, Rothman N *et al.* N-acetylation phenotype and genotype and risk of bladder cancer in benzidine-exposed workers. *Carcinogenesis.* 1993; **14**: 675-8.
180. Lan Q, Zhang L, Shen M *et al.* Polymorphisms in cytokine and cellular adhesion molecule gene and susceptibility to hematotoxicity among workers exposed to benzene. *Cancer Research.* 2005; **65**: 9574-81.
181. Lan Q, Zhang L, Shen M *et al.* Large-scale evaluation of candidate genes identifies associations between DNA repair and genomic maintenance and development of benzene hematotoxicity. *Carcinogenesis.* 2009; **30**: 50-8.
182. Lin YS, Kupper LL, Rappaport SM. Air samples versus biomarkers for epidemiology. *Occupational and Environmental Medicine.* 2005; **62**: 750-60.
183. Rappaport SM, Lyles RH, Kupper LL. An exposure-assessment strategy accounting for within- and between-worker sources of variability. *Annals of Occupational Hygiene.* 1995; **39**: 469-95.
184. De Bont R, van Larebeke N. Endogenous DNA damage in humans: A review of quantitative data. *Mutagenesis.* 2004; **19**: 169-85.
185. Yeh FS, Yu MC, Mo CC *et al.* Hepatitis B virus, aflatoxins, and hepatocellular carcinoma in Southern Guangxi, China. *Cancer Research.* 1989; **49**: 2506-9.
186. Qian GS, Ross RK, Yu MC *et al.* A follow-up study of urinary markers of aflatoxin exposure and liver cancer risk in Shanghai, People's Republic of China. *Cancer Epidemiology Biomarkers and Prevention.* 1994; **3**: 3-10.
187. Nieuwenhuijsen MJ. *Exposure assessment in occupational and environmental epidemiology.* Oxford: Oxford University Press, 2003.
188. Garcia-Closas M, Vermeulen R, Sherman ME *et al.* Application of biomarkers in cancer epidemiology. In: Fraumeni DSJF (ed.). *Cancer epidemiology and prevention,* 3rd edn. New York: Oxford University Press, 2006.
189. Vlaanderen J, Moore LE, Smith MT *et al.* Application of OMICS technologies in occupational and environmental health research. Current status and projections. *Occupational and Environmental Medicine.* 2010; **67**: 136-43.
190. Schulte PA, Hunter D, Rothman N. Ethical and social issues in the use of biomarkers in epidemiological research. IARC Scientific Publications, vol. 142. Lyon: International Agency for Research on Cancer, 1997: 313-18.
191. Guttmacher AE, Collins FS. Welcome to the genomic era. *New England Journal of Medicine.* 2003; **349**: 996-8.

SECTION THREE

Other systemic effects

86	Nephrotoxic effects of workplace exposures *Rema Saxena, Pearl Pai and Gordon M Bell*	1125
87	Neurotoxic effects of workplace exposures *Michael J Aminoff and Marcello Lotti*	1151
88	Hepatotoxic effects of workplace exposure *Thomas W Warnes and Alexander Smith*	1171
89	Workplace exposures and reproductive health *Jens Peter Bonde*	1196
90	Haemopoietic effects of workplace exposures: anaemias, leukaemias and lymphomas *Edward Gordon-Smith, Anthony Yardley-Jones and Atherton Gray*	1215

86

Nephrotoxic effects of workplace exposures

REMA SAXENA, PEARL PAI AND GORDON M BELL

Introduction	1125	Crystalline silica	1137
Heavy metals	**1125**	**Organic solvents and renal disease**	**1138**
Lead and renal disease	1126	Case reports and experimental studies	1138
Cadmium	1131	Case-control studies and progressive renal failure	1139
Mercury	1134	Cross-sectional studies	1139
Uranium	1136	Cohort studies	1141
Chromium	1136	Mechanisms of solvent-induced nephrotoxicity	1141
Beryllium	1136	Acknowledgements	1142
Arsenic	1137	References	1142
Bismuth, copper and gadolinium	1137		

INTRODUCTION

The worldwide acceptance rate for patients commencing renal replacement therapy (RRT) programmes is rising. This international increase is reflected in figures from the United Kingdom, but in some developed countries such as the United States, the acceptance rate has recently remained relatively stable.[1]

In the UK, the current overall annual acceptance rate of new patients starting renal replacement therapy (RRT) is approximately 113 per million.[2] After commencing dialysis, one year's dialysis treatment costs the National Health Service (NHS) between £20 000 and £25 000 per patient,[3] with a greater personal cost to the patient and their family. RRT overall, takes up >2 per cent of the total NHS budget.[4]

In the United States, between the combined years of 2001 to 2005, the incidence of reported end-stage renal disease from glomerulonephritis, secondary glomerulonephritis vasculitis, interstitial nephritis, pyelonephritis, hypertension and malignant renal tumours, was approximately 41.1 per cent.[5]

While immunological and vasculopathic associations are recognized in the causation of chronic kidney disease, occupational factors may also be relevant. In this regard, the nephrotoxicity of heavy metals has been studied for a long time, and evidence also links occupational organic solvent exposure with various kidney diseases.

This chapter reviews the renal effects of such workplace exposures.

HEAVY METALS

Metals are probably the oldest toxic materials known to man. Lead usage may have begun more than 4000 years ago when supplies were obtained as byproducts of silver smelting. Indeed, Hipprocrates in 370BC is credited with the first description of abdominal colic in a man who extracted metals. However, many of the metals of workplace concern today are only recently known to man. In 1817, cadmium was first recognized in ore containing zinc carbonate. Approximately 80 of the 105 elements in the periodic table are regarded as metals, 30 or so of which form compounds reported to produce toxicity in humans and of these only ten are known to be nephrotoxic. The renal toxicological profile of metals such as indium and tantalum, which are used increasingly in newer industries such as microelectronics, is unknown. With present day occupational and environmental standards, the acute and overt renal effects (such as acute renal failure) associated with exposures to lead and mercury are now uncommon. While there must be a full understanding of these well-recognized acute problems, conceptually what we now regard as the toxic effect of metals continues to broaden into the more subtle, chronic effects of long-term nephrotoxicity. In this respect, cause and effect may not always be obvious and allocating blame to particular agents can be difficult especially when there are small repeated exposures to one or more substances. Physicians interested in these nephrotoxic effects need to have an understanding of the metabolism of metals, including any renal cellular effects, and to recognize factors that might influence toxicity. Although treatment is clearly an important topic, prevention of toxicity through public health and worksite programmes, which include raising workers' awareness and adherence to control measures is of equal or perhaps greater importance. Increasingly, emphasis should be focused on the detection of early and possibly reversible biochemical indicators of toxicity, such as renal tubular dysfunction in cadmium toxicity.

LEAD AND RENAL DISEASE

As an occupational and environmental toxin, lead is one of the most widely studied. Its use and indeed suggestions of lead poisoning in lead workers and the general population, date back to ancient times. In the UK, effective control of working with lead goes back many years with the introduction of the Lead Regulations.[6]

Much of lead in the United Kingdom, comes from recycled scrap. Its uses in manufacturing have included electric batteries (27 per cent), electric cables (17 per cent), sheet, pipe, tubes (16 per cent), anti-knock in petrol (11 per cent), solder and alloys (9 per cent), pottery, plastic, glass, paint (4 per cent) and miscellaneous (15 per cent).[7]

Clinical lead poisoning still occurs in some industries (see Table 86.1)[8] as demonstrated in scaffolders involved in

Table 86.1 Industries using lead.

Industry
Smelting, refining, alloying and casting
Battery manufacture
Jewellery manufacture
Glass making
Manufacture of pigments and colours
Glazes and transfers in the pottery industry
Manufacture of inorganic and organic lead compounds
Shipbuilding repairing and breaking
Demolition industry
Painting of buildings and vehicles
Scrap industry
Vehicle radiator repair
Cable coverings manufacture
Use of lead alloys, e.g. manufacture of solder and on firing ranges
Metal reclamation industry

the renovation of previous lead painted structures with high levels of exposure. Other occupations at risk include workers in small/mobile workplaces where lead exposure may not be as obvious. Organic lead poisoning is still occasionally reported in tank cleaners who clean petrol storage tanks that have contained leaded petrol.[9]

In addition, children may be exposed to sources such as lead paint[10] and jewellery.

For over a century, an association between lead poisoning and renal disease has been recognized.[11–13]

The kidney is the first target organ of heavy metal toxicity and the extent of this renal damage depends on the nature, dose, route and duration of exposure.[14]

Four clinical manifestations of lead nephropathy are described: (1) acute lead nephropathy, (2) chronic progressive renal failure, (3) hypertension and (4) the presence of early markers of disturbed tubular function.

Acute lead poisoning

Acute lead poisoning results from short-term, but massive lead absorption and is associated with abdominal colic, encephalopathy, peripheral neuropathy and anaemia.

The major renal effect is disruption of the proximal tubular architecture and function,[15–18] resulting in aminoaciduria, phosphaturia and glycosuria, collectively known as the Fanconi syndrome.[19–21]

Histological changes include eosinophilic intranuclear inclusions in the proximal tubular cells, consisting of lead–protein complexes and mitochondrial swelling.[22–24]

This condition may result in children from repeated ingestion of inappropriate materials, such as lead paint chips.[19]

The blood lead level at which this tubular disorder develops is usually in excess of 150 μg/100 mL and has been induced experimentally in animals fed dietary lead.[25]

As with other forms of Fanconi syndrome, vitamin D-resistant rickets may develop and appears to be rapidly reversed following chelation therapy, which reverses both the tubular reabsorption defect and removes the inclusion bodies.[26]

Chronic, slowly progressive renal failure

This condition results from accumulating lead absorption, often from a recognized occupational source, although non-occupational causes have been identified, such as in childhood lead poisoning resulting from licking off the sweet-tasting lead paint, from the painted wooden verandas in Queensland.[27]

In adults, chronic lead nephropathy may present as chronic tubular interstitial nephritis and may develop several decades after the exposure.[28]

When lead is absorbed excessively, it is deposited mainly in the skeleton, from which it is slowly released once exposure ceases. This gradual release of lead over many years, may contribute to this delayed nephrotoxicity.[29]

Chronic exposure to high levels of lead results in irreversible changes in the kidney, including progressive renal interstitial fibrosis, dilatation of the tubules and tubular atrophy (Figure 86.1). These changes are accompanied by a reduction in glomerular filtration and azotaemia, but are non-specific and common to many other types of renal injury. Typically, renal failure is evident only after many years of excessive lead absorption and can then be associated with hypertension and gout.[30,31] Symptoms are subtle and patients often remain asymptomatic until significant reduction in renal function has occurred.[32]

As discussed by Ekong et al.[10] a blood lead level persistently above 70–80 μg/dL, is a recognized risk factor for chronic kidney disease.[29,33–35] However, concern remains as to whether lower levels of occupational exposure may also contribute to nephrotoxicity in view of the ongoing endogenous exposure from bone and environmental exposure, the burden of which increases with age. Those individuals with hypertension, diabetes, existing chronic kidney disease and those of low socioeconomic status appeared more susceptible, probably due to a higher lead exposure.[36,37]

As further illustrated by Ekong et al.,[10] research relating to the renal outcomes from occupational lead exposure has provided inconsistent results despite a large body of literature being available. This may be due to the smaller sample sizes and because the studies were often cross sections of currently employed workers, who were healthier than the general population. Few studies also included former workers. Furthermore, if renal function declined, workers who were followed in medical surveillance programmes were often removed from the source of the exposure. In other studies where exclusion criteria had been applied, the numbers excluded were not identified. Blood lead level rather than the cumulative measure has also been used and limitations existed due to the co-exposure with environmental cadmium.

Weaver et al.[38] reported an initial period of hyperfiltration following exposure, resulting in an inverse pattern of lead dose with serum creatinine before renal function declined in a group of young South Korean lead workers, but not in the older workers.

Khalil-Manesh et al.[35,39] have previously demonstrated hyperfiltration in animal models with low and high lead exposure. The more highly exposed animals went on to develop tubulointerstitial fibrosis with less severe renal damage observed in the lower exposed animals.

Hypertension

Hypertension is a significant risk factor for cardiovascular and cerebrovascular mortality.

Navas-Acien et al.[40] reviewed observational studies concerning lead exposure and cardiovascular end points using database searches and citations. They concluded that there was sufficient evidence to infer a causal relationship between lead exposure and hypertension.

Epidemiological studies in general population cohorts by Harlan,[41] Nash et al.,[42] Pocock et al.[43] and Schwartz,[44] suggested lead may elevate blood pressure in adults, at blood lead concentrations of <20 μg/dL, while studies utilizing measurements of lead in bone, such as those undertaken by Hu et al.[45] and Korrick et al.[46] found bone lead concentration to be a significant predictor of hypertension.

A pressor effect of lead at low dose has also been supported in animal investigations.[47–49]

Meta-analyses, however, including those of Nawrot et al.[50] and Staessen et al.[51] have only found a weak association between blood pressure and blood lead levels, while Schwartz[52] found inconsistent effects of blood lead levels on blood pressure. A review of the National Health and Nutrition Examination Survey III dataset[53] also failed to

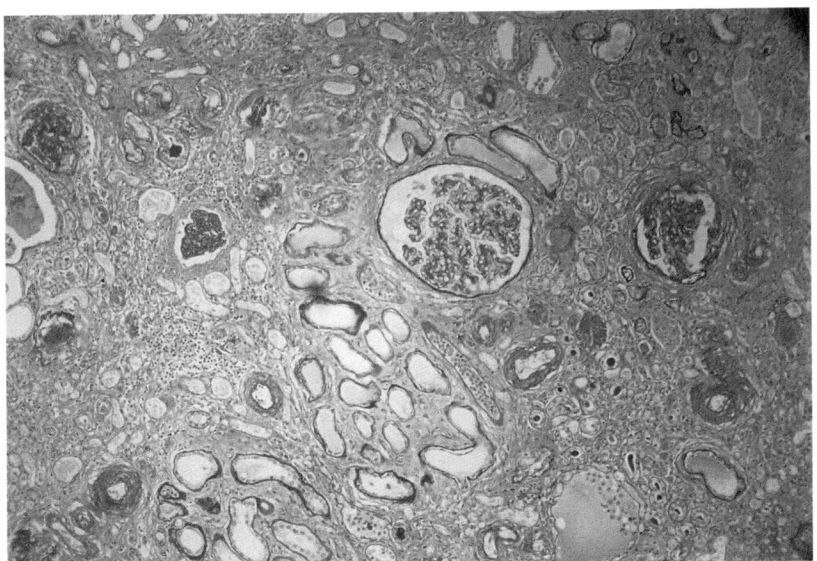

Figure 86.1 Autopsy section of a kidney of a patient exposed to lead in childhood through eating lead-based paint. The features are those of a marked focal interstitial fibrosis with focal tubular atrophy. Photograph kindly provided by Dr J Searle of the Brisbane Hospital, Brisbane, Australia.

show any consistent relationship between blood pressure and blood lead levels.

Two recent occupational studies have been described and were in favour of an association between lead and hypertension. Telisman et al.[54] followed 100 lead workers and 51 reference subjects. Variables including blood lead, delta-aminolaevulinic acid dehydratase (ALAD) activity, blood cadmium, erythrocyte protoporphyrin (EP), body mass index (BMI) and blood pressure were measured. ALAD and EP were used as an indicator of biologically active or chelatable lead.

Elevated levels of zinc protoporphyrin (ZPP) and decreased levels of ALAD represent markers of haem synthesis inhibition and have been shown to reflect biologically active lead by Fenga et al.[55] ZPP level in the blood is dependable on bone marrow lead during the preceding four months (red blood cell lifespan) and is unaffected by recent increases in the blood lead level. ALAD remains active in peripheral blood, thereby reflecting both current and long-term cumulative lead exposure.[56]

The ALAD gene codes for the ALAD enzyme. This requires eight zinc ions as cofactors for activation and catalyses the second step of haem synthesis, by the addition of two molecules of aminolaevulinic acid, to form porphobilinogen, the precursor of haem. Lead is thought to inhibit haem synthesis partly by inhibiting ALAD, via the displacement of a zinc ion. Consequently there are increased levels of aminolaevulinic acid in the plasma and urine.[57]

ALAD level activity is reduced in lead poisoning. This degree of ALAD inhibition may be used to indicate the degree of lead poisoning. ALAD remains active in peripheral blood and therefore reflects both current and cumulative lead exposure. It has been suggested that genetic polymorphism, such as those of ALAD and the vitamin D receptor genes, may modify led toxicokinetics and influence toxic risk to the kidney.[58–61]

In Telisman's study,[54] there was no significant difference in blood pressure between the two groups, which was thought to be due to the reference subjects having relatively high blood lead levels and body mass indices, but in the same subjects, a reduction in ALAD was significantly associated with increasing systolic blood pressure. Similarly, an increase in EP was associated with both an increase in systolic and diastolic blood pressures, after adjustment for confounding variables. This discrepancy was thought to be due to the fact that ALAD and EP better reflected biologically active or chelatable lead, rather than blood lead levels. The authors, therefore, concluded that long-term cumulative lead exposure could significantly increase blood pressure in moderately exposed male workers.

Fenga et al.[55] followed a group of 27 workers (mean length of employment 2.97 years), in a lead battery storage plant and measured a number of variables, including blood lead concentration, Zn-protoporphyrin (ZPP), BMI, ALAD activity and blood pressure. Although the numbers were small, the results showed that long-term occupational exposure was related to a slight increase in the systolic and diastolic blood pressure, in workers with a higher ($>15\,\mu g/dL$), but not with a lower blood lead.

The risk of lead-associated hypertension may be significantly reduced by preventative measures that lower chronic workplace lead exposure.

Early markers of disturbed renal function

Tubular dysfunction may be detected by the measurement of the excretion of tubular enzymes and microproteins which in turn can be used as early biomarkers of renal tubular dysfunction. Urinary N-acetyl-beta-D-glucosaminidase (NAG) for example, has been used as a marker of renal tubular dysfunction induced by lead in several studies,[62,63] including in work performed on rats.[64] Like beta-2 microglobulin (B2M), however, some studies have shown no effect on levels in the urine of lead workers, while other studies have found a rise.[65,66] Suggestions have also been made that urinary NAG is less useful following chronic lead exposure, due to age-related changes which occur at later stages.[67,68]

Diagnosis of lead nephropathy

Ingestion and inhalation are the principal routes of lead exposure and lead absorption.[69] Once absorbed, lead enters the bloodstream and is predominantly bound to erythrocyte proteins.[70–74] The average clearance half-life after a short-term limited exposure is 35 days.[73] As discussed by Hu et al.[75] clearance is via soft tissue and bone distribution, in addition to primarily, renal excretion. Faeces, sweat, hair and nails also excrete a small amount.

Blood lead levels measured in whole-blood specimens may be used as an indicator of circulating lead level. The level varies according to external lead exposure and lead mobilization from tissue stores and, therefore, is better suited to assessing acute lead exposure. On the other hand, lead tibia and patella levels provide an indication of the cumulative dose over decades and include the largest pool that is available for mobilization into the blood.

Non-invasive, in vivo x-ray fluorescence (XRF) instruments have been used to measure the bone lead levels, utilizing emitting x-rays at the bone (Figure 86.2). This, in turn, activates electrons in different electron shells and the lead atoms respond by fluorescing. The more the fluorescence, the more the photons that are counted and the greater the lead exposure. Two types of x-ray fluorescence exist. L-line stimulates electrons in the L electron shell, but measures lead in the subperiosteal bone only. K-line x-ray fluorescence stimulates electrons in the K shell and detects lead in the full thickness of the bone, hence is better for lead measurement. Validation of this procedure has been demonstrated. KXRF used for the in vivo measurement of lead in bone, allows estimation of retained cumulative

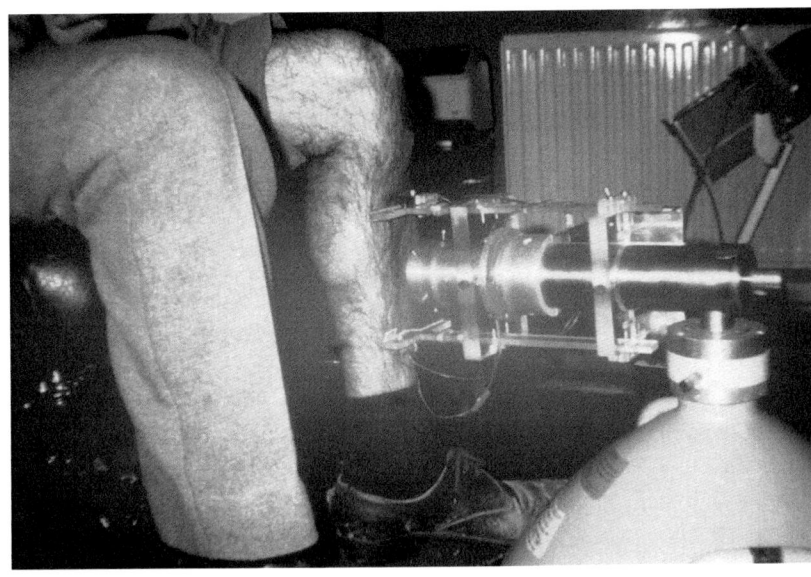

Figure 86.2 *In vivo* measurement of tibial bone lead by x-ray fluorescence.

lead dose in humans.[76] It is safe, non-invasive and has been used for more than three decades, both for research and, in certain circumstances, the practice of occupational and environmental medicine.[77]

The bulk of lead in bone is within compartments of cortical (more reliable and with a longer half-life) and trabecular bone, with only smaller amounts in bone tissue compartments which exchange rapidly with extracellular fluid and plasma. It has been suggested that in individuals with a peak lead exposure of many decades previously, tibia lead contributes little to the current blood lead levels due to its poor bioavailability. During physiological states, such as in pregnancy, post-menopausal osteoporosis and hyperthyroidism, greater circulating lead may derive from bone.[78–80]

Blood and bone lead levels provide the best measures for estimating recent and cumulative lead, respectively.

As an alternative to using KXRF, repeated and/or estimated measurements of blood lead over time may be used to calculate a cumulative blood lead index (CBLI).[81] This equates approximately to multiplying the average blood lead level by the number of years of exposure (as $\mu g \times$ years/dL), also called the IBL index. Several studies have supported correlation between CBLI and tibia lead.[81–86]

Finally, chelatable lead burden may be measured as lead excreted in the urine, collected over 4–24 hours, after the administration of intravenous ethylene diamine tetraacetic acid (EDTA) (Figure 86.3) or oral meso-2,3-dimercaptosuccinic acid (DMSA).[88] This measurement has been used in epidemiological studies, but there is debate whether this contributes further to studies that were measuring blood and bone lead.[89,90]

Current guidelines and recommendations

The measurement of whole blood lead level remains the standard method of monitoring lead-exposed workers at present. In the United Kingdom, the Control of Lead at

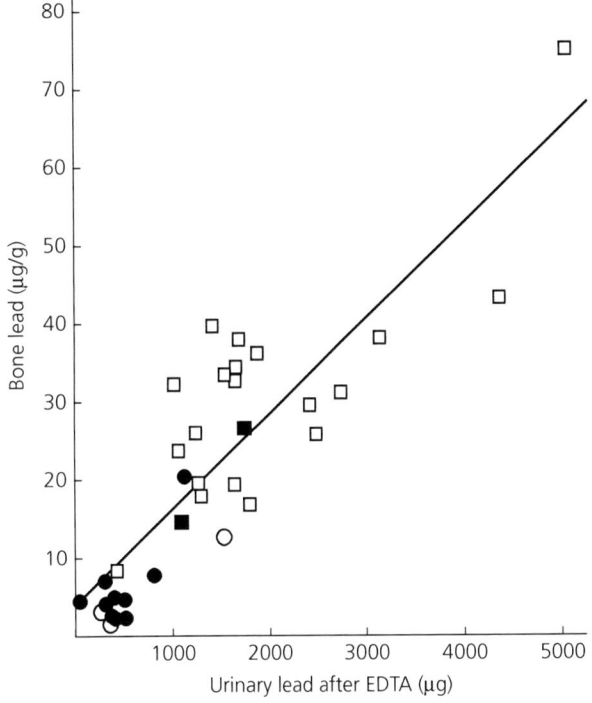

Figure 86.3 Relation between EDTA lead immobilization tests and transiliac bone lead in 35 at-risk patients, including 22 lead workers ($r = 0.87$). Reproduced from Ref. 87 with permission.

Work Regulations from 2000, has lowered the blood lead level for inorganic lead workers to 60 μg/100 mL, the threshold thought to cause proximal tubular injury.[32]

Results from studies, however, do vary concerning the blood lead level above which renal dysfunction occurs. Some show linear correlations between serum creatinine and blood lead level above 40 μg/100 mL, while others show no effect at levels less than 60 μg/100 mL.[32,91,92]

Germany has set a blood lead suspension limit of 40 μg/100 mL. In the United States, lead industries have introduced a voluntary programme to reduce blood lead levels to below 40 μg/100 mL. American legislation, however, suggests removing a worker if the level exceeds 60 μg/100 mL or if three levels taken over a six-month period exceed 50 μg/100 mL, until the level falls below 40 μg/100 mL.

Management

The management of lead nephropathy may be divided into primary and secondary prevention.

Primary prevention may be achieved by the following actions:

- by identifying susceptible groups, such as those individuals with pre-existing renal impairment, diabetes mellitus or with genetic predisposition and monitoring them more closely;
- by minimizing environmental exposure in general so that background lead levels other than industrial exposure are kept low;
- by minimizing industrial exposure and ensuring adequate monitoring at regular intervals (usually determined by baseline blood lead level and changes in exposure);
- by providing appropriate protective equipment;
- by ensuring appropriate personal hygiene.

Secondary prevention involves removing the exposed worker from the lead source and the use of chelation therapy.

Chelation therapy is used to reduce the blood lead level by increasing urinary lead excretion. These agents are organic compounds which link together metal ions and thereby enable their elimination from the body. The ideal chelating agents are water soluble and able to penetrate the cell membrane, having little effect on other metals.

Agents used include 2,3-dimercaprol (BAL) and its analogues meso-2,3-dimercaptosuccinic acid (DMSA) and sodium 2,3-dimercaptopropane (DMPS). D-penicillamine (DPA) and chelators belonging to the polyaminocarboxylic groups, such as derivatives of ethylene diamine tetra-acetic acid (EDTA) and diethylene triamine pentaacetic acid (DTPA), are also used.

Lin-Tan et al.[93] reported an improvement in renal function and a slowing in the progression of renal insufficiency with EDTA chelation in patients with chronic renal insufficiency secondary to environmental lead exposure.

In animals, DMSA chelation has also been shown to improve renal function, and to treat nephropathy[94] and hypertension,[95] associated with long-term exposure to low levels of lead. Foglieni et al.[96] have suggested in rat models that improvement in renal function may be the result of nitric oxide stimulation and a reduction in reactive oxygen species levels.

Previous animal studies suggested DMSA was not capable of chelating lead from the bones, but only from soft tissue.[97] Cory-Slechta et al.,[98] however, showed that lead could be mobilized from bone and kidney and redistributed initially to the brain and liver in rats. Levels in both brain and liver declined subsequently with calcium disodium EDTA injections, but no net loss from either tissue occurred over the five-day treatment period, despite a decline in blood lead levels.

The use of chelators may be associated with a number of side effects. For example, Kiran et al.[99] described how some of the EDTA derivatives could cause hypocalcaemia and renal side effects, such as tubular cell necrosis, haematuria, proteinuria (thought reversible once treatment had ceased). Powell et al.[100] has also described how chelation of endogenous essential metals could potentially occur.

DMPS and DMSA are considerably less toxic compared to older agents such as BAL, but newer agents including the monoisoamyl DMSA (MiADMSA), an ester of DMSA, have been developed further to optimize the effects.

Chelation therapy should be tailored to each individual patient, especially as controlled clinical trials have not been able to confirm consistent symptom improvement or a reduction in mortality in patients with lead encephalopathy.[101] In general, chelation therapy is used as the mainstay of treatment for acute lead nephropathy.

The use of combination chelating agents has been suggested. In addition to combining therapy with some naturally occurring antioxidants (vitamins), Swaran et al.[102] found co-administrating vitamin E during chelation with DMSA or MiADMSA in rats, had a beneficial role in reducing body lead burden. They also suggested that vitamin C therapy during chelation might reduce oxidative stress, but human studies on vitamin C and lead absorption have shown mixed results.

Kalia et al.[103] reinforced the potential importance of micronutrients, such as calcium, iron, zinc, selenium and copper, in reducing toxic metal absorption and as an adjunct in chelation therapy, to maintain essential metal status, but the excess and prolonged use of zinc might inadvertently cause the chelator to bind to the zinc instead.

Mortality

Several mortality studies (Table 86.2) have indicated an excess of death due to renal disease among cohorts of workers exposed to lead, but methodological problems related to the numbers of cases observed and the selection of controls or census data from the general population, may have limited their value.

Cardiovascular disease risk

Some mortality studies have suggested hypertensive cardiovascular disease[112] and cerebrovascular disease[111] are

Table 86.2 Mortality due to renal disease in cohorts exposed to lead.

Cohort (n)	Mortality due to renal dysfunction	No. patients with renal dysfunction	Ref.
7032	EM	21	Cooper and Gaffey[104]
241	EM	21	McMichael and Johnson[105]
1898	EM	19	Malcolm and Barnett[106]
57	EM	3	Davies[107]
4519	EM	20	Cooper et al.[108]
2300	EM	8	Cooper et al.[108]
1987	EM	9	Selevan et al.[109]
437	NEM	2	Gerhardsson et al.[110]
2276	NEM	11	Fanning[111]

NEM, no excess mortality; EM, excess mortality.

more frequent causes of death among lead workers in comparison with the general population.

The National Health and Nutrition Examination Survey (NHANES) provides an observational database and a snapshot of the health and nutritional status of the United States population, through physical examinations, clinical and laboratory tests and interviews. As part of the NHANES III study by Schober et al.,[113] mortality analysis was performed on 9757 general public participants above and including 40 years of age, who had had a blood lead level estimated. Blood lead levels as low as 5–9 μg/100 mL were associated with an increased risk of death from all causes, cardiovascular disease and cancer, but the significance of these findings was not clear.

Renal cell cancer

Conflicting results have been reported in the past concerning lead exposure and renal cancer risk. Some studies have suggested an increased risk,[33,114–116] while others have shown either a weak association or no association at all.[117–121] There were, however, limitations in some of these studies concerning numbers, follow-up time and lack of information regarding potential cofounders.

Conclusions

Lead is known to cause a range of renal diseases in exposed subjects. Excess lead is deposited mainly in the skeleton and can be released over a number of years following exposure cessation, resulting in delayed nephrotoxicity.

Cohort studies on lead-related renal outcomes have provided inconsistent results partly due to the small sample size, mixed exposure and the lack of a definitive early marker(s) of renal damage in lead exposure. An association with hypertension and increased mortality has also been suggested.

The diagnosis of lead toxicity is based on whole blood lead monitoring, as other measures are not widely available. Management should focus on identification of those individuals at increased risk of exposure and primary prevention. Newer forms of chelating agents and combination therapies have been used, but should be individually tailored to minimize side effects.

In Europe and the United States, the provision of lead-exposed workers with better protection, regular monitoring and personal hygiene provision, have all played a part in reducing lead absorption and clinical poisoning. Industries have also been moving away from lead-based materials. However, stringent monitoring and adherence to appropriate lead levels must be maintained for safety. There have been suggestions that the current blood lead guidelines, including in the United Kingdom, need to be revised to a lower recommended level. The European Scientific Committee on occupational exposure limits, for example, has suggested a reduction to 30 μg/100 mL.

Although such measures are being discussed in developed countries, in the developing world with the expansion of industry and the development of obesity and diabetes, we may see an increase in chronic lead nephropathy in the future.

CADMIUM

The use of cadmium in industry grew steadily after its discovery in 1817 by Strohmeyer. The first three cases of acute poisoning by cadmium were reported in 1858 by the Belgian physician, Sovet, in workers using silverware polishes containing cadmium carbonate. Following reports of Stephens in 1930 and Hardy and Skinner in 1947, Friberg described the clinical syndrome of cadmium nephrotoxicity with renal impairment and proteinuria in 1948. Further studies in Italy, Japan, Sweden and the UK confirmed these observations and defined the proteinuria as tubular in origin.[122,123]

Even though cadmium usage is much less than before, it is still used in the electroplating of other metals such as steel, iron, copper and as an alloy. In addition, it is being used in the printing and aircraft industry, pigments, dyes and in the electrodes of nickel/cadmium batteries. Some individuals may become acutely overexposed to this metal in the industry, but there is also evidence that continued low-grade cadmium exposure may result in progressive renal failure. Accordingly, efforts have been made to reduce its usage.

Metabolism and toxicity

The acute absorption of cadmium as dust or fume may induce a severe gastrointestinal disturbance or pulmonary oedema; chronic low-dose exposure may lead to a proximal renal tubular reabsorptive defect.

It has been suggested by Barbier et al.[124] that cadmium induces tubular toxicity, after accumulating in the renal cortex. The resulting renal effects have been supported by a large number of studies that demonstrated a variety of urinary abnormalities, including the increased excretion of proteins, enzymes, amino acids and calcium.[125,126]

Glomerular dysfunction has also been demonstrated in workers with heavy exposure to cadmium.[127–129] Animal experiments have suggested that cadmium may enhance the glomerular filtration of proteins, through a depletion of the glomerular polyanion involving sialic acid and its charge.[130–132] It has been suggested that subtle changes in glomerular permeability may occur, as manifested by the increased urinary excretion of transferrin and albumin and may precede the onset of proximal tubular impairment.[126] Roels et al.[129] suggested that glomerular impairment may occur as a result of the development of a degree of interstitial nephritis secondary to the tubular toxicity. Others have postulated that cadmium may be directly toxic to the glomerulus.[133,134]

Epidemiological studies of cadmium workers have revealed an increased risk of kidney stones in those with a high cadmium level.[135,136] Furthermore, there was a dose–response relationship between cumulative cadmium exposure and kidney stones.[135] One case report described a cadmium worker who went on to develop nephrolithiasis ten years after being exposed to cadmium fumes.[136] The authors concluded that in susceptible individuals, even minimal tubular lesions may predispose to stone formation. In male rats injected with cadmium, an increased incidence of stone formation was observed in the kidneys and bladder of these animals.[137]

The accumulation of cadmium in the liver induces the synthesis of a low molecular weight binding protein called 'metallothionein'.[138] In the kidney, cadmium is mostly bound to this protein. Cadmium toxicity is thought to be due to unbound cadmium ions. These free cadmium ions may have differing effects on the cells. Some of the mechanisms that have been postulated, include the blocking of the calcium transport in the cell,[139] lipid peroxidation of membranes[140,141] and depletion of metal cofactors for the metalloenzymes, caused by the displacement of essential metals from metallothionein.[142]

In rats, chronic cadmium exposure has been shown to cause metabolic acidosis, possibly due to an inhibition of renal bicarbonate reabsorption.[143] The same researcher went on to show how cadmium intoxication may impair the Na^+/H^+ exchange activity of the proximal tubular brush–border membrane and a reduction in Na^+/H^+ exchange-3 expression in the membrane, which facilitates the reabsorption of filtered bicarbonate.[144]

Diagnosis of renal dysfunction

MARKERS OF RENAL TUBULAR DYSFUNCTION

Tubular dysfunction is a salient feature of cadmium nephrotoxicity and tubular proteinuria is being used as a surrogate marker of cadmium nephrotoxicity.

Tubular proteinuria develops as a result of reduced tubular reabsorption of low molecular weight (LMW) proteins, which are usually taken up preferentially by the proximal renal tubules. In early tubular dysfunction, the urinary excretion of these LMW proteins is disproportionately increased compared with high molecular weight proteins and may be used as markers of early tubular dysfunction.

Even a slight reduction in tubular reabsorption, may result in a large increase in the urinary excretion of microproteins,[145,146] including urinary beta-2-microglobulin (B2M) and retinol binding protein (RBP). Urinary B2M, however, is unstable in acidic urine (pH <5.6), whereas urinary RBP is much more stable.

The normal level of urinary B2M/RBP is regarded as <300 µg/g creatinine. A B2M or RBP level of 300–1000 µg/g creatinine has been correlated with the development of incipient cadmium tubulopathy and a level of 1000–10 000 µg/g creatinine, with irreversible tubular proteinuria. Finally, a level of >10 000 µg/g creatinine, has been correlated with overt cadmium nephropathy, usually associated with a reduced glomerular filtration rate (GFR).[145]

Alpha-1-microglobulin is another LMW protein, but is considered a less sensitive marker of tubular dysfunction, due to its greater molecular weight.[146] However, some studies have suggested its use as a screening marker for environmental cadmium exposure.[147,148] Other tubular markers that have also been suggested include the urinary human Clara cell protein-CC16 or protein 1 in women.[149] The same protein is secreted by the prostate, reducing its sensitivity and specificity in men.

CADMIUM MEASUREMENT

Blood cadmium concentration falls rapidly after acute exposure and is, therefore, seldom used as the sole marker of acute toxicity. However, in subjects with a past history of high chronic exposure, blood cadmium level may increasingly reflect body burden rather than current exposure.[150]

In newly exposed workers, the concentration of cadmium in blood increases linearly to reach a plateau at about four months.[151] In workers currently exposed to cadmium, blood cadmium levels reflect mainly the uptake of the metal over the preceding few months. After an individual is removed from the exposure, the respective contributions of current exposure and body burden are progressively reversed. In cases of former cadmium workers with high levels of cadmium in tissues, the influence of the body burden becomes more prominent.[152]

In excessive acute exposure, urinary cadmium levels may be high, but in general, urinary cadmium is an indicator of cumulative body burden. As the renal cortical levels exceed 100–300 μg Cd/g of renal cortex, the urine cadmium level increases, either as a result of renal losses or failure to reabsorb filtered LMW cadmium complexes, because of the renal tubular dysfunction. The non-invasive technique of *in vivo* neutron activation analysis, enables more diagnostic precision without the need for biopsy analysis of cadmium.[153,154]

In workers moderately exposed to cadmium and in the general population, the urinary excretion of cadmium (expressed in terms of creatinine or as 24-hour urine output), is a reliable indicator of the body burden of cadmium.[154,155] Indeed, the level of urinary cadmium correlates better with the duration of exposure compared to blood cadmium. It was interesting that the urinary excretion of cadmium was found by a Belgian group to increase progressively with age, in parallel with the body burden, until the age of 50–60 years.[156] The measurement of metallothionein in the urine of cadmium workers may be used to provide information similar to urinary cadmium.[156,157]

In 1993, Roels *et al.*[158] recommended the use of different thresholds of cadmium urine concentration, to correlate with renal abnormalities. In their classifications, a urine cadmium concentration of 2 μg/g creatinine was associated with biochemical alterations. A urine cadmium concentration of 4 μg/g creatinine was linked to high molecular weight proteinurias and tubule antigen disturbance. Finally, at 10 μg/g creatinine of urine cadmium concentration, LMW proteinurias were observed. The latter was thought to be the threshold for developing microproteinuria, the critical effect predictive of a decline in renal function.[145]

In the past, there has been much debate as to whether cadmium-induced renal function was reversible. More recently, several clinical studies have supported the reversibility of tubular dysfunction. In one observational study of 32 male workers,[159] the evolution of cadmium-induced renal tubular dysfunction was observed. The results indicated that reversible tubular dysfunction occurred in those with urinary B2M levels between 300 and 1500 μg/g creatinine and those with urinary cadmium levels of less than or equal to 20 μg/g creatinine. In individuals with levels above these values, the cadmium-induced tubular dysfunction progressed, despite a reduction or cessation of the cadmium exposure. Similar reversibility of tubular dysfunction was observed in a cadmium factory where workers had been followed prospectively for four years.[160] During this time, the urinary tubular protein markers, blood and urinary cadmium levels were monitored and showed a reduction in the urinary LMW protein level as the exposure conditions improved.

Trzcinka-Ochocka *et al.*[161] similarly followed a group of 58 workers working in a nickel cadmium factory and after they had been removed from the cadmium exposure there was a general reduction in the tubular protein levels and urinary RBP. There was even some suggestion of reversibility in the rate of glomerular filtration rate decline, even in cases of relatively high past exposure.

Treatment

Once early renal tubular dysfunction is evident, the most important aspect in the management of cadmium tubular toxicity is the removal of the subject from further exposure.

As cadmium is tightly bound to metallothionein in the kidney and liver, finding an effective chelating agent is challenging. Nephrotoxicity can be produced by chelating agents that remove cadmium from the liver and then excreting it via the kidneys. The chelation and elimination through bile, is used in practice to remove cadmium from the liver. Sodium *N*-(4-methoxybenzyl)-D-glucamine dithiocarbamate, is one of the most effective chelating agents for removing cadmium from the liver and kidneys.[162] Even though the new chelating agents are more effective and less nephrotoxic, their use is mainly in acute rather than chronic cadmium exposure.

Current recommendation in the workplace

The Control of Substances Hazardous to Health Regulations (COSHH) requires employers: (1) to assess risk and to implement precautions to prevent or adequately control or reduce exposure to airborne cadmium below the workplace exposure limits (WEL) for long-term exposures equivalent to an eight-hour time-weighted average (TWA) reference period (0.03 mg/m^3 for cadmium sulphide and cadmium sulphide pigments and 0.025 mg/m^3 for the remaining cadmium compounds); (2) to maintain all fume and dust controls in appropriate working order; (3) to ensure the presence of a monitoring programme; and (4) to arrange any health surveillance as appropriate.[163,164]

In the United States, the Occupational Safety and Health Administration (OSHA) division of the Department of Labor, has recommended an action level for workplace exposure to cadmium of 2.5 μg/m^3 of air, calculated as an eight-hour TWA exposure. During any eight-hour working shift of a 40-hour working week, the permissible exposure limit is equivalent to a TWA concentration that must not exceed 5 µg/m³ of air for all cadmium compounds. In addition, other trigger levels for medical surveillance have been identified. A urinary cadmium level at or below 3 µg/g creatinine, a beta-2-microglobulin level at or below 300 µg/g creatinine and a blood cadmium level at or below 5 µg/L of whole blood, require only the minimum level of periodic medical surveillance. However, if these levels are exceeded, the employer is required to reassess the employee's occupational exposure to cadmium within two weeks and to correct any deficiencies within 30 days. The finding of a urine cadmium over 7 µg/g creatinine, or a whole blood cadmium over 10 µg/L, or a B2M level over 750 µg/g creatinine plus a urine cadmium over 3 µg/g creatinine, or a whole blood cadmium over 5 µg/L during either an initial or follow-up medical examination requires removing the employee from further cadmium exposure.[165]

PREVENTION

This mainly involves minimizing exposure through various strategies to reduce exposure to fume and dust and by providing adequate personal protective equipment, where appropriate, and maintaining a high standard of occupational hygiene measures.

PROGNOSIS

Although several studies have suggested the reversibility of cadmium-induced tubular dysfunction, the development of end-stage renal disease has been reported in a few heavily exposed cadmium workers.[166,167] A study[168] which included both cadmium-battery production workers and individuals residing in cadmium-polluted areas, also concluded that cadmium exposure contributed to the development of end-stage renal disease even at lower levels of exposure.

There was suggestive evidence of an increased risk of nephritis and nephrosis after high cadmium exposure,[169] but no statistical significance was reached in this or in the other studies regarding renal deaths.[170,171]

MERCURY

Most of the occupational health problems caused by mercury arise through its use in its elemental form. The high vapour pressure of elemental mercury results in potential exposure whenever the metal is used or handled. Although the skin is not a barrier to mercury, absorption occurs mainly via inhalation. Mercury readily crosses biological membranes and is rapidly oxidized to divalent mercury in the blood and within cells.

Mercury is mined in Russia, China and Almaden in Spain. Large-scale use of elemental mercury occurs in the chloralkali industry, although this is decreasing as newer technology takes over and provides other means for producing chlorine and sodium hydroxide. Elemental mercury is still used in temperature- and pressure-measuring equipment and in the manufacture of fluorescent and discharge lamps, as well as amalgams used in dentistry. Occupational exposure to elemental mercury is more widespread than exposure to mercury compounds. In the western hemisphere, there has been a general reduction in the use of mercury over two decades, especially in the chloralkali processes, where its use is expected to cease by 2010.[172]

Although mercury salts are widely used as toxins in animal experimental models of acute renal failure, mercury-related toxicity in humans is largely due to industrial or accidental exposure. The biotransformation to the organic salts, such as methyl, ethyl and phenoxyethyl mercury, may occur in industrial and agricultural processes.[173] These organomercurials can accumulate in proximal renal tubular cells where toxicity is determined by the intracellular interactions between the sulphydryl groups, lysosomes and phospholipid membranes.[173] The tubular toxicity has been associated with an increased leakage of tubular antigens and enzymuria[174] and biochemical alterations including a reduction of excretion of some eicosanoids and glycosaminoglycans at a low urinary pH.

Mercurous chloride (Hg_2Cl_2, calomel) is relatively non-toxic. It was widely used as a medicine until the twentieth century. In contrast, mercuric chloride ($HgCl_2$, corrosive sublimate) has a relatively high vapour pressure and water solubility, is highly nephrotoxic and is used to produce acute renal tubular necrosis in animal experiments. Similar toxicity is produced by both the phenyl and methoxymethyl mercuric salts.[175] The biological half-life of inorganic mercury that is retained within the kidney is approximately two months.[176]

Reversible proteinuria has been a recognized feature in workers with mercury exposure greater than 50 µg/m³. Many workers exposed to mercury have enhanced urinary mercury excretion without adverse renal effects.[177] The diagnosis of mercury-induced renal disease is currently based on a known exposure plus renal dysfunction.

An increased prevalence of proteinuria has been found in cross-sectional studies among exposed workers.[174,178,179] The same authors have reported increased urinary enzymuria indicative of an effect on the renal tubules.[174,180–182] These reported effects have generally been small and may be reversible with cessation of exposure,[183] but the long-term clinical significance of these findings is as yet unclear.

Urinary mercury and whole blood mercury levels have been used to assess the biological occupational exposure to mercury.[184,185] As detailed by Gompertz in 1982,[186] urinary mercury reflects the average exposure over the preceding two to four months, but this level can fluctuate in the day with a diurnal variation. Blood mercury tends to reflect exposure and uptake over the past few days. Unexposed subjects normally have a level of less than 5 µg/L or 5 µg/g creatinine, but the unexposed reference range is dependable on the dietary intake of mercury especially from fish. In the case of Sweden, such normal blood mercury values have been reported to be as high as 13 μg/L (65 nmol/L).[187]

Current recommendation in the workplace

In the United Kingdom, the biological values for inorganic mercury is limited to a urinary mercury level of 20 μmol/mol creatinine in the urine or 35 μg/g creatinine.[188] The long-term exposure limit of 0.025 mg/m^3 eight-hour TWA has been set for mercury and its inorganic divalent compounds.[189,190] A lower long-term exposure limit of 0.01 mg/m^3 eight-hour TWA has been set for alkaline mercury which is thought to be more toxic. In the United States, it has been suggested that the biological exposure index (BEI) for total inorganic mercury in the blood should be 15 μg/L.[191,192]

Clinical studies

Autopsy studies have shown that mercury from dental amalgam may result in increased amounts of mercury in the renal cortex to almost nine times the normal range and up to 433 ngHg/g of renal cortex, but no adverse effects have been identified from this source of exposure.[193] Accidental or suicidal ingestion of as little as 0.5 g of mercuric chloride can lead to typical oliguric acute renal failure with proximal tubular necrosis (Figure 86.4). The clinical picture in the first few days is dominated by gastrointestinal haemorrhage due to erosive gastritis. The prognosis for renal recovery is good with dialysis and supportive therapy.[194] The administration of intravenous DMPS (dimercapo-1-propane sulphonate) in the first 24–48 hours and before the development of oliguria may limit the extent of the renal failure.[194]

Nephrotic syndrome (proteinuria >3.5 g/day) has been reported sporadically following exposure to both elemental and organic mercury.[195] In children, the use of mercurial ointment or powder has been associated with the development of acrodynia or pink disease, but mercury exposure and the development of nephrotic syndrome has been rarely described in the occupational setting. In some individuals, mercury may be a triggering agent for immune reactions leading to proteinuria. In cases where renal diseases occur, membranous nephropathy is most commonly observed, although minimal change nephropathy and anti-glomerular basement membrane (GBM) antibody-mediated disease have also been described.[195] An increased prevalence of circulating anti-GBM antibody of the anti-laminin variety has been reported in male workers exposed to mercury vapour.[196] More recent studies have suggested that anti-double strand nuclear antibody (DNA) and total IgE may also play a role as their circulating concentrations have been shown to positively associate with the concentration of mercury in both urine and blood.[174]

It has been shown in both human and experimental animals[197] that the proteinuria associated with low or moderate exposure to mercury at work usually resolves following withdrawal from exposure. The immunopathological mechanism of the renal response in humans is not clear. The renal lesion in rats involves immune complex deposition, anti-GBM antibody deposition, complement and polyclonal B cell activation.[198] The lack of a dose–response curve in the development of renal disease in both humans and animals would indicate that this is an idiosyncratic response.

In an outbreak of chronic methyl mercury poisoning in 1956, several hundred adults ingested contaminated fish from the Minamata Bay in Japan[199] and went on to develop 'Minamata disease' which was predominantly a neurological disorder, with only minor renal involvement and low molecular weight proteinuria without albuminuria or renal failure.[199]

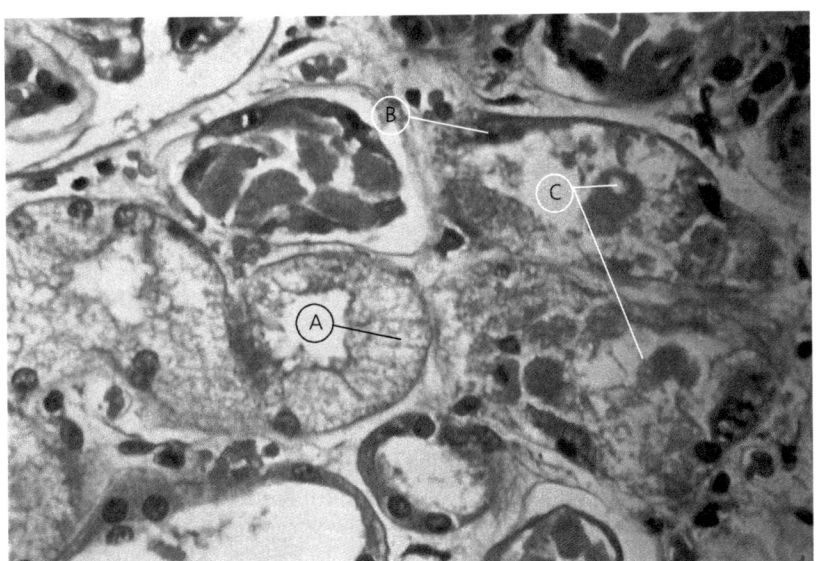

Figure 86.4 Renal biopsy of acute tubular necrosis occurring in a patient secondary to mercury toxicity. The renal tubular cells show varying stages of degeneration from frothy vacuolated cytoplasm (A) to loss of nuclei in tubular cells with dark pyknotic nuclei (B). Shedding of cells is seen into the tubular lumen with tubular cell casts surrounded by epithelial cells (C). Photograph kindly provided by Dr AR Morley of Newcastle University, Newcastle, UK.

Treatment of mercury toxicity

In managing acute, inorganic mercury poisoning treatment with chelators should be initiated after cessation of exposure. Thiol-based chelating agents, such as dimercaprol, DMPS and dimercaptosuccinic acid (DMSA), are used.[200,201] DMSA may be administered at a dose of 10 mg/kg orally, eight hourly for five days.

In cases of chronic poisoning, patient removal from the exposure source is the most important step taken to reduce or reverse proteinuria. The use of chelators may be considered in cases where there has been a high degree of exposure, but no other specific treatment is recommended.

URANIUM

Uranium is a naturally occurring heavy metal, used by the military and in the nuclear industry. Depleted uranium is a byproduct of uranium enrichment and enters the body through wounds, ingestion and inhalation. Toxicity occurs either through its chemical properties or its radioactivity.

The uranyl ion circulates bound to transferrin and is freely filtered at the glomerulus as the bicarbonate complex. This complex breaks down to UO which then binds to proteins and phospholipids in the proximal renal tubule, where it has a half-life of approximately one week.

Various animal experiments have been undertaken regarding uranium toxicity on the kidney. Banday et al.[202] recently demonstrated the specific alterations in the activities of metabolic and membrane enzymes and antioxidant defences following acute exposure in rats who were given a single nephrotoxic dose of uranyl nitrate, while Thiebault et al.[203] focused on cell death caused by uranium and suggested that DNA damage was reversible at low concentration (200–400 μmol/L), but became irreversible leading to cell death, at higher uranium concentrations.

Effects on the kidney from chronic uranium exposure are not as well established. Zhu et al.,[204] however, used animal experiments to demonstrate the renal effects of chronic exposure. They implanted depleted uranium (DU) fragments of three doses into rats and compared them with controls, which were implanted with biologically inert materials. Tissue samples were obtained at days 1 and 7 and months 3, 6 and 12. It was found that DU concentrations in the kidney peaked at 90 days post-implantation and although they then began to decrease slowly, remained at a relatively high level even at 360 days post-implantation. Changes in the basement membrane and proximal tubule were seen on electron microscopy and it was concluded that DU could accumulate in the kidneys for a long period, causing kidney injury.

Hodgson et al.[205] in a Health Protection Agency document, reviewed the scientific literature and suggested uranium concentrations at which kidney injury could occur. They concluded that acute exposures which led to concentrations of about 1 μg uranium per gram of kidney, has been associated with minor kidney dysfunction, while chronic levels which led to similar kidney dysfunction are less well established, probably below 0.3 μg uranium per gram of kidney.

Clinical nephrotoxicity has largely been confined to subjects employed in developing the atomic bomb (the Manhattan project) during the Second World War.[206] The acute tubular necrosis produced in animal models is thought to be similar in aetiology to that seen in these workers.

A worksite hazard study of renal toxicity in uranium mill workers demonstrated significantly increased urinary excretions of B2M, catalase and alkaline phosphatase, compared with non-exposed controls,[207] even though the abnormalities remained within the accepted normal range. The clinical significance of these findings remained unclear, however, as many workers had urine uranium levels in excess of the acceptable limit of 30 μg/L (126 nmol/L).

Recently, Vacquier et al.[208] reported on a cohort of 5086 uranium miners employed for at least one year between 1946 and 1990. The mean duration of follow up was just above 30 years. Cause of death was ascertained, radon exposure reconstructed for each year and exposure–risk relationships estimated. They observed a significant excess of kidney cancer deaths (standardized mortality ratio 2, 95 per cent confidence interval, 1.22–3.09). This was not associated with cumulative radon exposure.

CHROMIUM

Like many other heavy metals, chromium is selectively taken up by the proximal renal tubule, and acute tubular necrosis following massive absorption has been described. Although chronic renal failure due to long-term exposure to chromium has not been described, LMW proteinuria with increased urinary excretions of B2M and RBP have been reported in chromium workers.[209] A urine chromium of 10 μg/g creatinine (32 μmol/mol creatinine) has been suggested as a threshold for nephrotoxicity after the finding of proximal tubular enzymuria in workers exposed to ferrochromium.[210] Others[211] have not found any abnormalities in the urinary excretion of transferrin, albumin or RBP in platers exposed to hexavalent chromium and in whom urine chromium levels were less than 19 μg/g creatinine (61 μmol/mol creatinine).

BERYLLIUM

A syndrome similar to sarcoidosis may be induced by the long-term exposure to beryllium.[212] The common features include pulmonary fibrosis, hypercalcaemia and hypercalciuria. The cause of the hypercalcaemia is likely to be the same as in sarcoidosis and other granulomatous disease and is thought to be due to excessive extrarenal production of 1,25-dihydroxy vitamin D, although this is unproven.

Renal complications, such as interstitial nephritis, may rarely develop.

ARSENIC

Acute renal tubular necrosis may develop after exposure to arsine gas. Arsine is a powerful haemolytic agent. Within a few hours of inhalation, acute circulatory collapse and haemolysis accompanied by haemoglobinuria, jaundice and abdominal pain may occur.[213,214] Acute renal tubular necrosis sets in after a few days. Haemodialysis is required for renal support and removal of the arsenic haemoglobin complex by exchange transfusion may be life saving. Chronic renal failure may persist if the patient survives the acute illness. Similarly, persistent renal disease has been described following ingestion of illicitly distilled spirits (moonshine) contaminated with arsenic.[215]

BISMUTH, COPPER AND GADOLINIUM

Acute tubular necrosis has been described after the use of bismuth therapeutically[216] and after self-poisoning with copper sulphate.[217] However, neither metal has been observed to be nephrotoxic in the occupational environment. An unusual syndrome of nephrogenic systemic fibrosis has been observed in renal failure patients rarely after investigations by magnetic resonance imaging when a gadolinium-based agent has been included as contrast material.[218]

CRYSTALLINE SILICA

Exposure to crystalline silica is mainly through inhalation of dust containing quartz in mines, quarries and other sites (Figure 86.5).

In addition to silicosis, several studies have suggested an association between silica exposure and the development of renal disease. Some of the mechanisms that have been suggested include direct toxicity of the silica particles in the kidney, or indirectly through an autoimmune mechanism.[219, 220]

In a cohort of 2820 male ceramic workers in Lazio who entered a health surveillance programme between 1974 and 1987,[221] a retrospective assessment of the effect of cumulative exposure to silica on end-stage renal disease was undertaken. Six of the workers appeared in the kidney registry, giving rise to a relative risk of 1.87. The cumulative exposure was 0.2–3.8 mg/m^3 per year. Three of these six workers developed kidney failure as a result of glomerulonephritis. Two workers also suffered from silicosis, one of whom had a necrotizing glomerulonephritis and positive perinuclear antineutrophil cytoplasmic antibodies (p-ANCA). The researchers concluded that exposure to silica was associated with an increased risk of end-stage renal disease after a short or medium latency period, but

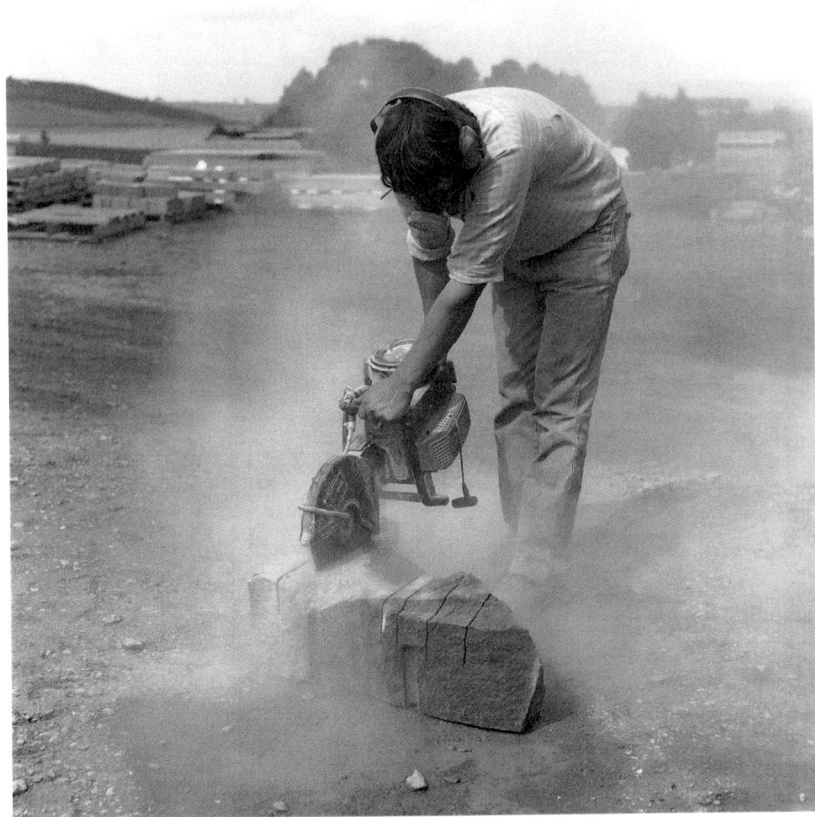

Figure 86.5 A stone cutter wearing respiratory protective equipment during potential exposure to silica dust.

this study was only able to detect those workers requiring dialysis. The long-term renal disease incidence was not studied.

An increase in end-stage renal disease cases was observed in a further cohort study of 4626 silica-exposed workers in the industrial sand industry in the United States.[222] However, the same researchers were unable to confirm a similar finding in 1328 workers with definite silicosis.[223] A combination of selection bias and the smaller number of cases in the second study, were possible limiting factors.

Several case–control and cohort studies have demonstrated an increase in ANCA-positive cases in those exposed to silica, but a definite association between silica exposure and ANCA-associated vasculitis has remained unproven. A recent population-based, case–control study carried out by Hogan et al.[224] attempted to evaluate the association of life-time silica exposure with the development of ANCA-small vessel vasculitis (SVV). A total of 129 case patients were enrolled. Their occupations were assessed and a silica exposure score was formulated before the groups were subdivided into none, low/medium or high life-time exposure. An increased risk for disease was found in those cases with high exposure, compared to those with no exposure. The authors concluded that a high life-time silica exposure was associated with ANCA-SVV. The same researchers carried out a further case controlled study in 2001[225] with results showing that 46 per cent of patients with ANCA-SVV had silica dust exposure, compared to 20 per cent of the controls. In a more recent study of 86 males exposed to silica dust in Bohemia,[226] there were no cases of ANCA-associated vasculitis, although there was an increase in ANCA positivity. It has been suggested that this increase in ANCA may have occurred as a result of endothelial damage caused by the generation of oxygen free radicals from phagocytes[227] and an increased interleukin-12 production. However, it is likely that other factors are required to induce systemic vasculitis.

An excess mortality from chronic non-malignant renal disease has been reported,[228] but not confirmed in a more recent cohort of 2670 sand workers.[229]

ORGANIC SOLVENTS AND RENAL DISEASE

Although the nitro-, amino- or chloro-derivatives of benzene have a known association with uroepithelial tumours, there is now a considerable body of evidence suggesting a role for organic solvent exposure in the development of non-neoplastic renal diseases.[230,231] The term organic 'solvent' refers to hydrocarbons, such as aliphatic, alicyclic, aromatic, halogenated hydrocarbons (carbon tetrachloride, trichloroethylene) and the commonly abused solvents toluene and xylene. Hydrocarbons are often used as solvents in industrial manufacturing practices because of their lipid solubility (Figure 86.6). Solvents are absorbed through the lungs, skin and gastrointestinal

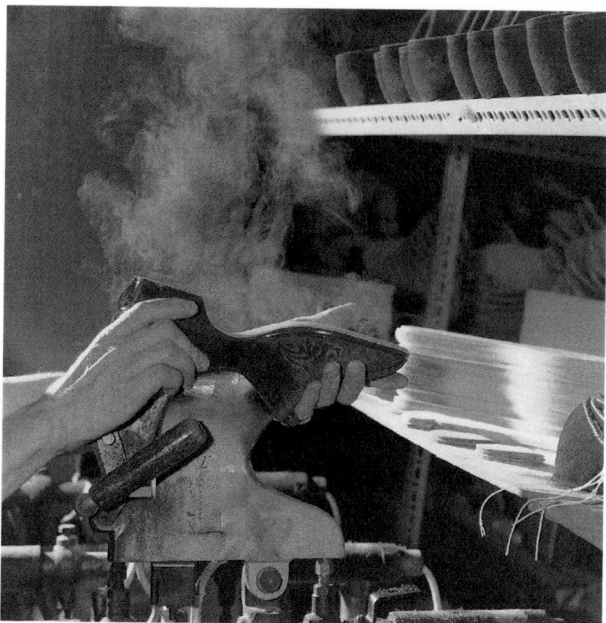

Figure 86.6 Solvent fumes during shoe manufacture.

tract[230,232] and are metabolized usually by cytochrome P450-dependent enzymes present in the liver, kidneys, lungs and other tissues.[233] Solvents are known to be neurotoxicants, affecting both the peripheral and central nervous systems.[234] However, occupational exposure to hydrocarbons with resulting nephrotoxicity is less well understood and in this section we review the evidence.

CASE REPORTS AND EXPERIMENTAL STUDIES

Case reports describe an association between organic solvent exposure and the development of acute tubular necrosis,[231] chronic tubulointerstitial damage[235] and different types of glomerulonephritis and Goodpasture's syndrome.[236–240] In parallel with these clinical observations, experimental studies in animals have identified organic solvent exposure as a factor in the development of both tubular[241,242] and glomerular lesions.[240,243–247] Thus, glomerular lesions similar to those found in Goodpasture's disease have been induced in rats exposed to petroleum vapours[240] and the nephrotic syndrome with severe glomerulonephritis and renal impairment, which is not dependent on either deposition of fibrin or coagulative mechanisms, has been induced in rats fed N,N¹ diacetylbenzidine (N,N¹-DAB).[243] Similarly, mesangial proliferative glomerulonephritis and tubulointerstitial disease, which again did not appear to be mediated by glomerular deposits of antigen–antibody complexes, has been described in rats after the administration of carbon tetrachloride.[246,247]

Long-term exposure to organic solvents is associated with proximal tubule cell apoptosis, a potential mechanism of progressive renal fibrosis and renal failure.[248]

CASE–CONTROL STUDIES AND PROGRESSIVE RENAL FAILURE

The majority of early case–control studies from different research groups reported a significantly greater exposure to organic solvents in patients with glomerulonephritis compared with control groups, and demonstrated evidence in favour of a possible role for chronic solvent exposure in the development of various types of glomerulonephritis, such as proliferative glomerulonephritis, membranous glomerulonephritis, post-streptococcal glomerulonephritis or rapidly progressive glomerulonephritis.

However, the evidence presented in some of the older studies may be criticized on one of the following grounds: (1) the unsatisfactory nature of the control group, (2) the possible bias of the unblinded interviewers, (3) the failure to consider recall bias, (4) failure to define a credible measure of solvent exposure, (5) the diversity of glomerular disease pattern and (6) the stage of disease studied.[249] More carefully performed studies had addressed these criticisms and generally now suggest that hydrocarbon exposure is more probably associated with progression of the disease and worsening renal function.[249–254]

A histopathological type of glomerulonephritis may be important in this association with clearly characterized risks of progression of renal failure associated with solvent exposure particularly among patients with membranous glomerulonephritis and IgA nephropathy[255] and possibly in patients with focal segmental glomerulosclerosis.[252]

A negative study failing to support this relation has been published,[256] but index patients within this study were not well characterized in terms of the histopathological diagnosis of glomerulonephritis. The most recent carefully controlled and characterized prospective case-controlled 'cohort' study of patients with glomerulonephritis further supported this association and noted that the risk incurred by organic solvent exposure and progressive renal failure was mediated only partly by baseline proteinuria.[255] This lends further credence to the concept that this progressive renal damage is mediated through concomitant tubular rather than glomerular injury.[251]

Nonetheless, it would be inappropriate to discount a carefully designed earlier study[257] where solvent exposure was significantly greater in patients with incipient (microalbuminuria) and overt (macroalbuminuria) diabetic nephropathy than those with no clinical evidence of nephropathy.[257] The suggestion of this study was that solvent exposure may also possibly play a role in the progression of diabetic nephropathy in patients with type I diabetes mellitus.

Histological evidence of tubulointerstitial damage in primary glomerular disorders would appear to correlate with severity of renal impairment and can predict the future outcome of renal disease.[258] This relationship between solvent exposure and morphological parameters of tubulointerstitial damage was carefully examined in 59 patients with biopsy-proven primary glomerulonephritis.[251] Solvent exposure correlated significantly with both relative interstitial volume, an index of tubulointerstitial damage, and serum creatinine, a marker of kidney function. Furthermore, solvent exposure was greater in patients with progressive renal failure compared with those with stable or improving renal function, suggesting a close and possibly causal relationship between occupational organic solvent exposure, concomitant tubular damage and progressive renal failure in patients with glomerulonephritis.

CROSS-SECTIONAL STUDIES

The rarity of glomerulonephritis in the general population makes a prospective cohort-analytic study of solvents in exposed populations logistically impossible.[259] Cross-sectional studies comparing parameters of renal dysfunction in solvent-exposed and matched non-exposed workers is feasible and the few such studies performed generally suggest an association between certain solvent exposures and renal damage.[260–267] Thus, in one study,[260] workers exposed to moderate amounts of styrene, toluene and a mixture of mainly aromatic compounds were found to have slight but significantly increased urinary excretions of erythrocytes, white/tubular epithelial cells and albumin compared with a non-exposed group. Likewise, workers mainly exposed to aliphatic and acyclic hydrocarbons were shown to have increased proteinuria and tubular enzymuria (lysozyme and β-glucuronidase) in the absence of albuminuria, findings which were indicative of tubular rather than glomerular dysfunction.[261] In a study of 20 000 workers, the prevalence of proteinuria was found to be higher in those exposed to hydrocarbons than in those who were not.[262] A significant shift of the cumulative frequency distribution of the urinary albumin concentration towards higher values has also been shown in workers exposed to styrene.[263]

Two other studies have used more sensitive markers of kidney damage. In one,[264] male oil refinery workers with exposures to hydrocarbons below the current US threshold limit values, were found to have significantly higher urinary excretions of albumin and (brush border) renal tubular antigen and a higher prevalence of circulating anti-laminin antibodies than a non-exposed group. In the other, the study population was classified into heavy, moderate and low hydrocarbon exposure groups (based on retrospective life-long hydrocarbon exposure scores using a method similar to that used in a recent study[268]) and the findings were compared with those of a control group.[265] The control group was unsatisfactory because 50 per cent of the controls had a past history of heavy metal exposure. Despite introducing this bias, the workers exposed to hydrocarbons were found to have an increase in the urinary excretion of glycosaminoglycans (a marker of glomerular basement membrane damage) and fractional albumin clearance.[265] The latter effect may have been secondary to an interaction between hypertension and hydrocarbon exposure.

Further studies have suggested that this interaction was significantly associated with abnormal proteinuria, an increased serum laminin concentration, albumin excretion rate and NAG activity. Furthermore, exposure to hydrocarbons seemed to accelerate the age-dependent decline in kidney function.[266] This contrasts with earlier studies from the same group suggesting that long-term moderate exposure to solvents did not entail a significant nephrotoxic risk.[267]

Similarly, two studies yielded contrasting conclusions about renal function in subjects occupationally exposed to perchloroethylene. In one,[269] no association could be found between exposure and renal outcome in workers exposed to perchloroethylene in dry cleaning shops. In the other, the findings were consistent with both glomerular and tubular dysfunction in workers exposed to low levels of perchloroethylene in dry cleaning (Figure 86.7) and indicated that solvent-exposed workers, especially dry cleaners, may need to be monitored for the possible development of chronic renal disease.[270]

In view of the ongoing controversy in this area of nephrology, we undertook one further such cross-sectional study in a car manufacturing plant with workers exposed to various solvents at their worksite.[271] The paint sprayers exposed to paint-based solvents had a significantly higher prevalence of renal impairment than the other groups (Figure 86.8) and a higher prevalence of abnormal total proteinuria and enzymuria than controls. Workers exposed to petroleum-based paints had a significantly higher prevalence of abnormal proteinuria, transferrinuria, tubular proteinuria and enzymuria, but albuminuria was similar in all groups. These results suggested that chronic solvent exposure may be associated with both clinical and subclinical renal dysfunction.

We have found evidence of endothelial activation and early basement-membrane disturbance resulting in autoantibody production as suggested by depressed serum laminin (marker of basement-membrane turnover) and elevated autoantibodies to laminin and Goodpasture's antigen (markers of anti-GBM antibody-mediated disease) in individuals occupationally exposed to paint and petroleum-based solvents (Figure 86.9).[272]

Unfortunately, there are no follow-up data on the renal outcome of these subjects. However, a recent study of a matched cohort of paint sprayers from a different car plant suggested that the proximal tubule damage mentioned above may be reduced by improved respiratory and skin protection at the worksite.[273]

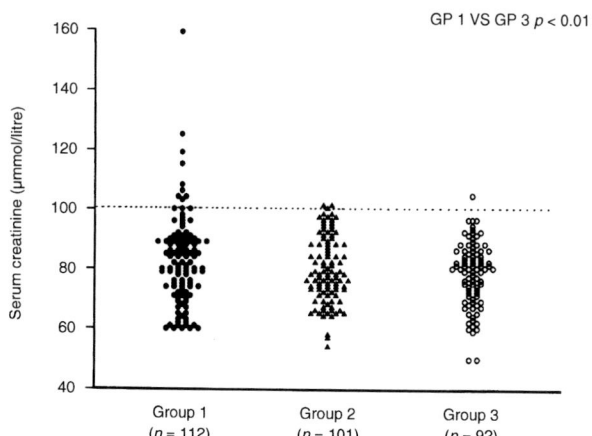

Figure 86.8 Dottogram of serum creatinine levels in three groups of workers in a car plant. Group 1 (paint sprayers) had a significantly different distribution from group 2 (transmission shop workers) and group 3 (body shop workers). Evidence of renal impairment was present in 11 per cent of group 1. The dotted line represents the upper reference limit derived from external controls. Reproduced from Ref. 250 with permission from Oxford University Press.

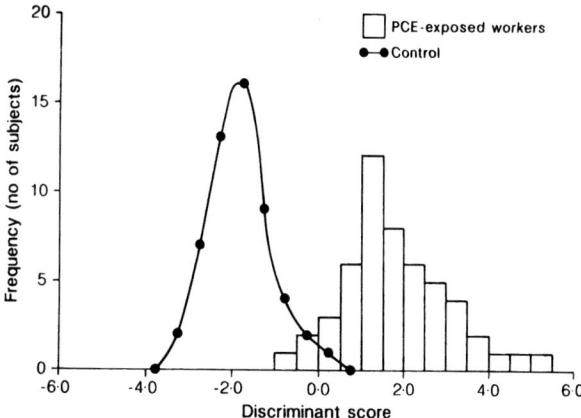

Figure 86.7 Distribution of workers exposed to perchloroethylene (PCE) and matched controls classified on the basis of 13 selected early markers of renal damage. According to discriminate function 87 per cent of subjects were correctly classified (χ^2 69.9, 13 df, $p < 0.001$). Reproduced from Ref. 270 with permission.

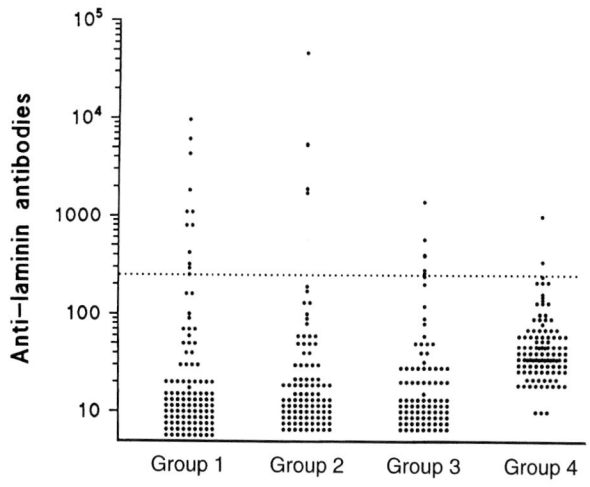

Figure 86.9 Distribution of levels of serum anti-laminin antibodies in three groups of workers in a car plant (group 1 paint sprayers, group 2 transmission workers, group 3 body shop workers and group 4 normal external controls). In group 1, there was approximately a six-fold increase in the proportion of subjects with anti-laminin antibody results compared with controls. Reproduced from Ref. 272 with permission from Oxford University Press.

COHORT STUDIES

A cohort study involves a sample of a population exposed to solvents who are compared with an age- and sex-matched cohort of unexposed individuals who are then followed for an outcome assessment, such as mortality due to renal failure (see Chapter 6). Such studies may offer valuable information in the investigation of the association between solvent exposure and glomerulonephritis. However, the diagnostic categories of 'nephritis and nephrosis' or 'genitourinary diseases' are likely to be invalid representations of renal mortality. Thus, in four large cohort studies of solvent-exposed workers, the risk of death (standardized mortality ratios) from renal causes was lower than otherwise expected in occupationally exposed cohorts.[274–277] The basic assumption for mortality studies is that the toxic effects are lethal. Such studies cast little light upon possible slight-to-moderate effects of exposure. Furthermore, the outcomes of 'register studies' are always difficult to interpret: diagnostic criteria may vary between and even within studies and the exposures are often vaguely or too generally defined. This may partly be explained by the influence of the well-documented healthy worker effect on non-cancer mortality frequently observed in occupational cohorts.[278] Moreover, mortality studies do not take into consideration those workers who take early retirement on health grounds (e.g. patients with end-stage renal failure requiring dialysis treatment), although the medical condition may eventually account for the individual's death.

MECHANISMS OF SOLVENT-INDUCED NEPHROTOXICITY

The mechanism underlying solvent-induced nephropathy remains speculative despite solvents being well-recognized tubulotoxins in both clinical and experimental settings.[241,248,272,279] Glomerulonephritis appears to be mainly an immune-mediated disease and there is experimental and clinical evidence of an immunosuppressive potential of various solvents.[280] Experimentally, solvent exposures have induced glomerular lesions in the presence of concomitant tubulointerstitial injury.[238,243–247,281,282] It is, therefore, possible to speculate that in susceptible individuals, low-grade tubular damage from chronic exposure to solvents may provoke local autoimmunity by releasing either sequestered or altered tubular and basement-membrane antigens (antibodies to proximal tubular antigens, laminin, Goodpasture's antigens) (Figure 86.9) with activation or damage of the overlying endothelium,[283] which results in the development of glomerulonephritis.[272] Autoimmunity may be favoured by the immunosuppressive effects of solvent exposure.[280] Furthermore, carbon tetrachloride nephrotoxicity can be inhibited by whole body irradiation exposed at each injection,[284] favouring the role of primary tubular damage and local autoimmunity in the possible pathogenesis of solvent-induced glomerulopathy.

An alternative hypothesis is that potentially glomerulotoxic immune factors arise independently of solvent exposure and that solvents merely facilitate the deposition of these mediators of immune damage in renal tissue.[285] However, occupational exposure to solvents is widespread and glomerulonephritis and tubular interstitial disease are infrequently seen, which could suggest the operation of as yet undefined possible genetic or idiosyncratic factors in this association.

Whatever the mechanism of solvent nephropathy, the observations serve to remind us that an occupational and recreational history should be obtained from patients with progressive renal failure and that they should receive counselling regarding relevant exposures. With improved means of reducing exposure to solvents in occupational settings (Figure 86.10), these risks should gradually reduce.

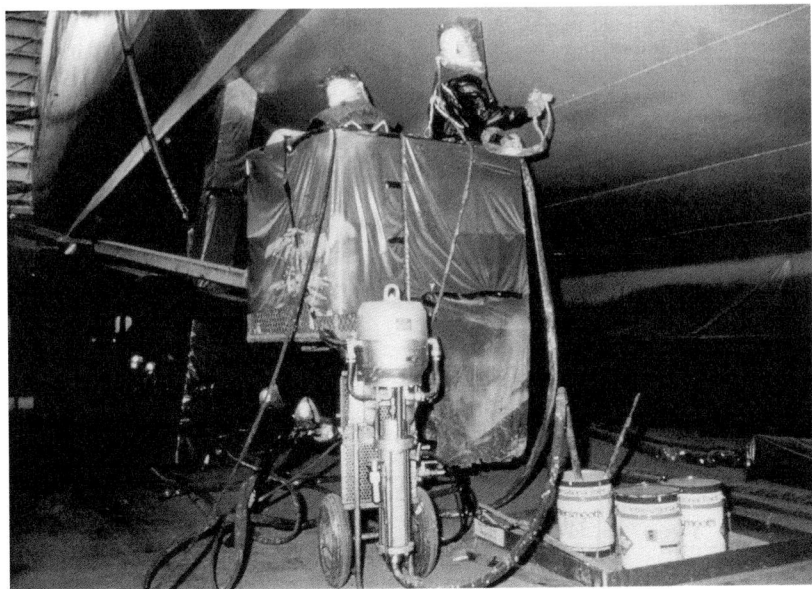

Figure 86.10 Boat paint sprayers with protective equipment and using air-fed masks.

> **Key points**
>
> - End-stage kidney failure is a personal and financial disaster for affected patients and an increasingly large cost burden for world healthcare programmes.
> - While immunological and vasculopathic associations are recognized in the causation of chronic kidney disease, occupational factors may be relevant and should be considered in all patients.
> - The nephrotoxicity of heavy metals has been studied for many years. Evidence also links occupational organic solvent exposure and progressive kidney failure.
> - Prevention of kidney toxicity from these agents through public health and work site programmes involving increasing awareness of risk and adherence to control measures provides more health benefit than limited treatment options.
> - Increasingly, emphasis should be focused on the detection and early and possibility reversible biochemical indicators of toxicity, such as renal tubular dysfunction in cadmium toxicity.

ACKNOWLEDGEMENTS

This chapter is updated from *Hunter's Diseases of Occupations*, 9th edn, Chapter 90, Nephrotoxic effects of workplace exposures by Gordon M Bell and Howard J Mason.

REFERENCES

1. Feest T. Epidemiology and causes of chronic renal failure. *Medicine*. 2007; **35**: 438-41.
2. Answell D, Feehally J, Feest T *et al*. UK renal registry report. Bristol: UK Renal Registry, 2007.
3. Department of Health. Second progress report on the Renal National Service Framework (NSF). London: Department of Health, May 2007.
4. Institute for Health and Clinical Excellence, National Institute for Health and Clinical Excellence. Chronic kidney disease: Early identification and management of chronic kidney diease in adults in primary and secondary care in the National Health Service (NHS) in England and Wales, January 2007.
5. US Renal Data System (USRDS) 2007 Annual data report: Atlas of chronic kidney disease and end stage renal disease in the United States. Bethesda, MD: National Institutes of Health, National Institute of Diabetes and Digestive and Kidney Diseases, 2007.
6. Lane RE. The care of the lead worker. 1949. *British Journal of Industrial Medicine*. 1949: **6**: 125-43.
7. Health and Safety Executive. Diseases from metals. Last accessed September 2009. Available from: www.hse.gov.uk.
8. Sen D, Wolfson H, Dilworth M. Lead exposure in scaffolders during refurbishment construction activity – an observational study. *Occupational Medicine*. 2002; **52**: 49-54.
9. Gidlow DA. Lead toxicity. *Occupational Medicine*. 2004; **54**: 76-81.
10. Ekong EB, Jaar BG, Weaver VM. Lead related nephrotoxicity: A review of the epidemiologic evidence. *Kidney International*. 2006; **70**: 2074-84.
11. Batuman V. Lead nephropathy, gout and hypertension. *American Journal of the Medical Sciences*. 1993; **305**: 241-7.
12. Bennett VM. Lead nephropathy. *Kidney International*. 1985; **28**: 212-20.
13. Ritz E, Wiecek A, Stoeppler M. Lead nephropathy. *Contributions to Nephrology*. 1987; **55**: 185-91.
14. Barbier O, Jacquillet G, Tauc M *et al*. Effect of heavy metals on, and handling by, the kidney. *Nephron. Physiology*. 2005; **99**: 105-10.
15. Goyer RA. The renal tubule in lead poisoning. Mitochondrial swelling and aminoaciduria. *Laboratory Investigation*. 1968; **19**: 71-7.
16. Goyer RA. Mechanisms of lead and cadmium nephrotoxicity. *Toxicology Letters*. 1989; **46**: 153-62.
17. Landrigan RJ. Toxicity of lead at low dose. *British Journal of Industrial Medicine*. 1989; **46**: 593-6.
18. Nolan CV, Shaikh ZA. Lead nephrotoxicity and associated disorders: Biochemical mechanisms. *Toxicology*. 1992; **73**: 127-46.
19. Chisolm JJ Jr, Harrison HC, Eberlein WR, Harrison HE. Aminoaciduria, hypophosphataemia and rickets in lead poisoning; study of a case. *American Journal of Diseases of Childhood*. 1995; **89**: 159-68.
20. Chisolm JJ Jr. Aminoaciduria as a manifestation of renal tubular injury in lead intoxication and a comparison with patterns of aminoaciduria seen in other diseases. *Journal of Pediatrics*. 1962; **60**: 1-17.
21. Hammond PB. Exposure of humans to lead. *Annual Review of Pharmacology and Toxicology*. 1977; **17**: 197-214.
22. Moore JF, Goyer RA, Wilson M. Lead induced inclusion bodies. Solubility, aminoacid content, and relationship to residual acidic nuclear proteins. *Laboratory Investigation*. 1973; **29**: 488-94.
23. Vyskocil A, Pancl J, Tusl M *et al*. Dose-related proximal tubular dysfunction in male rats chronically exposed to lead. *Journal of Applied Toxicology*. 1989; **9**: 395-9.
24. Cramér K, Goyer RA, Jagenburg R, Wilson MH. Renal ultrastructure, renal function and parameters of lead toxicity in workers with different periods of lead exposure. *British Journal of Industrial Medicine*. 1974; **31**: 113-27.

25. Goyer RA, Leonard DL, Bream PR, Irons TG. Aminoaciduria in experimental lead poisoning. *Proceedings of the Society for Experimental Biology and Medicine.* 1970; **135**: 767-71.
26. Goyer RA, Wilson MH. Lead-induced inclusion bodies: Results of ethylenediaminetetraacetic acid treatment. *Laboratory Investigation.* 1975; **32**: 149-56.
27. Henderson DA. The aetiology of chronic nephritis in Queensland. *Medical Journal of Australia.* 1958; **45**: 377-86.
28. Emmerson BT. Chronic lead nephropathy. *Kidney International.* 1973; **4**: 1-5.
29. Inglis JA, Henderson DA, Emmerson BT. The pathology and pathogenesis of chronic lead nephrotoxicity occurring in Queensland. *Journal of Pathology.* 1978; **124**: 65-76.
30. Batuman V, Maesaka JK, Haddad B et al. The role of lead in gout nephropathy. *New England Journal of Medicine.* 1981; **304**: 520-3.
31. Batuman V, Landy E, Maesaka JK, Wedeen RP. Contribution of lead to hypertension with renal impairment. *New England Journal of Medicine.* 1983; **309**: 17-21.
32. Loghman-Adham M. Renal effects of environmental and occupational lead exposure. A review. *Environmental Health Perspectives.* 1997; **105**: 928-38.
33. Steenland K, Selevan S, Landrigan P. The mortality of lead smelter workers: An update. *American Journal of Public Health.* 1992; **82**: 1641-4.
34. Weedon RP, Malik DK, Batuman V. Detection and treatment of occupational lead nephropathy. *Archives of Internal Medicine.* 1979; **139**: 53-7.
35. Khalil-Manesh F, Gonick HC, Cohen AH et al. Experimental model of lead nephropathy I. Continuous high-dose lead administration. *Kidney International.* 1992; **42**: 1192-203.
36. Muntner P, Menke A, De Salvo KB et al. Continued decline in blood lead levels among adults in the United States. The National Health and Nutrition Examination Surveys. *Archives of Internal Medicine.* 2005; **165**: 2155-61.
37. Centers for Disease Control and Prevention (CDC). Blood lead levels – United States 1999-2002. *MMWR Morbidity and Mortality Weekly Reports.* 2005; **54**: 513-16.
38. Weaver VM, Lee BK, Ahn KD et al. Associations of lead biomarkers with renal function in Korean lead workers. *Occupational and Environmental Medicine.* 2003; **60**: 551-62.
39. Khalil-Manesh F, Gonick HC, Cohen AH. Experimental model of lead nephropathy III. Continuous low-level lead administration. *Archives of Environmental Health.* 1993; **48**: 271-8.
40. Navas-Acien A, Guallar E, Silbergeld EK, Rothenberg SJ. Lead exposure and cardiovascular disease – a systematic review. *Environmental Health Perspectives.* 2007; **115**: 472-82.
41. Harlan WR. The relationship of blood lead levels to blood pressure in the US population. *Environmental Health Perspectives.* 1988; **78**: 9-13.
42. Nash D, Magder L, Lustberg M et al. Blood lead, blood pressure and hypertension in perimenopausal and postmenopausal women. *Journal of the American Medical Association.* 2003; **289**: 1523-32.
43. Pocock SJ, Shaper AG, Ashby D et al. The relationship between blood lead, blood pressure, stroke and heart attacks in middle-aged British men. *Environmental Health Perspectives.* 1988; **78**: 22-30.
44. Schwartz J. The relationship between blood lead and blood pressure in the NHANES II Survey. *Environmental Health Perspectives.* 1988; **78**: 15-22.
45. Hu H, Aro A, Payton M et al. The relationship of bone and blood lead to hypertension. The Normative Aging Study. *Journal of the American Medical Association.* 1996; **275**: 1171-6.
46. Korrick SA, Hunter DJ, Rotnitzky A et al. Lead and hypertension in a sample of middle-aged women. *American Journal of Public Health.* 1999; **89**: 330-35.
47. Fine BP, Vetrano T, Skurnick J, Ty A. Blood pressure elevation in young dogs during low-level lead poisoning. *Toxicology and Applied Pharmacology.* 1988; **93**: 388-93.
48. Gonick HC, Ding Y, Bondy SC et al. Lead-induced hypertension. Interplay of nitric oxide and reactive oxygen species. *Hypertension.* 1997; **30**: 1487-92.
49. Vaziri ND. Pathogenesis of lead-induced hypertension: Role of oxidative stress. *Journal of Hypertension.* 2002; **20** (Suppl.): 515-20.
50. Nawrot TS, Thijs L, Den Hond E et al. An epidemiological re-appraisal of the association between blood pressure and blood lead: A meta-analysis. *Journal of Human Hypertension.* 2002; **16**: 123-31.
51. Staessen JA, Bulpitt CJ, Fagard R et al. Hypertension caused by low-level lead exposure: Myth or fact? *Journal of Cardiovascular Risk.* 1994; **1**: 87-97.
52. Schwartz J. Lead, blood pressure and cardiovascular disease in men. *Archives of Environmental Health.* 1995; **50**: 31-7.
53. Den Hond E, Nawrot T, Staessen JA. The relationship between blood pressure and blood lead in NHANES III. National Health and Nutritional Examination Survey. *Journal of Human Hypertension.* 2002; **16**: 563-8.
54. Telisman S, Pizent A, Jurasovic J, Cvitkovic P. Lead effect on blood pressure in moderately lead-exposed male workers. *American Journal of Industrial Medicine.* 2004; **45**: 446-54.
55. Fenga C, Cacciola A, Martino LB et al. Relationship of blood lead levels to blood pressure in exhaust battery storage workers. *Industrial Health.* 2006; **44**: 304-9.
56. Goyer RA. Lead toxicity: current concerns. *Environmental Health Perspectives.* 1993; **100**: 177-87.
57. Kelada SN, Shetton E, Kaycmann RB, Khoury MJ. Delta-aminolevulinic acid dehydratase genotype and lead toxicity: A huge review. *American Journal of Epidemiology.* 2001; **154**: 1-13.
58. Wu MT, Kelsey K, Schwartz J et al. A delta-aminolevulinic acid dehydratase (ALAD) polymorphism may modify the relationship of low-level lead exposure to uricaemia and renal function: The normative aging study. *Environmental Health Perspectives.* 2003; **111**: 335-41.
59. Weaver VM, Schwartz BS, Ahn KD et al. Associations of renal function with polymorphisms in the delta-aminolevulinic acid dehydratase, vitamin D receptor and nitric oxide synthase genes in Korean lead workers. *Environmental Health Perspectives.* 2003; **111**: 1613-19.

60. Ye XB, Wu CER, Hua F et al. Association of blood lead levels, kidney function and blood pressure with D-aminolevulinic acid dehydratase and vitamin D receptor gene polymorphisms. *Toxicology Mechanisms and Methods*. 2003; **13**: 139–46.
61. Weaver VM, Lee BK, Todd AC et al. Effect modification by delta-aminolevulinic acid dehydratase, vitamin D receptor and nitric oxide synthase gene polymorphisms on associations between patella lead and renal function in lead workers. *Environmental Research*. 2006; **102**: 61–9.
62. Lim YC, Chia KS, Ong HY et al. Renal dysfunction in workers exposed to inorganic lead. *Annals of the Academy of Medicine, Singapore*. 2001; **30**: 112–17.
63. Lin T, Tai-Yi J. Benchmark dose approach for renal dysfunction in workers exposed to lead. *Environmental Toxicology*. 2007; **22**: 229–33.
64. Khalil-Manesh F, Gonick HC, Cohen AH. Experimental model of lead nephropathy. III. Continuous low-level lead administration. *Archives of Environmental Health*. 1993; **48**: 271–8.
65. Ong CN, Endo G, Chia KS. Evaluation of renal function in workers with low blood lead levels. In: *Occupational and environmental chemical hazards. Cellular and biochemical indices for monitoring toxicity*. Chichester: Ellis Horwood, 1987: 327–33.
66. Gennart JP, Bernard A, Lauwerys R. Assessment of thyroid, testers, kidney and autonomic nervous system function in lead-exposed workers. *International Archives of Occupational and Environmental Health*. 1992; **64**: 49–57.
67. Khalil-Manesh F, Gonick HC, Cohen AH et al. Experimental model of lead nephropathy. I. Continuous high-dose lead administration. *Kidney International*. 1992; **41**: 1192–203.
68. Chia KS, Keyaratnam J, Lee J et al. Lead-induced nephropathy: Relationship between various biological exposure indices and early markers of nephrotoxicity. *American Journal of Industrial Medicine*. 1995; **27**: 883–95.
69. White PD, Van Leeuwen P, Davis BD et al. The conceptual structure of the integrated exposure uptake biokinetic model for lead in children. *Environmental Health Perspectives*. 1998; **106** (Suppl. 6): 1513–30.
70. Bergdahl IA, Grubb A, Schütz A et al. Lead binding to delta-aminolevulinic acid dehydratase (ALAD) in human erythrocytes. *Pharmacology and Toxicology*. 1997; **81**: 153–8.
71. Church HJ, Day JP, Braithwaite RA, Brown SS. Binding of lead to a metallothionein-like protein in human erythrocytes. *Journal of Inorganic Biochemistry*. 1993; **49**: 55–68.
72. O'Flaherty EJ. Physiologically based models for bone-seeking elements. IV. Kinetics of lead disposition in humans. *Toxicology and Applied Pharmacology*. 1993; **118**: 16–29.
73. Rabinowitz MB. Toxicokinetica of bone lead. *Environmental Health Perspectives*. 1991; **91**: 33–7.
74. Simons TJ. Active transport of lead by the calcium pump in human red cell ghosts. *Journal of Physiology*. 1988; **405**: 105–13.
75. Hu H, Shih R, Rothenberg S, Schwartz BS. The epidemiology of lead toxicity in adults: Measuring dose and consideration of other methologic issues. *Environmental Health Perspectives*. 2007; **115**: 445–62.
76. Landrigan RJ, Todd AC. Direct measurement of lead in bone. A promising biomarker. *Journal of the American Medical Association*. 1994; **271**: 239–40.
77. Nie H, Howard HU, Chettle DR. Application and methodology of *in vivo* K x-ray fluorescence of Pb in bone (impact of KXRF data in the epidemiology of lead toxicity and consistency of the data generated by updated systems). *X-Ray Spectrometry*. 2008; **37**: 90.
78. Korrick SA, Schwartz J, Tsaih SW et al. Correlates of bone and blood lead levels among middle-aged and elderly women. *American Journal of Epidemiology*. 2002; **156**: 335–43.
79. Webber CE, Chettle DR, Bowins RJ et al. Hormone replacement therapy may reduce the return of endogenous lead from bone to the circulation. *Environmental Health Perspectives*. 1995; **103**: 1150–53.
80. Goldman RH, White R, Kales SN, Hu H. Lead poisoning from mobilisation of bone stores during thyrotoxicosis. *American Journal of Industrial Medicine*. 1994; **25**: 417–24.
81. Somervaille LJ, Chettle DR, Scott MC et al. In vivo tibia lead measurements as an index of cumulative exposure in occupationally exposed subjects. *British Journal of Industrial Medicine*. 1988; **45**: 174–81.
82. Armstrong R, Chettle DR, Scott MC et al. Repeated measurements of tibia lead concentrations by *in vivo* x-ray fluorescence in occupational exposure. *British Journal of Industrial Medicine*. 1992; **49**: 14–16.
83. Cake KM, Bowins RJ, Vaillancourt C et al. Partition of circulating lead between serum and red cells is different for internal and external sources of lead. *American Journal of Industrial Medicine*. 1996; **29**: 440–45.
84. Erkkilä J, Armstrong R, Riihimäki V et al. In vivo measurements of lead in bone at four anatomical sites: Long term occupational and consequent endogenous exposure. *British Journal of Industrial Medicine*. 1992; **49**: 631–44.
85. Hu H, Milder FL, Burger DE. The use of k x-ray fluorescence for measuring lead burden in epidemiological studies: High and low lead burdens and measurement uncertainty. *Environmental Health Perspectives*. 1991; **94**: 107–10.
86. McNeill FE, Stokes L, Brito JA et al. 109Cd K x-ray fluorescence measurements of tibial lead content in young adults exposed to lead in early childhood. *Occupational and Environmental Medicine*. 2000; **57**: 465–71.
87. Van de Vyver FL, D'Haese PC, Visser WJ et al. Bone lead in dialysis patients. *Kidney International*. 1988; **33**: 601–7.
88. Lee BK, Schwartz BS, Stewart W, Ahn KD. Provocative chelation with DMSA and EDTA: Evidence for differential access to lead storage sites. *Occupational and Environmental Medicine*. 1995; **52**: 13–19.
89. Dorsey CD, Lee BK, Bolla KI et al. Comparison of patella lead with blood lead and tibia lead and their associations with neurobehavioural test scores. *Journal of Occupational and Environmental Medicine*. 2006; **48**: 489–96.
90. Weaver VM, Lee BK, Todd AC et al. Associations of patella lead and other lead biomarkers with renal function in lead workers. *Journal of Occupational and Environmental Medicine*. 2005; **47**: 235–43.

91. Ehrlich R, Robins T, Jordaan E et al. Lead absorption and renal dysfunction in a South African battery factory. *Occupational and Environmental Medicine*. 1998; **55**: 453–60.
92. Gerhardsson L, Chettle DR, Englyst V et al. Kidney effects in long term exposed lead smelter workers. *British Journal of Industrial Medicine*. 1992; **49**: 186–92.
93. Lin-Tan DT, Lin JL, Yen TH et al. Long-term outcome of repeated lead chelation therapy in progressive non-diabetic chronic kidney diseases. *Nephrology, Dialysis, Transplantation*. 2007; **22**: 2924–31.
94. Cohen A, Bergamaschi E, Mutti A. Environmental model of lead nephropathy II. Effect of removal from lead exposure and chelation treatment with dimercaptosuccinic acid (DMSA). *Environmental Research*. 1992; **58**: 35–54.
95. Vaziri ND, Liang K, Ding Y. Increased nitric oxide inactivation by reactive oxygen species in lead-induced hypertension. *Kidney International*. 1999; **56**: 1492–8.
96. Foglieni C, Fulgenzi A, Ticozzi P et al. Protective effect of EDTA preadministration on renal ischaemia. *BMC Nephrology*. 2006; **7**: 5.
97. Flora SJ, Bhattacharya R, Vijayaraghavan R. Combined therapeutic potential of messo-2, 3-dimercaptosuccinic acid and calcium disodium edetate on the mobilisation and distribution of lead in experimental lead intoxication in rats. *Fundamental and Applied Toxicology*. 1995; **25**: 233–40.
98. Cory-Slechta DA, Weiss B, Cox C. Mobilisation and redistribution of lead over the course of calcium disodium ethylenediamine tetraacetate chelation therapy. *Journal of Pharmacology and Experimental Therapeutics*. 1987; **243**: 804–13.
99. Kiran K, Swaran JS, Flora SJ. Strategies for safe and effective therapeutic measures for chronic arsenic and lead poisoning. *Journal of Occupational Health*. 2005; **47**: 1–21.
100. Powell JJ, Burden TJ, Greenfield SM et al. Urinary excretion of essential metals following intravenous calcium diosodium edetate: An estimate of free zinc and zinc status in man. *Journal of Inorganic Biochemistry*. 1999; **75**: 159–65.
101. Kosnett MJ, Wedeen RP, Rothenberg SJ et al. Recommendations for medical management of adult lead exposure. *Environmental Health Perspectives*. 2007; **115**: 463–71.
102. Swaran JS, Flora SJA, Pande M, Mehta A. Beneficial effect of combined administration of some naturally occurring antioxidants (vitamins) and thiol chelators in the treatment of chronic lead intoxication. *Chemico-Biological Interactions*. 2003; **145**: 267–80.
103. Kalia K, Flora SJ. Strategies for safe and effective therapeutic measures for chronic arsenic and lead poisoning. *Journal of Occupational Health*. 2005; **47**: 1–21.
104. Cooper WC, Gaffey WR. Mortality of lead workers. *Journal of Occupational Medicine*. 1975; **17**: 100–7.
105. McMichael AJ, Johnson HM. Long term mortality profile of heavily exposed lead smelter workers. *Journal of Occupational Medicine*. 1982; **24**: 375–8.
106. Malcolm D, Barnett HAR. A mortality of lead workers 1925–1976. *British Journal of Industrial Medicine*. 1982; **39**: 404–10.
107. Davies JM. Long-term mortality study of chromate pigment workers who suffered lead poisoning. *British Journal of Industrial Medicine*. 1984; **41**: 170–8.
108. Cooper WC, Wong O, Kheifet S. Mortality among employees of lead battery plants and lead producing plants, 1947–1980. *Scandinavian Journal of Work and Environmental Health*. 1985; **11**: 331–45.
109. Selevan SG, Landrigan PJ, Stern FB, Jones JH. Mortality of lead smelter workers. *American Journal of Epidemiology*. 1985; **122**: 673–83.
110. Gerhardsson L, Lundstrom NG, Nordberg G, Wall S. Mortality and lead exposure: A retrospective cohort study of Swedish smelter workers. *British Journal of Industrial Medicine*. 1986; **43**: 707–11.
111. Fanning D. A mortality study of lead workers, 1926–1985. *Archives of Environmental Health*. 1988; **43**: 247–51.
112. Sharp DS, Becker CE, Smith AH. Chronic low level lead exposure. Its role in the pathogenesis of hypertension. *Medical Toxicology*. 1987; **2**: 210–32.
113. Schober SE, Mirel LB, Graubard BL et al. Blood lead levels and death from all causes, cardiovascular disease and cancer: Results from the NHANES III mortality study. *Environmental Health Perspectives*. 2006; **114**: 1538–41.
114. Mandel JS, McLaughlin JK, Schlehofer B et al. International renal cell cancer study. IV Occupation. *International Journal of Cancer* 1995; **61**: 601–5.
115. Cocco P, Hua F, Boffetta P et al. Mortality of Italian lead smelter workers. *Scandinavian Journal of Work and Environmental Health*. 1997; **23**: 15–23.
116. Pesch B, Haerting J, Ranft U et al. Occupational risk factors for renal cell carcinoma: Agent-specific results from a case control study in Germany. MURC Study Group. Multicentre urothelial and renal cell study. *International Journal of Epidemiology*. 2000; **29**: 1014–24.
117. Steenland K, Boffetta P. Lead and cancer in humans: Where are we now? *American Journal of Industrial Medicine*. 2000; **38**: 295–9.
118. Fu H, Boffetta P. Cancer and occupational exposure to inorganic lead compounds: A meta-analysis of published data. *Occupational and Environmental Medicine*. 1995; **52**: 73–81.
119. Lam TV, Agovino P, Niu X, Roche L. Linkage study of cancer risk among led-exposed workers in New Jersey. *Science of the Total Environment*. 2007; **372**: 455–62.
120. Rousseau MC, Parent ME, Nadon L et al. Occupational exposure to lead compounds and risk of cancer among men: A population-based case-control study. *American Journal of Epidemiology*. 2007; **166**: 1005–14.
121. Wong O, Harris F. Cancer mortality study of employees at lead battery plants and lead smelters, 1947–1995. *American Journal of Industrial Medicine*. 2000; **38**: 255–70.
122. Friberg L, Piscator M, Nordberg GF, Kjellstrom T. *Cadmium in the environment*, 2nd edn. Cleveland: CRC Press, 1994.
123. Lauwerys R, Bernard A, Roels HA et al. Characterisation of cadmium proteinuria in man and rat. *Environmental Health Perspectives*. 1984; **54**: 147–53.

124. Barbier O, Jacquillet G, Tauc M et al. Effect of heavy metals on, and handling by, the kidney. *Nephron. Physiology.* 2005; **99**: 105-10.
125. Roels H, Bernard AM, Cárdenas A et al. Markers of early renal changes induced by industrial pollutants. III. Application to workers exposed to cadmium. *British Journal of Industrial Medicine.* 1993; **50**: 37-48.
126. Bernard AM, Roels H, Cárdenas A, Lauwerys R. Assessment of urinary protein 1 and transferrin as early markers of cadmium nephrotoxicity. *British Journal of Industrial Medicine.* 1990; **47**: 559-65.
127. Järup L, Persson B, Elinder CG. Decreased glomerular filtration rate in solderers exposed to cadmium. *Occupational and Environmental Medicine.* 1995; **52**: 818-22.
128. Kido T, Nagawa K, Ishizaki M et al. Long-term observation of serum creatinine and arterial blood pH in persons with cadmium induced renal dysfunction. *Archives of Environmental Health.* 1990; **45**: 35-41.
129. Roels HA, Lauwerys RR, Buchet JP et al. Health significance of cadmium induced renal dysfunction: A five year follow up. *British Journal of Industrial Medicine.* 1989; **46**: 755-64.
130. Bernard A, Lauwerys R, Ouled Amot A. Loss of glomerular polyanion correlated with albuminuria in experimental cadmium nephropathy. *Archives of Toxicology.* 1992; **66**: 272-8.
131. Cardenas A, Bernard AM, Lauwerys RR. Disturbances of sialic acid metabolism by chronic cadmium exposure and its relation to proteinuria. *Toxicology and Applied Pharmacology.* 1991; **108**: 547-58.
132. Bernard AM, Amor AO, Lauwerys RR. Decrease of erythrocyte and glomerular membrane negative charges in chronic cadmium poisoning. *British Journal of Industrial Medicine.* 1988; **45**: 112-15.
133. Piscator M. Long-term observations on tubular and glomerular function in cadmium-exposed persons. *Environmental Health Perspectives.* 1984; **54**: 175-9.
134. Elinder CG, Edling C, Lindberg E et al. β_2-microglobinuria among workers previously exposed to cadmium: Follow-up and dose-response analyses. *American Journal of Industrial Medicine.* 1995; **8**: 553-64.
135. Järup L, Elinder CG. Incidence of renal stones among cadmium exposed battery workers. *British Journal of Industrial Medicine.* 1993; **50**: 598-602.
136. Trevisan A, Gardin C. Nephrolithiasis in a worker with cadmium exposure in the past. *International Archives of Occupational and Environmental Health.* 2005; **78**: 670-2.
137. Fahim MS, Khare NK. Effects of subtoxic levels of lead and cadmium on urogenital organs of male rats. *Archives of Andrology.* 1980; **4**: 357-62.
138. Shaikh ZA, Smith LM. Biological indicators of cadmium exposure and toxicity. *Experientia.* 1984; **40**: 36-43.
139. Järup L, Berglund M, Elinder CG et al. Health effects of cadmium exposure – a review of the literature and a risk estimate. *Scandinavian Journal of Work and Environmental Health.* 1998; **24** (Supp. 1): 1-51.
140. Sarkar S, Yadav P, Bhatnagr D. Lipid peroxidative damage on cadmium exposure and alterations in antioxidant system in rat erythrocytes: A study with relation to time. *Biometals.* 1998; **11**: 153-7.
141. Stacey NH, Cantilena LR Jr, Klaassen CD. Cadmium toxicity and liquid peroxidation in isolated rat hepatocytes. *Toxicology and Applied Pharmacology.* 1980; **53**: 470-80.
142. Petering DH, Loftsgaarden J, Scheider J, Fowler B. Metabolism of cadmium, zinc and copper in the rat kidney: The role of metallothionein and other binding sites. *Environmental Health Perspectives.* 1984; **54**: 73-81.
143. Ahn DW, Choi JK, Park YS. Renal acid-base regulation in cadmium-intoxicated rats. *Korean Journal of Physiology and Pharmacology.* 2002; **6**: 41-6.
144. Ahn DW, Chung JM, Kim JY et al. Inhibition of renal Na^+/H^+ exchange in cadmium-intoxicated rats. *Toxicology and Applied Pharmacology.* 2005; **204**: 91-8.
145. Bernard A. Renal dysfunction induced by cadmium: Biomarkers of critical effects. *Biometals.* 2004; **17**: 519-23.
146. Bernard A. The determination of β_2-microglobulin, retinol-binding protien and alpha 1-microglobulin in urine. In: *Biological monitoring of chemical exposure in the workplace.* Geneva: World Health Organization, 1996: 74-90.
147. Tohyama C, Kobayashi E, Saito H et al. Urinary alpha-1 microglobulin as an indicator protein of renal tubular dysfunction caused by environmental cadmium exposure. *Journal of Applied Toxicology.* 1986; **6**: 171-8.
148. Moriguchi J, Ezaki T, Tsukahara T et al. Comparative evaluation of four urinary tubular dysfunction markers, with special references to the effects of aging and correction for creatinine concentration. *Toxicology Letters.* 2003; **143**: 279-90.
149. Bernard AM, Thielemans NO, Lauwerys RR. Urinary protein 1 or clara cell protein: A new sensitive marker of proximal tubular dysfunction. *Kidney International.* 1994; **47**: S534-7.
150. Verschour M, Herber R, Van Hemmen J et al. Renal function of workers with low level cadmium exposure. *Scandinavian Journal of Work and Environmental Health.* 1987; **13**: 232-8.
151. Lauwerys R. Cadmium in man. In: Webb M (ed.). *Chemistry, biochemistry and biology of cadmium.* Amsterdam: Elsevier/North Holland, 1979: 433-45.
152. Roels H, Lauwerys R, Buchet JP et al. *In vivo* measurement of liver and kidney cadmium in workers exposed to this metal. *Environmental Research.* 1981; **26**: 217-40.
153. Roels H, Lauwerys RR, Dardenne AN. The critical level of cadmium in the human renal cortex: A re-evaluation. *Toxicology Letters.* 1983; **15**: 357-60.
154. Friberg L, Piscator M, Nordberg GF, Kjellstrom T. *Cadmium in the environment*, 2nd edn. Cleveland: CRC Press, 1994.
155. Fribeg L. Cadmium. In: Friberg L, Elinder CG, Kjellstrom T, Nordberg GF (eds). *Cadmium and health: A toxicological epidemiological appraisal*, vol 1. Boca Raton: CRC Press, 1984: 1-6.
156. Bernard A, Roels H, Buchet JP et al. Cadmium and health: The Belgium experience. In: Nordberg GF, Herber RFM, Alessio L (eds). *Cadmium in the human environment: Toxicity and carcinogenicity.* Lyons: International Agency for Research on Cancer, 1992: 15-33.

157. Roels H, Lauwerys R, Buchet JP et al. Significance of urinary metallothionein in workers exposed to cadmium. *International Archives of Occupational and Environmental Health*. 1983; **52**: 159–66.
158. Roels H, Bernard AM, Cardenas A et al. Markers of early renal changes induced by industrial pollutants. III. Application to workers exposed to cadmium. *British Journal of Industrial Medicine*. 1993; **50**: 37–48.
159. Roels HA, Van Assche FJ, Oversteyns M et al. Reversibility of microproteinuria in cadmium workers with incipient tubular dysfunction after reduction of exposure. *American Journal of Industrial Medicine*. 1997; **31**: 645–52.
160. Kawasaki T, Kono K, Dote T et al. Markers of cadmium exposure in workers in a cadmium pigment factory after changes in the exposure conditions. *Toxicology and Industrial Health*. 2004; **20**: 51–6.
161. Trzcinka-Ochocka M, Jakubowski M, Halatek T, Razniewska G. Reversibility of microproteinuria in nickle-cadmium battery workers after removal from exposure. *International Archives of Occupational and Environmental Health*. 2002; **75**: S101–6.
162. Goyer RA, Cherian MG, Jones MM, Reigart JR. Role of chelating agents for prevention, intervention and treatment of exposures to toxic metals. *Environmental Health Perspectives*. 1995; **103**: 1048–52.
163. Health and Safety Executive. Working with cadmium, are you at risk? IND G391. Bootle: Health and Saftey Executive, 2004.
164. Health and Safety Executive. Workplace exposure limits. Bootle: Health and Safety Executive, 2005.
165. Occupational Safety and Health Administration. Guidelines on cadmium. Washington DC: OSHA, 2003.
166. Friberg L, Elinder CG, Kjellstrom T, Nordberg GF. *Cadmium and health. A toxicological and epidemiological appraisal.* Boca Raton: CRC, 1986.
167. World Health Organization. Cadmium. Geneva: World Health Organization, 1992.
168. Hellström L, Elinder CG, Dahlberg B et al. Cadmium exposure and end stage renal disease. *American Journal of Kidney Disease*. 2001; **28**: 1001–8.
169. Armstrong BG, Kazantzis G. Prostatic cancer and chronic respiratory and renal disease in British cadmium workers: A case control study. *British Journal of Industrial Medicine*. 1985; **42**: 540–5.
170. Sorahan T, Adams RG, Waterhouse JA. Analysis of mortality from nephritis and nephrosis among nickel-cadmium battery workers. *Journal of Occupational Medicine*. 1983; **25**: 609–12.
171. Kazantzis G, Lam TH, Sullivan KR. Mortality of cadmium-exposed workers. A five year update. *Scandinavian Journal of Work and Environmental Health*. 1988; **14**: 220–3.
172. Health and Safety Executive. Mercury and its inorganic divalent compounds in air, Ref. 16/2. Bootle: Health and Safety Executive, April 2002.
173. Wedeen RP. Renal diseases of occupational origin. *Occupational Medicine*. 1992; **7**: 449–63.
174. Cardenas A, Roels H, Bernard AM et al. Markers of early renal changes induced by industrial pollutants. 1. Application to works exposed to mercury vapour. *British Journal of Industrial Medicine*. 1993; **50**: 17–27.
175. Magos L, Sparrow S, Snowden R. The comparative renal toxicology of phenyl mercury and mercuric chloride. *Archives of Toxicology*. 1982; **50**: 133–9.
176. Clarkson TW, Hursh JB, Sager PR et al. Mercury. In: Clarkson TW, Friberg L, Norberg GF, Sager PR (eds). *Biological monitoring of heavy metals*. New York: Plenum Press, 1988: 199–247.
177. Joselow M, Goldwater LJ. Absorption and excretion of mercury in man. *Archives of Environmental Health*. 1967; **15**: 155.
178. Foa V, Caimi L, Amante L et al. Patterns of some lysosomal enzymes in the plasma and of proteins in urine of workers exposed to inorganic mercury. *International Archives of Occupational and Environmental Health*. 1976; **37**: 115–24.
179. Roels H, Lauwerys R, Buchet JP et al. Comparison of renal function and psychomotor performance in workers exposed to elemental mercury. *International Archives of Occupational and Environmental Health*. 1982; **50**: 77–93.
180. Roels H, Gennart JP, Lauwerys R et al. Surveillance of workers exposed to mercury vapour: Validation of a previously proposed biological threshold limit value for mercury concentration in urine. *American Journal of Industrial Medicine*. 1985; **7**: 45–71.
181. Barregard L, Hultberg B, Schutz A, Sallsten G. Enzymuria in workers exposed to inorganic mercury. *International Archives of Environmental Health*. 1988; **61**: 65–9.
182. Ehrenberg RL, Vogt RL, Smith AB et al. Effects of elemental mercury exposure at a thermometer plant. *American Journal of Industrial Medicine*. 1991; **19**: 495–507.
183. Elligsen DG, Barregard L, Gaarder PI et al. Assessment of renal dysfunction in workers previously exposed to mercury at a Chloralkali plant. *British Journal of Industrial Medicine*. 1993; **50**: 881–7.
184. Foa V, Bertelli G. Mercury. In: Alessio L, Berlin L, Boni M, Roi R (eds). *Biological indicators for the assessment of human exposure to industrial chemicals*. Ispra: Commission of European Communities, 1986: 29–46.
185. BEI justification. Mercury – elemental and inorganic. *Applied Occupational and Environmental Hygiene*. 1990; 5–8.
186. Gompertz D. Biological monitoring of workers exposed to mercury vapour. *Journal of the Society of Occupational Medicine*. 1982; **32**: 141–5.
187. Langworth S, Eliner CG, Sundquist KG, Vesterberg O. Renal and immunological effects of occupational exposure to inorganic mercury. *British Journal of Industrial Medicine*. 1992; **49**: 394–401.
188. Health and Safety Executive. Workplace exposure limits HSC, EH40/2005. Bootle: Health and Safety Executive.
189. Health and Safety Executive. HSE guidance note EH65/19. Bootle: Health and Safety Executive.
190. Health and Safety Executive. HSE guidance note EH64, supplement. Bootle: Health and Safety Executive, 1995.
191. American Conference of Governmental Industrial Hygienists. TLVs and BEIs. Threshold limit values for

192. Occupational Safety and Health Administration. Mercury: OSHA standards. Washington DC: US Department of Labor, OSHA, 2007.
193. Nylander M, Friberg, Lind B. Mercury concentrations in the human brain and kidneys in relation to exposure from dental amalgam fillings. *Swedish Dental Journal.* 1987; **11**: 179-87.
194. Pai P, Thomas S, Hoenich N et al. Treatment of a case of severe mercuric salt overdose with DMPS and continuous haemofiltration. *Nephrology, Dialysis, Transplantation.* 2000; **15**: 1889-990.
195. Tubbs RR, Gerhardt GD, McMahon JT. Membranous glomerulonephritis associated with industrial mercury exposure. *American Journal of Clinical Pathology.* 1981; **77**: 409-13.
196. Lauwerys R, Bernard A, Roels H et al. Anti-laminin antibodies in workers exposed to mercury vapour. *Toxicology Letters.* 1983; **17**: 113-16.
197. Drueet P, Bernard A, Hirsch F. Immunologically mediated glomerulonephritis induced by heavy metals. *Archives of Toxicology.* 1982; **50**: 187.
198. Goldman M, Baran D, Druet P. Polyclonal activation and experimental nephropathies. *Kidney International.* 1988; **34**: 141-50.
199. Iesato K, Wakastin M, Wakashin Y. Renal tubular dsyfunction in Minimata disease. Detection of renal tubular antigen and β_2 microglobulin in the urine. *Annals of Internal Medicine.* 1977; **86**: 731-7.
200. Sallsten G, Barregard L, Schutz A. Clearance half life of mercury in urine after the cessation of long term occupational exposure: Influence of a chelating agent (DMPS) on excretion of mercury in urine. *Occupational and Environmental Medicine.* 1994; **51**: 337.
201. Bluhm RE, Bobbitt RG, Welch LW et al. Elemental mercury vapour toxicity, treatment and prognosis after acute, intensive exposure in chloralkali plant workers. Part I: History, neuropsychological findings and chelator effects. *Human and Experimental Toxicology.* 1992; **11**: 201.
202. Banday AA, Priyamvada S, Farooq N et al. Efect of uranyl nitrate on enzymes of carbohydrate metabolism and brush border membrane in different kidney tissues. *Food and Chemical Toxicology.* 2008; **46**: 2080-8.
203. Thiebault C, Carriere M, Milgram S et al. Uranium induces apoptosis and is genotoxic to normal rat kidney (NRK-52E) proximal cells. *Toxicological Sciences.* 2007; **98**: 479-87.
204. Zhu G, Xiang X, Chen X et al. Renal dysfunction induced by long-term exposure to depleted uranium in rats. *Archives of Toxicology.* 2009; **83**: 37-46.
205. Hodgson A, Pellow PGD, Stradling GN. HPA-RPD-025 - Influence of nephrotoxicity on urinary excretion of uranium. Last accessed September 2009. Available from: http://www.hpa.org.uk/webw/HPAweb&HPAwebStandard/HPAweb_C/1247816509891?p=1197637096018.
206. Dounce AL. The mechanism of action of uranium compounds in the animal body. In: Voegtlin C, Hodge HC (eds). *Pharmacology and toxicity of uranium compounds*, vol. 1. New York: McGraw-Hill, 1949: 951-91.
207. Thun MJ, Baker DB, Streeland K et al. Renal toxicity in uranium mill workers. *Scandinavian Journal of Work and Environmental Health.* 1985; **11**: 83-90.
208. Vacquier B, Caer S, Rogel A et al. Mortality risk in the French cohort of uranium miners: Extended follow-up 1946-1999. *Occupational and Environmental Medicine.* 2008; **65**: 597-604.
209. Weeden RP, Qian LF. Chromium-induced kidney disease. *Environmental Health Perspectives.* 1991; **92**: 71-4.
210. Wang X, Qin Q, Xu X et al. Chromium-induced early changes in renal function among ferrochromium-producing workers. *Toxicology.* 1994; **90**: 93-101.
211. Nagaya T, Ishikawa N, Hata H et al. Early renal effects of occupational exposure to low-level hexavalent chromium. *Archives of Toxicology.* 1994; **68**: 322-4.
212. Stoecklel JD, Hardy H, Weber AL. Chronic beryllium disease. Long-term follow-up of sixty cases and selective review of the literature. *American Journal of Medicine.* 1969; **46**: 545-61.
213. Fowler BA, Weissberg JB. Arsine poisoning. *New England Journal of Medicine.* 1974; **291**: 1171-84.
214. Gilberson A, Varizi ND, Mirahamadi K et al. Haemodialysis of acute arsenic intoxication with transient renal failure. *Archives of Internal Medicine.* 1976; **136**: 1303.
215. Gerhardt RE, Crecelis EA, Hudson JB. Moonshine related arsenic poisoning. *Archives of Internal Medicine.* 1977; **140**: 211-13.
216. Randall RE, Osheroff RJ, Bakerman S et al. Bismuth nephrotoxicity. *Annals of Internal Medicine.* 1972; **77**: 481-2.
217. Dash SC. Copper sulfate poisoning and acute renal failure (editorial). *International Journal of Artificial Organs.* 1989; **12**: 610.
218. Othersen JB, Maize JC, Woolson RF, Budisarlijevic MN. Nephrogenic systemic fibrosis after exposure to gadolinium in patients with renal failure. *Nephrology, Dialysis, Transplantation.* 2007; **22**: 3179-85.
219. Steenland K, Goldsmith DF. Silica exposure and autoimmune diseases. *American Journal of Industrial Medicine.* 1995; **28**: 603-8.
220. Parks CG, Conrad K, Cooper GS. Occupational exposure to crystalline silica and autoimmune disease. *Environmental Health Perspectives.* 1999; **107** (Suppl. 5): 793-802.
221. Rapiti E, Sperati A, Miceli M et al. End stage renal disease among ceramic workers exposed to silica. *Occupational and Environmental Medicine.* 1999; **56**: 559-61.
222. Steenland K, Sanderson W, Calvert GM. Kidney disease and arthritis in a cohort study of workers exposed to silica. *Epidemiology.* 2001; **12**: 405-12.
223. Steenland K, Rosenman K, Socie E, Valiante D. Silicosis and end-stage renal disease. *Scandinavian Journal of Work and Environmental Health.* 2002; **28**: 439-42.
224. Hogan SL, Cooper GS, Savitz DA et al. Association of silica exposure with anti-neutrophil cytoplasmic autoantibody small-vessel vasculitis: a population-based, case-control

study. *Clinical Journal of the American Society of Nephrology.* 2007; **2**: 290–9.
225. Hogan SL, Satterly KK, Dooley MA et al. Glomerular Disease Collaborative Network. Silica exposure in anti-neutrophil cytoplasmic autoantibody-associated glomerulonephritis and lupus nephritis. *Journal of the American Society of Nephrology.* 2001; **12**: 134–42.
226. Bartunková J, Pelclová D, Fenclová Z et al. Exposure to silica and risk of ANCA-associated vasculitis. *American Journal of Industrial Medicine.* 2006; **49**: 569–76.
227. Stratt P, Messuerotti A, Canavese C et al. The role of metals in autoimmune vasculitis: Epidemiological and pathogenic study. *Science of the Total Environment.* 2001; **270**: 179–90.
228. McDonald AD, McDonald JC, Rando RJ et al. Cohort mortality study of North American industrial sand workers. 1. Mortality from lung cancer, silicosis and other causes. *Annals of Occupational Hygiene.* 2001; **45**: 193–9.
229. McDonald JC, McDonald AD, Hughes JM et al. Mortality from lung and kidney disease in a cohort of North American industrial sand workers: An update. *Annals of Occupational Hygiene.* 2005; **49**: 367–73.
230. D'Haese PC, Elseviers MM, Yaqoob M, De Broe ME. Hydrocarbons, silicon containing compounds and pesticides. In: De Broe ME, Porter WM, Bennet WM, Verpooten GA (eds). *Clinical nephrotoxins*, 2nd edn. Amsterdam: Kluwer Academic Publishers, 2002: 545–58.
231. Yaqoob M, Bell GM. Organic solvents and renal disease. In: Holgate S (ed.). *Horizons in medicine*, No. 6. Oxford: Blackwell Science, 1995: 206–17.
232. Pederen LM. Biological studies in human exposure to and poisoning with organic solvents. *Pharmacology and Toxicology.* 1987; **3**: 1–38.
233. Clayton GD, Clayton EE (eds). *Industrial hygiene and toxicology*, vol. 27. New York: Wiley, 1981: 26.
234. Seaton A. Organic solvents and the nervous system: Time for reappraisal. *Quarterly Journal of Medicine.* 1992; **84**: 637–69.
235. Navarte J, Saba SR, Ramirez G. Occupational exposure to organic solvents causing chronic tubulo-interstitial nephritis. *Archives of Internal Medicine.* 1989; **149**: 154–9.
236. Anderson K. Acute nephritis due to turpentine absorbed by the skin. *British Medical Journal.* 1912; **3**: 881.
237. Cagnoli L, Cassanova S, Pasquali S et al. Relationship between hydrocarbon exposure and the nephrotic syndrome. *British Medical Journal.* 1980; **280**: 1068.
238. Beirne GJ, Brennan JT. Glomerulonephritis associated with hydrocarbon solvents. *Archives of Environmental Health.* 1972; **25**: 365–69.
239. Daniell WE, Couser WG, Rosenstock L. Occupational solvent exposure and glomerulonephritis. *Journal of the American Medical Association.* 1988; **259**: 2280–3.
240. Klavis G, Drommer W. Goodpasture's syndrome and the effects of benzene. *Archives of Toxicology.* 1970; **26**: 40–55.
241. Bruner RH. Pathological findings in laboratory animals exposed to hydrocarbon fuels of military interest. In: Mehlman MA, Hemstreet III CP, Thorpe JJ, Weaver NK (eds). *Renal effects of petroleum hydrocarbons.* Princeton, NJ: Princeton Scientific Publishers, 1984: 133–40.
242. Halder CA, Warne TM, Hatoum NS. Renal toxicity of gasoline and related petroleum naphthas in male rats. In: Mehlman MA, Hemstreet III CP, Thorpe JJ, Weaver NK (eds). *Renal effects of petroleum hydrocarbons.* Princeton, NJ: Princeton Scientific Publishers, 1984: 73–88.
243. Dunn TB, Morris HP, Wagner BP. Lipaemia and glomerular lesions in rats fed diets containing N-N diacetyl and tetramethyl-benzidine. *Proceedings of the Society for Experimental Biology and Medicine.* 1956; **91**: 105–7.
244. Harman JW, Miller EC, Miller JA. Chronic glomerulonephritis and nephrotic syndrome induced in rates by N, N-diacetylbenzidine. *American Journal of Pathology.* 1952; **28**: 529.
245. Harman JW. Chronic glomerulonephritis and nephrotic syndrome induced in rats with N, N-diacetylbenzidine. *Journal of Pathology.* 1970; **104**: 119–28.
246. Zimmerman SW, Norbach DH. Nephrotoxic effects of long-term carbon tetrachloride administration in rats. *Archives of Pathology and Laboratory Medicine.* 1980; **104**: 94–9.
247. Zimmerman SW, Norbach DH, Powers K. Carbon tetrachloride nephrotoxicity in rats with reduced renal mass. *Archives of Pathology and Laboratory Medicine.* 1983; **17**: 264–9.
248. Al-Ghamdi SS, Raftery MJ, Yaqoob MM. Toluene and p-xylene induced LLC-PK1 apoptosis. *Drugs and Chemical Toxicology.* 2004; **27**: 425–32.
249. Ravnskov U. Hydrocarbons may worsen renal function in glomerulonephritis. A meta-analysis of the case control studies. *American Journal of Industrial Medicine.* 2000; **37**: 599–606.
250. Yaqoob M, Stevenson A, Mason H, Bell GM. Hydrocarbon exposure and tubular damage: Additional factors in the progression of renal failure in primary glomerulonephritis. *Quarterly Journal of Medicine.* 1993; **86**: 661–7.
251. Yaqoob M, King A, McClelland P et al. Relationship between hydrocarbon exposure and nephropathology in primary glomerulonephritis. *Nephrology, Dialysis, Transplantation.* 1994; **9**: 1575–9.
252. Stengel B, Cenee S, Limasset J et al. Organic solvent exposure may increase the risk of glomerular nephropathies with chronic renal failure. *International Journal of Epidemiology.* 1995; **24**: 427–34.
253. Asal NR, Cleveland HL, Kaufman C et al. Hydrocarbons and chronic renal disease. *International Archives of Occupational and Environmental Health.* 1996; **68**: 229–35.
254. Ravnskov U. Hydrocarbon exposure may cause glomerulonephritis and worsen renal function: Evidence based on Hill's criteria for causality. *Quarterly Journal of Medicine.* 2000; **93**: 51–6.
255. Jacob S, Hery M, Protois J et al. Effect of organic solvent exposure on chronic kidney disease progression: The GN-Progress Cohort Study. *Journal of the American Society of Nephrology.* 2007; **18**: 274–81.

256. Fored CM, Nise G, Ejerblad E et al. Absence of association between organic solvent exposure and risk of chronic renal failure: A nationwide population-based case control study. *Journal of the American Society of Nephrology.* 2004; **15**: 180–6.
257. Yaqoob M, Patrick AW, McClelland P et al. Occupational hydrocarbon exposure and diabetic nephropathy. *Diabetic Medicine.* 1994; **11**: 789–93.
258. Cameron JS. Tubular and interstitial factors in the progression of glomerulonephritis. *Pediatric Nephrology.* 1992; **6**: 292–303.
259. Churchill DW, Fine A, Gault MH. Association between hydrocarbon exposure and glomerulonephritis: An appraisal of the evidence. *Nephron.* 1983; **33**: 169–72.
260. Askergren A, Allgen LG, Bergstrom J. Studies on kidney function in subjects exposed to organic solvents. 1. Excretion of albumin and beta-2-microglobulin in the urine. *Acta Medica Scandinavica.* 1981; **209**: 472–83.
261. Franchini I, Cavartorta A, Falzoi M et al. Early indicators of renal damage in workers exposed to organic solvents. *International Archives of Occupational and Environmental Health.* 1983; **52**: 1–9.
262. Brochard P, De Palmas J, Martini M et al. Étude de la prevalance des proteinuries dipistées chez des sujets exposé professionellment aux solvants. XXI International Congress Occupational Health, Dublin, September 1984.
263. Lauwerys R, Bernard A, Viau C, Buchet JP. Kidney disorders and haematotoxicity from organic solvent exposure. *Scandinavian Journal of Work and Environmental Health.* 1985; **11** (Suppl. 1): 83–90.
264. Via C, Bernard A, Lauwerys R et al. A cross-sectional survey of kidney function in oil refinery employeees. *American Journal of Industrial Medicine.* 1987; **11**: 177–87.
265. Hotz P, Pilliod J, Berode M et al. Glycosaminoglycans, albuminuria and hydrocarbon exposure. *Nephron.* 1991; **58**: 184–91.
266. Hotz P, Thielemans N, Bernard A et al. Serum laminin, hydrocarbon exposure and glomerular damage. *British Journal of Industrial Medicine.* 1993; **50**: 1104–10.
267. Vyskocil A, Popler A, Skutilova I et al. Urinary excretion of proteins and enzymes in workers exposed to hydrocarbons in a shoe factory. *International Archives of Occupational and Environmental Health.* 1991; **63**: 359–62.
268. Yaqoob M, Bell GM, Percy D, Finn R. Primary glomerulonephritis and hydrocarbon exposure: A case–control study and literature review. *Quarterly Journal of Medicine.* 1992; **83**: 409–18.
269. Solet D, Robins TG. Renal function in dry cleaning workers exposed to perchloroethylene. *American Journal of Industrial Medicine.* 1991; **20**: 601–14.
270. Mutti A, Alinovi R, Bergamaschi E et al. Nephropathies and exposure to perchloroethylene in dry cleaners. *Lancet.* 1992; **340**: 189–93.
271. Yaqoob M, Bell GM, McGregor AJ et al. Renal impairment due to hydrocarbon exposure. *Quarterly Journal of Medicine.* 1993; **86**: 165–74.
272. Stevenson A, Yaqoob M, Mason H et al. Biochemical markers of basement disturbances and occupational exposure to hydrocarbons and mixed solvents. *Quarterly Journal of Medicine.* 1995; **88**: 23–8.
273. Pai P, Stevenson A, Mason H, Bell GM. Occupational hydrocarbon exposure and nephrotoxicity: A cohort study and literature review. *Postgraduate Medical Journal.* 1998; **741**: 225–8.
274. Rushton L, Anderson MR. An epidemiologic survey of eight refineries in Britain. *British Journal of Industrial Medicine.* 1981; **38**: 225–34.
275. Kaplan SD. Update of a mortality study of workers in petroleum refineries. *Journal of Occupational Medicine.* 1986; **28**: 574–6.
276. Morgan RW, Kaplan SD, Gaffey WR. A general mortality study of production workers in the paint and coatings manufacturing industry. *Journal of Occupational Medicine.* 1981; **23**: 13–21.
277. Divine BJ, Barron V, Kaplan SD. Texaco mortality study. 1. Mortality among refinery, petrochemical and research workers. *Journal of Occupational Medicine.* 1985; **27**: 445–7.
278. Fox AJ, Collier PF. Low mortality rates in industrial cohort studies due to selection for work and survival in the industry. *British Journal of Preventive and Social Medicine.* 1976; **30**: 225–30.
279. Streicher HZ, Gabow PA, Moss AH et al. Syndromes of toluene sniffing in adults. *Annals of Internal Medicine.* 1981; **84**: 758–62.
280. Ravnskov U. Possible mechanisms of hydrocarbon associated glomerulonephritis. *Clinical Nephrology.* 1985; **23**: 294–98.
281. Glassock RJ, Edginton TS, Watson JI, Dixon FJ. Autologous immune complex nephritis induced with renal tubular antigen. *Journal of Experimental Medicine.* 1968; **127**: 573–87.
282. Shibita S, Yokoyama M. Nephritogenic glycoprotein. *Nephron.* 1990; **55**: 152–8.
283. Nishikawa K, Guo YJ, Miyasaka M et al. Antibodies to intercellular adhesion molecule 1/lymphocyte function-associated antigen 1 prevent crescent formation in rat auto-immune glomerulonephritis. *Journal of Experimental Medicine.* 1993; **177**: 667–77.
284. Ogawa M, Mori T, Mori Y et al. Study on chronic renal injuries induced by carbon tetrachloride: Selective inhibition of the nephrotoxicity by irradiation. *Nephron.* 1992; **60**: 68–73.
285. Yamamoto T, Wilson CB. Binding of anti-basement membrane after intratracheal gasoline instillation in rabbits. *American Journal of Pathology.* 1987; **126**: 497–505.

87

Neurotoxic effects of workplace exposures

MICHAEL J AMINOFF AND MARCELLO LOTTI

Introduction	1151	Organophosphate and carbamate insecticides	1160
Acrylamide	1152	Organochlorine pesticides	1161
Allyl chloride	1153	Pyrethroids	1161
1-Bromopropane	1153	Pesticides and parkinsonism	1161
Carbon disulphide	1154	Styrene	1162
Carbon monoxide	1154	Toluene	1162
Dimethylaminoproprionitrile	1155	Trichloroethylene	1163
Ethylene oxide	1155	Solvent mixtures	1163
Hexacarbon solvents	1156	Wartime exposure	1163
Metals	1156	Acknowledgement	1165
Methyl bromide	1159	References	1165

INTRODUCTION

Increasing numbers of chemical agents are being introduced into the occupational environment, and many of these agents are liable to produce neurotoxic effects manifested either as neurobehavioural changes or neurological deficits affecting cognition, motor control, sensation or autonomic function. Either the central or the peripheral nervous system, or both, may be damaged. This chapter will consider the main agents that have been implicated in the setting of workplace exposure. These may affect workers involved in the manufacture of potentially neurotoxic substances and those subject to industrial, agricultural, horticultural or military exposure.

A clinical or subclinical disturbance of function should be considered to have a neurotoxic basis only if certain basic criteria are satisfied. First, a temporal association should exist between toxin exposure and any clinical or other manifestations of neurological dysfunction. The tempo of the clinical disorder should be consistent with the biological effects and mechanisms of action of the presumed toxin. The course of the disorder should be arrested (sometimes after an interval during which mild progression occurs, the so-called 'coasting' phenomenon) when exposure to the putative toxin is discontinued. In some instances, it is possible to show that rechallenge (i.e. re-exposure to the likely toxin) leads to reappearance or exacerbation of the neurological disorder. Second, there should be no alternative explanation for the neurological dysfunction. Third, the manifestations of the presumed neurotoxic disorder should be similar to those in other cases of exposure to the same neurotoxin. Fourth, the presumed neurotoxic disorder should be biologically plausible, based on the known toxicity or effects of the toxin on biological systems. It may be possible to demonstrate a dose–response relationship in which the exposure dose is related to the development of the disorder or its severity. Fifth, it is sometimes possible to reproduce the presumed neurotoxic disorder experimentally under similar conditions of exposure in animals, thereby providing support for its aetiology, although a failure to reproduce it does not exclude the possibility of a neurotoxic disorder.

The assessment of neurotoxic effects poses a variety of problems, particularly with regard to the detection of mild or subclinical neurobehavioural disturbances related to chronic low-dose exposure or following a single episode of acute toxicity. Structured psychometric tests for investigating possible cognitive impairment are sensitive to focal disturbances in individual cortical regions. Potential confounding factors during testing, such as fatigue or exposure to alcohol and psychotropic drugs, have to be considered.

This also applies to the use of the electroencephalogram (EEG) and event-related evoked potential studies. For disturbances of motor function, quantitative tests of muscle strength and of coordination, body sway and balance are sometimes useful. Quantitative sensory testing may be helpful; a variety of modalities can be examined, including vibration and discriminative tactile sensibility, cold and warm thermal thresholds, and heat pain thresholds. Quantitative evaluation of autonomic (mainly cardiovascular) function is now a well-established procedure. Many of these tests are laborious and time-consuming, but less elaborate tests suitable for use in the field have been devised for some assessments.

Peripheral nerve function can be analysed using nerve conduction tests which assess function both in motor and sensory fibres. The sensitivity of measurements of motor and sensory nerve conduction velocity, in particular the former, is substantially greater than that for evoked muscle action potential and sensory nerve action potential amplitude. Strict temperature control during testing is vital. For the comparison of exposed workers with control subjects, the selection of appropriate control subjects is important. The use of sedentary office workers as controls for manual workers, for example, has led to erroneous conclusions, as manual workers frequently accumulate abnormalities of nerve conduction during their occupation as a consequence of repeated minor trauma or the development of subclinical entrapment neuropathies. Neuromuscular transmission and muscle function can be assessed by quantitative electromyography (EMG), but such testing is technically demanding.

Epidemiological studies involving case–control observations again demand scrupulous care in the selection of appropriate control subjects. For neurobehavioural observations, careful matching for age, sex, ethnic group and educational background is necessary. With these multiple problems in establishing a causal relationship between exposure to a particular neurotoxic agent and the occurrence of symptoms in a workforce, it is understandable that conflicting reports may arise, particularly as individual variations in susceptibility may complicate the issue. Animal experiments are not always informative because of interspecies differences, but may be crucial in clarifying the mechanism of action of toxic substances.

ACRYLAMIDE

Acrylamide polymers are used to separate solids from aqueous solutions in certain industries, and are constituents of adhesives and certain products, such as cardboard and moulded parts (see Chapter 42, Organic chemicals). The monomer, but not the polymer, is neurotoxic. Exposure typically occurs by inhalation or cutaneous absorption during the manufacture of the monomer or in the polymerization process. Acrylamide is also used for grouting in mines and tunnels; for this purpose, liquid monomer is pumped into the soil, where polymerization occurs after the addition of various catalysts, rendering the soil waterproof. Intoxication has occurred occasionally in workers involved in such grouting operations.[1] It is also used, for example, in manhole sealing operations. Typically, the powdered grout is mixed with water to produce an aqueous grout solution containing 10 per cent solids, to which an activator is added. A second solution is prepared consisting of an initiator or catalyst, such as ammonium persulphate. The solutions are mixed and injected where required; the acrylamide polymerizes and the cross-linking agent binds the polymer chain together, converting the mixture into a gel. During the liquid and gel phases of the grout operations, the grout is hazardous to workers because of the risk of dermal contact and absorption.

Occupational exposure may result in an encephalopathy, with confusion, hallucinations, poor concentration, drowsiness, and other changes, depending on the duration and severity of exposure. A length-dependent sensorimotor neuropathy also occurs and is typically associated with hyperhidrosis and redness and exfoliation of the skin,[2,3] and occasionally with urinary retention. Cerebellar disturbances may be conjoined.[4] Numbness of the feet is usually the earliest symptom. The tendon reflexes are lost at an early stage.

The neuropathy is arrested and may slowly reverse after discontinuation of exposure, but residual deficits – including sensory ataxia – are common. Histopathological studies show a distally predominant accumulation of neurofilaments in axons, and distal axonal degeneration in both the peripheral and central nervous systems. There is little secondary demyelination. On electrophysiological examination, maximal motor conduction velocity is normal or only slightly reduced, but compound muscle action potentials may be small and dispersed, with a prolongation in the distal motor latency.[2] These changes have been attributed to degeneration and subsequent regeneration of the distal parts of the motor axons. In keeping with an axonopathy, sensory nerve action potentials are reduced or absent[2,5] and this is the preferred electrophysiological means of monitoring workers who are at risk of developing the disorder.

More sophisticated electrophysiological studies have revealed that sensory fibres are more vulnerable than motor fibres, and large fibres more vulnerable than small ones.[6] Function is disturbed especially in the short, intramuscular segment of the large-diameter stretch receptor afferent axons from gastrocnemius.[7] Experimental studies have also indicated that sudomotor dysfunction occurs later than motor involvement and reflects damage to postganglionic sympathetic efferent nerve fibres.[8]

The pathogenesis of acrylamide neuropathy is unclear. Both fast and slow axonal transport systems are affected in acrylamide neuropathy. Impairment of fast axonal transport is probably responsible for the accumulation of tubulovesicular structures and of slow transport probably underlies the formation of neurofilamentous axonal swellings. The ability of the fast anterograde motor protein, kinesin, to interact with microtubules is affected; dynein–microtubule interactions (involved in retrograde transport) may similarly be impaired. There is also evidence of decreased presynaptic neurotransmitter release, perhaps related to impaired neurotransmitter uptake into synaptic vesicles.[9]

The effects on the nervous system are cumulative, and exposure must therefore be limited. Protective clothing (for example, gloves, head covering, face shield, goggles and overalls) limits dermal contact and a mask can be utilized to limit inhalation exposure. Bags of the monomer should carry warning labels about the means and hazards of exposure. Permissible airborne exposure limits of factory workers should be no more than $0.3 mg/m^3$ time-weighted average (TWA) according to recommendations of the Occupational Safety and Health Administration (OSHA) of the United States Department of Labor (American Conference of Governmental Industrial Hygienists (ACGIH) threshold limit value (TLV): $0.03 mg/m^3$ TWA and the National Institute for Occupational Safety and Health (NIOSH) recommended exposure limit (REL) $0.03 mg/m^3$ TWA). Myers and Macun[10] described the occurrence of acrylamide neuropathy in workers in a small factory in South Africa who were exposed to varying levels of acrylamide while manufacturing polyacrylamide flocculants. Logistic regression showed dose–response relationships of exposure with symptoms, abnormal sensation, weakness, gait disturbances and cutaneous abnormalities. Acrylamide-related abnormalities occurred in 67 per cent of those with exposure exceeding the recommended exposure level of NIOSH, compared with lesser exposure.

The encephalopathy and mild peripheral neuropathy resolve following cessation of exposure to acrylamide, but recovery is incomplete in patients with severe neuropathies. There is no specific treatment to hasten recovery.

ALLYL CHLORIDE

Allyl chloride, a chlorinated hydrocarbon, is a colourless, yellow or purple liquid with an unpleasant odour. It is used in the manufacture of epichlorohydrin which is employed for the manufacture of epoxy resins. It is also used in the production of glycerine insecticides and in the synthesis of polyacrylonitride. Precise information concerning risk of neurotoxicity in workers exposed to specific concentrations of allyl chloride is limited, but TLV is 1 ppm ($3 mg/m^3$ TWA) in many developed countries including the United States. Toxicity to the liver and kidney generally overshadows any neurotoxicity, but outbreaks of polyneuropathy have occurred in two factories in China in the absence of liver and kidney dysfunction. Subjects in one factory were exposed to allyl chloride at levels of $2.6–6650 mg/m^3$ for between 2.5 months and six years and most had a mixed sensorimotor polyneuropathy; electrophysiological studies showed neurogenic abnormalities in ten of the 19 subjects examined, so that the prevalence of neuropathy was 52.6 per cent. At the other factory, exposures were at $0.2–25.13 mg/m^3$ for 1–4.5 years; symptoms of workers were clinically milder and few abnormal neurological signs were present, but electrophysiological abnormalities of mild neuropathy were found in almost 50 per cent of subjects.[11] A central-peripheral distal axonopathy has been reproduced experimentally in mice.[12] A multifocal intra-axonal accumulation of neurofilaments preceded axonal degeneration.

The diagnosis is based on the occurrence of symptoms, signs and electrodiagnostic abnormalities indicative of neuropathy in subjects with known exposure to allyl chloride and no other identifiable cause of neuropathy. Management involves the discontinuation of exposure and supportive measures. Improvement may occur, but may be delayed for months. There is no specific treatment.

1-BROMOPROPANE

1-Bromopropane has replaced ozone-depleting solvents for degreasing and cleaning metal and optical instruments and as a glue solvent. Central and peripheral neurological disorders have recently been associated with occupational exposures to it for months or years, but the clinical picture is not consistent.[13–16] Features common to all reports include weakness of lower-extremity muscle groups, numbness, dysphagia and urinary difficulties. Diarrhoea is often present. Patients are unable to stand and some present with signs of a spastic paraparesis. Stretch reflexes may be normal, brisk or decreased, whereas vibration sense is always reduced. No involvement of cranial nerves has been described. Nerve conduction velocity and EMG studies are either normal or reveal a demyelinating or axonal neuropathy. Brain and spinal cord magnetic resonance imaging (MRI) may be normal or show increased T_2 signal in the periventricular white matter and at lumbar levels. Laboratory tests, including cerebrospinal fluid (CSF), are normal except for pseudo-hyperchloraemia. Since most autoanalysers react with all halide anions, hyperchloraemia in these patients masks high levels of blood bromide, reported as high as 12.5 mEq/L. Functional recovery is slow and poor.

No severe neurological symptoms have been observed in workers exposed to less than 170 ppm 1-bromopropane and having urinary 1-bromopropane levels lower than 120 ng/L,[17] but in another study mild signs of neurotoxicity were detected at environmental levels lower than 50 ppm.[18] The proposed limit of exposure in the United States is less than 10–25 ppm.

Conflicting results have also been reported in rats after inhalation of 1-bromopropane at similar dose levels and length of exposure. No neuropathological changes were found in one study,[19] whereas in another, ovoid debris of myelin was detected in tibial nerves together with swellings of preterminal axons in the nucleus gracilis.[20]

CARBON DISULPHIDE

Carbon disulphide has been used as a soil fumigant, in the manufacture of viscose rayon and cellophane films, in the cold vulcanization of rubber, in perfume production, and as a component in certain varnishes and insecticides (see Chapter 39, Gases). It has also been used as a solvent for rubber, wax resins, various oils and certain other chemicals. Toxicity may result from inhalation, ingestion and possibly skin contact, and is not confined to the nervous system. Heavy exposure may occur during the production of viscose rayon when spinning machines are opened, and while cutting and drying.

In the United States, the OSHA-enforceable standard (permissible exposure limit or PEL) for carbon disulphide in workplace air is 20 parts per million (ppm) averaged over eight hours of exposure, and NIOSH recommends that workroom air levels of carbon disulphide not exceed 1 ppm for a ten-hour work day, 40-hour work week. The ACGIH has assigned TLV of 10 ppm as a TWA for a normal eight-hour work day and a 40-hour work week. The findings of a recent study, however, suggested that the current TLV is insufficient to protect against the neurological effects of carbon disulphide and led to the recommendation that it be lowered.[21]

Inhalation exposure to concentrations above 400 ppm leads to narcosis. An encephalopathy may result from acute high exposure, with headache, irritability, uncontrollable anger, disrupted sleep, memory disturbances, mood swings, mania, depression, suicidal tendencies, confusion and other psychiatric manifestations.[22] Such symptoms may follow subacute exposure to levels in the order of 300 ppm, but are common also when workers are exposed chronically to concentrations averaging between 40 and 50 ppm; they are not to be expected at concentrations below 20 ppm.[23] Minor intellectual, affective or motor changes may only be revealed by neuropsychological testing.

Long-term exposure to carbon disulphide may lead to a variety of behavioural or psychiatric disturbances,[22] to extrapyramidal findings such as cogwheel rigidity, bradykinesia or dyskinesia, and to pyramidal deficits, such as a pseudobulbar palsy. A cerebellar syndrome may also occur, sometimes as a delayed manifestation of carbon disulphide exposure, perhaps as a consequence of concomitant age-related neuronal loss.[24] The pupillary and corneal reflexes may be lost, a retrobulbar optic neuropathy sometimes develops, and funduscopic examination may reveal a characteristic retinopathy with microaneurysms and punctate haemorrhages. In addition, there may be clinical or subclinical evidence of polyneuropathy.[25–27] Magnetic resonance imaging of the brain shows high signal intensities in the basal ganglia and subcortical white matter, suggesting small-vessel disease.[28] The neuropathy develops after exposure to levels of 100–150 ppm for several months or to lower levels for several years. It is histologically similar to the neuropathy produced by *n*-hexane, with focal axonal swellings and accumulations of neurofilaments.

There is no specific treatment for the neurological complications of carbon disulphide intoxication, but further exposure must be prevented and general symptomatic measures may be helpful. The peripheral neuropathy may persist at least for some years after cessation of exposure, showing evidence of central involvement.[28]

CARBON MONOXIDE

Carbon monoxide (CO) is an odourless, colourless gas derived from the incomplete combustion of carbon-containing materials (see Chapter 39, Gases). The noxious effects are the result of hypoxia. It binds tenaciously to haemoglobin to form carboxyhaemoglobin (COHb) and also impairs the dissociation of oxyhaemoglobin so that tissue hypoxia is greater than for a comparable degree of anaemia. It also binds to myoglobin, cytochrome oxidase, cytochrome P450, catalases and peroxidases. Elimination of carbon monoxide is increased by breathing pure oxygen or, more rapidly, by hyperbaric oxygen. Some is eliminated by conversion to carbon dioxide (CO_2).

Carbon monoxide poisoning may occur as a result of occupational exposure. The exhaust gases of internal combustion petrol engines contain carbon monoxide and may lead to occupational exposure in the workplace. Cases may certainly relate to industrial exposure, mainly in miners, garage employees and gas workers. The widespread misuse of equipment may lead to the appearance of outbreaks of carbon monoxide poisoning, as has occurred, for example, among Iowa farmers from the indoor use of pressure washers[29] or from the indoor burning of charcoal briquets.[30] A series of carbon monoxide (CO) poisonings has been reported in association with the industrial use of liquified petroleum gas-powered forklifts in inadequately ventilated warehouse and production facilities (in a plastic manufacturing plant, warehouse and embroidery company). Employees at these facilities developed symptoms of carbon monoxide poisoning, and in some the correct diagnosis was initially not made because of the non-specific nature of their symptoms, so that they were sent home untreated from the hospital.[31] Well-recognized industrial sources include catalytic cracking units in petroleum refineries and sintering of blast furnace feed in sintering plants. Carbon monoxide intoxication is also a major hazard for firefighters.

The current OSHA permissible exposure limit is 50 ppm (55 mg/m^3) as an eight-hour TWA concentration; NIOSH has established a recommended exposure limit of 35 ppm (40 mg/m^3) as an eight-hour TWA and 200 ppm (229 mg/m^3) as a ceiling; and the ACGIH has assigned a TLV of 25 ppm (29 mg/m^3) as a TWA for a normal eight-hour work day and 40-hour work week. The NIOSH limit is based on cardiovascular risks and the ACGIH limit on the risk of elevated carboxyhaemoglobin levels.

The consequences of acute exposure are highly variable. Cognitive or behavioural dysfunction is evident in most cases. Disorientation, excitement, apprehension or depression are seen in about 25 per cent of patients. Impaired consciousness is seen in about 66 per cent, ranging from lethargy, through stupor to coma. Affected individuals may show tremor, spasticity, rigidity, dyskinetic movements, exaggerated or depressed tendon reflexes and extensor plantar responses. Respiratory depression can lead to death. Localized neurological signs may be found, including evidence of focal cortical dysfunction. Generalized epileptic seizures may occur in the first or second week after intoxication.

Delayed deterioration is well described. Following a period of partial or apparently full recovery, after an interval of two to three weeks on average, a relapse occurs, sometimes abrupt in onset, with confusion, psychotic behaviour, focal cortical dysfunction and often an extrapyramidal syndrome of rigid parkinsonian type. These features may persist or subsequently improve.

Peripheral nerve involvement has been described. Sometimes, this has been focal or multifocal, presumably related to a combination of hypoxia and compression. A neuropathy with paranodal changes has been produced experimentally in rats.[32]

Pathologically, the central nervous system changes are typical of hypoxic/ischaemic damage, with focal or laminar necrosis of the cerebral cortex and neuronal loss in the hippocampus, cerebellar cortex and substantia nigra. Bilateral necrotic lesions of the globus pallidus are particularly characteristic. White matter lesions also occur, both diffuse and focal. The delayed deterioration is often associated with a diffuse subcortical leukoencephalopathy, but this is also seen in cases without a biphasic course and the pathology in patients with delayed deterioration after anoxia may be confined to grey matter.

Treatment of acute carbon monoxide poisoning consists of removal from the carbon monoxide-containing atmosphere, the administration of oxygen, with hyperbaric oxygen if available, and supportive measures including treatment of the metabolic acidosis. Prevention is important: the workplace should be screened for possible sources of exposure and likely hazardous features should be corrected. If motor vehicles are to be operated in confined spaces, adequate ventilation must be assured and carbon monoxide emissions assessed regularly. Various devices are available to monitor carbon monoxide levels in the work environment.

Adverse neurological effects of chronic low level carbon monoxide exposure are questionable. Stewart[33] concluded that visual perception was possibly marginally impaired at carboxyhaemoglobin levels of 5 per cent, but that cognitive function and the performance of complex motor tasks were not altered unless concentrations exceeded 10 per cent.

DIMETHYLAMINOPROPRIONITRILE

Dimethylaminoproprionitrile (DMAPN) has been used, along with acrylamide, in a grouting mixture. This combination is known to have caused peripheral neuropathy. It was then incorporated as a catalyst in the production of polyurethane foams. After its introduction in 1976–77, an unusual neuropathic syndrome developed in exposed workers, characterized primarily by autonomic involvement.[34] This began with difficulty with micturition and was followed by erectile dysfunction and sensory symptoms in the feet and hands. These symptoms were accompanied by insomnia and fatiguability. Examination showed distal sensory loss in the limbs and also in sacral dermatomes, slight distal weakness and depressed ankle jerks. Gradual recovery ensued, but urinary and sexual dysfunction sometimes persisted. Exposure had probably occurred by inhalation, but it may also have occurred through the skin. Nerve biopsy showed loss of both myelinated and unmyelinated axons. Nerve conduction studies showed minor abnormalities in some patients, which normalized several months after exposure had ceased. There are incomplete data concerning exposure levels during industrial use and the relation of exposure to safety.

ETHYLENE OXIDE

Ethylene oxide (EtO) is used mainly as a chemical intermediate in the manufacture of textiles, detergents, polyurethane foam, antifreeze, solvents and various other products, and as a fumigant and to sterilize heat-sensitive products, such as operating gowns used by hospital personnel and patients (see Chapter 39, Gases). Its byproduct, ethylene chlorohydrin (EtC), is considered to be highly toxic, but the mechanism of toxicity is unclear. The principal hazards are carcinogenicity and mutagenesis, rather than neurological. Chronic exposure (inhalation or transdermal) to ethylene oxide and ethylene chlorohydrin, however, has been reported to lead to peripheral neuropathy and mild cognitive impairment in operating department nurses and technicians,[35] although disposable operating gowns and drapes are now widely used. It has also been suggested that residual ethylene chlorohydrin in dialysis tubing after sterilization could contribute to the polyneuropathy encountered in patients receiving chronic haemodialysis.[36] It is known that neuropathy can be produced by exposure of rats to ethylene oxide.[37] This is a central-peripheral distal axonopathy that is diagnosed in humans on the basis of a history of exposure to a concentration deemed toxic, with improvement occurring on cessation of exposure. No specific treatment exists. The NIOSH REL is <0.1 ppm (<0.18 mg/m^3) TWA; 5 ppm (9 mg/m^3) ceiling, 10 min/day. The ACGIH TLV is 1 ppm (2 mg/m^3). Ethylene oxide is considered to be a human occupational carcinogen and workers should be exposed to levels that are as low as reasonably practicable.

HEXACARBON SOLVENTS

For a fuller discussion of hexacarbon solvents, see Chapter 42, Organic chemicals.

Methyl n-butyl ketone and n-hexane

Methyl n-butyl ketone is a solvent that has been used in the manufacture of vinyl and acrylic coatings and adhesives, and in the printing industry. In 1975, Allen et al.[38] reported an outbreak of polyneuropathy among workers in a plant producing plastic-coated and colour-printed fabrics. The temporal onset and cause of the outbreak correlated with exposure to methyl n-butyl ketone, which had recently replaced methyl isobutyl ketone, and new cases failed to appear after its elimination from the workplace. It has since become apparent that exposure via inhalation or skin contact to only small traces (a few ppm) of methyl n-butyl ketone is sufficient to lead to a neuropathy in exposed workers.[39]

n-Hexane is a solvent used in various paints, lacquers and printing inks. It is also used in the rubber industry and in glues, and exposure may occur in workers involved in manufacturing shoes or sandals, laminating processes and cabinet finishing. Exposure in the range of 500–2500 ppm leads to an insidiously progressive, distal, sensorimotor polyneuropathy, sometimes accompanied by visual impairment (due to optic neuropathy or maculopathy) or facial numbness.[40] n-Hexane has also been associated with the triggering of Leber hereditary optic neuropathy.[41] Tendon reflexes may show only mild changes. There is marked slowing of nerve conduction velocity and terminal motor latency, in addition to signs of denervation in affected muscles and small or absent sensory nerve action potentials. The neuropathy results from a disturbance of axonal transport, and is associated with giant, multifocal axonal swelling with accumulation of axonal neurofilaments, and with distal degeneration in both peripheral and central axons accompanied by secondary demyelination. Differential diagnosis may be difficult unless there is evidence of n-hexane exposure in an occupational setting. n-Hexane and methyl n-butyl ketone are metabolized to 2,5-hexanedione, the agent predominantly responsible for their neurotoxic effects. This γ-diketone structure reacts with lysine ε-amines to form pyrrole adducts to axonal neurofilaments and secondary cross-linking derivatives, hampering axonal transport.[42]

Acute exposure by inhalation to these hexacarbon solvents produces a pleasurable sense of euphoria, together with headache, unsteadiness, hallucinations and mild narcosis.[43] The inhalation for recreational purposes of certain glues has been associated with the development of the same sensorimotor polyneuropathy described above.[44]

The neurological deficit progresses for some months after occupational or recreational exposure is discontinued, and examination may show evidence of minor pyramidal dysfunction in addition to the neuropathy. Multimodality evoked potential studies have provided confirmatory evidence of central involvement at different levels of the nervous system (cord, brainstem and cerebral hemispheres) in workers exposed to n-hexane.[45]

Current ACGIH TLVs for n-hexane and methyl n-butyl ketone for occupational exposures are 50 and 5 ppm, respectively.

Methyl ethyl ketone

Methyl ethyl ketone is a solvent used in paints and lacquers, printer's ink and certain glues. Occupational exposure to methyl ethyl ketone has been monitored by measuring its concentration in the air of the working environment and also by determination of urinary levels at the end of a work shift. It was present with methyl n-butyl ketone in the mixture of chemicals that led to the outbreak of neuropathy referred to earlier. It has also been present with n-hexane in a number of compounds that have been inhaled for recreational purposes, with resulting development of a neuropathy. It is generally believed that methyl ethyl ketone does not itself cause a peripheral neuropathy, but that it may facilitate its development when exposure occurs to other hexacarbon solvents.[46–48]

Chronic occupational exposure to methyl ethyl ketone through both skin contact and inhalation has been associated in a single graphics worker with the development of multifocal myoclonus, ataxia and a postural tremor that resolved over one month after exposure to the work environment was discontinued.[49] Other similarly exposed workers were not affected, suggesting that individual susceptibility was an important factor. Ataxia and tremor, together with dysarthria, cognitive changes, headaches and respiratory difficulties, have also been reported in a labourer after acute exposure to a mixture of methyl ethyl ketone and toluene while spray-painting equipment in an enclosed, unventilated garage.[50]

METALS

Metals are covered in more detail in Chapters 12–38.

Aluminium

Aluminium causes both an acute fatal encephalopathy and a chronic progressive encephalopathy in subjects with chronic renal dysfunction.[51] Brain pathology is different from that in patients with Alzheimer's disease and is mainly non-specific.[52] Several epidemiological studies suggest, unconvincingly, associations between various environmental exposures to aluminium and sporadic Alzheimer's disease, amyotrophic lateral sclerosis and Parkinson's disease.

Epidemiological studies in workers exposed in an aluminium production foundry, during smelting and welding, showed no excess risk of neurological diseases. Overt manifestations of typical aluminium encephalopathy, such as seizures, myoclonus and speech disorders have not been reported in aluminium workers. However, several studies of occupational exposures reported small neurobehavioural changes in workers, although the results are controversial.[53–55] Whereas plasma aluminium levels below 10 mg/L are considered safe in dialysis patients, neurobehavioural performance was assessed in workers with average aluminium blood levels between 1 μg/L and 14 mg/L. However, the strongest positive correlations between impaired neuropsychological performance and aluminium blood levels were found at the lowest and highest levels; intermediate ones were not correlated.

Arsenic

Arsenic is a metalloid widely distributed in nature;[56] contaminated waters in certain areas of Southeast Asia currently cause most cases of arsenic poisoning in the world.[57] Exploiting the pro-apoptotic characteristics of arsenic, arsenic trioxide is used to induce remission in patients with acute promyelocytic leukaemia.[58] Occupational exposures may occur in the manufacture of paints, fungicides, wood preservatives and semiconductors; in gold mining, copper or lead smelting; and in pesticide spraying.

Acute arsenic poisoning after massive ingestion may cause haemorrhagic encephalopathy and the lethal dose is estimated to be around 100 mg.[59] The predominant neurological complication is peripheral neuropathy, which may rarely occur after repeated exposures. Neuropathy is inevitably accompanied by other manifestations of arsenic toxicity, including gastrointestinal illness, skin discolouration and anaemia, and begins with distal sensory symptoms, often painful, in the lower limbs and then in the hands; distal weakness follows. Following cessation of exposure, a prolonged gradual recovery may occur, but is usually incomplete. Electrophysiological features suggest a distal sensorimotor axonopathy,[60] but proximal demyelination may be conspicuous at an early stage.[61] However, pathological examination confirms axonal loss.[62] Urinary arsenic excretion exceeding 25 μg over 24 hours might indicate poisoning if the laboratory can distinguish toxic inorganic from non-toxic organic arsenic originating from seafood.[63] Levels between 0.1 and 0.5 mg/kg on a hair sample may also indicate chronic poisoning.

Arsenic causes oxidative stress and interferes with the function of numerous enzymes and of transduction cascades involving a variety of transcription factors.[64]

Despite numerous suggestions that include the use of dimercaptosuccinic acid (DMSA), there is no strong evidence to recommend specific chelating regimens for the treatment of chronic arsenic poisoning.[65]

Lead

Poisoning with lead is primarily related to inorganic lead compounds. Lead is widely employed industrially, and excessive exposure may therefore occur in a broad range of occupations. These include smelting, metal foundry work, battery manufacture and repair, demolition and ship-breaking, paint pigments and polyvinyl chloride manufacture, storage tank construction and repair, high technology industries, pottery production and railroad equipment repair, among many others. Nowadays, exposures are usually well controlled in major industries, but there are still industries in many less developed countries where clinical lead poisoning can occur. In occupational exposures, the current recommended permissible exposure limit to lead corresponds to 50 μg/m^3 in most countries, whereas blood lead limits may vary between 30 and 70 μg/dL. The clinical manifestations differ between children and adults and this discussion is confined to the latter.

Very few cases of lead encephalopathy, if any, have occurred in North America and Western Europe in recent years as a consequence of prolonged and extremely high exposures. Early features are mental confusion and reduced alertness, possibly progressing to coma and seizures if exposure continues. Pathological findings are non-specific.[66] Other signs of chronic lead poisoning associated with encephalopathy include neuropathy, autonomic dysfunction, microcytic hypochromic anaemia, nephropathy and hypertension.

Clinical lead neuropathy has also become a rarity. Lead neuropathy is predominantly motor in type, manifested by bilateral finger and wrist drop and bilateral foot drop. Distal sensory loss may also occur, but is less prominent. The tendon reflexes are depressed or lost. Other signs of chronic lead intoxication are always present, including anaemia and disturbances of haem metabolism, such as elevated erythrocyte protoporphyrins and urinary excretion of δ-aminolevulinic acid and coproporphyrins. Differential diagnosis includes porphyria, but blood lead levels higher than 90–100 μg/dL and a 24-hour urinary excretion of lead higher than 2 mg after a single intravenous dose of the chelator ethylenediamine tetra-acetic acid (EDTA) are discriminatory. Prognosis depends on the severity of weakness, but is usually good after removal from exposure.

Electrophysiological studies reflect axonal injury with compound muscle action potentials of reduced amplitude, normal or slightly slowed motor conduction velocities, and mildly prolonged distal latencies. Fibrillation potentials, polyphasic motor unit potentials and other signs of denervation are also characteristic of lead neuropathy. Pathological findings are poorly characterized. Whereas segmental demyelination is observed in animals,[67] nerve biopsy in human indicates an axonopathy[68] in accordance with the electrophysiological changes. The mechanism of lead neurotoxicity is unknown.

Treatment is aimed at reducing the body burden of lead,[69] but it is unclear whether chelation affords any benefit to patients with neuropathy. In cases with blood lead levels higher than 70–90 μg/dL, EDTA chelation is indicated with different time-schedules, depending on the amount of metal that can be successfully mobilized. Other chelators may also be used including meso-2,3-dimercaptosuccinic acid and penicillamine. However, caution should be exercised during chelation, because mobilization of lead from bone could possibly worsen toxicity.

Nerve conduction abnormalities are often reported in exposed workers with blood lead levels corresponding to 30–50 μg/dL, as well as an atypical purely sensory neuropathy in workers with blood levels above 40 μg/dL. These abnormalities of nerve conduction are of unclear significance and do not predict the occurrence of clinical neuropathy.[70]

There is increasing concern that cognitive function may be affected in workers with low exposures to lead, but study results are controversial. Meta-analyses of studies correlating blood lead levels and various neurobehavioural tests in exposed workers have reached opposite conclusions.[71–73] Whereas blood lead levels reflect recent exposures, other studies show correlations between cognitive impairment and cumulative lead exposure, as measured in various ways including assessments of lead in bone.[74] Patella and tibia bone lead concentrations were also associated with glial effects on the hippocampus when assessed by proton magnetic resonance spectroscopy.[75]

Suggestions have been made linking lead exposure to neurodegenerative disorders such as Parkinson's disease,[76] amyotrophic lateral sclerosis[77] and Alzheimer's disease[78] and to brain tumours,[79] but there is insufficient evidence to support these associations.

Manganese

Manganese is a heavy metal essential to a variety of physiological functions, but it is also a neurotoxicant. Possible sources of manganese intoxication are occupational exposures of miners, smelters, welders, manganese alloy producers, cell-battery factory workers, and farmers using manganese-containing fungicides.[80] An organic manganese compound is used to increase octane in fuel,[81] raising concern about the health effects of airborne manganese. Patients with liver failure may also suffer from manganese poisoning, since approximately 80 per cent of dietary manganese intake is cleared by biliary excretion.[82] Asymptomatic hepatitis infections may precipitate manganese neurotoxicity in exposed workers.[83]

The clinical picture of manganese-induced parkinsonism is well characterized.[84,85] The initial signs of neurotoxicity are usual behavioural and cognitive changes, including compulsive behaviour, accompanied by headache. Subsequently, a neurological syndrome resembling Parkinson's disease develops after long-term exposures above 27 mg/m³. Manganism is characterized by symmetric extrapyramidal abnormalities, including gait dysfunction, postural instability, bradykinesia, rigidity, masked facies, rest and intention tremor, micrographia and speech disturbances. Dystonic manifestations frequently occur, such as facial grimacing and plantar flexion of the foot ('cock-walk').

Magnetic resonance imaging (MRI), positron emission tomography (PET) and single-photon emission computed tomography (SPECT) are useful diagnostic tools for manganese-induced parkinsonism.[86] Because of the paramagnetic quality of manganese, a bilateral symmetrical increased signal intensity on T_1-weighted MRI is observed in the globus pallidus and midbrain in both manganese-intoxicated and asymptomatic manganese-exposed workers. As increased T_1-weighted signals disappear following withdrawal of exposure, they reflect manganese exposure and not necessarily manganism. [^{18}F]-dopa PET in manganese-intoxicated individuals is normal, suggesting that the nigrostriatal pathway is preserved. Similarly normal is the density of dopamine transporters, used as SPECT ligands, confirming the integrity of presynaptic nerve terminals of the nigrostriatal dopaminergic system.

Levodopa is generally unhelpful in the treatment of these patients.[87] This lack of effect, coupled with negative findings in PET/SPECT studies, suggests that the damage in manganese intoxication is primarily of pathways post-synaptic to the nigrostriatal system. There are some indications from the Chinese literature of effective long-term treatment of manganism with p-aminosalicylic acid, although the mechanism is unknown.[88] Upon removal from exposure, early neurobehavioural changes may be reversible, whereas manganese-induced parkinsonism often shows further progressive deterioration over five to ten years, until a plateau is reached.[89]

Pathological studies show neuronal loss and gliosis primarily affecting the globus pallidus, the substantia nigra pars reticularis, and to a lesser extent the striatum. Lewy bodies are not present and the substantia nigra pars compacta and other regions are usually intact.[84,90] Animal studies confirm the characteristics of manganese-induced parkinsonism.[91]

Distinction from Parkinson's disease is based upon medical history, clinical features, neuroimaging, sensitivity to levodopa and neuropathology.[84,85] The lack of a history of manganese exposure, an asymmetrical impairment, typical rest tremors, normal T_1-weighted MRI, decreased striatal uptake on PET/SPECT and, in particular, a good response to levodopa are indicative of Parkinson's disease. Concurrent alterations of MRI and PET/SPECT may indicate Parkinson's disease with incidental manganese exposure. The pathology of Parkinson's disease is characterized by degeneration of dopaminergic neurons in the substantia nigra pars compacta, intracytoplasmic Lewy bodies and a reduction in striatal dopamine. Degeneration also occurs in other regions, such as the locus ceruleus, Meynert nucleus and dorsal motor nucleus of the vagus. These pathological changes are absent in manganese-induced parkinsonism.

There is controversy concerning the neuropsychological effects of recurrent low-dose exposures to manganese, either occupational or environmental, because of inconsistent findings. Whereas several studies have shown poor performance on several cognitive tests,[92–94] others did not.[95–97] A recent meta-analysis of 19 studies on manganese-exposed workers concluded that low-dose manganese exposures are not associated with early neuromotor or cognitive dysfunction.[98] Exposure to low manganese doses, such as in welders,[99] has been suggested to be a risk factor for the early onset of Parkinson's disease.[100] However, a recent study[101] suggests that there is no relationship between welding and Parkinson's disease, and many reasons might account for a lack of association.[102,103]

Mercury

Occupational exposures to mercury vapour (Hg^0) may occur in chloralkali plants, mines, smelting, manufacturing of medical appliances and dental offices. Exposures to other forms of mercury, either inorganic or organic, may represent an environmental risk, but no longer an occupational one.

The main entry route of mercury is by inhalation, and since the brain is not protected from mercury vapour by the blood–brain barrier, deposition depends on the amount of unoxidized mercury that reaches the brain. Clinical manifestations of chronic mercury intoxication depend on the length and degree of exposure and are associated with air concentrations of mercury higher than $500\,\mu g/m^3$ and urinary mercury levels higher than $300\,\mu g/L$. Neurotoxicity will be common in the workplace at exposure levels to mercury vapour exceeding $50\,\mu g$ Hg/m^3.[104,105] Signs of chronic intoxication are erethism, tremor and stomatitis. Whereas the latter may also depend on oral hygiene, neurological signs are thought to be due to oxidation of Hg^0 to Hg^{2+}, which binds to thiol groups of proteins in the nervous system. The neurasthenic syndrome is characterized by non-specific symptoms and signs, such as insomnia, weakness, irritability, anxiety, loss of confidence and social withdrawal. Fine tremor initially involves the hands and originates centrally. Traditional clinical qualitative methods, as well as quantitative methods have been used to assess tremor in either intoxicated or exposed workers.[106] In milder cases, erethism and tremor regress slowly over a period of years following removal from exposure. Peripheral axonal sensorimotor polyneuropathy may also occur at levels of exposure similar to those causing neurasthenia and tremor, as evidenced clinically and electrophysiologically. Depending on severity and cumulative exposure to mercury, neuropathy may still be detected 20–35 years after the end of exposure.[107]

Although many studies have been conducted on low-level mercury exposure in workers, a specific no-observed-adverse-effect level has not been derived. A WHO panel suggested the following broad guidelines.[108] At exposures above $80\,\mu g$ mercury per m^3, corresponding to a urine mercury level of $100\,\mu g/g$ creatinine, there is high probability of developing classic neurological signs. Exposures in the range of 25 to $80\,\mu g$ mercury per m^3, corresponding to a urine mercury level of $30–100\,\mu g/g$ creatinine, increase the incidence in susceptible individuals of less severe neurotoxic effects, such as impaired psychomotor performance and tremor. The occurrence of non-specific subjective symptoms is also increased. At lower levels of exposure, there is no strong evidence of neurological effects.

Meso-2,3-dimercaptosuccinic acid is indicated in the treatment of mercury intoxication to remove the metal, but is unlikely to improve clinical signs.[109]

METHYL BROMIDE

Methyl bromide has been used as a fumigant, fire extinguisher, refrigerant and insecticide (see Chapter 39, Gases). Because of its high volatility, dangerous concentrations may accumulate in work areas and inhalation then leads to neurotoxicity. Clinical manifestations depend on dose and duration of exposure. Acute poisoning produces convulsions, pulmonary oedema, hyperpyrexia, coma and death. Other neurological manifestations of acute toxicity include psychosis, affective changes, ataxia, tremor and myoclonus.[110,111] Seizures may also occur following exposure to low concentrations, as may headache, nausea, dysarthria, confusion, hyperreflexia and visual abnormalities.[112]

Long-term exposure has been associated with a polyneuropathy[112,113] that may occur in the absence of systemic symptoms.[114] Paraesthesiae in the feet are followed by symmetric, distal sensory and motor deficits and areflexia. Gait ataxia may be conspicuous. Recovery to a variable extent occurs over the three to nine months following withdrawal from exposure. Visual disturbances and optic atrophy have also been reported.[115]

Cavanagh[111] related methyl bromide intoxication to altered glycolysis and pyruvate oxidation. The peripheral manifestations have been attributed to a distal axonopathy that reflects the altered metabolism of the neuronal perikaryon or an alteration of axonal transport.

A latent period of several hours or even one or two days may occur after exposure before the onset of symptoms, and victims may die without awareness that exposure to the odourless, colourless gas has even occurred. Chloropicrin is a common additive that leads to conjunctival and mucosal irritation, thereby warning of inhalation exposure to methyl bromide. Symptoms of toxicity may occur at a bromide level in the order of 3 mg/mL. With levels over 5 mg/dL, mental changes may lead to careless handling of the chemical by fumigators, and thus to even greater exposure.[116]

In the past, chelating agents, haemoperfusion and N-acetylcysteine[110] have been advocated for therapy, but their efficacy is uncertain. Otherwise, treatment is symptomatic and supportive. Clinical recovery may occur over a period of months. The OSHA PEL is 20 ppm ($80\,mg/m^3$).

ORGANOPHOSPHATE AND CARBAMATE INSECTICIDES

A large number of organophosphate (OP) and carbamate compounds are used as insecticides (see Chapter 43, Pesticides and other agrochemicals). Certain OPs have also been used as terrorism and chemical warfare agents. The use of OPs as drugs has been discontinued, but some carbamates, such as physostigmine, are still indicated in certain clinical contexts. Occupational exposures during spraying mainly occur through the skin, particularly in agricultural workers and in areas where insecticides are used to control vector-borne diseases.

These chemicals are inhibitors of acetylcholinesterase (AChE), causing an excess of acetylcholine at nerve endings. The degree and duration of AChE inhibition largely depend on the chemistry of the involved chemicals, which dictates rates of affinity, spontaneous reactivation and ageing of phosphorylated or carbamylated AChE.[109]

The clinical picture of acute OP and carbamate poisoning is characterized by cholinergic overstimulation throughout the body. Initial symptoms include anorexia, nausea and vomiting, abdominal pain and diarrhoea, hypersalivation, hyperlacrimation and excessive sweating, headache, dizziness and blurred vision. In most cases, these symptoms are associated with miosis, which may be the only sign in mild poisoning. More severe clinical signs include bronchoconstriction, muscle fasciculations, convulsions and coma. Death may occur because of respiratory failure or cardiac arrhythmias. Whereas the inhibition of AChE by carbamates is reversible, symptoms and signs of carbamate poisoning are less severe and of shorter duration.

Diagnosis is exclusively clinical. However, in severely ill patients with cardiorespiratory failure, an exposure to OPs may not initially be suspected and, conversely, patients with known exposure to OPs may present with unrelated illness. In such cases, signs of cholinergic overstimulation must be actively sought. There is usually a good correlation between the severity of signs and symptoms and the degree of AChE inhibition in red blood cells. However, this test has limited value in an emergency because severe OP poisoning requires prompt treatment and is inevitably associated with high AChE inhibition. Serial measurements of red blood cell AChE have no value in monitoring the clinical course of poisoning. Relatively lower levels of AChE inhibition in red blood cells, as well as the inhibition of plasma cholinesterase, may be difficult to interpret.[117]

Prompt treatment of poisoning by AChE inhibitors is not only life-saving, but will prevent a variety of neurological consequences due to prolonged hypoxia and seizures. Atropine is the cornerstone of treatment of OP and carbamate poisoning because it prevents the effects of acetylcholine by blocking its binding to muscarinic cholinergic receptors. Initial treatment of mild poisoning starts with 1-mg atropine intravenously and should be repeated every 10–20 minutes until clinical evidence of atropinization is achieved, and then maintained for 24–48 hours. If atropinization occurs rapidly, severe poisoning is unlikely. In severe cases, continuous intravenous atropine infusion may be required at a rate of 20 mg/hour. Atropine overdosage is unlikely and rarely serious.

Specific reactivators of phosphorylated AChE, such as oximes, are also indicated in OP poisoning, although their benefits have been questioned. However, data on the inefficacy of oximes are not convincing,[118] and this potentially life-saving therapy cannot be dismissed.[119,120] Therefore, treatment should be started with 1-g pralidoxime intravenously; if no improvement occurs, a second dose is given after 30 minutes or continuous infusion is commenced at the rate of 0.5 g/hour. Other oximes have different dosing regimens. Treatment with oxime is not recommended in carbamate and in moderate dimethoxy-OP poisonings, because rates of spontaneous reactivation of AChE are fast. Diazepam and supportive therapy are important.

Prognosis depends on the severity of poisoning and appropriateness of care. Pathology is non-specific unless severe hypoxia or convulsions occur. Although a variety of neurobehavioural changes have been reported several months after recovery from acute poisoning,[121–123] the significance of these effects is unclear. Contradictory results have been reported in studies of possible neurobehavioural effects of long-term low-level exposures to anticholinesterase agents.[123–125]

In 20–50 per cent of cases of severe OP poisoning, weakness of respiratory, neck and proximal limb muscles develops (the so-called 'intermediate syndrome').[126,127] The syndrome develops several hours after severe cholinergic overstimulation and is not a direct effect of AChE inhibition. Its pathogenesis is unknown, but the syndrome seems related to post-synaptic effects. Treatment is supportive and recovery time in surviving patients lasts up to 30–40 days.

Organophosphate-induced delayed polyneuropathy (OPIDP) is a rare toxic effect of certain OPs that, in the case of OP insecticides currently in use, occurs only after a severe episode of cholinergic toxicity.[128,129] Whether neuropathy may also follow a severe intoxication by carbamates is unsettled.[130] The usual initial complaint is of cramping muscle pain in the legs, followed by distal numbness and paraesthesias, beginning two to three weeks after acute poisoning. Progressive leg weakness then occurs, together with depression of the tendon reflexes. The arms and forearms may also be affected after severe exposures. This symmetrical, predominantly motor, neuropathy displays electrophysiological and histopathological features consistent with peripheral distal axonopathy. In time, there is complete functional recovery if spinal cord axons have been spared. Otherwise, irreversible pyramidal signs of central nervous system (CNS) involvement may become evident, particularly with severe exposures. There is no specific treatment for the disorder.

The mechanism of initiation of OPIDP is unknown, although the target has been identified. Neuropathy relates to inhibition of neuropathy target esterase (NTE) followed by ageing of the phosphoryl–NTE complex. Although these molecular changes occur within hours of exposure, little is known about subsequent events that lead to development of OPIDP.[131]

There is no evidence that long-term low-level exposures to OP insecticides causes OPIDP or any other type of neuropathy.[124]

ORGANOCHLORINE PESTICIDES

The chlorinated hydrocarbons constitute a wide range of chemicals[132] and include the organochlorine insecticide dichlorodiphenyltrichlorethane (DDT) and others, such as aldrin, dieldrin and lindane. They are only slowly degraded and persist for long periods in animals and in the environment. Decline in neurobehavioural functioning and increase of neuropsychological and psychiatric symptoms have been reported in retired DDT workers.[133] However, the significance of these findings is unclear because the interval since exposure was unknown. In fact, DDT neurotoxicity depends on its temporary action on voltage-dependent sodium channels. One member of this group, chlordecone (Kepone) was responsible for a major episode of industrial exposure in 1975 at a manufacturing plant in Hopewell, Virginia, and also environmental contamination through the James River which feeds into Chesapeake Bay.[134] Workers developed a neurological illness characterized by 'nervousness', opsoclonus, tremor, clumsiness for manual activities and mild gait ataxia.[135] Slight memory impairment was noticed. Slow but sometimes incomplete recovery occurred. Benign intracranial hypertension was observed in a small proportion of cases. Absorption was by inhalation of dust. The mechanism of neural damage was not established (see Chapter 43, Pesticides and other agrochemicals).

PYRETHROIDS

Synthetic pyrethroids are widely used insecticides. Occupational exposures may occur in professional sprayers, particularly in an agricultural setting and in tropical countries where these chemicals are used to control vector-borne diseases. Pyrethroids are safe insecticides because of their high selectivity for insects. Consequently, reports of poisoning are relatively few.[136] In mild cases of poisoning, symptoms may be non-specific and include dizziness, headache, anorexia, paraesthesias and fatigue; in more severe cases, muscle fasciculation, convulsions and coma occur. These effects may be caused by all pyrethroids.[137] A slowly progressive motor neuron disease indistinguishable from amyotrophic lateral sclerosis[138] has been reported after heavy and prolonged exposure to various pyrethroids. Partial improvement may occur a few weeks after cessation of exposure. However, the occurrence of weakness and the known mechanism of pyrethroid toxicity cast doubts on the aetiology of this disease.

The most common effect of pyrethroids is paraesthesias, in particular in the face and hands.[139] This is considered a local effect due to hyperexcitation of cutaneous sensory fibres, because there is no correlation between the occurrence of paraesthesias and urinary excretion of pyrethroids or their metabolites. Paraesthesias disappear within 24 hours and there is no specific treatment. Toxicity is purely functional and depends on pyrethroid action on voltage-dependent sodium channels, resulting in prolonged inward sodium currents that lead to repetitive firing and subsequently to membrane depolarization.[140]

PESTICIDES AND PARKINSONISM

Parkinson's disease (idiopathic parkinsonism) is one of the most common of the neurodegenerative diseases and becomes increasingly common with advancing age. Its pathogenesis is obscure, but both genetic and environmental factors have been implicated. Among environmental factors, pesticide exposure has been recognized for some time as an adverse risk factor for development of the disease, but it is difficult to establish this with certainty. Relevant environmental exposures may occur years before the development of clinical features of parkinsonism, and exposure to multiple potential toxins may lead to synergistic or additive effects.[141] Furthermore, the impact of any environmental factors may be genetically determined. Thus, persons exposed to pesticides or with polymorphisms in the cytochrome P-450 2D6 (*CYP2D6*) gene have only a slightly increased risk, whereas those with both have a greatly increased risk of parkinsonism.[142] Any toxin-mediated effect may remain subclinical until normal age-related cell loss reaches a certain critical level. Finally, the lack of precision in the available data, especially with regard to level of exposure, compounds the difficulties in interpreting studies. Most studies have examined exposure to any pesticide or to broad groups, such as insecticides or herbicides, and little information is available for specific agents or factors affecting exposure, such as protective clothing.[143]

Parkinsonism has developed in humans who took methyl phenyl pyridinium (MPTP) for recreational purposes. MPTP is a protoxin and is converted in the body to methylphenyl pyridinium (MPP), a toxin that causes selective degeneration of the dopaminergic nigrostriatal system, the cell population that degenerates in naturally occurring Parkinson's disease. MPP is structurally similar to paraquat, a herbicide. MPP inhibits mitochondrial complex I, as does rotenone, another pesticide. Various epidemiological studies have found a high risk of Parkinson's disease in relation to pesticide exposure, with odds ratios in the order of 2 to 7 depending on the study.[144–148] The risk relates to duration of pesticide exposure.[146–148] Thus, Petrovitch et al.,[148] in a prospective cohort study with 30-year follow up of Hawaiian plantation workers, found a relative risk for Parkinson's disease of 1.0, 1.7 and 1.9 for those who had worked on the plantation for 1–10, 11–20 and more than 20 years, respectively, compared to those who had never done plantation work. Kamel et al.[143] found that the incidence of Parkinson's disease was associated with cumulative days of pesticide use at enrolment, with personally applying pesticide more than half the time, and with certain pesticides.

Specific pesticides that have been incriminated include paraquat, organochlorine and carbamate derivatives. In Taiwan, where paraquat is widely used, the risk of developing Parkinson's disease was increased more than six times in those exposed for more than 20 years.[146] Animal studies support the belief that pesticides may be important in the aetiology of parkinsonism. Both rotenone and paraquat, for example, are toxic to nigrostriatal dopaminergic neurons. Case–control studies in humans have also related parkinsonism to farming, rural living and well-water consumption.[149]

At the present time, it is fair to conclude that pesticide exposure increases the risk of developing Parkinson's disease, but the mechanisms involved and risks with specific pesticides are not known and probably vary depending on genetic and other factors.

STYRENE

Styrene is used in the manufacture of reinforced plastic and certain resins (see Chapter 42, Organic chemicals). It is used especially in the construction of fibreglass-reinforced plastic boats and other articles, and significant occupational exposure may occur by contact and by inhalation. Exposure is often estimated using biological indices that are not specific for styrene, such as urinary mandelic acid or phenylglyoxylic acid concentration. Environmental measures of styrene may not reflect biological levels because there is considerable variation in styrene uptake and metabolism, depending on personal activities. Thus, both environmental and biological measures are required when exposure to styrene is being considered. Occupational exposure is typically not restricted to styrene, but also involves exposure to cleansing solvents and other chemicals, thereby complicating the interpretation of any disturbances that may arise in the workplace.

Concerns about the neurotoxicity of styrene have been underscored by its high lipid solubility. Acute changes in cognition, behaviour or level of consciousness occur at certain concentrations, but concerns regarding its safety in an industrial setting relate primarily to chronic, low-level exposure. A number of studies have been held to suggest that abnormalities in reaction time and psychomotor performance are induced by styrene at levels approaching current exposure standards, which range between 20 and 50 ppm in many countries. Following a critical analysis of this literature, Rebert and Hall[150] found that this contention was unjustified, relating to misinterpretation of the data or to type I statistical errors, or that confounding factors had invalidated the various studies. Indeed, no compelling evidence could be found by these authors of persisting neurological sequelae to long-term, low-level styrene exposure.

The inadequacies of these various studies merit emphasis. Rebert and Hall[150] noted that in many the documentation of exposure was poor and that the number of subjects studied was often very low when subgroups were considered, as when stratifying by level of exposure. Confounding factors were often problematic, demographic data and job characterization were usually incomplete, no attempt was made to validate self-reports of drug and alcohol use, and details of medication use were sparse. The potential effects of exposure to other chemicals were often neglected or minimized. Rarely was mention made of blinded procedures. A variety of statistical shortcomings was also conspicuous, including probable violation of certain statistical assumptions. The incidence of statistical significance was often overestimated because it was based on comparisons of non-independent measures and on multiple comparisons. In addition to these concerns, there was no general consistency in the literature and no clear indication of causal factors or biological mechanisms that might account for any real effects of styrene.

Several studies on occupational exposures have also suggested a relationship between inhaled styrene vapour and hearing loss. Evidence in rats indicates that styrene is harmful to the cochlea by causing hair cell degeneration.[151] Lawton et al.[152] reviewed the pertinent literature and concluded that the results are equivocal. In particular, investigations claiming styrene-induced hearing loss in exposed workers were affected by substantial shortcomings of experimental design and data analysis.

TOLUENE

Toluene is a solvent in paints and glues. It is also used to synthesize benzene, benzoic acid, nitrotoluene and other compounds. Exposure may occur in workers involved in laying linoleum or spraying paint, and in the printing industry (see Chapter 42, Organic chemicals).

The effects of exposure are primarily neurobehavioural. Chronic, high exposure may lead to cognitive changes, pyramidal tract findings, cerebellar ataxia, brainstem or cranial nerve disturbances, and tremor.[153] Bilateral visual loss from optic neuropathy has been described,[154] as also has ocular flutter or dysmetria and opsoclonus.[155] Cognitive abnormalities are characterized by disturbances of attention, memory and visuospatial function. Apathy and a flat affect are common. Cerebral magnetic resonance imaging may show diffuse abnormalities of the cerebral white matter, the degree of which correlates with neuropsychological impairment.[156] Diffuse cerebral atrophy and symmetric lesions in the basal ganglia and cingulate gyri have also been reported.[157]

The level and duration of exposure necessary to produce clinical evidence of neurotoxicity is uncertain, and it is not clear what neurobehavioural effects are produced by long-term, low-level exposure. Exposure to toluene at a level of 125 ppm may produce no neurological symptoms,[158,159] although minor abnormalities may be present on neurobehavioural studies.[160] At levels of 250 ppm, there may be insomnia, nervousness and intermittent stupor. A peripheral neuropathy does not occur with toluene.

Toluene may induce auditory damage in animals, but evidence in humans of toluene ototoxicity and of synergism with noise is less convincing.[161] Conficting results may be related to the intensity of exposure, with no ototoxicity or synergistic effects observed below 20 ppm toluene,[162,163] that is, the current ACGIH TLV.

TRICHLOROETHYLENE

Trichloroethylene was once used as an anaesthetic agent (see Chapter 42, Organic chemicals) and found widespread use as a dewaxing, degreasing and dry-cleaning agent. The solvent was present in paint removers and glues, but concerns over its toxicity have led to it being gradually replaced by safer solvents. Inhalation exposure to levels in the order of 50–200 ppm have led to changes in reaction time and performance on psychological tests in some but not other studies. At levels of exposure below 40 ppm, there is no convincing evidence of significant or long-term disturbances of cognitive function. The current permissible exposure limit (OSHA) is 100 ppm. With increasing exposure in an occupational setting, complaints of headache, fatigue, irritability, nausea and dizziness are common. Facial hyperaesthesia and masticatory weakness may result from dysfunction of the trigeminal nerve; other cranial nerves, such as the facial, optic and oculomotor, may also be affected. An autopsy study has shown fibre degeneration in the trigeminal nerve.[164] The reason for the susceptibility of the cranial nerves is unknown. A case–control study[165] and a mortality study[166] found weak associations between trichloroethylene exposures and risk of brain cancer. However, other studies did not show an increase of brain cancer incidence and mortality.[167–169]

SOLVENT MIXTURES

Prolonged, low-level, occupational exposure to mixtures of organic solvents occurs commonly, for example in house painters. Such exposure is reported to cause an encephalopathy or 'organic brain syndrome' characterized primarily by disturbances of memory, concentration and attention, and by changes in personality. However, the studies that form the basis of such claims generally fail to stand up to rigorous scientific scrutiny.[170–173] These studies, which have originated mainly from Scandinavia, are primarily epidemiological in nature. Objections to them include concerns that other factors, such as alcohol or drug/medication use or the lingering effect of acute exposure to solvents, may have been responsible for the encephalopathic features that were described. In addition, precise details concerning work conditions and extent of probable exposure to solvents were often not obtained or provided, or there was an over-reliance on subjective recall in determining the severity and duration of exposure. Moreover, factors known to influence the neuropsychological tests used to document the presence of an encephalopathy, such as educational background, age, stress and cultural factors, were not taken fully into account in certain uncontrolled studies. The use of controls from other workplace settings may have led to bias when comparisons were made. This is especially important when test and control populations differ in educational or other factors that may have been responsible for their original choice of occupation or if one group is prone to certain occupationally related non-toxic disorders, such as anxiety syndromes.

This is well exemplified by the study of Gade et al.[174] in which 20 solvent-exposed workers, mostly painters, were re-examined two years after they had originally been diagnosed with a chronic toxic encephalopathy.[175] Their performance on neuropsychological testing was unchanged, but the previous impression of significant cognitive decline could not be substantiated when comparison was now made to a non-exposed control group and allowance was made for the influence of age, educational background and level of intelligence.

The existence of a chronic encephalopathy characterized solely by cognitive, affective and personality changes in those exposed for long periods to low levels of organic solvents remains uncertain. No definite causal relationship has been established and the underlying mechanism for such an association is elusive.

It has been suggested that loss of colour vision may be part of the effects related to chronic exposure to organic solvents.[176] Although a recent review identified 13 studies investigating colour discrimination in workers and other subjects exposed to mixtures of solvents,[177] no conclusions can be drawn due to design limitations and methodological irregularities.

WARTIME EXPOSURE

Agent Orange and the Vietnam War

Over a ten-year period during the war in Vietnam, American forces sprayed millions of gallons of herbicides to strip vegetation that might conceal or provide sustenance for opposition forces. The preparation known as Agent Orange was used most commonly; more than 11 million gallons of Agent Orange were used before spraying was discontinued in 1971 because of concerns about long-term safety. Over the years since then, public concern has increased about the potential health hazards of exposure to Agent Orange. In addition to numerous scientific studies, various governmental reports have been published that bear on the issue.

Agent Orange contained 2,4,5-trichlorophenoxyacetic acid, and one of its contaminants was 2,3,7,8-tetrachlorodibenzo-p-dioxin (or TCDD) (see Chapter 42, Organic chemicals). Concerns have been raised that the exposure to the major TCDD-contaminated herbicides used in Vietnam was associated with the development of Hodgkin's or non-Hodgkin's lymphoma, soft-tissue sarcoma, chloracne and porphyria cutanea tarda and perhaps also of certain other neoplastic disorders.[178] Attention here is confined to the potential neurotoxicity of these agents.

The literature is voluminous, but much of it is methodologically flawed. Careful analysis of it has revealed no compelling evidence of an association between Agent Orange exposure and the development of cognitive or neuropsychological disorders or of chronic peripheral neuropathy.[178,179] Anecdotal reports suggest that peripheral neuropathy may develop acutely or subacutely following occupational exposure to herbicides,[180–182] although the possibility cannot be excluded that the neuropathy in these cases related not to the exposure but to other factors, such as development of the Guillain–Barré syndrome. There are no data on the development of an acute neuropathy following Agent Orange exposure in Vietnam.

Exposure of the local population to dioxin followed the chemical explosion that occurred in an industrial plant at Seveso in Italy, but there did not appear to be an increased risk of acute neuropathy[183] and the prevalence of peripheral neuropathy several years after the accident was not increased among those with heavy exposure to dioxin.[184,185]

In a recent report,[186] 15 workers who had been poisoned by 2,3,7,8 TCDD 35 years earlier were found to have changes in various combinations in their visual evoked potentials, EEG, colour vision, nerve conduction, SPECT and neurobehavioural responses. Interpretation of this report is hampered, however, by the limited number of subjects, lack of information on neurological status at the time of poisoning, lack of a control group and paucity of details concerning the examined parameters.

There is suggestive evidence that exposure to Agent Orange is associated with an increased risk of developing Parkinson's disease.

Gulf War syndrome

Soon after their return home, military personnel who took part in the Gulf War in 1990–91 reported higher rates of an array of symptoms and a decreased perception of well-being. However, despite numerous investigations, there is insufficient evidence to define a single neurological disease entity. An early cross-sectional epidemiological study on US veterans deployed in Iraq ranked neurological signs and symptoms in three different categories: impaired cognition, confusion-ataxia and 'arthroneuromyopathy', suggesting a spectrum of neurological injuries involving the central, peripheral and autonomic nervous systems.[187,188] In another small group of UK veterans, abnormalities of nerve conduction and cold thermal sensory threshold were reported.[189] However, a subsequent large study using quantitative sensory and autonomic function studies did not detect differences between UK veterans and controls.[190] Similar results were found in another controlled study, where no higher prevalence of polyneuropathy was found in US veterans deployed in the Gulf War when compared with non-deployed veterans.[191] The results of autonomic function studies are also controversial. In one study on male veterans affected by Gulf War illness, heart rate variability was significantly lower than controls,[192] whereas in another similar study this was not found.[193] However, in the latter study, heart-rate variability was reduced compared with controls both at night and during the day in female patients affected by Gulf War illness or with fibromyalgia.

Epidemiological studies on Gulf War veterans have revealed an increased incidence of amyotrophic lateral sclerosis,[194] particularly in young people diagnosed before the age of 45 years.[195] However, these reports have been criticized on methodological grounds, such as the small numbers of cases and the choice of reference statistics. It should be concluded that service in the Gulf War remains an uncertain trigger for amyotrophic lateral sclerosis.[196]

Although a high incidence of post-traumatic stress disorders is expected as a result of war-time events, contradictory results have been found in specific studies of Gulf War veterans, as well as in studies on the incidence of common mental disorders.[197–199]

Several environmental exposures to a variety of neurotoxic chemicals have been suggested to explain the aetiology of these chronic effects, including to pyridostigmine bromide (used as a prophylactic drug for nerve gas poisoning), organophosphates, insect repellants and other chemicals. However, expert committees concluded that there is inadequate or insufficient evidence to determine whether an association exists between exposures to drugs and chemicals and the observed effects.[200]

> **Key points**
>
> - A neurotoxic disorder should be considered if a temporal association exists between toxin exposure and any manifestations of neurological dysfunction.
> - The progression of a neurotoxic disorder is arrested by discontinuation of toxin exposure, but 'coasting' sometimes occurs, with mild progression continuing for a short interval after exposure is stopped.
> - Any presumed neurotoxic disorder must be biologically plausible, based on known toxicity or effects of the toxin on biological systems.
> - When comparing exposed workers with control subjects using quantitative testing techniques, the selected control subjects must be appropriate.

Note Added in Proof at Authors' Request

This chapter was delivered on time in December 2007. As publication has been delayed for reasons unconnected with the authors, more recent material is not included.

ACKNOWLEDGEMENT

The authors acknowledge the contribution of the late PK Thomas to this chapter in the previous (ninth) edition of this book.

REFERENCES

1. Kesson CM, Baird AW, Lawson DH. Acrylamide poisoning. *Postgraduate Medical Journal*. 1977; **53**: 16–17.
2. Fullerton PM. Electrophysiological and histological observations of peripheral nerves in acrylamide poisoning in man. *Journal of Neurology, Neurosurgery, and Psychiatry*. 1969; **32**: 186–92.
3. Garland TO, Patterson MWH. Six cases of acrylamide poisoning. *British Medical Journal*. 1967; **4**: 134–8.
4. He F, Zhang S, Wang H et al. Neurological and electroneuromyographic assessment of the adverse effects of acrylamide on occupationally exposed workers. *Scandinavian Journal of Work, Environment and Health*. 1989; **15**: 125–9.
5. Takahashi M, Ohara T, Hashimoto K. Electrophysiological study of nerve injuries in workers handling acrylamide. *Internationales Archiv für Arbeitsmedizin*. 1971; **28**: 1–11.
6. Sumner AJ, Asbury AK. Acrylamide neuropathy: Selective vulnerability of sensory fibers. *Archives of Neurology*. 1974; **30**: 419.
7. Sumner AJ, Asbury AK. Physiological studies of the dying-back phenomenon: Muscle stretch afferents in acrylamide neuropathy. *Brain*. 1975; **98**: 91–100.
8. Navarro X, Verdu E, Guerrero J et al. Abnormalities of sympathetic sudomotor function in experimental acrylamide neuropathy. *Journal of the Neurological Sciences*. 1993; **114**: 56–61.
9. Lopachin RM, Gavin T, Barber DS. Type-2 alkenes mediate synaptotoxicity in neurodegenerative diseases. *Neurotoxicology*. 2008; **29**: 871–82.
10. Myers JE, Macun I. Acrylamide neuropathy in a South African factory: An epidemiologic investigation. *American Journal of Industrial Medicine*. 1991; **19**: 487–93.
11. He FS, Zhang SC. Effects of allyl chloride on occupationally exposed subjects. *Scandinavian Journal of Work, Environment and Health*. 1985; **11** (Suppl. 4): 43–5.
12. He F, Jacobs JM, Scaravilli F. The pathology of allyl chloride neurotoxicity in mice. *Acta Neuropathologica*. 1981; **55**: 125–33.
13. Sclar G. Encephalomyeloradiculoneuropathy following exposure to an industrial solvent. *Clinical Neurology and Neurosurgery*. 1999; **101**: 199–202.
14. Ichihara G, Miller JK, Ziolkokwska A et al. Neurological disorders in three workers exposed to 1-bromopropane. *Journal of Occupational Health*. 2002; **44**: 1–7.
15. Majersik J, Caravati E, Steffens J. Severe neurotoxicity associated with exposure to the solvent 1-bromopropane (n-propyl bromide). *Clinical Toxicology*. 2007; **45**: 270–6.
16. Raymond LW, Ford MD. Severe illness in furniture makers using a new glue: 1-bromopropane toxicity confounded by arsenic. *Journal of Occupational and Environmental Medicine*. 2007; **49**: 1009–19.
17. Ichihara G, Li W, Ding X et al. A survey on exposure level, health status, and biomarkers in workers exposed to 1-bromopropane. *American Journal of Industrial Medicine*. 2004; **45**: 63–75.
18. Ichihara G, Li W, Shibata E et al. Neurologic abnormalities in workers of a 1-bromopropane factory. *Environmental Health Perspectives*. 2004; **112**: 1319–25.
19. Sohn YK, Suh JS, Kim JW et al. A histopathologic study of the nervous system after inhalation exposure of 1-bromopropane in rat. *Toxicology Letters*. 2002; **131**: 195–201.
20. Ichihara G, Kitoh J, Yu X et al. 1-Bromopropane, an alternative to ozone layer depleting solvents, is dose-dependently neurotoxic to rats in long-term inhalation exposure. *Toxicological Sciences*. 2000; **55**: 116–23.
21. Godderis L, Braeckman L, Vanhoorne M, Viaene M. Neurobehavioral and clinical effects in workers exposed to CS2. *International Journal of Hygiene and Environmental Health*. 2006; **209**: 139–50.
22. Huang CC, Chu CC, Chen RS et al. Chronic carbon disulfide encephalopathy. *European Neurology*. 1996; **36**: 364–8.
23. Putz-Anderson V, Albright BE, Lee ST et al. A behavioral examination of workers exposed to carbon disulfide. *Neurotoxicology*. 1983; **4**: 67–78.
24. Fonte R, Edallo A, Candura SM. Cerebellar atrophy as a delayed manifestation of chronic carbon disulfide poisoning. *Industrial Health*. 2003; **41**: 43–7.
25. Seppäläinen AM, Tolonen MT. Neurotoxicity of long-term exposure to carbon disulfide in the viscose rayon industry: A neurophysiological study. *Scandinavian Journal of Work, Environment and Health*. 1974; **11**: 145–53.
26. Peters HA, Levine RL, Matthews CG, Chapman LJ. Extrapyramidal and other neurologic manifestations associated with carbon disulfide fumigant exposure. *Archives of Neurology*. 1988; **45**: 537–40.
27. Chu CC, Huang CC, Cheng RS, Shih TS. Carbon disulfide-induced polyneuropathy in viscose rayon workers. *Occupational and Environmental Medicine*. 1995; **52**: 404–7.
28. Huang CC. Carbon disulfide neurotoxicity: Taiwan experience. *Acta Neurologica Taiwanica*. 2004; **13**: 3–9.
29. Centers for Disease Control and Prevention. Unintentional carbon monoxide poisoning from indoor use of pressure washers – Iowa, January 1992–January 1993. *Journal of the American Medical Association*. 1993; **270**: 2034–7.
30. Hampson NB, Kramer CC, Dunford RG, Norkool DM. Carbon monoxide poisoning from indoor burning of charcoal briquets. *Journal of the American Medical Association*. 1994; **27**: 52–3.
31. Centers for Disease Control and Prevention. Carbon monoxide poisoning associated with use of LPG-powered (Propane) forklifts in industrial settings – Iowa, 1998. *Morbidity and Mortality Weekly Report*. 1999; **48**: 1121–4.

32. Grunnet ML, Petajan JH. Carbon monoxide induced neuropathy in the rat. Ultrastructural changes. *Archives of Neurology*. 1976; **33**: 158–63.
33. Stewart RD. The effect of carbon monoxide on humans. *Journal of Occupational Medicine*. 1976; **18**: 304–9.
34. Pestronk A, Keogh J, Griffin JG. Dimethylaminoproprionitrile intoxication: A new industrial neuropathy. *Neurology*. 1979; **29**: 540–9.
35. Brashear A, Univerzagt FW, Farber MO et al. Ethylene oxide neurotoxicity: A cluster of 12 nurses with peripheral and central nervous system toxicity. *Neurology*. 1996; **46**: 992–8.
36. Windebank AJ, Blexrud MD. Residual ethylene oxide in hollow fiber hemodialysis units is neurotoxic in rats. *Annals of Neurology*. 1989; **26**: 63–8.
37. Ohnishi A, Inoue N, Tamamoto T et al. Ethylene oxide neuropathy in rats. Exposure to 250 ppm. *Journal of the Neurological Sciences*. 1986; **74**: 215–21.
38. Allen N, Mendell JR, Billmaier DJ et al. Toxic polyneuropathy due to methyl n-butyl ketone: An industrial outbreak. *Archives of Neurology*. 1975; **32**: 209–18.
39. Bos PMJ, de Mik G, Bragt PC. Critical review of the toxicity of methyl n-butyl ketone: Risk from occupational exposure. *American Journal of Industrial Medicine*. 1991; **20**: 175–94.
40. Yamamura Y. n-Hexane polyneuropathy. *Folia Psychiatrica et Neurologica Japonica*. 1969; **23**: 45–57.
41. Carelli V, Franceschini F, Venturi S et al. Grand rounds: Could occupational exposure to n-hexane and other solvents precipitate visual failure in Leber hereditary optic neuropathy? *Environmental Health Perspectives*. 2007; **115**: 113–15.
42. Spencer PS, Schaumburg HH, Sabri MI, Veronesi B. The enlarging view of hexacarbon neurotoxicity. *Critical Reviews in Toxicology*. 1980; **7**: 279–356.
43. Spencer PS, Couri D, Schaumburg HH. n-Hexane and methyl n-butyl ketone. In: Spencer PS, Schaumburg HH (eds). *Experimental and clinical neurotoxicology*. Baltimore: Williams and Wilkins, 1980: 456–75.
44. Korobkin R, Asbury AK, Sumner AJ, Nielsen SL. Glue-sniffing neuropathy. *Archives of Neurology*. 1975; **32**: 158–62.
45. Chang Y-C. Neurotoxic effects of n-hexane on the human central nervous system: Evoked potential abnormalities in n-hexane polyneuropathy. *Journal of Neurology, Neurosurgery, and Psychiatry*. 1987; **50**: 269–74.
46. Saida K, Mendell JR, Weiss HS. Peripheral nerve changes induced by methyl n-butyl ketone and potentiation by methyl ethyl ketone. *Journal of Neuropathology and Experimental Neurology*. 1976; **35**: 207–25.
47. Altenkirch H, Stoltenburg G, Wagner HM. Experimental studies on hydrocarbon neuropathies induced by methyl-ethyl-ketone (MEK). *Journal of Neurology*. 1978; **219**: 159–70.
48. Abou-Donia MB, Hu Z, Lapadula DM, Gupta RP. Mechanisms of joint neurotoxicity of n-hexane, methyl isobutyl ketone and O-ethyl O-4-nitrophenyl phenylphosphonothioate in hens. *Journal of Pharmacology and Experimental Therapeutics*. 1991; **257**: 282–9.
49. Orti-Pareja M, Jimenez-Jimenez FJ, Miguel J et al. Reversible myoclonus, tremor, and ataxia in a patient exposed to methyl ethyl ketone. *Neurology*. 1996; **46**: 272.
50. Welch L, Kirschner H, Heath A et al. Chronic neuropsychological and neurological impairment following acute exposure to a solvent mixture of toluene and methyl ethyl ketone (MEK). *Journal of Toxicology and Clinical Toxicology*. 1991; **29**: 435–45.
51. Willis MR, Savory J. Aluminium poisoning: Dialysis encephalopathy, osteomalacia, and anaemia. *Lancet*. 1983; **2**: 29–34.
52. Burks JS, Alfrey AC, Huddlestone J et al. A fatal encephalopathy in chronic haemodialysis patients. *Lancet*. 1976; **1**: 764–8.
53. Polizzi S, Pira E, Ferrara M et al. Neurotoxic effects of aluminium among foundry workers and Alzheimer's disease. *Neurotoxicology*. 2002; **23**: 761–74.
54. Buchta M, Kiesswetter E, Otto A et al. Longitudinal study examining the neurotoxicity of occupational exposure to aluminium-containing welding fumes. *International Archives of Occupational and Environmental Health*. 2003; **76**: 539–48.
55. Halatek T, Sinczuk-Walczak H, Rydzynski K. Prognostic significance of low serum levels of Clara cell phospholipid-binding protein in occupational aluminium neurotoxicity. *Journal of Inorganic Biochemistry*. 2005; **99**: 1904–11.
56. Oremland RS, Stoltz JF. The ecology of arsenic. *Science*. 2003; **300**: 939–44.
57. Bhattacharjee Y. Toxicology. A sluggish response to humanity's biggest mass poisoning. *Science*. 2007; **315**: 1659–61.
58. Zhu J, Chen Z, Lallemand-Breitenbach V, de The H. How acute promyelocytic leukaemia revived arsenic. *Nature Reviews. Cancer*. 2002; **2**: 705–13.
59. Ratnaike RN. Acute and chronic arsenic toxicity. *Postgraduate Medical Journal*. 2003; **79**: 391–6.
60. Le Quesne PM, McLeod JG. Peripheral neuropathy following a single exposure to arsenic. Clincal course in four patients with electrophysiological and histological studies. *Journal of the Neurological Sciences*. 1977; **32**: 437–51.
61. Donofrio PD, Wilbourn AJ, Albers JW et al. Acute arsenic intoxication presenting as Guillain-Barre-like syndrome. *Muscle and Nerve*. 1987; **10**: 114–20.
62. Ohta M. Ultrastructure of sural nerve in a case of arsenic neuropathy. *Acta Neuropathologica*. 1970; **16**: 233–42.
63. Moyer TP. Testing for arsenic. *Mayo Clinic Proceedings*. 1993; **68**: 1210–12.
64. Yoshito K, Daigo S. Arsenic: Signal transduction, transcription factor, and biotransformation involved in cellular response and toxicity. *Annual Review of Pharmacology and Toxicology*. 2007; **47**: 243–62.
65. Kalia K, Flora SJ. Strategies for safe and effective therapeutic measures for chronic arsenic and lead poisoning. *Journal of Occupational Health*. 2005; **47**: 1–21.
66. Pentschew A. Morphology and morphogenesis of lead encephalopathy. *Acta Neuropathologica*. 1965; **5**: 133–60.

67. Bouldin TW, Meighan ME, Gaynor JJ et al. Differential vulnerability of mixed and cutaneous nerves in lead neuropathy. *Journal of Neuropathology and Experimental Neurology*. 1985; **44**: 384–96.
68. Buchthal F, Behse F. Electrophysiology and nerve biopsy in men exposed to lead. *British Journal of Industrial Medicine*. 1979; **36**: 135–47.
69. Gracia RC, Snodgrass WR. Lead toxicity and chelation therapy. *American Journal of Health-System Pharmacy*. 2007; **64**: 45–53.
70. Thomson RM, Parry GJ. Neuropathies associated with excessive exposure to lead. *Muscle and Nerve*. 2006; **33**: 732–41.
71. Kosnett MJ, Wedeen RP, Rothenberg SJ et al. Recommendations for medical management of adult lead exposure. *Environmental Health Perspectives*. 2007; **115**: 463–71.
72. Balbus-Kornfeld JM, Stewart W, Bolla KI, Schwartz BS. Cumulative exposure to inorganic lead and neurobehavioural test performance in adults: An epidemiological review. *Occupational and Environmental Medicine*. 1995; **52**: 2–12.
73. Goodman M, LaVerda N, Clarke C et al. Neurobehavioural testing in workers occupationally exposed to lead: Systematic review and meta-analysis of publications. *Occupational and Environmental Medicine*. 2002; **59**: 217–23.
74. Shih RA, Hu H, Weisskopf MG, Schwartz BS. Cumulative lead dose and cognitive function in adults: A review of studies that measured both blood lead and bone lead. *Environmental Health Perspectives*. 2007; **115**: 483–92.
75. Weisskopf MG, Hu H, Sparrow D et al. Proton magnetic resonance spectroscopic evidence of glial effects of cumulative lead exposure in the adult human hippocampus. *Environmental Health Perspectives*. 2007; **115**: 519–23.
76. Coon S, Stark A, Peterson E et al. Whole-body lifetime occupational lead exposure and risk of Parkinson's disease. *Environmental Health Perspectives*. 2006; **114**: 1872–6.
77. Conradi S, Ronnevi LO, Nise G, Vesterberg O. Abnormal distribution of lead in amyotrophic lateral sclerosis – reestimation of lead in the cerebrospinal fluid. *Journal of the Neurological Sciences*. 1980; **48**: 413–18.
78. Monnet-Tschudi F, Zurich MG, Boschat C et al. Involvement of environmental mercury and lead in the etiology of neurodegenerative diseases. *Reviews on Environmental Health*. 2006; **21**: 105–17.
79. Rajaraman P, Stewart PA, Samet JM et al. Lead, genetic susceptibility, and risk of adult brain tumors. *Cancer Epidemiology, Biomarkers and Prevention*. 2006; **15**: 2514–20.
80. Levy BS, Nassetta WJ. Neurologic effects of manganese in humans: A review. *International Journal of Occupational and Environmental Health*. 2003; **9**: 153–63.
81. Kaiser J. Manganese: A high-octane dispute. *Science*. 2003; **300**: 926–8.
82. Hauser RA, Zesiewicz TA, Rosemurgy AS et al. Manganese intoxication and chronic liver failure. *Annals of Neurology*. 1994; **36**: 871–5.
83. Schaumburg HH, Herskovitz S, Cassano VA. Occupational manganese neurotoxicity provoked by hepatitis C. *Neurology*. 2006; **67**: 322–3.
84. Olanow CW. Manganese-induced parkinsonism and Parkinson's disease. *Annals of the New York Academy of Sciences*. 2004; **1012**: 209–23.
85. Cersosimo MG, Koller WC. The diagnosis of manganese-induced parkinsonism. *Neurotoxicology*. 2006; **27**: 340–6.
86. Kim Y. Neuroimaging in manganism. *Neurotoxicology*. 2006; **27**: 369–72.
87. Lu C, Huang C, Chu N, Calne DB. Levodopa failure in chronic manganism. *Neurology*. 1994; **44**: 1600–2.
88. Jiang YM, Mo XA, Du FQ et al. Effective treatment of manganese-induced occupational parkinsonism with p-aminosalicylic acid: A case of 17-year follow-up study. *Journal of Occupational and Environmental Medicine*. 2006; **48**: 644–9.
89. Huang CC, Chu NS, Lu CS et al. The natural history of neurological manganism over 18 years. *Parkinsonism and Related Disorders*. 2007; **13**: 143–5.
90. Yamada M, Ohno S, Okayasu I et al. Chronic manganese poisoning: A neuropathological study with determination of manganese distribution in the brain. *Acta Neuropathologica*. 1986; **70**: 273–8.
91. Aschner M, Guilarte TR, Schneider JS, Zheng W. Manganese: Recent advances in understanding its transport and neurotoxicity. *Toxicology and Applied Pharmacology*. 2007; **221**: 131–47.
92. Lucchini R, Selis L, Folli D et al. Neurobehavioral effects of manganese in workers from a ferroalloy plant after temporary cessation of exposure. *Scandinavian Journal of Work, Environment and Health*. 1995; **21**: 143–9.
93. Bowler RM, Roels HA, Nakagawa S et al. Dose-effect relationships between manganese exposure and neurological, neuropsychological and pulmonary function in confined space bridge welders. *Occupational and Environmental Medicine*. 2007; **64**: 167–77.
94. Mergler D. Neurotoxic effects of low level exposure to manganese in human populations. *Environmental Research*. 1999; **80**: 99–102.
95. Myers JE, teWaterNaude J, Fourie M et al. Nervous system effects of occupational manganese exposure on South African manganese mineworkers. *Neurotoxicology*. 2003; **24**: 649–56.
96. Bast-Pettersen R, Ellingsen DG, Hetland SM, Thomassen Y. Neuropsychological function in manganese alloy plant workers. *International Archives of Occupational and Environmental Health*. 2004; **77**: 277–87.
97. Deschamps FJ, Guillaumot M, Raux S. Neurological effects in workers exposed to manganese. *Journal of Occupational and Environmental Medicine*. 2001; **43**: 127–32.
98. Greiffenstein MF, Lees-Haley PR. Neuropsychological correlates of manganese exposure: A meta-analysis. *Journal of Clinical and Experimental Neuropsychology*. 2007; **29**: 113–26.
99. Racette BA, McGee-Minnich L, Moerlein SM et al. Welding-related parkinsonism: Clinical features, treatment, and pathophysiology. *Neurology*. 2001; **56**: 8–13.

100. Racette BA, Tabbal SD, Jennings D et al. Prevalence of parkinsonism and relationship to exposure in a large sample of Alabama welders. *Neurology*. 2005; **64**: 230–5.
101. Fored CM, Fryzek JP, Brandt L et al. Parkinson's disease and other basal ganglia or movement disorders in a large nationwide cohort of Swedish welders. *Occupational and Environmental Medicine*. 2006; **63**: 135–40.
102. Jankovic J. Searching for a relationship between manganese and welding and Parkinson's disease. *Neurology*. 2005; **64**: 2021–8.
103. McMillan G. Is electric arc welding linked to manganism or Parkinson's disease? *Toxicological Reviews*. 2005; **24**: 237–57.
104. Magos L, Clarkson TW. Overview of the clinical toxicity of mercury. *Annals of Clinical Biochemistry*. 2006; **43**: 257–68.
105. Clarkson TW, Magos L, Myers GJ. The toxicology of mercury – current exposures and clinical manifestations. *New England Journal of Medicine*. 2003; **349**: 1731–7.
106. Wastensson G, Lamoureux D, Sällsten G et al. Quantitative tremor assessment in workers with current low exposure to mercury vapor. *Neurotoxicology and Teratology*. 2006; **28**: 681–93.
107. Albers JW, Kallenbach LR, Fine LJ et al. Neurological abnormalities associated with remote occupational elemental mercury exposure. *Annals of Neurology*. 1988; **24**: 651–9.
108. World Health Organization. Environmental Health Criteria 118. Inorganic mercury. Geneva: WHO, 1991.
109. Bluhm RE, Bobbitt RG, Welch LW et al. Elemental mercury vapour toxicity, treatment, and prognosis after acute, intensive exposure in chloralkali plant workers. Part I: History, neuropsychological findings and chelator effects. *Human and Experimental Toxicology*. 1992; **11**: 201–10.
110. Hustinx WNM, van de Laar RTH, van Huffelen AC et al. Systemic effects of inhalational methyl bromide poisoning: A study of nine cases occupationally exposed due to inadvertent spread during fumigation. *British Journal of Industrial Medicine*. 1993; **50**: 155–9.
111. Cavanagh JB. Methyl bromide intoxication and acute energy deprivation syndromes. *Neuropathology and Applied Neurobiology*. 1992; **18**: 575–8.
112. De Haro L, Gastaut JL, Jouglard J, Renacco E. Central and peripheral neurotoxic effects of chronic methyl bromide intoxication. *Clinical Toxicology*. 1997; **35**: 29–34.
113. Cavalleri F, Galassi G, Ferrari S et al. Methyl bromide induced neuropathy: A clinical, neurophysiological, and morphological study. *Journal of Neurology, Neurosurgery, and Psychiatry*. 1995; **58**: 383.
114. Kantarjian AD, Sattar AS. Methyl bromide poisoning with nervous system manifestations resembling polyneuropathy. *Neurology*. 1963; **13**: 1054–8.
115. Chavez CT, Hepler RS, Straatsma BR. Methyl bromide optic atrophy. *American Journal of Ophthalmology*. 1985; **99**: 715–19.
116. Drawneek W, O'Brien MJ, Goldsmith HJ, Bourdillon RE. Industrial methyl-bromide poisoning in fumigators. *Lancet*. 1964; **2**: 855–6.
117. Lotti M. Cholinesterase inhibition: Complexities in interpretation. *Clinical Chemistry*. 1995; **41**: 1814–18.
118. Bismuth C, Inns RH, Marss TC. Efficacy, toxicity and clinical use of oximes in anticholinesterase poisoning. In: Ballantyne B, Marrs TC (eds). *Clinical and experimental toxicology of organophosphates and carbamates*. Oxford: Butterworth-Heinemann, 1992: 555–77.
119. Johnson MK, Vale JA, Marrs TC, Meredith TJ. Pralidoxime for organophosphorus poisoning. *Lancet*. 1992; **340**: 64.
120. Pawar KS, Bhoite RR, Pillay CP et al. Continuous pralidoxime infusion versus repeated bolus injection to treat organophosphorus pesticide poisoning: A randomised controlled trial. *Lancet*. 2006; **368**: 2136–41.
121. Rosenstock L, Keifer M, Daniell WE et al. Chronic central nervous system effects of acute organophosphate pesticide intoxication. The Pesticide Health Effects Study Group. *Lancet*. 1991; **338**: 223–7.
122. Roldán-Tapia L, Leyva A, Laynez F, Santed FS. Chronic neuropsychological sequelae of cholinesterase inhibitors in the absence of structural brain damage: Two cases of acute poisoning. *Environmental Health Perspectives*. 2005; **113**: 762–6.
123. Jamal GA, Hansen S, Julu PO. Low level exposures to organophosphorus esters may cause neurotoxicity. *Toxicology*. 2002; **181**: 23–33.
124. Lotti M. Low-level exposures to organophosphorus esters and peripheral nerve function. *Muscle and Nerve*. 2002; **25**: 492–504.
125. Solomon C, Poole J, Palmer KT et al. Neuropsychiatric symptoms in past users of sheep dip and other pesticides. *Occupational and Environmental Medicine*. 2007; **64**: 259–66.
126. Senanayake N, Karalliedde L. Neurotoxic effects of organophosphorus insecticides. An intermediate syndrome. *New England Journal of Medicine*. 1987; **316**: 761–3.
127. De Bleecker J, Van den Neucker K, Colardyn F. Intermediate syndrome in organophosphorus poisoning: A prospective study. *Critical Care Medicine*. 1993; **21**: 1706–11.
128. Lotti M. Clinical toxicology of anticholinesterase agents in humans. In: Krieger RI, Doull J (eds). *Handbook of pesticide toxicology*. San Diego: Academic Press, 2001: 1043–85.
129. Lotti M, Moretto A. Organophosphate-induced delayed polyneuropathy. *Toxicological Reviews*. 2005; **24**: 37–49.
130. Lotti M, Moretto A. Do carbamates cause polyneuropathy? *Muscle and Nerve*. 2006; **34**: 499–502.
131. Lotti M. The pathogenesis of organophosphate polyneuropathy. *Critical Reviews in Toxicology*. 1992; **21**: 465–88.
132. Evangelista De Duffard AM, Duffard R. Behavioral toxicology, risk assessment, and chlorinated hydrocarbons. *Environmental Health Perspectives*. 1996; **104** (Suppl. 2): 353–60.
133. van Wendel de Joode B, Wesseling C, Kromhout H et al. Chronic nervous-system effects of long-term occupational exposure to DDT. *Lancet*. 2001; **357**: 1014–16.
134. Cannon SB, Veazey Jr JM, Jackson RS et al. Epidemic kepone poisoning in chemical workers. *American Journal of Epidemiology*. 1978; **107**: 529–37.

135. Taylor JR, Selhorst JB, Calabrase VP. Chlordecone. In: Spencer PS, Schaumburg HH (eds). *Experimental and clinical neurotoxiciology*. Baltimore: Williams and Wilkins, 1980: 407-21.
136. Bradberry SM, Cage SA, Proudfoot AT, Vale JA. Poisoning due to pyrethroids. *Toxicological Reviews*. 2005; **24**: 93-106.
137. He F, Wang S, Liu L et al. Clinical manifestations and diagnosis of acute pyrethroid poisoning. *Archives of Toxicology*. 1989; **63**: 54-8.
138. Doi H, Kikuchi H, Murai H et al. Motor neuron disorder simulating ALS induced by chronic inhalation of pyrethroid insecticides. *Neurology*. 2006; **67**: 1894-5.
139. Le Quesne PM, Maxwell IC, Butterworth ST. Transient facial sensory symptoms following exposure to synthetic pyrethroids: A clinical and electrophysiological assessment. *Neurotoxicology*. 1981; **2**: 1-11.
140. Ray DE, Fry JR. A reassessment of the neurotoxicity of pyrethroid insecticides. *Pharmacology and Therapeutics*. 2006; **111**: 174-93.
141. DiMonte DA. The environment and Parkinson's disease: Is the nigrostriatal system preferentially targetted by neurotoxins? *Lancet*. 2003; **2**: 531-8.
142. Elbaz A, Levecque C, Clavel J et al. CYP2D6 polymorphism, pesticide exposure, and Parkinson's disease. *Annals of Neurology*. 2004; **55**: 430-4.
143. Kamel F, Tanner CM, Umbach DM et al. Pesticide exposure and self-reported Parkinson's disease in the Agricultural Health Study. *American Journal of Epidemiology*. 2006; **165**: 364-74.
144. Semchuk KM, Love EJ, Lee RG. Parkinson's disease and exposure to agricultural work and pesticide chemicals. *Neurology*. 1992; **42**: 1328-35.
145. Seidler A, Hellenbrand W, Robra BP et al. Possible environmental, occupational, and other etiologic factors for Parkinson's disease: A case-control study in Germany. *Neurology*. 1996; **46**: 1275-84.
146. Liou HH, Tsai MC, Chen CJ et al. Environmental risk factors and Parkinson's disease: A case-control study in Taiwan. *Neurology*. 1997; **48**: 1583-8.
147. Gorell JM, Johnson CC, Rybicki BA et al. The risk of Parkinson's disease with exposure to pesticides, farming, well water, and rural living. *Neurology*. 1998; **50**: 1346-50.
148. Petrovitch H, Ross W, Abbott RD et al. Plantation work and risk of Parkinson disease in a population-based longitudinal study. *Archives of Neurology*. 2002; **59**: 1787-92.
149. Priyadarshi A, Khuder SA, Schaub EA et al. Environmental risk factors and Parkinson's disease: A metaanalysis. *Environmental Research*. 2001; **86**: 122-7.
150. Rebert CS, Hall TA. The neuroepidemiology of styrene: A critical review of representative literature. *Critical Reviews in Toxicology*. 1994; **24**: S57-S106.
151. Yano BL, Dittenber DA, Albee RR, Mattsson JL. Abnormal auditory brainstem responses and cochlear pathology in rats induced by an exaggerated styrene exposure regimen. *Toxicologic Pathology*. 1992; **20**: 1-6.
152. Lawton BW, Hoffmann J, Triebig G. The ototoxicity of styrene: A review of occupational investigations. *International Archives of Occupational and Environmental Health*. 2006; **79**: 93-102.
153. Hormes JT, Filley CM, Rosenberg NL. Neurologic sequelae of chronic solvent vapor abuse. *Neurology*. 1986; **36**: 698-702.
154. Keane JR. Toluene optic neuropathy. *Annals of Neurology*. 1978; **4**: 390.
155. Lazar RB, Ho SU, Melen O, Daghestani AN. Multifocal central nervous system damage caused by toluene abuse. *Neurology*. 1983; **33**: 1337-40.
156. Filley CM, Heaton RK, Rosenberg NL. White matter dementia in chronic toluene abuse. *Neurology*. 1990; **40**: 532-4.
157. Ashikaga R, Araki Y, Miura K, Ishida O. Cranial MRI in chronic thinner intoxication. *Neuroradiology*. 1995; **37**: 443-4.
158. Antti-Poika M, Juntunen J, Matikäinen E et al. Occupational exposure to toluene: Neurotoxic effects with special emphasis on drinking habits. *International Archives of Occupational and Environmental Health*. 1985; **56**: 31-40.
159. Juntunen J, Matikäinen E, Antti-Poika M et al. Nervous system effects of long-term occupational exposure to toluene. *Acta Neurologica Scandinavica*. 1985; **72**: 512-17.
160. Foo SC, Jeyaratnam J, Koh D. Chronic neurobehavioural effects of toluene. *British Journal of Industrial Medicine*. 1990; **47**: 480-4.
161. Fuente A, McPherson B. Organic solvents and hearing loss: The challenge for audiology. *International Journal of Audiology*. 2006; **45**: 367-81.
162. Chang SJ, Chen CJ, Lien CH, Sung FC. Hearing loss in workers exposed to toluene and noise. *Environmental Health Perspectives*. 2006; **114**: 1283-6.
163. Schäper M, Demes P, Zupanic M et al. Occupational toluene exposure and auditory function: Results from a follow-up study. *Annals of Occupational Hygiene*. 2003; **47**: 493-502.
164. Buxton PH, Hayward M. Polyneuritis cranialis associated with industrial trichlorethylene poisoning. *Journal of Neurology, Neurosurgery, and Psychiatry*. 1967; **30**: 511-18.
165. Heineman EF, Cocco P, Gómez MR et al. Occupational exposure to chlorinated aliphatic hydrocarbons and risk of astrocytic brain cancer. *American Journal of Industrial Medicine*. 1994; **26**: 155-69.
166. Ritz B. Cancer mortality among workers exposed to chemicals during uranium processing. *Journal of Occupational and Environmental Medicine*. 1999; **41**: 556-66.
167. Blair A, Hartge P, Stewart PA et al. Mortality and cancer incidence of aircraft maintenance workers exposed to trichloroethylene and other organic solvents and chemicals: Extended follow up. *Occupational and Environmental Medicine*. 1998; **55**: 161-71.
168. Boice JD Jr, Marano DE, Fryzek JP et al. Mortality among aircraft manufacturing workers. *Occupational and Environmental Medicine*. 1999; **56**: 581-97.
169. Hansen J, Raaschou-Nielsen O, Christensen JM et al. Cancer incidence among Danish workers exposed to trichloroethylene. *Journal of Occupational and Environmental Medicine*. 2001; **43**: 133-9.

170. Grasso P, Sharratt M, Davies DM, Irvine D. Neurophysiological and psychological disorders and occupational exposure to organic solvents. *Food and Chemical Toxicology.* 1984; **22**: 819–52.
171. Grasso P. Neurotoxic and neurobehavioral effects of organic solvents on the nervous system. *Occupational Medicine.* 1988; **3**: 525–39.
172. Errebo-Knudsen EO, Olsen F. Organic solvents and presenile dementia (the painters' syndrome). A critical review of the Danish literature. *Science of the Total Environment.* 1986; **48**: 45–67.
173. Lees-Haley PR, Williams CW. Neurotoxicity of chronic low-dose exposure to organic solvents: A skeptical review. *Journal of Clinical Psychology.* 1997; **53**: 699–712.
174. Gade A, Mortensen EL, Bruhn P. 'Chronic painter's syndrome'. A reanalysis of psychological test data in a group of diagnosed cases, based on comparisons with matched controls. *Acta Neurologica Scandinavica.* 1988; **77**: 293–306.
175. Arlien-Soborg P, Bruhn P, Gyldensted C, Melgaard B. Chronic painters' syndrome: Chronic toxic encephalopathy in house painters. *Acta Neurologica Scandinavica.* 1979; **60**: 149–56.
176. Dick F, Semple S, Soutar A et al. Is colour vision impairment associated with cognitive impairment in solvent exposed workers? *Occupational and Environmental Medicine.* 2004; **61**: 76–8.
177. Lomax RB, Ridgway P, Meldrum M. Does occupational exposure to organic solvents affect colour discrimination? *Toxicological Reviews.* 2004; **23**: 91–121.
178. Institute of Medicine. Veterans and Agent Orange health effects of herbicides used in Vietnam. Washington DC: National Academy Press, 1994.
179. Institute of Medicine. Veterans and Agent Orange, update. Washington DC: National Academy Press, 1996.
180. Goldstein NP, Jones PH, Brown KR. Peripheral neuropathy after exposure to an ester of dichlorophenoxyacetic acid. *Journal of the American Medical Association.* 1959; **171**: 1306–9.
181. Berkley MC, Magee KR. Neuropathy following exposure to a dimethylamine salt of 2,4-D. *Archives of Internal Medicine.* 1963; **111**: 133–4.
182. Todd RL. A case of 2,4-D intoxication. *Journal of Iowa Medical Society.* 1962; **52**: 663–4.
183. Filippini G, Bordo B, Crenna P. Relationship between clinical and electrophysiological findings and indicators of heavy exposure to 2,3,7,8-tetrachlorodibenzo-p-dioxin. *Scandinavian Journal of Work, Environment and Health.* 1981; **7**: 257–62.
184. Barbieri S, Pirovano C, Scarlato G et al. Long-term effects of 2,3,7,8-tetrachlorodibenzo-p-dioxin on the peripheral nervous system. Clinical and neurophysiological controlled study on subjects with chloracne from the Seveso area. *Neuroepidemiology.* 1988; **7**: 29–37.
185. Assennato G, Cervino D, Emmett EA et al. Follow-up of subjects who developed chloracne following TCDD exposure at Seveso. *American Journal of Industrial Medicine.* 1989; **16**: 119–25.
186. Urban P, Pelclova D, Lukas E et al. Neurological and neurophysiological examinations on workers with chronic poisoning by 2,3,7,8-TCDD: Follow-up 35 years after exposure. *European Journal of Neurology.* 2007; **14**: 213–18.
187. Haley RW, Kurt TL, Hom J. Is there a Gulf War syndrome? Searching for syndromes by factor analysis of symptoms. *Journal of the American Medical Association.* 1997; **277**: 215–22.
188. Haley RW, Hom J, Roland PS et al. Evaluation of neurologic function in Gulf War veterans. A blinded case–control study. *Journal of the American Medical Association.* 1997; **277**: 223–30.
189. Jamal GA, Hansen S, Apartopoulos F, Peden A. The 'Gulf War syndrome'. Is there evidence of dysfunction in the nervous system? *Journal of Neurology, Neurosurgery, and Psychiatry.* 1996; **60**: 449–51.
190. Sharief MK, Priddin J, Delamont RS et al. Neurophysiologic analysis of neuromuscular symptoms in UK Gulf War veterans: A controlled study. *Neurology.* 2002; **59**: 1518–25.
191. Davis LE, Eisen SA, Murphy FM et al. Clinical and laboratory assessment of distal peripheral nerves in Gulf War veterans and spouses. *Neurology.* 2004; **63**: 1070–7.
192. Haley RW, Vongpatanasin W, Wolfe GI et al. Blunted circadian variation in autonomic regulation of sinus node function in veterans with Gulf War syndrome. *American Journal of Medicine.* 2004; **117**: 469–78.
193. Stein PK, Domitrovich PP, Ambrose K et al. Sex effects on heart rate variability in fibromyalgia and Gulf War illness. *Arthritis and Rheumatism.* 2004; **51**: 700–8.
194. Horner RD, Kamins KG, Feussner JR et al. Occurrence of amyotrophic lateral sclerosis among Gulf War veterans. *Neurology.* 2003; **61**: 742–9.
195. Haley RW. Excess incidence of ALS in young Gulf War veterans. *Neurology.* 2003; **61**: 750–6.
196. Rose MR. Gulf War service is an uncertain trigger for ALS. *Neurology.* 2003; **61**: 730–1.
197. Ismail K, Kent K, Brugha T et al. The mental health of UK Gulf war veterans: Phase 2 of a two phase cohort study. *British Medical Journal.* 2002; **325**: 576–81.
198. Stimpson NJ, Thomas HV, Weightman AL et al. Psychiatric disorder in veterans of the Persian Gulf War of 1991. Systematic review. *British Journal of Psychiatry.* 2003; **182**: 391–403.
199. Ishoy T, Knop J, Suadicani P et al. Increased psychological distress among Danish Gulf War veterans – without evidence for a neurotoxic background. The Danish Gulf War Study. *Danish Medical Bulletin.* 2004; **51**: 108–13.
200. Institute of Medicine. Gulf War and health. Washington DC: National Academy Press, 2000.

88

Hepatotoxic effects of workplace exposure

THOMAS W WARNES AND ALEXANDER SMITH

Introduction	1171	Specific occupational hepatotoxins	1180
Patterns of toxic liver injury	1172	Conclusions	1188
Treatment	1176	Acknowledgements	1189
Mechanisms of liver toxicity in model hepatotoxins	1176	References	1189

INTRODUCTION

A variety of classifications of hepatotoxic agents exists in the medical and toxicological literature based variously on the source and chemical nature of the toxicant,[1-3] the type of liver pathology produced[4,5] or on the toxic mechanisms involved.[6,7]

The liver is the first organ after the gut exposed to ingested chemicals, toxins and drugs, and its rich blood supply ensures that agents absorbed through the lungs and skin also reach the liver quickly and at high concentrations. It is thus easily injured by direct exposure to these agents. In addition, many xenobiotic compounds are actively removed from the bloodstream by the liver and detoxified by hepatic metabolic processes. However, in the course of detoxification, some are metabolized into even more toxic substances,[7] including free radicals.[8]

Due to increased awareness by workers, employers and physicians, traditionally recognized occupational hepatotoxins are now encountered much less frequently. However, a recent update to the *Pocket guide to chemical hazards* lists 228 industrial chemicals capable of causing liver injury.[9,10] Exposure is usually by inhalation or skin absorption. Occupational liver disease may occasionally present after an acute incident at work, and in these circumstances, diagnosis and identification of the toxic agent is relatively straightforward. In general, however, the diagnosis of occupational liver disease is rare in clinical practice and likely to be difficult. The patient may present with general symptoms of liver dysfunction or alternatively, an individual health check or routine workplace screen may have provided the initial clue to liver disease. However, the large functional reserve of the liver allows most cases of occupational liver injury to go undetected during many years of chronic exposure or until long after exposure has ceased and thus advanced liver disease may already be present and the occupational aetiology may be missed. Even when an occupational cause is suspected, it is usually difficult to quantify the level of exposure to a specific toxin, particularly when, with routine safety measures in place, exposure may have occurred in unpredictable ways, such as in machinery breakdown, during cleaning and maintenance, or as a result of accidental leakage.

It should be appreciated, furthermore, that abnormal liver function tests are found quite commonly in the general population not exposed to industrial chemicals.[11] The most common cause of abnormal liver function tests in the general population of Western countries is hepatic steatosis associated with obesity.[12,13] Gilbert's syndrome is present in 5 per cent of the population[14] and is diagnosed by the finding of indirect hyperbilirubinaemia in the absence of haemolysis. Serum gamma glutamyl transpeptidase (GGTP) may be a sensitive indicator of hepatotoxicity since it is a marker, among other things, of liver microsomal enzyme induction, but it is essentially non-specific.[11] Following the initial detection of an abnormality in liver function, a non-invasive screen should be carried out, including ultrasound scan of the liver, together with appropriate blood tests (Table 88.1 and Figure 88.1). These should permit diagnosis of metabolic, autoimmune and viral liver disorders, and if these have been excluded, then workplace exposure to chemicals needs to be carefully considered and liver biopsy may be required.

Chemicals and toxins can produce a wide spectrum of clinical presentations ranging from mildly abnormal liver function tests in asymptomatic patients, to fulminant liver

Table 88.1 Non-invasive screening of an individual with abnormal liver function tests.

Screening		
History	Workplace or environmental exposure	
	Alcohol, drug ingestion	
	Previous medical history	Hepatitis, jaundice
		Autoimmune disorders
		Liver or autoimmune disorders
	Family history	
Ultrasound scan	Steatosis	
	Chronic liver disease	
	Extrahepatic biliary obstruction	
	Infiltration	
	Venous abnormalities	Portal hypertension
		Portal or hepatic vein occlusion
	Tumours	
Immunology	Smooth muscle antibody	
	Anti-nuclear factor	Autoimmune hepatitis type 1
	Liver/kidney microsomal antibody (anti-LKM)	Autoimmune hepatitis type 2
	Antimitochondrial antibody (AMA)	Primary biliary cirrhosis (PBC)
Biochemistry	Serum iron, ferritin	Haemochromatosis
	Iron binding capacity	
	Serum caeruloplasmin	Wilson's disease
	α_1-Antitrypsin	α_1-antitrypsin deficiency
	α-Fetoprotein	Hepatoma
Viral screen	Hepatitis A antibody, IgM	Acute hepatitis A
	HbsAg	
	HB core antibody, IgM	Acute hepatitis B
	HB core antibody, IgG	Chronic hepatitis B
	HCV antibody	
	HCV-RNA by PCR	Hepatitis C

failure. The liver has only a limited number of ways of responding to chemical insults: these include steatosis, acute or chronic hepatitis, hepatocellular necrosis, cirrhosis, veno-occlusive disease, non-cirrhotic portal hypertension and hepatic neoplasia. Chemical compounds may have both hepatotoxic and carcinogenic potential. No classification of chemically induced hepatotoxicity is entirely satisfactory, since the response of the liver depends upon the dose, duration and route of the exposure, as well as on differing sensitivities of individuals to the particular chemical. Alcohol and drugs, such as anti-epileptics, as well as other chemicals such as dichlorodiphenyltrichloroethane (DDT), all increase hepatic microsomal enzyme activity and are degraded by specific cytochrome P_{450} isoforms. These agents can therefore increase the damage produced by hepatotoxins, such as carbon tetrachloride,[15] which are activated by the cytochrome P_{450} system.[7] In animals, repeated exposure to combinations of carbon tetrachloride and other agents, such as phenobarbitone and acetone, reliably produce cirrhosis,[16] and in some cases, hepatoma. Other drugs which the patient may be taking (e.g. cimetidine) may inhibit the cytochrome P_{450} system,[7] with secondary effects on the metabolism of chemical hepatotoxins. Phenothiazines (chlorpromazine, promazine and promethazine) have also been shown to inhibit the effect of CCl_4, possibly by membrane stabilization.[17]

The physician must therefore have a high index of suspicion regarding chemicals and toxins in the genesis of liver dysfunction and must be aware of the occupations which present a risk in this respect (Table 88.2), together with the wide range of industrial chemicals, elements and toxins which have been reported to produce hepatotoxicity (Table 88.3). This list is not exhaustive, but serves to indicate the wide range of substances which must be considered.

PATTERNS OF TOXIC LIVER INJURY

Acute injury

This may produce hepatocyte damage or cholestasis. Major elevations of the serum transaminase levels with marginal

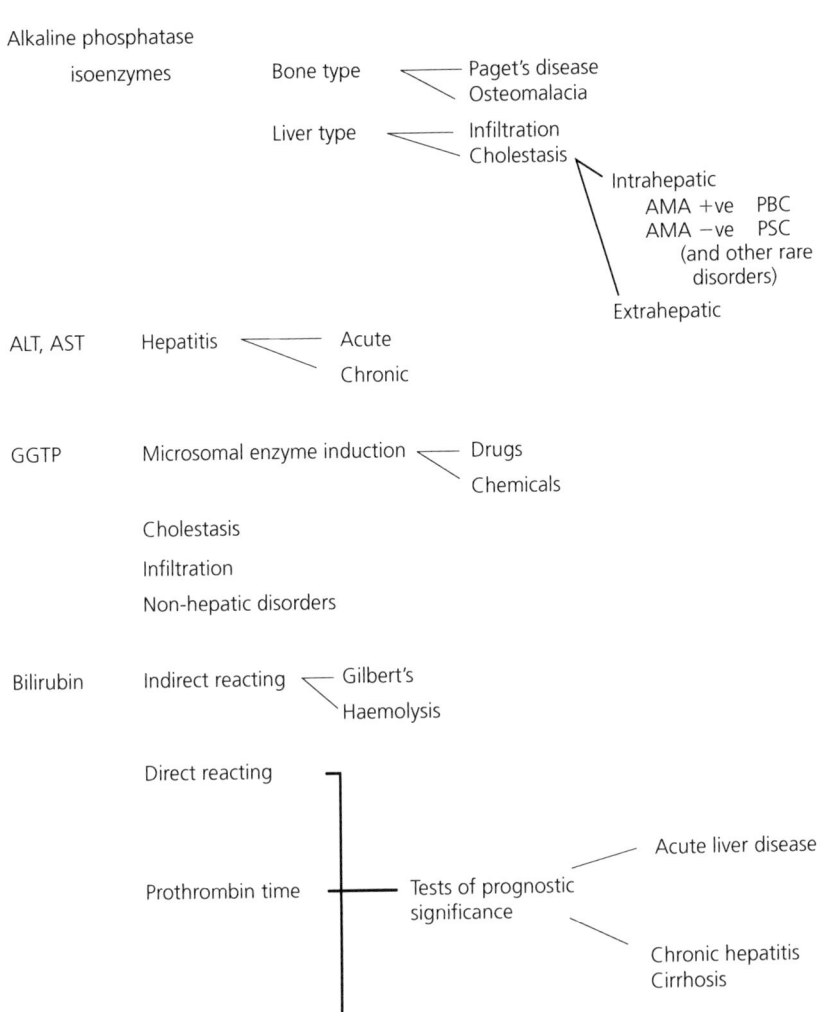

Figure 88.1 Disorders producing abnormal liver function tests (ALT). AST, aspartate aminotransferase; GGTP, γ-glutamyl transferase; PSC, primary sclerosing cholangitis.

elevation of alkaline phosphatase (ALP), are consistent with cytotoxic injury. Hepatomegaly may be present, but clinical signs of acute liver injury may be marginal, or similar to those found in symptomatic viral hepatitis. Clinically, cholestasis presents with pruritus, jaundice and elevation of the serum ALP and GGTP, with a much less impressive elevation of serum transaminase levels. The morphological findings are those of intracellular accumulation of bile or of canalicular bile deposits. Mixed hepatocellular and cholestatic forms of liver injury may be found, for example, that produced by exposure to methylene dianiline (4,4′-diaminodiphenylmethane)[18] a compound used in industry as an epoxy resin hardener, in the preparation of isocyanates, in the production of polyurethane and as an antioxidant in latex rubber. It was first identified as a liver toxin during an epidemic outbreak of jaundice in 84 inhabitants of the English town of Epping, who had eaten bread which had been made with flour that was inadvertently contaminated with methylene diamine during its transport to the bakery.[19] Jaundice was accompanied by elevation of serum ALP and transaminase levels. Needle biopsies showed cholestasis and hepatocellular damage. Recovery was rapid in most patients and none died. Re-exposure to methylene dianiline may cause recurrence of hepatitis, but the mechanism of action has not been extensively studied.[20]

Acute cytotoxic injury is indicated by steatosis and necrosis and these are often encountered together, for instance after intoxication with carbon tetrachloride (CCl_4). Yellow phosphorus steatosis may be microvesicular, macrovesicular,[21] or mixed; the type of steatosis is frequently characteristic for a number of chemicals. The chemical injury can also be classified according to its localization, since zonal damage often occurs in parallel with the activity of enzymes which mediate the metabolic activation of the chemical to the toxic metabolite. Thus, CCl_4 and dimethylnitrosamine produce centrilobular necrosis because cytochrome P_{450} is more abundant in Rappaport zone 3 (the centrizonal area).[22] It has been suggested that yellow phosphorus may produce periportal fibrosis,[23] but this claim has not been substantiated.

Acute liver injury may result in hepatic failure and death. However, if the patient recovers from the acute attack, the prognosis is good since complete recovery usually occurs.

Table 88.2 Occupations and chemical incidents associated with hepatotoxicity.

Industry	Process	
Aircraft industry	Manufacture and maintenance	Beryllium alloys
	Fuel handling	Kerosene
Car industry	Machine degreasing	See below
		Triorthocresyl phosphate
	Machine degreasing	See below
	Paint spraying	See below
Chemical industry/laboratory work	Acetone recycling	Acetone
	Acrylic fibre production	Acrylonitrile, dimethylacetamide
	Fruit paper production	Biphenyls
	Chlorine/acetaldehyde production	Mercury vapour
	Chemical production	Allyl chloride
		Benzidine/beta napthylamine
		Benzene
		$p\text{-}tert$ Butylphenol
		Dimethylformamide
Dry cleaning/machine degreasing		2,4,5-Trichlorophenol (TCP)
		Tetrachloroethylene
		Tetrachloromethane (chloroform)
		1,1,1-Trichloroethane
		Trichloroethylene
Environmental	Contaminated wheat	Hexachlorobenzene
	Contaminated bread	Methylenedianiline (Epping jaundice)
	Contaminated rice	Polychlorinated biphenyls (Yusho incident)
	Contaminated oil	Toxic oil syndrome (Spain)
	Vinyl chloride in environment	Vinyl chloride
	Contaminated wells	Arsenic
Electrical industry	Capacitor/transformer manufacture	Polychlorinated biphenyls (PCBs)
	Semiconductors	Selenium
Epoxy resin application		Methylenedianiline
		2-Nitropropane
Firework production		Phosphorus
GRP plastics manufacture		Styrene
Horticulture/gardening/pesticide production	Pesticide use	Carbamate insecticide (Isolan)
		Chlordecone (Kepone)
		Dichlorodiphenyl trichloroethane (DDT)
		Gamma hexachloro cyclohexane
		MCPA (2-methyl-4-chlorophenoxyacetic acid)
		Mucochloric acid
		Malathion
		Paraquat
		Pyramin
	Soil disinfection	Monobromoethane (methyl bromide)
Metal production/use	Beryllium ore reduction	Beryllium
	Fluorescent lamp manufacture	Beryllium
	X-ray tube manufacture	Beryllium
	Gold melting	Cadmium
	Chromium plating	Chromium
	Copper smelting/refining/working	Copper (plus contaminants arsenic, cadmium, iron, sulphur, zinc)
	Nickel alloy production	Nickel
Munitions work	(manufacture or disposal)	TNT (trinitrotoluene)
Neoprene application		Polychloroprene
Nursing		Cytostatic agents
Painting		1,2-Dichloroethane
		2-Nitropropane
		Xylene
Pharmaceutical industry		Trichloromethane (chloroform)
Plastic and rotogravure industry		Toluene
PVC production		Vinyl chloride
Refrigeration/air conditioning		Monochloromethane (methyl bromide)
Rocket industry		1,2-Dimethyl hydrazine
Rodent control		Phosphorus
Shoe-making		Toluene
Styrene polymerization		Styrene
Wine industry	Vintners	Arsenic
	Vineyard spraying	Bordeaux mixture (copper sulphate)
		Insecticide sprays (arsenic)

Table 88.3 Chemicals associated with liver disease.

Chemicals	
Haloalkanes	Carbon tetrachloride
	Trichloromethane (chloroform)
	Trichloroethane (methylchloroform)
	Tetrachloroethane
	Trichloroethylene
	Tetrachloroethylene (perchloroethylene)
Nitroparaffins	Nitromethane
	Nitroethane
	Nitropropane
Toluene	
Chlorinated napthalenes	
Nitroaromatics	Trinitrotoluene
	Nitrobenzene
Metals/metalloids	Copper
	Arsenic/arsine
	Beryllium
	Phosphorus
	Cadmium
	Selenium
	Chromium
	Lead
Pesticides and herbicides	Chlordecone
	Chlorophenoxy herbicides
	Paraquat
Polychlorinated biphenyls	
Vinyl chloride	
Methyl bromide	
Cytostatic agents	
Phthalate esters	

Chronic injury

Occasionally, long-term sequelae of acute intoxication eventually result in chronic liver disease, although this is much more commonly found after repeated or long-term exposure to chemicals. Chronicity is manifest by the presence of fibrosis in the liver. This is a consequence of the activation and transformation of hepatic stellate (Ito) cells into collagen-producing myofibroblasts. This activation can be induced by a number of factors, such as free radicals and cytokines.[24] Cirrhosis is frequently the end result with fibrous tissue disrupting the functional anatomy of the organ. The cirrhotic patient may be asymptomatic, or may present with hepatic decompensation associated with bleeding varices, ascites or encephalopathy. Cirrhosis has been reported after chronic exposure to arsenical pesticides[25] and to halogenated alkanes, such as carbon tetrachloride and chloroform.

Vascular lesions

Non-cirrhotic portal hypertension has been reported after exposure to vinyl chloride[26,27] and inorganic arsenicals[28,29] and usually presents with bleeding from gastric or oesophageal varices. Liver function tests may be normal or minimally disturbed. Splenomegaly, if present, is detected clinically and confirmed on ultrasound. The wedged hepatic vein pressure in such cases is either normal or only slightly raised, while the splenic pulp pressure is markedly elevated, indicating presinusoidal portal hypertension.

The histology shows enlargement and thickening of the portal vein branches with perisinusoidal fibrosis. In some cases, activation and proliferation of sinusoidal cells is seen. The liver histology closely resembles that found in idiopathic portal hypertension (Banti's syndrome) suggesting that this syndrome may sometimes result from unrecognized toxic injury. Occasionally, peliosis hepatis is seen in chemical liver injury, particularly with vinyl chloride. Both peliosis hepatis and non-cirrhotic portal hypertension can progress to hepatic angiosarcoma and this progression is well documented in vinyl chloride workers.

Malignant change

A wide range of chemicals has been shown to induce primary liver tumours in animal studies, but in humans, a causal relationship between primary liver tumours and previous exposure to a specific chemical has been shown convincingly for only a few compounds. Primary liver cancer is seen in association with arsenic[30] and vinyl chloride exposure,[31] but less commonly than angiosarcoma. Such tumours may present with right upper quadrant pain and weight loss. The diagnosis is made on abdominal ultrasound scan and confirmed on computed tomography (CT) scan, hepatic angiography and ultrasound-guided liver biopsy. Serum alphafetoprotein levels may be normal or raised. Dioxin has been shown to be a potent hepatocarcinogen in animal studies[32] and it has also been implicated in man,[33] although firm evidence is difficult to obtain.

Disturbances in porphyrin metabolism

Porphyrias can be acquired or can result from inborn metabolic errors of haem synthesis and they are characterized by increased urinary excretion of porphyrins or their precursors. Porphyria cutanea tarda (PCT) usually presents with photosensitive skin lesions, including bullae, hypertrichosis and hyperpigmentation, together with increased uroporphyrin excretion in the urine. Constitutional PCT is inherited in an autosomal dominant fashion and is characterized by a deficiency of uroporphyrinogen decarboxylase (UROD) in the liver, erythrocytes and other tissues, with a secondary elevation of aminolaevulinic acid synthetase (ALAS). Clinical presentation is precipitated by liver cell damage most often due to alcohol, oestrogens or hepatitis C; iron deposition in the liver is an important cofactor.

Acquired PCT occurs when UROD, particularly the liver enzyme, is inhibited by ingested agents. An outbreak of PCT in Turkey between 1956 and 1960 followed ingestion of bread contaminated with the fungicide hexachlorobenzene.[34] Between 3000 and 4000 people from several distinct genetic populations were affected, suggesting that there was no inherited predisposition. The time interval from ingestion to initial symptoms was about six months; these included weakness, loss of appetite and sensitivity to sunlight. A small number of patients were treated with EDTA, a heavy metal chelator, with reversal of skin symptoms and signs.[35,36] Exposure to vinyl chloride,[37] methyl chloride,[38] hexabromobenzene and polybrominated and polychlorinated biphenyls[39] may also cause acquired PCT. In animal studies, tetrachlorodibenzo-p-dioxin (TCDD), is the most porphyrinogenic substance known.[40] Following an explosion at a chemical plant near Seveso in Italy in 1976, the nearby population were exposed to TCDD. A brother and sister who were exposed to low levels developed overt PCT. They were part of a large family of 66 members who were also exposed, but showed no evidence of PCT. PCT in these two siblings developed on the background of a predisposing genetic defect resulting in UROD deficiency in erythrocytes and thus increased susceptibility to porphyria.[41] Thirteen of 60 other exposed individuals (22 per cent), not of the same family, developed coproporphyrinuria; UROD levels in erythrocytes were not decreased.[39] In the two patients with PCT, treatment with chloroquine resulted in remission of symptoms.[42]

Diagnosis of PCT depends on the finding of a characteristic isomeric distribution of porphyrins in the urine, stool and to a lesser extent plasma. Analyses are best performed in a specialized laboratory using the sensitive and specific technique of high pressure liquid chromatography (HPLC). Normal urine porphyrin content is 70 per cent coproporphyrin (70 per cent of which is isomer III), and 15 per cent uroporphyrin (90 per cent isomer I) with the remainder being 5-, 6- and 7-carboxylate porphyrins (all mostly isomer III). In PCT, urine contains mostly uroporphyrin (predominantly isomer I) and 7-carboxylate porphyrin (isomer III); 6-carboxylate porphyrin is mostly type III, while 5-carboxylate porphyrin and coproporphyrins are present as equal amounts of isomers I and III. These proportions hold for both familial and acquired PCT, although with hexachlorobenzene, more uroporphyrin III is present. Porphyrin excretion in faeces is increased, particularly isocoproporphyrin, and consists predominantly of type III isomers. The profile of porphyrins in plasma is similar to that in the urine. Total urinary porphyrins in patients exposed to chlorinated hydrocarbons without overt disease show no increase compared to controls, but the pattern of porphyrin distribution may be abnormal, indicating subclinical disease (PCT type A).[43]

Conventional treatment for porphyria is venesection. UROD inhibition by TCDD is prevented by an iron deficiency state. Venesection should be continued until urinary porphyrin concentration falls below 0.5 mg/L.

TREATMENT

Early identification of, and removal of the patient from, the offending chemical is the most important measure in treatment of acute hepatotoxicity since continued exposure to the toxic agent, especially if jaundice has appeared, may lead to acute liver failure. However, if the patient presents with symptoms of chronic liver injury, it is unlikely that exposure has been continuous and it may have been many years in the past.

Specific treatments or antidotes to hepatotoxins encountered in the workplace have been proposed, but they are largely experimental and none has been evaluated in controlled trials (Figure 88.2). Patients who develop acute liver failure, or complications of chronic liver disease, should be referred for specialized care on a Liver Unit. Management will generally be supportive and is aimed at detecting and addressing specific problems as they arise. Liver transplantation is an option for both acute or chronic liver disease, including malignancy, which is refractory to medical therapy.

MECHANISMS OF LIVER TOXICITY IN MODEL HEPATOTOXINS

The different processes resulting in hepatotoxicity can be illustrated by considering hepatotoxic mechanisms for four agents which are relatively well understood: carbon tetrachloride, vinyl chloride, hexachlorobenzene and dioxin (TCDD). While the dangers of these particular agents are now well appreciated and their use has been restricted and stringent controls applied, patients exposed in the past may still present with chronic problems. An understanding of the mechanisms established for these agents may also help in understanding how other established and novel hepatotoxins produce their effects.

Carbon tetrachloride

The various mechanisms resulting in CCl_4 hepatotoxicity have been extensively studied in the experimental animal (Figure 88.3).[6,7,44] Initially, direct lipid solvent injury to the hepatocyte and mitochondrial membranes produces altered cellular function. In adipose tissue, solvent effects lead to increased mobilization of triglyceride stores which then contributes to fat accumulation within the liver (steatosis).

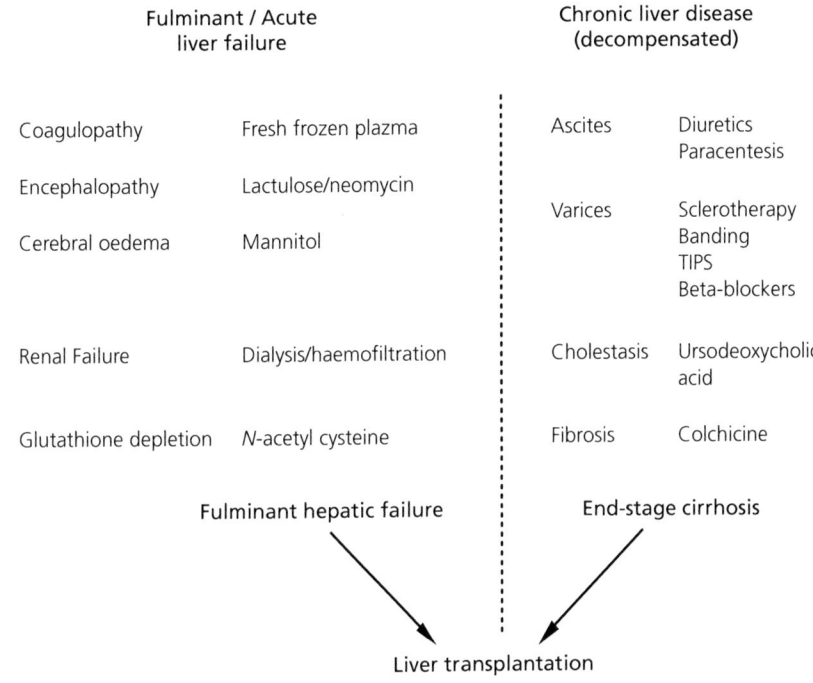

Figure 88.2 Treatment of occupational liver diseases. TIPS, transjugular intrahepatic portal-systemic shunt.

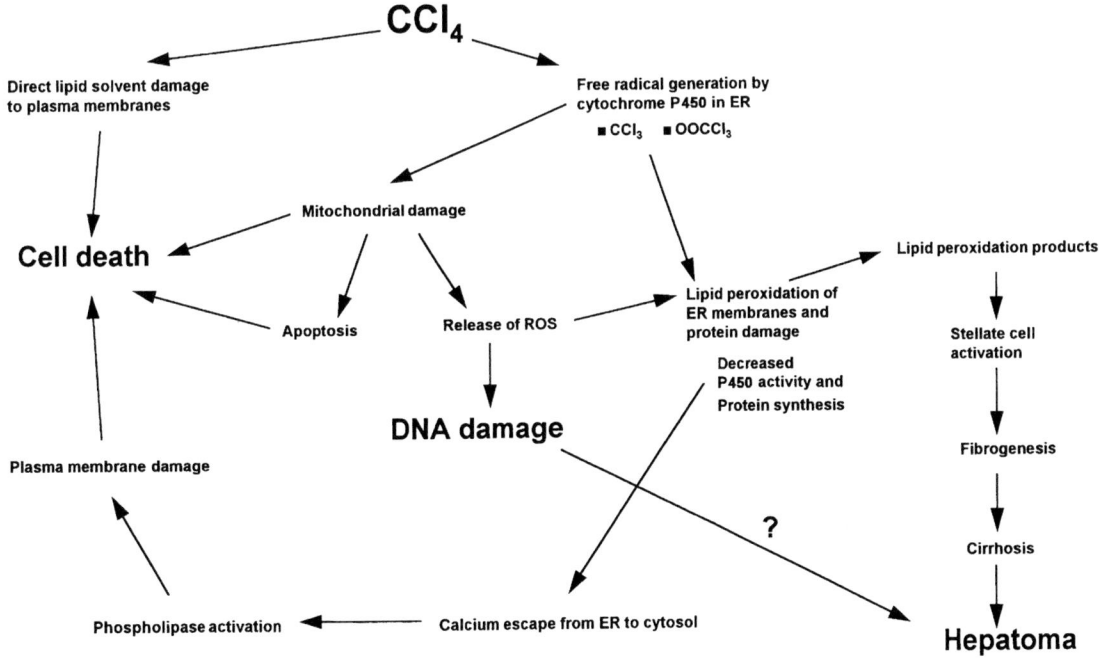

Figure 88.3 Mechanisms of carbon tetrachloride hepatotoxicity. ER, endoplasmic reticulum; ROS, reactive oxygen species.

A secondary effect, occurring after three hours of exposure to CCl_4, involves metabolic activation of CCl_4 by the cytochrome P_{450} system to the trichlorethyl radical ($\cdot CCl_3$) and then to the trichloromethylperoxy radical ($\cdot OOCCl_3$) in the presence of molecular oxygen.[45] The initial liver injury is centrizonal, due to the location of the cytochrome P_{450} enzyme. These free radicals derived from carbon tetrachloride initiate a chain reaction of lipid peroxidation within the endoplasmic reticulum by hydrogen abstraction from unsaturated fatty acids. Hepatic fibrogenesis leading to fibrosis and cirrhosis, may be triggered either directly by free radical-induced hepatocyte damage leading to Kupffer cell activation, and activation of stellate cells by cytokines or may be triggered by secondary activation of hepatic stellate cells by lipid peroxidation products, such as malondialdehyde or 4-hydroxy nonenal.[24,46] Concomitant with and/or subsequent to lipid peroxidation, other destructive processes occur in the endoplasmic reticulum. Carbon tetrachloride acts as a suicide substrate for cytochrome P_{450} leading to loss of enzyme activity. Damage to the rough endoplasmic reticulum also leads to decreased protein synthetic activity. Fat accumulation leading to steatosis is partly due to this decrease in protein synthesis, especially reduced synthesis of very low density lipoproteins (VLDL), which leads to a failure of the lipid export mechanism.[47,48]

Microsomal Ca^{2+}-ATPase, the pump responsible for sequestration of Ca^{2+} into the endoplasmic reticulum, is damaged by oxygen free radicals. Consequently, the intracellular free Ca^{2+} concentration is raised, thus activating a number of proteolytic enzymes, including phospholipases which are capable of propagating membrane disturbance at distant sites, and endonucleases which give rise to DNA strand breaks.[49]

Experimental studies have shown that carbon tetrachloride produces upregulation of genes involved in extracellular transport and cell signalling, as well as changes in regulation of genes involved in regulation of stress response and cell cycle.[50]

Vinyl chloride

Vinyl chloride metabolism occurs via different pathways depending on the level of exposure (Figure 88.4). At concentrations of less than 50 ppm, vinyl chloride monomer (VCM) is metabolized by alcohol dehydrogenase to produce chloroacetaldehyde and monochloroacetic acid, while at levels of more than 50 ppm, oxidation occurs by the peroxidase-catalase system to chloroacetaldehyde, and at concentrations of more than 250 ppm, it is metabolized by microsomal mixed function oxidase to chloroethylene oxide. Vinyl chloride and its reactive metabolites bind covalently to hepatic glutathione and are then hydrolysed and excreted in the urine as conjugates of cysteine. Both vinyl chloride and its metabolites produce hyperplasia of mesenchymal sinusoidal lining cells in the liver and spleen and also hyperplasia of hepatocytes. Hepatic stellate cell activation results in fibrosis and the end result is splenomegaly and portal hypertension; this fibrosis may be detectable by ultrasound scan. There is evidence that genetic polymorphism in the cytochrome P_{450}2E1 (CYP2E1) may be responsible for individual differences in

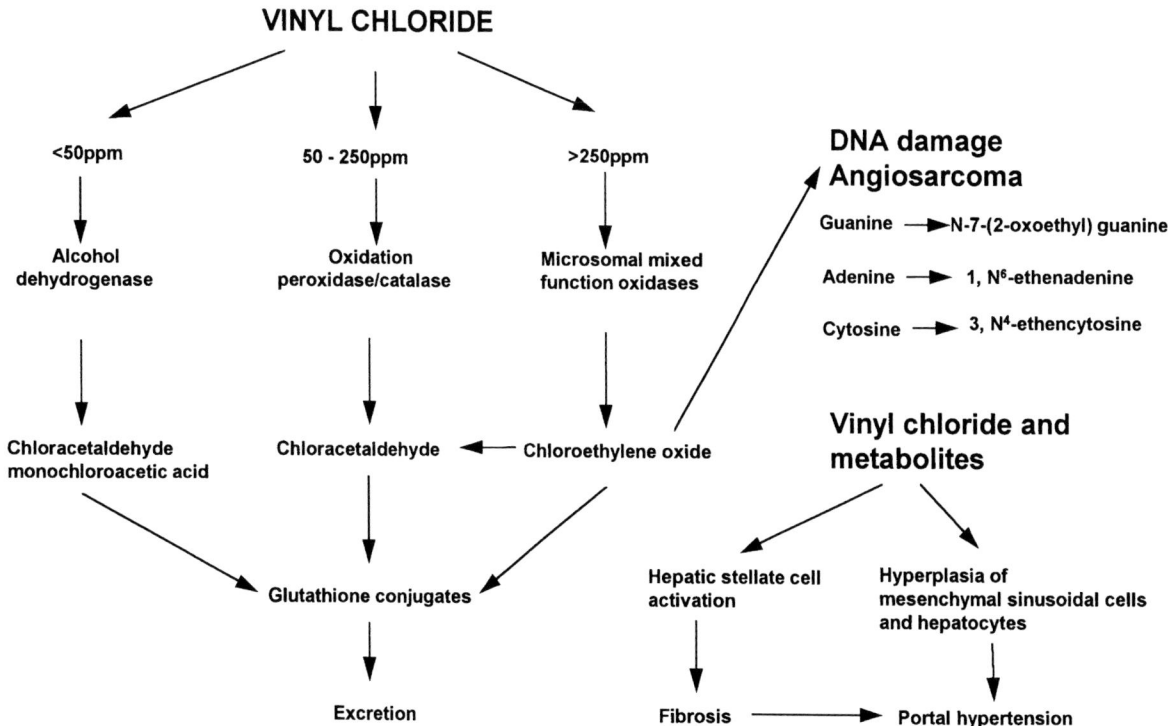

Figure 88.4 Mechanisms of vinyl chloride hepatotoxicity.

susceptibility to liver fibrosis associated with chronic VCM exposure[51] and to variable susceptibility to the carcinogenic effects of VCM in exposed groups of workers.[52] Liver ultrasonographic abnormalities increase as the cumulative exposure dose increases, although changes have been reported in VCM workers exposed within the current occupational health standards.[53] Similarly, exposure to low or moderate levels of VCM and ethylene dichloride may be associated with raised serum AST and ALT[54] although others have found that only GGT is associated with current VCM exposure.[55] In countries with a high incidence of viral hepatitis, there may be a synergistic effect of hepatitis B and C with occupational exposure to VCM and ethylene dichloride, in producing liver damage.[56] The metabolite chloroethylene oxide damages DNA bases and is thought to play a key role in the development of angiosarcoma. Female Chinese workers are at increased risk of chromosomal damage induced by VCM compared to males.[57]

Hexachlorobenzene

Hexachlorobenzene provides an excellent illustration of the mechanisms by which hepatic toxins may disturb haem synthesis and thereby produce acquired porphyria (Figure 88.5). This compound inhibits hepatic uroporphyrinogen decarboxylase and coproporphyrinogen oxidase and causes secondary coproporphyrinuria which may progress to uroporphyrinuria and to porphyria cutanea tarda. The $\cdot O^2$ radical may be involved in inhibition of uroporphyrinogen decarboxylase.[58]

Dioxin

2,3,7,8 Tetrachlorodibenzo-p-dioxin (TCDD) is the most fully investigated member of the very large polychlorinated dibenzo-p-dioxin family and is the most toxic synthetic compound known.[33] These compounds do not occur naturally, but are now ubiquitous in the environment. They are produced as contaminants during a variety of industrial synthetic reactions, such as the production of chlorinated phenols, during incineration of municipal and hospital wastes, from petrol and other fossil fuel combustion and during a host of other industrial processes. Dioxins are lipophilic and therefore accumulate in adipose tissue, skin, liver and breast milk in mammals, and have an extremely long half-life of between five and eight years in man. TCDD is immunotoxic and teratogenic and affects the gut, liver, skin and kidneys. Acute toxicity produces chloracne and death following a period of wasting. In chronic low-dose studies (as low as 0.1 µg/kg per day) TCDD acts as a potent carcinogen in many organs, including the liver.

A great deal is known about the mechanisms of TCDD toxicity, but many aspects remain uncertain.[33] TCDD, on entering the cell, binds to a specific aryl hydrocarbon (dioxin) receptor (AhR) (Figure 88.6). Binding of dioxin releases heat-shock protein 90 (HSP90) from the complex which can then bind an AhR nuclear translocator protein (Arnt). This allows the complex to enter the nucleus and interact with dioxin response elements (DREs), specific base sequences in the cell genome.[59] Binding to these sequences triggers expression of a number of genes including several cytochrome P_{450} genes and other enzymes.[60]

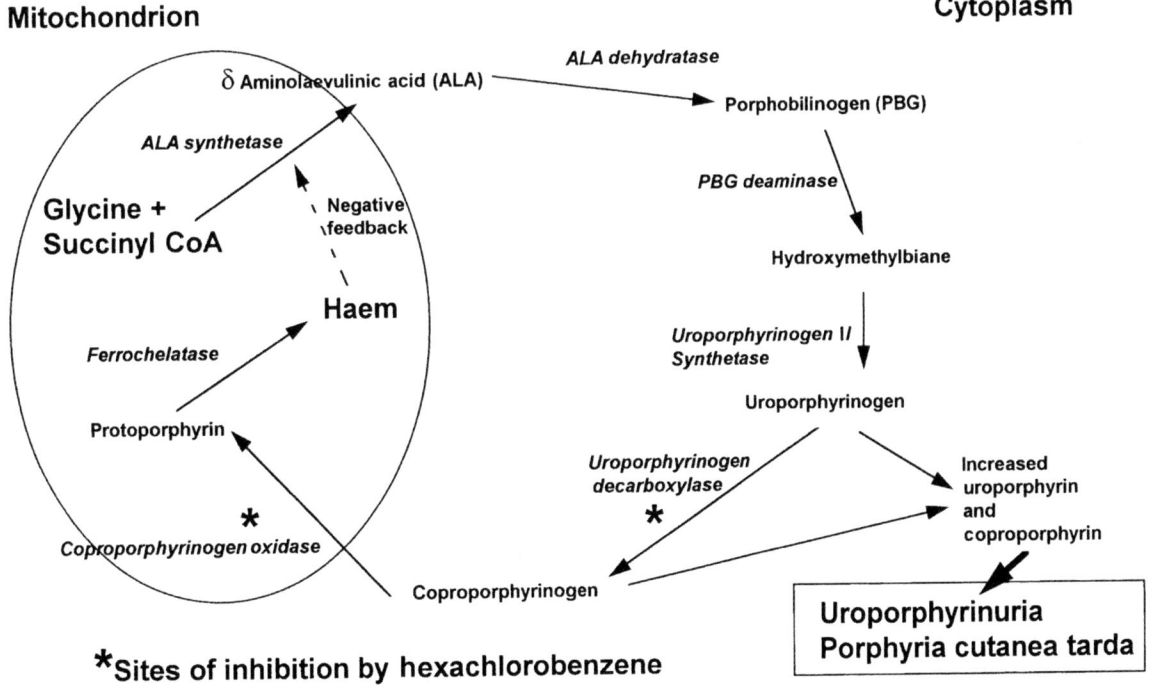

Figure 88.5 Disturbances of haem synthesis by hepatotoxins.

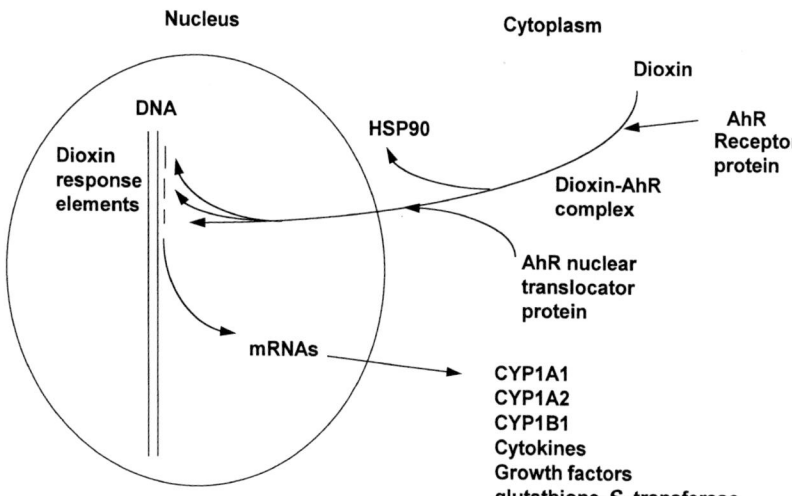

Figure 88.6 Proposed mechanisms of dioxin hepatotoxicity.

The mechanisms by which activation of these gene products result in the clinical problems associated with dioxin toxicity is still poorly understood, although effects on intracellular calcium levels, cytokine expression, and effects on oestrogen expression have all been proposed. Differences in the affinity of the AhR for dioxin in different species probably account for the enormous range (3000-fold) of sensitivity to dioxin in different species.

In laboratory animals, it is well established that dioxin is a potent hepatocarcinogen,[32] which can both initiate and promote carcinogenesis and produce cancers with exposures as low as 0.001 μg/kg per day. While TCDD does not itself modify DNA, it is a very effective tumour promotor, increasing cell turnover and fixing DNA defects which clonally expand to tumours. Initiation may arise following Ca^{2+}-triggered endonuclease DNA damage[49] or alternatively, free radical-induced DNA damage.

World concern over dioxin contamination was triggered by the Seveso incident in July 1976 when an explosion in an Italian chemical factory heavily contaminated the surrounding countryside and population. Bird and animal life in the area died. Human problems initially appeared to be limited to chloracne, but long-term follow-up studies have suggested an increased incidence of a variety of cancers, including hepatocellular carcinoma and cholangiocarcinoma.[33] However, no demonstrable hepatic injury or predisposition to liver cancer has been found in soldiers exposed to dioxin-contaminated herbicide (Agent Orange) used during the Vietnam war.[10,61]

SPECIFIC OCCUPATIONAL HEPATOTOXINS

The solvent controversy

Most industrial plants and businesses use solvents in some form or another. Evidence regarding their hepatotoxicity is conflicting. Abnormalities in liver function tests and histology have been reported in chemical industry workers and painters exposed to solvents,[62] but these studies lacked controls. The situation is further complicated by the fact that workers may be exposed to multiple agents.[63] Laboratory testing that is commonly used by clinicians (routine liver function tests) to detect liver toxicity may not be sensitive enough to detect early liver damage from industrial solvents and new methodologies are being developed in the diagnosis of solvent hepatotoxicity. Furthermore, clinical assessment must take account of synergism between the solvent or mixture of solvents concerned with medications, drugs of use and abuse, alcohol, nutrition and age of the individual concerned.[64]

Haloalkanes

CARBON TETRACHLORIDE (CCL_4, TETRACHLOROMETHANE)

Industrial accidents account for most cases of CCl_4 poisoning, the usual mechanism being the inhalation of fumes in a poorly ventilated environment. As little as 5 mL can produce the typical histological changes of hepatic necrosis and steatosis in zone 3. Within hours of an acute exposure, initial symptoms of headache, dizziness, confusion and blurred vision are found and these are followed by nausea, vomiting and diarrhoea.[65] Evidence of liver damage occurs 24–48 hours after exposure with tender hepatomegaly, increasing jaundice and a bleeding diathesis. In severe cases, ascites and coma can result. Death due to liver disease usually occurs within ten days of the onset of symptoms. The liver disease can last for three weeks, before recovery occurs, which in survivors, is rapid. The laboratory findings include marked elevation of the serum transaminase levels. Serum bilirubin rapidly rises, due to hepatocyte necrosis, haemolysis, destruction of the cytochrome P_{450} enzymes and decreased renal excretion of bilirubin. Liver histology shows centrilobular necrosis and steatosis. CCl_4 is no longer produced on a large scale in Western Europe or the United States and occupational exposure typically only occurs in countries that still allow its use.[44,64,66]

Treatment is supportive. In the experimental animal, carbon dioxide-induced hyperventilation has been shown to increase the pulmonary elimination of volatile hydrocarbons and to prevent CCl_4 toxicity. Prostacycline (prostaglandin I_2) is hepato-protective, even when given 24 hours after intoxication.[67] The mortality rate from CCl_4 poisoning is 10–25 per cent, most deaths occurring from renal failure. Hepatic causes of death account for one-quarter of the total, and occur in the first week after intoxication. If the patient survives, recovery is usually complete, but hepatic fibrosis and cirrhosis can ensue.

TRICHLOROMETHANE (CHLOROFORM)

This chemical was used in the community as a spot cleaning agent and formerly as an anaesthetic when death due to hepatic necrosis was occasionally reported.[68] Exposure is by inhalation. In acute chloroform poisoning, hepatotoxicity is associated with elevation of enzymes and in severe cases with coma. Empirical treatment with haemoperfusion, activated charcoal and N-acetylcysteine has been employed.[69] Some workers exposed daily for 12–48 months to moderately high levels of trichloromethane developed liver disorders. Subjects with pre-existing liver disease may be more sensitive to the effect of trichloromethane. Possible clinical presentations include jaundice, hepatomegaly and 'transaminitis' and cirrhosis is a possible sequel.

TRICHLOROETHANE

The most important isomer is 1,1,1-trichloroethane (methylchloroform) which is used extensively as an industrial degreasing agent. Experimental hepatotoxicity has been demonstrated in mice.[70] There are a number of isolated case reports of acute and chronic liver disease probably associated with exposure to this industrial solvent.[71–73] In man, presentation may be with ascites and hepatosplenomegaly, while the liver biopsy may show fibrosis, perivenular sclerosis of the central veins and subacute hepatic necrosis.[74] Occupational exposure has been associated with fatty liver and cirrhosis.[75] Patients with pre-existing chronic liver disease may be more sensitive to liver injury following exposure to very high levels of trichloroethane.

TETRACHLOROETHANE

This chlorinated hydrocarbon solvent is no longer used because of its hepatotoxicity, which was identified as a result of heavy exposures to workers in the First World War when it was used as 'dope' in aeroplane manufacture.[5] Absorption was mostly by inhalation, although occasionally ingestion and skin absorption occurred. Low-grade exposure produced hepatomegaly and a few patients became jaundiced. If the patient is removed from the contaminated environment, the liver recovers rapidly, but continued exposure can produce jaundice, hepatomegaly and ascites together with fulminant hepatic failure and subacute hepatic necrosis, both of which may be fatal.[76] The overall mortality rate was approximately 17 per cent. The histology is similar to that found with carbon tetrachloride and includes centrizonal necrosis, steatosis and bile duct proliferation. If exposure is prolonged, the patient may die of subacute hepatic necrosis often followed by post-necrotic fibrosis.[68]

TRICHLOROETHYLENE

Trichloroethylene was used in dry cleaning and as a degreasing agent in industry, but it has been replaced by less toxic chemicals. It is structurally similar to vinyl chloride. Severe liver injury can be seen in individuals who have sniffed solvents; they may develop raised serum transaminase levels associated with acute hepatic and renal failure.[77] Liver disease is rarely caused by occupational exposure, although fatal addiction at work may occur,[78] and acute hepatic failure has been described with degreasing. The liver histological changes include fatty liver, fibrosis and centrilobular necrosis, many of which have the potential for recovery after withdrawal from exposure. Trichloroethylene has been implicated as a probable cause of non-alcoholic steatohepatitis (NASH) in a patient suffering from chronic hepatitis C.[79]

TETRACHLOROETHYLENE (PERCHLOROETHYLENE)

This is probably the least hepatotoxic of the chlorinated hydrocarbons used as dry cleaning agents. Accidental exposure can produce central nervous system (CNS) depression, followed by hepatic and renal damage. Serum bilirubin, transaminases and ALP may be elevated; a variety of liver lesions has been described, including acute hepatitis and centrilobular necrosis.[80–82] Diagnosis is dependent on the history, supported by a chloroform-like odour of the solvent, which may be detected on the patient's breath for several hours after exposure. Repeated vapour exposures to high concentrations of tetrachloroethylene have produced hepatitis in experimental animals. Mild to moderate hepatic parenchymal changes were found on ultrasound scan in two-thirds of dry cleaners exposed to tetrachloroethylene, but only 19 per cent had a raised serum transaminase (ALT) level.[83]

N-Substituted amides

DIMETHYL ACETAMIDE

Acute toxicity of this solvent leads to raised serum transaminases and hepatomegaly, with focal necrosis on liver biopsy. More prolonged exposures are associated with microvesicular steatosis. Recovery after removal from the toxin may be incomplete.[84,85]

DIMETHYL FORMAMIDE

Acute exposure to dimethyl formamide (DMF) may be associated with raised AST and ALT levels and chronic exposure with microvesicular steatosis, while in severe cases hepatic necrosis can occur.[86,87] This widely used industrial solvent was incriminated in an outbreak of liver disease in workers coating fabric in poorly ventilated areas without appropriate skin protection: 62 per cent of workers tested had a raised serum AST or ALT and histology compatible with toxic hepatitis was found in the small number of patients biopsied.[88]

Nitro-paraffins

Nitromethane, nitroethane, 1-nitropropane and 2-nitropropane are used extensively in industry as solvents. Hepatotoxic effects may be underdiagnosed because 2-nitropropane (2-NP) is rarely used alone as a solvent and any toxicity is usually blamed on other chemicals. This chemical can produce acute liver failure.[89] Histology shows centrilobular necrosis, bile duct proliferation, cholestasis, steatosis and a mild inflammatory infiltrate in the periportal areas.[90] In one report,[91] two construction workers applied epoxy-resin coating to a water main in an under-ventilated underground vault; no protection was provided for their respiratory tracts or skin. One patient died of fulminant hepatic failure, while the other survived. 2-NP is also a hepatocarcinogen.

Acute liver damage produced by 2-NP in the experimental animal can be reduced by treatment with the antioxidant diphenyl diselenide.[92] The hepatotoxicity of this chemical is associated with lipid peroxidation and in the experimental animal at least, it can be reduced by pretreatment with either melatonin[93] or green tea infusion in drinking water.[94]

Toluene

Acute hepatocellular injury, with reversible renal failure, has been reported in a glue sniffer.[95] However, in a controlled study of car painters exposed to toluene, no increased hepatotoxicity was seen compared to controls.[96] 2,4,6-Trinitrotoluene (TNT) (see under Trinitrotoluene) is an important occupational and environmental pollutant which may be associated with toxic hepatitis, hepatomegaly and hepatocellular carcinoma. A recent study of TNT workers in an ammunition factory in China showed evidence of urinary mutagenicity and chromosomal abnormalities and monitoring of certain biomarkers may be of more value in assessing toxicity than chemical measurements of TNT metabolites in the air or on the skin.[97] The enormous production of munitions over the past century has led to large-scale discharge into the environment of water containing explosives and nitrated organic byproducts.[98]

Chlorinated napthalenes

A number of cases of acute yellow atrophy of the liver have occurred in workshops in which chlorinated napthalenes were used to impregnate electrical equipment. The average time of exposure varied from four to six months. The presentation is with general malaise followed by jaundice, associated with anorexia, dizziness, weight loss, vomiting and upper abdominal pain. Liver changes include necrosis, fibrosis and regeneration, which may be associated with acute enterocolitis together with pancreatitis. Hepatic decompensation was revealed by the presence of jaundice, ascites and oedema. Many patients who survived the acute insult developed subacute hepatic necrosis or macronodular cirrhosis.[99,100] Polychlorinated napthalenes induce the cytochrome P_{450} system and produce lipid peroxidation in the liver.[101] A study of workers in an electrical capacitor manufacturing plant, where chlorinated napthalenes were used with polychlorinated biphenyls (PCBs) and other chemicals, has shown a significantly increased mortality for liver and biliary tract cancer.[102]

Nitroaromatics

TRINITROTOLUENE

Trinitrotoluene (TNT) produced a considerable amount of hepatotoxicity in munitions workers in the First and Second World Wars, with an incidence of hepatotoxicity ranging from <0.01 to 5 per cent.[103] Since this time, the incidence of liver damage has been markedly decreased by improvement in industrial techniques. Absorption is largely through the skin, but inhalation, ingestion or mucus membrane exposure, may also result in significant absorption. The mechanism is unclear, but may be related to the production of a toxic intermediate. There appears to be a marked individual difference in susceptibility to the hepatotoxic effects of TNT. After a latent period of two to four months during the exposure period, the patient develops anorexia, weakness, nausea, vomiting and abdominal pain with hepatomegaly and jaundice. Some patients go on to develop fulminant hepatic failure, which may be fatal in up to 25 per cent. Others develop subacute hepatic failure with ascites and portal hypertension. These symptoms may be accompanied by extrahepatic manifestations, including rash, aplastic anaemia and methaemoglobinaemia. Some patients who survive chronic exposure may go on to develop macronodular cirrhosis.[104,105]

NITROBENZOATE

Nitrobenzoate has been used as a hepatotoxin in the experimental animal. Rare cases of liver damage have occurred in humans exposed to inhalation of toxic fumes during the production of aniline. It is also a potential human carcinogen.[10]

DINITROPHENOL

Dinitrophenol is used in the dye industry and in the manufacture of photographic developers, and workers may be exposed by inhalation or dermal contact. Rarely, it may cause cholestatic or necrotic liver injury.[106]

Aromatic hydrocarbon mixtures

Coke oven and byproduct workers may be exposed to emissions composed of polycyclic aromatic hydrocarbons and volatile organic compounds. Some of these are hepatotoxins. Workers most heavily exposed to coke oven emissions exhibit altered aminotransferase levels.[107]

Solvents and non-alcoholic steatohepatitis

In 1980, Ludwig et al.[108] described a series of patients who lacked a history of significant alcohol intake but in whom the liver histology resembled that of alcoholic liver disease. They termed this condition 'non-alcoholic steatohepatitis'. The main features on liver biopsy are steatosis (fatty liver), lobular inflammation, balloon degeneration of hepatocytes and Mallory bodies, with or without fibrosis.

It is recognized that NASH is the most common type of liver disease in affluent societies, affecting between 1 and 8 per cent of the population. Typically, it is asymptomatic, but in up to 16 per cent of cases, NASH may progress to advanced hepatic fibrosis and cirrhosis, sometimes associated with hepatic decompensation, and hepatocellular carcinoma may occasionally occur.[109]

Typically, NASH is associated with obesity, diabetes mellitus and hypertriglyceridaemia and recent studies from Brazil have clearly implicated solvents as a cause of NASH in petrochemical workers who lacked any alternative risk factors.[110] These Brazilian petrochemical workers were selected for study on the basis of having serum transaminase and/or GGTP levels at least 1.5 times the upper limit of normal in three or more determinations. They had been potentially exposed to a wide range of petrochemical products including acryonitrile, acetylene, benzene, carbon tetrachloride, chloroform, chloroethyl vinyl ether, dimethyl formamide, ethane, ethylene, hexane, methanol, toluene, trinitrotoluene, tetrachloroethane, vinyl chloride, styrene, xylene and hydrocarbon mists. The period of exposure was for at least five years. Improvement in liver enzyme tests occurred in workers removed from the industrial area. Further studies comparing such workers lacking alternative risk factors for NASH, with first, other workers exposed to petrochemicals who also presented with obesity, hyperlipidaemia or diabetes, and second, with NASH occurring in patients with risk factors other than petrochemicals, have characterized 'petrochemical NASH' as typically occurring in men younger than non-exposed individuals and histological evidence of cholestasis was more frequent. All exposed workers with NASH were asymptomatic. All subjects had elevated ALT, AST and GGTP levels and ultrasound scan showed steatosis. The mean time of work in the petrochemical industry was 15 ± 5.4 years. The liver histology characteristically showed relatively mild changes of steatohepatitis and fibrosis, but the long-term evolution of these changes has yet to be reported.[110–112] A lesion similar to NASH was reported from Spain in victims who had inadvertently consumed adulterated cooking oil[113] in the toxic oil syndrome epidemic in 1981.

STYRENE

Workers exposed to styrene when working with fibreglass-reinforced plastics, or boat and tank fabricators, may exhibit raised levels of direct-reacting bilirubin, alkaline phosphatase, ALT and AST, suggesting mild hepatic injury.[114]

SOLVENT MIXTURES

Workers are typically exposed to a single solvent, but mixtures of solvents are occasionally encountered, and sometimes in unusual environments. Thus, a study of asymptomatic craftsmen repairing shoes demonstrated abnormal liver function tests and it was suggested that periodic liver screening may be appropriate.[115] In car painters exposed to solvent mixtures in Brazil, measurement of serum bile acids appeared to be the most reliable measure of subclinical hepatotoxicity,[116] since elevated serum GGTP levels are often associated with obesity and alcohol consumption rather than occupational solvent exposure.[117,118]

MEDICOLEGAL ASPECTS OF SOLVENT HEPATOTOXICITY

While the liver biopsy appearances in individuals acutely exposed to high concentrations of solvents may be highly suggestive of toxic exposure, the more normal context is of chronic low-grade exposure and here the situation, from a medicolegal viewpoint, is much more complex. The liver has only a limited number of ways of responding to injurious agents, whether chemical, drug, viral, metabolic or autoimmune and the patterns of liver injury observed with these differing insults may overlap. The most common histological pattern with chronic, low-grade exposure to solvents appears to be NASH, which is undistinguishable from NASH due to other causes. Since the risk factors associated with NASH, such as overweight and obesity, hypertension, hyperlipidaemia and diabetes are so common and since the biopsy appearances in NASH may be similar to those seen in alcoholic liver disease, attribution of NASH to solvent exposure in a court of law is difficult. A successful outcome for the plaintiff is more likely if other causes of chronic liver disease can be excluded by the non-invasive liver screen (Table 88.1) and if the histology is compatible with NASH, especially if no other risk factors for NASH are present. The case is strengthened if it can be shown that suitable precautions and appropriate workplace environmental recommendations have not been followed. It is also likely that low level solvent exposure below recommended limits may act synergistically with other risk factors, such as alcohol consumption, overweight, hypertension and raised serum lipids or blood sugar, to cause NASH. However, while the synergism (the 'two-hit hypothesis')[119] is very likely from a medical point of view, it may be difficult to establish a causal link to liver damage in a court of law, due to the lack of a clear association between symptoms and liver damage (established by raised liver enzymes and liver biopsy) and also due to the lack of published information concerning the duration and levels of exposure to solvents required to produce NASH. However, this difficulty may be addressed by the new DNA microarray technology, in which samples of DNA from healthy persons are exposed to the chemical in question to determine which genes are affected (i.e. upregulated or downregulated). This is then used as a blueprint against which a claimant's DNA can be compared. This technique has already been used in courts in the United States in more than 20 cases involving chemicals as diverse as benzene and hexavalent chromium.[120,121]

Metals and metalloids

COPPER

With acute poisoning, jaundice as a result of liver injury and haemolysis occurs on the second or third day in about a quarter of patients. Elevated transaminases and hepatomegaly are also features.

Liver granulomas containing copper have been found in vineyard workers exposed to an antifungal spray called Bordeaux mixture which contained a 1–2 per cent aqueous copper sulphate solution.[122] The most common hepatic abnormality was a raised serum ALP; hepatomegaly was present in 40 per cent and one of seven patients biopsied had hepatic granulomata. Other features described in chronic occupational copper toxicity in vineyard sprayers include Kupffer cell proliferation, fibrosis, cirrhosis, portal hypertension and one case of angiosarcoma. While copper can be demonstrated in the liver histochemically, the gold standard for the diagnosis of liver disorders associated with increased hepatic copper is direct biochemical estimation by neutron activation analysis. Copper-induced hepatotoxicity is a multifactorial process involving the generation of reactive oxygen species that can affect biomolecules directly, with a consequent enhancement in membrane lipid peroxidation, DNA damage and protein oxidation.[123]

Acute copper toxicity is managed by gastric lavage to remove copper. Although penicillamine, a heavy metal chelator, is extremely effective in Wilson's disease,[124] there is no evidence that it is of benefit in acute copper poisoning.

ARSENIC

An outbreak of arsenic-induced liver disease in beer drinkers was reported from Manchester, England in 1900,[125] where the severity of the liver disease was proportional to the amount of arsenic in the beer. However, occupational exposure to arsenic has been most common in the production and use of pesticides. Up to 1942, when the use of these insecticides was banned, there was a significant incidence of cirrhosis in grape workers and vintners.[25] Exposure was in the form of oral ingestion via insecticide sprays and dust, which also led to high levels of residual arsenic in the wine. Occupational and environmentally induced liver disease secondary to arsenic exposure is exclusively chronic. Associated clinical features include pigmentation with spotty melanosis of the skin and hyperkeratoses of the palms of the hands and soles of the feet with tumours of the skin and other sites.[126]

Both organic and inorganic arsenicals cause necrosis of hepatocytes, injure sinusoidal and endothelial cells, and may cause obliteration and thrombosis of intrahepatic portal vein radicals. Although the number of cases of chronic liver disease in German vintners declined after 1942, the incidence of arsenical cirrhosis at autopsy continued to rise until the early 1950s due to the persistent effect of arsenic in the tissues, though alcoholism was likely to be a compounding factor in many cases.[25] Four patients with severe liver damage due to arsenic poisoning in the Mosel vintners died of cirrhosis, but milder forms of arsenic liver damage underwent healing with some degree of periportal scarring.[25] Chronic arsenic exposure can produce a variety of different patterns of liver injury, including steatosis, cirrhosis, non-cirrhotic portal hypertension, angiosarcoma and primary liver cancer.[127] A recent study of patients exposed to environmental arsenic for up to ten years, and noted to have hepatomegaly showed chronic inflammation, vacuolation and focal necrosis on liver biopsy, while cDNA microarray studies showed changed expression of genes involved in cell-cycle regulation, apoptosis and DNA damage response.[128] Similar studies have clarified the mechanism of arsenic-induced carcinogenicity.[129] The liver function tests in liver damage due to chronic arsenic poisoning are frequently normal, although bromosulphophthalein (BSP) retention may be present. Scalp hair arsenic levels may be raised and skin biopsy sometimes shows marked hyperkeratosis typical of chronic arsenic poisoning. On the other hand, analysis of tumour, liver, hair and other organs and tissues in a patient dying of haemangio-endothelial sarcoma due to arsenic poisoning showed no significant traces of arsenic.[127] In one case of non-cirrhotic portal hypertension, arsenic content on percutaneous liver biopsy, measured by neutron activation analysis, was markedly increased at 28 μg/g (normal being <0.25 μg/g dry liver).[28] The value of treatment with dimercaprol, a heavy metal chelator, is uncertain.[130]

Environmental arsenic poisoning has reached massive proportions in recent years in West Bengal and Bangladesh.[131] In an effort to supply clean drinking water to rural villages, thousands of tube wells have been sunk to allow use of subsurface water. Unfortunately, natural arsenic concentrations in this groundwater can reach very high levels and it is reported that over 220 000 people are now suffering from arsenic-related diseases. It is estimated that up to 90 million people in these areas are at risk. However, susceptibility to arsenic-induced liver diseases differs greatly between individuals, probably due to interindividual variations in arsenic metabolism.[132] Arsenite is an important cancer chemotherapeutic, but hepatotoxicity may limit its therapeutic value. Recent studies suggest that nitric oxide releasing prodrugs may reduce this hepatotoxicity.[133]

BERYLLIUM

Beryllium poisoning can produce a spectrum of hepatic abnormalities,[134] including hepatomegaly, focal or centrilobular necrosis, and granulomata which mimic those found in sarcoidosis, and contain beryllium.[135] In the past, exposures were primarily by inhalation; only rare case reports now occur due to significant improvements in industrial hygiene.

PHOSPHORUS

Acute poisoning is usually from suicidal intent, but hepatotoxicity from the manufacture of firecrackers has been reported.[136] Histological changes include microvesicular steatosis and necrosis,[5] while in the long term fibrosis may develop.[23] Diagnosis depends on the detection of a characteristic garlic odour on the breath, with phosphorescence of the stool.

CADMIUM

A wide spectrum of hepatotoxic effects, ranging from minor abnormality in liver function tests to necrosis or cirrhosis are found.[137] Increased hepatic cadmium concentrations have been implicated in the pathogenesis of cryptogenic liver disease in Japan.[138] Occupational hepatotoxicity has been reported in gold smelting.[1] In the experimental animal, cadmium damages hepatic mitochondria, increases lipid peroxidation, induces apoptosis, damages endothelial cells, activates Kupffer cells and induces collagen gene expression. Some of these pathological processes are prevented or modified by treatment with putrescine[139] or antioxidants, such as vitamin E or N-acetylcysteine.[140]

SELENIUM

At low concentrations, selenium is an essential trace element. At higher concentrations, acute hepatotoxicity can occur from accidental ingestion or inhalation of selenium dioxide or hydrogen selenide, resulting in steatosis.[141] In large quantities, and with chronic exposure, selenium can produce cirrhosis and, possibly, hepatic neoplasia.[142] In contrast, low plasma selenium levels are found in alcoholic liver disease[143,144] possibly resulting in oxidant stress, since glutathione peroxidase, an important factor in antioxidant defence, requires selenium as a cofactor.

CHROMIUM

The cytotoxic and genotoxic effects of chromium compounds depend on their valency and solubility. In vitro, kidney epithelial cells are ten times more sensitive towards Cr(VI) treatment than liver (Hep G2) epithelial cells, which explains the nephrotoxicity of this compound in vivo.[145]

However, chronic occupational exposure has been reported to produce hepatotoxicity in a chromium plating factory. Toxic hepatitis was accompanied by mild to moderate abnormalities in liver function tests.[146]

LEAD

Lead exposure occurs in workers involved in lead smelting and the manufacture of batteries, car radiators and pigments. Before 1977, when the lead content of paint was regulated, some construction workers had significant exposures. Lead inhibits enzymes involved in haem synthesis, interferes with certain energy and transport systems and may affect nucleic acid metabolism. While acute lead hepatotoxicity has not been reported, high blood levels (>75 mg/dL) were associated with liver injury in a series from Spain.[147] Liver biopsies showed centrilobular hepatitis with steatosis. Withdrawal from lead exposure led to rapid resolution of the liver dysfunction. In addition, chelation therapy appears to be of value.[10,147]

Pesticides and herbicides

This section includes herbicides, insecticides and fungicides which have different chemical structures and toxicities. Although the effects of acute pesticide poisoning are well known for the pesticides most commonly used, few data exist on the hepatic effects after long-term, low-dose exposure. Agricultural workers studied during the course of a spraying season in Spain showed mild elevations of serum AST levels, but no clinically significant hepatotoxicity.[148] The common pesticides associated with experimental hepatotoxicity are DDT, methoxychlor, chlordane, heptachlor, aldrin, dieldrin, lindane and chlordecone, but the evidence that they are hepatotoxic or hepatocarcinogenic in humans is conflicting. Acute hepatotoxicity has been reported after rare accidental ingestion of large amounts of DDT,[149] while centrizonal necrosis and hepatic failure after a single dose of 6 g of DDT has occurred. However, despite massive production, there is little evidence from the literature of poisoning in workers. Only minor elevations of AST and reductions in BSP excretion have been recorded. There has been no report of liver injury in the United States, despite exposure for 20 years with absorption of 500 times the daily ingestion of the average adult.[5] DDT induces hepatic mixed function oxidase which may result in production of hepatotoxic and hepatocarcinogenic metabolites from parent chemicals or drugs already in the environment or body.[150,151] Carcinogenicity in humans has been debated for years. However, no study has shown a definite risk of cancer in humans and the carcinogenic role of pesticides in the experimental animal is also disputed.

CHLORDECONE (KEPONE)

In the 1970s, chlordecone was detected in high concentrations in samples of blood, adipose tissue and liver from highly exposed factory workers at a kepone manufacturing plant in Virginia.[152,153] Many of the exposed factory workers had hepatomegaly and some had splenomegaly. Liver function tests were mostly normal and liver biopsy showed only non-specific changes. Two or three years after exposure ceased, there was no pesticide in the tissues, the liver and spleen were of normal size and the liver histology was normal.[154] There is evidence of potentiation of carbon tetrachloride hepatotoxicity by chlordecone in rats, which is both age and sex dependent.[155] Animals exposed to chlordecone develop liver cell injury and neoplastic changes,[156,157] but the ultimate effects of exposure in humans are unknown. Cohn et al.[153] reported on the use of cholestyramine to accelerate elimination of chlordecone following industrial exposure and toxicity. Chlordecone is no longer manufactured.

CHLOROPHENOXY HERBICIDES

In experimental animals, there is only minor evidence of hepatotoxicity[158] and the major effect on the liver appears to be induction of mixed function oxidases of the hepatic microsomes. Hepatotoxic effects have been attributed to 2,4,5-trichlorophenoxy acetic acid, but this toxicity is probably due to contamination with 2,3,7,8-tetrachlorodibenzo-p-dioxin. A major concern is a possible synergistic hepatotoxicity from two or more synthetic chemicals. Despite concurrent exposure to multiple organochlorine compounds, workers engaged in the manufacture or handling of mixtures of pesticides seldom manifest hepatotoxic effects.[159]

PARAQUAT

Paraquat (1,1'dimethyl 4,4'dipyridylium dichloride) is a powerful herbicide and toxicity is occasionally seen in manufacturers and gardeners. Accidental ingestion of as little as 2 g can produce shock, renal failure, pulmonary oedema and jaundice.[160,161] Toxicity may occur as a result of skin exposure or ingestion. Liver histology shows congestion with centrilobular necrosis, acidophilic bodies, steatosis, injury to the interlobular bile ducts and cholestasis. There may be two phases of hepatotoxicity; first, hepatocellular injury and then after two days, cholangiocellular damage.[161] Biochemical findings include raised serum bilirubin, transaminases and ALP. Paraquat induces hepatic lipid peroxidation and atypical necrosis (aponecrosis) and these processes, together with their high associated mortality rates, can be reduced in the experimental animal by pretreatment with vitamin E and selenium.[162,163]

Polychlorinated biphenyls

The manufacture of PCBs was banned in the 1970s due to their persistence in animal and human tissues and in the environment, but the liquids had become widely used as coolants and insulators in electrical systems. Skin absorption of PCBs in workers in the electrical manufacturing industry is followed by hepatic metabolism resulting in induction of the cytochrome P_{450} system and amino laevulinic acid (ALA) synthetase,[4,164–167] which may lead to porphyria (Figure 88.3). Abnormal liver function tests have been reported in workers exposed to PCBs,[168,169] but these reports have been poorly controlled and lack histology. Raised GGTP levels in serum may persist for up to two years after handling PCBs.[170] In general, raised enzyme levels correlate with serum PCB concentrations. PCBs can produce hepatocellular carcinoma in animals.[164] It is not clear whether they are direct carcinogens or whether carcinogenicity is associated with the metabolites, produced by cytochrome P_{450}. Two cases of hepatoma have been reported in autopsy examinations of patients from the Yusho epidemic in Japan in 1968,[171] in which about 10 000 people were affected[172,173] by consuming rice oil accidentally contaminated in the factory. The Taiwan epidemic of acute PCB toxicity known as Yucheng in 1979 also occurred after ingestion of contaminated rice oil.[174] In both cases, the major features were chloracne, conjunctivitis, neuropathy and oedema of the eyelids, while jaundice developed in 11 per cent.[175] Porphyria has also been reported.[176] Although elevated mortality from liver disease may occur in the short term, more recent studies have attributed the hepatotoxicity to contaminating dibenzofurans.[10,174] Epidemiological studies of the long-term effects of PCBs in humans have failed to show a significant increase in deaths from cirrhosis or hepatoma, but the long-term consequences of exposure are not known.

Vinyl chloride

This halogenated aliphatic hydrocarbon is structurally similar to trichloroethylene. Despite its known toxicity, it is still a vital component of the plastics industry in the manufacture of the widely used plastic polyvinyl chloride (PVC). Hepatotoxicity used to occur primarily by inhalation of vinyl chloride monomer (VCM) gas in workers manufacturing this chemical. Hepatic fibrosis, hepatosplenomegaly, non-cirrhotic portal hypertension, angiosarcoma and hepatocellular carcinoma have all been reported. Severe acute exposure in laboratory animals (more than 8000 ppm) produces hepatic necrosis 24–48 hours after exposure, associated with raised serum transaminases and GGTP levels.[5] Recovery is usually rapid and fulminant hepatic necrosis is rare. Histology shows isolated necrosis of hepatocytes with occasional polymorph infiltrate. In chronic exposure in workers, liver biopsy findings may be unremarkable, but in other patients, hepatic fibrosis is more marked, with extensive capsular and subcapsular fibrosis and portal fibrosis extending into the parenchyma and into the wall of portal vein branches.[177] Peliosis hepatis is occasionally seen. Non-cirrhotic portal hypertension, including nodular regenerative hyperplasia, has been reported and may be a precursor to angiosarcoma (ASL), a rare liver tumour in the general population. With the introduction of industrial measures designed to drastically reduce exposure in the United States, the United Kingdom and other European countries in 1974–75, when the toxicity of VCM became apparent, no cases of workers developing this tumour employed after that date are expected. By 1993, 173 cases had been documented in 14 countries[178] and the trend in UK experience[27] of the 20 cases diagnosed up to 1994 in workers exposed under the old factory conditions showed, at that time, no sign of decreasing (Figure 88.7). The authors calculated, based on duration of manufacture, age range and number of workers exposed and maximum latency of ASL, that a further 11–14 cases were likely to present. This study is also interesting in that all 20 of the UK cases of ASL came from only two of the seven factories in the UK producing VCM. In the two years following the publication of this paper, only two further cases were diagnosed by this group (personal communication). These findings may suggest a latent period of around 20 years.

The clinical features are those of a rapidly enlarging malignant liver tumour, although serum levels of α-fetoprotein (AFP) (a tumour marker associated with hepatocellular carcinoma) are usually normal. Metastases are unusual, but the prognosis is poor, the mean survival from presentation to death being 3.5 months (range 1.5–13). Most patients die from hepatic failure, although death from intraperitoneal haemorrhage may occur. VCM workers also have an increased incidence of hepatocellular carcinoma, especially if they are infected with the hepatitis B virus; serum AFP is frequently raised in such cases.[179]

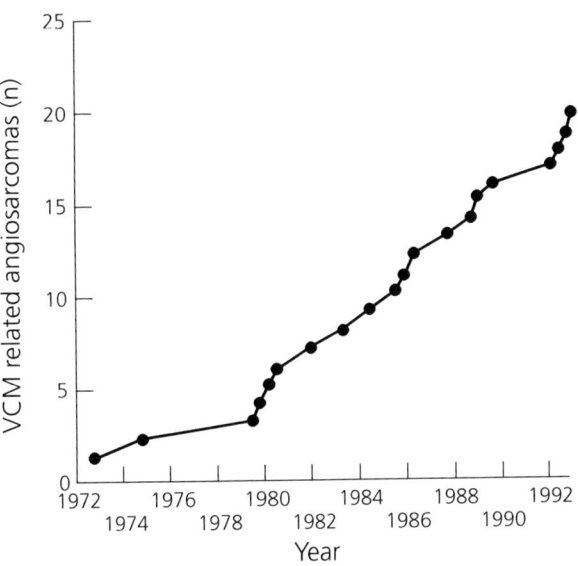

Figure 88.7 United Kingdom cumulative total of vinyl chloride monomer (VCM)-related angiosarcomas 1974–95. Reproduced from Ref. 27 with permission from the BMJ Publishing Group.

Under tight exposure controls for VCM workers, the value of screening with routine liver function tests is controversial. Thus, one group reported that serum ALP and GGTP were significantly elevated in workers exposed to VCM compared to controls, with no significant elevation in serum bilirubin, AST or ALT[180] and another group found that only GGTP was associated with current VCM exposure;[55] however, others reported that while relatively low levels of ethylene dichloride and VCM increase the risk of liver damage as demonstrated by raised serum ALT levels, GGTP was not associated with exposure to these chemicals.[54] Exposure to PVC or VCM may have a synergistic effect with chronic viral hepatitis B and C on liver damage produced by these viruses in high incidence countries for these infections as judged by raised serum aminotransferase activity.[56] However, liver function tests may fail to detect VCM-induced liver damage, while being of more value in suggesting steatosis or fibrosis due to non-occupational factors, such as alcohol intake, obesity and hyperlipidaemia.[181] Ultrasound examination of the liver is of value in detecting steatosis, but is generally considered to be less reliable in detecting the presence and extent of hepatic fibrosis. It has been employed, in conjunction with liver function tests, to screen VCM workers for liver damage[181,182] and in a large recent study was found to be of value in screening VCM workers; those exposed to 200 ppm for at least one year had a four-fold increased risk of periportal fibrosis.[183] Other screening tests advocated have included determination of fasting serum bile acids or low-dose indocyanine green clearance and measurement of urinary coproporphyrin excretion; however, none of these is widely used.

Methyl bromide

This is known to be hepatotoxic in both humans and animals. In one report,[184] intoxication simulated Reye's syndrome, but the liver histology merely showed hepatocyte swelling and sinusoidal congestion.

Cytotoxic drugs

Over 20 years ago, before the hazard became fully recognized, when tight exposure controls became instituted in hospitals, personnel working in oncology units or hospital pharmacies were at risk of developing insidious liver disease after chronic handling of cytotoxic drugs, including neomycin, vincristine, cyclophosphamide, doxorubicin, 5-fluorouracil and methotrexate.[185] Absorption is percutaneous or by inhalation. A free-radical based mechanism for the formation of active metabolites may explain the hepatotoxicity of some of these agents. Nurses handling these drugs can develop raised levels of gamma GT and ALP, while liver histology may show portal hepatitis, fibrosis and steatosis.[186] Increased mutagenicity in the urine of nurses handling these drugs has also been demonstrated.[187]

Phthalate esters

Both dioctyl phthalate and its isomer di-(2-ethyl hexyl) phthalate (DEHP) are plasticizers, which may be hepatotoxic[188,189] and hepatocarcinogenic[190,191] in the animal model. Dibutyl-phthalate is extensively used in industry and there is a high potential for human exposure in the workplace. In rats, it may cause hepatomegaly and cholestasis with elevated serum alkaline phosphatase levels.[192] However, there is no conclusive evidence for hepatotoxicity in humans.

CONCLUSIONS

It is now well established that oxidant stress plays an important pathogenic role in chronic liver disease in general[193–195] and in chemically induced liver disease in particular. In clinical practice, overt liver disease due to workplace exposure to hepatotoxins is nowadays rare, but is probably underdiagnosed and may be significantly more common than generally reported. The most important development in this area over the past few years has been the recognition that in patients with the histological appearance of NASH, but no evidence for the normally associated risk factors, certain solvent exposures can produce potentially serious chronic liver disease; in addition, synergistic interactions between solvent exposure and recognized risk factors for NASH such as obesity, hypertension, hyperlipidaemia and diabetes may increase the risk of liver damage.

However, exposure is often hard to quantify, and may occur some time prior to presentation of the liver disease. Furthermore, multiple agents may be implicated, making the actual toxic substance difficult to identify. Multiple agents which are themselves minimally toxic may act synergistically to produce injury. Safety procedures should be in place in the work environment which implies that reports of toxicity only occur when these measures break down and exposure becomes uncontrolled.

A number of difficulties complicate the diagnosis of occupational liver disease. The finding of abnormal liver function tests is relatively common in the general population, and elevations of serum GGTP are non-specific, while the interpretation of abnormal results can be complicated by the fact that alcoholism and drug ingestion may be denied. It has recently been shown that dramatically or intermittently elevated ALT levels may be of purely nutritional origin; especially when found in the absence of hepatic steatosis. Elevated ALT levels after a short overindulgent holiday can be caused not only by alcohol ingestion, but also by a higher than normal caloric intake than usual, particularly when this is associated with 'fast foods' combined with sedentary behaviour.[196,197] In addition, liver histology may be suggestive, but is never diagnostic, of occupational exposure to hepatotoxins.

Finally, proof of hepatotoxicity, even following acute exposure, is difficult to obtain. It would require (1) liver biopsy following the insult to characterize the damage; (2) the demonstration of recovery following removal of the hepatotoxin; and (3) most difficult, the demonstration (preferably including re-biopsy), of recurrence following re-exposure. In practice, these requirements are rarely, if ever, fulfilled.

In chronic liver disease, even when known causes are excluded, perhaps around 20 per cent of cases remain cryptogenic. In these, we are left to consider the possibilities of a novel, currently undiagnosable virus or occupational exposure to a hepatotoxin. Clearly, the latter is only likely to be diagnosed by a well-informed clinician who maintains a high index of suspicion, and who is aware of the new techniques, such as DNA microarray technology, now becoming available to clarify these issues.

> **Key points**
>
> - Diagnosis of occupational hepatotoxicity requires a high index of suspicion in the treating physician and a detailed history of possible exposure.
> - Although hepatotoxicity may occur after an acute exposure, it more commonly presents after chronic exposure or many years after exposure has ceased.
> - The liver only has a limited number of mechanisms to deal with hepatotoxins and the

- response of the liver will depend on the agent, duration and route of exposure.
- The hepatic response to hepatotoxins varies with genetic phenotype, with concurrent or subsequent exposure to prescribed drugs and alcohol and with the presence of other conditions, such as NASH, or its predisposing conditions, such as obesity and diabetes.
- Although routine workplace exposure to hepatotoxins in the developed world is now much less frequent due to increased awareness and health and safety legislation, exposure can still occur in less well-regulated industries, during accidental spills or escapes and particularly in the developing world.

ACKNOWLEDGEMENTS

We wish to acknowledge the assistance of Dr PM Smith and the late Dr FI Lee for their helpful discussions on the hepatotoxicity of vinyl chloride and for their permission to reproduce a figure from their paper[27] (reproduced as Figure 88.7). We also wish to acknowledge the assistance of Dr R Ede, of Hope Hospital, Manchester, for his advice on aspects of porphyrin metabolism and analysis. Finally, we would like to acknowledge the work of Dr Sanjiv Jain as a co-author of the earlier version of this chapter which appeared in the ninth edition of this textbook.

REFERENCES

1. Kahl R. Appendix 2. Liver injury in man ascribed to non-drug chemicals and natural toxins. In: McIntyre N, Benhamou JP, Bircher J et al. (eds). *Oxford Textbook of clinical hepatology*. Oxford: Oxford University Press, 1991.
2. Levy LS, Lee WR. Aliphatic chemicals (Chapter 9a). In: Raffle PAB, Adams PH, Baxter PJ, Lee WR (eds). *Hunter's Diseases of occupations*. London: Edwin Arnold, 1994.
3. Tar-Ching A. Aromatic chemicals (Chapter 9b). In: Raffle PAB, Adams PH, Baxter PJ, Lee WR (eds). *Hunter's Diseases of occupations*. London: Edwin Arnold, 1994.
4. Pond SM. Effects on the liver of chemicals encountered in the workplace. *Western Journal of Medicine*. 1982; **137**: 506–14.
5. Gitlin N. Clinical aspects of liver disease caused by industrial and environmental toxins. In: Zakim D, Boyer TD (eds). *Hepatology: A textbook of liver disease*, 3rd edn. Philadelphia: WB Saunders, 1996.
6. Kahl R. Toxic liver injury. In: McIntyre N, Benhamou JP, Bircher J et al. (eds). *Oxford textbook of clinical hepatology*. Oxford: Oxford University Press, 1991.
7. Dahm LS, Jones DP. Mechanisms of chemically induced liver disease. In: Zakim D, Boyer TD (eds). *Hepatology: A textbook of liver disease*, 3rd edn. Philadelphia: WB Saunders, 1996.
8. Dianzani MU. The role of free radicals in liver damage. *Proceedings of the Nutrition Society*. 1987; **46**: 43–52.
9. National Institute for Occupational Health and Safety. *Pocket guide to chemical hazards*. Washington DC: US Government Printing Office, US Department of Health and Human Services, Publication 97-140, 2004. Available from: www.cdc.gov/niosh/npg/npg.html.
10. Schiano TD, Hunt K. Occupational and environmental hepatotoxicity (Chapter 28). In: Boyer T, Wright T, Manns M (eds). *Zakim and Boyer's Hepatology*, 5th edn. Oxford: Elsevier, 2006.
11. Goddard CJR, Warnes TW. Raised liver enzymes in asymptomatic patients: Investigation and outcome. *Digestive Diseases*. 1992; **10**: 218–26.
12. Hultcrantz R, Glaumann H, Lindberg G, Nilsson LH. Liver investigation in 149 asymptomatic patients with moderately elevated activities of serum aminotransferases. *Scandinavian Journal of Gastroenterology*. 1986; **21**: 109–13.
13. Van Ness MM, Diehl AM. Is liver biopsy useful in the evaluation of patients with chronically elevated liver enzymes? *Annals of Internal Medicine*. 1989; **111**: 473–8.
14. Owens D, Evans J. Population studies on Gilbert's syndrome. *Journal of Medical Genetics*. 1975; **12**: 152–6.
15. Hasumura Y, Teschike R, Lieber CS. Increased carbon tetrachloride hepatotoxicity and its mechanism, after chronic ethanol consumption. *Gastroenterology*. 1974; **66**: 415–22.
16. Proctor E, Chatambra K. High yield of micronodular cirrhosis in the rat. *Gastroenterology*. 1982; **83**: 1183–90.
17. Zimmerman HJ, Mao R, Israsena S. Phenothiazine inhibition of carbon tetrachloride cytotoxicity *in vitro*. *Proceedings of the Society for Experimental Biology and Medicine*. 1966; **123**: 893–8.
18. Kopelman H, Scheuer PJ, Williams R. The liver lesion of the Epping Jaundice. *Quarterly Journal of Medicine*. 1966; **35**: 553–64.
19. Kopelman H, Robertson MH, Sanders PG, Ash I. The Epping jaundice. *British Medical Journal*. 1966; **1**: 514–16.
20. Bastian PG. Occupational hepatitis caused by methylenedianiline. *Medical Journal of Australia*. 1984; **141**: 553–5.
21. Diaz-Rivera RS, Collazo PJ, Pons ER, Torregrosa MV. Acute phosphorus poisoning. *Medicine*. 1950; **29**: 269–98.
22. Slater TF. Necrogenic action of carbon tetrachloride in the rat: A speculative mechanism based on activation. *Nature*. 1966; **209**: 36–40.
23. Greenburger NJ, Robinson WL, Isselbacher KJ. Toxic hepatitis after the ingestion of phosphorous with subsequent recovery. *Gastroenterology*. 1964; **47**: 179–83.
24. Britton RS, Bacon BR. Retinoids and oxyradicals in fibrogenesis. Therapeutic implications. In: Arroyo V, Bosch J, Bruguera M, Rodes J (eds). *Therapy in liver disease and the physiological basis of treatment*. London: Massoni, 1997.

25. Lüchtrath H. Cirrhosis of the liver in chronic arsenical poisoning of vintners. *German Medicine*. 1972; **2**: 127-8.
26. Smith PM, Crossley IR, Williams DMJ. Portal hypertension in vinyl chloride workers. *Lancet*. 1976; **2**: 602-4.
27. Lee FI, Smith PM, Bennett B, Williams DMJ. Occupationally related angiosarcoma of the liver in the United Kingdom, 1972-1994. *Gut*. 1996; **39**: 312-18.
28. Morris JS, Schmid M, Newman S et al. Arsenic and noncirrhotic portal hypertension. *Gastroenterology*. 1974; **64**: 86-94.
29. Chainuvati T, Viranuvatti V. Idiopathic portal hypertension and chronic arsenic poisoning. Report of a case. *Digestive Diseases and Sciences*. 1979; **24**: 70-3.
30. Jhaveri SS. A case of cirrhosis and primary carcinoma of the liver in chronic industrial arsenical intoxication. *British Journal of Industrial Medicine*. 1959; **16**: 248-50.
31. Evans DMD, Jones Williams W, Kung ITM. Angiosarcoma and hepatocellular carcinoma in vinyl chloride workers. *Histopathology*. 1983; **7**: 377-88.
32. Huff J, Lucier G, Tritscher A. Carcinogenicity of TCDD: Experimental, mechanistic and epidemiological evidence. *Annual Review of Pharmacology and Toxicology*. 1994; **34**: 343-72.
33. Whysner J, Williams GM. 2,3,7,8-tetrachlorodibenzo-p-dioxin. Mechanistic data and risk assessment. Gene regulation, cytotoxicity, enhanced cell proliferation and tumour promotion. *Pharmacology and Therapeutics*. 1996; **71**: 193-223.
34. Schmid R. Cutaneous porphyria in Turkey. *New England Journal of Medicine*. 1960; **263**: 397-8.
35. Peters H, Cripps D, Göcmen A et al. Turkish epidemic of hexachlorobenzene porphyria. *Annals of the New York Academy of Sciences*. 1987; **514**: 183-90.
36. Cripps DJ, Peters HA, Gocmen A, Dogramici I. Porphyria turcica due to hexachlorobenzene: A 20 to 30 year follow up study on 204 patients. *British Journal of Dermatology*. 1984; **111**: 413-52.
37. Doss M, Lange C-E, Veltman G. Vinyl chloride-induced hepatic coproporphyrinuria with transition to chronic hepatic porphyria. *Klinische Wochenschrift*. 1984; **62**: 175-8.
38. Chalmers JNM, Gillam AE, Kench JE. Porphyrinuria in a case of industrial methyl chloride poisoning. *Lancet*. 1940; **1**: 806-8.
39. Doss MO. Porphyrinurias and occupational disease. *Annals of the New York Academy of Sciences*. 1987; **514**: 204-18.
40. Goldstein JA, Hickman P, Bergman H, Vos JG. Hepatic porphyria induced by 2,3,7,8-tetrachloro dibenzo-p-dioxin in the mouse. *Research Communications in Chemical Pathology and Pharmacology*. 1973; **6**: 919-28.
41. Doss MO, Sauer H, von Tiepermann R, Colombi AM. Development of chronic hepatic porphyria (porphyria cutanea tarda) with an inherited uroporphyrinogen decarboxylase deficiency under exposure to dioxin. *International Journal of Biochemistry*. 1984; **16**: 369-73.
42. Strick JJTWA, Janssen MMT, Colombi AM. Incidence of chronic hepatic porphyria in an Italian family. *International Journal of Biochemistry*. 1980; **12**: 879-81.
43. Kappas A, Sassa S, Anderson KE. The porphyrias. In: Stanbury JB, Wyngaarden JB, Fredrickson DS et al. (eds). *The metabolic basis of inherited disease*, 5th edn. New York: McGraw-Hill, 1983.
44. Weber LW, Boll M, Stampfl A. Hepatotoxicity and mechanism of action of haloalkanes: Carbon tetrachloride as a toxicological model. *Critical Reviews in Toxicology*. 2003; **33**: 105-36.
45. Recknagel RO, Glende EA, Britton RS. Free radical damage and lipid peroxidation. In: Meeks RG, Steadman D, Bull RJ (eds). *Hepatotoxicology*. Boca Raton, FL: CRC Press, 1991.
46. Britton RS, Bacon BR. Role of free radicals in liver disease and hepatic fibrosis. *Hepato-Gastroenterology*. 1994; **41**: 343-8.
47. Recknagel RO. Carbon tetrachloride hepatotoxicity. *Pharmacological Reviews*. 1967; **19**: 145-208.
48. Judah JD, McLean AEM, McLean EK. Biochemical mechanisms of liver injury. *American Journal of Medicine*. 1970; **49**: 609-16.
49. McConkey DJ, Aw TY, Orrenius S. Role of Ca^{2+}-mediated endonuclease activation in chemical toxicity. In: Dekant W, Nawmann H-A (eds). *Tissue specific toxicity: Biochemical mechanisms*. London: Academic Press, 1992.
50. Harries HM, Fletcher ST, Duggan CM, Baker VA. The use of genomics technology to investigate gene expression changes in cultured human liver cells. *Toxicology In Vitro*. 2001; **15**: 399-405.
51. Hsieh HI, Chen PC, Wong RH et al. Effect of the CYP2E1 genotype on vinyl chloride monomer-induced liver fibrosis among polyvinyl chloride workers. *Toxicology*. 2007; **239**: 34-44.
52. Schindler J, Li Y, Marion MJ et al. The effect of genetic polymorphisms in the vinyl chloride metabolic pathway on mutagenic risk. *Journal of Human Genetics*. 2007; **52**: 448-55.
53. Zhu SM, Ren XF, Wan JX, Xia ZL. Evaluation in vinyl chloride monomer-exposed workers and the relationship between liver lesions and gene polymorphisms of metabolic enzymes. *World Journal of Gastroenterology*. 2005; **11**: 5821-7.
54. Cheng TJ, Huang ML, You NC et al. Abnormal liver function in workers exposed to low levels of ethylene dichloride and vinyl chloride monomer. *Journal of Occupational and Environmental Medicine*. 1999; **41**: 1128-33.
55. Du CL, Kuo ML, Chang HL et al. Changes in lymphocyte single strand breakage and liver function of workers exposed to vinyl chloride monomer. *Toxicology Letters*. 1995; **77**: 379-85.
56. Hsieh HI, Wang JD, Chen PC, Cheng TJ. Synergistic effect of hepatitis virus infection and occupational exposures to vinyl chloride monomer and ethylene dichloride on serum aminotransferase activity. *Occupational and Environmental Medicine*. 2003; **60**: 774-8.

57. Qiu Y, Zhu S, Liu J, Xia Z. Study of susceptibility of chromosomal damage induced by vinyl chloride monomer associated with genetic polymorphism in APE1, XRCC1 (article in Chinese with English abstract). *Wei Sheng Yan Jiu*. 2007; **36**: 132–6.
58. De Matteis F. Role of iron in the hydrogen peroxide-dependent oxidation of hexahydroporphyrin (porphyrinogen): A possible mechanism for the exacerbation by iron of hepatic uroporphyria. *Molecular Pharmacology*. 1988; **33**: 463–9.
59. Dennison MS, Fisher JM, Whitlock JP. The DNA recognition site for the dioxin-Ah receptor complex. *Journal of Biological Chemistry*. 1988; **263**: 1722–4.
60. Pratt WB. The role of the hsp-90 based chaperone system in signal transduction by nuclear receptors and receptor signalling via MAP kinase. *Annual Review of Pharmacology and Toxicology*. 1997; **37**: 297–324.
61. Frumkin H. Agent Orange and cancer: An overview for clinicians. *CA: A Cancer Journal for Clinicians*. 2003; **53**: 245–55.
62. Døssing M, Arlien-Søborg P, Milling Petersen L, Ranek L. Liver damage associated with occupational exposure to organic solvents in house painters. *European Journal of Clinical Investigation*. 1983; **13**: 151–7.
63. Døssing M, Ranek L. Isolated liver damage in chemical workers. *British Journal of Industrial Medicine*. 1984; **41**: 142–4.
64. Brautbar N, Williams J 2nd. Industrial solvents and liver toxicity: Risk assessment, risk factors and mechanisms. *International Journal of Hygiene and Environmental Health*. 2002; **205**: 479–91.
65. Nielsen VK, Larsen J. Acute renal failure due to CCl_4 poisoning. *Acta Medica Scandinavica*. 1965; **178**: 363–74.
66. Basu S. Carbon tetrachloride-induced lipid peroxidation: Eicosanoid formation and their regulation by antioxidant nutrients. *Toxicology*. 2003; **189**: 113–27.
67. Divald A, Uihelyi A, Jeney K et al. Hepatoprotective effects of prostacyclins on CCl_4-induced liver injury in rats. *Experimental and Molecular Pathology*. 1985; **42**: 163–6.
68. Willcox W. Toxic jaundice. *Lancet*. 1931; **2**: 57–63.
69. Choi SH, Lee SW, Hong YS et al. Diagnostic radio-opacity and hepatotoxicity following chloroform ingestion: A case report. *Emergency Medicine Journal*. 2006; **23**: 394–5.
70. McNutt NS, Amster RL, McConnell EE, Morris F. Hepatic lesions in mice after continuous inhalation exposure to 1,1,1-trichloroethane. *Laboratory Investigation*. 1975; **32**: 642–54.
71. Cohen C, Frank AL. Liver disease following occupational exposure to 1,1,1-trichloroethane: A case report. *American Journal of Industrial Medicine*. 1994; **26**: 237–41.
72. Xu ZJ, Zhang QH, Yang H. Clinical analysis of 19 patients with acute toxic hepatitis by 1,1,1-trichloroethane (in Chinese). *Zhonghua Gan Zang Bing Za Zhi*. 2003; **11**: 557.
73. Croquet V, Fort J, Oberti F et al. 1,1,1-trichloroethane-induced chronic active hepatitis (in French). *Gastroentérologie Clinique et Biologique*. 2003; **27**: 120–2.
74. Texter EC Jr, Grunow WA, Zimmerman HJ. Massive centrizonal necrosis of the liver due to inhalation of 1,1,1-trichloroethane. *Gastroenterology*. 1979; **76**: 1260 (Abstr.).
75. Thiele DL, Eigenbrodt EH, Ware AJ. Cirrhosis after repeated trichloroethylene and 1,1,1-trichloroethane exposure. *Gastroenterology*. 1982; **83**: 926–9.
76. Gurney R. Tetrachloroethane intoxication: Early recognition of liver damage and means of prevention. *Gastroenterology*. 1943; **1**: 1112–26.
77. Baerg RD, Kimberg DV. Centrolobular hepatic necrosis and acute renal failure in 'solvent sniffers'. *Annals of Internal Medicine*. 1970; **73**: 713–20.
78. James WRL. Fatal addiction to trichloroethylene. *British Journal of Industrial Medicine*. 1963; **20**: 47–9.
79. Caprioli F, Pometta R, Visentin S et al. 'Hepatitic flare', asthenia, peripheral polyneuropathy and diffuse liver steatosis in a hepatitis C virus asymptomatic chronic carrier. *Digestive and Liver Disease*. 2001; **33**: 359–62.
80. Meckler LC, Phelps DK. Liver disease secondary to tetrachloroethylene exposure. A case report. *Journal of the American Medical Association*. 1966; **197**: 662–3.
81. Stewart RD. Acute tetrachloroethylene intoxication. *Journal of the American Medical Association*. 1969; **208**: 1490–2.
82. Hughes JP. Hazardous exposure to some so-called safe solvents. *Journal of the American Medical Association*. 1954; **156**: 234–7.
83. Brodkin CA, Daniell W, Checkoway H et al. Hepatic ultrasonic changes in workers exposed to perchloroethylene. *Occupational and Environmental Medicine*. 1995; **52**: 679–85.
84. Marino G, Anastopoulos H, Woolf AD. Toxicity associated with severe inhalational and dermal exposure to dimethylacetamide and 1,2-ethanediamine. *Journal of Occupational Medicine*. 1994; **36**: 637–41.
85. Perbellini L, Princivalle A, Caivano M, Montagnani R. Biological monitoring of occupational exposure to N,N-dimethylacetamide with identification of a new metabolite. *Occupational and Environmental Medicine*. 2003; **60**: 746–51.
86. Luo JC, Kuo HW, Cheng TJ, Chang MJ. Abnormal liver function associated with occupational exposure to dimethylformamide and hepatitis B virus. *Journal of Occupational and Environmental Medicine*. 2001; **43**: 474–82.
87. Wrbitzky R. Liver function in workers exposed to N,N-dimethylformamide during the production of synthetic textiles. *International Archives of Occupational and Environmental Health*. 1999; **72**: 19–25.
88. Redlich CA, West AB, Fleming L et al. Clinical and pathological characteristics of hepatotoxicity associated with occupational exposure to dimethylformamide. *Gastroenterology*. 1990; **99**: 748–57.
89. Hine CH, Pasi A, Stephens BG. Fatalities following exposure to 2-nitropropane. *Journal of Occupational Medicine*. 1978; **20**: 333–7.
90. Skinner JB. The toxicity of 2-nitropropane. *Industrial Medicine*. 1947; **16**: 441–3.

91. Harrison R, Letz G, Pasternak G, Blanc P. Fulminant hepatic failure after occupational exposure to 2-nitropropane. *Annals of Internal Medicine*. 1987; **107**: 466-8.
92. Borges LP, Nogueira CW, Panatieri RB *et al*. Acute liver damage induced by 2-nitropropane in rats: Effect of diphenyl diselenide on antioxidant defenses. *Chemico-biological Interactions*. 2006; **160**: 99-107.
93. Kim SJ, Reiter RJ, Rouvier Garay MV *et al*. 2-Nitropropane-induced lipid peroxidation: Antitoxic effects of melatonin. *Toxicology*. 1998; **130**: 183-90.
94. Sai K, Kai S, Umemura T *et al*. Protective effects of green tea on hepatotoxicity, oxidative DNA damage and cell proliferation in the rat liver induced by repeated oral administration of 2-nitropropane. *Food and Chemical Toxicology*. 1998; **36**: 1043-51.
95. O'Brien ET, Yeoman WB, Hobby JAE. Hepatorenal damage from toluene in a glue sniffer. *British Medical Journal*. 1971; **2**: 29-30.
96. Kurppa K, Husman K. Car painter's exposure to a mixture of organic solvents. Serum activities of liver enzymes. *Scandinavian Journal of Environmental Health*. 1982; **8**: 137-40.
97. Sabbioni G, Sepai O, Norppa H *et al*. Comparison of biomarkers in workers exposed to 2,4,6-trinitrotoluene. *Biomarkers*. 2007; **12**: 21-37.
98. Lewis TA, Newcombe DA, Crawford RL. Bioremediation of soils contaminated with explosives. *Journal of Environmental Management*. 2004; **70**: 291-307.
99. Flinn FB, Jarvik NE. Actions of certain chlorinated napthalenes on the liver. *Proceedings of the Society for Experimental Biology and Medicine*. 1936; **35**: 118-20.
100. Flinn FB, Jarvik NE. Liver lesions caused by chlorinated napthalene. *American Journal of Hygiene*. 1938; **27**: 19-27.
101. Galoch A, Sapota A, Skrzypinska-Gawrysiak M, Kilanowicz A. Acute toxicity of polychlorinated naphthalenes and their effect on cytochrome P450. *Human and Experimental Toxicology*. 2006; **25**: 85-92.
102. Mallin K, McCann K, D'Aloisio A *et al*. Cohort mortality study of capacitor manufacturing workers, 1944-2000. *Journal of Occupational and Environmental Medicine*. 2004; **46**: 565-76.
103. McConnell WJ, Flinn RH. Summary of twenty-two trinitrotoluene fatalities in World War II. *Journal of Industrial Hygiene and Toxicology*. 1946; **28**: 76-82.
104. Livingston-Learmouth A, Cunningham BM. Observations on the effects of trinitrotoluene on women workers. *Lancet*. 1916; **2**: 261-4.
105. Martland HS. Trinitrotoluene poisoning. *Journal of American Medical Association*. 1917; **68**: 835-7.
106. Zimmerman HJ. Experimental hepatotoxicity. In: Zimmerman HJ (ed.). *Hepatotoxicity: The adverse effects of drugs and other chemicals on the liver*. Philadelphia: Lippincott Williams & Wilkins, 1999: 217.
107. Wu MT, Mao IF, Wypij D *et al*. Serum liver function profiles in coking workers. *American Journal of Industrial Medicine*. 1997; **32**: 478-86.
108. Ludwig J, Viggiano TR, McGill DB, Oh BJ. Nonalcoholic steatohepatitis: Mayo Clinic experiences with a hitherto unnamed disease. *Mayo Clinic Proceedings*. 1980; **55**: 434-8.
109. Farrell GC, George J, Hall PD *et al*. *Fatty liver disease: NASH and related disorders*. Oxford: Blackwell, 2005.
110. Cotrim HP, Andrade ZA, Parana R *et al*. Nonalcoholic steatohepatitis: A toxic liver disease in industrial workers. *Liver*. 1999; **19**: 299-304.
111. Brunt EM. Nonalcoholic steatohepatitis (NASH): Further expansion of this clinical entity. *Liver*. 1999; **19**: 263-4.
112. Cotrim HP, De Freitas LA, Freitas C *et al*. Clinical and histopathological features of NASH in workers exposed to chemicals with or without associated metabolic conditions. *Liver International*. 2004; **24**: 131-5.
113. Solis-Herruzo JA, Vidal JV, Colina F *et al*. Clinico-biochemical evolution and late hepatic lesions in the toxic oil syndrome. *Gastroenterology*. 1987; **93**: 558-68.
114. Brodkin CA, Moon JD, Camp J *et al*. Serum hepatic biochemical activity in two populations of workers exposed to styrene. *Occupational and Environmental Medicine*. 2001; **58**: 95-102.
115. Tomei F, Giuntoli P, Biagi M *et al*. Liver damage among shoe repairers. *American Journal of Industrial Medicine*. 1999; **36**: 541-7.
116. Nunes de Paiva MJ, Pereira Bastos de Siqueira ME. Increased serum bile acids as a possible biomarker of hepatotoxicity in Brazilian workers exposed to solvents in car repainting shops. *Biomarkers*. 2005; **10**: 456-63.
117. Fernández-D'Pool J, Oroño-Osorio A. Liver function of workers occupationally exposed to mixed organic solvents in a petrochemical industry. *Investigación Clínica*. 2001; **42**: 87-106.
118. Rees D, Soderlund N, Cronje R *et al*. Solvent exposure, alcohol consumption and liver injury in workers manufacturing paint. *Scandinavian Journal of Work and Environmental Health*. 1993; **19**: 236-44.
119. Day CP, James OF. Steatohepatitis: A tale of two 'hits'? *Gastroenterology*. 1998; **114**: 842-5.
120. Hawkes N. DNA test that could quickly solve thousands of sick workers' claims. *The Times*. September 17, 2008, p. 4.
121. Gavin IM, Gillis B, Arbieva Z, Prabhakar BS. Identification of human cell responses to hexavalent chromium. *Environmental and Molecular Mutagenesis*. 2007; **48**: 650-7.
122. Pimentel JC, Menezes AP. Liver granulomas containing copper in vineyard sprayer's lung. *American Journal of Respiratory Diseases*. 1975; **111**: 189-95.
123. Videla LA, Fernández V, Tapia G, Varela P. Oxidative stress-mediated hepatotoxicity of iron and copper: Role of Kupffer cells. *Biometals*. 2003; **16**: 103-11.
124. Sherlock S, Dooley J. *Diseases of the liver and biliary system*, 10th edn. Oxford: Blackwell, 1997.
125. Kelynack TN, Kirkby W, Delépine S, Tattersall CH. Arsenical poisoning from beer drinkers. *Lancet*. 1900; **1**: 1600-3.
126. Cowlishaw JL, Pollard EJ, Cowan AE, Powell LW. Liver disease associated with chronic arsenic ingestion. *Australia and New Zealand Journal of Medicine*. 1979; **9**: 310-13.

127. Regelson W, Kim U, Ospina J, Holland JF. Hemangioendothelial sarcoma of liver from chronic arsenic intoxication by Fowler's solution. *Cancer.* 1968; **21**: 514–22.
128. Lu T, Liu J, LeCluyse EL *et al.* Application of cDNA microarray to the study of arsenic-induced liver diseases in the population of Guizhou, China. *Toxicological Sciences.* 2001; **59**: 185–92.
129. Chen H, Liu J, Merrick BA, Waalkes MP. Genetic events associated with arsenic-induced malignant transformation: Applications of cDNA microarray technology. *Molecular Carcinogenesis.* 2001; **30**: 79–87.
130. Eagle H, Magnusson HJ. The systemic treatment of 227 cases of arsenic poisoning (encephalitis, dermatitis, blood dyscrasias, jaundice, fever) with 2,3 dimercaptopropanol (BAL). *American Journal of Syphilis, Gonorrhea, and Venereal Diseases.* 1946; **30**: 420–41.
131. Kumar S. Widescale arsenic poisoning found in South Asia. *Lancet.* 1997; **349**: 1387.
132. Schläwicke Engström K, Broberg K, Concha G *et al.* Genetic polymorphisms influencing arsenic metabolism: Evidence from Argentina. *Environmental Health Perspectives.* 2007; **115**: 599–605.
133. Qu W, Liu J, Fuquay R *et al.* The nitric oxide prodrug, V-PYRRO/NO, mitigates arsenic-induced liver cell toxicity and apoptosis. *Cancer Letters.* 2007; **256**: 238–45.
134. Sneddon IB. Berylliosis: A case report. *British Medical Journal.* 1955; **1**: 1448–50.
135. Prine JR, Brokeshoulder SF, McVean DE *et al.* Demonstration of the presence of beryllium in pulmonary granulomas. *American Journal of Clinical Pathology.* 1966; **45**: 448–54.
136. Marin GA, Montoya CA, Sierra JL, Senior JR. Evaluation of corticosteroid and exchange transfusion treatment in acute yellow phosphorous intoxication. *New England Journal of Medicine.* 1971; **284**: 125–8.
137. Singhal RL, Merali Z, Hrdina PD. Aspects of the biochemical toxicology of cadmium. *Federation Proceedings.* 1976; **35**: 75–80.
138. Sumino D, Hayakawa D, Shibata T *et al.* Heavy metals in normal Japanese tissues. Amounts of 15 heavy metals in 30 subjects. *Archives of Environmental Health.* 1975; **30**: 487–94.
139. Tzirogiannis KN, Panoutsopoulos GI, Demonakou MD *et al.* The hepatoprotective effect of putrescine against cadmium-induced acute liver injury. *Archives of Toxicology.* 2004; **78**: 321–9.
140. Shaikh ZA, Vu TT, Zaman K. Oxidative stress as a mechanism of chronic cadmium-induced hepatotoxicity and renal toxicity and protection by antioxidants. *Toxicology and Applied Pharmacology.* 1999; **154**: 256–63.
141. Schellman B, Raithel HJ, Schaller KH. Acute fatal selenium poisoning. *Archives of Toxicology.* 1986; **59**: 61–4.
142. Diplock AT. Metabolic aspects of selenium action and toxicity. *CRC Critical Reviews in Toxicology.* 1976; **4**: 219–26.
143. Korpela H, Kumpulainen J, Luoma PV *et al.* Decreased serum selenium in alcoholics as related to liver structure and function. *American Journal of Clinical Nutrition.* 1985; **42**: 147–51.
144. Dworkin B, Rosenthal WS, Jankowski RH *et al.* Low blood selenium in alcoholics with and without advanced liver disease. *Digestive Diseases and Sciences.* 1985; **30**: 838–44.
145. Dartsch PC, Hildenbrand S, Kimmel R, Schmahl FW. Investigations on the nephrotoxicity and hepatotoxicity of trivalent and hexavalent chromium compounds. *International Archives of Occupational and Environmental Health.* 1998; **71** (Suppl.): S40–5.
146. Pascale LR, Sheldon S, Waldstein MD *et al.* Chromium intoxication with special reference to hepatic injury. *Journal of the American Medical Association.* 1952; **149**: 1385–9.
147. Sanchez JA, de la Fuente JM, Castrillo JM *et al.* Hepatotoxidad por plomo inorganico: Resultados de 85 casos de saturnismo aguado. *Gastroenterología y Hepatología.* 1985; **8**: 246–50.
148. Hernández AF, Amparo Gómez M, Pérez V *et al.* Influence of exposure to pesticides on serum components and enzyme activities of cytotoxicity among intensive agriculture farmers. *Environmental Research.* 2006; **102**: 70–6.
149. Smith NJ. Death following accidental ingestion of DDT. *Journal of American Medical Association.* 1948; **136**: 469–71.
150. Fouts JR. Interaction of chemicals and drugs to produce effects on organ function. In: Lee DHK, Koten P (eds). *Multiple factors in the causation of environmentally induced disease.* New York: Academic Press, 1972.
151. Mitchell JR, Gillette JR. Drug–chemical interactions as a factor in experimentally induced disease. In: Lee DHK, Koten P (eds). *Multiple factors in the causation of environmentally induced disease.* New York: Academic Press, 1972.
152. Taylor JR, Selhorst JB, Houff SA *et al.* Chlordecone intoxication in man. 1. Clinical observations. *Neurology.* 1978; **28**: 626–30.
153. Cohn WJ, Boylan JJ, Blanke RV *et al.* Treatment of chlordecone (Kepone) toxicity with cholestyramine: Results of a controlled clinical trial. *New England Journal of Medicine.* 1978; **298**: 243–8.
154. Guzelian PS, Vranian J, Boylan JJ *et al.* Liver structure and function in patients poisoned with chlordecone (Kepone). *Gastroenterology.* 1980; **78**: 206–13.
155. Blain RB, Reeves R, Ewald KA *et al.* Susceptibility to chlordecone-carbon tetrachloride induced hepatotoxicity and lethality is both age and sex dependent. *Toxicological Sciences.* 1999; **50**: 280–6.
156. Anonymous. Report on carcinogenesis assay of technical grade chlordecone (Kepone). *American Industrial Hygiene Association Journal.* 1976; **37**: 680–1.
157. Eroschenko VP, Wilson WO. Cellular changes in the gonads, livers and adrenal glands of Japanese quail as affected by the insecticide Kepone. *Toxicology and Applied Pharmacology.* 1975; **31**: 491–504.

158. Rip JW, Cherry JH. Liver enlargement induced by the herbicide 2,4,5-trichlorophenoxyacetic acid (2, 4, 5-T). *Journal of Agricultural and Food Chemistry.* 1976; **24**: 245–50.
159. Deichmann WB, MacDonald WE. Organochlorine pesticides and liver cancer deaths in the United States, 1930–1972. *Ecotoxicology and Environmental Safety.* 1977; **1**: 89–110.
160. Bullivant CM. Accidental poisoning by paraquat: Report of two cases in man. *British Medical Journal.* 1966; **1**: 1272–3.
161. Mullick FG, Ishak KG, Mahabir R *et al.* Hepatic injury associated with paraquat toxicity in humans. *Liver.* 1981; **1**: 209–21.
162. Cheng WH, Quimby FW, Lei XG. Impacts of glutathione peroxidase-1 knockout on the protection by injected selenium against the pro-oxidant-induced liver aponecrosis and signaling in selenium-deficient mice. *Free Radical Biology and Medicine.* 2003; **34**: 918–27.
163. Nakagawa I, Suzuki M, Imura N, Naganuma A. Involvement of oxidative stress in paraquat-induced metallothionein synthesis under glutathione depletion. *Free Radical Biology and Medicine.* 1998; **24**: 1390–5.
164. Kimbrough RD. The toxicity of polychlorinated polycyclic compounds and related chemicals. *CRC Critical Reviews in Toxicology.* 1974; **2**: 445–98.
165. Nicholson WJ, Moore JA (eds). Health effects of halogenated aromatic hydrocarbons. *Annals of the New York Academy of Sciences.* 1979; **320**: 1–730.
166. Alvares AP, Fischbein A, Anderson KE, Kappas A. Alterations in drug metabolism in workers exposed to polychlorinated biphenyls. *Clinical Pharmacology and Therapeutics.* 1977; **22**: 140–6.
167. Alvares AP, Kappas A. The inducing properties of polychlorinated biphenyls on hepatic mono-oxygenases. *Clinical Pharmacology and Therapeutics.* 1977; **22**: 809–16.
168. Maroni M, Colombi A, Cantoni S *et al.* Occupational exposure to polychlorinated biphenyls in electrical workers. I. Environmental and blood polychlorinated biphenyls concentrations. *British Journal of Industrial Medicine.* 1981; **38**: 49–54.
169. Maroni M, Colombi A, Arbosti G *et al.* Occupational exposure to polychlorinated biphenyls in electrical workers. II. Health effects. *British Journal of Industrial Medicine.* 1981; **38**: 55–60.
170. Fischbein A. Liver function tests in workers with occupational exposure to polychlorinated biphenyls (PCBs): Comparison with Yusho and Yu-Cheng. *Environmental Health Perspectives.* 1985; **60**: 145–50.
171. Kikuchi M. Autopsy of patients with Yusho. *American Journal of Industrial Medicine.* 1984; **5**: 19–30.
172. Kuratsune M. An epidemiological study on 'Yusho' poisoning. *Fubuoka Acta Medica.* 1969; **60**: 403–10.
173. Kuratsune M, Yoshimura T, Matzusaka J *et al.* Epidemiologic study on Yusho, a poisoning caused by ingestion of rice oil contaminated with a commercial brand of polychlorinated biphenyls. *Environmental Health Perspectives.* 1972; **1**: 119–26.
174. Reggiani G, Bruppacher R. Symptoms, signs and findings in humans exposed to PCBs and their derivatives. *Environmental Health Perspectives.* 1985; **60**: 225–32.
175. Urabe H, Koda H, Asahi M. Current state of Yusho patients. *Annals of the New York Academy of Sciences.* 1979; **320**: 273–6.
176. Seki Y, Kawanishi S, Sano S. Mechanisms of PCB-induced porphyria and Yusho disease. *Annals of the New York Academy of Sciences.* 1987; **514**: 222–34.
177. Marsteller HJ, Lebach WK, Muller R *et al.* Chronic liver lesions in PVC (polyvinyl chloride) producing workers. *Deutsche Medizinische Wochenschrift.* 1973; **98**: 2311–14.
178. Forman D, Bennett B, Stafford J, Doll R. Exposure to vinyl chloride and angiosarcoma of the liver: A report of the register of cases. *British Journal of Industrial Medicine.* 1985; **42**: 750–3.
179. Du C-L, Wang JD. Increased morbidity odds ratio of primary liver cancer and cirrhosis of the liver among vinyl chloride monomer workers. *Occupational and Environmental Medicine.* 1998; **55**: 528–32.
180. Attarchi MS, Aminian O, Dolati M, Mazaheri M. Evaluation of liver enzyme levels in workers exposed to vinyl chloride vapors in a petrochemical complex: A cross-sectional study. *Journal of Occupational Medicine and Toxicology.* 2007; **2**: 6.
181. Maroni M, Fanetti AC. Liver function assessment in workers exposed to vinyl chloride. *International Archives of Occupational and Environmental Health.* 2006; **79**: 57–65.
182. Zhu SM, Ren XF, Wan JX, Xia ZL. Evaluation in vinyl chloride monomer-exposed workers and the relationship between liver lesions and gene polymorphisms of metabolic enzymes. *World Journal of Gastroenterology.* 2005; **11**: 5821–7.
183. Maroni M, Mocci F, Visentin S *et al.* Periportal fibrosis and other liver ultrasonography findings in vinyl chloride workers. *Occupational and Environmental Medicine.* 2003; **60**: 60–5.
184. Shield LK, Coleman TL, Markesbery WR. Methyl bromide intoxication: Neurologic features, including simulation of Reye's syndrome. *Neurology.* 1977; **27**: 959–62.
185. Knowles RS, Virden JE. Handling of injectable antineoplastic agents. *British Medical Journal.* 1980; **2**: 589–91.
186. Sotaniemi EA, Sutinen S, Arranto AJ *et al.* Liver damage in nurses handling cytostatic agents. *Acta Medica Scandinavica.* 1983; **214**: 181–9.
187. Falck K, Grohn P, Sorsa M *et al.* Mutagenicity in urine of nurses handling cytostatic drugs. *Lancet.* 1979; **1**: 1250–1.
188. Reddy JK, Warren JR, Reddy MK, Lalwani ND. Hepatic and renal effects of peroxisome proliferators: Biological implications. *Annals of the New York Academy of Sciences.* 1982; **386**: 81–110.
189. Moody DE, Reddy JK. Serum triglyceride and cholesterol contents in male rats receiving diets containing plasticizers and analogues of the ester 2-ethoxyethanol. *Toxicology Letters.* 1982; **10**: 379–83.

190. Warren JR, Lalwani ND, Reddy JK. Phthalate esters as peroxisome proliferator carcinogens. *Environmental Health Perspectives.* 1982; **45**: 35–40.
191. Kluwe WM, Haseman JK, Douglas JF, Huff JE. The carcinogenicity of dietary di-(2-ethoxyethyl) phthalate (DEHP) in Fischer 344 rats and B6C3F mice. *Journal of Toxicology and Environmental Health.* 1982; **10**: 797–815.
192. Marsman D. NTP technical report on the toxicity studies of dibutyl phthalate (CAS No. 84-74-2) administered in feed to F344/N rats and B6C3F1 mice. *Toxicity Report Series.* 1995; **30**: 1–G5.
193. Jain SK, Pemberton PW, Smith A *et al.* Oxidative stress in chronic hepatitis C: Not just a feature of late stage disease. *Journal of Hepatology.* 2002; **36**: 805–11.
194. Pemberton PW, Aboutwerat A, Smith A *et al.* Oxidant stress in type I autoimmune hepatitis: The link between necroinflammation and fibrogenesis? *Biochimica Biophysica Acta.* 2004; **1689**: 182–9.
195. Pemberton PW, Smith A, Warnes TW. Non-invasive monitoring of oxidant stress in alcoholic liver disease. *Scandinavian Journal of Gastroenterology.* 2005; **40**: 1102–8.
196. Marchesini G, Ridolfi V, Nepoti V. Hepatotoxicity of fast food? *Gut.* 2008; **57**: 568–70.
197. Kechagias S, Ernersson A, Dahlqvist O *et al.* Fast Food Study Group. Fast-food-based hyper-alimentation can induce rapid and profound elevation of serum alanine aminotransferase in healthy subjects. *Gut.* 2008; **57**: 649–54.

Workplace exposures and reproductive health

JENS PETER BONDE

Introduction	1196	Childhood cancer	1208
The range of adverse reproductive outcomes	1196	Risk assessment and clinical counselling	1208
Infertility	1196	Risk management	1209
Adverse pregnancy outcomes	1201	References	1210
Developmental toxicity	1208		

INTRODUCTION

Reproductive hazards in the workplace become an issue for the general practitioner, the obstetrician and the occupational health professional when pregnant women ask for advice on how to safely carry on their work. Similarly, infertility and adverse pregnancy outcomes are rather common, but causes are most often hard to identify. Infertile couples and affected families may be concerned about occupational exposures. There are several well-known examples of infertility, birth defects and other adverse reproductive outcomes that are caused by noxious exposures at the workplace. Therefore, there is a need for proper professional counselling. The purpose of this chapter is to help the reader undertake appropriate risk assessment as a basis for advising patients, families and workplaces.

THE RANGE OF ADVERSE REPRODUCTIVE OUTCOMES

The reproductive cycle can be divided into four phases, all of which are susceptible to disruption from occupational exposures: (1) gametogenesis and the sexual act in adult men and women; (2) prenatal development from fertilization through implantation, embryogenesis and fetal growth; (3) lactation and weaning; and (4) the prepubertal growth and development and sexual maturation. While direct occupational exposures are only likely in the first three reproductive phases, the adverse effects may be manifested in all four phases (Figure 89.1). Some effects are seen immediately as miscarriage related to intoxication with organic solvents, other effects may take months to develop as, for instance, reduced sperm count and infertility due to pesticide exposure and yet other effects may be latent for years as, for example, minor cognitive disturbances in school-age children following exposure to inorganic lead in the prenatal and early years of life.

Some biological processes of the reproductive cycle are more sensitive to environmental disruption as meiotic cell divisions and embryogenesis. In the following, the adverse reproductive end points are presented with a description of occurrence, mechanisms of action and occupational risk factors, while general approaches to clinical examination and risk assessment are outlined in concluding paragraphs.

INFERTILITY

Epidemiology

In the clinical setting, infertility is defined as the inability to become pregnant within one year of regular intercourse. This limit is of course arbitrary. In healthy young couples not using contraception, the probability to obtain a clinical recognized pregnancy within one menstrual cycle, the fecundability, is about 25 per cent.[1] The chance that healthy couples with normal fecundity do not become pregnant within one year because of bad luck is 3 per cent [$(1-0.25)^{12}$]. In contrast, subfertile couples may become pregnant within one year because of good luck. If, for instance, the fecundability is reduced to 50 per cent of the average, then $(1-(1-0.125)^{12}) = 80$ per cent will become pregnant within the first year of trying.

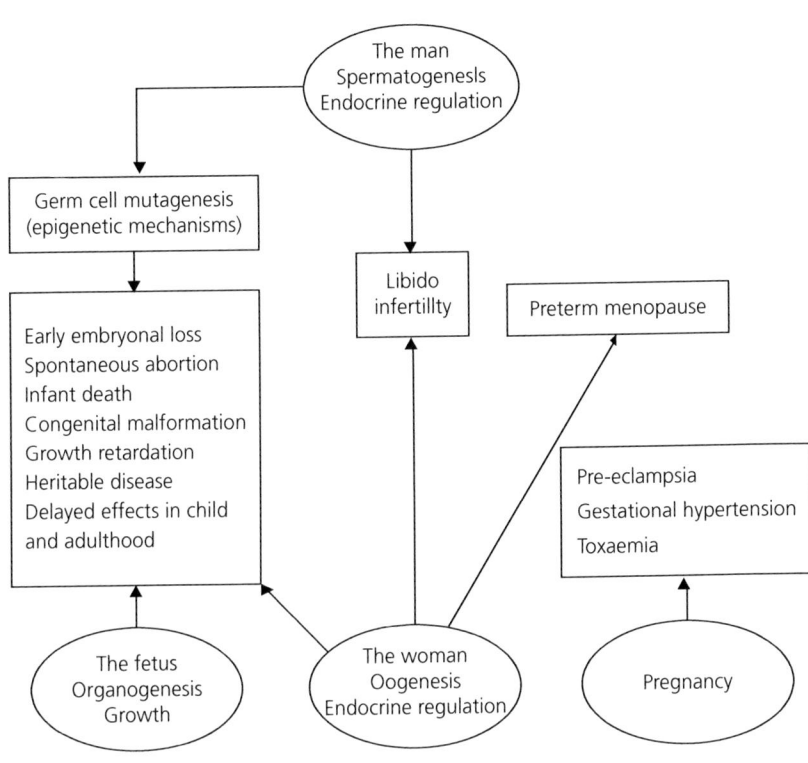

Figure 89.1 The range of short- and long-term adverse effects on reproductive function following exposure during the preconceptional, the prenatal and perinatal reproductive period.

The prevalence of infertility is in the range of 15–20 per cent in affluent countries[2] and some 6 per cent of children are conceived by artificial fertilization techniques. Clinical series indicate that female factors are involved in about 50 per cent of infertile cases and male factors in about 30 per cent.[3,4] The fecundity decreases substantially after 30 years of age among women, while male fecundity only declines moderately after 50 years of age. Tobacco smoking is known to reduce the fecundability among women with an average 30 per cent, but effects in adult men are limited.[5] Emerging evidence indicates that the male fetal gonad is highly sensitive to maternal smoking resulting in low sperm count after puberty.

Several reports indicate that sperm counts have declined in some regions during past decades. Increasing incidence of testicular cancer and possibly cryptorchidism and hypospadias parallels this trend. Since it is well established that testicular cancer has fetal origins, it has been hypothesized that all these conditions share a common prenatal aetiology.[6] Recent prospective studies demonstrate that the fecundability starts declining when sperm count gets lower than 40 million/mL (Figure 89.2).[7] Several surveys from various parts of Europe in the past ten years show that a sizeable proportion of men of fertile age have a sperm count below this limit (Figure 89.3).[8] Due to a lack of appropriate biological indices of female fecundity, little is known about regional or temporal shifts of fertility in women.

Mechanisms

Occupational exposures can adversely affect the male and the female reproductive systems at several levels that may

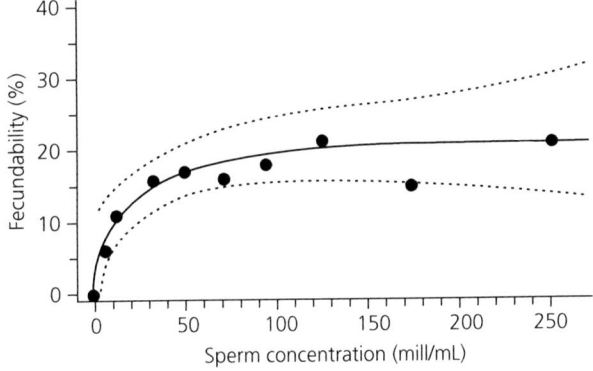

Figure 89.2 The fecundability as a function of sperm count in healthy men. Adapted with permission from Ref. 7.

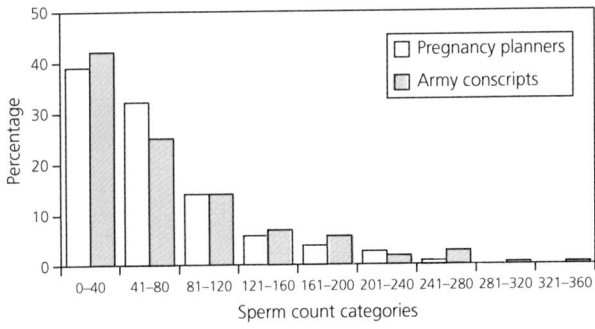

Figure 89.3 Distribution of sperm count in Danish men recruited from the general population.[114,115]

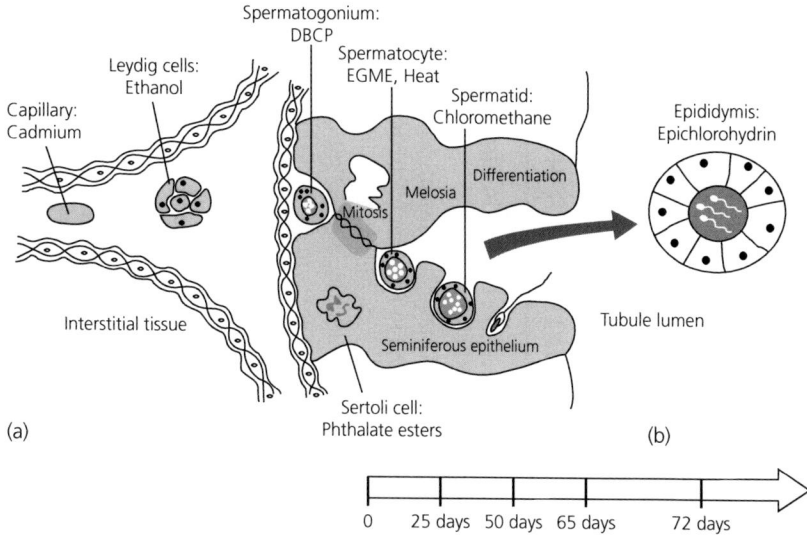

Figure 89.4 Site of action of male reproductive toxicants: (a) anatomic figure; (b) the seminiferous tubule.

cause inability to obtain fertilization or carry a fertilized ovum to a clinical pregnancy.

Spermatogenesis lasts 74 days in humans and can be damaged at any stage of differentiation resulting in impairment of number, structure, mobility and viability of sperm and causing loss of chromatin integrity and DNA damage (Figure 89.4). Exposure in the early stages of spermatogenesis most likely causes long-term effects while interference with the epididymal function results in transient effects if exposure is discontinued. The Sertoli cells of the testis are essential for proliferation and maturation of sperm and therefore Sertoli cell toxicants may cause severe impairment of semen quality. Other sites of action of the male reproductive system include neuro-endocrine control at the pituitary or testicular level (Leydig cells) and interference with epididymal and accessory sex gland function.

Dysfunction of the female reproductive system may be caused by disruption of the endocrine regulation of the menstrual cycle and impaired ovulation, tubular transport of the fertilized egg or implantation. The number of primordial gonocytes in the fetal gonad counts some two million at birth – a number that is reduced to 400 000 at puberty. It is often assumed that the oogenesis is less susceptible than the spermatogenesis to toxicants because oocytes are dormant and well protected in the ovary until the last few weeks before ovulation. However, it is known that polyaromatic hydrocarbons arising from combustion processes may cause destruction of oocytes in the ovarian stroma. Depletion of the pool of follicles may cause premature menopause.

Occupational risk of infertility

In 1977, it was incidentally discovered that the nematocide dibromochloropropane (DBCP) was causing severe oligospermia and a permanent inability to have children in some men.[9] So far, DBCP is the most well-established human reproductive toxicant conferred by occupational exposures. The compound is highly toxic to stem cells of the human seminiferous tubule and reproductive toxicity has also been seen in mice, rats and rabbits. The DBCP incident initiated heightened interest in reproductive hazards and during the past 30 years more than 100 occupational studies of semen quality and couple fertility have been undertaken. In general, cross-sectional semen studies have methodological limitations. Participation is most often low and selection bias may be introduced because control subjects seem to participate more often than exposed if they have experienced infertility.

The time-to-pregnancy approach to studies of couple fertility has become popular, but results needs cautious interpretation – first of all, because sexual behaviour and use of contraception has a strong impact on the end point and may vary between different occupational groups.[10] Examples of occupations and exposures that have been associated with subfertility in epidemiological studies are given in Table 89.1. In the following, certain selected exposures that may interfere with fertility are briefly reviewed.

IONIZING RADIATION

Healthcare and nuclear plant personnel, laboratory technicians, welding operators and radar technicians may be exposed to ionizing radiation at the workplace. The gonads are among the most radiosensitive tissues of the body. A temporary reduction in sperm count occurs after a radiation dose of 0.15 Gy, while single exposures above 2 Gy may cause permanent azoospermia.[11] Workplace exposure to gamma radiation is easy to monitor, while exposure to alpha and beta radiation by inhalation or ingestion of particles may easily escape recognition. However, at current occupational standards in industrial and research laboratories, exposure levels are far below the background radiation. If the usual exposure threshold of 15 mSv/year is not exceeded, reproductive effects seem unlikely.

Table 89.1 Occupational risk for infertility.

Occupational exposure	Men	Women
Anaesthetic gas		+
Dinitrotoluene and toluene diamine	+	
Metals		
Welding	+	
Chromium compounds		+
Cadmium		+
Lead	+*	
Manganese	(+)	
Mercury vapour (metallic)		+
Oral contraceptives and sexual hormones	+*	
Organic solvents		
Carbon disulphide	+*	
Chlorinated hydrocarbons	+	+
Ethylene glycol ethers	+	
Halogenated hydrocarbons	+	+
Ethoxy ethanol	+	
Persistent organochlorine compounds		
Polychlorinated biphenyls (PCB)	+*	+
p,p'-DDE (a DDT metabolite)	+	+
Dioxin	+	
Pesticides	+	+
Carbaryl	(+)	
Chloropren	+	
Dibromochloropropan	+*	
Ethylendibromide	+	
Para-tertiary butyl acid	(+)	
Plastic monomers		
Chloroprene	(+)	
Textile dyes	+	
Ionizing radiation, radium	+*	+*
Noise	(+)	+
Radar and microwaves	(+)	
Radiant heat	+*	

Occupational exposures that have been associated with reduced fertility or effects on biological indicators of reproductive function as semen quality or endocrine disruption. Substantial evidence of causal effects are indicated by an * and circumstantial evidence by (+).
References to original work are provided in reviews.[116–118]

HIGH FREQUENCY ELECTROMAGNETIC RADIATION

Exposure to high frequency electromagnetic radiation (HHF, 200 kHz–300 mHz, short waves or microwaves) is increasing because of widespread use of cellular phones. Occupational exposure occurs among military radar equipment operators and employees working with thermal plastic sealing, glue hardening, physiotherapy and telecommunication equipment. The apparent effect on semen quality of microwaves (100–300 000 mHz) reported in an earlier East European study may result from radiant heat associated with HHF exposure.[12] The significance of reduced semen quality observed in military radar equipment operators in the United States and Denmark is uncertain.[12–14] The effects observed in the small human populations are not seen in animal studies.

EXTREMELY LOW FREQUENCY ELECTROMAGNETIC RADIATION

There has been a tremendous increase in the population exposure to extremely low frequency electromagnetic radiation from household electrical equipment and power cables. Clues as to the possible significance for reproductive health may be obtained from occupational studies. Metal welders are among the highest exposed professionals because of the close proximity to power cables during electric arc welding. Comprehensive studies with full shift monitoring of electromagnetic fields provide no evidence that the endocrine profile or conventional semen characteristics are influenced by exposure to such fields.[15] Moreover, there is a paucity of experimental evidence indicating that we should expect any effects.

HEAT AND SEDENTARY BODY POSTURE

It is well known that elevation of the testis temperature impairs spermatogenesis.[16] Work in hot occupational environments and exposure to radiant heat among welders, foundry workers, ceramic workers and bakers may cause reduced sperm count.[17,18] Disruption of testicular heat regulation may cause delayed conception in taxi drivers.[19] Men sitting at work for eight hours a day have on average 0.7°C higher scrotal temperature during the day in comparison with employees with less than eight hours in the sedentary body position. An increase of scrotal temperature of this order of magnitude may be sufficient to impair spermatogenesis, but reduced sperm count seems not related to sedentary work.[20]

ORGANIC SOLVENTS AND GLYCOL ETHERS

Among the widely used volatile industrial organic solvents, it seems that carbon disulphide carries a risk to the male reproductive system.[21] This solvent is used in the viscose-rayon industry. High-level exposure in the workplace may cause reduced semen quality and disruption of endocrine homeostasis. Styrene is used in the manufacturing of reinforced plastic products as used in windmills and yachts. Manual laminating procedures often involve high exposure levels. There is limited evidence that inhalation of styrene may impair semen quality, but not time taken to conceive.[22,23] Animal as well as human data on reproductive effects of other widely used solvents such as toluene, xylene, benzene, carbon tetrachloride and trichlorethylene are limited.

Glycol ethers are solvents with low volatility, which increasingly have been used as substitutes for the highly volatile hydrocarbons in paints, adhesives, thinners, printing ink and anti-icing fluids. It has been estimated that two million workers are exposed to eight different glycol ethers

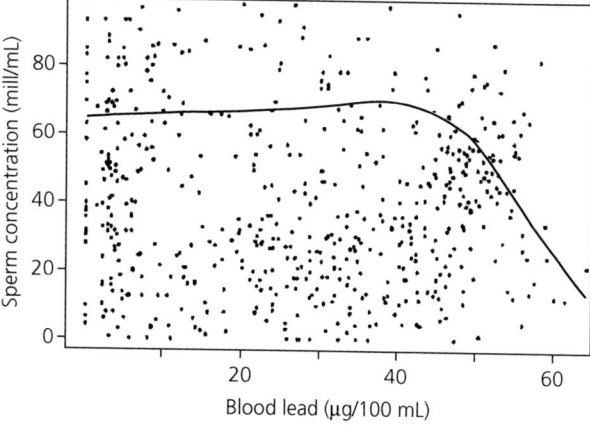

Figure 89.5 Concentration of sperm cells in fresh ejaculate in some 500 workers from the United Kingdom, Belgium and Italy, according to current blood lead level. No effects are observed below 45 μg lead/dL of blood. Adapted with permission from Ref. 32.

in the United States, including females in the semiconductor industry. Unequivocal reproductive toxicity of some of these compounds has been documented in laboratory rodents and a number of studies indicate reproductive effects in humans as well.[24] The solvent 2-bromopropane has specific effect on rat spermatogonia.[25] A small Korean study of electronic company workers exposed to this compound reported severely reduced sperm count.[26] Clearly, attention should be paid to this particular organic solvent for workers in the electronics industry.

INORGANIC LEAD

The reproductive toxicity of lead has been known for a long time. Several occupational surveys have linked exposure to inorganic lead in the exposure range of blood lead above 40–50 μg/dL to reduced sperm count and other signs of male reproductive toxicity,[27–29] although the literature is not entirely consistent.[30] The evidence in humans is supported by compelling evidence in mice, rabbits and some rat strains.[31] An international European study points to a threshold around 45 μg/dL below which effects on sperm count seem unlikely (Figure 89.5).[32] These findings are consistent with studies of delayed time to pregnancy not indicating effects in the lower exposure range below 50 μg/dL.[33] The lowest effect level of about 45 μg/dL of lead in blood is an average group threshold, which does not necessarily apply to all individual workers. The individual susceptibility could be influenced by genetic polymorphisms that modify the toxicokinetics of lead.[27]

METAL WELDERS

Several studies have demonstrated impaired semen quality, delayed time to conception and reduced fertility rate in metal welders,[34,35] but more recent studies have not corroborated earlier findings.[36,37] These apparent inconsistencies may be due to changing exposure levels. The risk is not related to welding stainless steel. Infertility of unknown aetiology in a welder exposed to high levels of welding fume particulates above 5–10 mg/m³ should prompt further evaluation of occupational risk.

PESTICIDES

Several pesticides have been studied in occupational settings after the reproductive toxicity of DBCP was recognized in 1977. European studies of wine yard workers, organic and conventional farmers and greenhouse workers exposed to low levels of a wide range of pesticides have not revealed an effect on fertility, except in greenhouse workers.[38–40] Other studies have found associations between pesticide exposure and fertility which may be explained by different exposure profiles and levels.[24,41–46] For the clinician, only limited information can be obtained from the epidemiological studies with poorly characterized exposures. In the individual case, emphasis must be on work history, exposure to specific chemicals and laboratory evidence (Box 89.1). Unfortunately, only few pesticides can routinely be measured in blood, urine or semen.

Male-mediated developmental toxicity

Animal studies have demonstrated how paternal exposure to mutagens and carcinogens before mating are capable of introducing heritable genomic changes. This can result in reproductive failures, such as miscarriage, congenital malformations and cancer in the offspring. By 1985, it was shown that exposure of male rats to cyclophosphamide causes post-implantation loss without interfering with fertility.[47] Aneuploid sperm is not a hereditable risk if they are disadvantaged at fertilization with respect to normal sperm cells. However, elegant studies demonstrated the absence of selection against aneuploid mouse sperm at fertilization.[48] Thus, the question about consequences of paternal exposures for pregnancy outcomes seems highly relevant, and since 1985 several synthetic chemicals have been found to induce genetic damage, that is transmitted to the offspring. In humans, treatment with cytotoxic drugs and tobacco smoking have been associated with increased frequency of aneuploidy in sperm cells,[49] but so far there is no clear evidence that developmental anomalies can be attributed to paternal smoking in spite of several findings suggesting such effects.[50] Many epidemiologic studies indicate an association between certain paternal occupational exposures and adverse pregnancy outcomes.[51] In most cases, positive findings obtained in one study have not been confirmed in other studies. However, a recent meta-analysis based on 14 studies selected by rigorous quality criteria concluded that occupational exposure to organic solvents is associated with an increased risk for neural tube defects, while associations with spontaneous abortion was less likely.[52] Inorganic lead has also been associated with male-mediated toxicity.[53]

Box 89.1 Extrapolation of animal data to human scenarios

Counselling of subfertile couples and pregnant women with regard to reproductive chemical hazards in the workplace is heavily reliant on reproductive toxicity testing in rodents because epidemiologic data are scanty or too crude to be useful. Therefore, the issue of extrapolation from animal studies to the human situation is important and briefly commented on here.

Reproductive toxicity testing was developed after the thalidomide catastrophe and includes single-generation and multiple-generation studies. The single-generation studies use the highest dose not causing maternal toxicity to detect teratogens and fetotoxic effects, while the costly multigeneration studies use low doses over long time periods.

In general, the similarities between rodents and humans are much stronger than the differences. It is therefore reasonable to assume that a reproductive effect that is observed in rodents will be seen in humans if exposure levels are relevant and toxicokinetics and mechanisms of actions are not irrelevant for humans. In particular, this is true for teratogens and compounds that directly interfere with spermatogenesis. When a compound increases the frequency of specific structural abnormalities following administration of doses that are not causing general toxicity of the mother animal (no signs of intoxication, intake of water and food and weight gain as in the reference group), structural defects are also likely to occur in humans, although the specific nature of the defects may differ from species to species. In particular, this is true if the structural defects are rare in the rodent species. For example, cleft palate is common in mice due to high cortisol levels in stress conditions, while such effects are not seen in humans. Resorptions, delayed ossifications, reduced fetal weight gain and increased occurrence of minor skeletal malformations are common in experimental animals following high doses that are associated with toxic effects in the mother animal. The importance of similar effects at dose levels that are not associated with maternal toxicity is uncertain and difficult to extrapolate to humans.

All known human teratogens cause structural abnormalities in at least one and most often several rodent species. On the other hand, there are several animal teratogens with unproven teratogenic effects in humans because data are lacking. One exception is acetylsalicyl acid, which is a teratogen in rodents but not in humans. Similarly, compounds disrupting specific steps of the spermatogenic cycle in rodents are also likely to produce similar effects in humans. Effects in humans have been observed at 2–10 per cent of the effective dose in rodents. Therefore, a safety factor of at least 100 is warranted.

It should be acknowledged that there are no appropriate animal models to predict subtle cognitive or behavioural effects following disruption of central nervous system development and likewise effects of physical strain, work postures and psychosocial strain cannot be predicted from animal studies.

Overall, it remains a prudent approach to regard any effect found in animals as likely to occur in humans until additional evidence might indicate otherwise.

It is obvious that epidemiological research in this field must overcome many difficulties and 'no evidence' cannot be taken as 'no effects'. The question about paternal exposures in pregnancy outcomes is often raised in clinical practice, but so far no confirmative answers can be given.

ADVERSE PREGNANCY OUTCOMES

Spontaneous abortion

It is estimated that up to 75 per cent of all fertilizations are lost and that 10–20 per cent of recognized pregnancies are terminated in spontaneous abortion (see p. 381 in Ref. 54). The probability of embryonal loss decreases with increasing gestational age (Figure 89.6). At least 30 per cent of recognized spontaneous abortions are chromosomally abnormal compared to 6 per cent in stillbirths and 0.6 per cent in live births (see p. 382 in Ref. 54). Chromosomal anomalies arise either before conception in male or female germ cells or at the time of fertilization, but are not caused by exposures taking place after this time. Maternal age above 30–35 years increases the risk of both chromosomally normal and abnormal spontaneous abortions. Other

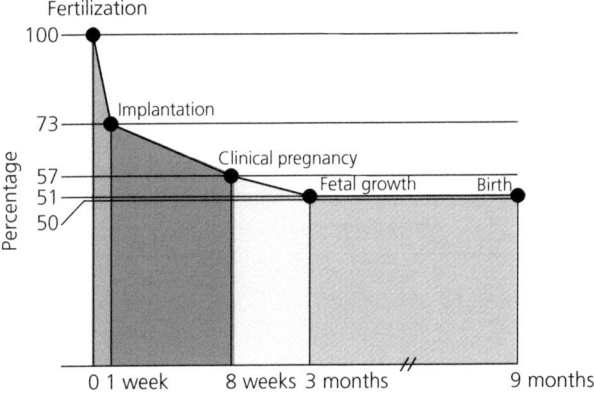

Figure 89.6 Embryonal loss from fertilization and through gestational ages.

indisputable known risk factors are surprisingly few and include earlier abortion, maternal smoking and use of intrauterine device (IUD).

Most epidemiological studies of occupational risk of spontaneous abortion are constrained by methodological limitations, which may explain that few hazards have been identified in spite of a quite large number of studies these

Table 89.2 Occupational exposures conferred during pregnancy associated with adverse pregnancy outcomes.

Occupation/exposure	Spontaneous abortion	Birth defect	Fetal growth retardation	Preterm birth	Other outcomes
Building painters	+				Childhood leukaemia
Dry cleaning	+	(+)			
Electronics industry	+				
Hospital workers	+		+		
Laboratory work	+	+			
Pharmaceutical industry	+	+			
Plast industry workers	+	(+)	+		Childhood malignancy
Textile industry	+		+		
Anaesthetic gases	+				
Antineoplastic agents	+				
Disinfectants	+				
Metals					
Arsenic					
Cadmium					
Inorganic lead	+	+			
Organic mercury					Mental retardation
Organic solvents	+*	+	+		Childhood malignancy
Pesticides	+	+			
Heat		+			
Ionizing radiation	+*	+*			
Microwaves	+				Changed sex ratio
Noise	+			+	Child hearing impairment
Physical exertion	+		+	+	
Mental strain		+*			
Infections	+*	+*	+*	+*	

Substantial evidence of causal effects are indicated by an asterix * and circumstantial evidence by (+).
References to original work are provided in reviews.[60,93,112,116,118–121]

past 25 years. Spontaneous abortion is a heterogeneous outcome and it is seldom possible to examine the risk of specific types of abortions – as, for instance, chromosomally normal or abnormal embryos. The risk of a specific type of fetal loss conferred by an occupational exposure must therefore be observed on top of the high frequency of background losses. Moreover, the observed frequency of spontaneous abortion is heavily dependent on whether or not early losses are ascertained and this may vary between occupational groups that are compared. In addition, many studies are difficult to interpret because of lacking information about type, level and time of exposure. These methodological limitations should be taken into account when considering Table 89.2 which lists a number of occupational exposures that have been associated with increased risk of spontaneous abortion and other adverse outcomes in several studies.

Birth defects

Congenital malformation occurs in 3–5 per cent of births. Causes are known in one-third of cases. Genetic defects account for 20 per cent, chromosomal aberrations for 5 per cent and diseases, lifestyle and environmental factors for 10 per cent of cases.[55] According to current knowledge, less than 1 per cent of birth defects are thought to be attributable to man-made chemicals (Tables 89.3 and 89.4).[56]

Teratogen refers to any agent that causes a structural abnormality following fetal exposure. Teratogens have seldom been identified by systematic epidemiologic studies. Most often, an increased occurrence of a particular malformation leads to the discovery of a teratogenic agent. For instance, Minamata disease, an encephalopathy that mimics cerebral palsy, was first recognized in villages surrounding Minamata Bay in Japan. This localized area of increased prevalence led to an investigation that pointed to methyl mercury as the offending agent. This compound was discharged into the bay by a local factory. Ingestion of contaminated fish during pregnancy was the primary cause for this devastating condition. Similar results followed the ingestion of grain laced with methyl mercury, which was used as a fungicide in Iraq.[57]

The sudden appearance of several cases of a rare disorder can also raise suspicions of teratogenicity. Cases of phocomelia in the early 1960s in Germany and Australia

Table 89.3 Reproductive hazards for pregnant women in selected occupations.

Occupation	Potential reproductive hazards	Councelling and comments
Dental assistants	Nitrous oxide, x-rays, creosol, chlorphenol, methacrylates. There are no data to indicate that mercury vapour from amalgam is teratogenic at exposure levels seen in dental clinics	Unless local exhaust and room ventilation is keeping nitrous oxide concentrations in ambient air at levels far below threshold limit values, pregnant women should be replaced
Electronics and semiconductor industry	Inorganic lead in solder tin, glycol ethers in adhesives	If local exhaust ventilation is adequate, soldering seldom causes measurable increase in blood lead. Skin absorption and inhalation of glycol ethers must be effectively ruled out
Greenhouse workers	Fungicides, insecticides, growth retardants	Pregnant women should not apply pesticides because of potential risk of high exposure and failure of protective equipment. Pesticide-treated cultures should not be handled until residue on leaves have disappeared (appropriate re-entry time). Use of gloves important to avoid skin absorption
Hair dressers	Dyes (includng toluene- and phenylenediamines), sprays, shampoos, permanent-wave solutions and perfumes	Use of gloves to avoid direct contact with dyes and local exhaust ventilation to clear room air for contaminants from sprays and permanent wave solutions are most often sufficient to ensure safe working conditions for pregnant women
Hospital staff	X-rays, strong magnetic fields antineoplastic drugs, anaesthetic gases, disinfectants, infections	Mixing and intravenous administration of antineoplastic drugs should be avoided. Open or semiclosed inhalation anaesthesia and work in insufficiently ventilated post-operative care units must be avoided
Laboratory technicians	Organic solvents, metals, pigments, pesticides, acrylamide, ionizing α- or β-emitters and many others	Exposures are complex and highly varaible depending on type of laboratory. A specific evaluation of each uniqe job task is warranted. If open handling of laboratory chemicals can be avoided and extraction, mixing and pipetting take place in ventilated hoods and closed benches conditions may be safe for pregnant women. Risk for spillage and unintended peak exposure should be considered
Painters in construction work	Organic solvents in paints, varnishes, fillers and adhesives	Use water-based rather than solvent-based products. Take care not to use water-based paints with low content of white spirit that may evaporate differentially and cause rather high exposure levels in ambient air. Work from ladder or scaffolds should be avoided in late pregnancy. If appropriate action is taken pregnant painters can most often continue work during pregnancy
Plastic extruders	Complex mixtures of organic compounds in low concentrations in ambient air	Irritation of mucus membranes is an indication of possible risk. Adequate control of process temperature important to avoid high exposure
Reinforced plastics laminating	Styrene, methylene chloride	Manual laminating is related to high exposures and use of airstream helmets and other protective outfit is necessary. Pregnant women should be replaced
Screen printing	Highly volatile organic solvents	In manual or semi-automatic screen printing, it is difficult to obtain sufficiently low exposure levels and replacement of pregnant women is advisable

Table 89.4 Causes of malformations.

Cause	Percentage
Unknown	65
Genetic	5
Mutations	15–20
Chromosomal abnormalities	5
Maternal conditions: Diabetes, alcoholism, drug addiction, nutritional deficiency	4
Maternal infections: Rubella, varicella, toxoplasmosis, herpes, cytomegalovirus, parvovirus B19, syphilis	3
Mechanical problems: Cord restriction, uterus malformation	1–2
Chemicals, drugs, radiation	<1%
Preconception exposures (excluding mutagens and infections)	<1%

Adapted with permission from Ref. 58

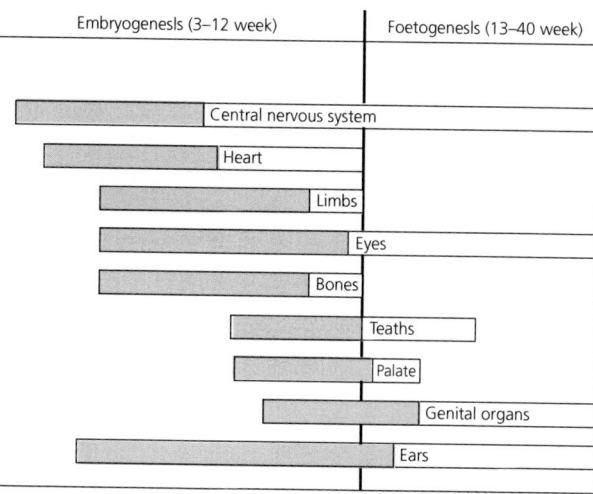

Figure 89.7 Embryogenesis and fetal development.

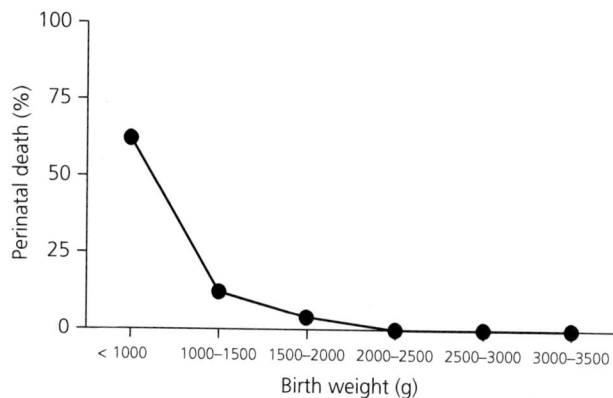

Figure 89.8 Perinatal mortality according to birth weight.

led to the identification of thalidomide as a human teratogen. Thalidomide was used to treat morning sickness, resulting in exposure at the stage in development when the embryo is most vulnerable, the first trimester.

Effects of teratogens follow an exposure–response relationship. There is a threshold below which no effect will be observed and both severity and frequency of malformations increase as the level of exposure increases.[58] Moreover, the time of exposure is important since certain stages of embryonic and fetal development are more vulnerable than others (Figure 89.7). Insults occurring from fertilization to early post-implantation most often results in an all-or-none response. Either the agent affects so many cells that the embryo is lost or so few cells that full repair from omnipotent remaining cells takes place. Otherwise, the embryonic stage (first trimester) is more vulnerable than the fetal period (second and third trimesters). Some malformations occur following exposure over a broad range of time as in microcephalia following ionizing radiation, while other malformations such as specific limb defects only occur after exposure during a narrow time period. Most teratogens are associated with a confined group of malformations that result after exposure during a critical period of embryonic development.

Growth retardation and preterm birth

The birth weight is a function of intrauterine growth, gestational age and genetic factors. Low birth weight is strongly related to perinatal mortality (Figure 89.8). The prevalence of children born before the 37th week of gestation is round 5–6 per cent in western countries and the prevalence of children with intrauterine growth retardation (IUGR, birth weight below the tenth percentile at the given gestational week) is slightly lower (3–5 per cent).

Occupational risk for adverse pregnancy outcomes

Women in gainful employment do not have less beneficial pregnancy outcomes than women with home employment.[59] An overview of the most common work-related reproductive hazards for the pregnant woman is given in Table 89.2. Table 89.3 provides an overview and comments on reproductive hazards in selected occupations. Epidemiologic research to date has not convincingly established any workplace exposure as a human teratogen.[60] However, in the aggregate, many studies suggest that some organic solvents, heavy metals and pesticides may cause malformations of several organ systems.[55] A more detailed description is provided below.

ANAESTHETIC GASES

A number of studies suggest that the risk of spontaneous abortion may be elevated among women exposed to anaesthetic gases.[61,62] A meta-analysis based on 19 studies concluded that exposure to anaesthetic gases a few decades ago was associated with a moderately elevated risk of spontaneous abortion.[63] However, reproductive toxicity has not been seen in animal studies using low-level exposure corresponding to concentrations measured in operating rooms. Working in modern operating theatres with closed anaesthetic systems and efficient exhaust ventilation, exposure to anaesthetic gases does not entail a risk if the equipment is properly maintained and exposure levels are controlled. This is contrary to mask anaesthesia in dental practice and among midwives and veterinarians, where high peak exposures to nitrous oxide can be encountered and deleterious effects in the first trimester cannot be excluded. Nitrous oxide is teratogenic in rats above 1000 ppm. Moreover, an increased risk of miscarriage was found in a large study of dental assistants that worked with nitrous oxide at least three hours per week without use of local exhaustion.[64] Precautions to protect midwives, nurses, dentists and dental assistants against exposure to nitrous oxide during pregnancy are warranted. This includes sufficient ventilation in post-operative care units where anaesthetic gas exposure from patient exhalations can result in ambient air concentrations exceeding threshold limit values.

PHARMACEUTICALS

Several pharmaceuticals including reproductive hormones, antineoplastic agents and certain immunosuppressive, antiviral and anti-inflammatory drugs exhibit reproductive toxicity in rodent studies. Antineoplastic drugs have received the most attention because mixing and intravenous administration may cause considerable exposure. A number of studies have reported increased risk of spontaneous abortion in nurses handling antineoplastic drugs. Given the well-established effects on cell growth by a variety of mechanisms, precautions must be taken to prevent skin contact or aerosol exposure to these agents. If it is not possible to comply with occupational safety standards, pregnant women should not handle antineoplastic drugs for other than oral administration. Results of studies performed in recent years in the Netherlands indicate that the risk for adverse pregnancy outcomes has not been eliminated.[65,66]

CLEANING AGENTS AND DISINFECTANTS

Soaps and ethanol solutions used for ordinary cleaning tasks are not considered a reproductive hazard, while high exposure to very reactive chemicals used to sterilize objects and surfaces, such as ethylene oxide, formaldehyde and glutaraldehyde have been associated with an increased risk of fetal loss in a few studies. The limited evidence precludes comprehensive risk assessment, but the available data and the reactive nature of the chemicals indicate that precautions should be taken to prevent overexposure of pregnant women.

ORGANIC SOLVENTS

Aliphatic and aromatic organic solvents readily pass the blood–placenta barrier. The concentration in fetal tissues may be the same or even higher than in maternal tissues. Several large and well-conducted studies indicate that high-level exposure to organic solvents during early pregnancy carries a risk for spontaneous abortion.[67,68] For instance, a Finnish study reported a nine-fold higher risk following first-trimester exposure to toluene in the shoe industry,[69] where high exposure levels are known to occur. Other data indicate that risk of miscarriage may be increased at exposure levels close to United States Occupational Safety and Health Administration (OSHA) permissible levels for toluene, xylene and formaldehyde.[70]

In several studies, birth defects have also been linked to organic solvent exposure during pregnancy. A study of women who received counselling because of concern about occupational solvent exposure reported a strongly elevated risk of subsequent birth defects.[71] This disturbing finding has not been corroborated in independent studies.

In general, data on magnitude of risk, exposure–response relations, no-effect levels, specificity of effects according to type of solvents and other details have not been clarified. Moreover, effects in humans are not strongly supported by studies in rodents. Reviews considering data on specific solvents, such as styrene, toluene, xylene and trichlorethylene have not been conclusive.[72,73] Considering the established neurotoxicity of organic solvents, it is remarkable that there is no evidence on neurobehavioural effects in children exposed during fetal life. High solvent exposure has also been linked to gestational hypertension and low birth weight.

Exposure during pregnancy should be kept at the lowest possible levels during the entire pregnancy. It should be kept in mind that permissible exposure levels for organic solvents are most often based upon irritant or neurotoxic effects that cannot be expected to provide sufficient protection against adverse pregnancy outcomes.

GLYCOL ETHERS AND THE SEMICONDUCTOR INDUSTRY

The reproductive toxicity of some ethylene glycol ethers has been well documented in animal studies. Increased risk of miscarriage has been observed in US semiconductor industries (see, for example, Ref. 74), but findings have not been corroborated by a British study.[75] Monomethyl and -ethyl ethers have caused malformations in many organs in several rodent species, but the epidemiological evidence is limited and is insufficient to allow conclusions with respect to risk for malformations in humans.[76]

INORGANIC LEAD

Maternal blood lead levels above 10 μg/dL have been linked to increased risk of gestational hypertension, spontaneous abortion and delayed cognitive capabilities in children. A prospective study of spontaneous abortion in Mexico used incidence-density analyses in order to achieve comparable opportunity for the outcome to occur among exposed and controls and observed a striking exposure–response relation between blood lead and spontaneous abortion at low exposure levels.[77] Blood lead levels in this range are far lower than permissible biological threshold values. Higher levels have been associated with reduced fetal growth. An increased risk of congenital malformations has also been suggested, but there is uncertainty with respect to specific malformations and exposure–response relationship.[78] Precautions to protect pregnant women from even low-level exposure are strongly justified by available evidence. Workplaces putting women of fertile age at risk from exposure to inorganic lead should develop practices to prevent exposure from the very early stages of pregnancy.

MERCURY AND OTHER METALS

Organic mercury causes severe disruption of fetal development of the brain as tragically encountered in Minamata Bay in Japan and other places in the 1950s. Exposure to methyl mercury is not usual in the occupational environment and there are no consistent indications that inorganic or metallic mercury are teratogens in humans.[79,80] Several studies among dental assistants with low-level elemental mercury exposure do not provide consistent data to indicate reproductive toxicity at these exposure levels. Other metals, such as nickel, arsenic, manganese and cadmium, have also been associated with reproductive toxicity in epidemiological studies, but the evidence is limited.[81]

PESTICIDES

Pesticides denote a large and heterogeneous group of chemicals that has toxicity to living organisms in common. Industrial workers engaged in manufacture and formulation of pesticides may be exposed through multiple pathways, while the predominant route of exposure among applicators in greenhouses and agriculture is through the skin. Spraying of pesticides also confers exposure through inhalation, unless the worker is adequately protected. Thousands of deaths are reported annually following acute intoxication in developing countries and high-level exposure in the occupational setting, as well as long-term low-level exposure of the general population continues to be of concern.

A large body of evidence in laboratory rodents suggests reproductive toxicity of some pesticides when given at exposure doses that are higher than those obtained from occupational exposure. In spite of numerous studies of birth defects in agricultural workers, the evidence is still inadequate to conclude whether some of these highly diverse compounds impose a risk for birth defects in humans.[82,83] Some pesticides have weak hormonal activity in *in vitro* and *in vivo* systems. In recent years, the hypothesis that endocrine disruption during fetal development may cause hypospadias and cryptorchidism attracted much attention.[84] Emerging evidence from environmental studies indicate that biopersistent organochlorines, such as dichlorodiphenyl-trichloroethane (DDT) and its main metabolite dichlorodiphenyl-dichloroethane (p,p'-DDE) may cause intrauterine growth retardation and miscarriage.[85,86]

HAIR DYES AND SPRAYS

Hairdressers, barbers and cosmetologists are exposed to a complex chemical environment of permanent and temporary hair dyes, hair sprays, shampoos, permanent-wave solutions and perfumes. Some constituents of dyes, such as toluene- and phenylenediamines, exhibit reproductive toxicity in laboratory animals. However, according to a 1993 IARC evaluation, no teratogenic effects were seen in rodents that were exposed by application of a number of hair dye formulations on the skin.[87] In general, ambient air measurements of volatile solvents as indicators of overall exposure have been very low (less than 10 ppm ethanol, acetone or diclormethane), but high peak exposure may occur and small amounts of toluenediamines have been measured in urine samples, which documents systemic uptake. A number of reproductive studies in the past two decades have reported slightly increased risk of miscarriage and birth defects, but findings are not entirely consistent.[88] Based upon a small number of cases, two studies indicated an increased risk of cleft palate[89] and thus there is need for additional research. However, potential hazards can be minimized by use of general and local exhaust ventilation and use of gloves to prevent skin absorption. With these precautions, job replacement is seldom needed.

OFFICE WORK

In the 1980s, video display terminals were suspected of causing adverse reproductive outcomes because of exposure to electromagnetic fields, but several large-scale epidemiological studies did not find an increased risk of spontaneous abortion nor any of an array of congenital defects.[90] This is a good example of how comprehensive reproductive epidemiology may help resolve widespread concern and fear related to introduction of new technologies.

IONIZING AND NON-IONIZING RADIATION

Genetic effects of ionizing radiation on male and female gametes before fertilization are mainly stochastic effects, while intrauterine effects in terms of miscarriage, stillbirth and birth defects are mainly deterministic effects.[58] A total dose during pregnancy of less than 1 mSv is not associated with increased risk of adverse pregnancy outcomes, but exposures should be kept as low as possible to protect the fetal gonads from stochastic genetic effects. For comparison, the average background exposure is in the range of 4 mSv/year. Exposures of hospital nurses above 0.5 mSv/year are unlikely if working conditions comply with current safety regulations.

Ultrasound and microwaves induce tissue damage because of hyperthermia at high exposure levels. Epidemiological studies have shown associations with miscarriage and changed sex ratio. Pregnant women should be protected from high exposures at the workplace. Very low frequency electromagnetic fields (video display terminals, welding, electric equipment) do not emit high enough energy to induce hyperthermia and biological effects have so far not been demonstrated.

NOISE

The fetal ear is sensitive to noise-induced damage from the 20th week of gestation.[91,92] Uterus and fetal fluids attenuate the sound level, but less so at low frequencies where resonance phenomena may even reinforce the sound pressure. Pregnant women should avoid very high exposure levels above 110 dB over eight hours and low frequency noise should be avoided at even lower exposure levels. In several studies, noise has been associated with miscarriage, preterm birth and growth retardation which has been attributed to high circulating cortisol levels related to continuous activation of the hypothalamic–pituitary–adrenal (HPA) axis. Noise exposure is, however, often correlated with several other risk factors, such as physical and mental strenuous work, which may confound observed associations.

PHYSICAL WORKLOAD

Strenuous work conditions have long been suspected to be associated with adverse pregnancy outcomes, in particular premature birth and intrauterine growth retardation. The metabolic demands of pregnancy and fetal growth may be in conflict with demands for blood flow, oxygen and nutrients needed in heavy physical work. Blood flow to the placenta and uterus may be redistributed and thus reduce oxygen and carbohydrate delivery resulting in restricted fetal growth and increased uterine contractility causing preterm birth. It is remarkable, however, that exercise in pregnancy is considered to be safe in healthy and well-nourished women.[93] An early review of epidemiological studies in the occupational setting found limited evidence for adverse pregnancy outcomes related to a number of individual ergonomic factors, such as prolonged standing, physical exertion and long work hours, while women exposed to several risk factors seemed at increased risk for giving preterm birth.[94] A more recent meta-analysis of a large number of studies addressing occupational risk for adverse pregnancy outcomes indicated an elevated risk of preterm delivery related to physically demanding work and prolonged standing (Figure 89.9).[95] This result, however, conflicts with the most recent findings.[96] More advanced assessment and ascertainment of exposure will probably be needed to get more exact knowledge and to establish

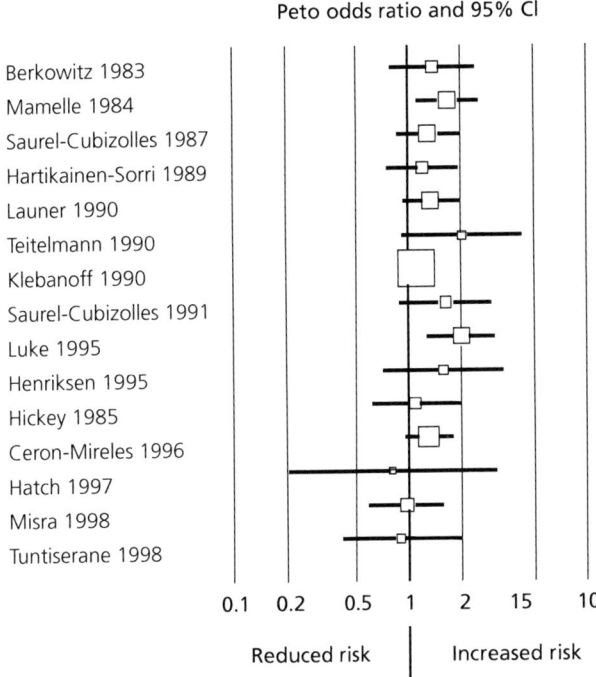

Figure 89.9 A meta-analysis of the risk of preterm delivery according to physical demanding work and prolonged standing. Data are adapted with permission from Ref. 89, where all studies cited in the figure can be found.

exposure–response relations, if any. At present, the evidence does not allow for highly specific or restrictive recommendations with respect to physical work conditions during pregnancy. In general, healthy and fit women are able to comply with physical work demands throughout pregnancy without posing a risk to the fetus. However, prolonged strenuous physical exertions, awkward postures and prolonged standing should be avoided and sufficient rest periods for the pregnant woman is warranted – in particular in the third trimester and in the presence of earlier pregnancy failures or if pregnancy complications develop.[97]

MENTAL STRAIN

Indications that psychosocial factors at the workplace have a bearing on adverse pregnancy outcomes are few.[98–100] However, severe emotional stress related to an unexpected loss of a child has been associated with an eight-fold increased risk of neural crest malformations if the event happened in the first trimester of pregnancy.[101] This finding indicates that stressful events, if sufficiently severe, may cause congenital malformations. Whether less severe psychosocial stressors put the pregnancy and fetus at risk seems plausible, but remains to be established.

SHIFT WORK

A large number of epidemiological studies have not demonstrated consistent associations between adverse pregnancy outcomes and rotating shift work or irregular work hours across different occupations and countries.[102] Nevertheless, several studies indicate that some forms of shift work are related to increased risk of spontaneous abortion, preterm birth and fetal growth retardation. Lack of consistency may be related to varying definitions of work schedules. At present, the strongest and most convincing evidence from a limited number of studies indicate that working a fixed night shift is associated with increased risk of spontaneous abortion.[96,103] The mechanisms involved may be related to disruption of circadian endogenous rhythm, but this explanation provides few clues on appropriate advice or whether monitoring of fetal growth is feasible if fixed night work cannot be avoided.

INFECTIONS

Several infectious diseases are severe reproductive hazards if infection takes place during the first trimester of pregnancy. However, immunization by natural infection or vaccination programmes and adherence to infection control procedures at hospitals and other workplaces strongly limit the occupational risk. Parvovirus B19 infection is of concern because only about two-thirds of women of fertile age are immune and infection in pregnancy is related to an increased risk of late fetal death. The annual seroconversion rate among susceptible women is about 10–15 per cent during epidemic periods and nursery school teachers have a three-fold increased risk for acquiring acute parvovirus B19 infection.[104] Since the risk of stillbirth following gestational infection is not negligible (1–5 per cent), susceptible nursery school teachers and day care workers should be replaced when pregnant – at least during periods with epidemics.[105] Prenatal infections with rubella, varicella, morbilli, hepatitis B, cytomegalovirus, immunodeficiency virus and toxoplasmosis are associated with severe developmental toxicity, but infections are seldom work-related.

DEVELOPMENTAL TOXICITY

Several prospective follow-up studies consistently indicate that exposure to inorganic lead during prenatal life cause subtle changes of behaviour and reduced learning capability that persists at least to school age.[106] Although studies of behaviour and cognitive function are expected to be highly sensitive to confounding by socioeconomic factors, the replication of findings in several well-defined independent studies have – together with biological plausibility of the findings – convinced the scientific community at large. Effects have been observed at low environmental exposures to lead in the blood lead range of 10–20 µg/dL – far lower than levels often encountered in industry. There is emerging evidence that polychlorinated biphenyls through interaction with thyroid function in prenatal life may cause delayed effects on cognitive function. Whether occupational exposure to organic solvents during pregnancy has a bearing on cerebral and cognitive development in the offspring is a question that surprisingly has never been addressed by reproductive epidemiology.

In follow-up studies of pregnant women who survived the A-bombing in Hiroshima and Nagasaki, it has been shown that ionizing radiation in weeks 8–15 is associated with increased risk of mental retardation.[107]

CHILDHOOD CANCER

The incidence of childhood cancer has been increasing in the United States.[108] Two in 1000 children develop malignant disease before 16 years of age, the most common cancers being leukaemia, brain tumours (medullo- and glioblastoma), kidney tumours (Wilms tumour) and retinoblastoma. The discovery that the synthetic oestrogenic drug diethylstilbestrol (DES) causes the extremely rare vaginal carcinoma in girls after puberty proves the concept of 'transplacental carcinogenesis'.[109] Likewise, testis tumours having their peak incidence at 30 years of age are derived from precursors that originate in prenatal life. Thus far, no parental occupational exposure has consistently been linked to malignant disease occurring in childhood or early adulthood.[108,110,111] There are, however, indications of increased risk of childhood leukaemia and nervous system cancer following maternal and paternal exposure to organic solvents, paints and pesticides.

RISK ASSESSMENT AND CLINICAL COUNSELLING

General and occupational health practitioners may be asked to provide an assessment of reproductive hazards and clinical advice in a variety of situations spanning couples planning a pregnancy, infertile couples and pregnant women through all gestational ages (Box 89.2).[112]

Box 89.2 Reproductive hazards

Established reproductive hazards include those for which substantial data in humans indicate reproductive effects at exposure levels occurring at the workplace or in the environment. Some compounds affect the fetus only at dose levels that approach maternal toxicity (for instance, metal mercury), while others cause adverse effects at otherwise subtoxic exposure levels (for instance, DBCP, PCB, inorganic lead).

Suspect hazards include those for which human data are limited, but animal data are substantial. The majority of chemicals in industrial use have not been thoroughly evaluated for reproductive toxicity.

The pregnant woman

The first step in the risk assessment is to delineate and specify potential harmful workplace exposures by taking occupational histories to assess the type, route, timing and level of the exposure. On many occasions, material safety data sheets (MSDS) and product labels may help to identify agents and ingredients of chemical products precisely. The MSDS may also provide information on human or experimental data suggestive of reproductive hazards, but most often fail to do so. However, practitioners can retrieve online reproductive toxicity data through one or more databases. Once the occupational history together with information from MSDS and reproductive toxicity databases indicate that the worker is exposed to an established or suspected reproductive hazard, the next step is to estimate exposure levels. The presence of a toxic agent in the workplace is not equivalent with exposures that imply absorption into the body and distribution to the target organ. An appropriate occupational history is of importance, but sometimes inspection of the workplace or even hygiene measurements may be needed to carry out a reliable estimate of exposure levels. Working with volatile organic solvents under a fume hood may reduce airborne exposure to very low levels, while the same work task on an unventilated bench could cause significant exposure. When accessing exposure levels, it should be kept in mind that the occupational exposure limits are not designed to protect specifically against reproductive risk. Thus, the risk assessment should be based upon no-observed effect levels in appropriate animal studies with appropriate safety factors of, for instance, 100 rather than on threshold limit values. A safety factor of 100 is based upon the fact that adverse effects have been observed in humans at 2–10 per cent of exposure levels in rodents and that variations of susceptibility within humans may be spanning one order of magnitude.

With the exception of inorganic lead, measurements of agents in blood or other tissues are seldom useful because of a lack of reference values for reproductive effects.

Sonographic imaging of fetal development is indicated if pregnant women have been exposed to teratogens or chemicals associated with fetal growth retardation in the relevant time period of gestation.

The subfertile couple

In infertile couples, the ovulatory function can be investigated by measurement of basal body temperature, preovulatory luteinizing hormone and surge in urine of midluteal serum progesterone levels. In addition, male reproductive function can be evaluated by semen analysis. When interpretating results of a semen analysis, the large day-to-day and week-to-week variation and the strong impact of sexual abstinence on sperm counts should be kept in mind. Sperm counts increase with duration of sexual abstinence up to six to eight days and then level off, but the period of abstinence only explains a minor part of the intra-individual variation which is also heavily influenced by factors related to semen collection. Determination of gonadotrophins in blood may help to discriminate between dysfunction of the testis (high gonadotrophin levels and low inhibin-B), insufficient function of the hypothalamus or pituitary (low gonadotrophins and inhibin-B) and androgen insensitive tissues (high LH and high testosterone). If the occupational history raises suspicion that one or more exposures at the workplace contribute to low semen quality, temporary replacement for three to six months can be associated with improvement of semen quality depending on type of insult (Box 89.3).

> **Box 89.3 Databases on reproductive toxicity**
>
> - IPCS/INCHEM (www.inchem.org). Toxicological monographs (criteria documents) from IPCS, WHO, IARC and ILO. Free online access to exhaustive information on exposures and compounds, but without any specific focus on reproductive toxicity.
> - Material safety datasheets (www.hazards.com/msds and www.siri.org/msds). Free information from the manufacturers, but no reproductive toxicity data.
> - Reprorisk® system of reproductive toxicity databases (www.micromedex.com/products/reprorisk).
> - Reprotext: Reviews of 850 chemicals
> - Reprotox (www.reprotox.org). Reviews of the scientific literature with interpretation of animal and human data. Catalogue of teratogenic agents: 2900 drugs original data, but no interpretation.
> - Teris teratogenic effects of 1100 drugs.
> - General information on exposure can be found in toxicological databases, such as TOXNET (www.toxnet.mlm.nih.gov).

RISK MANAGEMENT

The objectives of risk management are to eliminate existing risks, to reassure if no risk is anticipated and to ensure that no misleading statements may lead to harm.[113]

If the risk assessment is suggestive of a reproductive risk, this should be carefully communicated to the pregnant woman or the infertile couple. Appropriate actions include technical adjustments to reduce or eliminate exposure (for instance, closed artificial ventilation systems in operating theatres), use of protective devices (as gloves in hairdressers using dyes or greenhouse workers handling pesticide-treated cultures), change of job content so that specific tasks are avoided (as, for instance, use of acrylamide in the laboratory) or transfer to other jobs or departments. In a few countries, including Canada, Finland and Denmark, it is possible to obtain compensated pregnancy leave if a documented or suspected risk to the pregnancy or the fetus cannot be eliminated and replacement is not possible or feasible. Nevertheless, when a risk is clearly demonstrated, employees are in most countries obliged by law to undertake preventive measures or to offer other job tasks, replacement or leave. However, when the risk is less obvious because toxicity data are inadequate or exposure levels are low, employers may not be obliged to accommodate worker requests. In these instances, the risk communication is of particular importance so the decision finally made by the pregnant woman is as well informed as possible.

Agreed important principles for communication include honest and truthful answers to questions. However, it is also good practice to avoid to do harm by inappropriate information and to be aware of professional competence and limitations. Highly categorical advice is seldom justified.

Recommendation to terminate a pregnancy because of workplace exposures are almost never warranted – except perhaps accidental exposure to ionizing radiation above 0.3 Gy, rubella infection in the first trimester or severe anoxia.

Reduction of exposure to chemicals is clearly warranted when regulatory limits are exceeded or for even moderate exposure to agents known or suspected to be developmental hazards.

Rational advice to couples planning to become pregnant would be to ensure that blood lead levels are normalized before conception.

Key points

- Noxious exposures at the workplace are acknowledged risk factors for a range of adverse reproductive outcomes, including poor semen quality, menstrual disturbances, sexual dysfunction, infertility, spontaneous abortion, congenital malformation, preterm birth, fetal growth retardation, childhood cancer and impaired cognitive development during childhood.
- Occupational hazards include a wide range of toxicants, as well as physical, microbiological, ergonomic, night work and possibly psychosocial factors.
- The four reproductive cycles including gametogenesis, embryogenesis and fetal growth, lactation and prepubertal development are all susceptible to reproductive toxicants.
- Risk assessment should be based upon no-observed effect levels or benchmark doses in appropriate animal studies with appropriate safety factors because only few occupational exposure limits are designed to protect specifically against reproductive risks.

REFERENCES

1. Wilcox AJ, Weinberg CR, O'Connor JF et al. Incidence of early loss of pregnancy. *New England Journal of Medicine.* 1988; **319**: 189–94.
2. Juul S, Karmaus W, Olsen J. Regional differences in waiting time to pregnancy: Pregnancy-based surveys from Denmark, France, Germany, Italy and Sweden. The European Infertility and Subfecundity Study Group. *Human Reproduction.* 1999; **14**: 1250–4.
3. Evers JL. Female subfertility. *Lancet.* 2002; **360**: 151–9.
4. de Kretser DM. Male infertility. *Lancet.* 1997l; **349**: 787–90.
5. Ramlau-Hansen CH, Thulstrup AM, Aggerholm AS et al. Is smoking a risk factor for decreased semen quality? A cross-sectional analysis. *Human Reproduction.* 2007; **22**: 188–96.
6. Giwercman A, Carlsen E, Keiding N, Skakkebaek NE. Evidence for increasing incidence of abnormalities of the human testis: A review. *Environmental Health Perspectives.* 1993; **101** (Suppl. 2): 65–71.
7. Bonde JP, Ernst E, Jensen TK et al. Relation between semen quality and fertility: A population-based study of 430 first-pregnancy planners. *Lancet.* 1998; **352**: 1172–7.
8. Jorgensen N, Asklund C, Carlsen E, Skakkebaek NE. Coordinated European investigations of semen quality: Results from studies of Scandinavian young men is a matter of concern. *International Journal of Andrology.* 2006; **29**: 54–61.
9. Whorton D. Pesticides: Pesticide-induced infertility in male workers. Occupational Safety and Health Symposia 1978, Division of Technical Services, NIOSH (210-78-0053).
10. Bonde JP, Joffe M, Sallmen M et al. Validity issues relating to time-to-pregnancy studies of fertility. *Epidemiology.* 2006; **17**: 347–9.
11. Ogilvy-Stuart AL, Shalet SM. Effect of radiation on the human reproductive system. *Environmental Health Perspectives.* 1993; **101** (Suppl. 2): 109–16.
12. Lancranjan I, Maicanescu M, Rafaila E et al. Gonadic function in workmen with longterm exposure to microwaves. *Health Physics.* 1975; **29**: 381–3.
13. Hjollund NH, Bonde JP, Skotte J. Semen analysis of personnel operating military radar equipment. *Reproductive Toxicology.* 1997; **11**: 897.
14. Weyandt TB, Schrader SM, Turner TW, Simon SD. Semen analysis of military personnel associated with military duty assignments. *Reproductive Toxicology.* 1996; **10**: 521–8.
15. Hjollund NH, Skotte JH, Kolstad HA, Bonde JP. Extremely low frequency magnetic fields and fertility: A follow up study of couples planning first pregnancies. The Danish First Pregnancy Planner Study Team. *Occupational and Environmental Medicine.* 1999; **56**: 253–5.
16. Mieusset R, Bujan L. Testicular heating and its possible contributions to male infertility: A review. *International Journal of Andrology.* 1995; **18**: 169–84.

17. Figa-Talamanca I, Cini C, Varricchio GC et al. Effects of prolonged autovehicle driving on male reproduction function: A study among taxi drivers. *American Journal of Industrial Medicine.* 1996; **30**: 750–8.
18. Thonneau P, Ducot B, Bujan L et al. Heat exposure as a hazard to male fertility. *Lancet.* 1996; **347**: 204–5.
19. Bujan L, Daudin M, Charlet JP et al. Increase in scrotal temperature in car drivers. *Human Reproduction.* 2000; **15**: 1355–7.
20. Stoy J, Hjollund NH, Mortensen JT et al. Semen quality and sedentary work position. *International Journal of Andrology.* 2004; **27**: 5–11.
21. Vanhoorne M, Comhaire F, De Bacquer D. Epidemiological study of the effects of carbon disulfide on male sexuality and reproduction. *Archives of Environmental Health.* 1994; **49**: 273–8.
22. Kolstad HA, Bonde JP, Spano M et al. Sperm chromatin structure and semen quality following occupational styrene exposure. *Scandinavian Journal of Work and Environmental Health.* 1999; **25** (Suppl. 1): 70–3, discussion 76–8.
23. Kolstad HA, Bisanti L, Roeleveld N et al. Time to pregnancy for men occupationally exposed to styrene in several European reinforced plastics companies. *Scandinavian Journal of Work and Environmental Health.* 1999; **25** (Suppl. 1): 66–9, discussion 76–8.
24. Tielemans E, Burdorf A, te Velde ER et al. Occupationally related exposures and reduced semen quality: A case-control study. *Fertility and Sterility.* 1999; **71**: 690–6.
25. Omura M, Romero Y, Zhao M, Inoue N. Histopathological evidence that spermatogonia are the target cells of 2-bromopropane. *Toxicology Letters.* 1999; **104**: 19–6.
26. Kim Y, Jung K, Hwang T et al. Hematopoietic and reproductive hazards of Korean electronic workers exposed to solvents containing 2-bromopropane. *Scandinavian Journal of Work and Environmental Health.* 1996; **22**: 387–91.
27. Alexander BH, Checkoway H, van Netten C et al. Semen quality of men employed at a lead smelter. *Journal of Occupational Medicine.* 1996; **53**: 411–16.
28. Lancranjan I, Popescu HI, Gavanescu O et al. Reproductive ability of workmen occupationally exposed to lead. *Archives of Environmental Health.* 1975; **30**: 396–401.
29. Viskum S, Rabjerg L, Jorgensen PJ, Grandjean P. Improvement in semen quality associated with decreasing occupational lead exposure. *American Journal of Industrial Medicine.* 1999; **35**: 257–63.
30. Robins TG, Bornman MS, Ehrlich RI et al. Semen quality and fertility of men employed in a South African lead acid battery plant. *American Journal of Industrial Medicine.* 1997; **32**: 369–76.
31. Apostoli P, Kiss P, Porru S et al. Male reproductive toxicity of lead in animals and humans. ASCLEPIOS Study Group. *Occupational and Environmental Medicine.* 1998; **55**: 364–74.
32. Bonde JP, Joffe M, Apostoli P et al. Sperm count and chromatin structure in men exposed to inorganic lead: Lowest adverse effect levels. *Occupational and Environmental Medicine.* 2002; **59**: 234–42.
33. Joffe M, Bisanti L, Apostoli P et al. Time to pregnancy and occupational lead exposure. *Scandinavian Journal of Work and Environmental Health.* 1999; **25** (Suppl. 1): 64–5, discussion 76–8.
34. Bonde JP. Semen quality and sex hormones among mild steel and stainless steel welders: A cross sectional study. *British Journal of Industrial Medicine.* 1990; **47**: 508–14.
35. Mortensen JT. Risk for reduced sperm quality among metal workers, with special reference to welders. *Scandinavian Journal of Work and Environmental Health.* 1988; **14**: 27–30.
36. Hjollund NH, Bonde JP, Jensen TK et al. Semen quality and sex hormones with reference to metal welding. *Reproductive Toxicology.* 1998; **12**: 91–5.
37. Hjollund NH, Bonde JP, Jensen TK et al. A follow-up study of male exposure to welding and time to pregnancy. *Reproductive Toxicology.* 1998; **12**: 29–37.
38. Larsen SB, Giwercman A, Spano M, Bonde JP. A longitudinal study of semen quality in pesticide spraying Danish farmers. The ASCLEPIOS Study Group. *Reproductive Toxicology.* 1998; **12**: 581–9.
39. Thonneau P, Abell A, Larsen SB et al. Effects of pesticide exposure on time to pregnancy: Results of a multicenter study in France and Denmark. ASCLEPIOS Study Group. *American Journal of Epidemiology.* 1999; **150**: 157–63.
40. Abell A, Ernst E, Bonde JP. Semen quality and sexual hormones in greenhouse workers. *Scandinavian Journal of Work and Environmental Health.* 2000; **26**: 492–500.
41. de Cock J, Westveer K, Heederik D et al. Time to pregnancy and occupational exposure to pesticides in fruit growers in The Netherlands. *Occupational and Environmental Medicine.* 1994; **51**: 693–9.
42. Greenlee AR, Arbuckle TE, Chyou PH. Risk factors for female infertility in an agricultural region. *Epidemiology.* 2003; **14**: 429–36.
43. Petrelli G, Figa-Talamanca I. Reduction in fertility in male greenhouse workers exposed to pesticides. *European Journal of Epidemiology.* 2001; **17**: 675–7.
44. Rupa DS, Reddy PP, Reddi OS. Reproductive performance in population exposed to pesticides in cotton fields in India. *Environmental Research.* 1991; **55**: 123–8.
45. Sanchez-Pena LC, Reyes BE, Lopez-Carrillo L et al. Organophosphorous pesticide exposure alters sperm chromatin structure in Mexican agricultural workers. *Toxicology and Applied Pharmacology.* 2004; **196**: 108–13.
46. Tielemans E, van Kooij R, te Velde ER et al. Pesticide exposure and decreased fertilisation rates *in vitro*. *Lancet.* 1999; **354**: 484–5.
47. Trasler JM, Hales BF, Robaire B. Paternal cyclophosphamide treatment of rats causes fetal loss and malformations without affecting male fertility. *Nature.* 1985; **316**: 144–6.
48. Marchetti F, Lowe X, Bishop J, Wyrobek AJ. Absence of selection against aneuploid mouse sperm at fertilization. *Biology of Reproduction.* 1999; **61**: 948–54.

49. Harkonen K, Viitanen T, Larsen SB *et al.* Aneuploidy in sperm and exposure to fungicides and lifestyle factors. ASCLEPIOS Group. A European Concerted Action on Occupational Hazards to Male Reproductive Capability. *Environmental and Molecular Mutagenesis.* 1999; **34**: 39–46.
50. Savitz DA. Paternal exposure to known mutagens and health of the offspring: Ionizing radiation and tobacco smoke. *Advances in Experimental Medicine and Biology.* 2003; **518**: 49–57.
51. Savitz DA, Sonnenfeld NL, Olshan AF. Review of epidemiologic studies of paternal occupational exposure and spontaneous abortion. *American Journal of Industrial Medicine.* 1994; **25**: 361–83.
52. Logman JF, de Vries LE, Hemels ME *et al.* Paternal organic solvent exposure and adverse pregnancy outcomes: A meta-analysis. *American Journal of Industrial Medicine.* 2005; **47**: 37–44.
53. Silbergeld EK, Quintanilla-Vega B, Gandley RE. Mechanisms of male mediated developmental toxicity induced by lead. *Advances in Experimental Medicine and Biology.* 2003; **518**: 37–48.
54. Kline J, Stein Z, Susser M. *Conception to birth. Epidemiology of prenatal development.* Monographs in epidemiology and biostatistics, vol. 14. New York: Oxford University Press, 1989.
55. Maldonado G, Delzell E, Tyl RW, Sever LE. Occupational exposure to glycol ethers and human congenital malformations. *International Archives of Occupational and Environmental Health.* 2003; **76**: 405–23.
56. Brent RL. Addressing environmentally caused human birth defects. *Pediatrics in Review.* 2001; **22**: 153–65.
57. Al-Mufti AW, Copplestone JF, Kazantzis G *et al.* Epidemiology of organomercury poisoning in Iraq. I. Incidence in a defined area and relationship to the eating of contaminated bread. *Bulletin of the World Health Organization.* 1976; **53** (Suppl.): 23–36.
58. Brent RL, Beckman DA. Environmental teratogens. *Bulletin of the New York Academy of Medicine.* 1990; **66**: 123–63.
59. Marbury MC, Linn S, Monson RR *et al.* Work and pregnancy. *Journal of Occupational Medicine.* 1984; **26**: 415–21.
60. Sever LE. Congenital malformations related to occupational reproductive hazards. *Occupational Medicine.* 1994; **9**: 471–94.
61. Burm AG. Occupational hazards of inhalational anaesthetics. *Best Practice and Research. Clinical Anaesthesiology.* 2003; **17**: 147–61.
62. McGregor DG. Occupational exposure to trace concentrations of waste anesthetic gases. *Mayo Clinic Proceedings.* 2000; **75**: 273–7.
63. Boivin JF. Risk of spontaneous abortion in women occupationally exposed to anaesthetic gases: A meta-analysis. *Occupational and Environmental Medicine.* 1997; **54**: 541–8.
64. Rowland AS, Baird DD, Weinberg CR *et al.* Reduced fertility among women employed as dental assistants exposed to high levels of nitrous oxide. *New England Journal of Medicine.* 1992; **327**: 993–7.
65. Fransman W, Roeleveld N, Peelen S *et al.* Nurses with dermal exposure to antineoplastic drugs: Reproductive outcomes. *Epidemiology* 2007; **18**: 112–19.
66. Meijster T, Fransman W, van Hemmen J *et al.* A probabilistic assessment of the impact of interventions on oncology nurses' exposure to antineoplastic agents. *Occupational and Environmental Medicine.* 2006; **63**: 530–7.
67. Lindbohm ML. Effects of parental exposure to solvents on pregnancy outcome. *Journal of Occupational and Environmental Medicine.* 1995; **37**: 908–14.
68. McMartin KI, Chu M, Kopecky E *et al.* Pregnancy outcome following maternal organic solvent exposure: A meta-analysis of epidemiologic studies. *American Journal of Industrial Medicine.* 1998; **34**: 288–92.
69. Lindbohm ML, Taskinen H, Sallmen M, Hemminki K. Spontaneous abortions among women exposed to organic solvents. *American Journal of Industrial Medicine.* 1990; **17**: 449–63.
70. Taskinen H, Kyyronen P, Hemminki K *et al.* Laboratory work and pregnancy outcome. *Journal of Occupational Medicine.* 1994; **36**: 311–19.
71. Khattak S, Moghtader G, McMartin K *et al.* Pregnancy outcome following gestational exposure to organic solvents: A prospective controlled study. *Journal of the American Medical Association.* 1999; **281**: 1106–9.
72. Hardin BD, Kelman BJ, Brent RL. Trichloroethylene and dichloroethylene: A critical review of teratogenicity. *Birth Defects Research. Part A, Clinical and Molecular Teratology.* 2005; **73**: 931–55.
73. Watson RE, Jacobson CF, Williams AL *et al.* Trichloroethylene-contaminated drinking water and congenital heart defects: A critical analysis of the literature. *Reproductive Toxicology.* 2006; **21**: 117–47.
74. Correa A, Gray RH, Cohen R *et al.* Ethylene glycol ethers and risks of spontaneous abortion and subfertility. *American Journal of Epidemiology.* 1996; **143**: 707–17.
75. Elliott RC, Jones JR, McElvenny DM *et al.* Spontaneous abortion in the British semiconductor industry: An HSE investigation. Health and Safety Executive. *American Journal of Industrial Medicine.* 1999; **36**: 557–72.
76. Maldonado G, Delzell E, Tyl RW, Sever LE. Occupational exposure to glycol ethers and human congenital malformations. *International Archives of Occupational and Environmental Health.* 2003; **76**: 405–23.
77. Hertz-Picciotto I. The evidence that lead increases the risk for spontaneous abortion. *American Journal of Industrial Medicine.* 2000; **38**: 300–9.
78. Bellinger DC. Teratogen update: Lead and pregnancy. *Birth Defects Research. Part A, Clinical and Molecular Teratology.* 2005; **73**: 409–20.
79. Schuurs AH. Reproductive toxicity of occupational mercury. A review of the literature. *Journal of Dentistry.* 1999; **27**: 249–56.
80. Holson JF, DeSesso JM, Jacobson CF, Farr CH. Appropriate use of animal models in the assessment of risk during

80. prenatal development: An illustration using inorganic arsenic. *Teratology.* 2000, **62**: 51–71.
81. Anttila A, Sallmen M. Effects of parental occupational exposure to lead and other metals on spontaneous abortion. *Journal of Occupational and Environmental Medicine.* 1995; **37**: 915–21.
82. Garcia AM. Occupational exposure to pesticides and congenital malformations: A review of mechanisms, methods, and results. *American Journal of Industrial Medicine.* 1998; **33**: 232–40.
83. Nurminen T. Maternal pesticide exposure and pregnancy outcome. *Journal of Occupational and Environmental Medicine.* 1995; **37**: 935–40.
84. Giwercman A, Carlsen E, Keiding N, Skakkebaek NE. Evidence for increasing incidence of abnormalities of the human testis: A review. *Environmental Health Perspectives.* 1993; **101** (Suppl. 2): 65–71.
85. Longnecker MP, Klebanoff MA, Zhou H, Brock JW. Association between maternal serum concentration of the DDT metabolite DDE and preterm and small-for-gestational-age babies at birth. *Lancet.* 2001; **358**: 110–14.
86. Korrick SA, Chen C, Damokosh AI et al. Association of DDT with spontaneous abortion: A case-control study. *Annals of Epidemiology.* 2001; **11**: 491–6.
87. International Agency for Research on Cancer. Occupational exposures of hairdressers and barbers and personal use of hair colourants; some hair dyes, cosmetic colourants, industrial dyestuffs and aromatic amines. IARC Monographs on the Evaluation of Carcinogenic Risks to Humans. Lyon: IARC, 1993.
88. Zhu JL, Vestergaard M, Hjollund NH, Olsen J. Pregnancy outcomes among female hairdressers who participated in the Danish National Birth Cohort. *Scandinavian Journal of Work and Environmental Health.* 2006; **32**: 61–6.
89. Lorente C, Cordier S, Bergeret A et al. Maternal occupational risk factors for oral clefts. Occupational Exposure and Congenital Malformation Working Group. *Scandinavian Journal of Work and Environmental Health.* 2000; 26: 137–45.
90. Shaw GM. Adverse human reproductive outcomes and electromagnetic fields: A brief summary of the epidemiologic literature. *Bioelectromagnetics.* 2001; (Suppl. 5): S5–18.
91. Freeman S, Geal-Dor M, Sohmer H. Development of inner ear (cochlear and vestibular) function in the fetus-neonate. *Journal of Basic and Clinical Physiology and Pharmacology.* 1999; **10**: 173–89.
92. Querleu D, Renard X, Versyp F et al. Fetal hearing. *European Journal of Obstetrics, Gynecology, and Reproductive Biology.* 1988; **28**: 191–212.
93. Sternfeld B. Physical activity and pregnancy outcome. Review and recommendations. *Sports Medicine.* 1997; **23**: 33–47.
94. Marbury MC. Relationship of ergonomic stressors to birthweight and gestational age. *Scandinavian Journal of Work and Environmental Health.* 1992; **18**: 73–83.
95. Mozurkewich EL, Luke B, Avni M, Wolf FM. Working conditions and adverse pregnancy outcome: A meta-analysis. *Obstetrics and Gynecology.* 2000; **95**: 623–35.
96. Pompeii LA, Savitz DA, Evenson KR et al. Physical exertion at work and the risk of preterm delivery and small-for-gestational-age birth. *Obstetrics and Gynecology.* 2005; **106**: 1279–88.
97. Ahlborg G Jr. Physical work load and pregnancy outcome. *Journal of Occupational and Environmental Medicine.* 1995; **37**: 941–4.
98. Oths KS, Dunn LL, Palmer NS. A prospective study of psychosocial job strain and birth outcomes. *Epidemiology.* 2001; **12**: 744–6.
99. Croteau A, Marcoux S, Brisson C. Work activity in pregnancy, preventive measures, and the risk of preterm delivery. *American Journal of Epidemiology.* 2007; **166**: 951–65.
100. Dole N, Savitz DA, Siega-Riz AM et al. Psychosocial factors and preterm birth among African American and White women in central North Carolina. *American Journal of Public Health.* 2004; **94**: 1358–65.
101. Hansen D, Lou HC, Olsen J. Serious life events and congenital malformations: A national study with complete follow-up. *Lancet.* 2000; **356**: 875–80.
102. Nurminen T. Shift work and reproductive health. *Scandinavian Journal of Work and Environmental Health.* 1998; **24** (Suppl. 3): 28–34.
103. Zhu JL, Hjollund NH, Andersen AM, Olsen J. Shift work, job stress, and late fetal loss: The National Birth Cohort in Denmark. *Journal of Occupational and Environmental Medicine.* 2004; **46**: 1144–9.
104. Valeur-Jensen AK, Pedersen CB, Westergaard T et al. Risk factors for parvovirus B19 infection in pregnancy. *Journal of the American Medical Association.* 1999; **281**: 1099–105.
105. Cartter ML, Farley TA, Rosengren S et al. Occupational risk factors for infection with parvovirus B19 among pregnant women. *Journal of Infectious Diseases.* 1991; **163**: 282–5.
106. Bellinger DC. Lead. *Pediatrics.* 2004; **113**: 1016–22.
107. Otake M, Schull WJ. Radiation-related brain damage and growth retardation among the prenatally exposed atomic bomb survivors. *International Journal of Radiation Biology.* 1998; **74**: 159–71.
108. Colt JS, Blair A. Parental occupational exposures and risk of childhood cancer. *Environmental Health Perspectives.* 1998; **106** (Suppl. 3): 909–25.
109. Newbold RR, McLachlan JA. Transplacental hormonal carcinogenesis: Diethylstilbestrol as an example. *Progress in Clinical and Biological Research.* 1996; **394**: 131–47.
110. McKinney PA, Fear NT, Stockton D. Parental occupation at periconception: findings from the United Kingdom Childhood Cancer Study. *Occupational and Environmental Medicine.* 2003; **60**: 901–9.
111. Nasterlack M. Do pesticides cause childhood cancer? *International Archives of Occupational and Environmental Health.* 2006; **79**: 536–44.

112. Paul M. Occupational reproductive hazards. *Lancet.* 1997; **349**: 1385–8.
113. Ahlborg G Jr, Bonde JP, Hemminki K *et al.* Communication concerning the risks of occupational exposures in pregnancy. *International Journal of Occupational and Environmental Health.* 1996; **2**: 64–9.
114. Bonde JP, Hjollund NH, Jensen TK *et al.* A follow-up study of environmental and biologic determinants of fertility among 430 Danish first-pregnancy planners: Design and methods. *Reproductive Toxicology.* 1998; **12**: 19–27.
115. Andersen AG, Jensen TK, Carlsen E *et al.* High frequency of sub-optimal semen quality in an unselected population of young men. *Human Reproduction.* 2000; **15**: 366–72.
116. Bonde JP, Giwercman A. Occupational hazards to male fecundity. *Reproductive Medicine Reviews.* 1995; **4**: 59–73.
117. Kumar S. Occupational exposure associated with reproductive dysfunction. *Journal of Occupational Health.* 2004; **46**: 1–19.
118. Winker R, Rudiger HW. Reproductive toxicology in occupational settings: An update. *International Archives of Occupational and Environmental Health.* 2006; **79**: 1–10.
119. Shaw GM. Strenuous work, nutrition and adverse pregnancy outcomes: A brief review. *Journal of Nutrition.* 2003; **133**: 1718S–1721S.
120. Shi L, Chia SE. A review of studies on maternal occupational exposures and birth defects, and the limitations associated with these studies. *Occupational Medicine.* 2001; **51**: 230–44.
121. Taskinen HK. Effects of parental occupational exposures on spontaneous abortion and congenital malformation. *Scandinavian Journal of Work and Environmental Health.* 1990; **16**: 297–314.

90

Haemopoietic effects of workplace exposures: anaemias, leukaemias and lymphomas

EDWARD GORDON-SMITH, ANTHONY YARDLEY-JONES AND ATHERTON GRAY

Introduction	1215	Ionizing radiation	1224
Structure and function of the haemopoietic system	1215	Bone marrow failure	1224
Clinical evaluation	1218	Non-ionizing radiation	1225
Anaemia	1219	Other occupations and occupational agents	1225
Inherited disorders affected by occupational exposures	1220	Work-related issues resulting from treatment of haematological disease	1226
Lead and anaemia	1220	Case reports	1226
Bone marrow failure	1221	References	1227
Benzene and bone marrow failure	1222		
Other agents and aplastic anaemia	1224		

INTRODUCTION

The haemopoietic system is characterized by the proliferation and differentiation of cells which govern the delivery of oxygen to the tissues, the body's defence against infection and the maintenance of haemostasis. It is a system with a key physiological role and a high cell turnover which makes it sensitive to the influence of toxic agents which interfere with DNA replication and repair. In developed countries, many of the well-recognized causes of occupationally related disease, such as lead, benzene and ionizing radiation, are declining in incidence. However, in an increasingly complex globalized economy, with a migratory workforce operating in countries which have differing legislative controls, such diseases may still occur and it is important that an awareness of the effect of these exposures is maintained. Furthermore, the advent of new industries and processes carries the potential for producing substances with hitherto unrecognized haemopoietic effects.

In recent years, there have been extraordinary advances in the understanding of the molecular and genetic triggers of haematological diseases and these have allowed diagnoses to become more precise and treatments more focused. Treatment outcomes have improved and more patients, including those with occupational exposures, now have the option of returning to work. There is a need therefore to understand the issues concerning the long-term effects of some treatments and their impact on fitness for work. For all of these reasons the haemopoietic effects of workplace exposures are considered in this chapter as a distinct group.

STRUCTURE AND FUNCTION OF THE HAEMOPOIETIC SYSTEM

Stem cells and progenitor cells

The bone marrow stem cell has the capacity to renew itself as well as to produce progeny which proliferate and differentiate into mature cells. Stem cells are pluripotent which means that they are capable of forming colonies of progenitor cells (colony-forming units, CFU) which are multilineage (Figure 90.1), able to differentiate into red blood cells (erythrocytes), granulocytes and monocytes or platelets depending upon regulatory influences within the marrow. The stem cells also give rise to the cells of

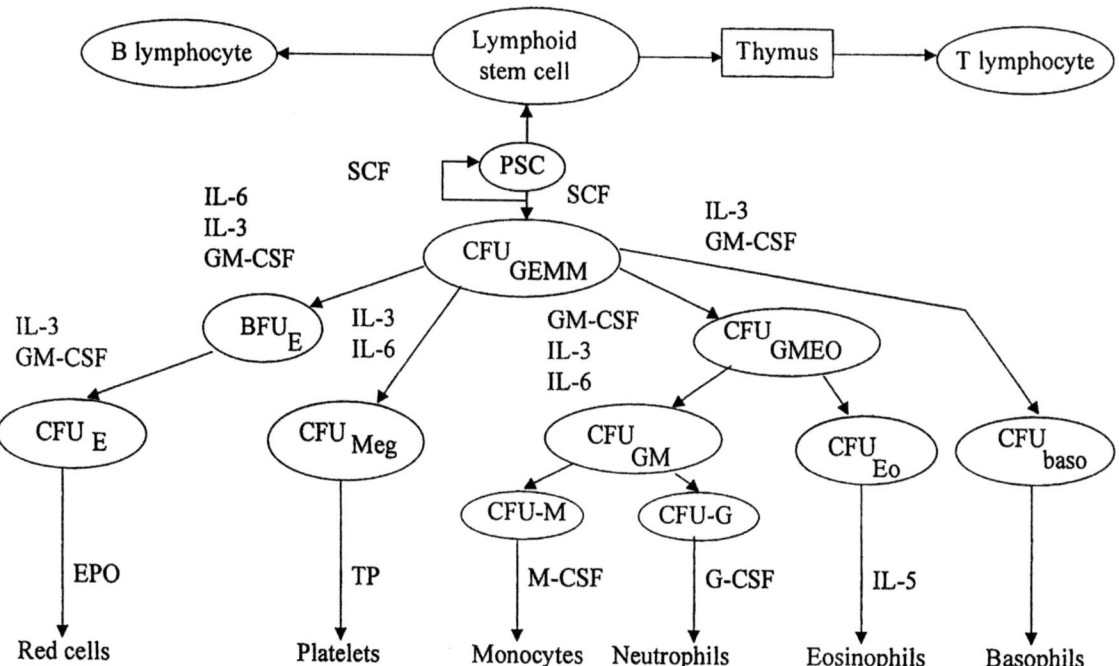

Figure 90.1 Maturation of haemopoietic cells. A simplified diagram of the maturation of haemopoietic cells from the pluripotent stem cell (PSC). baso, basophil; BFU, burst-forming unit; CFU, colony-forming unit; E, erythroid; Eo, eosinophil; GM, granulocyte, monocyte; GEMM, mixed granulocyte, erythroid, monocyte, megakaryocyte; MEG, megakaryocyte. Haemopoiesis is regulated by a family of glycoprotein growth factors with overlapping function and multiple sites of production. CSF, colony-stimulating factor; EPO, erythropoietin; IL, interleukin; SCF, stem cell factor; TP, thrombopoietin.

the immune system. As a consequence, it is not surprising that such a complex and rapidly proliferating system is sensitive to toxic effects at various stages. For example, inorganic lead and benzene exert their haematotoxic effects on erythropoiesis and progenitors, respectively, while ionizing radiation has the ability not only to damage dividing cells, but also resting cells including stem cells.

Regulation of haemopoiesis

As the bone marrow precursor cells (stem cells and progenitors) mature, they lose the capacity for self-renewal but increase their degree of differentiation before each cell division. It has been estimated that there are approximately 20 cell divisions in the maturation pathway and that one stem cell division is capable of producing one million mature blood cells. This is controlled by a complex array of interacting auxiliary cells, growth factors and extracellular matrix within the bone marrow stroma. The haemopoietic growth factors are glycoproteins which regulate the proliferation, differentiation and function of the blood cells. They act only at specific phases of cell maturation and either singly or in combination control the direction and rate of precursor cell differentiation. Many of them have now been cloned and are available for clinical use.

Circulating blood cells

The main circulating cells are the red blood cells (RBC), white blood cells including granulocytes, monocytes and lymphocytes, and platelets (thrombocytes). Red blood cells have a life span of 120 days. Granulocytes and monocytes have a short period in the circulation (about eight hours) before entering the tissues. Platelets have a life span of about ten days. The different life spans mean that toxic agents which acutely compromise cell production lead to a rapid fall in granulocytes and platelets, but anaemia may develop more slowly. Lymphocytes may survive and multiply in the circulation for prolonged periods and may reveal evidence of toxic damage after many years.

Red blood cells

Red blood cells (erythrocytes) transport oxygen from the lungs to the tissues and carbon dioxide in the opposite direction. To fulfil these functions, the erythrocyte is a deformable, biconcave disc, devoid of a nucleus and mitochondria, and contains functional haemoglobin (Hb) in high concentration. In order to maintain these characteristics, sources of energy and of reducing power are needed. Energy is generated as adenosine triphosphate (ATP) by the anaerobic glycolytic (Embden–Meyerhof, EM) pathway, 2 mol of ATP being produced from each mol of

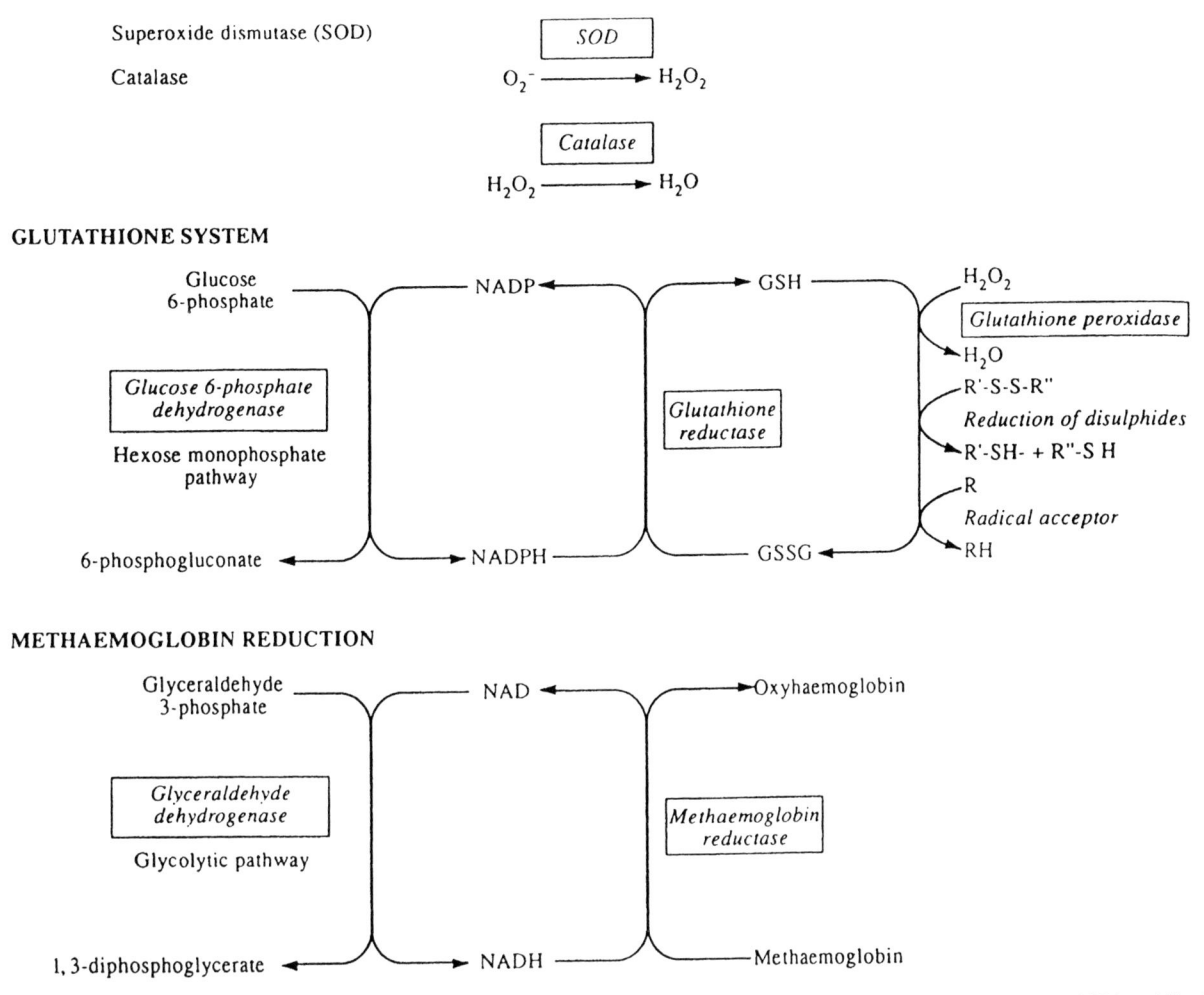

Figure 90.2 Principal reactions in the erythrocyte for the reduction of oxidized compounds. GHS, reduced glutathione; GSSG, oxidized glutathione; NADPH, reduced nicotinamide adenine dinucleotide phosphate; O_2^-, superoxide.

glucose (Figure 90.2). Reducing power, as reduced nicotinamide-adenine dinucleotide (NADH), is produced by the same pathway and as reduced nicotinamide-adenine dinucleotide phosphate (NADPH) by the hexose monophosphate (HMP) shunt (Figure 90.2). The role of the erythrocyte in oxygen carriage continuously exposes it to the risk of oxidative injury from endogenous substances (e.g. hydrogen peroxide, H_2O_2) often produced in response to infection, and exogenous oxidant drugs and chemicals. To counteract oxidant stress, the red cell has an array of protective antioxidants and redox defence mechanisms. These are largely a group of enzymes and co-factors catalysing reduction steps.

Haemoglobin is readily oxidized to methaemoglobin in which the ferrous iron (Fe^{2+}) is converted to the ferric state (Fe^{3+}) rendering the molecule incapable of oxygen transport. Methaemoglobin is mostly reduced by NADH:methaemoglobin reductase (cytochrome b_5 reductase) utilizing NADH derived from the EM pathway. Methaemoglobin-generating chemicals, such as aniline dyes and nitrobenzene, have a tendency to overwhelm even the normal erythrocyte's ability to reduce methaemoglobin to haemoglobin (Figure 90.2).

NADPH is a co-factor for glutathione reductase which maintains protein function by reduction of protein sulphydryl (-SH) groups, including those of haemoglobin, enzymes and the membrane. Glucose-6-phosphate dehydrogenase (G6PD) catalysing the first step in the HMP shunt is the only source of NADPH in red cells (Figure 90.2). Deficiency of NADPH results in the inefficient recycling of glutathione and, therefore, suboptimal protection against peroxides and slow reduction of disulphides. The red cells are therefore susceptible to added stress imposed by oxidant chemicals.

As molecular oxygen undergoes successive reductions, a number of reactive species, e.g. superoxide, hydrogen peroxide and hydroxyl radicals are generated. These have strong oxidizing potential and unless they are scavenged by enzymes in the red cells, such as superoxide dismutase, catalase and glutathione reductase, they may cause oxidative denaturation of haemoglobin, enzymes and other proteins, as well as membrane damage through lipid peroxidation. Which of these is the most important in damaging erythrocyte function depends on the type and origin of the oxidant stress and on the nature of the failure in reducing antioxidant protective mechanisms.

All of these defences against oxidant damage can be compromised by either congenital deficiency or impaired function of the relevant enzymes. Strong oxidizing agents, including some drugs and chemicals, however, may easily overwhelm these mechanisms resulting in oxidative haemolysis.

CLINICAL EVALUATION

History

An occupational history, as well as an accurate drug history, is part of the clinical evaluation of any patient presenting with a haematological disorder, but is particularly important in bone marrow failure syndromes, including aplastic anaemia, myelodysplastic syndrome and acute leukaemias. The latent interval between the onset of exposure and the clinical expression of disease may be many years, in which case a causal relation might well be overlooked. In these disorders, it is important that the occupational history encompasses both current and all previous employments, although the great majority of cases are not related to occupational exposure to potentially toxic substances. Anaemia, particularly haemolytic anaemia, may have a more rapid onset and potentially causative occupational exposure be more readily identified – providing such a possibility is thought about at the time.

Exposure dose, duration, peak levels as well as total, are each important but can be difficult to quantify. Dose determination may require particular techniques and expertise. Information on the use of personal protection (equipment and clothing) and general environmental control measures is essential in establishing whether a causal relation exists or not. Non-occupational environmental factors, such as the domestic or recreational use of pesticides and metals and the abuse or misuse of solvents, may also be relevant and should be recorded. Smoking history is important in cases of methaemoglobinaemia and carbon monoxide toxicity.

Inherited disorders may increase susceptibility to occupational risks so family and previous haematological histories are important. Drug records, both current and previous, are essential in establishing a possible occupational role. Particularly in bone marrow failure, multiple drug exposure may confound attempts to establish a precise causation. There are no tests which can be used to prove a particular causation, so aetiology is based on a number of circumstantial criteria; was the patient exposed to the potential cause, has the association been described before, and was the temporal relationship between exposure and presentation as expected in the causation of the disease?

Symptoms and signs

Symptoms of blood diseases relate mainly to deficiency of functioning blood cells. Anaemia is associated with fatigue, pallor and breathlessness on exertion. Slowly developing anaemia may be well tolerated down to very low levels of haemoglobin, whereas more acute anaemias produce effects early. Lack of granulocytes increases the risk of infection, but the susceptibility only becomes apparent at low levels (neutrophils $<0.5 \times 10^9$/L). Where occupational exposure is a potential risk to blood cell production, screening blood counts may be needed to identify problems before serious consequences arise. Easy bruising and haemorrhages are features of platelet deficiency, but again arise usually when there has been a marked reduction in number. Haemolytic anaemias due to increased RBC destruction present with mild acholuric jaundice with or without anaemia, depending on the rate of onset and destruction and the ability of the bone marrow to compensate for the increased loss. Obvious jaundice, particularly with bile in the urine, is suggestive of hepatic or biliary disease.

The bone marrow, spleen and the lymphatic system are the main organs associated with the haemopoietic system. Slight enlargement of the spleen, often detected only by ultrasound, is a feature of many anaemias including haemolytic anaemias when the spleen may be discovered on palpation. More marked enlargement, down to or below the umbilicus, is suggestive of lymphoma or myeloproliferative disorders such as myelofibrosis or chronic granulocytic leukaemia. Palpable lymph nodes raise the possibility of lymphoma. Systemic symptoms, such as fever and weight loss, are more usually features of leukaemia or lymphoma rather than aplastic anaemia or other types of marrow failure. It is important to elucidate all symptoms and signs involving other systems since many, if not all potentially toxic agents may affect other organs than the blood. Abdominal symptoms, neuropathies and liver abnormalities should be particularly examined.

Physical examination

Physical examination is important, but the signs of haematological disorders are often non-specific. Pallor may be noticed, but detection of anaemia by examination is notoriously difficult. Mouth ulcers and buccal haemorrhages may indicate low neutrophil counts or platelet levels, respectively. Petechial haemorrhages and more extensive bruising are also signs of thrombocytopenia. Jaundice, which may be mild, is suggestive of haemolysis. Certain occupational exposures may give rise to more specific physical signs, the detection of which should suggest the underlying diagnosis. These include central cyanosis caused by methaemoglobinaemia (nitrobenzene, aniline, aromatic amines); a blue line on the gingival margins (lead); peripheral neuropathy (arsenic, lead); plantar-palmar hyperkeratosis and transverse lines (Mee's lines) in the nail bed (arsenic); and acneiform eruptions (organochlorine compounds).

Laboratory investigation

Haematological diagnosis requires a full blood count with RBC indices and white blood cell differential, examination of the stained blood film and, where bone marrow damage is suspected, bone marrow aspirate and trephine. As with anaemias in general, those caused by workplace exposures, may be microcytic, normocytic or macrocytic. Lead poisoning characteristically produces a mild microcytic or normochromic anaemia, while haemolytic anaemias can be either normocytic or slightly macrocytic depending on the degree of reticulocytosis. Aplastic and myelodysplastic anaemias usually show a degree of macrocytosis. In general, the reticulocyte count should increase in response to anaemia and do so in proportion to its severity. This is particularly so when erythroid hyperplasia has had time to develop, as in chronic haemolysis. Failure of the reticulocyte count to increase in response to anaemia indicates impaired erythropoiesis. Investigation of haematological disorders is not discussed in detail, but examination of the blood film might reveal abnormalities which provide a clue to the underlying cause. Basophilic stippling of red cells (Figure 90.3) can be evidence of lead exposure, although the degree of stippling does not correlate with the body burden of lead. Heinz bodies (Figure 90.4) and other red cell inclusions are seen in haemolytic states associated with oxidant chemicals (aniline, naphthalene, nitrobenzene, nitrites and chlorates). These inclusions represent intracellular deposits of denatured globin and are also found in inherited haemoglobinopathies. Methaemoglobin is detected by changes in the Hb absorption spectra. Examination of the bone marrow requires not only histological review of the aspirate and trephine for dysplastic changes, but also cytogenetic analysis to look for acquired somatic mutations.

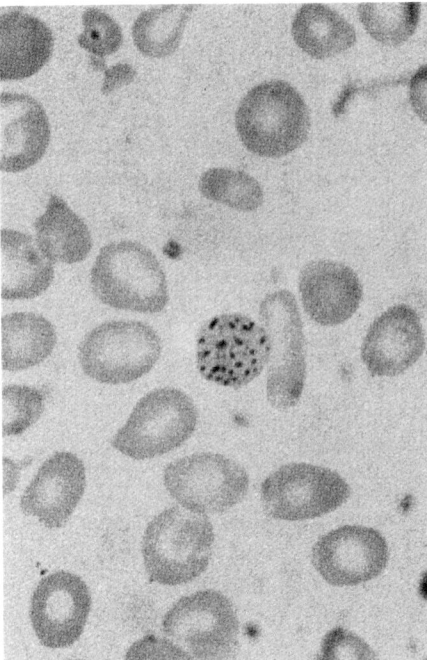

Figure 90.3 Basophilic stippling. From Ref. 66 with permission. See website (www.hodderplus.com/hunters) for colour plate.

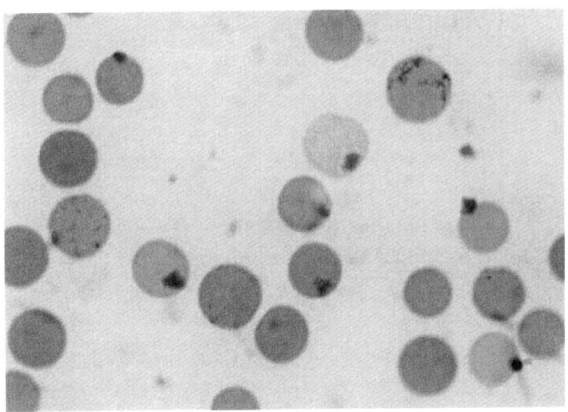

Figure 90.4 Heinz bodies. From Ref. 67 with permission. See website (www.hodderplus.com/hunters) for colour plate.

ANAEMIA

Anaemia is very common in many populations. It may be produced by dietary deficiency or malabsorption of iron, vitamin B_{12} or folic acid, chronic blood loss or an increased destruction of red blood cells – haemolytic anaemia. Occupational anaemias are mostly haemolytic.

Haemolytic anaemias

Haemolysis may be defined as that condition where the rate of red cell destruction is accelerated. The bone marrow normally responds to this change by increasing red cell production (erythroid hyperplasia), and theoretically this response can compensate for the excessive red cell destruction, even when the lifespan of the circulating cells is reduced from the normal 120 days to as few as 15–20 days. Anaemia develops when this compensatory mechanism fails to match the rate of haemolysis. Haemolytic anaemias may be due to intracellular defects of the membrane, haemoglobin or metabolic pathways or to extracellular events acting on the circulating red blood cells. The former are mainly inherited disorders, the latter acquired through many inherited disorders increase susceptibility to extracellular events. The excess destruction may take place in the reticuloendothelial system (extravascular haemolysis) or within the circulation (intravascular haemolysis).

Where haemolysis is attributable to occupational exposures, the clinical features are dependent on the agent and the route, duration and dose of the exposure. Anaemia may develop insidiously over a period of weeks or months, in which case pallor and mild jaundice may be the first indication of illness. Methaemoglobinaemia presents as central cyanosis. Acute intravascular haemolysis may occur following excessive oxidant stress and be accompanied by circulatory collapse, oliguria, haemoglobinuria, dyspnoea and generalized aching pains, especially in the loins and limbs.

Mechanisms of haemolysis

The most common mechanism of red cell damage in occupational medicine is oxidative attack which can be directed at the membrane of the red cell, the globin chains of the haemoglobin molecule or the haem group. The chemical may act as an oxidizing agent itself or it may interact with oxygen to form free radicals or peroxides. These are capable of oxidizing haem-bound ferrous iron to ferric iron with the formation of methaemoglobin which cannot serve as an oxygen carrier. This is a potentially reversible step, but if the oxidant stress is severe, the globin chains may denature and precipitate as inclusions known as Heinz bodies (Figure 90.4). These inclusions have an affinity with the red cell membrane which becomes damaged. Lipid peroxidation may also disrupt the integrity of the membrane. The damaged cells are then destroyed or fragmented in the reticuloendothelial system by the process of extravascular haemolysis. If the oxidant stress is greater there may be rapid red cell destruction with the clinical picture of intravascular haemolysis.

Acute intravascular haemolysis with methaemoglobinaemia is known to follow exposure to arsine, a highly toxic gas produced by the contact of acid with metals containing arsenic.[1,2] Chlorate also produces acute intravascular haemolysis, usually with acute renal failure.[3] Treatment for both arsine and chlorate poisoning is by red cell exchange transfusion.

INHERITED DISORDERS AFFECTED BY OCCUPATIONAL EXPOSURES

Glucose-6-phosphate dehydrogenase deficiency

Individuals with glucose-6-phosphate dehydrogenase (G6PD) deficiency have an increased susceptibility to oxidant chemicals. G6PD deficiency is an X-linked disorder common in much of Africa, Mediterranean countries and much of Southeast Asia, countries where falciparum malaria flourished. This diagnosis should be sought in any patient with acute haemolysis or recurrent haemolysis and especially where there is the likelihood of occupational exposure to oxidizing agents. Such individuals must avoid further exposure to oxidant chemicals, even though the exposure might be well within the relevant occupational exposure control values. Naphtha and naphtaline products produce acute intravascular haemolysis in G6PD-deficient subjects.[4]

Sickle cell disease

Sickle cell disease is common in parts of Africa, some parts of the Middle East around the Persian Gulf and occurs in small pockets in Greece. It is the result of inheriting the gene for HbS either in the homozygous state (HbS/S) or in combination with genes which deplete the normal HbA chains (HbS/β Thal; HbS/C). Patients suffer from recurrent painful crises and a number of other serious problems caused by the Hb in the red cells forming rigid structures which lead to non-deformable red cells and ischaemia. The process is aggravated by dehydration, fever, infection and cold. Hypoxia increases the precipitation of the Hb, so sufferers should avoid situations such as flying in unpressurized aircraft.[5] Heterozygotes (HbS/A) may have problems if hypoxia is severe.

Methaemoglobinaemia

Hereditary homozygous deficiency of the enzyme NADPH:methaemoglobin reductase is associated with benign congenital methaemoglobinaemia often with striking cyanosis. It is rare, but heterozygotes are asymptomatic unless exposed to oxidizing drugs or chemicals when cyanosis becomes apparent at much lower concentration of the agent than normal. Substances with the ability to induce the oxidation of the haem group leading to the formation of methaemoglobin include the aniline dyes, aromatic amines, nitro-substituted benzene compounds, and organic and inorganic nitrites and nitrates (see Chapter 42, Organic chemicals).[6–9] Methaemoglobin formation by itself does not necessarily lead to premature red cell destruction as shown by the absence of haemolysis in patients with methaemoglobinaemia induced by nitrites.

Some chemicals which produce methaemoglobinaemia have additional toxic effects which dominate the clinical presentation, for example methaemoglobinaemia produced by paraquat[10] is almost trivial in comparison with its effects on the lungs and other organ systems.

LEAD AND ANAEMIA

Chronic exposure to inorganic lead primarily affects erythropoiesis producing a combination of anaemia and bone marrow erythroid hyperplasia, an association best described by the term 'ineffective erythropoiesis'. The anaemia can be either microcytic or normochromic or mixed. Polychromasia may be noted on the blood film associated with slight elevation in the reticulocyte count and red cell survival is shortened. These are all features of haemolysis and reflect the inhibitory effect of lead on erythrocyte maturation and damage to the red cell membrane. The severity of the anaemia is poorly correlated with the degree of lead exposure, but is rarely seen at blood lead levels below 60 μg/100 mL in occupationally exposed groups. The anaemia of chronic lead exposure is characteristically persistent, unlike that of acute lead poisoning (see Chapter 23, Lead).

The bone marrow usually shows erythroid hyperplasia and may also be sideroblastic (ineffective erythropoiesis with typical ringed sideroblasts), but erythroid hypoplasia is also occasionally described.

Basophilic stippling (Figure 90.3) of red cells may be prominent, but it is not always found and correlates poorly with blood lead levels, haemoglobin and clinical symptoms. It is unusual when blood lead levels are below 80–100 μg/100 mL. With improved controls of current occupational exposures, this marker of lead poisoning is now a rare feature in the peripheral blood. In general, haematological parameters are neither sensitive nor specific in relation to blood lead levels, although there is a correlation between lead and Hb levels in environmentally exposed populations.[11] The mechanism of lead-induced anaemia involves reduced red cell production (ineffective erythropoiesis), as well as reduced red cell survival (haemolysis) (see Chapter 23, Lead).[12] The pathogenesis of the ineffective erythropoiesis is complex and not completely understood.

5-Aminolaevulinic acid (ALA) dehydratase is the enzyme most affected by lead, but the majority of the enzyme steps in the human biosynthetic pathway are inhibited by lead to some degree. The haemolytic component is due to both lead-induced structural alterations in the red cell membrane and impaired erythrocyte pyrimidine 5′-nucleotidase activity. Under normal conditions, this enzyme plays a prominent role in the cleavage of residual nucleotide chains that persist in the cell after nuclear extrusion. Deficiency, whether in the acquired or the congenital form, is usually associated with the presence of basophilic stippling which has been shown to result from the deposition of aggregates of ribosomal RNA. The accumulation of nucleotides inhibits the HMP shunt and this accelerates the rate of haemolysis. Lead may also impair globin chain synthesis. In view of its multiplicity of effects on the red cell, it is interesting that anaemia is a late sign of lead intoxication.[12] Biological effect monitoring techniques utilize the increase in substrate concentrations, such as urinary ALA and erythrocyte protoporphyrin, to screen for exposure. The general reduction in occupational exposures to the metal in developed countries has meant that patients with lead toxicity now more commonly present with non-haematological manifestations.

BONE MARROW FAILURE

In a number of disorders, failure of the bone marrow stem cells to produce adequate numbers or functional progenitors leads to inadequate circulating functional blood cells with consequent anaemia, risk of infection and defects of haemostasis. The disorders which may be generated by occupational exposures are aplastic anaemia, myelodysplastic syndromes (MDS) and acute myeloid leukaemia (AML).

Aplastic anaemia

Aplastic anaemia is a rare disease ($1–2 \times 10^6$ population/year in the West), defined by the presence of a peripheral blood pancytopenia and a hypocellular marrow. Remaining blood cells have more or less normal morphology (Figure 90.5a,b). The cause of the bone marrow failure lies in the pluripotent stem cells, but in some cases and at certain stages of the disease one of the cell lines may be more severely affected than the others. About 15 per cent of cases are thought to be triggered by exposure to drugs or chemicals, about 10 per cent follow a hepatitic illness and the great majority are idiopathic. Among the chemical and physical agents associated with aplastic anaemia are those which invariably cause aplasia given a sufficient dose (benzene, ionizing radiation) and those which only do so occasionally (arsenicals, gamma-benzene hexachloride and other insecticides, glycol ethers, carbon tetrachloride).[13] Hair dye containing paratoluenediamine and closely related compounds have been linked to several case reports of aplastic anaemia in non-occupationally exposed individuals having used the dye two to three weeks before the onset of symptoms.[14] In such case studies, it is difficult to be certain whether the dye was the aetiologic factor. Where a drug, chemical or virus has been identified as a likely cause of the marrow damage, the exposure is usually some 3–24 months before the effects of the pancytopenia become apparent. This is the idiosyncratic form of aplastic anaemia. Recurrent subclinical exposure to a myelotoxic agent, such as benzene, is associated with a much longer latent period. Cytogenetic abnormalities are uncommon[15] and the disease may remain stable for years or may evolve to a more malignant phase of myelodysplastic syndrome and/or acute myeloid leukaemia with the emergence of clonal cytogenetic abnormalities. Any age group may be affected, but there are peaks in young adults and in those over 50. In severe cases (neutrophils $<0.5 \times 10^9$/L, platelets $<20 \times 10^9$/L and reticulocytes $<20 \times 10^9$/L), the prognosis was very poor before the introduction of specific treatment with immunosuppression or stem cell transplantation. Five year survival following either treatment is of the order of 70 per cent, but patients treated with immunosuppression continue to have a high risk of developing abnormal clones, including MDS and AML.

becomes more common with increasing age. At one end of the spectrum, the syndrome overlaps with aplastic anaemia with a hypocellular marrow,[16] at the other end it merges with AML. There have been various classifications of the syndrome, the most recent being the WHO classification[17,18] and an International Prognostic Scoring System (IPSS) provides an important means of risk assessment for individual patients.[19] Cytogenetic abnormalities, cytopenias and the presence of leukaemic blasts are poor prognostic factors. MDS may arise some years after chemotherapy for other malignant haematological diseases, secondary MDS having a poor prognosis usually evolving into AML.

Acute myeloid leukaemia

This is not the place for a detailed discussion of AML. The disease may be stratified into good-, standard- and poor-risk groups according to a number of molecular and cytogenetic findings. AML may arise *de novo*, secondary to idiopathic MDS or aplastic anaemia or following chemo- and/or radiotherapy (treatment-associated AML (tAML)). Particular cytogenetic abnormalities are found in tAML following specific treatment schedules. Alkylating agents, such as melphalan and cyclophosphamide, are associated with abnormalities of chromosome 5 and 7; topoisomerase inhibitors, etoposide and doxorubicin, cause leukaemias with translocation at 11q23. Other anomalies are found with other therapeutic agents.

BENZENE AND BONE MARROW FAILURE

Benzene is volatile and readily absorbed by inhalation or through dermal contact. It was formerly used as a solvent in a wide variety of manufacturing processes involving leather, rubber, paint spraying and removing, dry cleaning, printing, batteries, linoleum and metal plating (see Chapter 42, Organic chemicals). Benzene itself is no longer used as a commercial solvent having been replaced by non-aromatic organic solvents, but it is still used in some chemical processes and is present in coal derivatives and petroleum fractions and distillates. Insecticides are often applied in petroleum-based media and in these cases the precise component which is causative in the development of aplastic anaemia (the insecticide or solvent) is often unclear.

The haematological effects of benzene exposure vary widely between individuals. An early stage of benzene toxicity is leukopenia, particularly lymphopenia,[20] which is reversible when exposure is withdrawn. More persistent exposure may lead to irreversible marrow damage though often with a latent period of 5–20 years. It is thought that metabolites of benzene are critical for its toxicity and variation in the metabolic pathway between individuals may account for some of the marked disparity in susceptibility to benzene in workers exposed to similar levels in the workplace.[21]

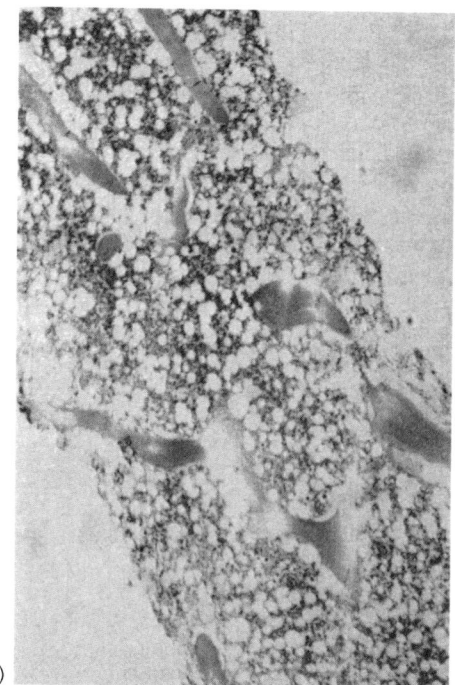
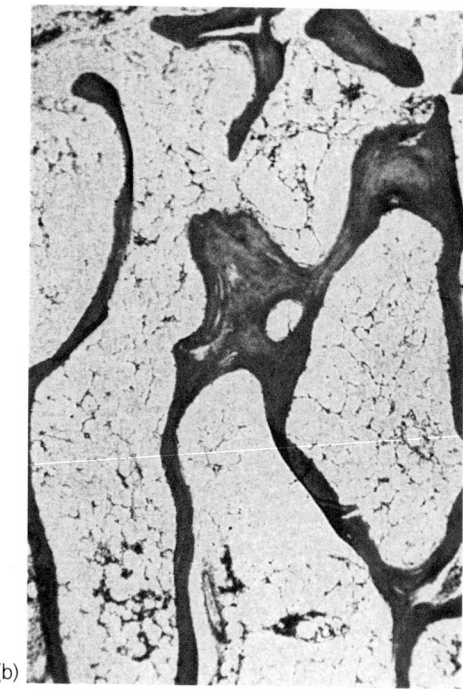

Figure 90.5 (a) Normal and (b) hypoplastic marrow. From Ref. 67 with permission. See website (www.hodderplus.com/hunters) for colour plate.

Myelodysplastic syndrome

Myelodysplasia implies abnormal morphology of blood cell progenitors in the marrow. MDS is a collection of bone marrow failure disorders with various abnormalities of some or all progenitor cell lines, often with cytogenetic abnormalities and variable cytopenias, and functional abnormalities in peripheral blood cells. The syndrome

Aplastic anaemia

The association of benzene with aplastic anaemia has been known about for nearly a century, but in countries where there are strict controls and substitution for other solvents has occurred, this is now rarely seen (see Chapter 42, Organic chemicals). Cases may still occur in developing countries and studies on exposed workers in China have been particularly illuminating for the epidemiology of benzene toxicity.[20,22] The incidence of aplastic anaemia in the general population is 1–2 per 10^6 per year: a six-fold increase was observed in one study on exposed Chinese workers[23] and as high as 15-fold in Italian shoe workers exposed to particularly high levels.[24]

Acute myeloid leukaemia and myelodysplastic syndrome

Malignant clonal disorders may arise after benzene exposure with or without an aplastic or intermediate phase. The incidence increases with the dose and duration of exposure.[25] Chronic exposure is more likely than acute poisoning to promote leukaemogenesis. Analysis of epidemiological studies suggests that there has to be a critical average concentration of benzene (>20 ppm) together with exposure for several years (more than six years)[26] before the increased risk of acquiring acute myeloid leukaemia becomes evident. Frequent short-term exposures at high levels (>100 ppm) may result in transient blood changes (leukocytosis, polymorphocytosis) with no apparent long-term effects. In contrast, repeated low-dose exposure above 20 ppm[27,28] results in cytopenias (anaemia, leukopenia and thrombocytopenia). The role of occasional high exposures in addition to long-term chronic exposures in the risk of developing acute myeloid leukaemia is a difficult area to explore given the lack of detail in historical occupational history data. Although removal of such exposed individuals from a benzene-containing environment usually results in the disappearance of such peripheral blood abnormalities over a period of months, the long-term risk of aplasia or leukaemia is not known.

Since the first suggestion in 1928 that benzene may be associated with leukaemia, several epidemiology studies have established that there is a specific causal relationship between the development of acute myeloid leukaemia and chronic exposure to benzene (see Chapter 42, Organic chemicals).[29]

The metabolism of benzene is complicated and gives rise to several reactive metabolites both in man and experimental animals which interact with a number of highly complex biological processes.[30] The profile of benzene metabolites produced is the result of a subtle interplay of oxidation and conjugation pathways and distribution of enzyme systems in the liver and other organs, as well as relative rates of perfusion in different organs and different species.[31] Experimental studies *in vivo* and *in vitro* suggest that the timing, duration and concentration of exposure to benzene metabolites (hydroquinone, catechol and muconaldehyde) are important independent factors in predicting potential leukaemogenic effects.[29] Furthermore, it has been shown that a greater number of these metabolites result from short-duration, high-level rather than from long-duration, low-level exposures.

The metabolites can cause chromosomal aberrations or deletions that can alter the regulation and function of gene expression and cell proliferation in the marrow. It is speculated that such effects may also play a role in the acute myeloid leukaemia induced by benzene in humans. The relationship of AML to benzene exposure bears some similarity to therapy-induced or secondary leukaemias in clinical practice and may indicate similar mechanisms of causation. Chromosomal aberrations involving chromosomes 5 and 7, either alone or in combination with other changes, are found in most patients with therapy-related myelodysplastic syndrome prior to the development of overt acute myeloid leukaemia[32] and similar characteristic chromosomal aberrations have been found in some patients with benzene-induced leukaemia that were cytogenetically monitored from shortly after the onset of symptoms through a pre-leukaemic phase and until death.[33] A cytogenetic analysis of therapy-related myelodysplasia/acute myeloid leukaemia, *de novo* acute myeloid leukaemia and refractory anaemia patients has revealed a critical region at band (5q31) that was deleted in all patients.[34,35] However, there does not appear to be a unique set of chromosome anomalies caused by benzene exposure different from that seen in *de novo* leukaemias.[36]

Epidemiological studies suggest that benzene concentrations of at least 20–25 ppm experienced over years, are necessary for the appearance of acute myeloid leukaemia in exposed individuals.[25] In the past, refinery workers have been a target population for such effects, but recent studies[37,38] have shown no consistently elevated risks in relation to acute myeloid leukaemia. This may be explained by lower levels of exposure.

Non-Hodgkin's lymphoma and other haematological malignancies

While experimental and epidemiological evidence is very strong for the association of benzene with aplastic anaemia, MDS and AML, that for non-Hodgkin's lymphoma (NHL) is less certain. Cytogenetic mutations in circulating lymphocytes may be present for years following benzene exposure.[39] Case–control studies have produced conflicting results, a finding reflected in review articles on benzene and NHL. Some studies suggest that organic solvents, including chlorinated hydrocarbons, may increase the risk of some types of NHL but not aromatic solvents such as benzene.[40] On the other hand, an Italian study[41] did find such an association. One difficulty is that NHL is a disparate collection of subtypes which may have very different triggers. Nonetheless, an occupational history should be obtained from patients with NHL particularly to identify heavy exposure.

OTHER AGENTS AND APLASTIC ANAEMIA

There have been several case reports implicating the organochlorine lindane as a cause of aplastic anaemia, agranulocytosis or bone marrow hypoplasia.[42–44] However, lindane exposure was only confirmed in two of the cases. There have been no reported cases following therapeutic use where dermal absorption was documented. Early epidemiological studies did not show an association.[45] A more recent case–control study did show an association for woodworm treatment and aplastic anaemia.[46] Many other agents involved in pesticides and organic solvents have been incriminated in aplastic anaemia cases. The difficulty is that there are no tests which can conclusively demonstrate such causality in individual cases and even in the rare disease only about 2–6 per cent have a potential association with these agents.[13]

IONIZING RADIATION

This is radiation that penetrates tissues and generates secondary ionizations. It includes neutrons, a-particles, electrons, x-rays and g-rays. It may be further classified into particles with high linear energy transfer which do not penetrate deeply, but generate relatively high levels of ionization and waves with low linear energy transfer, such as x-rays and γ-rays, which penetrate more deeply but generate less ionization (see Chapter 53, Ionizing radiations). Bone marrow is the most sensitive tissue to radiation exposure and with increasing doses thereafter the gastrointestinal tract, skin, lungs and other tissues become affected.

BONE MARROW FAILURE

Pancytopenia with an aplastic marrow is a prompt but reversible response to therapeutic doses of radiation. This is mainly caused by damage and apoptosis in the rapidly dividing progenitor cell pool, sensitive to radiation. Larger doses produce damage to the stem cell pool with delayed onset of pancytopenia and increased risk of malignant change. The severity of the injury is dependent on the type, quality, dose, dose rate and tissue distribution of the radiation. Radiation-induced bone marrow aplasia is now an uncommon occupational hazard owing to stringent controls of exposure and health surveillance procedures in the nuclear industry and in radiological medicine. Accidental exposure does, however, still occur.

Uniform whole-body irradiation with 1–10 Gy of low linear energy transfer radiation produces pancytopenia predisposing the recipient to infections and bleeding usually two to four weeks after the exposure. In human bone marrow, the total number of nucleated cells is reduced at day 1 by 10–20 per cent after 1–2 Gy, by 25–30 per cent after 3–4 Gy, by 50–60 per cent after 5–7 Gy and by a maximum of 80–85 per cent after 8–10 Gy. Whole body irradiation up to 10 Gy is administered under carefully determined conditions in haemopoietic stem cell transplants for acute leukaemias and other malignant disorders where the transplant rescues the patient from the irreversible stem cell loss. Resistant cells such as macrophages, stromal cells, vascular endothelium and some mature granulocytes and eosinophils remain.[47] Doses exceeding 30 Gy damage the marrow microenvironment such that it can no longer sustain haemopoiesis.

In radiation accidents, the exposure may be difficult or impossible to quantify, but such information is vital in planning management. Not only is the total dose difficult to estimate, but the variation of dose across the bone marrow may not be quantifiable. Stem cell transplantation is only rarely an option because an accidental whole body dose producing irreversible marrow damage is likely to be associated with lethal damage to non-haemopoietic organs. In an early attempt to rescue subjects exposed to accidental radiation exposure which rendered them severely pancytopenic, all five patients transplanted recovered their own marrow function.[48] The behaviour of haematological parameters can be useful in dosimetry estimations. The peripheral blood lymphocyte count is the most sensitive index of radiation injury and its fall is directly related to the whole body radiation dose up to doses of about 3 Gy. Neutrophils show an initial increase over the first few days after irradiation, then a dose-related fall. Between 10 and 15 days after a dose of 2–5 Gy, there is a second rise due to recovering haemopoiesis from precursor cell populations, followed by a second decline to about day 25. The time-course for platelet loss is similar to that for granulocytes, but usually there is no second rise. The severity of the thrombocytopenia is also a measure of the exposure dose.

Figure 90.6 shows data from accident cases, depicting the average time-courses for suppression and recovery of neutrophils, lymphocytes and platelets in man following irradiation.

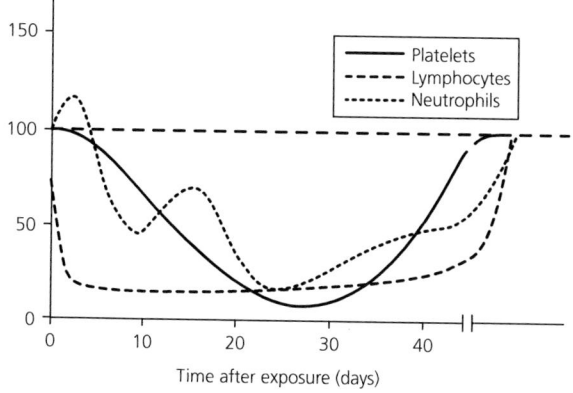

Figure 90.6 Effects of ionizing radiation on blood counts. Redrawn from Ref. 68 with permission.

Approximately three weeks after irradiation, patients become symptomatic as a result of the reduction in blood cell components. Where the radiation dose is less than 4–5 Gy, it is possible to support the individual with the use of blood and platelet transfusions and to treat infection with antibiotics appropriate to the pathogens isolated or suspected. If recovery is possible, it may be accelerated by the use of haemopoietic growth factors. Despite these measures, most victims (as found following the explosion at the Chernobyl nuclear power plant) receiving more than 5 Gy will not survive long enough for marrow function to recover.[49] This is not solely due to the marrow aplasia, but reflects the other injuries the patient may have suffered such as trauma, burns, inhalational effects, diarrhoea, and fluid and electrolyte depletion. Haemopoietic stem cell transplantation would seem the logical treatment for this group of patients, but is fraught with difficulties. These include the poor prognosis conferred by multiorgan damage, the inability to perform histocompatibility testing due to lymphocytopenia, the lack of compatible donors for most patients and the requirement for further immunosuppressive conditioning.

Leukaemia and MDS

The causal relationship between leukaemia and ionizing radiation is well documented and much of the risk estimates are based upon the incidence of acute myeloid leukaemia and myelodysplasia among the survivors of the Nagasaki and Hiroshima atomic bombs in 1945. There was also an increased incidence of chronic myeloid leukaemia with expression of the classical Philadelphia chromosome marker.[50]

The association of low level occupational exposures was established in studies on pioneering radiologists and radiation scientists[51] and led to changes in radiographic procedures (see Chapter 53, Ionizing radiations). Significant numbers of excess leukaemias – acute myeloid leukaemia, chronic myeloid leukaemia and acute lymphoblastic – have been reported in medical radiation workers in China during the period 1950–85.[52] The possibility that leukaemia and lymphoma could result from low level exposures to waste products from nuclear power plants has received extensive attention in the United Kingdom and elsewhere following the finding of geographic clusters of acute lymphoblastic leukaemia (ALL) around such plants.[53,54] Careful case–control studies did not confirm any link with the radiation from the plant and similar clusters are found with no nearby nuclear plant.

NON-IONIZING RADIATION

There is considerable debate regarding the possibility that the very low frequency waves of electromagnetic fields, such as those around electricity power lines,[55] household[56] and workplace appliances,[57] may have leukaemogenic effects. The profusion of population variables make such studies difficult to carry out and small effects may be present without being detectable. In addition, no clear distinction was made between the effects of electrical and magnetic fields. There is a view that while the risk may be small the populations at risk are large. Animal studies have not been helpful in elucidating any causative mechanisms and further studies are required (see Chapter 55, Extremely low frequency electric and magnetic fields).

OTHER OCCUPATIONS AND OCCUPATIONAL AGENTS

Leukaemias

There have been consistent reports of an increased risk of leukaemia in other occupational groups, such as electrical workers, printing workers and workers in the rubber industry. There is no indication of the agent that might be involved in these reports, but there is some speculation that benzene which was used as a solvent, especially in the rubber industry, might have been one of the factors.

Hodgkin's disease and non-Hodgkin's lymphoma

Several studies have indicated an increased risk of Hodgkin's disease in woodworkers with tasks ranging from the manufacturing of furniture to the installing of fences.[58,59] Eight of the studies showed an increased risk, although the studies involved different methods and were carried out in three countries. However, the consistency of the results would suggest that association is unlikely to be due to chance, but no specific factor in terms of causative agent linked the studies.

Studies in farmworkers have suggested an increased incidence of non-Hodgkin's lymphoma.[60] It has been speculated that possible farm risks would include elevated exposures to pesticides, agricultural chemicals, organic and inorganic dust, zoonotic pathogens and sunlight. The agricultural factor most prominently linked with non-Hodgkin's lymphoma has been exposure to phenoxyacetic acid herbicides[61,62] or insecticides.[63] Organophosphate pesticides are known to inhibit serine esterases, which are important in T cell and natural killer cell cytolytic activity and may play an important role in lymphomagenesis through an immunosuppressive mechanism.[64,65]

Finally, fungicides and fumigants have also been associated with increased risks of non-Hodgkin's lymphomas. One study[66] strengthened the hypothesis in relation to exposure to phosphated insecticides by showing a dose–response relationship which was also suggested for stannates, carbamates, chlorinated compounds and for DDT. Exposures to such a variety of chemicals make the identification of a causative agent extremely difficult. Nevertheless, the frequency with which such an association has been reported justifies a high index of suspicion.

WORK-RELATED ISSUES RESULTING FROM TREATMENT OF HAEMATOLOGICAL DISEASE

Major advances in the treatment of aplastic anaemia, acute leukaemia and lymphoma (whether due to occupational exposures or not) have meant that many more patients are being cured and are thus potentially able to return to work. This raises important questions of what is a safe working environment for such patients and what physical or mental limitations they might experience. As greater numbers of successfully treated patients are followed for longer periods of time, medical and social problems associated with the impact of the disease or its treatment have become apparent.

With improved medical technologies, it is likely that more people with chronic haematological or oncological diseases contracted through workplace exposures will enjoy improved therapy and be able to return to work. It is to be hoped that employers and their occupational health advisers will match the achievement with flexible and enlightened support and rehabilitation schemes.

CASE REPORTS

Case study 1: Pancytopenia

A 56-year-old expatriate plant manager at an overseas petrochemical refinery had a routine executive medical examination. He was asymptomatic and physical examination was normal. The results of the full blood count were as follows: haemoglobin 12.8 g/dL, mean corpuscular volume (MCV): 100 fL, white cell count: 5.5, neutrophils: 1.5, lymphocytes: 2.0, monocytes: 1.5, eosinophils: 0.5 (all $\times 10^9$/L) and platelets: 115 $\times 10^9$/L. He was given a copy of the results for his general practitioner and advised to make an appointment on his next visit home in four weeks time. The repeat full blood count showed identical results. In addition, it was commented that the blood film showed a mild pancytopenia and some dysplastic neutrophils. He was referred for a haematological opinion.

His current job was manager of a distillation plant at a refinery in the Far East. His career since leaving school had been in the oil refining business and he had had several jobs overseas. One of his first jobs was as a maintenance fitter with frequent exposures to hydrocarbon solvents, while carrying out routine and emergency repairs. He recalled a project about 20 years previously which lasted several weeks and involved work on a plant using mainly benzene. The refinery was in the tropics where he worked in enclosed areas, stripped to the waist. Little attention was given to personal protection and he was often breathing in an atmosphere heavily contaminated with various hydrocarbons. He had to have frequent rest periods to recover from acute inhalational effects.

Further investigations showed normal B_{12}, folate and iron levels. Renal and liver function tests were also normal. In view of the persisting pancytopenia, a bone marrow aspirate was performed and this showed hyperplasia with reduced numbers of megakaryocytes, dysplastic erythropoiesis and a blast count of 15 per cent (normal <5 per cent).

The diagnosis was myelodysplasia (French–American–British (FAB) classification: refractory anaemia with excess of blasts). Cytogenetic analysis of the marrow showed a complex karyotype and a clonal deletion of the long arm of chromosome 5. During subsequent follow up, the blood counts continued to decrease over a period of 12 months and he required regular blood transfusions to maintain the haemoglobin. Leukaemic blasts appeared in the peripheral blood and the bone marrow showed progression to acute myeloid leukaemia. There was no response to intravenous chemotherapy and he died following an intracranial haemorrhage six months after diagnosis.

COMMENTARY

This case illustrates the association between myelodysplasia, acute myeloid leukaemia and exposure to benzene. There continues to be debate about the risk posed by low-level exposures, but here acute high-level exposures occurred over a period of a few weeks. Both inhalational and dermal exposure was reported and no protective measures were taken. It would have been valuable to know whether any of the high exposures had any short-term effects on the haemopoietic system, such as pancytopenia or marrow hypoplasia, although the history was not suggestive of this.

The marrow showed evolution from myelodysplasia to acute myeloid leukaemia with characteristic biological and clinical features. These features are not diagnostic of benzene-related leukaemogenesis and are shared with other secondary leukaemias, such as those following chemotherapy. They are:

1. the long latent period lasting many years;
2. the complex chromosomal abnormalities particularly involving loss or interstital deletions of chromosomes 5 and 7;
3. the low remission rate in response to chemotherapy;
4. the poor prognosis.

Case study 2: Haemolytic anaemia

During the summer vacation, a 23-year-old, final year medical student presented to his general practitioner on a Friday evening with vague flu-like symptoms, headaches and a dry cough. He was a keen athlete and had noticed a decrease in his exercise tolerance over the previous week. Physical examination was unremarkable other than a comment in the general practitioner's notes that he looked 'pale and grey'.

The young man was told that it was probably a viral infection and was asked to return if there was no improvement in his symptoms. He felt better over the weekend, but the symptoms returned the following week and he noticed a consistent change in the colour of his urine. His partner, who was a nurse, thought that he looked slightly jaundiced, especially at the end of the day. He also felt increasingly tired and had several bouts of shivering.

The general practitioner confirmed the clinical impression of mild jaundice and requested a urine test and some haematological and biochemical investigations. The student was told to stay off work because of the possibility of infectious hepatitis or mononucleosis. After 48 hours, his symptoms had improved. The investigations showed a haemoglobin count of 10.1 g/dL, MCV: 102 fL, platelets: 395, white blood cell count: 8.5×10^9/L and normal differential count. The blood film was reported as showing polychromasia and increased numbers of irregularly contracted cells. Reticulocyte count was 4.5 per cent; direct antibody test was negative; haptoglobins were reduced. Bilirubin was 45 mmol/L with normal enzyme activities and normal renal function. The urine contained increased amounts of urobilinogen and urinary haemosiderin was detected on microscopy of the urinary deposit. Methaemoglobin levels in the blood were significantly raised.

On further questioning, the young man admitted he had taken a part-time job during his current vacation as laboratory assistant in a small chemical company. His main task was cleaning glassware in a washroom adjacent to the main laboratory with occasional deliveries to the pilot plant where the bulk of the glassware originated. He said the room was hot with little in the way of ventilation. Protective respiratory equipment and gloves were available, but he had not received any information or training in their use. He was unaware of what the chemicals were, although the odour from the glassware was unpleasant. He had noticed small residues of a viscous chemical in the glass containers. Skin contamination had occurred because of the high volume of washing that had been required recently.

Contact with the health and safety officer of the company revealed that the pilot plant was investigating a novel halogenated aniline compound. The health and safety data sheet revealed that the compound was likely to cause blood problems by inhalation or dermal exposure and warned of the specific risk of methaemoglobinaemia and haemolysis.

COMMENTARY

This case highlights the importance of all personnel involved in the handling of toxic substances being fully informed of the risks and safety procedures. This includes not only regular employees who are directly involved with the primary handling, but also casual staff and those who may be involved in cleaning and disposal. While the substance was labelled as hazardous on the containers from the manufacturers and full-time employees were aware of the risks, health and safety checks had not identified the individual illustrated in this case in its risk assessment.

The blood tests showed the pattern of increased red cell destruction (hyperbilirubinaemia, increased urinary urobilinogen, reduced haptoglobins, polychromasia, reticulocytosis) with evidence of intravascular haemolysis (haemoglobinuria, haemosiderinuria). The direct antibody test excluded an immunological mechanism of the increased red cell destruction and the presence of methaemoglobinaemia was consistent with oxidative haemolysis.

The patient's symptoms recovered completely within four to five days and his haematology profile had resumed its normal characteristics after ten days. The medical student continued with his studies and took an interest in toxicology.

Key points

- The bone marrow and blood are targets of assault from a number of toxic agents to which workers may be exposed.
- The bone marrow is particularly susceptible to agents which interfere with proliferation and differentiation of rapidly dividing cells.
- Benzene and radiation are two examples where excessive exposure may result in bone marrow failure syndromes, including aplastic anaemia, myelodysplastic syndrome and acute leukaemia.
- The latency of emergence of bone marrow failure from exposure may be several years. A careful and extensive occupational history is required in assessing bone marrow failure syndromes.
- Circulating red blood cells are particularly susceptible to agents which cause oxidative stress which may cause acute haemolytic anaemia and/or methaemoglobinaemia.

REFERENCES

1. McCarthy LJ, Danielson C, Houseworth J et al. Transfusion medicine illustrated. Black plasma resulting from inhalation of arsine gas. *Transfusion.* 2006; **46**: 1267.
2. Romeo L, Apostoli P, Kovacic M et al. Acute arsine intoxication as a consequence of metal burnishing perations. *American Journal of Industrial Medicine.* 1997; **32**: 211–16.
3. Eysseric H, Vincent F, Peoc'h M et al. A fatal case of chlorate poisoning: confirmation by ion chromatography of body fluids. *Journal of Forensic Science.* 2000; **45**: 474–7.

4. Santucci K, Shah B. Association of naphthalene with acute hemolytic anemia. *Academic Emergency Medicine.* 2000; **7**: 42–7.
5. Ware M, Tyghter D, Staniforth S, Serjeant G. Airline travel in sickle-cell disease. *Lancet.* 1998; **352**: 652.
6. Martinez MA, Ballesteros S, Almarza E et al. Acute nitrobenzene poisoning with severe associated methemoglobinemia: Identification in whole blood by GC-FID and GC-MS. *Journal of Analytical Toxicology.* 2003; **27**: 221–5.
7. Galluccio ST, Edwards NA, Caldicott DG, Greenwood JE. Methaemoglobinaemia: An explosive case. *Critical Care and Resuscitation.* 2007; **9**: 178–80.
8. Donovan JW. Nitrates, nitrites and other sources of methemoglobinemia. In: Haddad LM, Winchester JF (eds). *Clinical management of poisoning and drug overdose.* Philadelphia: Saunders, 1990, 1419–31.
9. Ewan AD, Atel AP, Aiyed HS. Acute methemoglobinemia: A common occupational hazard in an industrial city in western India. *Journal of Occupational Health.* 2001; **43**: 168–71.
10. Ng LL, Naik RB, Polak B. Paraquat ingestion with methaemoglobinaemia treated with methylene blue. *British Medical Journal.* 1982; **284**: 1445.
11. Fontana V, Baldi R, Franchini M et al. Adverse haematological outcome and environmental lead poisoning. *Journal of Exposure Analysis and Environmental Epidemiology.* 2004; **14**: 188–93.
12. Fonte R, Agosti A, Scafa F, Candura SM. Anaemia and abdominal pain due to occupational lead poisoning. *Haematologica.* 2007; **92**: e13–14.
13. Young NS, Alter BP. Drugs and chemicals. In: *Aplastic anemia acquired and inherited.* Philadelphia: WB Saunders, 1994: 100–32.
14. Hopkins JE, Manoharan A. Severe aplastic anaemia following the use of hair dye: Report of two cases and review of literature. *Postgraduate Medical Journal.* 1985; **61**: 1003–5.
15. Geary CG, Harrison CJ, Philpott NJ et al. Abnormal cytogenetic clones in patients with aplastic anaemia: Response to immunosuppressive therapy. *British Journal of Haematology.* 1999; **104**: 271–4.
16. Sloand EM. Hypocellular myelodysplasia. *Hematology-Oncology Clinics of North America.* 2009; **23**: 347–60.
17. Harris N, Jaffe E, Diebold J et al. World Health Organization classification of neoplastic diseases of the hematopoietic and lymphoid tissues: Report of the Clinical Advisory Committee meeting, Airlie House, Virginia, November 1997. *Journal of Clinical Oncology.* 1999; **17**: 3835–49.
18. Schiffer CA. World Health Organization and international prognostic scoring system: The limitations of current classification systems in assessing prognosis and determining appropriate therapy in myelodysplastic syndromes. *Seminars in Hematology.* 2008; **45**: 3–7.
19. Greenberg P, Cox C, Le Beau MM et al. International scoring system for evaluating prognosis in myelodysplastic syndromes. *Blood.* 1997; **89**: 2079–88.
20. Rothman N, Li GL, Dosemeci M et al. Hematotoxicity among Chinese workers heavily exposed to benzene. *American Journal of Industrial Medicine.* 1996; **29**: 236–46.
21. Nebert DW, Roe A, Vandale S et al. NAD(P)H:quinone oxidoreductase (NQ01) polymorphism, exposure to benzene, and predisposition to disease: a HuGE review. *Genetics in Medicine.* 2002; **4**: 62–70.
22. Qu Q, Shore R, Li G et al. Hematological changes among Chinese workers with a broad range of benzene exposures. *American Journal of Industrial Medicine.* 2002; **42**: 275–85.
23. Yin S-N, Hayes RB, Linet M et al. A cohort study of cancer among benzene exposed workers in China: Overall results. *American Journal of Industrial Medicine.* 1996; **29**: 227–35.
24. Paci E, Buiatti E, Seniori Costantini AS et al. Aplastic anemia, leukemia and other cancer mortality in a cohort of shoe workers exposed to benzene. *Scandinavian Journal of Work and Environmental Health.* 1989; **15**: 313–18.
25. Hayes RB, Yin S-N, Dosemeci M et al. Benzene and the dose-related incidence of hematologic neoplasms in China. *Journal of the National Cancer Institute.* 1997; **89**: 1065–71.
26. Schnatter AR, Nicolich MJ, Bird MG. Determination of leukemogenic benzene exposure concentrations: Refined analyses of the pliofilm cohort. *Risk Analysis.* 1996; **16**: 833–4.
27. Kipen HM, Cody RP, Crump KS et al. Haematologic effects of benzene: A 35-year longitudinal study of rubber workers. *Toxicology and Industrial Health.* 1988; **4**: 411–30.
28. Chang IW. Study on the threshold limit value of benzene and early diagnosis of benzene poisoning. *J Cath Med Coll.* 1972; **23**: 429–34.
29. Snyder R. Benzene and leukemia. *Critical Reviews in Toxicology.* 2002; **32**; 155–210.
30. Ross D. The role of metabolism and specific metabolites in benzene-induced toxicity: Evidence and issues. *Journal of Toxicology and Environmental Health A.* 2000; **61**: 357–72.
31. Yardley-Jones A, Anderson D, Park DV. The toxicology of benzene and its metabolism and molecular pathology in human risk assessment. *British Journal of Industrial Medicine.* 1991; **48**: 437–44.
32. Godley LA, Larson RA. Therapy-related myeloid leukemia. *Seminars in Oncology.* 2008; **35**: 418–29.
33. Van den Berghe H, Louwagie A, Broechaert-van Orshoven A et al. Chromosome analysis in two unusual malignant blood disorders presumably induced by benzene. *Blood.* 1979; **53**: 558.
34. Rowley JD, Golomb HM, Vardiman JW. Nonrandom chromosome abnormalities in acute leukaemia and dysmyelopoietic syndrome in patients with previously treated malignant disease. *Blood.* 1981; **58**: 759.
35. Le Beau MM, Albain KS, Larson RA et al. Clinical and cytogenetic correlations in 63 patients with therapy-related myelodysplastic syndromes and acute non-lymphocytic leukaemia. Further evidence for characteristic abnormalities of chromosomes Nos 5 and 7. *Journal of Clinical Oncology.* 1986; **4**: 325.
36. Zhang L, Eastmond DA, Smith MT. The nature of chromosomal aberrations detected in humans exposed to benzene. *Critical Reviews in Toxicology.* 2002; **32**: 1–42.
37. Rushton L, Romaniuk H. A case-control study to investigate the risk of leukemia associated with exposure to benzene in

38. Schnatter AR, Armstrong TW, Nicolich MJ et al. Risk of lymphohematopoietic malignancies and quantitative estimates of benzene exposure in Canadian marketing/distribution workers. *Occupational and Environmental Medicine.* 1996; **53**: 773–81.
39. Forni A. Benzene induced chromosome aberrations; a follow-up study. *Environmental Health Perspectives.* 1996; **104** (Suppl.): 459–63.
40. Mester B, Nieters A, Deeg E et al. Occupation and malignant lymphoma: A population-based case control study in Germany. *Occupational and Environmental Medicine.* 2006; **63**: 17–26.
41. Miligi L, Costantini AS, Veraldi A et al. Cancer and pesticides: An overview and some results of the Italian multicenter case-control study on hematolymphopoietic malignancies. *Annals of the New York Academy of Sciences.* 2006; **1076**: 366–77.
42. Vodopick H. Erythropoietic hypoplasia after exposure to gamma benzene hexachloride. *JAMA.* 1975; **234**: 850–51.
43. Loge JP. Aplastic anemia following exposure to benzene hexachloride (lindane). *JAMA.* 1965; **193**: 110–14.
44. Morgan DP, Stockdale EM, Roberts RJ et al. Anemia associated with exposure to lindane. *Archives of Environmental Health.* 1980; **35**: 307–10.
45. Samuels AJ, Milby TH. Human exposure to lindane: Clinical hematological and biochemical effects. *Journal of Occupational Medicine.* 1971; **13**: 147–51.
46. Muir KR, Chilvers CE, Harrison C et al. The role of occupational and environmental exposures in the aetiology of acquired severe aplastic anaemia: A case control investigation. *British Journal of Haematology.* 2003; **123**: 906–14.
47. International Atomic Energy Agency. *Manual on radiation haematology.* Vienna: IAEA, 1971.
48. Mathe G, Jeannet H, Pendic B. Transfusions et greffes de moelle osseuse homologue chez des humans iradies a haute dose accidentellement. *Revue Française d'Etudes Cliniques et Biologiques.* 1959; **4**: 226–30.
49. Champlin R. Bone marrow aplasia due to radiation accidents: Pathophysiology, assessment and treatment. *Baillière's Clinical Haematology.* 1989; **1**: 69–82.
50. Preston DL, Kusumi S, Tomonaga M et al. Cancer incidence in atomic bomb survivors. 3. Leukemia, lymphoma and multiple myeloma, 1950–1987. *Radiation Research.* 1994; **137** (Suppl.): S68–97.
51. Doll RS. Hazards of ionising radiation: 100 years of observations on man. *British Journal of Cancer.* 1995; **72**: 1339–49.
52. Wang J-X, Inskip PD, Boice JDJ et al. Cancer incidence among medical diagnostic X-ray workers in China, 1950 to 1985. *International Journal of Cancer.* 1995; **72**: 1339–49.
53. Gardner MJ, Snee MP, Hall AJ et al. Results of case-control study of leukaemia and lymphoma among young people near Sellafield nuclear plant in West Cumbria. *British Medical Journal.* 1990; **300**: 423.
54. Draper GJ, Little MP, Sorahan T et al. Cancer in the offspring of radiation workers: A record linkage study. *British Medical Journal.* 1997; **315**: 1181–8.
55. Miller AB, To T, Agnew DA et al. Leukemia following occupational exposure to 60-Hz electricity and magnetic fields among Ontario electric utility workers. *American Journal of Epidemiology.* 1996; **44**: 50–60.
56. Li CY, Theriault G, Lin RS. Epidemiological appraisal of studies of residential exposure to power frequency magnetic fields and adult cancers. *Occupational and Environmental Medicine.* 1996; **53**: 505–10.
57. Milham S Jr. Increased incidence of cancer in a cohort of office workers exposed to strong magnetic fields. *American Journal of Industrial Medicine.* 1996; **30**: 702–4.
58. Miller BA, Blair AE, Raynor HL et al. Cancer and other mortality patterns among United States furniture workers. *British Journal of Industrial Medicine.* 1989; **46**: 508–15.
59. Partanen T, Kauppinen T, Luukkonen R et al. Malignant lymphomas and leukemias and exposures in the wood industry: An industry based case referent study. *International Archives of Occupational and Environmental Health.* 1993; **64**: 593–6.
60. Blair A, Zahn SH. Cancer among farmers. *Occupational Medicine.* 1991; **6**: 335–54.
61. Cantor KP, Blair A, Everett G et al. Pesticides and other agricultural risk factors for non-Hodgkin's lymphoma among men in Iowa and Minnesota. *Cancer Research.* 1992; **52**: 2447–55.
62. Hoar SK, Blair A, Holmes FF et al. Agricultural herbicide use and risk of lymphoma and soft-tissue sarcoma. *JAMA.* 1986; **256**: 1411–17.
63. Zahm SH, Weisenburger DD, Babbitt PA et al. A case-control study of non-Hodgkin's lymphoma and the herbicide 2, 4-dichlorophenoxyacetic acid (2, 4-D) in Eastern Nebraska. *Epidemiology.* 1990; **1**: 349–56.
64. Thomas PT, Busse WW, Kerfvleit NI et al. Immunologic effects of pesticides. In: Baker SR, Wilkinson CR (eds). *The effects of pesticides on human health.* Advances in Modern Environmental Toxicology XVIII. Princeton, NJ: Princeton Scientific Publishers, 1990: 261–95.
65. Newcombe DS. Immune surveillance, organophosphorus exposure and lymphomagenesis. *Lancet.* 1992; **339**: 539–41.
66. Nanni O, Amadori D, Lugaresi C et al. Chronic lymphocytic leukaemias and non-Hodgkin's lymphomas by histological type in farming-animal breeding workers. *Occupational and Environmental Medicine.* 1996; **53**: 652–7.
67. Linch DC, Yates AP, Watts MJ (eds). *Colour guide to haematology.* Edinburgh: Churchill Livingstone, 1996.
68. Ballantyne B, Marrs T, Turner P. *General and applied toxicology,* vol. 2. London: Macmillan Press, 1993.

SECTION **FOUR**

Shift work

91 Shift work and extended hours of work 1233
Giovanni Costa, Simon Folkard and J Malcolm Harrington

Shift work and extended hours of work

GIOVANNI COSTA, SIMON FOLKARD AND J MALCOLM HARRINGTON

Introduction	1233	Preventive and compensatory measures	1239
Biological and social interference	1234	Medical surveillance	1240
Effects on health	1235	References	1242
Factors affecting tolerance to shift work and extended working hours	1238		

INTRODUCTION

The arrangement of working hours has become a crucial factor in work organization, and may vary with the economic and social consequences that can arise at different periods in the worker's life. Not only has the link between workplace and working times been broken (for example, through teleworking), but also the borders between working and leisure times are no longer fixed and rigidly determined by the normal working day. Working hours are extended to evening and night hours, as well as to the weekend, and hours of duty have become more and more variable (the '24-hour society').

In this context, shift work is the most common form of working time and enables round-the-clock activities not only in relation to rigid technological conditions (e.g. the chemical and steel industry, power plants) and necessary social services (e.g. hospitals, transportation, electricity, telecommunications), but also to support productive and economic choices (e.g. textile, paper, food, mechanical industry, banking), as well as the wider use of leisure time (e.g. entertainment). Shift work includes any arrangement of daily working hours that differs from standard day work. It is aimed at extending the organization's operational time from 8 hours up to 24 hours per day, by means of a succession of different teams of workers.

According to the results of the 3rd European Survey on Working Conditions outlined in Ref. 1, only 24 per cent of the working population (27 per cent of employed and 8 per cent of self-employed workers) were engaged in the so-called 'normal' or 'standard' day work, that is between 07.00–08.00 (7–8 a.m.) and 17.00–18.00 (5–6 p.m.), from Monday to Friday.[1] This means that the vast majority of workers are engaged in 'non-standard' working hours, including shift and night work, part-time work, weekend work, compressed work week, extended working hours, split shifts, on-call work, etc.

Working schedules can vary widely, in particular (1) duration of duty period (i.e. from 6 to 12 hours); (2) presence and extension of night work (i.e. between 24.00 (12 p.m.) and 05.00–06.00 (5–6 a.m.)); (3) permanent or rotating shift schedules (i.e. people work regularly on one shift or alternate periodically on different shifts); (4) continuous or discontinuous shift systems (i.e. all days worked or interruption on weekend); (5) start and finish time of the duty periods (i.e. between 04.00 (4 a.m.) and 07.00 (7 a.m.) in the morning, between 20.00 (8 p.m.) and 24.00 (12 p.m.) at night); (6) number of workers/crews who alternate during the working day (i.e. two, three or four shifts); (7) speed (i.e. 'fast', every one–two or three days, or 'slow', every 15–30 days) and direction of shift rotation (i.e. 'clockwise', morning–afternoon–night, or 'counter-clockwise', afternoon–morning–night; (8) number and position of rest days between shifts; (9) length of shift cycle (i.e. from six to nine days up to six months or more); (10) regularity/irregularity of the shift schedules.

According to the 4th European Survey on Working Conditions,[2] weekly working hours range from an average of 34 hours in the Netherlands to 55 hours in Turkey, and from a minimum of eight hours (as part-time work) to a maximum of 90 hours (as overtime work). Shift work, which includes night work, involves more than 17 per cent of the total working population, with large differences among the countries (from 6.4 per cent in Turkey to 33.5 per cent in Croatia).

In 2004, almost 15 percent of full-time salaried workers in the USA usually worked on alternating shifts including nights. In the United States, men were more likely than women to work such shifts (16.7 and 12.4 per cent, respectively); blacks were more likely than whites, Hispanics or Latinos, or Asians; and shift work decreased progressively with age.[3]

Extended working hours refers to working for longer than eight to nine hours per day, and 40 hours per week. According to the International Labour Organization, annual hours worked per person surpassed 1800 hours in 27 countries out of 52 monitored from 1996 to 2006, and 2200 hours in six Asian economies.[4] In the United States, almost one-third of the workforce regularly works more than the standard 40-hour week and one-fifth more than 50 hours.[3] In Europe, according to the 4th European Survey on Working Conditions, 16.9 per cent workers of the 27 EU member states worked 48 hours per week or more, ranging from 11.1 per cent in Luxembourg to 32.1 per cent in Turkey.[2]

Working irregular or extended hours may have negative consequences for health and well-being due to the stress derived from interference with psychophysiological functions and social life. The majority of the studies up to now have focused on shift work rather than on extended working hours since they are often confused. However, some recent studies have addressed this second aspect independently, with some contrasting results.[5,6]

BIOLOGICAL AND SOCIAL INTERFERENCE

Circadian rhythms and psychophysical conditions

It is commonly accepted that work efficiency at night is not the same as during the day. Man is a diurnal creature, synchronized to the 24-hour light/dark cycle, who is naturally awake and active during daylight and consequently resting and sleeping at night. This behaviour is determined by the regular oscillation of bodily functions ('circadian rhythms'). For example, core body temperature decreases during the night when people are asleep to a minimum of 35.5–36.0°C in the early hours of the morning, and increases during the waking day to reach a maximum (acrophase) of about 37.0–37.3°C at around 17.00 (5 p.m.). This rhythmicity is controlled by a strong endogenous oscillator (or body clock), located in the suprachiasmatic nuclei, and is influenced by environmental factors (synchronizers), such as work, activity, sleep, meals and, in particularly, light exposure.[7–9]

Night work forces the individual to change their normal sleep/wake cycle and to attempt to adjust to the nocturnal activity by a progressive phase shift of circadian rhythms that may be more or less complete depending on the number of successive night shifts. However, circadian rhythms very seldom show a complete inversion, rather there is a flattening of their amplitude and a dissociation between them due to differing rates of adjustment of the rhythms in the variables concerned. Indeed, even in permanent night workers, the vast majority show insufficient adjustment of their body clocks for it to be of any real benefit.[10] The general lack of circadian adjustment is due both to the continuous rotation through the different shifts on most shift systems, and to the fact that most individuals try to maintain a normal, day-oriented, social and family life during their free time and on rest days.

These rhythmic disturbances may have negative effects on health and well-being. In the short term, people may suffer from symptoms similar to those of jet lag and characterized by feelings of fatigue, sleepiness, insomnia, digestive troubles, and reduced mental ability and performance efficiency. In the longer term, such rhythmic disturbances may, often in combination with other factors, eventually result in the manifestation of a wide range of complaints and illnesses (see under Effects on health).[11–14]

Performance efficiency

Human error is often cited as an important factor in work-related accidents and depends on sleep and sleep-related factors, as well as on circadian rhythms in alertness and performance capabilities. Alertness can be substantially reduced by irregular rest/activity patterns and by prolonged physical and mental effort. In general, performance efficiency appears to parallel the circadian rhythm in body temperature, but it can peak earlier or later in the day depending on the demands of the task (e.g. physical, cognitive or memory-loaded), on the length of time that has elapsed since the individual's last proper sleep, and on their general level of arousal and motivation.

The dissociation of circadian rhythms in combination with the associated sleep deficit and fatigue may significantly impair work efficiency, in particular at night, making the worker more vulnerable to errors. This pattern has been reported for many groups of shift workers including train and truck drivers, nuclear power workers, nurses, switchboard operators and seamen. A 'post-lunch dip' has also been noted which appears to be only partially dependent on the meal itself, and which may also reflect 12-hour or shorter 'ultradian' rhythms in alertness and wakefulness superimposed on the 24-hour circadian cycle.[15,16]

In addition, sleepiness due to the truncation of sleep by an early start to the morning shift has been shown to cause a higher frequency of errors and accidents in train and bus drivers, while increased sleepiness and changes in electroencephalogram (EEG) ultradian rhythms (bursts of alpha and theta power density) have been recorded on the night shift, indicating a high propensity for the workers concerned to fall asleep 'on the job'.[17]

Family and social life

People engaged in shift work or extended working hours can face greater difficulties in their social lives since most activities are arranged according to the day-oriented rhythms of the general population. In addition, weekend work may interfere with various social activities, such as sports events, religious ceremonies, travel and entertainment. Shift workers thus face more difficulties in combining their time budgets (work hours, commuting and leisure times) with the complex organization of social activities, particularly when these require regular contacts and involve a great many people. Hence, shift work can lead to social marginalization.[18]

Shift work and extended working hours may also hinder the already complex coordination of family timetables, with the extent of any such hinderance depending on factors such as family composition and duties (e.g. marital status, number and age of children, housework, moonlighting and illnesses) and the organization of social services (e.g. school and shop hours and public transport). 'Time pressure' is a constant condition among those who have pressing family responsibilities (e.g. women with small children). These complaints may be further complicated when both partners have the same working conditions (i.e. as shift workers or with long working hours), and this can have negative effects on marital relationships, parental roles and children's education. Complaints from shift workers about family and social difficulties are more frequent than those related to biological adjustment, and are often the main cause of shift work intolerance.[19,20]

On the positive side, shift work can give more flexibility to those who enjoy solitary activities and to those who give a higher priority to family and domestic duties than to personal leisure. Consequently, shift work is sometimes popular since it provides greater opportunities to use daytime hours to meet particular needs (e.g. access to public offices), or simply allows longer spans of rest days between shift cycles. For this reason shift systems that include 'quick returns' (working two shifts in one day) and compressed working weeks (e.g. three or four days of 12 hours per day) are often preferred because of the longer spans of rest days, despite the clear negative effects of such systems on sleep and performance efficiency.

EFFECTS ON HEALTH

Sleep, chronic fatigue and psychoneurotic troubles

Sleep is the main function that is disrupted by shift work. Sleep duration is typically reduced before morning shifts, depending on their start time, and between night shifts because the individuals are trying to sleep when their body clocks expect them to be awake. People may have difficulty in falling asleep and remaining asleep during the day, while the environmental conditions (lighting and noise in particular) are also often far from ideal. Some interference occurs with the daytime sleeps between night shifts (in particular a reduction in stage 2 and rapid eye movement (REM) sleep, whereas slow wave sleep (SWS) sleep is unaffected, although irregularly distributed) and for the truncated night sleeps before morning shifts (again wih a loss of stage 2 and REM sleep due to the early wake up).[17,21,22]

The decreased length of main periods of sleep and early awakenings are strongly associated with increased sleepiness during the rest of the day and a higher recourse to napping. Naps may partially compensate for sleep deprivation and have a prophylactic effect in counteracting the fall in alertness if properly taken before or during the work shifts. The length of the nap seems less important (20 minutes and two hours may have the same value) than its temporal position in relation to the duty period.

Both homeostatic (time elapsed since prior sleep termination) and circadian (sleep/wake cycle) components interact in determining the extent of the reduction in alertness and psychophysical performance over the waking day, and even more so at night. This may be further aggravated by features of the work schedule, and in particular the number of night shifts in succession, the start time of morning shifts, and shorter rest periods between shifts (i.e. 'quick returns').

The disturbances of sleep can be both severe and long lasting, and may eventually lead to an increased incidence of symptoms of chronic fatigue, nervousness, persistent anxiety, and depression, which may require the administration of psychotropic drugs.[23] This has been confirmed in both cross-sectional and longitudinal survey studies using standardized psychological health questionnaires. Rather fewer studies have reported the incidence of those clinically diagnosed as suffering from psychological health problems, and those that have suffer from problems of adequate, matched control groups. Nevertheless, stress-related symptoms are relatively common in people working extended hours, particularly if associated with high work loads or monotonous, repetitive jobs. There is also some evidence that these symptoms may act as a risk or aggravating factor for other psychosomatic complaints or diseases including symptoms of gastrointestinal and cardiovascular health.

Digestive and metabolic disorders

Many shift workers complain of digestive disorders, reflecting on both the irregularity of meal timing and the poor quality of the food consumed, namely an increased consumption of prepacked meals and caffeinated drinks. Studies carried out over the last 50 years have shown that 20–75 per cent of night and shift workers, compared to 10–25 per cent of day workers, complain of disturbances of appetite, irregular bowel movements, constipation, dyspepsia, heartburn, abdominal pains and flatulence. In the longer term, many workers also develop more serious disorders, such as chronic gastritis, gastroduodenitis and peptic ulcers. A review of epidemiological studies found a generally higher prevalence of such disorders (from two to five times higher on average) amongst shift workers whose work schedule included night work.[24] However, improved diagnostic methods (endoscopy), better aetiopathological definition of peptic ulcer (i.e. *Helicobacter pylori*) and more appropriate therapies have recently changed the course of the disease, and hence its prevalence, as well as allowing people to continue shift working without major problems.

In recent years, an increased prevalence of metabolic disturbances in shift workers has also been emphasized.[25,26] It has been suggested that these may reflect several factors, and in particular (1) a mismatch of circadian rhythms of anabolic and catabolic phases; (2) changes in daily lifestyle (i.e. unbalanced diet, irregular timing of food intake, nibbling carbohydrates and increasing consumption of caffeinated or alcoholic drinks at night); and (3) disturbed sociotemporal patterns (i.e time pressure, work–non-work conflicts) with consequent higher stress levels.[27]

A higher prevalence of overweight and obesity and increased blood triglycerides levels has been found in several studies of both shift work[26–29] and extended hours,[30,31] whereas somewhat inconsistent findings have been reported for total and HDL cholesterol levels. With respect to glucose intolerance, a higher prevalence (two-fold) of type 2 diabetes in shift workers compared to day workers has been reported by two studies,[32,33] while a single study has reported an increased risk (RR = 3.73) for type 2 diabetes associated with a >50 hour/week overtime.[34]

Cardiovascular diseases

A number of epidemiological studies have indicated an association between shift work and cardiovascular diseases. More specifically, there is (1) an increased prevalence of cardiovascular risk factors among shift workers; (2) a higher morbidity due to cardiocirculatory and ischaemic heart diseases with increasing age and shift work experience; and (3) an increased relative risk of myocardial infarction in occupations with a high proportion of shift workers.[25,35]

It is worth noting that several possible confounding factors may also act as mediators or modifiers of the effect, such as age, smoking, diet and social class. The conclusion of a review of 17 cohort and longitudinal studies of shift work was that shift workers have a 40 per cent excess risk for cardiovascular disease compared to day workers, but that in the age group of 45–55 years, the relative risk rises to 1.6 in men and 3.0 in women.[36] Moreover, the relative risk for coronary heart disease increases to 2.3 when shift work is associated with obesity, and to 2.7 when associated with smoking (which alone has a RR of 1.6).[37] Furthermore, since smoking is often increased in shift workers, it can be viewed not only as a confounding variable, but also as an intermediary between shift work and ischaemic heart disease.[35,38]

With respect to extended hours, Japanese studies have indicated a two-fold increase of myocardial infarction in people working more than 60 hours per week[39] or 11 hours per day,[40] but the findings for hypertension have been inconsistent.[41]

Accidents

As mentioned under Biological and social interference (p. 1234), shift workers may be more prone to errors and work accidents due to reduced vigilance and performance capabilities, than their day-working counterparts. However, while some studies have reported a higher overall incidence of injuries and accidents on the night shift, others studies have found inconsistent effects.[24] These inconsistencies reflect a large number of potentially confounding factors, such as differences in the work sector studied or jobs examined, which may influence the relative risk of accidents. The most important factors relate to the manner in which work is organized on the different shifts. For example, maintenance and supervision are often largely confined to the day shift(s), while long, 'easy', runs of a particular job may be saved for the night shift. Furthermore, the day shift may be 'augmented' by permanent day workers, thus increasing the likelihood of accidents on the day shift. It is noteworthy that in the studies in which the a priori risk appeared to be constant across the 24-hour day, industrial injuries were higher on the night shift, and also showed a bigger increase over successive night shifts than over successive day shifts.[42–44]

Other studies have shown peaks in accidents at around 10.00–11.00 (10–11 a.m.) and 15.00–16.00 (3–4 p.m.) which probably reflect peaks in work activity since performance capabilities due to circadian rhythms should be relatively high at these times. There is, however, evidence that both long working hours and an early start time to the morning shift may be associated with an increased accident risk.[45] It is clear that careful attention needs to be paid to the potential accident risk when considering work schedules and other organizational factors. Indeed, it is noteworthy that the nuclear incidents at Three Mile Island and Chernobyl, the Bophal disaster, and many air accidents including the Challenger space shuttle, all occurred at night. Furthermore, in each case, shift scheduling and fatigue due to sustained operation were cited as important contributory factors.[46]

Absenteeism

Despite inconsistencies, a number of authors have cited the influence of aspects of shift scheduling on absenteeism rates, including the speed of rotation, the amount of overtime, and the shift start and finish times.[47,48] It should be noted that, in addition to the 'healthy worker effect', there are a number of reasons why shift workers may show lower absenteeism rates despite higher frequencies of complaints and illnesses. These may include (1) a higher solidarity with colleagues since an unexpected absence may cause more problems for shift handovers than for normal day work; (2) a higher threshold in the reporting of complaints and symptoms since shift workers more often accept them as 'part of the job' (e.g. digestive and sleep disorders); and (3) a higher punctuality rate since shift workers are less likely to have to travel to work during rush hours and have fewer problems accessing public offices during working hours. Finally, data on absenteeism are also inconsistent for extended work hours, probably due to confounding factors, such as motivation, work pacing and type of job.[41,49]

Women's reproductive function

There is good reason to assume that shift work may be a peculiar problem for women's health. This follows both from the potential disruption of their hormonal cycles and from the increased stress caused by the conflict between their irregular working schedules and their domestic duties. Disorders of the menstrual cycle, reproductive function and pregnancy outcomes have been reported in many groups of women shift workers, including a higher incidence of menstrual pains and abortion and interference with fetal development, such as premature births and/or low birthweight.[50–53] A meta-analysis of six studies carried out between 1987 and 1997 also suggested a weak but significant (RR = 1.24) association between extended working hours and preterm birth.[54] Women shift workers, especially those married with small children, may also have more difficulties in combining their irregular working schedules with their additional domestic duties, and may thus suffer more from sleep troubles and chronic fatigue than their male colleagues.[20,55] Indeed, some national legislation protects shift working women, e.g. exemption from night work when pregnant, and the possibility to transfer to day work during the first two to three years of age of their children.

Toxicological risk

Shift workers may be particularly susceptible to xenobiotics due to (1) potential fluctuations in the environmental concentrations of pollutants and a concomitant increase in risk at certain times of day; (2) the reduced interval between shifts; (3) pronounced circadian rhythms in the metabolism and excretion of toxic substances; and (4) the potentially detrimental consequences of circadian disturbances. Experimental chronotoxicology studies have demonstrated circadian rhythmicity in the activity and effectiveness of some toxic compounds (i.e. mercurials, cyanides and organophosphate pesticides), as well as variations in susceptibility after changes to the light–dark regimen. Thus, the balance between the 'biokinetics' of the substance and the 'chronoesthesy' of the biological system is more likely to be unfavourable at night when metabolic function is slowing down. This was dramatically demonstrated by the Bhopal disaster when, surprisingly, none of the night workers died from the vapours of methyl isocyanate, but thousands of inhabitants of the near villages died in their sleep. At the same time, thousands of cattle died while nocturnally active rats were observed to be scurrying around the corpses and carcasses.[56]

Risk assessment and biological monitoring should take into account circadian fluctuations in physiological responses (in terms of absorption, metabolism and excretion) and the consequent severity of the toxic effect. This should be evaluated not only with reference to environmental threshold limit values (TLVs) and biological exposure indices (BEI), but also for evening and night shifts, as has been suggested for prolonged, 12-hour shifts. Indeed, some studies have already shown a circadian excretion pattern of toxic substances or metabolites that can be used for better strategies in workers' biomonitoring.[57,58]

Mortality

Apart from the first negative report in 1949 (cited in Ref. 59), there have been only three well-controlled studies that have examined the mortality rates of shift workers. The first study was of 1578 deaths in 8603 male British industrial workers from 1956 to 1968.[60] The overall number of deaths was very close to that expected from national mortality rates, and no significant excess mortality was found in either the shift (722 versus 711.4) or ex-shift (120 versus 100.9) workers. Shift workers in some age groups had a significant excess (e.g. in those under 60 years old for artheriosclerotic heart diseases), but this was not consistent across work organizations and types of shift work. However, a recent re-analysis of the mortality rate ratios, adjusted for age, showed that former shift workers had a slight, but significantly, increased mortality risk compared with day workers (RR = 1.24; 95 per cent CI, 1.03–1.51).[61]

The second, Danish, study followed 1123 shift workers and 4084 day workers over a 22-year period. The relative death risk was 1.1 (95 per cent CI, 0.9–1.3) for shift workers after adjustment for age and social class.[62] The third study was based on a Swedish survey of 22 411 individuals between 1979 and 2000. The results, adjusted for age, stress, physical work load, disease at the outset of the study and smoking, showed no significant difference between shift and day workers in general, but an increased hazard ratio for female white-collar shift workers (HR = 2.61; 95 per cent CI, 1.26–5.41).[59]

With respect to extended hours, a Swedish survey of 2632 workers carried out from 1973 to 1996 reported that more than 5 hours/week overtime increased all-cause mortality in men (RR = 2.0) at 5-year follow up, and women (RR = 1.92) at 24-year follow up, when controlling for the other most important risk factors.[63]

Cancer and shift work

Several recent epidemiological studies have examined the association between cancer and shift work. A slightly higher incidence of breast cancer in women engaged in shift work, including night work has been reported in four studies of nurses (OR or RR 1.36–2.21), in four studies of flight attendants (standardized incidence ratio between 1.42 and 2.0), and in one study of sea radio and telegraph operators (OR = 1.5). These studies controlled for several important confounding factors (i.e. age, menarche, parity, menopausal status, family history, body mass index (BMI), contraceptives) but were limited with respect to the quantification of the exposure (both in terms of the definition of night work and the characteristics of the shift schedules), and with respect to the potential exposure to other proven carcinogens, i.e. antineoplastics, x-rays, cosmic radiation and electromagnetic fields).[64,65]

Possible explanations for such an association are based on perturbations of melatonin secretion and changes in gonadotropin axis resulting from the disruption of both dark–light exposure and sleep–activity patterns, with a consequent deregulation of circadian genes involved in cancer-related pathways (i.e. inactivation of *Per2* and inhibited expression of *Period* genes) and reduced immune defences (suppression of natural killer-cell activity and changes to the T-helper 1/T-helper 2 cytokine balance), such as has been found in rodents.[66]

The International Agency on Research on Cancer (IARC) recently classified 'shift work that involves circadian disruption' as 'probably carcinogenic to humans' (Group 2A) on the basis of 'limited evidence in humans for the carcinogenicity of shift-work that involves nightwork', and 'sufficient evidence in experimental animals for the carcinogenicity of light during the daily dark period (biological night)'.[67]

Ageing and shift work

Ageing is associated with a decreased ability to adjust to night work and an increase in sleep disturbances, such that night work may become less and less bearable with advancing age.[68] More difficulties have also been reported in changing from 8- to 12-hour shifts in those aged over 50 years.[69,70] Moreover, as people grow older, they tend to become more 'morning type', making it both more difficult to sleep during the day after night work, and more difficult to maintain alertness during the waking period.[71,72]

In general, health deterioration with increasing age may be more pronounced in shift workers than in day workers due to sleep problems and chronic fatigue, with a consequent reduction in work ability, and an increase in sick leave, sleep disorders and gastrointestinal and cardiovascular diseases.[73–76] Moreover, older people obviously suffer more health problems, quite independently of shift work, and these may hamper their adaptation and tolerance to irregular and/or extended hours. On the other hand, it should be noted that the greater experience of older workers may have resulted in their having better coping strategies and countermeasures. This is particularly true in terms of work commitment, regular life regimen, more satisfactory job positions, better housing conditions and fewer domestic constraints.

FACTORS AFFECTING TOLERANCE TO SHIFT WORK AND EXTENDED WORKING HOURS

It has been estimated that about 15–20 per cent of workers do not like shift work and suffer from serious problems that force them to leave, mainly due to circadian disruption and severe sleep problems. In contrast, around 10 per cent have no complaints since they are able to satisfactorily combine their personal attitudes and behaviours to their peculiar demands. The majority (70–75 per cent) simply tolerate shift work, showing various levels of (in)tolerance, that may be more or less manifested at different times and with different severity. Indeed, it is abundantly clear that a number of moderating variables, including individual differences, situational factors and social conditions, may significantly influence both the short-term circadian adjustment to, and the longer-term tolerance of night and shift work.[12,77,78]

Individual characteristics have been widely investigated in an attempt to determine which psychological and physiological factors are associated with either adverse health effects or a better tolerance, and hence may have important practical applications. Individuals who have a small amplitude of their circadian rhythms may have a less stable circadian structure (i.e. show larger phase shifts on abnormal work schedules) and may be more prone to internal desynchronization, thus having more long-term problems.[57,79] Morning types ('larks') and evening types ('owls') also differ in their circadian adjustment to night work: the former appear to be less tolerant to night work since they have an earlier phase of their circadian system, while the latter have a later circadian phase, face greater problems in waking up early in the morning, and may suffer from an even greater truncation of their night sleeps taken before morning shifts.

There are a number of other personality traits and/or behavioural characteristics, including neuroticism, locus of control, rigidity of sleeping habits and the ability to overcome drowsiness, that may influence the degree of circadian adjustment and hence have a potential impact on long-term tolerance. In addition, physical fitness can improve sleep, lessen fatigue and increase performance, and may thus improve tolerance to night work, as may a strong 'commitment to shift work', since this is associated with more stable sleep timings and other circadian behaviours.[80–83]

With respect to family and social conditions, marital status, number and age of children, living with old and/or ill people, housing location and comfort (e.g. rooms, protection from disturbing noises) have all been shown to influence tolerance to shift work.[84–86] For women in particular, the partner's job (whether a shift worker as well), the presence of small children, the organization of social services (i.e. school timetables, shop hours, public transport) and family support, are factors that may be important. It is well documented that married women with small children suffer from shorter and more fragmented sleep and from cumulative fatigue, and that they are obliged to significantly reduce their social relations and leisure activities.[55,87–89]

Absenteeism, work accidents, fatigue and the disruption of social and family life, are certainly enhanced by local factors, such as low social support, a lack of basic services, and long and uncomfortable commuting hours. Support from family and friends at home, and from co-workers and supervisors at work have been proved to enhance shift work adaptability and tolerance.[90,91] Indeed, many surveys in developing countries have shown that the effects of night work on health and safety are often aggravated by less than favourable social conditions (e.g. low nutrition, education and salary; poor housing, community services and social protection, labour market restrictions and discrimination), that are also often connected with poor working conditions (environmental pollution, heavy work) and long working hours.[92–95]

Even on the same work schedule, the cultural background and the socioeconomic conditions of each country or community may make the impact on health, safety and well-being quite different. In industrialized countries with high immigration levels, minority ethnic groups are often engaged in jobs with low pay and poor working conditions, including more shift and night work, with consequent negative effects on social integration.[96] Furthermore, the specific arangement of shift schedules is of paramount importance (see under Preventive and compensatory measures). The problem of tolerance to shift work is therefore multifaceted, with a high interindividual variability in terms of both clinical and temporal manifestations, due to the various complex interactions between personal characteristics, working and social conditions.

It is also noteworthy that the health troubles reported by shift workers are predominantly psychosomatic disorders that are quite common in the general population and have a multifactorial origin. They reflect the influence of several risk factors including genetic and family heritage, psychological characteristics, life styles, social conditions and intervening illnesses. Furthermore, their chronic degenerative nature makes their manifestation more likely to occur after long-term exposure and with increasing age. In this context, shift work may act as a further stress factor or a trigger as it combines conflicts between endogenous rhythms and social synchronizers with demanding working conditions and interferences with family and social life.

Consequently, the process of maladaptation, or intolerance, to shift work is variable in its speed of onset and intensity, depending on the differences in personal, working and social circumstances. Thus, health problems and disorders may manifest themselves at different life periods, with different degrees of severity and duration, and sometimes in an alternating or fluctuating way, thus further increasing the interindividual and intraindividual variability.[97,98]

It is, as yet, unclear as to the extent to which the disturbance of biological rhythms influences long-term tolerance. However, it is commonly presumed that circadian disturbances, including those of sleep, are the main causes of intolerance to night work in the first years of shift work, whereas longer-term intolerance may be more related to other personal, working and social circumstances. An important confounding factor in this respect, is the process of self-selection that occurs in shift workers. Most of the epidemiological studies in this field have been cross-sectional and have considered workforces in whom an unknown number of individuals may have previously left shift work because of illness or social problems. Indeed, longitudinal studies have found it virtually impossible to follow up the same sample of shift workers over a prolonged period, due either to transfers to day work because of problems, or to multiple change-overs from shift work to day work during the working life. This can lead to a serious underestimation of the problems associated with shift work, since the shift workers available for investigation are those who have 'survived' (i.e. there may be a 'healthy worker effect'). In contrast, studies of former shift workers may overestimate the complaints of shift workers on the whole.

Likewise, the equivocal or inconsistent association between extended working hours (i.e. 12-hour shifts) and health effects may be due, given the lack of prospective studies, to the fact that many other factors (i.e. job demands, workload and pacing, shift schedules, rest pauses, motivation, decision latitude, flexible times, commuting) may be confounded. This may underlie the conflicting findings that in some studies long working hours are not a problem, while in others they can have severe health effects, related to higher stress, sleep deficit and fatigue.[5,6,41,99,100]

PREVENTIVE AND COMPENSATORY MEASURES

Since shift and night work are risk factors for health and well-being, medical examinations should be carried out with the dual aims of giving the workers suggestions and guidelines on how best to cope with shift work, and of detecting the early signs of intolerance to night work.[101] The importance of this has been emphasized recently in international directives and recommendations. Thus the ILO Night Work Convention No. 171 and Recommendation No. 178 concerning Night Work (1990)[102,103] and the European Directive 2003/88/EC concerning 'certain aspects of the organisation of working time',[104] cover a number of specific measures for night workers, including health assessments prior to assignment to night work, at regular intervals thereafter, and in the case of any health complaints. They also state that night workers found to be unfit for night work for health reasons should be transferred, whenever possible, to day work.

Medical examinations should ensure an appropriate screening of workers who are going to be engaged in shift work in the first place, and then ensure that regular assessments of their continued suitability for night and shift work are conducted. With regard to the former, it should be emphasized that the ability to cope with a 'bad' shift schedule should not be used to 'select' shift workers. The primary aim should be to design shift schedules that minimize the potentially harmful consequences and to develop appropriate compensative measures. In this manner, disturbances to circadian rhythms, accumulation of a sleep debt and any marked interference with family and social life should be avoided, such that most people should be able to tolerate shift work without significant health impairment.

It would be totally inappropriate to develop a medical surveillance programme for people obliged to work an unfavourable shift system, because adoption of a better shift schedule would reduce the health complaints and the need for medical control or intervention. The main guidelines for designing better shift systems according to ergonomic criteria are:[105,106]

- Night work should be reduced as much as possible (i.e. diluting it among workers by increasing the number of crews).
- Night shifts should be carefully planned. The greater the number of night shifts in a row, the greater the circadian and sleep disturbance and the accumulation of fatigue.
- Rotating shifts are preferable to permanent night work. Although permanent shifts may reduce circadian disturbances they are not normally acceptable for social reasons. However, if safety is paramount, permanent night shifts may improve performance levels.
- Quickly rotating shift systems (that change every one, two or three days) are preferable to slowly rotating ones (changing every five or more days), since they minimize circadian disruption and any cumulative sleep debt.
- Clockwise rotation (morning–afternoon–night) is preferable to the counterclockwise (night–afternoon–morning) since it avoids 'quick returns' (e.g. morning and night shift on the same day). It also parallels the natural tendency of the circadian system to delay slightly.
- Duration of shifts should be set according to psychophysical demand, with a view to minimizing sleepiness and fatigue, particularly on the night shift, while proper rest pauses should be planned throughout the duty period.
- Early starts to the morning shifts should be avoided to reduce the truncation of the previous sleep and the consequent increase in sleepiness, fatigue, and the risk of errors and accidents.
- Extended work days (9–12 hours) should only be contemplated when the nature of the work, and the workload, are suitable (adequate breaks, no overtime) and the shift system is designed to minimize the accumulation of fatigue and the exposure to toxic substances.
- Shift system should be as regular as possible to allow people to better plan their family and social life, and their coping strategies.
- Rest days should follow night shifts to allow adequate recuperation, while continuous shift systems should include as many free weekends as possible, and allow at least two consecutive days off between shift cycles.
- It is also desirable, and advantageous in terms of health and well-being, to allow flexible working time arrangements, and to encourage workers' participation in designing tailor-made shift systems according to their needs and preferences.[107]

In addition to the ergonomic design of shift schedules, other countermeasures that can prove beneficial include the compensatory reduction of working hours for night work, the introduction of additional rest breaks (for meals and naps), the addition of supplementary rest-days or holidays, the improvement of canteen and transport facilities, the improvement of social services (i.e. child care facilities, extended school and shop hours), specific education and training courses for shift workers, financial support for improving housing condition (i.e. sleeping rooms), transfer to day work after a certain number of years on night work, and gradual or early retirement.

MEDICAL SURVEILLANCE

It is clear that some complaints or illnesses may be a contraindication for shift work, particularly when it is associated with other stress factors such as heavy work, heat, noise, monotony or high cognitive demands. Thus, the occupational health physician needs to carry out an evaluation of both the working conditions and the health status of the individuals before assigning people to shift and night work. In the light of various suggestions given by a number of authors and institutions, it appears reasonable to propose the following strategies for medical intervention:[11,108–110]

1. Consider exempting from night work all those suffering from severe complaints and disorders that could be connected to, or worsened by, shift work such as:
   a. chronic sleep disturbances;
   b. severe gastrointestinal diseases (e.g. peptic ulcer, chronic hepatic and pancreatic diseases, Crohn's disease);
   c. chronic heart diseases (e.g. myocardial infarction up to 12 months or with impaired heart function,

angina pectoris, hyperkinetic syndromes and severe hypertension);
d. brain injuries with sequelae and severe nervous disorders, and in particular chronic anxiety and depression;
e. epilepsy requiring medication since seizures can be encouraged by sleep deficit and the efficacy of the treatment can be hampered by irregular wake–rest schedules;
f. spasmophily (i.e. chronic idiopathic or constitutional tetany), as temporal changes can be a promoting factor of tetanic crisis;
g. insulin-dependent diabetes, thyroid (thyrotoxicosis and thyroidectomy) and suprarenal pathologies, since they require regular drug treatment that is strictly connected to the activity/rest periods;
h. chronic renal impairment, since the disruption of circadian rhythms can further impair renal functioning;
i. immunological disorders and cancers, to avoid further stress and facilitate medical treatment;
j. pregnancy, particularly if there is a known risk of miscarriage.
2. Evaluate carefully before assigning to night work people who are or who have:
a. over 45–50 years of age, as it becomes more difficult to sleep at irregular hours;
b. digestive troubles or chronic respiratory diseases (asthma and chronic obstructive bronchitis);
c. alcoholism or other drug addictions;
d. marked hemeralopia or visual impairment, which can make night work difficult or dangerous in case of reduced illumination;
e. women with small children (under six years);
f. long distance commuters.

Particular attention should also be also paid to those who score highly on scales of neuroticism, morningness or rigidity of sleeping habits. In contrast, some individual characteristics and preferences could be considered to predispose people towards shift work (see under Factors affecting tolerance to shift work and extended working hours, p. 1238).

Regular health checks should be aimed at detecting early signs of intolerance to night work which may require prompt organizational (e.g. change the shift schedule) and/or individual (e.g. improve coping strategies or transfer to day work) intervention. Such checks should focus primarily on sleeping times and troubles, eating and digestive problems, psychosomatic complaints, drug consumption, housing and commuting problems, workload, and out of job activities, preferably using standardized questionnaires[111] or check lists in order to facilite a comparison of the worker's health over the years. Furthermore, the use of sleep logs, diaries of daily activities, some rhythmometric recordings (e.g. body temperature, performance) or hormonal dosages (e.g. cortisol, melatonin) may be helpful in evaluating the level of an individual's (mal)adjustment.

Physicians should also bear in mind that shift work may worsen some disorders (e.g. sleep, digestive or nervous complaints) and hence hamper the efficacy of their pharmacological control, particularly when this requires a precisely timed administration and/or a stable life regimen, as is the case for diabetes, hypertension, asthma, hormonal pathologies, epilepsy and depression. In addition, people affected by seasonal affective disorders may encounter more difficulties in coping with night work, due to the lower exposure to bright light.[112]

The frequency of medical examinations should be set by the occupational physician and take into account factors concerning both the working conditions (e.g. shifts rotas, environmental conditions, workload, etc.) and aspects of the individual (e.g. age and health condition). Many authors have emphasized the importance of careful monitoring during the first year of assignment to night work, since it may be critical for the development of effective coping strategies. At each periodical check the individual's fitness for shift work should be re-evaluated if they complain of sleep, gastrointestinal, psychological or other related problems, or if they contracted any other illnesses that might hamper their psychophysical equilibrium and working capacity. Temporary exemption from night work should be considered in the case of transient health impairment or severe difficulties with family or social life.

It is also necessary to pay particular attention to older workers, for whom some specific recommendations can be given, such as the need to limit night work after 50 years of age, give such workers priority for transfer to their preferred shift (e.g. morning shifts), reduce work load (supplement crews), shorten working hours, increase rest pauses and increase the frequency of health checks (at least every two years).[113] In addition, long-term medical surveillance (e.g. over five years) should be organized for any individual who leaves night or shift work for health reasons since there is evidence that these individuals may have a higher prevalence of sleep, gastrointestinal and cardiovascular disorders for several years after leaving shift work.

It is also desirable to give workers information and guidelines on how best to cope with night and shift work.[114] Counselling and training should be carried out at both an individual and group level and educational programmes should be set up. They should deal with improving self-help strategies for coping, and in particular in relation to sleep hygiene, eating behaviour, stress management, physical fitness, housing conditions, transport facilities, out-of-work activities and proper exposure to bright light. Finally, the occupational health physicians should consider giving scientific and practical support to employers and trade unions in applying preventive and compensatory measures aimed at reducing the problems arising from night and shift work.[115]

> **Key points**
>
> - Work schedules that disrupt the normal sleep–wake cycle and the endogenous body clock are becoming increasingly common.
> - As well as disturbing sleep and family and social life, such schedules can result in impaired psychological and physical health and in an increased risk of injuries and accidents.
> - The health problems associated with abnormal work schedules include anxiety, depression, gastrointestinal disturbances, cardiovascular diseases, reproductive problems and possibly cancer.
> - There are substantial differences between individuals, associated with factors such as age, personality and health status, in their ability to tolerate shift work.
> - Designing better work schedules and providing good medical surveillance may minimize the adverse consequences of abnormal work schedules.

REFERENCES

1. Costa G, Åkerstedt T, Nachreiner F et al. Flexible work hours, health and well being: Results of the SALTSA project. *Chronobiology International*. 2004; **21**: 1–13.
2. Parent-Thirion A, Fernández Macías E, Hurley J, Vermeylen G. Fourth European Working Conditions Survey. Dublin: European Foundation for the Improvement of Living and Working Conditions, 2007. Available from www.eurofound.europa.eu.
3. US Bureau of Labor Statistics, Department of Labor. Occupational outlook handbook, 2005. Available from: www.bls.org.
4. International Labour Organization. Kilm 06. Geneva: International Labour Organization, 2007. Available from: www.ilo.org/public/english/employment/strat/kilm/download/kilm06.pdf.
5. Harrington JM. Health effects of shift work and extended hours of work. *Occupational and Environmental Medicine*. 2001; **58**: 68–72.
6. van der Hulst M. Long work hours and health. *Scandinavian Journal of Work, Environment and Health*. 2003; **29**: 171–88.
7. US Congress, Office of Technology Assessment. *Biological rhythms: Implications for the worker*. OTA-BA-463, Washington, DC: US Government Printing Office, 1991.
8. Folkard S, Waterhouse JM, Minors DS. Chronobiology and shift work: Current issues and trends. *Chronobiologia*. 1985; **12**: 31–54.
9. Roenneberg T, Kumar CJ, Merrow M. The human circadian clock entrains to sun time. *Currrent Biology*. 2007; **17**: R44–R45.
10. Folkard S. Do permanent night workers show circadian adjustment? A review based on the endogenous melatonin rhythm. *Chronobiology International*. 2008; **25**: 215–24.
11. Colquhoun WP, Costa G, Folkard S, Knauth P. *Shiftwork: Problems and solutions*. Frankfurt: Peter Lang, 1996.
12. Waterhouse JM, Folkard S, Minors DS. *Shiftwork, health and safety. An overview of the scientific literature 1978–1990*. London: Her Majesty's Stationery Office, 1992.
13. Cho K, Ennaceur A, Cole JC, Chang KS. Chronic jet lag produces cognitive deficits. *Journal of Neuroscience*. 2000; **20** (RC66): 1–5.
14. Rouch I, Wild P, Ansiau D, Marquie J-C. Shiftwork experience, age and cognitive performance. *Ergonomics*. 2005; **48**: 1282–93.
15. Monk TH, Folkard S, Wedderburn AI. Maintaining safety and high performance on shiftwork. *Applied Ergonomics*. 1996; **27**: 17–23.
16. Monk T. Shiftworker performance. *Occupational Medicine: State of Art Review*. 1990; **5**: 183–98.
17. Åkerstedt T. *Wide awake at odd hours*. Stockholm: Swedish Council for Work Life Research, 1996.
18. Colligan MJ, Rosa RR. Shiftwork effects on social and family life. *Occupational Medicine: State of Art Review*. 1990; **5**: 315–22.
19. Jansen NW, Kant I, Kristensen TS, Nijhuis FJ. Antecedents and consequences of work-family conflict: A prospective cohort study. *Journal of Occupational and Environmental Medicine*. 2005, **31**: 277–85.
20. Loudon R, Bohle P. Work/non-work conflict and health in shiftwork: relationships with family status and social support. *International Journal of Occupational and Environmental Health*. 1997; **3**: S71–S77.
21. Åkerstedt T. Shift work and disturbed sleep/wakefulness. *Occupational Medicine*. 2003; **53**: 89–94.
22. Tepas DI, Carvalhais AB. Sleep patterns of shiftworkers. *Occupational Medicine: State of Art Review*. 1990; **5**: 199–208.
23. Cole RJ, Loving RT, Kripke DF. Psychiatric aspects of shiftwork. *Occupational Medicine: State of Art Review*. 1990; **5**: 301–14.
24. Costa G. The impact of shift and night work on health. *Applied Ergonomics*. 1996; **27**: 9–16.
25. Knutsson A. Health disorders of shift workers. *Occupational Medicine*. 2003; **53**: 103–8.
26. Karlsson B, Knutsson A, Lindahl B. Is there an association between shift work and having a metabolic syndrome? Results from a population based study of 27485 people. *Occupational and Environmental Medicine*. 2001; **58**: 747–52.
27. Knutsson A, Bøggild H. Shiftwork and cardiovascular disease: Review of disease mechanisms. *Reviews on Environmental Health*. 2000; **15**: 359–72.
28. Ha M, Park J. Shiftwork and metabolic risk factors of cardiovascular diseases. *Journal of Occupational Health*. 2005; **47**: 89–95.
29. Karlsson B, Knutsson A, Lindahl B, Alfredsson L. Metabolic disturbances in male workers with rotating three-shift work. Results of the WOLF study. *International Archives*

of Occupational and Environmental Health. 2003; **76**: 424–30.
30. Nakamura K, Shimai S, Kikuchi S *et al.* Shift work and risk factors for coronary heart disease in Japanese blue-collar workers: Serum lipids and anthropometric characteristics. *Occupational Medicine*. 1997; **47**: 142–6.
31. Shields M. Long working hours and health. *Health Reports*. 1999; **11**: 33–48.
32. Koller M, Kundi M, Cervinka R. Field studies of shift work at an Austrian oil refinery. I. Health and psychosocial wellbeing of workers who drop out of shift work. *Ergonomics*. 1978; **21**: 835–47.
33. Mikuni E, Ohoshi T, Hayashi K, Miyamura K. Glucose intolerance in an employed population. *Tohoku Journal of Experimental Medicine*. 1983; **141**: 251–6.
34. Kawakami N, Araki S, Takatsuka N *et al.* Overtime, psychosocial working conditions, and occurrence of non-insulin dependent diabetes mellitus in Japanese men. *Journal of Epidemiology and Community Health*. 1999; **53**: 359–63.
35. Bøggild H, Knutsson A. Shiftwork and cardiovascular disease: Review of disease mechanisms. *Reviews on Environmental Health*. 2000; **15**: 359–72.
36. Bøggild H, Knutsson A. Shift work, risk factors and cardiovascular disease. *Scandinavian Journal of Work, Environment and Health*. 1999; **25**: 85–99.
37. Tenkanen L, Sjöblom T, Kalimo R *et al.* Shift work, occupation and coronary heart disease over 6 years of follow-up in the Helsinki Heart Study. *Scandinavian Journal of Work, Environment and Health*. 1997; **23**: 257–65.
38. van Amelsvoort L, Jansen N, Kant I. Smoking among shiftworkers: More than a confounding factor. *Chronobiology International*. 2006; **23**: 1105–13.
39. Liu Y, Tanaka H, The Fukuoka Heart Study Group. Overtime work, insufficient sleep, and risk of non-fatal acute myocardial infarction in Japanese men. *Occupational and Environmental Medicine*. 2002; **59**: 447–51.
40. Sokejima S, Kagamimori S. Working hours as a risk factor for acute myocardial infarction in Japan: Case-control study. *British Medical Journal*. 1998; **317**: 775–80.
41. Caruso CC, Hitchcock EM, Dick RB *et al.* Overtime and extended work shifts: Recent findings on illnesses, injuries, and health behaviors. Cincinnati, OH: US Department of Health and Human Services, Centers for Disease Control and Prevention, National Institute for Occupational Safety and Health, April 2004.
42. Smith L, Folkard S, Poole CJ. Increased injuries on night shift. *Lancet*. 1994; **344**: 1137–9.
43. Folkard S, Tucker P. Shiftwork, safety and productivity. *Occupational Medicine*. 2003; **53**: 95–101.
44. Folkard S, Lombardi DA. Modelling the impact of the components of long work hours on injuries and accidents. *American Journal of Industrial Medicine*. 2006; **49**: 953–63.
45. Folkard S, Robertson KA, Spencer MB. A fatigue/risk index to assess work schedules. *Somnology*. 2007; **11**: 177–85.
46. Price WJ, Holley DC. Shiftwork and safety in aviation. *Occupational Medicine: State of Art Review*. 1990; **5**: 343–77.
47. Fischer FM. Retrospective study regarding absenteeism among shiftworkers. *International Archives of Occupational and Environmental Health*. 1986; **58**: 301–20.
48. Kleiven M, Boggild H, Jeppesen HJ. Shift work and sick leave. *Scandinavian Journal of Work, Environment and Health*. 1998; **24** (Suppl. 3): 128–33.
49. Baker A, Heiler K, Ferguson SA. The effects of a roster schedule change from 8- to 12-hour shifts on health and safety in a mining operation. *Journal of Human Ergology*. 2001; **30**: 65–70.
50. Armstrong BG, Nolin AD, MacDonald AD. Work in pregnancy and birth weight for gestational age. *British Journal of Industrial Medicine*. 1989; **46**: 196–9.
51. Xu X, Ding M, Li B, Christiani DC. Association of rotating shiftwork with preterm births and low birth weight among never smoking women textile workers in China. *Occupational and Environmental Medicine*. 1994; **51**: 470–4.
52. Axelsson G, Rylander R, Molin I. Outcome of pregnancy in relation to irregular and inconvenient work schedules. *British Journal of Industrial Medicine*. 1989; **46**: 393–8.
53. Nurminen T. Shift work and reproductive health. *Scandinavian Journal of Work, Environment and Health*. 1998; **24** (Suppl. 3): 28–34.
54. Mozurkewich EL, Luke B, Avni M, Wolf FM. Working conditions and adverse pregnancy outcome: A meta-analysis. *Obstetrics and Gynecology*. 2000; **95**: 623–35.
55. Gadbois C. Women on night shift: Interdependence of sleep and off-job activities. In: Reinberg A, Vieux N, Andlauer P (eds). *Night and shift work: Biological and social aspects*. Oxford: Pergamon Press, 1981: 223–7.
56. Smolenski MH, Reinberg A. Clinical chronobiology: Relevance and applications to the practice of occupational medicine. *Occupational Medicine: State of Art Review*. 1990; **5**: 239–72.
57. Smolensky MH, Paustenbach DJ, Scheving LE. Biological rhythms, shiftwork, and occupational health. In: Cralley LJ, Cralley LV (eds.) *Patty's Industrial hygiene and toxicology*, vol 3B. New York: J Wiley & Sons, 1985: 175–312.
58. Goyal R, Krishnan K, Tardif R *et al.* Assessment of occupational health risk during unusual workshifts: Review of the needs and solutions for modifying environmental and biological limit values for volatile organic solvents. *Canadian Journal of Public Health*. 1992; **83**: 109–12.
59. Taylor PJ, Pocock SJ. Mortality of shift and day workers 1956–68. *British Journal of Industrial Medicine*. 1972; **29**: 201–7.
60. Knutsson A, Hammar N, Karlsson B. Shift workers' mortality scrutinized. *Chrobiology International*. 2004; **6**: 1049–53.
61. Bøggild H, Saudicani P, Hein HO, Gyntelberg F. Shift work, social class, and ischaemic heart disease in middle aged and elderly men: A 22 year follow up in the Copenhagen male study. *Occupational and Environmental Medicine*. 1999; **56**: 640–5.
62. Akerstedt T, Keklund G, Johansson S. Shift work and mortality. *Chronobiology International*. 2004, **6**: 1055–61.
63. Nylén L, Voss M, Floderus B. Mortality among women and men relative to unemployment, part time work, overtime work, and extra work: A study based on data from the

Swedish Twin Registry. *Occupational and Environmental Medicine*. 2001; **58**: 52-7.
64. Megdal SP, Kroenke CH, Laden F et al. Night work and breast cancer risk: A systematic review and meta-analysis. *European Journal of Cancer*. 2005; **41**: 2023-32.
65. Schernhammer ES, Kroenke CH, Laden F, Hankinson SE. Night work and risk of breast cancer. *Epidemiology*. 2006; **17**: 108-11.
66. Stevens RG. Circadian disruption and breast cancer: From melatonin to clock genes. *Epidemiology*. 2005; **16**: 254-8.
67. Straif F, Baan R, Grosse Y et al. on behalf of the WHO International Agency for Research on Cancer Monograph Working Group. Carcinogenicity of shift-work, painting, and fire-fighting. *Lancet Oncology*. 2007; **8**: 1065-6.
68. Costa G. Some considerations about aging, shift work and work ability. In: Costa G, Goedhard W, Ilmarinen J (eds.) *Assessment and promotion of work ability, health and well-being of ageing workers*. Amsterdam: Elsevier, 2005: 67-72.
69. Aguirre A, Heitmann A, Imrie A et al. Conversion from an 8-h to a 12-h shift schedule. In: Hornberger S, Knauth P, Costa G, Folkard S (eds.) *Shiftwork in the 21st century. Arbeitswissinschaft in der betrieblichen Praxis*, vol. 17. Frankfurt am Main: Peter Lang, 2000: 113-18.
70. Bourdouxhe MA, Queinnec Y, Granger D et al. Aging and shiftwork: The effects of 20 years of rotating 12-hour shifts among petroleum refinery operators. *Experimental Aging Research*. 1999; **25**: 323-9.
71. Härmä M, Hakkola T, Akerstedt T, Laitinen J. Age and adjustment to night work. *Occupational and Environmental Medicine*. 1994; **51**: 568-73.
72. Marquiè J, Foret J. Sleep, age and shiftwork experience. *Journal of Sleep Research*. 1999; **2**: 297-304.
73. Koller M. Health risk related to shift work. *International Archives of Occupational and Environmental Health*. 1983; **53**: 59-75.
74. Brugère D, Barrit J, Butat C et al. Shiftwork, age, and health: an epidemiological investigation. *International Journal of Occupational and Environmental Health*. 1997; **3**: S15-S19.
75. Derriennic F, Touranchet A, Volkoff S. *Age, travail, santé: Etudes sur les salariés âgés de 37 à 52 ans, Estev 1990*. Paris: Les Éditions Inserm, 1996.
76. Costa G, Sartori S. Ageing, working hours and work ability. *Ergonomics*. 2007; **50**: 1-17.
77. Costa G. Factor influencing health and tolerance to shift work. *Theoretical Issues in Ergonomics Science*. 2003; **4**: 263-88.
78. Härmä M. Individual differences in tolerance to shiftwork: A review. *Ergonomics*. 1993; **36**: 101-9.
79. Reinberg A, Andlauer P, De Prins J et al. Desynchronisation of the oral temperature circadian rhythm and intolerance to shift work. *Nature*. 1984; **308**: 272-4.
80. Härmä M. Ageing, physical fitness and shiftwork tolerance. *Applied Ergonomics*. 1996; **27**: 25-9.
81. Rosa R. Editorial: Factors for promoting adjustment to night and shift work. *Work and Stress*. 1990; **4**: 201-2.
82. Smith L, Norman P, Folkard S. Predicting shiftwork-related outcomes: Shiftwork locus of control and cyrcadian type. *Journal of Human Ergology*. 2001; **30**: 59-64.
83. Nachreiner F. Individual and social determinants of shiftwork tolerance. *Scandinavian Journal of Work, Environment and Health*. 1998; **24** (Suppl. 3): 35-42.
84. Bohle P, Tilley A. The impact of shift work on psychological well-being. *Ergonomics*. 1989; **32**: 1089-99.
85. Barton J, Aldridge J, Smith P. The emotional impact of shift work on the children of shift workers. *Scandinavian Journal of Work, Environment and Health*. 1998; **24** (Suppl. 3): 146-50.
86. Monk T, Folkard S. *Making shift work tolerable*. London: Taylor & Francis, 1992.
87. Presser HB. Shiftwork among American couples: The relevance of job and family factors. In: Haider M, Koller M, Cervinka R (eds). *Night and shiftwork: Long-term effects and their prevention*. Frankfurt: Peter Lang, 1986: 149-56.
88. Pisarski A. Effects of coping strategies, social support and work-non work conflict on shift workers health. *Scandinavian Journal of Work, Environment and Health*. 1998; **24** (Suppl. 3): 141-5.
89. Beerman B, Nachreiner F. Working shifts – different effects for women and men? *Work and Stress*. 1995; **9**: 289-97.
90. Pisarski A, Bohle P. Effects of supervisor support and coping on shiftwork tolerance. *Journal of Human Ergology*. 2001; **30**: 363-8.
91. Walker J. Social problems of shiftwork. In: S Folkard S, Monk T (eds). *Hours of work: Temporal factors in work scheduling*. Chichester: John Wiley & Sons, 1985: 221-5.
92. International Labour Organization. Night work. Report V/1. Geneva: International Labour Organization, 1988.
93. Ong CN, Kogi K. Shiftwork in developing countries: current issues and trends. *Occupational Medicine*. 1990; **5**: 417-28.
94. Kogi K, Ong CN, Catabong C. Some social aspects of shift work in Asian developing countries. *International Journal of Industrial Ergonomics*. 1989; **4**: 151-9.
95. Fischer FM. Shiftworkers in developing countries: Health and well-being and support measures. *Journal of Human Ergology*. 2001; **30**: 155-60.
96. Clark S. Shiftwork and leisure behaviour of ethnic and gender groups in the British textile industry. *Travail Humain*. 1990; **53**: 227-44.
97. Haider M, Cervinka R, Koller M, Kundi M. A destabilization theory of shiftworkers effects. In: Hekkens JM, Kerkhof GA, Rietveld WJ (eds). *Trends in chronobiology*. Oxford: Pergamon Press, 1988: 209-17.
98. Tepas D. Inter-individual vs intra-individual differences: An important distinction for shiftwork research. In: Hornberger S, Knauth P, Costa G, Folkard S (eds). *Shiftwork in the 21st century. Arbeitswissinschaft in der betrieblichen Praxis*, vol 17. Frankfurt: Peter Lang, 2000: 273-9.
99. Dahlgren A, Keklund G, Akerstedt T. Overtime work and its effects on sleep, sleepiness, cortisol and blood pressure in

an experimental field study. *Scandinavian Journal of Work, Environment and Health*. 2006; **32**: 318–27.
100. Spurgeon A, Harrington JM, Cooper CL. Health and safety problems associated with long working hours: A review of the current position. *Occupational and Environmental Medicine*. 1997; **54**: 367–75.
101. Kogi K. Improving shift workers' health and tolerance to shiftwork. *Applied Ergonomics*. 1996; **27**: 1–8.
102. International Labour Organization. Night Work Convention no 171. Geneva: International Labour Organization, 1990.
103. International Labour Organization. Night Work Recommendation no 178. Geneva: International Labour Organization, 1990.
104. European Parliament. Directive 2003/88/EC of the European Parliament and of the Council of 4 November 2003 concerning certain aspects of the organisation of working time. Official Journal L 299, 18/11/2003, 9–19.
105. Knauth P. Designing better shift systems. *Applied Ergonomics*. 1996; **27**: 39–44.
106. Knauth P, Hornberger S. Preventive and compensatory measures for shift workers. *Occupational Medicine*. 2003; **53**: 109–16.
107. Costa G, Sartori S, Akerstedt T. Influence of flexibility and variability of working hours on health and well-being. *Chronobiology International*. 2006; **23**: 1–13.
108. Koller M. Occupational health services for shift and night work. *Applied Ergonomics*. 1996; **27**: 31–7.
109. Scott AJ, LaDou J. Shiftwork: Effects on sleep and health with recommendations for medical surveillance and screening. *Occupational Medicine: State of Art Review*. 1990; **5**: 273–99.
110. Costa G. Guidelines for the medical surveillance of shiftworkers. *Scandinavian Journal of Work, Environment and Health*. 1998; **24** (Suppl 3): 151–5.
111. Barton J, Spelten E, Totterdell P *et al*. The Standard Shiftwork Index: A battery of questionnaires for assessing shiftwork related problems. *Work and Stress*. 1995; **9**: 4–30.
112. Koller M, Kundi M, Stidl H-G *et al*. Personal light dosimetry in permanent night and day workers. *Chronobiology International*. 1993; **10**: 143–55.
113. Härmä M, Kandolin I. Shiftwork, age and well-being: Recent developments and future perspectives. *Journal of Human Ergology*. 2001; **30**: 287–93.
114. Wedderburn A (ed.). *Guidelines for shiftworkers*. Bulletin of European Studies on Time No 3. Dublin: European Foundation for the Improvement of Living and Working Conditions, 1991.
115. Kogi K. Healthy shiftwork, healthy shiftworkers. *Journal of Human Ergology*. 2001; **30**: 3–8.

Index

Abbeystead (explosion) 269
abortion
   spontaneous 1201–2
   therapeutic, recommendation 1210
absence (from work)
   alcohol and 860–1
   shift work and 1236–7
   sickness see sickness
absorption 128
   gastrointestinal see gastrointestinal tract
   inhalation see inhalation
   light in ocular tissues 645
   metals 151–2
      lead 190
      manganese 203
      polonium 231–2
      uranium 244
   rate of 129
   see specific routes
abstinence in alcohol/drug abuse 866–7
acamprosate 866
accelerations, flying 595–6
   misinterpretations 601
acceptance and commitment therapy (ACT) 847
accidents
   'arising out of and in the course of employment' 97
   shift work and 1236
acclimatization 539
   high altitude 570, 572, 573, 575, 576
   thermal stress
      cold 529
      heat 534, 536
acetazolamide for altitude sickness
   preventive use 582
   therapeutic use 583
acetone 339
acetonitrile 352–3
2-acetylaminofluorene, biotransformation 134
acetylation status and bladder cancer 1113

acetyl-L-carnitine (ALCAR) in noise-related deafness 476
acetylcholinesterase inhibitors (anticholinesterases)
   nerve agent 315
   pesticides 396, 399, 401, 402, 404, 1160–1
      acute effects 404
      biological monitoring 61, 66, 415
      mechanisms of toxicity 397, 398–9
      treatment 410, 411
N-acetylcysteine (NAC) in noise-related deafness 476
acetylene 300, 322
N-acetylglucosaminidase, urinary 68
   lead and 1128
N-acetyltransferase 2 (NAT2)
   acetylation status and bladder cancer 1113
ACGIA see American Conference of Governmental Industrial Hygienists
acid(s), semiconductor production 447–448
acid anhydrides
   cyclic 362, 363
   sulphuric 288
acid gases 256
   skin burns 263
acid mists 288
acne
   chlorine/halogen 1067–8
   oil 1069
acoustic trauma 469–70
Acramin and 'Ardystil syndrome' 899
acrylamide 350–1
   neurotoxicity 351, 1152–3
acrylic acid esters 347–8
acrylonitrile 352–3
actinolite 994, 995
   dose–response and 1001
Actinomycetes and ventilation pneumonitis 980
action levels, lead 197–8

active noise control 472
active transport 128
acute lymphocytic leukaemia 1092
acute mountain sickness (AMS) 570–2, 574
   cerebral oedema progression from 575
   children 576
   females 576
   Lake Louise scoring system see Lake Louise acute mountain sickness score
   predisposition 578
   prevention 581–3, 585
   treatment 583–4, 585
acute myeloid leukaemia (AML) 1222
   benzene and 326, 327, 1223
   case report 1226
acute respiratory distress syndrome (ARDS; adult respiratory distress syndrome)
   gases 263
   welding 433
adaptation and habituation
   to cold 529
   to motion in flying 602–3
   to noise 465
   see also acclimatization
adhesive capsulitis (shoulder) 690, 690–1
adjustment disorder 813, 837
α-adrenoceptors, hand–arm vibration syndrome 492
Adson's test 503
adult life support in space 612–13
adult respiratory distress syndrome see acute respiratory distress syndrome
advanced life support systems, combat aircraft 596–7
adverse workplace events and psychological trauma 811–12
aerosols
   biological 438
   sampling, nanoparticles 914

aflatoxin and hepatocellular carcinoma 1114
African iron overload 186
afterdamp 268
age
　hearing loss and 471
　shift work and 1238
　ventilatory function 893–4
Agent Orange 1163–4
'aggregate' exposure 45
Agricola, Georgius 7, 8
agriculture and farming
　chemicals see pesticides
　dermatoses 1071
　extrinsic allergic alveolitis 970, 971
　lymphomas 1225
AIDS see human immunodeficiency virus
air
　as breathing mixture for divers 548–9
　compressed see compressed air work; diving
　flow obstruction/limitation 889–902
　　asthma 948–9
　　chronic 889–902
　　see also chronic obstructive pulmonary disease
　gases in 256
　　carbon monoxide 275–6
　　concentrations 254
　　outdoors see outdoor (ambient) air
　indoor see indoor environments
　manganese in 202–3
　measuring airborne exposure 45
　methane mixed with 269
　pollution see pollution
　quality guidelines for NO_2/SO_2, WHO 142
　radiation range in 624
　sampling 45
　in welding operator's breathing zone 423
　see also atmosphere
air conditioning systems
　aircraft 598
　buildings 923, 934
　　extrinsic allergic alveolitis and 928, 929, 980
　　humidifier fever and 929
　　Legionnaires' disease and 930
air pressure 545–624
air sickness 602–3
aircraft industry, hepatotoxic chemicals 1174
　see also flying

airway
　artificial, in space 612
　human (natural) see chronic obstructive pulmonary disease; respiratory tract; small airways dysfunction
Alcoholics Anonymous 866
alcohols 336–8
　ethyl see ethyl alcohol
aldehydes 338–9
Aldridge, Thomas 5
aldrin, conversion to dieldrin 134
aliphatic amines 355–6
aliphatic hydrocarbons 322–4
alkali(s), semiconductor production 447
alkaline phosphatase (ALP) 1173
alkanes 322
　halogenated, hepatotoxicity 1175, 1180–1
alkenes 322, 322–3
alkoxyalcohols see glycol ethers
alkyl amine gases 289–90
alkynes 32, 322
'all or none' diseases 92, 93
Allen's test 503
allergen(s) (allergenic antigens)
　asthma and 942, 943
　　respiratory surveillance in tertiary prevention 947
　byssinosis 961
　extrinsic allergic alveolitis and 971, 976
　IgE tests see immunoglobulin E tests
　indoor non-industrial 924
allergenicity
　acrylic/methacrylic acid esters 347
　ethanolamines 355
allergic alveolitis, extrinsic see extrinsic allergic alveolitis
allergic contact dermatitis 1063–4
　patch tests 1065–6
alloys 161
　aluminium see aluminium
　beryllium 162
　cobalt 175
　nickel see nickel
　semiconductors 444
allyl chloride 1153
alpha particles 624
altitude
　barometric pressure related to 592
　increased in, potential problems with 592–5
　see also flying; high altitude
aluminium 153–8, 1044–5, 1156–7
　alloys 153
　　beryllium–aluminium 162

　neurotoxicity 154–5, 1156–7
　pot room asthma in production of 283–4, 1043
　welding 153, 434–5
aluminium phosphide 295, 412
aluminium silicates 1011
alveolar concentration 131
alveolar echinococcosis 765
alveolar epithelial cells, type 1 138
alveolar macrophages and inorganic dusts 985
alveolitis
　cobalt-induced 176
　extrinsic allergic see extrinsic allergic alveolitis
Alzheimer's disease
　aluminium and 155
　electromagnetic fields and 669–70
amalgam, dental 215–16, 1134
American Conference of Governmental Industrial Hygienists (ACGIH)
　biological monitoring 58, 60
　arsenic 161
　exposure limits 40, 48
　manganese 208
　molybdenum 221
　phosphorus 225
　silver 235
　vanadium 247
American Industrial Hygiene Association's Emergency Response Planning Guidelines (ERPGs) 257, 258
Amiata, Mount 303
amides 348–51, 1181–2
　hepatotoxicity 1181–2
　N-substituted 1181–2
　semiconductor production 447
amines 353–6
　aliphatic 355–6
　aromatic see aromatic amines
　semiconductor production 447
　see also nitrosamines
δ-aminolaevulinic acid (ALA; 5-ALA) and lead 192, 196–7, 1128
δ-aminolaevulinic acid dehydratase (ALAD)
　deficiency 1221
　lead and 192, 197, 1221
δ-aminolaevulinic acid synthase (ALA synthase) and lead 192
ammonia 257, 288–9
amosite (brown asbestos) 26, 104, 991
　attribution of disease to exposure in case study 51–2

dose–response and 1001
amphetamine hydroxylation 133
amphiboles 990, 991, 993, 1001
    diffuse pleural thickening and 1002
    lung cancer and 1005
    mesothelioma and 1004
amyl nitrate
    cyanide poisoning 277, 278
    nitrile poisoning 353
t-amylmethylether (TAME) 341
amyotrophic lateral sclerosis and electromagnetic fields 670, 671
anaemia 1219–30
    aplastic *see* aplastic anaemia
    benzene 325
    haemolytic *see* haemolytic anaemia
    lead 1220–1
    naphthalene 332
    sickle cell *see* sickle cell anaemia
anaerobic fermentation 266–7
anaesthesia (general)
    gases used 298–301
        reproductive effects 1205
    at high altitude 581
    in space 612
anemometry 528
angiosarcoma (liver) and vinyl chloride 17, 26, 134, 368, 1096, 1187
anhydrides, acid *see* acid anhydrides
aniline 352–3, 353
    biological monitoring guidance values 61
animals
    as experimental models *see* laboratory studies
    infection naturally transmitted to human 750–70
    infection risk to workers with 741
anosmia, cadmium 168
anthophyllite 991
anthracene 332
anthrax (*B. anthracis*) 751–2
    bioterrorism 774–8
    historical perspectives 11–12
antibiotics
    anthrax (therapeutic and prophylactic) 753
    borreliosis 763
    brucellosis 755–6
    campylobacteriosis 761
    erysipeloid 763–4
    leptospirosis 758
    Mycobacterium marinum 764
    salmonellosis 760
    Streptococcus suis 758
    in tissue culture 790
    traveller's diarrhoea 743

antibodies
    monoclonal 785, 787
    serological testing *see* serological testing
anticholinesterases *see* acetylcholinesterase inhibitors
anticoagulant rodenticides 402
    acute effects 405–6
        management 412
antidotes
    cyanides 276, 277, 278, 317–18
    nitriles 353
    organophosphates 410, 411
    terrorist chemical attack 317–18
        nerve agents 315
        sarin 316
anti-emetics
    air sickness 603
    radiation casualties 640
anti-G straining manoeuvre (AGSM) 596
anti-G suits and trousers 596, 597
antigens
    allergenic *see* allergens
    fungal, cotton workers 960
antihistamines
    air sickness 603
    byssinosis 964
anti-inflammatory drugs, osteoarthritis 702
anti-knock agent *see* petrol
antimalarials 742
    aircrew, prophylaxis 607
antimony 159
    dust 1045
    semiconductor production 448
    see also stibine
antimony trihydride (stibine) 159, 295, 1042
antineoplastic agents *see* chemotherapeutic agents
antineutrophil cytoplasmic antibodies (ANCA) and silica 1024, 1025, 1137, 1138
antioxidants
    asthma susceptibility and 946
    noise-induced deafness 476
antiretrovirals in post-exposure prophylaxis 736
anxiety 812, 813
    case studies in management of 826, 827
    gassing 263
    phobic *see* phobia
    screening and treatment 847–8
    temporal association of work-related disability and 843

anylate choice 59–60
aplastic anaemia 1221, 1224
    benzene 1223
aqueous humor 647
arc welding 422–3
    burns 429
    particle emissions 425
    radiation 423, 424
archaeologists, viruses 744
Ardystil syndrome 899
argon 271
    breathing mixtures (divers) 549
argyria 234, 235
Arlidge, Thomas 12
Armstrong line 593
aromatic amines 353–5
    carcinogenicity 1089
        IARC classification 1083, 1084
aromatic hydrocarbons 324–31
    neurotoxicity 328–9, 330–1, 1162–3
    nitrogenated 1182–3
    polycyclic *see* polycyclic aromatic hydrocarbons
arrhythmias
    astronauts 610
    high altitude 579
arsenic 160–1, 1157, 1184–5
    biological monitoring guidance values 61
    carcinogenicity 161, 450, 1093
    hepatotoxicity 1184–5
    nephrotoxicity 294, 1137
    neurotoxicity 1157
    semiconductor production 448
arsine 294–5, 1042
    nephrotoxicity 294, 1137
    semiconductor production 448
arterial concentration of inhaled compounds, assessment 131
arthropathies, lead 193
    see also osteoarthritis; rheumatoid arthritis
artificial gravity in space 613
aryl hydrocarbon receptors and dioxins 1179, 1180
asbestos 102–4, 880–3, 990–1016
    attribution of disease to exposure 93, 95, 95, 1006
    in case study 51–2
    chronic obstructive pulmonary disease and 898, 996
    compensation schemes 102–4
    epidemiology of diseases 26, 1000–16
    health surveillance 996–7
    historical perspectives 16–18
    imaging of disease 880–3, 993, 995
    lung cancer and *see* lung cancer

asbestos (*Continued*)
  mesothelioma *see* mesothelioma
  mineral/fibre type 990–1, 1004–5
    malignancy and 1004–5, 1005
  nanotube behaviour compared with 906
  non-industrial and accidental exposure 996–7, 1005
  prevention of cancers due to 1104
  substitutes for 1104
    carcinogenicity 1088, 1104
  welding and exposures to 435
asbestosis (interstitial fibrosis) 991–2, 1000–1
  compensation 102
  diagnosis 991
  dose–response relationships 1001
  epidemiology 1000–1
  expert medical report 117
  latency 1001
  lung cancer and 994, 1006
  pathology 993
  pathophysiology 993
  prognosis 993
  radiology 880, 882, 883, 992
  signs and symptoms 991–2
ascertainment bias 95
Asiafreighter (arsine exposure) 294
aspartate aminotransferase, alcohol abuse 864–5
Aspergillus clavatus and malt-worker's lung 979
Aspergillus penicillium and *A. niger* in biotechnology 789
asphalt 335
asphyxiant gases 255, 268–78
  chemical 273–8
  simple 268–72
  welding 432–3
association
  in Bradford Hill criteria 91–2, 145
  causality and 144, 145
  measures of 78–9
  strength of 91–2
asthma incl. bronchial asthma (occupational) 310–13, 925–8, 941–57, 1042–3
  air pollutants and 144
    indoor non-industrial 925–8, 933
  COPD and 895–6
    asthma simulating COPD 891
  cyclic acid anhydrides and 362
  determinants 945–6
  diesel exhaust and 912
  epidemiology 944–5
  high altitude and 579, 580
  hydrogen sulphide and 292

identification and diagnosis 947–51
irritant gas-induced 264, 310–13
  isocyanates *see* isocyanates
  pot room asthma in aluminium production 283–4, 1043
management 951
mechanisms (pathogenesis) 943
metals 1042–3
  cobalt 176, 1042
  nickel 223–4, 1042–3
  tungsten 241
  vanadium 246, 1043
occupational groups and their agents as cause of 942–3
organic dusts and 941–57
outcome 951–2
pre-existing/exacerbated asthma vs 941
prevention 946–7
welders 434, 911, 1043
see also reactive airways dysfunction syndrome
asthma-like syndrome, aluminium smelting 154
astronauts *see* spaceflight
asustado 808
atelectasis, rounded, asbestosis 883, 992
atherogenesis and nanoparticles 908
atmosphere
  Earth's
    composition 265
    pressure 545–624
  spacecraft 608
  see also air; pollution
atom(s), radiation and 623–4
atomic weapons *see* nuclear weapon and atomic weapon explosions
atopy
  and asthma 946
  and byssinosis 960, 961–2
  and contact dermatitis 1065
atrial tachycardia, paroxysmal, high altitude 579
atropine
  AChE-inhibiting pesticides 315, 410, 1160
  sarin 316
attapulgite 1011
attributable fraction in exposed persons 79
attributable risk 78–9
attribution (of disease to cause/exposure) 51–4, 89, 92–4
  disease registers 94–5
  individual patients 94
    case study examples 51–4
attribution bias 95
audiometry 474, 477–80
  in noise-induced hearing loss 469

auditory brainstem response 477–8
autistic spectrum disorder 828
autodarkening welding filters 431, 658–9
autoimmune disease and silica 1024–5
autopsy, inorganic dust diseases 988
aviation *see* flying

Bacillus anthracis see anthrax
bacillus Calmette-Guérin (BCG) vaccination 739
back injury (incl. spine)
  aircraft accidents 605
  thermal stress and people with 540
  whole-body vibration 514–19
back pain, low (LBP) 715–24
  causes 717–18
  flying and 606
  historical treatment 715–16
  management and return to work 719–21
  non-specific 707, 719–20
  prevention 718–19
  prognosis 720
  whole-body vibration and 514–19
bacterial infections
  bioterrorism 774–8
  healthcare workers 739–40, 741
  zoonotic, presenting symptoms
    chest 751–6
    cutaneous 762–4, 764
    fever 754–6, 757–8
    gastrointestinal 759–61
bacterial toxins *see* toxins
bactericidal treatment of cotton 966
BADGE (bisphenol A diglycidyl ether) 361–2
bagassosis 979–80
balance problems (incl. vertigo)
  aircrew 601
  noise-induced 480
  styrene 327
Bantu siderosis 186
barium dust 1045
barometric pressure 545–624
Barr, Thomas 465
barrier creams 1067
basal cell carcinoma, UV-related 1092–3
  sun exposure 1071, 1093
  welding 423, 429
basal ganglia, manganism 206
basophilic stippling of red cells *see* red blood cells
batteries
  cobalt in 175
  NiCd 167
Bauer, George (Georgius Agricola) 7, 8
BCG vaccination 739

beat conditions 699
behavioural disorders *see* neurological problems; psychological disorders
behavioural management programmes, back pain 721
Békésy, G von 464, 467
Belgium, compensation schemes 105, 106
Bell, Dr JH 11–12
Beney Committee 101
bentonites 1036
benzene 325–7, 1222–4
    confusion with benzine 35
    haematological effects 325–6, 1222–4
        leukaemia and 326, 1092, 1223
    metabolism 134, 326–7
    monitoring 61, 326–7
    reducing exposure to 1104
    toluene (commercial) containing 36
benzidine 353, 354
benzine, confusion with benzene 35
benzo[a]pyrene 332
    biotransformation 134
benzodiazepines, organophosphate poisoning 411
bertrandite ore 162
beryllium 162–6, 1050–5, 1136–7, 1185
    carcinogenicity 164, 1051, 1087
    diagnosis 1052
    hepatotoxicity 1185
    lung disease (berylliosis) 1050–5
        acute 1051
        chronic 1051–2
        future research 1052
        imaging 883–4, 1051
        mechanisms 1050
        prevention 164, 1052
        treatment and follow-up 1052
    nephrotoxicity 1136–7
beta-agonist, altitude sickness prevention 582
beta particles 624
Beveridge Social Insurance and Allied Services Report 100
Bhopal disaster 253, 297, 364, 1237
bias 79, 90–2, 95
bicipital tendinitis 690
bile, copper excretion 181
bile acid measurements 69
bilirubin abnormalities, disorders producing 1173
bioaerosols 438
biochemical pesticides 396
biochemical tests in hepatotoxicity indicated by abnormal liver function tests 1172

biological degradation, protecting plant products from 395
biological effect
    early, cancer biomarkers 1112–13
    of shift work 1234–5
biological effect monitoring (BEM) 63–70
    biotechnology industry 795
    definition 56, 57, 63
    examples 63–4
    pesticides (incl. organophosphates) 66, 415–16, 417
biological exposure indices (BEIs) of the ACGIA 60
biological hazards
    biotechnology products 788–9
    semiconductor industry 449
biological methods of radiation detection 625
biological monitoring (BM) 56–73
    analyte choice 59–60
    chloroplatinate exposure 227
    definition 56, 57
    ethics 57–8
    interfering factors 59
    interpreting results 60–3
    legal framework 57
    pesticides 415
        acetylcholinesterase inhibition 61, 66, 415
    roles 57
    setting up BM programme 58–63
    silver 235
    strategy selection 58
    vanadium 247
biological plausibility 92, 145
biological tolerance values (BATs) 60
biologically relevant aerosol fraction 914
biomarkers 64–70
    of aggregate exposure 45
    alcohol abuse 69, 864–5
    carcinogenesis 68–9, 1111–15
    choice 60
    interfering factors and 59
    nephrotoxicity 68–9
        cadmium 168, 170, 1132
        lead 1128
    spinal loading and damage 718
biomass production 786
biomechanics *see* mechanical factors
biopsy
    hand–arm vibration syndrome 505
    lung, inorganic dust disease 987
        berylliosis 1051
    pleural, mesothelioma 993
biopsychosocial rehabilitation, back pain 721

biotechnology (incl. genetic modification) 782–98
    definitions 782
    development 783–4
    hazards 787–91
    low- vs high risk work 795
    products and applications 783, 786–7
    risk management 791–2
    surveillance 793–6
bioterrorism 773–81
biotransformation *see* transformation
biphenyls, polychlorinated (PCBs) 371–2, 1186
bipyridyl herbicides 399–400
    management of acute poisoning 411–12
bird-handlers/fanciers (incl. budgerigar's/pigeon's)
    C. psittaci 753
    extrinsic allergic alveolitis (bird-fancier's lung) 978–9
        diagnosis 977
        management 978
        outcome 977
birdstrike 599
bis(chloromethyl)ether 340
Bismarck, Otto von 14, 96
bismuth, nephrotoxicity 1137
bisphenol A 359–60
bisphenol A diglycidyl ether (BADGE) 361–2
bitumen 335
black damp 268
bladder cancer 108–90
    aluminium and 155
    aniline and 354
    biomarkers 68–9, 1113
    naphthylamines and 1089, 1101
    questionnaires on exposure evaluation 1110
blast trauma 469–70
blisters, frostbite 530
blood
    alcohol levels 860
    cadmium levels, assessment 1132–3
    hand–arm vibration syndrome and viscosity of 493
    lead levels, assessment 195, 196, 196–7, 1129
    mercury levels, assessment 1134–5
    nanoparticle translocation from lung to 907
    pesticide effects 398
blood-borne viral infections in healthcare workers 729–36
    clinical features and transmission risk to patients 733–4

blood-borne viral infections in healthcare workers (*Continued*)
    management 734–5
    prevention 735–6
blood cells 1216–18
    precursors of 1215–16
    radiation effects 626
    see also red blood cells; white cell count
blood pressure
    finger systolic, in hand–arm vibration syndrome 497, 505
    high *see* hypertension
blood tests
    hand–arm vibration syndrome 503
    radiation exposure 640
blood vessels *see* vascular system
blue asbestos (crocidolite) 16, 17, 26, 103, 991
body clock *see* circadian rhythms
bone manifestations/disorders
    astronauts (density loss) 610
    cadmium 169
    divers/compressed air workers (osteonecrosis) 553, 561–2, 566
    fluoride 282–3
    hand–arm vibration syndrome 502
bone marrow effects incl. failure 1221–2
    benzene 134, 1222–4
    ionizing radiation 626–7, 1224–5
        management 639, 1224, 1225
    lead 1221
boron compounds in semiconductor production, genotoxicity 451
boron hydride *see* diborane
boron trichloride 281
boron trifluoride 284
Borrelia and Lyme disease 762–3
botulism 776
bowel (intestine)
    barotrauma (divers) 551
    radiation effects 627
        management 640
    see also colorectal cancer
Boyle's law 548
Bradford Hill criteria 91–2, 145
brain
    damage/injury
        expert medical report 117
        with gases, hypoxic 265
    function, at high altitude 575–6
    imaging *see* neuroimaging
    MRI *see* magnetic resonance imaging
    nanoparticles 908
    oedema *see* oedema
    see also encephalitis; encephalopathy; neurological problems; neurotoxicity

brain cancer 1096–7
    electromagnetic fields and 666, 671
        in offspring of exposed parents 669
    epidemiology 1096–7
    radiofrequency fields and 676–7, 678
breast cancer 1097
    electromagnetic fields and 666
    epidemiology 1097
    radiofrequency fields and 677
    shift work and 1097, 1238
breath-hold diving 558
breath monitoring 130–1, 132
    see also exhaled breath condensate
breathing, flying 596, 597
breathing apparatus 49
breathing mixtures
    diving 548–9, 555, 558–9
    flying 593, 596–7
breathlessness *see* dyspnoea
British antilewisite (BAL) *see* dimercaprol
bromomethane (methyl bromide) 266, 296, 1159, 1188
1-bromopropane 1153–4
bromotrifluoromethane 287
bronchial asthma *see* asthma
bronchial carcinoma, asbestosis-related, imaging 883
bronchial hyper-reactivity and byssinosis 961–2
bronchiolitis obliterans/obstructive bronchiolitis 889, 892, 898–9
    gases 263
bronchitis (chronic industrial) 890–1
    asthma and, comorbid 890–1
    coal workers 1030
        disability benefit 1032
    cotton workers 964–5
        compensation 99–100
bronchoalveolar lavage
    beryllium 164, 1051
    extrinsic allergic alveolitis 929
    inorganic dust disease 986–7
bronchodilators, byssinosis 964
bronchopneumonia, high altitude, Kea 574
bronchoscopy, extrinsic allergic alveolitis 929
brown asbestos *see* amosite
brucellosis 754–6
    pulmonary, imaging 885
bubbles of gas
    at altitude 594
    diver's tissues/circulation 551, 552–3
bubonic plague 776
budgerigar-handlers *see* bird-handlers
building(s)
    for containment of genetically-modified organisms 794

    indoor pollution and management and prevention of exposures 933–4
    types of building 922
    see also indoor environments; sick building syndrome
building and construction industry
    dermatoses 1072
    lead 189
bullets, lead dust from 189
bullying 837
Bundibugyo ebolavirus 737
buoyancy and diving 554
burden of occupational disease, continuing 25–6
burn(s) *see* flash blindness and burns; skin; thermal trauma
burnout 844–5
burst lung, divers 550
1,3-butadiene 322, 324
2,3-butanedione 899
N-butane 301
butan-2-one (methyl ethyl ketone), biological monitoring guidance values 61
butoxyacetic acid (analyte) 61
butoxyethanol (ethylene glycol monobutyl ether) 344–5
    monitoring 61, 344
butoxyethylacetate 344, 345
1,2-butylene oxide 360–1
4-t-butylphenol 359
butyrlcholinesterase, plasma 66
byssinosis 890, 958–64
    acute 958–9
    chronic 959
    clinical features 962–3
    management 964
    pathogenesis and aetiology 959–61
    pathology 963
    physical examination 963
    prevention 965

cadmium 167–72, 896–7, 1131–4, 1185
    biological monitoring 64, 68
        guidance values 61
    chronic obstruction pulmonary disease and 896–7, 1042
    fumes/inhalation 167, 168, 170, 1041, 1042
    hepatotoxicity 1185
    metabolism 167–8, 1132
    nephrotoxicity 168–9, 170, 1131–4
    prevention of poisoning 1134
    prognosis with 1134
    recommendations 1133–4
    treatment of poisoning 1133

caeruloplasmin 181
caisson disease *see* decompression sickness
caisson work *see* compressed air work
calcific tendinitis 690
calcium
    bone, cadmium and 169
    lead mimicking metabolism of 192
    see also hypercalcaemia
calcium-channel blockers
    altitude sickness
        preventive use 583
        therapeutic use 583–4
    hand–arm vibration syndrome 507
calcium disodium edetate
    lead 194
    manganese 208
    mercury 218
calculi (stones), kidney, cadmium and 1132
calomel (mercurous chloride) 1134
Cameroon, Lake Nyos 270
campylobacteriosis 760–1
cancer 1081–121
    agents causing *see* carcinogen
    antineoplastic agents *see* chemotherapeutic agents
    clinical assessment 1100–3
    epidemiology 1081–111
        methodological issues in research 1104–11
        molecular 27
    prevention 1103–4
    shift work and 1097, 1237–8
    sites (organs/tissues) 1085–97
        bladder *see* bladder cancer
        liver *see* liver
        lung *see* lung cancer
        pleural *see* mesothelioma
        vascular system *see* lymphohaematopoietic cancers
    see also carcinogenesis *and specific histological types*
Caplan's syndrome 879, 1032
Cappadocia (Turkey), mesothelioma 1005, 1011
capsulitis, adhesive (shoulder) 690, 690–1
car industry, hepatotoxic chemicals 1174
carbamates 1160–1
    acute effects 404
        management 411
    mechanisms of toxicity 397–9
carbamathione in noise-related deafness 476
carbohydrate-deficient transferrin (CDT) 69, 865
carbon black 1037

carbon dioxide 269–71
    see also hypercapnia
carbon disulphide 374–6, 1154
    monitoring 61, 374–5
    neurotoxicity 374, 1154
carbon monoxide 273–8, 1154–5
    biological effect monitoring 64
    biological monitoring guidance values 61
    clinical features and acute poisoning 274–6
    in fires 260
    hypoxic brain injury 265
    neurotoxicity 275, 1154–5
    transfer factor, in extrinsic allergic alveolitis 974, 975
    welding 426, 427
carbon nanotubes (CNTs) 906
    pulmonary fibrogenicity 908
carbon particles, ultrafine, challenge 910
    see also carbon nanotubes
carbon tetrachloride (tetrachloromethane) 369–70, 1176–8, 1180–1
    hepatotoxicity 369, 1176–8, 1180–1
    pulmonary biotransformation 136
carbonic anhydrase inhibitors for altitude sickness
    preventive use 582
    therapeutic use 583
carbonless copy (self-copying) paper 925, 928
carbonyl fluoride 285
carbonyl sulphide 293
carboxyhaemoglobin 61, 64, 273–6, 1154
carboxylic acid and derivatives 346–7
carcinogen(s) 143–4, 1081–121
    ambient levels of 143–4
    asbestos
        laryngeal and gastrointestinal 1006–7
        respiratory tract *see* lung cancer; mesothelioma
    biological effect monitoring 65
    childhood cancer and *see* children
    chlorine 279
    electromagnetic fields 664–8, 671
        in offspring of exposed parents 669
    exposures to (general aspects)
        estimates of risk attributed to 1097–100
        evaluation 1109–11
        markers 1114–15
        models 1110–11
        prevalence estimates 1085
    IARC classification 1082–3, 1084
    indoor non-industrial sources 933

    industrial (in general) 26
        semiconductor production 449–50
    metals and metalloids 1043–4, 1083, 1084, 1086
        aluminium 155
        antimony 159
        arsenic 161, 450, 1093
        beryllium 164, 1051, 1087
        cadmium 169
        chromium 174, 1087
        cobalt 176, 177, 1043
        lead 1131
        manganese 203
        molybdenum 221
        nickel 223, 1086–7
        uranium 244
        vanadium 247
    most common (in EU) 1085
    nanoparticles 908
    organic chemicals 1083, 1084
        acrylamides 351
        acrylic acid esters 348
        acrylonitrile 352
        aniline 354
        aromatic hydrocarbon solvents 329
        benzene 326, 1092, 1104
        butoxyethanol 345
        carbon disulphide 375
        chlorinated hydrocarbons 366
        chlorophenoxy acid herbicides 401, 1111
        dimethylformamide 349
        dioxins 371
        ethylene oxide 360
        formaldehyde 338
        pesticides *see* pesticides
        polyaromatic hydrocarbons 333–4
        vinyl chloride 17, 26, 134, 368, 1096, 1187
    predicting unit risks for 143
    radiation 629–30
    radiofrequency fields 676–8
    silica 1022–4, 1087
    synthetic mineral fibres 1012
    welding 423, 429, 431, 435
    see also cancer; oncogenes *and specific carcinogens*
carcinogenesis, process of 27, 1111–15
    biomarkers 1111–15
carcinoma
    bronchial, asbestosis-related, imaging 883
    cutaneous *see* basal cell carcinoma; squamous cell carcinoma
    hepatocellular *see* hepatocellular carcinoma

cardiovascular system
    diving and 555
    electromagnetic fields and 670
    high altitude and disorders of 578–9
    noise stress-related disorders 481
    shift work and 1236
    space and microgravity and 609–10
    see also heart
cardiovascular toxicity
    cobalt 177
    lead 192, 1128–9, 1130–1
    nano- and ultrafine particles 904, 908–9
    of carbon 910
CAREX estimates 1085
Carozzi, Dr 15
carpal tunnel syndrome (median nerve entrapment at wrist) 497–9, 694–6
    clinical aspects 696
    epidemiology 695
    in hand–arm vibration syndrome 493, 497–9, 695–6
    MRI 505
    management 696
Carson, Rachel 18
cartilage and biomarkers in low back pain 718
CAS registry numbers 321
case–cohort studies 83–4
    cancer 1107
case–control studies 83, 87, 90
    cancer and carcinogens 1106–7
        bladder cancer and rubber industry 1090
        questionnaires 1109–10
        radiofrequency fields and cancer 676–7
    nephrotoxic organic solvents 1139
case–crossover studies 84
case definition 77–8
case formulation with psychological interventions 824–5, 829
case studies and reports
    attributing disease to exposure 51–4
    cancers, clinical assessment 1101–2
    haematological disorders 1226–7
    high altitude
        medical emergencies (Mauna Kea observatory) 574
        pre-existing conditions 579
    nephrotoxic organic solvent 1138
    psychological interventions 825–9
cast iron, manufacture 209
casualties of major radiation incidents and their treatment 636–7
    nuclear reactor accident 638–40

cataracts (lens opacities)
    infrared-induced 655
    radiation-induced 627
    radiofrequency field-induced 675–6
    UV-induced 649
catastrophic incidents see major incidents
category A agents (CDC) in bioterrorism 774
catering industry, dermatoses 1071
cause of disease 89–92
    attributing exposure as see attribution
    medical evidence 118
    probability of (concept of), with radiation 630
    public's perceptions of causality 144–5
    threats to interference of causation 90–2
CC16 (Clara cell protein) 66–7
CD4:CD8 T cell ratio and extrinsic allergic alveolitis 973
CDC laboratory biosafety guidance 774
cell
    division, pesticides affecting 398
    nanoparticles effects 909
    transmembrane transport see transport
cellosolves see glycol ethers
cellulitis (hand or knee), subcutaneous 699
cement ulcers/burns 1071
Centers for Disease Control laboratory biosafety guidance 774
central nervous system effects see neurological problems; neurotoxicity
cerebral oedema see oedema
cervical spondylosis 691
cervical syndrome 691
cestodes 765
Chadwick, Edwin 10
Chajnantor plateau observatory 581, 585
chance 79
charcoal, activated, pesticide poisoning 410
charcoal haemoperfusion and haemodialysis, thallium poisoning 237
charged particles 624, 625
Charles's law 548
chelatable lead burden, measurement 1129
chelation therapy
    arsenic 1157
    copper 181
    iron 186

    lead 194–5, 1130
    manganese 208
    mercury 218, 1136
    plutonium 636, 638
chemical(s) (foreign/exogenous - xenobiotics) 123–457
    agricultural see pesticides
    in biotechnology 790
    cautions with names of 35–6
    chronic obstructive pulmonary disease and 896
    cleaning, and asthma 928
    decomposition 36
    deliberate injury with see terrorism; warfare
    flying and exposure to 604
    hepatotoxic see hepatotoxicity
    impure 36
    nephrotoxic see nephrotoxicity
    neurotoxic see neurotoxicity
    obtaining further information on 36–7
    organic see organic compounds
    in semiconductor production 447–8
Chemical Abstracts Service (CAS) registry numbers 321
chemical asphyxiant gases 273–8
chemical industry, hepatotoxic chemicals 1174
chemotherapeutic (cytotoxic/antineoplastic) agents
    hepatotoxicity 1188
    in mesothelioma 994
    in tissue culture 790
Chernobyl 262, 627, 628, 629, 636, 637, 640, 1225
chest (thorax)
    compressions in space 612–13
    computed tomography see computed tomography
    infections see respiratory infections
    radiography (conventional/plain films) see X-ray radiography
chickenpox 738
children
    altitude illness 576
        scoring system 578
    copper overload syndromes 181
    iron toxicity 186
    labour, historical accounts 7, 10
    lead, neurobehavioural toxicity 193
    parental exposure and cancer risk to 1208
    electromagnetic fields 669
    see also developmental toxicity
chimney sweeping 1087
china clay (kaolin) pneumoconiosis 1033–4

chips (integrated/microprocessor) 445
Chlamydophila abortus 753
Chlamydophila psittaci see psittacosis
chloracetaldehyde 134
chloracne 1067–8
chloramines 279
chlorate salts 399, 412
chlordecone 36, 1161, 1186
chlorendic anhydride 363
chlorinated organic compounds
  see organochlorines
chlorine 257, 258, 264, 278–9
 hospital management 263, 264
 storage tank 258, 259
 warfare 314
chlorine trifluoride 284–5
chloroanilines 354–5
chlorobenzenes 370
chlorodifluoroethane 372, 374
chlorodifluoromethane 286, 372–3
chloroethane (ethyl chloride) 301
chloroethylene oxide (CEO) 369
chlorofluorocarbons (CFCs; freons) 265–6, 281, 286–7
chloroform (trichlormethane) 298, 369–70, 1181
chlorohydrocarbons (chlorinated hydrocarbons) 365–74
 IARC classification of carcinogenicity 1084, 1086
 neurotoxicity 366, 1153, 1161
 welding 427
chloromethane 296–7
chloromethylmethylether 340, 1087
chloropentafluoroethane 286
chlorophenols 358
chlorophenoxy acids *see* phenoxy acid herbicides
chloroplatinic acid and salts 226–7, 227
chloroquine 742
 aircrew, prophylaxis 607
chlorotetrafluoroethane 373
chlorotrifluoromethane 286
cholinergic pathways, insecticide effects 397, 404, 1160
 management 410–11
 see also acetylcholinesterase inhibitors; cholinesterase activity
cholinesterase activity 61
 see also acetylcholinesterase; butyrlcholinesterase
choroid 648
chromic acid, semiconductor production 448
chromium 173–4, 1136
 biological monitoring guidance values 61
 bronchial asthma and 1042–3
 carcinogenicity 174, 1087
 contact dermatitis 173, 1068
 hepatotoxicity 1185
 nasal septal perforation 173, 433
 nephrotoxicity 1136
 ulcers (chrome ulcers) chrome 173, 1071
 valency 152, 173, 174
 welding-related compounds of 425
chromophores, retinal 648, 649, 650
chromosomal aberrations and carcinogenesis 86, 1112, 1113
 benzene 1223
chronic disease/poisoning
 beryllium (CBD) 163–4
 manganese 203–6
 mercury 217–18, 218–19
chronic fatigue (syndrome) 841
 and shift work 1235
chronic lymphocytic leukaemia 1092
chronic obstructive pulmonary disease (COPD)/chronic airways obstruction 889–902
 definitions 889–90
 epidemiology 889–90
  population studies 899–900
 etiology/causes 893–900
  asbestos 898, 996
  attribution to 93–4, 95
  cotton workers 889–90, 964–5
  metal dusts/fumes 897–8, 1042
  naturally-occurring 895–6
  non-occupational factors 893–5
  welders 433–4, 898
 historical perspectives 890
 pathophysiology 892
 subacute onset 898–9
 uncertainties and controversies 890–1
chronic syndrome of organophosphate poisoning 407–8
chronobiology *see* circadian rhythms
chrysotile (white asbestos) 990–1
 case study in attribution of disease to exposure 51–2
 historical perspectives 17
 lung cancer and 1005
 mesothelioma and 1004–5
 substitutes 1104
cider, lead in 188
ciliary body 648
 and cancer 1238
circadian rhythms and shift work 1234
 and performance 1234
 and preventive measures 1240
 and tolerance 1238, 1239
 and toxicological risk 1237
cirrhosis
 alcoholic 861
 Indian childhood 181
civil law 113–14
 expert witnesses and 115–17
  court appearance 119, 120
Civil Procedure Rules (CPRs) 115–16
Clara cell 136
Clara cell protein (CC16) 66–7
clays
 china (kaolin) 1033–4
 fibrous 1011
cleaning chemicals
 asthma and 928
 dermatoses and 1072
 reproductive effects 1205
clearance 130
 see also elimination; excretion
climate and seasonal differences in environmental thermal stress in office workers 540
clostridium botulinum toxin 776
clothing, personal protective *see* personal protective equipment
clubbing of fingers, asbestosis 991
CMV (cytomegalovirus) 738–9
coal gas 268
coal tars and pitches, skin carcinoma 1093–4
coalworkers' diseases (incl. pneumoconiosis) 101–2, 879–80
 compensation 98, 101–2
 complicated 880, 1030–2
 COPD and 93–4
 Gough paper-mounted whole lung sections 989
 historical perspectives 7
 imaging 879–90
 simple 879, 1030
 see also fossil fuels
coatings (surface), welding 247
cobalt 175–9
 biological monitoring guidance values 61
 bronchial asthma 176, 1042
 carcinogenicity 176, 177, 1043
 tungsten carbide with *see* tungsten carbide
cobalt-60 (radioactive) 175
cochlea
 anatomy and physiology 461, 462
 hair cells *see* hair cells
 implants 476
 pathology (with noise) 466–7
 toughening (phenomenon) 476
 see also electrocochleography

Cochrane Collaboration
  and back pain 716
  and depression 848
coercion, substance abuse treatment 865–6
cognitive-behavioural therapy (CBT) 813, 819
  case studies 826, 827, 828
  chronic fatigue syndrome 841
  NICE recommendations 823
  toxic exposures and medically unexplained syndromes 841
  workplace incivility 816
  workplace phobia 812
cognitive effects
  aluminium 155
  of high altitude 575–6
  lead 1158
  of psychiatric illness 842–3
  radiofrequency fields 676
  see also neurological problems
cohort studies 81–2, 90
  cancer and carcinogens 1105–6
    bladder cancer and rubber industry 1090
    radiofrequency fields 677–8
  organic solvent nephrotoxicity 1141
  see also case–cohort studies
cold (exposure to; cold stress) 528–34
  assessment 528
  diving 555
  flying 597
  occupations with recognized challenges of 528
  performance effects 534
  personal protective equipment 541–2
  responses (=cold strain) 527
    assessment 528–9
  training in 539–40
  see also immersion
cold fingers or sensitivity in hand–arm vibration syndrome 496
  see also Raynaud's disease
cold injury 529–32
  liquefied gases 263
cold sensitization after freezing cold injury 531
cold urticaria 1071
colorectal cancer epidemiology 1096
colour vision, solvent mixtures affecting 1163
combined oestrogen and progestogen oral contraceptive and high altitude 576, 577
combustion reactions 258–60
  nanoparticles derived via (CDNPs) 903, 904, 907

commercial spaceflight 613
common employment 99
communicable diseases see infections
communicating
  to public about risk 144–7
  to workforce about biotechnology hazards 793
community, additional worker exposure in 49
community-based case–control studies of cancer 1106–7
comparison group in cohort studies of cancer 1106
compartmental models 129
compensation 37–8, 96–109
  Europe 97, 105–7
  extrinsic allergic alveolitis 978
  hearing loss, exaggeration of damage 476–7
  historical perspectives 12, 13, 14, 96, 97, 98–104, 107
  law see law
  post-traumatic distress syndrome 814
  soft tissue rheumatic conditions (upper limb) 698–9
    carpal tunnel syndrome 695, 696
    repetitive strain injury 697
  UK 97–105
  US 107–8
competency and alcohol 860
complement system and byssinosis 961
compliance, lung, asbestosis 993
compound(s), metal
  antimony 160
  arsenic 161
  beryllium 162
  cadmium 167, 169
  chromium 173, 174
  cobalt 176, 177
  copper 181
  gold 183
  inhalation injury 1041
  iron 185
  lead 188, 189, 190, 195
    organic see organic compounds
  manganese 202, 203, 207, 208
  mercury 214, 216, 217, 218
  molybdenum 221
  nickel 223
  phosphorus 225
  platinum group compounds 226, 227, 228
  silver 234, 235
  tin 238–9
  tungsten 241
  uranium 244
compound semiconductors 444

compressed air work (incl. tunnelling and caisson work) 547, 562–4
  assessing fitness for 565, 566–7
  bone necrosis 553, 561–2, 566
  decompression illness 564
  environment see environment
  historical perspectives 14
  legal issues 565
computed radiography 876
computed tomography (chest) 876–7
  asbestos exposure 881, 883, 992
    lung disease incl. cancer 883
    mesothelioma 882
  beryllium exposure 1051
  extrinsic allergic alveolitis 884, 974
  high-resolution see high-resolution CT
  silicosis 880
computers
  diving 558
  ergonomic problems with users of 702–3
concentrations
  of gas in air 254
  of nanoparticles
    particle mass 915
    particle number 914–15
    surface area 915–16
condensation particle counters (CPCs) 915, 916
confidence intervals 79–80
confidentiality 114
  history-taking and 38
confined (enclosed/poorly-ventilated) spaces, gassing 267–8
  carbon dioxide 269
  methane 269
confounding effects 80, 91
  case–control studies 83
  smoking and occupation and COPD 891–2
confounding in occupational cancer studies 1108
congenital malformations see developmental toxicity
congestive cardiomyopathy, cobalt 177
conjugation (phase 2) reactions 133, 135
conjunctivitis
  semiconductor industry 449
  UV/light-related 650–1
consciousness, loss while diving 555–6
conservation of energy, law of 526
consistency (in precautionary principle) 146
constitutional symptoms, decompression sickness 552

construction industry *see* building and construction industry
consultation distance and zones 258, 259
contact dermatitis 1062–9
　allergic *see* allergic contact dermatitis
　diagnosis 1064–5
　irritant *see* irritant contact dermatitis
　metals
　　aluminium 155
　　chromium 173, 1068
　　cobalt 177
　　nickel 223
　organics chemicals
　　acrylic/methacrylic acid esters 34
　　cyclic acid anhydrides 362
　　ethanolamines 355
　prevention 1065, 1067
　prognosis 1068–9
　protein 1069
　treatment 1067
contact lenses
　aircrew 600
　welders 431
contact urticaria 1069
containment measures in genetic modification 793, 794
contamination
　of cultures 789
　fish with mercury 215
　radioactive material 637, 637–8
　　external (skin) 617, 634, 636, 640
　welding and influence of contaminants on emissions 427
　see also decontamination
contingent employment 839
contraceptives, hormonal, and high altitude 576, 577
contributory negligence 99
control *see* prevention and control
Control of Industrial Major Accident Hazards (CIMAH) Regulations 258
Control of Major Accident Hazards (COMAH) regulations 258
Control of Substances Hazardous to Health (COSHH) regulations 36–7, 44
　biological monitoring 57
　cadmium 1133
Control of Vibration at Work Regulations (2005) 506, 520
controlled experimental studies
　non-randomized 81
　randomized 80–1
convulsions *see* seizures

cooling
　systems, for heat stress protection 541
　wet clothing causing 526
copper 1184
　beryllium alloyed with 162
　hepatotoxicity 1184
　iron interfering with intestinal absorption 186
　zinc interfering with metabolism of 250
Coriolis illusions 601
cornea
　anatomy 647
　UV damage (photokeratitis) 650–1
　welding 430
coronary artery (ischaemic heart) disease
　carbon ultrafine particles and 910
　high altitude and 578–9
　noise and 481
coronavirus, SARS *see* severe acute respiratory syndrome
cortical evoked response audiometry 479
corticosteroids (glucocorticoids)
　altitude sickness prevention 582
　berylliosis 1052
　see also dexamethasone; prednisone
Corti's organ *see* organ of Corti
COSHH regulations 36–7, 44
cosmetics, nanoparticles 906–7
cosmic radiation 625, 631–2
　space 608
costs
　and benefits (in precautionary principle) 146
　economic, of indoor non-industrial hazards 933
Cote d'Ivoire ebolavirus 737
cotton and flax and other textile workers 958–69
　diseases 958–69
　　chronic obstructive pulmonary disease 889–90, 964–5
　　compensation 99–100
　　prevention 965–6
　　measuring dust exposure 965
　　mortality and morbidity 958
　　see also byssinosis
cough, asbestosis 992
coumadin-derived rodenticides 405
counselling
　psychiatric disorders 816, 848
　reproductive 1201, 1208–9
　　specific occupations 1203
court, case going to 119–20
Coxiella burnetii see Q fever

crackles, inspiratory *see* inspiratory crackles
craft palsy 699
cramp, hand 698, 699
crashes, aircraft 604, 605
creatinine concentrations (and correction) 60
　cadmium 170
creosote 332, 333–4
cresol 359
　o-cresol (analyte) 62
Crimean Congo haemorrhagic fever 736
criminal law 113–14
crocidolite (blue asbestos) 16, 17, 26, 103, 991
Crohn's disease, high altitude 579
cross-coupled illusions 601
crossover studies
　case– 84
　randomized 81
cross-sectional surveys 84
　chronic obstruction pulmonary disease and ventilatory function 893–4
　organic solvent nephrotoxicity 1139–40
crude disease rates 78
cryolite 282
cryological (freezing cold) injury 529–31
cryptosporidiosis 761–2
crystalline silica *see* silica dust
CS gas 316
culture (cell and tissue)
　additives/media 790, 791
　contamination 789
culture and ethnicity
　shift work tolerance and 1239
　work stress and 808–9
cumulative exposure 44, 45
cupric acetoarsenite 160
cupric arsenite 160
cuproenzymes 180
cutis *see* skin
cyanide 276–8
　as nitrile metabolite 352
　poisoning 276–8
　　antidotes 276, 277, 278, 317–18
　　gold extraction 183
　　see also hydrogen cyanide
cyanogen 276
cyanogen bromide 277
cyanogen chloride 276, 277
cyanonitriles 277
cyclic acid anhydrides 362, 363
cyclohexane 322
cyclone sampler 45, 46
cyclopropane 299, 300
cystic echinococcosis 765

cytochrome P450 enzymes 132–3
   benzene and 326
   chloroform and carbon tetrachloride 369–70
   styrene and 330
cytogenetics *see* chromosomal aberrations
cytomegalovirus 738–9
Cytophaga 438
cytotoxic agents *see* chemotherapeutic agents

daily rhythmic activity *see* circadian rhythms
Dale Committee 101
Dalton's law 548
damages 117–18
dampness and moisture (indoor non-industrial) 923, 924
   asthma and 927
   prevention 933
Dangerous Trades (Thomas Oliver's) 12
dangerous trades, historical perspectives 11–12
dark-room disease 287
databases
   information on hazardous substances 37
      reproductive toxicity 1209
   for systematic reviews 86
Davy, Sir Humphrey 25, 268, 278, 298
DDT *see* dichlorodiphenyltrichloroethane
De Quervain's disease 694
de-acclimatization, heat stress 536
deafness *see* hearing loss; ototoxicity
dealkylation 135
death certificates 85
   see also mortality; post-mortem examination
Death, Valley of 271
decibels 460
   internationally agreed reference levels for calculation 460, 461
   measuring levels 471–2
decomposition, chemical 36
decompression (air pressure)
   divers
      planning 557
      procedures or tables 558
   flying, rapid 595
   tunnelling or caisson work 563–4
decompression (surgical)
   carpal tunnel 499
   De Quervain's disease 694
decompression sickness/illness (caisson disease)
   at altitude (incl. flying) 594

compressed air work 564
divers 551, 561
   reducing risk 557, 558
spacecraft 608
treatment 561, 564
decontamination
   pesticide 410
   terrorist attack 317
deep diving, breathing mixtures 559
deep frostbite 530
deep vein thrombosis risk, flying 607
defibrillators and electromagnetic fields 670
degreasing agents, hepatotoxic chemicals 1174
deltamethrin 403
demand–control–support model 836
dementia, dialysis 155
Denmark, compensation schemes 105
Denning, Lord 101
dental assistants, reproductive hazards 1203
dental technician's pneumoconiosis 1045
dentition (teeth)
   amalgam (for fillings) 215–16, 1135
   fluorosis 283
   yellowing with cadmium 169
dependence, drug and alcohol 859
depleted uranium *see* uranium
depression (low mood) 812–14
   case studies in management of 826, 827
   post-traumatic occurrence 837–8
   screening and treatment 847–8
   work ability and functional impairment in 842, 842–3
dermatitis (eczema) 49
   contact *see* contact dermatitis
   pustular, salmonellosis 760
dermis *see* skin
Descemet's membrane 647
desferroxamine, iron 186
designated treatment area, radiation accidents 638
deterministic effects of radiation 625, 626, 626–30
deterrent medication in substance abuse 866
detoxification 132–7
   example 133
   individual variation in enzyme activities 128
Deutsche Forschungsgemeinschaft (DFG), biological monitoring 58, 60, 65
   aluminium 155

developed countries *see* industrialized countries
developmental toxicity (incl. embryotoxicity/fetotoxicity/ teratogenicity and congenital malformations) 1200–1, 1202–4, 1208
   aromatic solvents 329
   carbon disulphide 375
   carbon monoxide 276
   dimethylacetamide 350
   electromagnetic fields 669
   ethylene oxide 360
   male-mediated 1200–1
   manganese 203
   methoxyethanol 342
   methyl mercury 215
   radiofrequency fields 678–9
dexamethasone in altitude sickness
   preventive use 582
   therapeutic use 583, 584
diabetes mellitus and high altitude 580
diacetyl 899
diagnosis 40–1
   biological effect monitoring and 64–70
   metal poisoning 152
      lead 194
      manganism 204–6
      mercury 218
dialysis and aluminium 155
diarrhoea
   radiation-related 640
   traveller's 742–3
   zoonoses 751, 759–62
Diatomaceous earth (kieselghur) 303, 1036
diatomite 1036
dibenzodioxins, polychlorinated 370
dibenzofurans, polychlorinated (PCDFs) 370, 371
diborane (boron hydride) 298
   semiconductor production 448
1,2-dibromochloropropane (DBCP) and infertility 1198
1,2-dibromotetrafluoroethane 286
3,4-dichloroaniline 355
1,4-dichlorobenzene 370
dichlorodifluoromethane 286, 287
dichlorodiphenyltrichloroethane (DDT) 396, 399, 404, 1161
   hepatotoxicity 1186
   neurotoxicity 1161
   reproductive toxicity 1206
dichlorofluoroethane 372, 374
dichlorofluoromethane 286

dichloromethane (methylene chloride) 274, 367–8
   biological monitoring guidance values 61
2,4-dichlorophenol 358, 359
dichlorosilane 281
1,2-dichlorotetrafluoroethane 286
dichlorotrifluoroethane 372–3
dicobalt edetate 277, 277–8
dieldrin, conversion from aldrin to 134
dienes 322, 323
diesel exhaust particles 905, 911–13
   bladder cancer 1089
   challenge tests 909–10
   epidemiological studies 911–13
dietary intake *see* ingestion
diethanolamine 355
diethyl ether 298
diethylene triamine pentoacetic acid (DTPA), plutonium 636, 638
N-diethylnitrosamine 357
differential diagnosis 41
Diffuse Mesothelioma Scheme (2008) 105
diffuse pleural thickening, asbestos-related 881, 995–6, 1002
   epidemiology 1002
   functional significance 996
   lung cancer and 103
   radiographic appearance 995
diffusion 128
diffusion charging aerosol surface area counter 915–16
1,1-difluoro-1-chloroethane 286
1,1-difluoroethyelene 286
digestive system *see* gastrointestinal tract
digit(s), hand *see* fingers
digital arteries
   in hand–arm vibration syndrome 492–3, 495, 496
   normal physiology 491
digital imaging 876
di-isocyanates 364
   asthma and
      chronic obstruction pulmonary disease and 896–7
      immunological tests 948
   biological monitoring guidance values 61
   see also isocyanates
dimercaprol/BAL (and derivatives)
   lead chelation 195, 1130
   mercury chelation 218
dimercaptopropane (DMPS), lead poisoning 1130
dimercaptosuccinic acid (DMSA)
   arsenic poisoning 1157
   lead poisoning 1130
   mercury poisoning 1159

dimethyl ether 300
N,N-dimethylacetamide (DMA; DMAA) 348, 349–50, 1181–2
   biological monitoring 61, 349–50
dimethylamine 289
dimethylaminoproprionitrile 1155
dimethylbenzene *see* xylene
dimethylformamide (DMF) 348–50
   hepatotoxicity 1182
   monitoring 61, 349–50
N-dimethylnitrosamine 357
2,2-dimethylpropane 300–1
dinitrophenol 1183
dioxins 1179–80
   as Agent Orange contaminant 1162–3
   chlorinated 370–2
   dioxan(e) and, confusion between 35–6
   exposure evaluation in cancer studies 1111
   mechanisms of hepatotoxicity 1179–80
diphenyl methane 4,4 diisocyanate (MDI; methylenediphenyl diisocyanate) 36, 364
'dippers' flu' 407
diquat 399, 400
   treatment of acute poisoning 411–12
direct radiography 876
direct-reading instruments 45, 46–7
directly standardized rates 78
disability (work)
   in expert report 119
   psychiatric disorders and 842–3, 844
   thermal stress and 540
disability benefit (in respiratory disease)
   coalworkers' pneumoconiosis 1032–3
   silicosis and lung cancer 1023
   smoking status and 37
disciplinary hearings, fitness to attend 811
disclosure of mental illness 839–40
discrimination with psychiatric disorders 839–40
disease(s)
   'all or none' 92, 93
   attributing exposure as cause of *see* attribution
   chronic *see* chronic disease
   compensation *see* compensation
   definition 28
   diagnosis 40–1
   industrial, historical perspectives 11–12
   measures of 77

   'more or less' 92, 93–4
   occupation affected by 39–40
   prescribed *see* prescribed disease
   prevention *see* prevention
   psychosocial risk factors for *see* psychosocial risk factors
   systemic *see* systemic disease
   see also exposure–disease paradigm; medical conditions
disease registers, attribution of disease 94–5
disinfectants, reproductive effects 1205
disorder, definition 28
disorientation, flying 601–2
dissatisfaction
   job 807
   with life 814, 815
distribution 128
   lead 190–1
   mercury 216–17
   volume of 130
disulfiram 866
diuretics, altitude sickness prevention 582
diurnal rhythms *see* circadian rhythms
diving 547–69
   assessing fitness for 565–6
   breathing mixtures 548–9, 555, 558–9
   current hazards and risks 559–61
   immersion-related pathophysiology 533, 554–5
   legal framework 565
   long-term health risks 561–2
   tasks 556–9
   thermal challenges 533, 555
Diving at Work Regulations (1997) 565
diving bells 557
DMPS (dimercaptopropane), lead poisoning 1130
DMSA *see* dimercaptosuccinic acid
DNA
   adducts 65
   hypermethylation, tumorigenesis and 1112
   manipulation/engineering (and recombinant DNA) 785
   hazards 792, 793
   sequence unchanged in epigenetic inheritance 138
   sequencing agents 790
   see also nucleic acid
doctors/physicians (incl. GPs)
   role in medicolegal report provision 114–17
   sickness absence and role of 810–11
   substance abuse 867–8

dodecane 36
dodecenyl succinic anhydride 363
Doll, Richard 16
doping, semiconductor 446, 448
dose
  ionizing radiation
    accidental exposure close to/at/above/well above limits 635–6
    lethal 626–7
    quantities 624–5
    threshold 626
  oral lethal, toxicity rating by 127
dose–response/exposure–response relationships 92
  asbestos-related diseases
    asbestosis 1001
    lung cancer 1005
    mesothelioma 1003–4
  asthma 945–6
  chemicals 127
    biological monitoring of dose–response line 63
  radiation 626
  silica-related diseases
    kidney damage 1024
    lung cancer 1022–3
    silicosis 1021–2
downsizing in organizations 839
downstream processing 787, 788
drinking and flying 604
  see also alcohol; water supply
driving, fitness after sickness to 39
driving licences and substance abuse 867
drugs
  abuse see substance abuse
  in alcohol abuse treatment 866
  altitude sickness
    preventive use 582
    therapeutic use 583–4
  as antidotes see antidotes
  in asthma 951
  in byssinosis 964
  flying 606–7
    for air sickness 603
    for fatigue and jet-lag 603–4
  frostbite 530
  gases acting like 255
  hand–arm vibration syndrome and 503
    differential diagnosis 498
    therapeutic use of drugs 507
  in osteoarthritis 701, 702
  see also antidotes; pharmaceuticals and specific (types of) drugs
dry bulb temperature 534, 535
dry cleaning, hepatotoxic chemicals 1174

drysuit 551, 554, 555
DTPA, plutonium 636, 638
Dupuytren's disease 698
  hand–arm vibration syndrome 493, 499–500, 698
dusts 939–1056
  IARC classification of carcinogenicity 1083, 1084, 1086
  inorganic see inorganic dust diseases
  measuring exposure 45, 46
  nuisance 905
  organic see organic dusts
  see also nanoparticles; powders
dyes
  hairdressing, reproductive toxicity 1206
  IARC classification of carcinogenicity 1083, 1084
dynamic model of sickness pathway 845–6
dynamics see kinetics
dyspnoea (breathlessness)
  asbestosis 991–2
  cadmium 168
  silicosis 1015

ear(s)
  anatomy and physiology 461–4
  barotrauma, divers 549
  protection 472–3
    aircraft 598
  toxicity see ototoxicity
ear drum see tympanic membrane
early biological effect, cancer biomarkers 1112–13
Ebola haemorrhagic fever 736, 737
echinococcosis 765
ecological studies 80, 81
ecological view of ill health 20
economic impact of indoor non-industrial hazards 933
ectoparasites 740–1, 1061
eczema see dermatitis
education (incl. information) and training
  manager, about psychiatric illness 847
  worker 49
    in back pain and its prevention 719, 721
    at high altitude 584–5
    noise 474–5
    pesticide operators 416
    shift/night work 1241
    in thermal stress management 539
effect (of disease) see biological effect monitoring; health; symptoms and signs

effect modification (in epidemiological studies) 80, 91
effort–reward imbalance 836
effusions, pleural, asbestos exposure 881, 996
ejection seats 605
elbow 692–3
  beat (subcutaneous cellulitis) 699
electric response audiometry 477–80
electric utility industry, electromagnetic fields 663, 677
electrocochleography 478
electrodiagnostic tests, hand–arm vibration syndrome 505
electrolyte disturbances in heat illness 537–8
electromagnetic fields (EMFs) 663–74
  acute effects 664
  extremely low frequency 663–74
  haematological effects 1225
  high-frequency 1199
  long-term effects 664–70
    reproductive 668–9, 1199, 1207
  nature 63
  occupational exposures 663–4
    electrical workers 663, 677
    welding 423–4
electromagnetic spectrum, non-ionizing radiation portion 644
electromyography in work activity (with related musculoskeletal disorders) 703
electron microscopy of nanoparticles 904
  personal samples 916
electron transport, pesticide effects 398
electronics industry
  dermatoses 1072
  reproductive hazards 1203
elemental semiconductors 444
elimination 129–30, 132–7
  half-lives 130
  in biological monitoring 59
  see also clearance; excretion
ELISPOT, beryllium 163
embolism (gas), pulmonary, divers 550
embryogenesis timelines 1204
embryotoxicity see developmental toxicity
emergency medical conditions
  at high altitude (Mauna Kea observatory) 574
  in space 611–13
emergency preparedness for bioterrorism 778–9
Emergency Response Planning Guidelines (ERPGs) of AMHI 257, 258

emesis *see* vomiting
emollients and moisturizers 1067
emotional distress *see* stress
emphysema 892
    cadmium 168
    coalworkers 1030
        disability benefit 1032
Employee assistance programmes (EAPs) 848
employers' duty
    to compensate 99
    noise management 474–5
employment *see* work
Employment Medical Advisory Service (EMAS) 18
Employment and Support Allowance (ESA) 818
encephalitis, rabies 765–6
encephalopathy
    metals
        aluminium 155, 1156–7
        arsenic 1157
        lead 193–4, 1157
        neurotoxicity 1157
    organic compounds
        acrylamide 1152, 1153
        aromatic solvents 328, 330–1
        carbon disulphide 1154
        carbon monoxide 1155
        solvent mixtures 1163
        white spirits 335
enclosed spaces *see* confined spaces
endocarditis, Q fever 754
endocrine effects
    lead 193
    pesticides 408–9
    see also hormones
endothelin (ET) and vibration-induced Raynaud's syndrome 493
    receptor antagonists in treatment 507
endothelium, corneal 647
endotoxins 438
    biotechnology processes and 789
    byssinosis and 959–60
        preventing exposure 966
endotracheal intubation in space 612
energy, law of conservation of 526
enterohaemorrhagic *E. coli* 761
enterotoxin-producing *E. coli* 742
entitlement to sickness absence, defining 810
environment(s)
    flying 597–9
    hepatotoxic chemicals and materials in 1174
    indoor *see* indoor environments; office
    noise pollution and EU policy 481–2

occupational/work 39
    exposure occurring at interface between person and 44
    pressure (divers and compressed air workers) 547–8
        physics 548–9
        physiology and pathophysiology 549–51
    risk to
        arsenic 1185
        biotechnology 791, 793
        gold 184
        iridium 228
        mercury 215
        osmium 229
        palladium 228
        platinum 227
        rhodium 228
        semiconductor materials 451
    space 608
    spacecraft 608–9
    thermally-challenging *see* thermal environments
    work, psychosocial 836–42
    zoonotic exposures 751
enzymes
    copper-containing 180
    detoxifying, individual variation in activities 128
    fungal, and byssinosis 961
    haem-containing 185
    lead-inhibited 191, 192
    liver *see* liver
    P450 *see* cytochrome P450 enzymes
    production (biotechnological) 787
epichlorohydrin 361
epicondylitis 692–3
'epidemic' of work stress 804–5
    see also pseudo-epidemics
epidemiology (general aspects) 25–6, 77–86
    in attribution of disease to exposure 51
    bias in studies 79, 90–2, 95
    cancer *see* cancer
    cause and effect in studies 90
    concepts and terminology 78–80
    design of studies 79–84
    explanations for discordant results 87
    interpretation of studies 79–80
    recent historical perspectives 19
epigenetics 138
    carcinogenesis and 1112
epileptic seizures *see* seizures
epithelium
    corneal 647
    lens 647
    retinal pigment 648
epoxidation 134

epoxide(s) 360–1
epoxide hydrolase (microsomal) and byssinosis 962
epoxybutane 360–1
equipment
    office *see* office environment
    personal protective *see* personal protective equipment
ergonomic problems 683–724
    back pain prevention and targeting of 718–19
    biotechnology industry 791
    semiconductor industry 449
erionite 1005, 1011
erysipeloid 763–4
erythrocytes *see* red blood cells
Escherichia coli
    enterohaemorrhagic 761
    enterotoxin-producing 742
    K12 789
essential metals 151–2
    chromium 173
    cobalt 175
    copper 180–1
    iron 185
    magnesium 199
    molybdenum 221
esters 347–8
ethane 301
ethanol *see* ethyl alcohol
ethanolamine 355
ethers 298, 300, 340–6
    glycol *see* glycol ethers
    see also bisphenol A diglycidyl ether; chloromethylmethylether
ethical issues
    biological monitoring (BM) 57–8
    information in history-taking 38
    substance abuse
        coercion to assess or treat 865
        testing 864
ethnicity *see* culture and ethnicity
ethoxyethanol and ethoxyethylacetate 343–4
ethyl acrylate 347
ethyl alcohol (ethanol - commonly called alcohol)
    abuse 859–70
        definitions 859
        diagnosing 861–5
        liver biomarkers 69, 864–5
        management/treatment 866–8
        medical profession 867–8
        prevention 868
        workplace problems 860–1
    flying and 604
    in methanol poisoning 337

ethyl chloride 301
ethylbenzene 325
ethylene 301, 322
ethylene dibromide 406
ethylene glycol 337–8
    as butoxyethanol metabolite 344
    as methoxyethanol metabolite 342
ethylene glycol ethers
    ethylene glycol monobutyl ether
        see butoxyethanol
    ethylene glycol monoethyl ether 343–4
    ethylene glycol monomethyl ether 342–3
    in semiconductor production 448
ethylene oxide 297–8, 360
    neurotoxicity 297, 1155
ethylenebisdithiocarbamate fungicides 408–9
ethylenethiourea 409
ethyne (acetylene) 300, 322
Europe (and the EU incl. directives)
    biological and social interference 1234–5
    biotechnology (incl. genetic modification) 783–4
    cancer epidemiology 1081–2, 1099
        numbers of deaths 1098, 1099
        ten most common carcinogenic exposures 1085
    cancer prevention 1103
    compensation schemes 97, 105–7
    diving 565
    environmental noise 481–2
    hand–arm vibration syndrome 505–6
    lead exposure 1131
    shift work (in survey) 1233
    tobacco smoke exposure indoors 926, 933
    whole-body vibration 513–14, 519, 519–20
European Centre of Ecotoxicology and Toxicology of Chemicals, biological monitoring and 57
evaporative loss in cold
    assessment 528
    protective garments and 541–2
Everest, Mount 570–1, 585–6
evidence-based occupational medicine 86–7
evoked response audiometry 477–80
examination *see* physical examination
excess relative risk (ERR), radiation exposure 630
excretion
    copper 181
    mercury 217
    see also clearance; elimination

exercises
    in back pain
        preventive 719
        therapeutic 720–1
    thermal challenges 526
    see also physical workload
exhaled breath condensate (EBC) 67
    cobalt 177
experimental studies
    Bradford Hill criteria 92
    controlled *see* controlled experimental studies
    see also laboratory studies
expert(s), carcinogen exposure evaluation by 1110
expert witness 113, 115–19
    in court 119–20
    reports 119, 120
        form 118–19
        purpose 117–18
exposure (to hazard), occupational 43–54
    attributing disease to *see* attribution
    to carcinogens *see* carcinogens
    control 44, 49–50
    determinants 47–8
    determining specific exposure 35–6
    diagnostic importance 40
    discordant results of epidemiological studies due to differences in 87
    effect/consequences *see* biological effect monitoring; effect; symptoms and signs
    extent 35
    gases 256–62
    kinetics of 130–2
    limits (OELs) 40, 44, 48
        acrylamide 1153
        carbon disulphide 1154
        carbon monoxide 1154–5
        iridium 228
        lasers and other light sources 653, 654, 657
        manganese 208
        osmium 229
        palladium 228
        platinum 227
        polonium 232
        rhodium 228
        silver 235
        spinal loading 718
        uranium 244
        vanadium 247
    measuring/quantifying levels of 43–9, 51
        cohort studies and 82
        holistic 48–9

        lead 195–7
        methods 45–9
        nanoparticles 914–16
        systemic exposure *see* biological monitoring
        vanadium 247
    monitoring *see* surveillance
    routes 44–5
        see also specific routes
    time sequence of effect after *see* time sequence
    variability 47–8
        see also biological exposure indices
exposure–disease paradigm 56
exposure–response relationships *see* dose–response relationships
external cardiac massage, immersion victims 533
external comparison group in cohort studies of cancer 1106
external ear (outer ear), anatomy and physiology 461
extractants, nucleic acid 790
extraction ratio 130
extra-vehicular activity (EVA) 609
extremely-low-frequency electromagnetic radiation 663–74
extrinsic allergic alveolitis (hypersensitivity pneumonitis) 928–9, 970–82
    acute/reversible 974–5
    causes 971
    chronic/irreversible 975
    clinical features 973–4
    compensation 978
    diagnosis and differential diagnosis 975–7
    epidemiology 970–1
    imaging 884–5, 974
    indoor non-industrial environments and 928–9
    management 977–8
    outcome 977
    pathology 971–3
    physiological features 974–5
    specific types 978–9
    subacute 975
eyes 644–62
    aircrew
        protection 599–600
        surgery 600
    anatomy 646–8
    chemicals affecting
        ammonia 289
        hydrogen sulphide 292–3
        silver 234

functions 644–6
ionizing radiation effects 627
light-induced effects/damage (incl. UV) 649–59
  acute 650–4
  chronic 654
  mechanisms 648–9
  nature (by spectral domain) 645
  protection see subheading below
  welding 423, 429–30
protection 656–9
  welders 431
radiofrequency field effects 675–6, 677
see also vision

face masks (respiratory protection) 50
facilitated diffusion 128
fact, witnesses of 114–15
factories, historical perspectives 6, 9, 10–12, 24
family life and shift work 1234–5
farmer's lung 971, 978
  diagnosis 976
  imaging 974
  immunopathology 973
  outcome 977
  see also agriculture and farming
FAST Alcohol Use Disorders Screening Test 862
fatigue/tiredness
  chronic see chronic fatigue
  in depression 842
  flying 603–4
Federal compensation schemes 107
females (women)
  high-altitude illness 576
  historical perspectives 7, 13–14
  postmenopausal, cadmium-associated osteomalacia 169
  of reproductive age
    epidemiology of infertility 1197
    lead suspension levels 196
    mechanisms of infertility 1198
    semiconductor industry and 450
    shift work and 1237
    see also pregnancy; reproductive effects
  see also sex
fence values (hearing assessment) 470–1
fermentation
  anaerobic 266–7
  in biotechnology 782
    ill-health incidents 789
    purification of products 788
  silage 291
ferritin 186
ferrochelatase and lead 192

fertility see reproductive effects
fettlers 1018
fetus
  developmental timelines 1204
  growth retardation 1202, 1204
  toxicity see developmental toxicity
FEV_1 see forced expiratory volume in 1 second
fever, zoonoses presenting with 751, 754–9
fibres see fibrous particles
fibromyalgia, repetitive strain injury as variant of 697–8
fibrosis, pulmonary
  aluminium 154
  asbestos see asbestosis
  in coalworker's pneumoconiosis, progressive massive 880, 1030–2
  cobalt 176
  in extrinsic allergic alveolitis 885, 977–8
  nanoparticles 908
  welders 434–5
fibrous particles and dusts/fibres 990–1013
  IARC classification of carcinogenicity 1083, 1084, 1086
  nanosized (high aspect ratio nanoparticles) 906
    sampling and measurement 914
  sampling 45
  synthetic/man-made 1012
    carcinogenicity 1088
    chronic obstruction pulmonary disease 896
film, radiographic
  exposure 876
  quality 875
    in ILO classification of pneumoconiosis 885
filter materials (light), protective 657–8
  welding 431, 658–9
filtration (transmembrane) 128
fingers
  clubbing in asbestosis 991
  systolic blood pressure in hand–arm vibration syndrome 497, 505
  see also cold fingers; fish-tank finger; pork finger; trigger finger; whale finger; white finger
Finland
  aluminium monitoring 155
  asthma incidence 944
  cancer
    job–exposure matrices (FINJEMs) 1110
    numbers of deaths 1098

compensation schemes 97, 105
indoor non-industrial environments
  asthma and 927, 928
  public health impact of hazards 933
fire, gas exposure 258–61
see also flammable gases
fire damp 268
fire fighters 260–1
  eye protection 658
first aid measures
  decompression sickness 553
  diving incidents 561
  gases 262–5
    hydrogen cyanide 276–7
  hydrofluoric acid poisoning 284
  pesticide poisoning 410
  welding-related eye damage 430
First World War 13, 14–15
fish
  decaying 266–7
  mercury contamination 215, 1135
fish-handler's disease 763
fish-tank finger 764
fishing industry, dermatoses 1072
fitness
  to attend disciplinary hearings 811
  to practice proceedings, expert witness 120–1
fitness to work (and its assessment)
  diving and compressed air work 565–6, 566–7
  flying 605–6
    as passenger 607
  on return
    after radiation exposure accident 636
    after sickness 39–40
  in thermal stress 539
five P model (case formulation with psychological interventions) 824–5
flammable gases 253
  characteristics 255
flash blindness and burns 655
  nuclear and atomic weapons explosions 599–600, 655
flax workers see cotton and flax and other textile workers
Flixborough (explosion) 253
flock-worker's lung 899
floristry, dermatoses 1073
fluids
  astronauts
    imbalances 609–10
    intravenous administration 611
  heat illness, replacement 537–8
fluorapatite 282

fluorescent lights 654
fluoride(s) 282–6, 302
    acute health effects 282
    biological monitoring guidance values 61
    chronic toxicity 282–3
    hydrolysis to hydrofluoric acid 284–6
fluorinated anaesthetics 299
fluorinated hydrocarbons 286–7
fluorine 281–4
    see also chlorofluorocarbons; hydrofluorocarbons
fluorodopa (in PET), manganism 206
fluoroform 286
flying 591–607
    accidents 604–5
    advanced life support systems 596–7
    environmental challenges 597–9
    exposure to chemicals 604
    fatigue and jet-lag 603–4
    fitness for see fitness
    food and drink 604
    gravitational stress 595–6, 597
    motion sickness 602–3
    pressure change 592–5
    radiation exposure 633
    spatial disorientation 601–2
    vision 599–601
folded lung (rounded atelectasis), asbestosis 883, 992
folliculitis, oil 1069
follow-up in epidemiological studies of cancer
    duration of 1107
    mortalities 1105
food
    dermatoses and handling of 1071
    flying and 604
    ingestion see ingestion
food technology, nanoparticles 906–7
footwear/shoe wear
    cold protection 541
    welding 431
forced expiratory volume in 1 second (FEV1)
    asthma 948–9
    byssinosis 963
    COPD 890, 893, 894
        coalworkers' 142
forearm problems 688, 693–6, 698, 699
foreign bodies in eye, welding 429–30
formaldehyde 338, 922
    solutions (formalin) 338
        impurities 36
formalin solution, impurities 36
formate 347
    methanol oxidized to 336–7

formic acid 346–7
fossil fuels, IARC classification of carcinogenicity 1083, 1084, 1086
foundry work, eye protection 656, 658
France
    asthma incidence 944
    compensation schemes 97, 105, 105–6
Francisella tularensis 776–7
free radicals (incl. reactive oxygen species) and oxidative stress
    cadmium 169
    CCl_4 and 136
    in cochlear noise-related injury 467, 476
    nanoparticles and 907–8, 909
    red blood cell protective mechanisms 1217–18
freezing cold injury 529–31
friction stir welding 423
frictional psoriasis 1062
'fright sickness' (*susto*) 807–8
frostbite 530–1
frostnip 530
frozen shoulder 690, 690–1
frusemide, altitude sickness prevention 582
fuel oils 335
    see also fossil fuels; jet fuel fumes
full coverage anti-G trousers 597
Fuller's earth 1036
fumes
    definition 254
    jet fuel 604
    metal 1040–2
        aluminium 154, 155
        beryllium 163
        cadmium/cadmium oxide 167, 168, 170, 1041, 1042
        copper 181
        lead oxide 189
        magnesium oxide 200
        manganese 202, 207
        zinc oxide 250, 437, 1040
        see also metal fume fever
    photocopiers and printers 925
    from welding see welding
functional impairment due to psychiatric disorder 842–3
functional restoration programmes, back pain 721
fungi
    byssinosis and
        fungal antigens 960
        fungal enzymes 961
    coalworkers' lungs infected with 1031
    extrinsic allergic alveolitis and 978, 979
    see also mould; yeast

fungi and byssinosis, see also mould; yeast
fungicides 401–2
    acute effects 405
    chronic effects 408–9, 409
furans, chlorinated 370–2

G force see gravitational stress
GABA and lead 192
gallium-67 imaging of lung 879
gamma-aminobutyric acid (GABA) and lead 192
gamma glutamyl transferase (GGT) 69, 1171, 1174
    alcohol abuse 864, 865
gamma rays 624
Gamow bag 584
ganglion cells, retinal 647–8
gardening see horticulture
gas(es) 261–313
    at altitude (incl. flying)
        bubbles in tissues/circulation 594
        expansion 592–3
    anaesthetic see anaesthesia
    in diving, bubbles in tissues/circulation 551, 552–3
    exposures 256–62
    industrial 261–313
        accident investigation 265
        characteristics of hazardous gases 255–6
        classification by health effects 255
        definitions 254–5
        first aid and treatment 262–5
        properties and effects 268–78
        semiconductor production 447, 448
    sampling 45
    welding emissions 426–7
gas embolism, divers 550
gas laws and pressure environments 548
gas welding 422–3
    principle components 425
gasoline 334
gasoline see petrol
gastric cancer epidemiology 1095–6
gastric lavage in pesticide poisoning 410
gastrointestinal tract (digestive system; gut)
    aluminium 154
    barotrauma (divers) 551
    biotransformation 135
    cadmium 167
    cancer
        asbestos and 1006–7
        epidemiology 1095, 1096
    copper, iron interfering with 186
    ionizing radiation effects 627
        management 640
    lead 190

metals (in general) absorbed in 152
pathogens causing infections
    intentional use 773
    zoonotic 752–3, 759–62
shift work and 1235–6
uranium 244
zinc absorption 249
    iron interfering with 186
see also diarrhoea; ingestion
gender *see* female; male; sex
gene(s), inserted, hazardous products from 791, 792
see also oncogenes; transgenes
general anaesthesia *see* anaesthesia
general damages 118
General Medical Council and expert witness immunity 120–1
general practitioners *see* doctors
genetic effects, radiation 630–1
genetic factors
    asthma 946
    byssinosis 962
genetic haematological disorders 1220
genetic modification *see* biotechnology
genetic polymorphisms *see* polymorphisms
genome-wide association studies and genome-wide interactions in cancer 1113, 1114
genotoxicity
    biological effect monitoring markers 65
    boron compounds (in semiconductor production) 451
    cobalt 176–7
    nanoparticles 908
    radiofrequency fields 678
geothermal power 302–3
German measles 739
germane 295
    from Earth 632
Germany
    cobalt carcinogenicity 177
    compensation in 105
    history 96
    Deutsche Forschungsgemeinschaft *see* Deutsche Forschungsgemeinschaft (DFG)
    lead exposure guidelines/recommendations 1129
    MAK values *see* MAK values
giant-cell interstitial pneumonitis, cobalt/hard metal 176, 1046
Giardia lamblia 742, 743
Gilbert's syndrome 1171

gingivitis, mercury 217
ginkgo biloba, altitude sickness prevention 583
glass fibres 1012
glass industry, eyewear 658
glasses *see* spectacles
glenohumeral joint 688
    restricted movement in frozen shoulder 690
gliomas and radiofrequency fields 676–7, 678
global dimensions *see* international dimensions
Global Initiative on Obstructive Lung Disease (GOLD) 890
globalization 19, 25
glomerular pathology
    cadmium 1132
    organic solvents 1139, 1141
gloves, cold protection 541
glucocorticoids *see* corticosteroids
glucose-6-phosphate dehydrogenase (G6PD) deficiency 1220
glucuronide conjugation products 135
glutaraldehyde 338–9
glutathione (GSH) 1217
    conjugation products 135
    in noise-related deafness 476
    in pulmonary detoxification 136–7
glycol ethers (cellosolves; alkoxyalcohols) 341–6
    reproductive effects 342, 343, 345, 346, 1199, 1205
    semiconductor production 448
glyphosate 412
goggles 658
    lasers 658
    night vision, aircrew 600–1
    welding 656, 657, 658
gold 183–4
GOLD (Global Initiative on Obstructive Lung Disease) 890
gold miners and silica and chronic obstruction pulmonary disease 898
golfer's elbow (medial epicondylitis) 692, 693
gonads *see* reproductive effects
Goodpasture's syndrome 1138
Gortex® garments 541
Gough paper-mounted whole lung sections 988, 989
gout, lead 193
government (state)
    history of intervention by 10–11
    policy *see* policies

grain workers and chronic obstruction pulmonary disease 895–6
granulomatous lung disease
    in extrinsic allergic alveolitis 972–3
    metals and 1045
        berylliosis 1051–2
gravimetric sampling of air 45
gravitational stress (incl. G force)
    flying 595–6, 597
    spacecraft
        launch 608
        re-entry 609
    see also microgravity
greenhouse workers, reproductive hazards 1203
Greenhow, Edward 10
grinders, silicosis 1017
grip strength and hand–arm vibration syndrome 500–2, 504
growth retardation, fetal 1202, 1204
Gulf War oil well fires 260
Gulf War syndrome 838, 840–1, 1164
    and depleted uranium 244, 841
gum disease (gingivitis), mercury 217
gut *see* gastrointestinal tract
gypsum 1037

Haber's rule 257
habituation *see* adaptation and habituation
haem
    enzymes containing 185
    synthesis 191, 192
        hepatotoxins and 1179
        lead and 192
haematological effects (incl. toxicity) 1215–29
    benzene *see* benzene
    case reports 1226–7
    clinical evaluation 1218–19
    ionizing radiation 626–7, 1224–5
    management 639
    lead 194, 1219, 1220–1
    methoxyethanol 342
    naphthalene 332–3
    semiconductor workers 451
    work-related issues resulting from treatment 1226
    see also lymphohaematopoietic cancers
haematopoietic system 1215–17
    cancers *see* lymphohaematopoietic cancers
    structure and function 1215–18
haemochromatoses 185–6, 186
haemodialysis, thallium poisoning 237

haemoglobin 1217
  adducts 60, 65
  carbon monoxide combining with (carboxyhaemoglobin) 61, 64, 273–6, 1154
  iron in 185
  see also methaemoglobin
haemoglobinopathies and high altitude 580
haemoglobinuria, arsine 294
haemolytic anaemia 1219–20
  case report 1226–7
haemolytic uraemic syndrome, enterohaemorrhagic E. coli 761
haemoperfusion, thallium poisoning 237
haemopoietic system see haematopoietic system
haemorrhagic fevers, viral 736–7
  bioterrorism 777
  zoonotic 756
hair cells (inner ear/cochlear)
  anatomy and physiology 463, 464
  damage 467
  otoacoustic emissions 479
hairdressing products
  dermatoses 1072
  reproductive hazards 1203, 1206
Haldane, John Scott 11, 25, 266, 268
half-lives, elimination see elimination
half-masks (respiratory protection) 50
Hall–Héroult process 283
halogenated anaesthetics 299
halogenated hydrocarbons 27, 286–7, 296–7, 365–74
  acne (=chloracne) 1069–70
  hepatotoxicity 1175, 1180–1
  welding 427
halothane 299, 300
Hamilton, Alice 15
hand
  beat (subcutaneous cellulitis) 699
  cramp 698, 699
  see also fingers
hand–arm vibration syndrome (with vibratory hand tools) 487–512
  classification 490
  clinical features 494–502
    carpal tunnel syndrome see carpal tunnel syndrome
    Dupuytren's disease 493, 499–500, 698
  diagnosis and tertiary case assessment 502–5
  differential diagnosis 497, 498
  epidemiology 489–90
  management of cases 506–7

pathophysiology 490–4
workplace health surveillance 505–6
hand–wrist tendinitis 694
hantavirus 756
hard metal 175
hard metal dust (and hard metal lung disease)
  cobalt (cobalt lung) 175, 176, 1045–6
  tungsten carbide and 241, 1045
HAV (hepatitis A virus) and travel 743
hazards
  definition and distinction from risk 35, 141
  exposure see exposure
  identification 141–2
  new 26–7
HBV see hepatitis B virus
HCV see hepatitis C virus
headaches, high altitude
  Mauna Kea 574
  treatment 583
headgear see helmets
health
  biotechnology and risks to 787–91
  diving and long-term effects on 561–2
  electromagnetic fields and 664–70
  gas effects on
    classification by 255
    irritant see irritant gases
  indoor non-industrial environments and 923–33
  ionizing radiation and see ionizing radiation
  radiofrequency fields and 675–9
  risk to see risk
  semiconductor industry and see semiconductor industry
  shift work and see shift work
  surveillance see surveillance
  welding and risks to see welding
  whole-body vibration effects on 514–19
  work affecting 38–9
  see also disease; fitness; medical conditions
Health and Safety at Work etc. Act (1974) 18
Health and Safety Executive (HSE) 18
  biological monitoring 60–1
  biotechnology (incl. genetic modification) 784
  cyanide poisoning 277
  diving 565
  Methods for Determination of Hazardous Substances 45

vibration
  hand–arm 506
  whole-body 520
  workplace exposure limits see workplace
health insurance see insurance
health outcomes investigation 77
  discordant results of epidemiological studies due to differences in 87
  other than illness or disease 86
health records see records
healthcare
  biotechnology in 783
  dermatoses in 1072–3
  see also veterinary care
healthcare workers/staff and medical personnel (incl. hospitals)
  infections in 729–41
  radiation exposure 633
    protection 638
  reproductive hazards 1203
  terrorist incident and risk to 318
  see also doctors
healthy lifestyle programmes 847
healthy worker effect in epidemiological studies of cancer 1107–8
hearing aids 475–6
hearing conservation programmes 471–5
hearing loss 464–9
  age-associated 471
  assessment 470–1, 474
  chemical-related see ototoxicity
  noise-induced 464–9
    diagnosis 469
    exaggeration 476–7
    management 475–6
    welding 431
heart
  arrhythmias see arrhythmias
  external massage after rescue from immersion 533
  see also coronary artery disease; myocardial infarction and entries under cardiovascular
heat (exposure to; heat stress) 534–8
  assessment 534–6
  diving, loss 555
  in fires 258
  flying 597–8
  occupations with recognized challenges of 528
  performance effects 538
  personal protective equipment 540–1
  responses to (=heat strain) 527–8
    assessment 536
    immediate consequences 536–8

testicular, and spermatogenesis 1199
training in 529
heat exhaustion 536
heat stroke 536
heaters, carbon monoxide from 273
    see also rewarming
heavy metals see metals
helicopters
    crashes and escape 605
    vibration 598
helium 271
helium–oxygen mixtures (helium),
    divers 549, 555, 558
helmets
    diving 556, 557
    noise-excluding 473–4
    welding 428, 431, 656, 657, 658–9
helminths 765
Henderson–Hasselbach equation 128
Hendra virus 756
henipavirus 756
Henry's law 548
hepatitis
    Q fever 754
    viral (in general), screening for 1172
    see also steatohepatitis
hepatitis A virus (HAV)
    sewage workers 744
    travellers 743
hepatitis B virus (HBV)
    in healthcare workers 729–31
        management 734
        prevention 735
        risk of transmission to patient 733
        risk of transmission to worker 732
        serological markers 732, 733
hepatitis C virus (HCV) in healthcare
    workers 729, 731
    management 734
    prevention 735
    risk of transmission to patient
        733–4
    risk of transmission to worker 732–3
hepatitis E virus 756–7
hepatocellular carcinoma
    aflatoxin and 1114
    epidemiology 1096
hepatotoxicity 1171–95
    biomarkers 69–70
        alcohol abuse 69, 864–5
    mechanisms 1176–80
    metals 1184–5
    organic chemicals 1175, 1176–84
        carbon tetrachloride 369, 1176–8,
            1180–1
        chloroform 369, 1181
        dimethylformamide 348, 1182

vinyl chloride 17, 26, 134, 368,
    1096, 1178–9, 1187
    treatment 1176, 1177
    see also liver
herbicides (weedkillers) 399–401,
    1185–6
    acute effects 405
        management 411–12
    carcinogenicity 401, 1111
    hepatotoxicity 1185–6
heredity see entries under genetic
herpes B virus 741
herpetic whitlow 739
heterocyclic nitrogen compounds
    356–7
HEV (hepatitis E virus) 756–7
hexacarbon solvents 369
    hepatotoxicity 1179
    neurotoxicity 1156
hexachlorobenzene 369, 1179
hexafluoroacetone 298
hexafluoroethane 286
hexahydrophthalic anhydride 363, 364
1,6-hexamethylenediisocyanate (HDI)
    364
    patch test 1066
n-hexane 322, 323–4
    biological monitoring guidance values
        61
    neurotoxicity 1156
2-hexanone, (methyl n-butyl ketone)
    340, 1156
hexavalent chromium 152, 173, 174
Hickman, Henry Hill 298
high altitude 570–90
    anaesthesia 581
    illness/sickness 570–8
        at-risk groups 578–80, 578–80
        not caused by high altitude 578
        prevention 581–3, 585
        treatment 583–4, 585
    rapid ascent by sea-level residents to
        578
    safe working 584–6
    sleep 580–1
    useful sources of information 586
high aspect ratio nanoparticles
    see fibrous particles
high-frequency electromagnetic
    radiation, reproductive effects
    1199
high-resolution CT 877–8
    asbestosis 883, 992
    extrinsic allergic alveolitis 884, 974
    silicosis 880
High Risk Offender Scheme (drink
    driving) 867

himic anhydride 363
hip
    osteoarthritis 701
    replacement, and flying 606
histamine and byssinosis 961
    see also antihistamines
histology examination of autopsy
    material, inorganic dust diseases
    988
historical perspectives 5–21, 24–5
    asbestos-related disease 1000
    back pain treatment 715–16
    bioterrorism 773
    cadmium exposure 1131
    chronic obstruction pulmonary
        disease 890
    compensation 12, 13, 14, 96, 97,
        98–104, 107
    eye protection 656
    flying 591
    gases
        from anaerobic fermentation 266
        anaesthetic 298–9
    high-altitude illness 570
    Hunter's own perspectives 6–7,
        13, 25
    job titles 35
    lead 11, 13, 15, 188–9
    manganism 204
    mercury 214–15
    noise-induced hearing loss 464–5
    pesticides 396–7
    phosphorus 11, 225
    psychological complaints 803
    warfare 14–16, 314
history-taking 33–40
    asthma diagnosis 948
    in attribution of disease to exposure
        51
    in expert report 118
    haematological disorders 1218
    hand–arm vibration syndrome 503
    hepatotoxic chemicals (after
        abnormal liver function tests)
        1172
    importance 38–40
    noise-induced hearing loss 469
    pregnant woman 1208–9
    relevant factors 34–8
    reliability of information 38
HIV see human immunodeficiency
    virus
HLA and asthma 946
Hodgkin's disease 1225–6
hogs see pig and hog farming
holistic exposure assessment 48–9
homeostasis, manganese 203

hormonal contraceptives and high altitude 576, 577
hormones
    bioengineered 786–7
    pesticide effects 398
    in tissue culture 790
    see also endocrine effects
horticulture and gardening
    dermatoses 1073
    hepatotoxic chemicals 1174
    reproductive hazards 1203
hospitals
    nuclear reactor accident casualties 640
    staff see healthcare workers
hot zone (terrorist chemical attack) 317
    drugs given in 317–18
hours worked 835–6
    extended see shift work and extended work hours
HSE see Health and Safety Executive
human immunodeficiency virus (HIV)
    in healthcare workers 729, 731
        management 734–5
        post-exposure prophylaxis 735–6
        risk of transmission to patient 734
        risk of transmission to worker 733
    in research laboratory workers 741
    serological tests 795
humidifier(s) 923, 924
    extrinsic allergic alveolitis and 928, 929
humidifier fever 929
    ventilation pneumonitis vs 980
humidity (indoors)
    non-industrial 924
    semiconductor production 449
Hunter, Donald 5–7, 12, 18, 20
    his own historical perspectives 6–7, 13, 25
hybridization (between organisms) 785
hydatid disease 765
hydrocarbons 329–36
    aliphatic 322–4
    aromatic see aromatic hydrocarbons
    halogenated see halogenated hydrocarbons
    mixtures of 334–6
    nitrogen-containing 348–57
hydrochloric acid
    hydrolysis to 280–1
    in semiconductor production 448
hydrochlorofluorocarbons (HCFCs) 265, 287
hydrofluoric acid
    first aid measures 284
    hydrolysis to 284–6
    in semiconductor production 448

hydrofluorocarbons (HFCs) 265–6, 281, 286, 372–6
hydrogen (gas) 273
    breathing mixtures (divers) 549
hydrogen bromide 281
hydrogen chloride 257, 280
    see also hydrochloric acid
hydrogen cyanide 257, 276–8
    in fires 260
    hypoxic brain injury 265
    terrorist attack 317–18
hydrogen fluoride 257
    acute health effects 282
    see also hydrofluoric acid
hydrogen halides (in general) 280–1
hydrogen iodide 281
hydrogen phosphide see phosphine
hydrogen selenide 294
hydrogen sulphide 257, 291–3
    hypoxic brain injury 265
hydrolysis 135
hydrothermal energy 302–3
hydroxocobalamin 278
N-hydroxy-2-acetylaminofluorene 134
hydroxylation 133, 134
1-hydroxypyrene (analyte) 62
hygiene practice
    nanoparticles 913–14
    welding 428
hyoscine, air sickness 603
hyperaemia after non-freezing cold injury 531
hyperbaric chambers with oxygen 263
    altitude sickness 584
    CO poisoning 275
hyperbaric oxygen, altitude sickness 584
hypercalcaemia, beryllium 1136
hypercapnia, divers 555
hyperkalaemia in heat illness 538
hypermethylation (DNA) and tumorigenesis 1112
hypersensitivity pneumonitis see extrinsic allergic alveolitis
hypersensitivity reactions see allergen; allergenicity; antigen; immune response; respiratory sensitization
hypertension
    portal 1175
    systemic
        cadmium 169
        high altitude and 579
        lead 1127–8
hyperthermia, divers 556
hypnotics, flying over time zones 603
hyponatraemia in heat illness 537–8
hypothermia
    immersion 532–4

    in divers 556
    land 532–3
hypoxia
    altitude (incl. flying) 593–4
    divers 555
    gases causing 262
        brain injury 265

IARC see International Agency for Research on Cancer
idiopathic copper toxicosis 181
illness/ill health
    definition 28
    ecological view 20
    measures of 77
    work-related, new wave of 27–8
illusions while flying 601
ILO see International Labour Organization
imaging 875–88
    brain see neuroimaging
    lung diseases 875–88
        asbestos-related 880–3, 993, 995
        beryllium-related 883–4, 1051
        extrinsic allergic alveolitis 884–5, 974
    see also specific modalities
immersion (cold) 532–4
    (patho)physiology 531, 532, 532–4
    divers 533, 554–5
    see also hypothermia
immune response (pathological incl. hypersensitivity)
    allergic contact dermatitis 1063–4
    asthma and 941, 943
    beryllium 163, 164, 1050–1
    byssinosis and 960–1
    chronic obstruction pulmonary disease causes and 895
    extrinsic allergic alveolitis and 971, 973
    mercury 1135
    organic solvent nephropathy and 1141
    silica 1024–5
    see also antibodies; antigens; autoimmune disease
immunity (immune system)
    astronauts 610
    pesticide effects 398, 406–7
immunity (legal term), expert witness 120–1
immunization
    active see vaccination; vaccines
    passive, hepatitis B in healthcare workers 735
immunocompromised persons, toxoplasmosis 858

immunoglobulin E tests 66, 67
   asthma (for respiratory sensitizers) 947, 948
   textile workers 960
immunoglobulin G tests 66
   cotton workers 960
   extrinsic allergic alveolitis 975, 976
immunological tests
   in asthma (for respiratory sensitizers) 947, 948
   in hepatotoxicity indicated by abnormal liver function tests 1172
impure chemicals 36
incapacity benefit 810–11
   government policy 817–18
incidence 78
   rates in cohort studies 82
incidence ratio, standardized (SIR), in cohort studies 82
incivility, workplace 816
Indian childhood cirrhosis 181
indirectly standardized rates 78
indium tin oxide 1045
individuals
   attribution of disease to exposure in *see* attribution
   characteristics and variations in susceptibility 137–8
     altitude sickness 578
     asthma 946
     cancer 1113–14
     shift work tolerance 1238–9
     variations in detoxifying enzyme activities 128
indoor environments (and indoor air), non-industrial 921–38
   changing the air 923, 933
   CO_2 levels as air quality measure 271
   gas exposures 256
   management and prevention of exposures 933–4
   sources of hazards 921–3
   see also confined spaces
Industrial Injuries Act (1946) 98, 100–1
Industrial Injuries Advisory Council 101
industrial injuries compensation, UK 97–8
Industrial Injuries Disablement Benefit (IIDB) 97, 97–8
Industrial Injuries Scheme (1946) 97
industrialized countries, cancer
   epidemiology 1081
   prevention 1103
industry
   hazards

carcinogens *see* carcinogens
   gases *see* gases
   hepatotoxic chemicals 1174
   historical perspectives 5–20
   lead 1126
   questionnaires for carcinogen exposure evaluation 1110
infections (and communicable/transmissible diseases) 725–70
   flying and exposure to risk 607
   from genetically-modified organisms 795
   healthcare worker *see* healthcare workers
   indoor non-industrial sources 930
   pregnancy outcome and 1208
   respiratory/pulmonary *see* respiratory infections
   in semiconductor industry 449
   see also biotechnology; bioterrorism; sepsis
infertility *see* reproductive effects
inflammatory response in lung
   in extrinsic allergic alveolitis 972–3
   granulomatous *see* granulomatous lung disease
   nanoparticles 907–8
     cardiovascular effects related to 908
   diesel exhaust 910, 912
information (for workers and managers) *see* education
information bias 91
infrared radiation, eye damage 654–5
   pathophysiology 645
   protective filter materials 657–8
infrasound 480
ingestion (incl. dietary intake) 49
   cadmium 167
   copper 181
   iron 185
   manganese 202
   measuring exposure via 44–5
   mercury 215, 216
   nickel 224
   radioactive material 632
   silver 234
   zinc 250
   see also food; gastrointestinal tract
inhalation (provocation) challenge
   asthma-causing agents 365, 949–51
   cotton extracts 960
   diesel exhaust particles 910
inhalation exposure and absorption
   aluminium 154
   beryllium 164
   chromium 174
   lead 190
   manganese 203

measuring 43–4, 44, 48
   dust 45
   mercury 216, 1041
     from dental amalgam 215–16
     treatment 218
   nickel 223
   zinc 250
   see also dusts; fumes; gases; powders
inhalation fevers 436–7
   metal fume *see* metal fume fevers
inhalation injury, metal compounds 1041
inhalation kinetics 130–1
inheritance *see entries under* genetic
injection exposure, measuring 45
injury, physical/mechanical *see* trauma
inner (internal) ear
   anatomy and physiology 462–3
   middle ear disease effects on 468
   noise-related damage 467, 475
inorganic dust diseases (incl. pneumoconiosis) 897–8, 983–1056
   chronic obstruction pulmonary disease and 897–8
   coalworkers *see* coalworkers' diseases
   extrinsic allergic alveolitis and 972
   fibrous *see* fibrous particles and dusts/fibres
   general aspects 985–9
     definition 985
     investigations and diagnosis 986
     pathogenesis 985–6
   hard metal (and associated disease) 175, 176
   ILO classification 880, 885–6, 987
   metals 1044–6
     aluminium 153, 154, 155, 1044–5
     beryllium *see* beryllium
     lead 189
   non-fibrous 1014–39
insecticide toxicity/poisoning 1160–1
   acute 404–5
     management 410–11
   lymphomas 1225–6
   mechanisms 397–9
insecurity, job 838–9
inspiratory crackles
   asbestosis 992
   extrinsic allergic alveolitis 974, 975, 976
Institute of Electrical and Electronic Engineers and MRI 670
Institute of Occupational Medicine total inhalable dust sampling head 45, 46
insulation, thermal, protective garments 541–2

insurance schemes (social and health) 97
    Europe 105, 106, 107
    historical background 13, 96, 100, 101, 102
    US 107
integrated chips 445
interactive effects in causation of cancer 1108–9
intermediate biomarkers in cancer 1112–13
'intermediate syndrome' (with organophosphates) 404
internal comparison group in cohort studies of cancer 1106
internal ear *see* inner ear
International Agency for Research on Cancer (IARC)
    classification of carcinogens 1082–3, 1084
        bladder cancer 1088
        lung cancer 1086
        skin cancer (non-melanocytic) 1093
    questionnaires on exposure evaluation 1110
International Commission on Non-Ionizing Radiation Protection and MRI 670
international dimensions/global aspects 19, 25
    historical perspectives in peace and war 14–16
International Labour Organization (ILO) and Office 15
    classification of pneumoconiosis 880, 885–6, 987
    asbestos-related disease 995
interspecies vs intraspecies susceptibility 128
interstitial lung disease
    metals 1044–6
        cobalt/hard metal 176, 1045–6
        welders 434, 911
intestine *see* bowel
intraocular lenses, aircrew 600
intraspecies vs interspecies susceptibility 128
intrauterine growth retardation 1202, 1204
investigations
    asthma 948–51
    contact dermatitis 1065–7
    inorganic dust diseases 986–7
iodine, radioactive
    prophylactic measures 640
    thyroid accumulation 627
IOM total inhalable dust sampling head 45, 46

ionic dissociation 128
ionizing radiation
    definition 624
    detection 625
    dose *see* dose
    factors influencing sensitivity to 631
    health effects 625–34
        haematological *see* haematological effects
        leukaemia 630, 631, 1092, 1225
        reproductive 627–8, 1198, 1206–7
    health surveillance 634–8
    legislation 632, 634
    natural background/sources 625
    occupational exposure 633
    nuclear reactor incidents 263
    physics 623–4
    protection 633–4
    semiconductor production 448–9
    sources and magnitude of exposure 631–2
    space 608
    welding 424
ipecacuana in pesticide poisoning, contraindicated 410
iridium 228
iris 648
iron 185–7
    manganese in manufacture of 204, 209
    see also siderosis
iron industry, chronic obstructive pulmonary disease 1042
irritant contact dermatitis 1062–3
    treatment 1067
irritant gases 253, 255, 278–98
    characteristics 255–6
    first aid and treatment 262
    health effects 257, 278–98
        asthma *see* asthma
        simple 278–94
irritant-induced asthma 943
    exposure–response relationships 945–6
ischaemic heart disease *see* coronary artery disease
isobutane 301, 322
isobutylene 301
isocyanates 36, 261, 297, 364–5
    asthma and 364, 364–5
        attribution to exposure in case study 53–4
    immunological tests 948
    see also di-isocyanates
isohexane (methylpentane) 322
isophorone diisocyanate (IPDI) 364
isopropyl alcohol in phenol poisoning 358

iso-strain model 836
Itai-itai disease 169
Italy, compensation schemes 106
Ivory Coast (Cote d'Ivoire) ebolavirus 737

Jamar grip test 500, 503, 504
Japan
    Minamata disease 215, 1135
    nerve agents in terrorism 316
jaw, phossy 225
jet fuel fumes 604
jet-lag 603–4
job–exposure matrices (JEMs) 1110
    electromagnetic fields 665
    see also work
joint involvement
    decompression sickness 552, 553
    hand–arm vibration syndrome 502
    see also arthropathies; osteoarthritis; rheumatic conditions; rheumatoid arthritis

K-line X-ray fluorescence, lead nephropathy 1128–9
kaolin workers' pneumoconiosis 1033–4
Kassmaul on mercury poisoning 214–15
Kehoe, Robert 189
Kepone® (chlordecone) 36, 1161, 1186
keratotomy, aircrew 600
kerosene 335
ketones 339–40
keyboards, computer 702–3
kidney
    accumulation and concentrations in
        cadmium 171
        mercury 217
    astronauts, dysfunction 610
    failure/dysfunction
        cadmium poisoning and its diagnosis 170, 1132–3
        lead poisoning (chronic) 1126–7, 1128
        organic solvents 1139
    toxicity *see* nephrotoxicity
    see also renal syndrome
kieselgahr 1036
KIM-1 (kidney injury molecule-1) 69
kinetics (dynamics) of chemicals 127–8
    aluminium 154
    arsenic 160–1
    of exposure 130–2
    lead 190–1
    manganese 203
    toxicokinetics 128–30
    see also metabolism
KL-6 (Krebs von den Lungen-6) 66

knee
    beat (subcutaneous cellulitis) 699
    osteoarthritis 699–701
Koch's postulates 91
Korean haemorrhagic fever 756
krypton 273
Kuwait (oil fires) 260

laboratory studies (incl. experimental/animal models)
    electromagnetic fields and cancer 668
    lead and renal damage 1127
    nanoparticles and nuisance dusts 905, 907
    organic solvents and renal damage 1138
    pesticide carcinogenicity 409
    phthalate esters and hepatotoxicity 1188
    radiofrequency fields and cancer 678
    reproductive toxicities, extrapolation to humans 1201
    vibration-induced neuropathology 492
laboratory tests
    haematological disorders 1219
    hand–arm vibration syndrome 503–5
    lead 194
    mercury 218
    radiation exposure 640
laboratory workers
    hepatotoxic chemicals 1174
    infections 741
    reproductive hazards 1203
    zoonotic 751
lagged analysis, epidemiological studies of cancer 1107
Lake Louise acute mountain sickness score
    calculating 576–8, 586–7
    Mauna Kea observatory 572–3
Lake Nyos (Cameroon) 270
laminating, reinforced plastic, reproductive hazards 1203
Lamp, safety 268
land-use planning and LUP SLOT 257
landfill gas 269
lanthanides 1045
laryngeal cancer 1095
    asbestos, and 1006–7
    epidemiology 1095
laryngeal mask airway in space 612
laryngeal spasm, ammonia 289
laser, ocular damage 649, 652–4

nature of 645
protection 656, 657, 658
laser in-situ keratomileusis (LASIK), aircrew 600
Lassa fever 736, 737
latency analysis, epidemiological studies of cancer 1107
lateral epicondylitis 692, 693
launch, spacecraft 608
Lavoisier 253
law (and legislation/regulations/guidelines/recommendations on safety) 111–21
    biological monitoring 57
    biotechnology (incl. genetic modification) 783–4
    cadmium exposure 1133–4
    cancer prevention 1103
    compensation 97
        UK 98, 99–101, 102, 104–5, 113, 114, 118, 120
    diving and compressed air work 565
    gases and 258
    history 10–11, 12, 13, 98, 99–101, 102
        US 18
    ionizing radiations 632, 634
    lead exposure 1129–30
    light damage prevention 656
    magnetic resonance imaging 670
    mercury exposure 1135
    noise exposure 474–5
    solvent hepatotoxicity and 1183
    substance abuse testing 864
    vibration
        hand–arm 505–6
        whole-body 513–14, 519, 519–20
lay perspectives on risk 144
L-dopa, manganism 205, 208
lead 36, 188–98, 1126–31, 1157–8, 1185
    acute poisoning 1126
    biochemical effects 191–2
    biological monitoring 57, 63–4
        guidance values 61
    cardiovascular disease risk 192, 1128–9, 1130–1
    chronic poisoning 1126–7
    distribution in body 190–1
    evaluating exposure 195–7
    haematological effects 194, 1219, 1220–1
    hepatotoxicity 1185
    historical perspectives 11, 13, 15, 188–9
    investigations of poisoning 194
    mortality 1130
    nephrotoxicity 192–3, 1126–31

neurotoxicity 193, 1157–8
organic see organic compounds
present day exposures 189
reproductive toxicity 193, 1200, 1206
treatment of poisoning 194–5, 1130
uptake 190
League of Nations and the International Labour Office 15
legal issues see law
Legge, Sir Thomas Morison 5, 11, 12, 12–13, 15, 24, 189
Legionnaires' disease 438, 930
legislation see law
lenses 647
    anatomy 647
    contact see contact lenses
    infrared-induced damage 655
    intraocular (implants), aircrew 600
    ionizing radiation-induced damage 627
    opacities see cataracts
    UV-induced damage 649
leptospirosis 69–70, 757–8
lethal dose (LD)
    ionizing radiation 626–7
    oral, toxicity rating by 127
leucocyanadin and byssinosis 960
leukaemia 1222, 1225
    benzene and 326, 1092, 1223
    electromagnetic fields and 665–6, 668, 671
        in offspring of exposed parents 669
    formaldehyde and 338
    ionizing radiation-related 630, 631, 1092, 1225
    radiofrequency fields and 677
    uranium and 244
leukocyte (white cell) count, semiconductor workers 451
leukoderma 1070
levodopa (L-dopa), manganism 205, 208
life support see adult life support; advanced life support systems
lifestyle programmes, healthy 847
lifting and back pain 717
light (optical radiation) 644–62
    ocular damage see eye
    see also infrared; ultraviolet
limb
    decompression sickness-related pain 552
    upper, problems 688, 692–9
Lind, James 9
lindane and aplastic anaemia 1224
lipid solubility 128
lipofuscin 649, 650

liquefied gases
   cold injury 263
   nitrogen and argon 272
   petrochemical 301–2
listeriosis 764
Liston, Robert 298
literature review in attribution of disease to exposure 51
lithium ion rechargeable batteries 175
Litvinenko, Alexander 232
liver 1171–95
   acute injury 1172–3
   alcoholic cirrhosis 861
   cadmium accumulation 170
      assessment 171
   cancer 1175
      epidemiology 1096
      vinyl chloride and 17, 26, 134, 368, 1096, 1178–9
   chemicals toxic to see hepatotoxicity
   chronic injury 1175
   enzymes 69, 133
      and alcohol abuse 864–5
   function tests, abnormal 1171, 1172
      disorders producing 1173
   patterns of toxic injury 1172–6
   pesticide effects 398
   see also hepatitis
loading, spinal (and back pain) 717, 718
   exposure limits 718
lobar pneumonia, welders 433
local exhaust (local extraction) ventilation 49
   welding 428
London smog 254, 288
longitudinal data, chronic obstruction pulmonary disease and ventilatory function 893–4
loop diuretics, altitude sickness prevention 582
Loudon 271
low-frequency electromagnetic radiation, extremely 663–74
low-molecular weight (LMW) proteinuria, cadmium 168, 170, 1132
Lujo virus 736
lumbar spine and whole-body vibration 518–19
lung 136–7
   anthrax 751, 775
   asthmatic complication of acute toxicity see reactive airways dysfunction syndrome
   biomarkers 66–7
   biotransformation in 136–7
   chronic obstructive disease see chronic obstructive pulmonary disease

compliance, asbestosis 993
divers 554
   barotrauma 549–50
   in decompression sickness 552–3
   long-term effects 562
echinococcosis 765
fibrosis see fibrosis
gases in
   causing acute injury 263
   ozone damage 290
   SO_2 causing chronic injury 288
hard metal disease see hard metal dust
imaging of diseases of 875–88
infections see respiratory infections
inflammation see pneumonitis
inhalation into see inhalation
inorganic dust damage
   pathogenesis 985–6
   post-mortem examination 988
metals absorbed in 151–2
   lead 190
nanoparticle translocation to other tissues 907
oedema see oedema
pesticide effects 398, 405
radiation effects 627
welding-related disorders 421–2, 432–5, 911
see also pulmonary syndrome and entries under pneumo-; respiratory
lung cancer 1085–8
   asbestos and 103–4, 994–5, 1005–6, 1087–8
      attribution 51–2, 93, 95, 1006
      compensation 103–4
      epidemiology 1005–6, 1087–8, 1108
      imaging 883
      pathogenesis 994
      smoking and 1005, 1109
   china clay and 1035
   metals and 1043–4
      aluminium 155
      beryllium 1051, 1087
      cadmium 169
      chromium 174, 1087
      cobalt (± tungsten carbide) 176, 1043–4
      nickel 223, 1086–7
      uranium 244
      vanadium 247
   radiogenic, sex and risk of 631
   silica and 1022–4, 1087
   smoking (involuntary) and 933
   welders 435
lung function/ventilatory function (and tests incl. spirometry)
   asthma 948–9

byssinosis 962, 963
   acute disease 929, 974–5
   chronic disease 975
chronic obstruction pulmonary disease and recognition of excessive decline 892–5
extrinsic allergic alveolitis, monitoring 978
inorganic dust diseases 987–8
   beryllium 1051
   in individual cases 988
welding fumes and 911
LUP SLOT 257
lupus erythematosus, systemic (SLE), silica and 1025
Luxembourg, compensation schemes 106
Lyme disease 762–3
lymphocyte proliferation test, blood beryllium 163
   see also T lymphocytes
lymphocytic leukaemia, acute and chronic 1092
lymphohaematopoietic cancers 1092, 1222, 1225–6
   benzene and 326, 1092, 1223–4
   case report 1226
   epidemiology 1092
   ethylene oxide 360
   phenoxy acid herbicides 401, 409
   radiofrequency fields 677
   see also Hodgkin's disease; leukaemia; non-Hodgkin's lymphoma
lymphomas see Hodgkin's disease; non-Hodgkin's lymphoma
lyssaviruses 765–6

machine degreasing, hepatotoxic chemicals 1174
McIntyre powder 154
macrophages and inorganic dusts 985
maculopathy, welding arc 430, 652
magnesium 199–200
magnesium phosphide 295
magnesium silicate, talc as form of 1035
magnetic fields see electromagnetic fields
magnetic resonance imaging 670
   brain
      carbon dioxide intoxication 374–5
      high altitude climbers 576
      manganism 205, 206–7, 208, 1158
      triethyltin intoxication 239
   exposures and risks 670
   in hand–arm vibration syndrome (median nerve entrapment) 505
   lung/thorax 878–9
mainstream tobacco smoke 922

major (mass/catastrophic) incidents
  gas exposure 256–7
  radiation exposure 636–7
  resilience to 815
MAK values 40, 155
  manganese 208
malaria 742
  aircraft and 607
Malaysian factories, possession states 808–9
male(s)
  developmental toxicity relating to male parent 1200–1
  fertility problems (incl. sperm) 1200–1
    dimethylformamide 348–9
    epidemiology 1197
    lead 193
    mechanisms 1198
    radiofrequency fields 679
    semiconductor industry 450–1
    testicular temperature and 1199
    welding 435
  see also sex
maleic anhydride 363
malodorous sulphur compounds 293
malt-worker's lung 979
mandelic acid (analyte) 62
manganese 201–12, 1158–9
  acute effects 203
  characteristics 210
  chronic effects 203–6
  deficiency 203
  health surveillance 208
  kinetics/metabolism 203
  metabolic activity 202
  mutagenicity/teratogenicity/carcinogenicity 203
  neurotoxicity 204, 206, 208, 1158–9
  sources 201
  treatment of poisoning 205, 208–9, 1158
  uses and sources of exposure 201–2
    welding 202, 207, 426
  workplace exposure limits 208
manganese chloride 202
manganese dioxide 202
manganese dipyridoxyl diphosphate 202
manganese ethylene-bis-dithiocarbamate 202
manganism 203–6
  brain imaging 205, 206–7, 208, 1158
  welders 426
manual metal arc welding 422
  particle emissions 425
manufactured nanoparticles (MNPs) 905, 907, 908, 909
Marburg virus 736–7, 737

marsh gas 268–9
masks (integrated circuit) 446
masks (respiratory protection) 50
Maslach Burnout Inventory 844–5
masons, silicosis 1017
mass incidents see major incidents
material safety data sheet (MSDS) 35, 37
  reproductive toxicity 1209
Mauna Kea observatory (Hawaii) 571–2
  individual susceptibility 578
  medical emergencies 574
  safe working 584
MCP-1 and diisocyanate asthma 948
Meadow, Professor, fitness to practice proceedings 120–1
measles 739
mechanical factors 683–724
  low back pain 717–18
media (communication) on health risks 147
media (culture/growth) 790, 791
medial epicondylitis 692, 693
median nerve compression at wrist see carpal tunnel syndrome
mediation 817
  counselling and 816
medical conditions/physical disorders
  comorbid with psychiatric disorders 845
  flying with 606
    passengers 607
  at high-altitude
    not caused by altitude 578
    pre-existing 578–80
  indoor (non-industrial) environment-related 925–33
  in shift workers, pre-existing
    exemption from night work 1240–1
    worsening 1241
  space, emergencies 611–13
  toxic exposures and medically unexplained conditions 840–1
  see also disease; health; systemic disease
medical contract cards 796
medical examination see physical examination
medical expert see expert witness
medical profession, historical perspectives 12–13
medical records see records
medical staff see doctors; healthcare workers
medical surveillance see surveillance
medicalization of work stress 804–6
medicine, nanoparticles in 906–7
medicolegal reports 113–21
  see also law
meerschaum 1011

melanin, eye 649, 650
melanoma, malignant
  electromagnetic fields and 667
  radiofrequency fields and 677
  semiconductor industry and 450
  sun exposure 1071
  welding (UV-related) 423, 429
    ocular 431
melatonin
  electromagnetic fields and 666–7
  jet-lag 603–4
  shift work and cancer and 1097, 1238
membrane, cell, transport across see transport
men see males
meningiomas and mobile phones 678
menstrual cycle control and high altitude 576, 577
mental health 799–856
  disorders see psychological disorders
mental stress see stress
mercaptans 293, 294
mercaptopropionyl glycine 219
mercurous chloride (calomel) 1134
mercury 36, 214–20, 1041, 1134–6, 1159
  acute inhalation injury 1041
  biological monitoring 62, 68
  current recommendations 1135
  nephrotoxicity 217, 218, 1134–6
  neurotoxicity 217, 217–18, 1159
  reproductive toxicity 1206
  treatment of toxicity 218, 1136, 1159
mesothelioma, asbestos-related 993–4, 1002–4, 1090–1
  peritoneal
    epidemiology 1004
    imaging 883
  pleural 102–3, 993–4, 1002–4, 1091–2
    attribution 95
    clinical assessment of case 1102
    compensation 98, 102–3
    epidemiology 26, 1002–4, 1090, 1091–2
    expert medical report 118
    historical perspectives 16
    imaging 881, 993
    pathology 993
    pleural plaques and risk of 995
    prognosis 994
    see also pleural disease
mesothelioma, non-asbestos-related 1005
  minerals 1005, 1011
  nanotubes 906
meta-analysis 86

metabolism
   red blood cell 1216–17
   shift work effects 1235–6
   thermal challenges and 527
   xenobiotics 131–2, 132–7
      cadmium 167–8, 1132
      chromium 173–4
      copper 180–1
      magnesium 199–200
      manganese 202
      organic chemicals *see text for specific chemicals*
      see also kinetics; transformation
metabolite production (in biotechnology) 786
metal(s) (incl. heavy metals) 149–250, 1040–9
   carcinogenic *see* carcinogens
   compounds *see* compounds
   diagnosis of poisoning *see* diagnosis
   dusts 1040–9
      chronic obstruction pulmonary disease 896–7, 1042
   essentiality vs toxicity 151–2
   fumes *see* fumes; metal fume fevers
   hepatotoxicity 1175, 1184–5
   nanoparticles 905
   neurotoxicity *see* neurotoxicity
   production, hepatotoxic chemicals 1174
   properties 151
   radioactive *see* radioactivity
   renal toxicity *see* nephrotoxicity
   reproductive toxicity *see* reproductive effects
   in semiconductor production 446, 447, 448
      deposition of atoms of 446
   welding *see* welding
metal active gas welding 423
   particle emissions 425
metal fume fevers 911, 1040–1
   copper 181
   magnesium 200
   manganese oxide 203
   vanadium and 247
   welding and 433, 437, 911
   zinc oxide 250, 437, 1040
metal inert gas welding 423
   particle emissions 425
metal oxide particles
   inhalation injury 1041
   welding 424
metal-workers' dermatoses 1073
metal-working fluids and extrinsic allergic alveolitis 979
metaldehyde 402, 412
metalloids 152

metallothionein 135
   cadmium and 168, 169
methaemoglobin (and methaemoglobinaemia) 1217, 1220
   aniline and 353
   chlorate salts and 412
   nitrogen oxides and 290, 291
methane 268–9, 322
   mines 268
   sewers 266
methanethiol (methyl mercaptan) 293, 294
methanol (methyl alcohol) 336–7
   methanal and, confusion between 36
methazolamide for altitude sickness, preventive use 582
Methods for Determination of Hazardous Substances (HSE's) 45
methoxyethanol 342–3
methoxyethylacetate 342
methoxypropanol 345–6
methyl alcohol *see* methanol
methyl benzene *see* toluene
methyl bromide 266, 296, 1159, 1188
methyl *n*-butyl ketone 340, 1156
methyl chloride 296–7
methyl ethyl ketone (MEK) 339–40
   biological monitoring guidance values 61
   n-hexane interactions with 323
   neurotoxicity 1156
methyl glycol ether in semiconductor production 448
methyl iso-butyl ketone (MiBK; 4-methylpentan-2-one) 340
   biological monitoring guidance values 62
   n-hexane interactions with 323
methyl isocyanate 297, 364
   Bhopal disaster 253, 297, 364, 1237
methyl mercaptan 293, 294
methyl mercury 214, 215, 216, 217, 218, 219
methyl methacrylate 347
methyl phenyl pyridinium (MPTP) 1161
methyl vinyl ether 300
N-methylacrylamide 350–1
methylation status (DNA) and tumorigenesis 1112
methylcyclopentadienyl manganese tricarbonyl 202
4,4'-methylene-bis-2-chloroaniline (MOCA) 353, 354–5
   biological monitoring guidance values 62
methylene chloride *see* dichloromethane

methylenedianiline (MDA) 354
   biological monitoring guidance values 62
methylenediphenyl diisocyanate (MDI) 36, 364
4,4-methylenediphenyl isocyanate 364
methylhexahydrophthalic anhydride 363, 364
methylhippuric acid (analyte) 62
N-methyl acetamide (analyte) 61
Methylophilus methylotrophus and *M. methanolica* in biotechnology 789
methylpentane (isohexane) 322
4-methylpentan-2-one *see* methyl iso-butyl ketone
2-methylpropane (isobutane) 301, 322
N-methylpyrrolidone 356
methyl-*tert*-butylether (MTBE) 340–1
methyltetrahydrophthalic anhydride 363, 364
N-methylthiobenzamide 136
Mexico City (explosion) 253
micas 1035–6
microbes *see* micro-organisms
α1-microglobulin and cadmium 1132
β2-microglobulin
   and cadmium 168, 169, 170, 1132
   and lead 1128
microgravity 609, 610
   medical emergencies in 611–13
   (patho)physiology 609–10
      methods of counteracting 613
   research and ground-based analogues 613
micronutrients
   essential, metals as *see* essential metals
   lead poisoning treatment 1130
micro-organisms/microbes
   in biotechnology 783, 785, 785–6
      risks and hazards and their management 788, 789, 791, 792, 793, 795, 796
   disease due to *see* bioterrorism; infections
   indoor non-industrial environments and dampness and 923
      extrinsic allergic alveolitis and 928
   inhalation fever 438
   as pesticides 395
   see also specific types
microprocessor chips 445
microsomal epoxide hydrolase and byssinosis 962
microwaves (short waves)
   eye damage 655
   reproductive effects 1199, 1207

middle ear
    anatomy and physiology 461–2
    barotrauma, divers 549
    effects of disease 468
migraine headaches, high altitude
        Mauna Kea 574
    treatment 583
miliaria rubra 538
military targets, gases at 254
    see also warfare
mill fever 958–9
Minamata disease 215, 1135
mineral dusts see inorganic dust diseases
mineral oils
    and lung cancer and chrysotile 1005
    and skin cancer 1093
mining
    coal see coalworkers' diseases
    dermatoses 1073
    gases 268
    gold 183
    historical perspectives 7, 7–8, 14
    manganese 201, 203, 207
    radon exposure 633
    silicosis risk 1017, 1022
miscarriage (spontaneous abortion) 1201–2
mists see vapours and mists
mitochondria and nanoparticles 909
mitral valve prolapse and high altitude 579
mobbing 837
mobile phones 676, 678
MOCA see 4,4'-methylene-bis-2-chloroaniline
moisture see dampness and moisture
moisturizers and emollients 1067
molecular mechanisms, carcinogenesis 27, 1112
molluscicides 402, 412
molybdenum 221–2
Mond process 224, 298
monitoring see biological monitoring; surveillance
monkeypox 764
monochloramine 279
monochloroacetic acid 346–7
monoclonal antibodies 785, 787
monocyte chemotactive protein-1 and diisocyanate asthma 948
monofilaments in assessment of hand–arm vibration syndrome 494, 503, 504
monomethylamine 289
montmorillonite 1036
Montreal Protocol and CFCs 265, 372
mood disorders see anxiety; depression

morbidity ratio, standardized 78
'more or less' diseases 92, 93–4
mortality (mortalities; deaths) 25–6
    alcohol 861
    asbestos, epidemiology 26
        lung cancer 1005, 1007
        mesothelioma 1003, 1091
    cancers (in general), Europe and North America, numbers 1098, 1099
    cotton workers 965
    in epidemiological studies 78
    firefighters 261
    high altitude 575, 579
        at Mauna Kea 584
    immersion 533
    lead poisoning 1130
    polonium 232
    proportional 85
    routine analyses 85–6
    shift work 1237–8
    silica-related lung cancer, risk 1023–4
    thallium 236
    welding (sudden) 429
    see also death certificates; lethal dose; post-mortem examination; suicide
mortality rates 78
    in cohort studies 82
    proportional 85, 86
mortality ratio, standardized (SMR) 78
    in cohort studies 82
    in risk of death assessment 85–6
Morton, William 298
Morvan's fibrillary chorea 204
mosquito control 395
motion sickness
    flying 602–3
    space 609
motor neurone disease (amyotrophic lateral sclerosis) and electromagnetic fields 670, 671
motor pathology, hand–arm vibration syndrome 492, 493
    assessment 504
mould (with dampness) 923, 924
    asthma and 927
    extrinsic allergic alveolitis and 978, 979
    prevention 933
moulders 1018
mountains see acute mountain sickness; high altitude
movement disorder, manganism 204, 206
MPTP (methyl phenyl pyridinium) 1161
trans-muconic acid 326, 327
muffs, ear 472–3
mukluk boots 542

multidisciplinary biopsychosocial rehabilitation, back pain 721
multidrug-resistant tuberculosis 740
multislice CT 877
muscarinic receptors, insecticide effects 404
    management 410–11, 411
muscle disease/disorders (incl. weakness)
    astronauts 610
    hand–arm vibration syndrome 493–4, 500–2
musculoskeletal disorders 687–712
    astronauts 610
    decompression sickness 552, 553
    indentifying 705–6
    lead 193
    preventing 706–7
    repeated movements and trauma 687–712
        hand–arm vibration syndrome 502
    risk factors and intervention studies 702–5
    welding 432
mushroom-worker's lung 979
mustard gas 314, 316
mutagenicity
    acrylamides 351
    manganese 203
    polyaromatic hydrocarbons 333
Mycobacterium marinum 764
Mycobacterium tuberculosis see tuberculosis
myelodysplasia and myelodysplastic syndrome 1222
    benzene and 1223
    case report 1226
myeloid leukaemia, acute see acute myeloid leukaemia
myocardial infarction (heart attack), work stressors associated with 840
    shift work 1236
myoglobin, iron in 185
Myvatn, Lake 303

N-substituted amides 1181–2
NADPH, red cell, and its deficiency 1217
NADPH:methaemoglobin reductase deficiency 1220
naltrexone 866
nanoparticles and ultrafine particles 903–20
    deliberate exposure (applications) 906–7
    exposure measurement 914–16
    in extrapulmonary sites 908–9
    risk assessment 913–14
    technology 784, 907–9

nanoparticles and ultrafine particles
(*Continued*)
  toxicology 904–9
    chamber studies 909–10
    epidemiological studies 910–13
  types and classification 904, 913
  welding 424, 904, 910–11
nanotubes 906
naphthacene 332
naphthalenes 332–3
  chlorinated 1182
naphthylamines 354
  bladder cancer 1089, 1101
α-naphthylthiourea (ANTU) 136
nasal cancers 1093–5
  epidemiology 1093–5
  formaldehyde 338
  nickel 223
  polyaromatic hydrocarbons 333
nasal challenge, diesel exhaust particles 909–10
nasal septal perforation, chromium 173, 433
nasal sinuses *see* paranasal sinuses
nasopharyngeal cancer epidemiology 1095
NAT2 acetylation status and bladder cancer 1113
National Health and Nutrition Examination Survey (NHANES)
  chronic obstruction pulmonary disease definition 890
  lead and cardiovascular disease risk 1131
National Health Insurance 13
National Institute for Health and Clinical Excellence (NICE) guidelines, psychological interventions 823–4
National Insurance (Industrial Injuries) Act (1946) 97
natural gas 268, 291
neck problems 688, 691–2
  welders 432
needle stick and sharps injuries 731–2
negligence, contributory 99
neon 273
nephrotic syndrome, mercury 1135
nephrotoxicity (renal/kidney toxicity) 1125–51
  ethylene glycol 337–8
  markers *see* biomarkers
  metals and metalloids 1125–37
    arsenic compounds 294, 1137
    cadmium 168–9, 170, 1131–4
    lead 192–3, 1126–31
    mercury 217, 218, 1134–6

    uranium 244, 1136
  organic compounds
    chloroform and carbon tetrachloride 369
    pesticides 398, 405
    solvents 1138–41
  silica 1024, 1137–8
nerve
  biopsy, hand–arm vibration syndrome 505
  conduction studies
    carpal tunnel syndrome 498, 499, 696
    lead poisoning 1158
nerve agents
  terrorism 315, 316
  warfare 314
nested case–control studies 83
  cancer 1107
neural reflexes, pulmonary, nanoparticles 908–9
neural retina 647–8
neuroborreliosis 763
neuroimaging (brain)
  high altitude climbers 576
  manganism 205, 206–7, 208, 1158
neurological
  problems/symptoms/dysfunction (physical causes to primarily CNS incl. neurobehavioural and cognitive effects)
    divers 562
      decompression sickness 551–2
    electromagnetic fields 669–70
    in hand–arm vibration syndrome 491–2, 497–9
      assessment 502–3, 505
      signs and symptoms 494–5, 502–3
    ionizing radiation 628
neuromuscular dysfunction, hand–arm vibration syndrome 493–4
neuropathy *see* peripheral neurotoxicity
neurotoxicity (of chemicals to primarily CNS incl. neuropsychiatric damage) 1151–70
  assessment for 1151–2
  biological effect monitoring markers 66
  carbon monoxide 275, 1154
  defining criteria 1151
  metals/metalloids 1156–9
    aluminium 154–5, 1156–7
    cadmium 169
    lead 193, 1157–8
    manganese 204, 206, 208, 1158–9
    mercury 217, 217–18, 1159
    thallium 236
    tin 239

  organic chemicals 1152–6, 1159–64
    acrylamides 351, 1152
    carbon disulphide 374, 1154
    chlorinated hydrocarbons 366, 1153, 1161
    ethylene oxide 297, 1155
    n-hexane 323, 1156
    methanol 336
    methyl *n*-butyl ketone 340, 1156
    methyl methacrylate 347–8
    pesticides *see subheading below*
    solvents 328–9, 330–1, 1153, 1156, 1162–3
    white spirits 335
  oxygen (divers) 548
  pesticides 397, 398, 399, 404, 405, 407–8, 411, 1160–2
    management 411
  smoke 261
  see also brain; peripheral neurotoxicity
neurotransmission and lead 192
neutrons 624
neutrophil gelatinase-associated lipocalin (NGAL) 68
NHANES *see* National Health and Nutrition Examination Survey
NICE guidelines, psychological interventions 823–4
nickel 223–4
  alloys 223, 225
    beryllium–nickel 163
  biological monitoring guidance values 62
  bronchial asthma 223–4, 1042–3
  carcinogenicity 223, 1086–7, 1093, 1094
  welding-related compounds of 425
nickel/cadmium batteries 167
nickel carbonyl 224, 298
nicotinamide adenine dinucleotide phosphate *see* NADPH
nicotinic junctions, insecticide effects 404
  management 410–11
nifedipine
  altitude sickness
    preventive use 583
    therapeutic use 583–4
  hand–arm vibration syndrome 507
night vision, aircrew 600–1
night work *see* shift work
9/11 (World Trade Center) attacks, firefighter deaths 261
Nipah virus 756
nitric oxide 257
  measurement 67
nitriles 352–3
  as herbicides 401

nitroaromatics, hepatotoxicity 1182–3
nitrobenzoate 1183
nitrogen (gas) 272
   narcosis, divers 548–9
nitrogen compounds, heterocyclic 356–7
nitrogen-containing hydrocarbons 348–57
nitrogen dioxide 257, 290–1
   WHO air quality guidelines 142
nitrogen oxides (in general) 290–1
   welding 426, 427
nitrogen trichloride 279
nitrogen trifluoride 286
nitroparaffins 1182
2-nitropropane 1182
N-nitrosamines 357
nitrosyl chloride 281
nitrous oxide 298–9, 300
   reproductive toxicity 1205
NMP22 Test Kit 68–9, 69
no adverse effect level (NOAEL) 142
nodules, pulmonary, in coalworker's pneumoconiosis 879
   in Caplan's syndrome 879, 1032
noise 49, 459–85
   aircraft 598
   hearing loss due to see noise
   measurement 471–2
   reduction measures 472–4
   semiconductor production 449
   systemic effects 481–2
   tinnitus due to 480
   vertigo due to 480
   welding 431
non-discrimination (in precautionary principle) 146
non-freezing cold injury 531–2
non-Hodgkin's lymphoma 1225–6
   and benzene 1223–4
   and electromagnetic fields 667
   and phenoxy acid herbicides 401, 409
   and radiofrequency fields 677
non-ionizing radiation see radiation
non-randomized controlled experiments 81
non-steroidal anti-inflammatory drugs (NSAIDs)
   altitude sickness-related headache 583
   osteoarthritis 702
nonylphenol 359–60
Nordic questionnaire 705–6
North America see United States and North America
Norway, compensation schemes 105
nose see rhinitis and entries under nasal
nuclear magnetic resonance imaging see magnetic resonance imaging

nuclear power reactors 638–40
   incidents 262–3, 638–40
   occupational doses 632
nuclear weapon and atomic weapon explosions 629, 630
   flash blindness 599–600, 655
nucleic acid extraction 790
nuisance dusts 905
nylon fibres 1012
Nyos, Lake (Cameroon) 270

obesity and overweight
   osteoarthritis and 702
   shift work and 1236
observational studies of disease causation 89–90
occupants, indoor air pollution by 922
occupation see work
occupational history see history-taking
Occupational Safety and Health Administration (OSHA) 37, 40
   cadmium exposure limits 1133–4
   vanadium dust exposure limits 247
ocular effects see eye
odds ratio 79
odour, bad, sulphur compounds 293
oedema, cerebral, high-altitude 573–5
   treatment 585
oedema, pulmonary
   cadmium 168
   chlorine 263, 264, 278, 279
   high-altitude (HAPO) 573, 574
      prevention 583
      treatment 585
   hydrogen sulphide 292
   immersion 554
   nitrogen dioxide 291
oestrogen and progestogen combined oral contraceptive and high altitude 576, 577
office environment (incl. equipment and materials) 925
   asthma and 928
   dermatoses and 1073
   reproductive hazards 1206
   sick building syndrome and 930
   thermal challenges 540
oil, see also fuel oils; mineral oils; petroleum oil; soluble oils
olfactory dysfunction, cadmium 168
Oliver, Thomas 5, 12
on-scene medical care in terrorist chemical attack 317
oncogenes 789, 795
opacities
   lens see cataracts

radiography, in ILO classification 880, 885
opencast coal mining exposures 1029
ophthalmic instruments, light from 651
ophthalmological effects see eye
opiate abuse, treatment 866
optical radiation see light
oral contraceptives and high altitude 576, 577
oral lethal dose (LD), toxicity rating by 127
ores
   beryllium 162
   magnesium 199
   manganese 201, 202, 207
   mining see mining
   platinum group metal-containing 226
   refining see refining
   vanadium 246
   zinc 249
orf 764–5
organ of Corti 462–3
   see also tissues and organs
organic compounds 321–94
   carcinogenic see carcinogens
   haematological disorders 1222–4
   lead in 188, 190, 195
      in petrol see petrol
   mercury 214, 215, 216, 217, 218
   nephrotoxicity see nephrotoxicity
   neurotoxicity see neurotoxicity
   reproductive toxicity see reproductive effects
   semiconductor production 447, 448
   tin 238–9
   volatile see volatile compounds
   welding close to 427
organic dusts 939–82
   toxic syndrome with pig or hog farming 267
organization
   as cause of psychiatric disorder
      in downsizing/retrenching/rightsizing in 839
      position in 835
   impact of psychiatric disorder on 843–5
   preventive strategies with psychiatric disorders 847
   see also workplace
organochlorines (chlorinated organic compounds) 27
   chlorinated naphthalenes 1182
   insecticidal 399
      acute effects 404
      carcinogenic effects 409
      management of acute poisoning 411
      neurotoxicity 366, 1153, 1161
      reproductive effects 1199

organophosphates/organophosphorus
   compounds 396, 404, 410–11,
   1160–1
  acute effects 404
   management 410–11
  attribution of Parkinson's disease to
   exposure in case study 52–3
  chronic effects 407–8
  mechanisms of toxicity 397, 402
  metabolism 133
  monitoring 66, 415, 415–16, 417
  neurotoxicity 397, 404, 407–8, 411,
   1160–1
  warfare 314
ornithosis 753
orthostatic intolerance, astronauts
   609–10
OSHA see Occupational Safety and
   Health Administration
osmium 229
osteoarthritis 699–702
  hand–arm vibration syndrome 505
osteofluorosis 282–3
osteomalacia, cadmium 169
osteonecrosis, dysbaric 553, 561–2, 566
otoacoustic emissions 479–80
otological effects of physical agents see
   hearing loss
ototoxicity of chemicals (incl. hearing loss)
  aromatic solvents 329
   styrene 329, 1162
   toluene 329, 1163
  chlorinated hydrocarbons 366
outdoor (ambient) air 265–6
  indoor air quality affected by 921–2
  pollution see pollution
outer ear, anatomy and physiology 461
Ovako Working Posture Analysing
   System 703–5
overload/overwork 815–16
overweight see obesity
Owen, Robert 9, 10
oxidation 134–5
  semiconductor production 447, 448
oxidative stress see free radicals
oximes
  AChE-inhibiting pesticides 315, 410,
   411, 1160
  sarin 316
oxygen
  at altitude, provision
   flying 593–4, 596–7
   high-altitude workers 581
  deficiency/depletion (in
   air/atmosphere) 266
   in confined spaces 267
   in fires 258

   nitrogen release and 272
   see also hypoxia
  divers
   enrichment of breathing mixtures
    with 558–9
   importance 548
   toxicity 548
   see also helium–oxygen mixtures
  excess in air/atmosphere 266
  reactive species see free radicals
  treatment with 262–3
   altitude sickness 583, 584
   CO poisoning 275
   cyanide poisoning 318
oxygen difluoride 285
ozone 289–90
  inhalational challenge with diesel
   exhaust particles and effects of
   910
  risk assessment 142
  welding 426

p53 (TP53) 27, 1112
P450 enzymes see cytochrome P450
   enzymes
pacemakers and electromagnetic fields 670
pain (musculoskeletal) 688–702, 703
  back see back pain
  decompression sickness 552, 553
  welders 432
painting
  dermatoses 1073
  hepatotoxic chemicals 1174
  reproductive hazards 1203
palladium 227–8
  fine particles 905
palygorskite 1011
pancreatic cancer epidemiology 1096
pancytopenia, case report 1226
paper, carbonless copy/self-copying 925,
   928
para-amino salicylic acid (PAS),
   manganese 208
Paracelsus 7, 8, 127
paraesthesias, pyrethroids 1161
paranasal sinuses
  at altitude (incl. flying) 593
  cancers 1093–5
   epidemiology 1093–5
   nickel 223, 1093, 1094
  divers, barotrauma 549
paraoxon, parathion metabolism to 133,
   134–5
paraquat 399–400, 1162, 1186
  acute effects 405
   management 411–12
  hepatotoxicity 1186

parasites
  ectoparasites 740–1, 1061
  zoonotic 758–9, 761–2, 765
parathion metabolism 133, 134–5
parental exposures
  cancer in offspring and see children
  developmental toxicity 1200–1
parietal pleural plaques, asbestos 995
Paris green 160
Parkinson's disease/idiopathic
   parkinsonism 1161–2
  manganese and
   distinction 205
   manganese as cause 207, 426, 1158
  pesticides and 408, 1161–2
   attribution to organophosphate
    exposure in case study 52–3
paronychia 739
paroxysmal atrial tachycardia, high
   altitude 579
participatory ergonomics in back pain
   prevention 718–19
particulate matter
  measuring exposure 45, 46
  ultrafine see nanoparticles and
   ultrafine particles
  welding see welding
parvovirus B19 739
  in pregnancy 1208
passengers, fitness to fly 607
past jobs, history-taking 33
patch tests (skin), allergic contact
   dermatitis 1065–6
pathogenic microbes see bioterrorism;
   infections
pathogenicity (of host microbes),
   accidental modification 792
pathology, definition 28
Pathways to Work programme 818
patients, healthcare worker infections
   transmitted to 733–4
peak (expiratory) flow (PEF)
  asthma 948–9
  byssinosis 963, 964
penicillamine
  copper 181
  lead 194
pensioning, disability, psychiatric
   disorders 844
pentachlorophenol 358, 359, 405
  endocrine effects 408
perceptions of risk (peoples') varying
   with specific risk 146
perchloroethene (tetrachloroethene;
   tetrachloroethylene) 366–7, 1140
perchloryl fluoride 285
performance

chronic alcohol use and 860
shift work and 1234
thermal challenges
  cold 534
  heat 538
perfusion pressure in hand–arm vibration syndrome 492
peripheral neurotoxicity (neuropathy and polyneuropathy)
  AChE-inhibiting pesticides 1160–1
  acrylamides 351, 1152–3
  allyl chloride 1153
  assessment for 1152
  biological effect monitoring markers 66
  cadmium 169
  ethylene oxide 297, 1155
  lead 193, 1157–8
  mercury 218
  methyl bromide 1159
  methyl n-butyl ketone 340, 1156
peritendinitis 693–4
peritoneal mesothelioma see mesothelioma
personal protective equipment (PPE) 37, 49–50
  contact dermatitis 1067
  ears see ears
  firefighters 541
  pesticides 413
  thermal stress 540–2
    cold immersion 533
  welding 428, 431
personal sampling, nanoparticles 914, 916
personality disorders 843
personality traits and shift work tolerance 1238
perstimulatory fatigue (adaptation to noise) 465
pesticides (and other agrochemicals) 395–420, 1160–2
  acetylcholinesterase-inhibiting see acetylcholinesterase inhibitors
  attribution of disease to exposure in case study 52–3
  biotransformation 133, 134
  carcinogenic 401, 409, 1083, 1084
    IARC classification 1083, 1084, 1086
  classification 395–6, 398–9
  lymphomas and 1225–6
  monitoring 61, 66, 412–16
  operators
    exposure 412–16
    training 416
  production (industry) 1174
  toxicity/poisoning
    acute effects 403–6
    chronic/long-term effects 406–9

  epidemiology 403
  hepatic 1174, 1185–6
  management of acute poisoning 409–12
  mechanisms 397–403
  neurological 397, 404, 407–8, 411, 1160–2
  oncological see carcinogenic (subheading above)
  reproductive 1199, 1200, 1206
petrochemicals, steatohepatitis 1183
petrol (gasoline), lead in (as anti-knock agent) 188, 189, 193, 195
  substitute for 202
petroleum gases, liquefied 301–2
petroleum oil
  folliculitis 1069
  Gulf War oil well fires 260
petroleum solvents 334, 335–6
phagocytosis 128
Phalen's test
  carpal tunnel syndrome 497–8, 696
  hand–arm vibration syndrome 497–8, 498, 499, 503
pharmaceuticals
  bioengineered 786–7
  dermatoses in production of 1072
  reproductive toxicity 1205
  see also drugs
phase 1 metabolism 133
phase 2 (conjugation) reactions 133, 135
phased return to work, psychiatric disorders 844
phenobarbitone detoxification 133
phenol 357–8
  derivatives 358–9
phenoxy acid herbicides (incl. chlorophenoxy acids) 400–1, 1186
  acute effects 405
    management 412
  carcinogenicity 409
    exposure evaluation 1111
  hepatotoxicity 1186
p-phenylenediaminephenylglycolic acid (PPD), prick test 1067
phenylglycolic acid (analyte) 62
phenylhydrazine 355
S-phenylmercapturic acid (analyte) 61
phobia/phobic anxiety
  work ability and 842
  workplace 812
phosgene 279–80
  warfare 314
phosphine (hydrogen phosphide) 295–6
  semiconductor production 448
phosphodiesterase inhibitors, altitude sickness prevention 582, 583

N-(phosphonomethyl)glycine (glyphosate) 412
phosphorus 225, 1185
  hepatotoxicity 1185
  historical perspectives 11, 225
phosphorus pentafluoride 285
phosphorus trifluoride 285
photochemical damage to eye 649
photochemical smog 290
photoconjunctivitis 650–1
photocopiers 925
photographic processing, dermatoses 1073
photokeratitis see cornea
photolithography 446, 451
photoreceptors 647
photorefractive keratotomy, aircrew 600
photoresist (silicon wafer coating) 446
photosensitization 655–6
phototoxicity, polyaromatic hydrocarbons 333
phototransduction 648
phthalates 922–3, 1118
phthalic anhydride 363, 364
physical agents (hazardous) 455–681
  biotechnology industry 791
  carcinogenic, IARC classification 1083, 1084, 1086
  indoor sources 922–3
  sick building syndrome and 932
  semiconductor production 448–9
Physical Agents Vibration Directive 505–6
  exposure action value (EAV) 506
physical containment, genetically-modified organisms 793, 794
physical disorders see disease; medical conditions
physical examination/medical examination
  in back pain prevention, pre-employment 719
  byssinosis 963
  haematological disorders 1218–19
  hand–arm vibration syndrome 503
  noise-induced hearing loss 469
  shift workers 1240, 1241
physical exercises see exercises
physical methods of radiation detection 625
physical properties 36
  beryllium 162
physical workload and pregnancy outcome 1207
physicians see doctors
physiological factors affecting biological monitoring 59

pig and hog farming
  organic dust toxic dust syndrome 267
  Streptococcus suis and 758
pigeon-handlers *see* bird-handlers
pigment(s), arsenic 160
pigment epithelium, retinal 648
pinocytosis 128
pipe systems, methane 269
piperazine 356
plague, bioterrorism 775–6
plants
  dermatoses associated with 1073
  genetically-modified 793
  products derived from
    pesticide 396
    protection from biological
      degradation 395
  see also greenhouse workers;
    herbicides; horticulture
plaster of Paris 1037
plastic extruders, reproductive hazards
  1203
plastic laminating, reinforced,
  reproductive hazards 1203
plasticizers 1188
  indoor non-industrial sources
    922–3
platinum 226–7
  bronchial asthma and complex salts of
    1042–3
platinum group metals 226–30
pleural disease, asbestos-related 95,
  880–2, 994–6, 1002–3
  attribution 95
  benign 994–6
  epidemiology 1002–3
  historical perspectives 16
  imaging 880–2, 992, 993
  malignant *see* mesothelioma
  see also mesothelioma
pleural features (incl. thickening/plaques/
    calcification)
  asbestosis 992, 994–6
  in ILO classification of
    pneumoconiosis 880, 885, 995
  see also effusions
plugs, ear 473
plutonium, internal exposure and
  contamination 636, 638
pneumoconiosis *see* inorganic dust
  diseases
pneumocytes (alveolar epithelial cells),
  type 1 138
pneumomediastinum, divers 550
pneumonia
  bronchial, high altitude 574
  lobar, welders 433

pneumonic plague 776
pneumonitis
  hypersensitivity *see* extrinsic allergic
    alveolitis
  metals 1041
    cobalt/hard metal 176, 1046
    manganese 203
    mercury 218
  ventilation 980
  welding 433
pneumothorax, divers 550
policies (incl. government)
  incapacity benefit and return to work
    817
  reporting of back pain to inform
    policy-making 719
  substance abuse 865
polishers, silicosis 1017
pollution
  air 256
    asthma in 144
    indoor *see* indoor environments
    SO$_2$ 287, 288
  noise *see* noise
polonium 231–3
polychlorinated biphenyls (PCBs)
  371–2, 1186
polychlorinated naphthalenes 1182
polycyclic aromatic hydrocarbons
  (PAHs) 332–4
  carcinogenicity
    bladder cancer 1089
    IARC classification 1083, 1084,
      1086
    lung cancer 1087
  monitoring 62, 63, 334
polyethylene glycol in phenol poisoning
  358
polymer fever 437–8
polymeric methylenediphenyl
  diisocyanate (polymeric MDI) 364
polymorphisms, genetic
  asthma susceptibility and 946
  detoxifying enzymes 128
  single nucleotide (SNPs), as cancer
    susceptibility markers 1113, 1114
polyneuropathy *see* peripheral
  neurotoxicity
polyphenols and byssinosis 960
polytetrafluoroethylene, inhalation of
  pyrolysis products 437–8
polyvinyl chloride (PVC) 302, 368, 369
  in fires 260
  indoor non-industrial sources 922–3
Pontiac fever 438, 930
popcorn worker's lung' 899
Popper, Karl, and causality 144

population(s) (in epidemiological
    studies)
  asthma 944–5
  chronic obstruction pulmonary
    disease 899–900
  samples 79
population attributable fraction 79
population-based interventions,
  psychiatric disorders 848
pork finger 763
porphyrins 1175–6
  disturbances 1175–6
  lead and 63–4, 192, 196, 197
  vanadium and 247
portable direct-reading instruments 46
portal hypertension 1175
positive pressure breathing, flying 596,
  597
positron emission tomography (PET),
  manganism 206, 1158
possession outbreak in factories 808–9
post-menopausal women, cadmium-
  associated osteomalacia 169
post-mortem examination, inorganic
  dust diseases 988
post-stimulatory fatigue 465–6
post-traumatic (dis)tress syndrome
    (PTSD) 811, 814
  gassing 263
  warfare 814, 838, 1164
posture
  observation and recoding 703–5
  sedentary, testicular temperature and
    1199
pot room asthma 283–4, 1043
potassium, heat illness-related
  disturbances 538
potassium permanganate 202, 203
pottery industry 1017–18, 1034
powders, aluminium 153, 154, 155
  see also dust; nanoparticles
pralidoxime, AChE-inhibiting pesticides
  410, 411, 1160
precarious employment 839
precautionary principle 146
precipitins, serum, extrinsic allergic
  alveolitis 976–7
predictive models of adverse effects 142
prednisone, berylliosis 1052
pre-employment examination in back
  pain prevention 719
pre-excitation syndrome, high altitude
  579
pregnancy 931–3, 1201–8
  carbon monoxide and 276
  indoor non-industrial environments
    and 931–3

loss/termination *see* abortion
manganese and 203
mercury and 219
occupational risk for adverse outcome 1204–8
risk assessment and clinical counselling 1208–9
VDUs and 668–9
see also developmental toxicity; reproductive effects
pre-launch, spacecraft 608
premature (preterm) birth 1202, 1204
prescribed disease 97, 98, 100–1
examples of prescription 101–4
present job, history-taking 33
presenteeism, sickness 843
pressure
barometric 545–624
perfusion, in hand–arm vibration syndrome 492
pressure breathing, flying 596, 597
preterm birth 1202, 1204
prevalence 78
prevention and control (of exposures and related diseases/disorders) 44, 49–50
asthma 946–7
back pain 718–19
berylliosis 164, 1052
blood-borne viral infections in healthcare workers 735–6
byssinosis 965–6
cadmium 1134
cancer 1103–4
contact dermatitis 1065, 1067
high-altitude sickness 581–3, 585
history 10–11, 24
indoor non-industrial exposures 933–4
lead nephropathy 1130
psychiatric disorders 847
astronauts 610–11
shift work-related problems 1239–40
silicosis *see* silicosis
silicotuberculosis 1017
substance abuse 868
welding processes 428
whole-body vibration 519–20
see also protection
previous jobs, history-taking 33
prick tests (skin) 1066
respiratory sensitizers 947
prickly heat 538
Priestley, Joseph 253, 269, 298
primaquine 742
primary prevention
cancer 1103–4

lead nephropathy 1130
psychiatric disorders 847
primates, infection risk to staff working with 741
printing processes, dermatoses 1073
prions 789, 795
probability
of causation (concept of), radiation 630
levels of, in accepting attribution of disease 92
professional bodies, expert witness immunity from powers of 120
progenitor cells, haemopoietic 1215–16
deficits in production 1221
progestogen-only contraceptives and high altitude 576, 577
promethazine, air sickness 603
propane 301, 322
prophylaxis *see* prevention
proportional mortality 78
rate (PMR), risk of death estimation 85, 86
proportionality (in precautionary principle) 146
propylene 301, 322
propylene glycol methylether 345–6
propylene oxide 360–1
n-propyl bromide (1-bromopropane) 1153–4
prospective cohort study 82
prostate cancer
cadmium and 169
electromagnetic fields and 667
protection
eyes 656–9
flying 599–600
from light 656–9
firefighters 260, 261, 541
flying
chemicals 604
eyes 599–600
fatigue and jet-lag 603–4
gravitational stress 596
noise 598
spatial disorientation 602
vibration 599
ionizing radiation 633–4
hospital staff 638
from psychological problems (individual's) 825
thermal stress 540–2
cold immersion 533
see also personal protective equipment
protein(s), bioengineered 786–7
protein contact dermatitis 1069

proteinuria
cadmium 168–9, 1132
mercury 1134, 1135
organic solvents 1139–40
Protocol for the Instruction of Experts to Give Evidence in Civil Claims 115–16
protozoan infections, zoonotic 758–9, 761–2
provocational testing by inhalation *see* inhalation challenge
Prussian blue with thallium poisoning 236–7
pseudo-epidemics of skin problems 1071
Pseudomonas aeruginosa in biotechnology 789
pseudotumours, pulmonary, asbestosis 883
psittacosis (*Chlamydophila psittaci* infection) 753
pulmonary disease, imaging 885
psoralens 655–6
psoriasis 1070
frictional 1062
psychological (psychiatric and behavioural) disorders 799–856
astronauts, and its prevention 610–11
chemical agents associated with
aluminium 155
cadmium 169
lead 193
manganese 206, 208
mercury 218
comorbid with physical disorders 845
effect of work on development of 833–6, 845–7
interventions targeting 847–8
effect on work ability incl. impaired function 842–3
evidence-based approach 833–56
expert witness 115
organizational effects 843–5
physical agents associated with
electromagnetic fields 669–70
radiofrequency fields 676
shift work and 1235
see also anxiety; mental health; neurological problems; neurotoxicity; stress
psychological interventions 823–31
case formulation 824–5, 829
case studies 825–9
limitations 829
psychomotor function and high altitude 575–6

psychosocial risk factors
  in low back pain
    for chronicity 720
    for occurrence 718
  for physical disorders (in general) 840–2
  for shift work intolerance 1238
psychosocial stress *see* stress
psychosocial work environment 836–42
psychosomatic disorders, shift workers 1239
psychotropic drugs
  abuse *see* substance abuse
  therapeutic use 813
PTFE, inhalation of pyrolysis products 437–8
public, communicating about risk to 144–7
public health
  indoor non-industrial hazards impacting on 933
  mosquito control 395
pulmonary artery gas embolism, divers 550
pulmonary syndrome, hantavirus 756
  see also lung
Purdue pegboard test, hand–arm vibration syndrome 494, 504
pustular dermatitis, salmonellosis 760
Puumala virus 756
PUVA (psoralens and UV-A) 656
pyrethrins and synthetic pyrethroids 399, 1161
  acute effects 405
    management 411
pyrexia (fever), zoonoses presenting with 751
pyromellitic dianhydride 363
pyrrolidones 356

Q fever (*Coxiella burnetii* infection) 754
  pulmonary imaging 885
quality assurance in biological monitoring 60
quantitative sensorineural tests (QSTs), hand–arm vibration syndrome 494, 505
quartz and related dusts 1014–15
  coalworker exposure 1029
questionnaires, carcinogen exposure evaluation 1109–10

rabies 765–6
radial keratotomy, aircrew 600
radiation 621–81
  ionizing *see* ionizing
  non-ionizing 644–81

  definition 644
  eye and *see* eye
  haematological effects 1225
  reproductive effects 1199, 1207
  in semiconductor production 449
  welding 423–4
radioactivity 623–4
  metallic elements 231–3, 243
  cobalt-60 isotope 175
radioallergosorbent test (RAST) 66
radiofrequency fields 675–9
radiographers 632–3
radiography *see* digital imaging; X-ray radiography
radiology *see* imaging
radionuclide studies of lung 879
radon 632
  lung cancer and 1043
  occupational doses 633
Ramazzini, Bernadino 7–9
randomization 80–1
randomized controlled experimental studies 80–1
randomized crossover studies 81
Rapid Upper Limb Assessment (RULA) technique 705
rare earth metals 1045
rare gases 271, 272
Ravenhill TH and altitude sickness 570, 571, 575
Raynaud's disease or phenomenon (RP)
  vibration-induced 491, 492–3, 495–7, 503
  treatment 507
  vinyl chloride 368
REACH initiative 1103
reactive airways dysfunction syndrome (RADS) 264, 310–13, 895
  chlorine 279
  clinical picture 311–12
  epidemiology 311
  pathology 312
  prognosis 312
  terminology and definitions 310–11
reactive oxygen species *see* free radicals
reassurance with ionizing radiation 635
reception centre for nuclear reactor accident victims 639–40
reconstruction algorithms in conventional vs high-resolution CT 877
records, medical/health
  in genetic modification work 796
  radiation overexposure 636
red blood cells (erythrocytes)
  destruction, accelerated *see* haemolytic anaemia
  pesticide effects 398

  stippling (basophilic) 1219
  lead 194, 1219, 1221
red flags, back pain 719
Reduced Earnings Allowance (originally Special Hardship Allowance; SHA) 97, 98–9, 100
reduction (reactions) 135
re-entry, spacecraft 609
refining
  aluminium 153
  gold 183
  manganese 202
  nickel 223
  platinum group metals 226, 227, 228, 229
  silver 235
  uranium 243
  vanadium 236
refractory materials manufacture 1017–18
regional cooling wear 541
registers (disease), attribution of disease 94–5
regulations *see* law
reinforced plastics laminating, reproductive hazards 1203
relative risk 79
renal cell cancer and lead 1131
renal syndrome, haemorrhagic fever with 756
  see also kidney; nephrotoxicity
repeated movements 687–712
repetitive strain injury (RSI) 696–8
reporting of back pain to inform policy-making 719
  see also medicolegal reports
reproductive effects/toxicity (incl. fertility) 1196–214
  counselling *see* counselling
  databases 1209
  epidemiology of infertility 1196–7
  mechanisms of infertility 1197–8
  metals 1, 1199, 1200, 1202, 1206
    lead 193, 1200, 1206
  organic compounds 1199, 1205, 1206
    carbon disulphide 375
    dimethylacetamide 350
    dimethylformamide 348–9
    glycol ethers 342, 343, 345, 346, 1199, 1205
    solvents 1199, 1199–200, 1205
  radiation 1206–7
    electromagnetic fields 668–9, 1199, 1207
    ionizing 627–8, 1198, 1206–7
    radiofrequency fields 678–9
  range of 1196

risk assessment 1208–9
risk management 1209–10
semiconductor production 450–1, 1203, 1205
shift work 1207–8, 1237
welding 435, 1200
see also developmental toxicity; females; males; pregnancy
research
cancer epidemiology, methodological issues 1104–11
future, berylliosis 1052
spaceflight health 613
see also laboratory studies; laboratory workers
resentment and sickness absence 816–17
resilience to catastrophic events 815
resistance, sickness absence as form of 806–7
resorcinol 359
respiratory disorders 871–1055
biomarkers 66–7
cotton workers 961–2, 962–3, 964–5
disability benefit see disability benefit
gases 263–4, 310–13
ammonia 289
chlorine 263, 278–9
hydrogen sulphide 292
nitrogen oxides 291
ozone 289, 290
sulphur dioxide 288
general issues 873–931
high altitude 573, 574
pre-existing 580
imaging 875–88
inorganic dust-related see inorganic dust disease
metals and metalloids
aluminium 154
cadmium 168
cobalt 176
manganese 203
mercury 218
nickel 223–4
tungsten 241
vanadium 246–7
organic compounds
cyclic acid anhydrides 362
dusts see organic dusts
isocyanates 53–4, 364, 364–5
welding 421–2, 432–5, 911
see also inhalation; inhalation fevers; lung and entries under pneumo-
respiratory distress syndrome, adult see acute respiratory distress syndrome
respiratory function see lung function
respiratory infections (chest/lung infections) 885

chronic obstruction pulmonary disease and 894
coalworkers 1031
imaging 885
ozone-related 289
semiconductor production 449
zoonotic 751, 751–6
see also severe acute respiratory syndrome
respiratory protection (incl. respirators) 49, 50
welding 428
respiratory sensitization
isocyanates 364
respiratory surveillance with 947
respiratory surveillance with respiratory sensitizing agents 947
respiratory tract (incl. airways)
astronauts 610
irritant gases in 255–6
Reston ebolavirus 737
retina 647–8
anatomy 646, 647–8
light-induced damage (incl. UV and infrared)
lasers 652–3
mechanisms 648–9
sunlight 651
welding arc 430, 652
light pathway in 648
light pathway to 644–5
retinol-binding protein (RBP) 64
and cadmium 168, 170, 1132
retirement, psychiatric disorders 844
retrenching in organizations 839
retrospective case-control studies 83
retrospective cohort studies 82
return to work (after sickness) 39–40, 817–18
back pain and 719–21
fitness see fitness
government policy 817–18
psychiatric disorders and 844
rewarming
frostbite 530
frostnip 530
immersion 533
non-freezing cold injury 531, 532, 533
rheumatic conditions/rheumatism
back pain attributed to (historical) 716
of upper limb 692–9
see also arthropathies
rheumatoid arthritis
coalworker' pneumoconiosis and (Caplan's syndrome) 879, 1032
silica and 1024–5
rhinitis, cyclic acid anhydrides 362

rhodium 228
rhodopsin 647, 648
rightsizing in organizations 839
riot control agents 316
risk 141–7
assessment/estimation 142–3
cancer attributed to occupational exposures 1097–110
nanoparticles 913–16
objective, with psychiatric disorders 834–6
psychosocial 841–2
reproductive hazards 1208
risk of mortality, methods 85–6
welding 428
attributable 78–9
communicating to public about 144–7
definition and distinction from hazard 35, 141
industrialization and 7–9
management
genetic modification 791–2
nanotechnology 913
reproductive 1209–10
relative 79
Roach–Schilling clinical grading, byssinosis 962
Robens Committee 18
rodent(s), leptospirosis 757, 758
rodenticides 402
acute effects 405–6
management 412
Roholm 283
Roos test 503
Rosen, George 5, 6
rotator cuff tendinitis 689, 689–90, 690
rotenone 1161, 1162
round atelectasis, asbestosis 883, 992
round-table mediation 817
routine surveillance see surveillance
rubber industry, bladder cancer 1089, 1090
rubella 739
rubeola (measles) 739
ruthenium 228–9

safety
alcohol and 860
at high altitude 584–6
historical perspectives 14, 15, 17, 18, 19
legislation see law
salmeterol, altitude sickness prevention 582
salmonellosis 759–60
salt depletion in heat illness 538
samples (population) 79

samples (specimens)
    analysis 60
    collection (sampling) 45–6, 658
        nanoparticles 914, 916
        time 58–9
        welding 427–8
    interpreting results 60–3
    serum, storage 795–6
Samuel Committee 99, 101
sarcoma, soft tissue, chlorophenoxy acid herbicides 401
    see also angiosarcoma
Sarcoptes scabiei 740–1
sarin
    terrorism 315
    Japan 316
    warfare 314
SARS see severe acute respiratory syndrome
satisfaction, job 845
    see also dissatisfaction
saturation diving 559, 566
scabies 740–1, 1062
scavenging of anaesthetic gases 299–300
scene of terrorist chemical attack, medical care 317
Scheele CW 278
Scheele's green 160
schizophrenia 843
Schweppes, Joseph 269
Scientific Committee on Occupational Exposure Limits (SCOEL) 40, 48
scientific developments (in precautionary principle) 146
scintigraphy (radionuclide studies) of lung 879
sclera 648
scleroderma
    lesions resembling 1070–1
        vinyl chloride 302, 307–8, 1070–1
    silica and 1025
SCOEL (Scientific Committee on Occupational Exposure Limits) 40, 48
Scottish law 113, 114
screen printing 1203
screening
    hepatotoxic chemicals 1171, 1172
    laser-induced eye damage 653–4
    psychiatric disorders 847–8
    substance abuse 865
        abuse 862, 865
scrotum
    cancer, clinical assessment of two cases 1101–2, 1102
    temperature, and infertility 1199

SCUBA 556
scurvy 9
secondary prevention
    asthma 947
    cancer 1104
    lead nephropathy 1130
section thickness in conventional vs high-resolution CT 877
sedentary work, thermal balance 526
seizures/convulsions, epileptic
    alcohol-related 860
    gases 263
    shift workers 1241
selection bias 91
selenium hepatotoxicity 1185
self-contained underwater breathing apparatus (SCUBA) 556
self-copying (carbonless copy) paper 925, 928
self-employed, compensation 97
Sellafield and leukaemia 631
semiconductor industry 444–53
    devices 445
    hazards 447–9
    health issues 449–51
        reproductive 450–1, 1203, 1205
    materials 444–5
    work processes in manufacture 445–7
sensory dysfunction in hand–arm vibration syndrome 491–2, 498, 499
    signs and symptoms 494–5
    tests 503, 504, 505
Seoul virus 756
sepiolite 1011
sepsis, radiation-related 639
serological testing/markers
    borreliosis 763
    brucellosis 755
    Coxiella burnetii 764
    hepatitis B infection 732, 733
    HIV 795
    leptospirosis 758
serum
    precipitins, extrinsic allergic alveolitis 976–7
    sample storage 795–6
severe acute respiratory syndrome (SARS) and coronavirus 737–8
    healthcare workers 737–8
    semiconductor industry 449
Seveso, dioxins 1180
sewage handing
    gases 267, 268
    infection risk 744
sewer gas 266
sex (gender)

    and high-altitude illness 576
    and mesothelioma deaths 1003
    and radiogenic cancer risk 631
    see also females; males
sex workers and infections 743–4
sharps injuries 731–2
sheep
    C. abortus 753
    orf 764
sheep dippers' flu 407
shielded arc welding 422
    gases 427
        asphyxia 432–3
    particle emissions 425
shift work (incl. nightwork) and extended work hours 1233–45
    breast cancer 1097, 1238
    factors affecting tolerance 1238–9
    health and 1235–8
        reproductive 1207–8, 1237
    preventive and compensatory measures 1239–40
    semiconductor industry 449
Shiga toxin-producing E. coli 761
shingles 738
shoes see footwear
short waves see microwaves
shoulder problems 688–91
    welders 432
sick building syndrome (SBS) 924, 925, 930–1
sick notes 810–11
sick role 807–8
sickle cell anaemia/disease 1220
    and high altitude 580
sickness absence 806–18, 843–4
    alcohol and 861
    defining entitlement 810
    as form of resistance 806–7
    short- vs long-term 843–4
sickness pathway/journey 845–7
sickness presence 843
siderosis 1044
    Bantu 186
    imaging 883
    welders 434
sidestream tobacco smoke 922, 925
sieverts and millisieverts 625
signs see symptoms and signs
silage fermentation 291
silane 293–4
sildenafil, altitude sickness prevention 583
Silent Spring 18
silica dust 1014–28
    diseases 1014–28, 1015–19

chronic obstruction pulmonary
disease 898
coalworkers 1029, 1032
comparative risks 1025–6
epidemiology 1021–8
malignant (carcinogenicity)
1022–4, 1087
renal 1024, 1137–8
see also silicosis
health surveillance of workers 1019
silicate minerals 1035–6
silicon tetrafluoride 282, 285
silicon wafer production 445–6
silicosis 880, 1014, 1015–19
acute 1015
aluminium used as prophylactic 154
chronic active 1015–16
chronic inactive 1016–17
coalworkers 1029, 1032
compensation 101
epidemiology 1021–2
historical perspectives 15
imaging 880
prevention 1017
mistaken belief with aluminium
154
risks in different occupations 1017–18
tuberculosis combined with 1016–17,
1019
silo-fillers' disease 291
silver 234–5
Simpson, Sir James 298
single nucleotide polymorphisms
(SNPs) as cancer susceptibility
markers 1113, 1114
single-photon emission computed
tomography (SPECT),
manganism 1158
sinuses, nasal see paranasal sinuses
skin (dermis; cutis) 132, 137, 1061–77
absorption via 132
mercury compounds 216
anthrax involving 751, 752, 775
biotransformation 137
hand/wrist
in hand–arm vibration syndrome
492, 493, 496, 505
normal physiology 491
injury/damage incl. burns
acid gases/vapours 263
cement 1071
hydrofluoric acid 284
ionizing radiation, prevention
640
phenol 358
UV radiation, welding 423
welding 429

lesions (in general)/dermatoses
1061–77
acrylamides 350
acrylic/methacrylic acid esters 347
beryllium 1051
chromium 173
cyclic acid anhydrides 362
decompression sickness 552
epidemiology 1061–2
mercury 216
nickel 223
occupations causing 1071–4
radiation 627, 629
silver 234
zoonoses 762–5
see also dermatitis
measuring exposure via 44
pesticide exposure 413
radiation contamination (=external
contamination) 634, 636, 637, 640
temperature in cold strain 527
measurement 529
skin cancers 1071, 1092–3
epidemiology 1092–3
polyaromatic hydrocarbons 333–4
semiconductor industry 450
sun exposure 1071, 1092–3
welding 423, 429
skin patch tests, allergic contact
dermatitis 1065–6
skin prick tests see prick tests
slate workers' pneumoconiosis 1033–4
sleep disturbances
air travel 603–4
high altitude 580–1
noise 481
shift work 1234, 1235
SLOT 257
small airways dysfunction,
asbestos-related 996
epidemiology 1000–1
small vessel vasculitis and silica 1025,
1138
smallpox 774, 775
smelting
aluminium 153, 154, 1044
lead 189
SO_2 exposure 288
smog
London 254, 288
photochemical 290
smoke (non-tobacco) 258, 260
firefighters and 260–1
smoking
asbestos and
asbestosis susceptibility and 1001
lung cancer and 1005, 1109

cessation, flying and 606
chronic obstruction pulmonary
disease and 891–2, 893
confounding and interactions 891–2
cotton dust and 890
history-taking of status 37
secondhand/environmental/
involuntary (indoors) 922, 925
and asthma 927
and cancer 933
in pregnancy 932
public health impact 933
Snow John 266, 298
social amplification of risk 146–7
social effects of shift work 1234–5
social environment and sick building
syndrome 932
social insurance see insurance
Soderberg process 283
sodium, disturbances see
hyponatraemia; salt depletion
sodium calcium edetate see calcium
disodium edetate
sodium chlorate and chlorate salts 399, 412
sodium metabisulphite 288
sodium thiosulphate 277, 278
soft tissue rheumatic conditions of
upper limb 692–9
soft tissue sarcoma, chlorophenoxy acid
herbicides 401
solar radiation see sunlight
solubility
alveolar concentration effects on 130,
131
gases 255–6
lipid 128
metals 152
soluble oils, dermatoses 1073
solvents (organic) 325–31, 1138–41
aromatic 324–31, 1162–3
hepatotoxicity 1183–4
hexacarbon see hexacarbon solvents
mixtures 1163, 1183
nephrotoxicity 1138–41
neurotoxicity 328–9, 330–1, 1153,
1156, 1162–3
for nucleic acid extraction 790
petroleum solvents 334, 335–6
pregnancy and non-industrial indoor
exposure to 932
reproductive effects 1199, 1199–200,
1205
in semiconductor production 447, 448
somatic structures see tissues and organs
somatoform and somatization disorders
840–1
somatogravic illusions 601

somatogyral illusions 601
soots and skin cancer 1093
sopite syndrome 609
sounds
   excessive *see* noise
   physics 459–61
   stimulation, effects 465–6
   see also decibels
spaceflight 607–13
   astronaut selection 611
   environments 608, 608–9
   extra-vehicular activity 609
   future of 613
   medical emergencies 611–13
   (patho)physiology 609–11
   pre-launch and launch 608
   re-entry 609
   research and ground-based analogues 613
spatial disorientation, flying 601–2
spatter, welding 424
special damages 118
Special Hardship Allowance (SHA – renamed the Reduced Earnings Allowance) 97, 98–9, 100
speciation, toxic metals 152
species, susceptibility within vs between 128
specific disease rates 78
specific gravity, urine 60
Specified Level of Toxicity (SLOT) 257
specimens *see* samples
spectacles (glasses) 656, 657, 658
   aircrew 600
sperm *see* males, fertility problems
spine
   cervical, symptoms relating to 691–2
   injury *see* back injury
spirit possession 808–9
spirometry *see* lung function
splenic enlargement 1218
spondylosis, cervical 691
spores, anthrax 751, 752
sputum examination, inorganic dust disease 986–7
squamous cell carcinoma (skin), UV-related 1092–3
   solar exposure 1071, 1093
   welding 423, 429
staff
   biotechnology containment measures and 794
   healthcare *see* healthcare workers
stainless steel *see* steel
stalinon 238–9, 239
standardized rates 78
   see also incidence ratio, standardized; mortality ratio, standardized
stannosis 238, 1045
   imaging 883
staphylococcal infections 741
State (US) compensation schemes 107–8
state *see* government
statistical significance 79
steam from geothermal power 302–3
steatohepatitis, non-alcoholic (NASH), solvents and 1183, 1184
steel industry (incl. stainless steel) 202
   chronic obstructive pulmonary disease 1042
   welding 425, 1043
stem cells, haemopoietic 1215–16
   deficits in production 1221
   transplantation following radiation accidents 1224, 1225
stereocilia 463, 464
   noise-related damage 467
sterilizing agents in biotechnology 790
steroids *see* corticosteroids
stibine 159, 295, 1042
stigma with psychiatric disorders 839–40
stochastic effects of radiation 625, 626, 629–30
Stockholm Workshop Scale, hand–arm vibration syndrome 487, 491, 495, 496
Stoffenmanager software tool 47
stomach *see* entries under gastric
stones, kidney, cadmium and 1132
straight-run white spirits 335
strain *see* stress and strain
strain
   thermal
      definition 525–6
      reduction 538–42
      see also cold; heat
Streptococcus suis 758
Streptomyces spp. in biotechnology 789
stress (psychosocial/mental) and strain, work 801–22, 836–7, 837
   biotechnology industry 791
   burnout due to 844–5
   as culture-bound syndrome 808–9
   discourse 804–5
   indoor non-industrial sources
      pregnancy and 932–3
      sick building syndrome and 931
   medical profession 867
   pregnancy outcome and 1207
   semiconductor production 449
   surveillance 809–10
   see also post-traumatic distress syndrome; strain

stress (thermal)
   definitions 525–6
   disability and 540
   see also cold; heat
stroma, corneal 647
styrene (vinyl benzene) 327–31, 1162, 1183
   biological monitoring guidance values 62
   hepatotoxicity 1183
   neurotoxicity 328, 1162
   ototoxicity 329, 1162
subcutaneous cellulitis, hand or knee 699
subfertility *see* reproductive effects
substance abuse 959–70
   definitions 859
   diagnosis 861–5
   management 865–6
      ingredients for successful treatment 866–7
   in medical profession 867–8
   prevention 868
succinic anhydride 363
Sudan ebolavirus 737
sugar cane and bagassosis 979–80
suicide 834–5
   aircraft crash 605
   drinking of copper solutions 181
   role of occupation in 834–5
sulphate conjugates 135
sulphur, malodorous compounds 293
sulphur-containing organic compounds 374–6
sulphur dioxide 257, 287–8
   WHO air quality guidelines 142
sulphur hexafluoride 285–6
sulphur mustard, warfare 314, 316
sulphur tetrafluoride 285
sulphur trioxide 288
sulphuric acid
   anhydride of 288
   mists 288
   SO_2 exposure in manufacture of 288
sulphuryl difluoride 286
sulphydryl (-SH; thio) groups
   lead affinity 191
   mercury affinity 216
sunglasses, aircrew 600
sunlight and solar radiation
   ocular damage
      acute 651–2
      chronic 654
   skin cancers 1071, 1092–3
   in space 608
   see also ultraviolet radiation
sunscreen, welding 431

superalloys 161
  cobalt in 175
superficial frostbite 530
superwarfarins 402, 405, 406
surface area
  body, pesticide exposure and 413
  concentrations of nanoparticles 915–16
surface coatings, welding 247
surface-supplied diving (SSD) 556–7
surgery
  decompressive see decompression
  eye, aircrew having had 600
  infection risk to healthcare workers 731–2
  osteoarthritis 702
  in space 612
surveillance/monitoring, workplace (health/medical) 84–6
  aluminium 155
  asbestos workers 996–7
  asthma 944, 947
  biotechnology 793–6
  chromium 174
  cobalt 177
  gold 183–4
  hand–arm vibration syndrome 505–6
  ionizing radiation 634–8
  manganese 208
  pesticides 61, 66, 412–16
  platinum group metals
    iridium 228
    osmium 229
    palladium 228
    platinum 227
    rhodium 228
    ruthenium 229
  psychological stress 809–10
  shift workers 1240–1
  silica workers 1019
  silver 235
  substance abuse 864
  vanadium 247
  welding 435–6
  whole-body vibration 520
Surveillance of Work and Occupational Respiratory Disease (SWORD) voluntary reporting scheme 95, 95
susceptibility
  biological effect monitoring and 64–70
  variations in 137–8
    individual see individuals
    intra- vs interspecies 128
suspension levels, lead 196, 197
susto 807–8

swallowing, hydrofluoric acid 284
sweat rate, required 535
Sweden, compensation schemes 97, 105
swimming pools, chlorine 279
SWORD (Surveillance of Work and Occupational Respiratory Disease) voluntary reporting scheme 95, 95
sympathetic nerves (and cutaneous circulation) 481
  hand–arm vibration syndrome 492
symptoms and signs (=effects)
  aniline poisoning 353
  asbestosis 991–2
  cervical spine problems 691–2
  diagnostic importance 40, 40–1
  in expert report 118–19
  haematological disorders 1218
  hand–arm vibration syndrome 494–5, 502
  heat exhaustion 537
  high-altitude illness 570, 573, 574, 575
  inorganic dust disease 986
  ionizing radiation 628, 629
  lead exposure
    inorganic 192
    organic 195
  in relation to activities, asking about 34
  sick building syndrome 931
  time between exposure and *see* time sequence
  see also biological effect monitoring; red flags; yellow flags
synthetic mineral fibres *see* fibrous particles
systematic review 86–7
systemic disease 1059–229
  hand–arm vibration syndrome and, differential diagnosis 498
  see also tissues and organs
systemic effects 1079–229
  fluoride 284
  gases (irritant and other) 294–8
  noise 481–2
systemic lupus erythematosus (SLE) and silica 1025
systemic sclerosis and silica 1025
  see also scleroderma
systolic blood pressure, finger, in hand–arm vibration syndrome 497, 505

T lymphocytes
  and beryllium 1050
  and extrinsic allergic alveolitis and 973
talc 1035

tanning, dermatoses 1073
tapeworms 765
task optimization (musculoskeletal disorder prevention) 706
technetium-99m imaging of lung 879
technological developments 26–7
  nanoparticles 784, 907–9
  see also biotechnology
teeth *see* dentition
Teflon® (PTFE), inhalation of pyrolysis products 437–8
telegraphist's cramp 699
Teleky, Ludwig 5, 6
temperature
  core
    in heat exhaustion 537
    in heat stroke 537
  fires 258
  measurement
    in cold stress and strain 528, 528–9
    in heat stress and strain 534–5, 536
  testicular, and infertility 1199
  see also cold; fever; heat; heaters *and* entries under thermal
temporal issues *see* time
tendinitis
  hand–wrist 694
  shoulder 689, 689–90, 691
  see also peritendinitis
tennis elbow (lateral epicondylitis) 692, 693
tenosynovitis 693–4
tension neck syndrome 692
teratogenicity *see* developmental toxicity
terrorism 254, 315–18
  aircraft crashes 605
  biological agents 773–81
tert-amylmethylether (TAME) 341
4-tert-butylphenol 359
tertiary prevention, asthma 947
tesla (T) and microtesla 663
testicles
  cancer
    and electromagnetic fields 667
    and radiofrequency fields 677
  temperature, and infertility 1199
tetrabromophthalic anhydride 363
tetracarbonylnickel (nickel carbonyl) 224, 298
2,3,7,8-tetrachlorodibenzodioxin (TCDD) 370, 371, 1179–80
  mechanisms of hepatotoxicity 1179–80
2,3,7,8-tetrachlorodibenzofuran 370
2,3,7,8-tetrachloro-p-dioxin 370
  as Agent Orange contaminant 1162–3

tetrachloroethene (tetrachloroethylene; perchloroethene) 366–7, 1140
　hepatotoxicity 1181
　nephrotoxicity 1140
tetrachloromethane *see* carbon tetrachloride
tetrachlorophthalic anhydride 363, 364
tetraethyl lead in petrol *see* petrol
1,1,1,2-tetrafluoroethane 286–7
tetrafluorohydrazine 285
tetrafluoromethane 286
tetrahydrophthalic anhydride 363
textile workers *see* cotton and flax and other textile workers
Thackrah, Charles Turner 9
thallium 236–7
theophylline, altitude sickness prevention 582
thermal aesthesiometry (TA) test, hand–arm vibration syndrome 494, 495, 500, 501
thermal environments (and their challenges) 525–44
　control 542–3
　divers 533, 555
　flying 597–8
　indoors (non-industrial) 923–4, 933–4
　occupations with recognized challenges 528
　physical and physiological principles (incl. thermoregulation) 526–7
　treatment 538–42
thermal trauma (incl. burns)
　cold 529–32
　light 648–9
　radiofrequency fields 675
Thermoactinomycetes sacchari and extrinsic allergic alveolitis 978, 979–80
thiol groups *see* sulphydryl groups
thiothiazolidine-4-carboxylic acid (analyte) 61
thoracic outlet syndrome 692
thorax *see* chest
thoriated (and thorium-free) tungsten electrodes 422, 424
Three Mile Island 262
threshold dose (ED_0) for deterministic effects of radiation 626
threshold limit values (TLVs) 40, 48
threshold shift (sound stimulation)
　permanent 466
　temporary 465–6
thrombosis, deep vein, flying and risk of 607
thrombotic thrombocytopenia purpura, enterohaemorrhagic *E. coli* 761

thyroid
　cobalt effects 177
　radiation effects 627
ticks and Lyme disease 762, 763
time
　of return to work with psychiatric disorders 844
　sampling 58–9
　work-related disability in depression and anxiety over 843
　see also circadian rhythms; hours worked
time sequence of exposure and effect (symptoms and signs) 34
　diagnostic importance 40–1
time-weighted average (TWA)
　electromagnetic fields 665
　inhalation exposure assessment 48
time-windows, epidemiological studies of cancer 1107
time zone changes 603
tin 238–40
　dusts *see* stannosis
　see also indium tin oxide
Tinel's test
　carpal tunnel syndrome 499, 696
　hand–arm vibration syndrome 498, 499, 503
tinnitus, noise-induced 480
tiredness *see* fatigue
tissues and organs (somatic structures) 1059–229
　biotransformation in, comparative ability 132, 133
　culture *see* culture
　gas bubbles *see* bubbles of gas
　light damage, mechanisms 648–9
　nanoparticle effects 907–9
　pesticide effects 398
　radiation effects 625–30
　vaporization at altitude 593
　welding 429–35
　see also systemic disease
tobacco smoke *see* smoking
toluene (methyl benzene) 327–31, 1162–3, 1182
　benzene in commercial preparations of 36
　hepatotoxicity 1182
　monitoring 62, 329
　neurotoxicity 328, 1162–3
　ototoxicity 329, 1163
toluene diisocyanate (TDI; tolylene diisocyanate) 36, 261, 364
　asthma and 943
　chronic obstruction pulmonary disease and 896

toluidines 354
tolylene diisocyanate *see* toluene diisocyanate
tooth *see* dentition
toxic exposures and medically unexplained conditions 840–1
toxic gases 253
　in fires 258
toxic shock syndrome, streptococcal 758
toxicity
　acute respiratory, asthmatic complication *see* reactive airways dysfunction syndrome
　biotechnological products 789
　biotransformation resulting in decreased *see* detoxification
　biotransformation resulting in increases, example 133
　pesticide *see* pesticide
　shift work and risk of 1237
　systemic *see* systemic effects
　see also specific (types of) compounds/materials etc.
toxicology
　general principles 127–40
　nanoparticle *see* nanoparticles
toxins, bacterial
　B. anthracis 752
　in biotechnology, accidental exposure 789
　bioterrorism 774, 776
　byssinosis and 959–60
　　preventing exposure 966
　Cytophaga 438
　enterohaemorrhagic *E. coli* 761
TP53 (tumour suppressor) gene 27, 1112
tracheal intubation in space 612
trade unions, historical perspectives 14
training *see* education
transfer factor for carbon monoxide in extrinsic allergic alveolitis 974, 975
transferrin
　aluminium binding 154
　carbohydrate-deficient (CDT) 69, 865
　iron binding 186
transformation (biotransformation)
　in biotechnology 787
　in human body 132–7
transgenes 787, 791, 793
transient otoacoustic emissions (TOAEs) 479–80
transmembrane transport *see* transport
transmissible diseases *see* infections

transport (transmembrane) 128
  manganese 203
  nanoparticles 909
trauma (physical incl. mechanical injury)
  acoustic/blast 469–70
  alcohol abuse and 865
  back see back injury
  barometric (divers) 549–50
  cold, liquefied gases 262
  cutaneous see skin
  flying (incl. crashes) 604, 605
  inhalation, metal compounds 1041
  ionizing radiation 640
  light see eye
  needle stick and sharps 731–2
  repeated 687–712
  welding 429, 429–31
  see also accidents
trauma (psychological) see post-traumatic distress syndrome; resilience; stress
travel and infections 742–3
treatment
  altitude sickness 583–4, 585
  asthma 951
  contact dermatitis 1067
  haematological disorders, work-related issues resulting from 1226
  hepatotoxic chemicals 1176, 1177
  metal exposure/poisoning 44
    arsenic 1157
    beryllium 1052
    cadmium 1133–4
    copper 181
    iron 186
    lead 194–5, 1130
    manganese 205, 208–9, 1158
    mercury 218, 1136, 1159
  methyl bromide 1159
  pesticide poisoning 409–12
  psychiatric disorders 847–8
    psychological methods see psychological interventions
  radiation casualties 636–8
    for bone marrow failure 1224, 1225
    nuclear reactor accident 639–40
  substance abuse
    coercion 865–6
    poor cooperation of failure 865–6
treatment area, designated, radiation accidents 638
tremolite 994, 1004
tremor, mercury 217
triazine herbicides 412
trichloroacetic acid (analyte) 62
trichloroethane 1181

trichloroethene see trichloroethylene
trichloroethylene (trichloroethene) 366–7, 1181
  biological monitoring guidance values 62
  hepatotoxicity 1181
  neurotoxicity 365, 366, 1163
trichloromethane (chloroform) 298, 369–70, 1181
2,4,6-trichlorophenol 358, 359
2,4,5-trichlorophenoxyacetic acid (in Agent Orange) 1163
1,1,2-trichloro-1,2,2-trifluoroethane 286
triethanolamine 355
triethyltin (TET) 238–9
trigger finger 694
trimellitic anhydride 363, 364
trimethylamine 289
trimethyltin (TMT) 238, 239
trinitrotoluene 1182
trivalent chromium 152, 173, 174
TSI Nanoparticle Surface Area Monitor 916
tuberculosis (*M. tuberculosis* infection) 90
  healthcare workers 739–40
  silicosis combined with 1016–17, 1019
  slate workers' pneumoconiosis risk of 1033
tubular damage/dysfunction (renal)
  cadmium 168, 169, 1132
  mercury 217, 218, 1135
  organic solvents 1139
tularaemia 776–7
tumour biomarkers 1111–12
  see also cancer; carcinogens
tungsten (wolfram) 241–2
tungsten arc (inert gas) welding 422–3
  particle emissions 425
  thorium-free electrodes 424
tungsten carbide, cobalt metal with 1045
  and lung cancer 176, 1043–4
tunnelling see compressed air work
Twin Towers (World Trade Center) attacks, firefighter deaths 261
twister's cramp 699
tympanic membrane (eardrum)
  perforation at high altitude 574
  temperature measurement 536
typhoidal salmonellae 760
typhus 9

ulcers (cutaneous) 1071
  chrome 173, 1071
  as frostbite sequelae, recurrent 531
ultrafine particles see nanoparticles and ultrafine particles

ultrasound
  auditory effects 480
  imaging with
    liver (after abnormal liver function tests) 1172
    lung 878
    in microgravity 611–12
  reproductive effects 1207
ultraviolet radiation
  ocular absorption 649
  ocular damage
    acute 650, 651
    pathophysiology 645
    protective filter materials 657–8, 658
    welding 423, 430
  psoralens and UV-A 656
  skin damage (incl. malignancy), welding 423, 429
  see also sunlight
Union Carbide pesticide plant in Bhopal 253, 297, 364, 1237
United States and North America
  biotechnology (incl. genetic modification) regulations 784
  cancer deaths 1098, 1099
  compensation schemes 107–8
  exposure data 40
  indoor non-industrial hazards
    asthma and 933
    tobacco smoke exposure 926
  International Labour Office and 15
  lead exposure guidelines/recommendations 1129–30, 1131
upper limb problems 688, 692–9
uranium 243–5, 1136
  depleted 243, 244, 245, 1136
    and Gulf War syndrome 244, 841
  nephrotoxicity 244, 1136
urinary bladder cancer see bladder cancer
urinary problems, astronauts 610
urine samples
  analytical result adjustments 60
  biological monitoring guidance values for common substances in 61–2
  cadmium levels, assessment 1132–3
  collection 58
  drug screening 865
  mercury levels, assessment 1134
  pesticides 415
  in radiation exposure 640
  renal biomarkers 68

urticaria
  cold 1071
  contact 1069
uterine cancer and radiofrequency fields 677

vaccination (active immunization)
  aircrew 607
  anthrax 753
  hepatitis A in travellers 743
  hepatitis B in healthcare workers 734, 735
  Q fever 764
  tuberculosis 739
vaccines, bioengineered 787
vaccinia virus 741, 774, 787, 795
valency (metals) 152
  chromium 152, 173, 174
  copper 180
  iron 185
  tin 238
van Allen belts 608
vanadium 246–8
  acute inhalation injury 1041
  asthma 246, 1043
vaporization of body tissues at altitude 593
vapours and mists
  definition 254
  inorganic acid 288
  protective garments permeable to 541
  sampling 45
  white spirit 335
  see also fumes
varicella zoster virus 738
variola virus (smallpox) 774, 775
vascular lesions, hepatic 1175
vascular system (arm/wrist/hand)
  hand–arm vibration syndrome-related phenomena 489, 492–3, 495–7
    clinical features 495–6
    treatment 507
    normal physiology 491
  see also entries under cardiovascular
vasculitis (ANCA-associated) and silica 1025, 1138
vasoconstriction, hand–arm vibration syndrome 491, 492, 493
vasodilation, hand–arm vibration syndrome 491, 492, 493
vasospasm in hand–arm vibration syndrome 490, 492, 495, 496
vectors (for genes/DNA) 785, 792–3, 793
venous thrombosis, deep, flying and risk of 607

ventilation (indoors) 49, 923, 933, 934
  local exhaust see local exhaust ventilation
  welding 428
  see also air conditioning
ventilation (physiological), function see lung function
ventilation pneumonitis 980
vermiculite 1036
verocytotoxin-producing E. coli 761
vertigo see balance problems
vestibular apparatus 462
  dysfunction see balance
veterinary care, dermatoses 1074
vibration 487–522
  aircraft 598–9
  hand–arm see hand–arm vibration syndrome
  see also white finger
vibrotactile threshold test (VTT), hand–arm vibration syndrome 494, 495, 501, 504, 505
video-assisted thoracoscopic surgery (VATS), mesothelioma 993
video display units see visual display units
video recording of work activities (with related musculoskeletal disorders) 703
Vietnam war, Agent Orange 1163–4
vinyl benzene see styrene
vinyl bromide 301
vinyl chloride 17, 18, 26–7, 302, 368–9, 1178–9, 1187
  angiosarcoma of liver and 17, 26, 134, 368, 1096, 1187
  epoxidation 134
  scleroderma-like lesions 302, 307–8, 1070–1
vinyl fluorides 302
N-vinylpyrrolidone 356
violence 837–8
viral infections
  archaeologists 744
  bioterrorism 774, 775, 777
  chronic obstruction pulmonary disease and 894
  healthcare workers 729–39
  laboratory research workers 741
  liver see hepatitis
  zoonotic, presentation 765–6
    cutaneous 764, 764–5
    fever 756–7, 759
viruses in biotechnology 785–6
visible light, pathophysiology of eye damage 645
vision 644–6

flying and 599–601
  mechanisms 644–6, 648
  solvent mixtures affecting 1163
  see also flash blindness
visors, aircrew 600
visual (video) display units (VDUs) 654
  musculoskeletal disorders 696
  prevention 706–7
  pregnancy and 668–9, 1206
vital status in cancer cohort studies 1105–6
vitamin B_{12} precursor (hydroxocobalamin) 278
vitamin D and cadmium 169
vitreous fibres, man-made 1012
vitreous humor 647
vocal cord dysfunction 264, 312
vocational driving licences and substance abuse 867
volatile compounds (incl. volatile organic compounds/VOCs)
  indoor non-industrial 922, 924–5
  pregnancy and 932
  inhalation kinetics 130–1
volcanic areas
  carbon dioxide 271
  hydrogen sulphide 292
volenti non fit injuria 99
volume of distribution 130
vomiting (emesis)
  agents inducing, in pesticide poisoning, contraindication 410
  radiation-related 640
VX 314, 315
VZV (varicella zoster virus) 738

warfare and military operations 314–15
  chemical agents 1163–4
  flying and exposure to chemicals in 604
  gases accidentally released 254
  historical perspectives 14–16, 314
  post-traumatic distress syndrome 814, 838, 1164
  somatoform and somatization disorders 840–1
warfarin 405
  see also superwarfarins
warming see rewarming
waste inactivation, biotechnology 794
water supply (incl. drinking water)
  copper 181
  manganese 202
  see also dampness; immersion
weapons, acoustic/blast trauma 469–70
weed killers see herbicides

weight loss
    asbestosis 992
    osteoarthritis, beneficial effects 702
    see also obesity
Weil's disease and leptospirosis 69–70, 757–8
welding (incl. fumes) 421–36, 910–11
    adverse health effects 429–35
        chronic obstructive pulmonary disease 433–4, 898
        metal fume fevers 433, 437, 911
        reproductive 435, 1200
        respiratory disorders (in general) 421–2, 432–5, 911, 1043
    of aluminium 153, 434–5
    control of exposures 428
    light damage 651, 652
        protection 656, 657, 658–9
    manganese in 202, 207, 426
    particles 424–6
        nano-sized 424, 904, 910–11
    principal processes 422–3
    sampling and analysis 427–8
    source/nature/variation of emissions 423–7
    steel 425, 1043
    surveillance 435–6
West Nile virus 758
wet bulb globe temperature index 534–5
wet clothing, cooling when wearing 526
wetness, diving 555
wetsuits 555
whale finger 763
wheeze, asbestosis 992
white asbestos see chrysotile
white cell count, semiconductor workers 451
white finger, vibration (VWF) 485, 698
    pathogenesis of neurosensory dysfunction 493
white phosphorus 225
white spirits 334, 335–6
whitlow, herpetic 739
WHO see World Health Organization
whole-body radiation exposure
    acute, effects 628
    chronic, effects 628–9
whole-body vibration 513–22
    control standards 519
    factors affecting exposures and control measures 519–20
    health effects 514–19
    measurements 514
    sources of exposure 514
    workplace surveillance 520
wind chill equivalent temperature 528, 529

wine, adulteration with lead 188
Wisconsin compensation schemes (1911) 107
withdrawal in substance abuse, medically-assisted 866
witnesses, of fact 114–15
Wolff–Parkinson–White syndrome, high altitude 579
wolfram see tungsten
wollastonite 1011–12
women see females
wood fuels, IARC classification of carcinogenicity 1083, 1084, 1086
woodworkers
    chronic obstruction pulmonary disease and wood dust 896
    dermatoses 1074
    lymphomas 1225
work (employment; job; occupation)
    asking about symptoms in relation to activities 34
    competency at, and alcohol 860
    definition 833
    disease affecting 39–40
    dissatisfaction 807
    health affected by 38–9
    overload 815–16
    psychiatric disorders and see psychological disorders
    return to see return to work
    satisfaction see dissatisfaction; satisfaction
    taking and recording information about 34
    title of job 34–5
Work Capability Assessment (WCA) 818
work-related illness, new wave of 27–8
Worker's Accident Insurance (Germany 1884) 96
Workmen's Compensation Acts (1897 and later) 98, 99–100
Workmen's Compensation (Silicosis) Act (1918) 101
workplace
    additional exposure outside of 48–9
    adverse events, and psychological trauma 811–12
    alcohol and competence and safety in 860
    asthma in, epidemiology studies 944
    in back pain prevention, improvements 718–19
    exposure limits (WELs - of the HSE) 44, 48
        gases 254–5
        manganese 208
        vanadium 247

incivility 816
phobia 812
surveillance see surveillance
see also organization
World Health Organization (WHO)
    air quality guidelines 142
    carcinogens, predicting unit risks 143
    noise-related disease 481–2
World Trade Center attacks, firefighter deaths 261
World War I 13, 14–15
worldwide dimensions see international dimensions
wrist problems 688, 694–6
writer's cramp 699

X-ray(s) 624
X-ray fluorescence, lead nephropathy 1128–9
X-ray radiography (conventional/plain films)
    chest, in lung diseases 875–6
        asbestos exposure 881, 882, 992, 993
        berylliosis 1051
        coalworker's pneumoconiosis 879, 880, 1030, 1031
        extrinsic allergic alveolitis 884, 974
        inorganic dust diseases (in general) 987
        silicosis 881
        slate workers' pneumoconiosis 1033
        stannosis 884
    hand–arm vibration syndrome 505
xenobiotics see chemicals
xenon 273
xylene (dimethylbenzene) 327–31
    measuring exposure 47
    monitoring 62, 330

yeasts in biotechnology 789
yellow flags, back pain chronicity 719
Yersinia pestis, bioterrorism 775–6
Yusho disease 371

Zaire ebolavirus 737
zeolites 1011
    mesothelioma 1005, 1011
zinc 249–50
    iron interfering with intestinal absorption 186
zinc chloride inhalation 437, 1041
zinc oxide fumes 250, 437, 1040
zinc protoporphyrin (ZPP)
    lead and 63–4, 192, 196, 197, 1128
    vanadium and 247
zoonoses 750–70